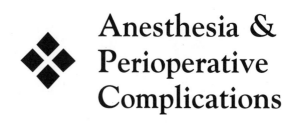

Anesthesia &
Perioperative
Complications

Visit our website at **www.mosby.com**

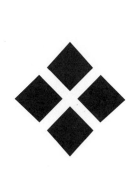

Anesthesia & Perioperative Complications

JONATHAN L. BENUMOF, M.D.
Professor of Anesthesia
Department of Anesthesiology
University of California, San Diego, School of Medicine
San Diego, California

LAWRENCE J. SAIDMAN, M.D.
Professor of Anesthesia
Department of Anesthesiology
Stanford University Medical Center
Stanford, California

SECOND EDITION

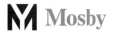 Mosby

St. Louis Baltimore Boston Carlsbad Chicago Minneapolis New York Philadelphia Portland
London Milan Sydney Tokyo Toronto

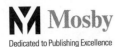

Dedicated to Publishing Excellence

Developmental Editor: Wendy Buckwalter
Project Manager: Patricia Tannian
Project Specialist: Suzanne C. Fannin
Design Manager: Gail Morey Hudson
Estimator: Dave Graybill
Cover Design: Maria Bellano

SECOND EDITION

Mosby, Inc.
A Harcourt Health Sciences Company
11830 Westline Industrial Drive
St. Louis, Missouri 63146

Printed in the United States of America
Composition by Graphic World, Inc.
Lithography/film by Graphic World, Inc.
Printing/binding by Maple Vail Book Manufacturing Group

Library of Congress Cataloging in Publication Data

Anesthesia and perioperative complications / [edited by] Jonathan L.
    Benumof, Lawrence J. Saidman.—2nd ed.
        p.   cm.
    Includes bibliographical references and index.
    ISBN 0-8151-2619-0
    1. Anesthesia—Complications.   2. Anesthetics—Side effects.
  I. Benumof, Jonathan   II. Saidman, Lawrence J.
    [DNLM: 1. Anesthesia—adverse effects.   2. Intraoperative Care—
  adverse effects.   3. Intraoperative Complications—etiology.
  4. Intraoperative Complications—prevention and control.   WO 245
  A5783 1999]
  RD82.5.A54   1999
  617.9'6041—dc21
  DNLM/DLC
  for Library of Congress   99-22920
                                                                CIP

99 00 01 02 03 / 9 8 7 6 5 4 3 2 1

Contributors

STEPHEN E. ABRAM, M.D.
Professor and Chair, Department of Anesthesiology
University of New Mexico School of Medicine
Albuquerque, New Mexico

JONATHAN M. ANAGNOSTOU, M.D.
Clinical Associate Professor of Anesthesia
Indiana University School of Medicine
Medical Director of Respiratory Care
Indiana University Hospital
Indianapolis, Indiana

JOHN L. ARD, Jr., M.D.
Assistant Professor of Anesthesiology
New York University Medical Center
New York, New York

JONATHAN L. BENUMOF, M.D.
Professor of Anesthesia, Department of Anesthesiology
University of California, San Diego, School of Medicine
San Diego, California

FREDERIC A. BERRY, M.D.
Professor of Anesthesiology and Pediatrics
University of Virginia Health Sciences Center
Charlottesville, Virginia

MARC H. BOIN, M.D.
Assistant Professor of Anesthesiology
University of Texas Medical School at Houston
Houston, Texas

JAY B. BRODSKY, M.D.
Professor of Anesthesiology
Stanford University School of Medicine
Stanford, California

LEVON M. CAPAN, M.D.
Associate Professor of Clinical Anesthesia
New York University School of Medicine
Associate Director, Anesthesia Service
Bellevue Hospital Center
New York, New York

ROBERT A. CAPLAN, M.D.
Clinical Professor of Anesthesiology
University of Washington School of Medicine
Staff Anesthesiologist
Virginia Mason Medical Center
Seattle, Washington

H.S. CHADWICK, M.D.
Associate Professor of Anesthesiology
University of Washington School of Medicine
Director, Obstetric Anesthesia
University of Washington Medical Center
Seattle, Washington

FREDERICK W. CHENEY, M.D.
Professor and Chair, Department of Anesthesiology
University of Washington School of Medicine
Attending Staff
University of Washington Medical Center and
    affiliated hospitals
Seattle, Washington

GREGORY CROSBY, M.D.
Associate Professor of Anaesthesia
Harvard Medical School
Brigham and Women's Hospital
Boston, Massachusetts

DEBORAH J. CULLEY, M.D.
Instructor of Anaesthesia
Harvard Medical School
Brigham and Women's Hospital
Boston, Massachusetts

NANCY JONES CUMMINGS, Esq.
Legal Counsel
Mayo Clinic Scottsdale
Scottsdale, Arizona

SYLVIA Y. DOLINSKI, M.D.
Assistant Professor
Department of Anesthesiology and Critical Care
Wake Forest University School of Medicine
Winston-Salem, North Carolina

JOHN H. EICHHORN, M.D.
Professor and Chairman, Department of Anesthesiology
University of Mississippi School of Medicine
Chairman, Department of Anesthesiology
University of Mississippi Medical Center
Jackson, Mississippi

JAMES B. EISENKRAFT, M.D.
Professor of Anesthesiology
Mount Sinai School of Medicine
Attending Anesthesiologist
The Mount Sinai Medical Center
New York, New York

JOHN PEDER ERICKSON, M.D.
Assistant Professor of Clinical Anesthesia
University of Chicago Pritzker School of Medicine
Chicago, Illinois
Medical Director, Midwest Medical Center
Palos Heights, Illinois

STEVEN M. FRANK, M.D.
Associate Professor of Anesthesiology
The Johns Hopkins University School of Medicine
Baltimore, Maryland

THOMAS J. GAL, M.D.
Professor of Anesthesiology
University of Virginia School of Medicine
Attending Anesthesiologist
University of Virginia Health Sciences Center
Charlottesville, Virginia

SIMON GELMAN, M.D., Ph.D.
Leroy D. Vandam/Benjamin G. Covino Professor
    of Anesthesia
Harvard Medical School
Chairman, Department of Anesthesiology
Perioperative and Pain Medicine
Brigham and Women's Hospital
Boston, Massachusetts

J.C. GERANCHER, M.D.
Assistant Professor of Anesthesia
Stanford University School of Medicine
Stanford, California

INGER GILLESBERG, M.D.
Research Associate, Department of Anesthesiology
University of Chicago Pritzker School of Medicine
Chicago, Illinois

RANDALL GOSKOWICZ, M.D.
Assistant Clinical Professor of Anesthesia
Director of Anesthesia for Liver Transplantation
Director of Residency Education
University of California, San Diego, School of Medicine
San Diego, California

CARIN HAGBERG, M.D.
Associate Professor of Anesthesiology
University of Texas Medical School at Houston
Staff Anesthesiologist
Hermann Hospital
Lyndon B. Johnson General Hospital
Houston, Texas

MEDHAT S. HANNALLAH, M.D., F.F.A.R.C.S.
Professor of Anesthesiology
Georgetown University Medical Center
Washington, District of Columbia

STEPHEN N. HARRIS, M.D.
Associate Professor of Anesthesiology
Director, Vascular Anesthesia
Co-Director, Intraoperative Echocardiography
Yale University School of Medicine
New Haven, Connecticut

QUINN H. HOGAN, M.D.
Associate Professor of Anesthesiology
Medical College of Wisconsin
Milwaukee, Wisconsin

GIRISH P. JOSHI, M.B., B.S., M.D., F.F.A.R.C.S.I
Associate Professor of Anesthesiology
University of Texas Southwestern Medical Center
Dallas, Texas

JERROLD H. LEVY, M.D.
Professor of Anesthesiology
Director of Cardiothoracic Anesthesiology
Emory University School of Medicine
Atlanta, Georgia

SPENCER S. LIU, M.D.
Clinical Assistant Professor of Anesthesiology
University of Washington School of Medicine
Staff Anesthesiologist, Virginia Mason Medical Center
Seattle, Washington

ROBERT J. LOWES, M.D.
Assistant Professor of Anesthesiology
Department of Anesthesiology
University of Texas Medical School at Galveston
Galveston, Texas

ANN C.P. LUI, M.D., M.Sc., F.R.C.P.C.
Assistant Professor of Anaesthesia
University of Ottawa Faculty of Medicine
Staff Anesthesiologist, Ottawa Hospital
Ottawa, Ontario, Canada

JOHN C. LUNDELL, M.D.
Fellow, Cardiothoracic Anesthesiology
Wake Forest University School of Medicine
Fellow, Cardiothoracic Anesthesia
Wake Forest Baptist Medical Center
Winston-Salem, North Carolina

SCOTT K. MAGNUSON, M.D.
Assistant Professor of Anesthesiology
University of California, San Diego, School of Medicine
San Diego, California

SANFORD M. MILLER, M.D.
Assistant Professor of Clinical Anesthesiology
Assistant Attending Anesthesiologist
New York University Medical Center
Associate Attending Anesthesiologist
Bellevue Hospital Center
New York, New York

DAVID M. MOSKOWITZ, M.D.
Clinical Assistant Professor of Anesthesiology
Division of Cardiothoracic and Vascular Anesthesia
Mount Sinai Medical Center
New York, New York

PHILLIP S. MUSHLIN, M.D., Ph.D.
Associate Professor of Anaesthesia
Harvard Medical School
Staff Anesthesiologist
Department of Anesthesiology, Perioperative, and
    Pain Medicine
Brigham and Women's Hospital
Boston, Massachusetts

JENNIFER E. O'FLAHERTY, M.D., M.P.H.
Assistant Professor of Anesthesiology
University of Virginia School of Medicine
Co-Medical Director, Virginia Ambulatory Surgery Center
Charlottesville, Virginia

NATHAN LEON PACE, M.D., M.Stat.
Professor and Vice Chairman, Department of Anesthesiology
University of Utah School of Medicine
Anesthesiologist, University of Utah Health Sciences Center
Salt Lake City, Utah

KAREN L. POSNER, Ph.D.
Research Associate Professor of Anesthesiology
Adjunct Research Associate Professor of Anthropology
University of Washington
Seattle, Washington

DONALD S. PROUGH, M.D.
Professor and Chairman, Department of Anesthesiology
University of Texas Medical School at Galveston
Galveston, Texas

DAVID L. REICH, M.D.
Professor of Anesthesiology
Co-Director of Cardiothoracic Anesthesia
Mount Sinai School of Medicine
New York, New York

ANNE T. ROGERS, M.B., Ch.B., F.R.C.P.C.
Associate Professor of Anesthesiology
Wake Forest University School of Medicine
Winston-Salem, North Carolina

MICHAEL F. ROIZEN, M.D.
Department of Anesthesiology and Critical Care Medicine
University of Chicago Pritzker School of Medicine
Chicago, Illinois

JOHN B. ROSE, M.D.
Assistant Professor of Anesthesiology and Pediatrics
University of Pennsylvania Health Systems
Associate Anesthesiologist, The Children's Hospital of
    Philadelphia
Philadelphia, Pennsylvania

STANLEY H. ROSENBAUM, M.D.
Professor of Anesthesiology, Internal Medicine, and Surgery
Yale University School of Medicine
New Haven, Connecticut

HENRY ROSENBERG, M.D.
Professor of Anesthesiology
Jefferson Medical College of Thomas Jefferson University
Philadelphia, Pennsylvania

BRIAN K. ROSS, M.D., Ph.D.
Associate Professor of Anesthesiology
University of Washington School of Medicine
Seattle, Washington

STEVEN ROTH, M.D.
Associate Professor of Anesthesia and Critical Care
Director, Neuroanesthesia
University of Chicago Pritzker School of Medicine
Chicago, Illinois

ROGER L. ROYSTER, M.D.
Professor and Vice Chairman, Department of
    Anesthesiology
Wake Forest University School of Medicine
Winston-Salem, North Carolina

LAWRENCE J. SAIDMAN, M.D.
Professor of Anesthesia, Department of Anesthesiology
Stanford University Medical Center
Stanford, California

RICHARD M. SOMMER, M.D.
Clinical Associate Professor of Anesthesiology
New York University School of Medicine
Attending Anesthesiologist
New York University Medical Center
Consultant, New York VA Medical Center
New York, New York

ROBERT K. STOELTING, M.D.
Professor and Chair, Department of Anesthesia
Indiana University School of Medicine
Indianapolis, Indiana

GALE E. THOMPSON, M.D.
Staff Anesthesiologist
The Mason Clinic
Seattle, Washington

METTE VEIEN, M.D.
Research Fellow, Department of Anesthesiology
Emory University School of Medicine
Atlanta, Georgia

MARK S. WALLACE, M.D.
Assistant Professor of Anesthesiology
University of California, San Diego, School of Medicine
Director, Pain Service
University of California, San Diego, Medical Center
San Diego, California

MEHERNOOR F. WATCHA, M.D.
Associate Professor of Anesthesiology and Pediatrics
University of Pennsylvania Health Systems
Associate Anesthesiologist
Children's Hospital of Philadelphia
Philadelphia, Pennsylvania

MICHAEL E. WEISS, M.D.
Clinical Associate Professor of Medicine
University of Washington School of Medicine
Seattle, Washington

RICHARD A. WIKLUND, M.D.
Associate Professor of Anesthesiology
Yale University School of Medicine
Medical Director, Preadmission Center
Yale-New Haven Hospital
New Haven, Connecticut

To

our colleagues

whose professional lives have been or will be
touched by an anesthetic-related complication.

Preface

When Mosby, Inc., the publishers of the first edition of *Anesthesia and Perioperative Complications,* asked us to consider preparing a second edition, we asked ourselves how we might improve on a product that had received very good reviews. Our responses were first, that all of the material retained from the first edition should be updated to reflect the state of anesthesia practice in 1999; second, that we should add chapters covering newly important subjects; and third, that we should recruit authors whose expertise in certain areas had emerged in the 7 years since the first edition had been published.

The results of our efforts are presented in this textbook, and a few comments are appropriate to convey the extent of the changes incorporated into the edition.

Of greatest importance is that this edition is remarkably different from the first. Although most of the chapter titles are the same as those in the first edition, nearly half of the chapters have authors new to this edition. In our opinion, this provides a fresh look at problems, the nature of which change over time, and reflects the most contemporary approach to issues of importance to patient care. In addition, we added a new section on complications related to surgery that are often attributed to anesthesia. For example, the chapters on abdominal surgery and surgically induced embolism describe the pathophysiology underlying the often severe hemodynamic changes associated with traction on the peritoneum and air or carbon dioxide embolism, respectively. At the same time, we retained the approach used in the first edition that identified complications related to specific anesthesia events or resulting from an insult to a system in the body and retained as well the section dealing with medicolegal considerations.

As before, we thank our authors without whose efforts this project would have never been completed. Our thanks go also to our editor, Wendy Buckwalter, whose gentle yet firm pressure kept us and our authors to the originally agreed upon timetable.

Jonathan L. Benumof
Lawrence J. Saidman

Contents

PART ONE

Complications of Specific Anesthetic Events

Chapter 1

Management of the Airway: Complications

Carin Hagberg
Marc H. Boin

Difficulty in managing the airway is the most important cause of major anesthesia-related morbidity and mortality. Adverse outcomes associated with respiratory events constituted the largest class of injury in the American Society of Anesthesiologists closed claims study.[1] Of the 1541 reported cases of problematic airway management, 522 (34%) were respiratory related and 85% resulted in death or brain damage. Most of the outcomes (72%) were thought to be preventable with better monitoring. Three mechanisms of injury accounted for three fourths of the adverse events: inadequate ventilation (38% of patients), esophageal intubation (18%), and difficult tracheal intubation (17%) (Table 1-1). Of note, most of these claims involved healthy young adults undergoing general anesthesia for nonemergency surgery.

In daily anesthetic practice, errors of omission are more common than errors of commission. Errors of omission include failure to recognize the magnitude of a problem, make appropriate observations, or act in a timely manner. Errors of commission, on the other hand, include such actions as trauma to the lips, nose, or laryngotracheal mucosa; forcing sharp instruments into areas in which they do not belong; or introducing air or secretions into regions of the body in which further complications will ensue. However, the primary goal of anesthesiologists is to ensure the safety and well-being of

Table 1-1. Distribution of claims for adverse respiratory events

Event	Number of cases	Percentage of 522 respiratory claims	Percentage of 1541 total claims
Inadequate ventilation	196	38	13
Esophageal intubation	94	18	6
Difficult tracheal intubation	87	17	6
Airway obstruction	34	7	2
Bronchospasm	32	6	2
Aspiration	26	5	2
Premature tracheal extubation	21	4	1
Unintentional tracheal extubation	14	3	1
Inadequate forced inspiratory pressure	11	2	1
Endobronchial intubation	7	1	<1
Total	522	100	34

Modified from Caplan RA, Posner KL, Ward RJ, et al: *Anesthesiology* 72:829, 1990.

their patients, and anesthesiologists are usually careful in performing the technical aspects of their jobs.

To minimize injury to the patient, the anesthesiologist should examine the patient's airway carefully, identify any potential problems, devise a plan that involves the least risk for injury, and have a backup plan immediately available. Common sense should prevail at all times. Complications should be evaluated for new insights that enable us to modify daily practice and minimize future problems. This chapter reviews the potential problems associated with airway management so that we may learn from the collective experience of our colleagues.

I. MASK VENTILATION

Mask ventilation is commonly used at the outset of administration of almost all general anesthetics. As benign as both the technique and the mask may seem, each has its own potential set of problems.

A. The sterilization process

Before any reusable mask is applied to a patient's face, it should be checked for leaks or pinhole defects in its air-filled bladder. If air or fluid is expressed from the bladder, the mask should be discarded immediately. A case report was published in which sterilizing solutions found access to the bladder of a reusable mask while it was being cleaned. Subsequent application of the mask to a patient's face resulted in extravasation of the cleaning fluid onto his cheeks. Some of that fluid leaked into his eyes, causing severe burning and irritation.[2] Another report identified a patient who contracted chemical conjunctivitis from glutaraldehyde on an anesthesia mask.[3] All reusable items applied to the skin of a patient should be completely free of residual cleansing agents. If the com-

mon cleaning solution, ethylene oxide, is not completely rinsed and aerated from reusable surfaces, it can cause serious mucosal injury. Water added to ethylene oxide forms ethylene glycol, an irritant. The presence of residual glutaraldehyde on an improperly rinsed laryngoscope blade has been implicated in causing massive tongue swelling and life-threatening allergic glossitis during otherwise uncomplicated administration of general anesthetic.[4] Care must also be taken to thoroughly rinse the suction channel of a fiberoptic bronchoscope after cleaning. Residual agents may drip out of the bronchoscope port into the larynx or trachea, causing severe chemical burns.

B. Mechanical difficulties

A mask is typically applied to a patient's face during induction of general anesthesia. During such placement, the air-filled bladder of the mask should be inspected to ensure that when gentle pressure is applied, no rigid parts of the mask are in direct contact with the bridge of the nose or mandible. Bruising and soft tissue damage may occur in these regions if they are subjected to excessive pressure. Care must be taken to avoid contact with the eyes to prevent corneal abrasions, retinal artery occlusions, or blindness. As induction proceeds, both firmer mask pressure and stronger lifting pressure on the angle of the mandible will be necessary to maintain a tight mask fit and secure an adequate airway. Pressure on the soft tissue of the submandibular region may obstruct the airway, especially in small children. In addition, excessive pressure on the mandible may damage the mandibular branch of the facial nerve, resulting in transient facial nerve paralysis.[5] Pressure from the rim of the mask on the mental nerves as they exit from the foramina has been implicated in causing lower-lip numbness in two patients.[6]

Occasionally, the base of the tongue may fall back into the oral pharynx during induction and obstruct the airway. Oropharyngeal airways must be gently inserted into the mouth to avoid injury, such as broken teeth or mucosal tears. Improper placement may cause worsened airway obstruction by forcing the tongue backward. Equal care should be given to the placement of nasopharyngeal airways to avoid nosebleeds and epistaxis.

During the course of induction, the lifting pressure applied to the angle of the mandible is sometimes sufficient to subluxate the temporomandibular joint. Patients may experience persistent pain or bruising at these points and may even have chronic dislocation of the jaw. These problems are not typical in small children but may be pronounced in adults. Positive airway pressure can force air into the stomach instead of the trachea. This may result in an exaggerated condition of gastric distention, causing more difficult ventilation and an increased propensity for regurgitation. Cricoid pressure can help reduce the amount of air being forced into the stomach and limit the likelihood of vomiting.

Numerous factors can make mask ventilation difficult or impossible, such as edentulous patients; patients with large tongues; full beards or excessive facial hair; heavy jaw muscles that resist mandibular subluxation; sleep ap-

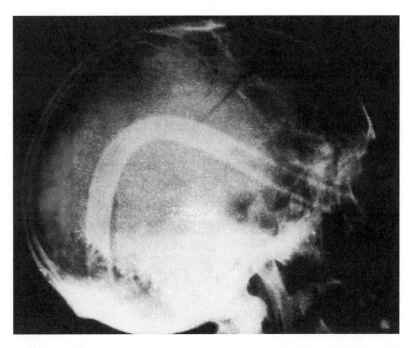

Fig. 1-1. Intracranial nasotracheal tube (computer enhanced). (From Horellow MF, Mathe D, Feiss P: *Anaesthesia* 33:73, 1978.)

nea; poor atlantooccipital extension; uncertain pharyngeal pathology, especially masses; and facial burns or deformities. In such cases, it may be best to avoid mask ventilation and immediately perform direct laryngoscopy or awake fiberoptic intubation. Patients with trauma to the pharyngeal mucosa may be at risk for subcutaneous emphysema. Patients who play wind instruments are also at risk because sufficiently high intrapharyngeal pressures can cause weakened soft tissue and laryngoceles in the lateral pharynx.

C. Prolonged ventilation

When a mask has been used for a long time, vulnerable parts of the face should be inspected for injury. The bridge of the nose and the area along the mandible are at particular risk for compromised blood flow.[7] Because mask ventilation offers no protection against silent regurgitation, the anesthesiologist should always be vigilant for any questionable airway noise, coughing, or bucking. Unlike opaque masks, transparent masks allow visualization of the mouth and early identification of vomitus. As noted, extra care should be taken to avoid undue pressure on the eyes or the orbits to avoid abrasions or injuries to the retinal artery. Whenever continuous positive airway pressure is applied to patients with basilar skull fractures, pneumocephalus may occur.[8,9] At least one published case report identified positive airway pressure as the cause of bilateral otorrhagia.[10]

II. NASAL INTUBATION
A. Cranial intubation

Nasotracheal intubations are potentially very hazardous. In the presence of basilar skull fractures or certain facial fractures (such as LeFort II or III fractures), the endotracheal tube may be inadvertently introduced into the cranial vault (Fig. 1-1).[11] Green, Wood, and Davis[12] reported a case of an uncomplicated nasotracheal intubation in which asystole occurred after the tube was introduced into the orbit. Substantial facial trauma and evidence of basilar skull fractures are usually considered to be contraindications for this technique. However, Bähr and Stoll[13] argued that if special care is taken, the complication rates of oral and nasal intubation do not differ. Nevertheless, if nasal intubation is going to be attempted in a patient with a known or suspected skull fracture, it should only be performed by using fiberoptic bronchoscopy and with extreme caution. Nasotracheal tubes may also dissect backward and run behind the posterior pharyngeal wall. Patients with an obstructed nasal passage secondary to convoluted turbinates are at increased risk for this complication.

B. Nasal injury

Nasal intubation may cause lacerations of the nasal mucosa, hemorrhage, and epistaxis. Nosebleeds are common but are relatively easy to prevent. It is paramount that the nasal mucosa be vasoconstricted before instrumentation. Some agents used for this purpose are 0.5% phenylephrine in 4% lidocaine, 4% cocaine, or 0.1% xylometazoline.[14] To minimize the chance of nasal injury, a small endotracheal tube that has been lubricated well and soaked in warm water (to increase its pliability) should be used. Minor bruising occurs in 54% of nasal intubations and most commonly involves the mucosa overlying the inferior turbinate and the adjacent septum.[15] Care should be taken to prevent an endotracheal tube from cutting into the pharyngeal mucosa and causing bleeding or creating a false submucosal passage. In addition, dislodgment of nasal polyps has been reported.[16] One case report cited complete obstruction of a nasotracheal tube caused by a fractured turbinate during intubation.[17] Rents in the pharyngeal mucosa can mature into retropharyngeal abscesses.[18] Should epistaxis occur, it is recommended that the endotracheal tube cuff be inflated and remain in the nostril to tamponade the bleeding.

Even in the absence of gross trauma, the mechanical damage to the superficial epithelial layers caused by nasal intubation results in mucociliary slowing in 65% of patients[19] and bacteremia in another 5.5%.[20] The most common organisms introduced into the blood are nasopharyngeal commensal organisms (e.g., *Streptococcus viridans*), which are known to cause endocarditis and systemic infection. Even short-term intubation has been reported to cause nasal septal and retropharyngeal abscesses. Acute otitis media has been reported to occur in 13% of nasally intubated neonates.[21] Paranasal sinusitis has also been reported, most commonly with nasal intubation for more than 5 days.[22,23] Infection may be related to sustained edema and occlusion of the sinus drainage pathways. Prompt diagnosis is critical, and paranasal sinusitis should be suspected in any patient with facial tenderness, pain, or purulent nasal discharge or in any nasally intubated patient who develops sepsis with no other obvious source.

Once the tube is secured in place in the trachea, care should be taken to ensure that it is also secured properly at the level of the nostril. Distortion of the nares can lead to ischemia, skin necrosis, or nasal adhesion.

C. Foreign bodies

The nostrils are common sites for entry of foreign bodies. Small children, who are renowned for placing small objects into their orifices, find that the nostrils are some of the most accessible sites. Smith, Timms, and Sutcliffe[24] reported a rhinolith that became dislodged during nasotracheal intubation. The mass was formed around the rubber tire of a toy car that the patient had placed in his nose 30 years earlier. Fortunately, the rhinolith caused no problems. However, during nasotracheal intubation, great potential exists to dislodge any similar foreign bodies, after which they may obstruct the endotracheal tube, pharynx, or trachea. If a nasal foreign body is known or suspected, it should be gingerly dislodged and advanced into the oral pharynx, if possible, where it can be retrieved before intubation.

III. ORAL INTUBATION
A. Insertion of the endotracheal tube

1. Anatomic requirements. Successful oral intubation requires four anatomic traits: adequate mouth opening, sufficient pharyngeal space (determined by visualization of the hypopharynx), compliant submandibular tissue (determined by measuring the thyromental distance), and adequate atlantooccipital extension.[25] If the patient's anatomy is compromised in any of these factors, intubation will be difficult at the very least.

The opening to the airway may prove inadequate because of facial scars, temporomandibular joint (TMJ) disease, macroglossia, or dental disease. Nasal intubation techniques, such as blind or fiberoptic approaches, may overcome this problem.

The pharyngeal space may be limited by tumors, abscesses, edema, or surgical or traumatic disruption. If the anatomy is distorted, the anesthesiologist must optimize viewing of the vocal cords. Awake intubation may be necessary and should be considered whenever the pharyngeal space is limited by these conditions. If direct laryngoscopy is performed, the patient should be placed in the proper "sniffing" position and a styletted endotracheal tube should be strongly considered. Every effort should be made to optimize visualization and identification of the pharyngeal structures.

The compliance of the submandibular space is critical to ensuring that the tongue will be easily placed out of the way to view the glottis. Compliance may be decreased by scarring, changes caused by radiation, or localized infections. Awake intubation or fiberoptic techniques should be strongly considered in these instances.

Extension of the atlantooccipital region is critical in lifting the epiglottis off the posterior pharyngeal wall during direct laryngoscopy. A fused, fixed, or unstable spine may be rigid enough to impede visualization of the glottic structures. Again, blind nasal or fiberoptic techniques should be considered.

2. Difficult intubation. Despite optimal positioning of the head and neck, the glottis is sometimes impossible to visualize, even in patients without any obvious predisposing features.[26-28] Risk factors for difficult tracheal intubation include male sex, age 40 to 59 years, and obesity.[25] White and Kander[26] identified several factors that should alert the anesthesiologist to a potentially difficult intubation (Fig. 1-2). These include a short muscular neck and a full set of teeth; a receding lower jaw with obtuse mandibular angles; protrusion of the upper incisors with reduced space between the angles of the mandible; a high-arched palate; and increased distance from the upper incisors to the posterior border of the mandibular ramus. They also identified several radiographic features that make direct laryngoscopy more difficult, such as increased posterior depth of the mandible (which limits submandibular displacement of the soft tissues); increased anterior depth of the mandible; reduced distance between the occiput and the C1 spinous process and in the C1-C2 interspinous gap (which narrows the limits of head extension); and reduced mobility of the mandible caused by TMJ dysfunction.

A chin-to-thyroid cartilage distance of less than three fingerbreadths (about 7 cm) hampers visualization of the glottis.[29] This is most likely because the soft tissues cannot be displaced into the submandibular space during direct laryngoscopy. In the absence of jaw measurements, the degree of difficulty of intubation may be predicted by performing a test described by Mallampati et al[30] and modified by Samsoon and Young.[31] The seated, awake patient is asked to open his or her mouth as wide as possible and maximally protrude his or her tongue without phonating. The ability to see the faucial pillars and uvula is then classified into one of four groups. The sensitivity and specificity for predicting a difficult intubation by viewing the pharyngeal structures exceed 81%; when combined with measurement of the thyromental distance measurement, the specificity increases to almost 98%.[29]

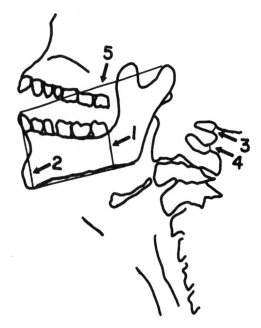

Fig. 1-2. Measurements relevant in assessing the difficulty of laryngoscopy in an adult. *1,* Increased posterior depth of the mandible; *2,* increased anterior depth of the mandible; *3,* reduction in the distance between the occiput and the spinous process of C1; *4,* reduction in the distance between the occiput and the C1-C2 interspinous gap; and *5,* effective mandibular length less than 3.6 times the posterior depth of the mandible. Effective mandibular length by itself, however, is no different in patients in whom laryngoscopy is difficult. (From White A, Kander PL: *Br J Anaesth* 47:468, 1975, as modified by Rosenberg H, Rosenberg HK: Airway obstruction and tracheal intubation. In Gravenstein N, Kirby RR, eds: *Complications in anesthesiology,* Philadelphia, 1996, Lippincott-Raven.)

Box 1-1 Miscellaneous causes of difficult
intubation

Enlarged tonsils and adenoids caused by inflammation
or tumors
  Lymphoma
Retropharyngeal abscess
Cystic hygroma
Retropharyngeal tumors
  Teratoma
  Neurofibroma
  Neuroblastoma
Nasopharyngeal meningoencephalocele
Myxedematous thickening of retropharyngeal soft tissues
Pharyngeal tumors
  Benign polyps
  Dermoids
  Teratomas
  Thyroglossal duct cysts
  Neuroblastoma
  Neurofibromas
  Hemangiomas
Laryngeal and upper tracheal tumors
  Papillomas
  Subglottic hemangiomas
Enlarged thyroid
Middle and lower tracheal compression
  Enlarged thyroid
  Mediastinal masses
    Teratoma
    Lymphoma
    Ectopic thyroid

Miscellaneous causes of difficult intubation are shown in Box 1-1.[32] Patients who proved difficult to intubate should be told of that fact so that they may notify future anesthesiologists. In addition, patients should be registered with the Medic Alert system.

3. Traumatic intubation

a. Spinal cord and vertebral column injury. When a patient's neck is fused as a result of ankylosing spondylitis, adequate neck extension may be impossible to obtain. Attempting to hyperextend the necks of these patients may result in cervical fractures and quadriplegia.[33] A head that is fixated in a cervical collar or halo does not allow neck extension and limits the successful use of direct laryngoscopy. A blind nasal or a fiberoptic intubation should be considered in these cases. If immediate intubation is necessary, a patient with an unstable neck resulting from an acute fracture may be supported by in-line cervical stabilization and carefully intubated, provided that the head is protected against excessive movement. Special attention should be given to patients with C1 or C2 fractures because any degree of extension might compromise spinal cord function. Ten percent to 25% of spinal cord injuries occur secondary to improper immobilization of the vertebral column after trauma.[34-36]

Hastings and Kelley[37] reported neurologic deterioration associated with direct laryngoscopy in a patient with a cervical spine injury. Several conditions, such as Down syndrome and rheumatoid arthritis, are associated with atlantoaxial instability.[38,39] Excessive neck extension in a patient with an undiagnosed Arnold-Chiari malformation may cause worsening of cerebellar tonsil herniation.[40] Whenever reasonable doubt about the degree of neck extension exists (regardless of the cause), a range-of-motion test and an assessment of neck extension should be performed before inducing anesthesia. Blind nasal and fiberoptic intubations should be considered in these cases to minimize injury.

b. Laryngotracheal trauma. Trauma to the larynx is not uncommon after endotracheal intubation. In one large study, 6.2% of patients sustained severe lesions, 4.5% had hematoma of the vocal cords, 1% had hematoma of the supraglottic region, and 1% sustained lacerations of the vocal cord mucosa.[41] Recovery is generally prompt with conservative therapy.[42] It is recommended that the larynx be inspected for injury before insertion of the endotracheal tube to document and treat any preexistent lesions. A small but significant number of patients sustain laryngeal injuries during short-term intubation.[42]

Arytenoid dislocation and subluxation have been reported.[43-46] Mitigating factors include traumatic and difficult intubations, repeated attempts at intubation, and attempted intubation with a lightwand stylet. These situations can usually be corrected easily but often require an ears, nose, and throat consultation.

The vocal process of the arytenoid is the most common site of injury caused by the endotracheal tube as it is positioned between the vocal cords. Granuloma formation most commonly occurs at this site. The degree of injury worsens as the size of the tube increases.[47] Granulations usually occur as a complication of long-term intubation but have been reported with short-term intubation.[48] Long-term intubation can also result in varying degrees of laryngeal edema and vocal fold ulcerations.[49,50]

Tracheal trauma is caused by various sources.[51] Injury may result from the endotracheal tube, the laryngoscope, the stylet, or related equipment. Predisposing factors include anatomic difficulties; blind or hurried intubation; inadequate positioning; poor visualization; or, most commonly, inexperience on the part of the intubator. The presence of an endotracheal tube may lead to edema, desquamation, inflammation, and ulceration of the airway.[52] The severity of the injury may be related to the duration of intubation, although this relation is not well established.[53] Any irritating stimulus, such as pressure from an oversized endotracheal tube, dry inhaled gases, allergic reactions to inhaled sprays, or chemical irritation from residual cleaning solutions, can initiate an inflammatory response and cause mucosal edema in the larynx or trachea. Edema after extubation limits the lumen diameter and increases airway resistance. Small children are most susceptible to this problem, in which a sudden increase in airway resistance results from laryngotracheobronchitis or croup. Almost 4% of children 1 to 3 years of age develop croup after tracheal intubation.[54,55] In addition, mechanical trauma may result from sharp objects within the trachea, such as a stylet tip that extends beyond the length of the endotracheal tube. One case of a bronchial rupture secondary to use of an endotracheal tube changer was reported.[56]

Endotracheal tube cuffs inflated to a pressure greater than that of the capillary perfusion (approximately 30 mm Hg) may devitalize the tracheal mucosa, leading to ulceration, necrosis, and loss of structural integrity. Ulceration will occur at even lower pressures in hypotensive patients. The need for increasing cuff volumes to maintain a seal is an ominous sign of tracheomalacia. To maintain an adequate airway seal in such patients, it may be necessary to use an uncuffed endotracheal tube and a throat pack. Massive gastric distention in an intubated patient may signal the presence of a tracheoesophageal fistula as the cuff progressively erodes into the esophagus.[57] Likewise, any patient with more than 10 ml of blood in the endotracheal tube without a known cause should be suspected of having a tracheocarotid fistula.[58] The various nerves in this region of the neck are also at risk. Erosion of the endotracheal tube into the paratracheal nerves may result in dysphonia, hoarseness, and laryngeal incompetence. Tracheomalacia results from erosion confined to the tracheal carti-

lages. It is imperative that the anesthesiologist inflate the cuff of the endotracheal tube only as much as necessary to ensure an adequate airway seal. In the presence of nitrous oxide during a lengthy surgical procedure, the pressure in the cuff should be periodically checked and limited to only the pressure necessary to maintain a seal. In the presence of 70% nitrous oxide, intracuff pressures take an average of 12 minutes to increase to levels that are potentially high enough to cause tracheal ischemia.[59]

c. Barotrauma. Barotrauma results from high-pressure distention of intrapulmonary structures. High-flow insufflation techniques in which small catheters are used distal to the larynx are most often associated with barotrauma. Such problems are common in microlaryngeal surgery in which jet ventilation is used.[60-64] Direct impingement of the catheter tip on the tracheal mucosa may also cause barotrauma.[62] Whenever air leaks into the peribronchial tissues, it can traverse into the subcutaneous space, the lung interstitium, or the pleural and pericardial cavities. The progressive accumulation of air may cause loss of pulmonary compliance; loss of ventilatory volume; or, if the accumulation is large enough, pericardial and pulmonary tamponade. Safety mechanisms should be in place to prevent high-pressure airflow in the event that intrapulmonary pressures become excessive. For diseased pulmonary tissue, the least possible airway pressure should be used to prevent parenchymal blowout. This advice also applies to patients with blunt thoracic trauma who have subcutaneous emphysema. Such patients should be presumed to have a bronchial leak until proven otherwise, and only low-pressure ventilation should be used until the lesions are located. In the presence of pneumothorax, chest tubes will help relieve the problem until it is corrected surgically.

d. Dental trauma. Dental injuries are one of the most common anesthesia-related malpractice claims reported,[65] with an overall incidence ranging from 1:100[66] to 1:1000 of all intubations[67] performed in the United States. A closed claims analysis done in the United States from 1978 to 1980 disclosed that broken teeth were among the most common complications during general anesthesia that resulted in litigation. Dental injuries are most common in small children, patients with periodontal disease (in which structural support is poor) or fixed dental work (such as bridges and capped teeth), and patients in whom intubation is difficult. All loose, diseased, chipped, or capped teeth must be noted in the chart before intubation,[68] and the patient must be advised of the risk of dental damage. Tooth protectors can be used, but they may be awkward and can obstruct vision.[69]

If a tooth is chipped or partially broken, the fragment should be located and retrieved. Unfortunately, it cannot be reaffixed to the original tooth. In the event that an entire tooth is avulsed, it should be retrieved and saved in a moist gauze or in normal saline without cleansing. Great care should be taken to ensure that any dislodged teeth or tooth fragments do not slip into the pharynx to later become lodged in the esophagus or the larynx. With rapid response from an oral surgeon or a dentist, an intact tooth can often be reimplanted and saved.[70]

e. Lip trauma. Lip injuries, which are typically found on the upper lip, include lacerations, hematomas, edema, and teeth marks. They are usually secondary to inattentive laryngoscopy, in which the lip is trapped between the laryngoscope blade and the teeth. Although these lesions are annoying to the patient, they are usually self-limited.

f. Damage to the uvula. Edema and necrosis of the uvula have been reported as rare complications of endotracheal intubation.[71,72] The trauma is postulated to result either from overzealous suctioning[73] or from direct pressure from the endotracheal tube.

g. Vocal cord paralysis. Numerous investigators have reported vocal cord paralysis after intubation with no other obvious source of injury.[74-77] One report associated vocal cord paralysis with use of ethylene oxide to sterilize endotracheal tubes.[78] Paralysis may be unilateral or bilateral. Hoarseness occurs with unilateral paralysis, whereas respiratory obstruction occurs with bilateral problems. The most likely source of injury is an endotracheal tube cuff that presses on the recurrent laryngeal nerve as it passes between the thyroid cartilage and the vocal process of the arytenoid cartilage.[75,76] Permanent voice change after intubation because of external laryngeal nerve trauma has been reported in up to 3% of patients undergoing surgery in sites other than the head or neck. However, vocal cord paralysis after intubation is usually temporary. Its incidence may be decreased by avoiding overinflation of the endotracheal tube cuff and by placing the endotracheal tube at least 15 mm below the vocal cords.[75]

Vocal cord paralysis may also have a central origin. One case was reported in which an infant with a Dandy-Walker cyst sustained left vocal cord paralysis after placement of a cystoperitoneal shunt.[79]

h. Other nerve injuries. Transient weakness, numbness, or paralysis of the tongue can occur after laryngoscopy, presumably because of pressure on the laryngeal or hypoglossal nerves.[80] One patient had loss of sensation in the tongue for 1 month after lingual nerve compression during difficult intubation.[81] Two other patients had signs of aspiration resulting from damage of the superior laryngeal nerve during difficult intubation.[82] This latter complication usually does not persist.

4. Esophageal intubation

a. Endotracheal tube placement. When visualization of the glottis is difficult, the endotracheal tube may inadvertently be introduced into the esophagus. Intubating the esophagus is not disastrous, but failing to detect and correct the condition is. Recognition of this error must be rapid to avoid the adverse effects of prolonged hypoxia. A closed claims analysis of adverse anesthetic events reported that 18% of respiratory-related claims involved esophageal intubation (see Table 1-1).[1] Preoxygenation can help alleviate this problem by allowing a longer apneic period for tracheal intubation and by delaying the onset of hypoxemia for up to 11 minutes. End-tidal CO_2 capnography is essential in confirming endotracheal placement of the tube. All other signs, such as bilateral breath sounds, chest wall movement, and absence of gastric sounds, are potentially misleading (Table 1-2).[83] Esophageal intubation can briefly produce an end-tidal

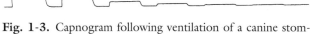

Fig. 1-3. Capnogram following ventilation of a canine stomach filled with 5% carbon dioxide. (From Good ML, Modell JH, Rush W: *Anesthesiology* 69:A266, 1988.)

Table 1-2. Methods of assessing endotracheal tube position

Technique	Documented failure
Direct cord visualization	None (gold standard)
End-tidal carbon dioxide measurement	None, but theoretically non–fail-safe (e.g., with cardiac arrest)
Fiberoptic bronchoscopy	None, but impractical
Video stethoscope	None, but impractical
Eschmann endotracheal tube changer	None, but cumbersome; traumatic and theoretically unreliable
Equal bilateral breath sounds	Yes
Symmetric bilateral chest wall movement	Yes
Epigastric auscultation and observation	Yes
Reservoir bag compliance and refilling	Yes
Presence of exhaled tidal volumes/respiratory effort	Yes
Normal ventilator function	Yes
Quality of air sound escaping around tube	Yes
Cuff palpation in neck	Yes
Chest radiography	Yes
Chest radiography	Yes
Tube condensation	No, but unreliable
Presence of gastric contents in the tube	No, but unreliable
Pulse oximetry	No, but relatively late

Modified from Birmingham PK, Cheney FW, Ward RJ: *Anesth Analg* 65:886, 1986.

CO_2 capnogram, but the waveform diminishes rapidly after 3 to 5 breaths[84] (Fig. 1-3). Excessive distention of the stomach with gas containing CO_2 may follow vigorous manual inflation while testing for correct tube placement.

It is recommended that a misplaced tube remain in place while the trachea is correctly intubated. This not only helps identify the correct orifice for intubation but also protects the trachea from invasion by regurgitated stomach contents. Once proper endotracheal intubation is achieved after an esophageal intubation, the stomach should be suctioned to minimize vomiting, gastric perforation, or compromise of ventilation.

b. Esophageal perforation and retropharyngeal abscess. Perforation of the esophagus has been reported on several occasions.[85-93] It seems most likely to occur when inexperienced clinicians handle emergency situations or when intubation is difficult. Perforation occurs most commonly over the cricopharyngeus muscle on the posterior esophageal wall, where the esophagus is narrowed and thin. Subcutaneous emphysema, pneumothorax, fever, cellulitis, cyanosis, throat pain, mediastinitis, empyema, pericarditis, and death can occur. Early detection and treatment of the condition are critical because the mortality rate of mediastinitis is more than 50%. An esophageal perforation should be suspected in any patient with a fever, sore throat, and subcutaneous emphysema following a history of difficult intubation.

A published case report identified a traumatic tracheal perforation through the esophagus. Intubation of the patient was difficult because of poor cervical neck extension. After several attempts, the tube was advanced into the trachea and its presence was confirmed by improved oxygen saturation. However, chest radiography after intubation revealed that the tube had gained access to the trachea by initially entering the esophagus and puncturing the walls of both the esophagus and the membranous trachea.[94]

5. Bronchial intubation

a. Use of an endotracheal tube. Bronchial intubation occurs often and is sometimes difficult to identify. Asymmetric chest expansion, unilateral absence of breath sounds (especially on the left side), and eventual arterial blood gas abnormalities are diagnostic features. If bronchial intubation goes undetected, it may lead to atelectasis, hypoxia, and pulmonary edema.[95] Transillumination of the neck with a lightwand[96] or direct visualization with a fiberoptic scope can assist in tube location. The endotracheal tube may also be deliberately advanced into a mainstem bronchus and withdrawn until bilateral breath sounds are auscultated.

The tip of the endotracheal tube may be moved during flexion or extension of the patient's head as the patient is positioned for surgery. Conrardy et al[97] showed that the tip of the endotracheal tube moved an average of 3.8 cm toward the carina when the neck was moved from full extension to full flexion. In some patients, this change was as great as 6.4 cm (Fig. 1-4).[97] It is easy to remember that the tip of the endotracheal tube moves in the same direction as the patient's nose. If the patient's neck is flexed, the nose is pointed downward and the endotracheal tube advances farther into the trachea. In addition, the tube moves away from the carina an average of 0.7 cm during lateral rotation of the head.

When inadvertent bronchial intubation is discovered, the tube should be withdrawn several centimeters and the lungs hyperinflated sufficiently to expand any atelectatic areas. In cases of chronic atelectasis, bronchoscopy may be required to remove the mucous plugs. This problem can be avoided by measuring the length of the endotracheal tube alongside the patient before intubation. The tip of the tube should ideally be at least 2 cm above the carina, which may be approximated at the sternal angle (of Louis) adjacent to the junction of the sternum with the second rib. In general, appropriate tube depths are 21 cm from the teeth in adult women and 23

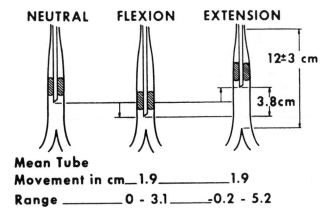

Mean Tube Movement in cm __1.9_____1.9

Range _____0 - 3.1_____-0.2 - 5.2

Fig. 1-4. The mean movement of an endotracheal tube with flexion and extension of the neck from a neutral position. The mean tube movement between flexion and extension is one-third to one-fourth the length of a normal adult trachea (12 ± 3 cm). (From Conrardy PA, Goodman LR, Lainge F, et al: *Crit Care Med* 4:8, 1976.)

cm in adult men.[98] If a cuffed tube is used, the cuff location can be found by squeezing the pilot balloon and feeling for the inflated cuff in the suprasternal notch.

b. Use of a double-lumen tube. Safe limits for the placement of double-lumen tubes have been outlined by Benumof et al.[99] Modern fiberoptic bronchoscopes have removed the guesswork surrounding endotracheal tube tip location. The double-lumen tube may be inserted blindly into the appropriate bronchus and followed by bronchoscopic confirmation of its position, or the bronchoscope may be inserted initially and used as a stylet over which the double-lumen tube is advanced. However, even in the best of hands, tracheobronchial injuries occur.[100] Bronchial rupture is a serious complication that requires immediate attention. Wagner, Gammage, and Wong[101] could not find a cause for the ruptured membranous trachea in one patient. Another case report identified a ruptured left mainstem bronchus, presumably caused by using too large a double-lumen tube for that patient.[102] One solution is to inflate the tracheal cuff and leave the nonintubated bronchial lumen open to the air. The intubated lung is then ventilated, and the bronchial cuff is inflated until the air leak disappears.[103]

6. Laryngospasm.

Reflex responses to stage II of anesthesia during intubation or extubation can be problematic. Laryngospasm can occur, in which the patient makes respiratory efforts but cannot move air in or out of the lungs. If direct laryngoscopy was performed, the vocal cords would be completely adducted. However, laryngospasm involves more than spastic closure of the vocal cords. An infolding of the arytenoids and the aryepiglottic folds occurs; these structures are subsequently covered by the epiglottis.[104] This explains why a firm jaw thrust can sometimes break the spasm—the hyoid is elevated, thereby stretching the epiglottis and aryepiglottic folds to open the forced closure. Positive mask pressure may help by distending the pharynx or vocal cords, but this technique is not always adequate.

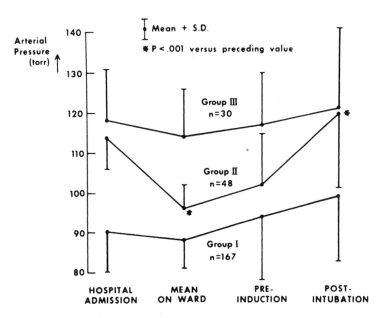

Fig. 1-5. Mean arterial blood pressure in response to hospital admission and endotracheal intubation in three groups of patients. A substantial increase in blood pressure occurred after intubation only in the group of patients who were hypertensive (blood pressure >140/90 mm Hg) at the time of admission but were otherwise normotensive during hospitalization. *SD*, Standard deviation. (From Bedford RF, Feinstein B: *Anesth Analg* 59:367, 1980.)

Treatment with a short-acting muscle relaxant, such as 10 to 20 mg of succinylcholine, may be necessary to break the spasm. The clinician should consider suctioning the stomach to relieve any entrapped air caused by the positive-pressure attempts once the spasm is broken and the patient can be ventilated.

7. Bronchospasm. Tracheal irritation from the endotracheal tube can cause bronchospasm that is sufficiently severe to prevent air movement throughout the lungs.[105] Approximately 80% of the measurable resistance to airflow occurs in the large central airways; the remaining 20% occurs in the smaller peripheral bronchioles.[106] The incidence of intraoperative bronchospasm is almost 9% with endotracheal intubation but is close to 0% with mask ventilation.[107] Poor correlation is seen with age, sex, duration or severity of reactive airway disease, duration of anesthesia, or the forced expiratory volume in 1 second.[107] Other factors that may contribute to bronchospasm include inhaled stimulants, release of allergic mediators, viral infections, exercise, or pharmacologic factors (including β-blockers, prostaglandin inhibitors, and anticholinesterases). The spasm can be treated with inhalation of epinephrine or isoproterenol or a β2-agonist (such as albuterol, metaproterenol, or terbutaline) or by deepening the level of a volatile anesthetic. As with laryngospasm, the best course is to avoid the condition altogether. In patients with reactive airway disease, ketamine[108] and inhaled anesthetics are ideal. A deep level of anesthesia should be achieved before airway instrumentation. A local anesthetic, such as 4% lidocaine, may be used to topically anesthetize the larynx and trachea, or lidocaine (1 to 2 mg/kg) may be injected intravenously before airway stimulation.[109]

Of equal concern in patients at risk for bronchospasm is the timing of extubation. These patients may be extubated either during deep anesthesia (if this approach can be used safely) or when they are fully awake and can protect their own airway reflexes. Although the degree of spasm in this condition is severe, it is usually self-limited and short-lived.

8. Hemodynamic changes. Direct laryngoscopy and tracheal intubation are both potent stimuli that may instigate an intense autonomic response.[110,111] Tachycardia, hypertension, arrhythmias, bronchospasm, and bronchorrhea are common; hypotension and bradycardia occur less often. All patients undergoing laryngoscopy while lightly anesthetized experience these responses to varying degrees. Patients with preexisting hypertension are even more at risk when they are under stress. Patients who are hypertensive (blood pressure >140/90 mm Hg) on admission to the hospital but are normotensive thereafter are most likely to develop severe hypertension after intubation (Fig. 1-5).[112]

Because many of these patients have coexisting cardiovascular disease and cannot meet increased myocardial oxygen demands, it is imperative that large hemodynamic responses be prevented. More than 11% of patients with myocardial disease develop some degree of myocardial ischemia during intubation.[113] The key element is to provide an adequate depth of anesthesia with either intravenous or inhalation agents before instrumentation of the airway. The sympathetic response may be further blunted directly by using β-blockers, narcotics, or vasodilators. Intravenous lidocaine (1.5 mg/kg) given 3 minutes before intubation is a useful adjunct.[114,115] Topical lidocaine sprayed directly on the vocal cords may also attenuate the response to intubation, especially if laryngoscopy is prolonged for more than 30 seconds.[116,117] Narcotics, especially fentanyl, are effective in blunting hemodynamic perturbations. A dose of 2 µg/kg of fentanyl will attenuate the autonomic changes, and 6 µg/kg will completely abolish them.[118,119] β-Blockers will blunt the increased heart rate and contractility associated with intubation. Esmolol (0.25 to 1 mg/kg) has the advantages of being β₁-selective and having a very short duration of action.[120] Labetalol (100 to 250 µg/kg) provides combined α- and β-blockade, which helps further diminish these responses, especially if it is given at least 3 minutes before intubation. Calcium-channel blockers, most notably verapamil, blunt the hypertension and tachycardia seen with intubation.[121] Vasodilators can prevent hypertension without depressing myocardial contractility. A small bolus of nitroglycerin[122] (50 µg) or nitroprusside[123] (50 to 100 µg) in a 70-kg adult briefly decreases the vascular tone. However, the exact dose required for each patient is so difficult to determine that these drugs are not commonly used for this purpose. Administration of an appropriate prophylactic dose of each of these drugs should be based on the response of the individual patient.

9. Coughing and bucking. Two additional adverse responses to intubation are coughing and bucking on the endotracheal tube.[124] Such responses are potentially hazardous in cases of increased intracranial pressure,[125] intracranial vascular anomalies, open-globe injuries, or ophthalmologic surgery[126] or in cases in which increased intraabdominal pressure could rupture an abdominal incision. Intubating a patient only when an adequate depth of anesthesia has been achieved will help prevent this reflex. Intravenous lidocaine, 1 to 2 mg/kg, will help suppress the cough response that occurs with endotracheal intubation.[127-129] In addition, the vocal cords may be sprayed with lidocaine to prevent their reactivity. The same conditions apply during emergence and extubation. Intravenous lidocaine may be given 3 to 5 minutes before extubation, and the patient may be extubated while still in the deep plane of anesthesia. A new, modified endotracheal tube is available that contains a small-bore channel incorporated into the tube's lesser curvature. This design permits the delivery of local anesthetic directly to the tracheal mucosa. A recent study found that administering topical lidocaine through this tube decreased the incidence of coughing on emergence without prolonging the emergence.[124] Regardless of the technique used, it is imperative that the laryngopharynx be completely cleared of foreign material and secretions before extubation is attempted.

10. Apnea. Apnea may be seen as a reflex response of tracheal irritation from the endotracheal tube. Extraneous reasons for the apnea— for example, if the patient is a premature or full-term neonate,[130] has had induction drugs or excessive narcotics, or has a reflux response to light levels of anesthesia—should be ruled out initially. If no central reason exists for the patient's lack of respiratory effort, mechanical ventilation can be initiated and spontaneous ventilation can be attempted later. Otherwise, the endotracheal tube may be removed, and by se-

curing a good mask fit, the patient's airway can be managed manually. The endotracheal tube may be replaced later if necessary.

11. Vomiting and aspiration. In any patient considered to have a full stomach, the likelihood of vomiting in response to irritation of the airway is increased, and aspiration of stomach contents is a constant concern. If the patient has not yet been intubated and vomits, the head should be turned immediately to the side and all gastric secretions should be suctioned or otherwise removed from the mouth. However, if the airway has already been secured, the endotracheal tube should be left in place and aggressive suctioning be performed around it. Once the patient is awake enough to respond to simple commands and can protect his or her own airway, the endotracheal tube may be removed.

The Sellick maneuver, or cricoid pressure, has removed much of the fear of emergency intubation. Cricoid pressure is effective in raising the pressure in the upper esophageal sphincter to a value greater than that found at rest, provided that at least 40 N of force (equivalent to 4.1 kg or 9 lb) is used.[131] Cricoid pressure has proven to be effective even in the presence of a nasogastric tube.[132] It is critical that the ease of intubation be assessed before inducing any patient with a potentially full stomach. Should any doubt exist about the success of an oral intubation, awake techniques should be considered. It is possible to completely obstruct the airway with cricoid pressure. Furthermore, reports have been published of airway obstruction during cricoid pressure as a result of lingual tonsils, lingual thyroid glands,[133] and undiagnosed laryngeal trauma.[134]

12. Injury to the eyes. Corneal abrasions are reported to be the most common eye complication that occurs during general anesthesia.[135] They are primarily caused by a facemask being placed on an open eye[136,137] or by the eyelids not being completely closed during anesthesia. Jewelry, identification cards, and loose-fitting watch bands have been implicated in scratching the eyeball.[138] In addition, a stethoscope hanging from the neck of a clinician can fall forward and strike the patient's eyes or forehead. Prevention consists of vigilance on the part of the anesthesiologist and application of adhesive tape over the closed eyelids. Some clinicians routinely apply lubricating ointment to the inside of the eyelids, although this has not been proven to increase efficacy. Although these injuries typically heal within 24 hours, they are usually painful and can lead to corneal ulceration. An immediate ophthalmologic consultation is recommended. Local anesthetics should not be applied because they can delay regeneration of the epithelium and may promote keratitis. Treatment consists of allowing the injured eye to rest by use of an eyepatch and applying an antibiotic ointment.

13. Sore throat. The incidence of sore throat after intubation is approximately 40% and is upward of 65% when blood is noted on the airway instruments.[139] Aggressive suctioning is probably a mitigating factor. The incidence is substantially higher in women and in patients undergoing thyroid surgery.[140] No correlation was seen with such factors as age, use of muscle relaxants, type of narcotic used, number of intubation attempts, or duration of intubation.[140] In one study, use of a beclomethasone inhaler (50 μg) was shown to prevent perioperative sore throat.[141] However, pain on swallowing usually lasts no more than 24 to 48 hours and can be relieved in part by having the patient breathe humidified air. Topical anesthesia, such as lidocaine jelly, applied to the endotracheal tube does not lessen the incidence of this problem and may actually worsen it.[142]

B. Maintenance of the endotracheal tube

1. Macroglossia. Massive tongue swelling, or macroglossia, has been reported in numerous instances. This condition occurs in both adult and pediatric patients.[143,144] Some cases occurred while a bite block was in place, some with an oral airway, and some with no protective device at all. The common denominator was that they all occurred when there was substantial neck flexion during endotracheal intubation and surgery was prolonged. Macroglossia is thought to occur secondary to obstructed venous and lymphatic drainage of the tongue, but this theory has not been substantiated. In each case, it was felt that the endotracheal tube may have severely compromised the circulation on the affected side of the tongue. Another report pointed out the sudden onset of tongue swelling after prolonged surgery to repair a cleft palate.[145] During this surgery, the tongue was retracted extensively, which may have led to postoperative swelling. Although this inflammation was not related to the use of anesthetic, the anesthesiologist should always be concerned about the potential for perioperative airway obstruction.

Macroglossia (occasionally to a life-threatening degree) has also been associated with angiotensin-converting enzyme inhibitors,. The edema shows an unusual predilection for the head and neck. Edema of the tongue is frequently the initial presentation, although the face, lips, floor of the mouth, pharynx, glottis, or larynx may be involved. Angioedema secondary to therapy with angiotensin-converting enzyme inhibitors usually begins spontaneously within hours to days after the medication has been started. However, one report identified an exacerbation of this problem only after the patient was exposed to tracheal intubation and general anesthesia.[146]

2. Airway obstruction. A patent airway is an absolute requirement for safe anesthesia. Airway obstruction can occur at any time during administration of a general anesthetic, particularly in prolonged surgeries or in patients with predisposing anatomic abnormalities. Airway obstruction should be considered whenever an intubated patient has diminished breath sounds associated with increasing peak inspiratory pressures. Such obstruction can result from diverse factors,[147] including a sharp bend or kink in the endotracheal tube; a tube that has been bitten closed; or a tube that is obstructed with mucus, blood, foreign bodies, or lubricant.[148] In one report, a tablet used for premedication was inhaled rather than swallowed and subsequently obstructed a tube.[149] The endotracheal tube may become warm with continued use during prolonged procedures; under these circumstances, the tube may kink and cause an obstruction.

Such kinking may seem to be a decrease in compliance and may be accompanied by wheezing. Many clinicians mistakenly treat the patient for bronchospasm when, in fact, the turbulent air movement comes from the endotracheal tube and not from the patient. At least two cases have been reported in which the plastic coating on a stylet sheared off and occluded the lumen of an endotracheal tube.[150,151] In another case, a tube was obstructed by the prominent knuckle of an aortic arch.[152] Nitrous oxide can cause expansion of gas bubbles trapped in the walls of an endotracheal tube, leading to airway obstruction.[153]

Even a reinforced anode wire tube is susceptible to problems. The anode tube can kink at the area between the end of the plastic adapter and the beginning of the support wire. In addition, the soft distal tip can fold backward into the tube and cause obstruction. Finally, although wire tubes have added reinforcement, patients can bite through them.[154,155]

The cuff of an endotracheal tube can also cause airway obstruction. An overinflated cuff may compress the bevel of the endotracheal tube against the tracheal wall, occluding its tip.[156] The cuff may also herniate over the tip of the tube and cause an obstruction.[157] When faced with any of these problems, the best solution is to pass a suction catheter or a fiberoptic bronchoscope down the lumen of the endotracheal tube and attempt to clear it. If the tube is totally obstructed, passage of a stylet may be tried. Total obstruction that cannot be remedied quickly requires removal of the tube, and the patient should be reintubated as rapidly as possible. It is recommended that the endotracheal tube and connecting hoses be supported and, if necessary, taped to prevent kinking caused by their own weight. Inspiratory gases should be humidified during long anesthesia to prevent tube obstruction from dried secretions.

Unusual causes of airway obstruction have been reported. In two patients, complete airway obstruction occurred secondary to achalasia and esophageal dilation. One of the patients was treated with aspiration of the esophagus,[158] and the other was treated with intravenous administration of nitroglycerin.[159]

Two cases of tension hydrothorax that caused airway obstruction during laparoscopic surgery have been reported. In the first, the patient had malignant ascites that, when combined with a pneumoperitoneum, led to such a rapid accumulation of pleural fluid that severe respiratory and cardiovascular compromise resulted.[160] The second case occurred during operative hysteroscopy when a large volume of glycine was absorbed through opened myometrial vessels under high intraabdominal pressure.[161] In each case, more than 1.5 L of clear fluid was drained once chest tubes were placed.

3. Disconnection and dislodgment. A common and serious complication of tracheal intubation is disconnection of the endotracheal tube from the remainder of the anesthesia circuit. This was identified as the most common critical incident in a study of anesthesia-related human errors and equipment failures.[162] A trained anesthesiologist will usually identify this problem immediately. The low-pressure alarm will sound first, and the patient's breath sounds will become absent. However, if the ventilator continues to function normally, the physician may be unaware of the nature of the problem. Disconnections are most likely to occur if the connections are made of dissimilar materials, if the patient's head is turned away from the anesthesiologist, or if the airway connections are hidden beneath the surgical drapes. Alarms to signal airway disconnection are included on all modern anesthesia machines; their signals should be taken seriously. It is recommended that connections between the endotracheal tube and the breathing circuit be checked and reinforced at the outset, before the anesthesiologist loses visual "control" of the airway. There should be no tension on the connections from the weight of the corrugated tubing or the drapes on the tubing. Furthermore, members of the surgical team should be discouraged from inadvertently leaning on any portion of the breathing circuit. The exact site of disconnection should be ascertained rapidly by checking each connection, beginning at the patient's airway and moving proximally back to the machine.[163] Nonetheless, it is imperative that the anesthesiologist have a prearranged plan in mind in the event that an airway is inadvertently disconnected or dislodged during surgery.

4. Circuit leaks. Leaks in an air delivery circuit can cause hypoventilation and dilution of the inspired gases by entry of room air into the system. With an ascending bellows system, such as that found in newer models of anesthesia machines, the bellows will not rise completely during exhalation. This situation indicates that the circuit leak exceeds the inflow of fresh gas. Older machines with a descending bellows system will not provide such a visual clue and will appear to function normally. The anesthesiologist should be vigilant at all times for signs of a potential circuit leak. The inspired oxygen concentration measured at the gas sampling port will be reduced because of dilution with room air, and the partial pressure of end-tidal CO_2 will increase. Cyanosis, a decrease in the oxygen saturation (SpO_2), or hypertension and tachycardia associated with hypercapnia may be the presenting signs, although each of these is typically a late finding.

5. Laser fires. Lasers are frequently used in the operating room to ablate benign and neoplastic tissues in the airway. One of the most catastrophic events associated with their use is an airway fire, which occurs when the laser ignites the endotracheal tube.[164-166] The risk that a laser beam will contact the wall of an endotracheal tube is 1:2.[167] Oxygen-rich inspired gas concentrations fuel brisk ignition of the plastic in the endotracheal tube and can fuel a fire in both directions. In essence, the endotracheal tube acts as a blowtorch; the fire is fed by the combustible walls of the tube and is intensified by the high rate of oxygen flow. The heat and fumes of the burning plastic my cause severe damage to the airway. Treatment consists of immediately disconnecting the circuit from the endotracheal tube and removing the burning tube from the airway. If the tube is not burning or if complete loss of the airway may occur with removal of the tube, leaving the tube in situ should be considered. The fire should be extinguished with saline, and the patient should be supported by facemask ventilation. The airway should

be evaluated for damage with bronchoscopy, and the appropriate supportive respiratory care should be given.

Numerous precautions can reduce the risk for an airway fire. If possible, placement of an endotracheal tube may be avoided altogether if air can be delivered through a ventilating laryngoscope, a jet ventilation system, or intermittent apneic ventilation. If a tracheostomy tube is in place, ventilation may occur distal to the site of laser surgery. Endotracheal tubes may be protected by wrapping them in noncombustible tapes; alternatively, red rubber or metal noncombustible tubes may be used. However, these techniques increase the potential for airway trauma or obstruction.[168,169] Most modern protective tapes are not 100% effective in the prevention of airway fires.[170] Cuff ignition can be minimized by filling the cuff with saline solution instead of air. Furthermore, should the cuff ignite and rupture, the saline will help extinguish the fire. Placing a dye in the saline, such as methylene blue, will further alert the anesthesiologist because in the event of a fire, steam that is the color of the dye will be emitted. Nitrous oxide should not be used because it easily supports combustion.[171] On the basis of laboratory simulations, it is recommended that inert gases, such as helium or nitrogen, be used instead of nitrous oxide and that concentrations of oxygen never exceed 40%.[172] Five centimeters of positive end-expiratory pressure with a forced inspiratory oxygen no greater than 40% prevents ignition of polyvinyl chloride components.[173]

6. Tracheal mucosal damage. A potential adverse consequence of tracheal intubation is erosion of the tracheal mucosa. Denuded tissue is eventually replaced with scar tissue, which ultimately retracts and leads to stenoses of the trachea, larynx, or nares. The incidence of granulomas has been reported to range from 1:800[174] to 1:20,000.[175] They are more common in women than in men and occur rarely in children. The most common site of erosion is along the posterior laryngeal wall, where granulation tissue easily overgrows. Side effects of granulomas include cough, hoarseness, and throat pain. The growths may be prevented by minimizing the trauma associated with laryngoscopy and intubation. When granulomas do occur, surgical excision is usually required.

Membranes and webs may eventually replace tracheal and laryngeal ulcers. These growths are commonly thick and gray. Care should be taken while intubating patients with such lesions because inadvertent detachment may result in respiratory obstruction or bleeding into the airway. With time, the inflammatory process associated with laryngeal ulcers may extend to the laryngeal cartilage. Should this occur, the cartilage may become inflamed (chondritis) or softened (chondromalacia).

Eroded vocal cords may adhere together, eventually forming synechiae. This is a potential problem whenever airflow between the vocal cords has been compromised as a result of tracheostomy.[176] Surgical correction is usually necessary.

Several months after prolonged tracheal intubation, tracheal stenosis and fibrosis may occur. This usually represents the end stage of a progression from tracheal wall erosion to cartilaginous weakening to healing with fibrosis formation.[51] Stenoses typically occur at the site of an inflated cuff, although they may occur at the location of the endotracheal tube tip. Symptoms include a nonproductive cough, dyspnea, and signs of respiratory obstruction. Dilation of the stenosis is curative if the stenosis is caught in its early stages. However, surgical correction may be necessary once the tracheal lumen has been reduced to 4 to 5 mm.[177,178]

C. Extubation of the endotracheal tube

1. Hemodynamic changes. Hemodynamic changes, including a 20% increase in heart rate and blood pressure, occur in most patients at the time of extubation.[179,180] Such changes, which are thought to result from catecholamine release in response to stimulation by the endotracheal tube, are usually transient and rarely require treatment. Although most patients tolerate these hemodynamic responses well, patients with cardiac disease,[113] pregnancy-induced hypertension,[181] and increased intracranial pressure[182] may be at particular risk for adverse effects. Patients with cardiac disease have shown decreased ejection fractions at the time of extubation.[183] Management consists of deep extubation or pharmacologic therapy. Deep extubation is appropriate for some patients but is inappropriate for patients with a difficult airway, those at high risk for aspiration, and those with compromised airway access. Pharmacologic strategies emphasize the importance of decreasing the heart rate, which is more likely than an increase in blood pressure to cause myocardial ischemia. β-Blockers seem to be the most successful at blunting the hemodynamic response to extubation. Esmolol, 1.5 mg/kg, given 2 to 4 minutes before extubation has been shown to prevent rapid increases in pulse and blood pressure associated with extubation.[184] Labetalol, 0.25 to 2.5 mg/kg, has also been used successfully.[182] Diltiazem, 0.1 to 0.2 mg/kg, has shown promise.[185] Finally, inconsistent results have been obtained with lidocaine and high-dose narcotics.[186]

2. Laryngospasm. Laryngospasm, a common cause of airway obstruction, is a protective reflex mediated by the vagus nerve. This reflex is an attempt to prevent aspiration of foreign bodies into the trachea. It may be provoked by movement of the cervical spine, pain, vocal cord irritation by secretions, or sudden stimulation while the patient is still in a light plane of anesthesia.[187]

The optimal course for treating laryngospasm is to avoid it in the first place. It is imperative that no saliva, blood, or gastric contents touch the glottis while the patient is lightly anesthetized. In cases in which laryngospasm is anticipated, the patient may undergo a deep extubation. The back of the mouth should be aggressively suctioned before emergence to remove any suspicious material from the posterior pharynx. A patient undergoing deep extubation should be placed on his or her side with the head down to keep the vocal cords clear of secretions during emergence. Because suctioning of the oropharynx does not adequately remove secretions around the vocal cords, it is best to extubate patients during a positive-pressure breath. The vigorous exhalation after extubation will help to remove any re-

maining secretions. Should a severe case of laryngospasm occur, the patient may require a small dose of succinylcholine (10 to 20 mg for an adult) to break the spasm, possibly followed by reintubation.[188]

3. Laryngeal edema. Laryngeal edema is an important cause of postextubation obstruction. This condition has various causes and is classified as supraglottic, retroarytenoidal, or subglottic.[189] Supraglottic edema most commonly results from surgical manipulation, positioning, hematoma formation, overaggressive fluid management, impaired venous drainage, or coexisting conditions (such as preeclampsia or angioneurotic edema). Retroarytenoidal edema typically results from local trauma or irritation. Subglottic edema occurs most often in children, particularly neonates and infants. Factors associated with development of subglottic edema include traumatic intubation, intubation lasting longer than 1 hour, bucking on the endotracheal tube, changes in head position, or tight-fitting tubes. Laryngeal edema usually presents as stridor within 30 to 60 minutes after extubation, although it may start as late as 6 hours postextubation. Regardless of the cause of laryngeal edema, management depends on the severity of the condition. Therapy consists of humidified oxygen, racemic epinephrine, head-up positioning, and occasionally, reintubation with a smaller endotracheal tube. The practice of administering parenteral steroids in the hope of reducing edema is controversial; studies are divided on their efficacy.[190]

4. Negative-pressure pulmonary edema. When airway obstruction occurs after extubation, negative-pressure pulmonary edema may occur in a spontaneously breathing patient. As a result of the obstruction, these patients generate sufficient negative intrapleural pressure that pulmonary edema occurs secondary to engorgement of the pulmonary vasculature and increased hydrostatic pressure in the pulmonary capillaries.[191] The condition is seen within minutes after extubation, typically presenting as a decrease in the SpO_2 along with production of pink, frothy sputum. Management involves removing the obstruction, supporting the patient with oxygen, monitoring the patient closely, and reducing the afterload with furosemide or morphine. Reintubation is rarely necessary; most cases resolve spontaneously without further complications.

5. Laryngotracheal trauma. Unlike trauma during intubation, airway trauma at the time of extubation is not well described. Arytenoid cartilage dislocation has been reported after both difficult and routine intubations.[42,192] Symptoms become apparent soon after extubation and may be mild (difficulty swallowing and voice changes) or major (complete airway obstruction). Management depends on the severity of the condition. Options include reintubation, arytenoid reduction, or tracheostomy. If laryngotracheal trauma is suspected, an otolaryngology consultation is warranted.

6. Airway compression. External compression of the airway after extubation may lead to obstruction. An excessively tight postsurgical neck dressing is a cause of external compression that is easily resolved. A more ominous situation is a rapidly expanding hematoma in close proximity to the airway. This may occur after certain surgeries, such as carotid endarterectomy, and must be quickly diagnosed and treated before total airway obstruction occurs.[193] Immediate surgical reexploration is indicated, although the airway concerns in these patients should be approached with extreme caution. To minimize airway distortion, general anesthesia should be avoided until the wound is evacuated under local anesthesia. However, even after surgical drainage, airway obstruction may occur as the result of venous or lymphatic congestion. Any use of muscle relaxants during anesthesia induction in these patients may result in catastrophe regardless of whether the wound was previously drained. Conservative options for managing the airway in this situation include awake fiberoptic intubation, surgical airways, or inhalation induction. Muscle relaxants should be avoided until the airway is secured.

External compression of the neck, such as chronic compression of a goiter, may also result from tracheomalacia.[194] This condition is usually seen after the goiter has been removed, although one case was reported in which the airway collapsed as soon as muscle relaxants were administered for induction.[195] Airway obstruction in these patients becomes apparent soon after extubation. Management includes reintubation, surgical tracheal support (stenting), or tracheostomy below the level of obstruction.

7. Aspiration. Pulmonary aspiration of gastric contents is a constant threat for any patient who has a full stomach or is at risk for postoperative vomiting. Laryngeal function is altered for at least 4 hours after tracheal extubation.[196] Depression of reflexes, along with the presence of residual anesthetic agents, places almost all recently extubated patients at risk. Aspiration is probably more prevalent than is currently thought. Most cases are so minor that they do not affect the patient's postoperative course. Perioperative problems, if they do occur, are usually attributed to such factors as atelectasis. Management consists of supportive measures. Depending on the extent of the aspiration, measures include supportive care, ranging from administration of oxygen through a nasal cannula to reintubation with mechanical ventilation and positive end-expiratory pressure.

8. Difficult extubation. Occasionally, endotracheal tubes are difficult to remove. Possible causes are failure to deflate the cuff, use of an oversized tube,[189] adhesion of the tube to the tracheal wall,[197] or transfixation of the tube by an inadvertent suture to a nearby organ.[198,199] In most cases, the problem arises from an inability to deflate the cuff, commonly as a result of failure in the cuff-deflating mechanism. Should this problem occur, the cuff should be punctured with a transtracheal needle. Forceful removal of an endotracheal tube with the cuff inflated may result in damage to the vocal cords.

IV. SPECIAL AIRWAY TECHNIQUES
A. Fiberoptic intubation

The fiberoptic bronchoscope can be used to achieve control of an airway when a difficult intubation is suspected. It combines direct vision with flexibility to view the pharynx when direct laryngoscopy is considered difficult or impossible. Use of the fiberoptic bronchoscope is not a quick

technique, and it probably should not be considered when speed is required. Although the device can be used in many different situations involving airway management, it also has several limitations and potential complications.

Intubation with a fiberoptic bronchoscope should not be attempted when the pharynx is filled with blood or saliva, when inadequate space exists within the oral cavity to identify pharyngeal structures, or when time is critical and creating a surgical airway is the priority. Relative contraindications include marked tissue edema, distortion of the oropharyngeal anatomy, narrowed nasal passages, soft tissue traction, or a severe cervical flexion deformity. The fiberoptic bronchoscope may be difficult to use if the operator is inexperienced, if topical anesthesia is inadequate, if light is not sufficient or the focus is not correct, if the lens is markedly fogged, or if an endotracheal tube cannot be passed over the bronchoscope.[200] While this device is being used, every effort should be made to provide a dry, bloodless field to promote success.

Potential complications associated with the fiberoptic bronchoscope include bleeding; epistaxis (especially if a nasal airway is attempted); laryngotracheal trauma; laryngospasm; bronchospasm; and aspiration of blood, saliva, or gastric contents. Another possible hazard is associated with the practice of insufflating oxygen through the suction channel. Although this technique can help to keep the tip of the bronchoscope clean and provide for a high volume of forced inspiratory oxygen, it can also result in high-pressure submucosal injection of oxygen should the tip cut into the pharyngeal mucosa. If this sequence occurs, the result may be pronounced subcutaneous emphysema of the pharynx, face, and periorbital regions.[201]

B. Retrograde wire intubation

Retrograde wire intubation is an excellent technique for securing a difficult airway. It can be used whenever anatomic limitations obscure the glottic opening. Because the technique is blind, it is important to exercise caution so as not to worsen any preexisting conditions. The method involves passing a wire cephalad from a puncture in the cricothyroid membrane until the wire protrudes from the mouth or nose. An endotracheal tube is then advanced over the wire and through the glottis until it reaches the point where the wire entered the trachea. The wire is then removed and the endotracheal tube is advanced further into the trachea. There are variations on the technique that will not be addressed, such as using the fiberoptic bronchoscope by passing the wire through the suction channel.

Although simple in concept, the basic technique has numerous problems and potential complications. The procedure takes some time to perform and should not be considered under emergency circumstances unless the practitioner is very experienced. The tip of the endotracheal tube has been known to get caught on the glottic structures and fail to enter the larynx. The problem may be alleviated somewhat by using a tapered dilator inside the endotracheal tube or by using an epidural catheter as the wire to assist with passing the endotracheal tube through the glottis. Bleeding may occur at the site of the tracheal puncture in quantities sufficient to cause a tracheal clot or airway obstruction. Cases of severe hemoptysis with resultant hypoxia, cardiopulmonary arrest, arrhythmias, and death following retrograde wire intubation have been reported.[202-206] Subcutaneous emphysema localized to the area of the transtracheal needle puncture is common but self-limited. In severe cases, the air may track back through the fascial planes of the neck, leading to tracheal compression with resultant airway compromise, pneumomediastinum, and pneumothorax.[207,208] Laryngospasm may result from irritation by the retrograde wire unless the vocal cords are anesthetized or relaxed. Other, less common complications include esophageal perforations, tracheal hematoma, laryngeal edema, infections, tracheitis, tracheal fistulas, trigeminal nerve injury, and vocal cord damage.[209,210]

C. Transtracheal jet ventilation

When a patient's condition deteriorates into a "cannot ventilate—cannot intubate" situation, lifesaving steps must be undertaken immediately or the patient will die. One emergency method is transtracheal jet ventilation (TTJV), which is accomplished by introducing a small percutaneous catheter into the trachea and insufflating the respiratory tract with high-pressure oxygen. Although this technique may be helpful in critical situations, life-threatening problems are associated with it.

To accomplish TTJV, a long, large-bore catheter is advanced through the cricothyroid membrane into the trachea. If this catheter is displaced from the trachea, subcutaneous emphysema, hypoventilation, pneumomediastinum, pneumothorax, severe abdominal distention, or death may result.[62] In a study of 28 emergency patients managed with TTJV, 2 developed subcutaneous emphysema and 1 developed mediastinal emphysema.[211] On the basis of normal skin compliance, a 4-inch catheter could be pulled from an intratracheal position into the subcutaneous space simply by applying traction to its proximal end. Thus the hub of the TTJV catheter must be continuously pressed firmly against the skin line.

Barotrauma is another potential complication of this technique.[212,213] Oxygen delivered through a transtracheal catheter must be able to escape the lungs freely or overdistention and pulmonary rupture may occur.[214,215] It is imperative that any changes in breath sounds, chest wall expansion, or hemodynamics be suspected as secondary to pneumothorax. In cases of total airway obstruction, the risk for pneumothorax is greatly increased because gas cannot escape from the lungs in a normal manner. Strong consideration should be given to placing a second transtracheal "egress" catheter in these circumstances. Laryngospasm can also impede the outward flow of oxygen from the trachea. This should be prevented by providing adequate local anesthesia to the neighboring structures or by relaxing the patient.[213] If the larynx is obstructed by a foreign body, only low-flow oxygen should be delivered until safe egress of gas is established.

Inadvertent placement of a gas delivery line into the gastrointestinal tract may also result in complications. In one case report, gas delivery introduced inadvertently into the stomach caused gastric rupture.[216] Other gastrointestinal complications include esophageal perforations, bleeding, hematoma, and hemoptysis.[217]

Damage to the tracheal mucosa may occur in patients who are managed with long-term TTJV, especially if the gas is not humidified.[218] The possibility of tracheal mucosal ulceration should be considered in any patient if nonhumidified TTJV is attempted through single-orifice catheters for a prolonged period.

D. Lighted stylets

The lighted stylet may be used to facilitate intubation under both local and general anesthesia. A light at the tip of a flexible stylet is used to transilluminate the soft tissues of the pharynx. The device can be used blindly or as an aid when direct laryngoscopy is difficult. It may also serve to confirm that the tip of an endotracheal tube is still within the cervical trachea and to establish that the tube has not been advanced too far.[219]

Because use of the lighted stylet is a blind technique, the pharyngeal pathologic condition cannot be visualized or avoided. This method should not be used in patients with suspected abnormalities of the upper airway, such as tumors, polyps, infections (e.g., epiglottitis or retropharyngeal abscess), trauma, or foreign bodies. The lighted stylet should also be used with caution in patients in whom transillumination of the anterior neck will be limited, such those with dark skin pigmentation, morbid obesity, or limited neck mobility. If placement of the stylet is difficult, the anesthesiologist should consider abandoning the technique for fear of worsening a pathologic process.

Several real and potential complications have been reported with the use of this device. Several cases have been reported in which the light fell off of the end of the stylet.[220-222] In another instance, the protective tubing was not removed from the stylet and thus had the potential to become dislodged within the trachea.[223] Finally, several cases of arytenoid subluxation have been reported with the use of this device.[44,224]

E. Lighted fiberoptic laryngoscopes

Numerous laryngoscope blades have been developed in an attempt to facilitate tracheal intubation. Two of the more recent additions to the collection are the lighted fiberoptic laryngoscopes: the Bullard laryngoscope and the Upsher laryngoscope. Both are rigid metal instruments that allow indirect viewing of the glottic structures via fiberoptic bundles. The small vertical dimension of these blades make them well suited for patients with restricted oral openings. In addition, because each portion of the blade is designed to match the anatomic airway, there is no need to manipulate the patient's head or neck to visualize the larynx. Thus these laryngoscopes are ideal for use in a patient with cervical spine pathologic conditions.

The greatest limitation of the Bullard and Upsher laryngoscopes is the lack of ease of use. Serious commitment and training are needed to become comfortable with these devices.[225] Passage of an endotracheal tube through the larynx takes slightly longer with a Bullard laryngoscope than with conventional fiberoptic bronchoscopy.[226] Awake intubations with these devices often do not fare well, possibly owing to poor visualization[227]; more investigation in this area is needed. Two cases of failed intubations with the Bullard laryngoscope were thought to be caused by an inability to trap the epiglottis.[228] A blade extender has been manufactured to help remedy this problem.

F. Laryngeal mask airway

The laryngeal mask airway (LMA), a device designed for upper airway management, serves as a cross between a facemask and an endotracheal tube. It is composed of a soft silicone tube that has been cut diagonally approximately 20 cm from its proximal end. The distal end is attached by an elliptical mask with an inflatable rim. Once the rim is inflated in the patient's posterior pharynx, its tip occludes the esophagus while the distal orifice fits snugly over the larynx. The proximal end of the LMA is then attached to a gas delivery system, and the patient is maintained with either spontaneous or controlled ventilation. With use of the LMA, muscle relaxation is unnecessary, laryngoscopy is avoided, and hemodynamic changes are minimized during insertion. Because the LMA is tolerated at a lighter depth of anesthesia than an endotracheal tube, its use may promote more rapid awakening and earlier discharge from the postanesthesia care unit.[229] The LMA has a clear advantage when laryngeal trauma must be minimized (e.g., in operatic singers); when a standard mask fit is impossible because of facial burns, delicate skin, or a full beard; when light planes of anesthesia are desired; or when a patient is scheduled for repeated surgeries. It has also proven valuable in situations in which mask ventilation is difficult and direct laryngoscopy is impossible[230] and may be used as a conduit for a fiberoptic intubation with a standard endotracheal tube. The device may be used in the American Society of Anesthesiologists Difficult Airway Algorithm in five different locations.[231]

Placing the LMA correctly can be very difficult. The mask may fold on itself either under or over its main axis. Pressure on the epiglottis can push the device down into the glottic opening or entrap it within the laryngeal inlet of the mask. In the worst case, the tip of the epiglottis can be folded into the vocal cords, inducing coughing and laryngospasm.[232] Excess lubricant can leak into the trachea, also promoting coughing or laryngospasm.[232] Regardless of the problems encountered in placing the LMA, airway patency is usually maintained.

Numerous complications are associated with the LMA. Perhaps the greatest limitation is the inability of the LMA to protect against pulmonary aspiration of gastric contents. Because the LMA does not isolate the trachea from the esophagus, its use is risky when the patient has a full stomach or when high airway pressures are necessary for positive-pressure ventilation. Furthermore, the pressure in the lower esophageal sphincter is much lower in patients breathing spontaneously with an LMA than in those breathing through a facemask or a Guedel airway.[233] In one series, the incidence of regurgitation of small amounts of gastric contents was as high as 25% in patients breathing spontaneously with an LMA.[234] Fortunately, most of the reported patients had favorable outcomes because the regurgitated material was not aspirated or because the aspiration was relatively mild.[235]

Several other complications of varying severity have been reported with the use of the LMA. The incidence of sore throat with this device is reported to be 7% to 12%, an incidence similar to that seen with oral airways.[236,237] The incidence of failed placement is 1% to 5%, although this tends to decrease with increasing operator experience.[238] The LMA cuff is permeable to nitrous oxide and carbon dioxide, which results in substantial increases in cuff pressure and volume during prolonged procedures.[239] Increased intracuff pressures may increase the incidence of postoperative sore throats or cause transient dysarthria. Several published case reports mention edema of the epiglottis, uvula, and posterior pharyngeal wall; at the worst, these conditions have led to airway obstruction.[240–242] Hypoglossal nerve paralysis,[243] postobstructive pulmonary edema,[244] and tongue cyanosis[245] have also been reported. Other problems with the LMA include dislodgment; kinking; and foreign bodies in the tube, leading to airway obstruction.[246]

G. Cuffed oropharyngeal airway

The cuffed oropharyngeal airway (COPA) is a new supraglottic airway device that combines a Guedel airway with a cuff at its distal end and a standard 15-mm adapter at its proximal end. This device was designed to displace the base of the tongue, elevate the epiglottis, and form an airtight seal in the proximal laryngopharynx.[247] Insertion of the device is relatively easy,[248,249] and it is well tolerated until emergence from anesthesia, when the patient is able to swallow and cough effectively.[249] In addition, the COPA has been found to be an effective adjunct to deep extubation at the end of surgery, when it helps diminish perioperative coughing and bucking.[250]

The COPA causes physiologic alterations and has clinical problems similar to those found with the LMA.[251] The COPA has a lower success rate than the laryngeal mask airway for first-time insertion, and experienced practitioners frequently require up to three attempts for successful placement.[247] The COPA also requires more frequent interventions during surgery (head lift and jaw thrust maneuvers) to maintain airway patency.[247,249,252] The LMA can maintain higher oropharyngeal leak pressures than the COPA, which may be a factor to consider during positive pressure ventilation.[247] Overall, the incidence of postoperative sore throat and coughing are similar for the COPA and the LMA; each condition occurs in less than 10% of patients and tends to resolve rapidly.[249]

Like the LMA, the COPA does not protect the airway from regurgitation and aspiration and is therefore contraindicated in nonfasting patients or in those who may have a full stomach.

H. Esophageal tracheal Combitube

The esophageal tracheal Combitube is an esophagotracheal double-lumen airway designed for emergency use when standard airway management measures have failed.[252,253] The device is inserted blindly into the mouth and advanced to preset markings. The distal tube is usually positioned within the esophagus at this point. A distal cuff is inflated within the esophagus, and a large-volume proximal cuff is inflated inside the pharynx. Ventilation is then attempted through the esophageal tube because esophageal intubation occurs in approximately 96% of insertions. If ventilation through this lumen fails, ventilation is attempted through the tracheal lumen.

The Combitube is not recommended for patients younger than 16 years of age or below 150 cm in height. Ideally, patients should not have intact gag reflexes. It should not be used in patients who are known to have ingested caustic substances. With the Combitube in the esophageal position, suctioning of the trachea is not possible, which may become a problem in patients with copious tracheal secretions. Finally, this device should not be used in patients with known esophageal disease or upper airway obstruction.[253]

Few complications have been reported with use of the Combitube. In two patients, the device was inserted too far, causing the large pharyngeal cuff to lie directly over the glottis and obstruct the upper airway.[254] This problem was easily resolved by partially withdrawing the Combitube until breath sounds were auscultated. Although tongue discoloration has been reported while the pharyngeal cuff was inflated, it usually resolves immediately without further adverse sequelae once the cuff is deflated. To date, no cases of esophageal perforation have been reported with the Combitube, in contrast to the problems experienced with its predecessor, the esophageal obturator airway.

I. Surgical airway

In cases in which tracheal intubation is impossible and a patient's airway is compromised, access to the trachea must be obtained rapidly. Under these circumstances, an emergency tracheostomy or cricothyroidotomy may be critical in saving a patient's life.[255] However, these procedures are associated with complications. The most severe complication is failure to establish an airway before brain damage or death results. These conditions occur either because the decision to progress to a surgical airway is not made soon enough or because the procedure is performed too slowly. If small blood vessels are transected during the early part of the surgery, the surgeon may focus on the hemorrhage and lose sight of the emergent need for airway access. If the surgical approach is too lateral, disruption of the major vessels of the neck may occur, causing the field to become so bloody that the anatomy will be impossible to identify. Approaching the neck through a region other than the cricothyroid membrane can also make the dissection difficult and tedious.

Accidental extubation occurs occasionally, most commonly in the early postoperative period. If the cannula is inadvertently removed from a fresh tracheostomy, it should be replaced as quickly as possible by the nearest health care worker. Skilled nurses and bedside equipment should be immediately available to address any such problems.

Bleeding is a complication of all surgeries, including airway access procedures. Minitracheostomy occasionally results in excessive bleeding into the airway, necessitating progression to a full surgical tracheostomy.[256] The inflated cuff of the formal tracheostomy prevents pul-

monary aspiration of blood. However, it is not uncommon for the patient to have such severe bleeding that he or she must return to the operating room. In rare cases, the innominate artery can rupture into the trachea because of excessive pressure from the tracheostomy tube, with resultant massive hemorrhage into the airway. Cardiothoracic surgeons should be consulted immediately for any episodes of sentinel bleeding.

If an air leak occurs and the cervical skin has healed around the tracheostomy tube, air can escape into the subcutaneous spaces of the neck, resulting in subcutaneous emphysema. If the condition goes unrecognized and the patient is maintained on high-pressure mechanical ventilation, the air may track to other locations. Air escaping into the paratracheal spaces can result in a pneumomediastinum. Furthermore, air released into the pleural cavity can result in a tension pneumothorax. Early recognition and treatment of subcutaneous emphysema will usually correct the problem, and the air will be reabsorbed.

Subglottic stenosis is a complication of long-term intubation. It usually results when the decision to progress to a tracheostomy is delayed too long. Tracheal stenosis is a complication of long-term tracheostomy. Such strictures can be treated with a Silastic stent or tracheal resection and repair. Subglottic stenoses are much more difficult to repair and frequently result in permanent speech impairment or laryngeal damage. If either of these types of stenoses are left untreated, they may eventually progress to granulomas, which require surgical excision.

A tracheostomy tube can cause tracheal erosion, particularly into the esophagus or the brachiocephalic artery. These tubes typically sit low in the trachea and are designed with a fixed curve. Because the tubes are relatively rigid and do not conform to the shape of the trachea, they can erode tissues at all contact points. Hoses connected to the tracheostomy may exert great leverage on the tube, causing further erosion at these same points. Furthermore, tube pressure can damage the skin at the insertion site.

V. CONCLUSION

This chapter has identified many of the challenges and complications that anesthesiologists may face when managing an airway. Errors may be technical or judgmental. By learning from the mistakes of the past, we may avoid them in the future. To minimize problems, we should anticipate them and devise a safe plan (as well as a backup plan) for each and every patient, maintain vigilance throughout all operative procedures, and use common sense at all times.

REFERENCES

1. Caplan RA, Posner KL, Ward RJ, et al: Adverse respiratory events in anesthesia: a closed claims analysis, *Anesthesiology* 72:828, 1990.
2. Durkan W, Fleming N: Potential eye damage from reusable masks, *Anesthesiology* 67:444, 1987 (letter).
3. Murray WJ, Ruddy MP: Toxic eye injury during induction of anesthesia, *South Med J* 78:1012, 1985.
4. Grigsby EJ, Lennon RL, Didier EP, et al: Massive tongue swelling after uncomplicated general anaesthesia, *Can J Anaesth* 37:825, 1990.
5. Glauber DT: Facial paralysis after general anesthesia, *Anesthesiology* 65:516, 1986.

6. Azar I, Lear E: Lower lip numbness following general anesthesia, *Anesthesiology* 65:450, 1986 (letter).

7. Smurthwaite GJ, Ford P: Skin necrosis following continuous positive airway pressure with a face mask, *Anaesthesia* 48:147, 1993.

8. Jarjour NN, Wilson P: Pneumocephalus associated with nasal continuous positive airway pressure in a patient with sleep apnea syndrome, *Chest* 96:1425, 1989.

9. Klopfenstein CE, Forster A, Suter PM: Pneumocephalus: a complication of continuous positive airway pressure after trauma, *Chest* 78:656, 1980.

10. Weaver LK, Fairfax WR, Greenway L: Bilateral otorrhagia associated with continuous positive airway pressure, *Chest* 93:878, 1988.

11. Horellou MF, Mathe D, Feiss P: A hazard of naso-tracheal intubation, *Anaesthesia* 33:73, 1978 (letter).

12. Green JG, Wood JM, Davis LF: Asystole after inadvertent intubation of the orbit, *J Oral Maxillofac Surg* 55:856, Aug 1997.

13. Bähr W, Stoll P: Nasal intubation in the presence of frontobasal fractures: a retrospective study, *J Oral Maxillofac Surg* 50:445, 1992.

14. O'Hanlon J, Harper KW: Epistaxis and nasotracheal intubation: prevention with vasoconstrictor spray, *Ir J Med Sci* 163:58, 1994.

15. O'Connell JE, Stevenson DS, Stokes MA: Pathological changes associated with short-term nasal intubation, *Anaesthesia* 51:347, 1996.

16. Binning R: A hazard of blind nasal intubation, *Anaesthesia* 29:366, 1974 (letter).

17. Politis C, Schiepers JP, Heylen R: Complete obstruction of a nasoendotracheal tube: a case report, *Acta Stomatol Belg* 93:13, 1996.

18. Hariri MA, Duncan PW: Infective complications of brief nasotracheal intubation, *J Laryngol Otol* 103:1217, 1989.

19. Elwany S, Mekhamer A: Effect of nasotracheal intubation on nasal mucociliary clearance, *Br J Anaesth* 59:755, 1987.

20. Dinner M, Tjeuw M, Artusio JF Jr: Bacteremia as a complication of nasotracheal intubation, *Anesth Analg* 66:460, 1987.

21. Halac E, Indiveri DR, Obregon RJ, et al: Complication of nasal endotracheal intubation, *J Pediatr* 103:166, 1983 (letter).

22. Willatts SM, Cochrane DF: Paranasal sinusitis: a complication of nasotracheal intubation: two case reports, *Br J Anaesth* 57:1026, 1985.

23. O'Reilly MJ, Reddick EJ, Black W, et al: Sepsis from sinusitis in nasotracheally intubated patients: a diagnostic dilemma, *Am J Surg* 147:601, 1984.

24. Smith WD, Timms MS, Sutcliffe H: Unusual complication of nasopharyngeal intubation, *Anaesthesia* 44:615, 1989 (letter).

25. Rose DK, Cohen MM: The airway: problems and predictions in 18,500 patients, *Can J Anaesth* 41(5 Pt 1):372, 1994.

26. White A, Kander PL: Anatomical factors in difficult direct laryngoscopy, *Br J Anaesth* 47:468, 1975.

27. Cass NM, James, NR, Lines V: Intubation under direct laryngoscopy, *BMJ* 2:488, 1956.

28. Benumof JL: Management of the difficult adult airway: with special emphasis on awake tracheal intubation, *Anesthesiology* 75:1087, 1991.

29. Frerk CM: Predicting difficult intubation, *Anaesthesia* 46:1005, 1991.

30. Mallampati SR, Gatt SP, Gugino LD, et al: A clinical sign to predict difficult tracheal intubation: a prospective study, *Can Anaesth Soc J* 32:429, 1985.

31. Samsoon GLT, Young JRB: Difficult tracheal intubation: a retrospective study, *Anaesthesia* 42:487, 1987.

32. Rosenberg H, Rosenberg HK: Airway obstruction and tracheal intubation. In Gravenstein N, Kirby RR, eds: *Complications in anesthesiology*, Philadelphia, 1996, Lippincott-Raven, p 219.

33. Salathé M, Johr M: Unsuspected cervical fractures: a common problem in ankylosing spondylitis, *Anesthesiology* 70:869, 1989.

34. Cloward RB: Acute cervical spine injuries, *Clin Symp* 32:3, 1980.

35. Podolsky S, Baraff LJ, Simon RR, et al: Efficacy of cervical spine immobilization methods, *J Trauma* 23:461, 1983.

36. Riggins RS, Kraus JF: The risk of neurologic damage with fractures of the vertebrae, *J Trauma* 17:126, 1977.

37. Hastings RH, Kelley SD: Neurologic deterioration associated with airway management in a cervical spine-injured patient, *Anesthesiology* 78:580, 1993.

38. Crosby ET, Lui A: The adult cervical spine: implications for airway management, *Can J Anaesth* 37:77, 1990.

39. Williams JP, Somerville GM, Miner ME, et al: Atlanto-axial subluxation and trisomy-21: another perioperative complication, *Anesthesiology* 67:253, 1987.

40. Dong ML: Arnold-Chiari malformation type I appearing after tonsillectomy, *Anesthesiology* 67:120, 1987.

41. Kambic V, Radsel Z: Intubation lesions of the larynx, *Br J Anaesth* 50:587, 1978.

42. Peppard SB, Dickens JH: Laryngeal injury following short-term intubation, *Ann Otol Rhinol Laryngol* 92(4 pt 1):327, 1983.

43. Frink EJ, Pattison BD: Posterior arytenoid dislocation following uneventful endotracheal intubation and anesthesia, *Anesthesiology* 70:358, 1989.

44. Gray B, Huggins NJ, Hirsch N: An unusual complication of tracheal intubation, *Anaesthesia* 45:558, 1990.

45. Debo RF, Colonna D, Deward G, et al: Cricoarytenoid subluxation: complication of blind intubation with a lighted stylet, *Ear Nose Throat J* 68:517, 1989.

46. Hiong YT, Fung CF, Sudhaman DA: Arytenoid subluxation: implications for the anaesthetist, *Anaesth Intensive Care* 24:609, 1996.

47. Bishop MJ, Weymuller EA Jr, Fink BR: Laryngeal effects of prolonged intubation, *Anesth Analg* 63:335, 1984.

48. Drosnes DL, Zwillenberg DA: Laryngeal granulomatous polyp after short-term intubation of a child, *Ann Otol Rhinol Laryngol* 99(3 Pt 1):183, 1990.

49. Alessi DM, Hanson DG, Berci G: Bedside videolaryngoscopic assessment of intubation trauma, *Ann Otol Rhinol Laryngol* 98(8 Pt 1):586, 1989.

50. Colice GL, Stukel TA, Dain B: Laryngeal complications of prolonged intubation, *Chest* 96:877, 1989.

51. van Klarenbosch J, Meyer J, de Lange JJ: Tracheal rupture after tracheal intubation, *Br J Anaesth* 73:550, 1994.

52. Kastanos N, Miro RE, Perez AM, et al: Laryngotracheal injury due to endotracheal intubation: incidence, evolution, and predisposing factors. A prospective long-term study, *Crit Care Med* 11:362, 1983.

53. Stauffer JL, Olson DE, Petty TL: Complications and consequences of endotracheal intubation and tracheotomy. A prospective study of 150 critically ill adult patients, *Am J Med* 70:65, 1981.

54. Jordon WS, Graves CL, Elwyn RA: New therapy for postintubation laryngeal edema and tracheitis in children, *JAMA* 212:585, 1970.

55. Pender JW: Endotracheal intubation in children: advantages and disadvantages, *Anesthesiology* 15:495, 1954.

56. Seitz PA, Gravenstein N: Endobronchial rupture from endotracheal reintubation with an endotracheal tube guide, *J Clin Anesth* 1:214, 1989.

57. Tessler S, Kupfer Y, Lerman A, et al: Massive gastric distention in the intubated patient: a marker for a defective airway, *Arch Intern Med* 150:318, 1990.

58. LoCicero J III: Tracheo-carotid artery erosion following endotracheal intubation, *J Trauma* 24:907, 1984.

59. O'Donnell JM: Orotracheal tube intracuff pressure initially and during anesthesia including nitrous oxide, *CRNA* 6:79, 1995.

60. Badran I, Jamal M: Pneumomediastinum due to Venturi system during microlaryngoscopy, *Middle East J Anesthesiol* 9:561, 1988.

61. Chang JL, Bleyaert A, Bedger R: Unilateral pneumothorax following jet ventilation during general anesthesia, *Anesthesiology* 53:244, 1980.

62. Egol A, Culpepper JA, Snyder JV: Barotrauma and hypotension resulting from jet ventilation in critically ill patients, *Chest* 88:98, 1985.

63. O'Sullivan TJ, Healy GB: Complications of Venturi jet ventilation during microlaryngeal surgery, *Arch Otolaryngol* 111:127, 1985.

64. Wetmore SJ, Key JM, Suen JY: Complications of laser surgery for laryngeal papillomatosis, *Laryngoscope* 95(7 Pt 1):798, 1985.

65. Rosenberg MB: Anesthesia-induced dental injury, *Int Anesthesiol Clin* 27:120, 1989.

66. Hyodo M, Masaki K, Kondo T: Statistical observation about the injury to the teeth caused by endotracheal intubation, *Masui* 20:1064, 1971.

67. Lockhart PB, Feldbau EV, Gabel RA, et al: Dental complications during and after tracheal intubation, *J Am Dent Assoc* 112:480, 1986.

68. Chadwick RG, Lindsay SM: Dental injuries during general anaesthesia, *Br Dent J* 180:255, 1996.

69. Aromaa U, Pesonen P, Linko K, et al: Difficulties with tooth protectors in endotracheal intubation, *Acta Anaesthesiol Scand* 32:304, 1988.

70. Quartararo C, Bishop MJ: Complications of tracheal intubation: prevention and treatment, *Semin Anesthesia* 9:119, 1990.
71. Krantz MA, Solomon DL, Poulos JC: Uvular necrosis following endotracheal intubation, *J Clin Anesth* 6:139, 1994.
72. Diaz JH: Is uvular edema a complication of endotracheal intubation? *Anesth Analg* 76:1139, 1993.
73. Bogetz MS, Tupper BJ, Vigil AC: Too much of a good thing: uvular trauma caused by overzealous suctioning, *Anesth Analg* 72:125, 1991.
74. Brandwein M, Abramson AL, Shikowitz MJ: Bilateral vocal cord paralysis following endotracheal intubation, *Arch Otolaryngol Head Neck Surg* 112:877, 1986.
75. Cavo JW Jr: True vocal cord paralysis following intubation, *Laryngoscope* 95:1352, 1985.
76. Lim EK, Chia KS, Ng BK: Recurrent laryngeal nerve palsy following endotracheal intubation, *Anaesth Intensive Care* 15:342, 1987.
77. Nuutinen J, Karja J: Bilateral vocal cord paralysis following general anesthesia, *Laryngoscope* 91:83, 1981.
78. Jones GOM, Hale DE, Wasmuth CE, et al: A survey of acute complications associated with endotracheal intubation, *Cleve Clin Q* 35:23, 1968.
79. Mayhew JF, Miner ME, Denneny J: Upper airway obstruction following cyst-to-peritoneal shunt in a child with a Dandy-Walker cyst, *Anesthesiology* 62:183, 1985.
80. Streppel M, Bachmann G, Stennert E: Hypoglossal nerve palsy as a complication of transoral intubation for general anesthesia, *Anesthesiology* 86:1007, 1997.
81. Teichner RL: Lingual nerve injury: a complication of orotracheal intubation. Case report, *Br J Anaesth* 43:413, 1971.
82. Aucott W, Prinsley P, Madden G: Laryngeal anaesthesia with aspiration following intubation, *Anaesthesia* 44:230, 1989.
83. Birmingham PK, Cheney FW, Ward RJ: Esophageal intubation: a review of detection techniques, *Anesth Analg* 65:886, 1986.
84. Sum-Ping ST, Mehta MP, Anderton JM: A comparative study of methods of detection of esophageal intubation, *Anesth Analg* 69:627, 1989.
85. Eldor J, Ofek B, Abramowitz HB: Perforation of oesophagus by tracheal tube during resuscitation, *Anaesthesia* 45:70, 1990.
86. Johnson KG, Hood DD: Esophageal perforation associated with endotracheal intubation, *Anesthesiology* 64:281, 1986.
87. Kras JF, Marchmont-Robinson H: Pharyngeal perforation during intubation in a patient with Crohn's disease, *J Oral Maxillofac Surg* 47:405, 1989.
88. Levine PA: Hypopharyngeal perforation: an untoward complication of endotracheal intubation, *Arch Otolaryngol* 106:578, 1980.
89. Majumdar B, Stevens RW, Obara LG: Retropharyngeal abscess following tracheal intubation, *Anaesthesia* 37:67, 1982.
90. Norman EA, Sosis M: Iatrogenic oesophageal perforation due to tracheal or nasogastric intubation, *Can Anaesth Soc J* 33:222, 1986.
91. a' Wengen DF: Piriform fossa perforation during attempted tracheal intubation, *Anaesthesia* 42:519, 1987.
92. Young PN, Robinson JM: Cellulitis as a complication of difficult tracheal intubation, *Anaesthesia* 42:569, 1987 (letter).
93. Gamlin F, Caldicott LD, Shah MV: Mediastinitis and sepsis syndrome following intubation, *Anaesthesia* 49:883, 1994.
94. Reyes G, Galvis AG, Thompson JW: Esophagotracheal perforation during emergency intubation, *Am J Emerg Med* 10:223, 1992.
95. Kramer MR, Melzer E, Sprung CL: Unilateral pulmonary edema after intubation of the right mainstem bronchus, *Crit Care Med* 17:472, 1989.
96. Mehta S: Guided orotracheal intubation in the operating room using a lighted stylet, *Anesthesiology* 66:105, 1987 (letter).
97. Conrardy PA, Goodman LR, Lainge F, et al: Alteration of endotracheal tube position: flexion and extension of the neck, *Crit Care Med* 4:7, 1976.
98. Owen RL, Cheney FW: Endobronchial intubation: a preventable complication, *Anesthesiology* 67:255, 1987.
99. Benumof JL, Partridge BL, Salvatierra C, et al: Margin of safety in positioning modern double-lumen endotracheal tubes, *Anesthesiology* 67:729, 1987.
100. Horie T, Higa K, Ken-Mizaki Y, et al: Tracheal rupture in a patient intubated with a double-lumen endobronchial tube, *Masui* 43:1366, 1994.
101. Wagner DL, Gammage GW, Wong ML: Tracheal rupture following the insertion of a disposable double-lumen endotracheal tube, *Anesthesiology* 63:698, 1985.
102. Hannallah M, Gomes M: Bronchial rupture associated with the use of a double-lumen tube in a small adult, *Anesthesiology* 71:457, 1989.
103. Benumof JL: Physiology of the open chest and one lung ventilation. In Benumof JL, ed: *Anesthesia for thoracic surgery,* ed 2, Philadelphia, 1994, WB Saunders.
104. Fink BR: Laryngeal complications of general anesthesia. In Orkin FK, Cooperman LH, eds: *Complications in anesthesiology,* Philadelphia, 1983, JB Lippincott.
105. Dohi S, Gold MI: Pulmonary mechanics during general anesthesia: the influence of mechanical irritation on the airway, *Br J Anaesth* 51:205, 1979.
106. Macklem PT, Mead J: Resistance of central and peripheral airways measured by a retrograde catheter, *J Appl Physiol* 22:395, 1967.
107. Kumeta Y, Hattori A, Mimura M, et al: A survey of perioperative bronchospasm in 105 patients with reactive airway disease, *Masui* 44:396, 1995.
108. Hirshman CA, Downes H, Farbood A, et al: Ketamine block of bronchospasm in experimental canine asthma, *Br J Anaesth* 51:713, 1979.
109. Brandus V, Joffe S, Benoit CV, et al: Bronchial spasm during general anesthesia, *Can Anaesth Soc J* 17:269, 1970.
110. Bedford RF: Circulatory responses to tracheal intubation, *Probl Anesthesia* 2:201, 1998.
111. Latorre F, Hofmann M, Kleemann PP, et al: Fiberoptic intubation and stress, *Anaesthetist* 42:423, 1993.
112. Bedford RF, Feinstein B: Hospital admission blood pressure: a predictor for hypertension following endotracheal intubation, *Anesth Analg* 59:367, 1980.
113. Edwards ND, Alford AM, Dobson PM, et al: Myocardial ischaemia during tracheal intubation and extubation, *Br J Anaesth* 73:537, 1994.
114. Abou-Madi MN, Keszler H, Yacoub JM: Cardiovascular reactions to laryngoscopy and tracheal intubation following small and large intravenous doses of lidocaine, *Can Anaesth Soc J* 24:12, 1977.
115. Tam S, Chuang F, Campbell M: Intravenous lidocaine: optimal time of injection before tracheal intubation, *Anesth Analg* 66:1036, 1987.
116. Hamill JF, Bedford RF, Weaver DC, et al: Lidocaine before endotracheal intubation: intravenous or laryngotracheal? *Anesthesiology* 55:578, 1981.
117. Stoelting RK: Circulatory changes during direct laryngoscopy and tracheal intubation: influence of duration of laryngoscopy with or without prior lidocaine, *Anesthesiology* 47:381, 1977.
118. Kautto UM: Attenuation of the circulatory response to laryngoscopy and intubation by fentanyl, *Acta Anaesthesiol Scand* 26:217, 1982.
119. Chen CT, Toung TJK, Donham RT, et al: Fentanyl dosage for suppression of circulatory response to laryngoscopy and endotracheal intubation, *Anesthesiology Review* 13:37, 1986.
120. Wang SC, Wu CC, Lin MS, et al: Use of esmolol to prevent hemodynamic changes during intubation in general anesthesia, *Acta Anaesthesiol Sin* 32:141, 1994.
121. Mikawa K, Nishina K, Maekawa N, et al: Comparison of nicardipine, diltiazem and verapamil for controlling the cardiovascular responses to tracheal intubation, *Br J Anaesth* 76:221, 1996.
122. Gallagher JD, Moore RA, Jose AB, et al: Prophylactic nitroglycerin infusions during coronary artery bypass surgery, *Anesthesiology* 64:785, 1986.
123. Stoelting RK: Attenuation of blood pressure response to laryngoscopy and tracheal intubation with sodium nitroprusside, *Anesth Analg* 58:116, 1979.
124. Gonzalez RM, Bjerke RJ, Drobycki T, et al: Prevention of endotracheal tube-induced coughing during emergence from general anesthesia, *Anesth Analg* 79:792, 1994.
125. Williams B: Cerebrospinal fluid pressure changes in response to coughing, *Brain* 99:331, 1976.
126. Donlon JV: Anesthesia and eye, ear, nose, and throat surgery. In Miller RD, ed: *Anesthesia,* ed 3, New York, 1990, Churchill Livingstone, p 2004.

127. Steinhaus JE, Gaskin I: A study of intravenous lidocaine as a suppressant of cough reflex, *Anesthesiology* 24:285, 1963.
128. Poulton TJ, James FM III: Cough suppression by lidocaine, *Anesthesiology* 50:470, 1979.
129. Yukioka H, Yoshimoto N, Nishimura K, et al: Intravenous lidocaine as a suppressant of coughing during tracheal intubation, *Anesth Analg* 64:1189, 1985.
130. Gerhardt T, Bancalari E: Apnea of prematurity. I. Lung function and regulation of breathing, *Pediatrics* 74:58, 1984.
131. Vanner RG, O'Dwyer JP, Pryle BJ, et al: Upper oesophageal sphincter pressure and the effect of cricoid pressure, *Anaesthesia* 47:95, 1992.
132. Salem MR, Joseph MJ, Heymann HJ, et al: Cricoid compression is effective in obliterating the esophageal lumen in the presence of a nasogastric tube, *Anesthesiology* 63:443, 1985.
133. Georgescu A, Miller JN, Lecklitner ML: The Sellick maneuver causing complete airway obstruction, *Anesth Analg* 74:457, 1992.
134. Shorten GD, Alfille PH, Gliklich RE: Airway obstruction following application of cricoid pressure, *J Clin Anesth* 3:403, 1991.
135. Gild WM, Posner KL, Caplan RA, et al: Eye injuries associated with anesthesia: a closed claims analysis, *Anesthesiology* 76:204, 1992.
136. Snow JC, Kripke BJ, Norton ML, et al: Corneal injuries during general anesthesia, *Anesth Analg* 54:465, 1975.
137. Batra YK, Bali IM: Corneal abrasions during general anesthesia, *Anesth Analg* 56:363, 1977.
138. Watson WJ, Moran RL: Corneal abrasion during induction, *Anesthesiology* 66:440, 1987 (letter).
139. Monroe MC, Gravenstein N, Saga-Rumley S: Postoperative sore throat: effect of oropharyngeal airway in orotracheally intubated patients, *Anesth Analg* 70:512, 1990.
140. Sanou J, Ilboudo D, Rouamba A, et al: Sore throat after tracheal intubation, *Cah Anesthesiol* 44:203, 1996.
141. el Hakim M: Beclomethasone prevents postoperative sore throat, *Acta Anaesthersiol Scand* 37:250, 1993.
142. Klemola UM, Saarnivaara L, Yrjola H: Post-operative sore throat: effect of lidocaine jelly and spray with endotracheal intubation, *Eur J Anesthiol* 5:391, 1988.
143. Mayhew JF, Miner M, Katz J: Macroglossia in a 16-month-old child after a craniotomy, *Anesthesiology* 62:683, 1985.
144. Teeple E, Maroon J, Rueger R: Hemimacroglossia and unilateral ischemic necrosis of the tongue in a long-duration neurosurgical procedure, *Anesthesiology* 64:845, 1986 (letter).
145. Patane PS, White SE: Macroglossia causing airway obstruction following cleft palate repair, *Anesthesiology* 71:995, 1989.
146. Kharasch ED: Angiotensin-converting enzyme inhibitor–induced angioedema associated with endotracheal intubation, *Anesth Analg* 74:602, 1992.
147. Blanc VF, Tremblay NAG: The complications of tracheal intubation: a new classification with a review of the literature, *Anesth Analg* 53:202, 1974.
148. Rosenberg H, Rosenberg HK: Airway obstruction and causes of difficult intubation. In Orkin FK, Cooperman LH, eds: *Complications in anesthesiology,* Philadelphia, 1983, JB Lippincott, p 125.
149. Ehrenpreis MB, Oliverio RM Jr: Endotracheal tube obstruction secondary to oral preoperative medication, *Anesth Analg* 63:867, 1984.
150. Cook WP, Schultetus RR: Obstruction of an endotracheal tube by the plastic coating sheared from a stylet, *Anesthesiology* 62:803, 1985.
151. Zmyslowski WP, Kam D, Simpson GT: An unusual cause of endotracheal tube obstruction, *Anesthesiology* 70:883, 1989 (letter).
152. Sapsford DJ, Snowdon SL: If in doubt, take it out: obstruction of tracheal tube by prominent aortic knuckle, *Anaesthesia* 40:552, 1985.
153. Populaire C, Robard S, Souron R: An armoured endotracheal tube obstruction in a child, *Can J Anaesth* 36(3 Pt 1):331, 1989.
154. Gemma M, Ferrazza C: "Dental trauma" to oral airways, *Can J Anaesth* 37:951, 1990 (letter).
155. McTaggart RA, Shustack A, Noseworth T, et al: Another cause of obstruction in an armoured endotracheal tube, *Anesthesiology* 59:164, 1983 (letter).
156. Wright PJ, Mundy JVB, Mansfield CJ: Obstruction of armoured tracheal tubes: case report and discussion, *Can J Anaesth* 35:195, 1988.
157. Treffers R, de Lange JJ: An unusual case of cuff herniation, *Acta Anaesthesiol Belg* 40:87, 1989.
158. Kendall AP, Lin E: Respiratory failure as presentation of achalasia of the esophagus, *Anaesthesia* 46:1039, 1991.
159. Westbrook JL: Oesophageal achalasia causing respiratory obstruction, *Anaesthesia* 47:38, 1992.
160. McConnell MS, Finn JC, Feeley TW: Tension hydrothorax during laparoscopy in a patient with ascites, *Anesthesiology* 80:1390, 1994.
161. Gallagher ML, Roberts-Fox M: Respiratory and circulatory compromise associated with acute hydrothorax during operative hysteroscopy, *Anesthesiology* 79:1129, 1993.
162. Cooper JB, Newbower RS, Kitz RJ: An analysis of major errors and equipment failures in anesthesia management: considerations for prevention and detection, *Anesthesiology* 60:34, 1984.
163. Raphael DT, Weller RS, Doran DJ: A response algorithm for the low-pressure alarm condition, *Anesth Analg* 67:876, 1988.
164. Snow JC, Norton ML, Saluja TS, et al: Fire hazard during CO_2 laser microsurgery on the larynx and trachea, *Anesth Analg* 55:146, 1976.
165. Ossoff ARG: Laser safety in otolaryngology: head and neck surgery—anesthetic and educational considerations for laryngeal surgery, *Laryngoscope* 99(suppl 48):1, 1989.
166. Hirshman CA, Smith J: Indirect ignition of the endotracheal tube during carbon dioxide laser surgery, *Arch Otolaryngol* 106:639, 1980.
167. Pashayan AG, Gravenstein N: High incidence of CO_2 laser beam contact with the tracheal tube during operations on the upper airway, *J Clin Anesth* 1:354, 1989.
168. Kaeder CS, Hirshman CA: Acute airway obstruction: a complication of aluminum tape wrapping of tracheal tubes in laser surgery, *Can Anaesth Soc J* 26:138, 1979.
169. Hirshman CA, Leon D, Porch D, et al: Improved metal endotracheal tube for laser surgery of the airway, *Anesth Analg* 59:789, 1980.
170. Sosis M, Dillon F: What is the safest foil tape for endotracheal tube protection during Nd-YAG laser surgery? A comparative study, *Anesthesiology* 72:553, 1990.
171. Wolf GL, Simpson JI: Flammability of endotracheal tubes in oxygen and nitrous oxide enriched atmosphere, *Anesthesiology* 67:236, 1987.
172. Pashayan AG, Gravenstein JS, Cassisi NJ, et al: The helium protocol for laryngotracheal operations with CO_2 laser: a retrospective review of 523 cases, *Anesthesiology* 68:801, 1988.
173. Pashayan AG, SanGiovanni C, Davis LE: Positive end-expiratory pressure lowers the risk of laser-induced polyvinyl chloride tracheal-tube fires, *Anesthesiology* 79:83, 1993.
174. Howland WS, Lewis JS: Postintubation granulomas of the larynx, *Cancer* 9:1244, 1956.
175. Snow JC, Harano M, Balough K: Postintubation granuloma of the larynx, *Anesth Analg* 45:425, 1966.
176. Kirchner JA, Sasaki CT: Fusion of the vocal cords following intubation and tracheostomy, *Trans Am Acad Ophthalmol Otolaryngol* 77:ORL88, 1973.
177. Geffin B, Bland J, Grillo HC: Anesthetic management of tracheal resection and reconstruction, *Anesth Analg* 48:884, 1969.
178. Webb WR, Ozdemir IA, Ikins PM, et al: Surgical management of tracheal stenosis, *Ann Surg* 179:819, 1974.
179. Bidwai AV, Bidwai VA, Rogers CR, et al: Blood pressure and pulse-rate responses to endotracheal extubation with and without prior injection of lidocaine, *Anesthesiology* 51:171, 1979.
180. Wohlner EC, Usubiaga LJ, Jacoby RM, et al: Cardiovascular effects of extubation, *Anesthesiology* 51:S194, 1979 (abstract).
181. Cooper RM: Extubation and changing endotracheal tubes. In Benumof JL, ed: *Airway management: principles and practice,* St Louis, 1996, Mosby, p 866.
182. Muzzi DA, Black S, Losasso TJ, et al: Labetalol and esmolol in the control of hypertension after intracranial surgery, *Anesth Analg* 70:68, 1990.
183. Coriat P, Mundler O, Bousseau D, et al: Response of left ventricular ejection fraction to recovery from general anesthesia: measurement by gated radionuclide angiography, *Anesth Analg* 65:593, 1986.
184. Dyson A, Isaac PA, Pennant JH, et al: Esmolol attenuates cardiovascular responses to extubation, *Anesth Analg* 71:675, 1990.

185. Mikawa K, Nishina K, Maekawa N, et al: Attenuation of cardiovascular responses to tracheal extubation: verapamil versus diltiazem, *Anesth Analg* 82:1205, 1996.
186. Paulissian R, Salem MR, Joseph NJ, et al: Hemodynamic responses to endotracheal extubation after coronary artery bypass grafting, *Anesth Analg* 73:10, 1991.
187. Rex MAE: A review of the structural and functional basis of laryngospasm and a discussion of the nerve pathways involved in the reflex and its clinical significance in man and animals, *Br J Anaesth* 42:891, 1970.
188. Chung DC, Rowbottom FJ: A very small dose of suxamethonium relieves laryngospasm, *Anaesthesia* 48:229, 1993.
189. Hartley M, Vaughan RS: Problems associated with tracheal extubation, *Br J Anaesth* 71:561, 1993.
190. Darmon JY, Rauss A, Dreyfuss D, et al: Evaluation of risk factors for laryngeal edema after tracheal extubation in adults and its prevention by dexamethasone: a placebo-controlled, double-blind, multi-center study, *Anesthesiology* 77:245, 1992.
191. Deepika K, Kenaan CA, Barrocas AM, et al: Negative pressure pulmonary edema after acute upper airway obstruction, *J Clin Anesth* 9(5):403, 1997.
192. Tolley NS, Cheesman TD, Morgan D, et al: Dislocated arytenoid: an intubation-induced injury, *Ann R Coll Surg Engl* 72:353, 1990.
193. O'Sullivan JC, Wells DG, Wells GR: Difficult airway management with neck swelling after carotid endarterectomy, *Anaesth Intensive Care* 14:460, 1986.
194. Geelhoed GW: Tracheomalacia from compressing goiter: management after thyroidectomy, *Surgery* 104:1100, 1988.
195. Wade JS: Cecil Joll lecture, 1979: respiratory obstruction in thyroid surgery, *Ann R Coll Surg Engl* 62:15, 1980.
196. Burgess GE III, Cooper JR Jr, Marino RJ, et al: Laryngeal competence after tracheal extubation, *Anesthesiology* 51:73, 1976.
197. Debain JJ, Le Brigand H, Binet JP: Quelques incidents et accidents de l'intubation trachéale prolongué, *Ann Otolaryngol Chir Cervicofac* 85:379, 1968.
198. Dryden GE: Circulatory collapse after pneumonectomy (an unusual complication from the use of a Carlens catheter): case report, *Anesth Analg* 56:451, 1977.
199. Lee C, Schwartz S, Mok MS: Difficult extubation due to transfixation of a nasotracheal tube by a Kirschner wire, *Anesthesiology* 46:427, 1977.
200. Ovassapian A: Fiberoptic tracheal intubation. In *Fiberoptic airway endoscopy in anaesthesia and critical care*, New York, 1990, Raven Press, p 57.
201. Bainton CR: Complications of managing the airway. In Benumof JL, ed: *Airway management: principles and practice*, St Louis, 1996, Mosby, p 895.
202. Kalinske RW, Parker RH, Brandt D: Diagnostic usefulness and safety of transtracheal aspiration, *N Engl J Med* 276:604, 1967.
203. Unger KM, Moser KM: Fatal complication of transtracheal aspiration: a report of two cases, *Arch Intern Med* 132:437, 1973.
204. Spencer CD, Beaty HN: Complications of transtracheal aspiration, *N Engl J Med* 286:304, 1972.
205. Schillaci CR, Iacovoni VF, Conte RS, et al: Transtracheal aspiration complicated by fatal endotracheal hemorrhage, *N Engl J Med* 295(9):48, 1976.
206. Hemley SD, Arida EJ, Diggs AM, et al: Percutaneous cricothyroid membrane bronchiography, *Radiology* 76:763, 1961.
207. Poon YK: Case history number 89: a life-threatening complication of cricothyroid membrane puncture, *Anesth Analg* 55:298, 1976.
208. Massey JY: Complications of transtracheal aspiration: a case report, *J Ark Med Soc* 67:254, 1971.
209. Sanchez A: Retrograde intubation technique. In Benumof JL, ed: *Airway management: principles and practice*, St Louis, 1996, Mosby, p 337.
210. Faithfull NS: Injury to terminal branches of the trigeminal nerve following tracheal intubation, *Br J Anaesth* 57:535, 1985.
211. Smith RB, Babinski M, Klain M, et al: Percutaneous transtracheal ventilation, *JACEP* 5:765, 1976.
212. Craft TM, Chambers PH, Ward ME, et al: Two cases of barotrauma associated with transtracheal jet ventilation, *Br J Anaesth* 64:524, 1990.
213. Schumacher P, Stotz G, Schneider M, et al: Laryngospasm during transtracheal high frequency jet ventilation, *Anaesthesia* 47:855, 1992.
214. Oliverio R Jr, Ruder CB, Fermon C, et al: Pneumothorax secondary to ball-valve obstruction during jet ventilation, *Anesthesiology* 51:255, 1979.
215. Smith RB, Schaer WB, Pfaeffle H: Percutaneous transtracheal ventilation for anesthesia: a review and report of complications, *Can J Anaesth* 22:607, 1975.
216. Braverman I, Sichel JY, Halimi P, et al: Complication of jet ventilation during microlaryngeal surgery, *Ann Otol Rhinol Laryngol* 103(8 Pt 1):624, 1994.
217. Benumof JL, Scheller MS: The importance of transtracheal jet ventilation in the management of the difficult airway, *Anesthesiology* 71:769, 1989.
218. Thomas T, Zornow M, Scheller MS, et al: The efficacy of three different modes of transtracheal ventilation in hypoxic hypercarbic swine, *Can J Anaesth* 35(suppl):61, 1988.
219. Mehta S: Transtracheal illumination for optimal tracheal tube placement: a clinical study, *Anaesthesia* 44:970, 1989.
220. Stone DJ, Stirt JA, Kaplan MJ, et al: A complication of lightwand-guided nasotracheal intubation, *Anesthesiology* 61:780, 1984.
221. Ellis DG, Jakymec A, Kaplan RM, et al: Guided orotracheal intubation in the operating room using a lighted stylet: a comparison with direct laryngoscopic technique, *Anesthesiology* 64:823, 1986.
222. Williams RT, Stewart RD: Transillumination of the trachea with a lighted stylet, *Anesth Analg* 65:542, 1986 (letter).
223. Moukabary K, Peterson CJ, Kingsley CP: A potential complication with the lightwand, *Anesthesiology* 81:523, 1994 (letter).
224. Szigeti CL, Baeuerle JJ, Mongan PD: Arytenoid dislocation with lighted stylet intubation: case report and retrospective review, *Anesth Analg* 78:185, 1994.
225. Cooper SD, Benumof JL, Ozaki GT: Evaluation of the Bullard laryngoscope using the new intubating stylet: comparison with conventional laryngoscopy, *Anesth Analg* 79:965, 1994.
226. Dyson A, Harris J, Bhatta K: Rapidity and accuracy of tracheal intubation in a mannequin: comparison of the fibreoptic with the Bullard laryngoscope, *Br J Anaesth* 65:268, 1990.
227. Saunders PR, Giesecke AH: Clinical assessment of the adult Bullard laryngoscope, *Can J Anaesth* 36:518, 1989 (abstract).
228. Cooper SD, Benumof JL, Ozaki GT: Evaluation of the Bullard laryngoscope using the new intubating stylet: comparison with conventional laryngoscopy, *Anesth Analg* 79:965, 1994.
229. Wilkins CJ, Cramp PG, Staples J, et al: Comparison of the anesthetic requirement for tolerance of laryngeal mask airway and endotracheal tube, *Anesth Analg* 75:794, 1992.
230. Pennant JH, White PF: The laryngeal mask airway: its use in anesthesiology, *Anesthesiology* 79:144, 1993.
231. Practice guidelines for management of the difficult airway: a report by the American Society of Anesthesiologists Task Force on Management of the Difficult Airway, *Anesthesiology* 78:597, 1993.
232. Brain AIJ: *The Intravent laryngeal mask instruction manual*, ed 2, Berkshire, UK, 1992, Brain Medical.
233. Rabey PG, Murphy PJ, Langton JA, et al: Effect of the laryngeal mask airway on lower oesophageal sphincter pressure in patients during general anaesthesia, *Br J Anaesth* 69:346, 1992.
234. Barker P, Langton JA, Murphy PJ, et al: Regurgitation of gastric contents during general anaesthesia using the laryngeal mask airway, *Br J Anaesth* 69:314, 1992.
235. Joshi GP, Smith I, White PF: Laryngeal mask airway. In Benumof JL, ed: *Airway management: principles and practice*, St Louis, 1996, Mosby, p 368.
236. Smith I, White PF: Use of the laryngeal mask airway as an alternative to a face mask during outpatient arthroscopy, *Anesthesiology* 77:850, 1992.
237. Alexander CA, Leach AB: Incidence of sore throats with the laryngeal mask, *Anaesthesia* 44:791, 1989 (letter).
238. Verghese C, Smith TG, Young E: Prospective survey of the use of the laryngeal mask in 2359 patients, *Anaesthesia* 48:58, 1993.
239. Marjot R: Pressure exerted by the laryngeal mask airway cuff upon the pharyngeal mucosa, *Br J Anaesth* 70:25, 1993.

240. Miller AC, Bickler P: The laryngeal mask airway: an unusual complication, *Anaesthesia* 46:659, 1991.

241. Lee JJ: Laryngeal mask and trauma to uvula, *Anaesthesia* 44:1014, 1989 (letter).

242. Marjot R: Trauma to the posterior pharyngeal wall caused by a laryngeal mask airway, *Anaesthesia* 46:589, 1991 (letter).

243. King C, Street MK: Twelfth cranial nerve paralysis following use of a laryngeal mask airway, *Anaesthesia* 49:786, 1994.

244. Ezri T, Priscu V, Szmuk P, et al: Laryngeal mask and pulmonary edema, *Anesthesiology* 78:219, 1993 (letter).

245. Wynn JM, Jones KL: Tongue cyanosis after laryngeal mask airway insertion, *Anesthesiology* 80:1403, 1994.

246. Conacher ID: Foreign body in a laryngeal mask airway, *Anaesthesia* 46:164, 1991 (letter).

247. Brimacombe JR, Brimacombe JC, Berry AM, et al: A comparison of the laryngeal mask airway and cuffed oropharyngeal airway in anesthetized adult patients, *Anesth Analg* 87:147, 1998.

248. Gerard A, Gouvitsos F, Boufflers E: Interest of the COPA (cuffed oropharyngeal airway) versus facial mask in emergency procedures, *Anesthesiology* 87(3A):A992, 1997 (abstract).

249. Maslowski D, Boufflers E, Reyford H, et al: Clinical evaluation of the COPA as a new device for airway management in gynecology, *Anesthesiology* 87(3A):A486, 1997 (abstract).

250. Cros AM, Boisson-Bertrand D, Colombani S, et al: Does COPA prevent agitation and respiratory incidents during recovery? *Anesthesiology* 87(3A):A472, 1997 (abstract).

251. Greenberg RS, Brimacombe JR, Berry A, et al: A randomized controlled trial comparing the cuffed oropharyngeal airway and the laryngeal mask airway in spontaneously breathing anesthetized adults, *Anesthesiology* 88:970, 1998.

252. Frass M, Frenzer R, Zdrahal F, et al: The esophageal tracheal combitube: preliminary results with a new airway for CPR, *Ann Emerg Med* 16:768, 1987.

253. Frass M: The Combitube: esophageal/tracheal double-lumen airway. In Benumof JL, ed: *Airway management: principles and practice,* St Louis, 1996, Mosby, p 444.

254. Green KS, Beger TH: Proper use of the Combitube, *Anesthesiology* 81:513, 1994 (letter).

255. Davidson TM, Magit AE: Surgical airway. In Benumof JL, ed: *Airway management: principles and practice,* St Louis, 1996, Mosby, p 513.

256. Wain JC, Wilson DJ, Mathieon DJ: Clinical experience with minitracheostomy, *Ann Thorac Surg* 49:881, 1990.

Chapter 2

Complications of Cardiovascular Monitoring

David L. Reich
David M. Moskowitz

As a result of the aging of the population and advances in surgical therapy, anesthesiologists are frequently confronted with elderly patients and those with disease. It is generally accepted that cardiovascular monitoring improves patient care and probably improves outcome. Although difficult to prove, a reasonable assumption is that appropriate hemodynamic monitoring reduces the incidence of major cardiovascular complications as long as the data obtained from the monitors are interpreted correctly and therapeutic interventions are implemented in a timely manner.

Many devices are currently available to monitor the cardiovascular system. These range from completely noninvasive devices, such as the blood pressure cuff and electrocardiogram (ECG), to invasive devices, such as the pulmonary artery catheter. In the past decade, transesophageal echocardiography (TEE), a minimally invasive technique, has gained popularity as an alternative to the pulmonary artery catheter. To make the best use of invasive monitoring systems, the potential benefits of the information obtained must outweigh the potential complications. In many critically ill patients, the benefits seem to outweigh the risks, which explains the increasing use of invasive monitoring techniques. This chapter reviews the complications associated with various forms of cardiovascular monitoring so that the clinician may make educated decisions on the basis of known benefits and risks.

I. ELECTRICAL HAZARDS OF CARDIOVASCULAR MONITORS
A. Microshock and macroshock

The application of large voltages or currents to skin or tissue represents a *macroshock*. All modern monitoring equipment in the operating room has electrically isolated connections; that is, there is no electrical connection between the isolated portion of the circuit (attached to the patient) and the electrical ground. However, faulty equipment may allow leakage of electrical current that could reach the patient through ECG electrodes or other conductive materials in contact with the patient's body. In one reported case, death from electrocution resulted when ECG electrodes inadvertently came into contact with a power cord.[1]

According to National Fire Protection Association (NFPA) standards, the upper threshold of electrical safety for external application is 50 mA.[2] Until 1984, all rooms used to conduct anesthesia were required to have an isolated power system to provide early warning of faulty leakage of current. This limit was set at 5 mA, which protects against macroshock but not microshock (discussed later). With the introduction of nonvolatile anesthetics, the NFPA made the isolated power system optional except in wet environments. Thus all patient monitoring equipment must be regularly inspected by biomedical engineering personnel for leakage of current.

The application of small amounts of electrical power to the heart represents a *microshock* (Fig. 2-1). The current may reach the heart by way of internal ECG leads, fluid-filled catheters, or internal equipment (Box 2-1). Reports of ventricular fibrillation caused by microshock are uncommon but do occur.[3] The NFPA standard for electrical contact with the heart is a maximal leakage of

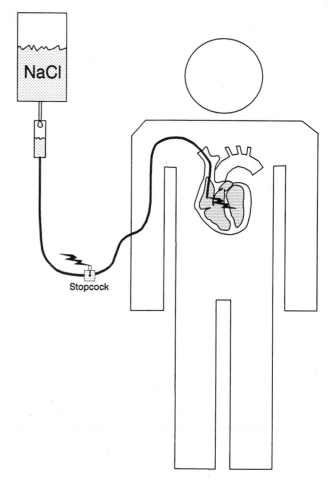

Fig. 2-1. Microshock is a potential hazard whenever a direct electrical connection to the heart exists. In the figure, a saline-filled central venous line serves as an electrical conductor from the stopcock to the heart. Microshock currents as low as 100 μA may result in ventricular fibrillation.

current of 10 μA. When pacing wires and intracardiac electrodes are used, they should always be covered with insulating material and should never be touched with bare hands.

B. Burns

Unipolar electrocautery is based on the principle that a high current density at the tip of the instrument (which has a small surface area) cauterizes the tissue. This current traverses the body and leaves by way of a *dispersal pad* (also known as a "return pad" or, incorrectly, a "grounding pad") with a large surface area. The large surface area ensures a low current density at the exit site with little production of heat. If the dispersal pad is faulty, the ECG lead may inadvertently become the grounding site for unipolar electrocautery. If this occurs, a burn will result because of the relatively small surface area of the lead (Fig. 2-2). This problem can be prevented by using electrically isolated monitoring equipment and preventing contact between ECG leads and wires and potentially grounded conductors, such as the metallic components of operating room tables.

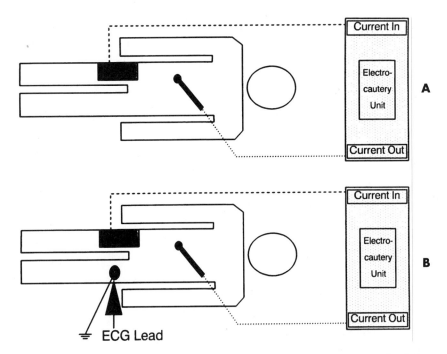

Fig. 2-2. A, Normally, current leaves the electrocautery device ("current out" of electro-cautery unit) and enters the patient through a small tip. The high current density at the instrument tip cauterizes the tissue. The current leaves the patient through the return pad ("current in" of electrocautery unit). The pad has a large surface area that allows a low current density and minimal heat generation. **B,** An ECG lead on the patient's thigh *(large arrow)* has inadvertently become grounded, short-circuiting the normal route through the return pad. The electrocautery current runs through the small surface area of the ECG lead, resulting in a burn from the high current density.

Box 2-1 Sources of microshock hazard

Echocardiographic leads
  Transcutaneous electrodes
  Esophageal electrodes
  Pacing wires
  Pulmonary artery catheter electrodes
Intravascular catheters filled with electrolyte solution (saline)
  Peripheral intravenous lines
  Central venous lines
  Pulmonary artery catheters
  Arterial lines
Internal equipment
  Endoscopic probes
  Transesophageal echocardiographic probes
  Esophageal temperature probes

II. PERIPHERAL INTRAVENOUS CATHETERS
A. Infection

Infection associated with use of intravenous (IV) catheters occurs for many reasons, including insertion through infected skin, poor aseptic technique during insertion or maintenance, sepsis with seeding of the catheter, and prolonged cannulation with colonization by skin flora. Lymphangitic streaks or cellulitis may result from catheter infection. Whenever infection at the cannulation site is identified, the catheter must be re-moved. The catheter is a foreign body that can never be sterilized with antibiotic therapy. Systemic antibiotic therapy may be required to eradicate the infection.

B. Phlebitis

The injection of irritating drugs, such as diazepam (in a vehicle of propylene glycol), potassium, or hypertonic fluids, sometimes results in phlebitis caused by a direct intimal injury. Physical signs include a tender vein with surrounding edema and erythema. The IV catheter must be removed, and antiinflammatory drugs may be administered. Antibiotic therapy is required if suppurative phlebitis is present.

C. Hematoma

Elderly patients with fragile veins and lax subcutaneous tissues and patients receiving glucocorticoid therapy are prone to developing hematomas during attempts at peripheral venous cannulation. Hematomas not only are painful and disfiguring but also may become infected. Pressure should be applied to prevent hematomas after unsuccessful cannulation. Conservative treatment involves using warm soaks or heating pads to accelerate the breakdown of extravasated blood.

Massive hematomas may occur if blood is extravasated during transfusions. This is especially dangerous when blood is administered under pressure to patients with precarious IV lines. Hematomas can exert pressure on the surrounding tissues, producing limb ischemia, or can serve as a nidus for infection.

D. Extravasation

Extravasation of caustic substances (e.g., vasopressors or thiopental) may result in tissue necrosis and skin sloughing. It is preferable to administer irritating drugs through large-bore IV lines with rapid flow of a concurrent intravenous fluid. An even better alternative is to administer these substances through a central venous line if possible.

III. NONINVASIVE BLOOD PRESSURE MONITORING

The proliferation of noninvasive devices for monitoring blood pressure has introduced the potential for a new set of complications. With these devices, a cuff is inflated to a suprasystolic pressure and slowly deflated to determine the blood pressure by the oscillometric method. A manufacturer-dependent algorithm measures the blood pressure. The rate of cuff deflation is directly proportional to the heart rate and rhythm.

Noninvasive blood pressure measurement techniques are advantageous in that they are technically easy to perform, generally accurate, and carry a negligible infectious risk. Furthermore, automated oscillometric machines allow the anesthesiologist to perform other tasks while the blood pressure is being measured. However, several risks remain. The innervation of the extremity is ischemic during cuff inflation. Improper cuff placement or prolonged or too-frequent cuff inflation may result in tissue ischemia, nerve damage, compartmental syndrome, or superficial thrombophlebitis.[4,5] Ecchymoses and petechial hemorrhages also may occur with high cuff pressures and in patients with excessive tissue at the point where the cuff is placed.

Several clinical situations may cause difficulties in obtaining noninvasive blood pressure measurements (Box 2-2). These situations impose a certain risk in that therapeutic interventions may be delayed while blood pressure measurements are awaited.

IV. INVASIVE ARTERIAL PRESSURE MONITORING
A. Sites (Box 2-3)

1. Radial and ulnar arteries. The ulnar artery provides the majority of blood flow to the hand in about 90% of persons.[6] The radial and ulnar arteries are connected by a palmar arch that provides collateral flow to the hand in the event of radial artery occlusion. Many anesthesiologists perform the Allen test before radial arterial cannulation. This is a popular bedside technique for assessing the adequacy of the collateral circulation to the palmar arch of the hand in the event that the radial artery becomes occluded during or after cannulation.

The Allen test is performed by occluding both the radial and ulnar arteries with compression and exercising the hand by the patient making and releasing a fist until it is pale. The ulnar artery is then released (with the hand open loosely), and the time until the hand regains its normal color is noted.[7] With normal collateral circulation, the color returns to the hand in about 5 seconds. If the hand takes longer than 15 seconds to return to its normal color, cannulation of the radial artery on that side of the body is somewhat controversial. The hand

---

Box 2-2 Causes of difficulty in obtaining noninvasive blood pressure measurements

Physiologic
Shock (hypotension or vasoconstriction)
Beat-to-beat variations in blood pressure (arrhythmia, hypovolemia, spontaneous or assisted ventilation, or rapidly changing blood pressure)
Irregular pulse rate

Anatomic
Conically shaped arm
Obese arm
Calcified brachial artery (lead-pipe syndrome)
Compression of artery (thoracic outlet syndrome, positioning, surgical manipulations, or surgical retraction)

Cuff compression variation
Movement (patient movement, shivering, or seizure)
External (person leaning on or moving the patient's arm)

Cuff-related
Incorrect size (especially with cuff that is too small; a cuff too large has minimal effects)
Incorrect application (cuff not snug enough, not squeezing all air out of the bladder before application, or kinking of cuff hoses)
Undetected (disconnected or leaking cuff, hose, or connectors)

Box 2-3 Sites for arterial cannulation

Radial artery
Ulnar artery
Brachial artery
Axillary artery
Femoral artery
Dorsalis pedis artery
Superficial temporal artery
Umbilical artery (in neonates)

---

may remain pale if the fingers are hyperextended or widely spread apart, even in the presence of normal collateral circulation.[8] Variations on the Allen test include use of a Doppler probe or pulse oximetry to assess collateral flow.[9-11]

The value of the Allen test has been challenged. Slogoff, Keats, and Arlund[12] cannulated the radial artery in 16 patients with poor ulnar collateral circulation (as assessed by using the Allen test) without any complications. In contrast, Mangano and Hickey[13] reported a case of hand ischemia requiring amputation in a patient with a normal preoperative result on the Allen test. Thus the predictive value of the Allen test is questionable. If the test demonstrates that the hand is dependent on the radial artery for adequate filling and other cannulation sites are not available, the ulnar artery may be selected.

2. *Brachial or axillary arteries.* The brachial artery lies medial to the bicipital tendon in the antecubital fossa, in close proximity to the median nerve. The rate of complications from percutaneous brachial artery catheter monitoring is lower than that following brachial artery cutdown for cardiac catheterization.[14] However, there is little (if any) collateral flow to the hand in brachial artery occlusion. Other sites should be chosen, if possible.

Brachial artery pressure tracings resemble those in the femoral artery and have less systolic augmentation than radial artery tracings.[15] In a study of 170 patients, brachial arterial pressure was found to reflect central aortic pressure more accurately than radial arterial pressures both before and after cardiopulmonary bypass.[16] Two reports of large series of perioperative brachial arterial monitoring have documented the safety of this technique.[14,17]

The axillary artery may be cannulated by using the Seldinger technique near the junction of the deltoid and pectoral muscles. This method has been recommended for patients who require long-term catheterization in the intensive care unit[18] and patients with peripheral vascular disease.[19] Because the tip of the catheter (which ranges in size from 15 to 20 cm) may lie in the aortic arch, use of the left axillary artery is recommended to minimize the chance of cerebral embolization during flushing. Arterial pressures measured in the axillary artery (via radial artery cannulation) more closely reflect central aortic blood pressure than do brachial arterial blood pressure measurements.[20]

3. *Femoral artery.* The femoral artery may be cannulated by using any of the techniques previously discussed. It is usually cannulated for monitoring purposes when other sites are not accessible or when other pulses are not palpable. The use of this site remains controversial because of the high rate of ischemic complications and pseudoaneurysm formation after diagnostic angiographic and cardiac catheterization procedures.[21] However, monitoring catheters are considerably smaller than diagnostic catheters, and the incidence of these complications should be much less with monitoring catheters. Use of this site is also less desirable in patients with peripheral vascular disease. Aortic inflow obstruction may decrease the arterial pressure in the femoral artery, or the femoral artery may have atheromatous plaques that could embolize and cause distal ischemia. The presence of atheromatous plaque may also make it more difficult to thread catheters in this artery.

The older literature stated that the femoral area was intrinsically dirty and that catheter sepsis and mortality were significantly increased with use of this site compared with other monitoring sites. More recent evidence suggests that femoral artery cannulation is safe but that long-term cannulation (>4 days) is associated with an 8% to 17% incidence of catheter-related infections.[22]

In patients undergoing thoracic aortic surgery, distal aortic perfusion (by using partial cardiopulmonary bypass, left heart bypass, or a heparinized shunt) may be performed during aortic cross-clamping to preserve spinal cord and visceral organ blood flow. In these situations, it may be preferable to measure the distal aortic pressure at the femoral or dorsalis pedis artery to optimize the distal perfusion pressure.[23] In repairs of aortic coarctation, simultaneous femoral and radial arterial monitoring may help to determine the adequacy of the surgical repair by documenting the pressure gradient following the repair. It is necessary to consult with the surgeon before cannulating the femoral vessels because these vessels may be used for extracorporeal perfusion or placement of an intraaortic balloon pump during surgery.

4. *Dorsalis pedis artery.* The dorsalis pedis is a relatively small artery that may be cannulated when other sites are not available. Because this artery is small, the incidence of failed cannulation is up to 20% and the incidence of thrombotic occlusion is around 8%.[24] In the dorsalis pedis artery, the systolic pressure is usually 10 to 20 mm Hg higher and the diastolic pressure is 15 to 20 mm Hg lower than in the radial or brachial arteries, but the mean arterial pressures are usually the same.[25,26] A modified Allen test may be performed by blanching the great toe during compression of the dorsalis pedis and posterior tibial arteries and releasing the pressure over the posterior tibial artery. These vessels probably should not be used in patients with diabetes or other peripheral vascular diseases.

5. *Superficial temporal artery.* The superficial artery is a branch of the external carotid artery that passes in front of the ear. It has a variable course that may be determined by using a Doppler probe. The artery may be tortuous and difficult to cannulate. The tip of the catheter must be positioned carefully so that embolization through the internal carotid to the cerebral circulation will not occur. This approach is not recommended in patients with carotid occlusive or cerebrovascular disease.

B. Doppler-assisted technique

In the Doppler-assisted technique, the artery is localized by using a Doppler flow probe. The direction of insertion of the percutaneous catheter is guided by the Doppler signals.[27,28] This technique may be especially useful in small children and infants. In adults, it may be helpful when palpation of the artery is difficult, such as in obese patients requiring femoral arterial cannulation.

C. Ultrasonography-guided arterial cannulation

Doppler-assisted techniques have been largely supplanted in clinical practice by two-dimensional ultrasonic methods. In the case of arterial catheterization, especially radial artery cannulation, a high-frequency ultrasonic transducer (e.g., 9 MHz) is required to visualize small structures in the near field. The artery is visualized in transverse section, and the catheter-over-needle assembly is advanced at a 30- to 60-degree angle, starting 5 to 15 mm distal to the ultrasonic transducer. The experienced clinician can see the artery and the catheter intersect within the ultrasonic imaging plane by using a triangulation technique. Commercial products that incorporate sterile needle guides are available to simplify the coordination of the needle insertion path with the ultrasonic imaging plane.

D. Surgical cutdown

In surgical cutdown, an incision is made in the skin overlying the artery, and the surrounding tissues are dissected away from the arterial wall. Proximal and distal ligatures are passed around the artery to control blood loss but are not tied down. Under direct vision, the artery is cannulated with a catheter-over-needle assembly. Alternatively, a small incision is made in the arterial wall to facilitate passage of the catheter.

E. Contraindications

1. Local infection. Placement of an arterial cannula through cellulitic or purulent tissue is likely to result in catheter sepsis. If signs of infection develop at an existing arterial cannulation site, the catheter must be removed and a cannulation site free of infection should be found. Strict aseptic technique is necessary during the insertion and maintenance of arterial cannulas.

2. Coagulopathy. Coagulopathy is a relative contraindication because it may result in hematoma formation during arterial cannulation at peripheral sites, such as the radial and dorsalis pedis arteries. However, the risk for formation of massive hematomas causing vascular or neurologic compromise is greater during attempts at axillary and femoral cannulation. This is because it is more difficult to apply direct pressure over the artery if attempts at cannulation fail or if the catheter is removed. Thus in patients receiving anticoagulant therapy, it is recommended that more peripheral arterial cannulation sites be used when this form of monitoring is required.

3. Proximal obstruction. Anatomic factors may lead to intraarterial pressure readings that markedly underestimate the central aortic pressure. The thoracic outlet syndrome and congenital anomalies of the aortic arch vessels will obstruct flow to the upper extremities. Aortic coarctation or severe atheromatous disease of the aorta and iliac vessels will diminish flow to the lower extremities. Arterial pressure distal to a previous arterial cutdown site may be lower than the central aortic pressure because of stenosis at the cutdown site.

4. Raynaud phenomenon. Radial and brachial arterial cannulation are contraindicated in patients with a history of Raynaud phenomenon or Buerger disease (thromboangiitis obliterans). This is especially important in the perioperative setting because hypothermia of the hand is the main trigger for vasospastic attacks in Raynaud phenomenon.[29] It is recommended that large arteries, such as the femoral or axillary artery, be used for intraarterial monitoring if indicated in patients with either of these diseases.

F. Surgical considerations

Several surgical maneuvers may interfere with intraarterial monitoring. During mediastinoscopy, the scope intermittently compresses the innominate artery against the manubrium. In this situation, in which damping of the arterial waveform is intermittent, it is advantageous to monitor radial artery pressure on the affected side and place a pulse oximeter on the opposite extremity. Thus the surgeon will be informed whenever compression of the innominate artery occurs.

The lateral decubitus position may compromise flow to the downward arm if an axillary roll is not properly positioned. In this situation, the damping may be prolonged; therefore it is best to monitor arterial pressure in a different extremity.

During descending thoracic aortic aneurysm repairs, the right radial, brachial, or axillary artery should be monitored because the left subclavian artery may be occluded during various phases of the procedure.

G. Complications of invasive arterial pressure monitoring

1. Risk for infection. One potential complication that is common to all forms of invasive monitoring is the risk for infection. Like intravenous catheters, arterial catheters may become infected by insertion through an infected skin site, poor aseptic technique during insertion or maintenance, sepsis with seeding of the catheter, or prolonged duration of cannulation with colonization by skin flora. Other factors associated with arterial catheter infection include nondisposable transducer domes, dextrose flush solutions, and duration of insertion.[30-32] Accessory factors, such as contaminated blood gas syringes, have also been linked with arterial catheter infections.[33]

2. Hemorrhage. The use of an intraarterial catheter carries the risk for exsanguination if the catheter or tubing assembly becomes disconnected. Use of a Luer lock connection instead of tapered connections and monitors with low-pressure alarms should decrease the risk for this complication.[34] Stopcocks are an additional source of occult hemorrhage because of the potential for loose connections or inadvertent changes in the position of the control lever that can open the system to the atmosphere.

3. Thrombosis and distal ischemia. Thrombosis of the radial artery after cannulation has been extensively studied. Factors that correlate with an increased incidence of thrombosis include prolonged duration of cannulation,[35] larger catheters,[36] and smaller radial artery size (i.e., a greater proportion of the artery is occupied by the catheter).[37] Other factors associated with thrombosis in adults (but not in children) include polypropylene catheters[38] and tapered catheters.[39] The incidence of thrombosis is not affected by the technique of cannulation[40] but is lowered with aspirin pretreatment.[41] To remove accumulated thrombus, Bedford[42] recommended removing arterial catheters by continuous aspiration of the catheter with a syringe during proximal and distal occlusion of the vessel.

The association between radial artery thrombosis and ischemia of the hand is less certain. As noted, the ability of the Allen test to predict hand complications after radial artery cannulation has been challenged.[12] Despite the widespread use of radial artery cannulation, hand complications are rarely reported. Slogoff, Keats, and Arlund[12] stated that in their experience, most ischemic complications occurred in patients who had had multiple embolic phenomena or were receiving high-dose vasopressor therapy with resultant ischemia in multiple extremities.

The hand should be closely examined at regular intervals in patients who have undergone axillary, brachial, radial, or ulnar arterial catheterization. Because thrombosis may appear several days after the catheter has been removed,[35] the examinations should be continued throughout the postoperative period. Recanalization of a thrombosed artery can be expected in an average of 13 days,[43] but the collateral blood flow may be tenuous during this period. Any evidence of hand ischemia should be aggressively investigated and promptly treated to prevent morbidity.[44]

The treatment plan should involve consultation with a vascular, hand, or plastic surgeon. Treatment of thrombosis has traditionally been conservative. However, use of fibrinolytic agents (such as streptokinase), stellate ganglion blockade, and surgical intervention should be considered.

4. Embolization. Flushing an arterial catheter forces particulate matter or air present in the catheter to move distally or proximally within the artery. Distal embolization may result in hand ischemia with tissue necrosis or loss of function. Forceful or prolonged flushing causes proximal embolization and may result in cerebral embolization. Cerebral embolization is most likely to originate in axillary or temporal sites but sometimes stems from brachial and radial catheters.[45] Emboli in the right arm are more likely than those in the left arm to reach the cerebral circulation because of the anatomy and direction of blood flow within the aortic arch. Other factors that influence the likelihood of cerebral embolization include the volume of flush solution, the rapidity of injection,[46] and the proximity of the intraluminal end of the catheter to the central circulation.

5. Skin necrosis. Necrosis of the skin over the volar aspect of the forearm after radial arterial cannulation has been reported in eight patients[47,48] and has led to full-thickness skin loss at that site. The necrosis presumably is due to thrombosis of the radial artery with proximal propagation of the thrombosis to involve the cutaneous branches of the radial artery.

6. Hematoma and neurologic injury. Hematoma formation may complicate any attempt at arterial puncture or cannulation and is particularly common in patients with coagulopathies. If a large hematoma develops, the resultant pressure may compress adjacent structures, especially if it forms in a fibrous sheath (such as the brachial plexus) or in a limited tissue compartment (such as the forearm[49]). If the arteries or veins are compressed, distal ischemia may occur. Compression of an adjacent nerve may result in neuropathy. Nerve damage is especially likely to occur if the nerve and artery lie in a limited tissue compartment, such as the fibrous sheath surrounding the brachial plexus. Hematoma formation should be prevented by the application of direct pressure following arterial punctures and, if possible, the correction of any underlying coagulopathy. Surgical consultation should be obtained if a massive hematoma forms or neurologic dysfunction develops. Surgical exploration and drainage may be necessary if conservative measures are ineffective.

Direct nerve injuries may also occur from needle trauma during attempts at arterial cannulation. Many arteries are located close to nerves. For example, the median nerve is close to the brachial artery, and the axillary artery lies within the brachial plexus sheath.

7. Late vascular complications. Traumatic arterial cannulation may cause partial disruption of the wall of an artery. As a result, a pseudoaneurysm may eventually form. The wall of a pseudoaneurysm is composed of fibrous tissue that continues to expand. If the pseudoaneurysm ruptures into a vein or if a vein and artery are injured simultaneously, an arteriovenous fistula results. The treatment for these lesions is surgical repair.[50]

8. Inaccurate pressure readings. Despite the great advantages of intraarterial monitoring, it does not always yield accurate pressure values. The monitoring system may be incorrectly zeroed and calibrated, or the transducers may not be set at the appropriate level relative to the zero point. The waveform will be dampened if the catheter is kinked or partially thrombosed or if there is air in the pressure tubing. This leads to underestimation of the systolic pressure and overestimation of the diastolic pressure, but the mean blood pressure should remain the same. Conversely, the waveform will be amplified (underdamped) if the pressure tubing is too long or the natural frequency of the transducer system is too low. This leads to overestimation of the systolic pressure and underestimation of the diastolic pressure. In patients with vasoconstriction and those in hypovolemic shock and after cardiopulmonary bypass surgery, the brachial and radial artery pressures may be substantially lower than the true central aortic pressure.

Another possible cause of inaccurate measurements is unsuspected arterial stenosis proximal to the arterial cannula, which occurs with the thoracic outlet syndrome, subclavian artery stenosis, or previous cannulation of the artery proximal to the current site. In Raynaud phenomenon, pressure readings from peripheral arteries will also be unreliable.

V. CENTRAL VENOUS PRESSURE MONITORING
A. Information system

Central venous pressure (CVP) catheters are used to measure the filling pressure of the right ventricle, estimate the intravascular volume status, and assess right ventricular function. The distal end of the catheter must lie within one of the large intrathoracic veins or the right atrium. Although water manometers have been used, an electronic system is preferred because it allows the observation of the right atrial waveform, which provides additional information. In any pressure-monitoring system, it is necessary to have a reproducible landmark (such as the midaxillary line) as a zero reference. This is especially important in monitoring venous pressures because small changes in the height of the reference point produce proportionately larger errors compared with arterial pressure monitoring.

B. Techniques

1. Conventional. Percutaneous central venous cannulation may be accomplished by catheter-through-the-needle, catheter-over-the-needle, or catheter-over-a-wire (Seldinger) techniques.[51] A modification of the Seldinger technique that may be used for internal jugular vein cannulation follows.

The vein is located by using a syringe attached to a small (22- to 25-gauge) finder needle. This reduces the risk for producing a large arterial puncture if the vein is difficult to locate. When venous blood is aspirated through the finder needle, the syringe and needle are withdrawn, leaving a small trail of blood on the drape to indicate the direction of the vein. Alternatively, the needle and syringe can be fixated and used as an identifying needle. A syringe attached to an 18-gauge IV catheter-over-needle is then inserted in an identical manner. When venous return is present, the whole assembly is lowered to prevent the needle from going through the posterior wall of the central vein and is advanced an additional 1 to 2 mm until the tip of the catheter is within the lumen of the vein. The catheter is then threaded into the vein.

Once the catheter is advanced into the vein, the needle is removed and an empty syringe is attached to the cannula to withdraw a sample of blood. To confirm that an artery has not been inadvertently cannulated, comparison of the color of the blood sample to an arterial sample drawn simultaneously is recommended.[52] If the results of this technique are inconclusive or an arterial catheter is not in place, the cannula may be attached to a transducer through sterile tubing to observe the pressure waveform. Another option is to attach the cannula to sterile tubing and allow blood to flow retrograde into the tubing. The tubing is then held upright as a venous manometer, and the height of the blood column is observed. If the catheter is in a vein, the blood will stop rising at a level consistent with the CVP and will show respiratory variation. A guidewire is then passed through the 18-gauge cannula, and the cannula is exchanged over the wire for a CVP catheter. The use of more than one technique to confirm the venous location of the catheter may provide additional reassurance of correct placement before cannulation of the vein with a larger cannula.

Considerations for selecting the site of cannulation include the experience of the operator, ease of access, anatomic anomalies, and the ability of the patient to tolerate the position required for catheter insertion. A controlled comparison of various techniques for internal jugular vein cannulation found no advantage to any particular technique.[53] The Trendelenburg position is frequently complicated by hypoxemia in patients undergoing cardiac surgery who are breathing room air.[54] However, this position is not necessary when venous distention is present in the supine position, as occurs in patients with right-sided heart failure.

2. Ultrasonography. Ultrasonography has been used to define the anatomic variations of the internal jugular vein.[55] Studies have demonstrated that two-dimensional ultrasonic guidance of internal jugular vein cannulation is helpful in locating the vein, permits more rapid cannulation, and decreases the incidence of arterial puncture.[56-59] Ultrasonography provides more precise data about the structural relation between the internal jugular vein and the carotid artery (Fig. 2-3). Troianos et al[60] found that in over 54% of patients, more than 75% of the internal jugular vein overlaid the carotid artery. Patients older than 60 years of age were more likely to have this type of anatomy. Alderson et al[61] found that the carotid artery coursed behind the internal jugular vein in 10% of pediatric patients. Sulek et al[62] observed greater overlap of the internal jugular vein and the carotid artery when the head was rotated 80 degrees compared with only 0 to 40 degrees. The data obtained from 2 and 4 cm above the clavicle did not differ, and the percentage of overlap was larger on the left side of the neck than on the right. Therefore rotating the patient's head to the side contralateral to the cannulation site may distort the normal anatomy in a manner that increases the risk for inadvertent carotid artery puncture.

Ultrasonography has also been used to show that the Valsalva maneuver increases the cross-sectional area of the internal jugular vein by approximately 25%[63] and that the Trendelenburg position increases it by approximately 37% (see Fig. 2-3).[64] Ultrasonic guidance of internal jugular vein cannulation is advantageous in many circumstances, such as in patients with difficult neck anatomy (e.g., a short neck or obesity), those who have had neck surgery, and those undergoing anticoagulation therapy.

C. Sites

1. Internal jugular vein. The right internal jugular vein is preferred by many anesthesiologists for CVP monitoring. Advantages of this technique include the high success rate that results from the usually constant relation of the anatomic structures; the short, straight course to the right atrium that almost always ensures right atrial or superior vena caval localization of the catheter tip; easy access from the head of the operating room table; and fewer complications than with subclavian vein catheterization. The technique is relatively contraindicated in patients with previous neck surgery or neck tumors and is absolutely contraindicated in patients with superior vena caval obstruction. If severe carotid occlusive disease is present, caution must be used in palpating for landmarks so as not to dislodge an atheromatous plaque and cause a stroke.

2. External jugular vein. Although the external jugular vein is another means of reaching the central circulation, the success rate with this approach is lower because of the tortuous path of the vein. In addition, a valve is usually present where the external jugular vein perforates the fascia to empty into the subclavian vein. One study, however, reported a success rate of 90% when a J wire was used to slide past obstructions into the central circulation.[65] The main advantage of this technique is that there is no need to advance a needle into the deeper structures of the neck.

3. Subclavian vein. The subclavian vein is readily accessible from the supraclavicular or infraclavicular approaches and has long been used for central venous access.[66] This approach has a higher success rate than the external jugular vein approach but a lower success rate than the right internal jugular vein approach. Cannulation of the subclavian vein is associated with a higher incidence of complications than the internal jugular vein approach, especially pneumothorax.[67-69] However, this may be the cannulation site of choice when central venous access is required for head and neck surgery. It is also useful for parenteral nutrition or for prolonged CVP access because the site is easier to maintain and well tolerated by patients.

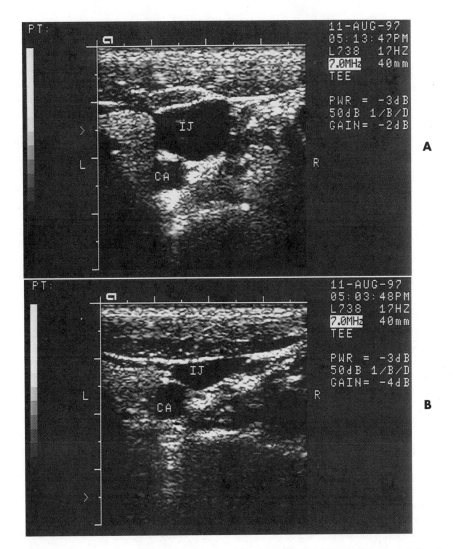

Fig. 2-3. Ultrasonographic images show the anatomic relation of the right internal jugular *(IJ)* vein and the carotid artery *(CA)*. With the Valsalva maneuver or Trendelenburg position **(A)**, the IJ vein becomes distended and circular. As gentle pressure is applied with the ultrasonographic probe **(B)**, the IJ vein is partially compressed and flattened anteriorly, whereas the CA size is unaffected. Compressibility during ultrasonic imaging is the most characteristic feature of the IJ vein.

4. Antecubital veins. The basilic and cephalic veins provide another route for central venous cannulation. The advantages of this approach are the low likelihood of complications and the ease of intraoperative access. The major disadvantage is that it is often difficult to ensure placement of the catheter in a central vein. Studies have indicated that blind advancement results in central venous cannulation in 59% to 75% of attempts.[70,71] Unsuccessful attempts result most frequently from failure to pass the catheter past the shoulder or from cannulation of the ipsilateral internal jugular vein. Turning the head to the ipsilateral side may help prevent internal jugular placement of the catheter.[72]

Artru and Colley[73] reported a high success rate (92%) for the placement of multiorificed catheters from the antecubital veins by using intravascular electrocardiography. These catheters are positioned at the junction of the superior vena cava and right atrium and are used for as-

piration of air emboli in patients undergoing neurosurgery. Because of problems inherent with intravascular electrocardiography, Mongan, Peterson, and Culling[74] devised a method for transducing the pressure waveform and identifying the point at which the catheter tip entered the right ventricle. They then calculated the distance required to withdraw three different types of air embolism–aspirating catheters to the junction of the superior vena cava and right atrium. Other investigators have used TEE to assist in the correct placement of these types of catheters.[75]

5. Femoral vein. The femoral vein is rarely cannulated in the adult patient for monitoring purposes. However, cannulation of this vein is technically simple, and the success rate is high. Cannulation should be done about 1 to 2 cm below the inguinal ligament. The vein typically lies medial to artery. Although the older literature reported a high rate of catheter sepsis and thrombophlebitis with this approach,[76,77] this may no longer be valid with disposable catheter kits and improved catheter technology.

In patients with superior vena caval obstruction, it is necessary to use the femoral vein for intravenous access and to obtain a true CVP measurement. The catheter should be long enough that the tip lies in the mediastinal portion of the inferior vena cava.

D. Contraindications

1. Absolute

a. Superior vena caval syndrome. Superior vena caval syndrome is a contraindication to the placement of a CVP catheter in the neck, subclavian area, or upper extremities. Venous pressures in the head and upper extremities are elevated by superior vena caval obstruction and do not reflect right atrial pressure. Medications administered in the obstructed venous circulation are delayed in reaching the central circulation through collateral vessels. Furthermore, rapid fluid administration into the obstructed venous circulation exacerbates the elevated venous pressures and causes more pronounced edema. Mild superior vena caval syndrome seen with ascending aortic aneurysms, however, does not seem to represent a contraindication to central venous cannulation of the upper body.

b. Infection at the site of insertion. Infection at the site of catheter insertion is an absolute contraindication to using that site to gain central venous access.

2. Relative

a. Coagulopathy. Coagulopathy predisposes to hemorrhagic complications of CVP catheter placement, such as airway obstruction from a neck hematoma, hemothorax, or hematoma collection with subsequent infection.

b. Newly inserted pacemaker wires. Newly inserted pacemaker wires may become dislodged or entangled during the insertion of CVP catheters. This could result in severe arrhythmias, especially if the patient is pacemaker dependent. In general, it is preferable to wait 4 to 6 weeks before placing a central line in a patient with newly inserted pacemaker wires.

E. Complications

The complications of central venous cannulation can be roughly divided into three categories: complications of vascular access, catheter insertion, or catheter presence (Box 2-4).

1. Arterial puncture. The reported incidence of inadvertent arterial puncture during central venous cannulation is 1.9% to 3.6%.[78-80] This occurs because all of the veins commonly used for cannulation (except the external jugular and cephalic veins) lie in close proximity to arteries and the venous anatomy varies considerably. Formation of localized hematomas is the usual consequence. The risk for this outcome may be minimized by using a small-gauge needle to locate the vein[81] or by using ultrasonographic guidance.

If the arterial puncture is large, direct pressure is not applied, or if the patient has a coagulopathy, a massive hematoma may form. In the neck, this may lead to upper airway obstruction requiring tracheal intubation. In the

arm or leg, venous obstruction may occur. If the artery is cannulated with a large-bore venous cannula, a surgical consultation may be required before its removal.[82] In some institutions, the introducer is removed by surgical cutdown, and the arterial puncture site is repaired.

Arteriovenous fistula from the carotid artery to the internal jugular vein has been reported following central venous cannulation.[83-85] Hemothorax may occur if the subclavian artery is lacerated during cannulation attempts. Symptoms of hypovolemia may predominate because of the large capacity of the pleural cavity. Hemothorax may also occur if an indwelling catheter erodes through a venous structure into the pleural cavity.

2. Pneumothorax. If the pleural cavity is entered and lung tissue is punctured during cannulation, pneumothorax may result. Tension pneumothorax may occur if air continues to accumulate owing to a ball-valve effect. Pneumothorax is most common with subclavian punctures and occurs only rarely with internal jugular vein cannulation.[86]

The treatment of pneumothorax depends on the patient's hemodynamic status. If the patient is in shock, has distended neck veins, and has a hyperresonant hemithorax, immediate therapy is indicated to relieve tension pneumothorax. A large-bore intravenous cannula may be placed through the second intercostal space, just above the superior border of the inferior rib, in the midclavicular line into the thoracic cavity. A rush of air will be detected, and the patient's clinical status will rapidly improve as the pressure within the hemithorax is relieved.

Box 2-4 Complications of central venous catheterization

Complications of vascular access
Arterial puncture
Hematoma
Arteriovenous fistula
Hemothorax
Chylothorax
Pneumothorax
Nerve injury
Brachial plexus
Stellate ganglion (Horner syndrome)
Emboli
Air
Catheter or wire shearing

Complications of catheter insertion
Cardiac perforation
Pericardial tamponade

Complications of catheter presence
Thrombosis
Thromboembolism
Infection
Sepsis
Endocarditis
Arrhythmias
Hydrothorax

Surgical consultation may then be obtained for placement of a chest (thoracostomy) tube.

3. Hydrothorax. If the catheter tip is placed extravascularly in the pleural cavity or erodes into this position, the fluid infused into the catheter will accumulate in the pleural cavity (a condition known as hydrothorax). The diagnosis is made by auscultation, percussion, and radiography of the chest. Pleurocentesis or placement of a thoracostomy tube may be necessary, and surgical consultation should be sought.

4. Chylothorax. Injury to the thoracic duct resulting in chylothorax has been reported after left internal jugular and left subclavian venous cannulation.[87] This injury generally occurs near the insertion site of the thoracic duct at the confluence of the left internal jugular and left subclavian veins (Fig. 2-4). Surgical consultation must be sought if this complication occurs. The chylous leak often persists despite conservative management (consisting of chest tube drainage and a low-fat diet). The consequences of a chronic chylothorax are nutrition depletion and possible immunosuppression. Fear of this complication is one of the major reasons for selecting right-sided internal jugular venous and subclavian venous cannulations.[88]

5. Pericardial effusion or tamponade. If the right atrium or right ventricle is perforated during central venous cannulation, pericardial effusion or tamponade may result. The likelihood of this complication is increased when inflexible guidewires; long, stiff dilators; or catheters are used. This complication has also been reported with use of an indwelling polyethylene catheter.[89] Modern flexible catheters and J-tipped guidewires have made this a rarely reported complication. Gravenstein

and Blackshear[90] evaluated the perforating aspects of central venous catheters in an in vitro model. An angle of incidence less than 40 degrees, single-orifice catheters, polyurethane catheters, silicone rubber catheters, and pigtail-tip catheters all greatly decreased the risk for perforation compared with more conventional catheters.

Oropello et al[91] claim that the dilators used in many central catheter kits may be a major cause of vessel perforation. They state that the dilator may bend the guidewire, creating its own path and causing it to perforate a vessel wall. In addition, several kits have dilators that are much longer than the catheters. In response to these problems, Oropello et al proposed an approach to maximize the safety of dilator use.

The physiology of fluid accumulation in the pericardial sac is such that sudden cardiovascular collapse occurs once a critical volume has been reached. This is explained by the compliance curve of the normal pericardium: The curve is flat until the critical volume is reached, then rises steeply with any further increase in volume.

If pericardial tamponade is imminent, immediate pericardiocentesis is indicated. A long needle attached to a syringe is directed through the skin at the junction of the xyphoid process and the sternum on the left side and is directed toward the left shoulder. The needle is advanced while suction is maintained with the syringe until free-flowing blood is obtained. An ECG electrode will show injury current (ST segment elevation) when the needle is within the pericardial sac. The withdrawal of small volumes of blood will result in marked hemodynamic improvement because of the nature of the pericardial compliance.

6. Venous air embolism. Venous air embolism is a potentially fatal complication that can occur when negative pressure in the venous system is open to the atmosphere. These conditions are met when patients are in the semi-upright or sitting position and the open end of the catheter is above the level of the right atrium or the patient generates a strong inspiratory effort. Paradoxical embolization is a risk if a patent foramen ovale or another intracardiac defect is present, such as an atrial or ventricular septal defect.

During central venous cannulation, air embolism can usually be prevented with positional maneuvers, such as the Trendelenburg position (which increases the venous pressure in the vessel). Once the central venous catheter has been placed, it is important to ensure that the catheter is firmly attached to its connecting tubing. If the subcutaneous tract has failed to close, air embolism may occur even after the catheter has been removed.[92,93]

Venous air embolism should be strongly considered when there is a sudden onset of tachycardia associated with pulmonary hypertension, systemic hypotension, and a sudden decrease in end-tidal carbon dioxide (if this measurement is available). A new murmur may be heard as a result of turbulent flow in the right ventricular outflow tract. Two-dimensional echocardiography (transesophageal or transthoracic) and precordial Doppler probe monitoring are highly sensitive methods of detecting air embolism.

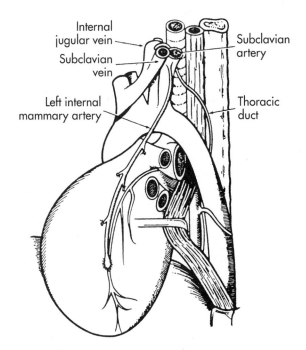

Fig. 2-4. The anatomic relation of the thoracic duct to the left internal jugular and subclavian veins is shown. (From Gratz I, Ashar M, Kidwell P, et al: *J Clin Monit* 10:185, 1994.)

Venous air embolism is most effectively treated by aspirating the air through a catheter positioned at the junction of the superior vena cava and the right atrium. An older (and probably less effective) method involves turning the patient to the left lateral decubitus position to move the embolus out of the right ventricular outflow tract.

7. Particulate embolism. Catheter or guidewire fragments may shear off and embolize to the right heart and pulmonary circulation when catheter-through-the-needle or Seldinger-type cannulation kits are used. Loss of a guidewire in the patient is also possible by not withdrawing a sufficient length of the wire to grasp it at the external end before inserting the catheter. Defective catheter manufacturing may also result in breakage and embolization. The position of the catheter fragment within the right-sided circulation will determine whether surgery or percutaneous transvenous techniques are necessary for its removal.[94,95]

The problems just discussed can almost always be avoided by using proper technique. A catheter must never be withdrawn through the inserting needle. Reinsertion of needles into standard (catheter-over-the-needle) IV cannulas is not recommended and should never be performed if the cannula is kinked or resistance is encountered. Likewise, guidewires should not be inserted through cannulas if blood return is not present or forcefully inserted if resistance is encountered. In addition, guidewires should not be withdrawn though inserting needles. During unsuccessful catheterization, the needle and catheter or needle and guidewire must be withdrawn simultaneously. The position of the catheter fragment within the circulation determines whether surgery or percutaneous techniques are best for its removal.[94]

8. Nerve injury. The brachial plexus, stellate ganglion, and phrenic nerve lie in close proximity to the internal jugular vein. These nerves may be injured during cannulation attempts. Paresthesias of the brachial plexus are not uncommon during attempts to localize the internal jugular vein. Horner syndrome has even been reported after internal jugular cannulation.[96]

Direct needle trauma is the most likely cause of paresthesias or motor deficits, and this risk is increased by the long-beveled needles used for vascular access.[97] Transient deficits may result from the deposition of local anesthetic in such locations as the brachial plexus, stellate ganglion, or cervical plexus. A large hematoma or pseudoaneurysm[98] may result in nerve injury after an inadvertent arterial puncture.

9. Arrhythmias. Transient atrial or ventricular arrhythmias commonly occur as the guidewire is passed into the right atrium or right ventricle during central venous cannulation with the Seldinger technique. This most likely results because the relatively inflexible guidewire causes extrasystoles as it contacts the endocardium. A case of ventricular fibrillation during guidewire insertion has been reported.[99] The same researchers reported a 70% reduction in the incidence of arrhythmias when guidewire insertion was limited to 22 cm.

Complete heart block has also occurred with guidewire insertion during central venous cannulation.[100] The patient was successfully managed by using a temporary transvenous pacemaker. This complication was previously reported with right heart and pulmonary artery catheterization (see following text) and most likely resulted from excessive insertion of the guidewire with impingement of the wire in the region of the right bundle branch. To avoid these complications, it is recommended that guidewire insertion be limited to the length necessary to reach the junction of the superior vena cava and right atrium. It is also imperative to monitor the patient appropriately (i.e., with ECG, pulse monitoring, or both) and to have resuscitative drugs and equipment immediately available when performing central venous catheterization.

VI. PULMONARY ARTERIAL CATHETERIZATION

A. Information system

The introduction of the flow-directed pulmonary artery catheter (PAC) has been a major advance in perioperative monitoring of patients. Since its introduction in the 1970s, the amount of information that can be obtained from critically ill patients has increased substantially.[101] Because increasing numbers of patients with multiple system organ dysfunction undergo surgical procedures, an understanding of the potential benefits and pitfalls of pulmonary artery catheterization is essential for anesthesiologists.

Tables 2-1 through 2-3 list the specific information that can be gathered with the PAC and the measurements of cardiovascular and pulmonary function that can be derived from this information. Special-purpose PACs for measurement of continuous cardiac output, continuous mixed venous oximetry, pacing, and thermodilution right ventricular ejection fraction are also available, further increasing the complexity of PAC monitoring.

Pulmonary capillary wedge pressure (PCWP) and pulmonary artery diastolic pressure are estimates of left atrial pressure, which in turn is an estimate of left ventricular end-diastolic pressure. Left ventricular end-diastolic pressure is an index of left ventricular end-diastolic volume (left ventricular preload). This curve is nonlinear and is affected by many factors, such as ventricular hypertrophy and myocardial ischemia.[102,103] Thus the PCWP and pulmonary artery diastolic pressure do

Table 2-1. Normal intracardiac pressures

Location	Mean intracardiac pressure (range) mm Hg
Right atrium	5 (1-10)
Right ventricle	25/5 (15-30)
Pulmonary artery (systolic/diastolic)	23/9 (15-30/5-15)
Mean pulmonary artery	15 (10-20)
Pulmonary capillary wedge	10 (5-15)
Left atrium	8 (4-12)
Left ventricular end-diastolic	8 (4-12)
Left ventricular systolic	130 (90-140)

not directly measure left ventricular preload and can be influenced by several factors (Fig. 2-5).

The patency of vascular channels between the distal port of the PAC and the left atrium is necessary to ensure a close relation between the PCWP and left atrial pressure. This condition is only met in the dependent portions of the lung (West zone III), where the pulmonary venous pressure exceeds the alveolar pressure.[104] Otherwise, the PCWP will reflect the alveolar pressure, not the left atrial pressure. Because positive end-expiratory pressure decreases the size of West zone III, it adversely affects the correlation between PCWP and left atrial pressures.[105] Of note, the adult respiratory distress syndrome seems to prevent the transmission of increased alveolar pressure to the pulmonary interstitium. This preserves the relation between PCWP and left ventricular end-diastolic pressure during the application of positive end-expiratory pressure.[106] Controversy remains over whether it is necessary or prudent to temporarily discontinue positive end-expiratory pressure to measure preload more accurately.[69,107]

B. Sites

The considerations for avoiding complications during the insertion of PACs are the same as those for CVP catheters (see Box 2-4). The right internal jugular approach remains the easiest because of the direct path between this vessel and the right atrium. The left subclavian approach is also good because the path to the right atrium and the pulmonary artery eventually follows the curvature of the PAC.

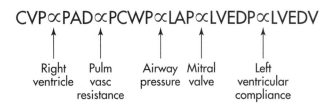

Fig. 2-5. The left ventricular end-diastolic volume *(LVEDV)* is related to left ventricular end-diastolic pressure *(LVEDP)* by left ventricular compliance. The LVEDP is related to the left atrial pressure *(LAP)* by the diastolic pressure gradient across the mitral valve. The pulmonary capillary wedge pressure *(PCWP)* is related to the LAP by pulmonary capillary resistance. The pulmonary artery diastolic pressure *(PAD)* is an estimation of the PCWP. The central venous pressure *(CVP)* will reflect the PAD if right ventricular function is normal.

Table 2-2. Derived hemodynamic values

Hemodynamic variable	Formula	Normal values
Cardiac index	CO/BSA	$2.8\text{-}4.2 \, 1 \cdot min^{-1} \cdot m^{-2}$
Stroke volume	$CO \cdot 1000/HR$	50-110 ml per heartbeat
Stroke index	SV/BSA	$30\text{-}65 \, ml \cdot m^{-2}$
Left ventricular stroke work index	$1.36 \cdot (MAP - PCWP) \cdot SI/100$	$45\text{-}60 \, gram\text{-}meters \cdot m^{-2}$
Right ventricular stroke work index	$1.36 \cdot (MPAP - CVP) \cdot SI/100$	$5\text{-}10 \, gram \, meters \cdot m^{-2}$
Systemic vascular resistance	$(MAP - CVP) \cdot 80/CO$	$900\text{-}1400 \, dynes/see \cdot cm^{-5}$
Systemic vascular resistance index	$(MAP - CVP) \cdot 80/CI$	$1500\text{-}2400 \, dynes/see \cdot m^2 \cdot cm^{-5}$
Pulmonary vascular resistance	$(MPAP - PCWP) \cdot 80/CO$	$150\text{-}250 \, dynes/see \cdot cm^{-5}$
Pulmonary vascular resistance index	$(MPAP - PCWP) \cdot 80/CI$	$250\text{-}400 \, dynes/sec \cdot m^2 \cdot cm^{-5}$

BSA, Body surface area; *CI,* cardiac index; *CO,* cardiac output; *CVP,* central venous pressure; *HR,* heart rate; *MAP,* mean arterial pressure; *MPAP,* mean pulmonary arterial pressure; *PCWP,* pulmonary capillary wedge pressure; *SI,* stroke index; *SV,* stroke volume.

Table 2-3. Oxygen delivery variables

Variables	Formula	Normal values
Arterial oxygen concentration	$(1.39 \cdot Hb = SaO_2) + (0.0031 \cdot PaO_2)$	18-20 ml/dl
Mixed venous oxygen concentration	$(1.39 \cdot Hb \cdot SvO_2) + (0.0031 \cdot PvO_2)$	13-16 ml/dl
Arteriovenous oxygen concentration difference	$CaO_2 - CvO_2$	4-5.5 ml/dl
Pulmonary capillary oxygen concentration	$(1.39 \cdot Hb \cdot ScO_2) + (0.0031 \cdot PcO_2)$	19-21 ml/dl
Pulmonary shunt fraction	$100 \cdot (CcO_2 - CaO_2)/(CcO_2 - CvO_2)$	2%-8%
Oxygen delivery	$10 \cdot CO \cdot CaO_2$	800-1100 ml/min
Oxygen consumption	$10 \cdot CO \cdot (CaO_2 - CvO_2)$	150-300 ml/min

From McGrath R: *Prog Cardiovasc Dis* 29:129, 1986.
CaO$_2$, Arterial oxygen concentration; *CcO$_2$,* pulmonary capillary oxygen concentration; *CO,* carbon monoxide; *CvO$_2$,* mixed venous oxygen concentration; *Hb,* hemoglobin; *PaO$_2$,* arterial partial pressure of oxygen; *PcO$_2$,* partial pressure of carbon dioxide; *PvO$_2$,* venous partial pressure of oxygen; *SaO$_2$,* arterial oxygen saturation; *ScO$_2$,* pulmonary capillary oxygen saturation; *SvO$_2$,* venous oxygen saturation.

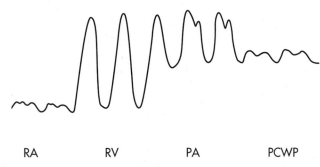

RA   RV   PA   PCWP

Fig. 2-6. The waveforms encountered during flotation of a pulmonary artery catheter from the venous circulation to the pulmonary capillary wedge pressure *(PCWP)* position are illustrated. Note the sudden increase in systolic pressure as the catheter enters the right ventricle *(RV)*, the sudden increase in diastolic pressure as the catheter enters the pulmonary artery *(PA)*, and the decrease in mean pressure as the catheter reaches the PCWP position. *RA,* Right atrium.

C. Flotation of the catheter

Passage of the PAC from the vessel introducer to the pulmonary artery can be accomplished by monitoring the pressure waveform from the distal port of the catheter or by using fluoroscopic guidance. Waveform monitoring is the more common technique for perioperative right-sided heart catheterization. First, the catheter tip must be advanced through the vessel introducer (which is about 15 cm in length) before inflating the balloon. The inflation of the balloon facilitates further advancement of the catheter through the right atrium and right ventricle into the pulmonary artery. The waveforms encountered are shown in Fig. 2-6.

The right atrial waveform is seen until the catheter tip crosses the tricuspid valve and enters the right ventricle. In the right ventricle, the systolic pressure increases suddenly, but the diastolic pressure changes little compared with the right atrial tracing. Arrhythmias, particularly premature ventricle complexes, usually occur at this point but almost always resolve without treatment once the catheter tip has crossed the pulmonic valve. The catheter is advanced rapidly through the right ventricle toward the pulmonary artery. A slight reverse Trendelenburg position and right lateral tilt facilitate passage of the catheter through the right ventricular cavity.[108]

As the catheter crosses the pulmonic valve, a dicrotic notch appears in the pressure waveform and the diastolic pressure increases suddenly. The pulmonary capillary wedge tracing is obtained by passing the catheter approximately 3 to 5 cm farther until the waveform changes in association with a decrease in the measured mean pressure. Deflation of the balloon results in reappearance of the pulmonary arterial waveform and an increase in the mean pressure.

The pulmonary arterial waveform should be continually monitored to be certain that the catheter does not float out into a constant wedge position. This may lead to pulmonary arterial rupture or pulmonary infarction. The PAC is covered with a sterile sheath that must be secured at both ends to prevent contamination of the ex-

---

> **Box 2-5** Indications for pulmonary artery catheter monitoring in patients undergoing anesthesia
>
> Major procedures involving large fluid shifts or blood loss in patients with coronary artery disease or decreased left ventricular function
> Procedures requiring cardiopulmonary bypass
> Patients undergoing surgery of the aorta requiring cross-clamping
> Patients with recent myocardial infarctions or unstable angina
> Patients with poor left-sided ventricular function (congestive heart failure) undergoing major surgery
> Patients in hypovolemic, cardiogenic, or septic shock or those with multiple organ failure
> Patients with massive trauma
> Patients with right-sided heart failure, chronic obstructive pulmonary disease, pulmonary hypertension, or pulmonary embolism
> Patients requiring high levels of positive end-expiratory pressure
> Hemodynamically unstable patients requiring inotropes or intraaortic balloon counterpulsation
> Patients undergoing hepatic transplantation
> Patients with massive ascites requiring major surgery

ternal portion of the catheter. Not infrequently, the PAC must be withdrawn a short distance because extra catheter in the right ventricle floats out more peripherally into the pulmonary artery over time as the catheter softens.

D. Indications

The operative procedures and medical conditions cited as indications for pulmonary arterial catheterization in the perioperative period remain controversial and vary by institution.[109,110] In a global sense, pulmonary arterial catheterization is indicated to assess volume status, measure cardiac output, measure mixed venous oxygen, and derive hemodynamic variables.[111] The American Society of Anesthesiologists Task Force on Pulmonary Artery Catheterization recently published practice guidelines that should be closely followed. In addition, we composed a list of relatively aggressive procedural indications (Box 2-5).

The ability of PACs to positively influence patient outcome has never been conclusively proven in large-scale prospective studies. Thus considerable controversy remains about the risk-to-benefit ratio of these catheters.[112,113] Many studies have reported no change or worsened outcome in patients who were monitored with PACs.[114-117] Major problems with studies of this type include design flaws and insufficient statistical power. The most common design flaw is a lack of therapeutic protocols, which introduces observer bias. Physician knowledge is another confounding variable, as was demonstrated in a multicenter study that indicated that competency in interpreting PAC-derived data was lacking in many patients and depended on diverse factors, including the level of training of the interpreter and the frequency of use.[118] In that study, as many as 47% of physicians could not correctly determine the PCWP to within 5 mm Hg.

Yet another problem with these studies is the clinical setting: operating room versus intensive care unit. Haupt et al[119] proposed that patients in the intensive care unit may have disease that is too far advanced to make invasive hemodynamic monitoring useful. Studies that have reported improved outcome used invasive hemodynamic monitoring to optimize perioperative oxygen delivery.[120-123] In a meta-analysis, Heyland et al[124] argue similarly that maximizing oxygen delivery is more effective in the perioperative setting (i.e., before the onset of irreversible organ damage) than in the long-term intensive care setting. In the subset of patients who had "intention to treat" before surgery, survival was improved.

Use of the PAC has contributed greatly to the understanding and care of patients with cardiac disease. It is impressive to observe large changes in the pulmonary arterial pressure and PCWP with almost no change in the CVP in some patients. In a prospective analysis of 62 consecutive pulmonary arterial catheterizations, Connors, McCaffree, and Gray[125] found that less than half of a group of clinicians correctly predicted the PCWP or cardiac output and more than 50% made at least one change to therapy on the basis of data from the PAC. Waller, Johnson, and Kaplan[126] showed that a group of experienced cardiac anesthesiologists and surgeons who were blinded to the information from the PAC during coronary artery bypass grafting were not aware of a problem during 65% of severe hemodynamic abnormalities. Likewise, Iberti and Fisher[127] showed that a group of physicians was unable to accurately predict hemodynamic data on clinical grounds and that 60% made at least one change in therapy and 33% changed their diagnosis on the basis of PAC data.

E. Contraindications

1. Absolute

a. Tricuspid or pulmonic valvular stenosis. It is unlikely that a PAC would be able to cross a stenotic valve, and if it did, it would worsen the obstruction to flow.

b. Right atrial or right ventricular masses (tumor or thrombus). The PAC may dislodge a portion of the mass, causing pulmonary or paradoxical embolization.

c. Tetralogy of Fallot. The right ventricular outflow tract is hypersensitive, and a PAC may induce a hypercyanotic episode ("tet spell") by eliciting spasm of the right ventricular infundibulum.

2. Relative

a. Severe arrhythmias. Transient atrial and ventricular arrhythmias are common during PAC placement in normal patients. The risk for inducing an arrhythmia in a patient who is prone to malignant arrhythmias must be weighed against the potential benefits of the information gained from PAC monitoring. The arrhythmias resolve without treatment once the catheter tip has passed through the right ventricle and crossed the pulmonary valve (see later discussion). Appropriate preparations must be undertaken to administer antiarrhythmic drugs; cardiopulmonary resuscitation; and electrical cardioversion or defibrillation, if required.

b. Coagulopathy. Obtaining central venous access in a patient with a coagulopathy has potential complications (as noted previously). In addition, the risk for endobronchial hemorrhage with inadvertent migration of the catheter or prolonged balloon inflation may be increased.

c. Newly inserted pacemaker wires. The catheter may displace newly inserted pacemaker wires during insertion or withdrawal. In approximately 4 to 6 weeks, the pacemaker wires become firmly embedded in the endocardium, and wire displacement becomes less likely.

F. Complications

Complications associated with PAC placement include almost all of those found in the section on CVP catheter placement (see Box 2-4). The only exceptions are atrial or ventricular perforation, which have never been reported with balloon-tipped catheters. Additional complications unique to the PAC are detailed here.

1. Arrhythmias. The most common complications associated with PAC insertion are transient arrhythmias, especially premature ventricular contractions.[78] Fatal arrhythmias have also been reported in rare instances.[128] Intravenous lidocaine has been used in attempts to suppress these arrhythmias, with mixed results.[129,130] However, a positional maneuver entailing a 5-degree head-up-and-right-lateral tilt was associated with a statistically significant decrease in malignant arrhythmias (compared with the Trendelenburg position) during PAC insertion.[108]

2. Complete heart block. Complete heart block may develop during pulmonary artery catheterization in patients with preexisting left bundle-branch block.[131,132] This potentially fatal complication most likely occurs because electrical irritability from the catheter tip causes transient right bundle-branch block as it passes through the right ventricular outflow tract. The incidence of right bundle-branch block was 3% in a prospective series of patients undergoing pulmonary artery catheterization.[133] However, in that series, none of the patients with preexisting left bundle-branch block developed complete heart block. In another study of 47 patients with left bundle-branch block, two developed complete heart block, but these patients had left bundle-branch block of recent onset.[134] It is imperative to have an external pacemaker immediately available or to use a pacing catheter when placing a PAC in patients with left bundle-branch block.

3. Endobronchial hemorrhage. Iatrogenic rupture of the pulmonary artery with endobronchial hemorrhage has become more common since the advent of PAC monitoring in the intensive care unit and the operating room. More than 30 cases have been recorded in the medical literature.[135] The incidence of pulmonary artery–induced endobronchial hemorrhage is 0.064% to 0.20%.[78,136] Hannan, Brown, and Bigman[137] reported a mortality rate of 46% in 28 patients with pulmonary artery–induced endobronchial hemorrhage and 75% in

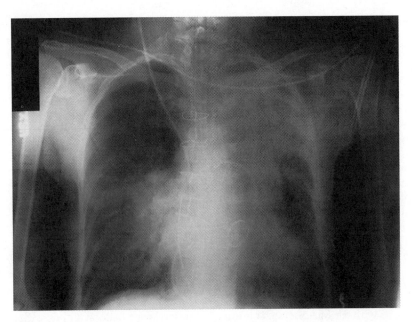

Fig. 2-7. A case of endobronchial hemorrhage caused by catheter-induced pulmonary artery rupture. A left-sided double-lumen endotracheal tube has been placed to protect the uninvolved lung.

anticoagulated patients. Out of these reports, several risk factors have emerged: advanced age, female sex, pulmonary hypertension, mitral stenosis, coagulopathy, distal placement of the catheter, and balloon hyperinflation.

It is important to consider the cause of the hemorrhage when forming a therapeutic plan. If the hemorrhage is minimal and a coagulopathy coexists, correction of the coagulopathy may be the only necessary therapy. Protection of the uninvolved lung is of prime importance. Tilting the patient toward the affected side or placement of a double-lumen endotracheal tube should protect the contralateral lung.[138] Strategies proposed to stop the hemorrhage include the application of positive end-expiratory pressure, placement of bronchial blockers,[139] use of rigid or flexible bronchoscopy, injection of clotted blood through the PAC, hyperinflation of the PAC balloon, and pulmonary resection.[140] If bleeding recurs, therapeutic embolization of the involved pulmonary artery may be useful.[141]

The clinician is clearly at a disadvantage unless the site of hemorrhage is known. Chest radiography will usually indicate the general location of the lesion (Fig. 2-7). A small amount of radiographic contrast dye may help to pinpoint the lesion if active hemorrhage is present. Even if the cause of endobronchial hemorrhage is unclear, the bleeding site must be unequivocally located before surgical treatment is attempted.

4. Pulmonary infarction. Pulmonary infarction is a rare complication of PAC monitoring. An early report suggested that the incidence of pulmonary infarction with PAC use was 7.2%.[142] However, continuously monitoring the pulmonary arterial waveform and keeping the balloon deflated when not determining the PCWP (to prevent inadvertent wedging of the catheter) were not standard practice at that time. Distal migration of PACs

may also occur during surgery because of the action of the right ventricle, uncoiling of the catheter, or softening of the catheter over time. Inadvertent catheter wedging occurs during cardiopulmonary bypass surgery because the size of the right ventricular chamber is diminished and the heart is retracted to perform bypass grafting. In addition, embolization of a thrombus formed on a PAC may result in pulmonary infarction.

5. Catheter knotting and entrapment. Knotting usually occurs as a result of coiling of the PAC within the right ventricle. Insertion of an appropriately sized guidewire under fluoroscopic guidance may aid in unknotting the catheter.[143] Alternatively, if no intracardiac structures are entangled, the knot may be tightened and withdrawn percutaneously along with the introducer.[144] If cardiac structures, such as the papillary muscles, are entangled in the knotted catheter, surgical intervention may be required. Placement of the catheter with the balloon deflated may increase the risk for passing the catheter between the chordae tendineae.[145] Sutures placed in the heart may inadvertently entrap the catheter. Such a case and the details of the percutaneous removal of the catheter have been described.[146]

6. Valvular damage. Withdrawal of the catheter with the balloon inflated may result in injury to the tricuspid[147] or pulmonic valves.[148] Septic endocarditis has also resulted from an indwelling PAC.[149]

7. Thrombocytopenia. Mild thrombocytopenia has been reported in dogs and humans with indwelling PACs.[150] This probably results from increased platelet consumption. Heparin-coated catheters may trigger heparin-induced thrombocytopenia, a rare disease that has been reported in one patient undergoing cardiac surgery.[151] This disease has high morbidity and mortality rates and is probably caused by an autoimmune response to heparin that results in thrombotic events and thrombocytopenia (induced by increased platelet consumption).[152]

8. Thrombus formation. The PAC is a foreign body that may serve as a nidus for thrombus formation. The thrombogenicity of these catheters seems to have been reduced by the introduction of heparin-bonded PACs.[153] However, introduction of high-dose aprotinin therapy may induce a hypercoagulable state that predisposes to thrombus formation on the catheter despite heparin bonding.[154] This phenomenon has also been reported with ε-aminocaproic acid therapy.[155] TEE can be a valuable tool for detecting and monitoring this complication.[156]

9. Incorrect placement. The catheter may pass through an interatrial or interventricular communication into the left side of the heart. It is then possible for it to enter the aorta through the left ventricular outflow tract. A similar complication has been reported in which the catheter crossed a surgically repaired tear in the superior vena cava into the left side of the heart.[157] This complication should be recognized by the similarity between the pulmonary arterial and systemic arterial waveforms. In a patient with an ascending aortic aneurysm, compression of the superior vena cava by the aneurysm may have led to traumatic placement of the PAC directly into the pulmonary vein.[158]

Venous cannula obstruction has occurred in a patient at the initiation of cardiopulmonary bypass when the PAC was repositioned at the start of surgery.[159,160] The temporal association with the abrupt loss of venous return and the negative pressure recorded on the distal lumen tracing indicated the cause of this complication. This stresses the importance of monitoring the pressure waveforms, even during cardiopulmonary bypass. Coronary sinus obstruction by a PAC has been reported.[161] Placement of the catheter in the liver has also been described. This was unrecognized because the wedged hepatic venous pressures sometimes mimic the pulmonary arterial pressure waveform.[162]

TEE has proven invaluable for confirming the proper placement of PACs. In many cases, TEE detected incorrect catheter placement and resulting complications.[156,158]

10. Catheter electrode detachment of pacing catheters. One type of multipurpose PAC contains five electrodes for bipolar atrial, ventricular, or atrioventricular sequential pacing. With appropriate filtering, the catheter may also be used for intracardiac electrocardiography. Intraoperative success rates of 80%, 93%, and 73% have been reported for atrial, ventricular, and atrioventricular sequential capture, respectively.[163] Electrode detachment has been reported twice with the multipurpose catheter: once with prolonged placement (60 hours)[164] and once during catheter withdrawal.[165]

11. Risk for perforation with pacing wires. The Paceport and A-V Paceport catheters (Baxter Edwards, Irvine, California) have lumina for the introduction of a ventricular wire (Paceport) or both atrial and ventricular wires (A-V Paceport) for temporary transvenous pacing. The success rate for ventricular pacing capture was 96% with the Paceport catheter.[166] The success rates for atrial

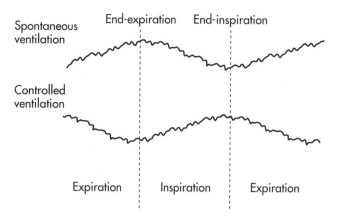

Fig. 2-8. Respiratory variation of the PCWP waveform during spontaneous and mechanical ventilation is shown. Inspiration is marked by negative mediastinal pressure in the spontaneously breathing patient and positive mediastinal pressure in the mechanically ventilated patient.

and ventricular pacing capture before cardiopulmonary bypass were 98% and 100%, respectively, in a study of the A-V Paceport catheter.[167] If the catheter were to move distally, as occurs during balloon inflation, the wire may perforate the right atrium or ventricle. Although this event has not yet been reported, it is recommended that the catheter not be inserted further and the balloon not be inflated once the pacing wires have been passed into the atrium or ventricle.

12. Erroneous interpretation of data. Malfunctions of the catheter and balloon can lead to spurious values for the PCWP and incorrect treatment of the patient. Shin, McAslan, and Ayella[168] reported eccentric inflation of the balloon with the catheter tip impinging on the pulmonary arterial wall. Five reviews[69,102,103,169,170] have pointed out many problems with clinical use of the PAC, including errors caused by human interpretation, ventilation modes (Fig. 2-8), compliance changes, ventricular interdependence, and technical problems.

"Catheter whip" is an artifact associated with long catheters, such as PACs. Because the tip of the catheter moves within the bloodstream of the cardiac chambers and great vessels, the motion of the fluid contained within the catheter is accelerated, causing artifactual pressure waves. These superimposed pressure waves may exceed 10 mm Hg in positive or negative deflections.

VII. MIXED VENOUS OXYGEN SATURATION

Monitoring the mixed venous oxygen saturation (SvO_2) is a means of providing a global estimate of the adequacy of oxygen delivery relative to the needs of the various tissues. The addition of fiberoptic bundles to PACs has enabled the continuous monitoring of SvO_2 by using reflectance spectrophotometry. The catheter is connected to a device that includes a light-emitting diode and a sensor to detect the light returning from the pulmonary artery. The SvO_2 is calculated from the differential absorption of various wavelengths of light by the saturated and desaturated hemoglobin.[171]

Continuous monitoring of SvO_2 has been complicated by artifacts caused by the vessel wall and clot formation on the catheter with loss of light intensity. A varying hematocrit may also introduce error, but not with all systems.[172] A study by Gettinger, DeTraglia, and Glass[173] demonstrated that a three-wavelength system (Opticath, Oximetrix, Inc., Mountain View, California) is more accurate than a two-wavelength system (Swan-Ganz, American Edwards Laboratories, Santa Ana, California). Data from a study by Bongard et al,[174] however, suggest that both systems function with acceptable accuracy and precision over wide ranges of SvO_2. Other investigators have also noted that values obtained with various fiberoptic catheter systems showed good agreement with in vitro (cooximetry) SvO_2 measurements.[175-178]

VIII. DETERMINATION OF CARDIAC OUTPUT

The cardiac output is the amount of blood pumped to the peripheral circulation by the heart each minute. This measurement reflects the status of the entire circulatory system because it is autoregulated by the tissues. The cardiac output is equal to the product of the stroke volume and the heart rate. Preload, afterload, heart rate, and contractility are the major determinants of the cardiac output. The measurement of cardiac output is of particular interest in patients with cardiac disease. This section briefly describes older methods, then focuses on current practices of cardiac output measurement.

A. Fick method

The Fick equation is derived from the concept that the amount of oxygen consumed by the tissues per unit of time is equal to the amount of oxygen extracted per unit of time from the circulation. Measurements must be taken at steady state because the Fick principle is only valid when oxygen uptake by the tissues equals that of the lungs.[179] The accuracy and reproducibility of the direct Fick cardiac output technique have been determined in various animal and human experiments and have usually been found to be high.

The major limitations of the direct Fick technique are related to errors in sampling and analysis, difficulty in obtaining oxygen uptake continuously in the operating room, the presence of bulky equipment surrounding the endotracheal tube, or the inability to maintain steady state hemodynamic and respiratory conditions.[180] To minimize sampling errors, one must ascertain that the venous blood is truly mixed venous blood and that the samples represent average rather than instantaneous samples.

The most serious errors in the measurement of cardiac output by the direct Fick technique result from changes in pulmonary volumes. Methods of determining oxygen consumption measure the uptake of oxygen by the lungs rather than by the blood. Because lung volumes can change, the oxygen consumption of the tissues is not necessarily measured. The use of calculated values for oxygen consumption is also fraught with errors, as Kendrick et al[181] demonstrated. They noted that differences between measured and assumed oxygen concentrations were often greater than 25% in either direction.

With the widespread availability of mass spectrometry, several investigators have attempted to continuously measure cardiac output by using the Fick principle.[182-187] Good correlations have usually been obtained in comparisons with thermodilution. In some studies, the reproducibility of the measurements was found to be better for the Fick method than for thermodilution. Some of the major obstacles encountered when using the Fick method were overcome in a study by Doi, Morita, and Ikeda,[188] who were able to measure cardiac output every 30 seconds and obtained good correlations compared with thermodilution (r = 0.961).

B. Thermodilution

The thermodilution method, done by using the PAC, is the current method of choice for measuring cardiac output in the clinical setting. With this technique, multiple cardiac outputs can be obtained at frequent intervals without blood withdrawal by using an inert indicator. A bolus of cold fluid is injected into the right atrium, and the resulting temperature change is detected by the thermistor in the pulmonary artery.[101,189] When thermal indicator is used, the modified Stewart-Hamilton equation is used to calculate cardiac output. Solution of this complex mathematical equation is performed by an analog computer, which integrates the area under the temperature-time curve. Cardiac output is inversely proportional to the area under the curve.

Since its introduction, thermal indicator has eliminated some but not all of the limitations associated with dye cardiac output techniques. Handling of the indicator is undoubtedly easier with thermal indicator than with dye indicator. The computer calibration procedures are greatly simplified, and blood withdrawal is not necessary. However, some common problems remain. Extrapolation of the tail end of the time-concentration curve remains essential. Various manufacturers have handled this problem differently, and inconsistencies can sometimes be observed when substituting one cardiac output computer for another.[190]

Erroneous cardiac output measurements still remain a major problem. The temperature-time curve is the crux of thermodilution, and any circumstances that affect this curve have consequences for the accuracy of the cardiac output measurement. Specifically, anything that results in less "cold" reaching the thermistor, more "cold" reaching the thermistor, or an unstable temperature baseline will adversely affect the accuracy of thermodilution.

Less "cold" reaching the thermistor results in overestimation of the cardiac output. This could be caused by injecting a smaller amount of indicator, indicator that is too warm, a thrombus on the thermistor, or partial wedging of the catheter. Conversely, underestimation of the cardiac output will occur if an excessive volume of injectate or injectate that is too cold is used to perform the measurement. Intracardiac shunts have unpredictable effects that depend on the anatomy and physiology of the individual patient. Surprisingly, in one report, large left-to-right shunts were found not to adversely affect the measurement of systemic cardiac output.[191]

Wetzel and Latson[192] observed variations of up to 80% in measured cardiac output when the rate of administration of intravenous crystalloid infusions caused fluctuations in baseline blood temperature. The rapid temperature decrease seen after hypothermic cardiopulmonary bypass surgery has been shown to result in underestimation of cardiac output by 0.6 to 2 L/min. In another study, the temperature decrease after cardiopulmonary bypass surgery was 0.14° C per minute.[193] Latson et al[194] also noted that the normal changes in the pulmonary artery that occur with each respiratory cycle seem to be exaggerated in the early phase after hypothermic cardiopulmonary bypass surgery. This may cause peak-to-peak errors of up to 50% in estimation of intermittent cardiac outputs if this procedure is initiated at different times during the ventilatory cycle. This effect was greatly decreased with thermal equilibration approximately 30 minutes after cardiopulmonary bypass.

Tricuspid regurgitation has generally been considered a source of error in cardiac output measurement by thermodilution. The scientific data, however, are contradictory. Some experimental reports indicate that tricuspid regurgitation does not impair the accuracy of thermodilution cardiac output compared with the Fick method[195] and electromagnetic flow probes.[196] However, Heerdt et al[197] reported that thermodilution cardiac output varied widely in both the direction and magnitude of error in comparison with Doppler and electromagnetic cardiac output in a single patient with acute tricuspid regurgitation.

Pulmonary arterial catheterization itself is not without problems, and as mentioned previously, the list of reported complications is long. In addition, measurement of cardiac output remains intermittent, and frequent measurements could lead to fluid overload. Furthermore, the need for repeated injections leads to the possibility of introducing air into the patient, with its attendant effects. Echocardiography and precordial Doppler imaging usually reveal a shower of air emboli during injections, but the risk for air embolism seems to be small. Approximately 30% of adults have a probe patent foramen ovale.[198] Thus paradoxical air embolism with systemic infarction can occur in these patients, and caution is recommended for all patients when measuring cardiac output with thermodilution.

Complications have also been attributed to the rapid injection of cold indicator into the right atrium. Nishikawa and Dohi[199] described slowing of the heart rate. In a prospective study, Harris et al[200] observed that with the use of iced injectate, patient heart rate decreased more than 10% in 22% of the measurements. In another study, Nishikawa and Dohi[201] found that slowing of the heart rate was more likely in patients with low cardiac index, low mean pulmonary arterial pressure, and high systemic vascular resistance.

Various attempts have been made to determine cardiac output continuously by using a thermal signal. Initial experiments focused on the use of intravascular heating devices.[202,203] Heating blood is inherently more risky than cooling it. However, the safety of the filamented PAC has been demonstrated when the level of heat is applied in a pulsatile manner in 15-second cycles.[204]

In vitro and in vivo studies have shown that continuous thermodilution cardiac outputs are reasonably accurate and precise.[205-207] However, Bottiger et al[208] found a poor correlation between intermittent and continuous thermodilution cardiac outputs (r = 0.273) in the first 45 minutes after cardiopulmonary bypass compared with cardiac output measurements obtained in more physiologically stable periods. Perhaps this observation is caused by the unstable thermal baseline after hypothermic cardiopulmonary bypass surgery (described in the previous section).

C. Transesophageal echocardiography

Echocardiography may be used to determine cardiac output by measuring flow through the heart valves. When TEE is used, the velocity-time integral of flow through the mitral valve is multiplied by the calculated valve area and a constant. This value is then multiplied by the heart rate to determine the cardiac output. Although the calculations are currently time consuming, the degree of accuracy has been promising.[209-211]

D. Thoracic bioimpedance

The first attempts at measuring cardiac output by thoracic electrical impedance date back to 1966, when Kubicek et al[212] presented an empiric equation for the calculation of left ventricular stroke volume. To measure thoracic electrical impedance, an alternating current of low amplitude and high frequency is introduced and simultaneously sensed by two sets of electrodes placed around the neck and xyphoid process. Ventilation and pulsatile blood flow induce changes in thoracic impedance. For the measurement of stroke volume, only the cardiac-induced pulsatile component of the total change in electrical impedance is analyzed because the respiratory component is filtered out.

It is questionable whether the accuracy of thoracic bioimpedance is adequate to justify its use as a clinical monitor of cardiac output. The potential problems with this monitoring system are similar to those encountered with ECG monitoring. A risk for macroshock is created by the multiple electrical connections needed to perform thoracic bioimpedance. These connections may also result in a burn if the return pad malfunctions during unipolar electrocautery.

IX. LEFT ATRIAL PRESSURE MONITORING

In left atrial pressure monitoring a catheter is placed in the right superior pulmonary vein (usually) and advanced into the left atrium. A Teflon-pledgetted purse-string stitch is made around the catheter to provide a surface for clotting on removal of the catheter. The catheter is brought out through the skin in the subxyphoid region and is sutured in place. It is important to maintain positive airway pressure or distend the left atrium by some method during insertion of the catheter to prevent entry of air into the pulmonary vein and the left side of the heart. A problem during insertion of the catheter in neonates is puncture of the right mainstem bronchus through the right superior pulmonary vein, with formation of a bronchopulmonary venous fistula.[213]

Left atrial pressure monitoring is highly informative but requires great caution. The possibility of air embolism to the coronary or cerebral circulations is always present, both on insertion and during continued use postoperatively in the intensive care unit. There is also the risk for clot formation on the catheter and subsequent embolization when the catheter is flushed or removed; therefore a continuous heparinized flushing system is necessary to avoid thrombus formation on the catheter tip after surgery. There is also a risk for bleeding after surgery when the left atrial pressure catheter is removed. It should therefore be removed while the chest tubes are still in place to diagnose and treat this problem. Other reported complications include catheter retention and prosthetic valve entrapment.[214]

With the wider application of PAC monitoring, left atrial pressure monitoring should probably be restricted to use in patients in whom PCWP measurements have been unsuccessful, are impractical, or are known to be inaccurate (e.g., in patients with pulmonary vascular disease or in small children). Continuous left atrial pressure monitoring is also useful in discontinuing cardiopulmonary bypass in high-risk patients. The catheter may also be used to infuse inotropic agents selectively into the systemic circulation to minimize the effects on the pulmonary circulation. The efficacy of this therapeutic maneuver has not been proven.

X. TRANSESOPHAGEAL ECHOCARDIOGRAPHY

Because of recent advances in ultrasound technology, anesthesiologists have been able to incorporate TEE into perioperative management. Echocardiography produces images of the heart and great vessels from which a wealth of information can be derived, such as detection of regional wall-motion abnormalities, indirect measurement of stroke volume, measurement of ejection fraction, and presence and degree of valvular disease or aortic disease. The clinical uses for TEE are expanding to areas outside of the cardiac operating room. Patients with substantial cardiovascular disease undergoing high-risk surgical procedures may benefit from TEE, which has improved management of myocardial ischemia and ventricular dysfunction.

A. Complications

Although TEE has been performed in thousands of patients, remarkably few reports of complications have been reported. The safety of intraoperative TEE has been proven by the extremely low incidence of major complications associated with its use and the transient nature of complications that do occur.[215] Absolute and relative contraindications to placement of the TEE probe are listed in Box 2-6. Complications of TEE may be grouped into three categories (Box 2-7): trauma to the airway and esophagus caused by probe contact with these structures, hemodynamic derangement caused by probe insertion and manipulation, and airway compromise.

Potential complications include damage to pharyngeal, laryngeal, esophageal, and gastric structures, resulting in perforation, laceration, abrasion, or hemorrhage. Additional risks include internal burns and microshock from the probe itself. O'Shea et al[216] evaluated the effects of TEE in animals by excising the entire esophagus after variable durations of continuous TEE use. They observed no significant mucosal or thermal injuries. In a human study, five of six patients had low contact pressure between the

---

Box 2-6 Contraindications to placement of the transesophageal echocardiography probe

Absolute

Esophageal
  Stricture
  Fistula
  Laceration
  Diverticulae
  Tumor
  Vascular ring (double aortic arch)
  Interruption
Recent suture lines

Relative

Symptomatic hiatal hernia
Esophagitis
Coagulopathy
Esophageal varices
Unexplained upper gastrointestinal bleeding
Cervical spine disease

Box 2-7 Complications of intraoperative transesophageal echocardiography

Direct trauma to the airway and esophagus

Esophageal bleeding
Dysphagia
Mallory-Weiss tear
Laryngeal discomfort
Vocal cord paralysis (usually transient)

Hemodynamic derangement caused by probe insertion and manipulation

Hypertension
Hypotension
Tachyarrhythmias
Bradyarrhythmias

Airway compromise

Endotracheal tube dislodgment
Tracheal compression (especially with double aortic arch or vascular ring anomalies)

---

transducer and the esophagus, but one patient had a significantly elevated (>60 mm Hg) contact pressure.[217]

Vocal cord paresis was attributed to intraoperative TEE in two patients who were undergoing craniotomies in the sitting position with marked cervical flexion.[218] One case report described a Mallory-Weiss tear caused by TEE in an elderly woman undergoing elective aortic valve replacement.[219] The resultant bleeding resolved spontaneously with correction of a coagulopathy, and the diagnosis was confirmed by endoscopy. Humphrey[220] described a patient in whom manipulations of the transesophageal transducer led to the undetected displacement of an esophageal stethoscope into the stomach. The missing stethoscope was discovered several weeks later and was removed by endoscopy.

Certain principles should be followed to decrease the already low rate of complications of TEE. The probe should be lubricated well before introduction and positioning. The tip of the probe should not be flexed or extended (retroflexed) for prolonged periods or forcefully manipulated at any time. The probe should remain in the neutral position during cardiopulmonary bypass because high-pressure contact in the presence of a low tissue perfusion pressure may result in tissue ischemia, possibly leading to tissue necrosis and ulceration. This form of monitoring should be avoided unless absolutely necessary in patients with esophageal problems.

By using the transgastric short-axis view at the midpapillary level, the ventricle can be roughly divided into four equal quadrants representing the three coronary artery circulations. The short-axis view of the left ventricle is actually a transgastric view. Thus it is reasonable to weigh the potential risks against the benefits of TEE in patients with gastric problems.

B. Incorrect interpretation

Complications related to the mechanical aspects of TEE have, fortunately, been very minimal. However, the complications related to incorrect interpretation have not yet been evaluated. These may become more common as echocardiography assumes a greater role in guiding anesthetic and surgical management. A series of recent reports have highlighted some of the difficulties and technical limitations that may be encountered when using color-flow Doppler technology to assess valvular function.

Stevenson[221] demonstrated that gain setting, pulse repetition frequency, and carrier frequency significantly affected the size of regurgitant valve lesions. Findings by Yoshida et al[222] suggest that with the introduction of highly sensitive techniques (such as color-flow Doppler), the limits of normality may need to be redefined. These investigators examined valvular function with transthoracic color-flow Doppler imaging in 211 apparently healthy volunteers. In their normal participants, prevalences of 38% to 45% for mitral regurgitation, 15% to 77% for tricuspid regurgitation, and 28% to 88% for pulmonary regurgitation were found. Regurgitant flow signals were never detected at the aortic valve. In an accompanying editorial, Sahn and Maciel[223] discussed the clinical implications of these observations and also indicated that the esophageal echocardiographic window significantly increases the sensitivity of color-flow Doppler imaging for intracardiac flow events. If TEE is used as a gold standard, the incidence of detectable valve regurgitation in healthy persons will increase substantially.

Although wall-motion abnormalities are sensitive indicators of myocardial ischemia,[224] their specificity and predictive value are less certain.[225] In one study, 20% of 156 high-risk patients developed new or worsened segmental wall-motion abnormalities.[226] However, these episodes correlated poorly with ECG changes and postoperative cardiac events. Difficulties also occur with interpretation of on-line

echocardiographic images and interobserver variability. Thus anesthetic or surgical management may be altered inappropriately on the basis of erroneous interpretations.

REFERENCES

1. Katcher ML, Shapiro MM: Severe burns and death associated with electronic monitors, *N Engl J Med* 317:56, 1987 (letter).
2. National Fire Protection Association: *1990 Edition of the National Electrical Code and Standard for Health Care Facilities*, Quincy, Mass, 1990, National Fire Protection Association.
3. McNulty SE, Cooper M, Staudt S: Transmitted radiofrequency current through a flow directed pulmonary artery catheter, *Anesth Analg* 78:587, 1994.
4. Celoria G, Dawson JA, Teres D: Compartment syndrome in a patient monitored with an automated blood pressure cuff, *J Clin Monit* 3:139, 1987.
5. Sy WP: Ulnar nerve palsy related to use of automatically cycled blood pressure cuff, *Anesth Analg* 60:687, 1981.
6. Mozersky DJ, Buckley CJ, Hagood CO Jr, et al: Ultrasonic evaluation of the palmar circulation: a useful adjunct to radial artery cannulation, *Am J Surg* 126:810, 1973.
7. Allen EV: Thromboangiitis obliterans: methods of diagnosis of chronic occlusive arterial lesions distal to the wrist with illustrated cases, *Am J Med Sci* 178:237, 1929.
8. Greenhow DE: Incorrect performance of Allen's test: ulnar-artery flow erroneously presumed inadequate, *Anesthesiology* 37:356, 1972.
9. Brodsky JB: A simple method to determine patency of the ulnar artery intraoperatively prior to radial-artery cannulation, *Anesthesiology* 42:626, 1975.
10. Nowak GS, Moorthy SS, McNiece WL: Use of pulse oximetry for assessment of collateral arterial flow, *Anesthesiology* 64:527, 1986 (letter).
11. Castella X: A practical way of performing Allen's test to assess palmar collateral circulation, *Anesth Analg* 77:1085, 1993.
12. Slogoff S, Keats AS, Arlund C: On the safety of radial artery cannulation, *Anesthesiology* 59:42, 1983.
13. Mangano DT, Hickey RF: Ischemic injury following uncomplicated radial artery catheterization, *Anesth Analg* 58:55, 1979.
14. Barnes RW, Foster E, Jansen GA, et al: Safety of brachial artery catheters as monitors in the intensive care unit: prospective evaluation with the Doppler ultrasonic velocity detector, *Anesthesiology* 44:260, 1976.
15. Pascarelli EF, Bertrand CA: Comparison of blood pressures in the arms and legs, *N Engl J Med* 270:693, 1964.
16. Bazaral MG, Welch M, Golding LAR, et al: Comparison of brachial and radial arterial pressure monitoring in patients undergoing coronary artery bypass surgery, *Anesthesiology* 73:38, 1990.
17. Gravlee GP, Wong AB, Adkins TG, et al: A comparison of radial, brachial, and aortic pressures after cardiopulmonary bypass, *J Cardiothorac Anesth* 3:20, 1989.
18. Gurman GM, Kriemerman S: Cannulation of big arteries in critically ill patients, *Crit Care Med* 13:217, 1985.
19. Yacoub OF, Bacaling JH, Kelly M: Monitoring of axillary arterial pressure in a patient with Buerger's disease requiring clipping of an intracranial aneurysm, *Br J Anaesth* 59:1056, 1987.
20. VanBeck JO, White RD, Abenstein JP, et al: Comparison of axillary artery or brachial artery pressure with aortic pressure after cardiopulmonary bypass using a long radial artery catheter, *J Cardiothorac Vasc Anesth* 7:312, 1993.
21. Eriksson I, Jorulf H: Surgical complications associated with arterial catheterization, *Scand J Thorac Cardiovasc Surg* 4:69, 1970.
22. Bedford RF: Invasive blood pressure monitoring. In Blitt CD, ed: *Monitoring in anesthesia and critical care medicine*, New York, 1989, Churchill-Livingstone.
23. Kopman EA, Ferguson TB: Intraoperative monitoring of femoral artery pressure during replacement of aneurysm of descending thoracic aorta, *Anesth Analg* 56:603, 1977.
24. Youngberg JA, Miller ED Jr: Evaluation of percutaneous cannulations of the dorsalis pedis artery, *Anesthesiology* 44:80, 1976.
25. Johnstone RE, Greenhow DE: Catheterization of the dorsalis pedis artery, *Anesthesiology* 39:654, 1973.

26. Husum B, Palm T, Eriksen J: Percutaneous cannulation of the dorsalis pedis artery: a prospective study, *Br J Anaesth* 51:1055, 1979.

27. Fukutome T, Kojiro M, Tanigawa K, et al: Doppler-guided "percutaneous" radial artery cannulation in small children, *Anesthesiology* 69:434, 1988 (letter).

28. Morray JP, Brandford GH, Barnes LF, et al: Doppler-assisted radial artery cannulation in infants and children, *Anesth Analg* 63:346, 1984.

29. Porter JM: Raynaud's syndrome. In Sabiston DC, ed: *Textbook of surgery*, Philadelphia, 1985, WB Saunders.

30. Band JD, Maki DG: Infection caused by arterial catheters used for hemodynamic monitoring, *Am J Med* 67:735, 1979.

31. Shinozaki T, Deane RS, Mazuzan JE Jr, et al: Bacterial contamination of arterial lines: a prospective study, *JAMA* 249:223, 1983.

32. Weinstein RA, Stamm WE, Kramer L: Pressure monitoring devices: overlooked source of nosocomial infection, *JAMA* 236:936, 1976.

33. Stamm WE, Colella JJ, Anderson RL, et al: Indwelling arterial catheters as a source of nosocomial bacteremia: an outbreak caused by *Flavobacterium* species, *N Engl J Med* 292:1099, 1975.

34. Pierson DJ, Hudson LD: Monitoring hemodynamics in the critically ill, *Med Clin North Am* 67:1343, 1983.

35. Bedford RF, Wollman H: Complications of percutaneous radial-artery cannulation: an objective prospective study in man, *Anesthesiology* 38:228, 1973.

36. Bedford RF: Radial arterial function following percutaneous cannulation with 18- and 20-gauge catheters, *Anesthesiology* 47:37, 1977.

37. Bedford RF: Wrist circumference predicts the risk of radial-arterial occlusion after cannulation, *Anesthesiology* 48:377, 1978.

38. Davis FM, Steward JM: Radial artery cannulation: a prospective study in patients undergoing cardiothoracic surgery, *Br J Anaesth* 52:41, 1980.

39. Downs JB, Rackstein AD, Klein EF Jr, et al: Hazards of radial-artery catheterization, *Anesthesiology* 38:283, 1973.

40. Jones RM, Hill AB, Nahrwold ML, et al: The effect of method of radial artery cannulation on postcannulation blood flow and thrombus formation, *Anesthesiology* 55:76, 1981.

41. Bedford RF, Ashford TP: Aspirin pretreatment prevents postcannulation radial-artery thrombosis, *Anesthesiology* 51:176, 1979.

42. Bedford RF: Removal of radial-artery thrombi following percutaneous cannulation for monitoring, *Anesthesiology* 46:430, 1977.

43. Kim JM, Arakawa K, Bliss J: Arterial cannulation: factors in the development of occlusion, *Anesth Analg* 54:836, 1975.

44. Vender JS, Watts DR: Differential diagnosis of hand ischemia in the presence of an arterial cannula, *Anesth Analg* 61:465, 1982.

45. Chang C, Dughi J, Shitabata P, et al: Air embolism and the radial arterial line, *Crit Care Med* 16:141, 1988.

46. Lowenstein E, Little JW III, Lo HH: Prevention of cerebral embolization from flushing radial-artery cannulas, *N Engl J Med* 285:1414, 1971.

47. Goldstein RD, Gordon MJV: Volar proximal skin necrosis after radial artery cannulation, *N Y State J Med* 90:375, 1990.

48. Wyatt R, Glaves I, Cooper DJ: Proximal skin necrosis after radial-artery cannulation, *Lancet* 1:1135, 1974.

49. Qvist J, Peterfreund R, Perlmutter G: Transient compartment syndrome of the forearm after attempted radial artery cannulation, *Anesth Analg* 83:183, 1996.

50. Freeark RJ, Baker WH: Arterial injuries. In Sabiston DC, ed: *Textbook of surgery*, Philadelphia, 1986, WB Saunders.

51. Reich DL, Kaplan JA: Hemodynamic monitoring. In Kaplan JA, ed: *Cardiac anesthesia*, ed 3, Orlando, 1993, Grune & Stratton.

52. Neustein S, Narang J, Bronheim D: Use of the color test for safer internal jugular vein cannulation, *Anesthesiology* 76:1062, 1992 (letter).

53. Metz S, Horrow JC, Balcar I: A controlled comparison of techniques for locating the internal jugular vein using ultrasonography, *Anesth Analg* 63:673, 1984.

54. Hensley FA Jr, Dodson DL, Martin DE, et al: Oxygen saturation during preinduction placement of monitoring catheters in the cardiac surgical patient, *Anesthesiology* 66:834, 1987.

55. Denys BG, Uretsky BF: Anatomical variations of internal jugular vein location: impact on central venous access, *Crit Care Med* 19:1516, 1991.

56. Gratz I, Afshar M, Kidwell P, et al: Doppler-guided cannulation of the internal jugular vein: a prospective, randomized trial, *J Clin Monit* 10:185, 1994.

57. Troianos CA, Jobes DR, Ellison N: Ultrasound-guided cannulation of the internal jugular vein: a prospective, randomized study, *Anesth Analg* 72:823, 1991.

58. Mallory DL, McGee WT, Shawker TH, et al: Ultrasound guidance improves the success rate of internal jugular vein cannulation: a prospective, randomized trial, *Chest* 98:157, 1990.

59. Denys BG, Uretsky BF, Reddy PS: Ultrasound assisted cannulation of the internal jugular vein: a prospective comparison to the external landmark-guided technique, *Circulation* 87:1557, 1993.

60. Troianos CA, Kuwik RJ, Pasqual JR, et al: Internal jugular vein and carotid artery anatomic relation as determined by ultrasonography, *Anesthesiology* 85:43, 1996.

61. Alderson PJ, Burrows FA, Stemp LI, et al: Use of ultrasound to evaluate internal jugular vein anatomy and to facilitate central venous cannulation in paediatric patients, *Br J Anaesth* 70:145, 1993.

62. Sulek CA, Gravenstein N, Blackshear RH, et al: Head rotation during internal jugular vein cannulation and the risk of carotid artery puncture, *Anesth Analg* 82:125, 1996.

63. van de Griendt EW, Muhiudeen I, Cassoria L, et al: The effects of Trendelenburg position and Valsalva maneuver on the cross-sectional area of the internal jugular vein, *Anesthesiology* 75:A423, 1991 (abstract).

64. Mallory DL, Shawker T, Evans RG, et al: Effects of clinical maneuvers on sonographically determined internal jugular vein size during venous cannulation, *Crit Care Med* 18:1269, 1990.

65. Blitt CD, Wright WA, Petty WC, et al: Cardiovascular catheterization via the external jugular vein: a technique employing the J-wire, *JAMA* 229:817, 1974.

66. Defalque RJ: Subclavian venipuncture: a review, *Anesth Analg* 47:677, 1968.

67. Wistbacka JO, Nuutinen LS: Catheter-related complications of total parenteral nutrition (TPN): a review, *Acta Anaesthesiol Scand* 82:84, 1985.

68. Herbst CA Jr: Indication, management, and complications of percutaneous subclavian catheters: an audit, *Arch Surg* 113:1421, 1978.

69. Kaufman B: Pitfalls of central hemodynamic monitoring, *Resident and Staff Physician* 30:27, 1992.

70. Kellner GA, Smart JF: Percutaneous placement of catheters to monitor "central venous pressure," *Anesthesiology* 36:515, 1972.

71. Webre DR, Arens JF: Use of cephalic and basilic veins for introduction of central venous catheters, *Anesthesiology* 38:389, 1973.

72. Burgess GE III, Marino RJ, Peuler MJ: Effect of head position on the location of venous catheters inserted via basilic veins, *Anesthesiology* 46:212, 1977.

73. Artru AA, Colley PS: Placement of multiorificed CVP catheters via antecubital veins using intravascular electrocardiography, *Anesthesiology* 69:132, 1988.

74. Mongan P, Peterson RE, Culling RD: Pressure monitoring can accurately position catheters for air embolism aspiration, *J Clin Monit* 8:121, 1992.

75. Roth S, Aronson S: Placement of a right atrial air aspiration catheter guided by transesophageal echocardiography, *Anesthesiology* 83:1359, 1995.

76. Burri C, Ahnefeld FW: *The caval catheter*, Berlin, 1978, Springer-Verlag.

77. Bansmer G, Keith D, Tesluk H: Complications following the use of indwelling catheters of the inferior vena cava, *JAMA* 167:1606, 1958.

78. Shah KB, Rao TLK, Laughlin S, El-Etr AA: A review of pulmonary artery catheterization in 6,245 patients, *Anesthesiology* 61:271, 1984.

79. Davies MJ, Cronin KD, Domaingue CM: Pulmonary artery catheterization: an assessment of risks and benefits in 220 surgical patients, *Anaesth Intensive Care* 10:9, 1982.

80. Sise MJ, Hollingsworth P, Brimm JE, et al: Complications of the flow-directed pulmonary artery catheter: a prospective analysis in 219 patients, *Crit Care Med* 9:315, 1981.

81. Jobes DR, Schwartz AJ, Greenhow DE, et al: Safer jugular vein cannulation: recognition of arterial puncture and preferential use of the external jugular route, *Anesthesiology* 59:353, 1983.

82. Eckhardt WF, Iaconetti D, Kwon JS, et al: Inadvertent carotid artery cannulation during pulmonary artery catheter insertion, *J Cardiothorac Vasc Anesth* 10:283, 1996.

83. Ortiz J, Zumbro GL, Dean WF, et al: Arteriovenous fistula as a complication of percutaneous internal jugular vein catheterization: case report, *Mil Med* 141:171, 1976.

84. Gobeil F, Couture P, Girard D, et al: Carotid artery–internal jugular fistula: another complication following pulmonary artery catheterization via the internal jugular venous route, *Anesthesiology* 80:230, 1994.

85. Robinson R, Errett L: Arteriovenous fistula following percutaneous internal jugular vein cannulation: a report of carotid artery-to-internal jugular vein fistula, *J Cardiothorac Anesth* 2:488, 1988.

86. Cook TL, Dueker CW: Tension pneumothorax following internal jugular cannulation and general anesthesia, *Anesthesiology* 45:554, 1976.

87. Khalil KG, Parker FB Jr, Mukherjee N, et al: Thoracic duct injury: a complication of jugular vein catheterization, *JAMA* 221:908, 1972.

88. Arditis J, Giala M, Anagnostidou A: Accidental puncture of the right lymphatic duct during pulmonary artery catheterization: a case report, *Acta Anaesthiol Scand* 32:67, 1988.

89. Friedman BA, Jurgeleit HC: Perforation of atrium by polyethylene CV catheter, *JAMA* 203:1141, 1968.

90. Gravenstein N, Blackshear RH: In vitro evaluation of relative perforating potential of central venous catheters: comparison of materials, selected models, number of lumens, and angles of incidence to simulated membrane, *J Clin Monit* 7:1, 1991.

91. Oropello JM, Leibowitz AB, Manasia A, et al: Dilator-associated complications of central vein catheter insertion: possible mechanisms of injury and suggestions for prevention, *J Cardiothorac Vasc Anesth* 10:634, 1994.

92. Green HL, Nemir P Jr: Air embolism as a complication during parenteral alimentation, *Am J Surg* 121:614, 1971.

93. Turnage WS, Harper JV: Venous air embolism occurring after removal of a central venous catheter, *Anesth Analg* 72:559, 1991.

94. Smyth NPD, Rogers JB: Transvenous removal of catheter emboli from the heart and great veins by endoscopic forceps, *Ann Thorac Surg* 11:403, 1971.

95. Akazawa S, Nakaigawa Y, Hotta K, et al: Unrecognized migration of an entire guidewire on insertion of a central venous catheter into the cardiovascular system, *Anesthesiology* 84:241, 1996 (letter).

96. Parikh RK: Horner's syndrome: a complication of percutaneous catheterization of internal jugular vein, *Anaesthesia* 27:327, 1972.

97. Selander D, Dhuner KG, Lundborg G: Peripheral nerve injury due to injection needles used for regional anesthesia: an experimental study of the acute effects of needle point trauma, *Acta Anaesth Scand* 21:182, 1977.

98. Nakayama M, Fujita S, Kawamata M, et al: Traumatic aneurysm of the internal jugular vein causing vagal nerve palsy: a rare complication of percutaneous catheterization, *Anesth Analg* 78:598, 1994.

99. Royster RL, Johnston WE, Gravlee GP, et al: Arrhythmias during venous cannulation prior to pulmonary artery catheter insertion, *Anesth Analg* 64:1214, 1985.

100. Eissa NT, Kvetan V: Guide wire as a cause of complete heart block in patients with preexisting left bundle branch block, *Anesthesiology* 73:772, 1990.

101. Swan HJC, Ganz W, Forrester JS, et al: Catheterization of the heart in man with the use of a flow-directed balloon-tipped catheter, *N Engl J Med* 283:447, 1970.

102. Raper R, Sibbald WJ: Misled by the wedge? The Swan-Ganz catheter and left ventricular preload, *Chest* 89:427, 1986.

103. Nadeau S, Noble WH: Misinterpretation of pressure measurements from the pulmonary artery catheter, *Can Anaesth Soc J* 33(3 Pt 1):352, 1986.

104. West JB: *Ventilation/blood flow and gas exchange,* ed 4, Oxford, 1970, Blackwell Scientific.

105. Shasby DM, Dauber IM, Pfister S, et al: Swan-Ganz catheter location and left atrial pressure determine the accuracy of the wedge pressure when positive end-expiratory pressure is used, *Chest* 80:666, 1981.

106. Teboul JL, Zapol WM, Brun-Buisson C, et al: A comparison of pulmonary artery occlusion pressure and left ventricular end-diastolic pressure during mechanical ventilation with PEEP in patients with severe ARDS, *Anesthesiology* 70:261, 1989.

107. Pinsky M, Vincent JL, De Smet JM: Estimating left ventricular filling pressure during positive end-expiratory pressure in humans, *Am Rev Respir Dis* 25:143, 1991.

108. Keusch DJ, Winters S, Thys DM: The patient's position influences the incidence of dysrhythmias during pulmonary artery catheterization, *Anesthesiology* 70:582, 1989.

109. Weintraub AC, Barash PG: A pulmonary artery catheter is indicated in all patients for coronary artery surgery. Pro: a pulmonary artery catheter is indicated in all patients for coronary artery surgery, *J Cardiothorac Anesth* 1:358, 1987.

110. Bashein G, Ivey TD: A pulmonary artery catheter is indicated in all patients for coronary artery surgery. Con: a pulmonary artery catheter is not indicated for all coronary artery surgery, *J Cardiothorac Anesth* 1:362, 1987.

111. Vender JS: Pulmonary artery and mixed venous monitoring: appropriate use. *1995 Annual Refresher Course Lectures* 144:1, 1995, American Society of Anesthesiologists, Chicago, Ill.

112. Robin ED: Defenders of the pulmonary artery catheter, *Chest* 93:1059, 1988.

113. Dalen JE, Bone RC. Is it time to pull the pulmonary artery catheter? *JAMA* 276:916, 1996 (editorial).

114. Ontario Intensive Care Study Group: Evaluation of right heart catheterization in critically ill patients, *Crit Care Med* 20:928, 1992.

115. Connors AF Jr, Speroff T, Dawson NV, et al: The effectiveness of right heart catheterization in the initial care of critically ill patients: SUPPORT Investigators, *JAMA* 276:889, 1996.

116. Gattinoni L, Brazzi L, Pelosi P, et al: A trial of goal-oriented hemodynamic therapy in critically ill patients: SvO₂ Collaborative Group, *N Engl J Med* 333:1025, 1995.

117. Tuman KJ, McCarthy RJ, Spiess BD, et al: Effect of pulmonary artery catheterization on outcome in patients undergoing coronary artery surgery, *Anesthesiology* 70:199, 1989.

118. Iberti TJ, Fischer EP, Leibowitz AB, et al: A multicenter study of physicians' knowledge of the pulmonary artery catheter: Pulmonary Artery Catheter Study Group, *JAMA* 264:2928, 1990.

119. Haupt M, Shoemaker W, Haddy F: Goal oriented hemodynamic therapy, *N Engl J Med* 334:799, 1996 (letter).

120. Shoemaker WC, Appel PL, Kram HB, et al: Prospective trial of supranormal values of survivors as therapeutic goals in high-risk surgical patients, *Chest* 94:1176, 1988.

121. Boyd O, Grounds RM, Bennett ED: A randomized clinical trial of the effect of deliberate perioperative increase of oxygen delivery on mortality in high-risk surgical patients, *JAMA* 270:2699, 1993.

122. Rao TLK, Jacobs KH, El-Etr AA: Reinfarction following anesthesia in patients with myocardial infarction, *Anesthesiology* 59:499, 1983.

123. Moore CH, Lombardo TR, Allums JA, et al: Left main coronary artery stenosis: hemodynamic monitoring to reduce mortality, *Ann Thorac Surg* 26:445, 1978.

124. Heyland DK, Cook DJ, King D, et al: Maximizing oxygen delivery in critically ill patients: a methodologic appraisal of the evidence, *Crit Care Med* 24:517, 1996.

125. Connors AF Jr, McCaffree DR, Gray BA: Evaluation of right heart catheterization in the critically ill patient without myocardial infarction, *N Engl J Med* 308:263, 1983.

126. Waller JL, Johnson SP, Kaplan JA: Usefulness of pulmonary artery catheters during aortocoronary bypass surgery, *Anesth Analg* 61:221, 1982.

127. Iberti T, Fisher CJ: A prospective study on the use of the pulmonary artery catheter in a medical intensive care unit: its effect on diagnosis and therapy, *Crit Care Med* 11:238, 1983 (abstract).

128. Sprung CL, Pozen RG, Rozanski JJ, et al: Advanced ventricular arrhythmias during bedside pulmonary artery catheterization, *Am J Med* 72:203, 1982.

129. Salmenperä, M, Peltola K, Rosenberg P: Does prophylactic lidocaine control cardiac arrhythmias associated with pulmonary artery catheterization? *Anesthesiology* 56:210, 1982.

130. Shaw TJI: The Swan-Ganz pulmonary artery catheter: incidence of complications, with particular reference to ventricular dysrhythmias, and their prevention, *Anaesthesia* 34:651, 1979.

131. Abernathy WS: Complete heart block caused by the Swan-Ganz catheter, *Chest* 65:349, 1974.

132. Thomson IR, Dalton BC, Lappas DG, et al: Right bundle-branch block and complete heart block caused by the Swan-Ganz catheter, *Anesthesiology* 51:359, 1979.

133. Sprung CL, Elser B, Schein RMH, et al: Risk of right bundle-branch block and complete heart block during pulmonary artery catheterization, *Crit Care Med* 17:1, 1989.

134. Morris D, Mulvihill D, Lew WYW: Risk of developing complete heart block during bedside pulmonary artery catheterization in patients with left bundle-branch block, *Arch Intern Med* 147:2005, 1987.

135. McDaniel DD, Stone JG, Faltas AN, et al: Catheter-induced pulmonary artery hemorrhage: diagnosis and management in cardiac operations, *J Thorac Cardiovasc Surg* 82:1, 1981.

136. Dhamee MS, Pattison CZ: Pulmonary artery rupture during cardiopulmonary bypass, *J Cardiothorac Anesth* 1:51, 1987.

137. Hannan AT, Brown M, Bigman O: Pulmonary artery catheter–induced hemorrhage, *Chest* 85:128, 1984.

138. Stein JM, Lisbon A: Pulmonary hemorrhage from pulmonary artery catherization treated with endobronchial intubation, *Anesthesiology* 55:698, 1981.

139. Purut CM, Scott SM, Parham JV, et al: Intraoperative management of severe endobronchial hemorrhage, *Ann Thorac Surg* 51:304, 1991.

140. Gourin A, Garzon AA: Operative treatment of massive hemoptysis, *Ann Thorac Surg* 18:52, 1974.

141. Carlson TA, Goldenberg IF, Murray PD, et al: Catheter-induced delayed recurrency pulmonary artery hemorrhage: intervention with therapeutic embolism of the pulmonary artery, *JAMA* 261:1943, 1989.

142. Foote GA, Schabel SI, Hodges M: Pulmonary complications of the flow-directed balloon-tipped catheter, *N Engl J Med* 290:927, 1974.

143. Mond HG, Clark DW, Nesbitt SJ, et al: A technique for un-knotting an intracardiac flow-directed balloon catheter, *Chest* 67:731, 1975.

144. Lipp H, O'Donoghue K, Resnekov L: Intracardiac knotting of a flow-directed balloon catheter, *N Engl J Med* 284:220, 1971.

145. Kainuma M, Yamada M, Miyake T: Pulmonary artery catheter passing between the chordae tendineae of the tricuspid valve, *Anesthesiology* 83:1130, 1995 (letter).

146. Lazzam C, Sanborn TA, Christian F Jr: Ventricular entrapment of a Swan-Ganz catheter: a technique for nonsurgical removal, *J Am Coll Cardiol* 13:1422, 1989.

147. Boscoe MJ, de Lange S: Damage to the tricuspid valve with a Swan-Ganz catheter, *BMJ* 283:346, 1981.

148. O'Toole JD, Wurtzbacher JJ, Wearner NE, et al: Pulmonary-valve injury and insufficiency during pulmonary-artery catheterization, *N Engl J Med* 301:1167, 1979.

149. Greene JF Jr, Fitzwater JE, Clemmer TP: Septic endocarditis and indwelling pulmonary artery catheters, *JAMA* 233:891, 1975.

150. Kim YL, Richman KA, Marshall BE: Thrombocytopenia associated with Swan-Ganz catheterization in patients, *Anesthesiology* 53:261, 1980.

151. Moberg PQ, Geary VM, Sheikh FM: Heparin-induced thrombocytopenia: a possible complication of heparin-coated pulmonary artery catheters, *J Cardiothorac Anesth* 4:226, 1990.

152. King DJ, Kelton JG: Heparin-associated thrombocytopenia, *Ann Intern Med* 100:535, 1984.

153. Mangano DT: Heparin bonding and long-term protection against thrombogenesis, *N Engl J Med* 307:894, 1982 (letter).

154. Böhrer H, Fleischer F, Lang J, et al: Early formation of thrombi on pulmonary artery catheters in cardiac surgical patients receiving high-dose aprotinin, *J Cardiothorac Anesth* 4:222, 1990.

155. Dentz ME, Slaughter TF, Mark JB: Early thrombus formation on heparin-bonded pulmonary artery catheters in patients receiving ε-aminocaproic acid, *Anesthesiology* 82:583, 1995.

156. Martens PR, Driessen JJ, Vandekerckhove Y, et al: Transesophageal echocardiographic detection of a right atrial thrombus around a pulmonary artery catheter, *Anesth Analg* 75:847, 1992.

157. Allyn J, Lichtenstein A, Koski EG, et al: Inadvertent passage of a pulmonary artery catheter from the superior vena cava through the left atrium and left ventricle into the aorta, *Anesthesiology* 70:1019, 1989.

158. Saad RM, Loubser PG, Rokey R: Intraoperative transesophageal and contrast echocardiographic detection of an unusual complication associated with a misplaced pulmonary artery catheter, *J Cardiothorac Vasc Anesth* 10:247, 1996.

159. Gilbert TB, Scherlis ML, Fiocco M, et al: Pulmonary artery catheter migration causing venous cannula obstruction during cardiopulmonary bypass, *Anesthesiology* 82:596, 1995.

160. Meluch AM, Karis JH: Obstruction of venous return by a pulmonary artery catheter during cardiopulmonary bypass, *Anesth Analg* 70:121, 1990 (letter).

161. Kozlowski JH: Inadvertent coronary sinus occlusion by a pulmonary artery catheter, *Crit Care Med* 14:649, 1986.

162. Tewari P, Kumar M, Kaushik S: Pulmonary artery catheter misplaced in liver, *J Cardiothorac Vasc Anesth* 9:482, 1995 (letter).

163. Zaidan JR, Freniere S: Use of a pacing pulmonary artery catheter during cardiac surgery, *Ann Thorac Surg* 35:633, 1983.

164. Macander PJ, Kuhnlein JL Jr, Buiteweg J, et al: Electrode detachment: a complication of the indwelling pacing Swan-Ganz catheter, *N Engl J Med* 314:1711, 1986 (letter).

165. Heiselman DE, Maxwell JS, Petno V: Electrode displacement from a multipurpose Swan-Ganz catheter, *Pacing Clin Electrophysiol* 9(1 Pt 1):134, 1986.

166. Mora CT, Seltzer JL, McNulty SE: Evaluation of a new design pulmonary artery catheter for intraoperative ventricular pacing, *J Cardiothorac Anesth* 2:303, 1988.

167. Trankina MF, White RD: Perioperative cardiac pacing using an atrioventricular pacing pulmonary artery catheter, *J Cardiothorac Anesth* 3:154, 1989.

168. Shin B, McAslan TC, Ayella RJ: Problems with measurement using the Swan-Ganz catheter, *Anesthesiology* 43:474, 1975.

169. Tuman KJ, Carroll GC, Ivankovich AD: Pitfalls in interpretation of pulmonary artery catheter data, *J Cardiothorac Anesth* 3:625, 1989.

170. Schmitt EA, Brantigan CO: Common artifacts of pulmonary artery pressures: recognition and interpretation, *J Clin Monit* 2:44, 1986.

171. Krouskop RW, Cabatu EE, Chelliah BP, et al: Accuracy and clinical utility of an oxygen saturation catheter, *Crit Care Med* 11:744, 1983.

172. van Woerkens EC, Trouwborst A, Tenbrinck R: Accuracy of a mixed venous saturation catheter during acutely induced changes in hematocrit in humans, *Crit Care Med* 19:1025, 1991.

173. Gettinger A, DeTraglia MC, Glass DD: In vivo comparison of two mixed venous saturation catheters, *Anesthesiology* 66:373, 1987.

174. Bongard F, Lee TS, Leighton T, et al: Simultaneous in vivo comparison of two- versus three-wavelength mixed venous (SvO_2) oximetry catheters, *J Clin Monit* 11: 329, 1995.

175. Reinhart K, Moser N, Rudolph T, et al: Accuracy of two mixed venous saturation catheters during long-term use in critically ill patients, *Anesthesiology* 69:769, 1988.

176. Scuderi PE, MacGregor DA, Bowton DL, et al: A laboratory comparison of three pulmonary artery oximetry catheters, *Anesthesiology* 81:245, 1994.

177. Pond CG, Blessios G, Bowlin J, et al: Perioperative evaluation of a new mixed venous oxygen saturation catheter in cardiac surgical patients, *J Cardiothorac Vasc Anesth* 6:280, 1992.

178. Armaganidis A, Dhainaut JF, Billard JL, et al: Accuracy assessment for three fiberoptic pulmonary artery catheters for SvO_2 monitoring, *Intensive Care Med* 20:484, 1994.

179. Jurado RA: Measurement of cardiac output by the direct Fick method. In Litwak RS, Jurado RA, eds: *Care of the cardiac surgical patient*, Norwalk, Conn, 1982, Appleton-Century-Crofts.

180. Guyton AC: The Fick principle. In Guyton AC, Jones CE, Coleman TG, eds: *Circulatory physiology: cardiac output and its regulation*, ed 2, Philadelphia, 1973, WB Saunders.

181. Kendrick AH, West J, Papouchado M, et al: Direct Fick cardiac output: are assumed values of oxygen consumption acceptable? *Eur Heart J* 9:337, 1988.

182. Heneghan CPH, Gillbe CE, Branthwaite MA: Measurement of metabolic gas exchange during anaesthesia: a method using mass spectometry, *Br J Anaesth* 53:73, 1981.

183. Heneghan CPH, Branthwaite MA: Non-invasive measurement of cardiac output during anaesthesia: an evaluation of the soluble gas uptake method, *Br J Anaesth* 53:351, 1981.

184. Davies G, Hess D, Jebson P: Continuous Fick cardiac output compared to continuous pulmonary artery electromagnetic flow measurements in pigs, *Anesthesiology* 66:805, 1987.

185. Davies GG, Jebson PJR, Glasgow BM, et al: Continuous Fick cardiac output compared to thermodilution cardiac output, *Crit Care Med* 14:881, 1986.

186. Rieke H, Weyland A, Hoeft A, et al: Continuous measurement of cardiac output based on the Fick principle in cardiac anesthesia, *Anaesthetist* 39:13, 1990.

187. Carpenter JP, Nair S, Staw I: Cardiac output determination: thermodilution versus a new computerized Fick method, *Crit Care Med* 13: 576, 1985.

188. Doi M, Morita K, Ikeda K: Frequently repeated Fick cardiac output measurements during anesthesia, *J Clin Monit* 6:107, 1990.

189. Forrester JS, Ganz W, Diamond G, et al: Thermodilution cardiac output determination with a single flow-directed catheter, *Am Heart J* 83:306, 1972.

190. Matthew EB, Vender JS: Comparison of thermodilution cardiac output measured by different computers, *Crit Care Med* 15:989, 1987 (letter).

191. Pearl RG, Siegel LC: Thermodilution cardiac output measurement with a large left-to-right shunt, *J Clin Monit* 7:146, 1991.

192. Wetzel RC, Latson TW: Major errors in thermodilution cardiac output measurement during rapid volume infusion, *Anesthesiology* 62:684, 1985.

193. Bazaral MG, Petre J, Novoa R: Errors in thermodilution cardiac output measurements caused by rapid pulmonary artery temperature decreases after cardiopulmonary bypass, *Anesthesiology* 77:31, 1992.

194. Latson TW, Whitten CW, O'Flaherty D, et al: Ventilation, thermal noise, and errors in cardiac output measurements after cardiopulmonary bypass, *Anesthesiology* 79:1233, 1993.

195. Hamilton MA, Stevenson LW, Woo M, et al: Effect of tricuspid regurgitation on the reliability of the thermodilution cardiac output in congestive heart failure, *Am J Cardiol* 64:945, 1989.

196. Kashtan HI, Maitland A, Salerno TA, et al: Effects of tricuspid regurgitation on thermodilution cardiac output: studies in an animal model, *Can J Anaesth* 34(3 Pt 1):246, 1987.

197. Heerdt PM, Pond CB, Blessios GA, et al: Inaccuracy of cardiac output by thermodilution during acute tricuspid regurgitation, *Ann Thorac Surg* 53:706, 1992.

198. Konstadt SN, Louie EK: Echocardiographic diagnosis of paradoxical embolism and the potential for right to left shunting, *Am J Card Imaging* 8:28, 1994.

199. Nishikawa T, Dohi S: Slowing of heart rate during cardiac output measurement by thermodilution, *Anesthesiology* 57:538, 1982.

200. Harris AP, Miller CF, Beattie C, et al: The slowing of sinus rhythm during thermodilution cardiac output determination and the effect of altering injectate temperature, *Anesthesiology* 63:540, 1985.

201. Nishikawa T, Dohi S: Hemodynamic status susceptible to slowing of heart rate during thermodilution cardiac output determination in anesthetized patients, *Crit Care Med* 18:841, 1990.

202. Barankay T, Jansco T, Nagy S, et al: Cardiac output estimation by a thermodilution method involving intravascular heating and thermistor recording, *Acta Physiol Acad Sci Hung* 38:167, 1970

203. Khalil HH, Richardson TQ, Guyton AC: Measurement of cardiac output by thermal dilution and direct Fick methods in dogs, *J Appl Physiol* 21:1131, 1966.

204. Yelderman M, Quinn MD, Mcknown RC: Thermal safety of a filamented pulmonary artery catheter, *J Clin Monit* 8:147, 1992.

205. Yelderman M: Continuous measurement of cardiac output with the use of stochastic system identification techniques, *J Clin Monit* 6:322, 1990.

206. Thrush D, Downs JB, Smith RA: Continuous thermodilution cardiac output: agreement with the Fick and bolus thermodilution methods, *J Cardiothorac Vasc Anesth* 9:39, 1995.

207. Yelderman M, Ramsay MA, Quinn MD, et al: Continuous thermodilution cardiac output measurements in intensive care unit patients, *J Cardiothorac Vasc Anesth* 6:270, 1990.

208. Bottiger BW, Rauch H, Bohrer H, et al: Continuous versus intermittent cardiac output measurement in cardiac surgical patients undergoing hypothermic cardiopulmonary bypass, *J Cardiothorac Vasc Anesth* 9:405, 1995.

209. Miller WE, Richards KL, Crawford MH: Accuracy of mitral Doppler echocardiographic cardiac output determinations in adults, *Am Heart J* 119:905, 1990.

210. Maslow A, Comunale ME, Haering JM, et al: Pulsed wave Doppler measurement of cardiac output from the right ventricular outflow tract, *Anesth Analg* 83:466, 1991.

211. Darmon PL, Hillel Z, Mogtader A, et al: Cardiac output by transesophageal echocardiography using continuous-wave Doppler across the aortic valve, *Anesthesiology* 80:796, 1994.

212. Kubicek WG, Karnegis JN, Patterson RP, et al: Development and evaluation of an impedance cardiac output system, *Aerosp Med* 37:1208, 1966.

213. Donahue PJ, Hansen DD, Mayer JE: A new complication of left atrial catheters, *J Cardiothorac Anesth* 3:757, 1989.

214. Carvalho R, Loures D, Brofman P, et al: Left atrial catheter complications, *J Thorac Cardiovasc Surg* 92:162, 1986 (letter).

215. Daniel WG, Erbel R, Kasper W, et al: Safety of transesophageal echocardiography: a multicenter survey of 10,419 examinations, *Circulation* 83:817, 1991.

216. O'Shea JP, Southern JE, D'Ambra MN, et al: Effects of prolonged transesophageal echocardiographic imaging and probe manipulation on the esophagus—an echocardiographic-pathologic study, *J Am Coll Cardiol* 17:1426, 1991.

217. Urbanowicz JH, Kernoff RS, Oppenheim G, et al: Transesophageal echocardiography and its potential for esophageal damage, *Anesthesiology* 72:40, 1990.

218. Cucchiara RF, Nugent M, Seward JB, et al: Air embolism in upright neurosurgical patients: detection and localization by two-dimensional transesophageal echocardiography, *Anesthesiology* 60:353, 1984.

219. Dewhirst WE, Stragand JJ, Fleming BM: Mallory-Weiss tear complicating intraoperative transesophageal echocardiography in a patient undergoing aortic valve replacement, *Anesthesiology* 73:777, 1990.

220. Humphrey LS: Esophageal stethoscope loss complicating transesophageal echocardiography, *J Cardiothorac Anesth* 2:356, 1988.

221. Stevenson JG: Two-dimensional color Doppler estimation of the severity of atrioventricular valve regurgitation: important effects of instrument gain setting, pulse repetition frequency, and carrier frequency, *J Am Soc Echocardiogr* 2:1, 1989.

222. Yoshida K, Yoshikawa J, Shakudo M, et al: Color Doppler evaluation of valvular regurgitation in normal subjects, *Circulation* 78:840, 1988.

223. Sahn DJ, Maciel BC: Physiological valvular regurgitation: Doppler echocardiography and the potential for iatrogenic heart disease, *Circulation* 78:1075, 1988.

224. Smith JS, Cahalan MK, Benefiel DJ, et al: Intraoperative detection of myocardial ischemia in high-risk patients: electrocardiography versus two-dimensional transesophageal echocardiography, *Circulation* 72:1015, 1985.

225. Thys DM: The intraoperative assessment of regional myocardial performance: is the cart before the horse? *J Cardiothorac Anesth* 1:273, 1987.

226. London MJ, Tubau JF, Wong MG, et al: The "natural history" of segmental wall motion abnormalities in patients undergoing non-cardiac surgery: S.P.I. Research Group, *Anesthesiology* 73:644, 1990.

Chapter 3

Complications of Neuraxial (Spinal/Epidural/Caudal) Anesthesia

J.C. Gerancher

Spencer S. Liu

"I don't want anybody messing with my spinal cord."

—One patient's refusal of epidural anesthesia in response to the anesthesiologist's recommendation that the technique be used for total knee arthroplasty

The rare, devastating complications of neuraxial anesthesia sometimes weigh so heavily in patients' assessment of risk that opportunities for readily and safely achievable benefits are lost. These complications are prominent in the anesthesia literature as well. Although most basic anesthesia texts include only one chapter on neuraxial anesthesia, much of the text of that chapter is usually devoted to complications, contraindications, and risk. Neither end of the needle is a comfortable place to be when complications occur; however, the incidence of complications with neuraxial anesthesia is similar to that of modern general anesthesia.[1,2] The increasingly well-understood pathophysiology of neuraxial anesthesia–related complications has encouraged prevention, as well as better assessment of risk. When complications do occur, they usually can be definitively diagnosed and treated.

As neuraxial anesthesia techniques have grown in popularity, the rare major complications, nerve injury and paralysis, have not been the only focus of attention. Be-

cause the minor and more common of complications—hypotension, postdural puncture headache, and urinary retention—have recently been better characterized, neuraxial techniques can be applied with less resultant morbidity in all facets of anesthesia and perioperative care. Thus a broader segment of our patients can reap the benefits of neuraxial anesthesia.

I. COMPLICATIONS OF TECHNIQUES
A. Spinal hematoma

Spinal hematoma after spinal, epidural, and caudal anesthesia was first described by Cooke in 1911.[3] Since then, it has occurred so rarely that its true incidence remains unknown and is unlikely to be revealed by prospective study or retrospective case series (such studies would require 1,000,000 patients).[4] However, two recent reviews[4,5] report on large case series that included a total of more than 1,000,000 patients who underwent spinal and epidural anesthesia without spinal hematoma formation. Meta-analysis of the data in these studies revealed a maximum incidence of spinal hematoma of 1:150,000 following epidural anesthesia and 1:220,000 following spinal anesthesia.[5]

Spinal hematoma results from bleeding and blood accumulation in the subarachnoid, subdural, or epidural spaces. During neuraxial anesthesia, the epidural space is the most common site of hematoma formation,[6] presumably because trauma causes bleeding of the epidural venous plexus. Hematoma formation results in neurologic symptoms when enough blood accumulates to cause spinal cord and nerve-root compression; early symptoms consist of back and radicular pain. When compression persists, nerve ischemia ensues and neurologic injury results. Later symptoms consist of lower-extremity motor weakness and bowel and bladder dysfunction. As blood accumulates, symptoms of weakness appear as ischemia develops over the course of several hours.

Risk factors for spinal hematoma include full anticoagulation at the time of neuraxial blockade (achieved with heparin or warfarin therapy), coagulopathy (disseminated intravascular coagulopathy, thrombocytopenia, or factor deficiency), and difficult or traumatic needle placement or catheter manipulation.[4] Spinal hematoma can occur spontaneously in the absence of trauma or neuraxial needle or catheter placement. In fact, spontaneous bleeding is the most frequent cause of spinal hematoma reported in the literature. Most reported spontaneous spinal hematomas have occurred during systemic anticoagulation therapy, although cases have occurred in the absence of any known deficit in coagulation.[7] Anticoagulation therapy immediately after lumbar puncture has been associated with spinal hematoma.[6] Five of 342 patients with acute cerebral ischemia developed spinal hematoma after diagnostic lumbar puncture and heparin-induced anticoagulation, whereas 0 of 342 patients undergoing diagnostic lumbar puncture alone developed spinal hematoma. Of the 5 patients who developed spinal hematoma, anticoagulation therapy was initiated within 1 hour of neuraxial needle placement, 4 had traumatic needle placement, and 4 were receiving concurrent aspirin therapy. However, three large case series, each reporting on approximately 1000 patients, described the safe use of systemic, full anticoagulation therapy following neuraxial blockade[8-10] in patients undergoing vascular or cardiac surgery. Taken together, these reports suggest that systemic anticoagulation therapy after neuraxial anesthesia is safe if administration of anticoagulants is delayed for 1 hour following neuraxial block and if drugs that affect platelet function are avoided while systemic anticoagulation therapy is being administered (see text that follows). Spinal anesthesia with small-gauge spinal needles should be considered in these situations. These types of needles may produce less vascular trauma and have been less frequently associated with spinal hematoma[4] than have large-gauge needles and epidural anesthesia with indwelling catheters. Manipulation and removal of epidural catheters during the nadir of anticoagulation seems prudent because spinal hematoma formation coincident with catheter removal has been reported.[4] Finally, postponement of surgery has been advocated when traumatic neuraxial needle placement occurs before planned full anticoagulation therapy.[8]

The classic symptom diagnostic of spinal hematoma is lower-extremity weakness within 24 hours of surgery after the appearance of severe back pain.[11] In practice, diagnosis by clinical criteria can be difficult. Presenting symptoms may be delayed for as long as 4 days. When neurologic symptoms do occur, they can be subtle, consisting initially of isolated radicular pain[12] or weakness alone.[4] Weakness in the recumbent postsurgical patient can easily be overlooked or attributed to postoperative epidural analgesia. For purposes of diagnosis, symptoms of pain and weakness usually appear as a relatively abrupt change when spinal hematoma is the cause. The most promising approach to diagnosing spinal hematoma seems to be a high degree of vigilance combined with early radiographic tests to rule out hematoma at the earliest suspicion. Complaints of back and radicular pain should be elicited and investigated. If a spinal hematoma is suspected, magnetic resonance imaging (MRI) is the test of choice for determining the presence and extent of an existent hematoma or for definitively ruling out the diagnosis. Gradient echo MRI is useful in definitively identifying the presence of blood in the compressing mass (Fig. 3-1).[11] Computed tomography and myelography can be used if MRI is not available.

Decompression by laminectomy and surgical evacuation of the hematoma is the treatment of choice when spinal hematoma is diagnosed. Recovery is most likely to result when the preoperative neurologic deficit is limited[7] and surgical treatment proceeds within 8 hours of diagnosis.[4] Although needle aspiration of blood[12] and spontaneous recovery[11] have been described, treatment should not be delayed. Even with surgical decompression within 8 hours of diagnosis, full recovery can be expected in only approximately half of patients affected by this complication.[4]

B. Epidural abscess

Epidural abscess associated with epidural catheterization was first described in 1974.[13] The incidence of abscess in neuraxial anesthesia is similar to that of spinal hematoma. A recent survey of more than 500,000 patients who underwent obstetric epidural anesthesia found one instance of epidural abscess and one instance of spinal hematoma.[14]

The pathophysiology of epidural abscess and spinal hematoma is similar in that both conditions are space-occupying lesions. Epidural abscess after neuraxial anesthesia is thought to result when bacteremic blood is introduced into the epidural space. The abscess causes back and radicular pain with spinal and nerve root compression, followed by ischemia, loss of motor function, and neurologic injury as the lesion persists. Epidural abscess, like spinal hematoma, has been reported more commonly from sources not related to neuraxial anesthesia.

Spontaneous abscess[15] resulting from bacteremia and hematologic spread is the type of epidural abscess most commonly reported in the literature. Spontaneous lesions have usually been reported in patients at risk for immunocompromise or hematologic infection, such as those with diabetes, chronic renal failure, cancer, herpes zoster, or rheumatoid arthritis; those undergoing steroid therapy; or those who use illicit intravenous drugs.[15] Patients with bacteremia who undergo neuraxial anesthesia may be at increased risk for epidural abscess compared with patients with bacteremia who do not undergo neuraxial blockade. Both experimental animals made bacteremic[16] and children with bacteremia studied retrospectively[17] have been reported to have a greater

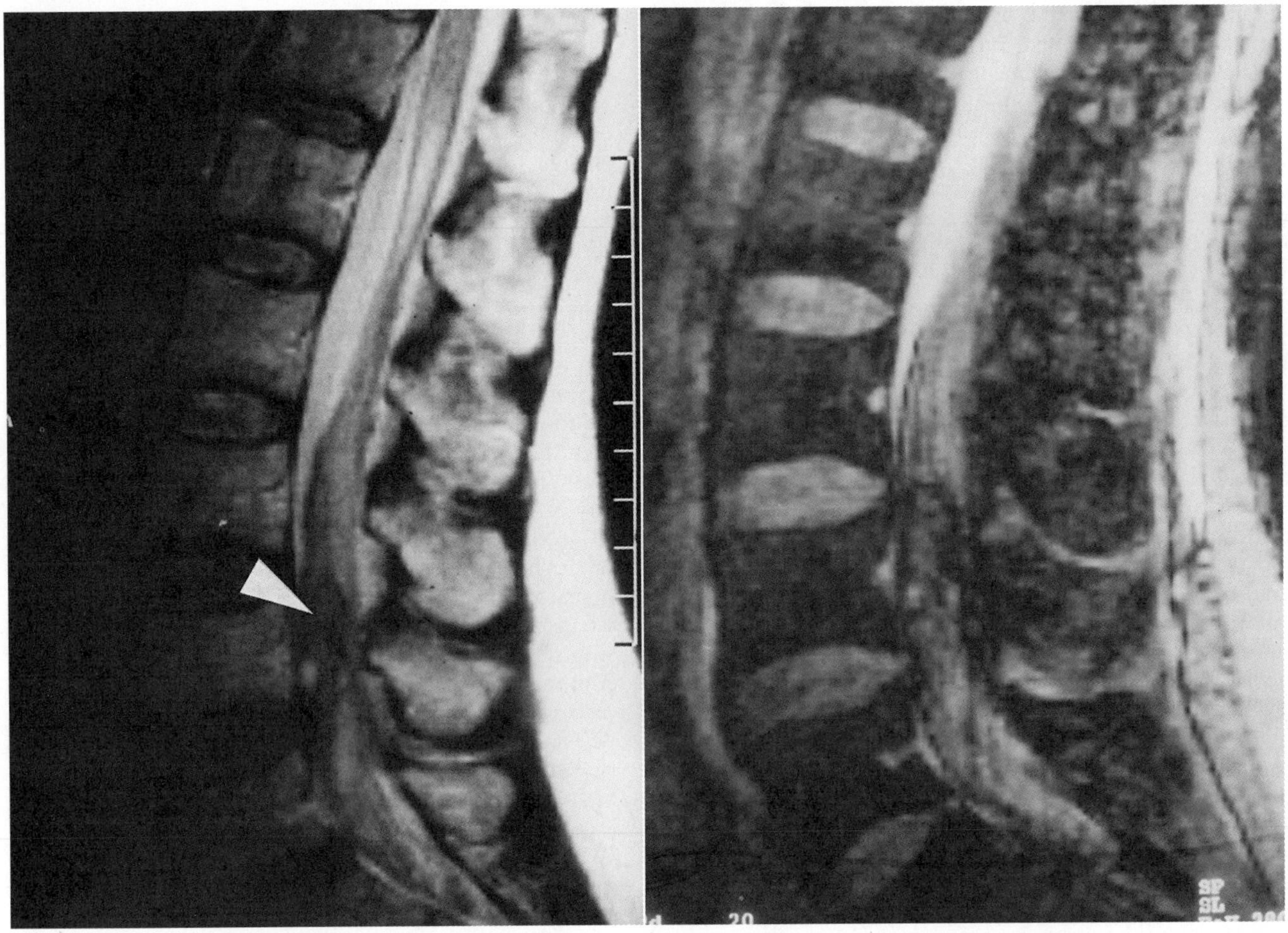

Fig. 3-1. A, Magnetic resonance image of a lumbar spinal hematoma. **B,** Confirmation of acute-subacute bleeding by gradient echo magnetic resonance imaging. (From Gerancher JC, Waterer R, Middleton J: *Anesthesiology* 86:490, 1997.)

incidence of meningitis when they undergo lumbar puncture while infected. On the other hand, obstetric patients with chorioamnionitis have safely had epidural analgesia without abscess formation despite occult bacteremia,[18] and results of a controlled study of diagnostic lumbar puncture in children with bacteremia[19] did not support an association between lumbar puncture and meningitis. A single dose of intravenous antibiotics before lumbar puncture was effective in preventing spinal infection in rats with bacteremia.[16] Taken together, these data suggest that fever is unlikely to increase a patient's risk for epidural abscess when neuraxial anesthesia is planned and that patients in whom bacteremia is strongly suspected may safely undergo neuraxial anesthesia after antibiotic therapy is started.

Immunocompromised patients may be at increased risk for epidural infection following neuraxial anesthesia. Patients with acquired immunodeficiency syndrome have experienced a high rate of catheter infection[20] during prolonged indwelling catheterization for chronic pain management, whereas parturients infected with human immunodeficiency virus undergoing brief epidural catheter placement did not.[21] Epidural abscess compli-

cating epidural steroid injection without catheter placement was recently reported.[22] In patients with preexisting or induced immune dysfunction, the risk for epidural abscess is likely to depend on the degree of immunocompromise and the duration of catheter placement.

Caudal anesthesia is the technique most often associated with epidural abscess; however, these infections have also been attributed to avoidable breaks in sterile technique.[23] Some practitioners advocate the use of bacterial filters on all epidural catheters,[24] whereas others have questioned their usefulness in preventing infection.[25] Local anesthetic solutions have been shown to be bacteriostatic and to remain free of bacteria even when prepared in syringes days in advance of use.[26] Ironically, contaminated multiple-use bottles of povidone-iodine have been implicated in epidemics of epidural abscess after neuraxial blockade.[27]

The clinical presentation of epidural abscess usually differs enough from that of spinal hematoma so that a differential diagnosis can be made.[23] Patients with epidural abscess usually present with fever, leukocytosis, and meningeal signs in addition to pain and weakness. In addition, purulence and erythema may be apparent at the site of block placement. Patients with epidural abscess usually present several days after neuraxial anesthesia, when the presentation of spinal hematoma is less likely.

The treatment of epidural abscess differs from that of spinal hematoma. Patients with epidural abscess should be treated aggressively with intravenous antibiotics. *Staphylococcus aureus* is the most common organism isolated, but therapy should be directed toward the organism causing bacteremia. Colonized caudal epidural catheters are more likely than lumbar catheters to harbor gram-negative bacteria. Both conservative management and percutaneous drainage have been successfully used in the management of epidural abscess. However, as with the management of spinal hematoma, early surgical evacuation is the treatment of choice.[28]

C. Neurologic injury

Both classic[29] and recent[30,31] studies of neuraxial techniques have found neurologic injury in the absence of a space-occupying lesion (such as spinal hematoma or epidural abscess). An incidence of approximately 1:2000 was found for permanent lumbar-sacral radiculopathies[30,31] following spinal and epidural anesthesia, whereas an incidence of approximately 1:1000 was found for transient, subjective, and isolated sensory deficits.[29]

The technique of neuraxial anesthesia itself has been implicated in the pathophysiology of these deficits. Trauma may occur with needle- or catheter-induced disruption of nerve fibers and may be further exacerbated by subsequent intraneural injection of anesthetic solutions into the spinal cord, cauda equina, or spinal nerve root. In a recent American Society of Anesthesiologists closed claims study, postoperative nerve injury was found to be a significant source of anesthesia-related claims.[32] The cause of injuries involving peripheral nerves after general and regional anesthesia was largely indeterminable. Despite extensive investigation, a cause was noted in only 21% of cases, and in only 15% of those cases was the injury related to anesthesia. However, 28% of lumbosacral nerve deficits were attributed to anesthesia; all of these deficits followed neuraxial anesthesia in which paresthesia or pain occurred after placement of a needle or catheter or injection of anesthetic.

In addition to having medicolegal implications, paresthesia may also be a risk factor for neurologic injury after neuraxial anesthesia. For example, in a retrospective review, paresthesia occurred in 6.3% of almost 5000 patients who underwent spinal anesthesia.[30] In this study, paresthesia during needle placement was found to significantly increase the risk for persistent paresthesia after surgery. In a recent prospective survey of more than 100,000 patients who underwent regional anesthesia, two thirds of instances in which neuraxial anesthesia resulted in nerve injury were complicated by paresthesia during block placement.[31] Clearly, not all paresthesias result in injury. Paresthesias occur in up to 60% of obstetric patients during placement of the epidural catheter,[33] and transient radicular pain without subsequent neurologic deficit has been described in 0.5% of thoracic epidural needle placements.[34]

When paresthesia occurs during administration of neuraxial anesthesia, we allow common sense to prevail. We reassess needle placement and cautiously proceed with catheter placement. Because patient feedback is important to our practice, we avoid neuraxial needle placement during general anesthesia or heavy sedation. When paresthesia occurs, we document its location for medicolegal reasons because paresthesias may radiate to sites other than that of postoperative neurologic injury.[29] Pediatric anesthesia represents an exception to our usual practice because neuraxial anesthesia is routinely and safely performed using general anesthesia in these patients.

The role of neuraxial anesthesia in postoperative peripheral nerve compression was recently investigated.[35] Postoperative lumbar epidural analgesia was not associated with a statistically significant increase in peroneal nerve palsy following total knee arthroscopy. However, palsies in patients with postoperative epidural analgesia were diagnosed later, were more severe, and were less likely to resolve completely. We recommend using opioids and low concentrations of local anesthetic in postoperative epidural infusions to minimize postoperative motor block, immobility, and, presumably, nerve injury.

Because postoperative nerve injuries are often subtle, they can be diagnosed at any time from resolution of neuraxial blockade to months after the surgical procedure.[29] As mentioned, nerve injury from trauma caused by placement of a neuraxial anesthetic is often impossible to differentiate from that related to the surgical procedure, positioning injury, stretch, and spontaneous occurrence. Diagnosis begins with careful documentation of the extent of sensory deficit, degree of motor impairment, and onset of symptoms. Physical examination can often distinguish a dermatomal (and therefore nerve root) pattern of deficit from a peripheral nerve deficit. Neurologic consultation and electromyographic testing is valuable for this purpose and can sometimes further differentiate spinal, cauda equina, and nerve root injuries. Determining the cause of nerve injury when possible is important from a medicolegal perspective and a quality assurance perspective; it may also be important for prognosis. Resolution can occur over 4 months after surgery, during which therapy consists of supportive measures, such as physical and occupational therapy.

D. Postdural puncture headache

Postdural puncture headache (PDPH) has been a complication of neuraxial anesthesia since 1898, when Bier and Hildebrandt produced a 100% incidence of this complication while performing spinal anesthesia on each other. Modern use of small-gauge, noncutting needles has reduced the incidence to 0.4% to 2%, even in young, ambulatory patients at greatest risk (Table 3-1).[36-43]

The pathophysiology of PDPH has been investigated for decades. Two aspects of its pathophysiology are evident: loss of cerebrospinal fluid through the dural puncture into the epidural space and resultant downward traction on intracranial vessels, which respond with painful vasodilatation. Pain is referred to the frontal region with trigeminal nerve stimulation, to the occiput with vagus and glossopharyngeal nerve stimulation, and to the neck with cervical nerve stimulation. Sixth cranial nerve palsy has accompanied PDPH, presumably because of abducens nerve traction.[44] Hearing loss has

Table 3-1. Incidence of postdural puncture headache (PDPH) varies per gauge and design of needle

Authors	Tip design	Gauge (needle orientation)	Population studied (no. of patients)	Incidence of PDPH (%)
Norris, Leighton, DeSimone[36]	Tuohy	18 (perpendicular)	OB-GYN (20)	73
Norris, Leighton, DeSimone[36]	Tuohy	18 (parallel)	OB-GYN (20)	30
Tourtellotte et al[37]	Quincke	22	Ambulatory (100)	36
Lynch, Arhelger, Krings-Ernst[38]	Whitacre	22	Ortho (100)	4
Neal et al[39]	Greene	22	GenOR (3.8)	3.8
Devcic et al[40]	Sprotte	24	OB-GYN (98)	4.2
Buettner[40a]	Quincke	25	Ortho (250)	7.8
Lambert et al[41]	Whitacre	25	OB-GYN (1000)	1.2
Lambert et al[41]	Quincke	26	OB-GYN (2400)	5.2
Lambert et al[41]	Quincke	27	OB-GYN (850)	2.7
Kang, Lee, Graf[42]	Whitacre	27	Ambulatory (250)	0.4
Dittmann et al[43]	Quincke	29	GenOR (1700)	2.5
Lambert et al[41]	Huber tip Weiss	Intended epidural	OB-GYN (21,000)	1.3

OB-GYN, Obstetrics-gynecology; *Ortho,* orthopedic surgery; *GenOR,* general surgery.

been attributed to cerebrospinal fluid leak after lumbar puncture and can occur with or without headache.[45]

Risk factors for PDPH are well understood, and prevention has been encouraged through alterations in technique and patient selection. The needle used during lumbar puncture is an important determinant of the incidence of PDPH. Use of pencil-tipped (Whitacre or Greene) and conical-tipped (Sprotte or Gertie Marx) spinal needles has dramatically reduced the incidence of PDPH compared with cutting-tipped (Quincke) needles of equal gauge. Presumably, the former types of needles, which are blunt, divide rather than cut fibers in their passage through the dura (Fig. 3-2, *A* and *B*).[46] If cutting-bevel needles are used, the incidence of headache is lower when the bevel is oriented parallel to the axis of the spine rather than perpendicular to it. However, although less cutting of longitudinally arranged dural fibers has been theorized, recent study of dural anatomy has not shown that the fibers are arranged so neatly.[47] Spinal needles are known to be deflected along their bevel during placement, and an alternative method of reducing the risk for PDPH is the formation of an oblique dural "flap." This technique has been postulated to reduce cerebrospinal fluid leak. Orientation of noncutting needles is not an issue in the prevention of PDPH, and headaches that do occur with use of these needles are of limited degree and duration.[44]

After tip design, needle gauge is the second most important factor determining the rate of PDPH. However, as needle diameter decreases, technical problems increase, along with the possibility of unrecognized and repeated lumbar punctures. This may contribute to an increased incidence of headache. It is probable that 25- and 27-gauge Whitacre needles represent the best compromise (see Table 3-1)[37-44] because the rate of PDPH associated with these needles is equal to the rate seen with epidural anesthesia.

PDPH rate is undoubtedly related to the experience and skill of the anesthesiologist. The rate of PDPH with 29-gauge Quincke needles was 2.5% among anesthesiology residents but 0.5% among their instructors.[43] Likewise, the rate of PDPH after epidural anesthesia depends on each practitioner's own rate of accidental dural puncture multiplied by the incidence of PDPH resulting from such a dural puncture. Therefore some experienced practitioners choose epidural over spinal anesthesia to avoid PDPH. However, the choice of epidural anesthesia over spinal or combined spinal-epidural anesthesia with appropriate needles should not be expected to significantly reduce the incidence of PDPH, regardless of practitioner experience. Caudal anesthesia carries an even smaller risk of accidental dural puncture compared with lumbar epidural anesthesia and may be an option for avoiding PDPH when clinically appropriate.

Risk factors for PDPH also include patient characteristics. Pregnancy, youth, and female sex have all been associated with an increased risk for PDPH. Old age and obesity may be protective. The incidence of PDPH after continuous spinal anesthesia has been small in morbidly obese parturients[48] and patients older than 65 years of age,[49] despite dural puncture with an 18-gauge epidural needle. Patients with a history of headache are no more likely than the general population to experience PDPH after lumbar puncture. Although advocated in the past, recumbency after spinal anesthesia, threading catheters through dural punctures after accidental dural puncture, using neuraxial opioids, choosing any one local anesthetic over other, and avoiding povidone-iodine skin preparation have not been shown to prevent PDPH.[44]

PDPH usually occurs 12 to 48 hours after dural puncture. Symptoms consist of bilateral, frontal, or occipital headache. The pain is usually throbbing and constant but is relieved when the patient is supine. Occasionally, the headache is associated with nausea, vomiting, and hearing and cranial nerve deficits. Postoperative and postpartum headaches are, unfortunately, very common. A bilateral, throbbing headache caused by caffeine with-

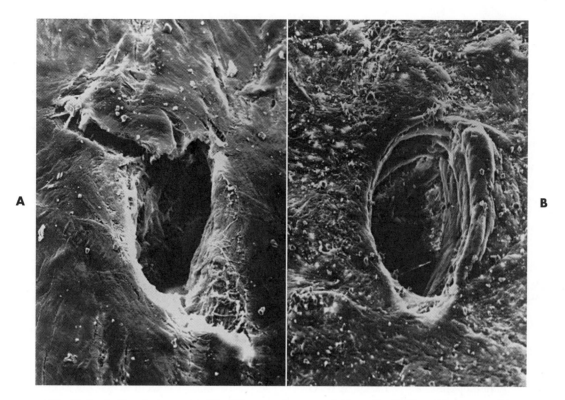

Fig. 3-2. A, Dural puncture with a 24-gauge Sprotte spinal needle. **B,** Dorsal puncture with a 26-gauge cutting spinal needle. (From Scott DB, Dittmann M, Clough DG, et al: *Reg Anesth* 18:213, 1993.)

drawal; migraine; or tension headache resulting from muscle contraction can share characteristics of PDPH. It is the postural component that distinguishes PDPH from these other varieties of headache. Thus if the patient has a history of disruption of normal caffeine ingestion, migraines, or frequent tension headaches, these causes should be considered when determining the source of the headache, whereas a known dural puncture should raise suspicion for PDPH. Muscle contraction headache occasionally accompanies PDPH, but the latter will have a postural component. Rare, life-threatening causes of headache, such as bacterial or viral meningitis, cerebral epidural hematoma, and cortical vein thrombosis, should be considered when severe postoperative or postpartum headache lacks a postural component. It is unusual for PDPH to last longer than 1 week if left untreated, but this condition may cause substantial discomfort. Only 42% of patients who have had PDPH would consider ever having spinal anesthesia again and would only have it if immediate treatment of the headache were available.[50]

Several treatment options are available for PDPH. Their use depends on the severity of symptoms, the degree to which symptoms interfere with recovery, and the patient's wishes. The most effective treatment available is an epidural blood patch. Autologous blood injected into the epidural space has been effective in promptly relieving 89% of PDPHs. However, PDPH recurs in as many as 11% of these initially therapeutic interventions. Treat-

ment of these headaches with repeated use of epidural blood patch can bring the effectiveness of this treatment to 97.5%.[51] Success probably depends on the timing of administration of the epidural blood patch,[52] the volume of blood administered,[53] and the size of the dural rent. The greatest success rate has been associated with administration of up to 15 ml of blood injected at or above the interspace of dural puncture more than 1 day after dural puncture.[53] Slow injection should be discontinued at the appearance of radicular discomfort. The mechanism by which an epidural blood patch cures PDPH is not fully understood but probably involves extrinsic compression on the cerebrospinal fluid space, increased subarachnoid pressure, relief of traction, tamponade of cerebrospinal fluid leakage, and eventual clotting of the dural rent with contact of blood and procoagulant cerebrospinal fluid. Subsequent failure of epidural blood patch therapy is thought to occur when the newly formed clot is dislodged. Epidural blood patch therapy is less effective when it is used as prophylaxis against anticipated PDPH.

The incidence of PDPH after accidental dural puncture is 18% with immediate, prophylactic administration of a blood patch and 76% without such treatment.[54] Reasons for this diminished effectiveness may include deposition of blood away from the site of dural puncture if a catheter technique is used or altered platelet function and dural structure with time.[54] Because a prophylactic epidural blood patch seems to decrease the incidence of postdural puncture headache, the technique is worth considering when epidural access proves to be difficult or late treatment of PDPH may be logistically difficult.

Epidural infusions of saline or dextran have been associated with immediate improvement of PDPH but are labor intensive, are only appropriate for inpatient therapy, and are associated with a high relapse rate.[44] Unfortunately, epidural blood patch therapy carries the same risks as the initial epidural placement and probably increases the risk for back pain, radicular pain, and fever. Conflicting data are available on the success of future epidural anesthesia after use of the epidural blood patch.[55] Because of these risks, less invasive treatment of PDPH is attractive.

Intravenous caffeine, oral medications (such as caffeine, butalbitol, and aspirin [Fiorinol]), and caffeinated beverages represent alternative and less invasive therapies for PDPH. These treatments are likely to be effective 50% of the time.[44] Sumatriptan, a serotonin receptor agonist and cerebral vasoconstrictor, has been advocated in the conservative management of PDPH.[56] We use conservative techniques when PDPH is mild, the risk for dural puncture during blood patch therapy is great, or the patient requests such treatments.

E. Backache

The 20% incidence of backache after surgery is similar to that found in the general population.[57] Backache following anesthesia seems to be related, at least in part, to needle entry with neuraxial anesthesia. After anesthesia, transient backache occurs frequently after epidural catheter placement (incidence of 30%),[58] less frequently after small-gauge spinal needle placement (11% to 13%), and still less frequently after general anesthesia (8%).[1]

Postoperative backache following neuraxial anesthesia probably has several causes. Trauma to intraspinous ligaments caused by spinal or epidural needles may result in postoperative pain; paraspinous muscle spasm is another potential cause. Use of any one type of spinal needle or the use of spinal introducer needles have not been associated with increased back pain, but multiple or difficult lumbar punctures result in more complaints of pain.[1] Lumbosacral ligamentous and nerve root stretch during neuraxial or general anesthesia are probably another part of the pathophysiology of backache because duration of surgical positioning has been correlated with pain. Local anesthetics and their additives also contribute to the pathophysiology of back pain. Agents, not techniques, are believed to be responsible for transient neurologic symptoms (also called transient radicular irritation [TRI]) and severe paralumbar pain (see following text).

Back pain of abrupt postoperative onset that is associated with radicular pain or is combined with muscle weakness may indicate spinal hematoma development, abscess formation, or neurologic injury. Pain of this character demands investigation to rule out such underlying pathologic processes. Fortunately, most backache is not pathologic, and neuraxial anesthesia does not result in chronic back pain.[57] Backache after neuraxial anesthesia is mostly mild and self-limited, resolving over 48 hours. Therapy usually consists of oral analgesics and reassurance. Although backache can be characterized as a minor complication of neuraxial anesthesia, in a recent investigation, fear of backache was the most common reason given by patients who refused neuraxial anesthesia.[58]

II. COMPLICATIONS OF ANESTHETIC AGENTS

Complications associated with neuraxial anesthesia have been attributed to the local anesthetics, opioids, and additives rather than the techniques used. Just as is the case with complications attributable to the technical aspects of neuraxial anesthesia, major complications caused by anesthetic agents occur rarely, and minor complications occur more commonly.

A. Local anesthetics

1. Central nervous system complications. Central nervous system complications can follow accidental systemic administration of local anesthetics during performance of epidural or caudal anesthesia. Such complications may occur with intravenous injection into the low-pressure venous plexus of the lumbar epidural space. Cannulation of one of these veins has been reported with an incidence as great as 9% during lumbar epidural block in obstetric patients.[59] During caudal anesthesia, high systemic concentrations of local anesthetic can result from cannulation of the sacral epidural plexus of veins as well as from sacral interosseus injection. Central nervous system reactions to local anesthetics depend on both the peak serum concentration of local anesthetic attained and the rapidity with which serum concentrations change. At low serum concentrations, local anesthetics are likely to produce mild excitatory responses, such as dizziness, perioral numbness, tinnitus, and a metallic taste in the mouth. These responses were shown to be highly reliable markers of intravascular injection in healthy, nonpremedicated volunteers who underwent intravenous administration of 100 mg of lidocaine and chloroprocaine.[60] Higher serum concentrations of local anesthetic cause blockade of the inhibitory pathways of the amygdala and unopposed facilitatory activity. Unopposed facilitation can result in generalized tonic-clonic seizures as brain concentrations increase. With further increases in brain concentrations of local anesthetics, both facilitatory and inhibitory pathways are blocked, and central nervous system depression results in somnolence, loss of consciousness, and, eventually, respiratory arrest.

Central nervous system depression without excitation is a common presenting symptom of intravenous local anesthetic toxicity when sedatives or opioids are administered concurrently.[61] Systemic administration of sedatives or opioids has two effects that modulate local anesthetic responses. First, by clouding the patient's sensorium, these agents interfere with the patient's ability to report the more subtle and subjective early effects of intravenous local anesthetic,[62] possibly allowing further administration of anesthetic. Sedatives can also cause depression of central nervous system excitation, and local anesthetic toxicity may first present as central nervous system depression. In addition, during neuraxial blockade, patients have been shown to have a greatly increased sensitivity to the hypnotic effect of sedatives[63] and to the respiratory depressant effects of opioids.[64] Deafferentation caused by conduction blockade has been hypothesized to account for this effect.[63] Therefore patients who are sedated before neuraxial blockade are likely to become more sedated once spinal or epidural anesthesia is established with local anesthetics.

Total spinal anesthesia can cause central nervous system complications in the absence of high serum concentrations of local anesthetics. Total spinal anesthesia (local anesthetic brain concentrations high enough to produce central nervous system depression, unconsciousness, and respiratory arrest) usually results from accidental spinal administration of large doses of local anesthetic intended for the epidural space. However, it has also occurred after spinal administration of standard doses of local anesthetics, most often when spinal anesthesia followed inadequate epidural block. Parturients seem to be at greater risk for this complication. The incidence of total spinal anesthesia in parturients undergoing cesarean section has been estimated to be 11% when spinal anesthesia follows unsuccessful epidural anesthesia compared with less than 1% with spinal anesthesia alone.[65] Conversely, epidural block following spinal anesthesia has proven to be safe during combined spinal epidural anesthesia. Possible mechanisms to explain total spinal blocks include an altered pressure gradient that favors transport of epidurally administered local anesthetics across the dural puncture, cephalad displacement of spinal fluid secondary to epidural compression, and increased sensitivity to local anesthetics in pregnancy.[65]

Central nervous system complications can be minimized with careful titration of local anesthetic. Incremental dosing of epidural catheters should follow test doses to rule out subarachnoid and intravenous administration.[61] A subarachnoid test dose should contain enough local anesthetic to produce limited spinal anesthesia in a timely manner (3 ml of 1.5% lidocaine[61]). Intravenous test dosing with epinephrine or local anesthetic is commonly used; use of isoproterenol, fentanyl, Doppler-detected air, and succinylcholine have also been advocated.[61]

The most reliable sign of a correctly placed epidural catheter is the presence of a discernible blockade. The interaction of systemic sedatives or opioids and neuraxial local anesthesia suggests that careful titration should guide the administration of these medications as well.

2. Cardiovascular complications. The incidence of cardiovascular complications ranges from 70% if relative hypotension following spinal anesthesia is considered, to rare for cardiac toxicity during epidural anesthesia with bupivacaine in parturients and in cases of unexplained cardiac arrest during spinal anesthesia in young, healthy patients.

Progressive hypotension can occur after neuraxial anesthesia. Blockade of lumbosacral sympathetic nerves results in vasodilation of the legs. Vascular pooling in the gut with low thoracic sympathectomy follows. Decreased heart rate with blockade of cardiac accelerator fibers follows with still higher levels of thoracic blockade. Although fluid pretreatment in various groups of patients has been shown to decrease the incidence and severity of hypotension,[66,67] it has not been shown to be effective in eliminating hypotension or the use of vasopressors in any group. Choosing the appropriate dose of spinal anesthesia for the location and duration of surgery is hampered

by wide individual variability in the duration and extent of surgical anesthesia obtained with any given dose of spinal local anesthetic. Techniques that allow for incremental titration of local anesthetic dose (epidural, combined spinal-epidural, and continuous spinal anesthesia) are important options in the care of critically ill patients in whom avoiding hypotension may be an especially important goal.

Severe cardiovascular complications can occur with unplanned systemic administration of local anesthetics. In the early 1980s, cardiac arrest in parturients during epidural anesthesia with 0.75% bupivacaine sensitized practitioners to the adverse hemodynamic effects of local anesthetics and to those of bupivacaine in particular. All local anesthetics are capable of producing hypotension, sinus bradycardia, and cardiovascular depression through their effects on vascular smooth muscle and the cardiac conduction system. The cardiac system is less susceptible than the central nervous system to the toxic effects of local anesthetics. Cardiovascular toxicity caused by bupivacaine differs from that caused by lidocaine in important ways. Bupivacaine is thought to produce cardiac toxicity by binding to sodium channels as rapidly as lidocaine but dissociating much more slowly. The result is accumulation of sodium-channel blockade in the cardiac conduction system, leading to more prominent reentry ventricular arrhythmias, development of torsades de pointes, and prolonged recovery from cardiac toxicity. In addition, the toxicity of bupivacaine is thought to result in part from effects at the brainstem that produce a potent, toxic interaction with the vasomotor centers of the medulla.[68] These characteristics were clinically evident when large doses of bupivacaine were given to parturients, who are especially susceptible to local anesthetic effects and toxicity.[69] Cardiac arrest was the presenting symptom of toxicity, followed by prolonged cardiovascular collapse and refractory arrhythmias.

Another uncommon cardiovascular complication of neuraxial anesthesia was suggested by the reviewers of the American Society of Anesthesiologist closed claims study.[70] In that study, 14 patients who experienced apparently sudden cardiac arrest during otherwise uneventful and hemodynamically stable spinal anesthesia were described. Even though these patients were young and healthy and despite evidence that their caregivers maintained appropriate standards of care, only one of the patients had functional neurologic recovery. The authors commented that "spinal anesthesia conducted under routine conditions and in a standard manner carries a poorly understood potential for sudden cardiac arrest and severe brain injury in healthy patients."[70] Other researchers have implicated respiratory depression, hypoxia, and sedation combined with a lack of vigilance as the cause of neuraxial anesthesia–related cardiac arrest. Subsequent case reports[71,72] described similar sudden cardiac arrests during spinal and epidural anesthesia that were treated without resultant morbidity (Fig. 3-3). Paradoxical Bezold-Jarish reflex—decreased ventricular filling and a vigorously contracting, empty ventricle reflexively triggering an abrupt decrease in heart rate during spinal sympathectomy—was thought to be the cause of these cardiac arrests.

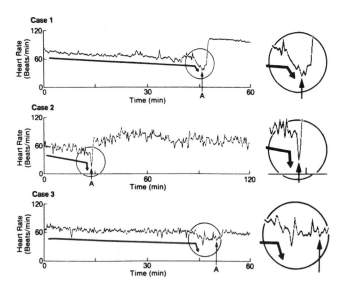

Fig. 3-3. The heart rate patterns of three patients during spinal anesthesia. Although the enlarged trend seems to indicate a sudden event, the entire trend reveals a gradual and progressive decrease in heart rate. (From Brown DL, Carpenter RL, Moore DC: *Anesthesiology* 68:971, 1988 [letter].)

Subsequent large-scale prospective studies of 1050 patients who underwent epidural anesthesia and 952 patients who underwent spinal anesthesia identified risk factors for bradycardia and hypotension during neuraxial anesthesia.[73,74] Risk factors for bradycardia during epidural anesthesia are female sex and use of a tourniquet. During spinal anesthesia, risk factors for bradycardia are a baseline heart rate less than 60 beats/min, American Society of Anesthesiologists physical status I, use of β-adrenergic blocking agents, and sensory block higher than the fifth thoracic dermatome. Risk factors for hypotension during epidural anesthesia are addition of epidural fentanyl, increased spread of sensory blockade, lack of tourniquet use, and use of carbonated lidocaine. During spinal blockade, risk factors for hypotension are sensory block higher than the fifth thoracic dermatome, age older than 40 years, baseline systolic blood pressure less than 120 mm Hg, use of combined spinal and general anesthesia, dural puncture cephalad to the L2-L3 interspace, and addition of phenylephrine to the local anesthetic spinal block. Recognition of these risk factors has focused attention on the importance of continued vigilance in the prevention of cardiovascular complications during neuraxial anesthesia.

3. Neurotoxicity. Neurotoxicity caused by neuraxial local anesthetics occurs rarely in clinical practice, but when it does, it manifests as cauda equina syndrome. Ferguson and Watkins[75] first characterized this syndrome after spinal anesthesia in 1937. They described a diffuse pattern of injury to the lumbosacral nerve roots that produced varying degrees of saddle anesthesia, bowel or bladder dysfunction, and paraplegia. More recently, local anesthetic neurotoxicity was implicated as a cause of cauda equina syndrome on two occasions. In the 1970s, several cases of cauda equina injuries occurred after

spinal administration of large volumes of chloroprocaine intended for the epidural space. Isolated nerve studies eventually implicated 0.2% sodium bisulfite and low pH as the most likely causes of these injuries.[76] Of note, chloroprocaine alone did not produce toxicity in these studies. These findings prompted the creation of the widely used, most current formulation of chloroprocaine containing ethylenediaminetetraacetic acid (EDTA).

More recently, reports of cauda equina syndrome following continuous spinal anesthesia prompted the report of a total of 12 cases in only 2 years. Maldistribution, sacral pooling, and exposure of the vulnerable cauda equina nerve roots to toxic concentrations of hyperbaric local anesthetic was hypothesized to account for these injuries.[77] Lidocaine, usually delivered in large, repeated doses as a 5% hyperbaric solution, was associated with all but one of these cases of cauda equina syndrome. These reports led to the recall of spinal microcatheters smaller than 24 gauge from the U.S. market in 1992.

As was the case with cauda equina syndrome after chloroprocaine administration, cauda equina syndrome following continuous spinal anesthesia heightened concern over local anesthetic neurotoxicity even though another factor (i.e., microcatheters and bisulfite) ultimately became the primary focus of attention. The neurotoxic potential of local anesthetic is a current topic of debate because evidence of lidocaine neurotoxicity has since accumulated. The 5% concentration of lidocaine used clinically has produced toxicity in isolated, desheathed amphibian nerves bathed in preparations in vitro,[78] whereas 1.5% lidocaine has not produced this effect. In addition, use of 5% hyperbaric lidocaine has caused persistent neurologic impairment in permanently catheterized rats, whereas use of 0.75% bupivacaine has not had this result.[79] In glass spinal models, concentrations equal to those producing toxicity in these in vitro studies are attainable even in the absence of a spinal catheter when 5% hyperbaric lidocaine is administered.[80]

The evidence for the toxicity of 5% hyperbaric lidocaine is, however, indirect and may not be clinically relevant. Desheathed amphibian nerves, permanently instrumented rats, and empirically constructed glass spinal models do not faithfully reproduce the clinical conditions in which 5% hyperbaric lidocaine has been used safely for 50 years in millions of patients undergoing spinal anesthesia. Clinically, 5% hyperbaric lidocaine has rarely been associated with toxicity. For example, single cases of cauda equina syndrome have been reported after lidocaine was administered repeatedly through a spinal (20-gauge epidural) macrocatheter[81] and after lidocaine was administered as a single injection through a pencil-point spinal needle.[82] A recent survey of practitioners who performed an estimated total of 40,000 spinal anesthetic procedures suggested an association between 5% hyperbaric lidocaine and toxicity.[31] In this survey, spinal administration of lidocaine was associated more often with permanent nerve injuries than was bupivacaine when placement of the spinal needle or catheter was uncomplicated by paresthesia but neurologic injury occurred.[31]

Investigations of the neurotoxic potential of lidocaine, long considered safe, continue. In the meantime, recommendations for variations in spinal anesthetic technique have been proposed in the hope of reducing maldistribution and local anesthetic neurotoxicity.[77,83] These recommendations include reducing the lidocaine dose to less than 60 mg, avoiding repeat dosing of failed blocks, decreasing the lidocaine concentration to 1.5%, using isobaric spinal solutions, diluting local anesthetic with aspirated cerebral spinal fluid, avoiding spinal epinephrine administration (see later discussion), and substituting bupivacaine for lidocaine whenever possible.

B. Opioids

1. Respiratory depression. As is the case for systemic administration of opioids, neuraxial administration of these substances has been associated with clinically evident respiratory depression. Retrospective surveys and prospective studies have estimated the incidence of respiratory depression at 0.09% to 0.9% for epidural and spinal morphine. These incidences are similar to incidences of 0.5% to 0.9% reported for opioids administered by intravenous patient-controlled analgesia, intramuscularly, and orally.[84] Respiratory depression induced by neuraxial administration of morphine differs qualitatively from that induced by intravenous, intramuscular, or oral administration of morphine. The onset of respiratory depression is bimodal and may be delayed as long as 24 hours after bolus injection of hydrophilic opioids (morphine or hydromorphone).[85] Immediate respiratory depression can occur after neuraxial administration of opioids when the doses are sufficiently large that systemic absorption of opioids can result in high blood concentrations and resultant respiratory depression. Immediate respiratory depression is therefore more common with epidural administration, in which boluses of morphine (up to 6 mg), fentanyl (up to 100 µg), and sufentanil (up to 50 µg) are often equal to therapeutic incremental intravenous doses. Delayed respiratory depression is also an important clinical concern when hydrophilic opioids are administered neuraxially. Six to 12 hours after bolus administration of hydrophilic opioids, cerebral spinal fluid transport cephalad to the ventral medulla produces peak cerebral spinal fluid concentrations of opioid at respiratory centers, resulting in a second peak in the incidence of respiratory depression.[85] As might be expected, immediate respiratory depression has not been described with the small doses of intrathecal hydrophilic opioid used clinically. Similarly, delayed respiratory depression has not been described following bolus administration of the short-acting lipophilic opioids fentanyl and sufentanil. Respiratory arrest after administration of intrathecal lipophilic opioids has been described but has occurred early in recovery while prominent local anesthetic spinal blockade was present.[86] Although large studies are lacking, lipophilic opioids are gaining popularity and have been used safely for outpatient anesthesia.

Several factors have been associated with risk for respiratory depression. The most important risk factor is the administration of an inappropriately large dose of opioid. Location of the epidural catheter, location of the surgical incision, and patient age have been advanced as important considerations in the choice of dose. Although the lipophilic opioids may seem to be a logical choice for

reduction of risk for respiratory depression, postoperative infusions of both lipophilic and hydrophilic opioids have resulted in similar degrees of respiratory depression.[84] Risk for respiratory depression is increased in older patients, those receiving other opioids or sedative hypnotics, those recovering from general anesthesia, those who have coexisting disease, and those who cannot tolerate opioids. Pregnancy and increased concentrations of progesterone may be protective.[85]

Respiratory depression following use of neuraxial opioids is characterized by gradually progressive somnolence and hypercarbia. Although slowing of respiration and a decreasing oxygen saturation have been classically described with delayed respiratory depression, these signs may be absent despite the presence of progressive, significant hypercarbia.[85] Monitoring after neuraxial opioid administration need not include continuous pulse oximetry but should include periodic assessment of sedation to monitor for somnolence along with respiratory rate. Naloxone and oxygen should be readily available for all patients receiving opioids for postoperative pain management; these substances are also effective treatment for the delayed respiratory depression seen with neuraxial opioids. What constitutes a minimum of safe monitoring following small doses of intrathecal or epidural opioids has not been determined. Therefore most institutions assess patients frequently (usually hourly) for as long as 24 hours.[87] Despite the similar incidence of respiratory depression following neuraxial administration of opioids and patient-controlled analgesia, most institutions maintain greater vigilance in monitoring patients who have received neuraxial opioids.

2. Nausea. The incidence of nausea after neuraxial administration of opioids is similar to that of systemic administration and varies clinically depending on agents used (usually a maximum of 30% with morphine and 20% with fentanyl) and the dose administered (usually a minimum of 10% with morphine and 5% with fentanyl).[85] Neuraxial opioids probably produce nausea by interacting with opioid receptors in the area postrema, delaying gastric emptying by a spinal cord opioid receptor–mediated effect and sensitizing the vestibular system to movement.[85] Risk factors for nausea include abdominal surgery and female sex. All known antiemetics have been used to treat nausea following neuraxial administration of opioids. Because many antiemetic agents have sedative properties, they must be used with caution in patients at risk for respiratory depression (see preceding text). As with all side effects complicating neuraxial administration of opioid, opioid receptor antagonists are effective in treatment of nausea but may also reverse analgesia. Small doses of naloxone and the partial agonist-antagonists nalbuphine and butorphanol have been used to treat nausea while preserving analgesia.

3. Pruritus. Pruritus may be the most common complication of neuraxial administration of opioids; it has been described in as many as 100% of obstetric patients receiving intrathecal sufentanil.[88] Pruritus is thought to occur with cephalad migration of neuraxially administered opioid and interaction with opioid receptors of the trigeminal nucleus in the medulla[85] or sensory neurons of the spinal cord,[88] promoting an itch response. Neuraxial opioids, unlike systemically administered opioids, do not promote histamine release. Despite this, antihistamines are commonly used and are often effective in treating pruritus caused by neuraxial opioids. In addition to the opioid receptor antagonists and mixed agonist-antagonists, low-dose propofol has been shown to be effective in the treatment of pruritus, although its mechanism of action is unknown.[89] A sitting posture combined with the addition of dextrose to sufentanil spinal anesthesia can greatly reduce pruritus presumably by limiting cephalad spread of opioid. Unfortunately, like many other treatments of neuraxial opioid complications, this approach also limits the effects of analgesia.[88]

4. Herpes reactivation. Neuraxial opioid administration and pruritus have been associated with reactivation of herpes simplex in pregnant patients. Reactivation of the virus is thought to result from opioid interaction with the trigeminal nucleus or mechanical irritation of sensory nerves in the face in patients with pruritis.[85] Because a high percentage of pregnant patients have peripartum recurrence of herpes simplex, the causal relation between neuraxial administration of opioids and herpes reactivation has been questioned.[90]

5. Urinary retention. The incidence of urinary retention has been difficult to characterize because most patients who have received neuraxial opioids also recover from surgery with urinary catheters. However, studies have suggested that the risk of urinary retention following epidural administration of morphine is approximately 50% in adults[85] and children.[91] Urinary retention is thought to be spinally mediated through opioid receptors. In contrast to the situation with hydrophilic opioids, addition of fentanyl to intrathecal lidocaine has been shown not to prolong recovery and time to urination.[92] Treatment of urinary retention with opioid receptor antagonist or mixed agonist-antagonists has been shown to reduce analgesia.

6. Neurotoxicity. Although some experimental and isolated clinical evidence of opioid-induced neurotoxicity exists, it has not been described in patients who received large doses of intrathecal morphine for prolonged periods.[85] Most opioids used clinically have been experimentally tested in animals that showed no signs of neurotoxicity.[93] Neuraxial administration of opioid formulations containing preservatives have resulted in neurologic injury in humans. Spinal morphine preparations and intravenous fentanyl and sufentanil preparations contain no preservatives, but many medications do contain potentially harmful preservatives.

C. Additive anesthetic agents

1. α₂-Adrenergic receptor agonists. Epinephrine has played an important role in enhancing the safety of neuraxial anesthesia. Epinephrine has been used clinically along with local anesthetics as a marker for intravascular injection, as a vasoconstrictor to limit systemic concentrations of local anesthetic, and as an adjuvant to prolong and enhance neuraxial anesthesia. Epinephrine prolongs both motor and lumbosacral sensory blockade in part by decreasing vascular uptake of local anesthetics. Along with clonidine, it produces antinociception through interaction with spinal α_2-adrenergic receptors.

Despite its role in enhancing safety, epinephrine has been associated with complications. For example, when used as a marker for intravascular injection, epinephrine can produce tachycardia and hypertension with unplanned intravascular administration. A recent analysis of the safety and cost of epinephrine administered as a test dose suggested that this use carries a poor risk-benefit ratio for patients at risk for coronary artery disease.[61] The use of epinephrine as an intravenous test dose has also been debated in obstetric anesthesia, in part because intravenous epinephrine causes a transient, dose-dependent reduction in uterine blood flow.[61] Epinephrine has been implicated as an aggravating factor in neurotoxicity caused by neuraxial local anesthetics[94] and in the reduction of spinal cord blood flow in cases of neurologic injury following spinal anesthesia.[95] However, in most clinical circumstances, the safety features of epinephrine outweigh these risks.

Unlike epinephrine, clonidine lacks prominent α_1- and β-adrenergic receptor activity, is not a marker of intravascular injection, and does not produce tachycardia or hypertension. It produces analgesia without the respiratory depression associated with neuraxial administration of narcotics and the prominent motor block associated with neuraxially administered local anesthetics. Instead, clonidine has been associated with dose-dependent sedation, hypotension, and bradycardia when administered orally, intravenously, epidurally, and intrathecally. These properties act as both assets and complicating factors in the clinical use of clonidine to prolong local anesthetic neuraxial blockade and to provide immediate postoperative analgesia.[96] Currently, clonidine is approved for epidural use for treatment of chronic pain.

Dexmedetomidine, another α_2-adrenergic receptor agonist, is more potent than clonidine and may have a more favorable side effect profile. This agent is currently being evaluated.

2. Cholinergic agents. Neostigmine is currently being evaluated in clinical trials as a promising spinally administered adjuvant to neuraxial blockade with local anesthetics. It provides analgesia by preventing breakdown of the acetylcholine synaptically released in descending analgesic pathways of the spinal cord in response to pain. During investigation in humans, neostigmine has greatly reduced postoperative narcotic requirements in a dose-dependent manner. Although this analgesia is promising, the trade-off has been a high incidence of nausea and vomiting.[97] Although neostigmine is not currently approved for spinal or epidural use, toxicity studies of its commercially available preparation suggest that it is safe for neuraxial use in humans.[98]

3. N-methyl-D-aspartate antagonists. Ketamine and amitriptyline have been used neuraxially in animals, in which their *N*-methyl-D-aspartate–antagonist properties have been shown to prevent hyperalgesia. These agents are not available for clinical use but are undergoing toxicity evaluation because they hold promise for the treatment of chronic pain and for use as preemptive analgesics.[97]

III. CONTROVERSIES IN NEURAXIAL ANESTHESIA–RELATED COMPLICATIONS

A. Lumbar back pain following epidural administration of chloroprocaine

Chloroprocaine with bisulfite and chloroprocaine with EDTA, the two local anesthetics associated most prominently with clinically evident neurotoxicity, have also been associated with clinically troublesome back and radicular pain following their use in neuraxial anesthesia. After chloroprocaine with bisulfite became associated with cauda equina syndrome, manufacturers substituted EDTA as an antioxidant in chloroprocaine formulations marketed in the United States (discussed previously). Reports of severe lumbar back pain, described as a deep, dull burning pain that began as the chloroprocaine epidural block wore off, appeared with use of the new formulation. This pain was severe enough to require epidural fentanyl treatment and lasted for as long as 24 hours. Low-pH commercial solutions, EDTA, skin infiltration with chloroprocaine, and large volumes of chloroprocaine seemed to be associated with this back pain. A prospective study[99] revealed that only EDTA-containing chloroprocaine solutions used in volumes greater than 25 ml were associated with a 60% incidence of lumbar back pain (compared with 0% following epidural anesthesia with lidocaine). The pain was not reduced by adjusting the pH of chloroprocaine solutions and was not associated with the use of chloroprocaine for skin infiltration. The definitive cause of this distinct type of pain remains controversial but may be soon resolved. The recent introduction of a newer formulation of preservative-free chloroprocaine may produce a smaller incidence of back pain than solutions that contain EDTA.

B. Transient neurologic symptoms following spinal administration of lidocaine

Transient neurologic symptoms (also called transient radicular irritation) have been only recently described as a complication of spinal anesthesia.[100] As with back pain associated with chloroprocaine, controversy has surrounded the cause of transient neurologic symptoms. The pain from this condition has been described as back pain with radiation to one or both legs and buttocks. It usually occurs within 24 hours of spinal anesthesia and resolves within 72 hours. Its severity has been rated as 2 to 6 out of 10 on a verbal rating scale.[101] A prospective study[101] found an incidence of 16% following administration of lidocaine and 0% following administration of bupivacaine in spinal anesthesia performed with small-gauge pencil-point spinal needles. The incidence of pain following knee arthroscopy was greater than that following inguinal hernia repair. Stretching of the cauda equina or sciatic nerve roots[101] has been offered as a contributing cause of transient neurologic symptoms, as has arachnoid membrane trauma,[102] musculoskeletal strain,[103] and toxicity from local anesthetic.

The causes of back pain after administration of chloroprocaine and lidocaine are not yet definitively elucidated. Because chloroprocaine and lidocaine have been clinically associated with cauda equina syndrome and because experimental evidence exists for neurotoxic potential of clinically used preparations, it is tempting to conclude that these specific types of back pain are another clinical manifestation of neurotoxicity. At this time, such a conclusion remains speculative and controversial.

C. Platelet function, deep venous thrombosis prophylaxis, and neuraxial techniques

Before surgery, approximately 40% of patients ingest medications that affect platelet function, including aspirin, acetaminophen, and nonsteroidal antiinflammatory drugs (NSAIDs).[104] These medications interfere with clot formation but do not affect prothrombin and partial thromboplastin times. In addition, prophylaxis of deep venous thrombosis in the form of subcutaneous low-dose unfractionated heparin; low-dose oral warfarin; and, most recently, low-molecular-weight heparin is commonly administered. Neuraxial anesthesia is often performed in patients who have received or will receive these medications perioperatively, even though antiplatelet therapy combined with neuraxial anesthesia has been associated with spinal hematoma.[7] Whether this association reflects the ubiquitous use of these medicines and therapies perioperatively or a true risk factor for spinal hematoma remains controversial.

Large case reviews (containing 1000 to 10,000 patients) are reassuring in that no incident of spinal hematoma following therapy with aspirin,[105] NSAIDs,[105] low-dose warfarin,[106] low-dose heparin,[107] or low-molecular-weight heparin[108] combined with neuraxial anesthesia has been found. However, these studies most likely show only that spinal hematoma remains a rare event despite the use of these medications, not necessarily that its incidence is unchanged. For example, two of these studies found an increased incidence of bloody epidural catheter placement and blood-tinged spinal fluid in patients receiving these medications, a finding already implicated as a risk factor for spinal hematoma after full anticoagulation therapy.[7]

Unlike the situation with full anticoagulation with heparin or warfarin, practitioners lack a meaningful monitor of anticoagulation when antiplatelet medications are administered. Although bleeding time is still used clinically, it has been shown to be useless as a screening measure of surgical bleeding[109] and is therefore unlikely to predict spinal hematoma formation in patients given antiplatelet medications. After subcutaneous low-dose heparin is administered, partial thromboplastin times increase in a large number of patients, but the timing of this effect varies greatly.[110] Anti–factor Xa activity can, in theory, be used to measure the anticoagulant effect of low-molecular-weight heparin. However, this test is not readily available, and guidelines for its use are not available at all. Thromboelastography is currently being investigated for use as a measure of platelet function.

Low-molecular-weight heparin preparations (such as enoxaparin) were recently approved for use in the United States, where it is used after total knee and hip arthroplasty beginning 12 hours after surgery but has been approved for preoperative use in abdominal surgery. The manufacturer does not recommend monitoring of anti–factor Xa activity. Since the introduction of low-molecular-weight heparins to the U.S. market in 1993, several cases of spinal hematoma have been reported following neuraxial anesthesia, prompting a recent review and publication of guidelines.[111] At the time of this writing, it seems safest to treat low-molecular-weight heparin with the same respect accorded unfractionated heparin infusions to avoid neuraxial bleeding. The benefits of neuraxial anesthesia should be weighed against the risk for spinal hematoma in the individual patient. Neuraxial anesthesia should be induced before enoxaparin administration, catheters should be removed at the nadir of therapeutic drug effect, spinal anesthesia should be chosen over epidural catheterization when possible, and a high level of vigilance for signs and symptoms of spinal hematoma must be maintained.[112]

D. Complications following thoracic and continuous spinal anesthesia

Compared with lumbar epidural catheterization, thoracic epidural and lumbar continuous spinal catheterization are regarded by some practitioners as inherently more difficult and fraught with complications, even though some basic anesthesia textbooks omit discussion of their safety and efficacy. The benefits of these two techniques are beyond the scope of this discussion. However, their safety has been the focus of several recent reviews. A retrospective and prospective study of more than 4000 patients[34] found that accidental dural puncture was the most common complication of thoracic epidural anesthesia, with a rate of 0.7%. This incidence not only confirmed previous experience with thoracic epidural catheterization but also produced an incidence of accidental dural puncture that was less than or equal to that found for lumbar epidural anesthesia in similar university teaching settings. Zero of 30 accidental dural punctures resulted in neurologic injury or PDPH, confirming our own anecdotal experience that PDPH is rare after thoracic dural puncture with epidural needles. Radicular paresthesia occurred with block placement in 0.5% of instances of thoracic anesthesia and resolved with needle or catheter removal. Postoperative nerve lesions were discovered in 0.6% of patients (adults who had been intravenously sedated) and consisted of peripheral nerve lesions (usually peroneal) not related to these paresthesias or to thoracic epidural anesthesia.

In contrast, thoracic epidural anesthesia has been safely induced in pediatric patients under general anesthesia. In a recent survey of more than 24,000 pediatric patients younger than 12 years of age who underwent regional anesthesia, thoracic epidural anesthesia was not associated with complications despite the concurrent use of general anesthesia for block placement in 89%.[113]

Unlike the situation for thoracic epidural anesthesia compared with lumbar epidural anesthesia, continuous spinal anesthesia has been associated with a greater incidence of postoperative complications than lumbar epidural anesthesia. The most serious of these complications was seen after the introduction of continuous spinal anesthesia 28-gauge microcatheters to the U.S. market. Four case reports of cauda equina syndrome[114] combined with reports to the U.S. Food and Drug Administration led to the 1992 recall of all microcatheters smaller than 24 gauge. As discussed, the local anesthetic agent used (5% hyperbaric lidocaine) in most of these cases of cauda equina syndrome has been implicated in the pathophysiology of this complication. Continuous spinal anesthesia with microcatheters (outside the United States) and macrocatheters (20-gauge epidural catheters) has been performed and has been subject to evaluation since 1992. Continuous spinal anesthesia seems to result in a higher incidence of difficulty in placing catheters spinally and in achieving adequate surgical anesthesia. Such technical problems have occurred with as many as 12% of microcatheter continuous spinal anesthetics.[112] In contrast, macrocatheters seem to reduce technical difficulties. In a university teaching program, a 100% rate of success was achieved with use of macrocatheters.[49] However, 6% of continuous spinal anesthetics required staff expertise to overcome technical difficulties in placing the needle or catheter, and 18% required a change in local anesthetic or baricity to achieve surgical anesthesia after placement.

The most common complication following continuous spinal anesthesia is PDPH. This condition has been reported to occur in approximately 1% of patients when groups including patients older than 65 years of age are examined.[49] In contrast, as many as 24% of obstetric patients have reported PDPH severe enough to require an epidural blood patch despite the use of microcatheters for continuous spinal anesthesia.[115] Studies of complications following continuous spinal anesthesia have been fewer and have included smaller numbers of patients than those examining spinal or epidural anesthesia. However, two of the largest trials of continuous spinal anesthesia revealed an approximate 0.5% incidence of persistent paresthesia after continuous spinal anesthesia using a macrocatheter technique.[49,115] This incidence seems to be much higher than that for other neuraxial techniques already discussed (1:2000, or 0.05%). This greater incidence of neurologic complications may be attributable to increased trauma during a technically difficult procedure, cumulative local anesthetic toxicity from a continuous technique, and selection of sicker patients at greater risk for postoperative nerve injury.

Despite the greater incidence of technical difficulty, PDPH, and persistent neurologic injury, we use continuous spinal anesthesia. We choose macrocatheters to minimize technical difficulties, choose patients older than 65 years of age to minimize the risk for postdural puncture headache, and choose clinical situations in which the benefit of a limited, dense spinal anesthetic clearly outweighs the risk for nerve injury.

IV. CONCLUSION

Our understanding of the complications associated with neuraxial anesthesia has grown greatly since Bier and Hildebrandt experienced the first postdural puncture headache. Along with this understanding has grown the popularity of neuraxial techniques and the application of these techniques to an increasingly broad segment of patients. Today, the practitioner of neuraxial anesthesia requires the knowledge to avoid rare, serious complications in critically ill patients and common, minor complications in healthy young outpatients. It is perhaps this latter population that represents the greatest challenge for the future.

REFERENCES

1. Standl T, Eckert S, Schulteam Esch J: Postoperative complaints after spinal and thiopentone-isoflurane anaesthesia in patients undergoing orthopaedic surgery: spinal versus general anaesthesia, *Acta Anaesthesiol Scand* 40:222, 1996.
2. Jellish WS, Thajil Z, Stevenson K, et al: A prospective randomized study comparing short- and intermediate perioperative outcome variables after spinal or general anesthesia for lumbar disk and laminectomy surgery, *Anesth Analg* 83:559, 1996.
3. Cooke J: Hemorrhage into the cauda equina following lumbar puncture, *Proc Path Soc Phil* 14:104, 1911.
4. Vandermeulen EP, Van Aken H, Vermylen J: Anticoagulants and spinal-epidural anesthesia, *Anesth Analg* 79:1165, 1994.
5. Tryba M: Epidural regional anesthesia and low molecular heparin: Pro, *Anasthesiol Intensivmed Notfallmed Schmerzther* 28:179, 1993.
6. Ruff RL, Dougherty JH Jr: Complications of lumbar puncture followed by anticoagulation, *Stroke* 12:879, 1981.
7. Foo D, Rossier AB: Preoperative neurological status in predicting surgical outcome of spinal epidural hematomas, *Surg Neurol* 15:389, 1981.
8. Rao TL, El-Etr AA: Anticoagulation following placement of epidural and subarachnoid catheters: an evaluation of neurologic sequelae, *Anesthesiology* 55:618, 1981.
9. Baron HC, LaRaja RD, Rossi G, et al: Continuous epidural analgesia in the heparinized vascular surgical patient: a retrospective review of 912 patients, *J Vasc Surg* 6:144, 1987.
10. Liem TH, Booij LH, Hasenbos MA, et al: Coronary artery bypass grafting using two different anesthetic techniques: Part 1: hemodynamic results, *J Cardiothorac Vasc Anesth* 6:148, 1992.
11. Gerancher JC, Waterer R, Middleton J: Transient paraparesis after postdural puncture spinal hematoma, *Anesthesiology* 86:490, 1997.
12. Solymosi L, Wappenschmidt J: A new neuroradiologic method for therapy of spinal epidural hematomas, *Neuroradiology* 27:67, 1985.
13. Ferguson JF, Kirsch WM: Epidural empyema following thoracic extradural block: case report, *J Neurosurg* 41:762, 1974.
14. Scott DB, Hibbard BM: Serious non-fatal complications associated with extradural block in obstetric practice, *Br J Anaesth* 64:537, 1990.
15. Kee WD, Jones MR, Thomas P, et al: Extradural abscess complicating extradural anaesthesia for caesarean section, *Br J Anaesth* 69:647, 1992.
16. Carp H, Bailey S: The association between meningitis and dural puncture in bacteremic rats, *Anesthesiology* 76: 739, 1992.
17. Teele DW, Dashefsky B, Rakusan T, et al: Meningitis after lumbar puncture in children with bacteremia, *N Engl J Med* 305:1079, 1981.
18. Goodman EJ, DeHorta E, Taguiam JM: Safety of spinal and epidural anesthesia in parturients with chorioamnionitis, *Reg Anesth* 21:436, 1996.
19. Shapiro ED, Aaron NH, Wald ER, et al: Risk factors for development of bacterial meningitis among children with occult bacteremia, *J Pediatr* 109:15, 1986.
20. Du Pen SL, Peterson DG, Williams A, et al: Infection during chronic epidural catheterization: diagnosis and treatment, *Anesthesiology* 73:905, 1990.
21. Hughes SC, Dailey PA, Landers D, et al: Parturients infected with human immunodeficiency virus and regional anesthesia: clinical and immunologic response, *Anesthesiology* 82:32, 1995.
22. Goucke CR, Graziotti P: Extradural abscess following local anaesthetic and steroid injection for chronic low back pain, *Br J Anaesth* 65:427, 1990.
23. Cousins M, Bridenbaugh P: *Neural blockade in clinical anesthesia and management of pain*, ed 2, Philadelphia, 1988, JB Lippincott.
24. James FM, George RH, Naiem H, et al: Bacteriologic aspects of epidural analgesia, *Anesth Analg* 55:187, 1976.
25. Abouleish E, Amortegui AJ: Millipore filters are not necessary for epidural block, *Anesthesiology* 55:604, 1981 (letter).
26. Driver RP Jr, Snyder IS, North FP, et al: Sterility of anesthetic and resuscitative drug syringes used in the obstetric operating room, *Anesth Analg* 86:994, 1998.
27. Birnbach DJ, Stein DJ, Murray O: Povidone iodine and skin disinfection before initiation of epidural anesthesia, *Anesthesia* 88:668, 1998.
28. Borum SE, McLeskey CH, Williamson JB, et al: Epidural abscess after obstetric epidural analgesia, *Anesthesiology* 82:1523, 1995.
29. Vandam L, Dripps R: Long-term follow-up of 10,098 spinal anesthetics. II. Incidence and analysis of minor sensory neurological defects, *Surgery* 38:463, 1955.
30. Horlocker TT, McGregor DG, Matsushige DK: A retrospective review of 4767 consecutive spinal anesthetics: central nervous system complications: Perioperative Outcomes Group, *Anesth Analg* 84:578, 1997.
31. Auroy Y, Narchi P, Messiah A, et al: Serious complications related to regional anesthesia: results of a prospective survey in France, *Anesthesiology* 87:479, 1997.
32. Kroll DA, Caplan RA, Posner K, et al: Nerve injury associated with anesthesia, *Anesthesiology* 73:202, 1990.
33. Sarna MC, Smith I, James JM: Paraesthesia with lumbar epidural catheters: a comparison of air and saline in a loss-of-resistance technique, *Anaesthesia* 45:1077, 1990.
34. Giebler RM, Scherer RU, Peters J: Incidence of neurologic complications related to thoracic epidural catheterization, *Anesthesiology* 86:55, 1997.
35. Horlocker TT, Cabanela ME, Wedel D: Does postoperative epidural analgesia increase the risk of peroneal nerve palsy after total knee arthroplasty? *Anesth Analg* 79:495, 1994.
36. Norris MC, Leighton BL, DeSimone CA: Needle bevel direction and headache after inadvertent dural puncture, *Anesthesiology* 70:729, 1989.
37. Tourtellotte WW, Henderson WG, Tucker RP, et al: A randomized, double-blind clinical trial comparing the 22 versus 26 gauge needle in the production of the post-lumbar puncture syndrome in normal individuals, *Headache* 12:73, 1972.
38. Lynch J, Arhelger S, Krings-Ernst I: Postdural puncture headache in young orthopaedic inpatients: comparison of a 0.33 mm (29-gauge) Quincke-type with a 0.7 mm (22-gauge) Whitacre spinal needle in 200 patients, *Acta Anaesthesiol Scand* 36:657, 1992.
39. Neal JN, Bridenbaugh LD, Mulroy MF, et al: Instance of postdural puncture headache is similar between 22 g, Greene and 26 g Quincke spinal needles, *Anesthesiology* 71:A678, 1989 (abstract).
40. Devcic A, Sprung J, Patel S, et al: PDPH in obstetric anesthesia: comparison of 24-gauge Sprotte and 25-gauge Quincke needles and effect of subarachnoid administration of fentanyl, *Reg Anesth* 18:222, 1993.
40a. Buettner J, Wresch KP, Klose R: Postdural puncture headache: comparison of 25-gauge Whitacre and Quincke needles, *Reg Anesth* 18:166, 1993.
41. Lambert DH, Hurley RJ, Hertwig L, et al: Role of needle gauge and tip configuration in the production of lumbar puncture headache, *Reg Anesth* 22:66, 1997.
42. Kang S, Lee Y, Graf J: Comparison of 25-g Whitacre, 27-g Whitacre, and 27-g Quincke needles for spinal anesthesia for ambulatory surgery patients, *Anesthesiology* 79:A33, 1993 (abstract).
43. Dittmann M, Schaefer RG, Renkl F, et al: Spinal anesthesia with 29 gauge Quincke point needles and postdural puncture headache in 2,378 patients, *Acta Anaesthesiol Scand* 38:691, 1994.
44. Neal J: Postdural puncture headache: prevention and treatment, *Prog Anesthesiology* 8:222, 1994.
45. Fog J, Wang LP, Sundberg A, et al: Hearing loss after spinal anesthesia is related to needle size, *Anesth Analg* 70:517, 1990.
46. Scott DB, Dittmann M, Clough DG, et al: Atraucan: a new needle for spinal anesthesia, *Reg Anesth* 18:213, 1993.
47. Celleno D, Capogna G, Costantino P, et al: An anatomic study of the effects of dural puncture with different spinal needles, *Reg Anesth* 18:218, 1993.
48. Bell E: Decreased incidence of postdural puncture headache in morbidly obese parturients following continuous spinal anesthesia using 17 gauge Tuohy needle, Society of Obstetrical Anesthesia and Perinatology 40th Annual Meeting:A85, 1997 (abstract).

49. Van Gessel E, Forster A, Gamulin Z: A prospective study of the feasibility of continuous spinal anesthesia in a university hospital, *Anesth Analg* 80:880, 1995.

50. Tarkkila PJ, Miralles JA, Palomaki EA: The subjective complications and efficiency of the epidural blood patch in the treatment of postdural puncture headache, *Reg Anesth* 14:247, 1989.

51. Abouleish E, Vega S, Blendinger I, et al: Long-term follow-up of epidural blood patch, *Anesth Analg* 54:459, 1975.

52. Loeser EA, Hill GE, Bennett GM, et al: Time vs. success rate for epidural blood patch, *Anesthesiology* 49:147, 1978.

53. Szeinfeld M, Ihmeidan IH, Moser MM, et al: Epidural blood patch: evaluation of the volume and spread of blood injected into the epidural space, *Anesthesiology* 64:820, 1986.

54. Colonna-Romano P, Shapiro B: Prophylactic epidural blood patch in obstetrics, *Anesthesiology* 69:A665, 1988 (abstract).

55. Blanche R, Eisenach JC, Tuttle R, et al: Previous wet tap does not reduce success rate of labor epidural analgesia, *Anesth Analg* 79:291, 1994.

56. Hodgson C, Roitberg-Henry A: The use of sumatriptan in the treatment of postdural puncture headache, *Anaesthesia* 52:808, 1997 (letter).

57. Macarthur AJ, Macarthur C, Weeks SK: Is epidural anesthesia in labor associated with chronic low back pain? A prospective cohort study, *Anesth Analg* 85:1066, 1997.

58. Seeberger MD, Lang ML, Drewe J, et al: Comparison of spinal and epidural anesthesia for patients younger than 50 years of age, *Anesth Analg* 78:667, 1994.

59. Verniquet AJ: Vessel puncture with epidural catheters: experience in obstetric patients, *Anaesthesia* 35:660, 1980.

60. Colonna-Romano P, Lingaraju N, Braitman LE: Epidural test dose: lidocaine 100 mg, not chloroprocaine, is a symptomatic marker of iv injection in labouring parturients, *Can J Anaesth* 40:714, 1993.

61. Mulroy MF, Norris MC, Liu SS: Safety steps for epidural injection of local anesthetics: review of the literature and recommendations, *Anesth Analg* 85:1346, 1997.

62. Moore JM, Liu SS, Neal JM: Premedication with fentanyl and midazolam decreases the reliability of intravenous lidocaine test dose, *Anesth Analg* 86:1015, 1998.

63. Ben-David B, Vaida S, Gaitini L: The influence of high spinal anesthesia on sensitivity to midazolam sedation, *Anesth Analg* 81:525, 1995.

64. Knill RL: Cardiac arrests during spinal anesthesia: unexpected? *Anesthesiology* 69:629, 1988.

65. Furst SR, Reisner LS: Risk of high spinal anesthesia following failed epidural block for cesarean delivery, *J Clin Anesth* 7:71, 1995.

66. Riley ET, Cohen SE, Rubenstein AJ, et al: Prevention of hypotension after spinal anesthesia for cesarean section: six percent hetastarch versus lactated Ringer's solution, *Anesth Analg* 81:838, 1995.

67. Buggy D, Higgins P, Moran C, et al: Prevention of spinal anesthesia-induced hypotension in the elderly: comparison between preanesthetic administration of crystalloids, colloids, and no prehydration, *Anesth Analg* 84:106, 1997.

68. Thomas RD, Behbehani MM, Coyle DE, et al: Cardiovascular toxicity of local anesthetics: an alternative hypothesis, *Anesth Analg* 65:444, 1986.

69. Clarkson CW, Hondeghem LM: Mechanism for bupivacaine depression of cardiac conduction: fast block of sodium channels during the action potential with slow recovery from block during diastole, *Anesthesiology* 62:396, 1985.

70. Caplan RA, Ward RJ, Posner K, et al: Unexpected cardiac arrest during spinal anesthesia: a closed claims analysis of predisposing factors, *Anesthesiology* 68:5, 1988.

71. Liguori GA, Sharrock NE: Asystole and severe bradycardia during epidural anesthesia in orthopedic patients, *Anesthesiology* 86:250, 1997.

72. Mackey DC, Carpenter RL, Thompson GE, et al: Bradycardia and asystole during spinal anesthesia: a report of three cases without morbidity, *Anesthesiology* 70:866, 1989.

73. Curatolo M, Scaramozzino P, Venuti FS, et al: Factors associated with hypotension and bradycardia after epidural blockade, *Anesth Analg* 83:1033, 1996.

74. Carpenter RL, Caplan RA, Brown DL, et al: Incidence and risk factors for side effects of spinal anesthesia, *Anesthesiology* 76:906, 1992.

75. Ferguson FR, Watkins KH: Paralysis of the bladder and associated neurological sequelae of spinal anaesthesia (cauda equina syndrome), *Br J Surg* 25:735, 1937.

76. Wang BC, Hillman DE, Spielholz NI, et al: Chronic neurological deficits and Nesacaine-CE: an effect of the anesthetic, 2-chloroprocaine, or the antioxidant, sodium bisulfite? *Anesth Analg* 63:445, 1984.

77. Drasner K: Lidocaine spinal anesthesia: a vanishing therapeutic index? *Anesthesiology* 87:469, 1997.

78. Lambert LA, Lambert DH, Strichartz GR: Irreversible conduction block in isolated nerve by high concentrations of local anesthetics, *Anesthesiology* 80:1082, 1994.

79. Drasner K, Sakura S, Chan VW, et al: Persistent sacral sensory deficit induced by intrathecal local anesthetic infusion in the rat, *Anesthesiology* 80:847, 1994.

80. Beardsley D, Holman S, Gantt R, et al: Transient neurologic deficit after spinal anesthesia: local anesthetic maldistribution with pencil point needles, *Anesth Analg* 81:314, 1995.

81. Drasner K, Rigler ML, Sessler DI: Cauda equina syndrome following intended epidural anesthesia, *Anesthesiology* 77:582, 1992.

82. Gerancher JC: Cauda equina syndrome following a single spinal administration of 5% hyperbaric lidocaine through a 25-gauge Whitacre needle, *Anesthesiology* 87:887, 1997.

83. Carpenter RL: Hyperbaric lidocaine spinal anesthesia: do we need an alternative? *Anesth Analg* 81:1125, 1995 (editorial).

84. Mulroy MF: Monitoring opioids, *Reg Anesth* 21(6 suppl):89, 1996.

85. Chaney MA: Side effects of intrathecal and epidural opioids, *Can J Anaesth* 42:891, 1995.

86. Cornish PB: Respiratory arrest after spinal anesthesia with lidocaine and fentanyl, *Anesth Analg* 84:1387, 1997.

87. Rawal N, Allvin R: Epidural and intrathecal opioids for postoperative pain management in Europe: a 17-nation questionnaire study of selected hospitals: Euro Pain Study Group on Acute Pain, *Acta Anaesthesiol Scand* 40:1119, 1996.

88. Gage JC, D'Angelo R, Miller R, et al: Does dextrose affect analgesia or the side effects of intrathecal sufentanil? *Anesth Analg* 85:826, 1997.

89. Borgeat A, Wilder-Smith OH, Suter PM: The nonhypnotic therapeutic applications of propofol, *Anesthesiology* 80:642, 1994.

90. Abouleish E: Intrathecal morphine as a cause for herpes simplex should be scratched out, *Anesthesiology* 75:919, 1991.

91. Dalens B, Tanguy A, Haberer JP: Lumbar epidural anesthesia for operative and postoperative pain relief in infants and young children, *Anesth Analg* 65:1069, 1986.

92. Liu S, Chiu AA, Carpenter RL, et al: Fentanyl prolongs lidocaine spinal anesthesia without prolonging recovery, *Anesth Analg* 80:730, 1995.

93. Sabbe MB, Grafe MR, Mjanger E, et al: Spinal delivery of sufentanil, alfentanil, and morphine in dogs: physiologic and toxicologic investigations, *Anesthesiology* 81:899, 1994.

94. Hashimoto K, Nakamura Y, Hampl K: Epinephrine increases the neurotoxic potential on intrathecally administered local anesthetic in the rat, *Anesthesiology* 85:A770, 1996 (abstract).

95. Rowlingson JC: Toxicity of local anesthetic additives, *Reg Anesth* 18:453, 1993.

96. Eisenach JC, De Kock M, Klimscha W: α_2-Adrenergic agonists for regional anesthesia: a clinical review of clonidine (1984-1995), *Anesthesiology* 85:655, 1995.

97. Eisenach JC: Three novel spinal analgesics: clonidine, neostigmine, amitriptyline, *Reg Anesth* 21:81, 1996.

98. Eisenach JC, Hood DD, Curry R: Phase I human safety assessment of intrathecal neostigmine containing methyl- and propyl-parabens, *Anesth Analg* 85:842, 1997.

99. Stevens RA, Urmey WF, Urquhart BL, et al: Back pain after epidural anesthesia with chloroprocaine, *Anesthesiology* 78:492, 1993.

100. Schneider M, Ettlin T, Kaufmann M, et al: Transient neurologic toxicity after hyperbaric subarachnoid anesthesia with 5% lidocaine, *Anesth Analg* 76:1154, 1993.

101. Pollock JE, Neal JM, Stephenson CA, et al: Prospective study of the incidence of transient radicular irritation in patients undergoing spinal anesthesia, *Anesthesiology* 84:1361, 1996.
102. Dahlgren N: Reply 2, *Acta Anesthesiol Scand* 40:864, 1996.
103. Naveira FA, Copeland S, Anderson M, et al: Transient neurologic toxicity after spinal anesthesia, or is it myofascial pain? Two case reports, *Anesthesiology* 88:268, 1998.
104. Horlocker TT, Wedel DJ, Offord KP: Does preoperative antiplatelet therapy increase the risk of hemorrhagic complications associated with regional anesthesia? *Anesth Analg* 70:631, 1990.
105. CLASP: A randomized trial of low-dose aspirin for the prevention and treatment of preeclampsia among 9364 pregnant women: CLASP (Collaborative Low-Dose Aspirin Study in Pregnancy) Collaborative Group, *Lancet* 343:619, 1994.
106. Odoom JA, Sih IL: Epidural analgesia and anticoagulant therapy: experience with one thousand cases of continuous epidurals, *Anaesthesia* 38:254, 1983.
107. Lowson SM, Goodchild CS: Low-dose heparin therapy and spinal anesthesia, *Anaesthesia* 44:67, 1989 (letter).
108. Bergqvist D, Lindblad B, Matzsch T: Low molecular weight heparin for thromboprophylaxis and epidural/spinal anesthesia: is there a risk? *Acta Anaesthesiol Scand* 36:605, 1992.
109. Rodgers RP, Levin J: A critical reappraisal of the bleeding time, *Semin Thromb Hemost* 16:1, 1990.
110. Cooke ED, Lloyd MJ, Bowcock SA, et al: Letter: monitoring during low-dose heparin prophylaxis, *N Engl J Med* 294:1066, 1976.
111. Horlocker TT, Heit JA: Low molecular weight heparin: biochemistry, pharmacology, perioperative prophylaxis regimens, and guidelines for regional anesthetic management, *Anesth Analg* 85:874, 1997.
112. Standl T, Eckert S, Schultz E: Microcatheter continuous spinal anaesthesia in the post-operative period: a prospective study of its effectiveness and complications, *Eur J Anaesthesiol* 12:273, 1995.
113. Giaufre E, Dalens B, Gombert A: Epidemiology and morbidity of regional anesthesia in children: a one-year prospective survey of the French-language society of Pediatric Anaesthesiologists, *Anesth Analg* 13:904, 1996.
114. Rigler ML, Drasner K, Krejcie TC, et al: Cauda equina syndrome after continuous spinal anesthesia, *Anesth Analg* 72:275, 1991.
115. Horlocker TT, MacGregor DG, Matsushige DK: Neurologic complications of 603 consecutive continuous spinal anesthetics using macrocatheter and microcatheter techniques: Perioperative Outcomes Group, *Anesth Analg* 84:1063, 1997.

Chapter 4

Complications of Nerve Blocks

Quinn H. Hogan
Stephen E. Abram

Perhaps no area of anesthesiology creates as passionate a controversy as does the choice between regional and general anesthesia. Arguments for the preferential use of regional anesthesia (instead of general anesthesia or in combination with it) emphasize diminished interference with circulatory and pulmonary function and beneficial influences on stress responses induced by extensive surgery. Detractors of regional anesthesia point out that modern general anesthesia can be safely administered to almost any patient and emphasize the risks of regional blocks. A balanced decision ultimately requires an appreciation of the nature and frequency of adverse outcomes from regional anesthesia. The calculation of risks and benefits is particularly critical when blocks are added to general anesthesia because this subjects the patient to the risks of both techniques.

The potential adverse outcomes associated with general and regional anesthesia differ qualitatively. Complications during general anesthesia (e.g., ventilatory failure or myocardial ischemia) are often at least in part due to the patient's coexisting disease and can be considered inevitable risks of anesthesia. With nerve blocks, complications (e.g., nerve injury or seizure) are in most cases the direct consequence of the actions of the anesthesiologist and therefore present a much more daunting responsibility. A further burden for anesthesiologists who perform nerve blocks is the still-common notion among physicians and patients that because general anesthesia is free of risk (except when bungled), why should one be subjected to the clear risk for needle-induced injury to nerves, vessels, and organs? This relative risk can be put into perspective by the information in other chapters in this book.

The most obvious and common complication of nerve block anesthesia is its failure, which often results in the patient being exposed to further risk. Additional blocks may be attempted, causing systemic concentrations of local anesthetic to increase further. Deeper sedation might be produced by supplementation with intravenous and inhaled drugs in an attempt to salvage an inadequate block, putting the patient at risk for hemodynamic and ventilatory complications,[1-3] especially if he or she has already been positioned in such a way that monitoring or airway management is impeded. Ultimately, the risks of general anesthesia might be added to those to which the patient was exposed during the failed block, increasing the total risk. In these ways, a failed block can initiate a sequence of events that generate further complications.

We first discuss the pathogenic mechanisms of complications during nerve blocks, after which each type of block is considered individually. Complications of spinal and epidural block are discussed in Chapter 3.

I. PATHOLOGIC PROCESSES INVOLVED IN COMPLICATIONS OF NERVE BLOCKS

A. Toxicity of injected solution

The goal of injection of local anesthetic is reversible neural dysfunction. The response is considered toxic if function fails to fully return. The rarity of neural injury after nerve block procedures demonstrates the safety of applying local anesthetics to nerves. It has become clear, however, that local anesthetics deviate from the defined ideal and may cause prolonged functional and structural changes in nerves and surrounding tissue. Local anesthetics produce various cytotoxic effects in cell cultures, including inhibition of cell growth, motility, and survival, as well as morphologic changes.[4] The extent of these effects is proportional to the length of time that the cells are exposed to the anesthetic solution (Fig. 4-1) and can occur with the usual clinical concentrations of local anesthetic concentrations. Cytotoxic changes are greater as concentrations of anesthetic increase (see Fig. 4-1). It is not clear how to extrapolate the pattern of these findings from cell cultures to that of nerves in vivo. The inhibition of cell growth and division in fibroblast cultures, however, may have direct relevance as the mechanism by which local anesthetics impede healing when injected into a wound.[5,6]

Myonecrosis caused by clinical concentrations of local anesthetics[7] has been recognized since 1959[8] and is characteristic of all local anesthetics that have been tested. Epinephrine and steroids intensify the effect of local anesthetics, which produces immediate, irreversible, and complete destruction of adult myocytes.[9] The molecular event that triggers myocyte toxicity from local anesthesia is a nonspecific increase in sarcoplasmic reticulum permeability to Ca^{2+} because of a direct action of local anesthetics on Ca^{2+}-release channels. This precipitates pathologic efflux of Ca^{2+} from the sarcoplasmic reticulum of mature myocytes into the myoplasm, resulting in cell death. Immature myocytes and neural elements lack an internal Ca^{2+} reservoir and are therefore spared. These cells regenerate new muscle, which is typically complete in 2 weeks. This action on Ca^{2+} channels takes place at local anesthetic concentrations typical of those found in tissue at the site of injection. A lower concentration, such as that which may circulate during an accidental intravenous local anesthetic injection, is unlikely to trigger this response. However, cocaine intoxication has been associated with malignant hyperpyrexia,[10,11] a condition with a cellular pathophysiology akin to that previously described.

Although experimental evidence for the widespread occurrence of myocyte toxicity following local anesthetic injection is convincing, clinically significant problems are only rarely recognized (Fig. 4-2). This may be in part because of the difficulty of examining deep sites of injection (e.g., psoas muscle), as well as rapid and complete recovery by the patient. Discomfort and dysfunction after injections performed for surgical anesthesia may be concealed by surgical pain. Inflammation develops only after 3 or 4 days, and atrophy takes longer to appear; thus

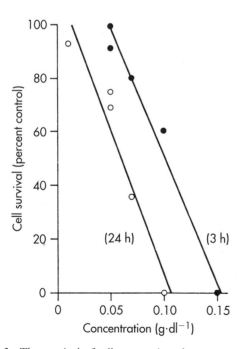

Fig. 4-1. The survival of cells grown in culture expressed as a percentage of control. Survival diminishes with increasing bupivacaine concentration and duration of exposure (in hours). (From Sturrock JE, Nunn JF: *Br J Anaesth* 51:273, 1979.)

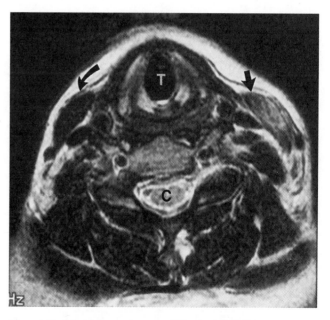

Fig. 4-2. Magnetic resonance (T2-weighted fast spin echo) axial image at the level of the sixth cervical vertebra of a patient who received repeated interscalene injections of bupivacaine for postoperative pain. An enlarged left sternocleidomastoid muscle *(straight arrow)* is evident, showing increased signal intensity compared with the normal right sternocleidomastoid muscle *(curved arrow)*. Biopsy revealed myonecrosis that probably was due to local anesthetic toxicity. *C,* Cord; *T,* trachea.

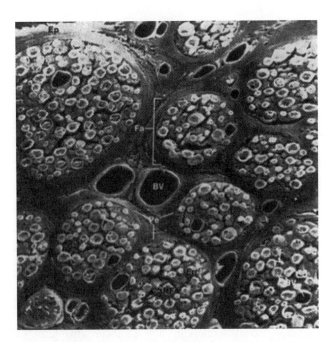

Fig. 4-3. The anatomy of a peripheral nerve as revealed by scanning electron microscopy. The nerve fibers *(NF)* are grouped into fascicles *(Fa)* by a perineural sheath *(Pe)*. Between and around the fascicles is the epineural connective tissue *(Ep)*. Blood vessels *(BV)* are found in the epineural tissue and in the endoneural space *(En)*, the area enclosed by perineurium. (From Kessel RG, Kardon RH: *Tissue and organs,* New York, 1979, WH Freeman.)

these events may be missed or not correlated to administration of anesthetic agents. There may be therapeutic efficacy for local anesthetic myotoxicity. Local anesthetic injection for treatment of trigger points in patients with myofascial pain may be effective through the generation of new muscle after destruction of diseased muscle.

Nerves may undergo cytotoxic changes following in vivo exposure to clinically used concentrations of local anesthetics. The exact site of deposition of the anesthetic plays an important role in determining the pathogenic potential of the drug. The outermost layer of a peripheral nerve, the epineurium (Fig. 4-3), is made of loose connective tissue in continuity at the intervertebral foramen with the dura of the nerve root. Within this inert supporting tissue, the individual axons are organized into fascicles by a surrounding sheath, the perineurium. The endoneurium within the fascicles provides the connective tissue between the axons. The perineurium includes multiple layers of metabolically active epithelium that control the endoneural milieu in the same manner as the pia-arachnoid does for the central nervous system.[12] By providing a diffusion barrier, the endothelium of the endoneural vessels and the perineurium act as a blood-nerve barrier for the fascicles.

After extrafascicular application of local anesthetics, the regulatory function of the perineurial and endothelial blood-nerve barrier is subtly compromised. The normally hypertonic endoneural fluid becomes hypotonic with the accumulation of edema, increased perineural permeability, and increased fluid pressures within the fascicles.[13] In addition, local anesthetics block fast axonal transport of cellular constituents,[14] probably through loss of axonal microtubules.[15] Inflammatory changes and injury to myelin and Schwann cells have been identified.[13,16,17] Greater concentrations of anesthetics produce axonal injury independent of edema formation and elevated endoneurial fluid pressure.[18] Ester local anesthetics may be somewhat more prone than amides to producing these changes,[16] although this idea is not supported by more recent data.[19] Local anesthetic–induced decrease in nerve blood flow may potentiate these direct cytotoxic effects.[20,21]

As with the effects of local anesthetics in cell cultures, the duration of exposure[22] and concentration of local anesthetic[23] is important in determining the incidence of local anesthetic-induced residual paralysis. The contribution of these changes after extrafascicular injections to clinical cases of nerve injury has not been determined, but it is prudent to use only the minimum necessary local anesthetic concentration. Because small-fiber neurons are more sensitive to chemical damage, the manifestations of nerve damage caused by local anesthetic include spontaneous paresthesias and deficits in pain and temperature perception but not loss of motor, touch, or proprioceptive function.[24]

There is less doubt about the clinical importance of neurotoxicity caused by local anesthetic when the drug is injected intrafascicularly (Fig. 4-4). Although axonal degeneration and a damaged blood-nerve barrier are inconsistent[25] or absent[26] after intrafascicular injection of saline alone, injection of lidocaine, 1%, and bupivacaine, 0.5%, results in evidence of axonal degeneration and barrier changes. Findings worsen progressively with increasing concentrations of both agents, especially when concentrations exceed the clinically used range.[25,26] Ester local anesthetics and carbonated lidocaine produce widespread and severe damage of nerve fibers and blood-nerve barriers when injected within the fascicles.[26] This evidence leads to the conclusion that the surrounding perineurium plays an important role in protecting the fascicular contents from the cytotoxic effects of local anesthetics.

In humans, nerve conduction studies may show neuropathy after intraneural injection of local anesthetics even in the absence of symptoms.[27] This disorder may emerge 1 week or more after the injection; thus it may not appear until well past the anesthesiologist's postoperative visit.

Intrathecal injection of local anesthetics anatomically resembles intrafascicular peripheral injection because the axons of the nerve roots are enclosed by only a frail and discontinuous pial layer.[28] Substances in the cerebrospinal fluid have ready access to the neural elements of the roots,[29] and awareness of the hazards of depositing high concentrations of local anesthetic into the subarachnoid space is increasing. These concerns are highlighted by the recent recognition in clinical settings that local anesthetics, particularly lidocaine, injected through

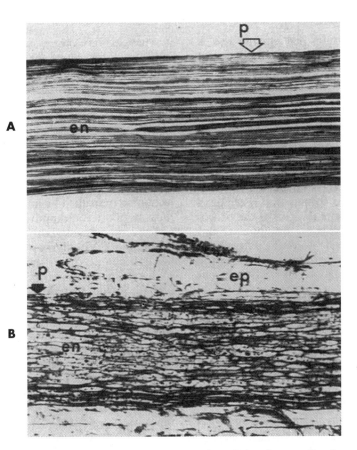

Fig. 4-4. A, Normal appearance of a peripheral nerve (longitudinal section). **B,** Twelve days after the intraperineurial injection of 0.5% bupivacaine with epinephrine, 5 μg/ml, the axons are fragmented and partially digested by Schwann cells. *en,* Endoneural space; *ep,* epineural connective tissue; *p,* perineurium. (From Selander D, Brattsand R, Lundborg G, et al: *Acta Anaesthesiol Scand* 23:127, 1979.)

very small intrathecal catheters can produce injury to the nerve roots of the cauda equina.[30,31] The catheter does not contribute directly to injury, but with a limited rate of injection, anesthetic solutions layer in high concentrations instead of mixing in the cerebrospinal fluid and becoming dilute.[32] Neural injury has been observed after spinal injection simply through a needle.[33] (This topic is discussed in greater detail in Chapter 3.)

More recently, further concern about local anesthetic toxicity has been raised by the description of transient radicular irritation in up to 40% of patients after spinal anesthesia.[34,35] This condition is frequently diagnosed following lidocaine injection but is rarely associated with bupivacaine use[34,35] and may follow injected doses of lidocaine as dilute as 2%.[36] The incidence of transient radicular irritation is not changed by reduction[37] or elimination[38] of glucose from lidocaine solutions. Cases of this condition have also been reported following spinal anesthesia with tetracaine[39] and mepivacaine.[40] It remains to be proved, however, that these events are actu-

ally associated with neural injury. The diagnosis of transient radicular irritation rests on back pain with radiation into the buttocks or legs, which is typical of deep somatic axial pain without nerve root involvement. No study has shown neural dysfunction in the many patients considered to have transient radicular irritation. Furthermore, the type of procedure strongly influences the frequency of this type of pain.[38] The generally low rate of neurotoxic injury during spinal anesthesia is evident in large reviews,[41,42] in which temporary sensory changes are found in about 1 in 1000 patients and permanent neurotoxic changes occur in about 1 in 20,000 patients.

Although animal models of intrathecal injection of local anesthetic have failed to show consistent changes in nerve structure, extensive functional impairment may occur even when the nerves retain a normal histologic appearance.[22,23] The mechanism of root injury from local anesthetic has not been fully resolved. Irreversible injury is evident after brief exposure to undiluted lidocaine, bupivacaine, and tetracaine at clinical concentrations,[43] and higher concentrations produce greater toxicity.[44] Consistent with clinical observations, lidocaine seems to have greater potential for toxicity than bupivacaine or tetracaine,[45] and its toxicity is potentiated by the addition of epinephrine.[46] Neurons are not killed because the resting membrane potential is intact after injury despite the inability to conduct an action potential.[38] The injury is not related to high concentrations of dextrose[43,47] and is not produced by blockade of voltage-gated sodium ion channels.[48] Injury to the spinal cord may also contribute to the generation of the cauda equina syndrome after local anesthetic injection.[23,49]

Additives to local anesthetic solutions may cause neuropathologic changes. Most notable is the injury caused by sodium bisulfite, an antioxidant added to preparations of chloroprocaine. In combination with low pH solutions, sodium bisulfite has a pronounced neurotoxic effect when administered intrathecally[50,51]; it is therefore no longer available in this formulation. Peripheral nerves seem to be more tolerant of the neurotoxic effects of bisulfite.[52] Bisulfite is also present in local anesthetic solutions containing epinephrine that is added before packaging. Even though no reports have implicated this mixture in a neurotoxic complication, it is probably best to avoid bisulfite by adding fresh epinephrine to the local anesthetic at the time of block administration.

The addition of epinephrine has been shown to increase the neurotoxicity of bisulfite-containing chloroprocaine solutions[16] and to increase the axonal degeneration that follows intrafascicular injection of bupivacaine.[25,26] Nerve blood flow, especially in the large epineural feeding arteries, is sensitive to the vasoconstrictive effect of injected epinephrine at usual clinical concentrations.[20] Because of these issues, epinephrine should be added to local anesthetic solutions only if prolongation of the block cannot be achieved by use of a different local anesthetic or if maximal doses have been used and systemic toxicity may result. Chlorocresol, an antimicrobial preservative added to multiuse vials, is neurotoxic and should not be used in nerve block solutions.

The general safety of local anesthetics has been demonstrated by years of safe clinical use. Rare complications can most often be attributed to circumstances in which nerves are exposed to high concentrations of drug for prolonged periods, such as repeated peripheral application or inadequate dilution of a large intrathecal dose of anesthetic. Additional factors, such as needle trauma or additives in the injected solution, or preexisting factors, such as diabetic vascular compromise,[53] may boost the manifestations of toxicity from the usual subclinical changes to a clinically relevant event.

B. Mechanical nerve damage

Injury to the nerve during needle insertion for nerve block anesthesia is an unavoidable risk. The interruption of the perineural tissue around the nerve fascicles breaches the blood-nerve barrier and produces edema of the nerve and herniation of the endoneural contents through the rent (Fig. 4-5). Fascicular injury is more likely to result from nerve contact with sharp-beveled needles than with a blunt-beveled needle[54]; likewise, a fine needle can be expected (e.g., 25-gauge) to penetrate the nerve more frequently than a larger (22-gauge) needle will. Needle-tip penetration of the nerve may not itself be the cause of clinical complications.[27,55] No functional change is evident in humans after the passage of a needle into the ulnar nerve if local anesthetic is not injected intraneurally.[27] In rats, no changes were observed in microscopic anatomy or in adequacy of diffusion barriers within the nerve after penetration of the fascicle with a needle and injection of saline solution[26] despite

the creation of intrafascicular pressures that transiently exceeded the nerve capillary perfusion pressure.[56] Nonetheless, the placement of a needle within a nerve is a source of concern because subperineurial injection of local anesthetic is likely to result in axonal degeneration.[25] Any injection accompanied by intense, lancinating pain must be aborted promptly.

The consequences of eliciting paresthesias during block procedures is not known. When the needle impinges on the nerve, some degree of nerve injury may occur, but this has not been proved. A clinical study by Selander, Edshage, and Wolff[57] contains the most pertinent information about paresthesias during nerve blocks. Symptomatic nerve lesions were apparent after surgery in 2.8% of patients in whom paresthesias were sought during axillary block and in 0.8% of patients in whom the injection was made on either side of the artery. However, close to half of the patients in whom a paresthesia was not sought nonetheless had one. The difference between the groups was not statistically significant, even though only patients who experienced paresthesias developed postblock neuropathy. It must be noted, however, that epinephrine was used uniformly in the paresthesia group but in only half of the artery group; in addition, sharp-pointed needles were used in all patients. In contrast, a study conducted in a nontraining situation[58] found that 3 of 835 patients (0.36%) who underwent brachial plexus block (done with the intention of producing paresthesia) developed postblock neuropathy. All three patients had multiple paresthesias during the block. A prudent approach would include the use of blunt needles

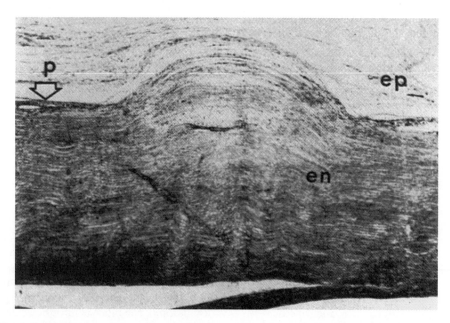

Fig. 4-5. Herniation of the endoneural contents through needle puncture of the perineurium. *en,* Endoneural space; *ep,* epineural connective tissue; *p,* perineurium. (From Selander D, Brattsand R, Lundborg G, et al: *Acta Anaesthesiol Scand* 23:127, 1979.)

and a gentle technique. If paresthesia is provoked, injection at this site should be done with no further needle advancement or with a slight withdrawal of the needle. Injection should be stopped immediately if it initiates or intensifies paresthesia. Seeking multiple paresthesias may be accompanied by an increased incidence of neuropathy because the initial deposit of local anesthetic may conceal needle contact with nerves. It is usually unwise to attempt a major nerve block in a patient who is unable to report a paresthesia, such as those who are deeply sedated or under general anesthesia.[59]

When catheters are left in close proximity to peripheral nerves for repeated dosing, irritation of the nerves may ensue. This complication is revealed when the pain subsides on removal of the offending catheter[60] and is rarely reported with modern catheters and cautious insertion.

Many investigators have advised against nerve blocks in confined fascial spaces, such as the ulnar nerve at the elbow or the peroneal nerve at the fibular head. There is concern that neuropathy is more likely to occur after these blocks either because of the pressure that develops in the enclosed space on injection of the anesthetic solution or because the nerve is fixed in position and is unable to recede from the encroaching needle. However, evidence of increased risk is generally lacking.

Other sources of neuropathy must be considered when evaluating nerve injury after a nerve block. Tourniquets may cause nerve damage either by ischemia or mechanical deformation. Distortion of the nerve under the tourniquet (Fig. 4-6) is the more likely mechanism of prolonged nerve dysfunction; even when ischemic periods last as long as 6 hours, ischemia alone fails to produce lasting structural changes in nerves,[61] and nerve function returns within 6 hours if the duration of ischemia is less than 2 hours.[62] However, the portion of the nerve under the proximal edge of the pneumatic cuff, where the mechanical distortion of the nerve is maximal, may suffer irreversible damage after 2 to 4 hours of tourniquet inflation.[63] Nerve damage can be minimized by using wide cuffs and inflation pressures that are just adequate for arterial occlusion[64] and by keeping inflation times as brief as possible. Alternating between the two cuffs of a double-cuff tourniquet may allow prolonged ischemia with diminished mechanical damage to the nerves because neither site is compressed for more than 1 hour.[65] With this arrangement, ischemic changes, such as tissue edema and sensory deficits, occur but resolve within 3 weeks, and permanent changes are rare. Large fibers represent the neural components that are most susceptible to both ischemic and mechanical damage. The main manifestations of tourniquet-induced neuropathy are motor loss and a diminished sense of touch, vibration, and position; preserved senses of heat, cold, and pain; and absence of spontaneous paresthesias.[66]

Special care must be used to avoid positioning injuries after nerve blocks because an anesthetized limb may be malpositioned without resulting pain. The most common upper-extremity injuries that result from malpositioning are ulnar damage, caused by direct pressure on the nerve at the elbow, and brachial plexus injury, caused by prolonged stretching of the plexus. Tension on the brachial plexus occurs when the arm is abducted excessively (more than 90 degrees) and is further increased by extension of the shoulder.[67] The most frequent lower-extremity injury caused by malpositioning is common peroneal nerve damage, which results from direct pressure over the fibular head. Other causes of postoperative neuropathy include deficits that predate the surgery, sur-

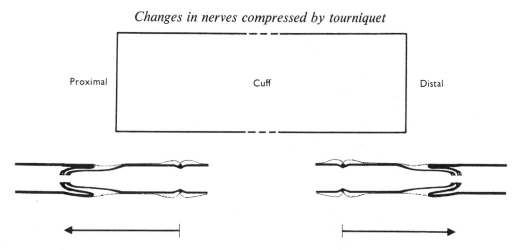

Changes in nerves compressed by tourniquet

Fig. 4-6. Nerve injury from tourniquets represented diagrammatically, showing maximal deformation at the margins of a tourniquet. A pressure gradient is created *(arrows),* causing intussusception of the node of Ranvier into the adjacent perinodal myelin sheath. (From Ochoa J, Fowler TJ, Gilliat RW: *J Anat* 113:433, 1972.)

gical injuries, and compression from compartment syndromes or casts. These considerations make careful pre-block neurologic examination of the limb imperative. If a neurologic deficit develops, early consultation with specialists for detailed neurologic and electrophysiologic diagnosis should be considered.

II. MISCELLANEOUS COMPLICATIONS RELATED TO PERFORMANCE OF NERVE BLOCKS
A. Systemic complications from local anesthetics

The physician must give close attention to the prevention of adverse systemic responses to the local anesthetic injected during nerve blocks. These blocks may be chosen to avoid the perceived greater risk of general anesthesia or major neuraxial block or may be performed away from the operating room for therapeutic or diagnostic purposes. The result may be a lessened expectation of systemic sequelae and a diminished preparedness to treat an adverse response. However, when large doses of local anesthetic are administered for nerve blocks, the patient must be monitored as attentively as he or she would be with general, spinal, or epidural anesthetic. In addition, resuscitation equipment and drugs must be immediately available.

In the setting of nerve blocks, toxic reactions may result early from intravascular injection of the drug or may be delayed until an extravascular bolus is absorbed. Many of the major nerves are in the vicinity of large vessels. Because failure to aspirate blood from the block needle does not ensure that the injectate will not enter a vessel, injection should proceed slowly and incrementally to allow the identification of intravascular injection before the full dose is administered. For example, if 30 ml of 1.5% lidocaine is to be injected, 6 ml might be injected at a time, with a wait of perhaps 1 minute between injections.

The peak serum concentration of local anesthetic and the likelihood of a resulting toxic response vary according to the dose of drug and site of injection.[68] Serum concentrations of anesthetic after intercostal blocks are the highest, probably because the drug is distributed throughout a large area by multiple small injections at different intercostal spaces and because the tissue is highly vascular. In contrast, the deposition of the same dose in a single mass, as with a lumbar sympathetic or celiac block, diminishes the exposure of the drug to absorption. Placement of the anesthetic solution into a sheathed enclosure or a fatty and minimally vascular tissue plane, as with brachial plexus blocks or sciatic-femoral blocks, results in the lowest blood concentration of anesthetic, provided that the injection is administered outside of the vessels.

The addition of epinephrine to local anesthetic solutions diminishes the peak blood concentration after nerve block procedures.[69] This effect is greatest with mepivacaine, prilocaine, and lidocaine, especially when these agents are used for intercostal and paracervical administration. Blood concentrations of etidocaine and bupivacaine after epidural block are not greatly affected by the addition of epinephrine, whereas most studies found a substantial diminution of plexus and peripheral nerve blocks with these drugs (although this effect was not as pronounced as that seen with the shorter-acting amides). The benefit of epinephrine for reducing blood concentrations of anesthetic must be weighed against the potential for increased neurotoxicity, as described earlier.

Although peak blood concentrations of local anesthetic are usually reached by 20 minutes after injection, it is important to realize that peak concentrations may occur up to 60 minutes after the injection.[69]

Because the performance of a nerve block may be stressful to patients,[24] sedation is commonly used. Benzodiazepines have been shown to increase the blood concentration of local anesthetic required to cause central nervous system toxicity[70,71] and would thus seem to protect the patient. Preventing central nervous system manifestations may, however, delay the discovery of blood concentrations of anesthetic high enough to cause cardiovascular toxicity, the threshold for which is not raised by benzodiazepines. More important, the early signs of toxicity require communication with the patient to elicit perceptions, such as circumoral numbness, dizziness, and tinnitus, as well as changes in speech and mental status. Identification of paresthesias also requires a responsive patient. For these reasons, aggressive sedation should be avoided in most nerve block procedures; the goal is a comfortable but responsive patient.

If local anesthetic is introduced into the arterial circulation of the brain, central nervous system toxicity can be prompt and profound. As little as 0.5 ml of 0.5% bupivacaine can cause a seizure if it is injected into the vertebral artery.[72,73] Other events may include loss of consciousness, transient blindness, aphasia, or hemiparesis.[74,75] The greatest risk for direct cerebrovascular administration of local anesthetics is through the vertebral or carotid arteries during blocks of the stellate ganglion, brachial plexus, and cervical plexus. However, it has been demonstrated in baboons that retrograde arterial flow can deliver local anesthetic to the brain arterial supply from forcible injections into the lingual, brachial, and femoral arteries.[76] Cardiopulmonary collapse after dental neural blockade may be due to passage of anesthetic through these routes.[77]

B. Vascular complications during nerve blocks

Because major vessels are often close to the desired target of the nerve block needle, vascular punctures are impossible to avoid with certainty. In most cases, such punctures are innocuous. Indeed, some techniques use the penetration of a major artery as the landmark to ensure effective needle placement, as in the transarterial technique of axillary brachial plexus blockade[78] and the transaortic technique of celiac plexus blockade.[79] Nonetheless, various complications may result from vascular punctures. Of greatest importance is the intravascular deposition of a portion of the injectate, causing high blood concentrations of local anesthetic and systemic toxicity. Direct toxicity to the vessels rarely results with a properly chosen injectate, but intraarterial injection of solutions with epinephrine may produce a transient vasospasm of the large arteries of the limb[80,81] and the microvasculature of the nerves, producing a sharp decrease in nerve blood flow.[82] Compartment syndromes have been reported when directly toxic solutions have been mistakenly injected during nerve block in the place of the desired local anesthetic solution.[83] Even when epinephrine is injected extravascularly, its action on distal terminal arteries may cause ischemia and tissue loss[84] and should be avoided at such sites as the digits, penis, ears, and, perhaps, the nose and ankle, depending on the adequacy of the patient's circulation.

The injection of solution into closed fascial spaces, such as the axillary sheath, may transiently produce intrasheath pressures greater than the mean arterial pressure.[85] In a similar manner, development of a carotid bruit may signal the compression of the vessel after an interscalene bolus injection.[86] There is no evidence that this mechanism produces vascular compromise. However, circulatory disturbance may result from vessel damage by the block needle. Case reports have documented the development of artery occlusion from subintimal administration of local anesthetic[87] and formation of pseudoaneurysm,[88,89] as well as venous narrowing and aneurysm formation after axillary block.[90] The absence of vascular occlusive complications in large series of regional anesthetics indicates that these complications are rare.[91] This optimistic view must be tempered by the knowledge that these problems may appear weeks after the block, making their incidence difficult to ascertain. The formation of hematomas after nerve blocks is well recognized.[24,92] Vascular punctures are common during nerve blockade, but hematomas are infrequent and are usually harmless, although they may occasionally contribute to nerve damage.[24]

The avoidance of vessel injury requires the use of needles no larger than 22 gauge. Insertion of the needle must be deliberate and gentle so as to penetrate vessels as few times as possible. A technique should be adopted in which the needle is advanced only in the axis of its shaft and is never moved laterally within the body, a movement that may cause lacerations from the needle tip. Redirection of the needle should take place only after the needle is withdrawn to the skin. When possible, firm pressure should be placed on the puncture site after blockade to minimize bleeding, especially if blood has been aspirated during the procedure. By comparing the patient's vital signs and vascular status after the block to those noted before the block, problems can be promptly identified and treated. Therapy for bleeding usually consists only of pressure to the area, but early surgical consultation may avoid tissue loss.

Anticoagulation presents a difficult decision for the physician considering nerve block injection. In the presence of full heparinization, nerve blocks may lead to problematic bleeding,[93] and other options should be chosen if possible. Heparin after nerve blockade is frequently administered without ill effects. However, one case report[94] implicated heparin administered after a subclavian perivascular brachial plexus block as a causative factor in the development of a hemothorax. Many patients undergoing nerve blocks have altered platelet function caused by nonsteroidal antiinflammatory drugs, such as aspirin. Although this is probably not a con-

traindication to nerve blocks in general, a rational approach would include careful consideration of the expected benefits of the nerve block; the relative desirability of alternative techniques; and other associated risk factors, such as anemia, vascular disease, and frail tissues that might exacerbate problems from vascular punctures. Blocks at sites where extravasation can be monitored directly and compression can be applied create less of a risk than blocks in which bleeding may not be apparent, such as celiac or intercostal blocks. A measurement of bleeding time may be useful in deciding whether to proceed. An even more uncertain relative contraindication is the use of small doses of subcutaneous heparin for pulmonary embolism prophylaxis. No simple rule can be applied as a substitute for a balanced judgment based on the nature of the block, the patient, and the disease.

C. Pulmonary complications

Any insertion of a needle into the chest or neck may lead to damage of the visceral pleura, initiating a slow leakage of air from the pulmonary parenchyma. Fear of causing pneumothorax discourages many anesthesiologists from using these blocks. However, this may be an overreaction. The incidence of pneumothorax in most studies is very low (as is enumerated in later discussions of individual blocks). The risk for pneumothorax accompanying the placement of an interpleural catheter is uncertain because studies differ greatly in their results. Obtaining a chest roentgenogram after such procedures as intercostal, supraclavicular, and stellate blocks is not necessary in most situations. Because the small needles used for nerve blocks cause slow leaks, a developing pneumothorax is likely to be missed by chest roentgenography done soon after the block. Six to 12 hours may elapse before intrapleural air accumulates and symptoms arise. In addition, because it is not necessary to treat small, asymptomatic pneumothoraces,[95] their discovery may be irrelevant. However, when a needle procedure in the chest is followed by chest pain, coughing, or shortness of breath, chest roentgenography should be done. With pneumothorax, physical examination may show hyperresonance or loss of breath sounds on the side where the procedure was done. The presence of subcutaneous emphysema is strong evidence of pneumothorax. Even less commonly, the chest may fill with blood from needle damage to an intercostal[93] or subclavian[94] artery or with chyle from damage to the thoracic duct.[96]

To minimize the risk for pneumothorax after nerve blocks, large needles and repeated deep probing should be avoided, and care should be used in patient selection. Agitated or coughing patients or those with emphysema are at increased risk for pneumothorax. General anesthesia may occasionally be administered after a block done by using needles near the pleura, perhaps after a failed block. In these cases, it is best to avoid the use of positive-pressure ventilation and nitrous oxide, both of which may expand any pneumothorax present. The bilateral use of blocks that carry a risk for pneumothorax is usually unwise. If patients are to be discharged home within 12 hours of a nerve block, procedures with a minimal risk for pneumothorax are desirable. For example, an epidural block may be a better choice than intercostal blocks, or an axillary block may be preferred to a supraclavicular block.

When pneumothorax is identified, treatment will depend on the extent of the lung collapse and the patient's condition. In the most common situation, collapse is less than 25% of the lung volume and reinflation is likely to be spontaneous. If the patient is not in distress, care should be conservative, with repeated chest roentgenography to confirm the lack of progression and attentive monitoring of the patient's condition. Larger accumulations are less likely to resolve,[97] especially when more than 50% of the lung has collapsed, and a surgeon should be consulted about placement of a chest tube. Discussion with the surgeon should include the fact that pulmonary air leaks caused by block needles are slow, and aggressive therapy with large thoracostomy tubes should therefore be tempered. If hemodynamic collapse follows a nerve block procedure near the lungs, a tension pneumothorax must be suspected, especially if the neck veins are distended and the trachea is deviated to the side opposite that in which the block was performed. On some occasions, the rapid onset of a cardiopulmonary crisis may preclude the performance of chest roentgenography. In this setting, decompression of the pneumothorax by passage of a large intravenous catheter in the second intercostal space at the midclavicular line may save the patient's life.

The proper expansion of the lungs depends on a complex interaction of diaphragm, intercostal, abdominal, and accessory muscle mechanics.[98] Interference with the motor nerves driving these muscles produces subtle deficits in mechanics that are well tolerated in healthy persons. Bilateral intercostal blocks from T6 to T12 result only in the minor loss in peak expiratory flows and endurance with no deficit in resting lung volumes or vital capacity.[99] The loss of a single phrenic nerve also produces changes in respiratory performance that are tolerable to most otherwise fit persons, as was shown in studies of phrenic paralysis after brachial plexus blocks above the clavicle in which the diaphragm was immobile but the patients were asymptomatic.[100-103] In healthy volunteers, only a slight increase in respiratory rate and decrease in partial pressure of blood oxygen is noted.[104] Healthy persons typically experience a 30% decrease in forced vital capacity and forced expiratory volume in 1 second,[105,106] even when efforts are made to limit block of the phrenic nerve by digital pressure above the site of injection[107] or by limitation of anesthetic dose.[108] Bilateral phrenic block can be expected to be less innocuous. Although a minimal change in tidal volume is seen after bilateral phrenic blocks in healthy volunteers and the decrease in vital capacity is reported to be similar to that after unilateral interscalene injection,[109] bilateral blockade is rarely indicated.

Even the unilateral loss of respiratory muscle activity is not always harmless, as case reports of respiratory distress after intercostal blocks[110,111] and brachial plexus blocks in the neck have shown.[112,113] Advanced emphysema is accompanied by flattening of the diaphragm and expansion of the anteroposterior dimensions of the chest, which diminish the ability of the diaphragm to expand the chest.[114] Because ventilation in patients with this condition is especially dependent on intercostal activity, they may be more susceptible to the adverse effects of intercostal paralysis. Decrements in ventilatory function after intercostal block are greatest in patients with preexisting pulmonary disease.[108]

Ventilatory motor interference should be considered a possibility whenever dyspnea follows a nerve block administered in the neck or an intercostal block. Unlike pneumothorax, ventilatory motor interference usually begins within 1 or 2 hours of the procedure. Phrenic block during interscalene injection develops either because of misplacement of the local anesthetic anterior to the anterior scalene muscle, which separates the phrenic nerve from the plexus, or, more commonly, because of the spread of anesthetic cephalad to the roots of C3 to C5. Confirmation of phrenic paresis requires radiographic or ultrasonographic examination. The frequency with which asymptomatic phrenic paresis is identified after brachial plexus blocks in the neck depends on the thoroughness of the radiologic study. Routine roentgenography showed phrenic involvement in 10% to 36% of patients,[101,115] whereas other studies showed incidences of 67% when fluoroscopy was used[102] and 80% when inspiratory and expiratory chest roentgenograms were compared.[100] Ultrasonography used to detect paradoxical diaphragm motion shows that all patients receiving intercostal blockade have phrenic paralysis.[116] Because diaphragm weakness is so common after these blocks, the real value in obtaining a chest roentgenogram is elimination of the alternative diagnosis of pneumothorax.

The risk for ventilatory motor block can be minimized by careful patient selection, cautious technique, use of solutions of anesthetic no more concentrated than necessary for an adequate result, and avoidance of the bilateral use of such blocks, especially those that carry the risk for phrenic block. The therapy for this complication is supplemental oxygen administration and ventilatory support until the motor block has resolved.

D. Undesired extension of blockade

Minute amounts of local anesthetic are needed to achieve a thorough block when the drug is placed in the immediate vicinity of the targeted axons. For example, 1 ml of 1% lidocaine produces a block when placed within the ulnar nerve of humans.[117] The requirement for doses of 5 to 60 ml for the various nerve blocks is attributable to the need to deliver the drug to the target nerve without requiring the perfection of needle placement that minimal doses would demand. For single nerves, such as the lateral femoral cutaneous nerve, an injection of 5 or 10 ml allows delivery from a pool of anesthetic by diffusion and bulk flow. For many blocks, large volumes are needed to reach nerves at a distance from the needle. Paratracheal stellate block anesthetizes the ganglion that resides at the T1 level by means of a needle placed at C6. Brachial plexus block at any level requires an adequate volume of injectate to reach the multiple components of the plexus; likewise, celiac block uses the bulk flow of a large injected volume to reach the entirety of the ganglion. Problems arise because the drug also travels to undesired destinations, causing blockade of neural components with pathologic as well as therapeutic consequences.

The long list of case reports in which local anesthetic reached unintended nerves proves the axiom, "If it can go wrong, it will," illustrated by the following examples.

Subarachnoid injection, often with a resulting total spinal anesthetic, may follow retrobulbar block,[118-120] brachial plexus block,[121-123] facet joint injection,[124] or intercostal block, especially when administered by the intrathoracic route during surgery.[125-129] In many of these patients, the presentation was cardiac arrest. In addition, postural headaches were reported in 3 of 24 patients receiving one or more thoracic paravertebral somatic nerve blocks; these were probably caused by dural puncture.[130]

Epidural spread of anesthetic can result from brachial plexus block,[131-134] intercostal block,[135] segmental somatic blocks[136] (Fig. 4-7), facet injections,[137,138] and injections at some distance from the neuraxis, such as femoral nerve blocks, especially if catheters are advanced from the site of entry.[139]

Spread to the paravertebral sympathetic chain may follow brachial plexus block[140] or intercostal block.[141-143] Spread to the contralateral sympathetic chain may occur during stellate ganglion block.[144] In contrast, somatic blockade can develop with injections of the lumbar sympathetic chain[145] (Fig. 4-8) or the cervicothoracic sympathetic chain.[146]

Finally, undesired peripheral nerve blocks may result from injection at other sites.[147-149]

Misplacement of needles may contribute to these undesired outcomes, as when an improperly angled needle enters a cervical neural foramen during interscalene block. However, accurate needle placement may still result in undesired blocks. Several pathways of undesired anesthetic effect are possible. As Macintosh and Mushin showed in 1947,[150] the paravertebral spaces communicate with the

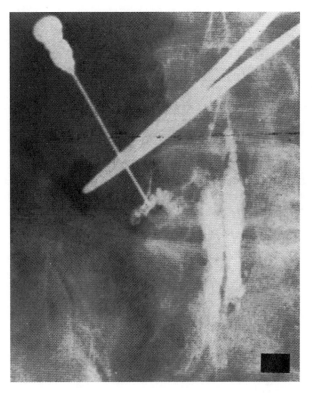

Fig. 4-7. Injection of a nerve root (in this case, the fifth lumbar) may not be selective unless small volumes of anesthetic are used. Spread of the drug to the epidural space is seen in this roentgenogram. (From Krempen JS, Smith B, DeFreest LJ: *Orthop Clin North Am* 6:311, 1975.)

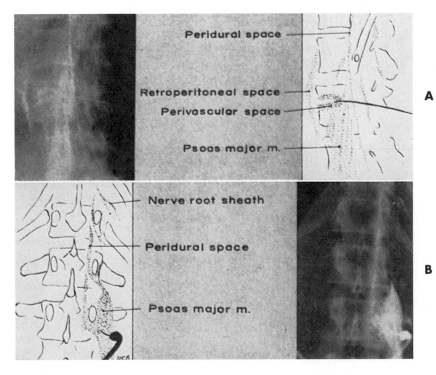

Fig. 4-8. Lateral (**A**) and posteroanterior (**B**) views of epidural spread of injectate after a lumbar paravertebral sympathetic block. Injections designed to produce differential blockade of the sympathetic nerves must be interpreted with caution because of the possibility of spillover into somatic nerves. (From Evans JA, Dobben GD, Gay GR: *JAMA* 200:93, 1967.)

epidural space (see Fig. 4-7) and with each other. In addition, the intercostal space allows passage of drugs into the paravertebral space.[151] By such communicating tissue planes, in other parts of the body as well, bulk flow of anesthetic may lead to blockade of undesired neural elements.

Passage of local anesthetic into the cerebrospinal fluid produces an extensive response. The common explanation is that drug injected into an extension of the subarachnoid space passes centrally through the neural foramen in the cerebrospinal fluid of the dural sleeve. It is certain that these extensions exist because they can be seen on myelography.[152] However, the usual termination of the subarachnoid space is at the dorsal root ganglion in or medial to the intervertebral foramen.[153] A more likely pathway leading to spinal anesthesia during peripheral nerve blocks is intraneural injection.[154,155] When injectate is introduced into the epineurium of peripheral nerves, only a localized bleb forms.[56] In contrast, when a solution is injected into a fascicle within a nerve, extensive subperineurial spread results, and the injectate eventually reaches the subpial and subarachnoid spaces (Fig. 4-9). The nerve fascicle is thus topographically an extension of the central nervous system, and it is fortunate that nerve fascicles are entered with difficulty.[27] When

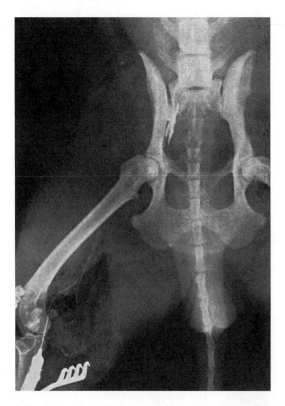

Fig. 4-9. Contrast medium injected into the endoneural space of a peripheral nerve in a dog. The medium flows proximally to the plexus and appears in the subarachnoid space and passes distally in another fascicle after rupture in the plexus. (From French JD, Strain WH, Jones GE: *J Neuropathol Exp Neurol* 7:47, 1948.)

spinal anesthesia results from a nerve block, the onset typically occurs within minutes of the injection.[59] It is important to realize, however, that the transit of local anesthetic to the cerebrospinal fluid may require 15 to 30 minutes, allowing delayed development of total spinal anesthesia.[155] Proper treatment of this event requires prompt ventilatory and hemodynamic support.

Because of the impossibility of limiting the spread of local anesthetics to the desired nerves only, the results of diagnostic nerve block procedures should be interpreted with caution. For example, the epidural spread of anesthetic injected into facet joints and near segmental nerves is common (see Fig. 4-7), as is the spread from sympathetic blocks to somatic nerves and vice versa. If a pain mechanism is diagnosed on the basis of a block that is in fact more extensive than is believed, inappropriate therapeutic procedures might be performed, including surgical ablations. This concern should encourage the use of small volumes of anesthetic when blocks are done for diagnosis.

E. Infections

The site of needle insertion for nerve blocks rarely becomes infected, although such cases have been reported after pudendal and paracervical blocks for obstetric procedures.[156,157] The low incidence of this complication may be in part attributable to the broad antimicrobial activity of local anesthetics.[158] As with many of the other complications of nerve blocks, because infections are rare and unexpected, the possibility might not be considered and early signs may be missed. Puncture sites should always be examined on subsequent days after a procedure for signs of inflammation.

F. Fetal complications

Obstetricians use pudendal and paracervical blocks to provide analgesia for labor and delivery. The advantage to the obstetrician is that specialized anesthesia training is not required for the use of these procedures. Paracervical block provides analgesia for uterine contractions and cervical dilatation, whereas pudendal block provides analgesia for perineal and vaginal distention.

Pudendal block is considered a safe and effective method of providing analgesia for vaginal delivery. The tissues injected are more vascular than the epidural space, and peak local anesthetic blood concentrations may be somewhat higher than those found in epidural analgesia. In addition, injection is generally performed close to delivery, when maternal blood concentrations of drug are near their peak. Despite the potential for fetal local anesthetic toxicity, reports of adverse reactions (either fetal or maternal) are rare, and blood concentrations of local anesthetic in the fetus are considerably lower than those seen in the mother.[159] Merkow et al[159] were unable to demonstrate substantial neurobehavioral depression among infants delivered after pudendal blocks with mepivacaine, chloroprocaine, or bupivacaine.

Paracervical block, in contrast, is associated with a large incidence of fetal bradycardia, ranging from 2% to 70%.[160] The incidence is related to the dose of local anesthetic. Although it has been postulated that the phenomenon may be caused by changes in uterine tone or blood flow, most of the evidence points to high fetal blood concentration of anesthetic as the cause.[161] Fetal concentrations of local anesthetic that exceed those in maternal blood have been documented,[161] leading to postulates that direct diffusion of drug into the uterine artery may occur. Direct uterine arterial injection and injection directly into the presenting part of the fetus may also occur with this block, leading to profound fetal toxicity or death.

III. COMPLICATIONS OF NEUROLYTIC BLOCKS

Ethanol and phenol are the agents used most extensively to produce neurolytic neural blockade. Alcohol causes extraction of phospholipids, cholesterol, and cerebrosides and precipitation of lipoproteins and mucoproteins.[162] The neurolytic effect of phenol is mainly the result of protein denaturation. When these drugs are administered in proximity to peripheral nerves, they cause axonal damage that results in wallerian degeneration. Less severe damage can result in local demyelination, producing a temporary neural deficit that recovers over days to weeks. Injury to the cell body of a neuron produces cell death and permanent loss of function. Damage to the optic nerve by neurolytic agents generally results in permanent blindness.

Alcohol and phenol affect other tissues as well and are capable of producing sclerosis of small blood vessels and local tissue irritation. Both drugs also have systemic effects; those of alcohol are well known. High blood concentrations of phenol produce toxicity similar to that of local anesthetics.

The complications of neurolytic blocks can be divided into four categories: damage to peripheral neural structures, spread to neuraxial structures, local tissue effects, and systemic effects.

A. Damage to peripheral nerves

Peripheral neurolytic blocks may produce unwanted effects if the drug spreads to adjacent peripheral nerves. The most devastating consequences involve damage to motor nerves, such as when the drug spreads to the facial nerve during trigeminal neurolytic block. Other examples include overflow of drug to the brachial plexus during stellate ganglion block; spread of drug to somatic nerve roots during celiac, splanchnic, or lumbar sympathetic blocks; and overflow of drug to the glossopharyngeal nerve during gasserian ganglion block.[163] Meticulous needle placement, use of a small test dose of local anesthetic, and use of small volumes of neurolytic agents should minimize such complications. A thorough knowledge of the anatomy of the peripheral nervous system is a prerequisite to performance of neurolytic blocks. Neurolytic agents should not be used around important motor nerves, such as the common peroneal nerve, damage to which may result in footdrop.

Another consequence of peripheral neurolytic block is neuropathic pain. Commonly termed *neuritis,*[164] this phenomenon is seen more commonly with alcohol than with phenol. It occurs sufficiently often to discourage many practitioners from using neurolytic agents on peripheral nerves. It may occur soon after the block or may come on weeks to months later as function in the blocked nerve returns. Denervation dysesthesia, also termed *anesthesia dolorosa,* is another potential consequence of neurolytic blockade. It results from loss of neural input from the affected area and may cause disruption of normal gating mechanisms in the dorsal horn or may lead to sensitization or spontaneous activity in dorsal horn neurons that are involved with nociceptive transmission. Unfortunately, prognostic local anesthetic blocks do not predict the occurrence of this problem. Denervation dysesthesia responds poorly to opioids but may be ameliorated by centrally acting drugs, such as tricyclic antidepressants or anticonvulsants.

Even when peripheral blocks are performed without apparent complications, untoward effects can result from loss of function of the blocked nerve. For instance, mandibular block may produce weakness of mastication. Block of the maxillary division of the trigeminal nerve can result in loss of corneal reflexes and keratitis.[165] Loss of sensation may result in repeated burns or injury to insensible areas, and some patients find the loss of sensation as distressing as their original pain.

B. Spread to neuraxial structures

The use of neurolytic agents in the epidural or subarachnoid space is recognized as a useful analgesic technique. However, the unintentional spread of neurolytic agents to these areas during attempted peripheral blocks may be devastating, especially because the volumes of drug used are generally higher than those used in neuraxial anesthesia. The resulting damage to the spinal cord and nerve roots may produce permanent or long-lasting sensory and motor block; bowel and bladder dysfunction; vasomotor instability; and, when blockade is extensive, paraplegia, quadriplegia, or death.

Neuraxial spread may occur whenever blocks are performed relatively near the posterior midline. Splanchnic, celiac, and lumbar sympathetic blocks have been associated with epidural and subarachnoid spread of drug, which results when the needle is placed too superficially and enters the neural foramen. Biplane fluoroscopy or computed tomography should be used whenever these blocks are performed with neurolytic agents. Other blocks associated with neuraxial spread are stellate ganglion block, paravertebral somatic root block, intercostal block, and facet rhizolysis. Subarachnoid spread of neurolytic agents can result from injection directly into the subarachnoid space or the dural root sleeve or from intraneural spread associated with intrafascicular injection.[56]

Subarachnoid injection is also a potential complication of certain cranial nerve blocks, such as gasserian ganglion block, and may result in permanent damage to other cranial nerves and vasomotor fibers

Surgical distortion of anatomy may lead to unexpected complications. One of the authors has seen subarachnoid spread of local anesthetic during a lesser occipital nerve block in a patient who had undergone craniotomy for acoustic neuroma. The needle apparently entered the dura through the craniotomy defect. Injection of lidocaine produced transient hypotension and loss of consciousness. The effect of such an injection with a neurolytic agent would be devastating.

C. Local tissue effects

Gangrene and slough of tissues has been reported to occur after neurolytic block, particularly after block of the infraorbital nerve.[166] The mechanism of slough after infraorbital block is unclear. Whenever alcohol or phenol is injected superficially, skin necrosis may occur, probably as a result of sclerosis of cutaneous blood vessels.

Pain, swelling, cellulitis, and abscess formation in the area of injection of neurolytic agents may occur. Histologic studies of lytic drug injection into muscles have shown the development of pallor and coagulation followed by necrosis, degeneration, and lymphocyte and macrophage infiltration.[167] New capillaries and fibroblasts appear in 7 to 10 days, and regeneration is complete in 2 to 3 weeks. Given the degree of tissue damage caused by neurolytic agents, one would expect substantial damage to organs injected with these drugs. Renal and ureteral damage can occur during neurolytic lumbar sympathetic block. Damage to these organs and spread of drug to other neural structures along a needle track can be reduced by clearing the needle of neurolytic agent with local anesthetic or saline before withdrawal.

D. Systemic effects

Ethanol has relatively little systemic effect, even in relatively large doses. Fifty milliliters of 50% ethanol, a dose commonly used for celiac plexus block, is roughly equivalent to 2 ounces of whiskey in its alcohol content. However, when alcohol metabolism is abnormal, as in patients taking disulfiram, even small quantities of alcohol can produce dramatic reactions related to accumulation of acetaldehyde. Symptoms include flushing, palpitations, headache, nausea, vomiting, and vertigo. Blood pressure may decrease precipitously. As little as 7 ml of alcohol may cause such reactions in patients taking disulfiram.[168] Acetaldehyde syndrome may also occur after alcohol blocks in patients deficient in aldehyde dehydrogenase[169] or in patients taking drugs that, like disulfiram, suppress aldehyde dehydrogenase activity. Carmofur, an antitumor agent, has been associated with acetaldehyde syndrome in patients who have undergone alcohol celiac plexus blocks.[170]

Use of large volumes of phenol or the intravascular injection of phenol produces systemic effects similar to those of local anesthetics. Increasing blood levels produce tinnitus and flushing[171]; high levels cause seizures, loss of consciousness, and hypotension.[164]

IV. COMPLICATIONS OF SPECIFIC BLOCKS

The following section describes the more common complications associated with specific types of blocks. Discussion is confined to blocks that are frequently used in practice.

Essentially all local anesthetic blocks can be associated with local anesthetic toxicity either through relative overdose or through intravascular injection. Discussion of the management of local anesthetic toxicity is found elsewhere in this book, and systemic reactions to local anesthetics are mentioned only for blocks that carry a particularly high risk for toxic reactions. Likewise, damage to a nerve by a block needle and local infection can result from any type of block. Again, discussion of such complications is confined to blocks for which such complications are particularly likely.

A. Cranial nerve blocks

1. Block of the trigeminal nerve and its branches. Block of the gasserian ganglion is now done infrequently. Injection of alcohol into the gasserian ganglion was at one time a common treatment for tic douloureux. In recent years, it has been found that many patients respond dramatically to anticonvulsants, particularly carbamazepine. In addition, microvascular decompression of the trigeminal nerve is used extensively in many institutions and has been shown to be highly effective in some series.[172] For patients who choose to undergo neural ablation, radiofrequency coagulation is more commonly used because it is more accurate and controllable.

Spread of drug in the cerebrospinal fluid surrounding the gasserian ganglion can result in involvement of other cranial nerves. Small quantities of local anesthetic injected into the adjacent subarachnoid space can produce widespread cranial nerve block and loss of consciousness.[165] Advancing the needle too far may produce damage to the third and sixth cranial nerves or to the substance of the brain itself (Fig. 4-10).

Injection of alcohol into the trigeminal ganglion is associated with various potentially serious problems. Anesthesia of the second division of the trigeminal nerve can result in keratitis and corneal ulceration through loss of corneal sensation and interference with corneal reflexes. An ophthalmologist should be consulted to help manage this complication. Blockade of paratrigeminal sympathetic fibers may cause ipsilateral Horner syndrome, whereas blockade of motor fibers to the masseter muscle can result in weakness of mastication.[173] Block of the oculomotor or abducens nerves will produce diplopia, which usually improves after a few days.[164] Other complications resulting from the spread of alcohol beyond the area of the ganglion include damage to the facial nerve with resulting paresis; involvement of the vestibular and auditory portions of the eighth nerve with dizziness, nausea, and nystagmus; hearing loss; and damage to the optic nerve. Injury to the glossopharyngeal nerve can result in dysphagia.

Denervation dysesthesia is a fairly common sequela to correctly performed gasserian ganglion alcohol block. This condition, which has been reported in about 10% of patients,[164] produces a constant burning sensation in the affected area. Herpes simplex of the lip, mucous membrane erosion of the mouth, and nasal ulceration are trophic disturbances that can occur after gasserian ganglion ablation.

Glycerol injection of the gasserian ganglion produces analgesia in many patients with tic but does not have the potential complications of alcohol injection.[174] The depth of anesthesia is less profound, but the original symptoms can recur weeks to months later.

Hemorrhage into the temporal fossa and cheek may result from puncture of vessels in the subtemporal re-

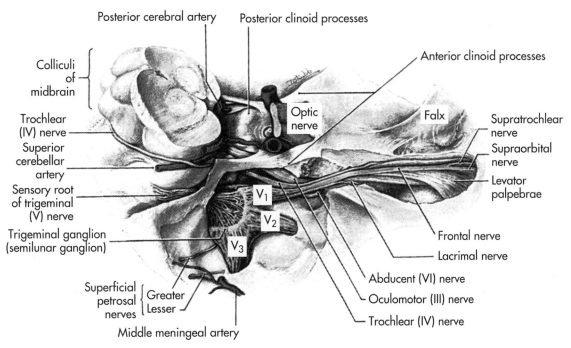

Fig. 4-10. Relation of the trigeminal ganglion to major intracranial neural and vascular structures. (From Grant JCB: *An atlas of anatomy,* ed 5, Baltimore, 1962, Williams & Wilkins.)

gion. Intraarterial injection of even small quantities of local anesthetic into the middle meningeal or carotid artery can produce central nervous system toxicity.

Supraorbital block with local anesthetic is likely to produce considerable swelling of the upper eyelid, but this complication is easily controlled with direct pressure. Injection of alcohol or phenol can produce slough of skin over the injection site. Because neurolytic agents can spread into the orbit, the volume of injectate should be kept low (less than 0.5 ml).

Block of the infraorbital area can be done at the level of the foramen rotundum or at the infraorbital foramen. Gangrene and slough at areas supplied by the nerve have been reported.[175] The cause of this complication is not known. One case of ocular muscle palsy after infraorbital alcohol block was reported.[176] In that patient, the nerve was injected under direct vision during a Caldwell-Luc procedure.

Intraarterial injection may result when the mandibular nerve is chosen for blocking because of proximity to the maxillary and middle meningeal arteries. Again, central nervous system toxicity can occur after injection of very small doses.

Neurolytic block of the mandibular nerve can produce weakness of mastication because this nerve contains motor branches to the masseter muscle. Facial nerve injury is a possible complication. One death related to carotid artery injury during the performance of this block has been reported.[177]

2. Glossopharyngeal nerve block. Bean-Lijewski[178] performed a prospective study to assess the efficacy of glossopharyngeal nerve block with 0.25% bupivacaine with epinephrine in controlling pain after tonsillectomy

in children. Local anesthetic was injected deep to the constrictor muscles into the lateral pharyngeal space. The study was interrupted because two of the first four children who received bupivacaine experienced life-threatening airway problems. Both of the 5-year-old children experienced airway obstruction soon after extubation and required emergency reintubation of the trachea. Pulmonary edema occurred in both cases. No mechanical reasons for obstruction were noted. Bean-Lijewski postulated that airway obstruction may have been associated with bilateral partial blockade of the recurrent laryngeal nerve, producing vocal cord adduction, or with blockade of the hypoglossal nerves, which causes loss of motor function of the tongue and upper pharyngeal muscles. Dyspnea and stridor associated with bilateral vocal cord adduction were documented in an adult patient after local infiltration for tonsillectomy.[179] Likewise, life-threatening upper-airway obstruction associated with hypoglossal nerve paralysis has been reported in an adult.[180] In the cases that occurred in the children who underwent tonsillectomy, one cannot say with assurance that the blocks were the cause of airway obstruction because this complication occurs occasionally in patients who undergo general anesthesia without regional block.

3. Retrobulbar block. Puncture of a vessel, particularly an artery, within the orbit may lead to serious problems because of increasing pressure within a relatively closed space. Hematoma formation initially produces palpebral edema and exophthalmus. As pressure increases, diplopia may occur. Eventually, vision may be compromised or lost because of pressure on the optic nerve or ophthalmic artery.

Injection of even minute amounts of local anesthetic into the ophthalmic artery may produce convulsions; this is due to retrograde spread of anesthetic within the ophthalmic artery to the internal carotid artery with subsequent rapid flow to the brain.[181] If a large dose of anesthetic is injected rapidly, the phase of central nervous system irritability may be bypassed with rapid development of apnea and hypotension and loss of consciousness.[182]

A life-threatening reaction can also result from spread of drug to the intracranial subarachnoid space. Spread of local anesthetic to the cerebrospinal fluid after retrobulbar block is well documented[118] and probably occurs through injection within the dural sheath of the optic nerve. Time to onset of central nervous system symptoms is generally several minutes as opposed to the instantaneous onset seen with intraarterial injection. Signs and symptoms of intracranial subarachnoid local anesthetic spread include drowsiness, blindness (including the contralateral eye), apnea, hemiplegia, aphasia, loss of consciousness, seizures, shivering, and cardiac arrest.[118] The practice of instructing the patient to look upward and medially during the block pulls the optic nerve forward, perhaps increasing the likelihood of subarachnoid spread.

Pulmonary edema has been reported after retrobulbar block. In one patient, pulmonary edema occurred 60 minutes after the block following completion of cataract surgery.[183] During surgery, the patient experienced partial block of the maxillary and mandibular divisions of the trigeminal nerve and some arterial desaturation, but no hypotension. The reporting authors considered this event neurogenic pulmonary edema, and they cited other, similar cases that followed retrobulbar blocks[184,185] and trigeminal nerve block.[186]

Two forms of neurogenic pulmonary edema have been described. One form is associated with massive sympathetic discharge and resulting left ventricular failure.[187] The other form is associated with normal pulmonary arterial pressures but increased pulmonary vascular permeability.[188]

Extraocular muscle palsies have been described after retrobulbar block.[189,190] They are generally thought to be related to myotoxicity caused by local anesthetic. Most patients recover, but these palsies persist in some patients, necessitating corrective strabismus surgery. The lowest effective concentration of drug should be selected to minimize the chance of this complication.

B. Occipital nerve block

In general, occipital nerve block carries little risk. The volume of anesthetic used in this procedure is small, and despite the high vascularity of the region, the risk for toxic reaction is low. Neuralgia of the greater or lesser occipital nerves is occasionally encountered in patients who have had posterior fossa craniotomy or removal of cerebellopontine angle tumors. If a bony defect exists at the site of the occipital block, it is possible for local anesthetic to spread to the intracranial subarachnoid space. Symptoms depend on the structures anesthetized, but hypotension, apnea, and loss of consciousness are likely. If the craniectomy defect is large, dura and perhaps brain could be herniated into the soft tissues of the occipital region, making injection into brain substance possible.

C. Cervical plexus block

The most likely serious complications of cervical plexus block are vertebral artery injection and subarachnoid injection. These complications can be minimized by cessation of injection if pain on injection occurs or if blood or cerebrospinal fluid is aspirated. Epidural spread may occur even with correct needle placement; this generally does not cause serious consequences unless high volumes and concentrations of local anesthetic are used. Epidural and subarachnoid block are more likely to occur if the needle angle is somewhat cephalad, allowing the needle to advance through the neural foramen.

Because the phrenic nerve arises from the cervical plexus, respiratory embarrassment related to phrenic blockade is a concern, particularly if bilateral cervical plexus block is contemplated.[165] However, even bilateral phrenic block is unlikely to produce serious respiratory embarrassment in the absence of preexisting pulmonary compromise.

D. Stellate ganglion block

The proximity of the carotid and vertebral arteries to the cervicothoracic sympathetic chain creates a substantial risk for central nervous system toxicity, which, as previously stated, can occur with very small doses. Seizures have been reported after injection of 15 mg of lidocaine.[72] Other central nervous system effects without convulsions have been reported after intraarterial injection. Szeinfeld, Laurencio, and Pallares[74] reported on a patient who had transient aphasia and blindness without seizure after injection of 2.5 mg of bupivacaine. Scott, Ghia, and Teeple[75] reported on a patient who experienced loss of consciousness followed by transient aphasia and hemiparesis, again without convulsions, after injection of 20 mg of lidocaine. Hematomas can form after puncture of a vessel in the neck with potential compromise of the airway. This complication is rare in the absence of coagulopathy.

The carotid artery lies superficial to the sympathetic chain but is retracted laterally during the performance of cervicothoracic sympathetic block. One should feel the carotid pulsation on the pads of the retracting fingers before needle insertion. The vertebral artery traverses the C7 transverse process and then enters a foramen to ascend behind the anterior tubercle of C6. Although the risk for intraarterial injection is moderate with a C7 approach, it is considerably less if the needle is positioned on the C6 anterior tubercle. However, the latter approach still carries some risk because the needle may slip off of the anterior tubercle during injection and, in a small percentage of patients, the vertebral artery may pass anterior to the C6 anterior tubercle[191] (Fig. 4-11).

Injection at the C7 level or deep to the C6 anterior tubercle may cause blockade of the adjacent nerve roots. Local anesthetic can spread from these locations to the brachial plexus and epidural space. Positioning the needle within the dural sheath of a nerve root may lead to subarachnoid spread. Such an injection of neurolytic agents will have devastating consequences (Fig. 4-12).

Pneumothorax is occasionally encountered after a C7 approach to the sympathetic chain but is very unlikely when the C6 approach is used. Hoarseness is often seen after stellate ganglion block. It has generally been attributed to recurrent laryngeal nerve block, and it would seem prudent to advise patients not to eat or drink until the hoarseness resolves because of the risk for aspiration. When contemplating performance of bilateral stellate block, the physician should wait a sufficient length of time to ensure that no hoarseness has occurred after the first side is done before attempting the second side. Bilateral tension pneumothorax can result from bilateral blocks; for this reason, some physicians are unwilling to block both sides in the same day.

Trauma to the thoracic duct has been reported after left stellate ganglion block.[96] The problem resolved after 5 days of pleural drainage. Patients should be followed carefully for several weeks because chyle may reaccumulate after initial resolution. Esophageal puncture can occur if the needle is angled medially. A bitter taste results without other symptoms. Leak of esophageal contents after needle puncture is unlikely.

A minor but annoying complication of stellate block is the occurrence of migraine headache in susceptible patients. A 35-year-old patient treated by one of the authors experienced severe migraines without aura, typical of her chronic intermittent headaches, that began almost immediately after stellate blocks performed for upper-extremity reflex sympathetic dystrophy. These occurred on two occasions, required intravenous opioids, and lasted several hours before subsiding completely. Lehmann, Warfield, and Bajwa[192] described a patient who developed new-onset classic migraines with aura that began the day after an otherwise uneventful stellate block. He continued to have intermittent bouts of mi-

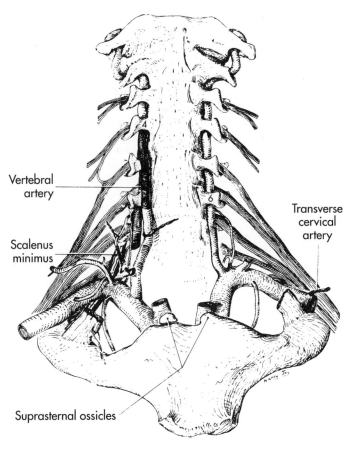

Fig. 4-11. Position of the vertebral artery with respect to the cervical anterior tubercles. The artery passes anterior to the C6 anterior tubercle in 6.4% of patients. (From Grant JCB: *An atlas of anatomy,* ed 5, Baltimore, 1962, Williams & Wilkins.)

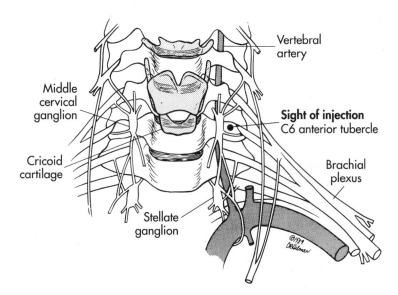

Fig. 4-12. Relation of the C6 anterior tubercle, the usual site of injection for cervicothoracic sympathetic block, to adjacent neural and vascular structures. Note that there is no anterior tubercle at C7 and that the chain lies even closer to the vertebral artery and roots of the brachial plexus at that level. (From Abram SE, Boas RA: Sympathetic and visceral nerve blocks. In Benumof JL, ed: *Clinical procedures in anesthesia and intensive care,* Philadelphia, 1991, JB Lippincott.)

graine over the next several months, after which they ceased spontaneously.

The risks of performing a neurolytic stellate ganglion block are considerable. The complications that occurred in a patient described by Superville-Sovak, Rasminsky, and Finlayson[193] illustrate the dangers of this procedure. After injection of 3 ml of 6% phenol in glycerin, the patient experienced hemiplegia, paralysis of one hemidiaphragm, and considerable reduction in vital capacity; eventually, the patient died. Autopsy revealed a spinal cord infarct in the distribution of the anterior spinal artery that involved one half of the spinal cord from C3 to C5, thrombosis of the vertebral artery, and direct neurolytic damage to the cervical cord and nerve roots. It would seem that few indications (if any) warrant exposing a patient to such devastating potential consequences.

E. Upper- and lower-extremity blocks

Neurologic dysfunction after extremity blocks can result from various causes, including preexisting, often unrecognized, neurologic deficits; nerve damage from surgical trauma; tourniquets; or malpositioning, as well as damage to a nerve during performance of a block. Preexisting neurologic problems should be documented by careful preoperative neurologic assessment. It is particularly important to assess preexisting nerve damage in trauma patients. The most common upper-extremity injuries that result from malpositioning are ulnar damage, caused by direct pressure on the nerve at the elbow, and brachial plexus injury, caused by stretching of the plexus. The most frequent lower-extremity malpositioning injury is common peroneal nerve damage, which results from direct pressure over the fibular head. Even when intraoperative positioning is managed properly, compression or malpositioning injuries may occur postoperatively while the block persists.

As discussed earlier in this chapter, injury to the brachial plexus can result from needle trauma. Most cases are probably associated with intraneural injection. Studies examining the consequences of eliciting paresthesias[57,194] have not clearly implicated this practice as a cause of neurologic damage. The overall incidence of nerve injury after axillary block is 0.4% to 5.5%.[24,57,58,194] The incidence of neurologic sequelae after continuous blocks was reported to be less than 1%.[195] No studies have been found that assess the incidence of nerve lesions occurring after interscalene or supraclavicular approaches. Persistent radiculopathy[196] and phrenic nerve damage[197] have been reported after interscalene block, and plexus injury has been reported after supraclavicular block.[198] Idiopathic brachial plexitis has been described in a patient who underwent total shoulder replacement under interscalene brachial plexus block.[199] The patient made an uneventful recovery from the block, but severe shoulder and arm pain and motor deficit in the hand began abruptly 18 hours after surgery. Magnetic resonance imaging failed to show a hematoma or any anatomic abnormality involving the brachial plexus. After 4 weeks, the patient recovered considerably. Electromyography showed abnormalities involving the entire ipsilateral brachial plexus and milder abnormalities involving the

contralateral plexus. The patient had complete neurologic recovery.

There are few published reports of neurologic damage after femoral plexus or sciatic blocks. Perhaps the preponderance of reports of injury after upper-extremity blocks reflects the much higher frequency with which this procedure is used. Born[200] reported neurologic deficits in 7 of 49 patients who underwent wrist or metacarpal blocks. Although the author attributed the complications to injection of bupivacaine into a confined space, it seems much more likely that the high complication rate was related to the use of 27-gauge needles, which probably predispose to intraneural injection. The safety of bupivacaine for wrist block is documented in a study by Nystrom et al,[201] who compared the incidence of neurologic complications from wrist block for 0.5% bupivacaine with that of 2% lidocaine in a double-blind, randomized trial. They reported only 1 patient of 71 who developed nerve damage unrelated to surgical manipulation; that patient received lidocaine. Block of the ulnar nerve within the ulnar groove at the elbow and the common peroneal nerve behind the fibular head are thought to be associated with a high frequency of neurologic damage, but little data on the subject are available.

Both arterial[87] and venous[202] insufficiency requiring vascular reconstruction have been reported after axillary block. These complications were thought to be related to needle trauma to the vessel wall.

Interscalene brachial plexus block is associated with essentially the same potential complications as stellate ganglion block, including vertebral artery injection; phrenic nerve block; recurrent laryngeal block; and epidural,[131] subdural,[203] and subarachnoid block. In one patient, subarachnoid block resulted in incomplete paralysis of slow onset with minimal need for cardiovascular or respiratory resuscitation.[204] Other patients have experienced total spinal anesthesia.[123,205]

Pneumothorax is the most common serious complication associated with supraclavicular block. The incidence ranges from 0.6% to 6%. Winnie[67] suggested that the subclavian perivascular approach is associated with a much lower incidence than that associated with more classical approaches. Risk is theoretically greater on the right side because of the higher dome of the lung on that side. It is also greater in tall, thin patients and in patients with emphysema. Mani et al[94] reported a case of hemopneumothorax after subclavian perivascular block in a patient who received heparin.

Relatively few cases of hemorrhagic complications occurring after extremity blocks have been reported, and those that have are usually associated with the use of anticoagulants. In addition to the case of hemopneumothorax previously mentioned,[94] Parziale, Marino, and Herndon[202] reported a case of compartment syndrome that followed a median nerve block at the elbow in a patient receiving warfarin. Hematoma formation without neurologic consequences has been reported[92] but was associated with neuropathic changes in two patients in Woolley and Vandam's series.[24] Johr[206] reported a case of femoral nerve compression by a hematoma after continuous femoral nerve block. The patient had been treated with dextran 70. Aida, Takahashi, and Shimoji[207] described two cases of renal capsular hematoma following lumbar plexus (psoas compartment) block. The condition was associated with severe low back pain and resolved spontaneously in both patients.

Anesthetic solutions containing epinephrine are not usually used in the digits owing to fear of producing gangrene, but published documentation to substantiate this fear is lacking. Similarly, warnings against the use of epinephrine for digital and penile blocks are common in regional anesthesia textbooks. It is not clear how common such injuries are or what concentrations of epinephrine are associated with them, but it seems prudent to avoid all vasoconstrictors in anesthetic solutions when performing blocks in the digits.

F. Intravenous regional anesthesia

The complications of intravenous regional anesthesia are related to the hazards of tourniquet inflation and local anesthetic toxicity. Because the duration of intravenous regional anesthesia is generally limited to 1.5 hours or less, the incidence of tourniquet-related nerve damage is very low. However, a case of permanent motor nerve damage was reported after an intravenous injection of regional anesthetic in a previously healthy young patient.[208] In that patient, the surgical procedure lasted only 50 minutes. If intravenous regional anesthesia is used for a surgical procedure for which a tourniquet is unnecessary, the risk associated with tourniquet use is added to the risk associated with anesthesia. Again, because of the relatively short period of tourniquet inflation, the release of accumulated metabolic products (such as lactic acid and potassium) at the time of cuff deflation is unlikely to cause problems. On the other hand, the reactive hyperemia that ensues can produce hemodynamic changes. Under most circumstances, such changes are insignificant. However, a sudden decrease in vascular resistance in the limb can cause a decrease in the subclavian artery pressure if there is proximal stenosis, resulting in reduced vertebral artery flow, a phenomenon termed *subclavian steal*. Carney and Anderson[209] described two cases of tourniquet-induced subclavian steal. One case occurred in a previously healthy 9-year-old patient who had permanent neurologic dysfunction. Although neither of these cases occurred after intravenous regional anesthesia, one of the authors has witnessed such cases and is aware of other patients in whom severe bradycardia and transient cortical blindness occurred after deflation of tourniquets that were used for intravenous regional anesthesia. Venous thrombosis is another reported complication of the use of an intraoperative tourniquet.[210]

Local anesthetic toxicity during intravenous regional block can occur at the time of tourniquet deflation or result from leaking of anesthetic beneath the cuff. Premature accidental cuff deflation is likely to cause acute local anesthetic toxicity if inflation occurs during the first 10 to 15 minutes, before the anesthetic has had time to diffuse out of the venous system into the tissues. There are very few reports of serious local anesthetic toxic reactions associated with the use of 0.5% lidocaine or prilo-

caine. However, Heath[211] reported that seven recorded deaths in the United Kingdom between 1979 and 1983 resulted from bupivacaine Bier blocks. In at least some of the recorded cases, 0.2% bupivacaine in a dose of 1.5 ml/kg of body weight was used, and early tourniquet inflation did not occur. The usual bupivacaine concentration for intravenous regional anesthesia is 0.25%, which is similar in potency and toxicity to 1% lidocaine or prilocaine. In light of the documented deaths associated with intravenous regional bupivacaine and the need for higher relative concentrations of the drug, it seems prudent to avoid its use altogether for this technique.

Toxic reactions related to leak of anesthetic under the cuff may occur when injection pressure exceeds cuff occlusion pressure. Davies, Wilkey, and Hall[212] reported that local anesthetic gained access to the general circulation in 13 of 52 patients. This is more likely to occur if arterial flow is not completely occluded and venous congestion occurs.[213] Systolic blood pressure seems to be an unreliable guide to determining tourniquet pressure, and it has been suggested that tourniquet pressure should be set at 100 mm Hg above occlusion pressure, the tourniquet pressure that abolishes arterial pulsation in the limb. Because exsanguination of the limb with an Esmarch bandage reduces the peak injection pressure,[214] it would be likely to reduce the risk of anesthetic leaking past the cuff. Even when exsanguination is carried out, toxic reactions can occur if large volumes of anesthetic are used. Rosenberg et al[215] reported a convulsion caused by local anesthetic in a 120-kg patient after injection of 80 ml of 0.25% bupivacaine. The tourniquet was set at 300 mm Hg, and the patient's blood pressure at the time of injection was 160/80 mm Hg. This report also illustrates the potential for local anesthetic toxicity with the use of bupivacaine.

G. Intercostal nerve blocks

Despite the fact that the intercostal spaces are fairly vascular, the reported incidence of systemic toxic reactions is low. Moore[216] described only five cases of convulsions resulting from local anesthetic among 17,000 patients. All five convulsions occurred in surgical patients who had bilateral blocks of the lower seven intercostal nerves. In a study of 10 patients who underwent bilateral intercostal blocks with 400 mg of bupivacaine (0.5% with epinephrine 3 μg/ml), Moore et al[217] found that mean peak arterial concentrations of anesthetic ranged from 1.7 to 4 μg/ml (mean, 3.3 μg/ml). Peak concentrations occurred 10 to 30 minutes after injection.

Pneumothorax is a recognized complication of intercostal block. The incidence of this complication depends on the skill of the anesthesiologist and the diligence with which one looks for subclinical cases. The reported incidence ranges from less than 0.1% in a series of 17,000 patients described by Moore[216] to 19%.[218] Clinically significant pneumothorax is probably caused either by rupture of an emphysematous bleb or by laceration of the visceral pleura by the needle. One may reduce needle trauma by asking the patient to hold his or her breath as the needle is walked off of the lower border of the rib and the anesthetic is injected.

Intraneural injection may result in spread of drug proximally to the subarachnoid space or spinal cord. Because the volumes of local anesthetic injected at any one intercostal space are generally low, the chances of developing a very high or total spinal block are relatively low. Two cases of subarachnoid block from the low thoracic level down were reported following intraoperative intercostal blocks performed during thoracotomy for thoracic diskectomy.[219] Both patients recovered without sequelae. If intraneural spread occurs with neurolytic agents, the resulting effect on the spinal cord may be devastating. It is therefore essential that great care be exercised and that small volumes be used in the performance of neurolytic intercostal block. As with other blocks, local bleeding may occur in anticoagulated patients[93] and may lead to substantial accumulation of blood in the pleural space.

H. Paravertebral somatic and sympathetic nerve blocks

Because of the proximity of the somatic nerve roots and the sympathetic chain in the lumbar and thoracic areas, the complications of paravertebral somatic and sympathetic nerve blocks will be considered together. The complications of cervical somatic root block are the same as those described for cervical plexus block.

The principal risk of these procedures is spread of drug to the epidural or subarachnoid space. This generally results from placement of the needle into the dural cuff, which extends over the nerve root. If small volumes of local anesthetic appropriate to diagnostic or prognostic nerve root blocks are used, the consequences of subarachnoid spread are minimal. If lumbar sympathetic block is performed by use of an approach that begins 8 to 10 cm lateral to the midline, the needle may enter the neural foramen, leading to epidural or subarachnoid spread. If large volumes are used, total spinal anesthesia may ensue.[220] Neurolytic lumbar sympathetic blocks can result in damage to somatic neural structures when needle positioning is faulty. In addition, the drug can spread posteriorly along the rami communicantes to the somatic roots even when needle position is satisfactory.[220]

We encountered one patient who developed a postlumbar puncture headache after an L3 paravertebral root block that resulted in subarachnoid spread of local anesthetic. Sharrock[130] reported on three cases of headache among 24 patients who underwent a total of 39 thoracic paravertebral somatic nerve blocks.

Pneumothorax is a potential complication of high lumbar and thoracic paravertebral blocks. There is little or no space between the thoracic sympathetic chain and the pleura. We treated a patient with an L1 nerve block who developed a 20% pneumothorax that resolved without intervention. DeKrey, Schroeder, and Buechel[221] described a fatal pneumothorax in a patient with severe pulmonary dysfunction.

Hematuria resulting from needle puncture of a kidney or ureter is occasionally encountered after lumbar sympathetic block. It is generally without serious consequences. However, injection of neurolytic agents into a kidney or ureter can produce substantial damage.

Kuzmarov et al[222] reported a case of ureteral damage requiring surgical repair that resulted from alcohol injected into the ureter during attempted sympathetic block.

Postsympathectomy limb pain, also referred to as sympathalgia, is commonly seen after surgical or neurolytic sympathectomy. In some series, it has occurred in almost every patient.[223] In sympathalgia, deep, boring pain sets in about 2 weeks after sympathectomy; this pain usually occurs in the anterior thigh and is often worse at night. The soft tissues of the thigh are very tender. The pain usually subsides spontaneously in several days to several weeks. The cause of this condition is unclear.

I. Celiac plexus and splanchnic nerve block

Celiac plexus block is associated with a low rate of complications. Even when neurolytic agents are used, the incidence of neurologic damage is low.[224] Brown, Bulley, and Quiel[225] observed no neurologic complications in a series of 136 patients. However, paraplegia has been reported with both alcohol and phenol,[226,227] and biplanar fluoroscopy or computed tomography should be used when this block is performed with neurolytic agents. In one case of transient paraplegia[228] and one case of permanent paraplegia[229] after alcohol celiac plexus block, it was postulated that spinal cord ischemia related to effects of the drug on the arterial supply to the cord was the cause of neurologic dysfunction. The case of permanent neurologic dysfunction was associated with intraoperative injection under direct vision anterior to the L1 vertebral body. It is unlikely that spread of the drug to the subarachnoid or epidural space occurred.

Pneumothorax is an occasional complication. It is somewhat more likely with splanchnic block because needle position is farther cephalad, at the T12 anterolateral border. Brown, Bulley, and Quiel[225] reported two cases of pneumothorax in their series of 136 celiac plexus blocks. Both resolved without need for thoracostomy.

Orthostatic hypotension occurs occasionally after celiac plexus block. It is more likely to occur if the needle position is retrocrural and close to the vertebral body, allowing spread of the drug to the lumbar sympathetic chain. Orthostatic hypotension is generally short-lived, even when neurolytic agents are used, and all the cases that we have encountered resolved within 48 hours. Transient diarrhea lasting 1 day to several days is fairly common after neurolytic celiac plexus block. A few cases of persistent diarrhea have been reported.[230,231]

Retroperitoneal fibrosis has been reported after repeated celiac plexus alcohol injections for chronic pancreatitis.[232] No apparent sequelae were noted except for the inability to continue treatment with these injections. Chest pain is common after celiac alcohol block and usually resolves within 1 hour. Pleural effusion is occasionally seen in the postblock period.[233]

J. Blocks of the perineum

Fetal complications of paracervical blocks are discussed earlier in this chapter. Both pudendal and paracervical blocks are associated with occasional retropsoas abscesses.[157,234] Retroperitoneal hematoma has been reported following pudendal block for vaginal delivery.[235]

As with epidural blocks, evidence indicates that pudendal blocks diminish the bearing-down reflex during labor and may prolong the second stage.[236]

As with digital nerve blocks, penile block with solutions containing epinephrine may lead to ischemia and gangrene of tissues distal to the block. This complication probably results from a combination of pressure on vessels by the injected solution and vasoconstriction of the small arteries by the epinephrine. Unlike the case with other areas of the body, no collateral flow is possible beyond the block.

REFERENCES

1. Caplan RA, Ward RJ, Posner K, et al: Unexpected cardiac arrest during spinal anesthesia: a closed claims analysis of predisposing factors, *Anesthesiology* 68:5, 1988.
2. Smith DC, Crul JF: Oxygen desaturation following sedation for regional analgesia, *Br J Anaesth* 62:206, 1989.
3. Ben-David B, Vaida S, Gaitini L: The influence of high spinal anesthesia on sensitivity to midazolam sedation, *Anesth Analg* 81:525, 1995.
4. Sturrock JE, Nunn JF: Cytotoxic effects of procaine, lignocaine and bupivacaine, *Br J Anaesth* 51:273, 1979.
5. Morris T, Tracey J: Lignocaine: its effects on wound healing, *Br J Surg* 64:902, 1977.
6. Bodvall B, Rais O: Effects of infiltration anaesthesia on the healing of incisions in traumatized and non-traumatized tissues, *Acta Chir Scand* 123:83, 1962.
7. Hogan Q, Dotson R, Erickson S, et al: Local anesthetic myotoxicity: a case and review, *Anesthesiology* 80:942, 1994.
8. Brun A: Effect of procaine, carbocaine and xylocaine on cutaneous muscle in rabbits and mice, *Acta Anaesthesiol Scand* 3:59, 1959.
9. Benoit PW, Belt WD: Destruction and regeneration of skeletal muscle after treatment with a local anaesthetic, bupivacaine (Marcaine), *J Anat* 107:547, 1970.
10. Loghmanee F, Tobak M: Fatal malignant hyperthermia associated with recreational cocaine and ethanol abuse, *Am J Forensic Med Pathol* 7:246, 1986.
11. Merigian KS, Roberts JR: Cocaine intoxication: hyperpyrexia, rhabdomyolysis and acute renal failure, *J Toxicol Clin Toxicol* 25:135, 1987.
12. Shanthaveerappa TR, Bourne GH: Perineural epithelium: a new concept of its role in the integrity of the peripheral nervous system, *Science* 154:1464, 1966.
13. Myers RR, Kalichman MW, Reisner LS, et al: Neurotoxicity of local anesthetics: altered perineurial permeability, edema, and nerve fiber injury, *Anesthesiology* 64:29, 1986.
14. Fink BR, Kennedy RD, Hendrickson AE, et al: Lidocaine inhibition of rapid axonal transport, *Anesthesiology* 36:422, 1972.
15. Byers MR, Fink BR, Kennedy RD: Effects of lidocaine on axonal morphology, microtubules, and rapid transport in rabbit vagus nerve in vitro, *J Neurobiol* 4:125, 1973.
16. Barsa J, Batra M, Fink BR, et al: A comparative in vivo study of local neurotoxicity of lidocaine, bupivacaine, 2-chloroprocaine, and a mixture of 2-chloroprocaine and bupivacaine, *Anesth Analg* 61:961, 1982.
17. Powell HC, Kalichman MW, Garrett RS, et al: Selective vulnerability of unmyelinated fiber Schwann cells in nerves exposed to local anesthetics, *Lab Invest* 59:271, 1988.
18. Kalichman MW, Powell HC, Myers R: Pathology of local anesthetic-induced nerve injury, *Acta Neuropathol* 75:583, 1988.
19. Kalichman MW, Moorhouse DF, Powell HC, et al: Relative neural toxicity of local anesthetics, *J Neuropathol Exp Neurol* 52:234, 1993.
20. Myers RR, Heckman HM: Effects of local anesthesia on nerve blood flow: studies using lidocaine with and without epinephrine, *Anesthesiology* 71:757, 1989.
21. Kalichman MW, Lalonde AW: Experimental nerve ischemia and injury produced by cocaine and procaine, *Brain Res* 22:34, 1991.
22. Li DF, Bahar M, Cole G, et al: Neurological toxicity of the subarachnoid infusion of bupivacaine, lignocaine or 2-chloroprocaine in the rat, *Br J Anaesth* 57:424, 1985.
23. Ready LB, Plumer MH, Haschke RH, et al: Neurotoxicity of intrathecal local anesthetics in rabbits, *Anesthesiology* 63:364, 1985.
24. Woolley EJ, Vandam LD: Neurological sequelae of brachial plexus nerve block, *Ann Surg* 149:53, 1959.
25. Selander D, Brattsand R, Lundborg G, et al: Local anesthetics: importance of mode of application, concentration and adrenaline for the appearance of nerve lesions: an experimental study of axonal degeneration and barrier damage after intrafascicular injection for topical application of bupivacaine (Marcaine), *Acta Anaesthesiol Scand* 23:127, 1979.
26. Gentili F, Hudson AR, Hunter D, et al: Nerve injection injury with local anesthetic agents: a light and electron microscopic, fluorescent microscopic, and horseradish peroxidase study, *Neurosurgery* 6:263, 1980.
27. Lofstrom B, Wennberg A, Wien L: Late disturbances in nerve function after block with local anaesthetic agents: an electroneurographic study, *Acta Anaesthesiol Scand* 10:111, 1966.
28. Parke WW, Watanabe R: The intrinsic vasculature of the lumbosacral spinal nerve roots, *Spine* 10:508, 1985.
29. Rydevik B, Holm S, Brown MD, et al: Diffusion from the cerebrospinal fluid as a nutritional pathway for spinal nerve roots, *Acta Physiol Scand* 138:247, 1990.
30. Rigler ML, Drasner K, Krejcie TC, et al: Cauda equina syndrome after continuous spinal anesthesia, *Anesth Analg* 72:275, 1991.
31. Schell RM, Brauer FS, Cole DJ, et al: Persistent sacral nerve root deficits after continuous spinal anaesthesia, *Can J Anaesth* 38:908, 1991.
32. Rigler ML, Drasner K: Distribution of catheter-injected local anesthetic in a model of the subarachnoid space, *Anesthesiology* 75:684, 1991.
33. Gerancher JC: Cauda equina syndrome following a single spinal administration of 5% hyperbaric lidocaine through a 25-gauge Whitacre needle, *Anesthesiology* 87:687, 1997.
34. Tarkkila P, Huhtala J, Tuominen M: Transient radicular irritation after spinal anesthesia with hyperbaric 5% lignocaine, *Br J Anaesth* 74:328, 1995.
35. Hampl KF, Schneider MC, Ummenhofer W, et al: Transient neurologic symptoms after spinal anesthesia, *Anesth Analg* 81:1148, 1995.
36. Hampl KF, Schneider MC, Pargger H, et al: A similar incidence of transient neurologic symptoms after spinal anesthesia with 2% and 5% lidocaine, *Anesth Analg* 83:1051, 1996.
37. Hampl KF, Schneider MC, Thorin D, et al: Hyperosmolarity does not contribute to transient radicular irritation after spinal anesthesia with hyperbaric 5% lidocaine, *Reg Anesth* 20:363, 1995.
38. Pollock JE, Neal JM, Stephenson CA, et al: Prospective study of the incidence of transient radicular irritation in patients undergoing spinal anesthesia, *Anesthesiology* 84:1361, 1996.
39. Sumi M, Sakura S, Kosaka Y: Intrathecal hyperbaric 0.5% tetracaine as a possible cause of transient neurologic toxicity, *Anesth Analg* 82:1076, 1996.
40. Lynch J, zur Nieden M, Kasper SM, et al: Transient radicular irritation after spinal anesthesia with hyperbaric 4% mepivacaine, *Anesth Analg* 85:872, 1997.
41. Horlocker TT, McGregor DG, Matsushige DK, et al: A retrospective review of 4767 consecutive spinal anesthetics: central nervous system complications: Perioperative Outcomes Group, *Anesth Analg* 84:578, 1997.
42. Auroy Y, Narchi P, Messiah A, et al: Serious complications related to regional anesthesia, *Anesthesiology* 87: 479, 1997.
43. Lambert LA, Lambert DH, Strichartz GR: Irreversible conduction block in isolated nerve by high concentrations of local anesthetics, *Anesthesiology* 80:1082, 1994.
44. Bainton CR, Strichartz GR: Concentration dependence of lidocaine-induced irreversible conduction loss in frog nerve, *Anesthesiology* 81:657, 1994.
45. Drasner K, Sakura S, Chan VWS, et al: Persistent sacral sensory deficit induced by intrathecal local anesthetic infusion in the rat, *Anesthesiology* 80:847, 1994.

46. Hashimoto K, Nakamura Y, Hampl KF, et al: Epinephrine increases the neurotoxic potential of intrathecally administered local anesthetic, *Anesthesiology* 85:A770, 1996 (abstract).
47. Sakura S, Chan VWS, Ciriales R, et al: The addition of 7.5% glucose does not alter the neurotoxicity of 5% lidocaine administered intrathecally in the rat, *Anesthesiology* 82:236, 1995.
48. Sakura S, Bollen AW, Ciriales R, et al: Local anesthetic neurotoxicity does not result from blockade of voltage-gated sodium channels, *Anesth Analg* 81:338, 1995.
49. Steele S, Montine T, Dentz M, et al: Histopathologic changes of cauda equina syndrome in a canine continuous spinal anesthesia model, *Anesthesiology* 79:A850, 1993 (abstract).
50. Gissen AJ, Datta S, Lambert D: The chloroprocaine controversy II: is chloroprocaine neurotoxic? *Reg Anaesth* 9:135, 1984.
51. Wang BC, Hillman DE, Spielholz NI, et al: Chronic neurological deficits and Nesacaine-CE—an effect of the anesthetic, 2-chloroprocaine, or the antioxidant, sodium bisulfite? *Anesth Analg* 63:445, 1984.
52. Covino B: Clinical pharmacology of local anesthetic agents. In Cousins MJ, Bridenbaugh PO, eds: *Neural blockade,* Philadelphia, 1988, JB Lippincott, p 130.
53. Kalichman MW, Calcutt NA: Local anesthetic-induced conduction block and nerve fiber injury in streptozotocin-diabetic rats, *Anesthesiology* 77:941, 1992.
54. Selander D, Dhuner KG, Lundborg G: Peripheral nerve injury due to injection needles used for regional anesthesia: an experimental study of the acute effects of needle point trauma, *Acta Anaesthesiol Scand* 21:182, 1977.
55. Moore DC: *Complications of regional anesthesia,* Springfield, Ill, 1955, Charles C Thomas, p 114.
56. Selander D, Sjostrand J: Longitudinal spread of intraneurally injected local anesthetics: an experimental study of the initial neural distribution following intraneural injections, *Acta Anaesthesiol Scand* 22:622, 1978.
57. Selander D, Edshage S, Wolff T: Paresthesiae or no paresthesiae? New lesions after axillary blocks, *Acta Anaesthesiol Scand* 23:27, 1979.
58. Winchell SW, Wolfe R: The incidence of neuropathy following upper extremity nerve blocks, *Reg Anaesth* 10:12, 1985.
59. Passannante AN: Spinal anesthesia and permanent neurologic deficit after interscalene block, *Anesth Analg* 82:873, 1996.
60. Ribeiro FC, Georgousis H, Bertram R, et al: Plexus irritation caused by interscalene brachial plexus catheter for shoulder surgery, *Anesth Analg* 82:870, 1996.
61. Tountas CP, Bergman RA: Tourniquet ischemia: ultrastructural and histochemical observations of ischemic human muscle and of monkey muscle and nerve, *J Hand Surg [Am]* 2:31, 1977.
62. Lundborg G: Structure and function of the intraneural microvessels as related to trauma, edema, formation and nerve function, *J Bone Joint Surg [Am]* 57:938, 1975.
63. Ochoa J, Fowler TJ, Gilliatt RW: Anatomical changes in peripheral nerve compressed by a pneumatic tourniquet, *J Anat* 113:433, 1972.
64. Moore MR, Garfin SR, Hargens AR: Wide tourniquets eliminate blood flow at low inflation pressures, *J Hand Surg [Am]* 12:1006, 1987.
65. Dreyfuss UY, Smith RJ: Sensory changes with prolonged double-cuff tourniquet time in hand surgery, *J Hand Surg [Am]* 13:736, 1988.
66. Mullick S: The tourniquet in operations upon the extremities, *Surg Gynecol Obstet* 146:821, 1978.
67. Winnie AP: *Plexus anesthesia,* vol 1, *Perivascular techniques of brachial plexus block,* Philadelphia, 1983, WB Saunders.
68. Covino B, Vassalo H: *Local anesthetics,* New York, 1976, Grune & Stratton, p 95.
69. Tucker GT, Mather LE: Properties, absorption, and disposition of local anesthetic agents. In Cousins M, Bridenbaugh PO, eds: *Neural blockade,* ed 2, Philadelphia, 1990, JB Lippincott.
70. Bernards CM, Carpenter RL, Rupp SM, et al: Effect of midazolam and diazepam premedication on central nervous system and cardiovascular toxicity of bupivacaine in pigs, *Anesthesiology* 70:318, 1989.
71. Torbiner ML, Yagiela JA, Mito RS: Effect of midazolam pretreatment on the intravenous toxicity of lidocaine with and without epinephrine in rats, *Anesth Analg* 68:744, 1989.
72. Korevaar WC, Burney RG, Moore PA: Convulsions during stellate ganglion block: a case report, *Anesth Analg* 58:329, 1979.
73. Kozody R, Ready LB, Barsa JE, et al: Dose requirement of local anaesthetic to produce grand mal seizure during stellate ganglion block, *Can Anaesth Soc J* 29:489, 1982.
74. Szeinfeld M, Laurencio M, Pallares V: Total reversible blindness following attempted stellate ganglion block, *Anesth Analg* 60:689, 1981.
75. Scott DL, Ghia JN, Teeple E: Aphasia and hemiparesis following stellate ganglion block, *Anesth Analg* 62:1038, 1983.
76. Aldrete JA, Romo-Salas F, Arora S, et al: Reverse arterial blood flow as a pathway for central nervous system toxic responses following injection of local anesthetics, *Anesth Analg* 57:428, 1978.
77. Tomlin PJ: Death in outpatient dental anaesthetic practice, *Anaesthesia* 29:551, 1974.
78. Cockings E, Moore PL, Lewis RC: Transarterial brachial plexus blockade using high doses of 1.5% mepivacaine, *Reg Anaesth* 12:159, 1987.
79. Ischia S, Luzzani A, Ischia A, et al: A new approach to the neurolytic block of the coeliac plexus: the transaortic technique, *Pain* 16:333, 1983.
80. Merrill DG, Brodsky JB, Hentz RV: Vascular insufficiency following axillary block of the brachial plexus, *Anesth Analg* 60:162, 1981.
81. Nishimura N, Morioka T, Sato S, et al: Effects of local anesthetic agents on the peripheral vascular system, *Anesth Analg* 44:135, 1965.
82. Selander D, Mansson L, Karlsson L, et al: Adrenergic vasoconstriction in peripheral nerves of the rabbit, *Anesthesiology* 62:6, 1985.
83. Hastings H II, Misamore G: Compartment syndrome resulting from intravenous regional anesthesia, *J Hand Surg [Am]* 12:559, 1987.
84. Moore DC: *Complications of regional anesthesia,* Springfield, Ill, 1955, Charles C Thomas, p 97.
85. Lennon RL, Linstromberg JW: Brachial plexus anesthesia and axillary sheath elastance, *Anesth Analg* 62:215, 1983.
86. Siler JN, Lief PL, Davis J: A new complication of interscalene brachial-plexus block, *Anesthesiology* 38:590, 1973.
87. Ott B, Neuberger L, Frey HP: Obliteration of the axillary artery after axillary block, *Anaesthesia* 44:773, 1989.
88. Groh GI, Gainor BJ, Jeffries JT, et al: Pseudoaneurysm of the axillary artery with median-nerve deficit after axillary block anesthesia: a case report, *J Bone Joint Surg [Am]* 72:1407, 1990.
89. Zipkin M, Backus WW, Scott B, et al: False aneurysm of the axillary artery following brachial plexus block, *J Clin Anesth* 3:143, 1991.
90. Restelli L, Pinciroli D, Conoscente F, et al: Insufficient venous drainage following axillary approach to brachial plexus blockade, *Br J Anaesth* 56:1051, 1984.
91. Stan TC, Krantz MA, Solomon DL, et al: The incidence of neurovascular complications following axillary brachial plexus block using a transarterial approach: a prospective study of 1,000 consecutive patients, *Reg Anesth* 20:486, 1995.
92. Moore DC: *Complications of regional anesthesia,* Springfield, Ill, 1955, Charles C Thomas, p 87.
93. Nielsen CH: Bleeding after intercostal nerve block in a patient anticoagulated with heparin, *Anesthesiology* 71:162, 1989.
94. Mani M, Ramamurthy N, Rao TLK, et al: An unusual complication of brachial plexus block and heparin therapy, *Anesthesiology* 48:213, 1978.
95. Moore DC: *Complications of regional anesthesia,* Springfield, Ill, 1955, Charles C Thomas, p 55.
96. Thompson KJ, Melding P, Hatangdi VS: Pneumochylothorax: a rare complication of stellate ganglion block, *Anesthesiology* 55:589, 1981.
97. Winnie AP: *Plexus anesthesia,* vol 1, *Perivascular techniques of brachial plexus block,* Philadelphia, 1983, WB Saunders, p 229.
98. Derenne JP, Macklem PT, Roussos C: The respiratory muscles: mechanics, control, and pathophysiology, part I, *Am Rev Respir Dis* 118:119, 1978.

99. Hecker BR, Bjurstrom R, Schoene RB: Effect of intercostal nerve blockade on respiratory mechanics and CO_2 raise chemosensitivity at rest and exercise, *Anesthesiology* 70:13, 1989.

100. Shaw WM: Paralysis of the phrenic nerve during brachial plexus anesthesia, *Anesthesiology* 10:627, 1949.

101. Harley N, Gjessing J: A critical assessment of supraclavicular brachial plexus block, *Anaesthesia* 24:564, 1969.

102. Knoblanche GE: The incidence and aetiology of phrenic nerve blockade associated with supraclavicular brachial plexus block, *Anaesth Intensive Care* 7:346, 1979.

103. Hickey R, Ramamurthy S: The diagnosis of phrenic nerve block on chest x-ray by a double-exposure technique, *Anesthesiology* 70:704, 1989.

104. Fujimura N, Namba H, Tsunoda K, et al: Effect of hemidiaphragmatic paresis caused by interscalene brachial plexus block on breathing pattern, chest wall mechanics, and arterial blood gases, *Anesth Analg* 81:962, 1995.

105. Urmey WF, McDonald M: Hemidiaphragmatic paresis during interscalene brachial plexus block: effects on pulmonary function and chest wall mechanics, *Anesth Analg* 74:352, 1992.

106. Pere P: The effect of continuous interscalene brachial plexus block with 0.125% bupivacaine plus fentanyl on diaphragmatic motility and ventilatory function, *Reg Anesth* 18:93, 1993.

107. Urmey WF, Grossi P, Sharrock NE, et al: Digital pressure during interscalene block is clinically ineffective in preventing anesthetic spread to the cervical plexus, *Anesth Analg* 83:366, 1996.

108. Urmey WF, Gloeggler PJ: Pulmonary function changes during interscalene brachial plexus block: effects of decreasing local anesthetic injection volume, *Reg Anesth* 18:244, 1993.

109. Eisele JH, Noble MIM, Katz J, et al: Bilateral phrenic-nerve block in man: technical problems and respiratory effects, *Anesthesiology* 37:64, 1972.

110. Cory PC, Mulroy MF: Postoperative respiratory failure following intercostal block, *Anesthesiology* 54:418, 1981.

111. Casey WF: Respiratory failure following intercostal nerve blockade, *Anaesthesia* 39:351, 1984.

112. Hood J, Knoblanche G: Respiratory failure following brachial plexus block, *Anaesth Intensive Care* 7:285, 1979.

113. Kayerker UM, Dick MM: Phrenic nerve paralysis following interscalene brachial plexus block, *Anesth Analg* 62:536, 1983.

114. Sharp JT, Goldberg NB, Druz WS, et al: Thoracoabdominal motion in chronic obstructive pulmonary disease, *Am Rev Respir Dis* 115:47, 1977.

115. Farrar MD, Scheybani M, Nolte H: Upper extremity block effectiveness and complications, *Reg Anaesth* 6:133, 1981.

116. Urmey WF, Talts KH, Sharrock NE: One hundred percent incidence of hemidiaphragmatic paresis associated with interscalene brachial plexus anesthesia as diagnosed by ultrasonography, *Anesth Analg* 72:498, 1991.

117. Albert J, Lofstrom B: Bilateral ulnar nerve blocks for the evaluation of local anaesthetic agents, *Acta Anaesthesiol Scand* 5:99, 1961.

118. Nicoll JMV, Acharya PA, Ahlen K, et al: Central nervous system complications after 6000 retrobulbar blocks, *Anesth Analg* 66:1298, 1987.

119. Rigg JD, James RH: Apnoea after retrobulbar block, *Anaesthesia* 44:26, 1989.

120. Wang BC, Bogart B, Hillman DE, et al: Subarachnoid injection: a potential complication of retrobulbar block, *Anesthesiology* 71:845, 1989.

121. Ross S, Scarborough CD: Total spinal anesthesia following brachial-plexus block, *Anesthesiology* 39:458, 1973.

122. Edde RR, Deutsch S: Cardiac arrest after interscalene brachial-plexus block, *Anesth Analg* 56:446, 1977.

123. Dutton RP, Eckhardt WF III, Sunder N: Total spinal anesthesia after interscalene blockade of the brachial plexus, *Anesthesiology* 80:939, 1994.

124. Goldstone JC, Pennant JH: Spinal anaesthesia following facet joint injection: a report of two cases, *Anaesthesia* 42:754, 1987.

125. Benumof JL, Semenza J: Total spinal anesthesia following intrathoracic intercostal nerve blocks, *Anesthesiology* 43:124, 1975.

126. Otto CW, Wall CL: Total spinal anesthesia: a rare complication of intrathoracic intercostal nerve block, *Ann Thorac Surg* 22:289, 1976.

127. Chester SC, Gutteridge GA: Subtotal spinal anaesthesia as a complication of intrathoracic intercostal nerve blocks, *Anaesth Intensive Care* 9:387, 1981.

128. Gallo JA Jr, Lebowitz PW, Battit GE, et al: Complications of intercostal nerve blocks performed under direct vision during thoracotomy: a repeat of two cases, *J Thorac Cardiovasc Surg* 86:628, 1983.

129. Sury MRJ, Bingham RM: Accidental spinal anaesthesia following intrathoracic intercostal nerve blockade, *Anaesthesia* 41:401, 1986.

130. Sharrock NE: Postural headache following thoracic somatic paravertebral nerve block, *Anesthesiology* 52:360, 1980.

131. Kumar A, Battit GE, Froese AB, et al: Bilateral cervical and thoracic epidural blockade complicating interscalene brachial plexus block: report of two cases, *Anesthesiology* 35:650, 1971.

132. Muravchick S, Owens WD: An unusual complication of lumbosacral plexus block: a case report, *Anesth Analg* 55:350, 1976.

133. Scammell SJ: Case report: inadvertent epidural anaesthesia as a complication of interscalene brachial plexus block, *Anaesth Intensive Care* 7:56, 1979.

134. Lombard TP, Couper JL: Bilateral spread of analgesia following interscalene brachial plexus block, *Anesthesiology* 58:472, 1983.

135. Middaugh RE, Menk EJ, Reynolds WJ, et al: Epidural block using large volumes of local anesthetic solution for intercostal nerve block, *Anesthesiology* 63:214, 1985.

136. Krempen JS, Smith B, DeFreest LJ: Selective nerve root infiltration for the evaluation of sciatica, *Orthop Clin North Am* 6:311, 1975.

137. Moran R, O'Connell D, Walsh MG: The diagnostic value of facet joint injections, *Spine* 13:1407, 1988.

138. Raymond J, Dumas JM: Intraarticular facet block: diagnostic test or therapeutic procedure? *Radiology* 151:333, 1984.

139. Singelyn FJ, Contreras V, Gouverneur JM: Epidural anesthesia complicating 3-in-1 lumbar plexus blockade, *Anesthesiology* 83:217, 1995.

140. Seltzer JL: Hoarseness and Horner's syndrome after interscalene brachial plexus block, *Anesth Analg* 56:585, 1977.

141. Skretting P: Hypotension after intercostal nerve block during thoracotomy under general anaesthesia, *Br J Anaesth* 53:527, 1981.

142. Purcell-Jones G, Speedy HM, Justins DM: Upper limb sympathetic blockade following intercostal nerve blocks, *Anaesthesia* 42:984, 1987.

143. Brown RH, Tewes PA: Cervical sympathetic blockade after thoracic intercostal injection of local anesthetic, *Anesthesiology* 70:1011, 1989.

144. Allen G, Samson B: Contralateral Horner's syndrome following stellate ganglion block, *Can Anaesth Soc J* 33:112, 1986 (letter).

145. Evans JA, Dobben GD, Gay GR: Peridural effusion of drugs following sympathetic blockade, *JAMA* 200:93, 1967.

146. Moore DC: Complications of regional anesthesia, Springfield, Ill, 1955, Charles C Thomas, p 53.

147. Sharrock NE: Inadvertent "3-in-1 block" following injection of the lateral cutaneous nerve of the thigh, *Anesth Analg* 59:887, 1980.

148. Huang KC, Fitzgerald MR, Tsueda K: Bilateral block of cervical and brachial plexuses following interscalene block, *Anaesth Intensive Care* 14:87, 1986.

149. Manara AR: Brachial plexus block: unilateral thoraco-abdominal blockade following the supraclavicular approach, *Anaesthesia* 42:757, 1987.

150. Macintosh RR, Mushin WM: Observations on the epidural space, *Anaesthesia* 2:100, 1947.

151. Nunn JF, Slavin G: Posterior intercostal nerve block for pain relief after cholecystectomy: anatomical basis and efficacy, *Br J Anaesth* 52:253, 1980.

152. Taveras JM, Wood EH: *Diagnostic neuroradiology*, vol 2, Baltimore, 1976, Williams & Wilkins, p 1144.

153. Shantha TR, Evans JA: The relationship of epidural anesthesia to neural membranes and arachnoid villi, *Anesthesiology* 37:543, 1972.

154. French JD, Strain WH, Jones GE: Mode of extension of contrast substances injected into peripheral nerves, *J Neuropathol Exp Neurol* 7:47, 1948.

155. Moore DC, Hain RF, Ward A, et al: Importance of the perineural spaces in nerve blocking, *JAMA* 13:1050, 1954.

156. Wenger DR, Gitchell RG: Severe infections following pudendal block anesthesia: need for orthopaedic awareness, *J Bone Joint Surg [Am]* 55:202, 1973.

157. Svancarek W, Chirino O, Schaefer G, et al: Retropsoas and subgluteal abscesses following paracervical and pudendal anesthesia, *JAMA* 237:892, 1977.

158. Schmidt RM, Rosenkranz HS: Antimicrobial activity of local anesthetics: lidocaine and procaine, *J Infect Dis* 121:597, 1970.

159. Merkow AJ, McGuinness GA, Erenberg A, et al: The neonatal neurobehavioral effects of bupivacaine, mepivacaine and 2-chloroprocaine used for pudendal block, *Anesthesiology* 52:309, 1980.

160. Hamilton LA Jr, Gottschalk W: Paracervical block: advantages and disadvantages, *Clin Obstet Gynecol* 17:199, 1974.

161. Ralston DH, Shnider SM: The fetal and neonatal effects of regional anesthesia in obstetrics, *Anesthesiology* 48:34, 1978.

162. Katy J, Joseph JW: Neuropathology of neurolytic and semidestructive agents. In Cousins MJ, Bridenbaugh PO, eds: *Neural blockade*, Philadelphia, 1982, JB Lippincott.

163. Moore DC: *Complications of regional anesthesia*, Springfield, Ill, 1955, Charles C Thomas.

164. Swerdlow M: Complications of neurolytic neural blockade. In Cousins MJ, Bridenbaugh PO, ed: *Neural blockade,* Philadelphia, 1982, JB Lippincott.

165. Murphy TM: Complications of neurolytic blocks. In Orkin FK, Cooperman LH, eds: *Complications in anesthesiology,* Philadelphia, 1983, JB Lippincott.

166. Macomber DW: Necrosis of nose and cheek secondary to treatment of trigeminal neuralgia, *Plast Reconstruct Surg* 11:337, 1953.

167. Mannheimer W, Pizzolato P, Adriani J: Mode of action and effects on tissues of long-acting local anesthetics, *JAMA* 154:29, 1953.

168. Hobbs WR, Rall TW, Verdoorn TA: Hypnotics and sedatives: ethanol. In Hardman JG, Limbird LD, eds: *Goodman & Gilman's: the pharmacological basis of therapeutics,* ed 9, New York, 1996, McGraw-Hill, p 361.

169. Noda J, Umeda S, Mori K, et al: Acetaldehyde syndrome after celiac plexus alcohol block, *Anesth Analg* 65:1300, 1986.

170. Noda J, Umeda S, Mori K, et al: Disulfiram-like reaction associated with carmofur after celiac plexus alcohol block, *Anesthesiology* 67:809, 1987.

171. Reid W, Watt JK, Gray TG: Phenol injection of sympathetic chain, *Br J Surg* 57:45, 1970.

172. Barker FG II, Jannetta PJ, Bissonette DJ, et al: The long-term outcome of microvascular decompression for trigeminal neuralgia, *N Engl J Med* 334:1077, 1996.

173. Crimeni R: Clinical experience with mepivacaine and alcohol in neuralgia of the trigeminal nerve, *Acta Anaesthesiol Scand* 24:173, 1966.

174. Hakanson S: Trigeminal neuralgia treated by the injection of glycerol into the trigeminal cistern, *Neurosurgery* 9:638, 1981.

175. Moore DC: *Complications of regional anesthesia,* Springfield, Ill, 1955, Charles C Thomas, p 121.

176. Morrison WV, Kalina RE: Ocular muscle palsy: results following alcohol injection of infraorbital nerve, *Arch Otolaryngol* 94:571, 1971.

177. Horowitz NH, Rizzoli HV: *Postoperative complications in neurosurgical practice,* Baltimore, 1967, Williams & Wilkins.

178. Bean-Lijewski JD: Glossopharyngeal nerve block for pain relief after pediatric tonsillectomy: retrospective analysis and two cases of life-threatening upper airway obstruction from an interrupted trial, *Anesth Analg* 84:1232, 1997.

179. Richardson GS: Bilateral abductor paralysis of vocal cords during local tonsillectomy, *Laryngoscope* 63:1197, 1953.

180. Levelle JP, Martinez OA: Airway obstruction after bilateral carotid endarterectomy, *Anesthesiology* 63:220, 1985.

181. Meyers EF, Ramirez RC, Boniuk I: Grand mal seizures after retrobulbar block, *Arch Ophthalmol* 96:847, 1978.

182. Rosenblatt RM, May DR, Barsoumian K: Cardiopulmonary arrest after retrobulbar block, *Am J Ophthalmol* 90:425, 1980.

183. Kwinten FA, de Moor GP, Lamers RJ: Acute pulmonary edema and trigeminal nerve blockade after retrobulbar block, *Anesth Analg* 83:1322, 1996.

184. Gray AT, Hynson JM: Pulmonary edema after nadbath and retrobulbar blocks, *Anesth Analg* 78:1177, 1994.

185. Elk JR, Wood J, Holladay JT: Pulmonary edema following retrobulbar block, *J Cataract Refract Surg* 14:216, 1988.

186. Wright RS, Feuerman T, Brown J: Neurogenic pulmonary edema after trigeminal nerve blockade, *Chest* 96:436, 1989.

187. Loughnan PM, Brown TC, Edis B, et al: Neurogenic pulmonary oedema in man: aetiology and management with vasodilators based on haemodynamic studies, *Anaesth Intensive Care* 8:65, 1980.

188. Colice GL, Matthay MA, Bass E, et al: Neurogenic pulmonary edema, *Am Rev Respir Dis* 130:941, 1984.

189. Rubin AP: Complications of local anesthesia for ophthalmic surgery, *Br J Anaesth* 75:93, 1995.

190. Rainin EA, Carlson BM: Postoperative diplopia and ptosis: a clinical hypothesis based on myotoxicity of local anesthetics, *Arch Ophthalmol* 103:1337, 1985.

191. Grant JCB: *An atlas of anatomy,* ed 5, Baltimore, 1962, Williams & Wilkins, p 567.

192. Lehmann LJ, Warfield CA, Bajwa ZH: Migraine headache following stellate ganglion block for reflex sympathetic dystrophy, *Headache* 36:335, 1996.

193. Superville-Sovak B, Rasminsky M, Finlayson MH: Complications of phenol neurolysis, *Arch Neurol* 32:226, 1975.

194. Plevak DJ, Linstromberg JW, Danielson DR: Paresthesia vs nonparesthesia: the axillary block, *Anesthesiology* 59:A216, 1983 (abstract).

195. Sada T, Kobayashi T, Murakami S: Continuous axillary brachial plexus block, *Can Anaesth Soc J* 30:201, 1983.

196. Barutell C, Vidal F, Raich M, et al: A neurological complication following interscalene brachial plexus block, *Anaesthesia* 35:365, 1980.

197. Bashein G, Robertson HT, Kennedy WF Jr: Persistent phrenic nerve paresis following interscalene brachial plexus block, *Anesthesiology* 63:102, 1985.

198. Lim EK, Pereira R: Brachial plexus injury following brachial plexus block, *Anaesthesia* 39:691, 1984.

199. Tetzlaff, JE, Dilger J, Yap E, et al: Idiopathic brachial plexitis after total shoulder replacement with interscalene brachial plexus block, *Anesth Analg* 85:644, 1997.

200. Born G: Neuropathy after bupivacaine (Marcaine) wrist and metacarpal blocks, *J Hand Surg [Am]* 9:109, 1984.

201. Nystrom A, Lindstrom G, Reiz S, et al: Bupivacaine: a safe local anesthetic for wrist blocks, *J Hand Surg [Am]* 14:495, 1989.

202. Parziale JR, Marino AR, Herndon JH: Diagnostic peripheral nerve block resulting in compartment syndrome: case report, *Am J Phys Med Rehabil* 67:82, 1988.

203. Tetzlaff, JE, Yoon HJ, Dilger J, et al: Subdural anesthesia as a complication of an interscalene brachial plexus block: case report, *Reg Anesth* 19:357, 1994.

204. Norris D, Klahsen A, Milne B: Delayed bilateral spinal anesthesia following interscalene brachial plexus block. *Can J Anaesth* 43:303, 1996.

205. Baraka A, Hanna M, Hammoud R: Unconsciousness and apnea complicating parascalene brachial plexus block: possible subarachnoid block, *Anesthesiology* 77:1046, 1992.

206. Johr M: A complication of continuous blockade of the femoral nerve, *Reg Anaesth* 10:37, 1987.

207. Aida S, Takahashi H, Shimoji K: Renal subcapsular hematoma after lumbar plexus block, *Anesthesiology* 84:452, 1996.

208. Larsen UT, Hommelgaard P: Pneumatic tourniquet paralysis following intravenous regional analgesia, *Anaesthesia* 42:526, 1987.

209. Carney AL, Anderson EM: Tourniquet subclavian steal: brainstem ischemia and cortical blindness—clinical significance and testing, *Adv Neurol* 30:283, 1981.

210. Kroese AJ, Stiris G: The risk of deep vein thrombosis after operations on a bloodless lower limb: a venographic study, *Injury* 7:271, 1976.

211. Heath ML: Bupivacaine toxicity and Bier blocks, *Anesthesiology* 59:481, 1983.

212. Davies JAH, Wilkey AD, Hall ID: Bupivacaine leak past inflated tourniquets during intravenous regional analgesia, *Anaesthesia* 39:996, 1984.

213. Davies JAH, Hall ID, Wilkey AD, et al: Intravenous regional anesthesia: the danger of the congested arm and the value of occlusion pressure, *Anaesthesia* 39:416, 1983.

214. Haasio J, Hiippala S, Rosenberg PH: Intravenous regional anesthesia of the arm: effect of the technique of exsanguination on the quality of anaesthesia and prilocaine plasma concentrations, *Anaesthesia* 44:19, 1989.
215. Rosenberg PH, Kalso EA, Tuominen MK, et al: Acute bupivacaine toxicity as a result of venous leakage under the tourniquet cuff during a Bier block, *Anesthesiology* 58:95, 1983.
216. Moore DC: Intercostal nerve block and celiac plexus block for pain therapy. In Benedetti C, Chipman CR, Moricca G, eds: *Advances in pain research and therapy: recent advances in the management of pain,* New York, 1984, Raven Press.
217. Moore DC, Mather LE, Bridenbaugh PO, et al: Arterial and venous plasma levels of bupivacaine following epidural and intercostal nerve blocks, *Anesthesiology* 45:39, 1976.
218. Chivers EM: Pulmonary complications following regional anesthesia for abdominal operations, *Br J Anaesth* 20:55, 1946.
219. Ghanayem AJ, Bohlman HH: Transient paraplegia from intraoperative intercostal nerve block after thoracic discectomy, *Spine* 19:1294, 1994.
220. Gay GR, Evans JA: Total spinal anesthesia following lumbar paravertebral block: a potentially lethal complication, *Anesth Analg* 50:344, 1971.
221. DeKrey JA, Schroeder CF, Buechel DR: Selective chemical sympathectomy, *Anesth Analg* 47:633, 1968.
222. Kuzmarov IW, MacIsaac SG, Sioufi, J, et al: Iatrogenic ureteral injury secondary to lumbar sympathetic ganglion blockade, *Urology* 16:617, 1980.
223. Litwin MS: Postsympathectomy neuralgia, *Acta Surg* 84:121, 1962.
224. Moore DC, Bush WH, Burnett LL: Celiac plexus block: a roentgenographic, anatomic study of technique and spread of solution in patients and corpses, *Anesth Analg* 60:369, 1981.
225. Brown DL, Bulley CK, Quiel EL: Neurolytic celiac plexus block for pancreatic cancer pain, *Anesth Analg* 66:869, 1987.
226. Cherry DA, Lamberty J: Paraplegia following coeliac plexus block, *Anaesth Intensive Care* 12:59, 1984.
227. Galizia EJ, Lahira SK: Paraplegia following coeliac plexus block with phenol: case report, *Br J Anaesth* 46:539, 1974.
228. Wong GY, Brown DL: Transient paraplegia following alcohol celiac plexus block, *Reg Anesth* 20:352, 1995.
229. Hayakawa J, Kobayashi O, Murayama H: Paraplegia after intraoperative celiac plexus block, *Anesth Analg* 84:447, 1997.
230. Dean AP, Reed WD: Diarrhoea: an unrecognized hazard of coeliac plexus block, *Aust N Z J Med* 21:47, 1991.
231. Chan VWS: Chronic diarrhea: an uncommon side effect of celiac plexus block, *Anesth Analg* 82:205, 1996.
232. Pateman J, Williams MP, Filshie J: Retroperitoneal fibrosis after multiple coeliac plexus blocks, *Anaesthesia* 45:309, 1990.
233. Fujita Y, Takaori M: Pleural effusion after CT-guided alcohol celiac plexus block, *Anesth Analg* 66:911, 1987.
234. Mercado AO, Naz JF, Ataya KM: Postabortal paracervical abscess as a complication of paracervical block anesthesia: a case report, *J Reprod Med* 34:247, 1989.
235. Kurzel RB, Au AH, Rooholamini SA: Retroperitoneal hematoma as a complication of pudendal block: diagnosis made by computed tomography, *West J Med* 164:523, 1996.
236. Langhoff-Roos J, Lindmark G: Analgesia and maternal side effects of pudendal block at delivery: a comparison of three local anesthetics, *Acta Obstet Gynecol Scand* 64:269, 1985.

Chapter 5

Complications of Pain Therapy

Mark S. Wallace
Scott K. Magnuson

I. COMPLICATIONS OF PHARMACOLOGIC THERAPIES

A. Systemic analgesics

1. Opioids. The opioids are currently our most potent pain relievers. They are derivatives of opium *(Papaver somniferum)* and include naturally occurring opium derivatives, partially synthetic derivatives of morphine, and synthetic compounds. The opioids have been included under the term *narcotic,* which is a misnomer. Use of the term *narcotic* by the U.S. Drug Enforcement Agency to include such drugs as cocaine has fostered misconceptions about long-term use of opioids. However, as long-term opioid use becomes more common, more complications will probably result.

The most common side effects of systemic opioid therapy are respiratory depression, nausea, constipation, and pruritus. Uncommon side effects include immune suppression, hepatotoxicity, subcutaneous reaction (with methadone), myoclonus, hyperalgesia and allodynia, pe-

ripheral edema, seizures (with meperidine), adverse reaction to monoamine oxidase (with meperidine), and delirium (with meperidine) (Box 5-1). With the exception of constipation, tolerance to the common side effects of the opioids is usually rapid.

Respiratory depression is the most serious side effect of opioid use, but it rarely occurs with the doses used in common daily practice. It is more likely to occur in opioid-naive patients, with very high doses of drug, and with methadone. One case report described a series of heroin addicts who died 3 days after starting methadone maintenance therapy. The third day correlated with the peak plasma concentration of the methadone; however, all of the patients had chronic hepatitis and one half had bronchopneumonia. In addition, other drugs were present on blood screening. Thus it is difficult to determine whether methadone was the actual cause of death.[1] If opioids are titrated appropriately, respiratory depression is rarely a problem.

Box 5-1 Complications of systemic opioids

Common
Respiratory depression
Nausea
Constipation
Pruritus

Uncommon
Immune suppression
Hepatotoxicity
Subcutaneous reaction (with methadone)
Myoclonus
Hyperalgesia and allodynia
Peripheral edema
Seizures (with meperidine)
Adverse reaction to monoamine oxidase (with meperidine)
Delirium (with meperidine)

Nausea and vomiting are less serious side effects of opioid use, but they may be substantial barriers to effective use of these agents. Acute nausea is due to the effects of opioids on the chemoreceptor trigger zone, vestibular system, and gastrointestinal system. Nausea and vomiting are uncommon in long-term opioid use because patients develop tolerance to these side effects. It is unclear whether chronic nausea is caused by a direct effect of opioids or by metabolites. Morphine, for example, has two metabolites that have been implicated in chronic nausea: morphine-6-glucuronide and morphine-3-glucuronide.[2-4] These metabolites most often accumulate in the presence of renal failure; however, with long-term morphine use, they can accumulate with normal renal function.

Patients receiving long-term opioid therapy will not develop tolerance to constipation; therefore an aggressive bowel regimen may be necessary. Constipation results from the activation of the mu receptor in the gastrointestinal tract. A prophylactic stool softener, a high-roughage diet, and adequate fluid intake is the most effective way to manage opioid-induced constipation. However, even with aggressive therapy, constipation can continue to be a major problem.[5] If the constipation goes untreated, severe impaction can occur, leading to bowel obstruction. Because opioid-induced constipation often responds poorly to aggressive bowel treatment, interest in oral opioid antagonists has grown. However, results have been mixed, and some patients have experienced loss of analgesia and the abstinence syndrome.[6-10] Pruritus is a minor side effect that most commonly occurs after intraspinal opioid therapy.

The mechanisms of several uncommon side effects of long-term systemic opioid therapy are not known. Myoclonus, a well-known side effect of opioid use, usually occurs with high doses of drug and resolves with cessation of therapy.[11-16] It may also be controlled with anti-

spasmodic agents.[17] Hyperalgesia and allodynia have also been reported with high doses of opioids; the mechanism of this side effect is probably similar to that of myoclonus.[18-20] Peripheral edema has been reported with both systemic and intraspinal opioid therapy.[21,22] The mechanism of this condition is unknown, but it responds poorly to diuretics and resolves with cessation of opioid therapy. Opioids have been shown to cause immunosuppression in preclinical studies, but the clinical significance of this effect is not known.[23-25] A retrospective study of 30 patients with acquired immune deficiency syndrome who were receiving long-term methadone therapy showed no evidence of immune suppression compared with matched controls (unpublished data). Hepatotoxicity has been reported with long-term opioid use, but this has only occurred in the presence of alcohol abuse.[26] Preclinical studies have shown that therapeutic doses of opioids are unlikely to result in hepatotoxicity.[27] In patients with terminal illness, it is common to deliver long-term opioid therapy subcutaneously; this method is well tolerated. Methadone is the only opioid that cannot be delivered by this route because of the possibility of a subcutaneous reaction.[28]

All opioids may induce seizures at high doses. However, meperidine is the only agent that can induce seizures at therapeutic levels. This is caused by its active metabolite normeperidine, which is seizurgenic.[29-32] Seizures occur more often with long-term opioid use and in the presence of renal failure.[33] Because meperidine has atropine-like effects, delirium may occur when this drug is used in combination with an anticholinergic agent.[34] In addition, meperidine has been reported to induce a syndrome characterized by tachycardia, increased blood pressure, arrhythmias, and hyperthermia in patients taking monoamine oxidase inhibitors.[35]

2. Nonopioid analgesics
a. Nonsteroidal antiinflammatory drugs. Nonsteroidal antiinflammatory drugs (NSAIDs) are some of the most common analgesics used for pain. The toxicity associated with NSAIDs constitutes about 72.6% of all toxicities caused by nonopioid analgesics, at a cost of $1.86 billion annually.[36] Side effects of NSAIDs are divided into gastrointestinal, hematologic, renal, and idiosyncratic.[37,38] The first three divisions are related to inhibition of prostaglandin synthesis; the mechanisms of idiosyncratic reactions are not known. As a group, the nonacetylated salicylates are less likely to cause side effects.

NSAIDs directly affect the gastric mucosa by causing localized irritation and indirectly affect the gastric mucosa secondary to a decrease in prostaglandin E_2 and prostaglandin I_2. These two substances protect the gastric mucosa; in their absence, gastric irritation and bleeding may occur. The risk for gastropathy is increased if the patient has a history of peptic ulcer disease or gastric bleeding, continued use of alcohol, increasing age, and high doses of NSAIDs.[39]

With the exception of aspirin, all NSAIDs reversibly inhibit platelet aggregation. Aspirin irreversibly inhibits platelet aggregation; therefore its effects last for the life span of the platelet. The effects of NSAIDs on platelet function vary according to the ratio of thromboxane to prostacyclin inhibition. These agents should be used cautiously in anticoagulated patients.[37]

Nephrotoxicity induced by NSAIDs is rare in healthy patients with normal renal function because renal blood flow and glomerular filtration are not prostaglandin dependent. However, in the presence of volume depletion or hepatic cirrhosis (or both), the risk for nephrotoxicity is substantial because renal function is dependent on normal prostaglandin levels. Nephrotoxicity manifests as hematuria, proteinuria, and the nephrotic syndrome. In addition, use of NSAIDs may lead to fluid retention, impaired responsiveness to diuretics, and hyperkalemia.[40]

Several rare, idiosyncratic side effects may result from NSAID use,[41-44] including dermatologic reactions, asymptomatic transaminasemia, and exacerbation of bronchospasm. Idiosyncratic reactions specific to certain NSAIDs include bone marrow toxicity (with phenylbutazone), central nervous system symptoms (with indomethacin), aseptic meningitis (with ibuprofen, sulindac, and tolmetin), and bilateral pulmonary infiltrates (with naproxen).

b. Acetaminophen. Acetaminophen is one of the most commonly used analgesics. The major serious side effect of this agent is hepatic necrosis, which usually occurs only with large doses. Fifty percent of adults develop severe hepatotoxicity with oral doses of 250 mg/kg of body weight, and almost 100% develop this condition with doses of 350 mg/kg.[45] However, in the setting of long-term use or alcohol abuse, the total daily dose of acetaminophen required for hepatic toxicity may be lower than the short-term dose.[46] Hepatic necrosis results from the formation of *N*-acetylbenzoquinoneimine, which reacts with the glutathione and sulfhydryl groups of proteins.[47] If long-term acetaminophen therapy is used, the total daily dose should be no more than 4 g.

Large doses of acetaminophen may also cause nephrotoxicity by mechanisms that are similar to those of hepatotoxicity. The renal manifestations are similar to those of acute tubular necrosis. The risk for nephrotoxicity increases in the presence of starvation, alcoholism, or medications that activate the P-450 system.[48]

c. Tramadol. Tramadol is a new analgesic that is gaining popularity in the United States. The most common side effects of this agent are nausea, somnolence, dizziness, vomiting, and headache. In long-term trials, nausea has been the most common side effect.[49]

3. Coanalgesics

a. Antidepressants. The side effects of antidepressants result from the anticholinergic, antihistaminic, antidopaminergic, and α_1-blocking activity of these agents. Because of this activity, the following side effects occur[50]:

- Anticholinergic effects, consisting of dry mouth, constipation, urinary retention, sedation, worsening of narrow-angle glaucoma
- Antihistaminic effects, consisting of sedation
- Antidopaminergic effects, consisting of dystonia
- α_1-Blockade, consisting of orthostatic hypotension
- Altered cardiac conduction through the His-Purkinje conduction system manifested by prolongation of the QRS complex

Table 5-1. Side effects unique to each antidepressant

Drug	Side effect
Amitriptyline	Weight gain
Amoxapine	Seizures, neuroleptic malignant syndrome
Fluoxetine	Occasional anxiety and nausea
Paroxetine	Nausea, sweating, dizziness, weakness, diarrhea, constipation, ejaculatory disturbances
Trazodone	Priapism
Maprotiline	Seizures

The side effects of the various antidepressants depend on the ratio of the different activities just mentioned. For example, tricyclic agents are more sedating than serotonin-specific reuptake inhibitors and atypical antidepressants. Of the tricyclic agents, amitriptyline is the most sedating, and desipramine is the least sedating. Table 5-1 lists side effects unique to each antidepressant.[51,52]

Antidepressant overdose occurs at a rate of approximately 250,000 to 500,000 incidents per year in the United States.[53,54] The presenting signs of overdose are related to the extreme manifestations of the intrinsic activity previously described. Extreme sedation, hypotension, and cardiac conduction defects are the most common presenting symptoms. Substantial overdose may result in coma, anticholinergic syndrome, adult respiratory distress syndrome, and seizures.[51]

b. Anticonvulsants. Because the anticonvulsants are chemically unrelated to one another, they all produce different side effects. Side effects that they have in common relate to the central nervous system and present as sedation, tremor, and ataxia.[51] With the exception of gabapentin, all anticonvulsants may cause cognitive and behavioral effects.[55,56] In addition, with the exception of clonazepam, all anticonvulsant agents produce nausea. Table 5-2 lists the side effects unique to each anticonvulsant.[51,57,58]

With the exception of clonazepam and gabapentin, overdose with any anticonvulsant may be fatal. Massive overdose may manifest as any combination of coma, seizures, respiratory failure, and cardiac conduction defects.[59,60]

c. Antiarrhythmic agents. Currently, mexiletine and tocainide are the only two oral antiarrhythmic agents used in management of chronic pain. They are structurally related to lidocaine and have side effects similar to those of lidocaine. The most common side effects are nausea, tremors, and irritability, which are dose related.[61] Tocainide produces the additional side effects of pulmonary fibrosis, agranulocytosis, and anemia.[62,63]

Overdose with antiarrhythmic agents may be fatal. Massive overdose may present as drowsiness, confusion, seizures, and respiratory arrest.[64] Cardiovascular toxicity manifests as progressive heart block, reduced cardiac contraction, hypotension, and asystole.[65] High doses of these agents are also proarrhythmic.

d. α_1-Antagonists and α_2-agonists. Orthostatic hypotension is the most common side effect of α_1-antagonists

Table 5-2. Side effects unique to each anticonvulsant

Drug	Side effects
Carbamazepine	Hematologic abnormalities
	Liver toxicity
Gabapentin	Weight gain
Phenytoin	Hirsutism
	Gingival hyperplasia
	Folic acid deficiency–induced neuropathy
	Vitamin K and D deficiency
	Hyperglycemia
Valproic acid	Transient alopecia
	Liver toxicity
	Weight gain

Table 5-3. Side effects of intraspinal opioids

Side effect	Incidence (%)
Respiratory depression	
Early	Rare
delayed	0.1-1
Sedation	
Nausea	5-50
Pruritus	10-75
Urinary retention	0-15
Reactivation of herpes simplex	3-14
Decreased muscle tone	0-5
Decreased gastrointestinal motility	50
Other	
Polyarthralgia	1-3
Amenorrhea	2.4
Peripheral edema	6.1

and α_2-agonists. The body fluids shift to compensate and eventually eliminate this side effect. Because of the decrease in blood pressure, a reflex tachycardia may result from use of α_1-antagonists. Because of its effects on the central nervous system, clonidine can result in sedation.

e. Antihistamines and muscle relaxants. Hydroxyzine is the only antihistamine with analgesic activity. Sedation is the most common side effect. Ataxia and disinhibition may also occur, and convulsions have been reported with high doses of hydroxyzine.[51]

The centrally acting skeletal muscle relaxants all have similar pharmacologic profiles. Drowsiness is the most common side effect, and headache, dizziness, blurred vision, nausea, and vomiting have been reported.[66] Chlorzoxazone has been reported to cause jaundice.[51]

B. Intraspinal analgesics

1. Opioids. Most of the side effects that occur with systemic delivery of opioids also occur with spinal delivery. However, the incidence and mechanism of these side effects differ. Table 5-3 lists the side effects of intraspinal opioid therapy.

a. Respiratory depression. Respiratory depression occurs almost exclusively with short-term intraspinal delivery of opioids; this effect is rarely seen with long-term intraspinal delivery. Respiratory depression after intraspinal administration of opioids may occur early or late. Early respiratory depression is thought to result from vascular redistribution, whereas late respiratory depression results from rostral spread in the cerebrospinal fluid. The more hydrophilic opioids clearly produce late respiratory depression by rostral spread; however, the exact mechanism of early depression is debatable. The route by which opioid reaches the brainstem is a point of controversy. Some believe that the drug is delivered directly to the brainstem by means of the vasculature, whereas others think that it goes first to the basivertebral venous system, then to the cisternal cerebrospinal fluid and to the brainstem.

When evaluating the respiratory effects of intraspinal opioids, one must differentiate between postoperative patients (who have a painful stimulus) and volunteers (who do not have a painful stimulus). In general, volunteers seem to have a dose response. Higher doses of epidural opioids cause a prolonged respiratory depres-

sion in volunteers that is not consistently seen in post-surgical patients. In addition, one study in which the same dose of diamorphine was given to the same patients before and after surgery showed that more profound early respiratory depression occurred before surgery.[67]

A painful stimulus can act for or against the development of respiratory depression. Pain stimulates respiration; however, it also inhibits the ability to breathe after thoracic and abdominal surgery, causing intrathoracic pressure to increase and drainage of the azygous system to be inhibited. In theory, this may increase blood flow through the basivertebral venous plexus and deliver more opioid to the brain. Intraabdominal procedures may also increase basivertebral flow by obstructing inferior vena cava flow. There are 25 case reports on respiratory depression after intraspinal opioids reported in the literature. In addition, there are 22 investigational studies on the effect of intraspinal opioids on respiration after surgery. Fifteen of the case reports and 14 of the investigational studies involve abdominal or thoracic surgery. Although the case reports demonstrate that respiratory depression can occur after intraspinal opioids, the investigational studies fail to demonstrate any significant respiratory depression in postoperative patients regardless of the site of surgery. However, it is difficult to extract from the literature the effects of surgical site on delayed respiratory depression because of the varying doses of opioid administered and varying ages of the patients.

Other factors contribute to delayed respiratory depression in postoperative patients. These include residual effects of parenteral opioids and sedatives (in 17 of 25 case reports and 8 of 22 investigational studies, patients received a sedative, an opioid, or both at some time before or after intraspinal administration of opioid) and residual effects of anesthesia. In addition, some studies showed respiratory depression immediately after surgery but before intraspinal opioid therapy in pediatric patients; this respiratory depression did not change significantly after opioid administration.[68,69]

There are no reports in the literature of delayed respiratory depression with lipid-soluble opioids. However, all opioids tend to cause early respiratory depression after epidural administration. Although only two investigations examined the respiratory effects of intrathecal morphine, neither produced early respiratory depression. The mechanism of this condition after epidural opioid therapy is controversial. Some investigators claim that early respiratory depression after epidural administration of opioids is due to rostral spread within the cerebrospinal fluid, whereas others claim that vascular redistribution is the cause. Some studies show peak cisternal concentration of opioids that are higher than peak plasma levels and claim that rostral spread is the mechanism, whereas others claim the reverse situation; that is, the opioid is absorbed systemically and delivered to the brainstem via the circulatory system. The problem of peak plasma concentrations of opioid that are lower than cisternal concentrations lies in the site of sampling. Plasma samples taken from an extremity will not reflect concentrations of opioid in the basivertebral system. Because the basivertebral system directly drains the site of opioid administration, plasma concentrations of opioid in this system will be very high and transfer a considerable quantity of opioid to the cisternal cerebrospinal fluid. This may explain the early peak cisternal concentrations and early respiratory depression seen with lipid-soluble agents. It has been shown that the epidural administration of lipid-soluble opioids result in early peak cisternal concentrations (10 minutes).[69a] Because lipid-soluble agents have limited rostral spread, bulk flow within the cerebrospinal fluid does not explain early peak cisternal concentrations after epidural administration of opioids.

The pharmacokinetics of epidural administration of a hydrophilic agent, such as morphine, differ slightly from those of lipid-soluble opioids. Substantial vascular absorption into the basivertebral plexus will occur; early delivery of the agent into the cisternal cerebrospinal fluid will then result in early respiratory depression. However, the drug will penetrate the dura and enter the cerebrospinal fluid. From there, bulk flow will move the drug rostrally to reach the cerebrospinal fluid at a time when plasma concentrations in the basivertebral plexus are negligible. This will result in a second increase in cisternal concentrations and delayed respiratory depression. Vascular redistribution results in early cisternal concentrations within the first hour. Between 1 and 2 hours, plasma concentrations of opioid within the basivertebral plexus decreases with a corresponding decrease in cisternal concentrations. As the opioid redistributes rostrally within the cerebrospinal fluid, a second increase in cisternal concentration occurs later, after 2 to 3 hours.

It is difficult to determine the exact mechanism of delayed respiratory depression after intrathecal morphine because in all of the published case reports, excessive doses of opioid (3 to 20 mg) in excessive volumes of fluid (3 to 10 ml) were used. In one exception, a patient only received 0.4 mg of drug; however, the volume of fluid was not stated, and the patient was elderly.[70] Intrathecal administration of opioids results in cerebrospinal fluid concentrations of drug more than 100 times greater than those that are found with epidural administration. These very high concentrations create a large concentration gradient that is more favorable for rostral spread of the drug in the cerebrospinal fluid. In addition, direct injection of the drug into the cerebrospinal fluid would create turbulence that could carry the drug rostrally to reach the brainstem early. The lack of case reports on early respiratory depression after intrathecal administration of morphine probably stems from the lack of recognition of this condition. Early respiratory depression is probably often mistaken as the residual effects of anesthesia. The lack of studies on the respiratory effects of intrathecal opioid therapy makes it difficult to describe the relation between the pharmacokinetics of intrathecally administered opioids and respiratory depression.

Identified risk factors for respiratory depression include old age, poor general condition, residual effects of general anesthesia, supplementary analgesia with epidural local anesthetics or parenteral opioid therapy, decreased pulmonary function, prolonged surgery in debilitated patients, and possibly, the spinal level at which opioids are administered. However, it is difficult to verify the relation between these factors and respiratory depression.

In summary, investigations of the effects of epidural opioid therapy on respiration show that both early and late respiratory depression may occur. Early respiratory depression is best explained by the delivery of agents (both lipid soluble and lipid insoluble) to the brainstem via the basivertebral plexus. Late respiratory depression is best explained by the rostral spread of the lipid-insoluble agents to reach the brainstem. Intrathecal injection of the lipid-soluble and lipid-insoluble opioids may result in early respiratory depression from the turbulent spread to the brainstem. However, late respiratory depression is best explained by the rostral spread in the cerebrospinal fluid. The lack of controlled studies makes it difficult to explain the exact mechanism of respiratory depression after intrathecal administration of opioids.

b. Sedation. Sedation may accompany respiratory depression and may signal impending respiratory depression. Many studies have noted less sedation with intraspinal opioid therapy than with systemic opioid therapy. Sedation most commonly occurs with prolonged infusions of the lipophilic agents; this represents vascular absorption and redistribution. The use of κ-selective agents is associated with deeper sedation.[71]

c. Nausea. The incidence of nausea varies widely but is more common with hydrophilic opioids (30% to 50% with morphine and hydromorphone) than with lipophilic agents (5% to 30% with fentanyl, sufentanil, and alfentanil)[72] Clearly nausea may occur secondary to vascular redistribution and rostral spread. In a 1982 study by Bromage et al,[73] nausea occurred about 6 hours after epidural administration of morphine in six of six volunteers. This most likely was due to rostral spread of the drug in the cerebrospinal fluid.[73] Early nausea most likely results from vascular redistribution.

The mechanism of the nausea is activation of the chemoreceptor trigger zone in the brainstem. Therefore the same principles discussed for respiratory depression apply for nausea.

d. Pruritus. Pruritus is an annoying side effect that occurs more commonly after administration of hydrophilic agents (40% to 75% of patients) than lipophilic agents (10% to 55% of patients).[72] Pruritus is often overlooked because many patients do not mention it. After administration of hydrophilic agents, pruritus is not only confined to the area of delivery of the opioid but also occurs on the face and neck. Thomas et al[74] demonstrated intense facial scratching in monkeys given morphine in the medullary dorsal horn. On this basis, they proposed that opioids act in the medullary dorsal horn to produce pruritus. Facial and neck itching probably represent rostral spread of the agent in the cerebrospinal fluid because lipophilic agents rarely cause itching in this area. The fact that lipophilic agents usually do not cause itching of the face and neck does not support delivery of the agent to the brainstem by means of the basivertebral plexus. If this system delivered agents to the brainstem, more pruritus of the face and neck would be evident.

Pruritus occurs much less frequently with systemic opioid therapy, which suggests a spinal mechanism for this side effect. Both excitatory and inhibitory mechanisms have been proposed. Shen and Crain[75] reported that low concentrations of morphine had an excitatory effect on cultured dorsal root ganglion cells in the mouse. It has also been proposed that opiates antagonize the inhibitory neurotransmitter glycine, which may lead to excitation of the dorsal horn cells.[76] It is unlikely that pruritus results from histamine release. Korsh et al[77] did not find increased plasma histamine concentrations in patients who had pruritus after epidural administration of 5 mg of morphine. Of note, antihistamines relieve pruritus in some patients.

e. Urinary retention. Urinary retention can occur with all opioids but seems to be more common with hydrophilic opioids (incidence of 10% to 15%) than with lipophilic agents (incidence of 0% of 5%).[72] The reason why hydrophilic agents cause a higher incidence of this side effect is not clear but may be associated with better penetrance of these agents into the dorsal horn. This better penetrance may occur because less drug binds to the myelin in the gray matter; thus more drug is available to reach the dorsal horn.[77a]

The mechanism of urinary retention of opioids is thought to be suppression of the micturition reflex through an action at the spinal level.[78] This autonomic reflex is inhibited by μ- and δ-agonists, but not κ-agonists.[79] Studies in humans show detrusor muscle relaxation with an increase in bladder capacity and a slight increase in external sphincter tone.[80] Although the exact mechanism of opioid actions on bladder function is not clear, there seems to be a vesicosphincteric dyssynergy.[81] Intraspinal opioid therapy has been shown to suppress the monosynaptic flexor reflexes involved in motor function.[82] This phenomenon results in a decrease in the spasticity seen in patients with spinal cord injury. This mechanism may be related to the suppression of the micturition reflex.

f. Reactivation of herpes simplex virus. Herpes simplex type I (labialis) has an estimated incidence of 3% to 35%.[83-85] A report on 4880 patients showed an incidence of 3.5%.[85] Herpes simplex reactivation has only been reported with use of morphine. Gieraerts et al[83] reported a correlation between facial pruritus and herpes simplex reactivation. This explains the lack of reactivation with lipophilic agents in that facial pruritus is not seen with these drugs. It is not clear whether the reactivation of the herpes is secondary to a direct effect of morphine on the trigeminal dorsal horn or ganglion or to facial scratching. It would be interesting to see whether the incidence would be decreased with aggressive treatment of pruritus.

g. Effect on motor function. Under normal circumstances, intraspinal administration of opioids does not affect motor function.[86] However, electrophysiologic studies have shown that intraspinal opioid therapy suppresses the monosynaptic flexor reflexes and antagonizes the motor neuron activity evoked by muscle stretch.[82,87] This side effect can be beneficial in the treatment of spasticity after spinal cord injury. Intraspinal administration of low doses of morphine has been shown to be effective in the treatment of spinal spasticity.[88]

h. Effect on gastrointestinal function. Systemic opioid therapy decreases gastrointestinal motility and may lead to constipation.[89,90] A similar effect has been shown after intraspinal delivery of μ- and δ-agonists in mice.[91] Although the effect of systemic opioid therapy on gastrointestinal function has been extensively studied, the effect of intraspinal delivery on gastrointestinal function has been poorly studied. One study in humans showed a delay in gastric emptying after thoracic epidural administration of 4 mg of morphine. The same dose administered intramuscularly did not produce this effect.[92] Therefore both human and animal studies indicate that intraspinal opioid therapy causes a delay in gastric emptying through a spinal mechanism.

i. Rare side effects. Other side effects that have been reported with intraspinal opioid therapy include polyarthralgia, amenorrhea, and peripheral edema.[93] The incidence and mechanism of these side effects are unknown.

2. Nonopioid analgesics. Other agents used intraspinally for pain management include clonidine, baclofen, and local anesthetics. Side effects reported with epidural administration of clonidine include hypotension, bradycardia, and withdrawal symptoms.[94] Side effects of baclofen—dizziness, somnolence, respiratory depression, and even coma—are for the most part related to central nervous system toxicity. Abrupt withdrawal of baclofen therapy may lead to seizures.[93] Long-term administration of local anesthetics may lead to reversible sensory and motor changes if excessive doses are used. The cauda equina syndrome has been reported after continuous spinal anesthesia using a small-bore catheter (28 gauge or smaller). In all patients, sacral block was initially restricted; to achieve an adequate depth of anesthesia, a dose of local anesthetic was administered that was greater than that usually used with a single-injection technique. The authors postulated that the combination of maldistribution and a relatively high dose of local anesthetic exposed neural tissue to a toxic concentration of anesthetic, leading to neural injury.[95] Since then, the

U.S. Food and Drug Administration removed small-bore catheters from the market. Local anesthetics in high concentrations have been shown to be neurotoxic.[96,97] The cauda equina syndrome has not been reported with the chronic delivery of local anesthetics by means of an implanted pump.

II. COMPLICATIONS OF SPINAL DIAGNOSTIC TECHNIQUES

A. Zygapophyseal (facet) and sacroiliac joint injections

The role of the facet and sacroiliac joints in back and neck pain is controversial. However, injection with local anesthetics and/or corticosteroids of these structures for the relief of pain is commonly performed. Although the benefits of this procedure are questionable, the risks are very low. Major complications that may result from incorrect needle placement include injury to the cord or nerve roots or inadvertent epidural, subdural, or subarachnoid placement of local anesthetic. Injection of the cervical facets may result in vertebral artery injection and seizure. Because of the course of the vertebral artery across the atlantoaxial joint, cervical facet injection is more likely when the lateral approach to this joint is used. Thus the block should always be performed from the posterior approach. However, care must be taken not to enter the joint too laterally because the vertebral artery may be entered.[98] Another possible side effect of upper cervical facet injection is ataxia and dizziness resulting from loss of the postural tonic neck reflexes.[99,100] Injection of the thoracic facet may result in pneumothorax. Use of fluoroscopy and careful attention to the anatomy should avoid these complications.[101]

B. Diskography

The complications listed for facet and sacroiliac joint injections also apply for diskography. The overall incidence of complications associated with diskography is 1.5%; diskitis is the most common.[102] Because of the poor blood supply to the central portion of the disk, risk for infection is, in theory, increased if bacteria are introduced into the disk. Because of this, diskitis can be very difficult to treat. Epidural abscess resulting from diskography has been reported.[103]

III. COMPLICATIONS OF NEUROLYTIC TECHNIQUES

Neurolysis involves the destruction of nervous tissue by surgical, chemical, thermal, or cryogenic means. It is usually indicated in patients with chronic pain and a limited life expectancy, most often because of cancer. Neurolysis has also been used to treat other chronic pain syndromes (Box 5-2), but this use is more controversial, and the relative risks of this treatment compared with the benefits must be carefully considered. Although cancer pain can be controlled with other means in most patients, almost 30% of patients require some sort of neurolytic blockade as a complete or adjunctive therapy.[104] Knowledge of the complications of neurolysis allows the physician to more adequately assess the suitability of a given procedure and to obtain proper informed consent from the patient.

A. Chemical neurolysis

Chemical neurolysis is most often performed with alcohol, phenol, or glycerol, although distilled water, ammonium salts, chlorocresol, and hypertonic saline have been used in the past. These chemicals are injected into the intrathecal, subdural, or epidural spaces; a nervous plexus or ganglion; or directly onto a peripheral nerve. Complications vary depending on the neurolytic agent used and the anatomic site of neurolysis.

Alcohol is one of the oldest and most commonly used neurolytic agents. Concentrations of 33% to more than 95% have been used. Alcohol leads to extraction of cholesterol, phospholipid, and cerebroside from nervous tissue and causes precipitation of lipoproteins and mucoproteins.[105] Wallerian degeneration ensues after injection onto peripheral nerves and with intrathecal injections.[106] When alcohol is injected onto peripheral nerves, the basal lamina around the Schwann tube is left intact, and regeneration of the nerve is possible. However, if the cell body is destroyed, regeneration is not possible.[107] Pain on injection caused by local irritation is common and can be blocked with the use of small amounts of local anesthetic injected before the alcohol. However, some patients develop neuralgias following alcohol injection that may persist from days to weeks.

Phenol first gained attention as a neurolytic agent after early reports suggested that this agent destroyed small motor fibers while sparing large ones.[108-110] However, subsequent studies found that low concentrations of phenol may have an effect similar to that of local anesthetics but concentrations sufficiently high to produce a prolonged response lead to nonselective destruction of nerve fibers similar to that seen with alcohol.[111-114] Phenol acts primarily through coagulation of proteins.[115] The degree of destruction produced by phenol is directly related to the concentration of the solution used. Injected intrathecally, phenol produces degeneration in the posterior columns and posterior nerve roots similar to that caused by alcohol. Peripheral application leads to segmental demyelination and wallerian degeneration. Regeneration after neurolysis with phenol occurs more rapidly with phenol than with alcohol. Phenol can be dissolved in water or glycerin but may be more potent in the aqueous solution. Reports that phenol may have greater affinity for vascular tissue than neurophospholipids have led some clinicians to favor alcohol over phenol for use in areas around major blood vessels, such as with celiac plexus neurolysis.[116]

Box 5-2 Indications for neurolysis

Cancer pain
Morton neuroma
Chronic pancreatitis
Chronic abdominal pain
Spinal cord spasticity
Trigeminal neuralgia
Peripheral vascular disease
Facet arthropathy

Glycerol has been used extensively since 1981 for facial pain, including trigeminal neuralgia and tic douloureux.[117-119] Histologic studies have shown the presence of inflammatory cells, myelin swelling, and axonolysis.[120] Burchiel and Russell[121] reported differential effects of glycerol on the electrophysiologic function of the nerve, but this has not been substantiated in histologic studies. Myelin destruction can occur weeks after administration of glycerol, suggesting that other events, such as compression of transperineural vessels leading to ischemia, may be at least partly responsible for the neurodestructive effects of this agent.

Knowing the mechanism of action of neurolytic agents helps to determine the possible complications associated with chemical neurolysis. Although all of the most commonly used neurolytic agents produce similar histologic results, the site of injection is the factor most directly related to the possible adverse consequences. If the neurolytic agent overflows into an area not intended for the block, catastrophic and long-lasting complications may result. The most common complaint with alcohol neurolytic blockade is pain on injection. Phenol, which has some local anesthetic properties, is associated with more comfort on injection. Pain on injection can be blocked by the use of small amounts of local anesthetics before injection.

Because of the risk for intravascular injection, repeated aspiration during injection should be performed. Intravascular injection of alcohol can produce acute intoxication and has been known to cause thrombosis of the vessel. Intravascular injection of phenol can produce a range of symptoms, including tinnitus, flushing, convulsions, cardiovascular depression, central nervous system depression, and renal damage.[122-125] Use of phenol carries a risk for cardiovascular toxicity; the mechanism of action remains unknown but may be related to the ability of phenol to produce sodium channel blockade in cardiac muscle.[126] Although cardiovascular toxicity is more frequent with dermal application of phenol, it has been reported with use of phenol in neurolytic blocks.[127]

Dermal swelling or cellulitis may occur after an injection of a neurolytic agent if the needle is removed without first being cleared. Patients with persistent pain in the area of injection may have an abscess or cellulitis caused by this mechanism. A small flush with saline or local anesthetic will prevent this complication.

Intrathecal neurolysis has been used extensively in the treatment of cancer and chronic nonmalignant pain syndromes with great success. However, the relative close proximity of sensory, motor, and autonomic nerve roots can result in complications. Positioning is key in performing a successful block, not only for targeting areas traversed by pain fibers but also for avoiding areas in which intrathecal neurolysis can lead to a poor outcome. Alcohol is hypobaric, whereas phenol is hyperbaric. Therefore while one administers an alcohol-based intrathecal neurolytic agent, the patient must be positioned with the dorsal nerve roots at the highest point. For phenol injection, the patients should be positioned with the dorsal nerve roots at the lowest point. Paresis, bladder dysfunction, bowel dysfunction, and dysesthesia have all been reported. Two older studies of intrathecal alcohol blocks revealed a total of 892 intrathecal alcohol blocks in 574 patients, causing 22 cases of bladder or muscle weakness (or both) and 4 cases of proprioceptive loss. Five of the 26 patients with complications had some permanent limb paralysis, and one of those five had permanent urinary incontinence.[128,129] Gerbershagen[130] reviewed reports of 2125 subarachnoid alcohol blocks leading to a total of 303 complications and found that most complications resolved within 4 months (Table 5-4). Likewise, Swerdlow[131] analyzed data from 300 patients receiving neurolytic blockade with phenol, chlorocresol, or both and found similar incidences of complications (Table 5-5).

In the cauda equina at the termination of the spinal cord (L1 to L2), the anterior and posterior roots are

Table 5-4. Complications in subarachnoid alcohol blocks

Complication	Duration transient no. (%)	Permanent no. (%)	Total no. (%)
Paresis or paralysis	92 (4.3)	18 (0.8)	110 (5.2)
Bladder dysfunction	137 (6.4)	16 (0.8)	153 (7.2)
Bowel disorder	8 (0.4)	3 (0.1)	11 (0.5)
Other	19 (0.9)	10 (0.5)	29 (1.4)
All (mean)	256 (12)	47 (2.2)	303 (14.3)

Data from Gerbershagen HY: *Acta Anaesthesiol Belg* 1:45, 1981.

Table 5-5. Complications of intrathecal neurolytic blockade using phenol and chlorocresol

Drug(s)	No. of patients	Complications						
		Bladder paresis no. (%)	Bowel paresis no. (%)	Muscle paresis no. (%)	Headache no. (%)	Paresthesia no. (%)	Numbness no. (%)	Total no. (%)
Phenol	145	7 (5)	1 (0.7)	4 (3)		1 (0.7)	4 (3)	17 (12)
Chlorocresol	138	10 (7)	1 (0.7)	7 (5)	1 (0.7)	1 (0.7)	4 (4)	25 (1)
Phenol and chlorocresol	17	3 (18)	1 (6)		1 (6)		1 (6)	6 (35)
All (mean)	300	20 (7)	3 (1)	11 (4)	2 (1)	2 (0.7)	9 (3)	48 (16)

Data from Swerdlow M: Intrathecal and extradural block and pain relief. In Swerdlow M, ed: *Relief of intractable pain,* Amsterdam, 1983, Elsevier.

closer to one another and the risk for lower-extremity paralysis is higher. Paralysis of intercostal muscles is usually well tolerated except in patients with severe respiratory disease.[132] Bladder dysfunction is possible with injections at or below the T10 vertebral level.

Epidural neurolysis has been used for the same indications as intrathecal neurolysis. Theoretical advantages include less cranial spread, less meningeal irritation, and the allowance for repeated injections if a catheter is left in place. An animal study of epidural phenol therapy, however, demonstrated poor control over the spread of neurolytic agents in the epidural space, with a high incidence of anterior root spread.[133] Efficacy rates are generally similar to those for intrathecal injections. Swerdlow[134] reported on 221 patients with cancer pain who received epidural injections of 6% to 10% phenol. Fifty-seven (26%) developed urinary incontinence; in 17 (8%), this condition persisted for longer than 2 weeks. Likewise, bowel incontinence was present immediately after neurolysis in 21 patients (10%) and lasted longer than 2 weeks in 8 (4%). Muscle weakness was seen in 14 patients (6%) initially and in 3 (1%) after 2 weeks. Bromage[135] discusses a series of 55 epidural neurolytic procedures using alcohol or phenol in which two patients had transient motor weakness, one after a thoracic block and one after a lumbar block. Two patients also developed transient urinary retention. Transient neuritis lasting 24 to 48 hours has also been reported following epidural neurolytic block with phenol in cancer patients.[136]

Celiac plexus neurolysis is very effective for treatment of abdominal pain, primarily of malignant origin, that involves the abdominal viscera. Approaches to the celiac plexus can be anterior, posterior, and intraabdominal (i.e., during surgery). These blocks have been performed both blind and with the aid of imaging techniques, such as computed tomography, fluoroscopy, and ultrasonography. Regardless of the approach and technique used, major complications can occur with this block. However, a review by Brown, Bulley, and Quiel[137] of 136 patients receiving neurolytic celiac plexus block for treatment of pancreatic cancer found no permanent neurologic complications, although two patients had pneumothorax. Reported complications include hypotension, subarachnoid injection, epidural injection, intraosseus injection, intrapsoas injection, retroperitoneal hematoma, and puncture of the viscera.[138] Further complications associated with neurolytic celiac plexus block include paralysis, dysesthesias, and sexual dysfunction. In a recent metaanalysis of complications of neurolytic celiac plexus block, common adverse effects were transient and included local pain (96% of patients), diarrhea (44%), and hypotension (38%).[139] A review of the major complications of neurolytic celiac plexus block (paraplegia and loss of bowel or bladder function) reported an incidence of 1 in 638 blocks.[140]

Hypotension results from spread of the neurolytic agent in the retroperitoneal space to the lumbar sympathetic plexus. Patients should have adequate intravascular access, and vasoactive drugs should be at hand in the event of severe hypotension. Gorbitz and Leavens[141] proposed that patients who experience exaggerated hypotension with a local anesthetic celiac plexus block should not be subjected to celiac plexus block with neurolytic agents.

Inadvertent intrathecal injection during celiac plexus block is more than a theoretical concern. Moore[142] reported on 3000 patients presenting for celiac plexus block of whom 18 had evidence of intrathecal injection. One case report described inadvertent intrathecal injection of alcohol that led to left lower-extremity paralysis and loss of anal and bladder sphincter function.[143] Paraplegia without intrathecal injection of neurolytics has also been reported.[144,145] One postulated mechanism is diffusion of the neurolytic agent onto the arterial supply of the spinal cord, also known as anterior spinal artery syndrome. Preclinical studies have shown sustained vasoconstriction in arterial smooth muscle with both alcohol and phenol.[146,147] Spread of neurolytics onto the somatic nerves can lead to persistent neuritis.[148]

A risk for hemorrhage is associated with celiac plexus block; this risk may be more pronounced in the setting of vascular prosthetic grafts. Gale et al[149] investigated the effect of alcohol and phenol on the tensile strength of Dacron and Gore-Tex prosthetic grafts in vitro. Alcohol and phenol caused substantial degradation of the Dacron grafts but only moderate degradation of the Gore-Tex grafts. These findings suggest that serious consideration should be given to alternative techniques of pain relief in patients with vascular prosthetic grafts in the immediate area of neurolytic blockade. Aortic pseudoaneurysm has also been reported as a complication of celiac plexus block.[150] Diarrhea is common after neurolytic celiac plexus block secondary to unopposed parasympathetic stimulation of the gut. This gradually resolves over days to weeks, although chronic diarrhea has been reported.[151] Hematuria can occur if the course of the needle is too lateral, resulting in puncture of the kidney.[142,143]

Other paravertebral sympathetic blocks have risks similar to those of celiac plexus block and risks that are unique to the anatomy of the area. Neurolytic lumbar sympathetic blocks have been associated with dysesthesias and paraplegia involving the lumbar dermatomes, most often L1 and L2. This may represent the anterior spinal artery syndrome (which is also seen in celiac plexus block).[152] Ureter laceration and puncture of the kidney have also occurred.[134] Genitofemoral and ilioinguinal neuralgia can be caused by spillover of the neurolytic agent or by needle tracking if the agent is not cleared from the needle before withdrawal. This is estimated to occur in 7% to 20% of lumbar neurolytic blocks and may take 5 weeks or more to resolve.[122,153] Ejaculatory dysfunction lasting 5 weeks following bilateral lumbar neurolytic blockade was reported by Baxter and O'Kafo.[154] Use of radiographic imaging techniques with a radiopaque solution while performing such blocks can reduce the incidence of these complications.

Thoracic sympathetic block is less commonly performed than celiac plexus or lumbar sympathetic block.

Pneumothorax, intercostal neuritis, and pleuritic chest pain are recognized complications.[155,156] Brown-Sequard paralysis may occur if the neurolytic agent reaches the spinal cord through inadvertent intrathecal injection.[156,157]

Stellate ganglion block with neurolytic agents can involve prolonged Horner syndrome. Spillage of the neurolytic agent onto the brachial plexus can cause upper-extremity motor weakness and neuralgias. Likewise, intravascular and intrathecal injection of the neurolytic agent are possible with this block.

Trigeminal neuralgia has been treated with chemical neurolysis of the gasserian ganglion with alcohol, although the use of glycerol or radiofrequency ablation has become favored on the basis of their safety. Stender[158] reported a mortality rate of 0.9% with blocks using alcohol to treat trigeminal neuralgia. Other complications include oculomotor palsy, abducens palsy, glossopharyngeal palsy, corneal anesthesia, facial anesthesia (cheek and nose), nasal ulceration, blindness (spillover onto the optic nerve), corneal ulceration (corneal reflex obtundation), and trigeminal motor weakness.[159,160] A review of 29 patients with trigeminal neuralgia treated by retrogasserian glycerol injection revealed the following complications: dysesthesia (81%), hypertension (70%), hypalgesia and hypesthesia (48%), headache (22%), ocular dysesthesia (11%), masseter weakness (7%), hyperalgesia (7%), and paroxysmal pain (7%).[161] Most of these complications resolved over 2 months, but dysesthesia and hypalgesia persisted longer than 8 weeks in 30% of the patients.

B. Radiofrequency lesioning

Radiofrequency ablation (RFA) dates back to the 1950s and has been used to treat a wide range of chronic pain syndromes at various anatomic sites (Box 5-3).

Lesioning involves the placement of an active electrode—the uninsulated tip of the radiofrequency needle—into the target tissue and passing a high-frequency alternating current through it. The electrical impedance of the surrounding tissue causes heat to be generated in the tissue itself. The size of the resulting lesion is primarily controlled by the size and temperature of the electrode tip, but time also plays a role: Equilibrium between the tissue and electrode occurs in about 60 seconds.

Skin burns at the dispersive electrode have been described. The recommendation is that a dispersing electrode of at least 150 cm² be used and placed on musculature as a low-impedance connection. Pain with lesioning is common and can be blocked with 1 or 2 ml of local anesthetic administered through the radiofrequency needle before injection. Lower-extremity numbness or motor weakness can occur with lumbar facet RFA; this stresses the importance of confirming accurate placement of the stimulating needle with both fluoroscopy and stimulation. Local anesthetic used before lesioning can find its way onto motor nerve roots and lead to immediate postprocedure numbness and weakness. This diagnosis is suggested by the rapid resolution of the symptoms over a period of hours. RFA of the lumbar facets, however, seems to be a safe procedure with relatively few complications. A review of 82 patients receiving unilateral and bilateral RFA for treatment of intractable mechanical low back pain found no complications.[162] Likewise, Shealy[163] reported on a series of more than 800 patients who underwent lumbar facet denervation without any neurologic complications.

Lumbar discogenic pain can be treated with RFA, most often of the rami communicans, although RFA of the disk itself is also performed. As with facet rhizotomy, there is a risk for sensory or motor deficit after RFA in this area if anterior roots are lesioned. Performance of the proper stimulation tests before lesioning will essentially eliminate this risk. Other complications include transient dysesthesias that can last for 2 to 4 weeks or postprocedure diskitis. Prophylactic antibiotics are usually recommended before RFA of the lumbar disk.

Gasserian ganglion RFA for treatment of trigeminal neuralgia has been very successful. RFA offers more controlled lesioning of the ganglion and trigeminal branches than does chemical neurolysis. Onofrio[164] reported on 140 patients with trigeminal pain who underwent percutaneous RFA of the gasserian ganglion. Complications included unintentional first-division analgesia in 10 patients, transient sixth nerve palsy in one, neuroparalytic keratitis in two, and anesthesia dolorosa in two. Broggi et al[165] found that RFA of the gasserian ganglion was effective and relatively safe. No patients in this series died, but 35% of patients had complications, including masseter weakness (10.5%), paresthesias (5.2%), anesthesia dolorosa (1.5%), ocular palsies (0.5%), corneal reflex impairment with keratitis (0.6%), and vasomotor rhinorrhea (0.1%).

Radiofrequency lesioning of the sphenopalatine ganglion is used for the treatment of cluster headaches, some migraines, and sphenopalatine neuritis. Reported complications include epistaxis, cheek hematoma, partial maxillary nerve ablation, and transient (<3 months) hypesthesia of the palate.[166]

The rami communicans may be blocked by RFA for treatment of diskogenic back pain. Thirty percent of patients experience postprocedure pain in the back or leg that persists for 2 to 3 weeks.[167]

Radiofrequency sympathetic block was the first radiofrequency procedure for the treatment of mechanical back pain, but this technique has largely been replaced by radiofrequency lesioning of the rami communicans. This block is associated with low morbidity, but 1% to 2%

Box 5-3 Clinical uses of radiofrequency lesioning

Facet joint arthropathy
Lumbar diskogenic pain
Lumbar ganglionostomy
Dorsal root ganglion
Stellate ganglion lesioning
Sphenopalatine ganglion
Trigeminal ganglion
Cordotomy
Sympathetic chain blocks
Sacroiliac joint pain

of patients experience the "overshoot" phenomenon—a hot, swollen, painful leg that usually resolves in less than 2 weeks but may persist for up to 8 months.[167]

Percutaneous RFA of the stellate ganglion has been used to treat upper-extremity pain caused by reflex sympathetic dystrophy. The same precautions used for local anesthetic blockade of the stellate ganglion must be observed.[168]

C. Cryoablation

It has long been known that application of cold results in anesthesia. Hippocrates (460 to 370 BC) used ice packs to anesthetize skin and superficial tissues before surgery. Baron Dominique Jean Larre, Napoleon's surgeon general, recognized that the frozen limbs of soldiers could be amputated without pain. Cryotherapy in the United States began in 1961 when Dr. Irvine Cooper developed a unit for use in neurosurgery. Contemporary cryotherapy probes operate on the Joule-Thomson effect, which states that heat is absorbed from surrounding tissues with the expansion of any gas. The probe is an enclosed system containing an inner tube and an outer tube. The inner tube delivers a gas (nitrous oxide or carbon dioxide) at high pressure to the tip of the probe, where it enters the larger outer tube and quickly loses pressure. This results in a rapid cooling of the probe tip to around $-70°$ C. Tissues surrounding the probe cool accordingly and become engulfed in an ice ball that varies in size depending on the probe size, freeze time, tissue permeability to water, and the proximity of vascular structures. The typical size of an ice ball is 3.5 to 5.5 mm. Cryoanalgesia results in a nerve block similar to that produced by local anesthetics. The nerve undergoes wallerian degeneration, but the epineurium and perineurium remain intact, allowing regeneration. The rate of regeneration determines the duration of analgesia. However, for reasons that are not entirely clear, persistent analgesia beyond the time necessary for regeneration is often seen. The therapeutic benefits of cryoanalgesia usually last from 2 weeks to 5 months. Clinical uses for cryoanalgesia in the pain clinic setting are listed in Box 5-4.

Because cryoablation does not damage the basal lamina of the nerve, neuroma formation is not an expected complication. The cryoprobe should be left in place and should not be removed before the ice ball has thawed completely. The ice ball may adhere to tissues and cause damage to other structures, including nerves and blood vessels, if it is removed too early. Freezing in the paravertebral space may involve the spinal cord or cause throm-

bosis of a spinal artery, possibly resulting in permanent neurologic deficit. Care should be taken to avoid placing the probe too superficially because full-thickness skin destruction may occur, resulting in a depigmented scar.[132]

IV. COMPLICATIONS OF IMPLANTABLE DEVICES

In general, morbidity from implanted intraspinal devices is uncommon; the risk for infection is greater with external systems than with implanted systems. Because pump catheter and spinal cord stimulator (SCS) leads are similar in size and structure the complications of these devices are similar and can be discussed together. Types of resultant morbidity can be divided into that associated with the catheter or lead system; that associated with the pump, port, or generator pocket; and complications of pump or generator systems.

A. Catheter- and lead-associated morbidity

The most serious complications of implanted intraspinal devices are related to the catheter or lead system. These complications include fibrosis or inflammation leading to pain on injection, neurologic problems secondary to fibrosis, infection, obstruction and altered diffusion kinetics of the drugs delivered, and catheter or lead malfunction.

1. Neurologic complications. Neurologic complications of placement of an intraspinal catheter or lead are rare. Most severe neurologic complications of epidural catheterization or lead placement result from epidural abscess or epidural fibrosis, but even these events are rare. Both of these phenomena are discussed later. Transient neurologic abnormalities after lumbar epidural blockade are much more common than permanent abnormalities (0.1% compared with 0.02%, respectively).[169,170] Paralysis associated with epidural anesthesia in the presence of spinal stenosis has been reported.[171] The mechanism of nerve injury in spinal stenosis may be related to the injection of fluid into a space of limited volume or the development of edema resulting in acute compression of the cauda equina at the level of the stenosis.[172]

2. Infection. Catheter or lead infection is a potentially serious but infrequent complication of implanted intraspinal devices. It is most common with externalized long-term catheters and in immunosuppressed patients. With externalized long-term catheters, the incidence of infection at the site of catheter insertion is higher than the incidence of nervous system infection (4.3% compared with <1%).[173-182] The incidence of SCS lead infection is 0% to 12% (mean, 5%).[183] The incidence of infection with short-term catheters and trial lead implantation is very low.[184,185] Rates of infection do not seem to differ for epidural and intrathecal catheters.[186] Infections may involve mild catheter colonization, deep paraspinous muscle infections, clinical meningitis, or epidural abscess. The catheter hub is regarded as the main point of entry for bacteria causing catheter colonization. However, hematogenous spread and tracking of bacteria from the insertion site may also occur. The most common microorganisms that have been isolated from intraspinal catheters include coagulase-negative staphylococci,

---

Box 5-4 Clinical uses of cryotherapy

Intercostal neuralgia
Painful neuroma
Facet joint arthropathy
Interspinous ligament pain
Diskogenic pain
Coccygodynia
Peripheral neuropathies
Head and neck pain

Staphylococcus aureus, and gram-negative bacilli. The latter two agents tend to cause more serious infections.

Although epidural abscess is rare, a few cases have been reported with long-term epidural catheters and SCS leads.[173, 187-190] *Staphylococcus aureus* is the most common bacterium isolated from epidural abscesses, followed by gram-negative rods. Rare organisms include mycobacteria, brucella, actinomyces, other fungi, echinococcus, and the Guinea worm. Whether epidural infection is acquired through hematogenous spread or through the catheter hub is controversial. It is believed that the initial step in hematogenous spread is minor trauma to the epidural fat leading to fat necrosis. The necrosed fat does not resist the infection and seeds bacteria from the blood during transient bacteremia.[191,192] However, even in the presence of infection, epidural catheters have been shown to be safe. Jakobsen, Christensen, and Carlsson[193] reported on a series of 69 patients who required an epidural catheter for repeated surgical treatment of abscesses or infected wounds. Twelve patients had their epidural catheters removed because of signs of local infections, but no serious infections occurred. The authors concluded that epidural catheters are relatively safe in this patient population.[193] However, these situations should be evaluated on a case-by-case basis. If epidural abscess is not diagnosed early, it may lead to paralysis. However, if there are no neurologic symptoms of abscess, it may be possible to treat the patient nonsurgically with antibiotics.[187] One case was reported in which an infected long-term epidural catheter was sterilized in vivo with intravenous antibiotic therapy.[194] In another case report, a patient developed staphylococcal meningitis after implantation of an intrathecal SynchroMed infusion pump. The meningitis was successfully treated with vancomycin administered through the implanted pump.[195]

Patient selection and strict aseptic technique are the most important factors in preventing catheter and lead infection. As mentioned previously, caution should be exercised when using intraspinally implanted devices in the immunocompromised or diabetic patient. Other methods that may be used to prevent catheter infection include antimicrobial dressings and the use of bacterial filters. Shapiro, Bond, and Garman[196] found a significant reduction in catheter colonization when a chlorhexidine dressing was used. Bacterial filters have been advocated to reduce infection rates. However, De Cicco et al[197] demonstrated a higher incidence of catheter hub colonization if the bacterial filters were changed too often. They concluded that these filters maintain function for at least 60 days and should not be changed frequently. Intermittent epidural aspiration should only be done if an infection is suspected. Frequent aspiration to monitor the presence of an infection may lead to an increased risk for contamination. Tunneling the catheter subcutaneously to exit at a site distant from the needle puncture site has been advised to reduce the incidence of catheter infection. This recommendation is based on the assumption that catheter colonization and intraspinal infections are caused by bacteria tracking along the catheter. However, studies have not supported this assumption and show that tunneling will reduce the incidence of catheter dislodgment but not catheter infection.[182,198] It has been suggested that local anesthetics are bactericidal and may prevent catheter infection; however, the concentrations commonly used probably have no effect.[199,200]

3. Fibrosis and inflammation. Although uncommon, both intrathecal and epidural catheters can become difficult to use for injection and may cause pain on injection.[201-205] In addition, altered diffusion kinetics of the drugs delivered in the epidural and intrathecal space may develop.[205,206] The common conclusion is that a local reaction to the catheter may cause the aforementioned observations. Animal studies have shown that a fibrous sheath develops around epidural catheters as early as 7 to 10 days after placement.[207-210] In humans, studies have shown that catheter encasement[211-213] may cause spinal cord compression necessitating surgical correction.[214,215] One study found an 11.6% incidence of back leakage from the insertion point with long-term catheters.[216] The incidence of epidural fibrosis secondary to catheter placement seems to be 0.5% to 19%.[201-202,213] Epidurography in patients with epidural fibrosis secondary to catheter placement shows encapsulation at the catheter tip.[202,212] One study of intrathecal catheters showed a 9.5% incidence of fibrosis.[217] The incidence of SCS lead fibrosis is unknown but is probably similar to that found with epidural catheters. Fibrosis of the SCS lead may result in inadequate stimulation or necessitate a higher amplitude to achieve adequate stimulation.

Review of the literature reveals a comparable cross-species epidural reaction to the catheter. The time courses of these reactions are 10 days for rats,[207] 7 to 14 days for dogs,[208] 30 days for sheep,[209] and 1 to 2 weeks for humans.[205,218-220] In general, the observed tissue reactions in the epidural space of dogs are similar to those that occur in other tissues (e.g., the mammary and intraperitoneal areas) in response to such foreign materials as intravascular catheters and pacemakers. Studies of the histopathology of long-term epidural catheters describe a nonspecific inflammation at the tissue-implant interface that is initially acute and progresses to a predominately chronic inflammation and, eventually, encapsulation. This reaction occurs most often at the tip, where biomechanical stresses are maximal.[69a]

Comparison of epidural reaction induced by different catheter materials shows that nylon and silicone catheters cause a greater tissue reaction than polyethylene catheters, although these differences are modest. The rank order seems to be nylon followed by silicone followed by polyethylene.[69a] Factors that influence this reactivity include net charge, smoothness, hydrophilicity, the possibility of outgassing of volatile agents used in sterilization, biomechanical factors, and susceptibility to infection. Occult infection has been hypothesized to cause encasement and capsular contracture of silicone breast prostheses. It has been shown that soaking breast prostheses in a 50-50 mixture of an iodine and saline solution and irrigating the wound with this solution decreases the chance of occult infection.[221,222] No study has examined the use of iodine solutions to sterilize intraspinal catheters or SCS leads.

Epidural reactivity has been more extensively studied than intrathecal reactivity, and the properties of the epidural space cannot necessarily be extended into the intrathecal space. Crul and Delhaas[223] looked at the differences between complications in cancer patients requiring epidural catheters and those requiring intrathecal catheters for pain control. During the first 20 days of treatment, a significant difference in the incidence of complications was observed between the epidural catheter group (8%) and the subarachnoid catheter group (25%). During the remainder of the treatment period, the complication rate increased to 55% in the epidural catheter group and decreased to 5% in the subarachnoid catheter group; this difference is significant. The most frequent complication in the epidural catheter group was obstruction and dislocation of the catheter, probably caused by the development of epidural fibrosis. The most frequent complication in patients with an intrathecal catheter was cerebrospinal fluid leak in the first 2 weeks. The authors concluded that the subarachnoid route is preferred for patients expected to live longer than 1 month.[223]

Several studies have examined the postmortem morphologic changes induced by neuraxial catheters. Ehring and Boekstegers[224] looked at the morphologic changes in the epidural space of a patient who received a 114-day infusion through a nylon epidural (Perifix) catheter (Braun Medical, Inc., Bethlehem, Pennsylvania) for cancer pain management. No macroscopic or histologic indication of inflammation was observed in the peridural space or spinal canal. The only alterations detected were nonspecific foreign-body reactions, such as an increase in foreign-body giant cells and single connective tissue adhesions.[224] This is consistent with a report on 15 patients with chronic pain who received long-term epidural or intrathecal morphine therapy through a nylon catheter. No reaction against the nylon catheter was seen, nor were there any neuropathologic findings related to the duration or cumulative dose of the intrathecal treatment. No new neurologic deficits could be attributed to intrathecal administration of the opiate-bupivacaine mixtures. The authors concluded that the neuropathologic and clinical neurologic findings in cancer patients treated with intrathecal morphine-bupivacaine mixtures seemed to be similar to those in animals and humans given intrathecal morphine or bupivacaine.[225] Although autopsy reports have failed to show significant reactions to agents delivered in the epidural space in humans, several reports in animals present contrary information. Larsen, Svendsen, and Andersen[226] showed that morphine causes a clinically significant inflammatory reaction in goats after epidural administration. This is important because epidural and intrathecal reactions to various agents may be species specific, and caution must be used when interpreting data from preclinical toxicology studies.

In summary, epidural fibrosis continues to be a minor problem in long-term catheterization and SCS lead placement. Most patients can undergo long-term catheterization without clinically significant fibrosis and altered drug delivery. Reactivity seems to be less pronounced in the intrathecal space, allowing for more prolonged drug delivery.

4. Malfunction. Previous studies of intrathecal delivery systems have found rates of catheter malfunction from 10% to 40%.[217] Catheter malfunction can be classified as (1) disconnection from the pump or port, (2) large-to-small catheter disconnect (if these types of catheters are involved), (3) kinks or holes, (4) breaks, and (5) dislodgments. Implantable infusion pumps have two locations at which the catheter may become disconnected: from the pump or port or from the large-to-small catheter disconnect. Over time, the catheters may develop a kink or hole or may break. Penn, York, and Paice[217] performed a prospective study of the reliability of thin- and thick-walled intrathecal catheters in 102 patients. Sixty percent of the patients had no catheter-related complications; the remaining patients had one to five complications. Because most of the complications occurred in the thin-walled Silastic catheter, the authors concluded that this type of catheter does not perform well and that larger, thick-walled catheters should be used. At present, most of the catheters in use are thick walled.

Lead electrode malfunction can also occur, necessitating lead replacement. A review of the literature shows a 0% to 75% (mean, 24%) incidence of electrode malfunction. The most common reason for lead malfunction is dislodgment of the electrode and loss of adequate paresthesia.[183] Other causes of lead malfunction include short circuit in the lead, loss of lead insulation resulting in electricity leakage, and lead disconnect.

B. Pump-, port-, or generator pocket–associated problems

Complications that can occur in the generator pocket include hematoma, seroma, infection, and capsule formation. Hematomas usually occur immediately after surgery. Meticulous care should be taken to control all bleeding before surgical incision closure because hematoma provides a nidus for infection and the pocket may require surgical exploration to evacuate the hematoma. Hematomas can be prevented by appropriately screening patients for coagulopathies before pump implantation.

Seromas may also develop around the pump or port. As with hematomas, seromas may increase the chance of infection in the presence of a foreign body. Seromas can be drained percutaneously; care should be taken to use strict aseptic technique. Seromas can be prevented by requiring the patient to wear an abdominal binder for 1 month after the implantation.

Infection may occur in the pump, generator pocket, or back incision. Not all wound infections require removal of the pump, generator, catheter, or lead, and if the infection is superficial, it can be treated with antibiotics. If an infection of the pocket is suspected, careful aspiration is useful to obtain a culture sample and measure sensitivity. If the infection is deep and severe (associated with fever and leukocytosis), the system should be removed. It may be necessary to leave the wound open in this case and allow it to close later. Consultation with an infectious disease specialist may be helpful.

The human body usually forms a fibrous capsule around any foreign object. With silicone breast implants, for example, this often leads to capsular contraction and pain.[227] A fibrous capsule may also form around implanted pumps, ports, or generators, and the patient may experience resultant pain. This complication rarely requires intervention; however, the system may have to be removed in some patients if the pain becomes severe.

C. Pump- and generator system–associated problems

Programmable pump complications can be categorized as filling errors, pump failure, programming errors, and torsion or flipping of a freely moveable pump.[93] Complications that may occur when filling the pump include inadvertent side port access, overfilling the pump, and inadvertent placement of drug in the pump pocket. Many intrathecal pumps contain a side port that gives direct access to the intrathecal space. If this side port is inadvertently opened when refilling the pump, a large dose of medication will be delivered directly into the cerebrospinal fluid, leading to overdose. The SynchroMed 8615 and 8615-S pumps (Medtronic, Minneapolis, Minnesota) and the Infusaid model 400 pump (Arrow International, Reading, Pennsylvania) contain side ports. The SynchroMed 8615-S pump has a screened side port that will only allow entry of a 25-gauge needle. This will prevent access by the usual 22-gauge Huber-type needle used for pump refill. In addition, the side ports of the SynchroMed 8615-S pump are located on the periphery of the pump, whereas the refill port is located in the center. The refill kits contain a template that can be used to locate the two different ports. The Arrow model 3000 pump (Arrow International, Reading, Pennsylvania) has a special bolus needle for bolus injection directly into the cerebrospinal fluid. The needle is designed with a sealed tip and a slot opening midway up the needle cannula. When the needle is inserted through the double-stacked septums within the pump, the closed tip is in contact with the needle stop, and the slot opening is automatically at the level of the bolus pathway, allowing bolus injection or infusion. If the pump is overfilled, the reservoir becomes overpressurized, which may lead to pump damage, pump failure, or drug overdose. Most pumps come with a manometer system to alert the physician or nurse of an overpressurized system. If the pump or port pocket is inadvertently accessed and the drug is deposited directly into the pocket, overdose may result. Most of the drugs used for intrathecal drug delivery are highly concentrated and may lead to very high plasma concentrations of drug and overdose.

Pump failure is most often caused by battery failure. The SynchroMed Infusion System is the only system that is battery operated. The normal battery life depends on the flow rate but is usually 3 to 5 years. The pump has a battery alarm that will alert the patient and physician when the battery is running low. When the battery fails, the entire pump must be replaced. By the time the battery requires replacement, most patients are receiving a stable flow rate and do not require many rate changes. At this point, it is may be more cost-effective to use one of the constant flow rate systems (Arrow or Infusaid) that are not battery operated. These systems are also less expensive than the SynchroMed pump; however, they have unique disadvantages that distinguish them from the SynchroMed pump that should be weighed. Another cause of pump failure is failure of the electronic telemetric receiving module, which prevents the pump from receiving programming instructions. This converts the pump to a constant flow system (like the Arrow and Infusaid systems). If the patient is at a stage where programmability is not important, the pump may be left in place and drug dosing may be adjusted by changing the drug concentration.

Programming errors can lead to inadequate pain relief, the abstinence syndrome, or drug overdose. Programming the pump to deliver a drug concentration that is higher than the actual drug concentration may lead to underdosing and increased pain or the abstinence syndrome. Programming the pump to deliver a drug concentration that is lower than the actual drug concentration may lead to drug overdose and death. The newer software that is available with Medtronic (Minneapolis, Minnesota) programmable pumps asks the programmer if the right choices have been made, which the programmer should carefully check. In addition, the software has certain constraints that do not allow extreme changes in drug concentration or delivery rate.

Pumps or ports that are not secured with sutures inside the pocket can flip or torque. Pumps that torque within the pocket may kink the catheter or pull the catheter out of the intrathecal space. If the pump flips on itself, it will be unable to be refilled or programmed. This problem usually is discovered at the time of refill when the pump cannot be accessed or programmed. If this happens, the pump will require surgical revision. Pumps and ports have anchors that can be sutured in the pocket, thus preventing this complication.

Generator failure is usually caused by battery failure. Other causes of generator failure include coming in contact with a magnet that may shut the generator off or generator short circuit.

V. MISCELLANEOUS TECHNIQUES
A. Epidural steroid injections

Epidural steroid injections are one of the most frequently performed pain management procedures. Although this technique has an impressive safety track record, complications can occur.

Arachnoiditis has not been reported in any patient who received only epidural steroid injections. There are, however, numerous reports of arachnoiditis following repeated subarachnoid injections of steroid preparations.[228-232] All of the corticosteroids commonly used for epidural steroid injections have been linked to the development of arachnoiditis. Four cases of aseptic meningitis after subarachnoid injection of steroids[228,233-235] and one case after epidural steroid injection have been reported.[236] The patient who underwent epidural steroid injection began to experience headache, lethargy, fever, and meningismus 48 hours after epidural injection of methylprednisolone. Examination of the cerebrospinal fluid revealed a high protein concentration and low glucose concentration, but cultures were negative. The patient's condition improved with a course of antibiotics. Similarly, four cases of bacterial meningitis have been reported: three occurred after subarachnoid injection of steroids,[237-239] and one occurred after epidural steroid injection.[239] Gram-positive organisms were cultured in the patient who underwent epidural steroid injection and in one of the patients who underwent subarachnoid steroid injection. Tuberculous meningitis and torula meningitis were isolated in the other two patients.

Six cases of epidural abscess as a complication of a single epidural injection of steroids have been cited.[240] Most of these cases involved patients who had diabetes mellitus as a risk factor.

Postdural puncture headache is a well-recognized complication of any epidural injection. Its incidence depends on the skill of the practitioner and the presence of altered anatomy, such as with previous back surgery, but is approximately 1%.[241]

One case of epidural hematoma after cervical epidural steroid injection that required emergent decompression has been reported.[242] Transient increases of radicular pain lasting 24 to 48 hours, also known as *steroid flare,* are seen in 5% to 10% of patients in the authors' experience. Simon et al[243] reported on a patient who had an allergic reaction to triamcinolone diacetate after epidural steroid injection. This was subsequently confirmed with skin testing. Retinal hemorrhage has been reported and may be secondary to a sudden increase in cerebrospinal fluid pressure following rapid injection of large volumes.[244] Siegfried[245] described a case of the complex regional pain syndrome after cervical epidural steroid injection in a patient with C3-4 and C4-5 herniated disks. Rare cases of the Cushing syndrome and steroid-induced myopathy have been reported.[246,247] Other complications include facial edema, buffalo hump, supraclavicular fat pads, skin bruising, scaly skin lesions, fluid retention, weight gain, hypertension, congestive heart failure, adrenal suppression, and irregular menses.[248]

B. Intravenous lidocaine infusions

Intravenous infusions of lidocaine have been used to treat multiple neuropathic pain states. They presumably act by decreasing the high-frequency firing of injured nerves that lead to facilitated pain states. The toxic side effects of local anesthetics have been well documented and relate mainly to central nervous system and cardiovascular toxicity. Local anesthetics vary considerably in their ability to cause toxic side effects; lidocaine is intermediate in its ability to cause toxicity.

The signs and symptoms of lidocaine toxicity are based on a dose-response relationship and correspond to increasing plasma concentrations of the drug (Table 5-6). Initially, patients describe feelings of light-headedness and dizziness, followed by signs of increasing central nervous system effects (visual or auditory disturbance, sedation, myoclonic twitching, and seizures) before manifesting cardiovascular depression.

The rate of injection and the rapidity with which plasma concentrations are achieved also correlate with toxicity.[249] The acid-base status of the patient markedly affects the

Table 5-6. Plasma concentration required for a specific lidocaine toxicity

Toxic effect of lidocaine	Plasma concentration (g/ml)
Numbness of tongue	3
Lightheadedness	4
Visual and auditory disturbances	7
Muscular twitching	8
Unconsciousness	10
Convulsions	12
Coma	14-16
Respiratory arrest	20
Cardiovascular depression	>25

toxicity profile of all local anesthetics.[250] Elevated partial pressure of carbon dioxide and decreased arterial pH have been associated with a lowered convulsive threshold.

Lidocaine decreases the maximum rate of depolarization without altering the resting membrane potential of cardiac muscle.[251] As plasma concentrations of lidocaine increase, the PR interval and QRS duration are prolonged on electrocardiography, reflecting an increased conduction time through various parts of the heart.[252] Very high concentrations of lidocaine (>25 μg/ml) will profoundly depress spontaneous pacemaker activity in the sinus node, resulting in sinus bradycardia and, possibly, sinus arrest. In addition, lidocaine, like all local anesthetics, can exert a negative inotropic effect. As little as 2 to 4 mg/kg can cause decreased contractility of the right ventricular myocardium in humans.[253] Lidocaine, compared with bupivacaine and etidocaine, has not been found to induce ventricular arrhythmias in both convulsive and supraconvulsive doses in awake animals.[254-257] Although enhanced cardiotoxicity during pregnancy has been documented with bupivacaine, it is not known whether pregnancy is associated with an increased risk for toxic side effects with other local anesthetics, including lidocaine. Like the convulsive threshold, acidosis and hypoxia can increase the central nervous system and cardiac toxicity with lidocaine.[258] Lidocaine produces a biphasic response on arteriolar smooth muscle. Nontoxic plasma concentrations cause vasoconstriction, and excessive plasma concentrations cause vasodilation. Allergic reactions to amino amide local anesthetics are very rare but have been reported.[259,260]

C. Phentolamine infusions

Phentolamine is an imidazoline derivative that produces a nonselective α-adrenergic blockade. It has been used as an outpatient diagnostic tool for sympathetically maintained pain. Phentolamine produces peripheral vasodilation with a resultant decrease in blood pressure. Baroreceptor-mediated increases in sympathetic stimulation and α_2-blockade resulting in increased norepinephrine release lead to an increase in heart rate and cardiac output. Patients with coronary artery disease, left ventricular dysfunction, or valvular disease may not be able to tolerate the increased myocardial demand, which predisposes them to angina and myocardial ischemia. However, in a retrospective review of 100 consecutive patients with known or suspected sympathetically mediated pain, intravenous administration of phentolamine did not result in any major complications.[261] The total doses used varied from 25 to 75 mg over 20 minutes after pretreatment with intravascular fluids and propranolol. Five patients developed transient minor complications, including sinus tachycardia, premature ventricular beats, dizziness, and wheezing.

D. Myofascial trigger-point injections

A myofascial trigger point is defined by Travell and Simmons[262] as a "hyperirritable spot, usually within a taut band of skeletal muscle or in the muscle's fascia, that is painful on compression and can give rise to characteristic referred pain, tenderness, and autonomic phenomena." Although the exact mechanism of a trigger point is unknown, it is proposed that trauma locally tears muscle fibers and sarcoplasmic reticulum, resulting in calcium release. This calcium release facilitates local contractile activity, and the ensuing increased metabolic activity creates byproducts that sensitize neighboring nociceptors. This high metabolic activity, documented by adenosine triphosphate depletion, produces "hot spots" seen on thermography. In addition to physical therapy, mobilization, and medications, trigger-point injection has been a mainstay in the treatment of myofascial pain.

With trigger-point injection, all of the resultant risks of any invasive procedure that violates the integrity of the skin are present, including risks for infection, bleeding, and hematoma. Pain with placement of the needle is common and may be reported as more severe in sensitized patients. Local anesthetic is commonly used, with or without steroid, but dry needling or acupuncture has been shown to be just as effective.[263] Because the volume of local anesthetic used is usually small, systemic toxicity is not a problem unless multiple sites are used with a subsequent large total volume of local anesthetic. Skeletal muscle irritation from local anesthetics has been reported[264,265]; the effect is more pronounced with more potent local anesthetics (such as bupivacaine and etidocaine) than with less potent local anesthetics (such as lidocaine). This effect is reversible within 2 weeks and is not associated with any clinical complaints of pain. However, postinjection soreness is not uncommon and has been reported to be higher in patients who underwent dry needling than in those who received a local anesthetic.[266]

The anatomic site of injection may also affect the associated morbidity. Pneumothorax has been reported in patients receiving trigger-point injections for myofascial pain involving the chest wall.[267]

E. Acupuncture

Acupuncture is one of the oldest forms of medical therapy and pain management; it dates back at least 2000 years. Its use is slowly being accepted into Western medical practices, although adequate, controlled, prospective studies on its efficacy are still lacking. Acupuncture has been used to treat numerous ailments and diseases, and acupuncture needles are often used for dry needling of trigger points.

Although acupuncture is considered by many to be safe and to have a low incidence of complications, complications do occur and may result in serious illness or death. Fainting with the needlestick is one of the most common events. It results from a vasovagal response and responds well to simple measures that favor adequate venous return to the heart and, occasionally, use of adrenergic agents.

Infectious complications can occur when needles are reused without appropriate sterilization. Hepatitis has been transmitted through acupuncture needles.[268,269] The use of disposable needles should essentially eliminate this risk. Bacterial endocarditis[270] and bacterial meningitis[271] have also been reported with acupuncture. A fatal case of staphylococcal septicemia has been reported in two patients,[272] whereas staphylococcal septicemia leading to disseminated intravascular coagulation has been reported in one patient.[273]

There have been numerous reports of pneumothorax after acupuncture.[274-278] Two of these case reports involved patients who underwent acupuncture for asthma. In both patients, bilateral pneumothorax resulted; one patient (a 15-year-old girl) narrowly avoided death, and the other (a 63-year-old woman) died.

Occasionally, a needle tip may break and remain lodged in the tissue. Although this generally poses no serious problems, needle migration has sometimes had serious adverse consequences. In one case, a 60-year-old woman who received embedded-type acupuncture needle treatment in 1975 presented in 1993 with a 3-week history of progressive motor and sensory disturbance of her right upper extremity. Computed tomography revealed that a needle had penetrated the medulla oblongata.[279] Three other case reports involving four patients demonstrated spinal cord and nerve root injury caused by needle migration.[280-282]

Cardiac tamponade as a result of direct acupuncture needle trauma has occurred in two patients, one of whom died.[283,284] Other adverse effects associated with acupuncture include lymphocytoma cutis,[285] hypotension,[286] perichondritis of the ear,[287-289] chronic osteomyelitis,[290] foreign body kidney stone,[291] activation of cutaneous herpes,[292] drop foot caused by direct nerve trauma,[293] bilateral psoas abscess,[294] and spinal epidural hematoma with subarachnoid hemorrhage.[295]

REFERENCES

1. Drummer OH, Opeskin K, Syrjanen M, et al: Methadone toxicity causing death in ten subjects starting on a methadone maintenance program, *Am J Forensic Med Pathol* 13:346, 1992.
2. Christrup LL: Morphine metabolites, *Acta Anaesthesiol Scand* 41(1 Pt 2):116, 1997.
3. Hagen NA, Foley KM, Cerbone DJ, et al: Chronic nausea and morphine-6-glucuronide, *J Pain Symptom Manage* 6:125, 1995.
4. Tiseo PJ, Thaler HT, Lapin J, et al: Morphine-6-glucuronide concentrations and opioid-related side effects: a survey in cancer patients, *Pain* 61:47, 1995.
5. Schoorl J, Zylicz Z: Laxative policy for terminal patients ineffective, *Ned Tijdschr Geneeskd* 141:823, 1997.
6. Cheskin LJ, Chami TN, Johnson RE, et al: Assessment of nalmefene glucuronide as a selective gut opioid antagonist, *Drug Alcohol Depend* 39:151, 1995.

7. Culpepper-Morgan JA, Inturrisi CE, Portenoy RK, et al: Treatment of opioid-induced constipation with oral naloxone: a pilot study, *Clin Pharmacol Ther* 52:90, 1992.

8. Latasch L, Zimmermann M, Eberhardt B, et al: Treatment of morphine-induced constipation with oral naloxone, *Anaesthesist* 46:191, 1997.

9. Yuan CS, Foss JF, O'Connor M, et al: Methylnaltrexone prevents morphine-induced delay in oral-cecal transit time without affecting analgesia: a double-blind randomized placebo-controlled trial, *Clin Pharmacol Ther* 59:469, 1996.

10. Yuan CS, Foss JF, Osinski J, et al: The safety and efficacy of oral methylnaltrexone in preventing morphine-induced delay in oral-cecal transit time, *Clin Pharmacol Ther* 61:467, 1997.

11. Glavina MJ, Robertshaw R: Myoclonic spasms following intrathecal morphine, *Anaesthesia* 43:389, 1988.

12. Kloke M, Bingel U, Seeber S: Complications of spinal opioid therapy: myoclonus, spastic muscle tone and spinal jerking, *Supportive Care Cancer* 2:249, 1994.

13. MacDonald N, Der L, Allan S, et al: Opioid hyperexcitability: the application of alternate opioid therapy, *Pain* 53:353, 1993.

14. Rozan JP, Kahn CH, Warfield CA: Epidural and intravenous opioid-induced neuroexcitation, *Anesthesiology* 83:860, 1995.

15. Sjogren P, Jensen NH, Jensen TS: Disappearance of morphine-induced hyperalgesia after discontinuing or substituting morphine with other opioid agonists, *Pain* 59:313, 1994.

16. Sylvester RK, Levitt R, Steen PD: Opioid-induced muscle activity: implications for managing chronic pain, *Ann Pharmacother* 29:1118, 1995.

17. Holdsworth MT, Adams VR, Chavez CM, et al: Continuous midazolam infusion for the management of morphine-induced myoclonus, *Ann Pharmacother* 29:25, 1995.

18. De Conno F, Caraceni A, Martini C, et al: Hyperalgesia and myoclonus with intrathecal infusion of high-dose morphine, *Pain* 47:337, 1991.

19. Jacobsen LS, Olsen AK, Sjogren P, et al: Morphine-induced hyperalgesia, allodynia and myoclonus—new side-effects of morphine? *Ugeskr Laeger* 157:3307, 1995.

20. Sjogren P, Jonsson T, Jensen NH, et al: Hyperalgesia and myoclonus in terminal cancer patients treated with continuous intravenous morphine, *Pain* 55:93, 1993.

21. Longwell B, Betz T, Horton H, et al: Weight gain and edema on methadone maintenance therapy, *Int J Addict* 14:329, 1979.

22. O'Conor LM, Woody G, Yeh HS, et al: Methadone and edema, *J Subst Abuse Treat* 8:153, 1991.

23. LeVier DG, Brown RD, Musgrove DL, et al: The effect of methadone on the immune status of B6C3F1 mice, *Fundam Appl Toxicol* 24:275, 1995.

24. Nair MP, Schwartz SA, Polasani R, et al: Immunoregulatory effects of morphine on human lymphocytes, *Clin Diagn Lab Immunol* 4:127, 1997.

25. Pacifici R, Di Carlo S, Bacosi A, et al: Macrophage functions in drugs of abuse-treated mice, *Int J Immunopharmacol* 15:711, 1993.

26. Jover R, Ponsoda X, Gomez-Lechon MJ, et al: Potentiation of heroin and methadone hepatotoxicity by ethanol: an in vitro study using cultured human hepatocytes, *Xenobiotica* 22:471, 1992.

27. Gomez-Lechon MJ, Ponsoda X, Jover R, et al: Hepatotoxicity of the opioids morphine, heroin, meperidine, and methadone to cultured human hepatocytes, *Mol Toxicol* 1:453, 1987-1988.

28. Bruera E, Fainsinger R, Moore M, et al: Local toxicity with subcutaneous methadone: experience of two centers, *Pain* 45:141, 1991.

29. Armstrong PJ, Bersten A: Normeperidine toxicity, *Anesth Analg* 65:536, 1986.

30. Clark RF, Wei EM, Anderson PO: Meperidine: therapeutic use and toxicity, *J Emerg Med,* 13:797, 1995.

31. Danziger LH, Martin SJ, Blum RA: Central nervous system toxicity associated with meperidine use in hepatic disease, *Pharmacotherapy* 14:235, 1994.

32. Stone PA, Macintyre PE, Jarvis DA: Norpethidine toxicity and patient controlled analgesia, *Br J Anaesth* 71:738, 1993.

33. Adair JC, Gilmore RL: Meperidine neurotoxicity after organ transplantation, *J Toxicol Clin Toxicol* 32:325, 1994.

34. Eisendrath SJ, Goldman B, Douglas J, et al: Meperidine-induced delirium, *Am J Psychiatry* 144:1062, 1987.

35. Meyer D, Halfin V: Toxicity secondary to meperidine in patients on monoamine oxidase inhibitors: a case report and critical review, *J Clin Psychopharmacol* 1:319, 1981.

36. McGoldrick MD, Bailie GR: Nonnarcotic analgesics: prevalence and estimated economic impact of toxicities, *Ann Pharmacother* 31:221, 1997.

37. Brooks PM: Side effects of non-steroidal anti-inflammatory drugs, *Med J Aust* 148:248, 1988.

38. Henry DA: Side effects of non-steroidal anti-inflammatory drugs, *Ballieres Clin Rheumatol* 2:425, 1998.

39. Hawkey CJ: Non-steroidal anti-inflammatory drugs and peptic ulcers, *BMJ* 300:278, 1990.

40. Murray MD, Brater DC: Adverse effects of nonsteroidal anti-inflammatory drugs on renal function, *Ann Intern Med* 112:559, 1990 (editorial).

41. O'Brien WM, Bagby GF: Rare adverse reactions to nonsteroidal antiinflammatory drugs, *J Rheumatol* 12:13, 1995.

42. O'Brien WM, Bagby GF: Rare adverse reactions to nonsteroidal antiinflammatory drugs, *J Rheumatol* 12:347, 1995.

43. O'Brien WM, Bagby GF: Rare adverse reactions to nonsteroidal antiinflammatory drugs (3), *J Rheumatol* 12:562, 1995.

44. O'Brien WM, Bagby GF: Rare adverse reactions to nonsteroidal antiinflammatory drugs: 4, *J Rheumatol* 12:785, 1995.

45. Ellenhorn MJ, Barceloux DG: *Medical toxicology: diagnosis and treatment of human poisoning,* New York, 1988, Elsevier Science, p 158.

46. Schueler L, Harper JL: Acetaminophen toxicity: report of case and review of the literature, *J Oral Maxillofac Surg* 53:1208, 1995.

47. Lewis RK, Paloucek FP: Assessment and treatment of acetaminophen overdose, *Clin Pharm Ther* 10:765, 1991.

48. Blakely P, McDonald BR: Acute renal failure due to acetaminophen ingestion: a case report and review of the literature, *J Am Soc Nephrol* 6:48, 1995.

49. Cossmann M, Kohnen C, Langford R, et al: Tolerance and safety of tramadol use: results of international studies and data from drug surveillance, *Drugs* 53:50, 1997.

50. Richelson E: Pharmacology of antidepressants in use in the United States, *J Clin Psychiatry* 43(11 Pt 2):4, 1982.

51. Haddox JD: Neuropsychiatric drug use in pain management. In Raj PP, ed: *Practical management of pain,* ed 2, St Louis, 1992, Mosby, p 636.

52. Wernicke JF: The side effect profile and safety of fluoxetine, *J Clin Psychiatry* 46(3 Pt 2):59, 1985.

53. Frommer DA, Kulig KW, Marx JA, et al: Tricyclic antidepressant overdose, *JAMA* 257:521, 1987.

54. Flomenbaum N, Price D: Recognition and management of antidepressant overdoses: tricyclics and trazodone, *Neuropsychobiology* 15(suppl 1):46, 1986.

55. Haider A, Tuchek JM, Haider S: Seizure control: how to use the new antiepileptic drugs in older patients, *Geriatrics* 51:42, 1996.

56. Reynolds EH, Trimble MR: Adverse neuropsychiatric effects of anticonvulsant drugs, *Drugs* 29:570, 1985.

57. Swerdlow M: Anticonvulsant drugs and chronic pain, *Clin Neuropharmacol* 7:51, 1984.

58. DeToledo JC, Toledo C, DeCerce J, et al: Changes in body weight with chronic, high-dose gabapentin therapy, *Ther Drug Monit* 19:394, 1997.

59. Hojer J, Malmlund HO, Berg A: Clinical features in 28 consecutive cases of laboratory confirmed massive poisoning with carbamazepine alone, *J Toxicol Clin Toxicol* 31:449, 1993.

60. Seymour JF: Carbamazepine overdose: features of 33 cases, *Drug Saf* 8:81, 1993.

61. Manolis AS, Deering TF, Cameron J, et al: Mexiletine: pharmacology and therapeutic use, *Clin Cardiol* 13:349, 1990.

62. Feinberg L, Travis WD, Ferrans V, et al: Pulmonary fibrosis associated with tocainide: report of a case with literature review, *Am Rev Respir Dis* 141:505, 1990.

63. Soff GA, Kadin ME: Tocainide-induced reversible agranulocytosis and anemia, *Arch Intern Med* 147:598, 1987.

64. Nelson LS, Hoffman RS: Mexiletine overdose producing status epilepticus without cardiovascular abnormalities, *J Toxicol Clin Toxicol* 32:731, 1994.

65. Denaro CP, Benowitz NL: Poisoning due to class 1B antiarrhythmic drugs: lignocaine, mexiletine and tocainide, *Med Toxicol Adverse Drug Exp* 4:412, 1989.

66. Elenbaas JK: Centrally acting oral skeletal muscle relaxants, *Am J Hosp Pharm* 37:1313, 1980.

67. Malins AF, Goodman NW, Cooper GM, et al: Ventilatory effects of pre- and postoperative diamorphine: a comparison of extradural and intramuscular administration, *Anaesthesia* 39:118, 1984.

68. Attia J, Ecoffey C, Sandouk P, et al: Epidural morphine in children: pharmacokinetics and CO_2 sensitivity, *Anesthesiology* 65:590, 1986.

69. Benlabed M, Ecoffey C, Levron JC, et al: Analgesia and ventilatory response to CO_2 following epidural sufentanil in children, *Anesthesiology* 67:948, 1987.

69a. Yaksh, TL: Personal communication, 1993.

70. Glass PSA: Respiratory depression following only 0.4 mg of intrathecal morphine, *Anesthesiology* 60:256, 1984.

71. Gregg R: Spinal analgesia, *Anesth Clin North Am* 7:79, 1989.

72. Grass JA: Fentanyl: clinical use as postoperative analgesic-epidural/intrathecal route, *J Pain Symptom Manage* 7:419, 1992.

73. Bromage PR, Camporesi EM, Durant PA, et al: Rostral spread of epidural morphine, *Anesthesiology* 56:431, 1982.

74. Thomas DA, Williams GM, Iwata K, et al: The medullary dorsal horn: a site of action of morphine in producing facial scratching in monkeys, *Anesthesiology* 79:548, 1993.

75. Shen K-F, Crain SM: Dual opioid modulation of the action potential duration of mouse dorsal root ganglion neurons in culture, *Brain Res* 491:227, 1989.

76. Ballantyne JC, Loach AB, Carr DB: Itching after epidural and spinal opiates, *Pain* 33:149, 1988.

77. Korsh J, Ramanathan S, Parker F, et al: Systemic histamine release by epidural morphine, *Anesthesiology* 67:A475, 1987 (abstract).

77a. Bernards C: Personal communication, 1993.

78. Tiseo PJ, Yaksh TL: The spinal pharmacology of urinary function: studies on urinary continence in the unanesthetized rat, *Ciba Found Symp* 151:91, 1990.

79. Durant PAC, Yaksh TL: Drug effects on urinary bladder tone during spinal morphine-induced inhibition of the micturition reflex in unanesthetized rats, *Anesthesiology* 68:325, 1988.

80. Rawal N, Mollefors K, Axelsson K, et al: An experimental study of urodynamic effects of epidural morphine and of naloxone reversal, *Anesth Analg* 62:641, 1983.

81. Drenger B, Magora F, Evron S, et al: The action of intrathecal morphine and methadone on the lower urinary tract in the dog, *J Urol* 135:852, 1986.

82. Jurna I: Inhibition of the effect of repetitive stimulation on spinal motoneurons of the cat by morphine and pethidine, *Int J Neuropharmacol* 5:117, 1966.

83. Gieraerts R, Navalgund A, Vaes L, et al: Increased incidence of itching and herpes simplex in patients given epidural morphine after cesarean section, *Anesth Analg* 66:1321, 1987.

84. Crone L-A, Conly JM, Storgard C, et al: Herpes labialis in parturients receiving epidural morphine following cesarean section, *Anesthesiology* 73:208, 1990.

85. Fuller JG, McMorland GH, Douglas MJ, et al: Epidural morphine for analgesia after caesarean section: a report of 4880 patients, *Can J Anaesth* 37:636, 1990.

86. Yaksh TL: Spinal opiate analgesia: characteristics and principles of action, *Pain* 11:293, 1981.

87. Krivoy W, Kroeger D, Zimmerman E: Actions of morphine on the segmental reflex of the decerebrate-spinal cat, *Br J Pharmacol* 47:457, 1973.

88. Erickson DL, Blacklock JB, Michaelson M, et al: Control of spasticity by implantable continuous flow morphine pump, *Neurosurgery* 16:215, 1985.

89. Kromer W: Endogenous and exogenous opioids in the control of gastrointestinal motility and secretion, *Pharmacol Rev* 40:121, 1988.

90. Konturek SJ: Opiates and the gastrointestinal tract, *Am J Gastroenterol* 74:285, 1980.

91. Porrecca F, Filla A, Burks TF: Spinal cord-mediated opiate effects on gastrointestinal transit in mice, *Eur J Pharmacol* 86:135, 1982.

92. Thoren T, Wattwill M: Effects on gastric emptying of thoracic epidural analgesia with morphine or bupivacaine, *Anesth Analg* 67:687, 1988.

93. Krames ES, Schuchard M: Implantable intraspinal infusional analgesia: management guidelines, *Pain Rev* 2:243, 1995.

94. Glynn C, O'Sullivan K: A double-blind randomised comparison of the effects of epidural clonidine, lignocaine and the combination of clonidine and lignocaine in patients with chronic pain, *Pain* 64:337, 1996.

95. Rigler ML, Drasner K, Krejcie TC, et al: Cauda equina syndrome after continuous spinal anesthesia, *Anesth Analg* 72:275, 1991.

96. Bainton CR; Strichartz GR: Concentration dependence of lidocaine-induced irreversible conduction loss in frog nerve, *Anesthesiology* 81:657, 1994.

97. Kalichman MW: Physiologic mechanisms by which local anesthetics may cause injury to nerve and spinal cord, *Reg Anesth* 18(suppl 6):448, 1993.

98. Bogduk N: Back pain: zygapophyseal blocks and epidural steroids. In Cousins MJ, Bridenbaugh PO, eds: *Neural blockade,* Philadelphia, 1988, JB Lippincott, p 935.

99. Bogduk N: Local anaesthetic blocks of the second cervical ganglion: a technique with an application in occipital headache, *Cephalgia* 1:41, 1981.

100. Bogduk N, Marsland A: On the concept of third occipital headache, *J Neurol Neurosurg Psychiatry* 49:775, 1986.

101. Masten TD, Fredrickson BE: Intra-articular facet block. In Thomas SB, ed: *Image-guided pain management,* Philadelphia, 1997, Lippincott-Raven, p133.

102. Guyer RD, Ohnmeiss DD, Mason SL, et al: Complications of cervical discography: findings in a large series, *J Spinal Disord* 10:95, 1997.

103. Connor PM, Darden BV II: Cervical discography complications and clinical efficacy, *Spine* 18:2035, 1993.

104. Ventafridda V, Tamburini M, Caraceni A, et al: A validation study of the WHO method for cancer pain relief, *Cancer* 59:850, 1987.

105. Rumsby MG, Finean JB: The action of organic solvents on the myelin sheath of peripheral nerve tissue. II. Short-chain aliphatic alcohols, *J Neurochem* 13:1509, 1966.

106. Bonica JJ, Buckley FP, Moricca G, et al: Neurolytic blockade and hypophysectomy. In Bonica JJ, ed: *The management of pain,* ed 2, Philadelphia, 1990, Lea & Febiger, p 1990.

107. Bonica J, Loeser J, Chapman C, et al: *The management of pain,* ed 2, Philadelphia, 1990, Lea & Febiger, p 1981.

108. Maher RM: Neurone selection in relief of pain, *Lancet* 1:16, 1957.

109. Iggo A, Walsh EG: Selective block of small fibers in the spinal roots by phenol, *Brain* 83:701, 1960.

110. Nathan PW, Sears TA: Effects of phenol in nervous conduction, *J Physiol (Lond)* 150:565, 1960.

111. Stewart WA, Lourie H: An experimental evaluation of the effects of subarachnoid injection of phenol-Pantopaque in cats, *J Neurosurg* 20:64, 1963.

112. Nathan PW, Sears TA, Smith MC: Effects of phenol solutions on the nerve roots of the cat: an electrophysiological and histological study, *J Neurol Sci* 2:7, 1965.

113. Smith MC: Histological findings following intrathecal injections of phenol solutions for the relief of pain, *Anaesthesia* 36:387, 1964.

114. Schaumburg HH, Byck R, Weller RO: The effect of phenol on peripheral nerves: a histological and electrophysiological study, *J Neuropathol Exp Neurol* 29:615, 1970.

115. Politis MJ, Schaumburg HH, Spencer PS: Neurotoxicity of selected chemicals. In Spencer PS, Schaumburg HH, eds: *Experimental and chemical neurotoxicity,* Baltimore, 1980, Williams & Wilkins.

116. Wood KM: The use of phenol as a neurolytic agent: a review, *Pain* 5:205, 1978.

117. Hakanson S: Trigeminal neuralgia treated by the injection of glycerol into the trigeminal cistern, *Neurosurgery* 9:638, 1981.

118. Lunsford LD, Bennett MH: Percutaneous retrogasserian glycerol rhizotomy for tic douloureux. Part I. Technique and results in 112 patients, *Neurosurgery* 14:424, 1984.

119. Sweet WH, Poletti CE, Macon JB: Treatment of trigeminal neuralgia and other facial pain by retrogasserian injection of glycerol, *Neurosurgery* 9:647, 1981.

120. Myers RR, Katz J: Neural pathology of neurolytic and semidestructive agents. In Cousins MJ, Bridenbaugh PO, eds: *Neural blockade in clinical anesthesia and management of pain,* ed 2, Philadelphia, 1988, JB Lippincott, p 1031.

121. Burchiel KJ, Russell LC: Glycerol neurolysis: neurophysiological effects of topical glycerol application on rat saphenous nerve, *J Neurosurg* 63:784, 1985.

122. Reid W, Watt JK, Gray TG: Phenol injection of the sympathetic chain, *Br J Surg* 57:45, 1970.

123. Benzon HT: Convulsions secondary to intravascular phenol: a hazard of celiac plexus block, *Anesth Analg* 58:150, 1979.

124. Felsenthal G: Pharmacology of phenol in peripheral nerve blocks: a review, *Arch Phys Med Rehabil* 55:1, 1974.

125. Goodman LS, Gilman A: *A pharmacological basis of therapeutics,* ed 4, London, 1970, Macmillan.

126. Zamponi GW, French RJ: Dissecting lidocaine action: diethylamide and phenol mimic separate modes of lidocaine block of sodium channels from heart and skeletal muscle, *Biophys J* 65:2335, 1993.

127. Gaudy JH, Tricot C, Sezeur A: Serious heart rate disorders following perioperative splanchnic nerve phenol nerve block, *Can J Anaesth* 40:357, 1993.

128. Derrick WS: Subarachnoid alcohol block for the control of intractable pain, *Acta Anaesthesiol Scand* 24:167, 1966.

129. Hay RC: Subarachnoid alcohol block in the control of intractable pain, *Anesth Analg* 41:12, 1962.

130. Gerbershagen HU: Neurolysis: subarachnoid neurolytic blockade, *Acta Anaesthesiol Belg* 1:45, 1981.

131. Swerdlow M: Intrathecal and extradural block and pain relief. In Swerdlow M, ed: *Relief of intractable pain,* Amsterdam, 1983, Elsevier.

132. Bonica JJ, Buckley FP, Moricca G, et al: Neurolytic blockade and hypophysectomy. In Bonica JJ: *The management of pain,* ed 2, Philadelphia, 1990, Lea & Febiger.

133. Katz JA, Sehlhorst S, Blisard KS: Histopathologic changes in primate spinal cord after single and repeated epidural phenol administration, *Reg Anesth* 20:283, 1995.

134. Swerdlow M: Complications of neurolytic neural blockade. In Cousins MJ, Bridenbaugh PO, eds: *Neural blockade in clinical anesthesia and management of pain,* ed 2, Philadelphia, 1988, JB Lippincott.

135. Bromage PR: *Epidural analgesia,* Philadelphia, 1978, WB Saunders.

136. Colpitt MR, Levy BA, Lawrence M: Treatment of cancer related pain with phenol epidural block, *Abstracts of 2nd World Congress on Pain,* p 147, 1978 (abstract).

137. Brown DL, Bulley CK, Quiel EL: Neurolytic celiac plexus block for pancreatic cancer pain, *Anesth Analg* 66:869, 1987.

138. Thompson GE, Moore DC: Celiac plexus, intercostal, and minor peripheral blockade. In Cousins MJ, Bridenbaugh PO, eds: *Neural blockade in clinical anesthesia and management of pain,* ed 2, Philadelphia, 1988, JB Lippincott.

139. Eisenberg E, Carr DB, Chalmers TC: Neurolytic celiac plexus block for treatment of cancer pain: a meta-analysis, *Anesth Analg* 80:290, 1995.

140. Davies DD: Incidence of major complications of neurolytic coeliac plexus block, *J R Soc Med* 86:264, 1993.

141. Gorbitz C, Leavens ME: Alcohol block of the celiac plexus for control of upper abdominal pain caused by cancer and pancreatitis: technical notes, *J Neurosurg* 34:575, 1971.

142. Moore DC: Celiac (splanchnic) plexus block with alcohol, *Adv Pain Res Ther* 2:357, 1979.

143. Leung JWC, Bowen-Wright M, Aveling W, et al: Coeliac plexus block for pain in pancreatic cancer and chronic pancreatitis, *Br J Surg* 70:730, 1983.

144. De Conno F, Caraceni A, Aldrighetti L, et al: Paraplegia following coeliac plexus block, *Pain* 55:383, 1993.

145. Wong GY, Brown DL: Transient paraplegia following alcohol celiac plexus block, *Reg Anesth,* 20:352, 1995.

146. Johnson ME, Sill JC, Brown DL, et al: The effect of the neurolytic agent ethanol on cytoplasmic calcium in arterial smooth muscle and endothelium, *Reg Anesth* 21:6, 1996.

147. Brown DL, Rorie DK: Altered reactivity of isolated segmental lumbar arteries of dogs following exposure to ethanol and phenol, *Pain* 56:139, 1994.

148. Jones RR: Technic for injection of splanchnic nerves with alcohol, *Anesth Analg* 36:75, 1957.

149. Gale DW, Valley MA, Rogers JN, et al: Effects of neurolytic concentrations of alcohol and phenol on Dacron and Gore-tex vascular prosthetic grafts, *Reg Anesth* 19(6):395, 1994.

150. Sett SS, Taylor DC: Aortic pseudoaneurysm secondary to celiac plexus block, *Ann Vasc Surg* 51:88, 1991.

151. Chan VW: Chronic diarrhea: an uncommon side effect of celiac plexus block, *Anesth Analg* 82:205, 1996.

152. Echenique EM, Gurutz LC: Reversible partial paraplegia after sympathetic lumbar block, *Neurologia* 10:101, 1995.

153. Cherry DA: Chemical lumbar sympathectomy, *Curr Concepts Pain* 2:12, 1984.

154. Baxter AD, O'Kafo BA: Ejaculatory failure after chemical sympathectomy, *Anesth Analg* 63:770, 1984.

155. White JC: Technique of paravertebral alcohol injection, *Surg Gynecol Obstet* 71:334, 1940.

156. Finneson BE: *Diagnosis and management of pain syndromes,* ed 2, Philadelphia, 1969, WB Saunders, p 239.

157. Molitch M, Wilson G: Brown-Sequard paralysis following a paravertebral alcohol injection for angina pectoris, *JAMA* 97:247, 1931.

158. Stender A: *Excerpta Medica International Congress series,* Washington, DC, 1961, p 36.

159. Henderson WR: Trigeminal neuralgia: the pain and its treatment, *BMJ* 1:7, 1967.

160. Miles J: Trigeminal neuralgia. In Lipton S, ed: *Persistent pain,* vol 2, London, 1980, Academic Press.

161. Igarashi S, Suzuki F, Iwasaki K, et al: Glycerol injection method for trigeminal neuralgia, *No Shinkei Geka* 13:267, 1985.

162. North RB, Han M, Zahurak M, et al: Radiofrequency lumbar facet denervation: analysis of prognostic factors, *Pain* 57:77, 1994.

163. Shealy CN: Facet denervation in the management of back and sciatic pain, *Clin Orthop* Mar-Apr(115):157, 1976.

164. Onofrio BM: Radiofrequency percutaneous gasserian ganglion lesions: results in 140 patients with trigeminal pain, *J Neurosurg* 42:132, 1975.

165. Broggi G, Franzini A, Lasio G, et al: Long-term results of percutaneous retrogasserian thermorhizotomy for "essential" trigeminal neuralgia: considerations in 1000 patients, *Neurosurgery* 26:783, 1990.

166. Sanders M, Zuurmond WW: Efficacy of sphenopalatine ganglion blockade in 66 patients suffering from cluster headache: a 12 to 70 month follow-up evaluation, *J Neurosurg* 7:876, 1997.

167. Sluijter ME: The use of radiofrequency lesions for pain relief in failed back patients, *Int Disabil Stud* 10:37, 1988.

168. Geurts JW, Stolker RJ: Percutaneous radiofrequency lesion of the stellate ganglion in the treatment of pain in upper extremity reflex sympathetic dystrophy, *The Pain Clinic* 6:17, 1993.

169. Dawkins CJM: Analysis of the complications of extradural and caudal block, *Anaesthesia* 24:554, 1969.

170. Usubiaga JE: Neurological complications following epidural anesthesia, *Int Anesthesiol Clin* 13:1, 1975.

171. Skoven JS, Wainapel SF, Willock MM: Paraplegia following epidural anesthesia, *Acta Neurol Scand* 72:437, 1985.

172. Yuen EC, Layzer RB, Weitz SR, et al: Neurologic complications of lumbar epidural anesthesia and analgesia, *Neurology* 45:1795, 1995.

173. Linnemann MU, Bulow HH: Infections after insertion of epidural catheters, *Ugeskr Laeger* 155:2350, 1993.

174. Holt HM, Andersen SS, Andersen O, et al: Infections following epidural catheterization, *J Hosp Infect* 30:253, 1995.

175. Pegues DA, Carr DB, Hopkins CC: Infectious complications associated with temporary epidural catheters, *Clin Infect Dis* 19:970, 1994.

176. Du Pen SL, Peterson DG, Williams A, et al: Infection during chronic epidural catheterization: diagnosis and treatment, *Anesthesiology* 73:905, 1990.

177. Aguilar JL, Roca G, Montes A, et al: [Experience with the Du Pen epidural catheter in chronic cancer pain], *Rev Esp Anestesiol Reanim* 39:183, 1992.

178. Yue SK, St. Marie B, Henrickson K: Initial clinical experience with the SKY epidural catheter, *J Pain Symptom Manage* 6:107, 1991.

179. Erdine S, Aldemir T: Long-term results of peridural morphine in 225 patients, *Pain* 45:155, 1991.

180. Bauer M, Knippenberger H, Kubli F, et al: The bacterial contamination of epidural catheters with areobe and anaerobe germs in obstetrics, *Geburtshilfe Frauenheilkd* 39:1054, 1979.

181. Hicks F, Simpson KH, Tosh GC: Management of spinal infusions in palliative care, *Palliat Med* 8:325, 1994.

182. Byers K, Axelrod P, Michael S, et al: Infections complicating tunneled intraspinal catheter systems used to treat chronic pain, *Clin Infect Dis* 21:403, 1995.

183. Turner JA, Loeser JD, Bell KG: Spinal cord stimulation for chronic low back pain: a systematic literature synthesis, *Neurosurgery* 37:1088, 1995.

184. Nickels JH, Poulos JG, Chaouki K: Risks of infection from short-term epidural catheter use, *Reg Anesth* 14:88, 1989.

185. Bevacqua BK, Slucky AV, Cleary WF: Is postoperative intrathecal catheter use associated with central nervous system infection? *Anesthesiology* 80:1234, 1994.

186. Nitescu P, Sjoberg M, Appelgren L, et al: Complications of intrathecal opioids and bupivacaine in the treatment of "refractory" cancer pain, *Clin J Pain* 11:45, 1995.

187. Kobayashi Y, Shiotani M, Oseto K, et al: Six cases of epidural abscess probably caused by epidural block and examination by gadolinium-MRI imaging, *Masui* 42:888, 1993.

188. Sollmann WP, Gaab MR, Panning B: Lumbar epidural hematoma and spinal abscess following peridural anesthesia, *Reg Anaesth* 10:121, 1987.

189. Strong WE: Epidural abscess associated with epidural catheterization: a rare event? Report of two cases with markedly delayed presentation, *Anesthesiology* 74:943, 1991.

190. Meglio M, Cioni B, Rossi GF: Spinal cord stimulation in management of chronic pain: a 9-year experience, *J Neurosurg* 70:519, 1989.

191. Hartstein GM, Robles JR: Epidural abscesses and hematomata, *Obstetr Anesth Dig* July:95-98, 1988.

192. Browder J, Meyers R: Infections of spinal epidural space: aspect of vertebral osteomyelitis, *Am J Surg* 37:4, 1937.

193. Jakobsen KB, Christensen MK, Carlsson PS: Extradural anaesthesia for repeated surgical treatment in the presence of infection, *Br J Anaesth* 75:536, 1995.

194. Hahn MB, Bettencourt JA, McCrea WB: In vivo sterilization of an infected long-term epidural catheter, *Anesthesiology* 76:645, 1992.

195. Bennett MI, Tai YM, Symonds JM: Staphylococcal meningitis following SynchroMed intrathecal pump implant: a case report, *Pain* 56:243, 1994.

196. Shapiro JM, Bond EL, Garman JK: Use of a chlorhexidine dressing to reduce microbial colonization of epidural catheters, *Anesthesiology* 73:625, 1990.

197. De Cicco M, Matovic M, Castellani GT, et al: Time-dependent efficacy of bacterial filters and infection risk in long-term epidural catheterization, *Anesthesiology* 82:765, 1995.

198. de Jong PC, Kansen PJ: A comparison of epidural catheters with or without subcutaneous injection ports for treatment of cancer pain, *Anesth Analg* 78:94, 1994.

199. Feldman JM, Chapin-Robertson K, Turner J: Do agents used for epidural analgesia have antimicrobial properties? *Reg Anesth* 19:43, 1994.

200. James FM, George RH, Naiem H, et al: Bacteriologic aspects of epidural analgesia, *Anesth Analg* 55:187, 1976.

201. Driessen JJ, de Mulder PH, Claessen JJ, et al: Epidural administration of morphine for control of cancer pain: Long-term efficacy and complications, *Clin J Pain* 5:217, 1989.

202. Arner S, Rawal N, Gustafsson LL: Clinical experience of long-term treatment with epidural and intrathecal opioids—a nationwide survey, *Acta Anaesthesiol Scand* 32:245, 1988.

203. DuPen SL, Peterson DG, Bogosian AC, et al: A new permanent exteriorized epidural catheter for narcotic self-administration to control cancer pain, *Cancer* 59:986, 1987.

204. Liew E, Hui YL: A preliminary study of long-term epidural morphine for cancer pain via a subcutaneously implanted reservoir, *Ma Tsui Hsueh Tsa Chi* 27:5, 1989.

205. Shigihara A, Suzuki M, Tase C, et al: Changes in analgesic levels, plasma concentrations and epidurogram during long-term continuous epidural block, *Masui* 44:994, 1995.

206. Samuelsson H, Nordberg G, Hedner T, et al: CSF and plasma morphine concentrations in cancer patients during chronic epidural morphine therapy and its relation to pain relief, *Pain* 30:303, 1987.

207. Durant P, Yaksh TL: Epidural injections of bupivicaine, morphine, fentanyl, lofentanil, and DADL in chronically implanted rat: a pharmacologic and morphologic study, *Anesthesiology* 64:43, 1986.

208. Sabbe MB, Grafe MR, Mjanger E, et al: Spinal delivery of sufentanil, alfentanil, and morphine in dogs: physiologic and toxicologic investigations, *Anesthesiology* 81:899, 1994.

209. Coombs DW, Colburn RW, DeLeo JA, et al: Comparative histopathology of epidural hydrogel and silicone elastomer catheters following 30 and 180 days implant in the ewe, *Acta Anaesthesiol Scand* 38:388, 1994.

210. Coombs DW, Colburn RW, DeLeo JA, et al: Testing an implantable intraspinal delivery device in the ewe, *Reg Anesth* 18:230, 1993.

211. Carl P, Crawford M, Ravlo O: Postmortem findings after long-term treatment of pain via an epidural catheter, *Ugeskr Laeger* 145:4001, 1983.

212. Cherry DA, Gourlay GK, Cousins MJ, et al: A technique for the insertion of an implantable portal system for the long term epidural administration of opioids in the treatment of cancer pain, *Anaesth Intensive Care* 13:145, 1985.

213. Aldrete JA: Epidural fibrosis after permanent catheter insertion and infusion, *J Pain Symptom Manage* 10:624, 1995.

214. Rodan BA, Cohen FL, Bean WJ, et al: Fibrous mass complicating epidural morphine infusion, *Neurosurgery* 16:68, 1985.

215. North RB, Cutchis PN, Epstein JA, et al: Spinal cord compression complicating subarachnoid infusion of morphine: case report and laboratory experience, *Neurosurgery* 29:778, 1991.

216. Auld AW, Maki-Jokela A, Murdoch DM: Intraspinal narcotic analgesia in the treatment of chronic pain, *Spine* 10:777, 1985.

217. Penn RD, York MM, Paice JA: Catheter systems for intrathecal drug delivery, *J Neurosurg* 83:215, 1995.

218. Hogan QH: Loculated? Encapsulated? Indented? *Pain* 53:241, 1993 (letter).

219. Takahashi H, Sato S, Tajima K, et al: Changes of epidurogram after long-term continuous epidural block, *J Jpn Soc Clin Anaesth* 11:38, 1991.

220. Nagaro T: The histopathological changes in the epidural space and changes in the effect of anesthetic after long-term continuous epidural block, *Masui* 35:227, 1986.

221. Landon B, Dobke M, Grzybowski J, et al: Enhanced activity of lysosomal β-galactosidase after silicone implantation: an experimental study in rats, *J Lab Clin Med* 121:742, 1993.

222. Virden C, Dobke M, Stein P, et al: Subclinical infection of the silicone breast implant as a possible cause of capsular contracture, *Aesthetic Plast Surg* 16:173, 1992.

223. Crul BJ, Delhaas EM: Technical complications during long-term subarachnoid or epidural administration of morphine in terminally ill cancer patients: a review of 140 cases, *Reg Anesth* 16:209, 1991.

224. Ehring E, Boekstegers A: Morphologic and histologic changes caused by continuous peridural analgesia in a cancer patient, *Reg Anesth* 9:46, 1986.

225. Sjoberg M, Karlsson PA, Nordborg C, et al: Neuropathologic findings after long-term intrathecal infusion of morphine and bupivacaine for pain treatment in cancer patients, *Anesthesiology* 76:173, 1992.

226. Larsen JJ, Svendsen O, Andersen HB: Microscopic epidural lesions in goats given repeated epidural injections of morphine: use of a modified autopsy procedure, *Acta Pharmacol Toxicol (Copenh)* 58:5, 1986.

227. Wallace MS, Wallace AM, Lee J, et al: Pain after breast surgery: a survey of 282 women, *Pain* 66:195, 1996.
228. Nelson DA, Vates TS Jr, Thomas Rosenbach Jr: Complications from intrathecal steroid therapy in patients with multiple sclerosis, *Acta Neurol Scand* 49:176, 1973.
229. Bernat JL, Sadowsky CH, Vincent FM, et al: Sclerosing spinal pachymeningitis: a complication of intrathecal administration of Depo-Medrol for multiple sclerosis, *J Neurol Neurosurg Psychiatry* 39:1124, 1976.
230. Ryan MD, Taylor TKF: Management of lumbar nerve root pain by intrathecal and epidural injections of depot methylprednisolone acetate, *Med J Aust* 2:532, 1981.
231. Roche J: Steroid-induced arachnoiditis, *Med J Aust* 140:281, 1984.
232. Carta F, Canu C, Datti R, et al: Calcification and ossification of the spinal arachnoid after intrathecal injection of Depo-Medrol, *Zentralbl Neurochir* 48:256, 1987.
233. Plumb VJ, Dismukes WE: Chemical meningitis related to intrathecal corticosteroid therapy, *South Med J* 70:1241, 1977.
234. Abram SE: Subarachnoid corticosteroid injection following inadequate response to epidural steroids for sciatica, *Anesth Analg* 57:313, 1978.
235. Gutknecht DR: Chemical meningitis following epidural injections of corticosteroids, *Am J Med* 82:570, 1987 (letter).
236. Morris JT, Knokol KA, Longfield RN: Chemical meningitis following epidural methylprednisolone injection, *Infect Med* 11:439, 1994.
237. Shealy CN: Dangers of spinal injections without proper diagnosis, *JAMA* 197:1104, 1966.
238. Roberts M, Sheppard GL, McCormick RC: Tuberculous meningitis after intrathecally administered methylprednisolone acetate, *JAMA* 200:894, 1967.
239. Dougherty JH Jr, Fraser RAR: Complications following intraspinal injections of steroids: report of two cases, *J Neurosurg* 48:1023, 1978.
240. Knight JW, Cordingley JJ, Palazzo MG: Epidural abscess following epidural steroid and local anaesthetic injection, *Anaesthesia* 52:576, 1997.
241. Warr AC, Wilkinson JA, Burn JMB, et al: Chronic lumbosciatic syndrome treat by epidural injection and manipulation, *Practitioner* 209:53, 1972.
242. Williams KN, Jackowski A, Evans PJD: Epidural haematoma requiring surgical decompression following repeated cervical epidural steroid injections for chronic pain, *Pain* 42:197, 1990.
243. Simon DL, Kunz RD, German JD, et al: Allergic or pseudoallergic reaction following epidural steroid deposition and skin testing, *Reg Anesth* 14:253, 1989.
244. Kushner FH, Olson JC: Retinal hemorrhage as a consequence of epidural steroid injection, *Arch Ophthalmol* 113:309, 1995.
245. Siegfried RN: Development of complex regional pain syndrome after a cervical epidural steroid injection, *Anesthesiology* 86:1394, 1997.
246. Boonen S, Van Distel G, Westhovens R, et al: Steroid myopathy induced by epidural triamcinolone injection, *Br J Rheum* 34:385, 1995.
247. Tuel SM, Meythaler JM, Cross LL: Cushing's syndrome from methylprednisolone, *Pain* 40:81, 1990.
248. Abram SE, O'Connor TC: Complications associated with epidural steroid injections, *Reg Anesth* 21:149, 1996.
249. Tucker GT, Boas RA: Pharmacokinetic aspects of intravenous regional anesthesia, *Anesthesiology* 34:538, 1971.
250. Englesson S: The influence of acid-base changes on central nervous system toxicity of local anesthetic agents. I. An experimental study in cats, *Acta Anaesthesiol Scand* 18:79, 1974.
251. Gettes LS: Physiology and pharmacology of antiarrhythmic drugs, *Hosp Pract (Off Ed)* 16:89, 1981.
252. Lieberman NA, Harris RS, Katz RI, et al: The effects of lidocaine on the electrical and mechanical activity of the heart, *Am J Cardiol* 22:375, 1968.
253. Harrison DC, Sprouse JH, Morrow AG: The antiarrhythmic properties of lidocaine and procaine amide; clinical and physiologic studies of their cardiovascular effects in man, *Circulation* 28:486, 1963.
254. Feldman HS, Arthur GR, Norway SB, et al: Cardiovascular effects of mepivacaine and etidocaine in the awake dog, *Anesthesiology* 61:A229, 1984 (abstract).
255. Kotelko DM, Shnider SM, Dailey PA, et al: Bupivacaine-induced cardiac arrhythmias in sheep, *Anesthesiology* 60:10, 1984.
256. Sage D, Feldman H, Arthur GR, et al: Cardiovascular effects of lidocaine and bupivacaine in the awake dog, *Anesthesiology* 59:A210, 1983 (abstract).
257. de Jong RH, Ronfeld RA, DeRosa RA: Cardiovascular effects of convulsant and supraconvulsant doses of amide local anesthetics, *Anesth Analg* 61:3, 1982.
258. Sage DJ, Feldman HS, Arthur GR, et al: Influence of lidocaine and bupivacaine on isolated guinea pig atria in the presence of acidosis and hypoxia, *Anesth Analg* 63:1, 1984.
259. Brown DT, Beamish D, Wildsmith JAW: Allergic reaction to an amide local anaesthetic, *Br J Anaesth* 53:435, 1981.
260. Reynolds F: Allergy reaction to an amide local anaesthetic, *Br J Anaesth* 53:901, 1981.
261. Shir Y, Cameron LB, Raja SN, et al: The safety of intravenous phentolamine administration in patients with neuropathic pain, *Anesth Analg* 76:1008, 1993.
262. Travell JG, Simmons DG: *Myofascial pain and dysfunction: the trigger point manual*, Baltimore, 1983, Williams & Wilkins.
263. Garvey TA, Marks MR, Wiesel SW: A prospective, randomized double-blind evaluation of trigger-point injection therapy for low-back pain, *Spine* 14:962, 1989.
264. Moore DC, Spierdijk J, VanKleef JD, et al: Chloroprocaine neurotoxicity: four additional cases, *Anesth Analg* 61:155, 1982.
265. Libelius R, Sonesson B, Stamenovic BA, et al: Denervation-like changes in skeletal muscle after treatment with a local anesthetic (Marcaine), *J Anat* 106:297, 1970.
266. Hong CZ: Lidocaine injection versus dry needling to myofascial trigger point: the importance of the local twitch response, *Am J Phys Med Rehabil* 73:256, 1994.
267. Shafer N: Pneumothorax following "trigger point" injection, *JAMA* 213:1193, 1970.
268. Schmid E, Hortling G, Kammuller H: Inoculation hepatitis caused by acupuncture: clinical cases studied over a 9-year period, *Fortschr Med* 102:862, 1984.
269. Li FP, Shiang EL: Acupuncture and possible hepatitis B infection, *JAMA* 243:1423, 1980 (letter).
270. Jefferys DB, Smith S, Brennand-Roper DA, et al: Acupuncture needles as a cause of bacterial endocarditis, *BMJ (Clin Res Ed)* 287:326, 1983.
271. Chen CY, Liu GC, Sheu RS, et al: Bacterial meningitis and lumbar epidural hematoma due to lumbar acupunctures: a case report, *Kao Hsiung I Hsueh Ko Hsueh Tsa Chih* 13:328, 1997.
272. Pierik MG: Fatal staphylococcal septicemia following acupuncture: report of two cases: occurrence of staphylococcal septicemia following acupuncture emphasizes need for thorough medical evaluation before such procedures, *R I Med J* 65:251, 1982.
273. Izatt E, Fairman M: Staphylococcal septicemia with disseminated intravascular coagulation associated with acupuncture, *Postgrad Med J* 53:285, 1977.
274. Schneider LB, Salzberg MR: Bilateral pneumothorax following acupuncture, *Ann Emerg Med* 13:643, 1984 (letter).
275. Carette MF, Mayaud C, Houacine S, et al: Treatment of an asthmatic crisis by acupuncture: probable role in the onset of pneumothorax with development to status asthmaticus, *Rev Pneumol Clin* 40:69, 1984.
276. Bodner G, Topilsky M, Greif J: Pneumothorax as a complication of acupuncture in the treatment of bronchial asthma, *Ann Allergy* 51:401, 1983.
277. Brettel HF: Acupuncture as a cause of death, *MMW Munch Med Wochenschr* 123:97, 1981.
278. Vilke GM, Wulfert EA: Case reports of two patients with pneumothorax following acupuncture, *J Emerg Med* 15:155, 1997.
279. Abumi K, Anbo H, Kaneda K: Migration of an acupuncture needle into the medulla oblongata, *Eur Spine J* 5:137, 1996.
280. Sasaki H, Abe H, Iwasaki Y, et al: Direct spinal cord and root injury caused by acupuncture: report of two cases, *No Shinkei Geka* 12:1219, 1984.

281. Shiraishi S, Goto I, Kuroiwa Y, et al: Spinal cord injury as a complication of an acupuncture, *Neurology* 29:1188, 1979.

282. Kondo A, Koyama T, Ishikawa J, et al: Injury to the spinal cord produced by acupuncture needle, *Surg Neurol* 11:155, 1979.

283. Kataoka H: Cardiac tamponade caused by penetration of an acupuncture needle into the right ventricle, *J Thorac Cardiovasc Surg* 114:674, 1997.

284. Halvorsen TB, Anda SS, Naess AB, et al: Fatal cardiac tamponade after acupuncture through congenital sternal foramen. *Lancet* 345:1175, 1995 (letter).

285. Bork K: Multiple lymphocytoma at the point of puncture as complication of acupuncture treatment: traumatic origin of lymphocytoma, *Hautarzt* 34:496, 1983.

286. Rajanna P: Hypotension following stimulation of acupuncture point, *J R Coll Gen Pract* 33:606, 1983.

287. Trautermann HG, Trautermann H: Perichondritis of the ear auricle after acupuncture, *HNO* 29:312, 1981.

288. Baltimore RS, Moloy PJ: Perichondritis of the ear as a complication of acupuncture, *Arch Otolaryngol* 102:572, 1976.

289. Allison G, Kravitz E: Auricular chondritis secondary to acupuncture, *N Engl J Med* 293:780, 1975 (letter).

290. Jones RO, Cross G III: Suspected chronic osteomyelitis secondary to acupuncture treatment: a case report, *J Am Podiatry Assoc* 70:149, 1980.

291. Aso Y, Murahashi I, Yokoyama M: Foreign body stone of the ureter as a complication of acupuncture, *Eur Urol* 5:57, 1979.

292. Chang TW: Activation of cutaneous herpes by acupuncture, *N Engl J Med* 291:1310, 1974 (letter).

293. Sobel E, Huang EY, Wieting CB: Drop foot as a complication of acupuncture injury and intragluteal injection, *J Am Podiatr Med Assoc* 87:52, 1997.

294. Garcia AA, Venkataramani A: Bilateral psoas abscesses following acupuncture, *West J Med* 161:90, 1994 (letter).

295. Keane JR, Ahmadi J, Gruen P: Spinal epidural hematoma with subarachnoid hemorrhage caused by acupuncture, *AJNR Am J Neuroradiol* 14:365, 1993.

Chapter 6

Equipment Failure: Anesthesia Delivery Systems

James B. Eisenkraft
Richard M. Sommer

Although uncommon, failure of the anesthesia delivery system may result in patient injury or death. More common than total failure of a delivery system component is operator error and misuse of the system. A sound understanding of anesthesia delivery systems is therefore essential for the safe practice of anesthesia.

Cooper, Newbower, and Kitz[1] found that approximately 30% of 1089 critical incidents during anesthesia were related to equipment failure, including breathing circuit disconnection, gas flow-control errors, loss of gas supply, leaks, misconnections, and ventilator malfunctions. Seventy incidents (6.4%) resulted in a "substantive negative outcome" for the patient; only 3 of the 70 were attributable to equipment failure. This confirmed the previous impression that human error is the dominant cause of anesthesia mishaps.[2] Although equipment failure is rarely the cause of death during anesthesia, critical incidents related to equipment are not infrequent and have prompted improvements in machine design and construction.[3]

Buffington, Ramanathan, and Turndorf[4] intentionally created five faults in a standard anesthesia machine and invited 190 attendees at a postgraduate assembly of the New York State Society of Anesthesiologists to identify them within 10 minutes. The average number of discovered faults was 2.2; 7.3% of participants found no faults, and only 3.4% found all five. The authors concluded that greater emphasis was needed in educational programs on the fundamentals of anesthesia machine design and detection of hazards.[4]

Kumar, Hintze, and Jacob[5] conducted a random survey of 169 anesthesia machines and ancillary monitors in 45 hospitals in Iowa. The machines ranged in age from 1 to 28 years (the oldest was made in 1958). Five machines had no backup source of oxygen, 60 had no functioning oxygen analyzer, and 15 leaked more than 500 ml of gas per minute (2 leaks were proximal, and 13 were distal to the common gas outlet [i.e., the patient circuit]). Fourteen of the 383 vaporizers tested did not meet the manufacturer's calibration standards, and 20 had been added downstream of the machine common gas outlet. Of the 123 machines with ventilators, 16 had no alarm for low airway pressure, and only 31 had a high-pressure alarm. Of the ventilators surveyed, 59% were of the hanging-bellows design and 41% of the standing-bellows design. Of the machines surveyed, 95.5% had a scavenging system, but in 24.3%, the scavenging circuit connectors were indistinguishable from the breathing circuit connectors—a potentially hazardous design.[5]

In 1993, the Australian Anaesthesia Patient Safety Foundation published the results of the Australian Incident Monitoring Study, which collected data on 2000 critical incidents.[6] Of these, 177 (9%) were due to general equipment failure, and 107 of these failures (60%) involved the anesthesia delivery system. Failures were related to problems with unidirectional valves, ventilator malfunction, gas or electric supply, circuit integrity, anesthesia vaporizers, absorbers, and pressure regulators.[6]

In 1997, Caplan et al[7] reported on the American Society of Anesthesiologists (ASA) Closed Claims Project, which investigated the role of anesthesia equipment

problems in adverse outcomes and malpractice litigation in the United States. Their analysis of 3791 claims arising from events that occurred from 1961 to 1994 found that gas delivery equipment problems accounted for 72 (2%) of all claims in the ASA Closed Claims Project database. Of these 72 claims, 39% were related to the breathing system, 21% to vaporizers, 17% to ventilators, 11% to gas tanks or gas lines, and only 7% to the anesthesia machine. Gas delivery equipment accounted for 34 of 1542 (7%) of all claims in the database before 1985 but only 18 of 1495 (1.2%) of claims since 1985. Although adverse outcomes caused by gas delivery equipment are rare and seem to be decreasing, the injuries that do occur are usually severe. Death or brain damage was the outcome in 76% of the 72 claims; therefore anesthesiologists cannot afford to be complacent about potential problems with the gas delivery system.[7]

In the ASA Closed Claims Study, initiating events in the 72 claims involving gas delivery equipment were circuit misconnections, disconnections, and delivery system errors. Claims involving misuse (i.e., human error) were 3 times more common than "pure" equipment failures (54 [75%] compared with 17 cases [24%]). Of the cases thought to be due to human error, 70% were considered to be the direct result of actions of the primary anesthesia provider; in the other 30%, misuse stemmed at least in part from the contributory actions of ancillary staff, such as technicians, nurses, and respiratory therapists. The predominant mechanisms of injury were hypoxemia, excessive airway pressure, and anesthetic agent overdose. In 78% of the 72 claims, it was thought that the use or better use of monitoring would have prevented an adverse outcome.[7]

In the study by Caplan et al,[7] 86% of the 72 claims resulted from events in the operating room and involved anesthesia gas delivery systems. With the recognition of how critical incidents and adverse outcomes can arise, anesthesia delivery systems have evolved considerably to the machines now available. This evolution demonstrates the application of the principles of risk reduction so that new delivery systems are designed to be safer.

Modern anesthesia delivery systems contain pneumatic, mechanical, and electronic components that are very reliable; thus unexpected equipment failure is rare in a system that has been well maintained and properly checked before use. Recognition of the importance of human error in critical incidents and of the limitations of human vigilance has led to a three-tier approach in the design of new delivery systems in the quest for increased safety.[8]

1. Where possible, anesthesia delivery systems are designed so that human error cannot occur. The introduction of keyed connections for gas tanks, gas lines, and vaporizers and fail-safe systems are examples. For example, it should be almost impossible to connect anything but an oxygen tank or line to the oxygen inlet of the machine.
2. If human error cannot be prevented, the system is designed to prevent such errors from causing injury. Examples of this are gas flow proportioning systems for nitrous oxide and oxygen that prevent a mixture containing less than 25% oxygen from

being accidentally set if nitrous oxide and oxygen are the only gases used. A high-pressure limiting device on the ventilator should prevent barotrauma if the ventilator is set to deliver an excessive tidal volume or pressure.

3. Because it is not always possible to prevent or correct for user error, the delivery system should be equipped with monitors and alarms that signal an operator error or an adverse condition that might be caused by an equipment failure or a change in the patient's condition.

The most current voluntary consensus standard describing the features of a modern machine was published by the American Society for Testing and Materials (ASTM) in March 1989. It describes the minimum performance and safety requirements necessary in the design of anesthesia machines for human use.[9] This standard supersedes the document published by the American National Standards Institute in 1979.[10] Use of a state-of-the-art delivery system that includes basic system monitors, together with adoption of *Standards for Basic Intraoperative Monitoring* (published by the ASA in 1986 and periodically updated[11]), is expected to enhance patient safety. However, absolute confirmation by demonstration of a statistically significant decrease in the number of adverse events may be difficult.[12]

Adverse outcomes resulting from anesthesia delivery systems are usually complex in origin and involve specific errors, failures, and sequences of events. Eichhorn[12] reviewed 70 anesthesia-related claims reported to the Harvard-affiliated hospitals malpractice insurance carrier from 1976 to 1988. Eleven major intraoperative accidents occurred, of which five were related to anesthesia equipment and involved user error. Eichhorn's report is especially valuable because it includes a brief synopsis of each major accident, which provides an understanding of how such events can occur and how they may be prevented with safety monitoring.[12]

Clearly the potential for development of delivery system–related problems is great, and equipment users may not be as educated as they should about detection of such problems. Complications of the anesthesia delivery system may be operator induced (misuse) or attributable to failure of a component. The approach taken in this chapter is to first trace the normal flow of gases and vapors from their storage containers through the various components of the delivery system and to consider the function of each gas and component. In this way, the effects of individual component failure will be more readily appreciated. The structure and function of the anesthesia delivery system are discussed in greater detail elsewhere.[13-15] Delivery system failure and operator error are then discussed in relation to the patient under the general categories of oxygenation, carbon dioxide, circuit pressures and volumes, anesthetic agent delivery, humidification of inhaled gases, and electrical failure. Finally, because prevention of failures or errors is clearly preferable to their occurrence, delivery system inspections and standards are discussed.

I. THE ANESTHESIA DELIVERY SYSTEM: STRUCTURE AND FUNCTION
A. Overview

The components of a modern basic anesthesia delivery system are depicted in Fig. 6-1. These include the anesthesia machine itself, which receives oxygen, nitrous oxide, and, perhaps, a third and fourth gas (such as helium, air, or carbon dioxide) delivered under pressure. A controlled mixture of oxygen and other gas or gases is delivered at a preset concentration and flow rate to a concentration-calibrated vaporizer, where a measured amount of a potent inhaled anesthetic agent may be added. The resulting fresh gas mixture of known composition and metered production rate leaves the anesthesia machine via the common gas outlet and flows to the patient circuit. The patient circuit is a minienvironment with which the patient makes respiratory exchange; the patient's arterial blood and brain equilibrate with the tensions of the gases in the circuit to produce the desired depth of anesthesia. The patient circuit also permits control of the tensions of carbon dioxide, oxygen, and other gases. An anesthesia ventilator bellows may be connected to the circuit, whereby the patient's lungs may be mechanically ventilated. Excess gases are vented from the anesthesia circuit through either the adjustable pressure-limiting (APL) valve (also known as a "pop-off" valve) or the ventilator pressure–relief valve. The vented gases enter the waste gas–scavenging system and are removed from the operating room, usually through the hospital suction system.

At present, the two largest U.S. manufacturers of anesthesia delivery systems (machines, ventilators, vaporizers, and scavenging systems) are North American Dräger (Telford, Pennsylvania) and Ohmeda (BOC

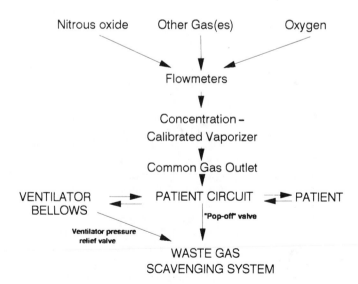

Fig. 6-1. A generic anesthesia delivery system. (From Eisenkraft JB: The anesthesia delivery system. In Longnecker DE, Tinker JH, Morgan GE, eds: *Principles and practice of anesthesiology,* ed 2, St Louis, 1998, Mosby.)

Health Care, Madison, Wisconsin).* The features of a basic anesthesia delivery system are reviewed with reference to North American Dräger and Ohmeda products where they differ substantially. The manufacturers' operator and service manuals represent the most comprehensive source of reference for any individual model of machine; therefore users are strongly encouraged to review the manuals relevant to their equipment.

B. Basic anesthesia machine

The flow arrangements of a basic two-gas anesthesia machine are shown in Fig. 6-2. The machine receives the

---

*In 1998, Ohmeda was purchased and renamed Datex-Ohmeda.

two basic gases, oxygen and nitrous oxide, from two supply sources, a tank or cylinder and a pipeline.

1. Oxygen. Oxygen tanks form a backup supply to the machine in case of pipeline failure. Machines are usually equipped with one or two E cylinders that hang on gas-specific oxygen yokes. The medical gas pin-indexed safety system ensures that the correct gas tank is mounted in the correct hanger yoke. The system consists of two pins in the yoke that fit into two holes in the tank valve. The two pins in the oxygen hanger yoke have a configuration that will match only the oxygen tank and should never be removed from the hanger yoke. Specific pin configurations exist for each of the medical gases supplied in small cylinders to prevent misconnections of gas supplies. A tank should therefore never be force-

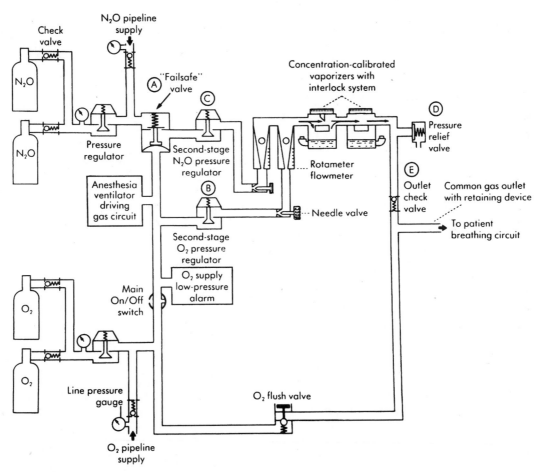

Fig. 6-2. Flow arrangements of a contemporary anesthesia machine. *A,* The fail-safe valve in Ohmeda machines is called a "pressure sensor shutoff valve"; in North American Dräger machines, it is called the "oxygen-failure protection device." *B,* A second-stage oxygen pressure regulator is used in Ohmeda (but not North American Dräger Narkomed) machines. *C,* A second-stage nitrous oxide pressure regulator is used in Ohmeda Modulus machines that have the Link-25 proportion limiting system but is not used in North American Dräger machines. *D,* Pressure-relief valve used in Ohmeda machines. In North American Dräger machines, excesses of pressure are relieved by a pressure-relief mechanism (e.g., that in the Vapor 19.1 vaporizer). *E,* An outlet check valve is used in Ohmeda machines (except Modulus II Plus and Modulus CD) but is not used in North American Dräger machines. (Modified from *"Check-out": a guide for preoperative inspection of an anesthesia machine,* Park Ridge, Ill, 1987, American Society of Anesthesiologists.)

fitted to a hanger yoke. In this way, only oxygen should enter the oxygen piping system of the machine.

Before a new oxygen tank is hung in the yoke, the plastic wrapper surrounding the tank valve should be removed, and the tank valve should be opened briefly so that the emerging oxygen will blow out any debris from the valve. If the wrapper is not removed before the tank is hung, a small plastic disk will lodge in the yoke inlet and may totally obstruct flow of oxygen from the tank.

Oxygen tanks are filled at the factory to a pressure of approximately 2000 psig at room temperature.[14] A full E cylinder of oxygen (internal volume of approximately 4.8 L) at a pressure of 2000 psig will produce approximately 660 L of gaseous oxygen at atmospheric pressure (14.7 psia, or 760 mm Hg).* If the oxygen tank pressure is 1000 psig, the tank is 50% full and will generate only 330 L (50% of 660 L) of gaseous oxygen. It is important to understand these principles when oxygen cylinders are used to supply the machine or to transport a ventilated patient. If the anesthesia machine is equipped with two E cylinders of oxygen, only one should be open at any time so that both tanks are not emptied simultaneously.

The hanger yokes for oxygen tanks and tanks of other gases contain a check valve to prevent leakage of gas through the yoke if no cylinder is hanging in place and the machine is being supplied by the pipeline or from a second oxygen tank (see Fig. 6-2). If two oxygen tanks are hanging, the check valve in each hanger yoke prevents transfilling of gas from one tank to the other. However, these check valves may leak; therefore if a yoke does not have a tank hanging in it, a yoke plug should be inserted. This prevents leakage of gas in the event of an incompetent check valve, which might otherwise cause depletion of the oxygen tank.

In many medical facilities, the oxygen pipeline is supplied from a bulk liquid source. Alarms and safety devices, including relief valves and shutoff valves, ensure the safe functioning of the bulk oxygen storage and pipeline systems. Pipeline oxygen is available in operating rooms through standard diameter-indexed gas-specific outlets or through manufacturer- and gas-specific quick connector outlets.[14]

Just as wall connectors are noninterchangeable among medical gases (e.g., a nitrous oxide hose connector cannot be connected to an oxygen outlet), quick connectors are manufacturer specific (e.g., Schraeder, Ohmeda, and Chemetron). At the machine end of the pipeline hose is a connector that is gas specific by a national standard.[13] The diameter-indexed safety system (DISS) specifies that the inlet connectors for the various medical gases must all differ in diameter. Occasionally, DISS fittings are used at wall gas outlets; however, because a wrench is usually needed to tighten the hose connector to the DISS fitting, these fittings are considered by some to be less convenient than the manufacturer gas-specific quick-connect fittings. The DISS and pin-indexed safety systems are de-

signed to ensure that the correct medical gas enters the correct part of the anesthesia machine.[16,17] It is possible, however, for tanks (E cylinders or bulk storage) to be filled with the wrong gas, thus allowing a hypoxic gas to enter the oxygen-designated parts of the machine. In one instance, the oxygen pipeline was connected to a bulk supply of nitrogen, with catastrophic results.[18]

Pipeline crossovers during hospital construction or maintenance may also result in failure of oxygen delivery.[19-21] Such crossovers may also occur in the tubing that connects the machine to the wall piped-gas supply. It is also possible for the gas supply to be contaminated by other chemicals. In one report, the solution used to clean the oxygen supply tubing between the delivery tanker and the hospital pipeline had not been flushed out and contaminated the gas supply. In this case, all of the hospital outlets had to be shut down, and patients were switched to tank supplies while the pipeline system was purged with fresh oxygen.[22] In another report, four deaths were attributed to an oxygen pipeline that had been flushed with trichloroethylene.[23]

Oxygen from the pipeline enters the high-pressure system of the machine at a pressure of 50 psig, whereas oxygen from a full tank supply enters the yoke at a pressure of around 2000 psig. The oxygen tank source is therefore regulated (i.e., oxygen passes through a pressure regulator) and enters the machine high-pressure system at a nominal pressure of 45 psig (see Fig. 6-2). Pressure regulators are valves that reduce a variable high-input pressure (in this case, 2000 psig) to a constant low-output pressure (in this case, 45 psig) for a given gas. Regulators can malfunction and may deteriorate with age. If excessively high pressure builds up, a pressure-relief valve in the regulator opens to vent gas to the atmosphere and protect the machine's high-pressure system from exposure to excessively high pressures.[14,24] If the regulator's diaphragm ruptures, oxygen at high pressure and velocity will flow to the atmosphere around the adjustment screw, causing a hissing noise. In this case, a new machine is needed because the leak is sufficiently large that even the oxygen supplied through the pipeline will be leaked (see Fig. 6-2). If the pressure loss is excessive, the low-oxygen-supply pressure alarm may also sound.

Once the supply from the oxygen tank has been checked, it should be turned off if the pipeline source is being used. If the oxygen tank remains on while the machine is being supplied from the pipeline, oxygen is drawn preferentially from the pipeline (50 psig) because the regulator that controls flow from the oxygen tanks will permit flow only when the pressure in the machine's high-pressure system decreases to less than 45 psig (see Fig. 6-2). However, the oxygen pipeline pressure at times may fluctuate to less than 45 psig; in this case, oxygen would be drawn from an open tank, and the backup tank supply would thus be unintentionally depleted.

Each pipeline inlet for each gas supplied to the machine has a check valve to prevent gas leakage if the pipeline is disconnected and the tanks are in use.[25] Malfunction of this valve during supply of the machine from the oxygen pipeline may interfere with oxygen supply to the machine.[26]

---

*psig, Pounds per square inch for gauge pressure; psia, pounds per square inch for absolute pressure. Thus 0 psig = 14.7 psia = 760 mm Hg pressure at sea level.

Oxygen entering the machine high-pressure system (i.e., all components upstream of the oxygen flow control valve) at a pressure of 45 psig (from the tank via the regulator) or 50 psig (from the pipeline) may flow or pressurize in at least five directions (see Fig. 6-2).

1. When the oxygen flush valve is opened, oxygen flows to the common gas outlet of the machine at a steady rate of 35 to 75 L/min.[9] Because the oxygen flush bypasses the vaporizers, high pressures in the patient circuit can accumulate (pipeline pressure up to 50 psig) when the flush is operated. Furthermore, the oxygen flush valve may stick in the open position.[27] Caution is therefore needed to prevent barotrauma when the oxygen flush is used.[28] Use of the oxygen flush to "drive" user-configured transtracheal jet ventilating systems from the machine common gas outlet is considered in a subsequent section.

2. If the oxygen pressure in the high-pressure system decreases (usually to <30 psig), an oxygen supply failure alarm is activated. In Ohmeda Modulus I, Modulus II, and Modulus Excel machines, a pressurized canister is used that emits an audible alarm for at least 7 seconds when the pressure falls below the threshold setting. In North American Dräger Narkomed[29] and Ohmeda Modulus II Plus and Modulus CD machines,[30] a pressure-operated electrical switch ensures a continuous audible alarm whenever the oxygen pressure in the high-pressure system falls below the threshold setting. Failure of the oxygen supply may be attributable to a pipeline interruption or malfunction, or the oxygen pipeline flow-control valve outside the operating room may have been turned off.[19-21]

   If the oxygen-supply alarm sounds during use of the oxygen pipeline, one of the oxygen backup supply tanks on the machine is opened and will restore supply pressure to the machine, silencing the alarm. When a backup tank is used to supply the machine with oxygen (or other gases), the lowest possible flow should be used to conserve oxygen. Thus if an oxygen-powered anesthesia ventilator is being used, it should be turned off and manual (bag) ventilation should be instituted or resumption of spontaneous ventilation by the patient should be considered, if feasible. Failure of the oxygen pipeline supply pressure will also activate alarms in the hospital so that the engineering or other departments responsible for supply and pipeline maintenance are alerted.[19]

3. Oxygen provides a power source for a pneumatically driven anesthesia ventilator.[29,30]

4. In fail-safe valves, oxygen pressurizes and holds open a pressure-sensor shutoff valve that decreases or interrupts the supply of nitrous oxide and other gases (such as helium or air) to their flow-control valves if the oxygen pressure in the high-pressure system falls below the threshold setting. This, in relation to nitrous oxide supply, is the so-called "fail-safe system" designed to prevent unintentional delivery of a hypoxic mixture to the flow-control valves.

   The fail-safe system differs between North American Dräger and Ohmeda machines. In Ohmeda machines, when the oxygen pressure in the machine's high-pressure system falls below 20 psig, the flow of nitrous oxide and all other gases to their flow-control valves is interrupted. The pressure-sensor shutoff valve on Ohmeda machines is an all-or-nothing threshold-based arrangement: It is open at oxygen pressures of 20 psig or more and is closed at pressures less than 20 psig.[30]

   The fail-safe valve in North American Dräger Narkomed machines is called the oxygen failure protection device (OFPD). There is one OFPD for each of the gases supplied to the machine.[29,31] As the oxygen supply pressure decreases, the OFPDs proportionately reduce the supply pressure of each of the other gases to their flow-control valves. The supply of nitrous oxide and other gases is completely interrupted (i.e., the OFPD totally closes) when the oxygen supply pressure falls below 12 ± 4 psig.[29] The "fail-safe system" ensures that at low or no oxygen supply pressures, only oxygen may be delivered to the common gas outlet of the machine and therefore to the breathing system. However, as long as the oxygen supply pressure in the machine's high-pressure system is adequate, other gases may flow to their flow-control valves. The fail-safe system does not require a flow of oxygen from its flow-control valve, only an adequate supply pressure to the oxygen flow-control valve. Thus a normally functioning fail-safe valve will permit flow of 100% nitrous oxide provided that the machine has an adequate oxygen supply pressure. The term *fail-safe system* may therefore be something of a misnomer because it does not ensure oxygen flow. It is a pressure-sensitive device, not a flow-sensitive device.

5. Oxygen flows to the flow-control valve (and then on to the flowmeter, or rotameter). Gas supply to the oxygen flow-control valves differs between Ohmeda and North American Dräger machines.

   In modern Ohmeda machines, the oxygen supply pressure to the flow-control valve is regulated to 14 psig by a second-stage regulator.[30] This regulator (see Fig. 6-2) ensures a constant supply pressure to the oxygen flow-control valve. Thus even if the oxygen supply pressure to the machine decreases to less than 45 to 50 psig, the flow set on the oxygen flowmeter will be maintained as long as it exceeds 14 psig. Without this second-stage oxygen regulator, if the oxygen supply pressure were to decrease, the oxygen flow would decrease at the flowmeter, and if another gas (such as nitrous oxide) were being used simultaneously, a hypoxic gas mixture could result at the level of the flowmeter.

   North American Dräger Narkomed anesthesia machines do not require a second-stage oxygen pressure regulator valve (see Fig.6-2).[29] These machines have OFPDs that create an interface between the supply pressure of oxygen in the machine's high-pressure system and that of nitrous oxide or any other gas.[29,31] A decrease in oxygen supply pressure and flow causes a proportionate decrease in the supply pressure of each of the other gases to their flow-control valves to prevent creation of a hypoxic gas mixture at the level of the flow-control valves (see the preceding discussion of the fail-safe system).

The use (in Ohmeda machines) or nonuse (in North American Dräger machines) of a second-stage oxygen regulator will affect the total gas flow emerging from the common gas outlet of the machine if the oxygen supply pressure were to decrease. In an Ohmeda machine, as long as the oxygen supply pressure exceeds 20 psig, all gas flows are maintained as set on the flow-control valves. In a North American Dräger Narkomed machine, if the oxygen supply pressure decreases from normal (45 to 50 psig), all gas flows decrease in proportion. A decrease in total gas flow from the common gas outlet may cause rebreathing, depending on the patient circuit in use; a Mapleson (rebreathing) system will be affected more than a system with carbon dioxide absorption (circle system).

2. Nitrous oxide. Like oxygen, nitrous oxide may be supplied from the pipeline at a pressure of 50 psig or from a backup E cylinder on the machine. Because it has a critical temperature* of 36.5° C (critical pressure, 1054 psig), nitrous oxide can exist as a liquid at room temperature (20° C).[32,33] E cylinders of nitrous oxide are factory filled to 85% to 95% capacity.[14] Above the liquid in the tank is nitrous oxide vapor; because the liquid agent is in equilibrium with its gas phase, the pressure exerted by the gaseous nitrous oxide is its saturated vapor pressure at the ambient temperature. At 20° C the saturated vapor pressure of nitrous oxide is 750 psig.[32,33] Overfilling of nitrous oxide cylinders with liquid nitrous oxide can result in potentially dangerous high pressures.[34]

A full E cylinder of nitrous oxide will generate approximately 1600 L of gas at 1 atm at sea level (14.7 psia). As long as some liquid nitrous oxide is present in the tank and the ambient temperature remains at 20° C, the pressure in the tank will remain at 750 psig.[20,29,30]

Nitrous oxide from the tank supply normally enters the hanger yoke at pressures of approximately 750 psig (at 20° C), then passes through a regulator that reduces this pressure to a nominal 45 psig at which it enters the machine's high-pressure system for nitrous oxide (see Fig. 6-2). The medical gas pin-indexed safety system is designed to ensure that only a nitrous oxide tank may hang in a nitrous oxide hanger yoke. As with oxygen, a check valve in each hanger yoke prevents back-leakage of nitrous oxide if no tank is hung in the yoke.

The nitrous oxide pipeline is supplied from bulk storage containers or banks of large tanks, usually H cylinders, each of which evolves 16,000 L of gas at atmospheric pressure.[14] The pressure in the nitrous oxide pipeline is regulated to 50 psig to supply the outlets (DISS or manufacturer-specific quick-connect design) in the operating room. After entering the machine's high-pressure system for nitrous oxide, the gas must flow past the "fail-safe" valve to reach the nitrous oxide flow-control valve and flowmeter.

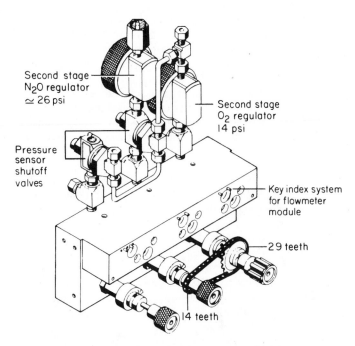

Fig. 6-3. The Ohmeda Link-25 proportion-limiting system, which ensures at least a 25% oxygen mixture at the level of the flow-control valves when oxygen and nitrous oxide are being used.[27,37] When the supply pressure to the second-stage oxygen regulator falls below a nominal 26 psig, the pressure sensors cause the supply of nitrous oxide and other gases to be shut off. (Modified from *Modulus II Plus anesthesia machine: preoperative checklists: operation and maintenance manual,* Madison, Wis, 1988, Ohmeda, BOC Healthcare.)

In Ohmeda Modulus anesthesia machines that have the Link-25 proportion-limiting system (see following text), a second-stage nitrous oxide regulator further reduces gas pressure so that nitrous oxide is supplied to its flow-control valve at a nominal pressure of 26 psig (Figs. 6-1 and 6-3). The actual downstream pressure of this regulator is adjusted at the factory or by a field service representative to ensure correct functioning of the proportioning system.

3. Flow-control valves and flowmeters. The proportions of oxygen and nitrous oxide and other medical gases supplied from the machine, as well as total gas flows delivered to the patient circuit, are adjusted by means of gas flow-control valves and are measured by flowmeters.[25,31,32] The flow-control valves represent the junction between the machine's high-pressure system and low-pressure system. The high-pressure system comprises those components upstream of the flow-control valves. The low-pressure system comprises those components downstream of the flow-control valves (i.e., between the valves and the machine's common gas outlet). The machine may have one flowmeter or two flowmeters (see Fig. 6-3) in series to measure the flow of each gas.[9,31] Two flowmeters in parallel for the same gas (e.g., low-flow and high-flow oxygen and nitrous oxide) are an obsolete arrangement and may be hazardous if a low flow of oxygen is set accidentally together with a high flow of

---

*Critical temperature is the highest temperature at which a gas may exist in liquid form. The pressure that must be applied to permit liquefaction of the gas at this temperature is the critical pressure.

nitrous oxide. The ASTM standard for anesthesia machines requires that machines have only one flow-control valve (knob) for each gas emerging at the common gas outlet.[9] If two flowmeters are present for a gas, the first permits accurate measurement of low flows, usually up to 1 L/min) and the other measures flows of up to 10 to 12 L/min. In North America, the oxygen flow-control valve and flowmeter are positioned on the right side of the flowmeter bank, downstream of the other flow-control valves and closest to the common gas outlet. In the event of a leak in one of the other flow-control valve tubes, this position is the one least likely to result in delivery of a hypoxic mixture at the common gas outlet.[35,36]

Flowmeters are precision instruments.[14,33,37] Flowmeter tubes are manufactured for specific gases, are calibrated with a unique float, and are made for use within a certain range of temperatures and pressures. Flowmeters are not interchangeable among medical gases, and if a gas passes through a flowmeter for which it was not calibrated, the flow shown would probably be incorrect. However, at low flows, the flow rates of gases with similar viscosities (such as 202-micropoise oxygen and 194-micropoise helium) would be read identically; likewise, at high flows, gases of similar density (such as nitrous oxide and carbon dioxide, both of which have molecular weights of 44) would be read identically.[13,37] Again, flow-control valves are not interchangeable among medical gases, and for the Ohmeda machines, they are key indexed so that they cannot be interchanged.[30]

Gas flow to the flowmeter tube is controlled by a touch- and color-coded knob that is linked to a needle valve.[25] In the United States, the oxygen flow-control knob is green, fluted, and larger than the other gas flow-control knobs. The nitrous oxide flow-control knob is blue, is not fluted, and is smaller than the other knobs. Flow-control knobs are now usually protected by a bar or some other device that prevents their settings from being accidentally changed when items are being arranged or are placed on the machine's table surface.

Anesthesia machine manufacturers offer, as an option, an oxygen flow that cannot be discontinued completely because either a stop is provided to ensure a minimum oxygen flow of 200 to 300 ml/min past the needle valve (Ohmeda)[25,30] or a gas-flow resistor is provided that permits a flow of 200 to 300 ml/min oxygen to bypass a totally closed oxygen flow-control needle valve (North American Dräger Narkomed).[29] In modern Narkomed machines, the minimum-oxygen-flow feature functions in the oxygen/nitrous oxide mode but not in the "all gases" mode.[29]

Flowmeters are also subject to failure. For example, a needle valve may break[38,39] or a stop mechanism for the flow-control knob may malfunction[40]; in either case, delivery of oxygen (or other gases) is prevented. Flow tubes are also subject to breakage and leakage.[14,33] Protection against breakage caused by external sources is offered by the plastic screen in front of the bank of flowmeter tubes.

4. Oxygen-ratio monitoring and proportioning systems. A major consideration in the design of modern anesthesia machines is the prevention of the delivery of a hypoxic gas mixture.[9] The "fail-safe" system described previously serves only to interrupt (Ohmeda) or proportionately reduce and ultimately interrupt (North American Dräger OFPD) the supply of nitrous oxide and other gases to their flow-control valves if the oxygen supply pressure to the machine is reduced. It does not prevent the delivery of a hypoxic mixture at the common gas outlet; thus, the term *fail-safe* is something of a misnomer.

In modern machines, the oxygen and nitrous oxide flow controls are physically interlinked either mechanically (Ohmeda)[30] or mechanically and pneumatically (North American Dräger)[29,31] so that a fresh gas mixture containing at least 25% oxygen is created at the level of the flowmeters when nitrous oxide and oxygen are used.

Ohmeda anesthesia machines use the Link-25 proportion-limiting control system to ensure an adequate percentage of oxygen in the gas mixture.[30] In Ohmeda Modulus machines with this system, a gear with 14 teeth is mounted on and is integral with the nitrous oxide flow-control spindle and a gear with 29 teeth is mounted and "floats" on a threaded oxygen flow-control valve spindle (see Fig. 6-3).[41] The two gears are connected by a precision stainless-steel-link chain. For every 2.07 revolutions of the nitrous oxide flow-control spindle, an oxygen flow-control spindle set to the lowest flow will rotate once (because of the 29:14 ratio of gear teeth). Because the gear on the oxygen flow-control spindle is thread-mounted so that it can float on the flow-control valve spindle (like a nut on a bolt), oxygen flow can be increased independently of nitrous oxide flow. However, regardless of the oxygen flow setting, if the flow of nitrous oxide is increased sufficiently, the gear on the oxygen spindle will engage with the oxygen flow-control knob, causing it to rotate and thereby increase oxygen flow.[37] If nitrous oxide flow is then decreased, the oxygen flow will remain high unless it is deliberately decreased by the user. The 75% nitrous oxide/25% oxygen proportion is completed because the nitrous oxide flow-control valve is supplied from a second-stage gas regulator that reduces nitrous oxide pressure to a nominal 26 psig before it reaches the flow-control valve, whereas the oxygen flow-control valve is supplied at a pressure of 14 psig from a second-stage oxygen regulator (see Figs. 6-2 and 6-3). The Link-25 system permits the nitrous oxide and oxygen flow-control valves to be set independently of one another, but if a nitrous oxide concentration of more than 75% is accidentally set, the oxygen flow is automatically increased to maintain at least 25% oxygen in the resulting gas mixture. This system thus increases the minimum flow of oxygen according to the nitrous oxide flow setting. Ohmeda Excel machines have a system that is similar in principle but has a 24:48 ratio of gear teeth.

It should be noted that the Link-25 system interconnects only the nitrous oxide and oxygen flow-control valves. If the anesthesia machine has flow-control valves for other gases, such as helium or air, a gas mixture containing less than 25% oxygen could be set at the level of the flowmeters.

In North America Dräger Narkomed machines, the oxygen-ratio monitoring controller (ORMC) (Fig. 6-4) serves to limit the flow of nitrous oxide according to the oxygen flow and create a mixture of at least 25% oxygen at the level of the flow-control valve.[29,31] At oxygen flow rates

Fig. 6-4. Oxygen-ratio monitor controller. See text for details of operation. (From Schreiber P: *Safety guidelines for anesthesia systems,* Telford, Pa, 1985, North American Dräger.)

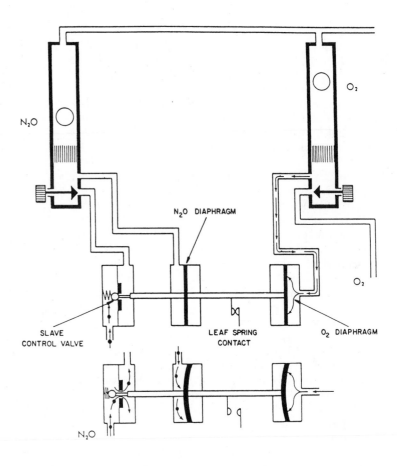

of less than 1 L/min, even higher concentrations of oxygen are delivered. In addition, when the Narkomed machine is used in the nitrous oxide/oxygen mode, an alarm is activated when the ORMC is functioning to prevent a hypoxic mixture. This does not occur when the machine is set to the "all gases" mode (that is, when air, helium, and other gases might be switched into the system).[29]

The ORMC works as follows (see Fig. 6-4). As oxygen flows past its flow-control valve and up the flowmeter tube, it encounters a resistor, which creates back-pressure that is applied to the oxygen diaphragm. As nitrous oxide flows past its flow-control valve and up its flowmeter tube, it also encounters a resistor, which causes back-pressure on the nitrous oxide diaphragm. The two diaphragms are linked by a connecting shaft, the ultimate position of which depends on the relative back-pressures (and therefore flows) of nitrous oxide and oxygen. The left-hand end of the connecting shaft controls the orifice of a slave valve, which in turn controls the supply pressure of nitrous oxide to its flow-control valve. When the oxygen flow is high, the shaft moves to the left and opens the slave flow-control valve. Conversely, if the flow of nitrous oxide is increased excessively, the shaft moves to the right, closing the slave valve orifice and limiting the supply pressure and thus the flow of nitrous oxide to its flow-control valve. When the ORMC is acting to prevent a hypoxic mixture, the leaf spring contacts (see Fig. 6-4) are closed, sounding an alarm. This alarm is disabled if the machine is in the "all gases" mode.[29]

Like the Link-25 system, the ORMC functions only between nitrous oxide and oxygen and does not provide interlinking of oxygen with other gases, such as air or helium, that the machine might also deliver. Thus if a third or fourth gas is in use, the proportioning systems afford no protection against creation of a hypoxic mixture. Although they are of elegant design, both the ORMC and Link-25 systems are subject to potential mechanical or pneumatic failure. In the case of the Link-25 system, breakage of the link chain[42] and incorrect mounting of the oxygen flow-control knob on its spindle causing late engagement of the floating gear and hence late increase in oxygen flow have been reported[41]; both of these malfunctions may result in hypoxic mixtures. Because of these limitations, one should not rely completely on a proportioning system. When one is setting gas flows, oxygen should always be increased first or decreased last, and the adequacy of flow and proportion of oxygen should always be confirmed by using the flowmeters. Furthermore, even if the systems are functioning correctly, they ensure adequacy of only more than 25% oxygen at the level of the flowmeter. An oxygen leak downstream of the flowmeters may result in a hypoxic gas mixture flowing from the common gas outlet.[31] A functional oxygen analyzer in the patient circuit with enabled low oxygen concentration alarm is therefore essential to detect and thereby facilitate correction of a potentially hypoxic mixture. The controlled flows of oxygen, nitrous oxide, and other gases are then mixed in the manifold at the top of

Table 6-1. Physical properties of potent volatile agents

Parameter	Halothane	Enflurane	Isoflurane	Methoxyflurane	Sevoflurane	Desflurane
Structure	CHBrClCF$_3$	CHFClCF$_2$OCHF$_2$	CF$_2$HOCHClCF$_3$	CHCl$_2$CF$_2$OCH$_3$	CH$_2$FOCH(CF$_3$)$_2$	CF$_2$HOCFHCF$_3$
Molecular weight	197.4	184.5	184.5	165.0	200	168
Boiling point at 760 mm Hg (°C)	50.2	56.5	48.5	104.7	58.5	23.5
SVP at 20° C (mm Hg)	243	175	238	20.3	160	664
Saturated vapor concentration at 20° C and 1 atm absolute (vol%)	32	23	31	2.7	21	87
MAC at 1 atm absolute (vol%)	0.75	1.68	1.15	0.16	1.7	6.0-7.25*
P$_{MAC1}$ (mm Hg)	5.7	12.8	8.7	1.22	12.9	46-55*
Specific gravity of liquid at 20° C	1.86	1.52	1.50	1.41	1.51	1.45
Vapor (ml) per liquid (g) at 20° C	123	130	130	145	120	143
Vapor (ml) per liquid (ml) at 20° C	226	196	195	204	182	207

From Eisenkraft JB: Anesthesia vaporizers. In Ehrenwerth J, Eisenkraft JB, eds: *Anesthesia equipment: principles and applications,* St Louis, 1992, Mosby.
*Age related.
SVP, Saturated vapor pressure; *MAC,* minimum alveolar concentration; *P$_{MAC1}$,* partial pressure at concentration of 1 MAC.

the flow-control valve bank and flow to a calibrated anesthesia vaporizer (see Fig. 6-2).

C. Anesthesia vaporizers

A vapor is the gas phase of an agent that is normally a liquid at room temperature and atmospheric pressure. Modern vaporizers facilitate the change of a liquid anesthetic into its vapor phase and add a controlled amount of this vapor to the flow of gases passing to the patient circuit.[13]

1. Regulating vaporizer output: measured-flow compared with variable-bypass vaporizers. The saturated vapor pressures at room temperature of the three most commonly used potent inhaled anesthetic agents—halothane, sevoflurane, and isoflurane—are 243, 160, and 238 mm Hg, respectively; these pressures far exceed those required clinically (Table 6-1). The vaporizer creates a saturated vapor that must be diluted by the bypass gas flow to create clinically useful concentrations. If this were not done, a lethal concentration of agent could be delivered to the patient circuit.

Modern anesthesia vaporizers for halothane, enflurane, isoflurane, and sevoflurane are concentration-calibrated and are of the variable bypass design.[9] In a variable-bypass vaporizer (such as the Tec series from Ohmeda and the Vapor 19.n series from Dräger), the total fresh gas flow from the anesthesia machine flow-control valves passes to the vaporizer. The vaporizer (Fig. 6-5) splits the incoming gas stream into a smaller flow, which enters the vaporizing chamber of the vaporizer to emerge with saturated vapor concentration of the agent, and a larger bypass flow that, when mixed with the vaporizing chamber output, results in the desired (or "dialed-in") concentration.[13,43]

VARIABLE BYPASS

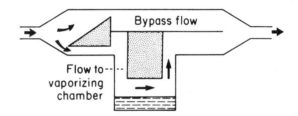

Fig. 6-5. Variable-bypass vaporizer. (From Eisenkraft JB: Vaporizers and vaporization of volatile anesthetics. In Eisenkraft JB, ed: *Progress in anesthesiology,* vol 2, San Antonio, Tex, 1988, Dannemiller Memorial Educational Foundation.)

In the almost-obsolete measured flow (non–concentration-calibrated) vaporizers, such as Copper Kettle (Foregger/Puritan-Bennett) or Verni-Trol (Ohmeda), a measured flow of oxygen is set on a separate flow-control valve to pass to the vaporizer, from which vapor at its saturated vapor pressure emerges (Fig. 6-6). This flow is then diluted by an additional measured flow of gases from other flow-control valves on the anesthesia machine. With this type of arrangement, several calculations are necessary to determine the anesthetic vapor concentration in the emerging gas mixture.

a. Measured-flow vaporizers. Although measured-flow vaporizers are no longer considered desirable[9] and are not mentioned in the ASTM F1161-88 standard, it is

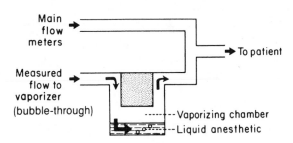

MEASURED FLOW VAPORIZER
(Copper Kettle, Verni-Trol)

Fig. 6-6. Measured-flow vaporizer (Copper Kettle or Verni-Trol). (From Eisenkraft JB: Vaporizers and vaporization of volatile anesthetics. In *Progress in anesthesiology,* vol 2, San Antonio, Tex, 1988, Dannemiller Memorial Educational Foundation.)

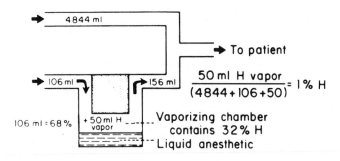

In practice main flow is set to 5 L/min, vaporizer flow is set to 100 ml/min and H output is 0.913%,

i.e., 47 ml H vapor diluted in (5000 + 100 + 47) ml

Fig. 6-7. Preparation of 1% (vol/vol) halothane *(H)* by a measured-flow vaporizer. (From Eisenkraft JB: Vaporizers and vaporization of volatile anesthetics. In *Progress in anesthesiology,* vol 2, San Antonio, Tex, 1988, Dannemiller Memorial Educational Foundation.)

helpful to review the function of a measured-flow vaporizer, such as the Copper Kettle.

Suppose that 1% (vol/vol) halothane is required at a total fresh gas flow rate of 5 L/min to the patient circuit (Fig. 6-7). To achieve this, the vaporizer would have to produce 50 ml of halothane vapor per minute (1% × 5000 ml).

In the vaporizing chamber, halothane vapor represents 32% (243 of 760 mm Hg) of the atmosphere, if one assumes that the temperature is kept constant at 20° C and saturated vapor pressure is therefore maintained at 243 mm Hg (see Table 6-1). If 50 ml of halothane vapor represents 32% of the total volume, the carrier gas (oxygen) must represent the other 68%, or 106 ml ([50/32] × 68); alternatively, this can be expressed as

$$\frac{243}{760} = \frac{50}{50 + Y}$$

where Y represents a carrier gas (oxygen) flow of 106 ml/min.

Thus if 106 ml/min of oxygen flows into a Copper Kettle vaporizer containing halothane, 156 ml/min of gas will emerge, of which 50 ml will be halothane vapor and 106 ml will be the oxygen that was supplied to the vaporizer. This vaporizer output of 156 ml/min must be diluted by an additional fresh gas flow of 4844 ml/min (5000 − 156 ml/min) to create a precise 1% halothane mixture (because 50 ml of halothane diluted in a total volume of 5000 ml = 1% halothane by volume).

In clinical practice, however, the anesthesiologist would probably set a flow of 100 ml/min to the Copper Kettle vaporizer and 5 L/min of fresh gas on the main flow-control valves, which would result in a vapor concentration that is a little less than 1% halothane:

$$\frac{243}{760} = \frac{x}{x + 100}$$

$$x = 47 \text{ ml}$$

$$\frac{47}{5147} = 0.91\%$$

where x represents the volume of halothane vapor produced by a vaporizer inflow of 100 ml/min of oxygen. Multiples of these values for flow (i.e., 100 ml/min for oxygen to the Copper Kettle; 5 L/min on the main flowmeters) are used to create other concentrations of halothane from a Copper Kettle vaporizer. Thus a gas flow of 100 ml/min to the vaporizer and a flow of 2500 ml/min on the main flow-control valves would produce approximately 2% halothane (1.78%).[43] It is important to realize that if oxygen flows only to the vaporizer and no diluent fresh gas flow is set on the main flow-control valves, lethal concentrations (approaching 32%) of halothane would be delivered to the anesthesia circuit, albeit at low flow rates.[13,43]

b. Variable-bypass (concentration-calibrated) vaporizers. In the preceding examples, it was necessary to calculate both the oxygen flow to the measured-flow vaporizer and the total diluent gas flow needed to produce the desired output concentration of vapor. This is inconvenient and may give rise to errors, but it is important to understand the principles underlying the calculations involved because such vaporizing systems may still be in use.

In the concentration-calibrated variable-bypass design, the vaporizer splits the total flow of gas arriving from the machine flow-control valves between a variable bypass and the vaporizing chamber containing the liquid anesthetic agent (see Fig. 6-5). The ratio of these flows, called the splitting ratio, depends on the anesthetic agent, the temperature, and the desired vapor concentration set to be delivered to the patient circuit. The splitting ratios for variable-bypass vaporizers used at 20° C are shown in Table 6-2.[43]

Concentration-calibrated vaporizers are agent-specific and should be used only with the agent for which the unit is designed and calibrated. To produce a 1% vapor concentration, a halothane vaporizer makes a flow split of 46:1, whereas an enflurane vaporizer makes a flow split of 28.7:1 (see Table 6-2). If an empty enflurane vaporizer

Table 6-2. Gas flow splitting ratios at 20° C*

	Halothane	Enflurane	Isoflurane	Methoxyflurane	Sevoflurane
1%	46:1	29:1	44:1	1.7:1	25:1
2%	22:1	14:1	21:1	0.36:1	12:1
3%	14:1	9:1	14:1	†	7:1

From Eisenkraft JB: Anesthesia vaporizers. In Ehrenwerth J, Eisenkraft JB, eds: *Anesthesia equipment: principles and applications,* St Louis, 1992, Mosby.

*Ratios are not given for desflurane, because the vaporizer for this agent (Ohmeda Tec 6) uses a different design from that used for the above agents.

†Maximum possible concentration is 2.7% at 20° C (see Table 6-1).

set to deliver 1% were filled with halothane, the halothane vapor emerging would exceed 1% (46/28.7 = 1.6%). An understanding of splitting ratios enables fairly accurate prediction of the concentration output of an empty agent-specific variable-bypass vaporizer that has been erroneously filled with an agent for which it was not designed (see following text).

2. Temperature compensation. Agent-specific concentration-calibrated vaporizers are located in the fresh gas pathway between the flow-control valves on the anesthesia machine and the common gas outlet. The vaporizers must be efficient and produce steady concentrations of agent over a fairly wide range of incoming gas flow rates. However, as the agent is vaporized and the temperature of the liquid decreases, the saturated vapor pressure and thus the vaporizing chamber output decrease. With a measured-flow vaporizer (e.g., Copper Kettle) or an uncompensated variable-bypass vaporizer, this would result in delivery of less anesthetic vapor to the patient circuit. For this reason, all vaporizing systems must be temperature compensated. This compensation may be done manually or automatically.[13,43]

Measured-flow vaporizers incorporate a thermometer that measures the temperature of the liquid agent in the vaporizing chamber. A lower temperature translates to a lower saturated vapor pressure in this chamber, and reference to the vapor pressure curves permits the user to reset either the vaporizer or diluent main gas flows or both to ensure correct output at the prevailing temperature. Such an arrangement can be tedious, but it ensures the most accurate and rapid temperature compensation. Modern variable-bypass vaporizers (such as Ohmeda Tec series vaporizers and the Dräger Vapor 19.1) have a temperature-sensitive valve in the bypass gas flow that performs automatic temperature compensation. When the temperature increases, the valve in the bypass opens wider to create a greater splitting ratio. More gas flows through the bypass, and less gas enters the vaporizing chamber. A smaller volume of a higher concentration of vapor emerges from the vaporizing chamber; when this vapor is mixed with an increased bypass gas flow, the vaporizer output is held reasonably constant when temperature changes are gradual and not extreme. Dräger Vapor 19.1 vaporizers are specified as accurate to ±15% of the concentration set on the dial when used within the

temperature range of +15° to +35° C at normal atmospheric pressure.[44] At temperatures outside this range, the resulting concentration increases beyond the upper tolerance limit despite continuing compensation. The boiling point of the potent volatile anesthetic agent must never be reached in the current variable-bypass vaporizers designed for halothane, enflurane, isoflurane, and sevoflurane because the vapor output concentration would be totally uncontrolled and lethal.

It is also important to recognize that any temperature-compensating mechanism has a certain amount of inertia. An increase in temperature would result in increased evaporation of liquid agent and therefore increased cooling (because of heat loss) of the remaining liquid. This would decrease the saturated vapor pressure of the agent. Changes in ambient temperature, unless they are drastic, usually do not result in major changes in vaporizer output. In Dräger Vapor 19.1 series vaporizers, a sudden change in temperature requires a compensation time of 6 min/° C to maintain output concentration within the limits stated previously.[44] In the case of an increase in temperature, vaporizer output would exceed that shown on the dial until compensation occurred.

In some older vaporizers (e.g., Fluotec Mark II, Ohio Medical [now Datex-Ohmeda], Madison, Wisconsin), the temperature-compensation valve was in the vaporizing chamber itself. Because the thymol preservatives added to halothane could cause this valve to stick, the temperature-compensating valve is situated in the bypass gas flow of modern vaporizers.[14]

3. Arrangement of vaporizers. Older anesthesia machines had up to three variable-bypass vaporizers arranged in series so that fresh gas passed through each vaporizer (through the bypass flow) to reach the common gas outlet of the anesthesia machine. Without an interlock system, which permits only one vaporizer to be in use at any one time, it was possible to have all three vaporizers on simultaneously. In addition to potentially causing an anesthetic overdose, the agent from the upstream vaporizer could contaminate the agent or agents in the downstream vaporizers. During subsequent use, the output of the downstream vaporizer would be contaminated. The resulting concentrations in the emerging gas and vapor mixture would be indeterminate and possibly lethal.[13,43]

With modern arrangements, only one vaporizer can be on at any time. The ASTM F1161-88 standard requires that to prevent cross-contamination of the contents of one vaporizer with agents from another, a system shall be provided that isolates the vaporizers from one another and prevents gas from passing through the vaporizing chamber of one vaporizer and then through that of another.[9] This specification is met by use of an interlock system. Contemporary North American Dräger and Ohmeda anesthesia machines incorporate manufacturer-specific interlock systems.[29,30]

4. Calibration and checking of vaporizer outputs. Vaporizers should be regularly serviced and their outputs checked to ensure that problems do not exist. The vaporizer is set to deliver a certain vapor concentration, and the actual output concentration is measured by an anesthetic-agent analyzer sampling gas via a connector

---

Box 6-1 Physical properties of desflurane

Formula: CF$_2$H—O—CFH—CF$_3$
Molecular weight: 168
Specific gravity: 1.45
Boiling point: 22.8° C at 760 mm Hg
Saturated vapor pressure: at 20° C = 669 mm Hg
Odor: ethereal
Preservative free
MAC: 6% to 7.25% (age-related)* at 760 mm Hg
P$_{MAC1}$: 46 to 55 mm Hg

Data courtesy Anaquest, Research and Development, Liberty Corner, New Jersey.
*From Rampil IJ, Lockhart SH, Zwass MS, et al: *Anesthesiology* 74:429, 1991.
MAC, Minimum alveolar concentration; *P$_{MAC1}$,* partial pressure at concentration of 1 MAC.

placed at the common gas outlet of the anesthesia machine.

Currently available, practical vapor-analysis methods include mass spectrometry, multiwavelength infrared spectroscopy, and laser-Raman spectroscopy. These three methods enable multiple agents to be identified and quantified in the presence of one another. Other technologies, such as single-wavelength infrared spectroscopy, photoacoustic spectroscopy, vibrating crystal, and refractometry, are accurate and reliable if only one agent is present and has been qualitatively identified to the analyzer. They are inaccurate in the presence of multiple agents. More detailed discussion of these technologies is provided elsewhere.[45]

5. The Ohmeda Tec 6 desflurane vaporizer. Desflurane (Suprane, Ohmeda) is a potent inhaled volatile anesthetic agent approved for use by the U.S. Food and Drug Administration (FDA) in 1992.[46,47] Its physical properties are shown in Box 6-1. With a saturated vapor pressure of 669 mm Hg at 20° C and a boiling point of 22.8° C at 1 atm, this agent is extremely volatile, which presents some problems with vaporization and production of controlled concentrations of vapor. Clearly this agent cannot be administered through the conventional variable-bypass vaporizers used for halothane, enflurane, isoflurane, and sevoflurane. If a variable-bypass vaporizer were filled with desflurane, an increase in temperature to more than 22.8° C would cause the desflurane to boil in the vaporizing chamber, resulting in uncontrolled desflurane output from the vaporizer. The consequences of misfilling contemporary agent-specific variable-bypass vaporizers with desflurane at 22° C have been predicted.[48] Thus an enflurane vaporizer set to deliver a minimum alveolar concentration (MAC) of 3 (approximately 5% enflurane) would deliver a MAC of 16 (approximately 96%) desflurane at 22° C.[48]

Ohmeda (Steeton, UK) designed the Tec 6 concentration-calibrated vaporizer for controlled administration of desflurane. It is designed to make the practical aspects of clinical administration of desflurane no different from those of other potent inhaled agents delivered with Ohmeda Tec series vaporizers.

The Tec 6 vaporizer heats liquid desflurane in a chamber (sump) to 39° C to produce vapor under pressure (approximately 1500 mm Hg or 2 atm absolute) analogous to having a reservoir of compressed gas in a tank (Fig. 6-8). The vapor leaves the sump via a variable-pressure regulating valve, the opening of which is continuously adjusted according to the output from a pressure sensor to ensure that the pressure of the desflurane vapor entering the rotary valve in the user-controlled concentration dial is the same as the pressure generated by the fresh gas inflow (from the anesthesia machine flowmeters) into a fixed restrictor. The concentration dial and rotary valve control the quantity of desflurane vapor added to the fresh gas flow so that the dialed-in concentration of desflurane emerges from the vaporizer outlet. Unlike other concentration-calibrated vaporizers (e.g., the Ohmeda Tec 5 and the Dräger Vapor 19.1), which are of variable-bypass design, no fresh gas enters the desflurane sump of the Tec 6.

The Tec 6 is calibrated by the manufacturer with 100% oxygen as the fresh gas. As the oxygen enters the vaporizer, it flows through a fixed restrictor (see Fig. 6-8). This device offers a fixed resistance, defined as change in pressure per unit change in flow. The resistance is approximately 10 cm H$_2$O/L/min over a wide range of gas flows. The back-pressure created by gas flowing through the fixed restrictor is therefore proportional to the main gas flow (as set on the machine flowmeters) and changes according to Poiseuille's law.[33] By sensing this back-pressure (by means of a pressure transducer) and by ensuring that the pressure of the desflurane vapor entering the variable restrictor is always made equal to this pressure (by means of the control electronics and variable-pressure control valve), the variable restrictor controls the concentration of desflurane (see Fig. 6-8).

Thus

$$\text{Resistance} = \Delta\,\text{Pressure}/\Delta\,\text{Flow}$$

The variable restrictor in the concentration dial (i.e., resistance$_{des}$) can therefore be calibrated in terms of desflurane concentration. However, the calibration of the variable restrictor is not linear.[49]

a. Design features of the Tec 6. In the Tec 6 vaporizer, the sump contains 450 ml desflurane when full (see Fig. 6-8).[46,47,49] Because the sump is pressurized to 1500 mm Hg, the agent level is sensed electronically and shown on a liquid crystal display rather than with the sight-glass used in variable-bypass vaporizers. When the vaporizer is energized by connecting the power cord to an electrical outlet, a heater in the sump heats the agent to 39° C and maintains that temperature by means of thermostatic controls. While the agent is being heated, the sump shutoff valve remains closed, and a solenoid locking device prevents the concentration dial from being switched to the on position. Once the vaporizer is operational (i.e., at 39° C), the dial lock is released, and when the dial is turned to on, the sump shutoff valve is opened, permitting desflurane vapor to flow to the pressure-regulating valve.

To prevent condensation ("rain out") of desflurane vapor, the heater in the sump is supplemented by heaters

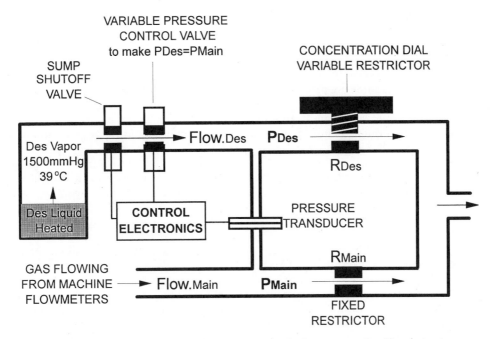

VARIABLE PRESSURE
CONTROL VALVE
to make PDes=PMain

SUMP
SHUTOFF
VALVE

CONCENTRATION DIAL
VARIABLE RESTRICTOR

Des Vapor
1500mmHg
39°C

Flow.Des   PDes

RDes

Des Liquid
Heated

CONTROL
ELECTRONICS

PRESSURE
TRANSDUCER

RMain

GAS FLOWING
FROM MACHINE
FLOWMETERS

Flow.Main   PMain

FIXED
RESTRICTOR

Fig. 6-8. Simplified schematic of the Ohmeda Tec 6 desflurane vaporizer illustrating its operating principles. P_{des}, Pressure of desflurane; P_{main}, pressure of main gas flow; R_{des}, resistance of variable restrictor in desflurane pathway; R_{main}, resistance of fixed restrictor in main gas pathway. (From Eisenkraft JB: The anesthesia delivery system. In Longnecker DE, Tinker JH, Morgan GE, eds: *Principles and practice of anesthesiology*, ed 2, St Louis, 1998, Mosby.)

in the rotary valve and in the vicinity of the pressure transducers that sense the back-pressures resulting from the main gas flow and flow of desflurane.

The Tec 6 vaporizer thus differs considerably from variable-bypass vaporizers. First, the fresh gas flow does not enter the vaporizing chamber. Second, the Tec 6 requires electrical power and incorporates sophisticated electronics to ensure normal operation. Third, it has a display panel to inform the user about its operational status. Finally, it has alarms that sound in the event of malfunction; if malfunction occurs, the sump shutoff valve closes.[50]

b. Filling system. Because of its high saturated vapor pressure, desflurane is supplied in plastic-coated glass bottles to which an agent-specific filling device is firmly attached. The vaporizer incorporates an agent-specific filling system that permits filling of the sump at any time, including when the vaporizer is in use. This may be important because desflurane has a low blood/gas partition coefficient.

During filling, the bottle is locked to the vaporizer filling system, and the high pressure of vapor in the sump at 39° C is transmitted to the interior of the bottle, which helps to drive liquid desflurane from the bottle into the sump. When filling is complete, the bottle is disconnected from the vaporizer filling system, and the valve on the bottle closes to avoid loss or spillage of agent. At this time, the bottle contains vapor at a pressure of 1500 mm Hg at 39° C. As the bottle and its contents cool to room temperature, the pressure in the bottle decreases toward atmospheric pressure (760 mm Hg at 22.8° C).

c. Effects of fresh gas composition on performance. The Tec 6 is calibrated at the factory by using 100% oxygen. Performance accuracy at 5 L/min of oxygen is specified as ±0.5% of delivered agent or ±15% of dial setting, whichever is greater.[50]

The Tec 6 uses back-pressure from gas flow through the fixed resistor to infer flow (see Fig. 6-8). If the viscosity of the gas flowing though the fixed resistor were to decrease, then the same flow would result in a lower back-pressure. This back-pressure is used to determine the pressure of desflurane upstream of the variable resistor in the concentration dial. A lower pressure results in a lower flow of desflurane vapor through the variable resistor.

Of the gases on the anesthesia machine, oxygen is the most viscous, and nitrous oxide is the least viscous. Thus changing the main gas flow composition from oxygen to oxygen/nitrous oxide decreases gas viscosity and therefore the output concentration of desflurane from that set on the dial. Differences between the actual concentration produced and the dial setting are greatest (up to 20% of dial setting) with high concentrations of nitrous oxide at low gas flow rates.[50,51] The clinical implications of this are minimal, however, because the anesthetic effect lost by the decrease in desflurane is offset by the anesthetic effect of the nitrous oxide.[50]

d. Effects of altitude on output. The Tec 6 vaporizer accurately delivers the dialed-in concentration of desflurane in terms of volume percent, even at altitudes above sea level. At sea level, 7% desflurane (MAC of 1) creates a partial pressure of desflurane (P_{des}) of 53 mm Hg (7% × 760 mm Hg) (see Table 6-1). At altitudes other than sea level, if the ambient pressure were 500 mm Hg, the same 7% desflurane would create a P_{des} of only 35 mm Hg (7% × 500), which is only 0.66 of the partial pressure at P_{MAC1}. To compensate for this decrease in potency output at increased altitude, a higher concentration must be set on the dial. Conversely, at higher ambient pressures, a dial setting for lower concentration would be indicated. Recommendations about how the dial setting should be changed at altitude are provided in the operator's manual.[50]

e. Interlock system. The Tec 6 vaporizer is manufactured by Ohmeda and can be mounted on an Ohmeda anesthesia machine with the patented Selectatec manifold. However, a version is also available for mounting on a North American Dräger Narkomed vaporizer exclusion system so that only one vaporizer can be in use at any one time.

D. Common gas outlet, outlet check valves, and pressure-relief valves

The fresh gas mixture produced by the settings of the flow-control valves for oxygen, nitrous oxide with or without other gases, and vapor from one concentration-calibrated vaporizer leave the machine through the common gas outlet. Ohmeda Modulus I, Ohmeda Modulus II, and Ohmeda Excel machines feature (1) an outlet check valve and (2) a pressure-relief valve, both located between the vaporizer and the common gas outlet (see Fig. 6-2).[13] The pressure-relief valve, as its name indicates, prevents the buildup of excessive pressures upstream of the outlet check valve. These components are located upstream from where the oxygen flush flow would join the machine low-pressure system to pass to the common gas outlet. The pressure-relief valve also prevents buildup of pressure in the anesthesia machine if the common gas outlet is obstructed. This may occur if the tubing connecting the common gas outlet to the anesthesia circuit becomes obstructed or kinked.

The purpose of the outlet check valve found only on Ohmeda Modulus I, Modulus II, and Excel anesthesia machines is to prevent reverse gas flow. In this situation, gas may flow back into the vaporizer ("pumping effect"), causing increased vaporizer output concentrations.

North American Dräger Narkomed machines do not require an outlet check valve because the Vapor 19.1 vaporizer design prevents any pumping effect. The Ohmeda Modulus II Plus and Modulus CD machines are equipped with Tec 4 or Tec 5 vaporizers, which incorporate a baffle system and a specially designed manifold to prevent the pumping effect; thus an outlet check valve is unnecessary on these machines. Nevertheless, the Modulus II Plus and Modulus CD machines have a pressure-relief valve that opens at 135 ± 15 mm Hg (2.2 psig)[30] (see Fig. 6-2). North American Dräger Narkomed machines do not require a separate pressure-relief valve. In these machines, pressure relief, if required, takes place through the Dräger Vapor 19.1 vaporizer when the pressure exceeds about 18 psig. The presence or absence of an outlet check valve and pressure-relief valve can be important when testing the low-pressure system of the anesthesia machine for leaks (see later discussion). In addition, if a transtracheal jet ventilation system has been configured to be connected

to the machine common gas outlet and ventilation is achieved by intermittent operation of the oxygen flush valve,[52,53] the driving pressure of such a system would be limited by the opening pressure of the pressure-relief valve. In the Ohmeda Modulus II Plus and Ohmeda Modulus CD machines, this driving pressure would be approximately 2.2 psig; in North American Dräger Narkomed machines equipped with Dräger Vapor 19.1 vaporizers, it would be 18 psig; and in Ohmeda Modulus II and Ohmeda Excel machines (which have outlet check valves) or North American Dräger Narkomed machines without vaporizers (which therefore do not have pressure-relief systems), it would be 45 to 55 psig, depending on whether the tank or pipeline oxygen supply to the machine was in use (see Fig. 6-2).[54]

The ASTM F1161-88 standard requires that machines have only one common gas outlet and that when the common gas outlet is connected to the breathing system by a fresh gas supply hose (the usual arrangement in most operating rooms), the common gas outlet must be equipped with a manufacturer-specific retaining device.[9] This retaining device helps prevent disconnection or misconnections between the machine common gas outlet and the patient circuit, which could result in patient injury.[30] A disconnection at that point may result in entrainment of room air, which might cause a hypoxic mixture in the circuit as well as failure of delivery of inhaled anesthetic.[55,56] North American Dräger Narkomed machines have a bar-type of retaining device, whereas Ohmeda machines have a spring-loaded bayonet-fitting retaining device.[29-31]

E. Anesthesia circuits

The anesthesia circuit represents a minienvironment with which the patient makes respiratory exchange. The fresh gas flow from the anesthesia machine delivers metered concentrations of oxygen, nitrous oxide, and inhaled anesthetic agent to the circuit, and gases are vented from the circuit to the scavenging system. In some arrangements, high fresh gas flow rates are used; as a result, the patient's inspired gas concentrations will approximate those in the fresh gas supply. Other circuits, such as the adult circle system, use lower fresh gas flow rates and rely on an absorption system for carbon dioxide. In the circle system, which uses low gas flow rates, the composition of the inspired gas may differ substantially from that of the fresh gas inflow.

Patient breathing circuits are generally composed of corrugated 22-mm tubing, a reservoir bag, and a connecting piece or elbow to the patient's airway. They may also include at least one valve. The way in which these items are arranged gives the resulting circuit its functional characteristics.[57] Incorrect arrangement of components may create circuit malfunction. Breathing systems are generally classified as *rebreathing,* which have no carbon dioxide absorption system (Mapleson classification circuits A through F), or *nonrebreathing,* which have a carbon dioxide absorber (such as a circle system).[49]

1. Rebreathing systems. Rebreathing systems, which are assigned letters according to the Mapleson classification, are discussed in more detail elsewhere (Fig. 6-9).[14,49,57-62] Because these systems do not have carbon

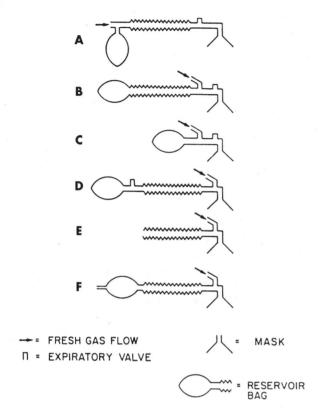

A

B

C

D

E

F

→ = FRESH GAS FLOW

Π = EXPIRATORY VALVE

= MASK

= RESERVOIR BAG

Fig. 6-9. The Mapleson classification of rebreathing systems. The Mapleson A circuit is also known as the Magill attachment. (From Conway CM: *Br J Anaesth* 57:649, 1985.)

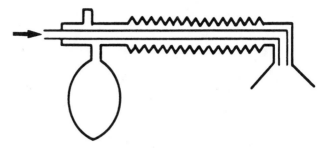

Fig. 6-10. Bain circuit, coaxial Mapleson D system.

dioxide absorbers, it is possible for the patient to inhale previously exhaled alveolar gas that contains carbon dioxide. The extent of rebreathing depends on the system anatomy, the patient's minute ventilation, pattern of ventilation, rate of fresh gas flow, and whether ventilation is spontaneous or controlled. An understanding of the functional characteristics of rebreathing systems is therefore essential to their appropriate use. Only the more commonly used systems, the coaxial Mapleson D (Bain circuit) and F (the Jackson-Rees modification of the Ayre T-piece system), are described here.

a. Coaxial Mapleson D system (Bain circuit). The coaxial Mapleson D system is shown in Fig. 6-10. Fresh gas from the anesthesia machine enters the inner (smaller-bore) tubing and is delivered to the patient end. Exhaled gas is carried through the outer tubing to the reservoir bag and pop-off valve. The outer tubing is usually made from transparent material so that the inner tubing may be inspected for kinking or disconnection. Clearly if the latter were to occur at the machine end, the whole system would become apparatus dead space and excessive rebreathing would result.

A ventilation nomogram shows that during controlled ventilation, the tension of carbon dioxide in the alveolar gas (P_{ACO_2}) can be estimated from a combination of fresh gas flow and minute ventilation ($\dot{V}_E$).[62] At high fresh gas flows, P_{ACO_2} becomes independent of fresh gas flow and dependent on $\dot{V}_E$. At a high $\dot{V}_E$, the P_{ACO_2} is in-

dependent of $\dot{V}_E$ and becomes dependent on fresh gas flow. The Bain circuit can thus be used to provide controlled rebreathing with hyperventilation, resulting in normal P_{ACO_2}. Because the pop-off valve in the Bain circuit is located close to the anesthesia machine, scavenging from the Bain circuit is not usually a problem.

A preuse check of the Bain circuit is essential to ensure that the inner gas delivery tube has not become disconnected. If this happens, rebreathing may result. Two inspection methods have been described. In one method,[63] the patient end of the whole system is occluded, the pop-off valve is closed, and the system is filled with oxygen until the reservoir bag is distended. The patient end is then unoccluded, and oxygen is flushed into the circuit through the inner tube. The high flow of oxygen produces a Venturi effect at the patient end of the circuit: the low pressure created at the end of the outer tubing draws oxygen along the outer tubing from the reservoir bag, causing the bag to deflate. If there is a disconnection or a leak in the inner tubing, flushing the circuit with oxygen would allow the high pressure to be transmitted from the inner to the outer tubing and the reservoir bag would remain inflated or distend further.[63] A second method[64] is to set a the oxygen flow-control valve for a flow of 50 ml/min and then occlude the distal (patient) end of the inner tube with the plunger of a small syringe. If the inner tube is intact, this sequence should cause the gas flow to cease and the oxygen flow-control valve bobbin to fall. The second test is preferred because if the inner tube has been omitted, the first test may not indicate that something is wrong.[14]

b. Mapleson F system (Jackson-Rees modification). The Mapleson F system is the Jackson-Rees modification of the Ayre T-piece (Mapleson E) system.[49,57,58] In this system (see Fig. 6-9), a two-tailed reservoir bag and a means of venting waste gases are added to the end of the expiratory limb tubing. The method of venting waste gases is usually via a valve with an adjustable orifice that is connected to a scavenging system.

The system functions like the Mapleson E system except that during exhalation, a mixture of exhaled and fresh gas collects in the bag, and on the next inspiration, the patient inhales fresh gas both from the machine common gas outlet and from the expiratory limb and bag. Addition of the two-tailed reservoir bag to the E system provides a means to qualitatively monitor ventilation

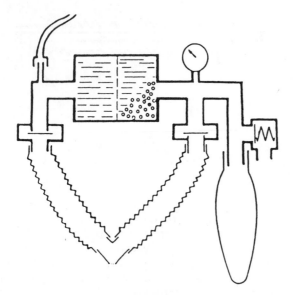

Fig. 6-11. Contemporary anesthesia circle system arrangement. (From Schreiber P: *Safety guidelines for anesthesia systems,* Telford, Pa, 1985, North American Dräger.)

during spontaneous breathing as well as to control ventilation by manually squeezing the reservoir bag. Prevention of rebreathing is achieved by use of fresh gas flows of two to three times minute ventilation.[58]

2. Circle system
a. Structure. In the circle system, the components form a circle into which fresh gas can enter and from which excess gas can leave. Several configurations are possible[60]; the usual arrangement of the components of a modern circle system is shown in Fig. 6-11. Fresh gas enters just upstream of the inspiratory unidirectional valve and, during inspiration, passes down the inspiratory limb of the circle to the Y-piece connector. During expiration, gas passes along the expiratory limb to the expiratory unidirectional valve. Just beyond the expiratory valve are the adjustable pressure-limiting valve and a reservoir bag. Gas then passes through a canister containing a carbon dioxide absorbent (e.g., soda lime) and emerges to rejoin fresh gas entering the circuit from the anesthesia machine just upstream of the inspiratory valve.

In the system described, rebreathing of carbon dioxide is prevented by the absorption of carbon dioxide from exhaled gas before it is reinspired. At high fresh gas flows, however, carbon dioxide absorption becomes unnecessary, and some older circle systems permit bypass of the absorber canister.[14] However, at lower fresh gas flows, carbon dioxide absorption is necessary. To this end, Eger[60] suggested the following three basic rules for preventing carbon dioxide rebreathing in a circle system:

1. A unidirectional valve must be situated between the reservoir bag and the patient on both the inspiratory and expiratory sides.
2. Fresh gas must not enter the system between the expiratory unidirectional valve and the patient.
3. The overflow valve must not be placed between the patient and the inspiratory unidirectional valve.

Incompetence of either of the unidirectional valves permits bidirectional gas flow in the corrugated patient tubing, leading to rebreathing of previously exhaled carbon dioxide.

The circle system is currently the most popular patient circuit in use in the United States. It has the advantages of permitting low fresh gas flows, reducing operating room pollution, and conserving heat and humidity. Disadvantages of the circle system include a somewhat complex design with multiple components that can malfunction or be arranged incorrectly.[31] In addition is the difficulty of predicting the inspired gas composition, particularly the concentration of inhaled anesthetic agent within the circle system, especially when low fresh gas flows are used. This may cease to be a problem, however, as monitoring of anesthetic and respiratory gas concentrations becomes more common.

b. Absorption of carbon dioxide. The carbon dioxide absorber is the central component in a circle system. Modern canisters are large, with a minimum gas space equal to the largest expected patient tidal volume. This design permits low gas flow rates and long dwell times; thus more complete removal ("scrubbing") of carbon dioxide can occur.[65] The two most commonly used carbon dioxide absorbents are soda lime (Sodasorb, Dewey and Almy Chemical Division, Lexington, Massachusetts)[65] and barium hydroxide lime (Baralyme, Chemetron Medical Division, Allied Health Care Products, Inc., St. Louis, Missouri).[14]

Absorptive surface area and flow of gas through the absorbent are a function of granule size. The smaller the size, the larger the surface area for absorption but the greater the resistance to gas flow. Conversely, large granules decrease absorptive surface area but offer less resistance to flow and may encourage channeling of gases through the absorbent, thereby decreasing carbon dioxide absorption.[65]

Indicators are added to the absorbent granules to show when they are becoming exhausted. These indicators are pH sensitive and are colorless when the absorbent is fresh but become colored when pH decreases. The most commonly used indicator is ethyl violet, which changes from colorless to purple as absorption proceeds.[14,65]

It has been reported that ethyl violet, the indicator added to Sodasorb, may be deactivated by fluorescent lighting and may even undergo temporal deactivation after a container of Sodasorb is opened, even if it is stored in the dark.[66] Such deactivation increases the hazard of using carbon dioxide absorption, but such a hazard would be offset by the use of continuous intraoperative capnography. The recommendation is that ultraviolet filters be used and additional ethyl violet be incorporated into Sodasorb to minimize the deactivation problem.[66]

The agent used for carbon dioxide absorption must be compatible with the anesthetic gases in use. The introduction of sevoflurane into clinical practice has generated controversy over its interaction with strong bases in carbon dioxide absorbents.[67] Sevoflurane reacts with carbon dioxide absorbents, decomposing to compound A, which is nephrotoxic in rats. High concentrations of compound A are more likely to occur with barium hy-

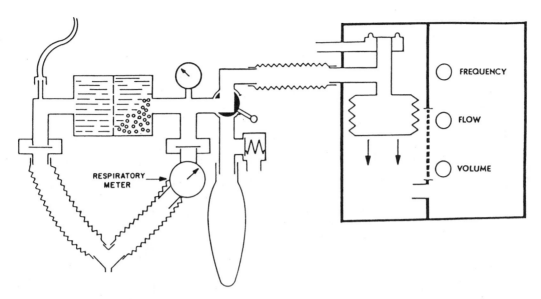

Fig. 6-12. A typical "bag-in-a-bottle" anesthesia ventilator. The reservoir bag and adjustable pressure-limiting valve are switched out of the circuit and replaced by a ventilator bellows (bag) in a bellows housing (bottle). (From Schreiber P: *Safety guidelines for anesthesia systems,* Telford, Pa, 1985, North American Dräger.)

droxide lime than with soda lime and are associated with lower fresh gas flow rates, greater absorbent temperatures (which are also associated with lower fresh gas flow rates), higher concentrations of sevoflurane, and increased carbon dioxide production. The MAC and number of hours of sevoflurane administration are the best predictors of compound A exposure during low-flow anesthesia. The nephrotoxicity of compound A in humans is controversial; until this issue is clarified, the FDA recommends that this agent be used at gas flow rates of 2 L/min or more to decrease compound A formation.[67]

Carbon monoxide toxicity is another potential hazard of the breakdown of potent inhaled agents by carbon dioxide absorbents. Desflurane, enflurane, and isoflurane have been found to interact with dry absorbent (barium hydroxide lime more so than soda lime) to produce carbon monoxide. This subject is addressed in a subsequent section.

F. Anesthesia ventilators

1. General considerations. Contemporary anesthesia ventilators, such as the North American Dräger AV-E and the Ohmeda 7000, 7800, and 7900 series, are examples of "bag-in-a-bottle" respirators.[68-70] Their basic principle of operation is that the reservoir bag of an anesthesia circle system is replaced by a bellows in a bellows housing, and the adjustable pressure-limiting valve is replaced by a ventilator pressure-relief valve. Inspiration occurs when compressed (driving) gas enters the bellows housing. The bellows is compressed, and the pressure-relief valve is held closed (Fig. 6-12). Gas in the bellows and fresh gas entering the patient circuit from the anesthesia machine are forced into the patient's lungs. At end-inspiration, the bellows housing ceases to be pressurized, the bellows refills (by gravity in the case of a hanging bellows [see Fig. 6-12]), and the pressure-relief

valve can open, venting excess patient circuit gas to the waste gas–scavenging system.

Anesthesia ventilators are also described as double-circuit ventilators because they have a driving-gas circuit and a patient circuit. The interface between these two circuits is the ventilator bellows. Although the North American Dräger AV-E and the Ohmeda models are double-circuit ventilators, their mechanisms of operation differ in certain details.

2. Ohmeda 7000. In the Ohmeda 7000 ventilator[68] (Fig. 6-13), the driving-gas supply (oxygen at a nominal pressure of 50 psig) passes to a pressure regulator, the output of which is set to 38 psig at a flow of 24 L/min. From here, the pressure-regulated oxygen flow passes to a block containing five solenoid flow-control valves connected in parallel. These valves are electronically opened during the inspiratory phase to direct oxygen flow through calibrated, tuned orifices. By controlling the duration of opening of each of the five solenoid valves, the control module determines the volume of oxygen that passes through into the collection chamber and enters the bellows housing. In the bellows housing, the oxygen exerts pressure on the bellows and displaces an equal volume of anesthesia gas mixture from the bellows into the patient circuit. This displaced volume is the tidal volume.

The Ohmeda 7000 ventilator uses a standing bellows that empties until the predetermined tidal volume has been delivered. During inspiration, the exhaust valve in the collection chamber is closed so that the driving gas does not escape. A ventilator pressure-relief valve located in the base of the bellows is held closed by the driving-gas pressure during inspiration so that gas passes from within the bellows to the patient circuit (see Fig. 6-13). Exhalation begins when the driving-gas exhaust valve, located in the control module, opens to permit the ventilation of driving gas from the bellows housing as this

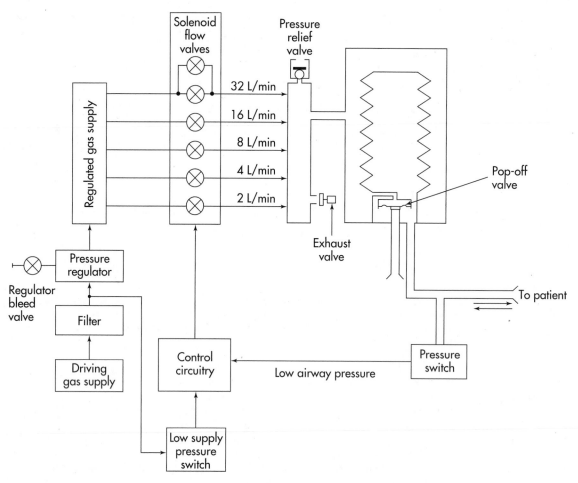

Fig. 6-13. The driving-gas circuit of the Ohmeda 7000 electronic anesthesia ventilator. (From *Ohmeda 7000 electronic anesthesia ventilator, service manual,* Madison, Wis, 1985, Ohmeda, The BOC Group.)

gas is displaced by the bellows refilling with anesthesia gases from the patient's lungs and fresh gas flow from the anesthesia machine. For the bellows to refill during exhalation, a slight positive pressure must be maintained in the patient circuit. The ventilator pressure-relief valve is therefore a positive end-expiratory pressure (PEEP) valve that exerts a pressure of about 2.5 cm H_2O on the gas contained within the patient circuit. At end-expiration, when the bellows has reached its limit of expansion and the circuit pressure has increased to more than 2.5 cm H_2O, the ventilator pressure-relief valve opens, and excess gas from the patient circuit is vented to the waste gas–scavenging system.

3. Ohmeda 7800 series. Ohmeda 7800 series ventilators[69] are very similar to the model 7000 ventilator but differ in certain features. The driving gas, oxygen at 50 psig, passes to a primary regulator of which the output is controlled to 26 psig. From here, the oxygen passes to a pneumatic manifold where its flowthrough into the bellows housing is controlled by a flow-control valve. This sophisticated valve varies the opening of a flow orifice according to the current supplied to the valve's coil, thereby controlling oxygen flow and volume of gas to

the bellows housing.[49,69] The ventilator controls of these two series also differ.

4. North American Dräger AV-E. The North American Dräger AV-E ventilator is also of double-circuit, pneumatically powered design.[29,49] A schema of this ventilator is shown in Fig. 6-14; the numbers in parentheses in the following description of its operation refer to the figure. The ventilator is powered by oxygen at a nominal driving pressure of 50 psig *(2).* When the ventilator switch *(3)* is turned on, oxygen pressure is supplied to a 1-psig switch *(4),* which is activated and energizes the electronic circuit. The respiratory rate *(7)* and inspiratory/expiratory ratio controls *(6)* are set as desired. Inspiration occurs when the solenoid valve *(9)* receives an electrical signal from the control unit *(5).* This signal remains active throughout inspiration and activates the solenoid valve *(9)* to allow oxygen at 50 psig to pass through it to activate the flow-control valve *(10).* Opening the flow-control valve allows oxygen that has passed through the adjustable flow regulator *(11)* to pass through the flow-control valve *(10)* to the Venturi nozzle *(13).* The inspiratory flow rate is adjusted by the flow regulator *(11)* (inspiratory flow-control knob), and the

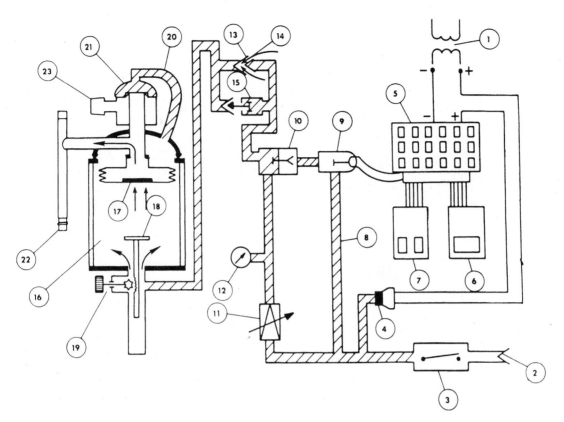

Fig. 6-14. The function of the North American Dräger AV-E ventilator during inspiration. (See text for details of operation.) *1*, Electric power supply (117 volts of alternating current); *2*, oxygen supply (50 psig); *3*, ventilator on/off switch; *4*, electrical supply on/off switch (1-psig pressure switch); *5*, printed circuit board; *6*, inspiratory/expiratory ratio control; *7*, frequency control; *8*, solenoid pilot pressure line; *9*, solenoid valve; *10*, flow-control valve; *11*, flow regulator; *12*, flow indicator gauge; *13*, Venturi nozzle; *14*, Venturi entrainment port; *15*, pilot actuator; *16*, bellows chamber; *17*, bellows; *18*, tidal-volume adjustment plate; *19*, tidal-volume control; *20*, relief-valve pilot line; *21*, ventilator relief valve; *22*, patient breathing system connector; *23*, waste gas–scavenging system connector. (Courtesy North American Dräger, Telford, Pa, 1986.)

flow rate is monitored on a flow-indicator gauge *(12)*. This indicator is really a pressure gauge that measures pressure downstream of the flow regulator. As the oxygen flows from the Venturi nozzle *(13)*, room air is entrained through the muffler and entrainment port *(14)*. The mixture of oxygen and entrained air is directed into the bellows chamber *(16)*. As pressure increases in the bellows chamber, the bellows is compressed and the anesthetic gases in the bellows are forced into the patient circuit through the breathing connector *(22)*. At the same time, driving-gas pressure from the bellows housing *(16)* is transmitted through the relief-valve pilot line *(20)* to hold the ventilator pressure-relief valve *(21)* closed as long as the bellows housing is under pressure (that is, throughout inspiration). In this model of ventilator, the bellows is normally emptied completely with each inspiratory cycle; thus the tidal volume is determined by the extent to which the bellows is allowed to expand during exhalation, which is in turn adjusted by the tidal-volume control knob *(19)* and bellows plate *(18)*. During the inspiratory pause, the oxygen continues

to flow from the Venturi nozzle *(13)*, but because the bellows is fully compressed, no further air is entrained and pressure is maintained in the bellows housing by the pressure of the oxygen jet from the Venturi nozzle. Meanwhile, the chamber *(16)* contains a mixture of air and oxygen.

Expiration (Fig. 6-15) begins when the electrical signal from the control unit *(5)* to the solenoid valve *(9)* stops. The solenoid valve is deactivated and closes, interrupting the supply of 50 psig of oxygen to the flow-control valve *(10)*, which therefore also closes. The preset oxygen flow from the flow regulator *(11)* is interrupted by the flow-control valve *(10)*, causing a pressure drop at the Venturi nozzle *(13)*, and no back-pressure is supplied to the pilot actuator *(15)*. The latter opens to vent gas from the bellows chamber *(16)* to be vented through the pilot actuator *(15)* and the entrainment port *(14)* of the Venturi nozzle *(13)*. As the pressure decreases in the bellows chamber *(16)*, the bellows *(17)* begins to refill. As long as pressure remains in the bellows chamber *(16)*, the ventilator pressure-relief valve *(2)* is pressurized and held closed.

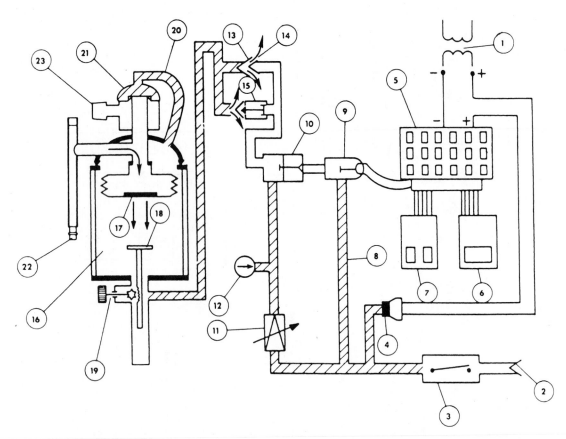

Fig. 6-15. The function of the North American Dräger AV-E ventilator during expiration. (See text for details of operation.) *1,* Electric power supply (117 volts of alternating current); *2,* oxygen supply (50 psig); *3,* ventilator on/off switch; *4,* electrical supply on/off switch (1-psig pressure switch); *5,* printed circuit board; *6,* inspiratory/expiratory ratio control; *7,* frequency control; *8,* solenoid pilot pressure line; *9,* solenoid valve; *10,* flow-control valve; *11,* flow regulator; *12,* flow indicator gauge; *13,* Venturi nozzle; *14,* Venturi entrainment port; *15,* pilot actuator; *16,* bellows chamber; *17,* bellows; *18,* tidal-volume adjustment plate; *19,* tidal-volume control; *20,* relief-valve pilot line; *21,* ventilator relief valve; *22,* patient breathing system connector; *23,* waste gas–scavenging system connector. (Courtesy North American Dräger, Telford, Pa, 1986.)

In the standing-bellows arrangement in Ohmeda ventilators and the standing-bellows version of the North American Dräger AV-E ventilator (Figs. 6-16 and 6-17), the ventilator pressure-relief valve applies about 2.5 cm of PEEP to the gas in the patient circuit. Once the standing bellows has reached its preset limit of expansion (the set tidal volume) and the patient circuit pressure exceeds 2.5 cm H_2O, the pressure-relief valve opens, permitting excess circuit gas to enter the waste gas–scavenging system.

In the North American Dräger AV-E ventilator, the ventilator pressure-relief valve is controlled by an external relief-valve pilot line (see Figs. 6-14 and 6-15, *20*), which is essentially a short piece of plastic tubing. Kinking of this line can cause malfunction of the ventilator.[71] Incompetence of the pressure-relief valve itself may result in patient hypoventilation.[71-73]

5. Design differences

a. Standing-bellows compared with hanging-bellows ventilators. Contemporary anesthesia ventilators are of the standing-bellows design; that is, they rise (fill by as-

cending) during exhalation and descend (empty) during inspiration. In the event of a disconnection, in which circuit pressure would become equal to atmospheric pressure, the bellows would not refill during exhalation.

In the hanging-bellows design (see Figs. 6-12 and 6-14), the bellows fills by gravity during exhalation so that the ventilator pressure-relief valve does not require a PEEP design. In the event of a patient circuit disconnection, room air would be entrained into the patient circuit through the leak and the bellows would refill, emptying through the leak on the next inspiration. For this reason, the standing-bellows design is preferred, although it is not required by the most recent standard describing specifications for anesthesia ventilators.[74]

b. North American Dräger compared with Ohmeda ventilators. In an Ohmeda ventilator, the gas entering the bellows housing is 100% oxygen (see Fig. 6-13), whereas in the North American Dräger AV-E ventilator, it is a mix-

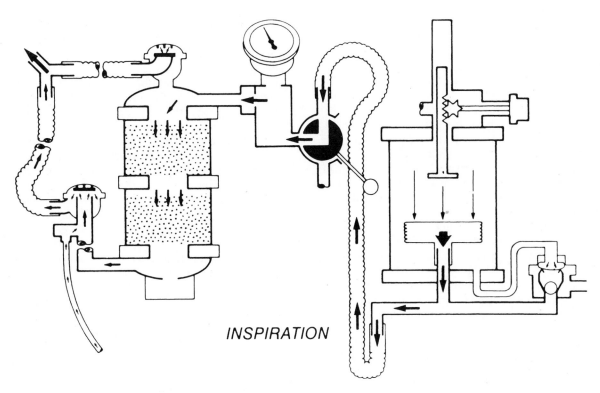

Fig. 6-16. North American Dräger AV-E standing-bellows ventilator showing events during inspiration. (Courtesy North American Dräger, Telford, Pa.)

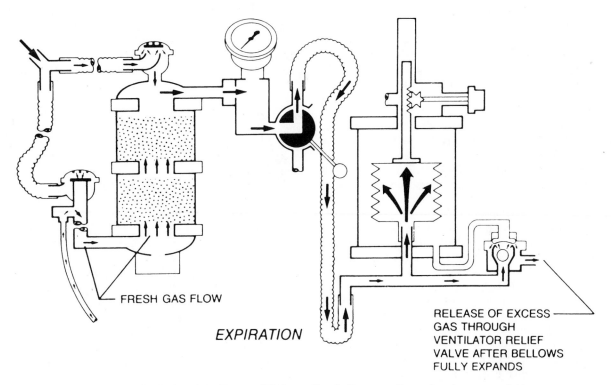

FRESH GAS FLOW

EXPIRATION

RELEASE OF EXCESS GAS THROUGH VENTILATOR RELIEF VALVE AFTER BELLOWS FULLY EXPANDS

Fig. 6-17. North American Dräger AV-E standing-bellows ventilator showing events during expiration. (Courtesy North American Dräger, Telford, Pa.)

ture of air and oxygen (see Figs. 6-14 and 6-15). In the event of a leak in the bellows, driving gas would enter the patient circuit and dilute the gases therein. This could cause oxygen enrichment with an Ohmeda ventilator but could cause a decrease in fractional inspired oxygen concentration (FIO_2) with a North American Dräger AV-E ventilator. Furthermore, a hole in the bellows of the Ohmeda ventilator would not alter the tidal volume because a driving-gas volume equal to tidal volume would enter the patient circuit. With the North American Dräger AV-E ventilator, because the driving gas flows throughout inspiration, a large volume of gas could enter the breathing system, increasing tidal volume and alveolar ventilation.

In the North American Dräger AV-E ventilator, the tidal volume is determined by setting the expansion limit of the bellows during expiration because the bellows is emptied completely during inspiration. The North American Dräger AV-E standing bellows (see Figs. 6-16 and 6-17) is graduated from 0 ml at the bottom to 2000 ml at the top of the housing. In the Ohmeda design, the bellows is graduated from 0 ml at the top to 1600 ml at the bottom of the bellows housing, because the tidal volume is displaced from the bellows by a metered volume of compressed oxygen from the ventilator control unit (see Fig. 6-13).

The North American Dräger AV-E ventilator uses a Venturi nozzle and a mixture of air and oxygen to compress the bellows. This economizes on the use of compressed oxygen. In Ohmeda ventilators, oxygen consumption is a little greater than the set minute ventilation.[75]

In Ohmeda ventilators, the circuit pressure-relief valve is flush mounted inside the bellows itself (see Fig. 6-13). The design does not use a relief-valve pilot line and is therefore not vulnerable to the effects of kinking of this line (see Fig. 6-14, 20).[71] A potential advantage of the exposed ventilator pressure-relief valve, however, is that its function can be observed if there is any concern; the Ohmeda valve, in contrast, is not normally visible for inspection.

Ohmeda ventilators incorporate a high pressure-relief valve in the driving-gas circuit (see Fig. 6-13). This may be preset to 65 cm H_2O (as in the Ohmeda 7000) or be adjustable (as in the Ohmeda 7800 series). In the 7800 series, when the pressure in the patient circuit exceeds the limit set by the user, the ventilator is automatically cycled to the exhalation mode. Most of the originally supplied North American Dräger AV-E ventilators do not have a pressure-limiting valve in the driving-gas circuit, although a retrofittable pressure-limit flow-control valve is available for certain ventilators (see the subsequent discussion of pressure and volume).

Because the Venturi nozzle of the North American Dräger AV-E ventilator requires entrainment of room air (see Figs. 6-14 and 6-15), a clean muffler is essential. If the muffler becomes blocked, air is no longer entrained and inspiration cannot be completed. If blockage of the muffler occurs during exhalation, gas cannot leave the ventilator bellows housing and the bellows remains compressed.[76]

6. Tidal volume considerations. Anesthesia ventilators (North American Dräger AV-E and Ohmeda 7000 and 7800 series) are designed to work in conjunction with an anesthesia circuit and a continuous-flow anesthesia machine. During inspiration, the ventilator pressure-relief valve is held closed so that gas in the bellows enters the patient circuit rather than the scavenging system (see Fig. 6-12). Meanwhile, fresh gas continues to enter the patient circuit from the anesthesia machine throughout the ventilatory cycle according to the flowmeter settings, which may result in additional tidal volume for the patient.

When setting the ventilator to achieve a certain delivered patient tidal volume, it is important to consider the rate of fresh gas flow from the anesthesia machine to the patient circuit.[77,78] Changing the fresh gas flow, respiratory rate, or inspiration/expiration ratio may have a profound effect on patient tidal volume, alveolar ventilation, and arterial carbon dioxide tension ($PaCO_2$).[78] The latter effect is illustrated in Fig. 6-18.

The additional minute ventilation to the circuit when one is using one of these models of anesthesia ventilator is approximated by the following formula:

$$\text{Additional minute ventilation} = (I/[I + E]) \times FGF$$

where I is inspiratory time, E is expiratory time, and FGF is the fresh gas flow rate. This result is divided by the respiratory rate to determine the potential augmentation of each ventilator bellows tidal volume. In terms of tidal volume actually delivered to the patient, this formula provides an approximation only. The actual augmentation of patient tidal volume also depends on the patient's total thoracic compliance compared with that of the anesthesia circuit components. If the patient's total thoracic compliance is low, additional fresh gas inflow from the machine may be accommodated mainly by compression within the circuit. Thus the following equation yields the patient minute ventilation *(MV):*

$$\text{Set MV} + (FGF \times I/[I + E]) - \text{Gas volume compressed in circuit at peak inspiratory pressure}$$

The last term can be calculated as the product of circuit compliance and peak inspiratory pressure. These considerations do not apply to intensive care unit ventilators that are designed to be minute volume dividers.

7. Positive end-expiratory pressure. The deliberate application of PEEP to the patient's airway is not uncommon during anesthesia. One may apply PEEP by adding a freestanding PEEP valve (such as a Boehringer valve, Wynnewood, Pennsylvania) between the expiratory limb of the circle and the expiratory unidirectional valve. Freestanding PEEP valves function well, but they may be used erroneously and can totally occlude the circuit if they are incorrectly placed in the inspiratory limb of the circle.[7,12,31]

North American Dräger and Ohmeda provide, as an option, PEEP valves that are built into their anesthesia delivery systems. These valves are purpose-designed and convenient and avoid the risk of erroneous valve placement. The position of a PEEP valve in the anesthesia cir-

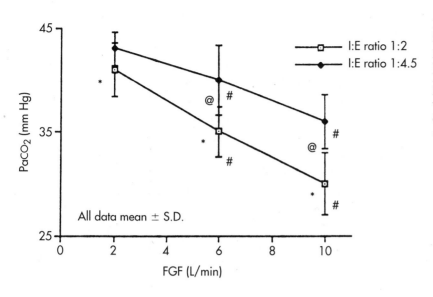

Fig. 6-18. Effect of fresh gas flow *(FGF)* and inspiratory/expiratory ratio *(I:E)* on $PaCO_2$ in patients ventilated with an anesthesia ventilator set to a constant tidal volume. Increasing FGF or the I:E ratio causes an increase in delivered tidal volume, an increase in alveolar ventilation, and a decrease in $PaCO_2$. (From Scheller MS, Jones BL, Benumof JL: *J Cardiothorac Anesth* 3:564, 1989.)

cuit deserves some consideration, however. At end-expiration, the part of the circuit between the PEEP valve and the inspiratory unidirectional valve will be at the PEEP determined by the PEEP valve setting. The remainder of the circuit is at 0 end-expiratory pressure (or +2.5 cm H_2O if a standing-bellows ventilator is used) (see Fig. 6-17). With the next inspiration, the emptying ventilator bellows must first compress gas in the patient circuit to the level set on the PEEP valve before any gas will flow past the inspiratory unidirectional valve to flow to the patient. If the tidal volume of the ventilator bellows is fixed, the additional compressible gas volume represents lost tidal volume for the patient. The closer the PEEP valve is to the ventilator bellows, the smaller the loss of tidal volume in the bellows to compression of gas in the circuit up to the set level of the PEEP. Thus once ventilator settings have been made without PEEP, the addition of a PEEP valve by the expiratory unidirectional valve will result in decreased minute ventilation for the patient.[79] This volume loss, attributable to compression of gas in the circuit, is greater with Ohmeda ventilators (series 7000 and 7800) than with the North American Dräger AV-E ventilator because a larger volume of compressible gas remains in an Ohmeda bellows at end-inspiration (total bellows volume of 1600 ml minus tidal volume), whereas almost no compressible gas remains in the AV-E bellows, which empties completely with each inspiration.[80]

The advantage of placing the PEEP valve near the expiratory unidirectional valve is that PEEP may be applied during spontaneous as well as mechanical ventilation (see Fig. 6-17).

8. Ohmeda 7900. The Ohmeda 7900 ventilator, introduced in 1996, incorporates features that address some of the limitations of the models of ventilators previously described.[70] This ventilator offers volume-controlled and pressure-controlled modes that are regulated through a closed-loop system that responds continuously to changes in delivered volume and airway pressure.

The ventilator receives data from a pair of pressure and flow sensors placed in the proximal respiratory and distal expiratory limbs of the breathing circuit. A pressure differential is measured across a variable-orifice flowmeter, and volume is determined by integrating flow with respect to time. The closed-loop feedback system (Smart Vent) compensates automatically for changes in fresh gas flow or the inspiratory/expiratory ratio; in other ventilators, these changes could alter the tidal volume. However, the feedback system cannot compensate for losses of compliance within the circuit.

The Ohmeda 7900 ventilator incorporates a valve that applies PEEP at the point where gas leaves the circuit (ventilator pressure-relief valve) to enter the waste gas–scavenging system. In this location, application of PEEP would have the least effect on tidal volume. Another feature is the integrated oxygen flush control. If the oxygen flush button is depressed during the inspiratory phase of ventilation, an electrical cut-out arrests inspiratory flow and causes the ventilator to cycle to exhalation. This feature provides some protection against barotrauma to the patient's lungs. Thus the Ohmeda 7900 offers features that address some of the limitations of its predecessors.

G. Waste gas–scavenging systems

Waste gases may leave the anesthesia circuit through the adjustable pressure-limiting valve or through the ventilator pressure-relief valve. In either case, tubing with an internal diameter of either 19 or 30 mm is used, compared with the 22-mm anesthesia circuit and ventilator tubing and the 15-mm common gas outlet and tracheal tube connectors (Fig. 6-19). The scavenging system interfaces with the hospital suction system to remove gas flow from the patient circuit.[49]

Scavenging systems may be open or closed. Closed systems use spring-loaded valves to ensure that excessively high or low pressures are not applied to the patient circuit

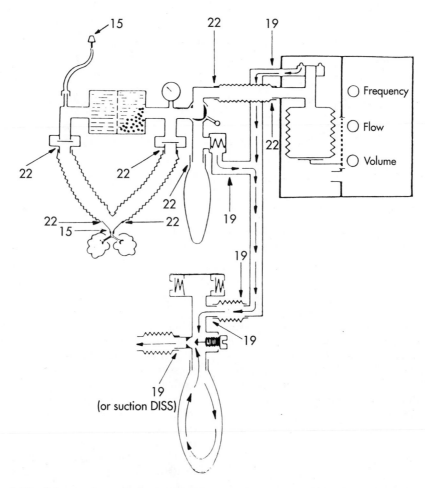

Fig. 6-19. Schema of anesthesia circuit and scavenging system tubing showing diameters in millimeters for hose connections. (See text for further explanation.) (From Schreiber P: *Safety guidelines for anesthesia systems,* Telford, Pa, 1985, North American Dräger.)

(Fig. 6-20).[49,81] Thus if the system is not connected to negative pressure (suction), excess pressure in the interface caused by gas entering it from the circuit would first cause distension of the interface reservoir bag, then the excess would be vented via the positive pressure–relief valve at about $+5$ cm H_2O. In the event that excessive suction might be applied to the circuit, the reservoir bag would first be sucked empty, then one (Ohmeda interface) or two (North American Dräger closed interface [see Fig. 6-20]) negative pressure–relief ("pop-in") valves (-0.25 to -1.80 cm H_2O), depending on the system, would open to preferentially draw in room air and minimize the potential application of negative pressure to the patient circuit.[81]

Open-reservoir scavenging interfaces are valveless (Fig. 6-21) and use continually open ports to provide pressure relief.[82] Waste gas from the circuit is directed to the bottom of the canister, and the hospital suction system aspirates gas from the bottom of the canister. In this type of interface, the reservoir canister contains the excess waste gas and thereby accommodates a range of waste gas flow rates from the patient circuit. Because this

type of interface depends on relief ports for pressure relief, care must be taken to ensure that these ports remain unoccluded at all times. Although the open reservoir system has the advantage of being valveless (valves can become stuck or malfunction), there is no visual indication that the system is functioning, whereas with the closed interface, the reservoir bag movement provides a constant indication of system function.

If the 19- or 30-mm tubing (see Fig. 6-19) connecting the adjustable pressure-limiting valve or the ventilator pressure-relief valve with the interface becomes occluded, pressure will build up in the patient breathing system. If the valves in a closed interface or the ports in an open interface become occluded, excesses of positive or negative pressure could develop in the circuit. Examples are discussed in a subsequent section.

H. Basic monitors and alarms

1. Oxygen analyzer and alarm. Anesthesia machines must be equipped with an analyzer that measures the oxygen concentration within the inspiratory limb of the anes-

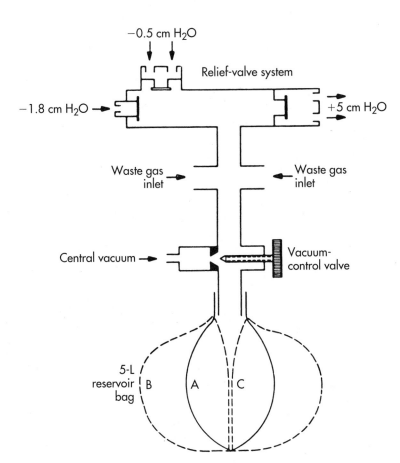

−0.5 cm H₂O

Relief-valve system

−1.8 cm H₂O →

→ +5 cm H₂O

Waste gas inlet

Waste gas inlet

Central vacuum →

Vacuum-control valve

5-L reservoir bag

B   A   C

Fig. 6-20. North American Dräger closed scavenger interface. (From Schreiber P: *Safety guidelines for anesthesia systems,* Telford, Pa, 1985, North American Dräger.)

thesia breathing system or within the fresh gas mixture.[9] The analyzer must be enabled and functioning whenever the anesthesia machine is capable of delivering an anesthetic gas mixture. It must sound a high-priority alarm when the measured oxygen concentration falls below the user-preset threshold.[9] Delivery-system oxygen analyzers are usually located near the inspiratory unidirectional valve. These analyzers (fuel cells) are specific for oxygen and are not "fooled" by other agents. Disasters associated with oxygen delivery failure or delivery of a hypoxic mixture would probably have been avoided if a functioning oxygen analyzer with alarm had been in use.[19,21]

Schreiber[31] stated that "the use of an oxygen analyzer with an anesthesia system is the single most important measure to prevent hypoxia." Furthermore, the ASA *Standards for Basic Intraoperative Monitoring* require monitoring of oxygen in the patient breathing system during induction of general anesthesia with an anesthesia machine.[11] An oxygen monitor and alarm system in the expiratory limb of a circle system with the alarm settings close to the expected expiratory oxygen concentration has been suggested as an effective backup system for detecting a disconnection.[83]

2. Monitoring of circuit pressures and volumes. The ASTM F1161-88 standard requires that an anesthesia machine be able to monitor breathing pressure as well as either exhaled volume or ventilatory carbon dioxide.[9]

The machine must be able to continually monitor pressure in the breathing system, and the pressure monitor must be designed to activate a visible and audible high-priority alarm when pressure in the system (1) exceeds a user-adjustable limit for high pressure and (2) exceeds a user-adjustable limit for continuing positive airway pressure for more than 15 ± 1 seconds. The latter alarm threshold should be adjustable between 10 and 30 cm H₂O. The pressure monitor and alarm must be enabled and function automatically whenever the anesthesia machine is in use.[9]

The *ASA Standards for Basic Anesthetic Monitoring*[11] require that when ventilation is controlled by a mechanical ventilator, a device that can detect disconnection of components of the breathing system should be in continuous use. The device must emit an audible signal when its alarm threshold is exceeded. This circuit low-pressure alarm is sometimes loosely termed the *disconnect alarm.* If the pressure in the circuit does not exceed the user-set minimum within a set period (usually 15 seconds, but this may be set at 60 seconds to allow a slow respiratory rate to be deliberately set on the ventilator), the alarm sounds. Modern circuit pressure monitors also sound an alarm when the pressure in the breathing system falls below −10 cm H₂O at any time (subatmospheric pressure alarm).

Modern delivery systems incorporate a mechanical pressure gauge that is usually mounted on the absorber,

Fig. 6-21. North American Dräger open-reservoir scavenging system. This interface uses continually open relief ports to provide positive and negative pressure relief (compare with the valves shown in Fig. 6-19). An adjustable needle valve regulates the waste gas exhaust flow, which is indicated on an un-calibrated flow-control valve. A flow-control valve reading halfway between the two white lines corresponds to a suction flow rate of about 25 L/min. (From *Open reservoir scavenger operator's instruction manual,* Telford, Pa, 1986, North American Dräger.)

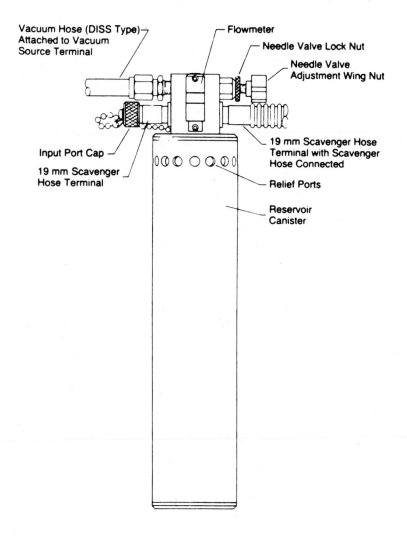

and the circuit pressure may be measured at that point (Fig. 6-22). In addition, pressure may be sensed at almost any point in the circuit and transmitted through pilot tubing to a remote electronic pressure monitor that incorporates audible and visible alarms. Ideally, pressure should be sensed at the patient connector, but water and sterilization problems make this site impractical.[31] Sensing pressure by the absorber may fail to detect abnormalities between the patient and the inspiratory and expiratory unidirectional valves. Thus if a freestanding PEEP valve were inserted between the expiratory limb of the circuit and the exhalation unidirectional valve, the PEEP would not be detectable by a pressure monitor sensing pressure by the absorber (see Fig. 6-22). Although the circle system is the most commonly used circuit, others (e.g., Bain or Mapleson F) may be used; pressure-monitoring adapters are available for use with these circuits.

The pressure monitoring and alarm connections in both the North American Dräger and Ohmeda absorber systems are self-sealing. If the pressure-monitoring sensor is disconnected from the absorber and the circle system is then used, the low-pressure alarm will be activated (because it senses atmospheric pressure) but the circuit pressure gauge will display normal pressures.

Monitoring of pressure at the absorber may also fail to detect a patient circuit disconnection during positive-pressure ventilation. Because the ventilator delivers its tidal volume in the proximity of the pressure alarm sensing point (see Fig. 6-22), the low-pressure alarm limit may be satisfied if not set to be sufficiently sensitive (i.e., just lower than the usual peak inspiratory pressure). It therefore is important to recognize where in the circuit the pressure gauge senses pressure and where the pressure monitoring and alarm system are sensing pressure, if they differ. The ASTM F1161-88 standard also requires monitoring of exhaled volume or ventilatory carbon dioxide.[9] An alarm is activated if the patient's exhaled volume falls below an operator-adjustable minimum. The monitor must be designed to be enabled and function automatically whenever the anesthesia machine is in use. When the volume monitor alarm is disabled, a low-priority alarm must be activated.

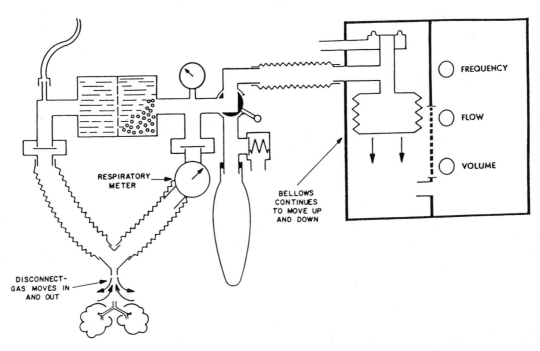

Fig. 6-22. Typical circle system connected to ventilator showing positions of pressure gauge (close to the absorber) and spirometer (expiratory limb of circle). With use of the hanging-bellows ventilator shown, a disconnect between the patient and the Y piece allows room air to be entrained during exhalation. This air is pulled through the respiratory meter, causing the meter to be fooled. (From Schreiber P: *Safety guidelines for anesthesia systems,* Telford, Pa, 1985, North American Dräger.)

Modern circle systems also incorporate a spirometer, which measures tidal and minute volumes; demonstrates reversal of gas flow if it should occur (because of incompetence of the exhalation unidirectional valve); and, if it is electronic, incorporates low and high alarm limits. Mechanical spirometers do not have an alarm. In North American Dräger systems, the spirometer is located on the absorber side (downstream) of the expiratory unidirectional valve. In Ohmeda systems, it is usually placed just upstream of the expiratory unidirectional valve. Thus in both systems, the gas volume flowing through the expiratory limb of the circuit (exhaled volume) is measured (see Fig. 6-22).

Monitoring exhaled volumes is valuable when a low-volume alarm limit can be set to be sensitive, that is, just less than the set ventilation parameters (including tidal volume, rate, fresh gas flow, and inspiratory/expiratory ratio). A disconnection in the patient circuit should result in a decrease in displayed tidal volume and minute volume. Unlike the pressure gauge, which senses pressure at the absorber, the spirometer will usually indicate flow problems in the patient circuit.

In the event of a circuit disconnection, a spirometer in the expiratory limb may be fooled if a hanging-bellows ventilator is being used. During exhalation, a weight in the hanging bellows causes it to descend, drawing room air in through the disconnection site and spirometer and into the descending bellows. Fig. 6-22 shows that fresh gas will also pass to the hanging bellows via the absorber;

thus if disconnection occurs, the decrease in the tidal volume reading compared with the tidal volume before the disconnection occurred is attributable to gas compressed in the patient circuit during exhalation. Unless the low-volume alarm limits have been set to be very sensitive, a spirometer in the expiratory limb of the circle will probably not detect a disconnection of the patient circuit with a hanging-bellows ventilator. In contrast, both the spirometer and the pressure monitor would detect a disconnection of the tubing between the ventilator and the breathing circuit.

As mentioned previously, the standing-bellows ventilator is preferred because a disconnection is more obvious (the bellows fails to fill on exhalation) and an expiratory spirometer is less likely to be fooled. However, it is possible for an expiratory limb spirometer to be fooled by a standing-bellows ventilator when there is a patient circuit disconnection. When the disconnection occurs, the standing bellows empties and falls to its bottom resting position as if the largest possible tidal volume had been delivered (see Fig. 6-16). At end-exhalation, the pressure in the driving-gas circuit is zero, but the empty bellows contains a residual volume of patient circuit gas. On the next inspiration, driving-gas pressure in the bellows housing increases, and the bellows is actively compressed, discharging some of the contained residual gas volume. With the next exhalation cycle, the bellows resumes its original unpressurized configuration and may aspirate gas from the patient circuit. Gas drawn through the spirometer and into the recoiling bellows will cause the spirometer to record a volume of as much as 140 ml, depending on the size of the bellows and the fresh gas flow from the anesthesia machine.[84] An inappropriately set low-volume alarm thus might record an adequate tidal volume and be fooled.

Although monitoring of pressure and exhaled volume are now required in modern delivery systems, it is apparent from the preceding discussion that not all ventilation or pressure problems are detectable when these monitors are used as currently configured. Detection is improved by "bracketing" the user-adjustable alarm-limit thresholds close to the patient's normal high and low pressures and volumes. Some older monitors had fixed alarm limits, and even some modern ones have default settings that may not provide adequate warning of problems in the circuit. Problems associated with alarm limits being set to be too insensitive are discussed further in a subsequent section. A novel pressure/flow sensor placed by the patient's airway might be an improvement over the current monitors because it can provide instantaneous measurements of flow, volume, and pressure at this important site.[85] This type of monitoring, called sidestream spirometry, is available from Datex-Ohmeda (Tewksbury, Massachusetts).

II. COMPLICATIONS
A. Hypoxemia

Hypoxemia, defined as a partial pressure of oxygen in the arterial blood (PaO_2) of less than 60 mm Hg, may be caused by problems in the patient or with the anesthesia delivery system. In the setting of adequate ventilation and normal or expected alveolar oxygen, the patient's pathosis is the cause of hypoxemia. A pulmonary pathosis may cause shunting, venous admixture, or (much less likely) diffusion defects. Pneumonia, atelectasis, pulmonary edema, pneumothorax, hemothorax, pyothorax, pulmonary embolism, alveolar proteinosis, and bronchospasm are some of the pathologic conditions that may cause hypoxemia; they are reviewed elsewhere in this book.

The anesthesia delivery system may cause hypoxemia by failing to deliver sufficient oxygen to the lungs, resulting in low alveolar oxygen levels. Apnea and severe hypoventilation are well-described causes of alveolar hypoxia. These problems can occur because of failure to initiate ventilation manually or mechanically or when disconnection exists in the breathing system even though ventilation is attempted. Delivery of a hypoxic gas mixture to the lungs is particularly problematic with regard to insufficient alveolar oxygen.

The anesthesia machine may be the source of delivery of a hypoxic mixture to the breathing system and, ultimately, to the patient. The only way to know qualitatively and quantitatively the oxygen composition of the gas mixture in the breathing system is to measure the oxygen concentration with an analyzer in the breathing system. If a gas other than oxygen is flowing through the oxygen flow-control valve, it may appear that oxygen is being delivered to the breathing circuit when, in fact, the circuit is receiving no oxygen at all.[42]

Oxygen analyzers have limitations. First, the oxygen analyzer must be properly calibrated, the alarm limits must be set, and the alarm must work. Second, the analyzer must actually be sampling the gases that the patient is breathing. An oxygen analyzer placed at the inspiratory unidirectional valve may show an adequate oxygen concentration, but the patient may not be receiving that gas if there is a circuit disconnection between the inspiratory valve and the patient. In those circumstances, the patient may not be receiving adequate oxygen, but the analyzer may not indicate that to the anesthesiologist. Finally, vigilant observation of the integrity of the breathing circuit and machine is required for safe patient care.

The oxygen pipeline may have a gas other than oxygen flowing through it. For example, the bulk liquid oxygen tank may be filled with liquid nitrogen.[86] The pipelines may be crossed so that nitrous oxide or another gas may be flowing through the oxygen pipeline. Inside the operating room, the hose from the wall nitrous oxide outlet may have an oxygen connector at the patient end. Connecting this to the oxygen inlet on the anesthesia machine would permit nitrous oxide to flow to the oxygen flow-control valve.[14,20,87-89] If such a situation is suspected, the oxygen pipeline connection to the machine should be disconnected and the reserve oxygen tank should be turned on. Failure to disconnect the pipeline gas (at 50 to 55 psig) will prevent the flow of tank oxygen, which is regulated to enter the machine at 45 psig (see section I.B.1).

A gas other than oxygen can flow from the oxygen cylinder yokes and through the oxygen flow-control valve to the breathing system. In a similar vein, an oxygen cylinder may be filled with a gas other than oxygen, and this cylinder may be attached to the oxygen yoke.[90] A nitrous oxide cylinder could be attached to an oxygen yoke if the pin-indexed system were defeated by removal of a pin or by placement of more than one washer between the yoke and the oxygen cylinder. Crossed pipes within the anesthesia machine could cause delivery of a gas other than oxygen to the oxygen flow-control valve.[91,92]

It is also possible for the oxygen flow-control valve not to deliver any gas to the patient.[93] The liquid oxygen tank and backup central supply cylinders may be empty, or the central system may be shut down for repairs or other purposes.[94] The pipeline system may not be connected from the wall to the anesthesia machine. The backup cylinders on the machine may be empty, absent, or turned off.[87] The oxygen flow-control valve or oxygen piping system in the machine may be obstructed, preventing the flow of oxygen to the flow-control valve.[39,40] The flow-control valve bobbin or flowmeter may become stuck because of static electricity, grit, or dirt, and it may appear that gas is flowing from the oxygen flow-control valve even when it is not.[31] In addition, a leak may exist in the flow-control valve tubes, which results in loss of the oxygen before it reaches the common gas outlet of the machine.[36,95-97] On older anesthesia machines, the nitrous oxide flow-control valve may be turned on without opening the oxygen flow-control valve. This type of problem should be prevented on anesthesia machines that have oxygen-ratio monitors and oxygen-flow controllers designed to prevent the delivery of a hypoxic mixture (see later discussion). However, one should not rely wholly upon these devices to prevent delivery of hypoxic mixtures.

The Ohmeda Link-25 system can be defeated if the oxygen flow-control needle valve is broken in the closed position or if the linkage between the flowmeter control valve fails.[38,41,98] This can result in a hypoxic mixture in the breathing circuit. In one case report involving this system, the set screws that secured the oxygen flow control knob to the threaded sleeve were loose. It is then possible to turn the oxygen knob counterclockwise to increase flow without causing an adequate increase in oxygen delivery. In this situation, not only did the oxygen flow fail to increase but the chain link system engaged, causing an unexpected and unwanted increase in nitrous oxide flow. The overall result was inadequate oxygen flow, unintended nitrous oxide flow, and the creation of a hypoxic gas mixture.[99] Hypoxic mixtures caused by failure of the North American Dräger ORMC (see Fig. 6-4) have not been reported in the anesthesia literature. In any event, it must be recognized that a fundamental limitation of all oxygen ratio monitor and controller systems is that they do not qualitatively analyze the gas that is flowing through the oxygen flow-control valve. For this reason, it is critical that the breathing circuit gas be continuously monitored with an oxygen analyzer.[31]

The anesthesia breathing system may contain a hypoxic mixture for many possible reasons. Valves in the circuit may be absent or incompetent, allowing rebreathing of exhaled gas that could become hypoxic if mixing with fresh gas was not sufficient. This is especially a problem if both the inspiratory and expiratory valves were missing in a circle breathing system. In Mapleson circuits, interruption or loss of fresh gas from the anesthesia machine may lead to severe rebreathing of a hypoxic mixture as the patient consumes the oxygen in the system and replaces it with carbon dioxide. Failure of the fresh gas supply from the anesthesia machine to the breathing circle will also result in a circle system that becomes progressively hypoxic as the patient uses up the oxygen. Disconnections between the anesthesia machine or vaporizer and the breathing circuit will also cause the system to become hypoxic.[56,100-102]

Leaks in the breathing circuit will cause fresh gases to be lost (see following text). If a hanging-bellows ventilator is used, the fresh gases may be replaced with room air that is entrained into the breathing system as the bellows falls during the exhalation phase of the ventilatory cycle. This would cause room air to be substituted for the desired breathing mixture.[55] A standing bellows would merely collapse if a substantial leak developed in the breathing system. Most important, leaks in the breathing system can result in severe hypoventilation or apnea. These leaks may occur in valve housings, in inspiratory or expiratory hoses, at connection sites, in ventilator hoses, or in pressure-relief valves; they may also be caused by subatmospheric pressure applied to the breathing system from a scavenger suction or a nasogastric tube that is in the trachea and applied to suction.[31,103]

A leak in the ventilator bellows will cause driving gas or gases to enter the breathing system. If air is the driving gas, the oxygen concentration in the breathing system will be reduced.[104]

During closed-system anesthesia, the flow of fresh gases from the anesthesia machine is adjusted so that the total flow into the breathing system equals the total uptake and other gas loss from the circuit. The circuit may become hypoxic or hyperoxic if it is not carefully monitored for oxygen concentration throughout the anesthetic. Hypoxic and hyperoxic mixtures occur because uptakes of oxygen and nitrous oxide change during the anesthetic. At first, nitrous oxide uptake is high, but as the anesthetic progresses, nitrous oxide uptake decreases. If a compensatory reduction in nitrous oxide flow is not made, the system concentration of oxygen will decrease and the patient will become hypoxemic.

B. Hyperoxia

An oxygen concentration that is higher than expected is a problem that the anesthesiologist rarely confronts. It is always attributable to administration of a gas mixture that contains more oxygen than is desired. In all circumstances, an accurate and properly positioned oxygen analyzer will detect this problem. Insufficient nitrous oxide, air, or helium administered from the nitrous oxide, air, or helium gas flow-control valves will cause the inspired oxygen concentration to increase. Leaks from any of these flow-control valves, inaccurate flow-control valves, and flow-control valves with stuck flowmeters may cause these gases to be lost or not administered, with a resultant increase in inspired oxygen. A leak in a hanging-bellows ventilator that causes entrainment or injection of driving gas from the bellows housing may cause the inspired oxygen concentration to increase if the oxygen content of the entrained gas is greater than that of the gas delivered from the common gas outlet.[104,105]

C. Hypercarbia (hypercapnia)

Hypercarbia, defined as an increase of the $PaCO_2$ to concentrations greater than 45 mm Hg, occurs when carbon dioxide production exceeds elimination. During anesthesia and surgery, patient factors and anesthesia-delivery system conditions may act individually or combine to produce hypercarbia.

Patients who are breathing spontaneously and are receiving inhaled or intravenous anesthetic agents may hypoventilate or become apneic because of the central respiratory depressant action of these agents. Airway obstruction caused by a central action of anesthetics or by neuromuscular blocking drugs prevents adequate gas exchange and results in hypercarbia and hypoxia. Pathosis of the central nervous system, high spinal cord, or phrenic nerve may cause hypoventilation or apnea and result in hypercarbia. Muscle relaxants (by blocking the neuromuscular junction) and high spinal or epidural anesthesia (by interfering with the transmission of neural output at the level of the spinal cord) result in apnea and hypercarbia.

Pulmonary pathosis in patients who are breathing spontaneously and in those who are mechanically ventilated can cause hypercarbia. Patients with substantial venous admixture will retain carbon dioxide if the minute ventilation is normal. However, hypercarbia is not a problem during one-lung anesthesia if the entire calculated minute ventilation is delivered to the ventilated lung and the pulmonary shunt is small.

Increased metabolic rate caused by fever, thyrotoxicosis, malignant hyperthermia, or hyperalimentation will result in increased carbon dioxide production. If this condition is not compensated for by an increase in alveolar ventilation equal to the increase in metabolic rate above the calculated normal, the result will be carbon dioxide retention and hypercarbia.

The anesthesia delivery system, through misuse, malfunction, or both, can cause hypercarbia. Apnea from failure to turn on a ventilator or failure to manually ventilate the patient will cause hypercarbia. Turning on the ventilator but failing to provide an adequate tidal volume and ventilatory rate to a patient with normal carbon dioxide production will result in increased $PaCO_2$. Leaks in the anesthesia machine, breathing circuit, or ventilator or failure to initially fill the ventilator bellows because of insufficient fresh gas flow from the anesthesia machine may lead to inadequate ventilation and hypercarbia.[31]

Insufficient fresh gas supply to the breathing circuit can be caused by failure of the central piped-gas system, valves that are closed to a particular operating room, leaks in the pipes, failure to connect the anesthesia machine to the piped-gas supply, or leaks in the hoses.[14,55,93] However, these problems are outside the anesthesia machine and can easily be overcome by use of the reserve gas cylinders on the anesthesia machine.

Within the machine, leaks may develop at the oxygen cylinder-yoke interface and in a cylinder mount if the check valve is absent and no other cylinder is present. Lack of a check valve on the pipeline system can create a large oxygen leak.[5] It is also possible for gas to leak from the pipes, flow-control valves, vaporizers, vaporizer selector switches, and vaporizer mounts on the anesthesia machine.[14,31,106-111]

The interface between the anesthesia machine and the breathing circuit may be a source of gas leakage.[55,56,100-102] Disconnection of the gas hose from the common gas outlet or the anesthesia circuit will cause a leak. A leak in that hose or from the other hoses in the breathing circuit may cause sufficient loss of gas volume to result in hypoventilation and hypercarbia. Disconnections and leaks of anesthesia circuit hoses, valve housings, tracheal tubes, ventilator hose, reservoir bag, ventilator bellows, and system-relief valves either in the ventilator or in the manual breathing system can reduce the breathing system volume and cause hypercarbia.[14,31,72,73,112-124] In addition, subatmospheric pressure in the breathing system, which may be caused by malfunction of the scavenger interface, sampling of gas for analysis of the breathing system contents, or suction on a nasogastric tube that was placed in the trachea, will cause gas to be lost from the breathing system and will result in a reduction in minute ventilation (see discussion of pressure and volume excesses). Gas flow from the machine to the circuit may also be prevented by obstruction of the piping system in the machine or in the hose to the circuit.[125-128]

The anesthesia ventilator can be the source of hypoventilation if it is set in such a way that it fails to deliver adequate alveolar minute ventilation. This may occur when the preset tidal volume is so small that only dead-space ventilation takes place. It may also occur with ventilators in which the tidal volume, respiratory rate, inspiratory/expiratory ratio, and flow of compressing gases into the bellows chamber can be independently set. With such ventilators (e.g., the North American Dräger AV-E), it is possible to set an adequate tidal volume and respiratory rate, but if the inspiratory time or driving-gas flow is not sufficient, the preset tidal volume may not be completely delivered, resulting in substantial hypoventilation. This problem can be prevented if one ensures that the ventilator bellows is adequately compressed and delivering the preset tidal volume before exhalation begins.

In patients with poor pulmonary compliance, the lungs may not be adequately ventilated even though adequate tidal volume and frequency are set on the ventilator. The bellows may fail to deliver the desired volume because the lungs are too stiff. In addition, a substantial volume may be lost to expansion of the compliant tubing of the breathing circuit when lung compliance is poor (see the section on considerations of tidal volume). When ventilators that are pressure cycled or have a high pressure limit are used for patients with poor pulmonary compliance, it is likely that the ventilator will cycle before delivering an adequate tidal volume. Each of these circumstances may result in hypercarbia because of hypoventilation.

The fresh gas flows from the anesthesia machine to the breathing circuit contribute to the tidal volume and minute ventilation. If the patient is normocarbic and these flows are significantly decreased, the result will be a decreased tidal volume, increased ratio of dead space to tidal volume, and increased $PaCO_2$.[77,78,129]

The carbon dioxide absorber is a common source of problems that result in hypoventilation or hypercarbia. Leaks from the absorber occur frequently when it is incorrectly closed. Absorbent granules may prevent the rubber gaskets from seating properly, or incorrectly applied gaskets may leak. Simply failing to return the absorber handle to the closed and locked position will cause a large gas leak.[130] Within the absorber, exhausted absorbent granules or channeling of gas flow through spent absorbent will allow recycling of exhaled gas and rebreathing of previously exhaled carbon dioxide. In addition, some (older) anesthesia circuits have a switch that allows the anesthetic gases to bypass the absorber and thereby permit rebreathing of carbon dioxide. Leaving the switch in the bypass position sets the stage for development of hypercarbia.

The anesthesiologist relies upon the color of the carbon dioxide absorbent to determine whether it has been exhausted. However, photodeactivation of the ethyl violet additive by fluorescent lights can give the false impression that the absorbent is fresh when it has in fact been exhausted. This can result in hypercarbia.[66] Some anesthesia machines are equipped to deliver carbon dioxide. Accidental or inappropriate delivery of carbon dioxide to the breathing circuit can cause hypercarbia to develop.[131,132] Sources for the delivery of carbon dioxide to the anesthesia machine and subsequently to the patient include bulk gas sources and cylinders that may be connected to the pipeline system or machine where other gases, such as oxygen and nitrous oxide, are meant to be connected. Capnography can be used to detect carbon dioxide in the fresh gas supply.

Problems within the breathing circuit may lead to rebreathing of exhaled gas before carbon dioxide has been removed. The result of these problems is an increase in apparatus dead space and dead-space ventilation. Inspiratory or expiratory unidirectional valves that are absent, broken, or malfunctioning in the open position will cause rebreathing of exhaled carbon dioxide. At normal total minute ventilation, the patient will become hypercarbic. Any large connecting tube, filter, adapter, or "artificial noses" placed between the Y piece of the breathing circuit and the patient will also increase dead-space ventilation.

The arrangement of the components of the circle system must be set in such a way that breathing of exhaled carbon dioxide is prevented (see description in previous section).[60] Although the circle system is designed to permit rebreathing of exhaled gas after absorption of carbon dioxide, valveless (Mapleson) breathing systems do not have carbon dioxide absorbers.[49] If these systems are used incorrectly, hypercarbia will result. The Mapleson A system (Magill attachment) is designed to be used in spontaneously breathing patients only. To prevent rebreathing, it is critical that the fresh gas flow rate be greater than 0.7 times the minute ventilation and that the hose between the patient and the reservoir bag be long enough to prevent carbon dioxide–laden exhaled gas from reaching the reservoir bag.[58,59]

The Mapleson B and C systems are designed so that rebreathing of exhaled carbon dioxide will always occur unless the fresh gas flow rate is equal to or greater than the peak inspiratory flow rate. In both systems, carbon dioxide accumulates in a blind pouch (see Fig. 6-9). Even at reasonable fresh gas flow rates, such as 1.5 to 2.5 times the minute ventilation, the patient's lungs must still be hyperventilated to prevent hypercarbia. Therefore when these systems are used, the patient's lungs must be hyperventilated and the fresh gas flow must exceed minute ventilation. If the patient breathes spontaneously, the work of breathing will be increased because of the increased minute ventilation resulting from rebreathing of exhaled carbon dioxide. Controlled ventilation does not impose any additional metabolic demands because no ventilatory work is done.[58,59]

The Mapleson D, E, and F systems are essentially T-piece systems, all of which function in a similar manner. Hypercarbia can be prevented by administration of fresh gas at 2.5 to 3 times the minute ventilation and provision of normal minute ventilation. Alternatively, smaller fresh gas flows can be used, but to prevent carbon dioxide accumulation, the patient's lungs must be hyperventilated. With all Mapleson systems, rebreathing and hypercarbia will occur if the fresh gas supply connection is disrupted. This disruption can be a particularly difficult problem with the Bain circuit because it may not be easy to detect a disconnected or kinked inner hose.[106,133,134]

Although uncommon, some machines may be equipped with a circle breathing system that does not have a carbon dioxide absorber. To prevent hypercarbia with this system, the fresh gas flows must be increased to 2 to 3 times the minute ventilation. Alternatively, the fresh flows can be set to 1.5 times the normal minute ventilation, and the patient's lungs can be hyperventilated to compensate for the partial rebreathing that will occur.

D. Hypocarbia (hypocapnia)

Unlike hypercarbia, hypocarbia results from hyperventilation to the point that carbon dioxide removal exceeds production. Physiologic circumstances that reduce the metabolic rate include sleep, general anesthesia, and hypothermia with general anesthesia. Therefore the predicted minute ventilation for an awake patient may produce hypocarbia in an unconscious or anesthetized patient.

Certain anesthesia machine–related situations can lead to unintended hyperventilation and resultant hypocarbia. The ventilator may be set to deliver substantially more than the required minute ventilation. This may occur by setting the ventilatory rate or tidal volume too high. Alternatively, the ventilator may be set correctly, but the contribution to ventilation of the fresh gas flow from the anesthesia machine may not have been considered.[64,113] Failure to recognize this may have clinically significant results in the patient with compliant lungs. Leaks into the breathing circuit from a North American Dräger AV-E ventilator bellows that has a hole in it will cause an augmentation of the tidal volume delivered and will hyperventilate the patient.[135] Leaks in the bellows may alter the exact gas mixture that the patient breathes and the minute ventilation because the gas that will be added to the breathing circuit will be the driving gas from the ventilator (air, oxygen, a mixture of air and oxygen, or some other gas).[104,105,136]

E. Circuit pressure and volume excesses

Adequate movement of gases between the delivery system and the patient's lungs is essential to anesthesia delivery and patient oxygenation and ventilation. Schreiber[31] described four basic causes of failure of this function:

1. Occlusion in the inspiratory or expiratory pathway
2. Insufficient amount of gas in the breathing system
3. Failure to initiate artificial ventilation when required
4. Disconnection in the breathing system during mechanical ventilation

1. Occlusions. The anesthesia system includes numerous tubes that may become occluded (see Fig. 6-18).[137] Such problems may occur outside the tube, within the wall of the tube, or within the lumen of the tube. Tubing misconnections are now less common since standard diameters were introduced. Nevertheless, even with adapters, misconnections are still possible. In general, circuit tubing connections are 22 mm in diameter, scavenging tubing (but not the scavenging reservoir bag mount) is 19 or 30 mm, and the common gas outlet and tracheal tube connectors are 15 mm.[31] Accessories added to the circuit may cause an obstruction. Filters placed in the circuit,[138] incorrectly connected humidifiers,[139] and manufacturing defects in tubing have been reported as causes of total occlusion of the breathing circuit.[14,140] A freestanding PEEP valve may cause obstruction if it is incorrectly placed in the inspiratory limb of a circle system.[7,31] The PEEP valves that use a weighted ball (such as those made by Boehringer) are designed to be mounted vertically on the expiratory side of a circle system. In one case, the weighted-ball PEEP valve was erroneously placed horizontally in the expiratory limb between the circuit and the exhalation unidirectional valve. At first, the circuit was unobstructed, but there was no PEEP. When the oxygen flush was operated, the metal ball was driven downstream, totally obstructing the PEEP valve and circuit and rendering ventilation of the patient impossible. Because of such potential user errors, freestanding PEEP valves are considered by many to be undesirable.[141-143] Bidirectional freestanding PEEP valves are available (e.g., Ambu Anesthesia PEEP valve [Ambu Inc., Linthium, Maryland]). If such a valve is accidentally reversed relative to the flow of gas, flow continues but the PEEP feature is bypassed.[144]

Although total occlusion of the breathing circuit should activate a pressure or volume alarm in most cases, depending on the system used, these alarms may be fooled when the tracheal tube is totally occluded.[12,103] Consider the hypothetical scenario of a breathing circuit with a pressure-monitoring system (such as the North American Dräger Pressure Monitor model DPMS) that incorporates three possible threshold settings for the breathing system low-pressure alarm (8, 12, and 25 cm H_2O) and a fixed setting of $+65$ cm H_2O for the high-pressure alarm limit threshold used with a North American Dräger Narkomed 2A anesthesia machine and ventilator. If the tracheal tube were to become totally obstructed (such as by kinking), pressure in the circuit would increase during inspiration, satisfying the low-pressure alarm, but unless the pressure reaches $+65$ cm H_2O, the high-pressure alarm will not sound. The peak pressure achieved in the circuit during inspiration depends on the inspiratory flow-control setting (which determines the driving pressure available to compress the bellows) and the fresh gas inflow rate from the anesthesia machine. At low inspiratory flow settings on the ventilator, the driving pressure of the North American Dräger anesthesia ventilator may be 50 cm H_2O or less, which, combined with normal rates of fresh gas inflow from the machine, may result in failure of peak inspiratory pressure to reach the high-pressure alarm threshold of $+65$ cm H_2O. During exhalation, excess gas is normally released from the patient circuit. The volume alarm may also be fooled in this situation, depending on its low-limit threshold setting. In the system described, the low-volume alarm threshold was fixed at 80 ml. The hypothetical scenario involved total failure to ventilate the patient's lungs. This situation would be immediately detectable by continuous capnometry; alternatively, pressure and volume alarms of which thresholds can be set close to the normal values for that particular patient can be used, or breath sounds can be continuously monitored.

Misconnections and obstructions may usually be prevented or detected by testing the breathing circuit before use with all accessories in place and in spontaneous, assisted, and controlled ventilation modes. Occasionally, an obstruction may develop because of failure of a component during use on a patient.[142]

2. Inadequate amount of gas in the breathing system. An insufficient volume of gas in the breathing system may be attributable to inadequate delivery or excessive loss. Inadequate delivery may be caused by failure of gas delivery to the machine or from the common gas outlet.[56,137] A decrease in oxygen supply pressure to the machine may cause a decrease in gas flows set at the flow-control valves. Flow setting errors may also occur. A disconnection, misconnection, or obstruction between the machine common gas outlet and the patient circuit has a similar effect.

Inadequate volume of gas in the circuit may be caused by excessive removal. In an active scavenging system, wall suction removes the waste gases from the scavenging interface. Excessive negative pressure may be applied to the circuit if the negative pressure–relief valve or valves on the interface become occluded.[145] A similar situation could arise with an open-reservoir scavenging system if the relief ports become occluded while suction is applied to the interface. A high subatmospheric pressure in the scavenging system may open the circuit adjustable pressure-limiting (APL) valve that transmits the subatmospheric pressure to the patient circuit. If a ventilator were being used, unrelieved excess negative pressure in the scavenging system would in most cases hold the ventilator pressure-relief valve to its seat, preventing it from opening on exhalation and causing high pressure to develop in the circuit.[146]

A sidestream sampling gas analyzer (such as a multiplexed mass spectrometer) connected to a patient circuit has been reported as the cause of excessive negative pressure in a breathing circuit in which the fresh gas flow of 50 ml/min during cardiopulmonary bypass was less than the mass spectrometer's gas sampling rate of 250 ml/min.[146] Sampling rates of commonly used gas analyzers vary from less than 50 ml/min to as high as 800 ml/min; therefore considerable potential exists for negative pressure to develop in the circuit if low fresh gas flow rates are used.[146]

Excess removal of gas by a sampling device during spontaneous ventilation creates a subatmospheric pressure in the circuit that in turn causes the APL valve to close, thereby preventing the negative pressure–relief valve or valves in the scavenging system from relieving the negative pressure in the circuit (see Fig. 6-18). During testing, maximum circuit subatmospheric pressure achieved by sidestream sampling devices ranged from -11 to -148 mm Hg. If such low pressures are transmitted to the patient's airway, barotrauma and cardiovascular dysfunction may result.[146]

Excessive volume loss resulting in negative pressures in the breathing system may occur if hospital suction is applied via the working channel of a fiberoptic bronchoscope that has been inserted into the system through an airway diaphragm adapter or if a suction catheter is accidentally advanced alongside the tracheal tube into the trachea.

Inadequate circuit volume and negative pressure may occur during spontaneous ventilation in the presence of a low rate of fresh gas flow and a reservoir bag that is too small (such as pediatric-sized bag used for an adult patient). During inspiration, the reservoir bag would collapse, and negative pressure would accumulate in the circuit. Circuit APL valves usually have a minimum opening pressure that is slightly greater than the pressure needed to distend the reservoir bag. If the bag were the correct size but noncompliant, or the APL valve had a low opening pressure, most of the gas would exit through the APL valve during exhalation rather than filling the bag. The net result would be an inadequate reservoir volume for the next inspiration.[31] Modern circuit-pressure monitors incorporate an audible and visible subatmospheric-pressure alarm that sounds when pressure is less than -10 cm H_2O at any time.[29,30]

3. Failure to initiate artificial ventilation. Failure to initiate artificial ventilation is usually attributable to operator error, such as forgetting to turn on the ventilator (e.g., after cardiopulmonary bypass), accidentally setting a respiratory rate of zero breaths per minute, failure to select the automatic setting for the ventilator at the manual/automatic selector switch in the circuit, or failure to connect the ventilator circuit hose to the patient circuit connector by the selector switch or at the bag mount.[31] Because some older circuit volume and pressure alarms must be deliberately enabled or are enabled only when the ventilator is on, these monitors may not detect forgetting to turn on the ventilator. In this respect, continuous capnography provides the most sensitive monitor of ventilation. If the delivery system incorporates a standing-bellows ventilator, failure to connect the ventilator tubing to the circuit will result in collapse of the bellows. With either bellows design, when a ventilator is turned on but the manual (bag) mode is selected at the selector switch, during inspiration the bellows will attempt to empty against a total obstruction, and failure of the bellows to empty will be readily observed (see Fig. 6-21). In this situation, failure to ventilate causes both the low-pressure and volume alarms to sound. Some older circle systems lack a manual/automatic selector switch, and the APL valve must be closed to initiate intermittent positive-pressure ventilation when the ventilator hose is connected to the bag mount. Failure to close the APL valve in this situation is another cause of failure to initiate intermittent positive-pressure ventilation.

Even if the breathing system incorporates a selector switch, the primary anesthesia ventilator sometimes fails, and a freestanding ventilator is brought in to provide intermittent positive-pressure ventilation. The foregoing considerations apply if the new ventilator is connected to the circuit via the bag mount connection; that is, the manual mode must be selected, and APL valve must be closed. In the North American Dräger AV-2 Plus ventilator, selecting the ventilator mode on the bag/ventilator switch in the circuit automatically turns on the ventilator and its alarms.

4. Leaks and disconnections in the breathing system. Breathing circuit disconnections and leaks are among the most common of anesthesia mishaps.[1,2,112,146] Anesthesia breathing systems contain numerous basic connections as well as supplementary ones as more monitors, humidifiers, and filters are added (see Fig. 6-18). Disconnec-

tions cannot be totally prevented, and the 15-mm connector between the patient and the circuit has been considered by some as a safety fuse to prevent unintentional extubation.[31] Circuit disconnections and their detection have been the subject of several reviews.* Cooper, Newbower, and Kitz[1] and Cooper et al[2] found that disconnection of the patient from the machine was responsible for 7.5% of critical incidents involving human error or equipment failure. Of these disconnections, about 70% occurred at the Y piece.[1,2]

The risk for disconnection is reduced by secure locking of connecting components, use of disconnect alarms (pressure monitors, volume monitors, and capnography), and user education. When a disconnection occurs, the anesthetist must systematically trace the flow of gases through the breathing system to look for the disconnection in the same manner as that used in the event of no-gas-flow or obstruction.[148]

The basic breathing system monitors of pressure and volume can detect most disconnections. Pressure monitors activate an alarm if the peak inspiratory pressure in the circuit fails to reach the threshold low setting. It is important that the alarm setting on the monitor be user adjustable and be capable of being set to a level just below the usual peak inspiratory pressure. Some monitors provide a continuous graphic display of the circuit pressure as well as of the alarm threshold or thresholds.[29] A response algorithm for the low-pressure alarm condition is described elsewhere.[149]

The circuit low-pressure alarm can be fooled if it is not set to be very sensitive. Thus a circuit disconnection at the Y piece combined with sufficient resistance at the patient connector end may not trigger the low-pressure alarm if inspiratory gas flow from the ventilator bellows is high enough and the low-pressure alarm threshold is crossed. Examples include unintended extubation of the trachea in a patient who has a small-diameter tracheal tube (where the tube connector offers high resistance to gas flow) or occlusion of the open patient connector by drapes.[31] A circuit low-pressure alarm that senses pressure in the absorber may be fooled if there is a high resistance between the inspiratory tubing connector and the Y piece, such as may be caused by a cascade humidifier in the inspiratory limb of the circle.[150] Humidifiers may also represent the source of a detectable leak in the anesthesia circuit.[122]

A circuit low-pressure alarm is less likely to be fooled when a standing-bellows ventilator is used because failure of the bellows to fill adequately during exhalation will result in lower peak pressures on the next inspiration. With hanging bellows, the peak inspiratory pressure will tend to be higher because the bellows fills completely during exhalation. A pressure alarm set to an inappropriately low threshold is therefore more likely to be fooled by a hanging-bellows ventilator.

Before the use of retaining devices at the common gas outlet, disconnections could occur at this site.[56] The diameter of the tubing connecting the common gas outlet

---

*References 1, 2, 12, 112, 147, 148.

to the circuit is relatively narrow and offers relatively high resistance to gas flow compared with the 22-mm circuit tubing. If a hanging-bellows ventilator were used with a large tidal volume setting, the resistance in the machine-to-circuit connector tubing might be such that during inspiration, the low-pressure alarm limit would be exceeded despite the leak.[56] During exhalation, room air would be entrained via the fresh gas inflow tubing to refill the bellows. A disconnection of this tubing may also lead to a hypoxic gas mixture in the circuit as air is entrained and oxygen is consumed. An oxygen analyzer with an appropriately set low-oxygen-concentration alarm in the patient circuit can detect this type of disconnection.

If, as is recommended, the circuit low-pressure alarm has been set to just below the peak inspiratory pressure, more false-positive alarms will be generated. Thus for a given ventilator setting of tidal volume, a decrease in fresh gas flow, inspiratory/expiratory ratio, or inspiratory flow rate or an increase in respiratory rate will decrease the peak inspiratory pressure, triggering the alarm. A false-positive alarm with appropriate response is preferable to a false-negative alarm (provided that it does not lead to permanent silencing of the alarm or monitor).

Leaks from the circuit other than those attributable to component disconnection may also result in inadequate exchange of gas between system and patient. Leaks may occur in any component because of cracking,[122] missing Luer lock nipples,[151] incorrect assembly,[119] or malfunction of a system component, particularly the ventilator pressure-relief valve.[71-73]

During inspiration, the ventilator pressure-relief valve is normally held closed by pressure from the driving-gas circuit from the bellows housing. If the pressure-relief valve is not held closed during inspiration, gas in the patient circuit exits to the scavenging system rather than being driven into the patient's lungs (see Fig. 6-19). Ventilator pressure-relief valve incompetence has been reported in connection with pilot-line disconnection or occlusion[113,152] and valve damage.[72,73] In such situations, appropriately set pressure and volume alarms detect the loss of volume from the circuit, but the source of the leak might be less obvious. If a closed-reservoir scavenging system is in use, one pinpoints the problem by observing the scavenging system reservoir bag.[113] The bag normally fills during exhalation (as gas is released from the patient circuit) and empties during inspiration, when the pressure-relief valve is closed (see Fig. 6-19). If the pressure-relief valve is incompetent, the scavenging system reservoir bag will fill during inspiration as the ventilator bellows empties its contained gas into the scavenging system and the scavenging reservoir bag empties during exhalation.[113]

Leaks and malfunctions in the patient circuit are sometimes first detected by an airway gas monitor capable of measuring nitrogen.[153] Application of negative pressure to the circuit by a malfunctioning scavenging system or intermittently by a hanging-bellows ventilator during exhalation may cause air to flow into the breathing system through a small leak that goes unrecognized by pressure, volume, or carbon dioxide monitoring.[153] A leak of room air or other gases into the patient circuit may result in dilution of the anesthesia gas mixture and, in the extreme case, awareness under anesthesia.[154] Leaks into the patient circuit may occur if the high pressure in the driving-gas circuit during inspiration forces driving gas into the patient circuit through a hole in the ventilator bellows. With an Ohmeda ventilator, the diluent gas would be the set tidal volume as 100% oxygen, but with a North American Dräger AV-E, it would be an indeterminate volume of an air/oxygen mixture.[135,155] A multigas or agent analyzer may detect such an event as a change in fraction of inspired oxygen, end-tidal carbon dioxide, or agent concentration. It may also be detectable as a change in peak inspiratory pressure, tidal volume, or minute volume.

5. High pressure in the breathing system. The anesthesia machine provides a continuous flow of gas to the patient circuit. Whenever the rate of circuit gas inflow exceeds the rate of outflow, excessive pressures may develop. If these pressures are transmitted to the patient's lungs, severe cardiovascular compromise, barotrauma, and pneumothorax may result.[156,157]

During spontaneous ventilation, high pressure may result from inadequate opening (or complete closure) of the APL valve, kinking or occlusion of the tubing between this valve and the scavenging interface, or malfunction of the interface (that is, no suction and obstruction of the interface positive-pressure relief valve). Because the patient circuit reservoir bag is "in circuit" during spontaneous ventilation, the bag will distend to accommodate the excess gas. Reservoir bags are highly distensible and limit the maximum circuit pressure to approximately 45 cm H_2O. Nevertheless, such an airway pressure could produce hypotension by inhibiting venous return. Increases in circuit pressure will be more rapid when the fresh gas inflow rate is high (e.g., during prolonged use of the oxygen flush).[28]

Excessive circuit pressures may occur during use of an anesthesia ventilator. Thus during inspiration, the ventilator pressure-relief valve is normally held closed; during expiration, it opens to vent excess gas to the scavenging system. The effects of fresh gas flow, inspiratory/expiratory ratio, and respiratory rate on tidal volume, alveolar ventilation, and, by inference, circuit pressure have been discussed in detail. Selection of a high inspiratory gas flow rate on the ventilator will be associated with increased peak pressures in the circuit.

Ventilator malfunctions resulting in excessive circuit pressures have been reported. Failure of the ventilator to cycle from inspiration to expiration causes driving gas to continue to enter (North American Dräger) or enter but not leave (Ohmeda) the bellows housing.[28] This causes the ventilator pressure-relief valve to remain closed and excess gas to build up pressure within the circuit. The increase in pressure is limited by the pressure of the driving gas in the bellows housing. In North American Dräger ventilators, the pressure of the driving gas in the bellows housing depends on the setting of the inspiratory flow-control knob.[31,71]

Other reported causes of failure of the ventilator pressure-relief valve to open normally include mechanical obstruction of the driving-gas exhaust system (North American Dräger AV-E muffler)[76]; kinking of a ventilator pressure-relief valve pilot line during inspiration[71]; and diffusion of nitrous oxide into the space between the two pieces of rubber constituting the relief valve diaphragm, causing insidious PEEP.[158] Even with normal ventilator function, high pressures in the circuit may be caused by occlusion of the tubing between the ventilator pressure-relief valve and the scavenging system or obstruction of the scavenging interface positive pressure-relief valve (see Fig. 6-19). In such cases, as the pressure in the patient circuit increases, the ventilator bellows empties less completely and may even become distorted.

High pressures arising in the circuit are detected by the circuit pressure monitor, which incorporates two types of alarms.[31] A continuing pressure alarm usually sounds when the circuit pressure remains in excess of +15 cm H_2O for more than 10 seconds. A high-pressure alarm sounds whenever the circuit pressure exceeds the threshold limit, which, in modern monitors, is set by the user but has a default setting of 50 to 65 cm H_2O, depending on the unit. When either of these alarms is activated during mechanical ventilation, a problem with the ventilator circuit should be suspected. Circuit pressure can be immediately relieved by disconnecting the patient from the circuit at the Y piece or by selecting the manual (bag) mode and relieving pressure by the APL valve. The incorporation of safety relief valves into the circuit as a protection against high pressures has not been popular because these devices limit the ability to ventilate the lungs of a patient with poor total thoracic compliance.[31]

As protection against excessive pressures in the patient circuit during mechanical ventilation, circuit pressure-limiting devices are available from Ohmeda and North American Dräger. Ohmeda 7800 series ventilators incorporate an inspiratory high-pressure limit so that when the selected threshold (pressure measured in the patient circuit downstream of the inspiratory unidirectional valve) is exceeded, the ventilator cycles to expiration, the pressure in the driving-gas circuit decreases to zero, and excess gas in the patient circuit is discharged to the scavenging system via the ventilator pressure-relief valve.[68] Basic North American Dräger AV-E ventilators are not pressure-limited, but a pressure-limit control is available and may be retrofitted to certain standing-bellows AV-E units.[159] The AV-E's pressure-limit control device senses the pressure in the patient circuit at the bellows; whenever the threshold high-pressure limit is exceeded, a valve opens in the driving-gas circuit (bellows housing) to release excess driving gas to the atmosphere, thereby limiting driving-gas pressure so that patient circuit pressure does not exceed the set limit for the remainder of the inspiration. The time cycling (inspiratory/expiratory ratio) of the AV-E is thus maintained,[159] in contrast with the Ohmeda 7800 series ventilators.[68] Both the North American Dräger and the Ohmeda approaches to limiting pressure in the patient circuit require a normally functioning ventilator pressure-relief valve, because it is through this valve (the opening pressure of which is controlled by the pressure in the driving-gas circuit) that the patient circuit is relieved of excess gas and pressure. If the pressure-relief valve or its outflow path becomes obstructed, neither the North American Dräger nor the Ohmeda pressure-limiting mechanisms would be effective in relieving pressure in the patient circuit.

F. Anesthetic agent dose and administration problems

Patient complications can result from overdose or underdose with an anesthetic agent or from administration of an incorrect agent. The chances of vaporizer malfunction resulting in anesthetic overdose or underdose are perhaps greater with a rebreathing system than with a circle system. In the former system, high flows of fresh gas are delivered directly to the patient's airway, whereas in the latter system, there is a greater discrepancy between delivered and inspired agent concentrations unless high flows are used.

1. Liquid agent in the fresh gas piping. Lethal overdose with an anesthetic agent may occur when excessive amounts of saturated vapor or liquid agent enter the fresh gas delivery system.[160] The former situation is more likely to occur with a measured-flow vaporizer arrangement (Copper Kettle or Verni-Trol) because errors in calculation or flow setting can easily arise. In addition, some older model vaporizers can be overfilled so that excess liquid could enter the fresh gas delivery system. Modern vaporizers are concentration calibrated and are designed to prevent overfilling.[9]

Tilting or tipping of a vaporizer may cause liquid agent to enter the fresh gas or bypass lines. Such an occurrence could result in lethal concentrations of vapor being delivered to the common gas outlet of the machine and to the patient circuit. One milliliter of a potent volatile liquid agent will produce approximately 200 ml of vapor at 20° C (see Table 6-1).[45] If 1 ml of liquid halothane entered the common gas tubing and evaporate, at a temperature of 20° C, 11 L of fresh gas would be required to dilute the resulting vapor to a concentration of 2% or a MAC of approximately 3. It is easy to appreciate how a relatively small volume of liquid agent in the wrong place can have a profound effect on a patient.

If a vaporizer has been tilted or tipped and there is concern that liquid agent may have leaked into the fresh gas delivery system, the patient should be immediately disconnected from the breathing system. The vaporizer should then be purged with a high flow of oxygen from the flow-control valve (not the oxygen flush, which bypasses the vaporizer) with the vaporizer dial set to a high concentration. If any doubt still exists about the safe function of the vaporizer, it should be withdrawn from clinical service until it is certified by an authorized service representative as safe for use. Additional caution is needed with a halothane vaporizer that has been tipped. Liquid halothane contains thymol, a sticky preservative that does not evaporate; thus thymol entering the flow-control and temperature-compensating parts of a vaporizer could cause vaporizer malfunction even after the halothane has been flushed out of these parts.

Modern vaporizers are mounted on the back bar of the anesthesia machine. Ohmeda Tec 4 and Tec 5 vaporizers are designed to be easily mounted on or removed from Selectatec series mounted manifolds.[161,162] Because they are designed to be removable, Tec vaporizers incorporate an antispill mechanism that prevents liquid agent from entering the bypass sections.[161,162] Dräger Vapor 19.1 vaporizers are not designed to be easily removable and are more permanently mounted on North American Dräger Narkomed machines.[44] Only authorized personnel should remove these vaporizers. These vaporizers do not incorporate an antispill mechanism; the risk for spillage is in theory minimized by the "permanent" mounting. Nevertheless, spillage of liquid agent could occur in such vaporizers if the whole Narkomed machine were tilted or even laid on its side. This may occur if the machine overhangs an electrically powered operating table that is being raised.

Vaporizers in the United States may be of the funnel-fill or key-fill design, whereas the latter design is mandatory in Canada. Overfilling of key-fill design vaporizers has been described. Key-fill systems are designed to be used with (1) a gas-tight joint between the bottle of anesthetic liquid and the corresponding agent-specific vaporizer and (2) the vaporizer dial turned to the off position during filling. Correct use of the key-fill system prevents overfilling by two mechanisms. First, intake of gas into the bottle of anesthetic liquid ceases when the maximum safe level of liquid agent in the vaporizing chamber has been reached. Second, when the vaporizer is off, the gas space at the top of the vaporizing chamber is sealed, thereby preventing overfilling. Slow filling of a key-fill vaporizer has led to such incorrect practices as speed filling. Such practices include loosening of the seal between the bottle and the vaporizer, which permits direct unlimited entry of room air into the bottle (rather than only the gas in the vaporizing chamber) and turning the vaporizer dial to the on position. Such a double-fault condition permits an excessive amount of room air to enter the agent bottle and therefore an excessive amount of liquid anesthetic agent to enter the vaporizer. This practice is reported to have caused anesthetic overdose and other adverse outcomes.[163,164]

2. Concentration dial design. Overdose with an anesthetic agent may also occur if a vaporizer delivers unexpectedly high but not lethal concentrations of agent. In modern vaporizers, concentration is increased when one turns the dial counterclockwise.[9] However, in some older vaporizers, turning the dial clockwise increases agent concentration. Some machines may still be equipped with the older design or a combination of the two designs, which might present a hazard if the dial is turned inappropriately. It is therefore important that the anesthetist deliberately observe the dial and calibration settings when changing a vaporizer dial concentration setting (Fig. 6-23).

3. Incorrect filling of vaporizers

a. Single agent. Overdose or underdose with an anesthetic agent can occur if an agent-specific vaporizer is filled wholly or partially with an incorrect agent.[44] If an empty concentration-calibrated variable-bypass vaporizer designed for one agent is filled with an inappropriate agent, the vaporizer concentration output may be erroneous.[165,166] At room temperature, the vaporizing characteristics of halothane and isoflurane are almost identical to those of enflurane and sevoflurane. Currently, this problem really applies only to interchanging halothane or isoflurane with enflurane or sevoflurane (see Table 6-1).

A more dangerous situation would be created if a vaporizer designed for methoxyflurane (an agent with a sat-

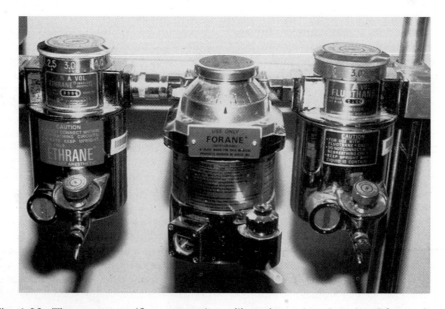

Fig. 6-23. Three agent-specific concentration-calibrated vaporizers in series. Of note, there is no interlock system, and the outer vaporizers (Foregger) produce an increase in concentration when the dial is rotated clockwise. In the center vaporizer, which is of contemporary configuration, counterclockwise dial rotation increases output concentration.

urated vapor pressure of 20.3 mm Hg at 20° C) were filled with halothane, enflurane, sevoflurane, or isoflurane (see Table 6-1). A methoxyflurane vaporizer filled with halothane and set to deliver 1% methoxyflurane (6 MAC of methoxyflurane) would deliver 14.8% (approximately 20 MAC) halothane. If the vaporizer is set to deliver 1 MAC (0.16%) of methoxyflurane, it produces a flow split of 16:1, similar to that of a halothane or isoflurane variable-bypass vaporizer set to deliver 2.7% (see Table 6-2). Because methoxyflurane has almost completely disappeared from clinical use, such errors are now unlikely to occur.

The outputs of erroneously filled variable-bypass vaporizers are shown in Table 6-3. Erroneous filling affects the output concentration and, consequently, the MAC or potency output of the vaporizer.[165] Thus an enflurane vaporizer set to 2% (1.19 MAC) but filled with halothane will deliver 3.21% (4.01 MAC) of halothane, or 3.3 times the anticipated potency of anesthetic output (see Table 6-3).[165] Because enflurane and sevoflurane have similar saturated vapor pressures at 20° C and similar MACs, filling an enflurane vaporizer with sevoflurane or a sevoflurane vaporizer with enflurane is predicted to have the fewest consequences.[167]

Erroneous filling of vaporizers may be prevented by paying careful attention to the agent used and the vaporizer. Agent-specific keyed-filling mechanisms, analogous to the pin-indexed system for medical gases, are available as options on modern vaporizers.[14,44,161,162] Liquid anesthetic agents are available in bottles that have an agent-specific collar. Agent-specific filling devices have one end that fits the collar on the agent bottle and another end that fits only the vaporizer designed for that agent. These filling devices, although well intentioned, have not gained much popularity in the United States. Thus agents are not always supplied in agent-specific collared bottles, and even the problem of erroneous fitting of a collar to a bottle has been reported.[168] The ASTM F1161-88 standard states that the vaporizer filling mechanism should be fitted with a permanently attached standard, agent-specific keyed-filling device to prevent accidental filling with the wrong agent.[9] As mentioned previously, the key-fill design is mandatory in Canada, where incorrect use of key-fillers has been reported to cause adverse outcomes.[165]

Agent-specific filling devices assume even greater importance with desflurane, which has a saturated vapor pressure of 669 mm Hg at 20° C and a boiling point of 22.8° C (see Box 6-1). Filling a variable-bypass vaporizer (e.g., the Ohmeda Tec 4 or Tec 5 or the Dräger Vapor 19.1) with desflurane may result in very high concentration outputs of this agent. An isoflurane variable-bypass vaporizer that is set to deliver 1% isoflurane (0.87 MAC) but is filled with desflurane will deliver approximately 13% desflurane (2.6 MAC) at 20° C. A small increase in temperature would result in a drastically increased output concentration and could become uncontrolled and potentially lethal if the desflurane were to boil. Andrews, Johnston, and Kramer[48] presented a mathematical model that demonstrates the potential for desflurane overdose in such a situation. To prevent such an occurrence, desflurane is supplied in bottles equipped with an agent-specific filling device that can only be used to fill a desflurane vaporizer.

b. Mixed agents. Perhaps a more likely scenario is that an agent-specific vaporizer is partially filled with the correct agent but is topped up with an incorrect agent.[165] This situation is more complex; the vaporizer output is more difficult to predict, and large errors in vapor delivery may occur. When mixed, halothane, enflurane, and isoflurane do not react chemically but do influence the extent of each other's ease of vaporization.[169] For example, halothane facilitates the vaporization of both enflurane and isoflurane and, in the process, is itself more likely to vaporize.[169] The clinical consequences depend on the potencies of each of the mixed agents as well as the delivered vapor concentrations. If a halothane vaporizer that is 25% full is refilled to 100% with isoflurane and set to deliver 1%, the halothane output is 0.41% (0.51 MAC), and the isoflurane output is 0.9% (0.78 MAC) (Table 6-4).[165] In this case, the output potency of 1.29 MAC is close to the expected 1.25 MAC (1% halothane).

On the other hand, an enflurane vaporizer that is 25% full and is set to deliver 2% (1.19 MAC) enflurane, which is then filled to 100% with halothane, has an output of 2.43% (3.03 MAC) halothane and 0.96% (0.57 MAC) enflurane

Table 6-3. Oxygen output of erroneously filled vaporizers at 22° C

Vaporizers	Liquid	Setting (%)	Output (%)	Output (MAC)*
Halothane	Halothane	1.0	1.00	1.25
	Enflurane	1.0	0.62	0.37
	Isoflurane	1.0	0.96	0.84
Enflurane	Enflurane	2.0	2.00	1.19
	Isoflurane	2.0	3.09	2.69
	Halothane	2.0	3.21	4.01
Isoflurane	Isoflurane	1.5	1.50	1.30
	Halothane	1.5	1.56	1.95
	Enflurane	1.5	0.97	0.57

From Bruce DL, Linde HW: *Anesthesiology* 60:342, 1984.
*MAC, Minimum alveolar concentration in vol%.

Table 6-4. Vaporizer output after incorrect refilling from 25% full to 100% full

Vaporizer	Setting%	Refill liquid	Halothane %	Halothane MAC*	Enflurane %	Enflurane MAC	Isoflurane %	Isoflurane MAC	Total MAC
Halothane	1.0	Enflurane	0.33	0.41	0.64	0.38	—	—	0.79
	1.0	Isoflurane	0.41	0.51	—	—	0.90	0.78	1.29
Enflurane	2.0	Halothane	2.43	3.03	0.96	0.57	—	—	3.60
Isoflurane	1.5	Halothane	1.28	1.60	—	—	0.57	0.50	2.10

From Bruce DL, Linde HW: *Anesthesiology* 60:342, 1984.
*MAC, Minimum alveolar concentration in vol%.

(see Table 6-4).[165] This represents a total MAC of 3.6, or more than twice that intended. In any event, erroneous filling of vaporizers must be avoided, and if erroneous filling is suspected, the vaporizer must be emptied and, if necessary, serviced, purged, and refilled with the correct agent.

4. Simultaneous use of more than one vaporizer. Modern anesthesia vaporizers incorporate an interlock system to prevent simultaneous use of more than one vaporizer and agent.[9] Older anesthesia machines had up to three variable-bypass vaporizers arranged in series such that fresh gas passed through each vaporizer (albeit via the bypass flow) to reach the common gas outlet of the anesthesia machine. Without an interlock device, which would have permitted only one vaporizer to be in use at any time, it was possible to have all three vaporizers on simultaneously (see Fig. 6-22). Apart from potentially causing anesthetic overdose, the agent from the upstream vaporizer could contaminate the agent or agents in those downstream.[170,171] During subsequent use, the output of the downstream vaporizer would be contaminated; as a result, the concentration and results of the emerging gas and vapor mixture would be indeterminate and possibly lethal. With in-series arrangements, care must be taken to ensure that only one vaporizer is on at any time, and to minimize risk to the patient if cross-contamination occurs, the sequence of vaporizers from upstream to downstream should be such that the agent that has the lowest saturated vapor pressure is upstream (that is, farthest from the patient). The most appropriate in-series sequence would therefore be methoxyflurane, sevoflurane, enflurane, isoflurane, and halothane; halothane would be closest to the common gas outlet of the anesthesia machine. Because the use of vaporizer safety interlocking devices is widespread, the foregoing strategy may be of historical interest only.

Although vaporizer interlock systems are a desirable (and now standard) safety feature on modern machines,[9] failures of these systems have been reported with variable-bypass vaporizers[111,127,172,173] as well as the Ohmeda Tec 6 desflurane vaporizer. Failure may make it possible for more than one vaporizer to be on at one time.[172] Exclusion of the selected vaporizer has been described with a Selectatec system.[173] It is therefore important that the anesthetist check the interlock system periodically for correct function.

The good intentions of the vaporizer interlock system can also be defeated if a freestanding vaporizer is used in series with the fresh gas flow but downstream of the common gas outlet. Such arrangements, configured by the user, are potentially dangerous and should not be used.[174] Freestanding vaporizers are still used, however, on cardiopulmonary bypass machines, in veterinary facilities, and in laboratories. Such vaporizers can be hazardous because they are easily tipped (liquid agents can enter the vaporizer bypass, resulting in overdose). In addition, reversal of gas flow direction through a variable-bypass vaporizer can profoundly affect its performance, depending on the model of vaporizer. Reversal of the gas inflow and outflow connections to a freestanding vaporizer in clinical practice has been reported to result in delivery of dangerously high concentrations of anesthetic agent.[175,176] Ohmeda Tec series vaporizers may be mounted on cardiopulmonary bypass machines by using a specially designed bracket and vaporizer manifold available from the manufacturer; the gas inflow and outflow connections are clearly labeled.

5. Pumping effect. Measured-flow vaporizers and other older concentration-calibrated vaporizers were subject to the so-called "pumping effect," which may result in increased output concentrations, during mechanical ventilation when low fresh gas flow rates were in use. The explanation for this effect is that during positive-pressure ventilation, increases in pressure in the vaporizer cause bypass gas to enter the vaporizing chamber of the vaporizer, thereby increasing vapor output.[14] Recent vaporizing systems are designed to be compensated for or protected against the pumping effect.[44,161,162] In older Ohmeda anesthesia machines, vaporizer protection is afforded by an outlet check valve located just upstream of the common gas outlet (see Fig. 6-2), which prevents increases in pressure in the patient circuit from being transmitted back into the machine and to the vaporizer. Some older vaporizers (such as the Ohio Ethrane vaporizer, Ohio Medical, Madison, Wisconsin) incorporated a check valve in the vaporizer outlet.[55] Contemporary variable-bypass vaporizers (the Ohmeda Tec 4 and Tec 5 and Dräger Vapor 19.1) use baffles or other design features rather than check valves to prevent the pumping effect.[16,160-162]

If an anesthesia machine is used for a patient who is susceptible to malignant hyperthermia, it has been recommended that the vaporizers be removed and that the machine be flushed with oxygen at 10 L/min for 5 minutes. In addition, the fresh gas outlet hose should be replaced, and a new disposable circle should be used.[177] However, others have disagreed with some of these recommendations.[178]

6. Anesthetic agent underdose. Anesthetic agent underdose may also occur, resulting in light anesthesia, patient movement, or even awareness. Perhaps the most common cause of this problem is the user forgetting to turn the vaporizer on. In some early vaporizer exclusion systems (North American Dräger Vapor, Ohio Selectatec), the vaporizer dial could be turned on while the vaporizer was excluded from the gas delivery system. In recent systems, the exclusion mechanism is activated only when the vaporizer is turned on, avoiding this potential problem.[29,161,162]

7. Ohmeda Tec 6 desflurane vaporizer. As noted in a previous section, the Ohmeda Tec 6 vaporizer differs substantially from the variable-bypass vaporizer used for agents other than desflurane. Because of this, different problems might be expected to result from malfunctions of the various electronic and mechanical components. Reported problems include delivery of vapor concentrations greater than those set on the dial and problems with the interlock system in models designed to be mounted on North American Dräger anesthesia machines.[179-183]

8. Miscellaneous malfunctions. An internal malfunction of the vaporizer may result in unintentional delivery of high concentrations of anesthetic vapor. Regular checking of function and calibration of output are therefore essential. Such checking should ideally be performed in the usual-use environment of the vaporizer. The output of Ohmeda Tec 4 vaporizers has been found to be accurate in the proximity of a 1.5 Tesla magnet in a magnetic resonance imaging suite.[184,185]

Although numerous design features have helped make contemporary vaporizing systems safer for the patient, an agent-specific analyzer should ideally be used in the patient circuit to monitor inhaled concentrations.[186] Various units using different technologies are available, all of which incorporate alarm features.

G. Humidification problems

Humidification of the inspired gases is desirable because it (1) prevents heat loss caused by evaporation of water from the tracheobronchial tree, (2) maintains moisture in the conducting airways and thereby facilitates ciliary function, and (3) prevents water loss from the patient by evaporation. Humidity can be provided by heat and moisture exchange devices that are attached to the tracheal tube[187,188] and by moistening the inside of the breathing tubes and reservoir bag with water before use. In addition, unheated water vaporizers can be used to provide moisture to the patient. However, a system that does not use heat will cool as evaporation takes place and will therefore generate less humidity.[14]

Heated humidifiers (vaporizers) are devices through which the inspired gases are passed to become saturated with water at the temperature of the humidifier. The dry gases either bubble through the humidifier or pass over or blow by the surface of the water. Heat is usually provided by electricity. The advantage of this type of system is that the inspired gases become saturated with water at

a higher temperature. However, as the gas cools on leaving the humidifier, condensation will occur in the tubing and the amount of humidity delivered to the patient will decrease. The condensation problem can be managed by heating the gases in the inspiratory hose either externally or internally with a heating wire. Keeping the distance from the humidifier to the patient as short as possible will also decrease the amount of condensation.

Another technique is to heat the humidifier to a temperature higher than body temperature so that as the inspired gases cool in the inspiratory tubing, they enter the tracheal tube at the desired temperature. Care must be taken when using this technique to avoid burning the patient's tracheobronchial tree. It is therefore mandatory to monitor the temperature of the inspired gases at the tracheal tube to ensure that the gases are not too hot. Because the gases that are delivered to the patient have a maximum relative humidity of 100%, there is little chance that the patient will be overloaded with fluid when a heated humidifier is used.[14]

Hazards associated with the artificial nose (heat and moisture exchanger) include misconnection, obstruction, and disconnection.[189,190] A heated humidifier may cause bulk delivery of water to the patient, thermal trauma to the airway, obstruction of the breathing circuit, and electrical and fire hazards. These devices are powered by electricity, and thermostat failure may cause superheating of the gases in the humidifier, resulting in softening of the plastic inspiratory tubing.[14,191] Softening of the inspiratory hose may in turn lead to complete occlusion of the inspiratory hose and thereby prevent the patient's lungs from being ventilated. One can avoid this problem by making sure that the gas flow through the humidifier is initiated before the humidifier is turned on.[139] Other hazards, such as erroneously filling the humidifier with a liquid other than water, will create a hazard that is determined by the chemical used and the amount of exposure that the patient receives.

Humidity can also be provided with a nebulizer technique. Nebulizers create droplets of water through a jet of gas over the surface of the water or by ultrasonic means. Unlike the heated vaporizer, the nebulizer creates three hazards. It can act as a nidus for bacterial transmission, respiratory resistance may increase, and the patient may become overhydrated. Therefore extreme care should be taken in cleaning the nebulizer, sterile water must be used, and the amount of water delivered must be carefully monitored. In addition, because of the risk for increased respiratory resistance, nebulizers should probably not be used in patients who are breathing spontaneously.

When using heated humidifiers or nebulizers, the anesthesiologist should guard against fluid overload, thermal injury, additional sites of disconnection within the breathing circuit, obstruction to gas flow, burning of the equipment because of electrical malfunction, shock hazards, and risk for transmission of infection via the nebulizer.[14,191]

H. Electrical failures

Before the late 1970s, most anesthesia machines were completely mechanical or pneumatic and had no electrical components. These machines consisted of a gas piping system, regulators, valves, flow-control valves, vaporizers, and a ventilator that was completely pneumatic. Pneumatically or battery-powered monitoring and alarm systems were attached to the machine.

During the 1980s, anesthesia machines were redesigned to include electrical systems that control the ventilator, alarm system, and integrated monitors (e.g., the North American Dräger Narkomed 2B).[192] This type of machine is equipped with a power cord and accepts an electrical input of 90 to 130 volts at 50 to 60 Hz. There are four electrical outlets on the anesthesia machine into which additional equipment can be plugged. It also has a battery backup system consisting of a 12-volt rechargeable battery; this system is activated when the alternating current (AC) to the machine fails.

Before using the machine, the operator should check the status of the AC power supply and the charge on the battery. Use should not be started if the power has failed or the battery is not charged. A discharged battery takes 16 hours to recharge.[192]

The main on/off switch on the machine turns on the electrical supply and mechanically opens the flow of gases to their flow-control valves and flowmeters. Even if the electrical system failed completely, the flow of gas to the flowmeter would not be interrupted. If the AC power failed, the battery backup system would take over. However, the backup battery provides power only to the ventilator control circuits, the monitors built into the machine, and the alarm system. Any peripheral device that is plugged into the AC receptacles in the machine will lose power when AC power to the machine fails.

The backup battery system will provide power for at least 30 minutes. When the battery voltage decreases to 10 volts, all electrical power to the anesthesia machine ceases in order to prevent the battery from deeply discharging. At that point, the ventilator will stop and the monitors and alarms in the machine will cease to function. Patient ventilation must be performed manually until the power is restored.[192]

Some electrical problems are common. The main on/off switch on the anesthesia machine may be left in the on position and the power cord may be disconnected from the wall. This will result in discharge of the battery, and the machine will deliver gases when turned on, but no electrical monitors or alarms will function until the battery can be recharged. Alternatively, the power cord from the machine may be plugged into a receptacle that is built into the machine. In this circumstance, the machine is not powered by the external AC power supply and runs off of the battery system only. Any other device that is plugged into the other receptacles will not receive power.

The North American Dräger Narkomed 2B anesthesia machine incorporates three circuit breakers. They are associated with the primary AC power supply, the battery, and the convenience receptacles. When the circuit breaker for the convenience receptacles is in the open (tripped) position, the receptacles will not be energized. In this case, the source of the tripping of the circuit breaker should be sought, and the breaker should be reset.[192]

Hospitals are required to have backup electrical power supplies so that electricity is supplied in the event of a primary power source failure. However, all power to an operating room can be lost if both the primary and backup systems fail or if the terminal power distribution (wires and circuit breakers) fails.[193] These problems can be dealt with and overcome by the use of uninterruptible power supplies (backup batteries) located in the operating room. However, these power supplies are limited in their storage capacity and therefore in their ability to deliver electrical power. Heath care organizations must determine how much emergency power in the form of batteries is desirable and how much money should be spent on this resource.

When the AC power supply to the operating room fails completely, all electrical equipment that does not have a backup battery will cease to function. Electrically powered patient monitors will cease to function unless AC power can be restored. In addition, important life-support devices, such as the cardiopulmonary bypass machine, will also stop and will require either manual or battery power to maintain artificial circulation. Finally, the operating room lights may fail during total loss of electricity; this problem must be managed with flashlights.[194,195]

I. Other potential complications

Monitoring of the anesthesia breathing system to assess function of the delivery system assumes that any failure will be detectable as an abnormality of pressure, volume, flow, or gas composition and that the commonly used monitoring systems will detect such abnormalities. Although this is true for most failures, scenarios continue to be reported in which state-of-the-art monitoring failed to detect an abnormality or potential hazard.

1. Carbon monoxide accumulation. Several instances of carbon monoxide accumulation in the breathing system during enflurane, isoflurane, and desflurane anesthesia have been reported. Carbon monoxide poisoning usually occurred in the first patient to undergo general anesthesia on a Monday morning after the anesthesia machine had been unused over the 2-day weekend.[196,197] In one study, the reported incidence of intraoperative carbon monoxide exposure was 4.4 per 1000 of the first patients of the day and 2.6 per 1000 total patients.[198] The toxic effects of carbon monoxide have been described elsewhere and depend on the concentration of carbon monoxide and duration of exposure.[199] Carbon monoxide poisoning can result from the reaction of desflurane, enflurane, and isoflurane with dry Baralyme and soda lime.[199] When they contain standard amounts of water, these absorbents generate no carbon monoxide, whereas very high concentrations of carbon monoxide can result when these absorbents are dry.[199]

Halothane and sevoflurane do not seem to react with dry or wet absorbent agents to produce carbon monoxide.[199] Factors leading to carbon monoxide formation include higher temperature of the absorbent agent, drier absorbent, and higher concentration of anesthetic agent. Risk is greater with use of barium hydroxide lime than with soda lime and with use of the following agents (listed in descending order of risk): desflurane, enflurane, and isoflurane.[199] It is believed that in the reported clinical cases, continued flow of dry gas through the carbon dioxide absorbent over 26 to 48 hours caused the absorbent to lose moisture. When the machine was used with desflurane, enflurane, or isoflurane (usually on a Monday morning), carbon monoxide was produced, causing increased carboxyhemoglobin concentrations.[199]

Intraoperative detection of carbon monoxide in the breathing system or in the anesthetized patient is difficult because commonly used respiratory gas monitors do not monitor carbon monoxide.[200,201] If carbon monoxide poisoning is suspected, an arterial blood sample should be sent for laboratory hemoximetry.

If the carbon dioxide absorbent agent in the circle system is known or suspected to be desiccated, it should not be used. One should avoid the use of high fresh gas flow rates for prolonged periods, consider changing the carbon dioxide absorbent on Monday mornings, and change the absorbent or add water to it if the machine was left for days with gas flowing.[202] Thus although monitoring the breathing system for the presence of carbon monoxide is not generally feasible, it should be possible to prevent carbon monoxide poisoning because the causes of carbon monoxide generation in breathing circuits are understood.

2. Radiofrequency interference and cellular telephones. Several reports describe how the radiation emitted by portable transmitting devices (e.g., cellular telephones and walkie-talkies) may interfere with the function of microprocessor-controlled electronic equipment, particularly sophisticated ventilators and monitors.[203] The Emergency Care Research Institute recommends that health care facilities proscribe the use of transmitting devices in operating rooms, intensive care units, and other critical care areas.[204] An awareness of this potential problem is becoming increasingly important as anesthesia delivery and monitoring systems become more computer dependent.

III. PREVENTION OF COMPLICATIONS
A. Preuse check of the anesthesia delivery system

The purpose of preuse check of the anesthesia delivery system is to ensure that all of the necessary equipment is present and functioning as expected before induction of anesthesia. The usefulness of this is self-evident; moreover, it is supported by anesthesia literature that describes anesthesia machine malfunctions that could have been discovered before induction if the equipment had been checked thoroughly.[205] The FDA's *Anesthesia Apparatus Checkout Recommendations,*[206] published in August 1986, stated that "this checkout, or a reasonable equivalent, should be conducted before administering anesthesia. This is a guideline which users are encouraged to modify to accommodate differences in equipment design and variations in local clinical practice. Such local modifications should have appropriate peer review. Users should refer to the operator's manual for special procedures or precautions." However, a 1991 study showed that anesthesia practitioners could not detect 70% of cases of machine faults despite use of the 1986 FDA recommendations.[207] The checklist was revisited, and a revised version was published in 1993 (Appendix 6-1, p. 155).[208] Many anesthesia departments have

adopted these recommendations without modification, whereas others have modified them to suit their needs. Whichever approach is taken, it is critical that the machine be carefully inspected and checked before use. A study by Olympio, Goldstein, and Mathes[209] found that anesthesia apparatus checkout procedures improved after intensive training sessions, although high rates of compliance were not achieved.

When the delivery system is checked before the start of anesthesia, it is desirable to arrange it in the way it will be used during surgery. Moving the machine after anesthesia has begun, modifying the breathing circuit with a humidifier, or adding other components can affect the performance of the anesthesia delivery system. Inspecting the machine under the conditions in which it will be used during surgery will minimize this type of problem.[71] However, the preoperative equipment check does not guard against intraoperative equipment failure. The anesthesiologist must be vigilant in monitoring of equipment performance and must be ready to intervene in any hazardous situation.

The generic FDA Anesthesia Apparatus Checkout Recommendations are self-explanatory (see Appendix 6-1). Of particular note is item 1, which states that backup ventilation equipment should be available and functioning. Thus the mere presence of a self-inflating resuscitation bag is not enough; it must also be tested to ensure that it can develop pressure sufficient to ventilate the patient's lungs.

With reference to item 5 ("perform leak check of machine low-pressure system"), it has been reported that the negative-pressure leak test is the most sensitive for detecting leaks in the low-pressure system (i.e., the components located between the flowmeter control valves and the common gas outlet) of all anesthesia delivery systems.[210] Although some have recommended the adoption of this test as the universal low-pressure leak test,[211] leak-check procedures recommended by the machine manufacturer in the operator's manual should also be heeded. North American Dräger describes a positive-pressure leak check for Narkomed machines,[29] whereas Ohmeda recommends a negative-pressure leak check for the recent Modulus and Excel machines.[30]

Item 13 requires that the alarm limits of all monitors be checked, calibrated, and set. The volume settings of all audible alarms should be set so that they are appropriate for the conditions under which the machine will be used. If the room is noisy (e.g., during orthopedic surgery), greater volume settings will be required so that the sound of the alarm will command the attention of the anesthesiologist.

B. Anesthesia machine standards and obsolescence

The American National Standards Institute Z-79.8 standard, approved in 1979, greatly improved the design and safety features of the anesthesia machines produced in the subsequent decade.[9] The ASA Committee on Equipment and Standards examined the issue of aging anesthesia gas machines, beginning with a panel on anesthesia machine obsolescence at the 1988 ASA meeting.[212]

In March 1989, the ASA Board of Directors approved the following policy submitted by the Committee on

Equipment and Standards: "The age of an anesthesia gas machine has not been demonstrated to be a factor in anesthetic mishaps. An anesthesia gas machine, however, which no longer functions as designed and is not modified to meet acceptable levels of performance and monitoring should not be used. Each anesthesia department should establish a protocol to ensure that all anesthesia staff members are qualified in the operation of each type of gas machine, ventilator, and monitor before use."[213]

The most recent anesthesia machine standard is the ASTM F1161-88.[9] Contemporary North American Dräger Narkomed and Ohmeda machines far exceed this standard, and both companies offer an evaluation program with a view to upgrading or replacing older equipment that may no longer be considered acceptable.

A list of the important aspects of the recent ASTM F1161-88 standard follows. Numbers in parentheses refer to sections in the standards document. Users are encouraged to review the original document for further details.[6]

1. Flow control (section 9.1). Only one flow-adjustment control for each gas delivered to the common gas outlet shall be provided. Thus banks of flow-control valves in parallel with separate high- and low-flow controls for the same gas are now undesirable. Some new anesthesia machines include separate flow-control and delivery nipples for oxygen. This does not violate the standard because oxygen is not being delivered to the common gas outlet.

2. Concentration-calibrated vaporizers (section 12.1). All vaporizers located within the fresh gas circuit shall be concentration-calibrated. Control of the vapor concentration shall be provided by means of calibrated knobs or dials (12.1.1). Measured-flow vaporizers (Copper Kettle and Verni-Trol) are not mentioned and therefore are no longer considered up-to-date.

3. Common gas outlet (section 13.1.1). When the common gas outlet is connected to the breathing system by a fresh gas supply hose, the common gas outlet shall be provided with a retaining device. The outlet should have a manufacturer-specific fitting.

4. Alarms (section 16). Monitor alarms should be categorized as high, medium, or low priority. The alarms should be distinguishable audibly and visually, and the operator response should be immediate, prompt, or at least display awareness, according to clinical priority and appropriateness. Present machines should therefore incorporate an integrated and prioritized alarm system.

5. Oxygen supply precautions (section 17). The machine must be designed so that whenever the oxygen supply pressure is reduced from normal (manufacturer

specified) and until flow ceases, the set oxygen concentration shall not decrease at the common gas outlet. The oxygen concentration in the anesthesia circuit shall be measured, and the analyzer will sound a high-priority alarm when the concentration falls below the preset threshold. The machine is designed so that the oxygen analyzer is enabled and functioning whenever the machine is capable of delivering an anesthetic mixture.

6. Ventilatory monitoring (section 18). The anesthesia machine shall have breathing pressure monitoring as well as either exhaled volume or ventilatory carbon dioxide monitoring. The alarms associated with these monitors are to be enabled and function automatically whenever the machine is in use.

Refer to the original document for further information and for the rationale for the stated requirements.[9]

IV. CONCLUSIONS

Misuse or component failure of the anesthesia delivery system may cause complications to the patient.[7,214] Delivery systems continue to evolve as more is learned about patient safety and as design and monitoring features are added.[214] Clearly a basic understanding of the structure and function of these systems will enhance patient safety by avoiding misuse, facilitating troubleshooting, or allowing the use of alternative techniques if a component fails. All locations in which anesthesia is performed should have an adequate backup tank supply of oxygen and a functioning, self-inflating resuscitation bag immediately available for use in the event of a total machine failure.

From their review of the ASA closed claims project database, Caplan et al[7] were not able to specifically address the question of whether older anesthesia machines are more likely to be associated with gas delivery equipment-related malpractice claims. Anesthesia machine obsolescence is a controversial issue[8,215-217] that may become more so with increasing concerns about cost containment. It is estimated that 40,000 anesthesia machines are in use in the United States; their average age is 7 years.[218] Machines are generally purchased with a 10- to 15-year replacement cycle, but there may be economic pressure to extend this period, leading to a potential increase in the number of machines in use that lack desirable safety design features. Although some states (in particular, New York and New Jersey) have implemented regulation with regard to the practice of anesthesiology, as of 1998 only New Jersey has published regulations for requirements for anesthesia equipment, safety, maintenance, and inspection.[219]

Anesthesia Apparatus Checkout Recommendations, 1993

This checkout, or a reasonable equivalent, should be conducted before administration of anesthesia. These recommendations are only valid for an anesthesia system that conforms to current and relevant standards and includes an ascending bellows ventilator and at least the following monitors: capnograph, pulse oximeter, oxygen analyzer, respiratory volume monitor (spirometer), and breathing system pressure monitor with high and low pressure alarms.

This is a guideline which users are encouraged to modify to accommodate differences in equipment design and variations in local clinical practice. Such local modifications should have appropriate peer review. Users should refer to the operator's manual for the manufacturer's specific procedures and precautions, especially the manufacturer's low pressure leak test (step #5).

Emergency Ventilation Equipment
*1. **Verify Backup Ventilation Equipment Is Available and Functioning**

High Pressure System
*2. **Check Oxygen Cylinder Supply**
   a. Open O_2 cylinder and verify at least half full (about 1000 psi).
   b. Close cylinder.
*3. **Check Central Pipeline Supplies**
   a. Check that hoses are connected and pipeline gauges read about 50 psi.

Low Pressure System
*4. **Check Initial Status of Low Pressure System**
   a. Close flow control valves and turn vaporizers off.
   b. Check fill level and tighten vaporizers' filler caps.
*5. **Perform Leak Check of Machine Low Pressure System**
   a. Verify that the machine master switch and flow control valves are OFF.
   b. Attach "Suction Bulb" to common (fresh) gas outlet.
   c. Squeeze bulb repeatedly until fully collapsed.
   d. Verify bulb stays fully collapsed for at least 10 seconds.
   e. Open one vaporizer at a time and repeat 'c' and 'd' as above.
   f. Remove suction bulb, and reconnect fresh gas hose.
*6. **Turn on Machine Master Switch and All Other Necessary Electrical Equipment**
*7. **Test Flowmeters**
   a. Adjust flow of all gases through their full range, checking for smooth operation of floats and undamaged flowtubes.
   b. Attempt to create a hypoxic O_2/N_2O mixture and verify correct changes in flow and/or alarm.

Scavenging System
*8. **Adjust and Check Scavenging System**
   a. Ensure proper connections between the scavenging system and both APL (pop-off) valve and ventilator relief valve.
   b. Adjust waste gas vacuum (if possible).
   c. Fully open APL valve and occlude Y-piece.
   d. With minimum O_2 flow, allow scavenger reservoir bag to collapse completely and verify that absorber pressure gauge reads about zero.
   e. With the O_2 flush activated, allow the scavenger reservoir bag to distend fully, and then verify that absorber pressure gauge reads <10 cm H_2O.

Breathing System
*9. **Calibrate O_2 Monitor**
   a. Ensure monitor reads 21% in room air.
   b. Verify low O_2 alarm is enabled and functioning.
   c. Reinstall sensor in circuit and flush breathing system with O_2.
   d. Verify that monitor now reads greater than 90%.
10. **Check Initial Status of Breathing System**
   a. Set selector switch to "Bag" mode.
   b. Check that breathing circuit is complete, undamaged and unobstructed.
   c. Verify that CO_2 absorbent is adequate.
   d. Install breathing circuit accessory equipment (e.g., humidifier, PEEP valve) to be used during the case.
11. **Perform Leak Check of the Breathing System**
   a. Set all gas flows to zero (or minimum).
   b. Close APL (pop-off) valve and occlude Y-piece.
   c. Pressurize breathing system to about 30 cm H_2O with O_2 flush.
   d. Ensure that pressure remains fixed for at least 10 seconds.
   e. Open APL (pop-off) valve and ensure that pressure decreases.

Manual and Automatic Ventilation Systems
12. **Test Ventilation Systems and Unidirectional Valves**
   a. Place a second breathing bag on Y-piece.
   b. Set appropriate ventilator parameters for next patient.
   c. Switch to automatic ventilation (Ventilator) mode.
   d. Fill bellows and breathing bag with O_2 flush and then turn ventilator ON.
   e. Set O_2 flow to minimum, other gas flows to zero.
   f. Verify that during inspiration bellows delivers appropriate tidal volume and that during expiration bellows fills completely.
   g. Set fresh gas flow to about 5 L/min.
   h. Verify that the ventilator bellows and simulated lungs fill, *and empty* appropriately without sustained pressure at end expiration.
   i. *Check for proper action of unidirectional valves.*
   j. Exercise breathing circuit accessories to ensure proper function.

---

*If an anesthesia provider uses the same machine in successive cases, these steps need not be repeated or may be abbreviated after the initial checkout.

k. Turn ventilator OFF and switch to manual ventilation (Bag/APL) mode.

l. Ventilate manually and assure inflation and deflation of artificial lungs and appropriate feel of system resistance and compliance.

m. Remove second breathing bag from Y-piece.

Monitors

13. Check, Calibrate, and/or Set Alarm Limits of All Monitors

- Capnometer
- Pulse Oximeter
- Oxygen Analyzer

- Respiratory Volume Monitor (Spirometer)
- Pressure Monitor with High and Low Airway Alarms

Final Position

14. Check Final Status of Machine

a. Vaporizers off

b. APL valve open

c. Selector switch to "Bag"

d. All flowmeters to zero

e. Patient suction level adequate

f. Breathing system ready to use

REFERENCES

1. Cooper JB, Newbower RS, Kitz RJ: An analysis of major errors and equipment failures in anesthesia management: considerations for prevention and detection, *Anesthesiology* 60:34, 1984.
2. Cooper JB, Newbower RS, Long CD, et al: Preventable anesthesia mishaps: a study of human factors, *Anesthesiology* 49:399, 1978.
3. Sykes MK: Incidence of mortality and morbidity due to anaesthetic equipment failure, *Eur J Anaesthesiol* 4:198, 1987.
4. Buffington CW, Ramanathan S, Turndorf H: Detection of anesthesia machine faults, *Anesth Analg* 63:79, 1984.
5. Kumar V, Hintze MS, Jacob AM: A random survey of anesthesia machines and ancillary monitors in 45 hospitals, *Anesth Analg* 67:644, 1988.
6. Webb RK, Currie M, Morgan CA, et al: The Australian Incident Monitoring Study: an analysis of 2000 incident reports, *Anaesth Intensive Care* 21:520, 1998.
7. Caplan RA, Vistica MF, Posner KL, et al: Adverse anesthetic outcomes arising from gas delivery equipment: a closed claims analysis, *Anesthesiology* 87:741, 1997.
8. Schreiber PJ: Con: there is nothing wrong with old anesthesia machines and equipment, *J Clin Monit* 12:39, 1996.
9. American Society for Testing and Materials: *Minimum performance and safety requirements for components and systems of anesthesia gas machines F1161-88,* Philadelphia, 1989, American Society for Testing and Materials.
10. American National Standards Institute: *Minimum performance and safety requirements for components and systems of continuous flow anesthesia machines for human use,* ANSI Z79.8-1979, New York, 1979, American National Standards Institute.
11. *Standards for basic anesthetic monitoring,* Park Ridge, Ill, 1996, American Society of Anesthesiologists.
12. Eichhorn JH: Prevention of intraoperative anesthesia accidents and related severe injury through safety monitoring, *Anesthesiology* 70:572, 1989.
13. Eisenkraft JB: The anesthesia machine. In Ehrenwerth J, Eisenkraft JB, eds: *Anesthesia equipment: principles and applications,* St Louis, 1992, Mosby, p 27.
14. Dorsch JA, Dorsch SE: *Understanding anesthesia equipment,* ed 3, Baltimore, 1994, Williams & Wilkins.
15. Petty C: *The anesthesia machine,* New York, 1987, Churchill Livingstone.
16. *Diameter-index safety system,* CGA V-5, New York, 1978, Compressed Gas Association.
17. *Compressed gas cylinder valve outlet and inlet connections,* CGA V-1, New York, 1977, Compressed Gas Association.
18. Holland R: Wrong gas disaster in Hong Kong, *Anesthesia Patient Safety Foundation Newsletter* 4:26, 1989.
19. Eichhorn JH: Medical gas delivery systems, *Int Anesthesiol Clin* 19:1, 1981.
20. Feeley TW, McClelland KJ, Malhotra IV: The hazards of bulk oxygen delivery systems, *Lancet* 1:1416, 1975.
21. Sprague DH, Archer GW Jr: Intraoperative hypoxia from an erroneously filled liquid oxygen reservoir, *Anesthesiology* 42:360, 1975.
22. Gilmour IJ, McComb C, Palahniuk RJ: Contamination of a hospital oxygen supply, *Anesth Analg* 71:302, 1990.
23. Moss E: Hospital deaths reportedly due to contaminated oxygen, *Anesthesia Patient Safety Foundation Newsletter* 11:13, 1996.
24. Bowie E, Huffman LM: *The anesthesia machine: essentials for understanding,* Madison, Wis, 1986, Ohmeda, The BOC Group.
25. Heine JF, Adams PM: Another potential failure in an oxygen delivery system, *Anesthesiology* 63:335, 1985 (letter).
26. Varga DA, Guttery JS, Grundy BL: Intermittent oxygen delivery in an Ohmeda Unitrol Anesthesia Machine due to a faulty O-ring check valve assembly, *Anesth Analg* 66:1200, 1987 (letter).
27. Bailey PL: Failed release of an oxygen flush valve, *Anesthesiology* 59:480, 1983 (letter).
28. Sprung J, Samaan F, Hensler T, et al: Excessive airway pressure due to ventilator flow control valve malfunction during anesthesia for open heart surgery, *Anesthesiology* 73:1035, 1990 (letter).
29. *Narkomed 3 anesthesia system, operator's instruction manual,* Telford, Penn, 1986, North American Dräger.

30. *Modulus II Plus anesthesia machine, preoperative checklists, operation and maintenance manual,* Madison, Wis, 1988, Ohmeda, The BOC Group.
31. Schreiber P: *Safety guidelines for anesthesia systems,* Telford, Penn, 1985, North American Dräger.
32. Rau JL, Rau MY: *Fundamental respiratory therapy equipment,* Sarasota, Fla, 1977, Glenn Educational Medical Series.
33. Parbrook GD, Davis PD, Parbrook EO: *Basic physics and measurement in anesthesia,* ed 2, Norwalk, Conn, 1986, Appleton-Century-Crofts.
34. Meyer RM, Ferderbar PJ: Liquid full nitrous oxide cylinders, *Anesthesiology* 78:584, 1993.
35. Eger EI II, Hylton RR, Irwin RH, et al: Anesthetic flow meter sequence: a cause for hypoxia, *Anesthesiology* 24:396, 1963.
36. Williams AR, Hilton PJ: Selective oxygen leak: a potential cause of patient hypoxia, *Anaesthesia* 41:1133, 1986.
37. Sykes MK, Vickers MD, Hull CJ: *Principles of measurement for anesthetists,* Philadelphia, 1981, FA Davis.
38. Khahil SN, Neuman J: Failure of an oxygen flow control valve, *Anesthesiology,* 73:355, 1990 (letter).
39. Beudoin MG: Oxygen needle valve obstruction, *Anaesth Intensive Care* 16:130, 1988 (letter).
40. Rung GW, Schneider AJL: Oxygen flow control valve failure on the North American Dräger Narkomed 2A anesthesia machine, *Anesth Analg* 65:209, 1986.
41. Richards C: Failure of a nitrous oxide–oxygen proportioning device, *Anesthesiology* 71:997, 1989 (letter).
42. Abraham ZA, Basagoitia J: A potentially lethal anesthesia machine failure, *Anesthesiology* 66:589, 1987 (letter).
43. Eisenkraft JB: Anesthesia vaporizers. In Ehrenwerth J, Eisenkraft JB, eds: *Anesthesia equipment: principles and applications,* St Louis, Mosby, 57, 1993.
44. *Operating manual,* Vapor 19.1, Lübeck, Germany, 1986, Drägerwerk.
45. Eisenkraft JB, Raemer DB: Monitoring gases in the anesthesia delivery system. In Ehrenwerth J, Eisenkraft JB, eds: *Anesthesia equipment: principles and applications,* St Louis, 1993, Mosby, p 201.
46. Andrews JJ, Johnston RV Jr: The new Tec 6 desflurane vaporizer, *Anesth Analg* 76:1338, 1993.
47. Weiskopf RB, Sampson D, Moore MA: The desflurane (Tec 6) vaporizer: design, design considerations and performance evaluation, *Br J Anaesth* 72:474, 1994.
48. Andrews JJ, Johnston RV Jr, Kramer GC: Consequences of misfilling contemporary vaporizers with desflurane, *Can J Anaesth* 40:71, 1993.
49. Eisenkraft JB: Anesthesia delivery system. In Longnecker DE, Tinker JH, Morgan GE, eds: *Principles and practice of anesthesiology,* ed 2, St Louis, 1998, Mosby, p 1011.
50. *Tec 6 vaporizer operation and maintenance manual,* Madison, Wis, 1992, Ohmeda, BOC Health Care.
51. Johnston RV Jr, Andrews JJ, Deyo DJ, et al: The effects of carrier gas composition on the performance of the Tec 6 desflurane vaporizer, *Anesth Analg* 79:548, 1994.
52. Benumof JL, Scheller MS: The importance of transtracheal jet ventilation in the management of the difficult airway, *Anesthesiology* 71:769, 1989.
53. Delaney WA, Kaiser RE Jr: Percutaneous transtracheal jet ventilation made easy, *Anesthesiology* 74:952, 1991 (letter).
54. Gaughan SD, Benumof JL, Ozaki JGT: Can an anesthesia machine flush valve provide for effective jet ventilation? *Anesth Analg* 76:800, 1993.
55. Capan L, Ramanathan S, Chalon J, et al: A possible hazard with use of the Ohio Ethrane vaporizer, *Anesth Analg* 59:65, 1980.
56. Ghanooni S, Wilks DH, Finestone SC: A case report of an unusual disconnection, *Anesth Analg* 62:696, 1983.
57. Magee PT: Anesthetic breathing systems. In Eisenkraft JB, ed: *Progress in anesthesiology,* vol 4, San Antonio, Tex, 1990, Dannemiller Memorial Educational Foundation.
58. Sykes MK: Rebreathing circuits, a review, *Br J Anaesth* 40:666, 1960.
59. Conway CM: Anaesthetic breathing systems, *Br J Anaesth* 57:649, 1985.

60. Eger EI II: Anesthetic systems: construction and function. In *Anesthetic uptake and action,* Baltimore, 1974, Williams & Wilkins, p 206.

61. Bain JA, Spoerel WE: Flow requirements for a modified Mapleson D system during controlled ventilation, *Can Anaesth Soc J* 20:629, 1973.

62. Seeley HF, Barnes PK, Conway CM: Controlled ventilation with the Mapleson D system: a theoretical and experimental study, *Br J Anaesth* 49:107, 1977.

63. Pethick SL: Correspondence, *Can Anaesth Soc J* 22:115, 1975.

64. Seed RF: A test for coaxial circuits, *Anaesthesia* 32:676, 1977.

65. *The Sodasorb manual of carbon dioxide absorption,* Lexington, Mass, 1962, Dewey and Almy Chemical Division of WR Grace & Co.

66. Andrews JJ, Johnston RV Jr, Bee DE, et al: Photodeactivation of ethyl violet: a potential hazard of Sodasorb, *Anesthesiology* 72:59, 1990.

67. Kharasch ED: Inhalation anesthetic toxicity: current controversies, In *48th Annual refresher course lectures and clinical update program,* Park Ridge, Ill, 1997, American Society of Anesthesiologists.

68. *Ohmeda 7000 electronic anesthesia ventilator, service manual,* Madison, Wis, 1985, Ohmeda, The BOC Group.

69. *Ohmeda 7810 electronic anesthesia ventilator, service manual,* Madison, Wis, 1989, Ohmeda, The BOC Group.

70. *Ohmeda 7900 ventilator: operation and maintenance manual,* Madison, Wis, 1997, Ohmeda, BOC Health Care.

71. Eisenkraft JB: Potential for barotrauma or hypoventilation with the Dräger AV-E ventilator, *J Clin Anesth* 1:452, 1989.

72. Khalil SN, Gholston TK, Binderman J, et al: Flapper valve malfunction in an Ohio closed scavenging system, *Anesth Analg* 66:1334, 1987.

73. Sommer RM, Bhalla GS, Jackson JM, et al: Hypoventilation caused by ventilator valve rupture, *Anesth Analg* 67:999, 1988.

74. American Society for Testing and Materials: *Standard specification for ventilators intended for use during anesthesia, F1101-90,* West Conshohocken, Penn, 1990, American Society for Testing and Materials.

75. Raessler KL, Kretzman WE, Gravenstein N: Oxygen consumption by anesthesia ventilators, *Anesthesiology* 69:A271, 1988 (abstract).

76. Roth S, Tweedie E, Sommer RM: Excessive airway pressure due to a malfunctioning anesthesia ventilator, *Anesthesiology* 65:532, 1986.

77. Gravenstein N, Banner MJ, McLaughlin G: Tidal volume changes due to the interaction of anesthesia machine and anesthesia ventilator, *J Clin Monit* 3:187, 1987.

78. Scheller MS, Jones BR, Benumof JL: The influence of fresh gas flow and inspiratory/expiratory ratio on tidal volume and arterial PCO_2 in mechanically ventilated surgical patients, *J Cardiothorac Anesth* 3:564, 1989.

79. Elliott WR, Harris AE, Philip JH: Positive end-expiratory pressure: implications for tidal volume changes in anesthesia machine ventilation, *J Clin Monit* 5:100, 1989.

80. Pan PH, van der Aa JJ: Anesthesia ventilator performance, delivered tidal volume, and PEEP, *Anesthesiology* 73:A420, 1990 (abstract).

81. *Narkomed 2A anesthesia machine, technical service manual, operating principles,* Telford, Penn, 1989, North American Dräger.

82. *Open Reservoir Scavenger operator's instruction manual,* Telford, Penn, 1986, North American Dräger.

83. Knaack-Steinegger R, Thomson DA: The measurement of expiratory oxygen as a disconnection alarm, *Anesthesiology* 68:70:343, 1989.

84. Gravenstein JS, Nederstigt JA: Monitoring for disconnection: ventilators with bellows rising on expiration can deliver tidal volumes after disconnection, *J Clin Monit* 6:207, 1990.

85. Merilainen P, Hanninen H, Tuomaala L: A novel sensor for routine continuous spirometry of intubated patients, *J Clin Monit* 9:374, 1993.

86. Bernstein DB, Rosenberg AD: Intraoperative hypoxia from nitrogen tanks with oxygen fittings, *Anesth Analg* 84:225, 1997.

87. Feeley TW, Hedley-Whyte J: Bulk oxygen delivery systems: design and dangers, *Anesthesiology* 44:301, 1976.

88. O'Connor CJ Jr, Hubin KF: Bypassing the diameter-indexed safety system, *Anesthesiology* 71:318, 1989 (letter).

89. Anderson B, Chamley D: Wall outlet oxygen failure, *Anaesth Intensive Care* 15:468, 1987 (letter).

90. Jawan B, Lee JH: Cardiac arrest caused by an incorrectly filled oxygen cylinder: a case report, *Br J Anaesth* 64:749, 1990.

91. Bonsu AK, Stead AL: Accidental cross-connection of oxygen and nitrous oxide in an anaesthetic machine, *Anaesthesia* 38:767, 1983.

92. Heath ML: Accidents associated with equipment, *Anaesthesia* 39:57, 1984.

93. Lacoumenta S, Hall GM: A burst oxygen pipeline, *Anaesthesia* 38:596, 1983 (letter).

94. Carley RH, Houghton IT, Park GR: A near disaster from piped gases, *Anaesthesia* 39:891, 1984.

95. Hanning CD, Kruchek D, Chunara A: Preferential oxygen leak: an unusual case, *Anaesthesia* 42:1329, 1987 (letter).

96. Moore JK, Railton R: Hypoxia caused by a leaking rotameter: the value of an oxygen analyser, *Anaesthesia* 39:380, 1984, (letter).

97. Cole AG, Thompson JB, Fodor IM, et al: Anaesthetic machine hazard from the Selectatec block, *Anaesthesia* 38:175, 1983 (letter).

98. Goodyear CM: Failure of nitrous oxide–oxygen proportioning device, *Anesthesiology* 72:397, 1990 (letter).

99. Gordon PC, James MFM, Lapham H, et al: Failure of the proportioning system to prevent hypoxic mixture on a Modulus II Plus anesthesia machine, *Anesthesiology* 82:598, 1995 (letter).

100. Rossiter SK: An unexpected disconnection of the gas supply to a Cape Waine 3 ventilator, *Anaesthesia* 38:180, 1983 (letter).

101. Henshaw J: Circle system disconnection, *Anaesth Intensive Care* 16:240, 1988 (letter).

102. Horan BF: Unusual disconnection, *Anaesth Intensive Care* 15:466, 1987 (letter).

103. Eisenkraft JB: Complications of the anesthesia gas delivery system. In Schwartz AJ, Matjasko MJ, Otto CW, eds: *ASA refresher course lectures,* vol 26, Philadelphia, 1998, Lippincott-Raven, p 45.

104. Ripp CH, Chapin JW: A bellow's leak in an Ohio anesthesia ventilator, *Anesth Analg* 64:942, 1985 (letter).

105. Spoor J: Ventilator malfunction, *Anaesth Intensive Care* 14:329, 1986 (letter).

106. Berner MS: Profound hypercapnia due to disconnection within an anaesthetic machine, *Can J Anaesth* 34:622, 1987.

107. McQuillan PJ, Jackson IJ: Potential leaks from anaesthetic machines: potential leaks through open Rotameter valves and empty cylinder yokes, *Anaesthesia* 42:1308, 1987.

108. Bamber PA: Safety hazard with cylinder yoke on a Boyle's machine, *Anaesthesia* 41:1260, 1986 (letter).

109. Jablonski J, Reynolds AC: A potential cause (and cure) of a major gas leak, *Anesthesiology* 62:842, 1985 (letter).

110. Jove F, Milliken RA: Loss of anesthetic gases due to defective safety equipment, *Anesth Analg* 62:369, 1983 (letter).

111. Pyles ST, Kaplan RF, Munson ES: Gas loss from Ohio Modulus Vaporizer Selector-Interlock Valve, *Anesth Analg* 62:1052, 1983 (letter).

112. Sara CA, Wark HJ: Disconnection: an appraisal, *Anaesth Intensive Care* 14:448, 1986.

113. Eisenkraft JB, Sommer RM: Flapper valve malfunction, *Anesth Analg* 67:1131, 1988 (letter).

114. Poulton TJ: Unusual corrugated tubing leak, *Anesth Analg* 65:1365, 1986 (letter).

115. Nelson RA, Snowdon SL: Failure of an adjustable pressure limiting valve, *Anaesthesia* 44:788, 1989 (letter).

116. Cooper MG, Vouden J, Rigg D: Circuit leaks, *Anaesth Intensive Care* 15:359, 1987 (letter).

117. Hutchinson BR: An unusual leak, *Anaesth Intensive Care* 15:355, 1987 (letter).

118. Ferderbar PJ, Kettler RE, Jablonski J, et al: A cause of breathing system leak during closed circuit anesthesia, *Anesthesiology* 65:661, 1986.

119. Raja SN, Geller H: Another potential source of a major gas leak, *Anesthesiology* 64:297, 1986 (letter).

120. Brown MR, Burris WR, Hilley MD: Breathing circuit mishap resulting from Y-piece disintegration, *Anesthesiology* 69:436, 1988 (letter).

121. Colavita RD, Apfelbaum JL: An unusual source of leak in the anesthesia circuit, *Anesthesiology* 62:208, 1985 (letter).

122. Lamarche Y: Anaesthetic breathing circuit leak from cracked oxygen analyzer sensor connector, *Can Anaesth Soc J* 32:682, 1985 (letter).

123. Miller DC, Collins JW, Wallace L: Failure of the expiratory valve on a Bain system, *Anaesthesia* 43:992, 1988 (letter).

124. Robblee JA, Crosby E, Keon WJ: Hypoxemia after intraluminal oxygen line obstruction during cardiopulmonary bypass, *Ann Thorac Surg* 48:575, 1989.

125. Wan YL, Swan M: Exotic obstruction, *Anaesth Intensive Care* 18:274, 1990 (letter).

126. Boscoe MJ, Baxter RC: Failure of anaesthetic gas supply, *Anaesthesia* 38:997, 1983 (letter).

127. Hogan TS: Selectatec switch malfunction, *Anaesthesia* 40:66, 1985.

128. Milliken RA, Bizzarri DV: An unusual cause of failure of anesthetic gas delivery to a patient circuit, *Anesth Analg* 63:1047, 1984 (letter).

129. Ghani GA: Fresh gas flow affects minute volume during mechanical ventilation, *Anesth Analg* 63:619, 1984 (letter).

130. Birch AA, Fisher NA: Leak of soda lime seal after anesthesia machine check, *J Clin Anesth* 1:474, 1989 (letter).

131. Nunn JF: Carbon dioxide cylinders on anaesthetic apparatus, *Br J Anaesth* 65:155, 1990 (editorial).

132. Razis PA: Carbon dioxide: a survey of its use in anaesthesia in the UK, *Anaesthesia* 44:348, 1989.

133. Sims C, Cullingford DW: Kinking of the Mera-F-Circuit, *Anaesth Intensive Care* 16:243, 1988 (letter).

134. Hewitt AJ, Campbell W: Unusual damage to a Bain system, *Anaesthesia* 41:882, 1986 (letter).

135. Waterman PM, Pautler S, Smith RB: Accidental ventilator-induced hyperventilation, *Anesthesiology* 48:141, 1978.

136. Neufeld PD, Walker EA, Johnson DL: Survey on breathing system disconnexions, *Anaesthesia* 41:438, 1986 (letter).

137. Goldman JM, Phelps RW: No flow anesthesia, *Anesth Analg* 66:1339, 1987 (letter).

138. Koga Y, Iwatsuki N, Takahashi M, et al: A hazardous defect in a humidifier, *Anesth Analg* 71:712, 1990 (letter).

139. Shroff PK, Skerman JH: Humidifier malfunction: a cause of anesthesia circuit occlusion, *Anesth Analg* 67:710, 1988 (letter).

140. Spurring PW, Small LFG: Breathing circuit disconnexions and misconnexions: review of some common causes and some suggestions for improved safety, *Anaesthesia* 38:683, 1983.

141. Arellano R, Ross D, Lee K: Inappropriate attachment of PEEP valve causing total obstruction of ventilation bag, *Anesth Analg* 66:1050, 1987 (letter).

142. Anagnostou JM, Hults S, Moorthy SS: PEEP valve barotrauma, *Anesth Analg* 70:674, 1990 (letter).

143. Cooper JB: Unidirectional PEEP valves can cause safety hazard, *Anesthesia Patient Safety Foundation Newsletter* 5:28, 1990.

144. Lee D: PEEP safety cited, *Anesthesia Patient Safety Foundation Newsletter* 5:21, 1990.

145. Sharrock NE, Leith DE: Potential pulmonary barotrauma when venting anesthetic gases to suction, *Anesthesiology* 46:152, 1977.

146. Mushlin PS, Mark JB, Elliott WR, et al: Inadvertent development of subatmospheric airway pressure during cardiopulmonary bypass, *Anesthesiology* 71:459, 1989.

147. McEwen JA, Small CF, Jenkins LC: Detection of interruptions in the breathing gas of ventilated anaesthetized patients, *Can J Anaesth* 35:549, 1988.

148. Adams AP: Breathing system disconnections, *Br J Anaesth* 73:46, 1994.

149. Raphael DT: An algorithmic response for the breathing system low pressure alarm condition. In Eisenkraft JB, ed: *Progress in anesthesiology*, vol 10, San Antonio, Tex, 1997, Dannemiller Memorial Educational Foundation.

150. Slee TA, Pavlin EG: Failure of low pressure alarm associated with the use of a humidifier, *Anesthesiology* 69:791, 1988.

151. Needleman S, Kaplan RF: Unusual source of air leak in a pediatric anesthesia breathing circuit, *Anesth Analg* 81:654, 1995 (letter).

152. Choi JJ, Guida J, Wu W-H: Hypoventilatory hazard of an anesthetic scavenging device, *Anesthesiology* 65:126, 1986 (letter).

153. Lanier WL: Intraoperative air entrainment with Ohio Modulus Anesthesia Machine, *Anesthesiology* 64:266, 1986.

154. Baraka A, Muallem M: Awareness during anaesthesia due to a ventilator malfunction, *Anaesthesia* 34:678, 1979 (letter).

155. Longmuir J, Craig DB: Inadvertent increase in inspired oxygen concentration due to defect in ventilator bellows, *Can Anaesth Soc J* 23:327, 1976.

156. Dean HN, Parsons DE, Raphaely RC: Case report: bilateral tension pneumothorax from mechanical failure of anesthesia machine due to misplaced expiratory valve, *Anesth Analg* 50:195, 1971.

157. Sears BE, Bocar ND: Pneumothorax resulting from a closed anesthesia ventilator port, *Anesthesiology* 47:311, 1977.

158. Henzig D: Insidious PEEP from a defective ventilator gas evacuation outlet valve, *Anesthesiology* 57:251, 1982 (letter).

159. *Pressure limit control, operator's instruction manual*, Telford, Penn, 1988, North American Dräger.

160. Kopriva CJ, Lowenstein E: An anesthetic accident: cardiovascular collapse from liquid halothane delivery, *Anesthesiology* 30:246, 1969.

161. *Tec 5 continuous flow vaporizer, operation and maintenance manual*, Steeton, UK, 1989, Ohmeda.

162. *Tec 4 continuous flow vaporizer, operation manual*, V5, Steeton, UK, 1987, Ohmeda.

163. Hardy JF: Vaporizer overfilling, *Can J Anaesth* 40:1, 1993 (editorial).

164. Sinclair A, van Bergen J: Vaporizer overfilling, *Can J Anaesth* 40:77, 1993 (letter).

165. Bruce DL, Linde HW: Vaporization of mixed anesthetic liquids, *Anesthesiology* 60:342, 1984.

166. Chilcoat RT: Hazards of mis-filled vaporizers: summary tables, *Anesthesiology* 63:726, 1985 (letter).

167. Abel M, Eisenkraft JB: Performance of erroneously filled sevoflurane, enflurane and other agent-specific vaporizers, *J Clin Monit* 12:119, 1996.

168. Riegle EV, Desertspring D: Failure of the agent-specific filling device, *Anesthesiology* 73:353, 1990 (letter).

169. Korman B, Ritchie IM: Chemistry of halothane-enflurane mixtures applied to anesthesia, *Anesthesiology* 63:152, 1985.

170. Murray WJ, Zsigmond EK, Fleming P: Contamination of in-series vaporizers with halothane-methoxyflurane, *Anesthesiology* 38:487, 1973.

171. Dorsch SE, Dorsch JA: Chemical cross-contamination between vaporizers in series, *Anesth Analg* 52:176, 1973.

172. Silvasi DL, Haynes A, Brown ACD: Potentially lethal failure of the vapor exclusion system, *Anesthesiology* 71:289, 1989.

173. Cudmore J, Keogh J: Another Selectatec switch malfunction, *Anaesthesia* 45:754, 1990.

174. Marks WE, Bullard JR: Another hazard of free-standing vaporizers: increased anesthetic concentration with reversed flow of vaporizing gas, *Anesthesiology* 45:445, 1976.

175. Railton R, Inglis MD: High halothane concentrations from reversed flow in a vaporizer, *Anaesthesia* 41:672, 1986 (letter).

176. Gregg AS, Jones RS, Snowdon SL: Flow reversal through a Mark III halothane vaporizer, *Br J Anaesth* 71:303, 1993.

177. Beebe JJ, Sessler DI: Preparation of anesthesia machines for patients susceptible to malignant hyperthermia, *Anesthesiology* 69:395, 1988.

178. Cooper JB, Philip JH: More on anesthesia machines and malignant hyperthermia, *Anesthesiology* 70:561, 1989 (letter).

179. Abdi S, Acquadro MA: Technical failure of desflurane vaporizer Tec 6, *Anesthesiology* 83:226, 1995 (letter).

180. Lockey D, Purcell-Jones G: A problem with a desflurane vaporizer, *Anaesthesia* 50:574, 1995 (letter).

181. Viney JP, Gartrell AD: Incorrectly adjusted vaporizer exclusion system, *Anesthesiology* 81:781, 1994 (letter).

182. Riddle RT: Tec 6 recall, *Anesthesiology* 81:791, 1994 (letter).

183. Riddle RT: Medical device recall alert, *Anesth Analg* 79:808, 1994 (letter).

184. Rao CC, Brandl R, Mashak JN: Modification of Ohmeda Excel 210 anesthesia machine for use during magnetic resonance imaging, *Anesthesiology* 71:A365, 1989 (abstract).

185. Rao CC, Krishna G, Emhardt J: Anesthesia machine for use during magnetic resonance imaging, *Anesthesiology* 73:1054, 1990 (letter).

186. Munshi C, Dhamee S, Bardeen-Henschel A, et al: Recognition of mixed anesthetic agents by mass spectrometer during anesthesia, *J Clin Monit* 2:121, 1986.

187. Bickler PE, Sessler DI: Efficiency of airway heat and moisture exchangers in anesthetized humans, *Anesth Analg* 71:415, 1990.

188. Turner DA, Wright EM: Efficiency of heat and moisture exchangers, *Anaesthesia* 42:1117, 1987 (letter).

189. Bengtsson M, Johnson A: Failure of a heat and moisture exchanger as a cause of disconnection during anaesthesia, *Acta Anaesthesiol Scand* 33:522, 1989.

190. Prasad KK, Chen L: Complications related to the use of a heat and moisture exchanger, *Anesthesiology* 72:958, 1990 (letter).

191. Ward CF, Reisner LS, Zlott LS: Murphy's law and humidification, *Anesth Analg* 62:460, 1983.

192. *Operators manual, North American Dräger Narkomed 2B,* Telford, Penn, 1988, North American Dräger.

193. *National electrical code 1993, 70-539,* Quincy, Mass, 1993, National Fire Protection Association.

194. Greenhalgh DL, Thomas WA: Blackout during cardiopulmonary bypass, *Anaesthesia* 45:175, 1990 (letter).

195. Welch RH, Feldman JM: Anesthesia during total electrical failure, or what would you do if the lights went out? *J Clin Anesth* 1:358, 1989.

196. Moon R, Meyer A, Scott D, et al: Intraoperative carbon monoxide toxicity, *Anesthesiology* 73:A1049, 1990 (abstract).

197. Moon R, Ingram C, Brunner EA, et al: Spontaneous generation of carbon monoxide within anesthetic circuits, *Anesthesiology* 75:A873, 1991 (abstract).

198. Baum J, Sachs G, Dreisch C: Carbon monoxide generation in carbon dioxide absorbents, *Anesth Analg* 81:144, 1995.

199. Fang ZX, Eger EI II, Laster MJ, et al: Carbon monoxide production from degradation of desflurane, enflurane, isoflurane, halothane, and sevoflurane by soda lime and Baralyme, *Anesth Analg* 80:1187, 1995.

200. Woehlck HJ, Dunning M, Ghandi S, et al: Indirect detection of intraoperative carbon monoxide exposure by mass spectrometry during isoflurane anesthesia, *Anesthesiology* 83:213, 1995.

201. Woehlck HJ, Dunning M, Nithipatikom K, et al: Mass spectrometry provides warning of CO exposure via trifluoromethane, *Anesthesiology* 84:1489, 1996.

202. Baxter PJ, Kharasch ED: Rehydration of desiccated Baralyme prevents carbon monoxide formation from desflurane in an anesthesia machine, *Anesthesiology* 86:1061, 1997.

203. Sprung J, Siker D, Koch R, et al: Disruption of an infrared capnograph monitor by hand-held radio transceivers, *Anesthesiology* 83:1352, 1995.

204. Medical equipment interference from cellular phones gets hospital industry attention, *Technology for Anesthesia* 15:5, 1994.

205. Crosby WM: Checking the anaesthetic machine, drugs, and monitoring devices, *Anaesth Intensive Care* 16:32, 1988.

206. U.S. Food and Drug Administration: *Anesthesia apparatus checkout recommendations,* Rockville, Md, 1986, U.S. Food and Drug Administration.

207. March MG, Crowley JJ: An evaluation of anesthesiologists' present checkout methods and the validity of the FDA checklist, *Anesthesiology* 75:724, 1991.

208. U.S. Food and Drug Administration: Anesthesia apparatus checkout recommendations, 1993, *Federal Register* 59, no 131:35373, July 11, 1994.

209. Olympio MA, Goldstein MM, Mathes DD: Instructional review improves performance of anesthesia apparatus checkout procedures, *Anesth Analg* 83:618, 1996.

210. Targ AG, Andrews BW: A new device to check the anesthesia machine low pressure system, *Anesthesiology* 79:629, 1993 (letter).

211. Myers JA, Good ML, Andrews JJ: Comparison of tests for detecting leaks in the low pressure system of anesthesia gas machines, *Anesth Analg* 84:179, 1997.

212. Lees DE: Old anesthesia equipment target of study, panel, *Anesthesia Patient Safety Foundation Newsletter* 4:13, Park Ridge, Ill, 1989, American Society of Anesthesiologists.

213. ASA Committee on Equipment and Standards: Annual report, Park Ridge, Ill, 1989, American Society of Anesthesiologists.

214. Eisenkraft JB: A commentary on anesthesia gas delivery equipment and adverse outcomes, *Anesthesiology* 87:731, 1997 (editorial).

215. Arens JF: Pro: there is nothing wrong with old anesthesia machines and equipment, *J Clin Monit* 12:37, 1996.

216. Eichhorn JH: Medicolegal and risk management aspects of anesthesia equipment. In Ehrenwerth J, Eisenkraft JB, eds: *Anesthesia equipment: principles and applications,* St Louis, 1993, Mosby.

217. Gravenstein JS: To "obsolete" old equipment or not? *Anesthesia Patient Safety Foundation Newsletter* 11:13, 1996.

218. Riddle RT: Personal communication, August 1997.

219. Subchapter 18: anesthesia 21 *New Jersey Register* 21:503, Feb 21, 1989.

Chapter 7

Complications of Drugs Used in Anesthesia

Jonathan M. Anagnostou
Robert K. Stoelting

I. **Inhaled Anesthetics**
   A. Volatile Drugs
      1. Central nervous system complications
      2. Respiratory complications
      3. Cardiovascular complications
      4. Renal complications
      5. Uterine complications
      6. Carbon monoxide
      7. Malignant hyperthermia
      8. Drug interactions
   B. Nitrous Oxide
II. **Intravenous Anesthetics**
   A. Barbiturates
      1. Cardiovascular effects
      2. Respiratory effects
   B. Benzodiazepines and Antagonist
   C. Propofol
   D. Etomidate
   E. Ketamine
III. **Drugs Used in Psychiatric Disorders**
   A. Antipsychotic Agents
   B. Tricyclic Antidepressants
   C. Monoamine Oxidase Inhibitors
   D. Selective Serotonin Reuptake Inhibitors
IV. **Opioid Agonists**
   A. Morphine
   B. Meperidine
   C. Fentanyl
   D. Sufentanil
   E. Alfentanil
   F. Remifentanil
   G. Neuraxial Opioids
V. **Opioid Antagonist: Naloxone**
VI. **Opioid Agonist-Antagonists**
   A. Butorphanol
   B. Nalbuphine
   C. Pentazocine
   D. Buprenorphine
VII. **Local Anesthetics**
   A. Lidocaine
   B. Mepivacaine
   C. Bupivacaine
   D. Ropivacaine
   E. Prilocaine
   F. Etidocaine
   G. Chloroprocaine
   H. Cocaine
   I. Tetracaine
   J. Benzocaine
VIII. **Neuromuscular Blockers**
   A. Depolarizing Neuromuscular Relaxants: Succinylcholine

   B. Nondepolarizing Neuromuscular Relaxants
      1. *d*-Tubocurarine
      2. Metocurine
      3. Pancuronium
      4. Atracurium
      5. *cis*-Atracurium
      6. Vecuronium
      7. Rocuronium
      8. Mivacurium
      9. Doxacurium
      10. Pipecuronium
IX. **Cholinesterase Inhibitors**
X. **Anticholinergic Agents**
XI. **Vasoactive Drugs**
   A. Catecholamines
      1. Epinephrine
      2. Norepinephrine
      3. Isoproterenol
      4. Dopamine
      5. Dobutamine
   B. Noncatecholamine Inotropic Agents
      1. Amrinone
      2. Digitalis
      3. Ephedrine
      4. Mephentermine
      5. Metaraminol
   C. Selective β_2-Receptor Agonists
   D. Vasopressors
      1. Phenylephrine
      2. Methoxamine
   E. Vasodilators
      1. Nitroprusside
      2. Nitroglycerin
      3. Hydralazine
      4. Minoxidil
      5. Diazoxide
      6. Adenosine
      7. Nitric oxide
   F. β-Adrenergic Receptor Blockers
   G. α-Adrenergic Receptor Blockers
      1. Phentolamine
      2. Phenoxybenzamine
      3. Prazosin
   H. Mixed Adrenergic Antagonists: Labetalol
   I. Ganglionic Blockers: Trimethaphan
   J. Central Sympatholytics
      1. Clonidine
      2. Methyldopa
      3. Reserpine
XII. **Calcium-Channel Blockers**
   A. Verapamil
   B. Nifedipine

161

This chapter discusses side effects of drugs commonly encountered in anesthetic practice. Our purpose is not to restate the pharmacology of these drugs but to concentrate on the potentially harmful properties that are most relevant to perioperative patient care. Clearly, pharmacologic effect that might be acceptable in one clinical circumstance may be very undesirable in another. For example, the tachycardia produced by pancuronium might be acceptable in an otherwise healthy young adult, whereas this same effect in an elderly patient with severe atherosclerotic coronary artery disease may lead to myocardial ischemia.

Tables 7-1 and 7-2 (see end of chapter) serve as rapid reference tools that list adverse effects and drug interactions. The text provides additional details and explanations of the material presented in the tables. For certain drugs, other chapters provide more detailed explanations, although many important adverse effects are listed in the tables in this chapter for rapid reference.

I. INHALED ANESTHETICS
A. Volatile drugs

Although many of the side effects of the volatile drugs are similar, these drugs have clinically significant differences. These differences are best illustrated by comparisons at equivalent minimum alveolar concentrations (MACs); statements about qualitative differences among agents are made with this understanding. (For a discussion of the hepatotoxic complications of volatile anesthetics, see Chapter 20.)

1. Central nervous system complications. Isoflurane causes electrical silence on electroencephalography at a MAC of more than 2.[1,2] In contrast, enflurane causes high-voltage and high-frequency rates of activity on electroencephalography that may progress to spike-and-wave activity, especially at a MAC of more than 2 and during periods of hyperventilation in which the partial pressure of carbon dioxide in the arterial blood ($PaCO_2$) is less than 30 mm Hg.[3] These events may accompany myoclonic patient movements indistinguishable from seizures. Amitriptyline may enhance the seizure activity seen with enflurane.[4] Electrical seizures have been reported during induction of sevoflurane anesthesia in two children with epilepsy.[5]

All of the available volatile anesthetic drugs may increase cerebral blood flow; halothane causes a larger increase than isoflurane.[6] In animals, the effects of desflurane and seveoflurane on cerebral blood flow are similar to those of isoflurane.[7,8] However, in patients with intracranial mass lesions, desflurane at a MAC of 1.1 increases cerebrospinal fluid pressure, whereas isoflurane does not.[9] Increases in intracranial pressure parallel the increases in cerebral blood flow. These effects may be blunted by hyperventilation to a $PaCO_2$ of 30 mm Hg; however, in the case of halothane, it seems that the hyperventilation must precede administration of the drug to be effective.[10] In patients with intracranial tumors, substantial increases in intracranial pressure with administration of isoflurane have been reported despite hyperventilation.[11]

2. Respiratory complications. The state of general anesthesia induces respiratory changes, such as decrease in lung volumes and alteration in diaphragmatic function. In addition, the volatile anesthetics depress the normal responses to hypercarbia in a dose-dependent manner.[12] The depressant effects of sevoflurane on ventilation are similar to those of halothane at a MAC of 1.1 but are greater at a MAC of 1.4.[13]

The inhaled anesthetics can irritate the airways. In volunteers, sevoflurane and halothane were the least irritating agents.[14] This irritation may produce coughing or laryngospasm during inhalation induction of general anesthesia.[15] Of the available volatile agents, desflurane is perhaps the most irritating to the airway, although premedication with fentanyl and midazolam may attenuate this irritation.[16]

3. Cardiovascular complications. In the absence of surgical stimulation, all of the volatile anesthetics decrease blood pressure in a dose-dependent manner, albeit by somewhat different mechanisms.[6] All of these agents have myocardial depressant properties; halothane and enflurane have more pronounced effects than other drugs. Isoflurane decreases peripheral vascular resistance; at a MAC of less than 2, cardiac output is maintained, stroke volume is decreased, and heart rate is increased with this agent. Desflurane also decreases blood pressure and peripheral vascular resistance and increases heart rate. Sevoflurane decreases blood pressure via a decrease in peripheral vascular resistance; the heart rate remains stable.[17] When desflurane and halothane were administered without adjuvant analgesics to healthy young adult volunteers, abrupt increases in the MAC of 0.5 to 1 in the inhaled concentrations of these agents produced increases in heart rate and blood pressure; larger absolute changes were observed with desflurane.[18] Halothane decreases in blood pressure via depression of cardiac output do not substantially change peripheral resistance. Enflurane decreases both cardiac output and peripheral resistance while causing a dose-dependent increase in heart rate. The volatile agents may sensitize the heart to the cardiac arrhythmic effects of epinephrine; halothane is the most sensitizing of these agents.[19] (See Chapter 11 for further discussion of the arrhythmogenic properties of the volatile anesthetics.)

The issue of ischemia associated with the use of various volatile anesthetics remains controversial. It has been suggested that isoflurane may produce coronary steal in patients with coronary artery disease by dilating nondiseased coronary vessels and thereby diverting flow from ischemic areas of myocardium.[20] Although this seems plausible, isoflurane may actually improve tolerance to pacing-induced ischemia.[21] Moreover, if hemodynamic factors that affect myocardial oxygen balance (i.e., heart rate and blood pressure) are controlled, ischemia is not a problem for most patients with coronary artery disease who receive isoflurane during anesthesia.[22,23] In one study, desflurane used alone compared with sufentanil in patients undergoing coronary artery bypass grafting was associated with a greater incidence of myocardial ischemia during induction, although no differences between the agents in terms of postoperative myocardial infarction or cardiac death were observed.[24] However, another investigation of patients undergoing coronary artery bypass grafting found no difference in the incidence of ischemia in patients anesthetized with desflurane and low-dose (10 μg/kg) fentanyl and those given high-dose fentanyl (50 μg/kg) and midazolam.[25] In cardiac patients undergoing noncardiac surgery, a recent investigation found that sevoflurane and isoflurane did not differ in terms of the incidence of perioperative ischemia and adverse cardiac events.[26]

4. Renal complications. Methoxyflurane, enflurane, and sevoflurane are metabolized in the body to produce fluoride ions. Free fluoride ions may be toxic to the kidneys; renal dysfunction manifests as a decreased concentrating ability.[27] Prolonged anesthesia with enflurane (9.6 hours at a MAC of 1) may produce a renal concentrating defect,[28] but a shorter exposure (2.7 hours at a MAC of 1) does not.[29] Compared with enflurane, metabolism of methoxyflurane produces fluoride in potentially nephrotoxic concentrations with smaller doses.[27] Halothane,[28] isoflurane,[30] and desflurane[31] are not metabolized to fluoride in amounts great enough to be nephrotoxic.

In addition to the metabolic production of fluoride, sevoflurane reacts with carbon dioxide absorbents to produce a vinyl ether known as compound A (CH_2F—O—C[=CF_2] [CF_3]). Compound A produces renal injury in rats with a threshold for injury on the order of 150 ppm/hr (50 ppm for 3 hours).[32] Exposure to compound A can be minimized with higher rates of fresh gas inflow, which "wash out" the compound from the breathing circuit. The package insert for sevoflurane (Abbott Laboratories, Chicago, Illinois) recommends a fresh gas inflow of at least 2 L/min when this agent is used and recommends against the use of sevoflurane in patients with preexisting renal dysfunction. In a recent comparative study of adult volunteers given either sevoflurane or desflurane at a MAC of 1.25 at a fresh gas inflow rate of 2 L/min, 4 to 8 hours of sevoflurane (but not desflurane) administration produced biochemical evidence of transient renal tubular and glomerular injury (e.g., urinary albumin and α-glutathione-S-transferase).[33] Exposures to compound A of more than 160 ppm/hr and average serum fluoride concentrations higher than 50 μmol/L were documented in the sevoflurane group. Conversely, a study of similar design that involved only sevoflurane found lower concentrations of compound A and fluoride along with clinically insignificant increases in α-glutathione-S-transferase concentration and no change in urinary albumin excretion.[34] The contradictory findings and conclusions of these two well-publicized human studies remain to be fully explained. Although the mechanism and clinical significance of compound A nephrotoxicity remain controversial,[32,34,35] a case of suspected sevoflurane-induced nonoliguric renal failure in a patient without preexisting renal dysfunction was recently reported.[36]

5. Uterine complications. The volatile inhaled agents produce uterine relaxation, which may increase intraoperative uterine bleeding in the pregnant patient.[37] This effect can be minimized by limiting the dose of volatile drug to a MAC of 0.6 or less.[38]

6. Carbon monoxide. When the volatile anesthetics desflurane, isoflurane, and enflurane are exposed to dry carbon dioxide absorbents, such as soda lime and barium hydroxide lime, carbon monoxide is produced.[39] Little carbon monoxide is produced with halothane or sevoflurane. Although clinically significant intraoperative carbon monoxide poisoning is rare, a carboxyhemoglobin concentration of more than 30% has been reported during inhaled anesthesia with desflurane.[40] Carbon dioxide absorbents normally contain at least 10% to 15% water by weight; however, this water can be removed by the prolonged flow of dry gases through the absorbent. Interventions to avoid the use of dried-out carbon dioxide absorbents during inhaled anesthesia have been shown to reduce the risk for intraoperative carbon monoxide exposure. These include turning off gas flows when anesthesia machines are not in use and replacing absorbent canisters whenever dessication is suspected.[41] In addition, adding water to dessicated barium hydroxide lime has been shown to decrease carbon monoxide production from desflurane in a single anesthesia machine.[42]

7. Malignant hyperthermia. Volatile anesthetics, especially when administered with succinylcholine, are the drugs most frequently implicated in triggering malignant hyperthermia in susceptible patients.[43] Sevoflurane was associated with documented malignant hyperthermia in at least one case,[44] and desflurane was shown to trigger the syndrome in a swine model.[45]

8. Drug interactions. Many drugs decrease the MAC of the volatile anesthetics, and the dose of volatile anesthetic should be altered accordingly to avoid an anesthetic overdose. Among the MAC-lowering drugs are opioids and opioid agonist-antagonists,[46] benzodiazepines,[47] nitrous oxide,[48] lidocaine,[49] clonidine,[50] reserpine, and methyldopa.[51] Epinephrine[19] and other β-adrenergic receptor agonists[52] are associated with cardiac arrhythmias in the presence of halothane and, to a lesser extent, enflurane and isoflurane. The myocardial depression produced by the volatile anesthetics may be more pronounced when β-adrenergic receptor blockers[53] or calcium-channel blockers are used.[54] Halothane is associated with significant cardiac arrhythmias when it is administered to patients receiving theophylline[55] or the combination of pancuronium and a tricyclic antidepressant.[56] In patients receiving amiodarone, volatile anesthetics may be associated with heart block and sinus arrest or with bradycardia resistant to atropine.[57-59]

B. Nitrous oxide

Respiratory drive in response to carbon dioxide is not depressed, and the $PaCO_2$ does not increase in adults breathing nitrous oxide alone.[43] However, hypoxic ventilatory drive is blunted.[60] Nitrous oxide may increase cerebral blood flow and intracranial pressure,[61] but probably to a lesser degree than the volatile anesthetics.

Although nitrous oxide produces mild sympathetic stimulation when it is administered to a patient receiving one of the volatile anesthetics,[62-64] substantial cardiovascular depression (decreased cardiac output and increased cardiac filling pressures) may occur when nitrous oxide is used concomitantly with an opioid anesthetic.[65] Nitrous oxide alone, even in an analgesic dose of 40%, can cause myocardial depression in patients with occlusive coronary artery disease.[66] Pulmonary arterial pressures may increase with nitrous oxide administration, especially in patients with preexisting pulmonary hypertension.[67]

Inhibition of methionine synthetase, an enzyme involved in DNA synthesis, has been found with exposure to nitrous oxide.[68,69] Nitrous oxide oxidizes the cobalt in vitamin B_{12} to an inactive state,[68] thus inhibiting the activity of methionine synthetase and preventing the conversion of methyltetrahydrofolate to tetrahydrofolate, a compound required for DNA synthesis. This effect is probably responsible for several complications of nitrous oxide. Megaloblastic anemia may follow prolonged (many hours) administration,[70] and megaloblastic changes may be seen in critically ill patients after as little as 5 hours of exposure.[71] These changes are reversible on discontinuation of nitrous oxide administration. Chronic nonmedical abuse of nitrous oxide is associated with anemia and neurologic damage that usually manifest as polyneuropathy.[72] Nitrous oxide is teratogenic in animals if exposure occurs early in pregnancy.[73] The significance of this finding in humans is unknown, although studies have failed to demonstrate an increased incidence of birth defects in children born to women exposed to nitrous oxide anesthesia during the first or second trimester of pregnancy.[74,75]

Complications can result from nitrous oxide in closed spaces in the body because nitrous oxide diffuses into and out of closed body cavities faster than nitrogen does. This causes expansion of distensible spaces or increases in the pressure in nondistensible ones.[76] For example, the bowel may become distended during abdominal surgery, and a preexisting pneumothorax may greatly increase in size to become a tension pneumothorax.[77] Similarly, a venous air embolism may enlarge.[78] During middle ear surgery, middle ear pressure may increase,[79] and tympanic membrane rupture has occurred.[80] Dislodgment of a tympanic membrane graft may follow the development of negative middle ear pressure on discontinuation of nitrous oxide after the closure of the previously open middle ear; this occurs because the nitrous oxide diffuses out of the closed space faster than nitrogen diffuses into it.

II. INTRAVENOUS ANESTHETICS
A. Barbiturates

Although almost all of the barbiturates have somewhat similar side effects, the ultra–short-acting agents are of the most interest to anesthesiologists. Thiopental is probably the archetypical drug in this class, although thiamylal and methohexital are also commonly used and have adverse effects similar to those of thiopental.[81] Use of barbiturates should be avoided in patients with acute intermittent porphyria because acute exacerbations of the disorder may result.[82] The effects of barbiturates may be exaggerated in patients taking monoamine oxide inhibitors (MAOIs), and prolonged sedation may follow thiopental administration in patients taking tricyclic antidepressants.[83]

1. Cardiovascular effects. The doses of barbiturates used in induction of anesthesia cause a moderate (10% to 20%) decrease in blood pressure that is attributable mainly to a decrease in peripheral vascular tone with venous pooling. A baroreceptor-mediated compensatory increase in heart rate occurs, and cardiac output may fall because of decreased preload.[84] Hypotension may be severe in hypovolemic patients.[85] Occasional phlebitis may follow thiopental administration; this is more of a problem with the 5% than with the 2.5% solution of the drug.[86] Extravascular injection may cause tissue sloughing, and intraarterial injection of thiopental may result in thrombosis and permanent neurovascular damage.[87]

2. Respiratory effects. The ultra–short-acting barbiturates are potent respiratory depressants, and apnea usually accompanies the doses used for anesthetic induction with these drugs.[88] Respiratory depression with thiopental is potentiated by the presence of other central nervous system depressants, especially the opioids.[89] With a smaller dose or before the peak effect of an induction dose, hypersensitivity to airway stimulation may occur, with the potential for laryngospasm.[90]

B. Benzodiazepines and antagonist

Although the benzodiazepines produce only a mild decrease in respiratory drive when they are used for sedation in healthy patients,[91] apnea may be induced in patients with preexisting pulmonary disease or in those receiving other central nervous system depressants, such as opioids.[92] When used in larger doses for induction of anesthesia, midazolam often induces apnea.[93] Cardiovascular side effects are usually mild and consist of small decreases in blood pressure, peripheral vascular tone, and cardiac output.[94,95] However, on occasion, even a small dose of diazepam may induce hypotension.[96] Compared with diazepam, induction doses of midazolam produce a greater decrease in blood pressure because greater decreases in peripheral vascular tone result.[97] Hypovolemia accentuates this hypotensive effect.[98] The aqueous preparation of diazepam may cause pain on intravenous injection and phlebitis.[99] The benzodiazepines often produce anterograde amnesia; this effect may be more profound with midazolam.[100] This effect can be advantageous, as during cardiac anesthesia, or a complication, as for a mother during delivery of her child.[101] Maternal intake of diazepam during pregnancy has been associated with fetal anomalies.[102]

Interactions of the benzodiazepines with other drugs include potentiation of their sedative effects by other central nervous system depressants and modification of their elimination. Alcohol accentuates the central nervous system depressant effects of diazepam because it enhances systemic absorption of this drug.[103] Diazepam in doses up to 0.2 mg/kg of body weight decreases the MAC of halothane.[47] Cimetidine delays the hepatic clearance of diazepam but not midazolam or lorazepam.[81] When added to large doses of opioid anes-

thetic in patients undergoing cardiac surgery, benzodiazepines may cause substantial decreases in cardiac output and blood pressure.[104]

Flumazenil is a specific benzodiazepine-receptor antagonist. When used to reverse benzodiazepine effects, flumazenil should be titrated because it may cause anxiety, agitation, and rarely, seizures.[105] In patients with head injury who are sedated with benzodiazepines, flumazenil may increase intracranial pressure.[106]

C. Propofol

Propofol may cause pain on injection, especially when it is administered via a small vein.[107] Other bothersome side effects include coughing, hiccups, and involuntary skeletal muscle movements. Seizure-like episodes associated with propofol anesthesia have been reported. These may or may not represent primary cortical seizure activity,[108] and, conversely, propofol has been advocated as a treatment for status epilepticus.[109] Nausea and vomiting occur somewhat less frequently following propofol administration than thiopental administration.[107] Acute pancreatitis following the use of propofol in patients undergoing nonabdominal surgery was recently reported[110]; however, this association has been challenged by representatives of the manufacturer, Zeneca Pharmaceuticals (Wilmington, Delaware).[111] Cardiovascular depression and hypotension following propofol use can be pronounced in patients with coronary artery disease.[112] Heart block has been reported with propofol administration.[113] It should be emphasized that propofol is packaged in a vehicle that supports bacterial growth, and clinical infections have been associated with its use.[114] The drug should be handled using strict aseptic technique and should be used promptly once a vial is opened.

D. Etomidate

In contrast to propofol, etomidate is generally associated with cardiovascular stability.[115] Pain on injection and phlebitis occur more often with etomidate than with thiopental.[116] Etomidate causes cerebral vasoconstriction and decreases intracranial pressure.[117] Although anticonvulsant activity has been documented in animals,[118] etomidate may activate seizure foci in humans.[119] Myoclonic movements not associated with epileptiform activity on electroencephalography occur in up to one third of patients; this incidence may be decreased by pretreatment with an opioid or a benzodiazepine.[81] Etomidate increases the respiratory rate while decreasing tidal volume but may also cause apnea.[120] Significant adrenocortical suppression may occur, especially with prolonged administration, as when the drug is used for sedation in a critical care setting.[121] The incidence of postoperative nausea and vomiting is higher with etomidate than with thiopental.[122]

E. Ketamine

Ketamine is a direct myocardial depressant in vitro[123] but increases sympathetic tone in vivo, causing an increase in heart rate and blood pressure.[124] In critically ill patients in whom endogenous catecholamines may be depleted, ketamine can cause clinically significant decreases in blood pressure.[125] Ventilation is usually not depressed, but apnea can occur, especially in the presence of other central nervous system depressants.[126] The airway reflexes are usually well maintained with ketamine, but this phenomenon is not reliable.[127] Ketamine often increases oropharyngeal secretions, an effect that may be blunted by pretreatment with an antisialagogue, such as glycopyrrolate.[81] Ketamine is a potent cerebral vasodilator and can substantially increase intracranial pressure.[128,129] Transient cortical blindness (the mechanism of which is not known) has been associated with this drug. Emergence delirium occurs in 5% to 30% of patients. This phenomenon is more likely to occur with anticholinergic or droperidol premedication, in patients younger than 16 years of age, in women, and in patients with a psychiatric history; the incidence is decreased with benzodiazepine premedication.[126] In patients receiving tricyclic antidepressants, ketamine may induce hypertension and cardiac arrhythmias.[83] Hypotension may result from use of ketamine in a patient under halothane anesthesia.[123,124]

III. DRUGS USED IN PSYCHIATRIC DISORDERS

A. Antipsychotic agents

So-called antipsychotic agents often used by anesthesiologists include the phenothiazines and the butyrophenones. The most common adverse effects of these drugs are related to their cholinergic effects and include dry mouth, blurred vision, urinary retention, and tachycardia.[130] Orthostatic hypotension is relatively frequent, and the blood pressure may decrease because of peripheral α-adrenergic receptor blockade, especially during hypovolemia. Cardiac side effects may include prolongation of the PR and QT intervals and the QRS complex on electrocardiography. Preexisting heart block may be exaggerated. Sudden death from a cardiac arrhythmia has been reported with large doses of phenothiazine.[131] Possible central nervous system complications include disorientation, hallucinations, and extrapyramidal effects, such as dystoias, akathisia, and tardive dyskinesia (after prolonged therapy).[130] Droperidol may also be associated with dysphoric reactions, which can be so intense that they cause the patient to refuse surgery.[132] Antipsychotic agents interfere with hypothalamic thermoregulation, an effect that can lead to hypothermic complications[133] but may be useful in treating postoperative shivering. Antipsychotic drugs decrease the seizure threshold[134]; thus, these drugs should be used with extreme caution (if at all) in patients with parkinsonism because they may worsen symptoms of the disease. Antipsychotic agents have minimal respiratory effects but can potentiate the respiratory depression of opioids.[135]

The neuroleptic malignant syndrome has been associated with antipsychotic agents, usually early in the course of therapy.[136] This syndrome is clinically similar to malignant hyperthermia but is probably mediated by a somewhat different mechanism. Symptoms include fever, diaphoresis, dyspnea, skeletal muscle rigidity, tremors, and altered consciousness. Associated features may include tachycardia, cardiac arrhythmias, blood pressure changes, leukocytosis, and elevated concentrations of plasma creatine phosphokinase and hepatic transaminase. Risk factors appear to be high ambient temperature, malnutrition, dehydration, and physical exertion. The mortality rate associated with the neuroleptic malignant syndrome is high (approximately 20%). Treatment is symptomatic and includes discontinuation of antipsychotic medication, intravenous fluids, and cooling of the patient.[137] Bromocriptine (2 to 20 mg intravenously every 8 hours) and dantrolene sodium have been reported to help resolve the syndrome.

B. Tricyclic antidepressants

Tricyclic antidepressants have clinically significant anticholinergic adverse effects, including nausea and vomiting, drying of mucous membranes, and difficulty with urination.[130] Sedation, tremor, and seizures can occur. Cardiovascular complications include orthostatic hypotension and cardiac arrhythmias.[138] Overdose with tricyclic antidepressants is a potentially life-threatening condition that causes delirium, respiratory depression, seizures, cardiac arrhythmias, and cardiac arrest.[139] Serious ventricular arrhythmias have occurred in patients receiving tricyclic antidepressants during halothane anesthesia and in the presence of pancuronium.[83] Tricyclic antidepressants potentiate the central nervous system depressant effects of opioids.[140]

C. Monoamine oxidase inhibitors

Complications of MAOIs include orthostatic hypotension, hepatotoxicity, and serious drug interactions.[141] Overdose with these compounds produces a syndrome of sympathetic nervous system hyperactivity, including blood pressure liability, agitation, hyperpyrexia, and seizures.[142] The MAOIs potentiate the depressant effects of ethanol, barbiturates, and opioids[143] and may prolong the action of succinylcholine.[144] Hypertension, convulsions, and fever may occur if meperidine is administered to a patient receiving an MAOI.[145] Administration of sympathomimetic compounds, especially indirect-acting agents, is exaggerated in the presence of MAOIs. Hypotension in this setting is best treated by reduced doses of a direct-acting sympathomimetic agent, such as phenylephrine.[146] It has been traditionally recommended that treatment with MAOIs be discontinued for 2 weeks before elective surgery to avoid intraoperative hemodynamic instability; however, reports of stable anesthetic courses in these patients has led to the questioning of this recommendation.[147]

D. Selective serotonin reuptake inhibitors

Although selective serotonin reuptake inhibitors are generally considered to have fewer side effects than most older psychiatric drugs, problems have been reported. Hyponatremia caused by the inappropriate secretion of antidiuretic hormone has been associated with fluoxetine, sertaline, paroxetine, and fluvoxamine.[148] In addition, selective serotonin reuptake inhibitors are known to inhibit cytochrome P-450 enzymes and may inhibit the metabolism of drugs that are substrates of P-450 (e.g., diazepam, phenytoin).[149]

IV. OPIOID AGONISTS

A. Morphine

Morphine is the prototypical opioid agonist to which all other opioids are compared. Central nervous system complications of morphine use include respiratory depression, apnea, nausea, and vomiting.[150] Opioids have a sedative effect, but amnesia is not reliable, and intraoperative awareness may accompany the use of large doses of an opioid as the sole anesthetic agent.[151] Because euphoria and a feeling of well-being accompany morphine use, the drug has a high potential for abuse.

Potential adverse cardiovascular effects of morphine include a decrease in peripheral vascular tone and hypotension resulting from histamine release.[152] These effects are especially pronounced in hypovolemic patients. Sinus bradycardia secondary to central vagal stimulation may accompany administration of large doses of morphine.[153]

Morphine causes constipation and spasm of the sphincter of Oddi.[154] Gastric emptying is delayed, and in patients with gastroesophageal reflux, the severity of disease symptoms is increased. This may increase the risk of aspiration during anesthesia.[155]

B. Meperidine

Meperidine causes less biliary spasm than morphine does.[154] It is hemodynamically well tolerated in the healthy patient, but a large dose of meperidine (2 to 10 mg/kg intravenously) causes clinically significant cardiovascular depression, including decreased peripheral vascular resistance, cardiac output, and blood pressure.[156] In contrast to morphine, meperidine can cause tachycardia[156] perhaps because of its structural similarity to atropine. Like morphine, meperidine causes histamine release.[157] When meperidine is administered in the presence of MAOIs, its effects may be considerably potentiated. In addition, a severe reaction consisting of convulsions, high fever, and hypotension may occur.[145]

C. Fentanyl

Like the other opioids, fentanyl is a potent respiratory depressant. Fentanyl may cause delayed respiratory depression occurring 30 to 60 minutes after apparent initial recovery from the effects of the drug.[158] Large doses of fentanyl can produce chest wall rigidity, making ventilation of the lungs difficult. This rigidity may be prevented by pretreatment with a nondepolarizing neuromuscular blocker or by administration of a volatile anesthetic.[159] In contrast to morphine, fentanyl is not likely to decrease peripheral vascular tone or blood pressure; however, fentanyl is more likely to induce bradycardia.[160] Unlike morphine, fentanyl does not cause histamine release.[157]

D. Sufentanil

The complications of sufentanil are similar to those seen with fentanyl. Sufentanil may cause hypotension and bradycardia when large doses are used for induction of anesthesia.[161] Chest wall rigidity and delayed respiratory depression have occurred with sufentanil.[162]

E. Alfentanil

The adverse effects of alfentanil are similar to those of fentanyl. When used in large doses (125 to 150 mg/kg) for induction of anesthesia in patients undergoing coronary artery bypass procedures, alfentanil may cause a substantial decrease in blood pressure; this decrease may be greater than that produced by fentanyl or sufentanil.[163]

F. Remifentanil

The ultra–short-acting character of remifentanil allows this agent to be rapidly titrated via continuous intravenous infusion. Side effects usually abate with reduction of dose or discontinuation of the infusion. When used as an adjuvant drug during general anesthesia, remifentanil may be associated with bradycardia and hypotension. When used for analgesia in the immediate postoperative period, bolus doses or rapid increases in infusion rates may produce muscle rigidity and respiratory depression.[164]

G. Neuraxial opioids

The epidural or intrathecal administration of an opioid can produce adverse effects that differ somewhat from those seen after intravenous injection of the same drug. Respiratory depression after epidural administration of morphine occurs in a biphasic manner; an early phase occurs within the first hour after injection, and a later phase occurs about 6 to 12 hours thereafter. More lipid-soluble opioids may be associated with a lower incidence of delayed respiratory depression. Other complications of neuraxial administration of opioids include pruritus, nausea, and urinary retention. These complications are reversible with naloxone therapy.[165] Intrathecal administration of sufentanil for analgesia during labor may produce mild to moderate hypotension.[166] Sleep apnea may be a risk factor for respiratory depression with neuraxial administration of opioid.[167]

V. OPIOID ANTAGONIST: NALOXONE

Naloxone is the prototypical opioid antagonist. When used to reverse the depressant effects of opioids, naloxone may cause hypertension, tachycardia, cardiac arrhythmias, and pulmonary edema.[168] These complications are believed to be caused by a centrally mediated catecholamine release that accompanies the sudden "pharmacologic arousal." Careful titration of small intravenous doses of naloxone to reverse respiratory depression while maintaining analgesia should minimize this problem.[169] Naloxone can also produce nausea and vomiting, a complication that may also be attenuated by slow administration.[169]

VI. OPIOID AGONIST-ANTAGONISTS

As a rule, the opioid agonist-antagonists have side effects similar to those seen with the true opioids. The respiratory depression seen with these compounds reaches a ceiling effect beyond which additional doses do not produce additional depression.[155] However, clinically significant hypoventilation can occur.[170] Dysphoria is relatively common with opioid agonist-antagonists, an effect that limits the potential for abuse. These compounds are less likely than the pure agonist drugs to cause biliary spasm.[154] The antagonist properties of these agents may blunt the analgesic effects of subsequently administered true agonists[170] and may precipitate symptoms of opioid withdrawal in opioid-dependent patients.[171]

A. Butorphanol

Side effects of butorphanol include sedation, diaphoresis, nausea, vomiting, and dysphoric reactions, including hallucinations.[171] Butorphanol may cause clinically significant increases in pulmonary arterial pressure with increased myocardial oxygen demand.[172]

B. Nalbuphine

Dysphoric reactions with nalbuphine are uncommon, although dizziness, nausea, and vomiting may occur.[173] In contrast to butorphanol, nalbuphine does not increase pulmonary arterial pressure and myocardial work.[174]

C. Pentazocine

Common adverse effects of pentazocine include dizziness, diaphoresis, nausea, and vomiting.[175] Pentazocine increases the heart rate, the pulmonary and systemic arterial blood pressures, and the left ventricular filling pressure.[176] Although dysphoric reactions occur with pentazocine use, this agent does have some potential for abuse.[175]

D. Buprenorphine

The respiratory depression observed with buprenorphine use may be difficult to treat because it is not easily reversed by naloxone therapy.[177] Doxapram has been suggested as an alternative pharmacologic treatment.[178] The cardiovascular effects of buprenorphine are similar to those of morphine. As with the other agents in this class, sedation and nausea occur, but dysphoria is uncommon.

VII. LOCAL ANESTHETICS

Most complications of local anesthetics are attributable to a high blood concentration of drug secondary to inadvertent intravascular injection.[179] In general, as the blood concentration of drug increases, the patient may experience circumoral numbness, restlessness, tinnitus, and blurred vision. Drowsiness may occur with the amide local anesthetics. At even greater blood concentrations of drugs, seizures followed by central nervous system depression, apnea, and cardiovascular collapse occur. If the blood concentration of local anesthetic increases rapidly, overt seizures may be the initial symptom. Local anesthetics can interfere with neuromuscular transmission and may potentiate the effects of neuromuscular blocking drugs.[180] (See Chapter 11 for a discussion of local anesthetics and cardiac arrhythmias.)

True allergic reactions to local anesthetics are rare, probably accounting for less than 1% of all adverse reactions.[181] A patient's reaction is often termed an allergy when, in fact, it is due to a toxic blood concentration of the local anesthetic or is a reaction to the epinephrine in the local preparation. Many of the allergic reactions that occur with use of a local anesthetic are responses to preservatives, such as methylparaben, and not to the local anesthetic itself.[182] With the ester local anesthetics, p-aminobenzoic acid (PABA) is often the offending compound. This substance is a metabolite of the ester local anesthetics; therefore cross-sensitivity between these agents is to be expected. Because PABA is a common ingredient in many commercial sunscreen preparations, it might also be wise to avoid ester local anesthetics in a patient who reports an allergy to sunscreens. Patients who are allergic to esters do not seem to have increased risk for allergic responses to amide local anesthetics.[183]

A. Lidocaine

In addition to causing central nervous system toxicity, high concentrations of lidocaine can produce profound myocardial depression.[184] Atrioventricular conduction may be slowed, and heart block may be induced.[185] Lidocaine depresses the ventilatory response to hypoxia at clinically relevant plasma concentrations.[186] The systemic toxicity produced by lidocaine may be enhanced in the presence of hyperkalemia.[187] The combination of therapeutic concentrations of lidocaine and mexiletine have resulted in neurotoxicity.[188]

B. Mepivacaine

Although it is similar to lidocaine in most respects, mepivacaine causes neonatal depression when it is used for epidural anesthesia because it produces a greater and longer-lasting fetal blood concentration.[189]

C. Bupivacaine

Bupivacaine seems to be more cardiotoxic than most other local anesthetics and more likely to produce cardiac arrhythmias.[190] This cardiotoxicity may be even more pronounced in pregnancy.[191] (See Chapters 11 and 24.)

D. Ropivacaine

Ropivacaine is similar to bupivacaine in many respects but produces less intense motor block and has less cardiac toxicity.[192]

E. Prilocaine

Prilocaine has been associated with methemoglobinemia that is probably mediated through its metabolite o-toluidine.[193]

F. Etidocaine

Like bupivacaine, etidocaine seems to be more cardiotoxic than other, less potent local anesthetics.[190] Etidocaine used for peridural anesthesia can be associated more with profound motor blockade than with sensory blockade, an effect that may cause the patient substantial psychiologic stress.[194]

G. Chloroprocaine

The rapid plasma hydrolysis of chloroprocaine accounts for the very low systemic toxicity associated with this agent.[195] Neurologic deficits have been reported after inadvertent subarachnoid injection of chloroprocaine; this effect may be caused by the sodium bisulfite used as a preservative rather than by the drug itself.[196]

H. Cocaine

The toxic effects of cocaine stem mainly from its ability to block catecholamine reuptake both in the central nervous system and systemically.[197] Potential cardiovascular complications include tachycardia, peripheral vasoconstriction, hypertension, myocardial ischemia, cardiac arrhythmias, and death. Potential adverse effects to the central nervous system include restlessness, headache, nausea, convulsions, coma, and respiratory failure secondary to medullary depression. In smaller doses, cocaine produces feelings of well-being and euphoria and is a drug with great potential for abuse.

I. Tetracaine

Relative to its local anesthetic potency, tetracaine may have high intravenous toxicity compared with other local anesthetics.[194]

J. Benzocaine

Benzocaine is a local anesthetic principally used for topical anesthesia. It may cause clinically significant methemoglobinemia.[198]

VIII. NEUROMUSCULAR BLOCKERS

A. Depolarizing neuromuscular relaxants: succinylcholine

Possible adverse effects of succinylcholine include increases in intraocular, intracranial, and intragastric pressure.[199] These effects may be blunted but not abolished by pretreatment with a small dose of a nondepolarizing relaxant, such as *d*-tubocurarine or metocurine. Myalgias, especially of the neck, back, and abdomen, occur frequently after succinylcholine administration; these effects may also be attenuated by similar pretreatment. The potassium concentration in the patient's serum increases after succinylcholine is administered, but this is not blocked by pretreatment with a nondepolarizing relaxant.[200] This increase in serum potassium concentration may be sufficient to cause cardiac arrhythmias and even cardiac arrest in patients with severe burns, upper motor neuron lesions, skeletal muscle atrophy caused by denervation, and severe intraabdominal infections.[201] Sustained skeletal muscle contraction has also been described in patients with myotonic dystrophy and myotonia congenita.[202] Myoglobinuria can occur after administration of succinylcholine to normal pediatric patients.[203] Administration of succinylcholine with a volatile anesthetic is the classic means of triggering malignant hyperthermia in susceptible patients.[43] Cardiac arrhythmias may be induced by succinylcholine (see Chapter 11 for further details).

Prolonged paralysis can occur in the presence of drugs that interfere with pseudocholinesterase, the plasma enzyme that degrades succinylcholine, and in patients with abnormal or deficient pseudocholinesterase activity.[199] Compounds that may prolong the action of succinylcholine by this mechanism include certain insecticides, echothiophate eye drops, trimethaphan, and certain chemotherapeutic agents, such as cyclophosphamide. Prolonged neuromuscular blockade with features of depolarizing blockade (phase II block) can also occur with larger doses of succinylcholine or in patients with deficient pseudocholinesterase activity.[204] Prolongation of succinylcholine-induced neuromuscular block has also been reported in patients taking cimetidine.[205]

B. Nondepolarizing neuromuscular relaxants

One of the most dangerous complications of the nondepolarizing neuromuscular blockers is inadequate antagonism (reversal) or recovery from their skeletal muscle–relaxant effects. The resultant inability to support the airway leads to hypoventilation, hypercarbia, and hypoxemia, most often in the postanesthesia care unit.[206] Long-term use of nondepolarizing neuromuscular blockers (days to weeks) may be associated with prolonged skeletal muscle weakness, and monitoring of peripheral nerve twitch response in such cases is highly recommended.[207] Awareness is also a potential complication of nondepolarizing agents used in the intensive care unit; thus adequate sedation must be ensured.

1. *d*-Tubocurarine. The neuromuscular blocker *d*-tubocurarine decreases peripheral vascular tone and blood pressure by histamine release and some blockade of autonomic ganglia.[208]

2. *Metocurine.* The side effects of this agent are similar to those of *d*-tubocurarine but are of lesser magnitude.[209]

3. *Pancuronium.* In contrast to *d*-tubocurarine, pancuronium increases heart rate, cardiac output, and blood pressure by increasing plasma catecholamine concentrations and selective vagal blockade.[208] These cardiovascular effects may precipitate myocardial ischemia in patients with atherosclerotic coronary artery disease. Patients receiving digoxin may be at increased risk for cardiac arrhythmias after pancuronium administration.[210]

4. *Atracurium.* With larger doses (>2 times ED95) and rapid intravenous administration, atracurium causes histamine release with resultant cutaneous flushing and decreases in peripheral vascular tone and blood pressure.[211] In mechanically ventilated neurosurgical patients, a bolus dose of atracurium may produce modest transient decreases in cerebral perfusion pressure.[212]

5. *cis*-Atracurium. This *cis* isomer of atracurium is approximately 4 times as potent as atracurium and is largely devoid of cardiovascular side effects at bolus doses up to 8 times ED95.[213]

6. *Vecuronium.* Vecuronium is remarkably devoid of cardiovascular side effects even at larger doses, although some believe that vecuronium may magnify the bradycardia produced by opioids.[214]

7. *Rocuronium.* At doses up to 4 times ED95 (1.2 mg/kg), rocuronium causes no clinically significant hemodynamic changes or histamine release.[215]

8. Mivacurium. Mivacurium is metabolized by plasma cholinesterase and may have prolonged effects in patients with atypical or reduced levels of this enzyme. Histamine release may accompany rapid (<10 to 15 seconds) or large-dose (3 times ED95) administration.[216,217]

9. Doxacurium. Doxacurium has no clinically relevant cardiovascular and histamine-releasing side effects.[218]

10. Pipecuronium. Pipecuronium is a steroid-based relaxant that like doxacurium, is essentially devoid of histamine-releasing and cardiovascular side effects.[219]

IX. CHOLINESTERASE INHIBITORS

The cholinesterase inhibitors include neostigmine, pyridostigmine, edrophonium, and physostigmine. Their effects and complications are largely related to their anticholinesterase activity, which leads to accumulation of acetylcholine at various cholinergic sites throughout the body.[201] Possible adverse effects of the cholinesterase inhibitors include bradyarrhythmias, atrioventricular nodal block, peripheral vasodilatation, excess salivation, sweating, increased gastrointestinal motility, increased bladder tone, and bronchoconstriction. The muscarinic side effects of these agents are minimized by the concurrent administration of an anticholinergic agent. In larger doses, the cholinesterase inhibitors may produce skeletal muscle weakness.[220] Neostigmine and pyridostigmine cause pronounced inhibition of plasma cholinesterase and can greatly prolong the action of a subsequently administered dose of succinylcholine.[221] The ophthalmic anticholinesterase drugs used in the treatment of glaucoma (echothiophate, isoflurophate, and demecarium bromide) produce a similar effect. Physostigmine crosses the blood-brain barrier and produces central nervous system stimulation, an effect that has been used therapeutically.[222]

X. ANTICHOLINERGIC AGENTS

The anticholinergic drugs are competitive muscarinic receptor blockers, and their adverse effects are largely predictable on that basis. These include bradycardia (with small doses), tachycardia, dry mouth, photophobia, blurred vision, urinary retention, dry skin, fever, and changes in mental status.[223] Intravenous administration of atropine has been reported to induce ventricular tachycardia and fibrillation.[224] Bronchial secretions are reduced; this drying effect can lead to mucous plugging.[225] In patients with narrow-angle glaucoma, scopolamine may cause a deleterious increase in intraocular pressure; thus its use in these patients has been discouraged.[226] Atropine may produce the central anticholinergic syndrome, which consists of restlessness, mental status changes, and hyperpyrexia.[227] Scopolamine may also produce this syndrome but more commonly causes sedation and amnesia. Glycopyrrolate does not cause central nervous system complications because it does not readily cross the blood-brain barrier. Ipratropium bromide is a newer anticholinergic drug administered by inhalation for the treatment of bronchospastic disorders. Because ipratropium is poorly absorbed, it rarely produces systemic complications.[225]

XI. VASOACTIVE DRUGS
A. Catecholamines

The complications of catecholamines are largely an extension of their pharmacologic effects. Clinically significant hypertension may be induced with epinephrine, norepinephrine, and dopamine if the dose is not carefully titrated.[228] Catecholamines may exacerbate digitalis-associated cardiac arrhythmias, perhaps by intracellular shifting of potassium.[229]

1. Epinephrine. Epinephrine can cause clinically significant tachycardia and cardiac arrhythmias,[83] especially in the presence of halothane.[19] This drug may induce myocardial ischemia, especially in patients with preexisting cardiac disorders.[83] Epinephrine should not be added to local anesthetics for "ring blocks" of digits because the intense localized vasoconstriction caused by this catecholamine produces ischemia and necrosis of the digit.[194]

2. Norepinephrine. The intense α-adrenergic receptor effects of norepinephrine may produce ischemia of the extremities, particularly when this agent is administered in larger doses and in patients with peripheral vascular disease.[230] Metabolic acidosis can be induced by this peripheral vasoconstriction, and vasoconstriction and increased afterload may exacerbate myocardial ischemia.[231] Extravasation of norepinephrine may cause local tissue necrosis and sloughing. Prompt infiltration of the area of extravasation with a solution of 0.5% to 1% phentolamine may minimize local tissue loss.

3. Isoproterenol. The intense β-adrenergic receptor effects of isoproterenol may produce tachycardia, cardiac arrhythmias, and hypotension because of peripheral vasodilation.[228] Myocardial oxygen demand is increased, and myocardial ischemia may be exacerbated.

4. Dopamine. In small doses (less than 3 mg/kg/min), dopamine may decrease blood pressure in the presence of hypovolemia because of renal and mesenteric vasodilatation by stimulation of dopaminergic receptors. At larger doses, stimulation of β_1-adrenergic receptors may produce tachycardia, tachyarrhythmias, increased myocardial oxygen consumption, and myocardial ischemia.[232] At doses greater than 15 to 20 mg/kg/min, the α-adrenergic receptor effects of prolonged dopamine therapy can lead to limb ischemia and gangrene.[233] Inadvertent subcutaneous infiltration may produce local tissue necrosis; this may be treated in the same manner as that described for norepinephrine. Nausea and vomiting often occur when dopamine is administered to the awake patient. Clinically significant hypertension may result if dopamine is given to a patient with pheochromocytoma.

Dopamine may adversely interact with certain drugs. For example, MAOIs may greatly enhance the hypertensive response to dopamine,[130] just as the initial effect of bretylium does.[234] Administration of dopamine to a patient receiving phenytoin may induce hypotension.[235]

5. Dobutamine. Because of its β-adrenergic receptor-stimulating properties, dobutamine can produce tachycardia, cardiac arrhythmias, and myocardial ischemia. Blood pressure may decrease somewhat if the cardiac output does not increase in proportion to the decrease in peripheral vascular resistance. Nausea, headache, and skeletal muscle tremors are other potential adverse effects of dobutamine.[228]

B. Noncatecholamine inotropic agents

1. Amrinone. In addition to its positive inotropic effects, amrinone decreases systemic vascular resistance and cardiac filling pressures.[236] Hypotension may be a significant problem, especially in the presence of hypovolemia. Amrinone should be used only for short-term therapy because prolonged administration of the drug can cause thrombocytopenia and gastrointestinal disturbances. Milrinone has pharmacologic properties similar to those of amrinone; however, it has not been associated with gastrointestinal or thrombocytopenic complications.[237]

2. Digitalis. Complications of digitalis are very common; they occur in up to 20% of patients.[238] A wide range of cardiac arrhythmias have been described with digitalis toxicity; the most common rhythm disturbances include paraoxysmal atrial tachycardia with atrioventricular block, accelerated junctional rhythms, premature atrial and ventricular contractions, and ventricular tachycardia. High degrees of atrioventricular block may also occur.[239] Digitalis causes constriction of the coronary and mesenteric vasculature and may produce myocardial and gastrointestinal ischemia. Other problems that may complicate digitalis therapy include gastrointestinal disturbances (anorexia, nausea, and vomiting), visual disturbances (blurred vision and color vision changes), and mental status changes (confusion, delirium, and psychosis). The potential for complications with digitalis is increased in patients with hypokalemia, hypercalcemia, and hypomagnesemia. Pain and local irritation occur with extravasation of digitalis preparations. Adverse reactions to digitalis are more common and severe when the drug is administered intravenously.

3. Ephedrine. Ephedrine is a mixed direct- and indirect-acting α- and β-adrenergic receptor agonist with adverse effects similar to but much less frequent and severe than those of epinephrine.[240] Ephedrine crosses the blood-brain barrier and may cause agitation and tremors.

4. Mephentermine. Like ephedrine, mephentermine is a mixed-acting drug with α- and β-adrenergic receptor–stimulating properties and similar side effects. In contrast to ephedrine, mephentermine mildly decreases uterine blood flow.[241]

5. Metaraminol. Metaraminol produces more intense vasoconstriction than ephedrine and may cause reflex bradycardia.[232] Metaraminol is stored in postganglionic sympathetic nerve terminals as a false transmitter, and abrupt discontinuation of therapy with this drug after a few hours may result in hypotension. It substantially decreases uterine blood flow in pregnancy.[241]

C. Selective β_2-receptor agonists

Used mainly as bronchodilators and to halt contractions in premature labor, selective β_2-adrenergic receptor agonists are less likely than the nonselective β-agonists to cause cardiac stimulation. Selective β_2-agonists in common use include terbutaline, metaproterenol, albuterol, isoetharine, and ritodrine. Potential adverse effects include tachycardia, cardiac arrhythmias, and hypokalemia caused by a shift of potassium into cells.[232,242] When used in the management of premature labor, β_2-agonists may also induce hypertension, pulmonary edema, and deterioration of glucose control in diabetic mothers.[243]

D. Vasopressors

1. Phenylephrine. Phenylephrine increases blood pressure mainly by direct α-adrenergic stimulation. Potential complications include hypertension if phenylephrine is administered in too large a dose and reflex bradycardia with a resultant decrease in cardiac output.[244] Phenylephrine decreases renal, splanchnic, and uterine blood flow.

2. Methoxamine. Like phenylephrine, methoxamine is a direct-acting α-adrenergic agonist that induces similar side effects.[83] Methoxamine reduces renal blood flow to a greater extent than norepinephrine in equipotent doses.

E. Vasodilators

1. Nitroprusside. Nitroprusside is an arteriodilator and venodilator and may rapidly induce hypotension and reflex tachycardia. Such effects can produce myocardial ischemia, infarction, or stroke.[245] Nitroprusside inhibits hypoxic pulmonary vasoconstriction, and hypoxemia may occur.[246] Other adverse effects of nitroprusside include nausea, restlessness, intracranial hypertension, and rarely, methemoglobinemia.[245] The degradation of nitroprusside in the body produces cyanide, which is converted by hepatic and renal rhodanase to thiocyanate. Hypothermia does not interfere with the nonenzymatic liberation of cyanide from nitroprusside, but the enzymatic conversion of cyanide to thiocyanate is slowed.[247] Both cyanide and thiocyanate in sufficient concentrations produce toxicity, although the latter agent is somewhat less dangerous. Features of thiocyanate toxicity include nausea, tinnitus, changes in mental status, hyperreflexia, skeletal muscle spasms, and convulsions. Cyanide binds to cytochrome *c*, thus blocking aerobic metabolism. Cyanide toxicity may be recognized by resistance to the drug, progressive metabolic acidosis, and increased mixed venous oxygen saturation. To minimize toxicity, the dosage of nitroprusside should be limited to 8 mg/kg/min in the short term or 0.5 mg/kg/hr for infusions longer than 3 hours.[248] In addition to supportive care, hemodialysis may be required for the management of thiocyanate toxicity. Treatment of cyanide toxicity includes stopping nitroprusside therapy and administering of thiosulfate (150 mg/kg intravenously); this acts as a sulfur donor for the rhodanase system to bind cyanide. If cyanide toxicity is imminently life threatening, sodium nitrite (5 mg/kg intravenously) may be given to convert hemoglobin to methemoglobin, which binds cyanide to form cyanmethemoglobin. Use of hydroxycobalamin has also been advocated because it combines with cyanide to form cyanocobalamin. Hydroxycobalamin infusion (25 mg/hr) has been used for prevention of cyanide toxicity during nitroprusside therapy.[249]

2. Nitroglycerin. Although it is a more prominent venodilator than arteriodilator, intravenous nitroglycerin may induce clinically significant hypotension[250] and may cause hypoxemia because of ventilation-perfusion mismatch.[251] Headache is a frequent complication of nitroglycerin therapy; methemoglobinemia occurs rarely. In contrast to nitroprusside, nitroglycerin does not produce reflex tachycardia.

3. Hydralazine. A direct arteriolar smooth-muscle dilator, hydralazine causes a decrease in systemic vascular resistance and blood pressure, which induces reflex tachycardia and increases myocardial work. This effect may exacerbate angina pectoris in susceptible patients, and it has been recommended that hydralazine be used with a β-adrenergic blocker to blunt the reflex tachycardia. The onset of maximal action of hydralazine is 20 to 30 minutes, and overshoot hypotension sometimes occurs. Other adverse effects of hydralazine include headache, cutaneous flushing, and after prolonged therapy, a lupus-like syndrome.[252,253]

4. Minoxidil. Minoxidil is an arterial vasodilator with complications similar to those of hydralazine, except that no lupus-like syndrome has been described.[253] Pericardial effusion has occurred with minoxidil therapy. Minoxidil also promotes hair growth, which may be viewed as a complication or, more recently, as a therapeutic effect.

5. Diazoxide. A potent vasodilator chemically related to the thiazide diuretics,[252] diazoxide may cause reflex tachycardia and precipitate anginal symptoms in patients with coronary artery disease. Other possible complications include fluid retention, hyperglycemia, orthostatic hypotension, and pain (if the drug is extravasated).

6. Adenosine. Used as a vasodilator and for treatment of supraventricular tachycardia, adenosine may cause hypotension and heart block.[254]

7. Nitric oxide. Inhaled nitric oxide has been used experimentally as a specific pulmonary vasodilator in certain critically ill patients. It is critical to closely control and monitor inhaled nitric oxide therapy because overdose, resulting in pulmonary edema and methemoglobinemia, may be rapidly fatal.[255] Nitric oxide has been reported to interfere with platelet function and produce prolonged bleeding in healthy volunteers[256] but not in patients with acute respiratory distress syndrome.[257]

F. β-Adrenergic receptor blockers

Propranolol is the prototypical β-blocker. Other common nonselective β-blockers include timolol, pindolol, and nadalol. Propranolol competitively antagonizes both β_1 (cardiac) and β_2 (noncardiac) receptors, and its adverse effects are largely predictable on that basis. Propranolol may induce hypotension, bradycardia, bronchospasm, and congestive heart failure in susceptible patients.[258] Raynaud's phenomenon may be precipitated in patients with peripheral vascular disease as a result of blockade of the vasodilatory effect of β_2-receptors. Abrupt cessation

of β-blocker therapy is associated with a rebound sympathetic nervous system hyperactivity with worsening of the patient's underlying disorder (such as angina pectoris or hypertension). In diabetic patients, β-blockers may mask the adrenergically mediated signs of hypoglycemia, such as tremor and sweating, and may prolong hypoglycemia by interfering with epinephrine-induced glycogenolysis. Timolol may produce bradycardia and increased airway resistance even when administered as eye drops.[259] Propranolol crosses the blood-brain barrier and may produce depression, lethargy, and rarely, psychotic reactions.[253] Nadolol does not readily enter the central nervous system and is much less likely to cause these central nervous system complications. Pindolol is a nonselective β-antagonist with some intrinsic β-agonist activity. It is less likely to cause bradycardia, and larger doses can produce increases in blood pressure.[260]

The selective β_1-adrenergic receptor antagonists include metoprolol, atenolol, and esmolol. It should be recognized that these compounds are only relatively β_1 selective and may exhibit β_2-adrenergic receptor blocking effects with larger doses.[261] These drugs are much less likely than the nonselective β-blockers to cause peripheral, metabolic, and bronchospastic complications.

General anesthesia is usually well tolerated in patients receiving β-antagonists, and therapy with these drugs should be continued to the time of surgery because rebound phenomena can occur with abrupt withdrawal.[262] Additive cardiac depressant effects when volatile anesthetics are administered to patients receiving β-blockers are less prominent with isoflurane than with enflurane or halothane.[53] Timolol eye drops have been reported to cause clinically significant intraoperative bradycardia.[263]

G. α-Adrenergic receptor blockers

1. Phentolamine. A nonselective α-adrenergic receptor antagonist, phentolamine produces peripheral vasodilation and decreases in blood pressure through reflex sympathetic cardiac stimulation. Potential complications include tachycardia, cardiac arrhythmias, exacerbation for angina, abdominal pain, and diarrhea.[264]

2. Phenoxybenzamine. Like phentolamine, phenoxybenzamine is a nonselective α-adrenergic receptor antagonist and has similar adverse effects. Orthostatic hypotension may be prominent with this drug.[264]

3. Prazosin. Prazosin is a selective α_1-adrenergic antagonist that decreases blood pressure by peripheral vasodilatation. Because α_2-receptor–mediated inhibition of norepinephrine release remains intact, prazosin causes less reflex tachycardia than phentolamine.[83] Other complications of prazosin include dry mouth, lethargy, vertigo, orthostatic hypotension, and syncope. Syncope most frequently occurs on initiation of therapy.[264]

H. Mixed adrenergic antagonists: labetalol

Labetalol acts as a selective α_1-adrenergic receptor antagonist and a nonselective β-adrenergic receptor antagonist. Peripheral resistance, cardiac output, and usually heart rate are decreased.[265] Potential complications include orthostatic hypotension, fatigue, and nausea.

Bronchospasm seems to be less of a problem with labetalol than with the other nonselective β-antagonists. Anesthetized patients are somewhat more sensitive to the hypotensive effects of labetalol. Clinical experience indicates that incremental intravenous administration of 5 to 10 mg is helpful in avoiding overshoot hypotension.

I. Ganglionic blockers: trimethaphan

Trimethaphan is a ganglionic blocker used to control blood pressure.[266] It decreases peripheral vascular tone, cardiac preload, and cardiac output. Tachycardia may occur because of parasympathetic ganglionic blockade. Urinary retention and decreases in gastrointestinal motility to the point of ileus may be produced. Unlike nitroprusside, trimethaphan does not increase intracranial pressure, but cerebral blood flow is decreased. Trimethaphan inhibits plasma cholinesterase, and this effect may prolong the action of succinylcholine.[267] In large doses, trimethaphan may cause histamine release.

J. Central sympatholytics

1. Clonidine. Adverse effects of clonidine include dry mouth, skin rashes, and constipation.[247] Sedation is a common side effect, and the MAC of volatile anesthetics is reduced in the presence of clonidine.[50] Abrupt discontinuation of clonidine therapy can result in clinically significant rebound hypertension.[268]

Recently, the α_2-adrenergic agonist action of clonidine has been used in regional analgesia. For this purpose, clonidine is administered epidurally or intrathecally. Side effects include bradycardia, hypotension, and dose-dependent sedation.[269]

2. Methyldopa. Methyldopa therapy causes sedation with a reduction in MAC.[51] Hepatic dysfunction with fever and malaise may complicate therapy, and fatal hepatic necrosis attributable to methyldopa has been described. Coombs-positive hemolytic anemia and orthostatic hypotension may also occur.[252] Like clonidine therapy, abrupt discontinuation of methyldopa therapy is associated with rebound hypertension.[268]

3. Reserpine. Dry mouth, sedation, orthostatic hypotension, and bradycardia are complications of reserpine therapy.[253] Reserpine depletes central nervous system catecholamines and increases sensitivity to direct-acting sympathomimetics while blunting the response to indirect-acting ones.

XII. CALCIUM-CHANNEL BLOCKERS

Calcium-channel blockers differ in their relative effects on the heart and peripheral vasculature. Their potential complications differ accordingly. Therapy with calcium-channel blockers should be continued preoperatively when it is used to treat cardiovascular disorders. Abrupt discontinuation of therapy with these drugs has been reported to exacerbate the patient's underlying condition. Sudden withdrawal of nifedipine therapy has been associated with hypertensive crisis and exacerbation of rest angina.[270,271] Nonetheless, there are potentially adverse drug interactions of specific relevance to anesthesia. Because they are myocardial depressants and vasodilators,

calcium-channel blockers should be carefully titrated when administered to patients receiving volatile anesthetics, particularly in the presence of preexisting cardiac disease.[272] Calcium-entry blockers may potentiate the effects of neuromuscular blocking agents.[273] Verapamil has been reported to enhance the toxicity of several other drugs, including digoxin, carbamazepine, and the oral hypoglycemics.[274]

A. Verapamil

The adverse effects of verapamil are mainly extensions of its therapeutic actions. Myocardial depression and hypotension may occur, particularly in patients with preexisting myocardial dysfunction.[275] Verapamil can produce atrioventricular heart block, especially in the presence of underlying sick-sinus syndrome.[276] Verapamil may speed the ventricular response rate in patients with a preexcitation syndrome, such as Wolff-Parkinson-White syndrome.[277] Caution is advised if verapamil is used in the presence of a β-blocker because complete heart block can occur.[278] Dizziness, nausea, headache, constipation, and hepatic dysfunction are other possible side effects of verapamil. Verapamil has been reported to induce respiratory failure when administered intravenously to a patient with Duchenne muscular dystrophy, possibly because of a neuromuscular blocking effect.[279]

B. Nifedipine

Unlike verapamil, nifedipine has little effect on cardiac conduction and has a greater effect in decreasing peripheral vascular tone.[54] This may cause hypotension with reflex tachycardia. Nifedipine can induce myocardial depression in patients with aortic stenosis or preexisting ventricular dysfunction. A recent review questioned the use of sublingual nifedipine to treat hypertensive emergencies because an association with hypotension, myocardial ischemia, cerebral ischemia, and some deaths was reported.[280]

C. Diltiazem

The cardiovascular effects of diltiazem are intermediate in character between those of nifedipine and verapamil.[281] Reflex tachycardia is not a problem, but bradycardia may occur.

D. Nicardipine

Nicardipine is similar to nifedipine in its cardiovascular effects. Vasodilatation producing hypotension and reflex tachycardia may occur.[282]

XIII. HISTAMINE BLOCKERS

Histamine blockers may be classified according to whether they antagonize primarily H_1- or H_2-receptors. The potential adverse effects of these two drug classes differ substantially.

A. H_1-blockers

The H_1-receptor antagonists represent a chemically diverse group of compounds. Diphenhydramine and promethazine are probably of most interest to anesthesiologists. In general, adverse effects of these antihistamines include sedation, dizziness, and the anticholinergic effects of dry mouth and increased heart rate.[283] Rapid intravenous injection of H_1-blockers may cause a decrease in blood pressure. Antihistamine poisoning may lead to seizures, coma, and cardiovascular collapse. Promethazine enhances the sedative effects of opioids.[284]

B. H_2-blockers

Cimetidine is the model H_2-blocker. Blockade of H_2-receptors decreases gastric acidity as a desired therapeutic effect, although this breakdown of the gastric acid barrier has been alleged to predispose to infection.[285] Cimetidine crosses the blood-brain barrier and can produce sedation, confusion, and even coma, especially in elderly patients.[286] Rapid intravenous administration of cimetidine frequently induces a decrease in blood pressure and has been reported to cause bradycardia, heart block, and cardiac arrest.[287] A reversible interstitial nephritis with an increase in serum creatinine concentration occurs in about 3% of patients who receive long-term therapy with H_2-blockers. Mild increases in serum transaminase and alkaline phosphatase concentrations have also been described. Gynecomastia may be induced in some male patients. Neutropenia and thrombocytopenia occur rarely with cimetidine and are usually reversible upon discontinuation of therapy.[288] Cimetidine reduces hepatic blood flow and decreases the elimination of drugs metabolized by cytochrome P-450 enzymes (such as lidocaine, propranolol, and diazepam).[283] Pretreatment with cimetidine may also prolong the neuromuscular block caused by a bolus dose of succinylcholine.[205]

Newer H_2-blockers, such as ranitidine and famotidine, may have fewer side effects than cimetidine.[289] Ranitidine is less likely to cause sedation than cimetidine, and neither ranitidine nor famotidine seem to alter hepatic metabolism of drugs. Bradycardia has been reported with intravenous administration of ranitidine.[290]

XIV. ANTACIDS

Although the use of antacids is remarkably safe, complications can occur.[291] Antacids increase gastric fluid volume[292] and delay gastric emptying,[293] and all antacids except aluminum hydroxide may produce a metabolic alkalosis in patients with renal failure. If aspirated into the lungs, particulate antacids produce a granulomatous pulmonary reaction that may be as damaging as acid aspiration.[294]

A. Aluminum hydroxide

The most common complication of aluminum hydroxide administration is constipation. Hypophosphatemia may occur as aluminum binds with phosphates in the intestinal tract, and because these aluminum phosphates are not absorbed, phosphate loss ensues. With this hypophosphatemia, calcium absorption increases, and hypercalciuria with nephrolithiasis may follow.[295] Hypomagnesemia is another potential adverse effect of aluminum hydroxide therapy. In patients with renal failure, the accumulation of aluminum to toxic concentrations has been reported.[296]

B. Calcium carbonate

Hyperphosphatemia and hypercalcemia may occur with use of calcium carbonate, especially in the presence of renal failure. Acid rebound is common because calcium promotes increased secretion of gastric acid.[297] Hypercalcemic alkalosis with an increase in serum creatinine and blood urea nitrogen concentrations (the milk-alkali syndrome) occurs rarely after prolonged calcium carbonate therapy.

C. Sucralfate

Sucralfate, although it is not an antacid, is a complex of aluminum hydroxide and sucrose sulfate. Like aluminum hydroxide, its main complication is constipation.

D. Sodium bicarbonate

Although sodium bicarbonate is a very potent acid-neutralizing agent, its effect on gastric pH is short lived, and the large amount of sodium absorbed may cause great difficulty for patients with hypertension or congestive heart failure.

E. Sodium citrate

Sodium citrate is associated with few adverse effects. Aspiration of 0.3 M of sodium citrate causes less pulmonary damage than that caused by particulate antacids.[294] The "complications" of poor palatability is lessened considerably in commercial preparations containing citric acid (such as Polycitra and Bicitra [Baker Norton Pharmaceuticals, Miami, Florida]).

XV. DIURETICS
A. Loop diuretics

Loop diuretics (furosemide, bumetanide, and ethacrynic acid) are potent drugs that may substantially alter the body's fluid and electrolyte balance. Hypovolemia, hyponatremia, and hypokalemia can be problems with these drugs. The volume depletion caused by loop diuretics can be severe and even result in death.[298] Uric acid concentrations are increased, and precipitation of acute attacks of gout is possible in susceptible persons. Ototoxicity occurs with a high peak blood concentration of these drugs, and rapid injection should be avoided. Ethacrinic acid may be more ototoxic than furosemide. The chemical structure of furosemide is similar to that of the sulfonamides, and cross-allergic responses occur. Blood pressure may decrease after intravenous administration of furosemide because of increased venous capacitance with a decrease in cardiac preload. Interstitial nephritis has been reported with furosemide.[299] Lithium clearance is decreased by the loop diuretics, and elevation of lithium levels may occur with perioperative use of furosemide.[300] Furosemide may enhance the relaxant effect of nondepolarizing neuromuscular blockers.[301]

B. Thiazides

Thiazide diuretics may cause a hypochloremic, hypokalemic metabolic alkalosis and, like loop diuretics, may increase serum concentrations of uric acid.[299] These drugs decrease carbohydrate tolerance and can elevate serum glucose concentrations in diabetic patients. Rashes are common. Other reported complications of thiazide therapy include purpura, photosensitive dermatitis, antibody-induced thrombocytopenia, bone marrow depression, and necrotizing vasculitis.[299]

C. Potassium-sparing diuretics

Potassium-sparing diuretics can seriously elevate serum potassium concentrations, especially in renal failure. In addition, spironolactone may produce nausea in men and women and gynecomastia in men.[299]

D. Osmotic diuretics

Osmotic diuretics (mannitol and urea) transiently increase extracellular fluid volume[302] and may exacerbate congestive heart failure. Hyponatremia can occur because of the sodium-losing diuresis of these drugs. Urea produces a clinically significant incidence of venous thrombosis, and tissue necrosis may occur with extravasation of urea solutions.

E. Carbonic anhydrase inhibitors

Large doses of carbonic anhydrase inhibitors (such as acetazolamide) may cause paresthesias and drowsiness.[299] Acetazolamide is teratogenic in animals and has been associated with osteomalacia when combined with phenytoin.

XVI. ANTICOAGULANTS, THROMBOLYTICS, AND ANTIFIBRINOLYTICS

The chief danger of use of any of the anticoagulants and thrombolytic agents is hemorrhage.[303] Although the incidence of this complication may be minimized by appropriate hematologic monitoring, bleeding can occur despite maintenance of coagulation within the desired therapeutic range. Anticoagulation is a strong relative contraindication to spinal or epidural anesthesia because of the risk for peridural hematoma. Hemorrhagic complications seem to be more frequent in elderly women.

A. Heparin

A small short-term decrease in platelet count may accompany heparin therapy in up to one third of patients.[304] This is usually of little clinical significance; however, severe thrombocytopenia may occur in less than 1% of heparin-treated patients. Platelet counts usually approach normal values on discontinuation of therapy. Paradoxically, some patients may display thrombotic diathesis during heparin therapy because of a decrease in antithrombin III activity.[305] Necrosis of the skin and subcutaneous tissues has been attributed to heparin.[306] Serum transaminase concentrations increase in many patients during heparin therapy.[307] Hyperkalemia may occur, especially in patients with diabetes or renal insufficiency.[308] Heparin is highly protein bound and may displace other drugs (e.g., diazepam or propranolol) from protein-binding sites, thereby increasing free plasma concentrations of these agents.[309]

Use of low-molecular-weight heparins (e.g., enoxaparin, dalteparin, ardeparin, and danaparoid) used to prevent perioperative deep venous thrombosis may increase the risk for peridural hematomas in patients undergoing spinal or epidural anesthesia or lumbar puncture. The U.S. Food and Drug Administration (FDA) issued a public health advisory on December 15, 1997, stating that it had received more than 30 reports of epidural and spinal hematomas associated with the use of these drugs and spinal and epidural anesthesia, including reports of permanent neurologic injury. Most of these reports involved elderly women, and the FDA's report indicated an increased risk with the use of indwelling epidural catheters and drugs that affect hemostasis (e.g., nonsteroidal antiinflammatory drugs and other anticoagulants).

B. Coumarin derivatives (oral anticoagulants)

Coumarin derivatives are associated with serious teratogenic effects when administered to pregnant women in the first trimester. In addition, these drugs cross the placenta and produce a high risk for fetal hemorrhage.[310] Like heparin, coumarin may cause skin necrosis.[306] Concomitant administration of salicylates or phenylbutazone substantially increases the risk for hemorrhagic complications.[311]

C. Thrombolytics

In contrast to the traditional anticoagulants, which prevent formation of new clot, the thrombolytic agents (streptokinase, urokinase, and tissue plasminogen activators) enhance the conversion of plasminogen to plasmin and thus the lysis of existing clot.[312] This pharmacologic action explains the greater risk for hemorrhage with these drugs than with heparin.[312] Fever is a common side effect of these drugs, and allergic responses are more prevalent with streptokinase than with urokinase or tissue plasminogen activators. Aminocaproic acid antagonizes the thrombolytic effect of these drugs and may be used to treat overdose with thrombolytic drug overdose.[306]

D. Protamine

Although protamine is usually administered to neutralize the effects of heparin, it has intrinsic anticoagulant properties.[313] Intraoperative bleeding has been attributed to protamine excess when this drug is used to reverse heparin anticoagulation; this effect may be caused by inhibition of platelet aggregation.[314] Protamine may be associated with clinically significant histamine release, especially if it is administered rapidly, producing cutaneous flushing, bronchoconstriction, hypotension, and tachycardia. Patients with limited cardiac reserve may be more susceptible to protamine-induced hypotension.[315] Protamine has been reported to increase pulmonary vascular resistance.[316] Allergic reactions to protamine seem to be more likely in patients receiving protamine-containing insulin preparations[317] and, possibly, in patients who are allergic to fish (protamine is a fish-derived product).

E. Aprotinin

The nonspecific protease inhibitor aprotinin has been implicated in producing a relatively high incidence of anaphylactic reactions; an even higher incidence (up to 4%) occurs with reexposure to the drug within 6 months.[318] Aprotinin has also been alleged to cause thrombotic complications,[319] and one recent multicenter study of patients undergoing cardiac valve surgery found an increased incidence of postoperative renal dysfunction in diabetic patients given aprotinin.[320]

F. Lysine analogs

The most commonly used specific antifibrinolytic drugs include the lysine analogs ϵ-aminocaproic acid and tranexamic acid. Thrombotic complications are rare with these agents, although hematuria may be a contraindication because of the potential for urinary tract clot formation, renal colic, and obstructive uropathy.[321] Thrombus formation on pulmonary artery catheters has also been reported following use of ϵ-aminocaproic acid.[322]

XVII. ANTIPLATELET AGENTS
A. Aspirin

Aspirin's antiplatelet effect may prolong bleeding time for several days and may cause excessive intraoperative bleeding.[323] Symptoms of salicylate toxicity include headache, tinnitus, confusion, drowsiness, nausea, and hyperventilation.[324]

B. Dipyridamole

Complications of dipyridamole therapy include dizziness, abdominal distress, headache, and rashes.[303]

C. Dextrans

Used as volume expanders and antiplatelet agents, dextran 40 and dextran 70 have been associated with severe anaphylactoid reactions.[325] Dextran 40 may cause acute renal failure,[326] especially if administered to hypovolemic patients, because it is filtered by the kidney and may increase urine viscosity to the point of tubular obstruction. Dextran 70 may produce a bleeding diathesis.[327]

XVIII. ANTIARRHYTHMIC AGENTS

The complications of lidocaine, calcium-channel blockers, digitalis, adenosine, and β-adrenergic antagonists are covered elsewhere in this chapter.

A. Procainamide

In addition to its membrane-stabilizing effects, procainamide has ganglion-blocking properties. Vasodilatation and hypotension may occur after procainamide administration, particularly after rapid intravenous injection.[327] Procainamide slows impulse conduction through the heart, causing widening of the QRS complex and prolongation of the PR and QT intervals on echocardiography, which may be premonitory signs of heart block or cardiac arrest. Negative inotropic effects of procainamide can be pronounced in patients with preexisting myocardial dysfunction.[328] Fever, agranulocytosis, and a lupus-like syndrome may also be complications of procainamide therapy. Procainamide may enhance the neuromuscular blockade of nondepolarizing muscle re-

laxants[329] and may induce substantial muscle weakness in myasthenic patients.[330]

B. Quinidine

Gastrointestinal upset (nausea, vomiting, and diarrhea) are the most frequent side effects of quinidine. On echocardiography, prolongation of the QRS complex and QT interval occur with higher blood concentrations of drug, and serious ventricular arrhythmias, including ventricular tachycardia (torsade de pointes) and ventricular fibrillation, may result. Quinidine has α-adrenergic blocking properties and can cause hypotension, which can be severe if the drug is administered intravenously. Hypokalemia exacerbates quinidine-induced cardiac arrhythmias. A high blood concentration of quinidine may produce tinnitus and vertigo similar to that seen in salicylate toxicity. Fever, hepatic dysfunction, and thrombocytopenia are immunologically mediated complications of quinidine therapy.[328] Quinidine enhances the muscle-relaxant effects of the depolarizing and nondepolarizing neuromuscular blockers[331] and increases the plasma concentration of digoxin.[328]

C. Bretylium

Release of endogenous norepinephrine as a result of administration of bretylium may cause initial tachycardia and hypertension; however, bretylium subsequently produces an adrenergic block, which can lead to hypotension and bradycardia.[332] Nausea and vomiting may also occur with use of bretylium.[233]

D. Phenytoin

Phenytoin (diphenylhydantoin) has anticonvulsant and antiarrhythmic properties. When phenytoin is administered by rapid intravenous infusion, transient high blood concentrations of drug may induce nystagmus, dizziness, hypotension, heart block, and asystole. Long-term therapy is associated with gingival hyperplasia, peripheral neuropathy, hyperglycemia, skin rashes, megaloblastic anemia, and hepatitis.[328]

E. Disopyramide

The complications of disopyramide include anticholinergic effects (dry mouth and urinary retention), myocardial depression, and conduction abnormalities.[328] Congestive heart failure can be induced by disopyramide when administered in the presence of preexisting myocardial dysfunction.[333]

F. Amiodarone

Administration of the antiarrhythmic drug amiodarone may be accompanied by bradycardia and lengthening of the QT interval on echocardiography.[334] Vasodilatation, hypotension, heart block, and sinus arrest can complicate amiodarone therapy,[335] and severe bradycardia with sinus arrest has occurred in patients under general anesthesia.[336] Bradycardia resulting from amiodarone therapy seems to be resistant to atropine and may require β-adrenergic therapy with isoproterenol or insertion of an artificial pacemaker. Long-term therapy with amiodarone is sometimes associated with hyperthyroidism or hypothyroidism, photosensitivity, neuropathies, and hepatotoxicity. Amiodarone may greatly elevate plasma concentrations of digoxin.[337]

G. Mexiletine

A class 1-B antiarrhythmic agent, mexiletine has side effects similar to those of lidocaine. Seizures have been reported with mexiletine,[338] and neurotoxicity has been reported with the combination of mexiletine and lidocaine at "therapeutic" blood concentrations.[188]

XIX. SELECTED ANTIBIOTICS

Most patients receive antibiotic therapy after surgery, and anesthesiologists frequently administer these drugs at the request of the surgeon. Therefore we discuss the antibiotic-induced complications of greatest importance to the practice of anesthesia.

A. Penicillins and cephalosporins

The most common adverse reactions to penicillins and cephalosporins are allergy related.[339] Most of these reactions are skin rashes, but bronchospasm, angioedema, and anaphylaxis also occur. Despite the common β-lactam structure, the cross-sensitivity between penicillins and cephalosporins is not absolute but is estimated to occur in up to 10% of patients with a penicillin allergy.[340] Patients who are allergic to penicillin may experience anaphylaxis in response to cephalosporin use.[341] In light of this incidence of cross-sensitivity, the administration of a cephalosporin to a patient with a history of a life-threatening reaction to a penicillin must be considered carefully.

B. Aminoglycosides

Aminoglycosides may cause ototoxicity and nephrotoxicity, especially in high blood concentrations.[342,343] Rapid intravenous administration of these drugs is best avoided to prevent high peak blood concentrations, which may induce demonstrable ototoxicity with a single injection of aminoglycoside.[344] The effects of the nondepolarizing neuromuscular blockers may be potentiated.[345] Skeletal muscle weakness has been reported and may be pronounced in patients with myasthenia gravis.[346]

C. Vancomycin

Rapid intravenous infusion (less than 60 minutes) of vancomycin can be associated with cutaneous flushing, bronchospasm, and profound hypotension caused by histamine release and, possibly, direct myocardial depression. Skin rashes, ototoxicity, and, rarely, nephrotoxicity are other complications of vancomycin therapy.[347]

D. Amphotericin B

Serious adverse effects are common with amphotericin B, an antifungal agent. During infusion of amphotericin B, fever, chills, and malaise occur frequently, and hypotension is not uncommon. Renal toxicity is common. Anemia, thrombocytopenia, hypokalemia, and seizures can also occur with use of amphotericin B.[348,349]

XX. MISCELLANEOUS DRUGS

A. Metoclopramide

Metoclopramide stimulates upper gastrointestinal motility and can cause abdominal pain and cramping.[350] The drug should not be used in patients with bowel obstruction or perforation because increases in intraluminal gastrointestinal pressures may cause or increase intraperitoneal spillage of bowel contents. Extreme restlessness (akathisia) can occur with higher blood concentrations of metoclopramide,[351] especially in children, elderly patients, and patients with renal failure. Metoclopramide may cause extrapyramidal reactions and sedation and may increase the extrapyramidal and sedative effects of other drugs. Other complications of metoclopramide therapy occur mainly with long-term therapy and include dysphoria, agitation, oral or periorbital edema, dry mouth, and cutaneous rashes.

B. Theophylline

Adverse effects of theophylline therapy include nausea and vomiting, headache, restlessness, agitation, seizures, tachycardia, and cardiac arrhythmias.[352,353] Cardiac arrhythmias may be more frequent or severe when theophylline is combined with β-agonists or halothane anesthesia.[55,353] Avoidance of intravenous administration of theophylline through a central line has been suggested to minimize exposure of the heart to high drug concentrations.[354] Monitoring the blood concentration of theophylline is useful in avoidance of toxicity.

C. Pentoxifylline

When it is used to improve capillary blood flow in patients with peripheral vascular disease, pentoxifylline therapy rarely causes complications; however, these complications include cardiac arrhythmias, hypotension, and angina.[355]

D. Doxapram

Doxapram may induce hypertension, tachycardia, vomiting, sweating, fever, and convulsions.[356]

E. Dantrolene

When dantrolene is administered for prophylaxis against malignant hyperthermia, it can induce dizziness, nausea, blurred vision, diarrhea, and sedation.[357] Skeletal muscle weakness is a common subjective complaint and can be clinically significant in patients with preexisting muscular disorders.[358] Hepatitis after long-term therapy with dantrolene is not uncommon[359]; however, hepatic dysfunction with short-term administration has not been reported.

F. Ketorolac

Ketorolac is a nonsteroidal antiinflammatory drug. When administered in the perioperative period, it has been associated with increased bleeding following tonsillectomy[360] but not after mastectomy.[361] Ketorolac has been reported to cause acute renal failure[362] and gastric ulceration.[363]

G. Ondansetron

Used as an antiemetic, ondansetron rarely causes clinically significant complications. However, when it was administered in a large (32-mg) intravenous dose over 15 minutes in healthy adults, ondansetron was found to prolong the QTc interval on electrocardiography.[364] Cardiac arrhythmias have been reported with use of ondansetron plus metoclopramide.[365] Psychiatric disturbances have also been described following ondansetron therapy.[366]

Table 7-1. Drug complications

Pharmaceutical class	Drug	Complications and adverse effects
Inhaled anesthetics	Halothane	Myocardial depression, hypotension, arrhythmias, respiratory depression, hepatotoxicity, increased intracranial pressure, uterine relaxation
	Enflurane	Myocardial depression, hypotension, tachycardia, arrhythmias, respiratory depression, "seizures," increased intracranial pressure, nephrotoxicity, hepatotoxicity, uterine relaxation
	Isoflurane	Vasodilatation, hypotension, myocardial depression, tachycardia, arrhythmias, respiratory depression, increased intracranial pressure, possible hepatotoxicity, uterine relaxation
	Desflurane	Vasodilatation, tachycardia (especially with abrupt increases in concentration), hypotension, airway irritation, increased intracranial pressure, respiratory depression
	Sevoflurane	Vasodilatation, hypotension, myocardial depression, possible nephrotoxicity (with compound A and fluoride)
	Nitrous oxide	Expansion of closed spaces in the body, increased intracranial pressure, decreased hypoxic respiratory drive, myocardial depression, increased pulmonary arterial pressure, megaloblastic anemia, neurotoxicity (with long-term exposure)
Intravenous anesthetics	Barbiturates	Hypotension, vasodilatation, tachycardia, respiratory depression, phlebitis, tissue damage with extravasation or arterial injection
	Benzodiazepine antagonist (flumazenil)	Respiratory depression, vasodilatation, amnesia, phlebitis, pain on injection (diazepam); anxiety, agitation seizures (with flumazenil)
	Propofol	Hypotension, heart block, pain on injection, myoclonus, hiccups, support of bacterial growth
	Etomidate	Pain on injection, myoclonus, activation of seizure foci, adrenal suppression, nausea
	Ketamine	Tachycardia, arrhythmias, increased secretions, increased intracranial pressure, emergence delirium, transient cortical blindness, flashbacks
Drugs used in psychiatric disorders	Phenothiazines and butyrophenones	Dry mouth, blurred vision, urinary retention, tachycardia, orthostatic hypotension, heart blocks, arrhythmias, disorientation, dysphoria, impaired thermoregulation, lowered seizure threshold, neuroleptic malignant syndrome
	Tricyclics	Dry mouth, nausea, tremor, seizures, arrhythmias, orthostatic hypotension
	Monoamine oxidase inhibitors	Orthostatic hypotension, hepatotoxicity, seizures, fever
	Selective serotonin reuptake inhibitors	Hyponatremia (inappropriate secretion of antidiuretic hormone)
Opioid agonists	Morphine	Respiratory depression, nausea, vasodilatation, hypotension, bradycardia, biliary spasm, urinary retention, delayed gastric emptying
	Meperidine	Respiratory depression, cardiovascular depression, hypotension, tachycardia, biliary spasm, nausea
	Fentanyl	Respiratory depression, chest wall rigidity, bradycardia
	Sufentanil	Similar to those of fentanyl; hypotension

Table 7-1. Drug complications—cont'd

Pharmaceutical class	Drug	Complications and adverse effects
	Alfentanil	Similar to those of fentanyl; hypotension
	Remifentanil	Similar to those of fentanyl; hypotension
	Spinal or epidural administration of neuraxial opioids	Respiratory depression (early and delayed), pruritis, urinary retention, nausea, somnolence, mild hypotension (intrathecal sufentanil in laboring parturients)
Opioid antagonist	Naloxone	Hypertension, tachycardia, arrhythmias, pulmonary edema, nausea, vomiting
Opioid agonist-antagonists	Butorphanol	Respiratory depression, diaphoresis, nausea, dysphoria, increased pulmonary arterial pressure
	Nalbuphine	Respiratory depression, dizziness, nausea
	Pentazocine	Respiratory depression, dysphoria, nausea, tachycardia, increased pulmonary arterial pressure, hypertension
	Buprenorphine	Respiratory depression, nausea, cardiovascular effects similar to those of morphine
Local anesthetics	All	Tinnitus, agitation, blurred vision, drowsiness, seizures, coma, cardiovascular collapse
	Ester-type local anesthetics	Cross-sensitivity to *p*-aminobenzoic acid
	Lidocaine	Arteriolar vasodilatation, myocardial depression, heart blocks, respiratory depression
	Mepivacaine	Similar to those of lidocaine; fetal depression
	Bupivacaine	Cardiotoxicity, lesser margin between central nervous system and cardiac toxicity
	Ropivacaine	Similar to those of bupivacaine but less cardiotoxic
	Prilocaine	Methemoglobinemia
	Etidocaine	Similar to those of bupivacaine
	Chloroprocaine	Neutrotoxicity with subarachnoid use (it is not known whether the drug or the preservative causes this effect)
	Cocaine	Tachycardia, hypertension, myocardial ischemia, arrhythmias, agitation
	Tetracaine	Possibility of relatively high intravenous toxicity for anesthetic potency
	Benzocaine	Methemoglobinemia
Depolarizing relaxant	Succinylcholine	Increased intracranial and intraocular pressures, myalgias, hyperkalemia, myoglobinuria, arrhythmias, sustained muscle contractions, triggering of malignant hyperthermia
Nondepolarizing relaxants	All	Respiratory embarrassment (incomplete reversal), weakness with prolonged use in the intensive care unit
	d-Tubocurarine	Vasodilatation, histamine release, hypotension
	Metocurine	Adverse effects are similar to *d*-tubocurarine but of lesser magnitude
	Pancuronium	Tachycardia, hypertension, arrhythmias
	Atracurium	Histamine release, vasodilatation, hypotension, transient decreased cerebral perfusion pressure (in ventilated neurosurgical patients)
	Vecuronium	Potentiation of opioid-induced bradycardia
	Mivacurium	Cutaneous flushing, hypotension, prolonged block in peudocholinesterase-deficient patients
Cholinesterase inhibitors	All	Bradycardia, heart blocks, vasodilatation, salivation, abdominal cramping, bronchoconstriction, skeletal muscle weakness (with large doses)
	Physostigmine	Agitation
Anticholinergic drugs	Atropine	Bradycardia (with small doses), tachycardia, arrhythmias, photophobia, blurred vision, urinary retention, dry skin, fever, mental status changes, thickening of bronchial secretions, increased intraocular pressure (in narrow-angle glaucoma)
	Scopolamine	Similar to those of atropine, except this drug produces sedation and amnesia

Continued.

Table 7-1. Drug complications—cont'd

Pharmaceutical class	Drug	Complications and adverse effects
	Glycopyrrolate	Similar to those of atropine, but this drug produces less tachycardia and no central nervous system effects
	Ipratropium	Inspissated bronchial secretions, systemic effects rare (not absorbed with inhalation)
Catecholamines	Epinephrine	Tachycardia, arrhythmias, myocardial ischemia, hyperglycemia, hypertension
	Norepinephrine	Hypertension, peripheral ischemia, arrhythmias, tissue necrosis with extravasation
	Isoproterenol	Tachycardia, arrhythmias, vasodilatation, hypotension, myocardial ischemia
	Dopamine	Hypotension (with small doses), tachycardia, arrhythmias, myocardial ischemia, peripheral ischemia (with large doses), tissue necrosis with extravasation, hypertension, nausea, vomiting
	Dobutamine	Tachycardia, arrhythmias, hypotension, nausea, headache, muscle tremors
Noncatecholamine inotropes	Amrinone	Vasodilatation, hypotension, gastrointestinal upset, thrombocytopenia
	Milrinone	Vasodilatation, hypotension
	Digitalis	Arrhythmias, heart block, myocardial and bowel ischemia, nausea, vomiting, visual disturbances, mental status changes, tissue irritation on extravasation
	Ephedrine	Similar to those of epinephrine but are less severe; tremor and agitation may also occur
	Mephentermine	Similar to those of ephedrine; decreases uterine blood flow in the parturient
	Metaraminol	Hypertension, bradycardia, hypotension if prolonged infusion is abruptly stopped
Selective β_2-adrenergic receptor agonists	All	Tachycardia, arrhythmias, hypokalemia; when used in premature labor, may also cause hypertension, pulmonary edema, and worsening of diabetic control
Vasopressors	Phenylephrine	Hypertension, bradycardia
	Methoxamine	Similar to those of phenylephrine; decreased renal perfusion
Vasodilators	Nitroprusside	Hypotension, tachycardia, myocardial ischemia, nausea, restlessness, intracranial hypertension, hypoxemia Cyanide toxicity—metabolic acidosis Thiocyanate toxicity—tinnitus, mental status changes, muscle spasms, convulsions
	Nitroglycerin	Hypotension, headache, methemoglobinemia, hypoxemia
	Hydralazine	Hypotension, tachycardia, headache, cutaneous flushing, lupus-like syndrome
	Minoxidil	Similar to hydralazine, pericardial effusion; no lupus-like syndrome
	Diazoxide	Hypotension, tachycardia, myocardial ischemia, hyperglycemia, pain on extravasation
	Adenosine	Hypotension, heart block
	Nitric oxide	Methemoglobinemia, pulmonary edema
β-Adrenergic receptor blockers	Nonselective (e.g., propranolol)	Bradycardia, hypotension, bronchospasm, congestive heart failure (in susceptible patients), Raynaud's phenomenon, exacerbation of hypoglycemia in diabetic patients, lethargy, fatigue
	Nadolol	Same as above, except lesser central nervous system problems
	Pindolol	Same as above, except less bradycardia; hypertension (larger doses)
	Timolol	Same as above; eye drops may cause intraoperative bradycardia

Table 7-1. Drug complications—cont'd

Pharmaceutical class	Drug	Complications and adverse effects
	Selective β_1-adrenergic receptor antagonists (e.g., metoprolol)	Same as those of nonselective β-blockers, but bronchospasm, Raynaud's phenomenon, and exacerbation of hypoglycemia in diabetic patients are less likely
α-Adrenergic receptor blockers	Phentolamine	Vasodilatation, hypotension, tachycardia, arrhythmias, myocardial ischemia, abdominal pain, diarrhea
	Phenoxybenzamine	Similar to those of phentolamine
	Prazosin	Same as those of phentolamine but less tachycardia; also dry mouth, lethargy, vertigo, syncope (especially with the first dose)
Mixed adrenergic blocker	Labetalol	Bradycardia, hypotension, fatigue, nausea, bronchospasm
Ganglionic blocker	Trimethaphan	Vasodilatation, hypotension, tachycardia, urinary retention, ileus, histamine release (with large doses)
Central sympatholytics	Clonidine	Sedation, dry mouth, skin rash, constipation, rebound hypertension with abrupt discontinuation of therapy
	Clonidine (neuraxial administration)	Hypotension, bradycardia, sedation
	Methyldopa	Sedation, hepatotoxicity, anemia, orthostatic hypotension, rebound hypertension
	Reserpine	Dry mouth, sedation, orthostatic hypotension, bradycardia
Calcium-channel blockers	Verapamil	Myocardial depression, hypotension, heart blocks, dizziness, nausea, headache, hepatotoxicity, accelerated heart rate (in preexcitation syndromes)
	Nifedipine	Vasodilatation, hypotension, tachycardia, myocardial depression, rebound hypertension, angina
	Diltiazem	Bradycardia, hypotension, myocardial depression
	Nicardipine	Similar to those of nifedipine
Histamine$_1$-blockers	All	Sedation, dizziness, dry mouth, tachycardia, seizures, hypotension (with rapid intravenous injection)
	Promethazine	Same as above, plus tissue necrosis on extravasation or arterial injection
Histamine$_2$-blockers	Cimetidine	Sedation, confusion, coma, hypotension (with intravenous injection), bradycardia, heart block (with intravenous injection), nephritis, neutropenia, thrombocytopenia
	Ranitidine	Same as those of cimetidine, except no heart block or central nervous system effects
	Famotidine	Same as those of ranitidine
Antacids	Aluminum hydroxide	Constipation, hypophosphatemia, nephrolithiasis, hypomagnesemia, aluminum toxicity (in renal failure), granulomatous reaction (if aspirated)
	Calcium carbonate	Hypercalcemia, hyperphosphatemia, acid rebound, milk-alkali syndrome, granulomatous reaction (if aspirated), metabolic alkalosis
	Sodium bicarbonate	Metabolic alkalosis, sodium overload (in congestive heart failure)
	Sodium citrate	Poor ability to taste, damage if aspirated (but less than that seen with particulate antacids)
Diuretics	Furosemide	Vasodilatation, hypotension, hypovolemia, hyponatremia, hypokalemia, ototoxicity, interstitial nephritis, hyperuricemia
	Ethacrynic acid	Same as those of furosemide, except increased ototoxicity
	Thiazides	Hypochloremia, hypokalemia, hyperuricemia, metabolic alkalosis, hyperglycemia, thrombocytopenia, rashes
	Spironolactone	Hyperkalemia, nausea
	Mannitol	Hyponatremia, transient increased vascular volume, fluid shift
	Urea	Same as those of mannitol; venous thrombosis, tissue necrosis if the drug is extravasated

Continued.

Table 7-1. Drug complications—cont'd

Pharmaceutical class	Drug	Complications and adverse effects
	Acetazolamide	Drowziness, metabolic acidosis, rashes, paresthesias
Anticoagulants	Heparin	Bleeding, thrombocytopenia, cutaneous necrosis, paradoxical hypercoagulability, increased hepatic enzymes, neuropathy, alopecia
	Low-molecular-weight heparin (e.g., enoxaparin)	Spinal or epidural hematoma with a spinal or epidural procedure
	Coumarin	Bleeding, teratogenicity, skin necrosis
	Protamine	Histamine release, vasodilatation, hypotension, bronchoconstriction, tachycardia, increased pulmonary arterial pressure
Thrombolytics	Streptokinase	Bleeding, fever, allergic reactions
	Urokinase, tissue plasminogen activators	Same as those of streptokinase, except fewer allergic responses
Antifibrinolytics	Aprotinin	Anaphylaxis (especially on reexposure), thrombotic events, possible renal dysfunction in diabetic patients
	ε-Aminocaproic acid, tranexamic acid	Catheter thrombosis, urinary obstruction (in patients with hematuria)
Antiplatelet drugs	Aspirin	Prolonged bleeding times, tinnitus, nausea, confusion, hyperventilation
	Dipyridamole	Dizziness, headache, abdominal distress, rashes, vasodilatation, hypotension (with intravenous injection)
	Dextrans	Anaphylaxis, acute renal failure (with dextran 40), bleeding diathesis (with dextran 70)
Antiarrhythmic drugs	Lidocaine	*See* local anesthetics
	Verapamil	*See* calcium-channel blockers
	Adenosine	*See* vasodilators
	Procainamide	Vasodilatation, hypotension, heart block, myocardial depression, fever, agranulocytosis, lupus-like syndrome, muscle weakness (in myasthenic patients)
	Quinidine	Gastrointestinal disturbances, ventricular arrhythmias, hypotension, tinnitus, vertigo, fever, thrombocytopenia, hepatotoxicity
	Bretylium	Tachycardia, hypertension, bradycardia, hypotension, nausea, vomiting
	Phenytoin	Nystagmus, dizziness, hypotension, heart blocks, asystole, gingival hyperplasia, hepatitis, hyperglycemia, rashes, peripheral neuropathy, anemia
	Disopyramide	Myocardial depression, heart block, dry mouth, urinary retention
	Amiodarone	Bradycardia, heart block, vasodilatation, hypotension, thyroid dysfunction, hepatotoxicity, neuropathy
	Mexiletine	Seizures
Antibiotics	Penicillins and cephalosporins	Skin rashes, angioedema, anaphylaxis, up to 10% incidence of cross-reactivity
	Aminoglycosides	Ototoxicity, nephrotoxicity, skeletal muscle weakness
	Vancomycin	Bronchospasm, hypotension, flushing, ototoxicity, nephrotoxicity, possible myocardial depression
	Amphotericin B	Fever, hypotension, nephrotoxicity, hypokalemia, thrombocytopenia, anemia, seizures
Miscellaneous drugs	Metoclopramide	Abdominal cramps, restlessness, extrapyramidal reactions, sedation, dysphoria, rashes
	Theophylline	Nausea, vomiting, headache, agitation, tachycardia, arrhythmias, seizures
	Pentoxifylline	Arrhythmias, hypotension, angina
	Doxapram	Hypertension, tachycardia, vomiting, fever, convulsions
	Dantrolene	Dizziness, nausea, diarrhea, sedation, muscle weakness, hepatitis (with long-term use)
	Ketorolac	GI complications, renal dysfunction, possible increased postoperative bleeding (with certain procedures)
	Ondansetron	Psychiatric disturbances, possible cardiac arrhythmias

Table 7-2. Selected drug interactions

Drug	Combination	Adverse interaction
Volatile anesthetic	Nitrous oxide	Increased depth of anesthesia (i.e., decrease in minimum alveolar concentration)
	Opioids (including agonist-antagonists)	Increased depth of anesthesia
	Benzodiazepines	Increased depth of anesthesia
	Lidocaine	Increased depth of anesthesia
	Clonidine	Increased depth of anesthesia
	Methyldopa	Increased depth of anesthesia
	Reserpine	Increased depth of anesthesia
	Epinephrine and other β-adrenergic receptor agonists	Arrhythmias are greatest with halothane
	β-Adrenergic receptor blockers	Myocardial depression
	Calcium-channel blockers	Myocardial depression
	Timolol (ophthalmic)	Bradycardia
	Amiodarone	Bradycardia, heart block
Halothane	Theophylline	Arrhythmias
	Pancuronium plus a tricyclic antidepressant	Arrhythmias
Nitrous oxide	Opioids	Myocardial depression
Barbiturates	Central nervous system depressants	Increased respiratory depression
Benzodiazepines	Central nervous system depressants	Increased respiratory depression
	Alcohol	Increased drug absorption
	Opioids (large doses)	Myocardial depression
Diazepam	Cimetidine	Decreased diazepam clearance
	Selective serotonin reuptake inhibitors	Decreased diazepam clearance
Ketamine	Tricyclic antidepressants	Hypertension arrhythmias
	Halothane	Hypertension, arrhythmias, hypotension (myocardial depression)
Antipsychotics	Opioids	Potentiation of opioid sedation
Tricyclic antidepressants	Opioids	Potentiation of opioid sedation
	Halothane plus pancuronium	Hypertension, arrhythmias
	Ketamine	Hypertension, arrhythmias
Monoamine oxidase inhibitors	Succinylcholine	Prolonged muscle relaxation
	Barbiturates	Increased sedation
	Opioids	Increased sedation
	Alcohol	Increased sedation
	Meperidine (and, perhaps, other opioids)	Hypertension, seizures, hyperpyrexia
	Sympathomimetics	Exaggerated sympathomimetic response
Selective serotonin reuptake inhibitors	Diazepam	Decreased clearance of diazepam
	Phenytoin	Decreased clearance of phenytoin
Naloxone	Opioids	Hypertension, arrhythmias, pulmonary edema ("sudden arousal")
Opioid agonist-antagonists	Opioids	Blunting of opioid analgesia
	Opioids (in physical dependency)	Precipitation of opioid withdrawal
Flumazenil	Benzodiazepines	Anxiety, agitation, seizures, increased intracranial pressure (patients with head injury)
Local anesthetics	Neuromuscular blockers	Enhanced muscle relaxation
Lidocaine	Mexiletine	Neurotoxicity
Succinylcholine	Halothane	Classic combination that triggers malignant hyperthermia

Continued.

Table 7-2. Selected drug interactions—cont'd

Drug	Combination	Adverse interaction
	Cholinesterase inhibitors	Prolonged neuromuscular block
	Echothiophate, isoflurophate (ophthalmic)	Prolonged neuromuscular block
	Trimethaphan	Prolonged neuromuscular block
	Cyclophosphamide	Prolonged neuromuscular block
	Cimetidine	Prolonged neuromuscular block
Nondepolarizing neuromuscular blockers	Aminoglycoside antibiotics	Enhanced muscle relaxation
Pancuronium	Digoxin	Arrhythmias
Vecuronium	Potent opioids (sufentanil, fentanyl)	Possible enhanced opioid bradycardia
β-Adrenergic receptor agonists	Digoxin	Arrhythmias
Dopamine	Bretylium	Hypertension on initiating bretylium therapy
	Phenytoin	Hypotension
Direct-acting sympathomimetics	Reserpine	Enhanced sympathomimetic effect
Clonidine	Central nervous system depressants	Increased sedation, especially with neuraxial administration of clonidine
Verapamil	β-Adrenergic receptor blockers	Heart block
	Digoxin	
	Carbamazepine	Enhanced toxicity
	Oral hypoglycemic agents	Enhanced toxicity
Calcium-channel blockers	Neuromuscular blockers	Enhanced muscle relaxation
Promethazine	Opioids	Enhanced sedation
Cimetidine	Lidocaine, propranolol, diazepam, and other hepatically metabolized drugs	Decreased elimination of other drug
Furosemide	Lithium compounds	Elevated lithium concentrations
	Neuromuscular blockers	Enhanced muscle relaxation
	Sulfonamides	Allergic cross-sensitivity
Heparin (including low-molecular-weight and fractionated heparins)	Certain protein-bound drugs (e.g., diazepam, propranolol)	Elevated free plasma concentrations of other drug
	Salicylates, nonsteroidal antiinflammatory drugs	Increased bleeding diathesis
Coumarin	Salicylates, phenylbutazone	Increased bleeding diathesis
Protamine	Isophane insulin suspension, possibly fish	Allergic cross-sensitivity
Procainamide	Neuromuscular blockers	Enhanced muscle relaxation
Quinidine	Neuromuscular blockers	Enhanced muscle relaxation
Amiodarone	Digoxin	Increased blood concentrations of digoxin
	Volatile anesthetics	Bradycardia, sinus arrest
Aminoglycosides	Neuromuscular blockers	Enhanced muscle relaxation
Metoclopramide	Opioids	Impairment of the gastric emptying effect of metoclopramide
	Anticholinergics	Impaired gastric emptying

REFERENCES

1. Kavan EM, Julien RM: Central nervous system's effects of isoflurane (Forane), *Can Anaesth Soc J* 21:390, 1974.
2. Eger EI II, Stevens WC, Cromwell TH: The electroencephalogram in man anesthetized with Forane, *Anesthesiology* 35:504, 1971.
3. Neigh JL, Garman JK, Harp JR: The electroencephalographic pattern during anesthesia with ethrane: effects of depth of anesthesia, PaCO$_2$, and nitrous oxide, *Anesthesiology* 35:482, 1971.
4. Sprague DH, Wolf S: Enflurane seizures in patients taking amitriptyline, *Anesth Analg* 61:67, 1982.
5. Komatsu H, Taie S, Endo S, et al: Electrical seizures during sevoflurane anesthesia in two pediatric patients with epilepsy, *Anesthesiology* 81:1535, 1994.
6. Stevens WC, Kingston HGG: Inhalation anesthesia. In Barash PG, Cullen BF, Stoelting RK, eds: *Clinical anesthesia*, ed 3, Philadelphia, 1996, Lippincott-Raven.
7. Lutz LJ, Milde JH, Milde LN: The cerebral functional, metabolic, and hemodynamic effects of desflurane in dogs, *Anesthesiology* 73:125, 1990.
8. Scheller MS, Nakakimura K, Fleischer JE, et al: Cerebral effects of sevoflurane in the dog: comparison with isoflurane and enflurane, *Br J Anaesth* 65:388, 1990.
9. Muzzi DA, Losasso TJ, Dietz NM, et al: The effect of desflurane and isoflurane on cerebrospinal fluid pressure in humans with supratentorial mass lesions, *Anesthesiology* 76:720, 1992.
10. Adams RW, Cucciara RF, Gronert GA, et al: Isoflurane and cerebrospinal fluid pressure in neurosurgical patients, *Anesthesiology* 54:97, 1981.
11. Grosslight K, Foster R, Colohan AR, et al: Isoflurane for neuroanesthesia: risk factors for increases in intracranial pressure, *Anesthesiology* 63:533, 1985.
12. Eger EI II: *Desflurane (Suprane): a compendium and reference*, Rutherford, Pa, 1993, Healthpress Publishing Group.
13. Doi M, Ikeda K: Respiratory effects of sevoflurane, *Anesth Analg* 66:241, 1987.
14. Doi M, Ikeda K: Airway irritation produced by volatile anaesthetics during brief inhalation: comparison of halothane, enflurane, isoflurane and sevoflurane, *Can J Anaesth* 40:122, 1993.
15. Sloan NH, Conard PF, Karsunky PK, et al: Sevoflurane versus isoflurane: induction and recovery characteristics with single-breath inhaled inductions of anesthesia, *Anesth Analg* 82:528, 1996.
16. Kelly RE, Hartman GS, Embree PB, et al: Inhaled induction and emergence from desflurane anesthesia in the ambulatory surgical patient: the effect of premedication, *Anesth Analg* 77:540, 1993.
17. Ebert TJ, Harkin CP, Muzi M: Cardiovascular responses to sevoflurane: a review, *Anesth Analg* 81(suppl 6):S11, 1995.
18. Ebert TJ, Muzi M: Sympathetic hyperactivity during desflurane anesthesia in healthy volunteers: a comparison with isoflurane, *Anesthesiology* 79:444, 1993.
19. Johnston RR, Eger EI II, Wilson C: A comparative interaction of epinephrine with enflurane, isoflurane, and halothane in man, *Anesth Analg* 55:709, 1976.
20. Reiz S, Ostman M: Regional coronary hemodynamics during isoflurane–nitrous oxide anesthesia in patients with ischemic heart disease, *Anesth Analg* 64:570, 1985.
21. Tarnow J, Markschies-Hornung A, Schulte-Sasse U: Isoflurane improves the tolerance to pacing-induced myocardial ischemia, *Anesthesiology* 64:147, 1986.
22. Moffit EA, Barker RA, Glenn JJ, et al: Myocardial metabolism and hemodynamic responses with isoflurane anesthesia for coronary artery surgery, *Anesth Analg* 63:252, 1984.
23. Tuman KJ, McCarthy RJ, Spiess BD, et al: Does choice of anesthetic agent significantly alter outcome after coronary artery surgery? *Anesthesiology* 70:189, 1989.
24. Helman JD, Leung JM, Bellows WH, et al: The risk of myocardial ischemia in patients receiving desflurane versus sufentanil anesthesia for coronary artery bypass graft surgery, *Anesthesiology* 77:47, 1992.
25. Parsons RS, Jones RM, Wrigley SR, et al: Comparison of desflurane and fentanyl-based anaesthetic techniques for coronary artery bypass surgery, *Br J Anaesth* 72:430, 1994.

26. Ebert TJ, Kharasch ED, Rooke GA, et al: Myocardial ischemia and adverse cardiac outcomes in cardiac patients undergoing noncardiac surgery with sevoflurane and isoflurane: Sevoflurane Ischemia Study Group, *Anesth Analg* 85:993, 1997.
27. Berman ML, Holaday DA: Inhalation anesthetic metabolism and toxicity. In Barash PG, Cullen BF, Stoelting RK, eds: *Clinical anesthesia*, ed 3, Philadelphia, 1989, JB Lippincott.
28. Mazze RI, Calverley RK, Smith NT: Inorganic fluoride nephrotoxicity: prolonged enflurane and halothane anesthesia in volunteers, *Anesthesiology* 46:265, 1977.
29. Cousins MJ, Greenstein LR, Hitt BA, et al: Metabolism and renal effects of enflurane in man, *Anesthesiology* 44:44, 1976.
30. Mazze RI, Cousins MJ, Barr GA: Renal effects and metabolism of isoflurane in man, *Anesthesiology* 40:536, 1974.
31. Sutton TS, Koblin DD, Gruenke LD, et al: Fluoride metabolites after prolonged exposure of volunteers and patients to desflurane, *Anesth Analg* 73:180, 1991.
32. Gonsowski CT, Laster MJ, Eger EI II, et al: Toxicity of compound A in rats: effect of 3-hour administration, *Anesthesiology* 80:556, 1994.
33. Eger EI II, Gong D, Koblin DD, et al: Dose-related markers of renal injury after sevoflurane versus desflurane anesthesia in volunteers, *Anesth Analg* 85:1154, 1997.
34. Bito H, Ikeda K: Closed-circuit anesthesia with sevoflurane in humans: effects on renal and hepatic function and concentrations of breakdown products with soda lime in the circuit, *Anesthesiology* 80:71, 1994.
35. Kharasch ED, Thorning D, Garton K, et al: Role of renal cysteine conjugate β-lyase in the mechanism of compound A nephrotoxicity in rats, *Anesthesiology* 86:160, 1997.
36. Tung A, Jacobsohn E: A case of nonoliguric renal failure after general anesthesia with sevoflurane and desflurane, *Anesth Analg* 85:1407, 1997.
37. Munson ES, Embro WJ: Enflurane, isoflurane, and halothane and isolated human uterine muscle, *Anesthesiology* 46:11, 1977.
38. Warren TM, Datta S, Ostheimer GM, et al: Comparison of the maternal and neonatal effects of halothane, enflurane, and isoflurane for cesarean delivery, *Anesth Analg* 62:516, 1983.
39. Fang ZX, Eger EI II, Laster MJ, et al: Carbon monoxide production from degradation of desflurane, enflurane, isoflurane, halothane, and sevoflurane by soda lime and Baralyme, *Anesth Analg* 80:1187, 1995.
40. Lentz RE: Carbon monoxide poisoning during anesthesia poses puzzles, *J Clin Monit* 11:66, 1995.
41. Woehlck HJ, Dunning M III, Connolly LA: Reduction in the incidence of carbon monoxide exposures in humans undergoing general anesthesia, *Anesthesiology* 87:228, 1997.
42. Baxter PJ, Kharasch ED: Rehydration of dessicated Baralyme prevents carbon monoxide formation from desflurane in an anesthesia machine, *Anesthesiology* 86:1061, 1997.
43. Nelson TE, Flewellen EH: Current concepts: the malignant hyperthermia syndrome, *N Engl J Med* 309:416, 1983.
44. Ducart A, Adnet P, Renaud B, et al: Malignant hyperthermia during sevoflurane anesthesia, *Anesth Analg* 80:609, 1995.
45. Wedel DJ, Gammel SA, Milde JH, et al: Delayed onset of malignant hyperthermia induced by isoflurane and desflurane compared with halothane in susceptible swine, *Anesthesiology* 78:1138, 1993.
46. Murphy MR, Hug CC Jr: The enflurane sparing effect of morphine, butorphanol, and nalbuphine, *Anesthesiology* 57:489, 1982.
47. Perisho JA, Buechel DR, Miller RD: The effect of diazepam (Valium) on minimum alveolar anesthetic requirement (MAC) in man, *Can Anaesth Soc J* 18:536, 1971.
48. Saidman LJ, Eger EI: Effect of nitrous oxide and of narcotic premedication on the alveolar concentration of halothane required for anesthesia, *Anesthesiology* 25:302, 1964.
49. DiFazio CA, Neiderlehner JR, Burney RG: The anesthetic potency of lidocaine in the rat, *Anesth Analg* 55:818, 1976.
50. Bloor BC, Flacke WE: Reduction in halothane anesthetic requirement by clonidine, an alpha-adrenergic agonist, *Anesth Analg* 61:741, 1982.

51. Miller RD, Way WL, Eger EI II: The effects of alpha-methyl-dopa, reserpine, guanethidine, and iproniazid on minimum alveolar anesthetic requirement (MAC), *Anesthesiology* 29:1153, 1968.

52. Thiagarajah S, Grynsztejn M, Lear E, et al: Ventricular arrhythmias after terbutaline administration to patients anesthetized with halothane, *Anesth Analg* 65:417, 1986.

53. Foex P: Alpha- and beta-adrenoceptor antagonists, *Br J Anaesth* 56:751, 1984.

54. Reves JG, Kissin I, Lell WA, et al: Calcium entry blockers: uses and implications for anesthesiologists, *Anesthesiology* 57:504, 1982.

55. Roizen MF, Stevens WC: Multiform ventricular tachycardia due to the interaction of aminophylline and halothane, *Anesth Analg* 57:738, 1978.

56. Edwards RP, Miller RD, Roizen MF, et al: Cardiac effects of imipramine and pancuronium during halothane and enflurane, *Anesthesiology* 50:421, 1979.

57. Navalgund AA, Alifimoff JK, Jakymec AJ, et al: Amiodarone-induced sinus arrest successfully treated with ephedrine and isoproterenol, *Anesth Analg* 65:414, 1986.

58. Liberman BA, Teasdale SJ: Anaesthesia and amiodarone, *Can Anaesth Soc J* 32:629, 1985.

59. Eger EI II: Respiratory effects of nitrous oxide. In Eger EI, ed: *Nitrous oxide,* New York, 1985, Elsevier.

60. Knill RL, Clement JL: Variable effects of anaesthetics on the ventilatory response to hypoxaemia in man, *Can Anaesth Soc J* 29:93, 1982.

61. Hendriksen HT, Jorgensen PB: The effect of nitrous oxide on intracranial pressure in patients with intracranial disorders, *Br J Anaesth* 45:486, 1973.

62. Smith NT, Eger EI II, Stoelting RK, et al: The cardiovascular and sympathomimetic responses to the addition of nitrous oxide to halothane in man, *Anesthesiology* 32:410, 1970.

63. Dolan WM, Stevens WC, Eger EI II, et al: The cardiovascular and respiratory effects of isoflurane–nitrous oxide anaesthesia, *Can Anaesth Soc J* 21:557, 1974.

64. Smith NT, Calverly RK, Prys-Roberts C, et al: Impact of nitrous oxide on the circulation during enflurane anesthesia in man, *Anesthesiology* 48:345, 1978.

65. McDermott RW, Stanley TH: The cardiovascular effects of low concentrations of nitrous oxide during morphine anesthesia, *Anesthesiology* 41:89, 1974.

66. Eisele JH, Reitan JA, Massumi RA, et al: Myocardial performance and N₂O analgesia in coronary artery disease, *Anesthesiology* 44:16, 1976.

67. Schulte-Sasse U, Hess W, Tarnow J: Pulmonary vascular responses to nitrous oxide in patients with normal and high pulmonary vascular resistance, *Anesthesiology* 57:9, 1982.

68. Koblin DD, Watson JE, Deady JE, et al: Inactivation of methionine synthetase activity by nitrous oxide in mice, *Anesthesiology* 54:318, 1981.

69. Royston D, Nunn JF, Weinbren HK, et al: Rate of inactivation of human and rodent hepatic methionine synthetase by nitrous oxide, *Anesthesiology* 68:213, 1988.

70. O'Sullivan H, Jennings F, Ward K, et al: Human bone marrow biochemical function and megaloblastic hematopoesis after nitrous oxide anesthesia, *Anesthesiology* 55:645, 1981.

71. Amess JAL, Burman JF, Rees GM, et al: Megaloblastic haematopoiesis in patients receiving nitrous oxide, *Lancet* 2:339, 1978.

72. Layzer RB, Fishman RA, Schafer JA: Neuropathy following abuse of nitrous oxide, *Neurology* 28:504, 1978.

73. Lane GA, DuBoulay PM, Tait AR, et al: Nitrous oxide is teratogenic, halothane is not, *Anesthesiology* 55:A252, 1981 (abstract).

74. Crawford JS, Lewis M: Nitrous oxide in early human pregnancy, *Anaesthesia* 41:900, 1986.

75. Aldridge LM, Tunstall ME: Nitrous oxide and the fetus: a review and the results of a retrospective study of 175 cases of anaesthesia for insertion of Shirodkar suture, *Br J Anaesth* 58:1348, 1986.

76. Eger EI: *Anesthetic uptake and action,* Baltimore, 1974, Williams & Wilkins.

77. Jastak JT, Donaldson D: Nitrous oxide, *Anesthesia Progress* 38:142, 1991.

78. Munson ES, Merrick HC: Effect of nitrous oxide on venous air embolism, *Anesthesiology* 27:783, 1966.

79. Casey WF, Drake-Lee AB: Nitrous oxide and middle ear pressure: a study of induction methods in children, *Anaesthesia* 37:896, 1982.

80. Owens WD, Gustave F, Sclaroff A: Tympanic membrane rupture with nitrous oxide anesthesia, *Anesth Analg* 57:283, 1978.

81. Wood MW: Intravenous anesthetic agents. In Wood MW, Wood AJJ, eds: *Drugs and anesthesia: pharmacology for anesthesiologists,* ed 2, Baltimore, 1990, Williams & Wilkins.

82. Stoelting RK, Dierdorf SF, McCammon RL: Metabolism and nutrition. In *Anesthesia and co-existing disease,* ed 2, New York, 1988, Churchill Livingstone.

83. Durrett LR, Lawson NW: Autonomic nervous system physiology and pharmacology. In Barash PG, Cullen BF, Stoelting RK, eds: *Clinical anesthesia,* Philadelphia, 1989, JB Lippincott.

84. Sonntag H, Hellberg K, Schenk HD, et al: Effects of thiopental (Trapanal) on coronary blood flow and myocardial metabolism in man, *Acta Anaesthesiol Scand* 19:69, 1975.

85. Graves CL: Management of general anesthesia during hemorrhage, *Int Anesthesiol Clin* 12:1, 1974.

86. O'Donnell JF, Hewitt JC, Dundee JW: Clinical studies on induction agents: 28: a further comparison of venous complications following thiopentone, methohexitone, and propanidid, *Br J Anaesth* 41:681, 1969.

87. Stone HH, Donnelly CC: The accidental intra-arterial injection of thiopental, *Anesthesiology* 22:995, 1961.

88. Dundee JW, Wyant GM: *Intravenous anesthesia,* Edinburgh, 1974, Churchill Livingstone.

89. Helrich M, Eckenhoff JE, Jones RE: Influence of opiates on the respiratory response of man to thiopental, *Anesthesiology* 17:459, 1956.

90. Harrison GA: The influence of different anesthetic agents on the response to respiratory tract irritation, *Br J Anaesth* 34:804, 1962.

91. Power SJ, Morgan M, Chakrabarti MK: Carbon dioxide response curves following midazolam and diazepam, *Br J Anaesth* 55:837, 1983.

92. Greenblatt DJ, Allen MD, Noel BJ, et al: Acute overdosage with benzodiazepine derivatives, *Clin Pharmacol Ther* 21:497, 1977.

93. Reves JG, Fragen RJ, Vinik HR, et al: Midazolam: pharmacology and uses, *Anesthesiology* 62:310, 1985.

94. Rao S, Sherbaniuk RW, Prasad K, et al: Cardiopulmonary effects of diazepam, *Clin Pharmacol Ther* 14:182, 1973.

95. McCammon RL, Hilgenberg JC, Stoelting RK: Hemodynamic effects of diazepam and diazepam–nitrous oxide in patients with coronary artery disease, *Anesth Analg* 59:438, 1980.

96. Falk RB Jr, Denlinger JK, Nahrwold ML, et al: Acute vasodilation following induction of anesthesia with intravenous diazepam and nitrous oxide, *Anesthesiology* 49:149, 1978.

97. Samuelson PN, Reves JG, Kouchoukos NT, et al: Hemodynamic responses to anesthetic induction with midazolam or diazepam in patients with ischemic heart disease, *Anesth Analg* 60:802, 1981.

98. Adams P, Gelman S, Reves JG, et al: Midazolam pharmacodynamics and pharmacokinetics during acute hypovolemia, *Anesthesiology* 63:140, 1985.

99. Korttila K, Aromaa U: Venous complications after intravenous injection of diazepam, fluintrazepam, thiopentone and etomidate, *Acta Anaesthesiol Scand* 24:227, 1980.

100. McClure JH, Brown DT, Wildsmith JAW: Comparison of the IV administration of midazolam and diazepam as sedation during spinal anesthesia, *Br J Anaesth* 55:1089, 1983.

101. Camann W, Cohen MB, Ostheimer GW: Is midazolam desirable for sedation in parturients? *Anesthesiology* 65:441, 1986.

102. Saxen I, Saxen L: Association between maternal intake of diazepam and oral clefts, *Lancet* 2:498, 1975 (letter).

103. Gyermek L: Clinical effects of diazepam prior to and during general anesthesia, *Curr Ther Res* 17:175, 1975.

104. Stanley TH, Bennett GM, Loeser EA, et al: Cardiovascular effects of diazepam and droperidol during morphine anesthesia, *Anesthesiology* 44:255, 1976.

105. Amrein R, Leishman B, Bentzinger C, et al: Flumazenil and benzodiazepine antagonism: actions and clinical use in intoxications and anaesthesiology, *Med Toxicol Adverse Drug Exp* 2:411, 1987.

106. Chiolero RL, Ravussin P, Anderes JP, et al: The effects of midazolam reversal by RO 15-1788 on cerebral perfusion pressure in patients with severe head injury, *Intensive Care Med* 14:196, 1988.
107. Smith I, White PF, Nathanson M, et al: Propofol: an update on its clinical use, *Anesthesiology* 81:1005, 1994.
108. Sutherland MJ, Burt P: Propofol and seizures, *Anaesth Intensive Care* 22:744, 1994.
109. Kuisma M, Roine RO: Propofol in prehospital treatment of status epilepticus, *Epilepsia* 36:1241, 1995.
110. Leisure GS, O'Flaherty J, Green L, et al: Propofol and postoperative pancreatitis, *Anesthesiology* 84:224, 1996.
111. Goodale DB, Suljada-Petchel K: Pancreatitis after propofol administration: is there a relationship—reply, *Anesthesiology* 84:236, 1996.
112. Profeta JP, Guffin A, Mikula S, et al: The hemodynamic effects of propofol and thiamylal sodium for induction in coronary artery surgery, *Anesth Analg* 66:S142, 1987.
113. James MFM, Reyneke CJ, Whiffler K: Heart block following propofol: a case report, *Br J Anaesth* 62:213, 1989.
114. Bennett SN, McNeil MM, Bland LA, et al: Postoperative infections traced to contamination of an intravenous anesthetic, propofol, *N Engl J Med* 333:147, 1995.
115. Tarnow J, Hess W, Klein W: Etomidate, alfathesin and thiopentone as induction agents for coronary artery surgery, *Can Anaesth Soc J* 27:338, 1980.
116. Schou Olesen A, Huttel MS, Hole P: Venous sequelae following the injection of etomidate or thiopentone IV, *Br J Anaesth* 56:171, 1984.
117. Moss E, Powell D, Gibson WRM, et al: Effect of etomidate on intracranial pressure and cerebral perfusion pressure, *Br J Anaesth* 51:347, 1979.
118. Wauquier A: Profile of etomidate: A hypnotic, anticonvulsant and brain protective compound, *Anaesthesia* 38(suppl):26, 1983.
119. Gancher S, Laxer KD, Krieger W: Activation of epileptogenic activity by etomidate, *Anesthesiology* 61:616, 1984.
120. Morgan M, Lumley J, Whitwam JG: Respiratory effects of etomidate, *Br J Anaesth* 49:233, 1977.
121. Wagner RL, White PF, Kan PB, et al: Inhibition of adrenal steroidogenesis by the anesthetic etomidate, *N Engl J Med* 310:1415, 1984.
122. Horrigan RW, Moyers JR, Johnson BH, et al: Etomidate versus thiopentone with and without fentanyl: a comparative study of awakening in man, *Anesthesiology* 52:362, 1980.
123. Schwartz DA, Horwitz LD: Effects of ketamine on left ventricular performance, *J Pharmacol Exp Ther* 194:410, 1975.
124. Tweed WA, Minuck M, Mymin D: Circulatory responses to ketamine anesthesia, *Anesthesiology* 37:613, 1972.
125. Pedersen T, Engbaek J, Klausen NO, et al: Effects of low-dose ketamine and thiopentone on cardiac performance and myocardial oxygen balance in hight-risk patients, *Acta Anaesthesiol Scand* 26:235, 1982.
126. White PF, Way WL, Trevor AJ: Ketamine—its pharmacology and therapeutic uses, *Anesthesiology* 56:119, 1982.
127. Taylor PA, Towey RM: Depression of laryngeal reflexes during ketamine anesthesia, *BMJ* 2:688, 1971.
128. Takeshita H, Okuda Y, Sari A: The effects of ketamine on cerebral circulation and metabolism in man, *Anesthesiology* 36:69, 1972.
129. Bidwai AV, Stanley HT, Graves CL, et al: The effects of ketamine on cardiovascular dynamics during halothane and enflurane anesthesia, *Anesth Analg* 54:588, 1975.
130. Drugs for psychiatric disorders, *Med Lett Drugs Ther* 25:45, 1983.
131. Stoelting RK, Dierdorf SF, McCammon RL: Psychiatric illness. In *Anesthesia and co-existing disease*, ed 2, New York, 1988, Churchill Livingstone.
132. Lee CM, Yeakel AE: Patient refusal of surgery following Innovar premedication, *Anesth Analg* 54:224, 1975.
133. Shader RI, DiMascio A: *Psychotropic drug side effects: chemical and theoretical perspectives*, Baltimore, 1970, Williams & Wilkins.
134. Itil TM: Effects of psychotropic drugs on qualitatively and quantitatively analyzed human EEG. In Clark WG, del Giudice J, eds: *Principles of psychopharmacology,* ed 2, New York, 1978, Academic Press.
135. Kaufman JS: Drug interactions involving psychotherapeutic agents. In Simpson LL, ed: *Drug treatment of mental disorders,* New York, 1976, Raven Press.
136. Caroff SN: The neuroleptic malignant syndrome, *J Clin Psychiatry* 41:79, 1980.
137. Guze BH, Baxter LR: Current concepts: neuroleptic malignant syndrome, *N Engl J Med* 313:163, 1985.
138. Kosanin R: Anesthetic considerations in patients on tricyclic antidepressant therapy, *Anesthesiol Rev* 8:38, 1981.
139. Vohra J, Burrows GD: Cardiovascular complications of tricyclic antidepressant overdosage, *Drugs* 8:432, 1974.
140. Jaffe JH, Martin WR: Opioid analgesics and antagonists. In Gilman AG, Goodman LS, Rall TW, et al, eds: *The pharmacological basis of therapeutics,* New York, 1985, Macmillan.
141. Stack CG, Rogers P, Linter SP: Monoamine oxidase inhibitors and anaesthesia: a review, *Br J Anaesth* 60:222, 1988.
142. Baldessarian RJ: *Chemotherapy in psychiatry: principles and practice,* rev ed, Cambridge, Mass, 1985, Harvard University Press.
143. Janowsky EC, Risch C, Janowsky DS: Effects of anesthesia on patients taking psychotropic drugs, *J Clin Psychopharmacol* 1:14, 1981.
144. Bodley PO, Halwax K, Potts L: Low serum pseudocholinesterase levels complicating treatment with phenlzine, *BMJ* 3:510, 1969.
145. Brown TCK, Cass NM: Beware—the use of MAO inhibitors is increasing again, *Anaesth Intensive Care* 7:65, 1979.
146. Boakes AJ, Laurence DR, Teoh PC, et al: Interactions between sympathomimetic amines and antidepressant agents in man, *BMJ* 1:311, 1973.
147. Hirshman CA, Lindeman K: MAO inhibitors: must they be discontinued before anesthesia? *JAMA* 260:3507, 1988.
148. Liu BA, Mittmann N, Knowles SR, et al: Hyponatremia and the syndrome of inappropriate secretion of antidiuretic hormone associated with the use of selective serotinin reuptake inhibitors: a review of spontaneous reports, *Can Med Assoc J* 155:519, 1996.
149. Richelson E: Pharmacokinetic drug interactions of new antidepressants: a review of the effects on the metabolism of other drugs, *Mayo Clin Proc* 72:835, 1997.
150. Martin WR: Pharmacology of opioids, *Pharmacol Rev* 35:283, 1983.
151. Hilgenberg JC: Intraoperative awareness during high dose fentanyl–oxygen anesthesia, *Anesthesiology* 54:341, 1981.
152. Rosow CE, Moss J, Philbin DM, et al: Histamine release during morphine and fentanyl anesthesia, *Anesthesiology* 56:93, 1982.
153. Wood M: Opioid agonists and antagonists. In Wood MW, Wood AJJ, eds: *Drugs and anesthesia: pharmacology for anesthesiologists,* ed 2, Baltimore, 1990, Williams & Wilkins.
154. Radnay PA, Brodman E, Mankikar D, et al: The effect of equianalgesic doses of fentanyl, morphine, meperidine and pentazocine on common bile duct pressure, *Anaesthetist* 29:26, 1980.
155. Murphy MR: Opioids. In Barash PG, Cullen BF, Stoelting RK, eds: *Clinical anesthesia,* Philadelphia, 1989, JB Lippincott.
156. Stanley TH, Liu WS: Cardiovascular effects of meperidine–N$_2$O anesthesia before and after pancuronium, *Anesth Analg* 56:669, 1977.
157. Flacke JW, Flacke WE, Bloor BC, et al: Histamine release by four narcotics: a double-blind study in humans, *Anesth Analg* 66:723, 1987.
158. Becker LD, Paulson BA, Miller RD, et al: Biphasic respiratory depression after fentanyl-droperidol or fentanyl alone used to supplement nitrous oxide anesthesia, *Anesthesiology* 44:291, 1976.
159. Moldenhauer CC, Hug CC Jr: Use of narcotic analgesics as anaesthetics, *Clin Anaesthesiol* 2:107, 1984.
160. Bennet GM, Stanley TH: Comparison of the cardiovascular effects of morphine-N$_2$O and fentanyl-N$_2$O balanced anesthesia in man, *Anesthesiology* 51:S102, 1979.
161. Monk JP, Beresford R, Ward A: Sufentanil: a review of its pharmacological properties and therapeutic use, *Drugs* 36:286, 1988.
162. Chang J, Fish KJ: Acute respiratory arrest and rigidity after anesthesia with sufentanil: a case report, *Anesthesiology* 63:710, 1985.
163. Miller DR, Wellwood M, Teasdale SJ, et al: Effects of anaesthetic induction on myocardial function and metabolism: a comparison of fentanyl, sufentanil and alfentanil, *Can J Anaesth* 35(3 pt 1):219, 1988.

164. Schuttler J, Albrecht S, Breivik H, et al: A comparison of remifentanil and alfentanil in patients undergoing major abdominal surgery, *Anaesthesia* 52:307, 1997.

165. Cousins MJ, Mather LE: Intrathecal and epidural administration of opioids, *Anesthesiology* 61:276, 1984.

166. Cohen SE, Cherry CM, Holbrook RH Jr, et al: Intrathecal sufentanil for labor analgesia—sensory changes, side effects, and fetal heart rate changes, *Anesth Analg* 77:1155, 1993.

167. Ostermeier AM, Roizen MF, Hautkappe M, et al: Three sudden postoperative respiratory arrests associated with epidural opioids in patients with sleep apnea, *Anesth Analg* 85:452, 1997.

168. Smith G, Pinnock C: Naloxone—paradox or panacea? *Br J Anaesth* 57:547, 1985 (editorial).

169. Longnecker DE, Grazis PA, Eggers GWN Jr: Naloxone for antagonism of morphine-induced respiratory depression. *Anesth Analg* 52:447, 1973.

170. Jasinski DR: Human pharmacology of narcotic antagonists, *Br J Clin Pharmacol* 7(suppl 3):287S, 1979.

171. Vandam LD: Drug therapy: butorphanol, *N Engl J Med* 302:381, 1980.

172. Popio KA, Jackson DH, Ross AM, et al: Hemodynamic and respiratory effects of morphine and butorphanol, *Clin Pharmacol Ther* 23:281, 1978.

173. Errick JK, Heel RC: Nalbuphine: a preliminary review of its pharmacological properties and therapeutic efficacy, *Drugs* 26:191, 1983.

174. Lee G, Low RI, Amsterdam EA, et al: Hemodynamic effects of morphine and nalbuphine in acute myocardial infarction, *Clin Pharmacol Ther* 29:576, 1981.

175. Brogden RN, Speight TM, Avery GS: Pentazocine: a review of its pharmacological properties, therapeutic efficacy and dependence liability, *Drugs* 5:6, 1973.

176. Lee G, DeMaria A, Amsterdam EA, et al: Comparative effects of morphine, meperidine and pentazocine on cardiocirculatory dynamics in patients with acute myocardial infarction, *Am J Med* 60:949, 1976.

177. Heel RC, Brogden RN, Speight TM, et al: Buprenorphine: a review of its pharmacological properties and therapeutic efficacy, *Drugs* 17:81, 1979.

178. Stoelting RK: Opioid agonists and antagonists. In *Pharmacology and physiology in anesthetic practice*, Philadelphia, 1987, JB Lippincott.

179. Mather LE, Cousins MJ: Local anesthetics and their current clinical use, *Drugs* 18:185, 1979.

180. Matsuo S, Rao DBS, Chaudry I, et al: Interaction of muscle relaxants and local anesthetics at the neuromuscular junction, *Anesth Analg* 57:580, 1978.

181. Brown DT, Beamish D, Wildsmith JAW: Allergic reaction to an amide local anaesthetic, *Br J Anaesth* 53:435, 1981.

182. Nagel JE, Fuscaldo JT, Fireman P: Paraben allergy, *JAMA* 237:1594, 1977.

183. Aldrete JA, Johnson DA: Allergy to local anesthetics, *JAMA* 207:356, 1969.

184. Edouard A, Berdeaux A, Langloys J, et al: Effects of lidocaine on myocardial contractility and baroreflex control of heart rate in conscious dogs, *Anesthesiology* 64:316, 1986.

185. Collinsworth KA, Kalman SM, Harrison DC: The clinical pharmacology of lidocaine as an antiarrhythmic drug, *Circulation* 50:1217, 1974.

186. Gross JB, Caldwell CB, Shaw LM, et al: The effect of lidocaine infusion on the ventilatory response to hypoxia, *Anesthesiology* 61:662, 1984.

187. Avery P, Redon D, Schaenzer G, et al: The influence of serum potassium on the cerebral and cardiac toxicity of bupivacaine and lidocaine, *Anesthesiology* 61:134, 1984.

188. Christie JM, Valdes C, Markowsky SJ: Neurotoxicity of lidocaine combined with mexiletine, *Anesth Analg* 77:1291, 1993.

189. Scanlon JW, Brown WU Jr, Weiss JB, et al: Neurobehavioral responses of newborn infants after maternal epidural anesthesia, *Anesthesiology* 40:121, 1974.

190. de Jong RH, Ronfeld RA, DeRosa RA: Cardiovascular effects of convulsant and supraconvulsant doses of amide local anesthetics, *Anesth Analg* 61:3, 1982.

191. Morishima HO, Pedersen H, Finster M, et al: Bupivacaine toxicity in pregnant and nonpregnant ewes, *Anesthesiology* 63:134, 1985.

192. McCLure JH: Ropivacaine, *Br J Anaesth* 76:300, 1996.

193. Climie CR, McLean S, Starmer GA, et al: Methaemoglobinaemia in mother and foetus following continuous epidural analgesia with prilocaine: clinical and experimental data, *Br J Anaesth* 39:155, 1967.

194. Scott DB, Cousins MJ: Clinical pharmacology of local anesthetic agents. In Cousins MJ, Bridenbaug PO, eds: *Neural blockade in clinical anesthesia and management of pain,* Philadelphia, 1980, JB Lippincott.

195. Tucker GT: Pharmacokinetics of local anesthetics, *Br J Anaesth* 58:717, 1986.

196. Wang BC, Hillman DE, Spielholz NI, et al: Chronic neurological deficits and Nesacaine-CE—an effect of the anesthetic, 2-chloroprocaine, or the antioxidant, sodium bisulfite? *Anesth Analg* 63:445, 1984.

197. Cregler LL, Mark H: Medical complications of cocaine abuse, *N Engl J Med* 315:1495, 1986.

198. Severinghaus JW, Xu FD, Spellman MJ Jr: Benzocaine and methemoglobin: recommended actions, *Anesthesiology* 74:385, 1991 (letter).

199. Durant NN, Katz RL: Suxamethonium, *Br J Anaesth* 54:195, 1982.

200. Stoelting RK, Peterson C: Adverse effects of increased succinylcholine dose following *d*-tubocurarine pretreatment. *Anesth Analg* 54:282, 1975.

201. Lebowitz PW, Ramsey FM: Muscle relaxants. In Barash PG, Cullen BF, Stoelting RK, eds: *Clinical anesthesia,* Philadelphia, 1989, JB Lippincott.

202. Mitchell MM, Ali HH, Savarese JJ: Myotonia and neuromuscular blocking agents, *Anesthesiology* 49:44, 1978.

203. Ryan JF, Kagen LJ, Hyman AI: Myoglobinemia after a single dose of succinylcholine, *N Engl J Med* 285:824, 1971.

204. Katz RL, Ryan JF: The neuromuscular effects of suxamethonium in man, *Br J Anaesth* 41:381, 1969.

205. Kambam JR, Dymond R, Krestow M: Effect of cimetidine on duration of action of succinylcholine, *Anesth Analg* 66:191, 1987.

206. Mecca RS: Postoperative recovery. In Barash PG, Cullen BF, Stoelting RK, eds: *Clinical anesthesia,* ed 2, Philadelphia, 1992, JB Lippincott.

207. Shapiro BA, Warren J, Egol AB, et al: Practice parameters for sustained neuromuscular blockade in the adult critically ill patient: an executive summary: Society of Critical Care Medicine, *Crit Care Med* 23:1601, 1995.

208. Stoelting RK: The hemodynamic effects of pancuronium and *d*-tubocurarine in anesthetized patients, *Anesthesiology* 36:612, 1972.

209. Stoelting RK: Hemodynamic effects of dimethyltubocurarine during nitrous oxide–halothane anesthesia, *Anesth Analg* 53:513, 1974.

210. Bartolone RS, Rao TLK: Arrhythmias following muscle relaxant administration in patients receiving digitalis, *Anesthesiology* 58:567, 1983.

211. Basta SJ, Ali HH, Savarese JJ, et al: Clinical pharmacology of atracurium besylate (BW 33A): a new non-depolarizing muscle relaxant, *Anesth Analg* 61:723, 1982.

212. Schramm WM, Papousek A, Michalek-Sauberer A, et al: The cerebral and cardiovascular effects of *cis*-atracurium and atracurium in neurosurgical patients, *Anesth Analg* 86:123, 1998.

213. Lein AC, Belmont MR, Abalos A, et al: The cardiovascular effects and histamine-releasing properties of 51W89 in patients receiving nitrous oxide/opioid/barbiturate anesthesia, *Anesthesiology* 82:1131, 1995.

214. Starr NJ, Sethna DH, Estafanous FG: Bradycardia and asystole following the rapid administration of sufentanil with vecuronium, *Anesthesiology* 64:521, 1986.

215. Levy JH, Davis GK, Duggan J, et al: Determination of the hemodynamics and histamine release of rocuronium (Org 9426) when administered in increasing doses under N_2O/O_2–sufentanil anesthesia, *Anesth Analg* 78:318, 1994.

216. Savarese JJ, Ali HH, Basta SJ, et al: The clinical neuromuscular pharmacology of mivacurium chloride (BW B1090U): a short-acting nondepolarizing ester neuromuscular blocking drug, *Anesthesiology* 68:723, 1988.

217. Savarese JJ, Ali HH, Basta SJ, et al: The cardiovascular effects of mivacurium chloride (BW B1090U) in patients receiving nitrous oxide–opiate–barbiturate anesthesia, *Anesthesiology* 70:386, 1989.

218. Dresner DL, Bastá SJ, Ali HH, et al: Pharmacokinetics and pharmacodynamics of doxacurium in young and elderly patients during isoflurane anesthesia, *Anesth Analg* 71:498, 1990.

219. Larijani GE, Bartkowski RR, Azad SS, et al: Clinical pharmacology of pipecuronium bromide, *Anesth Analg* 68:734, 1989.

220. Payne JP, Hughes R, AL Azawi SA: Neuromuscular blockade by neostigmine in anaesthetized man, *Br J Anaesth* 52:69, 1980.

221. Sunew KY, Hicks RG: Effects of neostigmine and pyridostigmine on duration of succinylcholine action and pseudocholinesterase activity, *Anesthesiology* 49:188, 1978.

222. Bidwai AV, Stanely TH, Rogers C, et al: Reversal of diazepam-induced postanesthetic somnolence with physostigmine, *Anesthesiology* 51:256, 1979.

223. Weiner N: Atropine, scopolamine and related antimuscarinic drugs. In Goodman AG, Gilman A, eds: *The pharmacologic basis of therapeutics,* New York, 1980, Macmillan.

224. Cooper MJ, Abinader EG: Atropine-induced ventricular fibrillation: case report and review of the literature, *Am Heart J* 97:225, 1979.

225. Gross NJ, Skorodin MS: Anticholinergic, antimuscarinic bronchodilators, *Am Rev Respir Dis* 129:856, 1984.

226. Garde JF, Aston R, Endler GC, et al: Racial mydriatic response to belladonna preparations, *Anesth Analg* 57:572, 1978.

227. Flacke WE, Flacke JW: Cholinergic and anticholinergic agents. In Smith NT, Corbascio AN, eds: *Drug interaction in anesthesia,* Philadelphia, 1986, Lea & Febiger.

228. Zaritsky AL, Chernow B: Catecholamines and sympathomimetics. In Chernow B, Lake CR, eds: *The pharmacologic approach to the critically ill patient,* Baltimore, 1983, Williams & Wilkins.

229. Packer M, Gottlieb SS, Kessler PD: Hormone-electrolyte interactions in the pathogenesis of lethal cardiac arrhythmias in patients with congestive heart failure: basis of a new physiologic approach to control of arrhythmia, *Am J Med* 80:23, 1986.

230. Tarazi RC: Sympathomimetic agents in the treatment of shock, *Ann Intern Med* 81:364, 1974.

231. Sobel BE, Braunwald E: The management of acute myocardial infarction. In Braunwald E, ed: *Heart disease: a textbook of cardiovascular medicine,* Philadelphia, 1984, WB Saunders.

232. Weiner N: Norepinephrine, epinephrine, and the sympathomimetic amines. In Gilman AG, Goodman LS, Rall TW, et al, eds: *The pharmacological basis of therapeutics,* New York, 1985, Macmillan.

233. Golbranson FL, Lurie L, Vance RM, et al: Multiple extremity amputations in hypotensive patients treated with dopamine, *JAMA* 243:1145, 1980.

234. Anderson JL: Bretylium tosylate: profile of the only available class III antiarrhythmic agent, *Clin Ther* 7:205, 1985.

235. Bivins BA, Rapp RP, Griffin WO Jr, et al: Dopamine-phenytoin interaction: a cause of hypotension in the critically ill, *Arch Surg* 113:245, 1978.

236. Rutman HI, LeJemtel TH, Sonnenblick EH: Newer cardiotonic agents: implications for patients with heart failure and ischemic heart disease, *J Cardiothorac Anesth* 1:59, 1987.

237. Young RA, Ward A: Milrinone: a preliminary review of its pharmacologic properties and therapeutic use, *Drugs* 36:158, 1988.

238. Chung EK: *Digitalis intoxication,* Baltimore, 1969, Williams & Wilkins.

239. Smith TW, Antman EM, Freidman PL, et al: Digitalis glycosides: mechanisms and manifestations of toxicity: part II, *Prog Cardiovasc Dis* 26:495, 1984.

240. Smith NT, Corbascio AN: The use and misuse of pressor agents, *Anesthesiology* 33:58, 1970.

241. Ralston DH, Shnider SM, DeLorimier AA: Effects of equipotent ephedrine, metaraminol, mephentermine and methoxamine, on uterine blood flow in the pregnant ewe, *Anesthesiology* 40:354, 1970.

242. Hurlbert BJ, Edelman JD, David K: Serum potassium levels during and after terbutaline, *Anesth Analg* 60:723, 1980.

243. Speilman FJ, Herbert WN: Maternal cardiovascular effects of drugs that alter uterine activity, *Obstet Gynecol Surv* 43:516, 1988.

244. Hug CC, Kaplan JA: Pharmacology—cardiac drugs. In Kaplan JA, ed: *Cardiac anesthesia,* New York, 1979, Grune & Stratton.

245. Cohn JN, Burke LP: Nitroprusside, *Ann Intern Med* 91:752, 1979.

246. Mookherjee S, Keighley JF, Warner RA et al: Hemodynamic, ventilatory and blood gas changes during infusion of sodium nitroferricyanide (Nitroprusside), *Chest* 72:273, 1977.

247. Moore RA, Geller EA, Gallagher JD, et al: Effect of hypothermic cardiopulmonary bypass on nitroprusside metabolism, *Clin Pharmacol Ther* 37:680, 1985.

248. Tinker JH, Michenfelder JD: Sodium nitroprusside: pharmacology, toxicology and therapeutics, *Anesthesiology* 45:340, 1976.

249. Cottrell JE, Casthely P, Brodie JD, et al: Prevention of nitroprusside-induced cyanide toxicity with hydroxycobalamin, *N Engl J Med* 298:809, 1979.

250. Hill NS, Antman EM, Green LH, et al: Intravenous nitroglycerin: a review of pharmacology, indications, therapeutic effects and complications, *Chest* 79:69, 1981.

251. Weygandt GR, Kopman EA, Bauer S, et al: The cause of hypoxemia induced by nitroglycerin, *Am J Cardiol* 43:427, 1979.

252. Ziegler MG: Antihypertensives. In Chernow B, Lake CR, eds: *The pharmacologic approach to the critically ill patient,* Baltimore, 1983, Williams & Wilkins.

253. Husserl FE, Messerli FH: Adverse effects of antihypertensive drugs, *Drugs* 22:188, 1981.

254. Owall A, Gordon E, Lagerkranser M, et al: Clinical experience with adenosine for controlled hypotension during cerebral aneurysm surgery, *Anesth Analg* 66:229, 1987.

255. Clutton-Brock J: Two cases of poisoning by contamination of nitrous oxide with higher oxides of nitrogen during anaesthesia, *Br J Anaesth* 39:388, 1967.

256. Hogman M, Frostell C, Arnberg H, et al: Bleeding time prolongation and NO inhalation, *Lancet* 341:1664, 1993 (letter).

257. Samama CM, Diaby M, Fellahi JL, et al: Inhibition of platelet aggregation by inhaled nitric oxide in patients with acute respiratory distress syndrome, *Anesthesiology* 83:56, 1995.

258. Shand DG: Drug therapy: propranolol, *N Engl J Med* 293:280, 1975.

259. Zimmerman TJ, Kooner KS, Morgan KS: Safety and efficacy of timolol in pediatric glaucoma, *Surv Ophthalmol* 28(suppl):262, 1983.

260. Frishman WH: Drug theapy: pindolol: a new β-adrenoceptor antagonist with partial agonist activity, *N Engl J Med* 308:940, 1983.

261. Koch-Weser J: Drug therapy: metoprolol, *N Engl J Med* 301:698, 1979.

262. Miller RR, Olsen HG, Amsterdam EA, et al: Propranolol-withdrawal rebound phenomenon: exacerbation of coronary events after abrupt cessation of antianginal therapy, *N Engl J Med* 293:416, 1975.

263. Mishra P, Calvey TN, Williams NE, et al: Intraoperative bradycardia and hypotension associated with timolol and pilocarpine eye drops, *Br J Anaesth* 55:897, 1983.

264. Weiner N: Drugs that inhibit adrenergic nerves and block adrenergic receptors. In Gilman AG, Goodman LS, Rall TW, et al, eds: *The pharmacological basis of therapeutics,* ed 7, New York, 1985, Macmillan.

265. Wilson DJ, Wallin JD, Vlachakis ND, et al: Intravenous labetalol in the treatment of severe hypertension and hypertensive emergencies, *Am J Med* 75:95, 1983.

266. Vickers MD, Schneiden H, Wood-Smith FG: Cardiovascular drugs (trimethaphan camsylate). In *Drugs in anaesthesia practice,* ed 6, London, 1984, Butterworth & Co.

267. Wilson SL, Miller RN, Wright C, et al: Prolonged neuromuscular blockade associated with trimethaphan: a case report, *Anesth Analg* 55:353, 1976.

268. Drugs for hypertension, *Med Lett Drugs Ther* 29:1, 1987.

269. Eisenach JC, De Kock M, Klimscha W: Alpha-2 adrenergic agonists for regional anesthesia: a clinical review of clonidine (1984-1995), *Anesthesiology* 85:655, 1996.
270. Bursztyn M, Tordjman K, Grossman E, et al: Hypertensive crisis associated with nifedipine withdrawal, *Arch Intern Med* 146:397, 1986.
271. Gottlieb SO, Ouyang P, Achuff SC, et al: Acute nifedipine withdrawal: consequences of preoperative and late cessation of therapy in patients with prior unstable angina, *J Am Coll Cardiol* 4:382, 1984.
272. Merin RG: Calcium channel blocking drugs and anesthetics: is the drug interaction beneficial or detrimental? *Anesthesiology* 66:111, 1987.
273. Durant NN, Nguyen N, Katz RL: Potentiation of neuromuscular blockade by verapamil, *Anesthesiology* 60:298, 1984.
274. Verapamil for hypertension, *Med Lett Drugs Ther* 29:37, 1987.
275. Chew CY, Hecht HS, Collett JT, et al: Influence of severity of ventricular dysfunction on hemodynamic responses to intravenously administered verapamil in ischemic heart disease, *Am J Cardiol* 47:917, 1981.
276. McGoon MD, Vlietstra RE, Holmes DR Jr, et al: The clinical use of verapamil, *Mayo Clin Proc* 57:495, 1982.
277. Gulamhusein S, Ko P, Carruthers SG, et al: Acceleration of the ventricular response during atrial fibrillation in the Wolff-Parkinson-White syndrome after verapamil, *Circulation* 65:348, 1982.
278. Singh BN, Ellrodt G, Peter CT: Verapamil: a review of its pharmacological properties and therapeutic use, *Drugs* 15:169, 1978.
279. Zalman F, Perloff JK, Durant NN, et al: Acute respiratory failure following intravenous verapamil in Duchenne's muscular dystrophy, *Am Heart J* 105:510, 1983.
280. Grossman E, Messerli FH, Grodzidei T, et al: Should a moratorium be placed on sublingual nifedipine capsules given for hypertensive emergencies and pseudoemergencies? *JAMA* 276:1328, 1996.
281. Chaffman M, Brogden RN: Diltiazem: a review of its pharmacological properties and therapeutic efficacy, *Drugs* 29:387, 1985.
282. Dougall HT, McLay J: A comparative review of the adverse effects of calcium antagonists, *Drug Saf* 15:91, 1996.
283. Stoelting RK: Histamine and histamine receptor antagonists. In *Pharmacology and physiology in anesthetic practice,* Philadelphia, 1987, JB Lippincott.
284. Keats AS, Telford J, Kurosu Y: "Potentiation" of meperidine by promethazine, *Anesthesiology* 22:34, 1961.
285. Cristiano P, Paradisi F: Can cimetidine facilitate infections by the oral route? *Lancet* 2:45, 1982 (letter).
286. Schentag JJ, Cerra FB, Calleri G, et al: Pharmacokinetic and clinical studies in patients with cimetidine-associated mental confusion, *Lancet* 1:177, 1979.
287. Shaw RG, Mashford ML, Desmond PV: Cardiac arrest after intravenous injection of cimetidine, *Med J Aust* 2:629, 1980.
288. McGuigan JE: A consideration of the adverse effects of cimetidine, *Gastroenterology* 80:181, 1981.
289. Zedis JB, Friedman LS, Isselbacher KJ: Ranitidine: a new H₂ receptor antagonist, *N Engl J Med* 309:1368, 1983.
290. Camarri E, Chirone E, Fanteria G, et al: Ranitidine-induced bradycardia, *Lancet* 2:160, 1982 (letter).
291. Stoelting RK: Gastric antacids, stimulants, and antiemetics. In *Pharmacology and physiology in anesthetic practice,* Philadelphia, 1987, JB Lippincott.
292. Schmidt JF, Schierup L, Banning AM: The effect of sodium citrate on the pH and the amount of gastric contents before general anaesthesia, *Acta Anaesthesiol Scand* 28:263, 1984.
293. O'Sullivan GM, Bullingham RE: Noninvasive assessment by radiotelemetry of antacid effect during labor, *Anesth Analg* 64:95, 1985.
294. Gibbs CP, Schwartz DJ, Wynne JW, et al: Antacid pulmonary aspiration in the dog, *Anesthesiology* 51:380, 1979.
295. Cooke N, Teitelbaum S, Avioli LV: Antacid-induced osteomalacia and nephrolithiasis, *Arch Intern Med* 138:1007, 1978.
296. Alfrey AC, LeGendre GR, Kaehny WS: The dialysis encephalopathy syndrome: possible aluminum intoxication, *N Engl J Med* 294:184, 1976.
297. Clayman CB: The carbonate affair: chalk one up, *JAMA* 244:2554, 1980 (editorial).
298. Plumb VJ, James TN: Clinical hazards of powerful diuretics: furosemide and ethacrynic acid, *Mod Concepts Cardiovasc Dis* 47:91, 1978.
299. Weiner IM, Mudge GH: Diuretics and other agents employed in the mobilization of edema fluid. In Gilman AG, Goodman LS, Rall TW, et al, eds: *The pharmacological basis of therapeutics,* ed 7, New York, 1985, Macmillan.
300. Havdala HS, Borison RL, Diamond BI: Potential hazards and applications of lithium in anesthesiology, *Anesthesiology* 50:534, 1979.
301. Miller RD, Sohn YJ, Matteo RS: Enhancement of *d*-tubocurarine neuromuscular blockade by diuretics in man, *Anesthesiology* 45:442, 1976.
302. Warren SE, Blantz RC: Mannitol, *Arch Intern Med* 141:493, 1981.
303. O'Reily RA: Anticoagulant, antithrombotic, and thrombolytic drugs. In Gilman AG, Goodman LS, Rall TW, et al, eds: *The pharmacological basis of therapeutics,* New York, 1985, Macmillan.
304. Cipolle RJ, Rodovold KA, Seifert R, et al: Heparin-associated thrombocytopenia: a prospective evaluation of 211 patients, *Ther Drug Monit* 5:205, 1983.
305. Kakkar VV, Bentley PG, Scully MF, et al: Antithrombin III and heparin, *Lancet* 1:103, 1980 (letter).
306. Deykin D: Current status of anticoagulant therapy, *Am J Med* 72:659, 1982.
307. Nielsen HK, Husted SE, Koopman HD, et al: Heparin-induced increase in serum levels of aminotransferases: a controlled clinical trial, *Acta Med Scand* 215:231, 1984.
308. Edes TE, Sunderrajan EV: Heparin-induced hyperkalemia, *Arch Intern Med* 145:1070, 1985.
309. Wood AJJ, Robertson D, Robertson RM, et al: Elevated plasma free drug concentrations of propranolol and diazepam during cardiac catheterization, *Circulation* 62:1119, 1980.
310. Hall JG, Pauli RM, Wilson KM: Maternal and fetal sequelae of anticoagulation during pregnancy, *Am J Med* 68:122, 1980.
311. Peterson CE, Kwaan HC: Current concepts of warfarin therapy, *Arch Intern Med* 146:581, 1986.
312. Goldhaber SZ, Buring JE, Lipnick RJ, et al: Pooled analyses of randomized trials of streptokinase and heparin in phlebographically documented acute deep venous thrombosis, *Am J Med* 76:393, 1984.
313. Jaques LB: Protamine—antagonist to heparin, *Can Med Assoc J* 108:1291, 1973.
314. Ellison N, Edmunds LH Jr, Colman RW: Platelet aggregation following heparin and protamine administration, *Anesthesiology* 48:65, 1978.
315. Michaels IAL, Barash PG: Hemodynamic changes during protamine administration, *Anesth Analg* 62:831, 1983.
316. Lowenstein E, Johnston WE, Lappas DG, et al: Catastrophic pulmonary vasoconstriction associated with protamine reversal of heparin, *Anesthesiology* 59:470, 1983.
317. Stewart WJ, McSweeney SM, Kellett MA, et al: Increased risk of severe protamine reactions in NPH insulin–dependent diabetics undergoing cardiac catheterization, *Circulation* 70:788, 1984.
318. Dietrich W, Spath P, Ebell A, et al: Prevalence of anaphylactic reactions to aprotinin: analysis of two hundred forty-eight reexposures to aprotinin in heart operations, *J Thorac Cardiovasc Surg* 113:194, 1997.
319. Ray MJ, Marsh NA, Mengerson K: A brief review of studies evaluating the adverse effects of aprotinin therapy in aortocoronary bypass surgery, *Thromb Haemost* 77:1038, 1997 (letter).
320. D'Ambra MN, Akins CW, Blackstone EH, et al: Aprotinin in primary valve replacement and reconstruction: a multicenter, double-blind, placebo-controlled trial, *J Thorac Cardiovasc Surg* 112:1081, 1996.
321. Schultz M, van der Lelie H: Microscopic haematuria as a relative contraindication for tranexamic acid, *Br J Haematol* 89:663, 1995.
322. Dentz ME, Slaughter TF, Mark JB: Early thrombus formation on heparin-bonded pulmonary artery catheters in patients receiving ε-aminocaproic acid, *Anesthesiology* 82:583, 1995.

323. Davies DW, Steward DT: Unexplained excessive bleeding during opeation: role of acetyl salicylic acid, *Can Anaesth Soc J* 24:452, 1977.

324. Brenner BE, Simon RR: Management of salicylate intoxication, *Drugs* 24:335, 1982.

325. Thompson WL: Rational use of albumin and plasma substitutes, *Johns Hopkins Med J* 136:220, 1975.

326. Feest TG: Low molecular weight dextran: a continuing cause of acute renal failure, *BMJ* 2:1300, 1976.

327. Lima JJ, Goldfarb AL, Conti DR, et al: Safety and efficacy of procainamide infusions, *Am J Cardiol* 43:98, 1979.

328. Bigger TJ, Hoffman BF: Antiarrhythmic drugs. In Gilman AG, Goodman LS, Rall TW, et al, eds: *The pharmacological basis of therapeutics*, New York, 1985, Macmillan.

329. Roden DM, Woosley RL: Antiarrhythmic drugs. In Wood MW, Wood AJJ, eds: *Drugs and anesthesia: pharmacology for anesthesiologists*, ed 2, Baltimore, 1990, Williams & Wilkins.

330. Kornfeld P, Horowitz SH, Genkins G: Myasthenia gravis unmasked by antiarrhythmic agents, *Mt Sinai J Med* 43:10, 1976.

331. Miller RD, Way WL, Katzung BG: The potentiation of neuromuscular blocking agents by quinidine, *Anesthesiology* 28:1036, 1967.

332. Koch-Weser J: Drug therapy: bretylium, *N Engl J Med* 300:473, 1979.

333. Podrid PJ, Schoeneberger A, Lown B: Congestive heart failure caused by oral disopyramide, *N Engl J Med* 302:614, 1980.

334. Heger JJ, Prystowsky EN, Jackman WM, et al: Amiodarone: clinical efficacy and electrophysiology during low-term therapy for recurrent ventricular tachycardia or ventricular fibrillation, *N Engl J Med* 305:539, 1981.

335. Liberman BA, Teasdale SJ: Anaesthesia and amiodarone, *Can Anaesth Soc J* 32:629, 1985.

336. Navalgund AA, Alifimoff JK, Jakymec AJ, et al: Amiodarone-induced sinus arrest successfully treated with ephedrine and isoproterenol, *Anesth Analg* 65:414, 1986.

337. Moysey JO, Jaggarao NSV, Grundy EN, et al: Amiodarone increases plasma digoxin concentrations, *Br Med J (Clin Res Ed)* 282:272, 1981.

338. Frank SE, Snyder JT: Survival following severe overdose with mexiletine, nifedepine, and nitroglycerin, *Am J Emerg Med* 9:43, 1991.

339. Idsoe O, Guthe T, Willcox RR, et al: Nature and extent of penicillin side-reactions, with particular reference to fatalities from anaphylactic shock, *Bull World Health Organ* 38:159, 1968.

340. Mandell GL, Sande MA; Penicillins, cephalosporins, and other beta-lactam antibiotics. In Gilman AG, Goodman LS, Rall TW, et al, eds: *The pharmacological basis of therapeutics*, New York, 1985, Macmillan.

341. Scholand JF, Tennenbaum JI, Cerilli GJ: Anaphylaxis to cephalothin in a patient allergic to penicllin, *JAMA* 206:130, 1968.

342. Gary NE, Buzzeo L, Salaki RP, et al: Gentamicin-associated acute renal failure, *Arch Intern Med* 136:1101, 1976.

343. Meyer RD: Amikacin, *Ann Intern Med* 95:328, 1981.

344. Wilson P, Ramsden RT: Immediate effects of tobramycin on human cochlea and correlation with serum tobramycin levels, *BMJ* 1:259, 1977.

345. Sokoll MD, Gergis SD: Antibiotics and neuromuscular function, *Anesthesiology* 55:148, 1981.

346. Holtzman JL: Gentamicin and neuromuscular blockade, *Ann Intern Med* 84:55, 1976 (letter).

347. Geraci JE, Hermans PE: Vancomycin, *Mayo Clin Proc* 58:88, 1983.

348. Bennett JE: Chemotherapy of systemic mycoses (part 1), *N Engl J Med* 290:30, 1974.

349. Bennett JE: Chemotherapy of systemic mycoses (part 2), *N Engl J Med* 290:320, 1974.

350. Schulze-Delrieu K: Drug therapy: metoclopramide, *N Engl J Med* 305:28, 1981.

351. Bateman DN, Davies DS: Pharmacokinetics of metoclopramide, *Lancet* 1:166, 1979 (letter).

352. Van Dellen RG: Clinical pharmacology: series on pharmacology in practice: 4: theophylline: practical application of new knowledge, *Mayo Clin Proc* 54:733, 1979.

353. Stirt JA, Sullivan SF: Aminophylline, *Anesth Analg* 60:587, 1981.

354. Wood MW: Drugs and the respiratory system. In Wood MW, Wood AJJ, eds: *Drugs and anesthesia: pharmacology for anesthesiologists*, ed 2, Baltimore, 1990, Williams & Wilkins.

355. Pentoxifylline for intermittent claudication, *Med Lett Drugs Ther* 26:103, 1984.

356. Mark LC: Analeptics: changing concepts, declining status, *Am J Med Sci* 254:296, 1967.

357. Britt BA: Dantrolene, *Can Anaesth Soc J* 31:61, 1984.

358. Watson CB, Reierson N, Norfleet EA: Clinically significant muscle weakness induced by oral dantrolene sodium prophylaxis for malignant hyperthermia, *Anesthesiology* 65:312, 1986.

359. Davidoff RA: Pharmacology of spasticity, *Neurology* 28(9 pt 2):46, 1978.

360. Judkins JH, Dray TG, Hubbell RN: Intraoperative ketorolac and posttonsillectomy bleeding, *Arch Otolaryngol Head Neck Surg* 122:937, 1996.

361. Bosek V, Cox CE: Comparison of analgesic effect of locally and systemically administered ketorolac in mastectomy patients, *Ann Surg Oncol* 3:62, 1996.

362. Quan DJ, Kayser SR: Ketorolac induced acute renal failure following a single dose, *J Toxicol Clin Toxicol* 32:305, 1994.

363. Maliekal J, Elboim CM: Gastrointestinal complications associated with intramuscular ketorolac tromethamine therapy in the elderly, *Ann Pharmacother* 29:698, 1995.

364. Boike SC, Ilson B, Zariffa N, et al: Cardiovascular effects of IV granisetron at two administration rates and of ondansetron in healthy adults, *Am J Health Sys Pharm* 54:1172, 1997.

365. Baguley WA, Hay WT, Mackie KP, et al: Cardiac arrhythmias associated with the intravenous administration of ondansetron and metoclopramide, *Anesth Analg* 84:1380, 1997.

366. Mitchell KE, Popkin MK, Trick W, et al: Psychiatric complications associated with ondansetron, *Psychosomatics* 35:161, 1994.

Chapter 8

Perioperative Nerve Injury

Anne C.P. Lui
Gale E. Thompson

Despite the common tendency to link perioperative nerve injury to either the anesthetic or the anesthesiologist, the mechanisms of nerve injury are often obscure. Our primary goal in this chapter is to emphasize the great diversity of possible etiologic factors. An almost imperative corollary to our goal is to emphasize that each case of nerve injury has a temporal perspective. The term *perioperative* must be construed to mean preoperative, intraoperative, and postoperative. The preoperative period may be measured in days, months, or years and implies that preexisting disease processes may have contributed to what finally becomes overtly manifest as an intraoperative event. Likewise, the postoperative perspective must be days in duration because nerve injuries may either be induced in that period or become objectively or subjectively apparent only after more acute postsurgical problems are resolved. Careful analysis of any case may reveal multiple possible etiologic factors at different times. Such analysis is important from the medical standpoint of prevention as well as for the legal implications. Although some authors[1] opine that perioperative nerve injuries should never happen, there is good reason

to question whether they are always preventable or whether some of the commonly used prophylactic measures are even rational or effective.

From the patient's perspective there is perhaps nothing more irritating than to come to the hospital for a "successful" surgical procedure and then to go home with a totally unexpected nerve deficit in an area of the body far removed from the site of surgery. In our experience the significance of the nerve injury is often compounded by the patient's vocation. For example, an auctioneer developed a vocal cord paralysis after tracheal intubation and a carpenter was awarded $60,000 for an ulnar neuropathy of his hammering hand after hernia repair. Similarly distressed was a karate instructor who developed a long thoracic nerve injury after kidney surgery. An even more ominous case involved a pianist who suffered bilateral ulnar nerve deficits during the course of two separate abdominal operations. Finger contractions developed and ultimately resulted in amputations. The court awarded her roughly $50,000.

Legal action is common in cases of nerve injury. The doctrine of *res ipsa loquitur* is applied in many instances. Defending such a case is a considerable challenge.

Dornette has written a good summary of the origins, elements, and pertinent case histories of the *res ipsa* doctrine.[2] The Committee on Professional Liability of the American Society of Anesthesiologists (ASA)[3,4] found nerve damage to be the second most common anesthetic injury (15%) in their review of 1541 closed malpractice claims related to anesthetic care. Even when anesthetic care was judged to be appropriate, payment was made in 45% of claims. The median payment for disabling nerve injury was $56,000, as compared to a median payment of $225,000 for claims for other types of disabling injury. Because 92% of these cases occurred between 1975 and 1985, they probably do not reflect current settlement amounts. In addition, closed claims analysis is retrospective and provides no information about incidence because the population from which these claims were drawn is unknown. However, a few historical data points establish the incidence of perioperative nerve injury at about 0.1%. This number has important implications for informed consent.

I. HISTORICAL PERSPECTIVE

It appears that the first association of anesthesiology with nerve injury was a report by Budinger[5] from Vienna in 1894. He described several cases of nerve injury following chloroform anesthesia. Interestingly, trichloroethylene and nitrous oxide have also been considered to induce metabolic changes that could be neurotoxic. Although these general anesthetic agents were first incriminated, the pendulum has now swung far more toward the implication of regional anesthesia as a potential cause of nerve injury. In the first half of the twentieth century, some of the problems obviously were attributable to impurities of injected drugs or unsterile techniques in performing nerve blocks. Such problems have sometimes achieved considerable notoriety and sensationalism, such as the famous *Woolley and Roe*[6] case in England. Reverberations from that judgment cast a pall over the use of spinal anesthesia in that country for many years. Likewise, Kennedy, Effron, and Perry's inflammatory article[7] "The Grave Spinal Cord Paralysis Caused by Spinal Anesthesia" did little to promote the use of regional anesthesia and certainly perpetuated the notion that regional anesthesia is one of the primary causes of perioperative nerve injury. Today the association of cauda equina syndrome with continuous spinal anesthesia has resurrected fears of neurotoxicity from local anesthetics.[8]

Dhunér[9] authored one of the reports on the incidence of nerve injury in 1950. This study, from the Karolinska Institute in Sweden, reported 31 nerve palsies in 30,000 operations, for an incidence of 0.1%. Dhunér was critical of spinal anesthesia and wrote, "It is well known that analgesia and even spinal puncture may produce cord or nerve damage." Of 31 neuropathies described by Dhunér, 26 were in the upper extremity. Eleven involved the brachial plexus, seven the radial nerve, and eight the ulnar nerve. There were five cases of lower extremity neuropathy, and each involved the common peroneal nerve. Of the patients with peroneal nerve palsies, four had received subarachnoid block with dibucaine. One of the patients with peroneal nerve palsy received only general anesthesia, so Dhunér was forced to conclude that "other factors may be responsible."

In 1973 Parks[10] reported 72 nerve palsies in 50,000 general surgery patients. Here again, the incidence was about 0.14%. Of these patients, only 3 out of 72 had received spinal anesthesia. Parks added a new perspective on etiology by suggesting that muscle relaxants may increase the potential for nerve injury. Sixty-three of the 72 patients received muscle relaxants, and the impression was that this sometimes allowed abnormal stretching or positioning of extremities, with consequent nerve damage.

We have also obtained data about nerve injuries through mechanisms of the quality assurance program at Virginia Mason Clinic. Through educational efforts we have gradually increased sensitivity to the problem and devised methods of data collection. During the first 3 years of this study, we were somewhat surprised to find 30 nerve injuries in a series of 26,167 surgical patients (0.11% incidence). By 1988 we had identified a total of 67 perianesthetic neuropathies in 65 patients. One interesting finding was the high incidence of underlying disease in patients who developed perioperative neuropathy. Of the 65 patients, 35 had significant medical problems, as depicted in Table 8-1. Thirteen of our cases did not receive a major anesthetic, and six of these occurred in obstetric patients. Other cases included a median nerve palsy after intravenous use of vasoactive drugs, a brachial plexus palsy after infiltration of an intravenous catheter through which intravenous pyelogram dye had been injected, median nerve trauma related to angioplasty needle insertion, and a vocal cord paralysis after subclavian vein cannulation.

II. ANATOMIC CONSIDERATIONS

The peripheral nervous system consists of cranial nerves III to XII, spinal roots, autonomic ganglia, nerve plexuses, and peripheral nerves in a complex network of efferent and afferent fibers. The neuron is the key conducting unit of the nervous system. It is made up of the cell body (perikaryon) and a cytoplasmic extension called the axon. The life of the axon depends on continuity with the cell body. Thus axoplasmic transport of macromolecules from the cell body down the entire axon (which can be as much as 1 to 2 m in length) can pose special prob-

Table 8-1. Significant underlying medical problems in 65 neuropathy patients

Disease	Number of patients
Diabetes mellitus	7
Alcohol abuse	5
Severe peripheral vascular disease	6
Preexisting neuropathy	4
Renal failure	4
Hypothyroidism	2
Morbid obesity	4
Hepatic failure	2
Nelson's disease	1

Courtesy Quality Assurance Program, Virginia Mason Clinic, Seattle, Washington.

lems. This transport system is vital for normal growth and regeneration of the axon, for maintaining the integrity of the axonal membrane and its conducting properties, and for supplying precursors of the cell's neurotransmitters. Three kinds of transport are recognized: fast axon transport, which is calcium dependent and probably occurs along neurotubules, carrying enzymes, polypeptides, polysaccharides, and neurosecretory granules to the nerve terminals; slow axon transport, which occurs at rates of 1 to 50 mm/day and may correlate with the bulk flow of axoplasm; and retrograde axon transport, which conveys trophic factors back to the cell body. Examples of clinical correlates that illustrate defects in each of these transport systems support the belief that the transport system dictates the survival and welfare of the axon and to some degree the structures it innervates.[11]

A. Spinal roots

There are 31 pairs of spinal nerves, each formed by a dorsal root and a ventral root that arise from the spinal cord. These spinal nerve roots can be damaged by direct trauma (penetrating injuries, fracture or dislocation of the spine), indirect trauma (such as traction injuries of the brachial plexus or lumbosacral plexus), or lesions encroaching on the intervertebral foramen (osteophytes, tumor of the spine, intervertebral disk disease). The cauda equina begins immediately below the conus medullaris at the first lumbar vertebrae in adults (or the third lumbar vertebrae at birth). The nerve roots (L2 to S5) of the cauda equina provide sensory, motor, and autonomic innervation to most of the lower extremity, the pelvic floor, and the sphincters. The cauda equina syndrome consists of low back pain, saddle anesthesia, chronic paraplegia, and sphincter and sexual dysfunction. There are many causes of cauda equina syndrome, including compression of the nerve roots by tumor, herniated disk, or spinal stenosis; infectious, inflammatory, or immune-mediated causes; ischemic insults or venous infarctions; and traumatic lesions such as electric shock or radiation.[12]

B. Peripheral nerves

Peripheral nerve fibers originate from sensory, motor, or autonomic cell bodies in the dorsal ganglia or ventral horn of the spinal cord. The cytoplasm of the neuron extends beyond the central nervous system as the axon. Surrounding the axon of many fibers are variable layers of myelin produced by a single Schwann cell. A layer of connective tissue called the endoneurium encloses each fiber. Bundles of fibers form fascicles (or funiculi) wrapped in connective tissue known as perineurium. Several fascicles, encased in more connective tissue called the epineurium, form the peripheral nerve. Peripheral nerves can be classified by fiber size: larger myelinated A fibers, smaller preganglionic sympathetic myelinated B fibers, and small unmyelinated C fibers (Table 8-2). In addition to nutrient supply from the neuron, blood vessels along the course of the nerve also contribute to the fibers' nutrition. These blood vessels, called vasa nervorum, run a longitudinal course with numerous anastomoses and are called epineurial, interfascicular perineurial, and intrafascicular arteries, arterioles, and capillaries.

Table 8-2. Classification of peripheral nerve fibers by size and conduction velocity

Type	Diameter (μm)	Conduction velocity (m/sec)
Aα	13-22	80-120
Aβ	8-13	40-80
Aγ	4-8	15-40
Aδ (pain)	2-6	5-30
B	1-3	3-15
C (pain)	1-2	1-2

The histologic anatomy of the nerve partly determines the susceptibility to injury. Nerve trunks containing numerous small fibers with abundant perineurium are less vulnerable to compression injuries than those composed of large fibers with little supporting connective tissue. Furthermore, partial injury to a nerve with many small fibers results in less significant deficit than the same injury to a nerve with a few large fibers.[13] Anatomic location is another factor that predisposes certain nerves to injury. Nerves that are superficially located are in direct contact with bone or may cross areas of fibrous tissue, where they are susceptible to damage by compression. Increased tension is placed on a nerve that crosses joints, especially in the extensor aspect. Thus the radial nerve in the spiral groove of the humerus, the common peroneal nerve at the head of the fibula, the ulnar nerve behind the medial condyle, and the supraorbital nerve are all superficial structures that are prone to compression against bone. Extreme flexion, abduction, and external rotation of the thighs in the lithotomy position compress the femoral nerve against the fibrous inguinal ligament, which may lead to femoral nerve palsy. Chronic friction is yet another etiologic factor; examples include the ulnar nerve as it crosses the medial intermuscular septum in the forearm, the median nerve in the carpal tunnel, and the lateral femoral cutaneous nerve as it pierces the fascia lata or as it passes through the inguinal ligament.

Even when similar nerves are equally injured, the clinical disability may differ. For example, Sunderland and Swaney[14] suggest that in injury of the recurrent laryngeal nerve, the nerve supply to the adductor and abductor mechanisms are often equally damaged. However, the adductor muscle mass, three times that of the abductor mass, results in greater adductor tone, so there is a tendency to midline drift of the paralyzed vocal cords.

C. Individual nerves

1. Optic and facial nerves. Although the optic nerve is not part of the peripheral nervous system, strictly speaking, it is discussed here in the context of nerve injuries to the face area. The optic nerve may be damaged in the presence of ocular compression by an improperly placed horseshoe headrest with the patient in the prone position. The superficial orbital nerves are not protected by soft tissue padding and can easily be compressed against the orbital rim by underlying or overlying objects such as the endotracheal tube connector. The incidence of anterior ischemic optic neuropathy following open heart surgery is less than 0.5% and

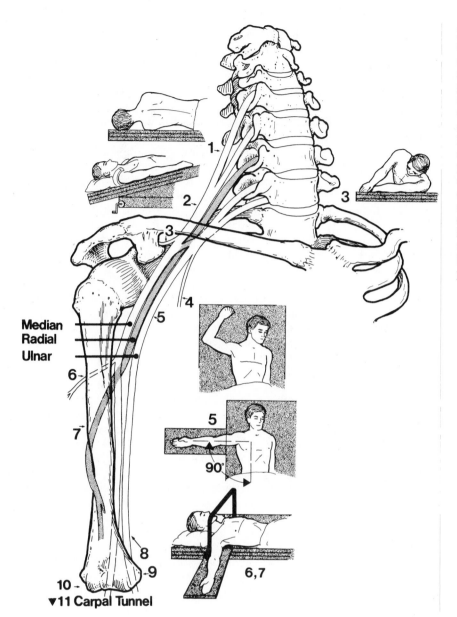

Fig. 8-1. Locations and causes of injury to brachial plexus and nerves of the upper extremity. *1,* Impingement or traction of nerve roots; *2,* impingement of brachial plexus between clavicle and first rib; *3,* traction of supraclavicular nerve; *4,* traction of long thoracic nerve; *5,* traction or compression of brachial plexus by head of humerus in abduction; *6,* compression of axillary nerve against humerus; *7,* compression of radial nerve against humerus; *8,* compression of ulnar nerve against medial supracondylar ridge; *9,* traction or compression of ulnar nerve across medial epicondyle; *10,* median neuropathy from intravenous infiltration or direct needle trauma; *11,* carpal tunnel syndrome caused by hyperextension of wrist or tightly applied strap over wrist.

can be associated with prolonged cardiac bypass time, low hematocrit, excessive perioperative body weight gain, and the use of epinephrine and amrinone.[15] The facial nerve can be compressed against the ramus of the mandible during maneuvers to maintain a patent airway or by a mask strap.

2. Spinal accessory nerve. The spinal accessory nerve is a pure motor nerve that innervates the sternocleidomastoid and the trapezius. The most common cause of spinal accessory nerve injury is iatrogenic, usually relating to biopsy of a lymph node or excision of a benign tumor.[16] Cases of spinal accessory nerve injury have also been reported following carotid endarterectomy,[17] rhytidectomy,[18] and internal jugular vein cannulation.[19]

3. Long thoracic nerve. Long thoracic nerve palsies that develop after anesthetics for surgical procedures have been reviewed by Martin.[20] Mechanisms of injury include direct trauma to the posterior triangle of the neck, compression by shoulder braces in the Trendelenburg position, or traction injuries in which the angle of the neck and shoulder is increased or the shoulder is dis-

placed downward, as by a fully loaded knapsack. Prolonged exertion at the shoulder can also selectively injure the long thoracic nerve, as after practice at grenade throwing, archery, or tennis. There is a high incidence of idiopathic onset, and Foo and Swann[21] use the term *neuralgic amyotrophy* to describe cases of isolated long thoracic nerve palsy.

4. Brachial plexus. Nerve roots C5 to T1 form the brachial plexus. These roots invaginate the dura in a funnel shape as they leave the spinal cord. The dura continues along each nerve root and eventually blends with the epineurium. The roots can be compressed in the presence of a narrowed intervertebral foramen during hyperextension, lateral flexion, or rotation of the cervical spine. Under increasing tension, the nerve roots may be more susceptible to injury than the peripheral nerve as a result of a lower tensile strength and lesser amount of epineurial and perineurial connective tissue. The plexus can also be injured in other ways, such as direct trauma, vascular injury, and lesions associated with bone and joint injury (Fig. 8-1).[22]

The trunk of the plexus can be compressed between the clavicle and the first rib or between the scalenus anterior and scalenus medius muscles, as in thoracic outlet syndrome or cervical rib syndrome. Of particular importance to the physician positioning an unconscious patient is that hyperabduction of the arm, with the shoulders posteriorly displaced and forced downward, reduces the costoclavicular space. In this position the subclavian artery is also occluded by the costoclavicular compression, and the absence of the radial pulse warns of potential nerve compression. Postanesthetic palsies may be attributable to stretch[23] or compression of the plexus for prolonged periods. The plexus is stretched when the neck is extended and flexed to the opposite side or when the arm is in any extreme position, particularly when abducted and externally rotated. This position causes bowing of the cords of the plexus against the head of the humerus. Improperly placed shoulder braces used to support the patient in the Trendelenburg position can force the shoulders downward, stretching the plexus, or can injure the nerves by direct compression. Similar traction and compression injuries are seen in the neuropathies associated with prolonged abnormal positioning in the comatose patient from drug overdose[24] or the asphyxiated patient in "crowd-crush" disasters (Fig. 8-2).[25] The Erb-Duchenne palsy describes involvement of the upper trunk of the brachial plexus (C5 to C6) and is the most common presentation. This injury can occur with recreational backpacking, in firearm recoil palsy, and in contact sports such as wrestling and football.

A case of idiopathic brachial neuritis, presenting 12 hours after an uneventful anesthetic for hysteroscopy, has been reported. The authors found elevated ganglioside antibody titers that may help differentiate postoperative idiopathic brachial neuritis from traction and compression causes of brachial neuropathy.[26]

Nerve palsies in the newborn occur in about 1 in 857 deliveries.[27] Brachial plexus palsies are the most common and are associated with shoulder dystocia or difficult breech with an obstructed aftercoming head. Also in breech deliveries where the arms are fully abducted or when the arms are adducted but forcibly pulled downward to help deliver the head, there is risk of compression and traction injuries to the plexus.

The annual incidence of brachial plexus neuropathy is 1.64 in 100,000. After total shoulder arthroplasty, the incidence is 4%. The postulated mechanism of injury is traction on the plexus during the operation.[28]

5. Ulnar nerve. Ulnar nerve entrapment is the second most common entrapment neuropathy (the first is carpal tunnel syndrome). Major etiologic factors are acute or recurrent compression, inherent anatomic deformities impeding nerve mobility, or lesions within the cubital tunnel. The ulnar nerve may be constricted by a taut aponeurosis, particularly with elbow flexion. Recurrent subluxation of the nerve may contribute to ulnar neuropathy. The ulnar nerve is particularly susceptible to damage at its superficial position as it passes behind the epicondyle of the humerus. Repeated pressure from resting the elbow on a hard surface may precipitate injury, especially if the ulnar groove is shallow. In the comatose or anesthetized patient, injury to the nerve is often the result of either an overstretched nerve in a hyperflexed elbow or direct compression of the nerve against a hard object such as an armboard or side rail of the operating room table (Fig. 8-3). Supination of the forearm moves the epicondylar area away from direct contact with the hard surface. Tomlinson et al[29] prospectively studied 335 patients undergoing cardiac surgery and found an incidence of 4.8% of brachial plexus injury related to traction from the median sternotomy. Specifically, the ulnar nerve is the most common clinically identifiable site of nerve injury after use of a sternal retractor. The incidence of nerve injury with different retractors is not known. Merchant, Brown, and Watson[30] report ulnar neuropathy with clinical changes in 15% and subclinical changes in 40% of patients having coronary artery bypass surgery. Interestingly, subclinical changes occurred in 33% of limbs studied preoperatively with electrophysiologic

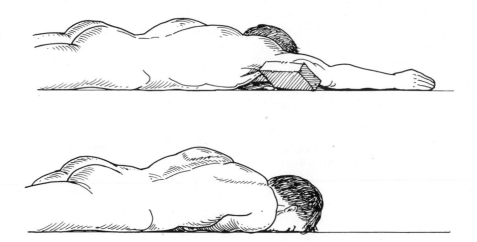

Fig. 8-2. The patient with trauma or drug overdose may have sustained nerve injury before arrival in the operating room. A compressed extremity may undergo compartmental pressures up to 225 mm Hg from body weight alone.

methods. Three cases of ulnar neuropathy associated with the use of automatically cycled blood pressure cuffs have been reported.[31] The ASA Closed Claims Project found that ulnar neuropathy represented one third of all nerve injuries (5% of all claims) and that the file contained information specifically stating that the arm was padded in 18% of these patients.[4] Preventive measures did not prevent injuries.

In a retrospective review of 1,129,692 diagnostic and noncardiac surgical procedures attended by an anesthesia care team, the rate of developing ulnar neuropathy was 1 in 2729. In patients who developed ulnar neuropathy, 70% were male, 9% of cases were bilateral, and neuropathy occurred even when precautions and padding were documented.[32] Based on this study, an assessment of relative risk was determined statistically. Using multivariate analysis, the following factors were associated with an increased risk of ulnar neuropathy: male gender, increasing age (35% increase in risk per decade), extremes of weight (body mass index [BMI] higher than 37 or lower than 24), and hospital stay exceeding 14 days. Of note was the lack of association of nerve injury to patient position during the surgery, duration of surgery, or type of anesthetic administered. The majority of neuropathy first presented more than 24 hours postoperatively. Fewer than 10% of the initial symptoms were noted in the postanesthetic recovery unit.

Stoelting concludes that ulnar neuropathy is not always preventable[33] and that the cause of the problem is beyond the control, and therefore the liability, of the anesthesiologist.[34] Historically, the liability for perioperative ulnar neuropathy, based on data from the ASA Closed Claims Project amounts to a median payment of $17,500 (range $1400 to $330,000).[35]

6. Radial nerve. Radial nerve damage is usually the result of prolonged, unyielding pressure on the arm where the nerve spirals around the humerus. There are many specific causes of radial nerve palsy in this region: injection injuries, tourniquet palsy, crutch palsy, Saturday night palsy, drug overdose, and birth palsy. There has also been a report of radial nerve palsy from the use of an automatic blood pressure monitor.[36]

7. Median nerve. Compression of the median nerve at the wrist causes carpal tunnel syndrome. A reported prevalence of carpal tunnel syndrome is 220 per 100,000, but the incidence of carpal tunnel syndrome is increased among electronic parts assemblers, frozen-food processors, musicians, and dental hygienists. The incidence among shellfish packers, for example, is 200 times higher than in the general population.[37]

8. Lumbosacral plexus. The lumbosacral plexus is well protected in the psoas muscle, and indirect traction injury on the plexus is very unlikely. Because there is limited movement of the lumbar vertebral column, this usually poses little threat to adjacent nerve roots. At the ala of the sacrum, however, the trunk of the plexus is in direct contact with bone against which it can be compressed. The posterior division of L4-L5 and S1 is in proximity to the bony pelvis. Compression of the plexus in this region can result in exclusive involvement of the common peroneal component and a clinical picture of foot drop, with accompanying sensory changes. The lumbosacral trunk may be injured in the mother during difficult forceps delivery or may be compressed by the fetal head or buttocks. The lumbosacral plexus is often affected in diabetic radiculoplexus neuropathy and idiopathic lumbosacral plexus neuropathy.[38] The sacral roots can also be compressed by space-occupying lesions such as tumor or

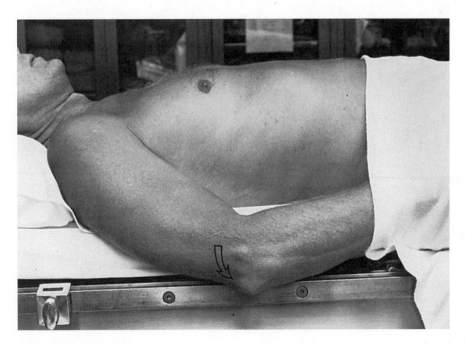

Fig. 8-3. Positioning of the arm showing the ulnar nerve compressed against the side rail of the operating room table *(arrow)*.

aneurysms in the sacral hollow, where the nerves are minimally protected by a thin layer of piriformis muscle.

9. Femoral nerve. The femoral nerve lies between the psoas and iliacus muscle. Compression injuries by retractors during pelvic surgery are the result of direct pressure or indirect compression of the nerve within the iliopsoas furrow from a laterally displaced psoas. The lithotomy position places the nerve at risk of compression under the inguinal ligament. The absence of a femoral pulse below the inguinal ligament may suggest nerve compression.

10. Lateral femoral cutaneous nerve. The lateral femoral cutaneous nerve may also be compressed in the lithotomy position. More common is idiopathic meralgia paresthetica (*meralgia* is "thigh" in Greek), a condition that is rarely disabling. Interesting, however, is its appearance during pregnancy; perhaps factors yet unknown can increase the susceptibility to entrapment neuropathies. Other sources of injury include soft tissue contusion medial to the anterior superior iliac spine from seat-belt injury, braces, or belts, or various diseases involving the pelvis or gut such as appendicitis, diverticulitis, or tumors.

11. Sciatic nerve. The sciatic nerve is superficial as it passes beneath the lower border of the gluteus maximus before it continues underneath the long head of the biceps femoris. It is vulnerable to direct compression when the patient is seated on a firm surface. Furthermore, flexion of the hip stretches the nerve as it comes around between the ischial tuberosity and the greater trochanter of the femur. This bony relationship places the nerve at risk for injury with trauma to the hip joint as well as in certain surgical operations on the hip and femur. The mechanism of injury may be a result of manipulation of the hip joint to facilitate surgery, leakage of methylmethacrylate (particularly from the acetabular component), or hematoma or postoperative scarring involving the sciatic nerve. The lithotomy position may also overstretch and damage the sciatic nerve, with the common peroneal component being the more vulnerable. Injection injuries may occur anywhere along the gluteal area where the sciatic nerve lies.

12. Peroneal nerve. The superficial branch of the common peroneal nerve is prone to injury where it lies superficially and in direct contact with bone as it wraps around laterally to the head and neck of the fibula. This nerve can be damaged by pressure from a tight plaster cast or when forced against leg braces used for the lithotomy position (Fig. 8-4). Warner et al[39] retrospectively reviewed 198,461 cases performed in the lithotomy position at the Mayo Clinic between 1957 and 1991. The rate of developing a neuropathy that persisted for more than 3 months was 1 in 3608 (total of 55 cases). Of the 55 cases, 43 involved the common peroneal nerve, 8 the sciatic nerve, and 4 the femoral nerve. Risk factors identified using multivariate analysis were lithotomy position lasting more than 4 hours, patients with BMI lower than 20, and smoking within 30 days of the procedure.

A much higher incidence of peroneal nerve palsy has been reported in total knee arthroplasties. In a recent retrospective review of 10,361 consecutive total knee arthroplasties, 32 peroneal nerve palsies were documented. Epidural analgesia for postoperative pain control, previous laminectomy, and preoperative valgus deformity were significantly associated with postoperative peroneal nerve palsy in this group of patients.[40] These

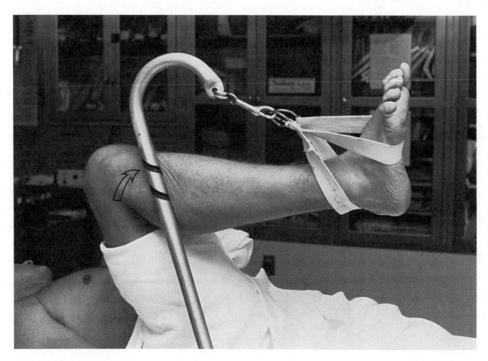

Fig. 8-4. Positioning of the lower extremity showing the superficial branch of the common peroneal nerve compressed against the leg braces used for the lithotomy position *(arrow)*.

authors postulate that decreased proprioception and sensation in patients receiving epidural analgesia resulted in suboptimal positioning, causing nerve injury.

Additional mechanisms for injury include crossing the leg in the seated position and compressing the nerve against the lower knee. The Japanese kneeling position can compress the nerve between the tendon of the biceps femoris, the lateral head of the gastrocnemius, and the head of the fibula. A case of peroneal nerve palsy after sequential pneumatic compression for prophylaxis of deep venous thrombosis has been reported.[41]

III. ETIOLOGIC FACTORS

A. Pressure changes, ischemia of nerves, and position-related injuries

The normal function and viability of the nerve fiber depends on the availability of oxygen and nutrients supplied through the vasa nervorum, as previously described. Oxygen supply to the nerve can be compromised by hypoxia or by pressure on the nerve trunk because of compression, traction, stretch, or friction injuries.

1. Compression neuropathy. Compression neuropathy is the result of nerve damage caused by mechanical pressure. A classic example is prolonged external compression of the radial nerve against the humerus, resulting in Saturday night palsy. Other external forces include tourniquet compression, crush injuries, obstetric nerve injuries, and a tight plaster cast compressing the peroneal nerve against the fibular neck. Nerves may also be compressed by adjacent internal structures such as callus around a healing fracture site; fibrous bands, tumors, or displaced bone; and edema, blood extravasation, or hematoma. The type of nerve damage from mechanical injury ranges from transient reversible changes to chronic pain syndromes and permanent paralysis. One classification of localized nerve injuries proposed by Seddon[42] introduced the terms *neuropraxia, axonotmesis,* and *neurotmesis.* Neuropraxia is a clinical entity that correlates with mild nerve injury associated with motor paralysis and only partial sensory loss. Spontaneous and rapid recovery usually ensues within days or weeks. Axonotmesis is best illustrated by the injury caused when a nerve is crushed with forceps, resulting in axonal interruption but intact neuronal stroma. Wallerian degeneration follows with distal denervation, and finally recovery occurs by axonal regeneration. Neurotmesis refers to partial or complete transection of the nerve.

Sunderland[43] based his classification of nerve injuries on the anatomy of the nerve trunk in relation to the endoneurium, perineurium, and epineurium. Thus he arrived at five degrees of injury: conduction abnormality in the axon, interruption of the axon alone, loss of endoneural continuity, disruption of the perineurium and funiculi, and complete loss of continuity of the nerve trunk.

The pathologic condition of a pressure-induced nerve lesion depends on the magnitude, duration, and rate of application of the compressive force. An acute, transient, deforming force can result in a temporary characteristic pattern of conduction block corresponding to a first-degree injury (or neurapraxia) at one end of the injury

scale to a fifth-degree injury with complete nerve transection (neurotmesis) at the other end. The former represents the mildest degree of compression lesion and correlates with studies using sphygmomanometer cuff pressures sufficient to obliterate arterial flow without damage to the nerve fibers. More persistent compression results in focal demyelination caused by local ischemia, and recovery occurs by remyelination. This is consistent with the time to clinical recovery of the Saturday night palsy of 6 to 8 weeks.[44] However, recovery may be delayed for up to 5 months as a result of axonal compression by adjacent cellular edema. A slowly applied persistent deforming force on a nerve fiber leads to axonal thinning, segmental demyelination, wallerian degeneration, and characteristic bulbous paranodal swellings such as that seen in the median nerve in the carpal tunnel syndrome. The pathophysiologic mechanism involved in these lesions remains controversial. Both direct mechanical damage[45] and chronic ischemia[46] have been proposed as the primary cause.

2. Traction and stretch injury. Traction and stretch injury has been the subject of research for over one and a half centuries. The peripheral nerve behaves as plastic material with individual variations in elasticity, ability to withstand maximum elongation, tensile strength, and susceptibility to breaking forces. These variations are attributable to the different tissue components of the nerve. Extension of any nerve involves a primary elongation, but further stretching is resisted by the perineurium with the resultant decrease in cross-sectional area, raising of intraneural pressure, and compression of the vasa nervorum. Lundborg and Rydevik[47,48] have shown that circulatory compromise occurs with as little as 8% elongation, and complete ischemia occurs at 15% elongation.

3. Ischemia. Ischemia is the common end point to both compressive and stretch injuries. When ischemia is the sole cause of nerve injury, pathologic changes appear later than in injury arising from a compressive-ischemic mechanism.[49] Fink and Cairns[50] studied the action potential of A and C fibers under various oxygen tensions and found that the A potential declines progressively with reduction in oxygen tension below 20 mm Hg, whereas C potential remains almost unaffected even at zero oxygen tension. These results show that myelinated A fibers depend on aerobic metabolism, whereas the C fibers are resistant to hypoxemia and rely on glycolytic metabolism for energy. This is consistent with observations of ischemic nerve injury in which motor function and tactile sensations are lost long before pain transmission is affected.

Peripheral vascular diseases associated with neuropathies may involve either large or small arteries. Large arteries can be occluded by emboli (associated with cardiac disease, subacute endocarditis, air, tumor, and so on), thromboangiitis obliterans, arteriosclerosis, Volkmann's ischemia, and vasospasm. Diseases of the arteriae nervorum include polyarteritis nodosa, amyloid, diabetes, and typhus. Various hematologic disorders such as sickle cell disease, polycythemia, macroglobulinemia, cryoglobulinemia, thrombocytopenia, hemophilia, and the use of anticoagulants can also lead to nerve ischemia. Common sites for these neuropathies are in the watershed areas in the midarm and midthigh. The pathologic condition is one of patchy nerve fiber degeneration, with a centripetal distribution.

Vascular occlusion of the vasa nervorum may cause neuropathic complications of burn patients, which are often undiagnosed. The most common abnormality is mononeuritis multiplex. Other possible causes include direct thermal injury or disseminated neurotoxin.[51]

B. Regional anesthesia

Regional anesthesia has been notorious for causing nerve damage. As stated earlier, such notoriety is not always deserved. However, the potential for needle or catheter trauma, instillation of neurotoxic drugs, drug additives, or contaminants, and the possible failure to appreciate preexisting nerve injury, vascular abnormality, or other disease may contribute to neuropathy. Neurologic complications may also coincide temporally with, but not be directly caused by, the regional anesthetic. For example, the incidence of ulnar nerve injury following regional anesthesia is 1 in 3005, compared with 1 in 2518 following general anesthesia.[32]

The incidence of permanent neurologic sequelae after spinal anesthesia is less than 1 in 10,000.[52] A similar incidence is reflected in a recent prospective survey in France of 40,640 patients undergoing spinal anesthesia, in which three cases of neurologic deficit lasting more than 3 months were reported.[53] In the pediatric population, regional anesthesia is associated with less than 1 in 10,000 incidence of transient paresthesia, and no permanent neurologic deficit, as reported in a prospective multicenter study involving 85,412 procedures.[54] Transient neurologic complication is noted in 0.5% and sensory cauda equina syndrome in 0.2% of 603 patients undergoing continuous spinal anesthesia.[55] The maximal risk of persistent nerve injury following epidural (thoracic or lumbar) catheterization for postoperative analgesia in 4227 surgical cancer patients has been calculated in a prospective study at 0.07%.[56] A similar risk exists for thoracic epidural anesthesia. The incidence of transient neurologic complication (all spontaneously resolved) is estimated to be 0.6% ($n = 24$) in a study of 4185 patients receiving a thoracic epidural. Of the 24 affected patients, 14 had peroneal nerve palsy. All of the 14 patients with peroneal nerve palsy were operated on in the lithotomy position.[57] Based on studies to date, regional anesthesia techniques are not associated with an increased risk of permanent neuropathy.

Another area of current controversy is transient neurologic symptoms (also known as transient radicular irritation [TRI]; see Chapter 3). Transient neurologic symptoms are clinically defined as pain or dysesthesia involving the gluteal area or legs following resolution of spinal anesthesia but within 24 hours of surgery. The incidence of transient neurologic symptoms was 16% for lidocaine and 0% for bupivacaine in one prospective study of 159 patients.[58] There is no difference in the incidence between patients receiving 5% hyperbaric lidocaine and 2% isobaric lidocaine. The phenomenon appears to be aggravated by positional stretching of lumbosacral roots

in the lithotomy position or during knee arthroscopy. Although transient neurologic symptoms are felt to be manifestations of the neurotoxicity of the local anesthetic, no data indicate that such manifestations are restricted to lidocaine or to local anesthetics alone. In a prospective study of 160 patients, transient neurologic symptoms occurred in 1.3% of patients receiving tetracaine and in 12.5% when phenylephrine was added to the tetracaine.[59] Although all transient neurologic symptoms resolve over time, the symptoms are not entirely benign and may require opioid analgesics or even readmission to the hospital for management.

1. Needle trauma. Injections may cause nerve damage by several mechanisms including direct needle trauma, intraneural injection, deposition of toxic material in the perineural space, vasospasm, or thrombosis. Needle trauma can occur with passage of the needle through a nerve fascicle. The extent of the injury may depend on whether the needle bevel enters parallel or transverse to the nerve fibers.[60] When the needle is inserted parallel to the nerve fibers, only slitlike fiber separation is seen. Transverse insertion of the needle results in more extensive fascicular injury, larger puncture sites, stretch, distortion, and herniation of nerve fibers. Damage to diffusion barriers from needle puncture, damage to neural blood vessels and resultant hematoma, edema, degeneration, and disruption of the nerve fiber can cause delayed recovery or even permanent deficits. Although the frequency of puncture lesions is greater with a long beveled needle than with a short 45-degree beveled needle, nerve injuries induced by short beveled needles are more severe and take longer to repair.[61] This leaves open the debate on the optimum needle bevel for peripheral nerve blocks.

Intramuscular injections in the gluteal area may be associated with direct trauma to the underlying nerve or injection of vasoactive or crystalline drugs into the inferior gluteal artery, causing ischemia to the sciatic nerve or lumbosacral plexus. Likewise, nerve injury may result from attempted blood draw or intravenous or arterial cannulation.

2. Intraneural injection. Intraneural injection causes a rise in intrafascicular pressure and initiates a compression-ischemia injury. The anoxic nerve fiber may then be vulnerable even to agents with low neurotoxicity.[62] The pathologic condition appears as fragmentation and swelling of the axon, swelling of the fascicles with separation of fibers, endoneural edema, and hemorrhage.

3. Local anesthetic toxicity. There is now clear evidence that local anesthetics, in the absence of additives, detergents, or antiseptics and independent of pH, osmolality, lipid solubility, or dissociation constants, can cause cytotoxic changes to nerves in vitro. The extent of nerve injury appears to depend on concentration, not dosage. In spinal anesthesia, the final concentration of local anesthetic is determined by the amount of drug injected and the volume of cerebrospinal fluid in which the drug is distributed.[63] This may explain Pollock et al's findings[58] of similar incidence of transient neurologic symptoms in patients receiving 5% and 2% lidocaine for spinal anesthesia. The relative potency for nerve injury is the same as the relative potency for producing nerve conduction block.

The mechanism of local anesthetic–induced nerve injury is unclear. There is evidence to support direct injury to the Schwann cell or the axon or indirect effects caused by alterations in nerve microenvironment. Nerves treated with local anesthetic in vitro undergo demyelination secondary to Schwann cell injury, but the predominant lesion is axonal degeneration. Furthermore, local anesthetics alter both blood flow and permeability characteristics of the interstitium surrounding the nerve. Changes in permeability can disrupt ionic gradients across the neurolemma. Local anesthetic applied to a nerve in vitro causes reduction in blood flow, with resultant ischemic injury. One of the mechanisms of reduced nerve blood flow may be related to prostaglandin metabolism and may be prevented with acetylsalicylic acid. The ischemic hypothesis may explain why patients with compromised blood flow (e.g., diabetic patients) are predisposed to nerve injury.[64] In Warner et al's study,[39] diabetes is a risk factor for perioperative neuropathy only with univariate analysis, not when multivariate analysis is used.

4. Local anesthetic additives. Nerve damage can occur when the local anesthetic is carried in a medium containing neurotoxic additives such as sodium bisulfite.[65] The injury may be further exacerbated by the presence of epinephrine in the solution. Intrathecally administered agents must be screened carefully for neurotoxic potential. Although ketamine has attractive analgesic potential when administered intrathecally, the preservative chlorobutanol, found in ketamine solution, induces severe spinal cord lesions in experimental rabbits,[66] making the solution unsuitable for intrathecal administration.

C. Toxic neuropathies

The neurotoxic effects of metals, pharmaceutical products, and environmental and biologic substances have been reviewed recently.[67]

1. Drugs. A prudent guideline is that just about any drug or its additives has the potential to produce neurotoxicity. Each of the following parenteral agents can result in nerve damage: antimicrobials (sulfa drugs, penicillin, methicillin, tetracycline, erythromycin, streptomycin, chloramphenicol, ethambutol, metronidazole, nitrofurantoin, isoniazid), salicylates, vitamin K, alcohol, paraldehyde, promazine, barbiturates, magnesium sulfate, colchicine, typhoid vaccine, chemotherapeutic agents (vincristine, vinblastine, cisplatin, docetaxol, paclitaxel), phenytoin, perhexiline, hydralazine, antidysrhythmics (amiodarone), antilipemic drugs (bezafibrate), clioquinol, dapsone, disulfiram, methaqualone, glutethimide, thalidomide, FK 506 (a new immunosuppressant replacing cyclosporin in organ transplantation), and botulinum toxin. Arterial spasm can lead to ischemic neuropathy after intravenous injection of vasoactive drugs. For example, chronic use of amphetamine results in necrotizing angiitis and mononeuritis multiplex.

2. Anesthetic agents

a. Nitrous oxide. Whether nitrous oxide as used in anesthesia has neuropathic potential is unclear. There have been clinical reports of neuropathy associated with abuse of nitrous oxide; however, a contaminant may have been the etiologic agent. Dyck et al[68] were unable to demonstrate nitrous oxide neurotoxicity in rats.

b. Trichloroethylene. Trichloroethylene is not neurotoxic, but its metabolite, dichloroacetylene, causes a neuropathy mainly affecting the fifth cranial nerve.[69] This neuropathy usually becomes evident 8 to 48 hours after exposure and the patient may take 18 months to recover. The pathology of the lesion has not been studied.

3. Alcoholic neuropathy. Alcoholic neuropathy is one of the most common neuropathies in North America and is invariably associated with high alcohol intake and dietary deficiencies. Thiamine deficiency plays a major role, but the direct toxic effects of alcohol, as well as multiple nutritional deficiencies, cannot be excluded. Both large and small fibers of the peripheral nervous system are affected in alcoholic polyneuropathy. Clinical findings include hypoesthesia, hyperalgesia, and paradoxic sensation. Heart rate variability has been used to assess alcohol-induced toxicity of the autonomic nervous system. An increase in heart rate caused by decreased parasympathetic activity is commonly seen, even though both the sympathetic and parasympathetic nervous systems are involved.

4. Household, industrial, and agricultural poisons. Household, industrial, and agricultural poisons associated with peripheral neuropathy include acrylamide, hexacarbons, carbon disulfide, organophosphates, carbamate insecticides, arsenic, lead, mercury, thallium, and ethylene oxide. Sensorimotor polyneuropathies in workers exposed to ethylene oxide sterilizers have been reported.[70] Occupations involving exposure to chemical solvents, neurotoxic metals and gases, and pesticides may be the cause of neuropathy.

D. Neuropathies associated with systemic diseases

1. Metabolic disorders. Up to 50% of insulin-dependent diabetic patients have symptomatic neuropathy. Nerve biopsies of patients with neuropathy reveal prominent intraneural microangiopathy and endothelial hyperplasia, consistent with a reduction in intraneural oxygen tension. Other proposed mechanisms include disturbed lipid and carbohydrate metabolism, which alters cellular composition, accumulation of sorbitol, and deficiency of myoinositol. There is also increasing evidence that an inflammatory or immune-mediated vasculitis that induces ischemic nerve fiber degeneration is the cause for certain types of diabetic neuropathy. Carpal tunnel syndrome is common in diabetes mellitus, suggesting repetitive shear forces, anatomic factors, and stiffness of connective tissue as additional inciting factors.[71]

Uremic neuropathy is associated with long-standing severe renal failure. The exact pathogenesis is unknown and is probably multifactorial. Main features of this neuropathy include axonal degeneration with segmental demyelination.

2. Nutritional deficiencies. Deficiencies of the B and E vitamin groups are well-known causes of neuropathy. Deficiencies of thiamine, vitamin B_{12}, nicotinamide, and pyridoxine (as in isoniazid-induced neuropathy) have been well documented to cause peripheral nerve damage. Thiamine deficiency in Western society may occur in patients with impaired nutrition (such as those with gastrointestinal disease or AIDS).[72] In Cuba an epidemic outbreak of peripheral neuropathy at a cumulative incidence of 461 in 100,000 was reported in 1992 to 1993. The risk factors include smoking, alcohol consumption, lower B-vitamin intake, weight loss (even without overt malnutrition), and excessive sugar consumption. The symptoms responded to vitamin B and folate supplements.[73]

Starvation after gastric bypass for morbid obesity can result in a demyelinating polyneuropathy with severe sensory ataxia.[74]

3. Infectious causes of neuropathy. Guillain-Barré syndrome, Lyme disease, diphtheria, and leprosy are some infectious diseases associated with neuropathy.

Neurologic disorders relating to human immunodeficiency virus (HIV) infection can involve the entire neuraxis, including the peripheral nerves. In the 1990s HIV replaced syphilis as the "great masquerader." The most common peripheral neuropathy associated with HIV infection is distal symmetric polyneuropathy that presents with burning feet as the chief complaint. The association is related at least in part to vitamin B_{12} deficiency. Other peripheral neuropathies associated with HIV infection are as follows:

- Inflammatory demyelinating polyneuropathy has similar clinical presentation as Guillain-Barré syndrome.
- Multiple mononeuropathy may be caused by an autoimmune mechanism or be secondary to opportunistic infections such as cytomegalovirus.
- Progressive polyradiculopathy may have symptoms similar to those of cauda equina syndrome.
- Autonomic neuropathy may cause orthostatic hypotension, diarrhea, and urinary dysfunction, and occurs more often in the late stages of infection. Neuropathy may be secondary to chemotherapeutic treatment, antiviral agents, zidovudine, and other neurotoxic drugs.[75,76]

4. Critical illness polyneuropathy. Approximately 70% of adult patients with sepsis have peripheral neuropathy on electrophysiologic studies, but 30% are asymptomatic.[77] There is a spectrum of presentation. Flaccid quadriplegia with inability to separate from ventilatory support despite full cardiopulmonary recovery is the common presentation. Critical illness polyneuropathy is a common cause of neuromuscular ventilatory failure in critically ill patients regardless of the primary cause. Facial and paraspinal muscle weaknesses are prominent. Upon recovery, residual weakness may involve the peroneal nerve.[78] Critical illness polyneuropathy has also been reported in pediatric patients. The cause of the neuropathy has not been elucidated, but it may be associated with the systemic inflammatory response syndrome.[79]

5. Others. Other systemic disorders that may have associated peripheral neuropathy include hypothyroidism, acromegaly, systemic lupus erythematosus, sarcoidosis, amyloidosis, and lymphoproliferative disease. Carcinomatous neuropathy may result from direct nerve compression by the tumor mass, tumor infiltration of nerves, paraneoplastic syndromes (most often seen in prostate, breast, and lung cancer), or irradiation of the tumor.

E. Nerve injuries in athletes

Athletes may acquire nerve injury through acute injury or chronic injury secondary to repetitive microtrauma or nerve entrapment. Repetitive shoulder motions that cause traction on the nerve, such as hyperabduction, may produce suprascapular neuropathy. Sports such as weightlifting predispose to this type of neuropathy. Axillary nerve injury may result from anterior shoulder dislocation. Weightlifters may develop musculocutaneous nerve palsy. Posterior interosseous nerve entrapment is common in tennis players. Baseball pitchers are prone to ulnar neuritis. Compression of the ulnar and median nerves at the wrist is seen in bicyclists. The bicycle seat may compress the pudendal nerves. Acute femoral neuropathies have been described in activities involving hyperextension of the hip (e.g., gymnastics, dance, football, basketball, long-jumping). The mechanism of injury may be iliopsoas hematoma and subsequent compression of the femoral nerve injury. The common peroneal nerve as it wraps around the fibula just below the knee is vulnerable to impact from hockey pucks, soccer kicks, and football clipping injuries. Compression lesion of the posterior tibial nerve by repetitive dorsiflexion of the ankle results in tarsal tunnel syndrome, common among runners and mountain climbers.[80]

F. Occupational palsies

Certain posturing of the limb or recurrent use can result in nerve injuries. Suprascapular nerve entrapment can be caused by recurrent loading of the affected shoulder with heavy weights. The long thoracic nerve can be affected in plasterers and painters. Operating a pneumatic hammer may injure the axillary nerve or produce carpal tunnel syndromes. A survey of dentists revealed a 29% prevalence of upper extremity neuropathy, suggesting the possibility of an occupational concern.[81] Compression of the ulnar nerve at the cubital fossa can occur in motorists who rest their elbows for prolonged periods on the car window ledge. Intense repeated pronation of the forearm can precipitate a friction injury of the median nerve as it passes between the two heads of the pronator teres. Occupations that require repeated hand movements (e.g., gardening, dressmaking, meatpacking, baking, hairdressing, and instrumental music) can result in median nerve paralysis. The deep palmar branch of the ulnar nerve can be injured in the hypothenar eminence in shoemakers from pushing an awl and in cyclists (from pressure on the handlebars). Vocational stress is the most common cause of carpal tunnel syndrome.

Peripheral nerve problems occur in 22.5% of musicians, including professional performers, students, teachers, and amateurs.[82] The majority of the peripheral nerve disorders fall into the category of compression neuropathies. The most common diagnosis is thoracic outlet syndrome based on the following clinical criteria: pain in the forearm; dysesthesia involving the ulnar, and sometimes radial, aspects of the forearm; and symptoms reproducible by hyperabduction or internal rotation with downward traction of the shoulder. The thoracic outlet syndrome is more common in women, by a ratio of 2:1. The injury tends to involve the left arm of string players and the right arm of keyboard instrumentalists. Carpal tunnel syndrome is the second most common neuropathy observed in musicians, who may complain of loss of dexterity in the affected hand and pain and paresthesia in the distribution of the median nerve. The third most common nerve disorder is ulnar neuropathy at the elbow. Sustained flexion of the elbow together with repetitive finger movement (as in the left hand of the string instrumentalist) appears to cause more nerve injury than repetitive elbow movement (as in the bowing action of the right hand). Cervical radiculopathy, digital neuropathy, and entrapment of the radial nerve are also described.

G. Congenital neuropathy

Anomalous anatomy may restrict nerve mobility, as in the ulnar nerve entrapment neuropathy, or impinge on nerves such as the brachial plexus in patients with cervical rib syndrome. Aside from mechanical causes, there are many forms of hereditary neuropathy that can be classified into motor, sensory, and autonomic involvement. A patient with hereditary liability to pressure palsies may present with a perioperative neuropathy. Hereditary liability to pressure palsies is an autosomal dominant disorder, affecting mainly those of German or Dutch descent.[83] The condition becomes manifest in the second or third decade. The nerves involved are the usual ones susceptible to compression injury. Neuropathy with delayed recovery develops after apparently minor insult or may develop spontaneously. Other congenital neuropathies may affect the autonomic (e.g., Shy-Drager syndrome or familial dysautonomia), sensory, or motor neurons.

Recurrent attacks of brachial neuritis may be inherited as an autosomal dominant trait known as hereditary recurrent brachial neuropathy. The history consists of familial tendency to brachial neuritis, unexplained vocal cord paralysis, or lumbosacral plexus lesions.

Some inherited neuropathies are associated with underlying genetic metabolic disorders, such as mucopolysaccharidosis, Krabbe's disease (deficiency of galactosylceramide β-galactosidase), and Refsum's disease (syndrome of chronic neuropathy, ichthyosis, deafness, and retinitis pigmentosa).

IV. DIAGNOSIS AND EVALUATION

Peripheral neuropathy is a vast topic with multiple etiologic mechanisms that include congenital predisposition, anatomic variations, underlying disease, occupational or recreational activities that precipitate or exacerbate nerve injuries, and exposure to neurotoxic drugs or chemicals, as discussed in this chapter. The diagnosis of a new onset perioperative neuropathy must be made in the context of the complete differential diagnosis of all peripheral neuropathies. A complete history is an essential first step in diagnosis.

The initial presentation of a patient's nerve injury may be dramatic or subtle. At times it is obvious that a patient has a nonfunctional limb, loss of sensation, or pain. In other situations the neuropathy either develops slowly or goes unrecognized in the midst of other signs and symptoms that prevail on the postoperative scene. Whatever the situation, it behooves physicians and nurses to be as objective as possible in their written descriptions. A record is being formed with each comment, and the medicolegal implications are great. Truth and objectivity are to be greatly desired; there is no room for implication, innuendo, and hasty defensive or offensive judgments. If the site of nerve trauma or disease is obvious, it is quite likely that some of the initial pain symptoms will arise from nerve endings of pain fibers in adjacent tissues. However, there is no known mechanism for an axon to announce its own site of injury. In many instances the site of nerve trauma is unclear, and sometimes it can never be defined precisely despite an array of potentially diagnostic tests. In general, the sites of more peripheral lesions can be identified with greater precision than those of more central lesions because simple tests or neurologic examination provide sufficient evidence. More involved tests must be used to document spinal cord, nerve root, or proximal plexus injury sites, and sometimes the patient (or the physician) may be reluctant to allow further investigation into what is already a frustrating, unexpected, and irritating new event in life. The physician must recognize that many diagnostic approaches can produce morbidity, and a judgment must be made about the ultimate value of precise localization. Before committing the patient to a battery of invasive tests, first question whether the investigations will be helpful to therapy, to future prophylaxis, or in identifying causation.

One might wonder why pain should so often be a component of the symptom complex after isolated peripheral nerve injury. Shouldn't there be a loss of sensation or motor function? In reality, the genesis of pain is a complex matter. Loeser[84] has defined four general mechanisms: sensitization of peripheral terminals, pathophysiology of primary afferent fibers, crosstalk between fibers, and dorsal horn physiologic changes. These concepts are fascinatingly revealing of contemporary neuroscience research, but thus far there is no simple explanation to offer most patients about the cause, management, or future course of their pain.

The initial evaluation of any perioperative neuropathy should entail a careful history and physical examination. Consultation to a neurologist can provide objective documentation. Follow-up examinations are equally important to define the time course and morbidity from the injury. Specific diagnostic tests may also be indicated at various times. If the differential diagnosis should include epidural or central neuraxonal hematoma, a computerized tomographic scan or magnetic resonance imaging examination should be performed immediately. The electromyogram[85] should also be considered early if there is any hint of preexisting nerve damage. However, it must be remembered that degeneration potentials are unlikely until 3 weeks after injury. Therefore, if present, they would signify that the nerve lesion existed before the operation. Nerve conduction studies are sometimes helpful in localizing the precise site of injury along the course of a nerve. Some nerves are more easily mapped than others, so the site of injury can be predicted with greater certainty. Nerve conduction studies are difficult with deep or paravertebral segments of the nerve. There is also some debate about what constitutes "abnormal," though a motor nerve conduction velocity below 40 m/sec would generally be of concern. The amplitude of the compound muscle action potential can be determined from surface electrodes over certain muscles, and this potential can be quantified and compared with an opposite extremity. It may also be quantified as one moves the stimulating electrode farther away from the muscle along the course of the nerve in an inching technique. This is another way in which the precise site of a nerve lesion may be determined. Sensory evoked responses may also give comparative data between the same nerve in opposite extremities or between different nerves in one extremity. The latency and form of these evoked responses can be quantified.

V. PREVENTION AND TREATMENT

Like many diseases, peripheral nerve injuries are better prevented than treated. However, as we understand more about preexisting subclinical neuropathies and mechanisms of injury, this seemingly obvious precept may not be true or practical in application. With regard to surgical positioning, some operations become increasingly complex during their course and may force intraoperative changes in the patient's body position. Previously cushioned areas of the body may then become vulnerable to pressure from the table, armboards, surgical retraction devices, or displaced or crumpled pads. In fact, some pads sold as protective devices (as for the elbow) have little scientific background to support their use, and one might wonder whether they might even contribute to ischemic neuropathy when tightly applied. Perhaps the best prophylaxis against surgical positioning injuries is for the anesthesiologist (and, one would hope, the surgeon and operating room nurses) to periodically imagine themselves to be the patient and ask, "Would I be comfortable in this position?" It is appropriate to periodically reassess pressure points and perhaps rearrange cushions or body position within reasonable and tolerable limits.[86] While the anesthesiologist is doing this to nonsurgical areas, the surgeon must likewise reevaluate the duration and application of pressures applied to the surgical wound. Choosing a postoperative analgesic regimen that minimizes sedation may avoid unnecessary crush injury. In patients receiving postoperative epidural analgesia, a light local anesthetic and opioid infusion are recommended to attain minimal motor block and avoid pressure palsy.[87]

Regional anesthesia is fraught with potential complications, as elucidated earlier in the chapter. However, the low incidence of permanent neurologic deficit reported in the literature attests to the safety of regional anesthesia when performed by anesthesiologists with knowledge of the subject.

It is obvious that the diabetic, uremic, alcoholic, or cachectic surgical patient might require a special degree of awareness. Optimal metabolic control may contribute to restoration of normal nerve function if a clinical neuropathy does occur. However, the prevention of chronic diabetic complications by rigid metabolic control is not always achievable. Overaggressive insulin treatment may precipitate hypoglycemia, further exacerbating neuropathic states. Alternative therapeutic approaches have been considered. Aminoguanidine, aldose reductase inhibitors, vasodilators, radical scavengers, and neurotrophic factors are being tested for prevention of the pathogenesis of diabetic neuropathy.[88] Steroid therapy may facilitate healing if there is associated connective tissue disease such as rheumatoid arthritis, lupus erythematosus, scleroderma, or any of various vasculitides. Carcinomatous neuropathy may respond to chemotherapy, radiation therapy, tumor removal, or decompression in some instances; however, the treatment itself can cause nerve injury. Pyridoxine can reverse isoniazid-induced neuropathy, and beriberi and pellagra (50% incidence of neuropathy) are responsive to dietary thiamine, niacin, tryptophan, or other essential amino acids. Adjustments of dosages of antidysrhythmic and antilipemic drugs can avert neuropathic effects. Methylcobalamin is being investigated for reducing acrylamide toxicity. Analogs of adrenocorticotropic hormone and neurotrophic factors are used to control the neurotoxicity of Taxol and cisplatin.[67] There are many potential sites and mechanisms where nerve damage can occur. Nerve growth factor (NGF) has neurotrophic and neuroprotective effects. Early studies on recombinant NGF show promise in its use for treating peripheral neuropathies, particularly the toxic neuropathies and diabetic neuropathies.[89] Immunotherapy may be effective for neuropathies with autoimmune pathogenesis such as those associated with connective tissue diseases (systemic lupus erythematosus, rheumatoid arthritis) and infections (HIV, Lyme disease, Guillain-Barré, diphtheria).

Frustratingly simplistic is the adage that time is a major contributor to healing. Neither time nor other treatment will cure all neuropathies, and dogmatic statements about appropriate therapy must be viewed with skepticism. Protection from recurrent injury or compression and avoidance of repetitive injurious activity are a first step to treating the problem. Physical therapy can provide passive and active exercises to minimize contracture deformities.[90] Occupational and physical therapists can also encourage and advise the patient about compensatory ways to accomplish basic tasks such as walking, eating, or buttoning a shirt. They can also assess techniques designed to reduce static and dynamic loading while increasing the capacity of the muscular apparatus to withstand the stress of the occupation, sport, or instrument playing. Attention to such details will certainly enhance rapport. Surgical intervention is sometimes indicated in the treatment of perioperative neuropathies. This is obvious in the case of an epidural hematoma and is probably indicated where other postsurgical or anticoagulant-induced hematoma has produced ischemic nerve injury. Cubital tunnel decompression, reconstructive nerve repair, and other surgical interventions appear to be useful for some patients with ulnar neuropathy, but there are few criteria at present to predict which patients will benefit. In Warner, Warner, and Martin's study,[32] 18 patients had transposition decompression of the postoperatively affected ulnar nerve, and only 10 patients showed improvement following transposition. Even if a "cure" results, there is still reason to question cause and effect. Likewise, surgery itself may lead to abnormal scarring, intraneural fibrosis, or impairment of nerve blood supply. Warner, Warner, and Martin[32] also report a disturbing persistence (beyond a year) of motor and sensory deficits in 41% of the patients with postoperative ulnar neuropathy. In 6% of the patients, motor and sensory functions returned but persistent pain remained the chief complaint. There is still much to be learned about mechanisms of injury,[91] appropriate and effective preventive measures, and appropriate and effective therapeutic modalities.

REFERENCES

1. Britt BA, Gordon RA: Peripheral nerve injuries associated with anaesthesia, *Can Anaesth Soc J* 11:514, 1964.
2. Dornette WHL: Compression neuropathies: medical aspects and legal implications, *Int Anesth Clin* 24:201, 1986.
3. Cheney FW, Posner K, Caplan RA, et al: Standard of care and anesthesia liability, *JAMA* 261:1599, 1989.
4. Kroll DA, Caplan RA, Posner K, et al: Nerve injury associated with anesthesia, *Anesthesiology* 73:202, 1990.
5. Budinger K: Über Lähmungen nach Chloroformnarkosen, *Arch Klin Chir* 47:121, 1894.
6. Cope RW: The *Woolley and Roe* case, *Anaesthesia* 9:249, 1954.
7. Kennedy F, Effron AS, Perry G: The grave spinal cord paralysis caused by spinal anesthesia, *Surg Gynecol Obstet* 91:385, 1950.
8. Rigler ML, Drasner K, Krejcie TC, et al: Cauda equina syndrome after continuous spinal anesthesia, *Anesth Analg* 72:275, 1991.
9. Dhunér KG: Nerve injuries following operations: a survey of cases occurring during a six year period, *Anesthesiology* 11:289, 1950.
10. Parks BJ: Postoperative peripheral neuropathies, *Surgery* 74:348, 1973.
11. Dyck PJ, Low PA, Stevens JC: Diseases of peripheral nerves. In Joynt RJ, ed: *Clinical neurology,* Philadelphia, 1988, JB Lippincott.
12. Jaradeh S: Cauda equina syndrome: a neurologist's perspective, *Reg Anesth* 18:473, 1993.
13. Sunderland S: *Nerves and nerve injuries,* ed 2, Edinburgh, 1978, Churchill-Livingstone.
14. Sunderland S, Swaney WE: The intraneural topography of the recurrent laryngeal nerve in man, *Anat Rec* 114:411, 1952.
15. Shapira OM, Kimmel WA, Lindsey PS, et al: Anterior ischemic optic neuropathy after open heart operations, *Ann Thorac Surg* 61:660, 1996.
16. Donner TR, Kline DG: Extracranial spinal accessory nerve injury, *Neurosurgery* 32:907, 1993.
17. Yagnik PM, Chong PS: Spinal accessory nerve injury: a complication of carotid endarterectomy, *Muscle Nerve* 19: 907, 1996.
18. Blackwell KE, Landman MD, Calcaterra TC: Spinal accessory nerve palsy: an unusual complication of rhytidectomy, *Head Neck* 16:181, 1994.
19. Burns S, Herbison GJ: Spinal accessory nerve injury as a complication of internal jugular vein cannulation, *Ann Intern Med* 125:700, 1996.
20. Martin JT: Postoperative isolated dysfunction of the long thoracic nerve: a rare entity of uncertain etiology, *Anesth Analg* 69:614, 1989.
21. Foo CL, Swann M: Isolated paralysis of the serratus anterior: a report of 20 cases, *J Bone Joint Surg* 65B:552, 1983.
22. Leffert RD: *Brachial plexus injuries,* Edinburgh, 1985, Churchill-Livingstone.
23. Jackson L, Keats AS: Mechanism of brachial plexus palsy following anesthesia, *Anesthesiology* 26:190, 1965.
24. LaForce FM: Crush syndrome after ethanol, *N Engl J Med* 284:1104, 1971.
25. Leech P, Cuthbert H: Brachial plexus lesions associated with traumatic asphyxia, *Br J Surg* 59:539, 1972.
26. Fibuch EE, Mertz J, Geller B: Postoperative onset of idiopathic brachial neuritis, *Anesthesiology* 84:455, 1996.
27. Rubin A: Birth injuries: incidence, mechanism and end results, *Obstet Gynecol* 23:218, 1964.
28. Lynch NM, Cofield, Silbert PL, et al: Neurologic complications after total shoulder arthroplasty, *J Shoulder Elbow Surg* 5:53, 1996.
29. Tomlinson D, Hirsch I, Kodali S, et al: Protecting the brachial plexus during median sternotomy, *J Thorac Cardiovasc Surg* 94:291, 1987.
30. Merchant RN, Brown WF, Watson BV: Peripheral nerve injuries in cardiac anesthesia, *Can J Anaesth* 37:S152, 1990
31. Sy WP: Ulnar nerve palsy possibly related to use of automatically cycled blood pressure cuff, *Anesth Analg* 60:687, 1981.
32. Warner MA, Warner ME, Martin, JT: Ulnar neuropathy: incidence, outcome, and risk factors in sedated or anesthetized patients, *Anesthesiology* 81:1332, 1994.
33. Stoelting RK: Postoperative ulnar nerve palsy: is it a preventable complication? *Anesth Analg* 76:7, 1993.
34. Stoelting RK: Brachial plexus injury after median sternotomy: an unexpected liability for anesthesiologists, *J Cardiothorac Vasc Anesth* 8:2, 1994.
35. Caplan RA, Posner KL, Cheney FW: Perioperative ulnar neuropathy: are we ready for shortcuts? *Anesthesiology* 81:1321, 1994.
36. Bickler PE, Schapera A, Bainton CR: Acute radial nerve injury from use of automatic blood pressure monitor, *Anesthesiology* 73:186, 1990.
37. Dawson DM: Entrapment neuropathies of the upper extremities, *N Engl J Med* 329:2013, 1993.
38. Evans BA, Stevens JC, Dyck PJ: Lumbosacral plexus neuropathy, *Neurology* 31:1327, 1981.
39. Warner MA, Martin JT, Schroeder DR, et al: Lower-extremity motor neuropathy associated with surgery performed on patients in a lithotomy position, *Anesthesiology* 81:6, 1994.
40. Idusuyi OB, Morrey BF: Peroneal nerve palsy after total knee arthroplasty: assessment of predisposing and prognostic factors, *J Bone Joint Surg* 78:177, 1996.
41. Pittman GR: Peroneal nerve palsy following sequential pneumatic compression, *JAMA* 261:2201, 1989.
42. Seddon HJ: Three types of nerve injury, *Brain* 66:237, 1943.
43. Sunderland S: A classification of peripheral nerve injuries producing loss of function, *Brain* 68:56, 1951.
44. Trojaborg W: Rate of recovery in motor and sensory fibers of the radial nerve: clinical and physiological aspects, *J Neurol Neurosurg Psychiatry* 33:625, 1970.
45. Fullerton PM, Gilliatt RW: Pressure neuropathy in the hind foot of the guinea pig, *J Neurol Neurosurg Psychiatry* 30:18, 1967.
46. Ochoa J, Marotte L: The nature of the nerve lesion caused by chronic entrapment in the guinea-pig, *J Neurol Sci* 19:491, 1973.
47. Lundborg G, Rydevik B: Effects of stretching the tibial nerve of the rabbit, *J Bone Joint Surg* 55B:390, 1973.
48. Lundborg G: Structure and function of the intraneural microvessels as related to trauma, edema formation and nerve function, *J Bone Joint Surg* 57A:938, 1975.
49. Lundborg G: Limb ischemia and nerve injury, *Arch Surg* 104:631, 1972.
50. Fink BR, Cairns AM: A bioenergetic basis for peripheral nerve fiber dissociation, *Pain* 12:307, 1982.
51. Marquez S, Turley JJ, Peters WJ: Neuropathy in burn patients, *Brain* 116:471, 1993.
52. Vandam LD, Dripps RD: Long-term follow-up of patients who received 10,098 spinal anesthetics. IV. Neurological disease incident to traumatic lumbar puncture during spinal anesthesia, *JAMA* 172:1483, 1960.
53. Auroy Y, Narchi P, Messial A, et al: Serious complications related to regional anesthesia: results of a prospective survey in France, *Anesthesiology* 87:001, 1997.
54. Giaufré E, Dalens B, Gombert A: Epidemiology and morbidity of regional anesthesia in children: a one-year prospective survey of the French-Language Society of Pediatric Anesthesiologists, *Anesth Analg* 83:904, 1996.
55. Horlocker TT, McGregor DG, Matsushige DK, et al: Neurologic complications of 603 consecutive continuous spinal anesthetics using macrocatheter and microcatheter techniques, *Anesth Analg* 84:1063, 1997.

56. De Leon-Casasola OA, Parker B, Lema MJ, et al: Postoperative epidural bupivacaine-morphine therapy: experience with 4,227 surgical cancer patients, *Anesthesiology* 81:368, 1994.
57. Giebler RM, Scherer RU, Peters J: Incidence of neurologic complications related to thoracic epidural catheterization, *Anesthesiology* 86:55, 1997.
58. Pollock JE, Neal JM, Stephenson CA, et al: Prospective study of the incidence of transient radicular irritation in patients undergoing spinal anesthesia, *Anesthesiology* 84:1361, 1996.
59. Sakura S, Sumi A, Sagaguchi Y, et al: The addition of phenylephrine contributes to the development of transient neurologic symptoms after spinal anaesthesia with 0.5% tetracaine, *Anesthesiology* 87:771, 1997.
60. Selander D, Dhuner KG, Lundborg G: Peripheral nerve injury due to injection needles used for regional anesthesia, *Acta Anaesthesiol Scand* 21:182, 1977.
61. Rice ASC, McMahon SB: Peripheral nerve injury caused by injection needles used in regional anesthesia: influence of bevel configuration, studies in a rat model, *Br J Anaesth* 69:433, 1992.
62. Selander D, Brattsand R, Lundborg G, et al: Local anesthetics: importance of mode of application, concentration and adrenaline for the appearance of nerve lesions, *Acta Anaesthesiol Scand* 23:127, 1979.
63. Lui ACP, Munhall RJ, Winnie AP, et al: Baricity and the distribution of lidocaine in a spinal canal model, *Can J Anaesth* 38:522, 1991.
64. Kalichman MW: Physiologic mechanisms by which local anesthetics may cause injury to nerve and spinal cord, *Reg Anesth* 18:448, 1993.
65. Wang BC, Hillman DE, Spielholtz NI, et al: Chronic neurologic deficits and Nesacaine-CE: an effect of anesthetic, 2-chloroprocaine, or the antioxidant, sodium bisulfite? *Anesth Analg* 63:445, 1984.
66. Malinovsky JM, Lepage JY, Cozian A, et al: Is ketamine or its preservative responsible for neurotoxicity in the rabbit? *Anesthesiology* 78:109, 1993.
67. Mizisin AP, Powell HC: Toxic neuropathies, *Curr Opin Neurol* 8:367, 1995.
68. Dyck PJ, Grina LA, Lambert EH, et al: Nitrous oxide neurotoxicity studies in man and rat, *Anesthesiology* 53:205, 1980.
69. Buxton PH, Hayward M: Polyneuritis cranialis associated with industrial trichloroethylene poisoning, *J Neurol Neurosurg Psychiatry* 30:511, 1967.
70. Kuzuhara S, Kanazawa I, Nakanishi T, et al: Ethylene oxide polyneuropathy, *Neurology* 33:377, 1983.
71. Dyck PJ, Gianni C: Pathologic alterations in the diabetic neuropathies of humans: a review, *J Neuropathol Exp Neurol* 55:1181, 1996.
72. Kril JJ: Neuropathology of thiamine deficiency disorders, *Metab Brain Dis* 11:9, 1996.
73. Roman GC: An epidemic in Cuba of optic neuropathy, sensorineural deafness, peripheral sensory neuropathy and dorsolateral myeloneuropathy, *J Neurol Sci* 127:11, 1994.
74. Feit H, Glasberg M, Ireton C, et al: Peripheral neuropathy and starvation after gastric partitioning for morbid obesity, *Ann Intern Med* 96:453, 1982.
75. Price RW: Neurologic complications of HIV infection, *Lancet* 348:445, 1996.
76. Simpson DM, Olney RK: Peripheral neuropathies associated with human immunodeficiency virus infection, *Neurol Clin* 10:685, 1992.
77. Bolton CF: Neuromuscular complications of sepsis, *Intensive Care Med* 19:S58, 1993.
78. Hunt EF, Fogel W, Krieger D, et al: Critical illness neuropathy: clinical findings and outcomes of a frequent cause of neuromuscular weaning failure, *Crit Care Med* 24:1328, 1996.
79. Bolton CF: Sepsis and the systemic inflammatory response syndrome: neuromuscular manifestations, *Crit Care Med* 24:1408, 1996.
80. Lorei MP, Hershman EB: Peripheral nerve injuries in athletes: treatment and prevention, *Sports Med* 16:130, 1993.
81. Stockstill JW, Harn SD, Strickland D, et al: Prevalence of upper extremity neuropathy in clinical dentist population, *J Am Dent Assoc* 124:67, 1993.
82. Lederman RJ: Neuromuscular problems in the performing arts, *Muscle Nerve* 17:569, 1994.
83. Meier C, Mull C: Hereditary neuropathy with liability to pressure palsies, *J Neurol* 228:73, 1982.
84. Loeser JD: Peripheral nerve disorders. In Bonica JJ, ed: *The management of pain*, Philadelphia, 1990, Lea & Febiger.
85. Brailliar F: Electromyography: its use and misuse in peripheral nerve injuries, *Orthop Clin North Am* 12:229, 1981.
86. Martin JT: *Positioning in anesthesia and surgery*, ed 2, Philadelphia, 1987, WB Saunders.
87. Horlocker TT, Cabanela ME, Wedel DJ: Does postoperative epidural analgesia increase the risk of peroneal nerve palsy after total knee arthroplasty? *Anesth Analg* 79:495, 1994.
88. Gries FA: Alternative therapeutic principles in the prevention of microvascular and neuropathic complications, *Diabetes Res Clin Pract* 28:S201, 1995.
89. Riaz SS, Tomlinson DR: Neurotrophic factors in peripheral neuropathies: pharmacological strategies, *Prog Neurobiol* 49:125, 1996.
90. Mubarak SJ, Hargens AR: *Compartment syndromes and Volkmann's contracture*, Philadelphia, 1981, WB Saunders, p 168.
91. Dawson DM, Krarup C: Perioperative nerve lesions, *Arch Neurol* 46:1355, 1989.

Chapter 9

Why Monitoring During Anesthesia Has Unintended and Undesirable Consequences

Nathan Leon Pace

A monitor is more than a box of motors, a video tube, and circuits; it has an associated collection of interfacing cables, cords, couplings, hoses, sensors, and transducers. This monitoring ensemble produces numbers and graphics that describe the physiologic state of a patient and the body's response to the trespasses of surgery and to anesthesia care activities (drugs, fluids, breathing, and so forth). This monitoring ensemble can also abrade, burn, constrict, compress, crush, fibrillate, incise, infarct, obstruct, perforate, and shock human tissues. Such injuries can result not only from a defective machine (electrical shock from an improperly grounded electrocardiograph) but also from one without malfunction (pulse oximeter sensor burn). The injuries can be the consequence of the placement or insertion of a sensor (nosebleed from a nasopharyngeal temperature probe) or coupling tubing (radial artery thrombosis after arterial catheterization). Because many monitor boxes are heavy, injuries can also result from a monitor falling onto a patient. Although these complications are important, this chapter is not intended to explore in detail complications from defective machines, improperly secured monitors, or the associated vascular access procedures, nor is the function or operation of monitors discussed at length.

Other perioperative monitoring complications can be inferred from the lore of operating room anesthesia.

Story 1. A toddler is anesthetized with halothane for lengthy ear surgery. After induction, mechanical ventilation is started with an inhaled halothane concentration of greater than 2%. Monitors include an automatic oscillometric blood pressure cuff and a big-toe pulse oximeter probe. Five minutes later the oximeter fails to display oxygen saturation readings. The resident spends the next 10 minutes repositioning the oximeter probe without success. Controlled ventilation and the inspired halothane concentration continue unchanged. The attending anesthesiologist returns and recognizes the impending cardiovascular collapse; pulse oximetry readings and measurable blood pressure return as halothane concentration is lowered rapidly.

Story 2. In the midst of abdominal aortic resection, the anesthesia resident draws an arterial blood sample from an indwelling arterial catheter but omits resetting the stopcock to reestablish circulation-to-transducer continuity. A few minutes later the sudden discovery of a normal electrocardiograph waveform and an absent pressure pulse prompt the diagnosis of pulseless electrical activity. Increasing doses of vasoactive drugs are administered, and the surgeons notice increasing blood leak through the aortic graft suture line.

Story 3. Several recovery room nurses spend 20 minutes exchanging electrocardiograph cables, leads, and skin patches before recognizing cardiac arrest as the cause of a flat line pattern.

These stories indicate a broader class of medical mishaps or unintended consequences that could just as well be considered a perioperative complication, such as a burn from an electrocardiograph electrode. A brief list of the broad groupings of perioperative complications would thus be quite inclusive (Box 9-1). The wide scope of perioperative complications reinforces the axiom that the risk of monitoring is merited only if control of the monitored variable improves patient care. Cost constraints provide further motivation for a judicious choice of monitors. The purchase of monitors that provide useless information leaves less capital available for useful monitors.

Box 9-1 General categories of monitoring complications

Monitors and their interfacing devices can damage human tissues.

Time and attention spent collecting and contemplating variables only tenuously or ambiguously related to patient physiology and pathophysiology detract from attention to useful physiologic variables.

Anesthesiologists are already confronted with an overload of data. Additional monitors may decrease vigilance.

Complex or tedious monitor operations and apparent or real monitor malfunctions can distract attention from patient status.

The drugs and procedures of anesthesia each have a set of risks; one must consider the harmful consequences of therapies chosen to control and manipulate variables that are either erroneous or uninterpretable.

I. INVESTIGATION OF MONITORS AND UNDESIRABLE PERIOPERATIVE CONSEQUENCES

Since the addition of the first devices to aid the anesthesiologist's primary senses, there have been arguments about the merits of monitoring. This debate continues today and usually focuses on the improvement in patient care to be expected.[1,2] However, as forcefully argued by Keats, increased use of monitoring is not synonymous with better patient care and may actually impair care.[3]

Technology assessment is the attempt to establish formal, structured means of resolving the uncertainty about the technology, new and old, of medicine.[4-7] The argument about the role of anesthesia monitoring is thus part of a larger effort encompassing all medicine.[8] In turn, the question, "What are the complications of monitoring?" is part of the debate about the merits of monitoring, and it warrants continued technology assessment.[9] The methods of technology assessment should be applied to all aspects of anesthesia monitoring, from the most complex device to the simplest esophageal stethoscope.[10]

The goal of this chapter is to examine the types of evidence used to judge monitor performance and then review the evidence concerning commonly used monitors and their complications. The management of complications of monitoring is not discussed. Similar approaches for judging the diagnostic ability of imaging technology[11] and for weighing evidence about the effectiveness of critical care monitoring devices[12] have been published. There is already considerable evidence published in medical and engineering journals to answer some of these questions. These reports can be grouped into three broad categories of evidence.

A. Data reliability

Monitors are used to measure physiologic variables. A patient is the signal generator. The signals are of two types: electrical potentials and everything else. Electrical potentials include the electrocardiogram, electroencephalogram, and electromyogram readings and evoked potentials. The others include pressures, gas tensions, flows, saturations, and displacements. Monitor function proceeds from data (signal) acquisition to data processing and finally to data presentation and display.[13] The electrical potentials can be acquired directly by electrodes; the other signals require transducers to generate an electrical potential. Transducers are generally well engineered and are very rugged and robust; the same can be said for the electronics of the monitor box. However, the signal can always be corrupted with noise caused by the improper attachment of the sensor (electrode or transducer) to the patient. Microprocessor-based monitors have provided extensive data processing and improved the data display dramatically. However, this same technology can yield displays and numbers whose origin in the raw variable is not clear. For example, the preparation of data for presentation often includes an averaging of the signal over real time; many algorithms are available for this averaging.[14] These different algorithms applied to the same signal do not produce the same displayed values. With the ever greater degree of variable processing, it is important to confirm the reasonableness of the raw data transformations.

Some monitors are developed with the expectation that their readings will be interchangeable with data provided by an existing monitor; the hope of the monitor developer is to provide a monitor that is less expensive or has more timely results or has less risk. To prove the interchangeability of the new and old monitor data, simultaneous measurements from old and new are obtained in patients. Until recently researchers have mistakenly analyzed these numbers by calibration statistical techniques (linear regression and correlation). Statisticians have now convinced researchers that comparison statistical techniques (mean difference and variability) should be used.[15-18]

Understanding the variation between measurements focuses in succession on several key points. First, we need to know the repeatability of a measurement over a short period of time in the same subject. With most of the variables obtained by our monitors, successive measurements cannot be obtained with a sufficiently short interval to eliminate physiologic variation. Only the combined physiologic variation and measurement error can be estimated. Bland and Altman[15] recommend calculating a coefficient of repeatability that is the 95% range for the difference in two repeated measurements. A change from one occasion to another in a subject should be greater than this coefficient of repeatability to be attributed to a real alteration in patient state (Box 9-2). Experienced anesthesiologists have long avoided an overinterpretation of changes of such magnitude in hemodynamic variables.

Next, comparison between devices is specified by a measure of bias and a measure of scatter or variability (Box 9-3). The mean difference, also known as bias, between new and old values shows whether the new method overestimates or underestimates values obtained by the old method. Besides desiring a small or zero bias, the values of the two devices must bunch close together so that the values of new and old are interchangeable.[15]

Box 9-2 Distinguishing variability between sequential measurements

1. Suppose that systolic blood pressure is measured every 5 minutes for 1 hour during a period of stable anesthesia and surgery in a homogenous group of anesthetized patients.
2. Calculate the standard deviation (SD) of these systolic blood pressures for each patient. Using these individual SDs, calculate the pooled within-subject standard deviation (SD_{pooled}) for the group of patients.
3. Calculate the 95% range for the difference in two repeated measurements by the formula $2 \times \sqrt{2} \times SD_{pooled}$. Then the difference between two successive measurements of blood pressure in a similar patient must be greater than $2 \times \sqrt{2} \times SD_{pooled}$ to be considered a change in systolic blood pressure beyond the variability imposed by physiologic variation and measurement error.
4. For example, if SD_{pooled} = 5 mm Hg, then $2 \times \sqrt{2} \times SD_{pooled} \approx 14$ mm Hg. Under these conditions of variability, if systolic pressure is now 120 mm Hg and when repeated is 130 mm Hg, one cannot be certain that a change in systolic blood pressure has occurred.

Box 9-3 Determining interchangeability of measurements by different devices

1. Suppose that systolic blood pressure is measured simultaneously by two different devices every 5 minutes for 1 hour during a period of stable anesthesia and surgery in a homogenous group of anesthetized patients. Device 1 is a new blood pressure monitor being compared with device 2, the standard blood pressure monitor.
2. Create two new variables from each pair of blood pressure measurements. The difference in pressure is blood pressure$_{device1}$ − blood pressure$_{device2}$, denoted as pressure$_{difference}$. The average pressure is (blood pressure$_{device1}$ + blood pressure$_{device2}$)/2, denoted as pressure$_{average}$.
3. Calculate the mean ($\bar{x}_{pooled}$), pooled standard deviation (SD_{pooled}), and pooled standard error (SE_{pooled}) of pressure$_{difference}$ for all measurements.
4. The bias (mean difference between devices) is assessed by $\bar{x}_{pooled}$. The expectation should be that there is no bias ($\bar{x}_{pooled}$ = 0) between the two devices. The statistical test of bias uses the SE_{pooled}. Suppose that $\bar{x}_{pooled}$ = 5 mm Hg and that this is statistically different from zero. Then device 1 systematically overestimates device 2 by 5 mm Hg.
5. The variability of the measurements of the two devices is assessed by calculating the 95% range for the limits of agreement by the formula $\bar{x}_{pooled} \pm 2 \times SD_{pooled}$. If the difference between a pair of measurements by device 1 and device 2 lies within this range, then the values for device 1 and device 2 are considered indistinguishable. Within this range lie 95% of the differences between device 1 and device 2.
6. For example, if $\bar{x}_{pooled}$ = 2 mm Hg and SD_{pooled} = 7.5 mm Hg, then the 95% range for the limits of agreement = $2 \pm 2 \times 7.5$ mm Hg = −13 mm Hg to +17 mm Hg. Under these conditions, a systolic blood pressure of 155 mm Hg by device 1 and a systolic blood pressure of 140 mm Hg by device 2 (difference = 15 mm Hg) must be considered indistinguishable.
7. If differences in values of device 1 versus device 2 within this 95% range for the limits of agreement have no clinical importance or biologic relevance, then the values from device 1 and device 2 are interchangeable. Thus if considered clinical judgment holds that a systolic blood pressure variation of −13 mm Hg to +17 mm Hg from actual pressure is unimportant, then device 1 and device 2 can function interchangeably. Otherwise, device 1 is not interchangeable with device 2.

There is a surprisingly large degree of variability in most studies comparing two anesthesia monitors.

Graphically, bias and variability can be revealed by a scatter plot. Instead of plotting new values against old values in a regression plot, two new variables are created (see Box 9-3). For each pair of new and old values, a new number pair (the difference and the average) is calculated. This difference-average pair is plotted as well as horizontal control lines denoting bias and variability (Fig. 9-1). This is known as the Bland-Altman plot, after the two English statisticians who popularized its use. The Bland-Altman plot should also be inspected for any variation in the bias along the range of values.

B. Data interpretability

The typical medical test is a laboratory assay or procedure result that classifies patients into categories (e.g., having a myocardial infarction vs. not having a myocardial infarction by changes in enzyme concentration or ST segment depression). In the last two decades statisticians and experts in medical decision making have expanded the understanding of diagnostic tests.[19] Useful guidelines for interpreting reports about diagnostic tests have appeared.[20,21] This is one element of the development of evidence-based medicine. Each of our operating room monitors is also a diagnostic system in that each allows diagnoses such as inadequate anesthesia, hypovolemia,

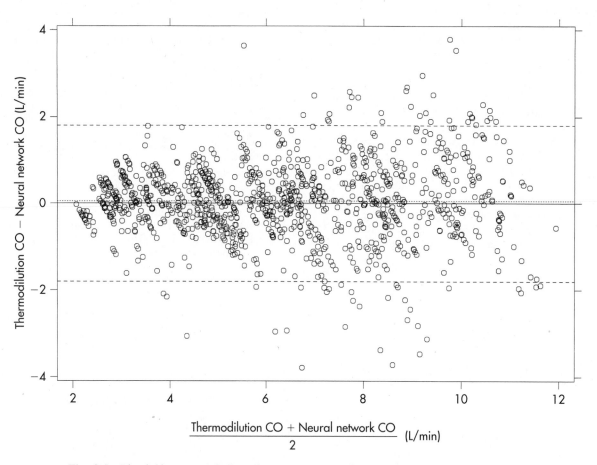

Fig. 9-1. Bland-Altman comparison plot, a comparison (bias and scatter) of two cardiac output measurement methods: thermodilution and a new neural network method. To compare the two methods, one makes a scatter plot of the difference versus average value for the 1127 pairs of values. The mean of the differences is the bias or offset between the two methods; for this plot the mean difference is 0.05 L/min, represented by the *horizontal dotted line*. The *horizontal solid line* at 0 represents perfect identity between values obtained by the two methods. This bias (0.05 L/min) does not reach statistical significance. The *horizontal dashed lines* are the lower and upper bounds of the 95% limits of agreement (−1.75 L/min to +1.85 L/min). For data within this range, values of the two monitors are indistinguishable. The width of the limits of agreement determines the interchangeability of the measurement methods. Most anesthesiologists would find a variation in cardiac output of 3.6 L/min clinically important. Because the range of the 95% limits of agreement is 3.6 L/min, the two methods cannot be considered interchangeable. Also, as average cardiac output increases, the scatter of points outside the 95% limits of agreement increases; the variability of the two measurements increases with higher cardiac output.

ischemia, and hypoxia. Instead of being used once or twice per operating room visit, our diagnostic systems are used repeatedly or continuously during anesthesia.

Monitoring is thus more than just measuring[13]; monitoring implies the analysis and interpretation of data. A monitor uncovers undesirable conditions that call for corrective action. This interpretation can proceed only with a firm grasp of physiology. One way to interpret the variable is by comparing its value with an expected range of acceptable values. How to derive at this acceptable range is not a trivial matter. For example, an increase in heart rate of 10 beats/min or more might be thought sufficient to necessitate more anesthesia, whereas a much larger increase (more than 30 beats/min) or a heart rate greater than 130 beats/min could also be interpreted as indicating hypovolemia, necessitating fluid and blood infusion.

Diagnostic systems are usually not perfect and sometimes confuse noise with the particular signal that reveals disease or organ dysfunction.[22] The performance of a monitor is established by its application to a group of test patients in whom the specified event might occur; a standard method is used to confirm or refute the diagnosis of the event in question. The selection of patients and the application of the standard method (sometimes denoted the gold standard) are critical for this performance test.[23] This set of performance data (observed frequencies of each cell) is tabulated in a two-way contingency table (Table 9-1). Several diagnostic measures can be derived from this two-way table (Table 9-2). These diagnostic measures can be derived from signal detection theory or Bayesian considerations. The measures of test efficacy most often cited are the sensitivity and specificity. The proportion of diseased patients who are correctly classified is called the sensitivity, or true positive ratio, and the proportion of nondiseased patients correctly classified is the specificity, or true negative ratio. The ideal diagnostic test would have a sensitivity and specificity of 1.0. It was believed that these two measures were independent of the prevalence of the disease being identified. Clinician researchers thought that Bayes's theorem required such constancy, whereas statisticians thought such constancy had been empirically demonstrated[19]; neither is true. For example, Hlatky et al[24] empirically demonstrated that the sensitivity and specificity of exercise electrocardiography for detecting coronary disease vary with clinical history, extent of disease, and other variables. This reaffirms that the type of patients being tested (also known as case mix or spectrum bias) must be explicitly defined in the study and use of diagnostic tests.[23]

Two other measures, the positive and negative predictive values (see Table 9-2), are used to calculate the accuracy of the test in a particular patient group. The pos-

Table 9-1. Two-way truth table

		Disease (reality)		
		Positive = disease = $D+$	Negative = no disease = $D-$	ROW TOTALS
Test results	Yes = positive test = $R+$	TP	FP	TP + FP
	No = negative test = $R-$	FN	TN	FN + TN
	COLUMN TOTALS	TP + FN	FP + TN	TP + FP + FN + TN = N

TP, True positive; FP, false positive; FN, false negative, TN, true negative.

Table 9-2. Derivation of diagnostic measures

Diagnostic measure	Alternative name	Probability notation	Formula
True positive ratio	Sensitivity	$P(R+|D+)$	$= TP/(TP + FN)$
True negative ratio	Specificity	$P(R-|D-)$	$= TN/(FP + TN)$
Positive predictive value		$P(D+|R+)$	$= TP/(TP + FP)$
Negative predictive value		$P(D-|R+)$	$= TN/(FN + TN)$
Positive test likelihood ratio	Risk ratio	$P(R+|D+)/P(R+|D-)$	$= SE/(1 - SP)$
Negative test likelihood ratio	Risk ratio	$P(R-|D+)/P(R-|D-)$	$= (1 - SE)/SP$

$P(X+|Y+)$ is the notation for conditional probability (i.e, the probability that X is true given that Y is true).
SE, Sensitivity; SP, specificity.

itive predictive value is the proportion of patients who test positive who actually have the disease. The predictive values depend explicitly on the prevalence of disease and the performance measures of the test. Two new diagnostic measures are now in use: test likelihood ratios (LRs). A patient has a pretest and posttest probability of the target disorder. The pretest probability can be assessed from a clinical impression. Test LRs are not probabilities. Rather, they indicate how much a given test result will raise or lower the pretest probability.[25] An LR of 1 means that pretest and posttest probabilities are identical. Calculating the posttest probability for a range of pretest probabilities is very instructive about the real meaning of a diagnostic test (Box 9-4).

It is an obvious oversimplification to consider a diagnostic system (including anesthesia monitors) as providing only a binary yes-or-no answer. The amount (in millimeters) of ST-segment depression necessary to assert the existence of myocardial ischemia is an obvious example. The measures of the diagnostic test (sensitivity and specificity) obviously change depending on the diagnostic cut point. A test measure that accommodates alternative diagnostic cut points is the relative operating characteristics (ROC) curve[22]; it is also known as a receiver operating characteristics curve because of its initial use in signal detection analysis. This is a plot of the true positive ratio (sensitivity) versus the false positive ratio (1 − specificity) for all possible diagnostic cut points (Fig. 9-2). The area under the curve is the measure of performance. If the curve follows the line of identity (diagonal line), the area is 0.5; such a test has no discriminating ability. An area of 1.0 indicates perfect discrimination; the curve follows the left and upper axes. ROC curves are appearing regularly in reports of the diagnostic properties of monitoring devices.

C. Data efficacy and effectiveness

The consequences of using an anesthesia monitor are the ultimate test of that monitor.[26] How does the monitor influence treatment? Can the monitored variables be manipulated by therapeutic changes? Does the change in treatment alter patient morbidity and mortality? How often does it harm the patient? The paradigm of the scientific process is collecting observations during events under experimental control. Statisticians recommend that the importance of evidence be ranked or weighted by the experimental design used in collecting observations (Box 9-5). As in proving the efficacy of a new drug, the multiple-center, randomized controlled trial (RCT) of patient outcome is the standard for proving the efficacy of a monitor. In the RCT, two or more cohorts of patients randomly assigned to care by different monitoring methods are observed. Very few RCTs of perioperative monitoring have been performed. A distinction must be made between efficacy and effectiveness. Efficacy is the monitor at its best under ideal circumstances; effectiveness is the monitor used under ordinary clinical circumstances. Even if efficacy is demonstrated, effectiveness is not ensured. Some monitors are too unstable to be used as anything other than a research device.

Box 9-4 Use of test likelihood ratios

1. Suppose that a new test for recovery from muscle relaxants classifies patients as having low, medium, or high strength. A clinical trial of extubation has the following results:

Test result	Extubation trial		
Strength	Succeed	Fail	Likelihood ratio
High	30	3	7.84
Medium	6	6	0.78
Low	1	20	0.04
Totals	37	29	

Using the conditional probability notation from Table 9-2, it is easy to extend the calculation of positive test likelihood ratio (LR) to a test that classifies patients into more than two groups. For example, for the test result High: LR $= P(R+ |D+)/P(R+ |D-) = (30/37)/(3/29) = 0.8108/0.1034 = 7.84$.

2. One can show the effect of the LR on posttest probability for different possible pretest probabilities. A critical assumption is that the test properties shown are relevant for patients with various pretest probabilities.

Pretest probability of successful extubation (%)	Test result	LR	Posttest probability of successful extubation (%)
70	High	7.84	95
70	Medium	0.78	65
70	Low	0.04	9
20	High	7.84	66
20	Medium	0.78	16
20	Low	0.04	1

Pretest probability is first converted to odds: probability/(100 − probability). The odds are multiplied by LR. The product is then converted back to a probability: 100 × product/(product + 1). Thus for a pretest probability of 70%, the odds are 70/(100 − 70) = 2.33. The product of odds and LR is 2.33 × 7.84 = 18.29. The posttest probability is 100 × 18.19/19.29 = 95%.

3. Clearly the posttest probability of successful extubation can go up considerably (20% to 66%), remain nearly unchanged (70% to 65%), or drop dramatically (70% to 9%). The test result cannot be considered in isolation from the pretest probability.

One of the choices when one is designing an RCT of anesthesia monitors is whether the experimenter should prescribe how the data are to be used. One can depend on the clinical wisdom of the attending physician, derived from accepted principles of physiology, pharmacology, and practice experience, to interpret and use the monitor data appropriately; this allows clinical decisions based not just on the monitored variables of experimen-

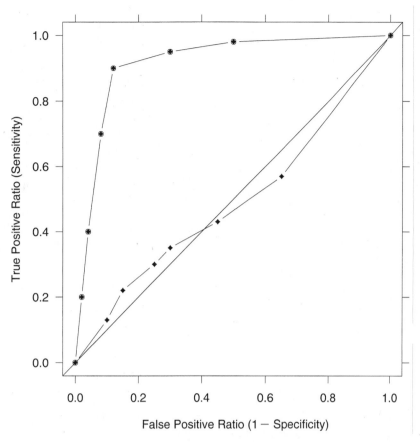

Fig. 9-2. A relative operating characteristics (ROC) curve is a plot of the true positive ratio (sensitivity) and the false positive ratio (1 − specificity) for all possible cut points of a diagnostic test. The area under the ROC curve is the measure of performance. If the curve follows the line of identity *(diagonal line)*, the area is 0.5; such a test has no discriminating ability. An area of 1.0 indicates perfect discrimination; such a curve follows the left and upper axes. The top curve reflects a very good test; its area is greater than 0.9. The curve that wanders above and below the line of identity reflects a test or monitor with no diagnostic power.

Box 9-5 Weighting the value of types of evidence

MOST VALUABLE
1. Multiple-center randomized controlled trial
2. Single-center randomized controlled trial
3. Nonrandomized trial with concurrent controls
4. Nonrandomized trial with historical controls
5. Case series
6. Case report
LEAST VALUABLE

---

tal interest, but also on patient history, physical examination, and laboratory tests. Such decision making may also be amorphous, without focus, difficult to explicitly formulate, and difficult to replicate consistently. Alternatively, the care of patients could be constrained by predetermined algorithms for interpretation of the monitor data and changes in therapy; because of the complexities

of physiology and pathophysiology, the prescription of how to interpret and respond to a monitored variable almost always is rather general, regardless of the intention to control patient care rigidly. This method is precise but ignores alternative multivariate reasoning and inarticulate decisions. Both choices present difficulties in planning, accomplishing, and interpreting the study. And in all RCTs, human error can add so much additional variability that making any conclusions is impossible.[27]

The premier role of the RCT has tended to obscure the importance of the observational study; this is the nonrandomized trial with concurrent controls (level 3 evidence in Box 9-5).[28] Epidemiologists also call this the natural experiment: two or more cohorts being observed, but the assignment to monitoring method not being under experimental control. Although such evidence is never definitive in the same way as RCT evidence is, sometimes it is the only or the initial evidence. Anesthesiologists have been important participants in notable natural experiments. Following the London cholera epidemic of 1854, the great anesthesiologist and epidemiologist John Snow estimated the relative mortality from drinking impure water[29]: "The proportion of fatal attacks to each 10,000 houses was as follows: Southwark and Vauxhall 71, Lambeth 5. The cholera was therefore fourteen times as fatal at this period, amongst persons having the impure water of the Southwark and Vauxhall Company, as amongst those having the purer water from Thames Ditton." This difference in mortality helped elucidate the mode of spread of cholera. The National Halothane Study was a very large natural experiment of hepatitis following anesthesia.[30]

Because RCTs of outcome are so difficult to accomplish, other alternatives have been sought. Surrogate end points can be the focus of the RCT.[31] An example might be chronically elevated blood pressure as a surrogate for stroke. A surrogate end point correlates with the end point of interest (death, stroke, and so forth) but can be measured with less expense or at an earlier time. Most clinical studies of monitors report variables such as blood pressure and heart rate with the apparent hope that the reported values will function as surrogate end points. Unfortunately, there is little validation in anesthesia for surrogate end points. Meta-analyses of existing, usually smaller reports are being attempted as replacements for large-scale RCTs.[32] Another alternative is to examine existing databases collected for other purposes, such as hospital mortalities or insurance claims. For anesthesia, this is being attempted through the review of closed malpractice claims of U.S. insurance carriers.[33]

An almost universal problem in discussing the complications of monitors is the inability to calculate an incident rate. Some organizations, such as the Emergency Care Research Institute (ECRI) (Plymouth Meeting, Pennsylvania), maintain databases of complications reported in journals, to the Food and Drug Administration, and to equipment manufacturers; the ECRI also presents its own interpretations and recommendations. The Food and Drug Administration, through its MedWatch program, provides electronic and printed reports of safety issues with medical devices. Observational studies are published for selected series of patients at self-reporting institutions. The generalizability of these reports, usually from academic medical centers, is difficult to assess. Some complications are obviously difficult to define. There is no database that maintains a comprehensive record of such complications. Medical journals publish only the first few case reports of each type of complication associated with a monitor. It is just as hard to determine patient exposure. There is no inventory of what monitors are used in all the operating rooms of the country. One must depend on cross-sectional sample surveys to determine how widespread monitor use is. Neither the number of incidents of complications nor the tally of patient exposures to the monitor is generally available.

The importance of demonstrating an improvement in outcome is being reaffirmed by examples of failed monitors. Intrapartum fetal heart rate monitoring became common in the United States during the past 25 years. It was anticipated that an early warning of the presence of fetal hypoxia by changes in the fetal heart rate pattern would allow immediate intervention to save the fetus.

Neither fetal wastage nor neonatal salvage has been improved by this monitor, which prompted a dramatic increase in the incidence of cesarean delivery.[34] Anesthesia researchers must overcome the inertia and difficulties that have prevented many definitive outcome studies of anesthesia monitors. If RCTs are not possible, then appropriate observational studies should be performed to guide clinical policy development.

II. COMMONLY USED MONITORS

In a chapter that can offer only some highlights of the evidence concerning anesthesia monitors, not all monitors can be discussed. The main emphasis is on commercially available, commonly used devices. Electrocardiography and anesthesia machines with their failure detection devices are discussed elsewhere. The narrative proceeds variable by variable rather than monitor by monitor. With the continuing explosion of biomedical literature, this presentation can highlight only some of the evidence and makes no pretense of including all citations.

A. Vascular pressure

In addition to providing anesthesia, our ultimate concern is maintaining homeostasis by ensuring the transport of oxygen and substrate to tissues. Blood pressure is measured in the hope that it is an indicator of this flow. Actually two types of pressure are monitored: those that distend and fill the heart and those generated by the heart to cause flow. The true driving force for flow is the difference in fluid energy between the aorta (left heart) and the right atrium and between the pulmonary artery and the left atrium (right heart). Fluid energy is the summation of pressure energy, gravitational potential energy, and kinetic energy:

$$E = P + \rho gh + \rho v^2/2$$

where:

P = pressure energy
ρ = fluid density
g = acceleration caused by gravity
h = height above reference point
v = fluid velocity

In systemic arteries, kinetic energy ($\rho v^2/2$) is a negligible fraction of total fluid energy; in the atria and pulmonary artery, kinetic energy can be a large fraction of total fluid energy. The importance of kinetic energy is illustrated by Bernoulli's principle, in which fluid flows against a pressure gradient but not against the total energy gradient.

The first recorded vascular pressures were obtained invasively by a fluid-filled manometer. Today fluid-filled catheters are used to measure both driving and filling pressures but are attached to transducers. Pressure waveforms are essentially low-frequency sound, with most energy in the frequency range below 10 to 20 cycles per second (Hz). To transduce or "hear" and display this pressure waveform faithfully, the intravascular catheter, connecting tubing, stopcocks, transducer, and monitor amplifier must have certain characteristics that describe the dynamic response. The fluid-filled catheter-transducer system is idealized by a model of a mass hooked to a spring. Derived from this model are differential equations with parameters, the natural frequency, f_n, and the damping coefficient zeta, ζ, describing model behavior. Measurements of the real physical system can be made to calculate these parameters; such parameter estimators have been used very successfully in understanding catheter-transducer system performance.[35,36]

If any of the frequencies of fluid vibrations in the catheter-transducer system is close to f_n, the amplitude of the vibrations increases and the peaks and valleys (systolic and diastolic) of the pressure pulse are exaggerated. As long as the natural frequency is above 20 Hz there is little distortion. The fluid vibrations die away with time, like a bouncing ball rebounding less with each bounce. Damping describes the bouncing of the ball. For the catheter-transducer system, ζ describes how long the vibrations reverberate. Excessively high or low damping will distort the pulse pressure. The continuous-flush device may be used to determine whether adequate fidelity exists in the catheter-transducer system. In the flush test the 300 mm Hg pressure at which the flush fluid is maintained is directed against the transducer membrane as almost a square-wave pulse by momentary activation of the rapid-flush mechanism. An adequate pressure waveform is present if the termination of the square wave results in one undershoot on the pressure trace followed by a small overshoot; care must be taken to purge all air from the catheter transducer assemblage before performing the flush test.[37]

1. Invasive driving pressures. The arterial pressure pulse is very complex, composed of both a pressure wave that is propagated from the heart at a velocity of 5 to 10 m/sec and a flow element that travels more slowly at a velocity of 0.3 to 0.5 m/sec in the aorta.[38,39] It is generated by the contraction of the ventricle and sustained by the viscoelastic properties of the arteries. The pressure pulse is greatly changed as it travels distally, being both amplified and modified; the flow velocity drops dramatically.

Systemic arterial pressure is obtained from catheters placed in an artery, usually in an extremity and most often in the radial artery. Arterial catheters are end-hole tubes, always placed with the catheter tip facing upstream. The measured pressure is thus a summation of pressure and kinetic energy. However, even if flow is tripled or more, kinetic energy is still a very small percentage of pressure energy. Catheters advanced through the right side of the heart into the pulmonary artery are also end-hole catheters, but the tip faces downstream. The measured pressure is the pressure energy minus some fraction of the kinetic energy. Within the pulmonary artery the total driving energy has a large kinetic component; when cardiac output increases threefold, kinetic pressure becomes one half of total systolic energy. Pulmonary artery pressure (PAP) so measured is not necessarily an adequate estimator of driving energy.

a. Reliability. Reliability of invasive pressures depends largely on the fidelity of the catheter-transducer-monitor system. With the nearly universal availability of inexpensive, single-use transducers, one can rely on the transducer being within 1% of the transducer sensitivity, which has been fixed at 5.0 μV/V/mm Hg; calibration tests of transducers are no longer necessary.[40] The blood pressure

monitor itself adds a small additional error and variability to measurement but is usually of little consequence.[40] Before one interprets the pressure, the transducer must also be referenced to zero. By convention, pressures are referenced to atmosphere at the right atrial level.

The more complicated the plumbing connecting catheter and transducer, the more likely it is that the dynamic system response will be degraded. Long, narrow connecting tubing and the pulmonary arterial catheter itself decrease f_n and increase ζ. On the other hand, if tubing is short and stiff and there are no air bubbles, f_n will increase and ζ will decrease. Improper damping and a low natural frequency do not impair measurement of mean pressure, only of systolic and diastolic pressure.

b. Interpretability. Although there are published normal ranges of systemic and pulmonary arterial pressures, the use and interpretation of pressure and pressure changes depends on the patient, the surgery, and the clinical circumstances. Other uses of invasive blood pressure have been attempted. The arterial and pulmonary arterial pressure pulse has been integrated to derive cardiac output. This has always proved less reliable than standard methods of cardiac output determination. The systemic arterial waveform has been analyzed to obtain systemic vascular resistance; ratios of systolic and diastolic pressure have been integrated over time to predict endocardial ischemia. It seems pointless to attempt such derivations from radial arterial pressure waveforms because there is too much variability and distortion of the pressure pulse as it travels from the aortic arch to the periphery. As one example, the dicrotic notch seen in the pressure waveform in a peripheral artery is probably not related to aortic closure.[41] In fact, even the mean pressure in the radial arterial may be unreliable after cardiopulmonary bypass; there can be a discrepancy of 10 to 30 mm Hg between central and peripheral mean pressure for 30 or more minutes.[42] Anesthesiologists have long noted that if blood or fluid loss is not replaced, the systemic arterial pressure is more variable during controlled ventilation. During mechanical inspiration, systolic arterial pressure increases (denoted Δup); during exhalation, systolic arterial pressure decreases (Δdown). With hypovolemia Δdown widens, as confirmed in animal and human experiments. Whether this variability is a useful measure of volume status during clinical care is not known.[43]

c. Usefulness. Despite the widespread use of radial arterial catheterization, nearly universal for all critically ill patients and for all patients having cardiac, vascular, and neurologic surgery, no formal study of the usefulness of invasive systemic pressures is available. The same is true for PAPs. Radial artery catheters have become such an integral part of anesthesia care that it is difficult to conceive of circumstances that would motivate the initiation of a formal RCT. Radial artery catheters are also inserted to allow frequent, repetitive sampling of arterial blood. The consequences of this phlebotomy and proof of the usefulness of such sampling are beyond the scope of this review.

What is available are summarized patient experiences compared with historical controls. Rao, Jacobs, and El-Etr[44] compared the myocardial reinfarction rate in pa-

---

Box 9-6 Side effects and complications of arterial and pulmonary arterial catheterization

Arrhythmias
Embolism (air, catheter fragment, thrombus)
Hemorrhage (disconnection, ventricular or great vessel rupture)
Infection (skin site, bacteremia, sepsis)
Pain
Pneumothorax
Tissue damage (endocarditis, local hematoma, nerve injury, pulmonary infarction, vessel thrombosis)

Box 9-7 Artifacts in pulmonary arterial occlusion pressure measurements

Incomplete wedging
Inconsistent maintenance of zero reference level
Overwedging (herniation of balloon to cover catheter tip)
Patient position
Rapidly varying intrathoracic respiratory pressure changes
Slow response and update times of monitor digital displays

---

tients anesthetized between 1977 to 1982 with that of similar patients treated from 1973 to 1976. The reinfarction rate for those anesthetized within the first 3 months after the primary infarction fell from 36% to about 6%. In the earlier period only a small minority of patients had radial arterial catheterization and almost none had pulmonary arterial catheterization; in the later period these monitors were used almost universally. But there were other differences as well. The increase in the use of β-adrenergic receptor blocking drugs and the decrease in the use of vasopressors were just as dramatic. Which (if any) of these differences was responsible for the change in outcome is unknowable from this report. Studies of pulmonary artery catheter filling pressures are discussed later in this chapter.

d. Complications. Arterial and pulmonary arterial catheterization produces nontrivial complications (Box 9-6). A variety of reports provide reasonable estimation of rates for this form of monitoring. Overall, serious complications occur at low rates for both types of catheterization.[45,46] Because it is easy to obtain artifactual pressure readings, the potential for making adverse therapeutic choices is great. These choices include all activities used to influence hemodynamics: fluid infusion, blood transfusion, diuresis, vasoconstrictor or vasodilator infusion, sympathomimetic and sympatholytic administration, ventilatory changes, and administration of anesthetic drugs. Mistakes in therapeutic choices involving erroneously measured pressures or misinterpreted pressures are a common part of the anesthesia experience.

2. Filling pressures. Filling pressures are of two kinds: those reflecting right ventricular end-diastolic pressure (RVEDP) and those reflecting left ventricular end-diastolic pressure (LVEDP).[47,48] These two pressures are not ordinarily obtained by intravascular catheters terminating in either ventricle. Rather, RVEDP and LVEDP are estimated from pressures measured elsewhere. Central venous catheters (tip advanced to the region of the right atrium) often have been placed in operative patients in the last three decades; central venous pressure (CVP) is measured and used to estimate RVEDP. However, most central venous catheters are placed not for pressure measurements but for other purposes, such as fluid administration (parenteral alimentation, cancer chemotherapy, vasoactive drugs, and so on) and blood access (hemodialysis, phlebotomy).

Before 1970, LVEDP could be estimated only by retrograde catheterization of the aorta or by direct placement during open chest surgery of a catheter into the left atrium to measure left atrial pressure (LAP). Since that time a practical balloon-flotation pulmonary arterial catheter has been used to obtain estimates of LVEDP. When a pulmonary arterial catheter is advanced into the pulmonary artery, eventually the tip wedges and occludes a small arterial branch, stopping blood flow. The motionless blood beyond the catheter tip becomes an extension of the fluid column within the catheter lumen. This stationary column of blood terminates at the confluence of small pulmonary veins coming from adjacent lung segments. If the patency of the fluid column is ensured, the catheter tip pressure will be in equilibrium with the downstream pressure. The advantage of the balloon catheter is the possibility of inflating the balloon and allowing blood flow temporarily to advance the catheter tip occluding an artery; catheter manipulation (advancement and withdrawal) is avoided. This measurement is called pulmonary artery occlusion pressure (PAOP) and is an estimate of LAP and LVEDP.

a. Reliability. The initial motivation for measuring CVP was the hope that it would allow estimation of RVEDP and that RVEDP and LVEDP would change in parallel; thus a variable of the right side of the heart was expected to describe events in the left side of the heart. Numerous studies have confirmed that although RVEDP and LVEDP might be similar in health, there is often little agreement during critical illness or surgery. This poor correlation led to the rapid growth in the use of balloon-flotation catheters. The actual measurement of PAOP requires considerable attention because many artifacts are possible (Box 9-7). Most of these can be minimized by strict attention to details of measurement.[49,50] Particularly important is the elimination of respiratory artifact, which can usually be eliminated easily during anesthesia by a momentary interruption of ventilation. Strictly speaking, three criteria should be met to ensure that a true PAOP has been obtained: the phasic pulmonary artery waveform should change, mean PAP should fall, and the PO_2 of a blood sample drawn through a wedged catheter should be higher than that of mixed venous blood. Anesthesiologists usually skip the third criterion.

b. Interpretability. Clinicians usually work with the assumption that the greater the ventricular filling, the greater the flow produced (Starling Law of the Heart). Traditionally, clinical signs and symptoms were used to assess ventricular filling. It is clear that the sicker the patient becomes, the less accuracy the clinician will have in estimating PAOP from signs and symptoms; the rate of correctly predicting PAOP was only 30% in one study of critically ill patients.[51] In this same study, therapy was altered in half of the patients after pulmonary arterial catheterization. Clinicians use filling pressure to estimate ventricular filling. The use of PAOP to estimate LVEDP has the further hidden assumptions that the pressures PAOP, pulmonary venous pressure (PVP), LAP, and LVEDP are nearly identical:

$$PAOP \approx PVP \approx LAP \approx LVEDP$$

These identities are likely to be true during health, but physiology is altered during critical illness and the interventions to maintain homeostasis. Positive end-expiratory pressure (PEEP) can make interpretation of PAOP difficult in two ways. First, the actual distending pressure of a cardiac chamber is the inside pressure minus the outside pressure, also called the transmural pressure. With PEEP the true transmural filling pressure is reduced to the extent that lung parenchyma transmits airway pressure to the juxtacardiac region. There is no feasible clinical method to measure juxtacardiac pressure. PAOP during PEEP produces an overestimation of transmural filling pressure. Second, because the pulmonary capillaries are flaccid and collapsible, PAOP equals PVP only if PVP exceeds alveolar pressure; otherwise PAOP reflects alveolar pressure. This is an example of the vascular waterfall phenomenon.[52] The relationship between PVP and PAOP is complex and depends on hydrostatic pressure gradients in the lung and the alveolar pressure (PEEP). The measurement of PAOP also depends on the random migration of the catheter tip during balloon inflation to dependent or less dependent lung segments. PAOP is in equilibrium with PVP and LAP only if the catheter tip lodges in the West functional zone III.[53] Although some pragmatic rules have been given to interpret PAOP in the face of PEEP, ultimately the presence of a PAOP to PVP discrepancy or the effect of PEEP on transmural pressure cannot be determined by common clinical measurements. A temporary removal of PEEP is also not a solution; removal of PEEP causes its own changes in left ventricular events.

A near equality of LAP and LVEDP does not always exist. Mitral valve stenosis and insufficiency make LAP exceed LVEDP. LAP may also underestimate LVEDP. With conditions impairing left ventricular distensibility, atrial contraction contributes a much greater fraction to diastolic filling. LVEDP becomes greater than LAP, sometimes by as much as 10 mm Hg.[54]

Even if PAOP perfectly reflects LVEDP, there are reasons to be suspicious of an easy interpretation. The Starling law as usually expressed relates ventricular volume, not pressure, to the force of contraction. Using PAOP to estimate left ventricular end-diastolic volumes (LVEDV) requires that the pressure-volume relationship be reasonably linear and fairly constant. An elevated PAOP that reflects overdistention of a healthy heart may indicate normal or reduced filling in a ventricle stiffened by hypertrophy or injury. There is considerable evidence that during and after cardiopulmonary bypass,[55] abdominal aortic surgery,[56] and sepsis and acute myocardial disease[57] PAOP is unreliable. It is likely that even changes in

PAOP are fundamentally ambiguous in those or similar situations. There has been some attempt to use increases in PAOP during anesthesia to diagnose myocardial ischemia. This was interpreted to be a reflection of ischemia-induced myocardial wall stiffening. Others have found a PAOP increase to have little (15%) positive predictive value of myocardial ischemia during anesthesia.[58]

Fluid flux into the lung from the pulmonary microvascular is modeled by the Starling equation; one of the four variables in this equation is pulmonary capillary pressure (PCP). It is obvious that PCP is intermediate between PAP and PVP; PAOP must be an underestimation of PCP. Attempts have been made to look at the initial PAOP waveform decay during occlusion to estimate PCP; there appear to be many confounding factors preventing this from being a clinically useful measurement.[59]

The ability of physicians to do useful things with a pulmonary arterial catheter requires specific knowledge of human physiology. Several surveys of physician knowledge have been published. In 1997 the responses of more than 1000 critical care specialists (anesthesiologists, internists, pediatricians, and surgeons) were tallied.[60] Significant deficits in knowledge appeared. One third could not identify the PAOP waveform in a clearly marked tracing. One third incorrectly identified the constituent elements of the equation for oxygen transport. Even larger knowledge deficits were seen in an earlier report presenting the same questionnaire to a more diverse group of physicians.[61]

c. Usefulness. Many skeptical voices have been raised against the common use of balloon-flotation catheters. One physician went so far as to write that the overuse of these catheters had become a cult.[62] The specialty of anesthesiology promulgated practice guidelines,[63] and this debate has continued within anesthesia for two decades.[64-66] In 1987 and 1990, two large observational studies compared mortality following acute myocardial infarction.[67,68] Both use retrospective data gathering and reported increased mortality in those with right heart catheterization (RHC). Both reports were criticized for the well-known limitations of observational studies. An observational study of perioperative use also appeared at this time. Tuman et al[69] found no difference in morbidity and mortality in 1094 patients having coronary artery surgery, half managed with and half managed without RHC. This controversy peaked in 1996 with the publication of an observational study that found higher mortality in critically ill patients whose care included RHC.[70] The experimental methodology of the 1996 report by Connors et al[70] is not easily rejected. As a byproduct of the Study to Understand Prognoses and Preferences for Outcomes and Risks of Treatments (SUPPORT), prospectively collected data on almost 6000 patients treated at five medical centers were analyzed for the effect of RHC; the severity of illness of these patients is reflected by the approximately 33% 30-day mortality. Because RHC was not randomly allocated to SUPPORT patients, there was adjustment for treatment selection bias by both case matching and multiple variable regression analysis. The specific findings for the RHC group included higher mortality at 30, 60, and 180 days, longer intensive care unit stays, and greater hospital costs. Like other medical controversies, these apparent adverse effects were well reported in the U.S. national media, including the call by Connors et al and others for further RCTs and even a moratorium on further catheter use.[71]

In response, the defenders of RHC organized a consensus conference under the auspices of the Society of Critical Care Medicine to rebut these negative findings.[72] A product of this conference was a meta-analysis of the 16 RCTs of RHC published through 1997[73]; overall, no benefit was found from RHC in studies including medical, surgical, and trauma patients. The consensus conference posed the question, "Does management with pulmonary artery catheters improve patient outcomes?" for about 20 medical conditions, including myocardial infarction, aortic surgery, and respiratory failure. Despite the absence of benefit of RHC in the RCTs[73] and the harm from RHC suggested by the observational studies,[67,68,70] their consensus was that outcome was improved in 7 conditions (including acute myocardial infarction), improved outcome was uncertain in 11 conditions, and outcome was not improved in only 3 conditions[72]; "expert opinion" appears to have played the greatest role in this vote of confidence for RHC.[74] This absurd consensus statement has been criticized harshly.[75]

d. Complications. Tissue damage from balloon-flotation catheters is listed briefly (see Box 9-6). The variety of suboptimal or erroneous treatment decisions possible seems endless.[76] Most revolve around the administration or diuresis of fluids and the administration of inotropic drugs. Any positive effects on outcome from valid PAOP data can be negated easily by the all-too-common invalid PAOP data.

3. Noninvasive driving pressures. The oldest noninvasive or indirect method of obtaining blood pressure is direct palpation of an artery.[77] Direct palpation is a continuous measurement, but it cannot easily be quantitated or replicated between observers. Nevertheless, a quick touching of an artery can provide one with a reality check in deciding whether a monitor or a patient is in trouble. Other methods for noninvasive blood pressure measurement can be grouped together by principle of measurement.

All occlusive cuff methods involve an inflatable cuff wrapped around an extremity to collapse large blood vessels. It is believed that cuff and arterial transmural pressure are equal at the point at which the vessel's lumen just opens. Lumen opening during cuff deflation can be determined in numerous ways (Box 9-8). Until 20 or so

years ago auscultatory detection was the standard noninvasive method in the operating room. Low-frequency Korotkoff sounds produced by flow turbulence are auscultated through their five phases during cuff deflation. The first and last audible sounds mark systolic and diastolic pressure. Oscillometric methods actually predate the use of Korotkoff sounds, but the original, purely mechanical devices were not popular. Automatic oscillometric monitors became successful because of built-in inflation pumps and software to control, measure, and display repeated blood pressure determinations.

Fundamentally different are transcutaneous pulse-recording methods. These attempt to provide continuous, directly calibrated pulse recordings. The Penaz method (Finapres) places a small cuff around a finger; incorporated within the cuff is a photoplethysmograph.[78] The photoplethysmograph measures finger volume; a computer software–driven pump applies varying amounts of cuff pressure (counterpulsation) to keep finger volume constant and allow maximal arterial pulsation. The varying cuff pressure is a continuous measure of arterial pressure. Another transcutaneous pulse-recording method is arterial tonometry.[79] This requires an adequately sized, superficial artery overlying a bony structure. The principle is similar to that of ocular tonometry. A special transducer is applied over the center of the artery with sufficient force to distort the vessel. If this position is carefully maintained, the normal contract stress between transducer and skin in the small area directly over the artery approximates arterial pressure. Automated tonometers that intelligently locate the transducer skin contact point are now becoming available. High-fidelity tonometry blood pressure monitoring offers rigorous pulse wave analysis.[39]

a. Reliability. An array of difficulties cause artifact in noninvasive blood pressure measurement. All occlusive cuff methods are susceptible to a mismatch of cuff and extremity (Box 9-9)[80]; a cuff of insufficient width will produce overestimation of pressure by 5 mm Hg or more. A mismatch of cuff and finger is also possible with the Finapres. Auscultatory measurement is very dependent on observer hearing, sight, and skill. Arterial tonometry is exquisitely sensitive to body motion misaligning transducer and artery.

There are more troubling difficulties in the basic meaning of occlusive blood pressures. It has been determined that the oscillometric cuff pressure at the time of maximum oscillations corresponds with mean pressure.[81] Yet none of the algorithms for derivation of oscillometric pressures has been made public; the user does not know the exact meaning of the displayed pressures. The empirically observed consequence of the different algorithms of oscillometric blood pressure devices is that

---

Box 9-8 Detection of arterial opening with occlusive cuff methods

Doppler changes in flow
Korotkoff sounds
Oscillometry
Palpation
Plethysmography
Skin flushing

Box 9-9 Occlusive cuff blood pressure errors

Cuff loosely applied: high reading
Cuff too narrow: high reading
Cuff too wide: low reading

blood pressure measurements by devices from different manufacturers are not interchangeable.[82]

For 50 years, comparisons of invasive and noninvasive measurements have been published. Bruner et al[83] summarized these efforts in stating that "the values yielded by direct and indirect measurement did not necessarily correlate. Different investigators found different degrees of noncorrelation; the variations were unpredictable and defied easy rationalization." The Association for the Advancement of Medical Instrumentation (AAMI, Arlington, Virginia) has standards for evaluating the performance of noninvasive blood pressure monitors.[84] All noninvasive methods have been compared with invasive pressures. The relationships are sometimes marvelously precise and other times very tenuous for Finapres methods[85] and tonometry methods.[86]

b. Interpretability. See the discussion of invasive driving pressures.

c. Usefulness. Inspired by the turn-of-the-century competition between medical students Codman and Cushing to give the best anesthesia care, repetitive auscultatory blood pressure determinations as a standard practice spread throughout the community of anesthesiologists at the beginning of the twentieth century.[87] This practice seems so reasonable that it has never been questioned seriously. This practice still seems plausible when one considers the dramatic effects on hemodynamics of current anesthetic drugs and the devastating possible trespasses of surgical tissue manipulation. Yet the recently published Multicenter Study of General Anesthesia provides an interesting perspective on the usefulness of blood pressure.[88,89] About 17,000 patients were randomly assigned to receive either halothane, enflurane, isoflurane, or fentanyl for elective surgery. Hypertension was more common and hypotension less common with fentanyl than with the three inhalational drugs, but there was no difference in death or other severe morbidity (stroke, myocardial infarction) between these anesthetics.

Do we really know whether and when blood pressure monitoring makes a difference? The Australian Incident Monitoring Study (AIMS) exhaustively reviewed 2000 incidents submitted by anesthesiologists. In an analysis of blood pressure monitoring it was noted that although pulse oximetry, capnography, and ventilator disconnection alarms were more useful in detecting incidents, blood pressure monitoring detected 12% of incidents.[90] Some of these incidents were nearly catastrophic, such as an anesthetic vaporizer set too high. Mangano[91] reviewed and summarized an enormous quantity of literature, concluding that hypotension and tachycardia were predictors of perioperative cardiac morbidity; hyperten-

sion was indeterminate as a predictor of perioperative cardiac morbidity. The American Society of Anesthesiologists (ASA) Standards for Basic Anesthetic Monitoring direct that arterial blood pressure should be determined every 5 minutes[92]; there is no reason to reject this standard.

Cooper[93] has argued that the automated devices should replace auscultatory measurements because they would be more reliable in detecting problems. An interesting study of anesthesia residents showed that the use of automatic noninvasive blood pressure devices during the maintenance phase of anesthesia appeared to decrease vigilance.[94] If monitors do decrease vigilance, no matter what their convenience and continual data production, their use might not be desirable. This point awaits clarification as part of ongoing attempts to automatically record, store, and display data without decreasing vigilance.[95]

d. Complications. All occlusive cuff measurements can leave an extremity ischemic for long periods if cuff inflation is too frequent or cuff deflation is too slow. This ischemia may produce nerve palsy[96] and an acute compartment syndrome with muscle necrosis.[97] The small finger cuff used by the Penaz method remains constantly inflated above venous pressure and produces fingertip venous stasis, swelling, hypoxemia, and acidemia; transient finger numbness and fingertip pressure blisters have been noted.[98] Direct tissue injury is certainly rare compared to that seen with invasively obtained driving pressures. Because it is very easy to obtain artifactual pressure readings, the potential for making adverse therapeutic choices is as great as or greater than with invasive pressures.

B. Respiratory gas monitoring

Intraoperative capnography is strongly encouraged by the ASA[92] and is now common. Besides carbon dioxide (CO_2), other respiratory and anesthetic gases are routinely measured. A variety of methods are available for gas measurement (Table 9-3). Their physical principles can be summarized briefly (Box 9-10). Infrared absorption monitoring was originally limited to CO_2 detection and lacked volatile agent specificity, whereas these monitors are now mated with a rapid responding paramagnetic oxygen analyzer and use polychromatic techniques to specify the volatile agent. The respiratory gas is usually drawn from the breathing circuit by a pump and sent to the analyzer (sidestream); some infrared analyzers have been sufficiently miniaturized to mount the detector directly in the ventilatory gas stream (in-line). Originally mass spectrometers, which were too costly, were installed at a central site and sequentially sampled the operating suites by long sam-

Table 9-3. Properties of respiratory gas monitors

Analyzer type	Sampling	Gases	Volatile agent specificity
Infrared absorption	Sidestream/in-line	CO_2, N_2O, volatile anesthetics	Yes
Mass spectroscopy	Sidestream	O_2, CO_2, N_2, N_2O, volatile anesthetics	Yes
Paramagnetic analysis	Sidestream	O_2	No
Raman spectroscopy	Sidestream	O_2, CO_2, N_2, N_2O, volatile anesthetics	Yes

---

Box 9-10 Physical principles of gas monitors

Infrared absorption: Infrared analyzers emit one or more wavelengths of infrared light and measure light absorption.

Mass spectroscopy: The mass spectrometer uses electrostatic and magnetic fields to spread gases into a spectrum according to their mass-to-charge ratios for measurement by ion current detectors.

Paramagnetic analysis: The oxygen molecule has magnetic properties from unpaired electrons; this is known as paramagnetism. Interaction of the sampled gas with a magnetic field is proportional to the concentration of oxygen.

Raman spectroscopy: The gas sample is illuminated by coherent photons that interact and excite the molecules; some photons are re-emitted at a lower energy and frequency. The frequency shift between incident and scattered light is specific for each gas.

---

pling lines. All types of analyzers are now available as solo units. All capnometers have software with breath detection algorithms to detect inspired and expired peak values.

a. Reliability. Gas monitors in general have an enviable record of providing reliable data.[99] Their accuracy is satisfactory (within a few tenths of a percent of standard reference samples for all measured gases when frequent automatic self-calibration is used to compensate for drift), and they maintain excellent repeatability. Precision is also good for all measured gases. Time-shared mass spectrometers cannot provide continuous monitoring of all patients; the most recent data may be several minutes old. In-line analyzers have optical windows in the sensor for the transmission of light through the gas stream; being close to the endotracheal tube, these windows are easily coated with secretions. There is a degradation in performance of all infrared analyzers, sidestream and in-line, when the optics are contaminated. All sidestream analyzers may be disabled by water drops or secretions in the sampling line that prevent aspiration of sample gas. All sidestream analyzers may provide factitious values if inspired gas can be entrained and mixed with expired gas near the sampling port; end-tidal CO_2 (PET_{CO_2}) is underestimated.

The 10% to 90% rise time, the response of the sensor to a change in gas concentration, varies from about 50 to 500 ms for different analyzers. This is preceded by a delay phase of several seconds for sidestream analyzers as gas flows from the patient to the sensor. The maximum breathing rate that can be measured accurately depends on the rise time. As rise time exceeds 600 ms, respiratory rates above 20 breaths per minute have artifactually high inspired CO_2 (PI_{CO_2}) and low PET_{CO_2}.[100]

b. Interpretability. In health, arterial CO_2 (Pa_{CO_2}) is kept in a carefully controlled range near 40 mm Hg. Under anesthesia, Pa_{CO_2} may be allowed to vary from 25 to 65 mm Hg or higher with little apparent consequence as long as coexisting hypoxemia is prevented. There is no clear PET_{CO_2} cutoff point at which ventilation should be

increased or decreased. Because PET_{CO_2} is used to estimate Pa_{CO_2}, the Pa_{CO_2}-to-PET_{CO_2} difference (gradient) is of great importance. Unfortunately this gradient increases with increasing dead space secondary to any increased ventilation-perfusion mismatching. Induction of anesthesia by itself without pulmonary disease worsens ventilation-perfusion matching. Although attempts have been made to use prolonged expiratory pauses to reduce the Pa_{CO_2}-to-PET_{CO_2} difference,[101] the degree of dead space cannot be determined from the PET_{CO_2} alone.

PET_{CO_2} does have an interesting potential as a predictor of the restoration of a spontaneous heartbeat during resuscitation from cardiac arrest. CO_2 delivery to the lung depends on cardiac output; an increasing PET_{CO_2} is consistent with improving cardiac output by external chest compression or internal cardiac massage. In a human study, those who were resuscitated had a higher PET_{CO_2} in the early phases of advanced cardiac life support than did those who could not be resuscitated. A cutoff point of 10 mm Hg of PET_{CO_2} had a very high sensitivity and specificity.[102]

The gases oxygen (O_2) and nitrous oxide (N_2O) are measured principally to detect failure of gas delivery to or within the anesthesia machine. Because nitrogen (N_2) is so insoluble, it is quickly washed out of the body during anesthesia with the common use of mixtures of O_2 and N_2O. Detection of N_2 during anesthesia thus has a straightforward interpretation; either air has entered the breathing circuit through a leak or venous air embolism is occurring.

Volatile anesthetics (currently halothane, enflurane, isoflurane, desflurane, and sevoflurane) are given by titration; the minimum alveolar concentration (MAC) provides only an estimate of the appropriate anesthetizing concentration for any given patient. The low therapeutic index of volatile anesthetics and their severe myocardial depression require constant vigilance. Nevertheless, within the range of 0% to 2.5% (up to 6% for desflurane), no inspired concentration is absolutely contraindicated for all patients. Even higher inspired concentrations may be used temporarily to decrease the time to achieve anesthetizing concentrations in the brain. The agent-specific analyzers can certainly detect the misfilling of a vaporizer; analyzers can identify a vaporizer that is out of calibration.

c. Usefulness. Capnography is used for two main purposes: to detect catastrophes and to adjust ventilation. The former seems the most important. Catastrophes are usually episodes of hypoventilation signaled by absent CO_2 in the capnogram; they result from esophageal intubation, tracheal extubation, anesthesia circuit disconnection, endotracheal tube obstruction, ventilator malfunction, and patient apnea. No better way of detecting these catastrophes is available.[103] Another catastrophe is heralded by the sudden drop in PET_{CO_2} during constant minute ventilation; this may warn of massive dead space effect from venous embolism (air, fat, thrombus, amniotic fluid) to the pulmonary artery. Although no RCT has been performed, the likely efficacy of capnography is suggested by the review of closed malpractice claims.[33] About 30% of the negative outcomes were believed to have been preventable by additional monitoring; in one half of that 30%, capnography and pulse oximetry were the monitors of greatest likely use. Arguments about the degree of usefulness of capnography for more than catastrophe detection continue.[104,105]

Inspiratory O_2 and N_2O from the gas analyzers provide a redundancy for the machine-mounted in-circuit O_2 sensor. The usefulness of N_2 measurements to detect venous air embolism is confirmed in animal studies, but its clinical results have been discussed only in case reports.[106] Detection of breathing circuit leaks and disconnections is also claimed to be feasible.

Again, no RCT has confirmed the efficacy of using intraoperative measurements of the volatile anesthetics. Large surveys of patient outcome do indicate that they may have a role. In one such report of over 150,000 anesthetic cases, half of the cardiac arrests were identified as resulting from an overdose of volatile anesthetics.[107]

d. Complications. There are almost no reports of direct patient injury from respiratory gas monitors, although the in-line analyzers can become hot enough to cause burns. Because respiratory gas monitoring requires the interposition of a sampling port near the mask or endotracheal tube, there is an increased chance for a breathing circuit disconnection. Of course, the gas monitor will apprehend its own disconnection. Misapplication of monitoring data also seems unlikely to harm the patient. Sudden changes in PET_{CO_2} will only increase vigilance. The analyzers cannot develop a failure state in which normal CO_2 waveforms are displayed unless there is gas movement.

C. Blood flow

Measurement of cardiac output is an integral part of the anesthesia care of many patients. Historically, measurement of flow by the Fick principle came first and is still considered the standard. Derived from conservation of mass considerations, the basic relationship states that arterial oxygen transport equals mixed venous oxygen transport plus oxygen consumption. Formally this is written as

$$\dot{Q} \times Ca_{O_2} = \dot{Q} \times C\overline{v}_{O_2} + \dot{V}_{O_2} \Rightarrow \dot{Q} = \frac{\dot{V}_{O_2}}{Ca_{O_2} - C\overline{v}_{O_2}}$$

where the time derivatives Q and $\dot{V}_{O_2}$ are cardiac output and oxygen consumption, and Ca_{O_2} and $C\overline{v}_{O_2}$ are arterial and mixed venous oxygen content. Algebraic manipulation produces the solution for cardiac output.

Usually mixed expired gases must be collected for several minutes to obtain an average oxygen consumption. This is a steady-state determination of average flow during the time of expired gas collection. The awkwardness of the oxygen-consumption measurement and the need to obtain a mixed venous blood sample has kept Fick determinations in use as a research tool.

Several rapid-injection indicator dilution methods derive flow by the conservation of mass or energy principle. Initial use of this measurement technique used the actual intravenous injection of a green dye. It is now most commonly implemented by the addition of a thermistor to a pulmonary arterial catheter and the use of a bolus of cool

or cold fluid (usually 10 ml normal saline) as the injectate; negative calories (temperature decrease) are the indicator. Temperature at the catheter tip after bolus injection exhibits a temperature fall and then a return to a baseline value. The conservation of heat principle, analogous to conservation of mass, allows derivation of the Stewart-Hamilton equation, which can be written as

$$\dot{Q} = \frac{K \times M}{\int_0^T C(t)dt}$$

where K is an empirical constant, M is the mass of indicator (quantity of negative calories), and $C(t)$ is the time-varying indicator concentration (temperature changes). A dedicated microprocessor integrates the temperature change over time and calculates cardiac output. The terminal portion of integration is an extrapolation. Temperature measurement is truncated or stopped before return to baseline temperature is complete; this is done to avoid recirculation artifacts and minimize the effect of pulmonary artery temperature fluctuations. The derived flow is an averaged value over the several heartbeats of temperature integration. Clinical use of thermodilution methods mandates an average of triplicate determinations obtained over a several-minute period.

Two other techniques of flow measurement are also available: thoracic bioimpedance and various types of continuous-wave and pulsed Doppler ultrasonography. Both are less invasive than Fick and indicator dilution methods and offer the promise of continuous cardiac output. With each heartbeat the volume of blood within the thorax varies temporally with the cardiac cycle. Blood has the highest conductivity of any body tissue (lowest impedance, denoted Z, to the flow of electricity), so the conductivity of the entire thorax varies with the cardiac cycle; conductivity also varies with blood flow velocity. Four pairs of surface electrocardiogram electrodes are placed on the neck and chest. Two of the electrodes inject an alternating milliampere current into the body; the other two measure changes in electrical potential and impedance. Stroke volume is a quadratic or cubic function of an idealized thoracic dimension, maximum rate of change of impedance, baseline impedance, and ventricular ejection time; several different functional relationships for estimating stroke volume are in use. A typical equation is of the following form:

$$\dot{Q} = HR \times SV_{bioimpedance} = HR \times \frac{f(L) \times T \times dZ/dt}{Z_{baseline}}$$

Bioimpedance monitors average a string of heartbeats and display the cardiac output.

High-frequency, inaudible sound (above 2 MHz) can be aimed through the body by ultrasound transducers, which are combined transmitters and receivers. As the sound is reflected back toward the transducer by the internal structures of the body, objects that are moving change the frequency of the reflected sound in proportion to the velocity of the moving object; this is called the Doppler effect. If the velocity of aortic blood flow is measured, cardiac output can be determined from the equation

$$\dot{Q} = HR \times SV_{doppler} = HR \times CSA \times \int V(t)dt$$

where the heart rate *(HR)* and aortic cross-sectional area *(CSA)* are multiplied by the time integral of aortic root blood velocity. There are many variations on the implementation of this monitor. The transducer is usually placed in the suprasternal notch, but esophageal probes have been developed. Both continuous and pulsed Doppler scanners are used. The number of heartbeats averaged to calculate cardiac output also varies. In some systems CSA is measured; in others nomograms adjust CSA values for gender, age, height, and weight.

a. Reliability. To obtain thermodilution cardiac output, one must use an empirical constant that adjusts for the injectate volume, injectate temperature, catheter size, and the particular monitor; current monitors automatically select the correct constant.[108] Error is added if actual injectate temperature and volume vary from the predetermined values. Numerous studies show little difference between using room temperature and cold injectate. Automatic injectors that consistently deliver the solution over a fixed interval do not reduce variability.[109] Intracardiac shunts and valvular regurgitation of the right side of the heart may prevent accurate thermodilution measurement because the injectate may not mix properly or even pass the thermistor.

A thermodilution value varies somewhat depending on when in the respiratory cycle the injection is made. The usual convention is to start injection during the end-expiratory pause; this improves the precision of repeated determinations.[110] Because blood flow varies during the respiratory cycle because of complex interactions between intrathoracic pressure, ventricular filling, and ventricular emptying, the values from end-expiration, though precise, are biased. These values would not necessarily reflect a time-weighted average over the several beats of a complete respiratory cycle.

In general the reproducibility of thermodilution values is good; Stetz et al[111] summarized nine studies of the thermodilution method. The average triplicate value has to change only about 6% to 15% between measurement sessions to imply a change in patient hemodynamics. Stetz et al[111] also compiled 11 studies that compared thermodilution cardiac outputs to the Fick or dye dilution method. Although these reports did not use proper bias and precision measures, the overall impression was an interchangeability of thermodilution with older methods. However, the thermodilution method does systematically overestimate cardiac output during low flow.[112]

The biggest reliability issue for Doppler cardiac outputs is the value of aortic CSA used in the calculation. The aorta is not a cylinder, its shape and area change with every heartbeat, and its area depends on aortic pressure. Error is added by the assumption that CSA is constant. Many refinements of empirical bioimpedance equations have been attempted. All such equations are empirically derived and make simplifying assumptions of a symmetric thorax and constancy of blood resistivity among the various circulatory parts. Reports on these

two methods have not generally included reproducibility data. After the initial enthusiastic reports for each new variation of Doppler and bioimpedance methods, other authors conduct comparison trials with thermodilution methods.[113] Certainly for perioperative use, these follow-up studies have failed to validate the interchangeability of these noninvasive methods with the thermodilution method.[114-116]

b. Interpretability. Like most physiologic variables, cardiac output can vary widely during anesthesia without apparent adverse consequences. Cardiac output is one of those variables that reflects the balance between ongoing surgical trauma (i.e., the stress of surgery) and the suppression by anesthetic drugs of the hormonal and metabolic response to that stress. During and after anesthesia is the stress response good or bad? If it is good, under what circumstances? If bad, how bad? This issue has not been resolved.[117] Until it is, one will have difficulty deciding whether any particular cardiac output value is too high, too low, or just right.

Certain variables are derived from cardiac output and vascular pressures. Systemic vascular resistance (SVR) and pulmonary vascular resistance (PVR) are calculated by a variation on Ohm's law; driving pressure minus filling pressure is divided by flow. Because left ventricular systolic performance is inversely related to the force opposing ventricular fiber shortening, a clinically obtainable measure of this opposition, called left ventricular afterload, is desirable. Clinicians have used SVR to adjust vasodilator drug infusion in hopes that they were rationally manipulating afterload. Unfortunately, SVR is not related to ventricular afterload.[118] SVR does reflect peripheral vasomotor tone. Blood ejection from the heart is pulsatile; Ohm's law is inappropriate. The real afterload is a complex mixture of ventricular geometry, pressure changes, flow acceleration, and the elasticity and viscosity of the aorta. Similar problems interfere with the interpretation of PVR. Changes in PVR cannot easily distinguish among vasodilation, vascular recruitment, or rheologic changes.[119] Some researchers have advocated the abandonment of PVR as now calculated.[120]

c. Usefulness. Clinicians have long noted that survivors of critical illness have a robust response to the stress of massive blood loss, elective surgical trauma, multiple accidental trauma, sepsis, and burns. In a 1985 report 220 critically ill patients were compared for variables of hemodynamics and oxygen delivery (oxygen delivery being cardiac output times arterial oxygen content) by their survivor status; all flow and oxygen delivery variables were indexed by body surface area.[121,122] Fifty percent of survivors had cardiac index values greater than 4.5 L/min/m² and oxygen delivery greater than 650 ml/min/m². Nonsurvivors had lower values, yet still within the range considered typical of good health. These results suggested that a hyperdynamic state with supranormal oxygen delivery was necessary for survival of such patients and that those destined to die for want of a robust response to stress could be made into survivors by manipulating hemodynamics and oxygen transport with fluids and drugs, all guided by repeated measurement of hemodynamics and flow with RHC. Shoemaker et al[123] tested this hypothesis by studying 88 high-risk general surgery patients. Three groups were created; one received CVP monitoring and the other two had thermodilution balloon-flotation catheters placed. In one of the thermodilution groups, a detailed protocol to create a hyperdynamic circulatory state by the transfusion of blood and the use of vasoactive drugs was followed. This latter group had a 4% death rate; the other two lost 23% and 33% of their patients.

Later attempts to replicate this success have had mixed results. The largest study attempted included over 750 patients with all types of critical illness.[124] In the hyperdynamic group, fluids, inotropic drugs, vasodilator drugs, and vasopressor drugs were all used to raise flow. Mortality (about 60% at 6 months) was unaffected by the hyperdynamic protocols. A meta-analysis of nine RCTs reported through 1995 showed no benefit of supranormal values.[125] In one of these RCTs mortality was higher in the supranormal group (54% vs. 34%).[126] Despite the initial enthusiasm for producing the hyperdynamic state, it is an unproven therapy.

d. Complications. For thermodilution outputs the risks are those of the balloon-flotation catheter with one addition. The repetitive injection of aliquots of saline presents opportunities for contamination and bacterial growth in the injectate. Patients may unexpectedly be inoculated with microbes. If prefilled syringes of injectate or bags or bottles of injectate are kept for 24 hours at room temperature, about 15% have positive cultures for skin organisms.[127] There seem to be no reports of complications with the two noninvasive output methods. The Doppler method as implemented in an esophageal probe seems to have the potential for oral, pharyngeal, and esophageal trauma.

Whether clinicians are giving frequent unnecessary fluid challenges and inotropic infusions because of erroneous flow measurements is not known because no one reports such information. Considering the disparity between the usual clinical interpretations and the real meaning of SVR and PVR, one must conclude that patients benefit from therapies chosen to manipulate resistance despite the measurement, not because of it. One must wonder whether other clinical clues really provide the basis for the chosen therapies.

D. Near-infrared spectroscopy

Over a century ago hemoglobin, a chromophore, was identified as the main carrier of oxygen; also discovered was that the absorption of light by a hemoglobin solution changed as oxygen was added.[128] The measurement of hemoglobin concentration is by spectroscopy (also called spectrophotometry and optical spectrometry); the extinction (absorbance) of red and near-infrared (NIR) light (600 to 1000 nm) transmitted through a hemoglobin solution is proportional to the concentration of the hemoglobin, the thickness of the solution (pathlength traveled by the photons), and the extinction coefficient of the hemoglobin. Denoting the intensity of incident light and transmitted light as $I_{incident}$ and $I_{transmitted}$, the concentration of hemoglobin as C, the pathlength as D, and the extinction coefficient as ϵ, the transmission of light is described by the Lambert-Beer law (an exponential function):

$$I_{transmitted} = I_{incident} \exp^{(-D \times C \times \epsilon)}$$

Each hemoglobin species (reduced [HHb], oxyhemoglobin [O_2Hb], methemoglobin [MetHb], carboxyhemoglobin [COHb], and so forth) has a unique extinction pattern. If a blood specimen is transilluminated with a known intensity of one distinct wavelength for each hemoglobin species present and the intensity of transmitted light at each wavelength is measured, a system of simultaneous equations based on the Lambert-Beer law allows calculation of the concentration of each hemoglobin species if the pathlength and extinction coefficients are known.

The product of pathlength, concentration, and extinction coefficient is a unitless number. Consider the ratio $I_{incident}/I_{transmitted}$ as this product decreases from -1 to -10. $I_{incident}/I_{transmitted}$ is 37% at -1 and 0.005% at -10. By the exponential nature of the Lambert-Beer law, measuring the change in light intensity rapidly outstrips the sensitivity of light detectors as pathlength increases. Although in laboratory instruments one can carefully control and minimize the width of the chamber through which light is shone, monitors must be applied in varying circumstances. The problems of measuring change in light intensity because of long pathlengths and light scattering and the determination of pathlength have crucially affected the development and application of NIR spectroscopy in monitors.

By assuming that methemoglobin and carboxyhemoglobin are present in negligible quantities, one can simplify in vivo oximeters to include light emitters and detectors for only two wavelengths (usually 660 nm [red] and 940 nm [NIR]). A specific, calibrated light-emitting diode is used to generate each wavelength. Two forms of oximetry have been incorporated as anesthesia monitors: an external pulse oximeter and an intravascular venous oximeter. Still in an earlier stage of clinical use is an external tissue oximeter of cerebral metabolism that uses multiple wavelengths. Externally applied oximeters are possible because skin, water, and soft tissues are transparent to red and NIR light.

1. Pulse oximetry. There is an unchanging and constant component of red and NIR light transmission through any tissue: extinction by skin, soft tissue, bones, and venous and capillary blood varying slowly.[129-131] The hemoglobin in arterial blood makes only a small contribution to light extinction. Serendipitously, it was noted that there are pulsatile variations in light transmission that are caused by pulsatile arterial blood volume changes. This pulsatile change in extinction is also a function of arterial saturation and can be called the pulsatile component. For each wavelength (660 and 940 nm), the ratio of constant to pulsatile extinction is calculated; this is called the pulse-added absorbance. The pulse oximeter determines the ratio of pulsatile change in light extinction at the two wavelengths to allow estimation of saturation (pulse-added absorbance$_{660}$/pulse-added absorbance$_{940}$). Because the optics of the tissue between emitter and detector are not ideal (do not satisfy all the conditions of the Lambert-Beer law), this estimation is derived from empirical calibration curves obtained in human volunteers. Pulse oximetry saturation is denoted SpO_2 and represents the functional saturation of hemoglobin available for oxygen binding:

$$SpO_2 = 100 \times O_2Hb/(O_2Hb + HHb)$$

Clearly SpO_2 might be different from the oxyhemoglobin percentage obtained from a multiwavelength spectrometer:

$$So_2 = 100 \times O_2Hb/(O_2Hb + HHb + MetHb + COHb)$$

a. Reliability. Considering the number of assumptions inherent in pulse oximetry, one might expect limitations. Many studies have compared pulse oximetry with in vitro oximetry. Unfortunately, most used calibration statistical methods. Kelleher[132] and Tremper and Barker[131] very usefully tabulated the results of these numerous studies, including bias and precision when it was derived. In the range of oxygen saturations from 70% to 100%, the bias is generally small (1% to 2%), as is the range of agreement (-4% to 5%); this bias and precision are compatible with the manufacturer's claims. There are ongoing attempts to improve the signal captured by the pulse oximeter.[133]

Although the presence or absence of other hemoglobins cannot be determined by pulse oximetry, COHb and MetHb can interfere with SpO_2 accuracy because both species absorb light in the red to NIR spectrum. With increasing COHb, SpO_2 falls much more slowly than the oxyhemoglobin percentage falls. The presence of COHb is treated by the pulse oximeter as if it were a mixture of 90% O_2Hb and 10% HHb.[134] MetHb can cause both an overestimation and an underestimation of SpO_2; as MetHb increases, SpO_2 settles toward 85% regardless of the actual oxyhemoglobin percentage.[135] Accuracy at very low saturations (less than 70%) is problematic; this is understandable because SpO_2 is estimated from empirical calibrations during which severe hypoxemia is not induced. In general, saturation is underestimated and precision deteriorates at values below 70%.[136]

Users of pulse oximeters are familiar with many other circumstances in which SpO_2 is unavailable or cannot be trusted (Box 9-11).[137] It is also important to remember that the response time of the monitor to actual changes in saturation is mostly a function of the circulation time to the sensor site. Although probes on the ear can respond in 10 seconds, finger and toe locations take 20 to 30 and 40 to 80 seconds, respectively.

b. Interpretability. Ensuring adequate oxygen transport, especially to the brain and heart, is one of the anesthesiologist's primary concerns. SpO_2 is monitored to avoid and correct hypoxia. Whether SpO_2 is interpretable depends on the exact expectations placed on it. If the detection of a large, rapid fall in saturation from the 90% range is the goal, SpO_2 serves well as a catastrophe alarm. If instead the goal is to determine the safety of mild hypoxemia after anesthesia at discharge from the postanesthesia care unit (PACU), SpO_2 is of little help.[138] Although there are research devices capable of measuring tissue oxygen status (high-energy phosphate concentrations by magnetic resonance spectroscopy and cy-

Box 9-11 Other limitations of pulse oximetry causing absent or low SpO_2 reading

Low pulse-amplitude states
Hypotension
Ischemia
Vasoconstriction
Hypothermia

Dyes
Methylene blue
Indigo carmine
Nail polish

Other
Motion artifact
Shivering
Electrocautery
Excessive ambient light

tochrome redox state by NIR spectroscopy), there has been no systematic clinical study of the minimum level of SpO_2 associated with maintenance of sufficient cerebral tissue oxygen delivery.

c. Usefulness. Several well-conducted studies show that low saturation is often missed without the aid of pulse oximetry. This may occur during preinduction placement of monitoring catheters,[139] anesthesia,[140] transport to the PACU,[141] care within the PACU,[142] and during sleep following surgery.[143] These reports have changed anesthesia and PACU practices. For example, continuous postoperative O_2 therapy is now common in the PACU and this O_2 therapy is often continued upon transfer from the PACU to the hospital ward.

In the largest RCT ever conducted of a monitoring technology in the operating room and PACU, five Danish hospitals randomly allocated elective and emergent adult surgical patients to either have or not have pulse oximetry monitoring.[144,145] This clinical trial occurred just as pulse oximetry was being disseminated into anesthesia care in Denmark. Hospital morbidity and mortality were recorded; serious events occurred in about 10% of patients. Myocardial ischemia (as defined by angina or ST segment depression) was detected more often in the control group (12 patients in the oximetry group vs. 26 patients in the control group), but had no postoperative consequences. Several changes in PACU care were observed in association with the use of pulse oximetry. These included increased use of supplemental oxygen at discharge and increased use of naloxone. The two groups did not differ significantly in cardiovascular, respiratory, neurologic, or infectious complications and had equal numbers of in-hospital deaths.

Although the failure of this enormous research effort to prove a monitor useful brought dismay, no voices have called for abandonment of pulse oximetry.[146] Pulse oximetry remains the most practical method to fulfill the ASA standard of quantitative assessment of blood oxygenation

---

Box 9-12 Treatments for arterial desaturation

Correct equipment failure
Improve distribution of ventilation (airway suctioning, patient positioning)
Increase functional residual capacity (PEEP)
Increase inspired oxygen
Increase ventilation
Lower oxygen consumption

---

during anesthesia.[92] With the greater recognition of the frequency of desaturation and the resultant changes in practice management, no other outcome study of sufficient size for adequate statistical power is now possible. Other attempts to justify pulse oximetry have included economic analysis of the cost of operating room catastrophes (death and brain damage) compared with the cost of oximeters.[147,148] It is being claimed that since the adoption of monitoring standards in Massachusetts there have been few or no anesthesia deaths and hypoxic brain injuries as a result of better monitoring including pulse oximetry.[149] Finally, the AIMS analysis found that pulse oximetry detected 9% of incidents and could have detected 60% had the incidents not been detected by other monitors.[150]

d. Complications. Remarkably few patient injuries have been reported from pulse oximeters. These have consisted of burns and ischemic skin necrosis.[151] Also, pulse oximetry does not seem to decrease overall vigilance or produce distractions. If desaturation is noticed, the treatment is ordinarily straightforward and includes one or more of the treatments listed in Box 9-12. Even if this desaturation is fictitious, these routine patient care activities, as usually instituted during anesthesia, have little associated risk.

2. Mixed venous oximetry. Fiberoptic bundles have been implanted in pulmonary artery catheters, terminating at the catheter tip, to provide mixed venous oximetry; this at least triples the cost of the catheter.[152,153] This is a reflectance spectroscopy. Red and NIR light is transmitted through part of the bundles, and the reflected light is conducted back to light detectors through the remaining bundles. Mixed venous oxygen saturation is displayed continuously by the monitor. Because fewer than four wavelengths of light are used, assumptions about the absence of other hemoglobin species must be made. There are two mixed venous oximeters available, one using two wavelengths and the other using three wavelengths. Because the catheter tip is embedded in flowing blood, pulse oximetry methods are not necessary. The derived saturation is empirically calculated because it depends on Hb concentration, blood velocity, and other factors. An in vitro calibration before insertion and repeated in vivo recalibrations are necessary because the monitor performance drifts over time.

a. Reliability. Compared to pulse oximetry, fewer studies comparing in vivo mixed venous saturations to bench oxygen saturations have been performed. There

does appear to be a difference in the stability of accuracy and precision between the two- and three-wavelength catheters. A 1988 report found the bias of the two wavelength devices to increase over time[154]; this problem appears to have been corrected, according to a 1995 report.[155] In vivo oximetry certainly appears to face the same problems as pulse oximeters in the presence of MetHb and COHb.[135]

b. Interpretability. A rewriting of the Fick equation is the usual method for interpreting mixed venous saturation ($S\bar{v}O_2$):

$$S\bar{v}O_2 \propto C\bar{v}O_2 = CaO_2 - \frac{\dot{V}O_2}{\dot{Q}}$$

Assuming that CaO_2 is constant, $S\bar{v}O_2$ is proportional to the balance of oxygen uptake and cardiac output. Sometimes there is the further assumption that oxygen consumption is constant; then $S\bar{v}O_2$ is hyperbolically proportional to flow. Because $S\bar{v}O_2$ is about 70% to 75% in healthy persons, values less than that are said to reflect failing physiologic compensations for maintaining oxygen delivery during anemia, hypovolemia, sepsis, fever, and so on. It is particularly hoped that $S\bar{v}O_2$ will provide an early warning of hemodynamic changes.

A careful examination of these and other assumptions reveals that interpretation of mixed venous oxygen is fraught with uncertainty. The use of $S\bar{v}O_2$ is an example of the use of arteriovenous concentration differences with the assumption that arterial concentration is constant.[156] Oxygen transport should probably be modeled as a nonlinear, nonstationary system. Mixed venous blood is the combined flow of venous blood from all parts of the body; mixed venous oxygen content is the average of oxygen content of these flows, averaged in proportion to the amount of blood from an organ, as expressed by the equation

$$S\bar{v}O_2 \propto C\bar{v}O_2 = \frac{\sum_{i=1}^{n} C\bar{v}O_{2i} \times \dot{Q}_i}{\sum_{i=1}^{n} \dot{Q}_i}$$

Any $C\bar{v}O_2$ and by extension any $S\bar{v}O_2$ can be derived from an infinite number of combinations of flows and oxygen consumptions within and between organs, flows and oxygen consumptions that can change dramatically and quickly with anesthesia and critical illness. No particular $S\bar{v}O_2$ value is proof of adequate oxygen transport to any specific organ. These objections to facile interpretation are not merely theoretical but are based on empirical observations. Threshold values of $S\bar{v}O_2$ that result in death or organ failure have not been demonstrated.[157,158] Changes in $S\bar{v}O_2$ correlate poorly with changes in cardiac output in some studies.[159]

c. Usefulness. In the debate about efficacy, enthusiasts of the use of mixed venous pulmonary arterial balloon catheters have published testimonials to their clinical applicability.[160] The high cost of this technology has prompted several clinical trials. In one case series (coronary artery surgery) compared to historical controls at the same institution[161] and in two randomized controlled clinical trials (coronary artery surgery and critical illness),[162,163] the availability of $S\bar{v}O_2$ did not improve outcome but did increase the cost of care. These studies suffer from their small size and the lack of a firm protocol for the interpretation and use of the data.

The targeted hyperdynamic approach to critical illness can also be applied by monitoring $S\bar{v}O_2$ and targeting therapy to keep it normal or elevated. The goal-oriented hemodynamic therapy trial of Gattinoni et al[124] included a control group and two hyperdynamic groups, one titrated by monitoring flow and the other titrated by monitoring $S\bar{v}O_2$; the $S\bar{v}O_2$ group had no better survival than the control or the flow group. Considering the basic ambiguity of $S\bar{v}O_2$, one is skeptical that there will ever be such a successful demonstration.

Another proposed use of continual $S\bar{v}O_2$ monitoring is to continuously update calculated values of oxygen consumption by a reverse Fick equation:

$$\dot{V}O_2 = \dot{Q} \times (CaO_2 - C\bar{v}O_2) \propto \dot{Q} \times (SpO_2 - S\bar{v}O_2) \times Hb$$

Assuming some constancy of hemoglobin and ignoring dissolved oxygen, thermodilution flow measurements along with pulse oximetry and mixed venous oximetry values can be plugged into this equation. Unfortunately, the error in these measurements is summed and propagated in the calculation of oxygen consumption; the errors are so large that this continual oxygen consumption is not useful.[164]

d. Complications. There seem to be no tissue injuries other than those from any pulmonary arterial catheter.

3. Cerebral oximetry. Oxygen is the final electron acceptor at the terminal enzyme (cytochrome *c* oxidase) of oxidative phosphorylation in the mitochondrion; 90% of oxygen is used there.[128] The redox (oxidation reduction) potential at *c* oxidase defines the sufficiency of oxygen transport to the mitochondria.[165] This enzyme is also a chromophore. If sufficient different wavelengths of NIR light are shown through or reflected from the cerebral cortex, the absolute and relative concentrations of oxyhemoglobin versus reduced hemoglobin and oxidized *c* oxidase versus reduced *c* oxidase can be determined noninvasively.[166]

a. Reliability. Although much initial development used transmission spectroscopy across the heads of infants and small animals, adult craniums are too thick to allow sufficient light transmission. An alternative approach has been to place the light emitter and detector adjacent to each other (several centimeters apart) and use reflectance spectroscopy. From the Lambert-Beer equation (see page 223), the pathlength of light must be known to determine the absolute concentration of chromophores. This has remained a fundamentally difficult, only partially solved problem. Two different types of devices have resulted from the difficulty with pathlength. Some instruments are intended to be monitors of concentrations of the chromophores (cerebral oxyhemoglobin, reduced hemoglobin, and oxidized c oxidase); Wahr et al[128] reviewed the various attempts to estimate light pathlength and calculate concentrations in a large number of animal and human studies. Cerebral chromophore

concentration monitors remain research devices. By ignoring light pathlength, in vivo saturation monitors of the relative concentration of cerebral oxyhemoglobin (regional cerebral saturation or $rScO_2$) have been produced; cerebral oximeters are possible because pathlength cancels out in the ratio of absorbances. Such monitors based on reflectance spectroscopy are available for clinical use.

b. Interpretability. Because the bulk of cerebral cortical blood (70% to 80%) is venous, values from cerebral oximetry are a highly weighted average of partially desaturated hemoglobin; any relative change in the volume of venous or arterial blood will change measured $rScO_2$ even if no change in arterial oxygen saturation has occurred. The absorption of NIR is by blood in both the scalp and the cerebral cortex. Changes in scalp blood flow will change $rScO_2$ even if the cerebral cortex has had no change in oxygen delivery or oxygen use. In an attempt to eliminate contamination of the estimated $rScO_2$ by scalp blood flow, the INVOS monitor (Somanentics, Troy, Michigan) uses three adjacent probes over the scalp: one emitter and two detectors.[167] The detector closest to the light source is considered to reflect scalp contamination; the light attenuation at the near detector is subtracted from light attenuation measured at the more distant detector to derive $rScO_2$. However, one report revealed normal $rScO_2$ in patients with complete absence of cerebral blood flow, suggesting that the dual detectors cannot eliminate contamination of the $rScO_2$ value by scalp blood flow.[168]

In any case, there is no standard measurement to serve as a referent for cerebral oximetry. Attempts have been made to compare cerebral oximetry to related variables such as jugular venous oxygen saturation in healthy volunteers during hypoxia. Although $rScO_2$ had an excellent linear correlation with jugular venous oxygen saturation for each subject, the slopes and intercepts vary so widely among subjects as to negate its value as a monitor.[169]

c. Usefulness. No RCTs have been conducted of the use of cerebral oximetry. It is disturbing to note that a case series has been published in which cerebral oximeter probes placed on dead adults (some with the brain removed) found $rScO_2$ in the normal range.[170] Unless this discrepancy can be resolved, current devices for cerebral oximetry will be abandoned.

d. Complications. Although skin burns seem possible, no adverse effects have been reported. One must wonder about erroneous treatment decisions made possible by a monitor that cannot distinguish the living from the dead.

E. Neuromuscular function

In 1954 Beecher and Todd[171] reviewed deaths during 600,000 anesthetic sessions, concluded that the use of curare increased mortality sixfold, and recommended that it not be used for trivial reasons. Since then the complexity of the neuromuscular junction and the potent actions of neuromuscular blocking drugs have been richly explored. Seventy to 80% of the acetylcholine receptors of the neuromuscular junction must be occupied before loss of neuromuscular function is detected.[172] The neuromuscular junction has both prejunctional and postjunctional acetylcholine receptors; this explains differential effects of neuromuscular blocking drugs.[173] There is great individual variation in the response to neuromuscular blocking drugs.[174] Muscles have different sensitivity to neuromuscular blocking drugs (from least to most: respiratory, facial, thenar, pharyngeal).[175]

A few years after the report by Beecher and Todd, equipment to test neuromuscular function objectively during anesthesia was created and recommended.[176] A supramaximal electrical stimulus (50 to 60 milliamperes) is applied to a peripheral nerve; the muscle enervated is observed for the evoked contraction. The stimulus is applied by needle electrodes, disposable skin pads, or direct contact. The most commonly used nerves are the ulnar and a branch of the facial with observation of the abductor pollicis and orbicularis oculi, respectively. A single stimulus is typically 0.2 ms in duration. The stimulation is most commonly applied as a single impulse at 0.1 Hz, four consecutive impulses at 2 Hz (train-of-four or TOF), or repetitive 5-second bursts at 50 to 100 Hz (tetanic stimulation). A variant of tetanic stimulation called double-burst stimulation consists of several short bursts of tetanic stimulation.[177] The contraction can be evaluated by visual examination, tactile examination, force transduction (thenar muscles), accelerometry (piezoelectric transducer on thumb), and electromyography (thenar or facial muscles). A single stimulation is observed for the strength of twitch; the ratio of the fourth twitch to the first twitch is calculated for the TOF; with tetanic stimulation, the resulting tetany is observed for fade with time. Nerve stimulation is applied to allow one to judge and titrate the onset and continuation of paralysis and the restoration of neuromuscular function at the termination of anesthesia.[178,179]

a. Reliability. Two aspects of reliability are important: the function of the nerve stimulator and the method of contractile assessment. Nerve stimulators are rugged, compact, well-packaged instruments. Most offer a variety of preprogrammed stimulation patterns; some are now incorporated with assessment and recording devices. It is hard to find a systematic comparison of nerve stimulators. The force transduction mechanomyogram is the standard measurement of contraction, but the equipment requires excessive care and attention to be a useful clinical monitor. Visual and tactile examination are the most common methods of evaluation, but quantification is difficult; tactile assessment has been shown to lack accuracy.[180] Electromyography requires the amplification of very-low-level

electrical signals, needs considerable signal processing, and is vulnerable to electrical surgical interference, but in some studies it appears interchangeable with mechanomyograms.[181] Accelerometry is an easily applied new method not requiring special positioning of the thumb and showing very good precision with the mechanomyogram.[182]

Several circumstances produce unreliable data. Direct placement of the stimulating electrodes over the muscle must be avoided. Direct muscle stimulation is possible even with total acetylcholine receptor blockade. Immediately after a tetanic stimulation the single or multiple twitch responses will be increased (posttetanic facilitation) for 10 or so minutes. The degree of blockade increases with falling temperature; if a temperature differential exists between the extremities and the core, misleading information is obtained.[183]

b. Interpretability. The evaluation of neuromuscular block after succinylcholine is simple, with all responses being abolished for 5 to 20 minutes with the usual intubating dosage. Use of nondepolarizing drugs is more complicated. Waud and Waud,[172] Ali and Savarese,[178] and Viby-Mogensen[179] have synthesized animal and clinical studies to relate receptor occupancy, stimulus response, and clinical consequences; a compilation of their findings roughly indicates the patterns of response (Table 9-4). Because of the differential sensitivity of skeletal muscles, these tests on peripheral muscles may not always allow adequate prediction of abdominal relaxation; clinical observation of the surgical field is still necessary. A considerable controversy remains, namely, what test performance should be achieved to predict safe extubation at the termination of induced paralysis.[184] A typical criterion has been the achievement of a TOF ratio of 70%.[185] Some recent work suggests that a TOF ratio less than 90% leaves the patient with dysfunctional swallowing, at risk for aspiration.[185a] Even a sustained head lift may be necessary to allow one to predict successful airway maintenance and airway protection.[186] The latter is obviously difficult to assess consistently in patients emerging from anesthesia.

c. Usefulness. It is well documented that patients who have been paralyzed during anesthesia with nondepolarizing neuromuscular blocking drugs show a high frequency of clinically significant residual paralysis if a nerve stimulator is not used to allow assessment of neuromuscular function.[187] The use of nerve stimulators has become quite common over the last 20 years. But as with

Table 9-4. Correlation of nerve stimulator responses, receptor occupancy, and clinical relaxation with nondepolarizing neuromuscular blocking drugs

Receptor occupancy (%)	0.1-Hz single twitch (% control)	2 Hz TOF ratio (%)	5-sec 50-Hz tetanic stimulation	Clinical consequence
50	100	100	Sustained	Sustained head life
70-75	100	~70	Sustained	Normal vital capacity
80	20-80	0-40	Fade	Normal tidal volume
90-95	0	0	Minimal response	Surgical relaxation

TOF, Train-of-four.

other monitors, no clinical trials have been performed to prove greater patient safety. Large epidemiologic surveys no longer identify patients receiving paralyzing drugs as having a higher mortality.[188] Although the ASA Closed Claim Study does not identify residual paralysis as a cause of respiratory complications[189] or identify nerve stimulators as a monitor that might have prevented a mishap,[33] the likely explanation is that their use is already sufficiently widespread to have reduced to a low level this source of complications. Finally, in an observational analysis of patients receiving pancuronium during major surgery, patients with a TOF less than 0.7 following tracheal intubation had more postoperative pulmonary complications (risk ratio for pneumonia/atelectasis = 3.5).[190]

d. Complications. Although nerve stimulators inject electrical current into the body, their complications are rarely mentioned. A small full-thickness burn under a disposable skin electrode has occurred.[191] The balance between information and complications is very favorable.

F. Temperature

Being homeothermic, humans maintain a body temperature near 37° C by muscular activity, changes in metabolism, sweating, vasomotor redistribution, and behavioral activities.[192] This thermoregulation is controlled from the hypothalamic region. During general anesthesia thermoregulation is dramatically degraded and body temperature depends much more on environmental conditions. Protective devices in the operating room against heat loss by conduction, radiation, convection, and evaporation include insulation, fluid warmers, airway heat exchangers, forced-air blankets, and radiant lights.

Body temperature is measured by contact and noncontact methods. The former methods include glass thermometers, thermistors, thermocouples, and liquid crystals. The radiant heat (infrared photons) emitted by the body can give temperature without contact. Temperature is measured in the nose, mouth, rectum, tympanic membrane, bladder, heart, pulmonary artery and muscle, and at multiple skin sites including the axilla, big toe, and forehead.

a. Reliability. All methods available are accurate to ±0.3° C or better. Most physiologic monitors now incorporate temperature monitoring by thermistor or thermocouple methods and provide digital displays with precision to 0.1° C. Their response time to temperature change is quite rapid and depends mostly on the heat mass of the temperature probe itself. Self-contained liquid crystal strips applied to the skin are the least accurate and slowest responding method used during anesthesia.

b. Interpretability. Most core temperature change, up or down, during anesthesia is a consequence of initial heat redistribution caused by anesthesia-induced vasodilation,[193] surgical conditions (exposure, skin preparation solutions, and open body cavities) and environmental changes (cool rooms and multiple layers of insulating covers). Specialized surgery (cardiopulmonary bypass and neurosurgery) may require the induction of a hypothermic state. In animal experiments, mild hypothermia provides some cerebral protection. Although lacking human RCTs, the intentional cooling of patients (33° to

34° C) to produce a mild hypothermia for cerebral vascular surgery is now common at many hospitals.[194]

Anesthesia may be requested to allow patients to tolerate the deliberate production of hyperthermia. Of course, the rare genetic disorder malignant hyperthermia is always possible.

The interpretation is simple. After the initial heat redistribution, if temperature is up, so is body heat content and vice versa. The solutions are also simple: Reduce heat production and increase heat loss, or reduce heat loss and add heat. The distinction between passive warming causing hyperthermia and the active process of malignant hyperthermia is suggested when one considers the rate of temperature increase (slow for the former and fast for the latter). Additional diagnostic methods are used if malignant hyperthermia is suspected.

Not totally resolved in clinical monitoring is the question of which temperature is the best to monitor. Tympanic membrane temperature probably best allows prediction of thermoregulatory activity of the body.[195] There are temperature gradients throughout the body; the central heat core of the body is the brain, thorax, and abdomen.[196] Tympanic, nasopharyngeal, and esophageal are usually considered to be the best estimates of core temperature. Yet on occasion core temperature can be misleading about the heat content of the body. During the rewarming of cardiopulmonary bypass, these core temperatures rapidly return to 37° C, whereas rectal and bladder temperature recover more slowly. Complicated surgical procedures require temperature monitoring at multiple sites.

Skin temperature (skin liquid crystals or temperature probes placed on the skin) can be useful, but because of temperature gradients between core and periphery, it cannot provide the same information as other temperatures can.

c. Usefulness. The well-known effects of hypothermia on anesthetic requirements, volatile anesthetic uptake and elimination, and drug metabolism provide very persuasive reasons to monitor every patient's temperature. Also, the devastating consequences of unrecognized malignant hyperthermia require 100% recognition of that condition.

In the last decade, convincing evidence has accumulated that even mild hypothermia during surgery has adverse effects. An RCT of patients having total hip arthroplasty created a normothermic group and a mild hypothermic (~35° C) group; blood loss in the hypothermic group was about 500 ml higher than in the normothermic group.[197] Another RCT divided 300 patients undergoing abdominal, thoracic, or vascular surgical procedures into two groups, one allowed to cool to about 35.4° C and the other kept at 36.7° C; all patients either had coronary artery disease or were at high risk for coronary artery disease. Morbid cardiac events (unstable angina or ischemia, cardiac arrest, or myocardial infarction) were twice as likely in the hypothermic group.[198] Still another RCT found a threefold higher incidence of surgical wound infections in hypothermic (about 2° C cooler) patients undergoing colorectal surgery[199]; this study engendered considerable controversy about experimental design and methods.

d. Complications. All temperature probes can abrade or puncture the tissue into or against which they are placed. Because temperature probes are usually reusable, cross-infection between patients is possible if the probe is not cleaned properly. Epistaxis is common with nasopharyngeal temperature monitoring, but is usually a self-limiting injury. Of particular concern is the perforation of the tympanic membrane, which occurs on occasion with tympanic thermometry during anesthesia.[200] Because the probe is usually inserted after anesthesia is induced, the patient cannot complain when the probe is inserted too deeply. The risk of tympanic perforation discourages most anesthesiologists from the use of this monitoring site. Considering the minimal morbidity evident in published reports, the existing near-universal use of temperature monitoring, and the great importance of temperature control, temperature monitoring seems likely to continue.[92]

III. MORE SPECIALIZED MONITORS

The previously discussed monitors are accessible to every anesthesiologist. Many are used universally; others have or have had proponents arguing for standard use in all patients. The invasive pressure methods have been taught routinely by training programs for at least 20 years. The cost of equipment is within the budget of most hospitals; the insertion and application of interfacing devices and monitor use are common skills.

Other monitoring methods are much more specialized; these are imaging of the heart and recording of cerebral blood flow velocity,[201] jugular venous bulb oxygen saturation,[202] and brain electrical activity. Although all have emerged from pure research use, clinical use is not universal. The use of these monitors is not a common skill; there is a real concern about the training process. Equipment costs can range from $30,000 to $200,000, several orders of magnitude higher than some of the previously discussed monitors. Most institutions have found it effective to provide full-time technician support for some of these devices; this is not the case for other perioperative monitoring technologies. There is a very extensive literature for these methods. Only limited comments are presented here to highlight a few aspects of their perioperative role.

A. Cerebral electrical activity

For the last 30 years recording of central nervous system activity has gradually moved from the physiology laboratory and the electroencephalographer's office to the operating room.[203] This move resulted from the development of better electronics, microprocessors, and signal-averaging software. The operating room is a hostile environment for the detection, amplification, and processing of the very-low-voltage scalp potentials; numerous sources of electrical noise can overwhelm the detection of physiologic signals. Because most intraoperative monitoring uses processed rather than raw electroencephalograms (EEGs), it is vital to remember that the computer software can process junk signals just as well as the real thing. The monitoring environment process is also unfriendly because three clinical events

(cerebral hypoxia, hypothermia, and deep anesthesia) produce much the same result: a decreased frequency and a decreased amplitude of cerebral electrical potentials.

In general terms there are three potential applications for intraoperative EEGs: determination of anesthetic depth, detection of cerebral ischemia, and titration of barbiturate infusion to produce burst suppression. A fourth application, seizure recognition during epilepsy surgery, is superspecialized and actually uses electrocorticography; a fully trained electroencephalographer performs this monitoring. Analog EEG (strip-chart recorder) has proved too difficult for use by anesthesiologists in the operating room for most purposes. Processed EEGs showing the amplitudes of bands of frequency activity are now available with a variety of devices that use several algorithms to extract analog EEG features. Good electrode placement with low-impedance pathways is always critical.

Anesthetic depth determination would be used to avoid light anesthesia with awareness, to prevent needless deep anesthesia, and to titrate deep anesthesia to increase brain resistance to ischemia or hypoxia. The analog EEG has been used extensively to uncover EEG patterns associated with inhalation and intravenous anesthetics. Similarly, processed EEG has been studied for the same purpose; there is a great diversity of patterns by dosage within inhalation and intravenous drugs and between inhalation and intravenous drugs.[204] Many attempts have been made to use the 95% spectral edge frequency to judge anesthetic depth. There are EEG patterns for restricted circumstances (certain drugs, certain patients) that allow identification of light anesthesia,[205] but these patterns have no universality for all patients and all possible drug combinations.[206] The basic problem is the inability to relate consciousness mechanistically to electrical activity; only empirical correlations are available.[207]

A new type of EEG processing has generated considerable interest. This processing derives an index of the phase coupling of the EEG and is called the bispectral (BIS) score.[208] In volunteer subjects the BIS score predicts response to verbal commands during sedation[209] and correlates well with loss of consciousness for intravenous and inhalation anesthetics.[210] However, the BIS score does not forewarn of movement or hemodynamic changes. The BIS monitor, unlike most other monitors of cerebral electrical activity, is easily set up and used. Outcome studies with the BIS monitor are awaited.

Sufficiently deep anesthesia will produce electrical silence. It is hoped that this suppression of EEG would reflect a condition of brain protection, the ability of the central nervous system to tolerate longer periods of hypoxia with full recovery.[211] Some attempts have been successful; others have not. After successful resuscitation from cardiac arrest, some patients remained in a coma; an attempt to improve survival by using high-dose barbiturate therapy was not successful.[212] Nussmeier, Arlund, and Slogoff[213] titrated barbiturate therapy during cardiopulmonary bypass by EEG monitoring and reduced neuropsychiatric complications. The use of routine EEG monitoring during heart surgery to detect cerebral hypoxia and ischemia remains controversial. Some centers report routine EEG use during carotid artery surgery to determine the necessity of shunting during carotid artery cross-clamping.[214]

Event-related activity of the central nervous system can be detected by repeated stimulation of a sensory system and averaging of the EEG to show pathway-specific electrical activity. Evoked potentials (EVPs) are very-low-voltage signals produced by somatosensory, auditory, or visual field stimulation.[215] Five hundred to 1000 stimuli are required to generate an EVP. Specialized equipment and technical support are necessary for EVP monitoring. Somatosensory EVPs are the most commonly used during anesthesia. The evidence for their usefulness has been extensively reviewed by Gugino and Chabot.[216] The use of somatosensory EVPs in spinal surgery is now routine, although questions remain about their sensitivity and specificity. To monitor dorsal horn integrity, monitoring of motor EVPs is being tried during spinal surgery. Magnetic transcranial stimulation consists of stimulating the cerebral cortex by magnetic fields; motor EVPs are recorded from the epidural space, nerves, or muscle groups.[217] Anesthetic agents can considerably modify all EVPs, hampering interpretation. The role of EVPs in aortic and carotid surgery is less well defined.

If needle electrodes are used, EEGs and EVPs would have the risk of cross-infection. Other complications are not reported. Improperly obtained or interpreted cerebral electrical signals have obvious possibilities for prompting mistakes. For example, the failure to recognize loss of dorsal column pathway function during surgical distraction of the spinal column could leave a patient paraplegic.

B. Cardiac imaging

Echocardiography uses sound waves in the 2.5- to 5-MHz range to penetrate tissue.[218-221] Piezoelectric crystals emit these high-frequency sound waves; the same or another set of crystals receive the reflected sound waves. The time delay of the echo specifies the distance of a structure from the emitter, the intensity of the echo is proportional to tissue density, and any Doppler shift in the reflected signal provides information about velocity. By mechanical or electronic means, echo probes scan a 90-degree sector; computer software generates a two-dimensional image or tomographic slice through tissue from the reflected sound. By repeated imaging of the heart, a series of images can be displayed to provide a real-time slice of the beating heart. If Doppler measurement is used, color-flow mapping of blood velocity can be superimposed on the two-dimensional image.

Initial cardiac imaging used a transthoracic approach. This provided diagnostic images of valve lesions, heart size, and so on; intraoperative use was not practical. With the miniaturization of electronic components, the Doppler probe was mounted on a flexible gastroscope and advanced blindly down the esophagus to provide a transesophageal retrocardiac view of the heart, known since as transesophageal echocardiography (TEE). The depth of the probe down the esophagus and its angulation provide several distinct views, including a basal short-axis view of the outflow tracts and valves, a long-axis view of all four chambers, and a short-axis cross-section of the left ventricle. A main emphasis of intraoperative use has been continuous visualization of the left ventricle short axis for assessment of global ventricular function, contractile indices, left ventricular filling, and regional ventricular function.

In just 15 years TEE has become an invaluable tool in the operating room. A task force of anesthesiologists has created practice guidelines concerning training in and use of TEE.[222] The TEE Task Force classified use of TEE into three categories by weight of evidence or expert opinion. An example of category I (the strongest evidence) was intraoperative use in valve repair. An example of category III (little current scientific support) was intraoperative monitoring for emboli during orthopedic procedures. Most importantly, the TEE Task Force specified objectives for basic and advanced training in TEE, including both cognitive and technical skills.

Among the initial hopes for TEE monitoring was real-time observations of regional wall motion for the early detection of myocardial ischemia.[223] As a segment of ventricular wall becomes ischemic, the contraction of that segment progressively changes within seconds from normal motion to hypokinesis, followed by akinesis, then dyskinesis. The sudden development of segmental wall motion abnormalities (SWMAs) is thought to be the earliest and most sensitive detector of ischemia.[224] Yet this issue is not fully resolved, with questions remaining about the reliability, interpretability, and usefulness of this technology for detection of ischemia.[224] For example, during acute hypovolemia new SWMAs may develop in the absence of myocardial ischemia.[225]

Reports of complications with intraoperative TEE are rare but should be similar to those associated with flexible gastroscopy. Esophageal perforation secondary to a difficult esophageal intubation would be the most feared event. The TEE Task Force summarized reports of adverse effects; serious morbidity such as esophageal injury or bleeding, vocal cord paralysis, arrhythmias, hypotension, seizures, and cardiac arrest occur in less than 3% of TEE examinations. Minor complications of lip bruises (13%), hoarseness (12%), and dysphagia (2%) from TEE are more common.

It is unknown how often erroneous interpretations lead to mistaken therapy changes. Because new SWMAs do not necessarily indicate myocardial ischemia, unnecessary therapies may be instituted to treat a nonexistent ischemia. Also of concern is the increased workload inherent in TEE monitoring by the anesthesiologist. One study suggested a decrease in vigilance because of TEE monitoring.[226]

IV. CONCLUSION

There is a clear dilemma for anesthesiologists with respect to the complications caused by perioperative monitoring. The tissue injuries produced by most monitors are well understood. The immediate consequences of therapy chosen mistakenly because of a monitored variable are more or less predictable. Yet it is hard to pin down with assurance the benefits of monitoring in terms of patient morbidity and mortality. One must be skeptical about one's clinical impressions of monitoring because of the enormous variability in patient physiologic behavior. Formal studies using rigorous methods are necessary. Without a firm estimate of benefits, no reasonable model can be written to balance risks and benefits. There is no better example of this conundrum than the continuing controversy about balloon-flotation pulmonary arterial catheters, a monitoring device introduced in 1970. The specialty of anesthesiology still lacks certainty in most monitoring choices.

REFERENCES

1. Moyers J: Monitoring instruments are no substitute for careful clinical observation, *J Clin Monit* 4:107, 1988.
2. Pierce EC, Jr: Monitoring instruments have significantly reduced anesthetic mishaps, *J Clin Monit* 4:111, 1988.
3. Keats AS: Anesthesia mortality in perspective, *Anesth Analg* 71:113, 1990.
4. Banta HD, Thacker SB: The case for reassessment of health care technology. Once is not enough, *JAMA* 264:235, 1990.
5. Fuchs VR, Garber AM: The new technology assessment, *N Engl J Med* 323:673, 1990.
6. Guyatt G, Drummond M, Feeny D, et al: Guidelines for the clinical and economic evaluation of health care technologies, *Soc Sci Med* 4:393, 1986.
7. Mosteller F, Burdick E: Current issues in health care technology assessment, *Int J Technol Assess Health Care* 5:123, 1989.
8. Pace NL: Technology assessment of anesthesia monitors, *J Clin Monit* 8:142, 1992.
9. Byrick RJ, Cohen MM: Technology assessment of anaesthesia monitors: problems and future directions, *Can J Anaesth* 42:234, 1995.
10. Cooper JO, Cullen BF: Observer reliability in detecting surreptitious random occlusions of the monaural esophageal stethoscope, *J Clin Monit* 6:271, 1990.
11. Fryback DG, Thornbury JR: The efficacy of diagnostic imaging, *Med Decis Making* 11:88, 1991.
12. Coalition for Critical Care Excellence, Consensus Conference on Physiologic Monitoring Devices: Standards of evidence for the safety and effectiveness of critical care monitoring devices and related interventions, *Crit Care Med* 23:1756, 1995.
13. Hope CE, Morrison DL: Understanding and selecting monitoring equipment in anaesthesia and intensive care, *Can Anaesth Soc J* 33:670, 1986.
14. Ream AK: Mean blood pressure algorithms, *J Clin Monit* 1:138, 1985.
15. Bland JM, Altman DG: Statistical methods for assessing agreement between two methods of clinical measurement, *Lancet* 1:307, 1986.
16. Bland JM, Altman DG: Comparing methods of measurement: why plotting difference against standard method is misleading, *Lancet* 356:1085, 1995.
17. Chinn S: The assessment of methods of measurement, *Stat Med* 9:351, 1990.
18. LaMantia KR, O'Connor T, Barash PG: Comparing methods of measurement: an alternative approach, *Anesthesiology* 72:781, 1990.
19. Kraemer HC: *Evaluating medical tests: objective and quantitative guidelines*, Newbury Park, Calif, 1992, Sage.
20. Jaeschke R, Guyatt G, Sackett DL, et al: Users' guides to the medical literature. III. How to use an article about a diagnostic test: A. Are the results of the study valid? *JAMA* 271:389, 1994.
21. Jaeschke R, Guyatt G, Sackett DL, et al: Users' guides to the medical literature. III. How to use an article about a diagnostic test: B. What are the results and will they help me in caring for my patients? *JAMA* 271:703, 1994.
22. Swets JA: Measuring the accuracy of diagnostic systems, *Science* 240:1285, 1988.
23. Begg CB: Biases in the assessment of diagnostic tests, *Stat Med* 6:411, 1987.
24. Hlatky MA, Pryor DB, Harrell FEJ, et al: Factors affecting sensitivity and specificity of exercise electrocardiography, *Am J Med* 77:64, 1984.
25. Jaeschke RZ, Meade MO, Guyatt GH, et al: How to use diagnostic test articles in the intensive care unit: diagnosing weanability using f/Vt, *Crit Care Med* 25:1514, 1997.
26. Pace NL: But what does monitoring do to patient outcome? *Int J Clin Monit Comput* 1:197, 1985.
27. Arnstein F: Catalogue of human error, *Br J Anaesth* 79:645, 1997.
28. Duncan PG: That was then, this is now! The value of observing change, *Anesth Analg* 86:225, 1998.
29. Snow J: *On the mode of communication of cholera*, London, 1855, Churchill.
30. Bunker JP, The Subcommittee on the National Halothane Study of the Committee on Anesthesia, National Academy of Sciences National Research Council: Summary of the national halothane study, *JAMA* 197:775, 1966.
31. Prentice RL: Surrogate endpoints in clinical trials: definition and operational criteria, *Stat Med* 8:431, 1989.
32. Irwig L, Tosteson ANA, Gatsonis C, et al: Guidelines for meta-analyses evaluating diagnostic tests, *Ann Intern Med* 120:667, 1994.
33. Tinker JH, Dull DL, Caplan RA, et al: Role of monitoring devices in prevention of anesthetic mishaps: a closed claim analysis, *Anesthesiology* 71:541, 1989.
34. Freeman R: Intrapartum fetal monitoring: a disappointing story, *N Engl J Med* 322:624, 1990.
35. Fry DL: Physiologic recording by modern instruments with particular reference to pressure recording, *Physiol Rev* 40:753, 1960.
36. Kleinman B: Understanding natural frequency and damping and how they relate to the measurement of blood pressure, *J Clin Monit* 5:137, 1989.
37. Kleinman B, Powell S, Gardner RM: Equivalence of fast flush and square wave testing of blood pressure monitoring systems, *J Clin Monit* 12:149, 1996.
38. Weiss BM, Pasch T: Measurement of systemic arterial pressure, *Curr Opin Anaesthesiol* 10:459, 1997.
39. O'Rourke MF, Gallagher DE: Pulse wave analysis, *J Hypertens* 14:S147, 1996.
40. Gardner RM: Accuracy and reliability of disposable pressure transducers coupled with modern pressure monitors, *Crit Care Med* 24:879, 1996.
41. Schwid HA, Taylor LA, Smith NT: Computer model analysis of the radial artery pressure waveform, *J Clin Monit* 3:220, 1987.
42. Pauca AL, Hudspeth AS, Wallenhaupt SL, et al: Radial artery-to-aorta pressure difference after discontinuation of cardiopulmonary bypass, *Anesthesiology* 70:935, 1989.
43. Rooke GA: Systolic pressure variation as an indicator of hypovolemia, *Curr Opin Anaesthesiol* 8:511, 1995.
44. Rao TLK, Jacobs KH, El-Etr AA: Reinfarction following anesthesia in patients with myocardial infarction, *Anesthesiology* 59:499, 1983.
45. Shah KB, Rao TLK, Laughlin S, et al: A review of pulmonary artery catheterization in 6,245 patients, *Anesthesiology* 61:271, 1984.
46. Slogoff S, Keats AS: On the safety of radial artery cannulation, *Anesthesiology* 59:42, 1983.
47. O'Quin R, Marini JJ: Pulmonary artery occlusion pressure: clinical physiology, measurement, and interpretation, *Am Rev Respir Dis* 128:319, 1983.
48. Tuman KJ, Carroll GC, Ivankovich AD: Pitfalls in interpretation of pulmonary artery catheter data, *J Cardiothorac Anesth* 3:625, 1989.
49. Groom L, Frisch SR, Elliott M: Reproducibility and accuracy of pulmonary artery pressure measurement in supine and lateral position, *Heart Lung* 19:147, 1990.
50. Schmitt EA, Brantigan CO: Common artifacts of pulmonary artery and pulmonary artery wedge pressures: recognition and interpretation, *J Clin Monit* 2:44, 1986.
51. Eisenberg PR, Jaffe AS, Schuster DP: Clinical evaluation compared to pulmonary artery catheterization in the hemodynamic assessment of critically ill patients, *Crit Care Med* 12:549, 1984.

52. Permutt S, Riley RL: Hemodynamics of collapsible vessels with tone: the vascular waterfall, *J Appl Physiol* 18:924, 1963.

53. West JB, Dollery CT, Naimark A: Distribution of blood flow in isolated lung: relation to vascular and alveolar pressures, *J Appl Physiol* 19:713, 1964.

54. Rahimtoola SH, Ehsani A, Sinno MZ, et al: Left atrial transport function in myocardial infarction: importance of the booster pump function, *Am J Med* 59:686, 1975.

55. Hansen RM, Viquerat CE, Matthay MA, et al: Poor correlation between pulmonary arterial wedge pressure and left ventricular end-diastolic volume after coronary artery bypass graft surgery, *Anesthesiology* 64:764, 1986.

56. Kalman PG, Wellwood MR, Weisel RD, et al: Cardiac dysfunction during abdominal aortic operation: the limitations of pulmonary wedge pressures, *J Vasc Surg* 3:773, 1986.

57. Calvin JE, Driedger AA, Sibbald WJ: Does the pulmonary capillary wedge pressure predict left ventricular preload in critically ill patients? *Crit Care Med* 9:437, 1981.

58. van Daele ME, Sutherland GR, Mitchell MM, et al: Do changes in pulmonary capillary wedge pressure adequately reflect myocardial ischemia during anesthesia? A correlative preoperative hemodynamic, electrocardiographic, and transesophageal echocardiographic study, *Circulation* 81:865, 1990.

59. Dawson CA, Bronikowski TA, Linehan JH, et al: On the estimation of pulmonary capillary pressure from arterial occlusion, *Am Rev Respir Dis* 140:1228, 1989.

60. Trottier SJ, Taylor RW: Physicians' attitudes toward and knowledge of the pulmonary artery catheter: Society of Critical Care Medicine membership survey, *New Horiz* 5:201, 1997.

61. Iberti TJ, Fischer EP, Leibowitz AB, et al: A multicenter study of physicians' knowledge of the pulmonary artery catheter, *JAMA* 264:2928, 1990.

62. Robin ED: The cult of the Swan-Ganz catheter: overuse and abuse of pulmonary flow catheters, *Ann Intern Med* 103:445, 1985.

63. The American Society of Anesthesiologists Task Force on Pulmonary Artery Catheterization: Practice guidelines for pulmonary artery catheterization, *Anesthesiology* 78:380, 1993.

64. Keats AS: The Rovenstein Lecture, 1983: cardiovascular anesthesia—perceptions and perspectives, *Anesthesiology* 60:467, 1984.

65. Lowenstein E, Teplick R: To (PA) catheterize or not to (PA) catheterize—that is the question, *Anesthesiology* 53:361, 1980.

66. Tuman KJ, Roizen MF: Outcome assessment and pulmonary artery catheterization: why does the debate continue? *Anesth Analg* 84:1, 1997.

67. Gore JM, Goldberg RJ, Spodick DH, et al: A community-wide assessment of the use of pulmonary artery catheters in patients with acute myocardial infarction, *Chest* 92:721, 1987.

68. Zion MM, Balkin J, Rosenmann D: Use of pulmonary artery catheters in patients with acute myocardial infarction, *Chest* 98:1331, 1990.

69. Tuman KJ, McCarthy RJ, Spiess BD, et al: Effect of pulmonary artery catheterization on outcome in patients undergoing coronary artery surgery, *Anesthesiology* 70:199, 1989.

70. Connors AF Jr, Speroff T, Dawson NV, et al: The effectiveness of right heart catheterization in the initial care of critically ill patients, *JAMA* 276:889, 1996.

71. Dalen JE, Bone RC: Is it time to pull the pulmonary artery catheter? *JAMA* 276:916, 1996.

72. Pulmonary Artery Catheter Consensus Conference Participants: Pulmonary artery catheter consensus conference: consensus statement, *Crit Care Med* 25:910, 1997.

73. Ivanov RI, Allen J, Sandham JD, et al: Pulmonary artery catheterization: a narrative and systematic critique of randomized controlled trials and recommendations for the future, *New Horiz* 5:268, 1997.

74. Sibbald WJ, Keenan SP: Show me the evidence: a critical appraisal of the Pulmonary Artery Catheter Consensus Conference and other musings on how critical care practitioners need to improve the way we conduct business, *Crit Care Med* 25:2060, 1997.

75. Fink MP: The flow-directed, pulmonary artery catheter and outcome in critically ill patients: have we heard the last word? *Crit Care Med* 25:902, 1997.

76. Connors AF Jr: Right heart catheterization: is it effective? *New Horiz* 5:195, 1997.

77. Carroll GC: Blood pressure monitoring, *Crit Care Clin* 4:411, 1988.

78. Boehmer RD: Continuous real-time, noninvasive monitor of blood pressure: Penaz methodology applied to the finger, *J Clin Monit* 3:282, 1987.

79. Drzewiecki GM, Melbin J, Noordergraaf A: Arterial tonometry: review, analysis, *J Biomech* 16:141, 1983.

80. Manning DM, Kuchirka C, Kaminski J: Miscuffing: inappropriate blood pressure cuff application, *Circulation* 68:763, 1983.

81. Geddes LA, Voelz M, Combs C, et al: Characterization of the oscillometric method for measuring indirect blood pressure, *Ann Biomed Eng* 10:271, 1982.

82. Kaufmann MA, Pargger H, Drop LJ: Oscillometric blood pressure measurements by different devices are not interchangeable, *Anesth Analg* 82:377, 1996.

83. Bruner JMR, Krenis LJ, Kunsman JM, et al: Comparison of direct and indirect methods of measuring arterial blood pressure I, II, III, *Med Instrum* 14:11, 1981.

84. White WB, Berson AS, Robbins C, et al: National standard for measurement of resting and ambulatory blood pressures with automated sphygmomanometers, *Hypertension* 21:504, 1993.

85. Pace NL, East TD: Simultaneous comparison of intra-arterial, oscillometric and Finapres monitoring during anesthesia with automated sphygmomanometers, *Anesth Analg* 73:213, 1991.

86. Weiss BM, Spahn DR, Rahmig H, et al: Radial artery tonometry: moderately accurate but unpredictable technique of continuous non-invasive arterial pressure measurement, *Br J Anaesth* 76:405, 1996.

87. Beecher HK: The first anesthesia records (Codman, Cushing), *Surg Gynecol Obstet* 71:689, 1940.

88. Forrest JB, Cahalan MK, Rehder K, et al: Multicenter study of general anesthesia. II. Results, *Anesthesiology* 72:262, 1990.

89. Forrest JB, Rehder K, Goldsmith CH, et al: Multicenter study of general anesthesia. I. Design and patient demography, *Anesthesiology* 72:252, 1990.

90. Cockings JGL, Webb RK, Klepper ID, et al: Blood pressure monitoring applications and limitations: an analysis of 2000 incident reports, *Anaesth Intens Care* 21:565, 1993.

91. Mangano DT: Perioperative cardiac morbidity, *Anesthesiology* 72:153, 1990.

92. House of Delegates: *Standards for basic anesthetic monitoring,* Park Ridge, Ill, 1996, American Society of Anesthesiologists.

93. Cooper JB: Toward prevention of anesthetic mishaps, *Int Anesthesiol Clin* 22:167, 1984.

94. Kay J, Neal M: Effect of automatic blood pressure devices on vigilance of anesthesia residents, *J Clin Monit* 2:148, 1986.

95. Loeb RG: Manual record keeping is not necessary for anesthesia vigilance, *J Clin Monit* 11:9, 1995.

96. Bickler PE, Schapera A, Bainton CR: Acute radial nerve injury from use of an automatic blood pressure monitor, *Anesthesiology* 73:186, 1990.

97. Celoria G, Dawson JA, Teres D: Compartment syndrome in a patient monitored with an automated blood pressure cuff, *J Clin Monit* 3:139, 1987.

98. Northwood D: Morbidity after use of the Finapres blood pressure monitor, *Anaesthesia* 44:1010, 1989.

99. Walder B, Lauder R, Zbinden AM: Accuracy and cross-sensitivity of 10 different anesthetic gas monitors, *J Clin Monit* 9:364, 1993.

100. Brunner JX, Westenskow DR: How the rise time of carbon dioxide analysers influences the accuracy of carbon dioxide measurements, *Br J Anaesth* 61:628, 1988.

101. Tavernier B, Rey D, Thevenin D, et al: Can prolonged expiration manoeuvres improve the prediction of arterial PCO_2 from end-tidal PCO_2? *Br J Anaesth* 78:536, 1997.

102. Cantineau JP, Lambert Y, Merckx P, et al: End-tidal carbon dioxide during cardiopulmonary resuscitation in humans presenting mostly with asystole: a predictor of outcome, *Crit Care Med* 24:791, 1996.

103. Birmingham PK, Cheney FW, Ward RJ: Esophageal intubation: a review of detection and techniques, *Anesth Analg* 65:886, 1986.

104. Block FE: A carbon dioxide monitor that does not show the waveform is worthless, *J Clin Monit* 4:213, 1988.

105. Polaheimo MPJ: A carbon dioxide monitor that does not show the waveform has value, *J Clin Monit* 4:210, 1988.

106. Sprung J, Whalley D, Schoenwald PK, et al: End-tidal nitrogen provides an early warning of slow, ongoing venous air embolism, *Anesthesiology* 85:1203, 1996.

107. Keenan RL, Boyan CP: Cardiac arrest due to anesthesia: a study of incidence and causes, *JAMA* 253:2372, 1985.

108. Nishikawa T, Dohi S: Errors in the measurement of cardiac output by thermodilution, *Can J Anaesth* 40:142, 1993.

109. Nelson LD: Automatic vs manual injections for thermodilution cardiac output determinations, *Crit Care Med* 10:190, 1982.

110. Stevens JH, Raffin TA, Mihm FG, et al: Thermodilution cardiac output measurement: effects of the respiratory cycle on its reproducibility, *JAMA* 253:2240, 1985.

111. Stetz CW, Miller RG, Kelly GE, et al: Reliability of the thermodilution method in the determination of cardiac output in clinical practice, *Am Rev Respir Dis* 126:1001, 1982.

112. van Grondelle A, Ditchey RV, Groves BM, et al: Thermodilution method overestimates low cardiac output in humans, *Am J Physiol* 245:H690, 1983.

113. Moore FA, Haenel JB, Moore EE: Alternatives to Swan-Ganz cardiac output monitoring, *Surg Clin North Am* 71:699, 1991.

114. Clarke DE, Raffin TA: Thoracic electrical bioimpedance measurement of cardiac output: not ready for prime time, *Crit Care Med* 21:1111, 1993.

115. Siegel LC, Shafer SL, Martinez GM, et al: Simultaneous measurements of cardiac output by thermodilution, esophageal Doppler, and electrical impedance in anesthetized patients, *J Cardiothorac Anesth* 2:590, 1988.

116. Spahn DR, Schmid ER, Tornic M, et al: Noninvasive versus invasive assessment of cardiac output after cardiac surgery: clinical validation, *J Cardiothorac Anesth* 4:46, 1990.

117. Roizen MF: Should we all have a sympathectomy at birth? Or at least preoperatively? *Anesthesiology* 68:482, 1988.

118. Lang RM, Borow KM, Neumann A, et al: Systemic vascular resistance: an unreliable index of left ventricular afterload, *Circulation* 74:1114, 1986.

119. Borback MS: Problems associated with the determination of pulmonary vascular resistance, *J Clin Monit* 6:118, 1990.

120. McGregor M, Sniderman A: On pulmonary vascular resistance: the need for more precise definition, *Am J Cardiol* 55:217, 1985.

121. Bland RD, Shoemaker WC: Probability of survival as a prognostic and severity of illness score in critically ill surgical patients, *Crit Care Med* 85:91, 1985.

122. Bland RD, Shoemaker WC, Abraham E, et al: Hemodynamic and oxygen transport patterns in surviving and nonsurviving postoperative patients, *Crit Care Med* 13:85, 1985.

123. Shoemaker WC, Appel PL, Kram HB, et al: Prospective trial of supranormal values of survivors as therapeutic goals in high-risk surgical patients, *Chest* 94:1176, 1988.

124. Gattinoni L, Brazzi L, Pelosi P, et al: A trial of goal-oriented hemodynamic therapy in critically ill patients, *N Engl J Med* 333:1025, 1995.

125. Heyland DK, Cook DJ, King D: Maximizing oxygen delivery in critically ill patients: a methodologic appraisal of the evidence, *Crit Care Med* 24:517, 1996.

126. Hayes MA, Timmins AC, Yau EH, et al: Elevation of systemic oxygen delivery in the treatment of critically ill patients, *N Engl J Med* 330:1717, 1994.

127. Burke KG, Larson E, Maciorowski L, et al: Evaluation of the sterility of thermodilution room-temperature injectate preparations, *Crit Care Med* 14:503, 1986.

128. Wahr JA, Tremper KK, Samra S, et al: Near-infrared spectroscopy: theory and applications, *J Cardiothorac Vasc Anesth* 10:406, 1996.

129. Lindberg LG, Lennmarken C, Vegfors M: Pulse oximetry: clinical implications and recent technical developments, *Acta Anaesthesiol Scand* 39:279, 1995.

130. Severinghaus JW, Kelleher JF: Recent developments in pulse oximetry, *Anesthesiology* 76:1018, 1992.

131. Tremper KK, Barker SJ: Pulse oximetry, *Anesthesiology* 70:98, 1989.

132. Kelleher JF: Pulse oximetry, *J Clin Monit* 5:37, 1989.

133. Pollard V, Prough DS: Signal extraction technology: a better mousetrap? *Anesth Analg* 83:213, 1996.

134. Barker SJ, Tremper KK: The effect of carbon monoxide inhalation on pulse oximeter signal detection, *Anesthesiology* 67:599, 1987.

135. Barker SJ, Tremper KK, Hyatt J: Effects of methemoglobinemia on pulse oximetry and mixed venous oximetry, *Anesthesiology* 70:112, 1989.

136. Severinghaus JW, Naifeh KH, Koh SO: Errors in 14 pulse oximeters during profound hypoxia, *J Clin Monit* 5:72, 1989.

137. Severinghaus JW, Spellman MJ Jr: Pulse oximeter failure thresholds in hypotension and ischemia, *Anesthesiology* 73:532, 1990.

138. Fairley HB: Changing perspectives in monitoring oxygenation, *Anesthesiology* 70:2, 1989.

139. Hensley FA Jr: Oxygen saturation during preinduction placement of monitoring catheters in the cardiac surgical patient, *Anesthesiology* 66:834, 1987.

140. Raemer DB, Warren DL, Morris R, et al: Hypoxemia during ambulatory gynecologic surgery as evaluated by the pulse oximeter, *J Clin Monit* 3:244, 1987.

141. Tyler IL, Tantisira B, Winter PM, et al: Continuous monitoring of arterial oxygen saturation with pulse oximetry during transfer to the recovery room, *Anesth Analg* 64:1108, 1985.

142. Morris RW, Buschman A, Warren DL, et al: The prevalence of hypoxemia detected by pulse oximetry during recovery from anesthesia, *J Clin Monit* 4:16, 1988.

143. Kurth CD: Postoperative arterial oxygen saturation: what to expect, *Anesthesiology* 80:1, 1995.

144. Moller JT, Johannessen NW, Espersen K, et al: Randomized evaluation of pulse oximetry in 20,802 patients. II. Perioperative events and postoperative complications, *Anesthesiology* 78:445, 1993.

145. Moller JT, Pedersen T, Rasmussen LS, et al: Randomized evaluation of pulse oximetry in 20,802 patients. I. Design, demography, pulse oximetry failure rate, and overall complication rate, *Anesthesiology* 78:436, 1993.

146. Eichhorn JH: Pulse oximetry as a standard of practice in anesthesia, *Anesthesiology* 78:423, 1993.

147. Caplan RA, Ward RJ, Posner K, et al: Unexpected cardiac arrest during spinal anesthesia: a closed claims analysis of predisposing factors, *Anesthesiology* 68:5, 1988.

148. Whitcher C, Ream AK, Parsons D, et al: Anesthetic mishaps and the cost of monitoring: a proposed standard for monitoring equipment, *J Clin Monit* 4:5, 1988.

149. Brahams D: Anaesthesia and the law: monitoring, *Anaesthesia* 44:606, 1989.

150. Runciman WB, Webb RK, Barker L, et al: The pulse oximeter: applications and limitations—an analysis of 2000 incident reports, *Anaesth Intens Care* 21:543, 1993.

151. Murphy KG, Secunda JA, Rockoff MA: Severe burns from a pulse oximeter, *Anesthesiology* 73:350, 1990.

152. Kupeli IA, Satwicz PR: Mixed venous oximetry, *Int Anesthesiol Clin* 27:176, 1989.

153. Schweiss JF: Mixed venous hemoglobin saturation: theory and application, *Int Anesthesiol Clin* 25:113, 1987.

154. Karis JH, Lumb PD: Clinical evaluation of the Edwards Laboratories and Oximetrix mixed venous oxygen saturation catheters, *J Cardiothorac Anesth* 2:440, 1988.

155. Bongard F, Lee TS, Leighton T, et al: Simultaneous in vivo comparison of two- versus three-wavelength mixed venous (SvO_2) oximetry catheters, *J Clin Monit* 11:329, 1995.

156. Zierler KL: Theory of the use of arteriovenous concentration differences for measuring metabolism in steady and non-steady states, *J Clin Invest* 40:2111, 1961.

157. Astiz ME, Rackow EC, Kaufman B, et al: Relationship of oxygen delivery and mixed venous oxygenation to lactic acidosis in patients with sepsis and acute myocardial infarction, *Crit Care Med* 16:655, 1988.

158. Schlichtig R, Cowden WL, Chaitman BR: Tolerance of unusually low mixed venous oxygen saturation: adaptions in the chronic low cardiac output syndrome, *Am J Med* 80:813, 1986.

159. Magilligan DJ Jr, Teasdall R, Eisinminger R, et al: Mixed venous oxygen saturation as a predictor of cardiac output in the postoperative cardiac surgical patient, *Ann Thorac Surg* 44:260, 1987.

160. Norfleet EA, Watson CB: Continuous mixed venous oxygen saturation measurement: a significant advance in hemodynamic monitoring? *J Clin Monit* 1:245, 1985.

161. Larson LO, Kyff JV: The cost-effectiveness of Oximetrix pulmonary artery catheters in the postoperative care of coronary artery bypass graft patients, *J Cardiothorac Anesth* 3:257, 1989.

162. Jastremski MS, Chelluri L, Berney KM, et al: Analysis of the effects of continuous on-line monitoring of mixed venous oxygen saturation on patient outcome and cost-effectiveness, *Crit Care Med* 17:148, 1989.

163. Pearson KS, Gomez MN, Moyers JR, et al: A cost/benefit analysis of randomized invasive monitoring for patients undergoing cardiac surgery, *Anesth Analg* 69:336, 1989.

164. Woda RP, Dzwonczyk RD, Orlowski JP, et al: Effect of measurement error on calculated variables of oxygen transport, *J Appl Physiol* 80:559, 1996.

165. Cohen PJ: The metabolic function of oxygen and biochemical lesions of hypoxia, *Anesthesiology* 37:148, 1972.

166. Jobsis FF: Noninvasive infrared monitoring of cerebral and myocardial oxygen sufficiency and circulatory parameters, *Science* 198:1264, 1997.

167. McCormick PW, Stewart M, Goetting MG, et al: Noninvasive cerebral optical spectroscopy for monitoring cerebral oxygen delivery and hemodynamics, *Crit Care Med* 19:89, 1991.

168. Gomersall CD, Joynt GM, Gin T, et al: Failure of the INVOS 3100 cerebral oximeter to detect complete absence of cerebral blood flow, *Crit Care Med* 25:1252, 1997.

169. Henson LC, Calalang C, Temp JA, et al: Accuracy of a cerebral oximeter in healthy volunteers under conditions of isocapnic hypoxia, *Anesthesiology* 88:58, 1998.

170. Schwarz G, Litscher G, Kleinert R, et al: Cerebral oximetry in dead subjects, *J Neurosurg Anesthesiol* 8:189, 1996.

171. Beecher HK, Todd DP: *A study of the deaths associated with anesthesia and surgery,* Springfield, Ill, 1954, Charles C Thomas.

172. Waud BE, Waud DR: The relation between response to "train-of-four" stimulation and receptor occlusion during competitive neuromuscular block, *Anesthesiology* 37:413, 1972.

173. Bowman WC: Prejunctional and postjunctional cholinoreceptors at the neuromuscular junction, *Anesth Analg* 59:935, 1980.

174. Matteo RS, Spector S, Horowitz PE: Relation of serum *d*-tubocurarine concentration to neuromuscular blockade in man, *Anesthesiology* 41:440, 1974.

175. Paloheimo MP, Wilson RC, Edmonds HL Jr, et al: Comparison of neuromuscular blockade in upper facial and hypothenar muscles, *J Clin Monit* 4:256, 1988.

176. Christie TH, Churchill-Davidson HC: The St. Thomas's Hospital nerve stimulator in the diagnosis of prolonged apnoea, *Lancet* 1:775, 1958.

177. Engbaek J, Ostergaad J, Viby-Mogensen J: Double burst stimulation (DBS). A new pattern of nerve stimulation to identify residual neuromuscular block, *Br J Anaesth* 62:274, 1989.

178. Ali HH, Savarese JJ: Monitoring of neuromuscular function, *Anesthesiology* 45:216, 1976.

179. Viby-Mogensen J: Clinical assessment of neuromuscular transmission, *Br J Anaesth* 54:209, 1982.

180. Dupuis JY, Martin R, Tessonnier JM, et al: Clinical assessment of the muscular response to tetanic nerve stimulation, *Can J Anaesth* 37:397, 1990.

181. Kopman AF: The dose-effect relationship of metocurine: the integrated electromyogram of the first dorsal interosseous muscle and the mechanomyogram of the adductor pollicis compared, *Anesthesiology* 68:604, 1988.

182. May O, Nielsen K, Werner MU: The acceleration transducer: an assessment of its precision in comparison with a force displacement transducer, *Acta Anaesthesiol Scand* 32:239, 1988.

183. Thornberry EA, Mazumdar B: The effect of change of temperature on neuromuscular monitoring in the presence of atracurium blockade, *Anaesthesia* 43:447, 1988.

184. Miller RD: How should residual neuromuscular blockade be detected? *Anesthesiology* 70:379, 1989.

185. Brand JB, Cullen DJ, Wilson NE, et al: Spontaneous recovery from nondepolarizing neuromuscular blockade: correlation between clinical and evoked responses, *Anesth Analg* 56:55, 1977.

185a. Eriksson LI, Sundman E, Olsson R, et al: Functional assessment of the pharynx at rest and during swallowing in partially paralyzed humans: simultaneous videomanometry and mechanomyography of awake human volunteers, *Anesthesiology* 87:1035, 1997.

186. Pavlin EG, Holle RH, Schoene RB: Recovery of airway protection compared with ventilation in humans after paralysis with curare, *Anesthesiology* 70:381, 1989.

187. Viby-Mogensen J, Jorgensen BC, Ording H: Residual curarization in the recovery room, *Anesthesiology* 50:539, 1979.

188. Cohen MM, Duncan PG, Tate RB: Does anesthesia contribute to operative mortality? *JAMA* 260:2859, 1988.

189. Caplan RA, Posner KL, Ward RJ, et al: Adverse respiratory events in anesthesia: a closed claims analysis, *Anesthesiology* 72:828, 1990.

190. Berg H, Viby-Mogensen J, Roed J, et al: Residual neuromuscular block is a risk factor for postoperative pulmonary complications: a prospective, randomised, and blinded study of postoperative pulmonary complications after atracurium, vecuronium and pancuronium, *Acta Anaesthesiol Scand* 41:1095, 1997.

191. Cooper JB, DeCesare R, D'Ambra MN: An engineering critical incident: direct current burn from a neuromuscular stimulator, *Anesthesiology* 73:168, 1990.

192. Young CC, Sladen RN: Temperature monitoring, *Int Anesthesiol Clin* 34:149, 1996.

193. Matsukawa T, Sessler DI, Sessler AM, et al: Heat flow and distribution during induction of general anesthesia, *Anesthesiology* 82:662, 1995.

194. Wass CT, Lanier WL: Hypothermia-associated protection from ischemic brain injury: implications for patient management, *Int Anesthesiol Clin* 34:95, 1996.

195. Benzinger M: Tympanic thermometry in surgery and anesthesia, *JAMA* 209:1207, 1969.

196. Cork RC, Vaughan RW, Humphrey LS: Precision and accuracy of intraoperative temperature monitoring, *Anesth Analg* 62:211, 1983.

197. Schmied H, Kurz A, Sessler DI, et al: Mild hypothermia increases blood loss and transfusion requirements during total hip arthroplasty, *Lancet* 347:289, 1996.

198. Frank SM, Fleisher LA, Breslow MJ, et al: Perioperative maintenance of normothermia reduces the incidence of morbid cardiac events: a randomized clinical trial, *JAMA* 277:1127, 1997.

199. Kurz A, Sessler DI, Lenhardt R: Perioperative normothermia to reduce the incidence of surgical-wound infection and shorten hospitalization. Study of Wound Infection and Temperature Group, *N Engl J Med* 334:1209, 1996.

200. Wallace CT, Marks WE Jr, Adkins WY, et al: Perforation of the tympanic membrane: a complication of tympanic thermometry during anesthesia, *Anesthesiology* 41:290, 1974.

201. Kahn RA, Slogoff FB, Reich DL, et al: Transcranial Doppler ultrasonography: what is its role in cardiac and vascular surgical patients? *J Cardiothorac Vasc Anesth* 9:589, 1995.

202. Robertson CS, Cormio M: Cerebral metabolic management, *New Horiz* 3:410, 1995.

203. Mahla ME: The electroencephalogram in the operating room, *Semin Anesth* 16:3, 1997.

204. Muzzi D, Cucchiara RF: Brain monitoring with the electroencephalogram, *Semin Anesth* 8:93, 1989.

205. Rampil IJ, Matteo RS: Changes in EEG spectral edge frequency correlate with the hemodynamic response to laryngoscopy and intubation, *Anesthesiology* 67:139, 1987.

206. Dwyer RC, Rampil IJ, Eger EI II: The electroencephalogram does not predict depth of isoflurane anesthesia, *Anesthesiology* 81:403, 1994.

207. Mori K: The EEG and awareness during anaesthesia, *Anaesthesia* 42:1153, 1987.

208. Sigl JC, Chamoun NG: An introduction to bispectral analysis for the electroencephalogram, *J Clin Monit* 10:392, 1994.

209. Kearse LA, Rosow C, Zaslavsky A, et al: Bispectral analysis of the electroencephalogram predicts conscious processing of information during propofol sedation and hypnosis, *Anesthesiology* 88:25, 1998.

210. Glass PS, Bloom M, Kearse L, et al: Bispectral analysis measures sedation and memory effects of propofol, midazolam, isoflurane, and alfentanil in healthy volunteers, *Anesthesiology* 86:836, 1997.
211. Michenfelder JD: A valid demonstration of barbiturate-induced brain protection in man—at last, *Anesthesiology* 64:140, 1986.
212. Abramson NS: Randomized clinical study of thiopental loading in comatose survivors of cardiac arrest, *N Engl J Med* 314:397, 1986.
213. Nussmeier NA, Arlund C, Slogoff S: Neuropsychiatric complications after cardiopulmonary bypass: cerebral protection by a barbiturate, *Anesthesiology* 64:165, 1986.
214. Chemtob GA, Kearse LA Jr: The use of electroencephalography in carotid endarterectomy, *Int Anesthesiol Clin* 28:143, 1990.
215. Nicholas JF, Samra SK: Sensory evoked potentials, *Semin Anesth* 16:14, 1997.
216. Gugino V, Chabot RJ: Somatosensory evoked potentials, *Int Anesthesiol Clin* 28:154, 1990.
217. Kalkman CJ: Motor evoked potentials, *Semin Anesth* 16:28, 1997.
218. Cahalan MK, Litt L, Botvinick EH, et al: Advances in noninvasive cardiovascular imaging: implications for the anesthesiologist, *Anesthesiology* 66:356, 1987.
219. Daniel WG, Mugge A: Transesophageal echocardiography, *N Engl J Med* 332:1268, 1995.
220. Joffe II, Jacobs LE, Lampert C, et al: Role of echocardiography in perioperative management of patients undergoing open heart surgery, *Am Heart J* 131:162, 1996.
221. Sarier KK, Konstadt SN: Echocardiography for the anesthesiologist, *Int Anesthesiol Clin* 34:57, 1996.
222. Task Force on Perioperative Transesophageal Echocardiography: Practice guidelines for perioperative transesophageal echocardiography: a report by the American Society of Anesthesiologists and the Society of Cardiovascular Anesthesiologists Task Force of Transesophageal Echocardiography, *Anesthesiology* 84:986, 1996.
223. Clements FM, de Bruijn NP: Perioperative evaluation of regional wall motion by transesophageal two-dimensional echocardiography, *Anesth Analg* 66:249, 1987.
224. Smith JS, Cahalan MK, Benefiel DJ, et al: Intraoperative detection of myocardial ischemia in high-risk patients: electrocardiography versus two-dimensional transesophageal echocardiography, *Circulation* 72:1015, 1985.
225. Seeberger MD, Cahalan MK, Rouine-Rapp K, et al: Acute hypovolemia may cause segmental wall motion abnormalities in the absence of myocardial ischemia, *Anesth Analg* 85:1252, 1997.
226. Weinger MB, Herndon OW, Gaba DM: The effect of electronic record keeping and transesophageal echocardiography on task distribution, workload, and vigilance during cardiac anesthesia, *Anesthesiology* 87:144, 1997.

PART TWO

The Causes of Systemic Complications

Chapter 10

Causes and Consequences of Impaired Gas Exchange

Thomas J. Gal

I. **Overall Gas Exchange**
   A. Carbon Dioxide Elimination
     1. Fundamental determinants of carbon dioxide tensions
     2. Causes of hypercapnia
       a. Hypercapnia with normal lung function
       b. Hypercapnia with impaired lung function
     3. Physiologic consequences of abnormal carbon dioxide tensions
       a. Hypercapnia
       b. Hypocapnia
   B. Oxygenation
     1. Alveolar gas composition
     2. Causes of hypoxemia
       a. Normal lung function
       b. Abnormal lung function
     3. Physiologic consequences of hypoxemia
II. **Impaired Gas Exchange Associated with Anesthesia**
   A. Alterations in Respiratory Mechanics
   B. Alterations in Intrapulmonary Gas Distribution
     1. Further alterations in the intrapulmonary distribution of ventilation in the lateral position
   C. Inhibition of Hypoxic Pulmonary Vasoconstriction
   D. Alterations in the Control of Breathing

     1. Carbon dioxide sensitivity
     2. Sensitivity to hypoxia
     3. Response to acidosis
     4. Ventilatory indices of chemosensitivity
       a. Carbon dioxide response
       b. Hypoxic response
     5. Effects of anesthetics on respiratory control
       a. Inhaled anesthetics
       b. Intravenous agents
III. **Other Contributing Causes of Impaired Gas Exchange**
   A. Pulmonary Edema
   B. Pulmonary Embolism
   C. Bronchospasm
   D. Pulmonary Aspiration of Gastric Contents
   E. Pneumothorax
   F. Influence of Chronic Disease States on Gas Exchange
     1. Cardiac disease
     2. Renal disease
     3. Hepatic disease
     4. Obesity
     5. Pulmonary disease
       a. Restrictive disease
       b. Obstructive disease

Abnormalities of gas exchange are reflected by the gas composition of the arterial blood. This composition is expressed as a weighted average of all the gas-exchanging units in the lungs. In the blood leaving each alveolus, the oxygen (O_2) and carbon dioxide (CO_2) tensions depend on the composition of the alveolar gas and the efficiency with which the incoming pulmonary blood flow equilibrates. Anesthetic drugs and techniques appear to significantly alter this process, and the effects are often further compounded by preexisting disease and other acute events. The purpose of this discussion is to provide some insight into the nature and mechanism of the alterations in normal gas exchange and to examine some of the physiologic consequences.

I. OVERALL GAS EXCHANGE
A. Carbon dioxide elimination

1. Fundamental determinants of carbon dioxide tensions. The CO_2 removed by alveolar ventilation is constantly added to the alveolar gas from the pulmonary cir-

culation. The CO_2 tension in the arterial blood (Pa_{CO_2}) is the net result of the balance between the metabolic rate of CO_2 production by body tissues ($\dot{V}_{CO_2}$) and the rate at which the lungs excrete CO_2 via alveolar ventilation ($\dot{V}_A$). Pa_{CO_2} is directly proportional to $\dot{V}_{CO_2}$ and inversely proportional to $\dot{V}_A$. This relationship can be expressed as

$$Pa_{CO_2} = K \times \dot{V}_{CO_2}/\dot{V}_A$$

The proportional constant *(K)* is equal to 0.863 when $\dot{V}_{CO_2}$ is expressed in milliliters per minute as a dry gas at standard temperature and pressure (STPD) and $\dot{V}_A$ is expressed in liters per minute as a saturated gas at body temperature and pressure (BTPS). The *K* value allows simultaneous conversion of concentration to partial pressure and corrects for units that conventionally express the gas volumes.

This equation simply states that under the ideal conditions of a steady state, the CO_2 output is matched by the alveolar ventilation. If $\dot{V}_A$ is depressed for some reason,

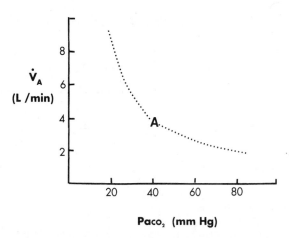

Fig. 10-1. CO_2 excretion hyperbola describing the reciprocal relationship between alveolar ventilation $(\dot{V}_A)$ and arterial CO_2 tension (Pa_{CO_2}). The curve assumes a constant CO_2 production. Under normal resting conditions the relationship lies at point *A*. (From Gal TJ: Respiratory physiology during anesthesia. In Kaplan JA, ed: *Thoracic anesthesia,* ed 2, New York, 1990, Churchill Livingstone.)

Pa_{CO_2} must rise in proportion to this decrease in $\dot{V}_A$. This inverse relationship between $\dot{V}_A$ and Pa_{CO_2} is described by a rectangular hyperbola (Fig. 10-1). In many clinical settings, however, this simple relationship is modified by other factors that result in a rise of Pa_{CO_2} above normal (more than 46 mm Hg) to produce hypercapnia.

2. Causes of hypercapnia

a. Hypercapnia with normal lung function. Endogenous CO_2 production may increase with such conditions as fever, sepsis, seizures, hyperthyroidism, and total parenteral nutrition with a very high glucose intake.[1] Unless ventilation is increased accordingly, CO_2 elevations may occur in such patients.

Occasionally, nonmetabolic sources for CO_2 may be present. For example, an increase in Pa_{CO_2} may be observed following CO_2 instillation for laparoscopy. Similarly, transient elevations in Pa_{CO_2} occur after administration of sodium bicarbonate if ventilation is not allowed to increase.[2] More common and perhaps more dangerous is an increased CO_2 in the inspired gas. Whether this results from anesthetic mishaps such as failure of soda lime absorber, incompetent values in the circle system, or merely from breathing in confined spaces, a new steady state will be achieved. This new Pa_{CO_2} will be defined by the quantity of CO_2 in the inspired air, the CO_2 generated by metabolism, and the relative changes in alveolar ventilation.

How the system responds to a decrease in alveolar ventilation is a crucial determinant of how adequately CO_2 is eliminated. Alveolar hypoventilation may result in hypercapnia whether or not respiratory system disease is present. The responsiveness of the respiratory control system to CO_2 is an important determinant of Pa_{CO_2}. This respiratory controller is affected by a wide variety of disease states and drugs. These are discussed in more detail later in the chapter. Signals arising in the respiratory

controller must produce a response in the respiratory system bellows. If the respiratory muscles are weak or easily fatigued, the respiratory drive will not be translated into adequate ventilation. Similarly, if the muscles must overcome an increased mechanical workload because of decreased compliance or increased resistance of the respiratory system, CO_2 retention may occur also.

b. Hypercapnia with impaired lung function. Retention of carbon dioxide occurs more commonly when there is disturbance of the gas exchange function of the lung. Net effective alveolar ventilation can be decreased even if total ventilation is increased. This situation results either because significant portions of the lung are not perfused and function as a dead space or disease is severe enough to significantly affect the matching of ventilation and perfusion.

The alveolar ventilation, which determines Pa_{CO_2}, cannot be measured directly but must be derived from another volume, the minute volume ($\dot{V}_E$). The alveolar ventilation differs from this volume of air, which moves in and out of the lungs each minute by an amount of gas that does not participate in the exchange of CO_2 with the blood. This volume of gas is usually called the physiologic dead space. However, some have preferred to call this wasted ventilation because this portion of each breath is literally wasted with respect to its contribution to gas exchange.

A portion of this dead space gas is contained in the conducting airways from the mouth and nose down to the terminal bronchioles and is called the anatomic dead space. In a normal adult, this consists of about one third the volume of each breath. The anatomic dead space (V_D) is larger in males than females presumably because of body size and lung volume. The anatomic V_D is larger in older men than younger men because of the increase in end-expiratory lung volume (functional residual capacity [FRC]) seen with advancing age. In general, anatomic V_D is affected by changes in airway caliber and increased with increasing lung volume. The average increase appears to be 2 to 3 ml per 100-ml lung volume increase.[3] Other factors that influence the size of the upper airway affect V_D. These include positioning of the neck and jaw and the presence of artificial oral airways. Finally, tracheal intubation, which decreases the volume of the upper airway, and tracheostomy, which bypasses the upper airway, also decrease anatomic V_D.

The other portion of the physiologic dead space, the alveolar dead space, may be defined as the part of the inspired gas that passes through the conducting airways to mix with gas at the alveolar level but does not actively participate in gas exchange. The alveolar dead space results from a lack of effective perfusion of the airspaces to which inspired gas is distributed. Factors such as reduced cardiac output, hypovolemia, hypotension, and pulmonary embolism tend to reduce pulmonary blood flow. Thus they increase the alveolar dead space fraction and impair CO_2 excretion.

The sum of the combined anatomic and alveolar components, the physiologic dead space, cannot be measured directly but can be calculated from CO_2 tensions in simultaneously collected samples of mixed expired air (Pe_{CO_2}) and arterial blood (Pa_{CO_2}). The formula used to calculate the fraction of wasted ventilation per breath or, more specifically, the ratio of physiologic dead space (V_D) to tidal volume (V_T) is a modification of the classic Bohr equation proposed by Enghoff. In this equation alveolar CO_2 tension (PA_{CO_2}) is replaced by Pa_{CO_2}. The expired gas is a mixture of dead space gas and that from the gas-exchanging compartment. Because dead space gas contains essentially no CO_2, the quantity of CO_2 expired should come entirely from the gas-exchanging compartment.

$$V_T \times P_{ECO_2} = (V_T - V_D) \times Pa_{CO_2}$$

Amount of CO_2 Amount expired from
expired   gas-exchanging compartment

By solving for V_D/V_T this can be expressed as

$$\frac{V_D}{V_T} = \frac{Pa_{CO_2} - P_{ECO_2}}{Pa_{CO_2}}$$

Typical values for V_D/V_T in healthy subjects are about 0.30, so that nearly one third of the inspired V_T does not participate in gas exchange. In diseased lungs, V_D/V_T increases and values greater than 0.75 may be observed.

The concept of dead space (V_D) and ventilation-perfusion ($\dot{V}_A/\dot{Q}$) mismatch involves a continuum in which V_D implies the most extreme mismatch in which the $\dot{V}_A/\dot{Q}$ ratio reaches infinity. If such a large increase in $\dot{V}_A/\dot{Q}$ mismatch cannot be compensated for by increasing ventilation, Pa_{CO_2} will necessarily rise. A less common malfunction of CO_2 excretion results when large areas of right-to-left shunt and low $\dot{V}_A/\dot{Q}$ areas are present. Here the CO_2 in mixed venous blood enters the arterial system without the opportunity for excretion via a ventilated alveolus. Again, ventilation must increase to compensate for this inefficiency in CO_2 excretion.

Hypercapnic patients with chronic obstructive pulmonary disease (COPD) tend to breathe more rapidly and shallowly than their normocapnic counterparts. The shallow breathing pattern with reduced tidal volumes does not reflect a reduced neural drive to breathe. The tidal volume is reduced primarily by a decreased inspiratory time associated with the rapid rates. This appears to be related largely to the sense of inspiratory effort. As breathing effort increases, the sensation of excessive effort by the respiratory center causes a reduction in the size of each breath. Although the shallower breaths avoid the sensation of effort and dyspnea and prevent fatigue, they do not provide for adequate gas exchange, and arterial CO_2 tension usually increases. The end point of respiratory failure is commonly believed to result from fatigue of the respiratory muscles. Rather than the result of fatigue, hypercapnia provides patients with COPD with an economical breathing strategy to eliminate CO_2 using far less energy than their normocapnic counterparts.[4]

3. Physiologic consequences of abnormal carbon dioxide tensions

a. Hypercapnia. There are no specific clinical diagnostic signs of hypercapnia. The varied signs and symptoms include headache, nausea, sweating, flushing, restlessness, tachypnea with marked hypercapnia (more than 90 mm Hg), and unconsciousness. These reflect the actions of CO_2 on the respiratory cardiovascular and central nervous system (CNS) functions.

Whenever CO_2 elimination is less than its production, Pa_{CO_2} increases. When a new Pa_{CO_2} steady state occurs, CO_2 excretion must equal production. If the ventilatory response to CO_2 (increased $\dot{V}_E$) is insufficient, Pa_{CO_2} will continue to rise further until severe hypercapnia (Pa_{CO_2} above 90 mm Hg) ensues and depresses respiration. The ventilatory response to CO_2, so characteristic in the awake patient, is blunted but not completely eliminated during general anesthesia.

Hypercapnia may affect respiratory gas exchange by its mild effect on pulmonary vasoconstriction[5] or by depression of diaphragmatic function.[6] In addition, the reduced alveolar ventilation associated with increased Pa_{CO_2} may be inadequate to deliver oxygen to the alveoli to replace that taken off by the pulmonary blood flow. Thus the oxygen tension in the alveoli (PA_{O_2}) decreases and in turn reduces Pa_{O_2}. This secondary effect of hypercapnia is also associated with a shift of the oxyhemoglobin dissociation curve to the right. The rightward shift further decreases oxygen saturation at any given Pa_{O_2}. However, this decreased affinity of hemoglobin for oxygen does facilitate unloading of oxygen from blood to tissues at a higher Pa_{O_2}.

Many of the circulatory effects of hypercapnia appear to enhance oxygen delivery and CO_2 removal at the tissue level. The direct effect of CO_2 and the accompanying acidosis on the heart and blood vessels is to depress the function of smooth and cardiac muscle. The result is decreased cardiac contractility and, in most vascular beds, vasodilation. The one exception is the pulmonary circulation, which tends to constrict.

In healthy people the direct effects of CO_2 are modified by those of central sympathetic stimulation, which result in tachycardia, mild hypertension, and increased myocardial contractility. With disease states that depress autonomic responsiveness and with most anesthetics, most of this sympathetic stimulation is suppressed and the direct depressant effects of acidosis on the tissues are manifest.

Hypercapnia affects CNS function by its stimulating effect on breathing. The excess CO_2 also acts on the CNS vascular bed to produce vasodilation. In the presence of cerebral pathology, the vasodilation within the closed cranial space may produce dangerous increases in intracranial pressure. Higher CO_2 tensions depress general neuronal activity and produce a state of unconsciousness not unlike that of general anesthesia.

b. Hypocapnia. Alveolar hyperventilation from any cause results in decreased CO_2 tension (hypocapnia). This hypocapnia may decrease cardiac output by decreasing sympathetic activity, ionized calcium, or coronary blood flow. At the same time, a leftward shift of the oxyhemoglobin dissociation curve (increased affinity for O_2) results in reduced ability to give up O_2 at the tissue level. This necessitates an increased cardiac output to maintain the same rate of O_2 delivery. Vasoconstriction of cerebral and spinal cord vessels may also have undesirable effects. To add to this, hypocapnia may further increase oxygen consumption in the face of a decreased tissue oxygen supply.

Hypocapnia also decreases ionized calcium and serum potassium concentrations. The latter, for example, changes about 1.5 mEq/L with each 10 mm Hg change in $PaCO_2$ as a result of altered potassium distribution between intracellular and extracellular spaces.[7]

Further abnormalities in gas exchange may result from reductions in CO_2 tension. Disturbances in $\dot{V}/\dot{Q}$ matching may develop if hypocapnia inhibits hypoxic pulmonary vasoconstriction (HPV). Local increases in airway resistance may also occur in normal patients and those with lung disease.[8] This bronchoconstriction appears to be a response to the reduction in alveolar CO_2 tension, which is analogous to the vascular response to reduced alveolar O_2 tension.

Some of the physiologic impact of hypocapnia relates to the difference in time course for CO_2 concentrations associated with acute hyperventilation as opposed to hypoventilation. The $PaCO_2$ tends to decrease far more rapidly during hyperventilation than does a similar increase in $PaCO_2$ during hypoventilation. Following hyperventilation, 50% of the decrease in $PaCO_2$ occurs in about 3 minutes, whereas a 50% increase in $PaCO_2$ takes nearly 20 minutes to occur following a decrease in ventilation. During complete apnea, $PaCO_2$ rises 8 to 15 mm Hg in the first minute or so and exhibits a subsequent linear increase of about 3 mm Hg/min.

B. Oxygenation

Whenever the supply of oxygen to the tissue does not meet metabolic demands, hypoxia results. Hypoxia has been variously subdivided into hypoxic, stagnant, anemic, and histotoxic types. Stagnant hypoxia is produced when blood flow to the tissues is reduced, whereas anemic hypoxia results from a decreased oxygen-carrying capacity because of low hemoglobin or binding of hemoglobin with other substances (e.g., carbon monoxide). If the cell is unable to use oxygen to produce energy, the term *histotoxic hypoxia* is applied. Such hypoxia can result from cyanide toxicity and, unlike the other forms of hypoxia, is characterized by an increase in mixed venous oxygen tension because tissues cannot use the oxygen presented to them.

By far, the most common variant of hypoxia encountered clinically is hypoxic hypoxia. This is associated with an abnormally low arterial oxygen tension (PaO_2), which is called hypoxemia. The causes of hypoxemia are many and varied and must take into account factors such as inspired O_2 concentration, alveolar CO_2 tension, barometric pressure, patient age, and the presence of lung disease.

1. Alveolar gas composition. The alveolar gas content is influenced by the matching of ventilation and blood flow and by the composition of the mixed venous blood. First and foremost, however, the composition of gas in the alveoli depends on the content of the inspired gas. The partial pressure of each gas in this inspired mixture is proportional to the fractional concentration of the gas. As gases enter the respiratory tract, they are warmed to body temperature and humidified. Thus it is necessary to take into account the partial pressure exerted by water vapor (PH_2O) at body temperature, which is usually 47 mm Hg. Thus the fraction concentration of oxygen in the inspired air (FIO_2), which is expressed as a dry gas, can be used to calculate the inspired oxygen tension (PIO_2) within the trachea:

$$PIO_2 = FIO_2(P_B - 47) \text{ mm Hg}$$

Table 10-1. Typical partial pressures (mm Hg) for respiratory gases during normal air breathing ($FIO_2 = 0.2$)

	Atmosphere	Trachea	Alveoli
O_2	150	150	100
CO_2	0	0	40
H_2O^*	20	47	47
N_2	590	563	573
Total	760	760	760

*Water vapor pressure varies with relative humidity and ambient temperature. Partial pressures of oxygen (PO_2) and nitrogen (PN_2) change accordingly.

For clinical purposes, it is sufficient to use the standard barometric pressure (P_B) at sea level, 760 mm Hg, to calculate PIO_2. Thus in a subject breathing room air,

$$PIO_2 = 0.21(760 - 47) = 150 \text{ mm Hg}$$

There are differences in gas composition between ambient air and that in the trachea and the alveoli. The total pressure of gas in the trachea and alveoli is equal to the atmospheric pressure (Table 10-1). Because there is no exchange of nitrogen within the respiratory tract, the partial pressure of nitrogen is the same in the alveoli and trachea. However, the oxygen tension in the alveoli (PAO_2) will be less than the PIO_2 in the trachea because CO_2 is added to the alveoli from mixed venous blood. The PAO_2 therefore differs from the PIO_2 by an amount directly related to the quantity of CO_2 added. If the CO_2 volume added by the blood equals the oxygen taken up by the blood, than PAO_2 may be calculated simply as

$$PAO_2 = PIO_2 - PACO_2$$

Usually, the ratio of CO_2 produced to the O_2 consumed, the respiratory exchange ratio (R), is less than 1.0. If one assumes that R approximates 0.8 and also assumes that ideal $PACO_2$ can be estimated by arterial CO_2 tension ($PaCO_2$), the alveolar gas equation can be simplified for clinical uses as

$$PAO_2 = PIO_2 - PaCO_2/0.8$$

2. Causes of hypoxemia
a. Normal lung function. When there is no impairment of lung function, hypoxemia may result from a variety of factors that include low inspired O_2 concentration (FIO_2), hypoventilation, decreased cardiac output, increased oxygen consumption, a shift in the O_2 hemoglobin dissociation curve, and decreased hemoglobin concentration. By far, the most dangerous but easily correctable cause of hypoxemia is a low FIO_2. Any decrease in inspired O_2 concentration below that of normal ambient air results in hypoxemia. The alveolar oxygen tension is increased or decreased by an amount determined by the PO_2 of the inspired gas if other factors remain constant. The alveolar-to-arterial O_2 difference $P(A-a)O_2$ however, is not increased.

The PAO_2 can also be decreased by a diminished alveolar ventilation, whether caused by airway obstruction or drug-induced depression of breathing. The simplified alveolar air equation suggests that as CO_2 tension in-

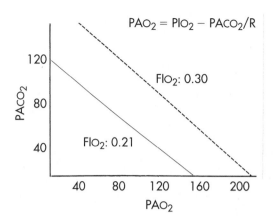

Fig. 10-2. O_2 and CO_2 diagram based on the simplified alveolar air equation for ambient air ($FIO_2 = 0.21$). Values at sea level (atmospheric pressure = 760 mm) are indicated by the solid line and those for an enriched O_2 mixture ($FIO_2 = 0.30$) are indicated by the dotted line. An R value of 0.8 was used to calculate both lines.

creases, PAO_2 will decrease by a similar amount. Thus unless FIO_2 is increased above 0.21, hypoxemia can result from hypoventilation. Again, as in the case of decreased FIO_2, the $P(A-a)O_2$ will not increase.

The effect of increasing FIO_2 from 0.1 to 0.30 is shown in Fig. 10-2. It is apparent that at high $PACO_2$ values (90 mm Hg) associated with marked hypoventilation but not apnea, an FIO_2 of 0.30 will provide a safe PAO_2 to avoid the hypoxemia that would occur with room air (0.21), assuming a normal $P(A-a)O_2$. The improvement in PAO_2 at any ventilation or $PACO_2$ is about 64 mm Hg. Thus at the high $PACO_2$ associated with marked hypoventilation, an FIO_2 of 0.30 appears to be the maximum O_2 concentration required to correct the hypoxemia present with the ambient air.

PAO_2 can be influenced by a decrease in cardiac output, which, in the absence of other changes, may temporarily increase PAO_2 because less blood flows through the lungs to remove O_2 from the alveolar gas. More important, the reduced cardiac output is associated with increased tissue O_2 extraction, which results in a reduced O_2 content in the mixed venous blood. As the blood passes through the lungs with its reduced O_2 content, the resultant PaO_2 is lower than that with a normal cardiac output. Abnormal O_2 transport because of decreased hemoglobin concentration or rightward shifts of the oxyhemoglobin dissociation curve and increased metabolic rate also can lead to increased O_2 extraction by tissues and a similar reduction in mixed venous arterial oxygen tensions.

b. Abnormal lung function. When hypoxemia occurs in the presence of a normal or increased PAO_2, it can result only from disturbances in the normal gas exchange function of the lung. This interference with the lung's ability to oxygenate blood consists of three basic abnormalities:
- Diffusion: an impaired movement of gas (O_2) from alveolus to capillary
- Shunt: the presence of channels (extrapulmonary and pulmonary) that allow venous blood to bypass the normal gas exchange units in the lung

- Ventilation-perfusion mismatch: poor matching of blood and gas at the alveolar level

(1) DIFFUSION ABNORMALITY. Normally O_2 and CO_2 equilibrate between blood and gas phases in far less time than it takes the red cells to traverse the pulmonary capillary network. Thus diffusion limitation plays a very small role in normal gas exchange at rest unless FIO_2 is reduced, as at high altitude. During vigorous exercise, however, some patients can develop a decreased PaO_2 because the increased velocity of blood flow through the pulmonary capillaries shortens the time available for diffusion equilibrium. Although this abnormal diffusion can be caused by thickening of the air-blood interface (alveolar-capillary block), it more commonly results from a reduction in pulmonary capillary blood volume. The latter state differs from the thickened membrane in that as capillaries are destroyed or obstructed, others are recruited and the flow velocity through these remaining vessels increases. Thus with severe disease (e.g., emphysema) the time available for gas exchange at rest may be as short as with exercise, and equilibration of gas fails to occur adequately. This failure can be offset easily by increasing the driving pressure for O_2 (i.e., the PAO_2) with oxygen-enriched mixtures.

(2) SHUNTS. Another interference with ideal gas exchange occurs in the form of right-to-left shunts. Normally, a small amount of venous blood bypasses the right ventricle and empties directly into the left atrium. The anatomic shunt represents venous return from pleural, bronchial, and thebesian veins, accounting for as much as 5% of total cardiac output. Right-to-left shunts of greater magnitude occur with cyanotic congenital heart disease.

In addition to these discrete anatomic pathways, a shunt effect may be produced by normal vessels that perfuse areas of lung that are not ventilated because the airways are closed or the conducting airways are obstructed. The term *shunt effect* or *venous admixture* is generally applied to these lung units, whose ventilation is maximally decreased (but some ventilation is still present) compared to the amount of perfusion. The venous admixture is manifest clinically by hypoxemia, which is responsive to increased inspired O_2 concentration. In diseases associated with major areas of lung without ventilation (absolute shunt) or in the case of the anatomic shunts, the hypoxemia is refractory to O_2 administration.

(3) VENTILATION-PERFUSION IMBALANCE. The distribution of ventilation and pulmonary blood flow is neither uniform nor proportionate, even in normal lungs. This nonuniform distribution or $\dot{V}_A/\dot{Q}$ results in impaired gas exchange. The primary effect of $\dot{V}_A/\dot{Q}$ mismatch is an impairment of oxygenation. The high PaO_2 of lung regions with high $\dot{V}_A/\dot{Q}$ ratios produces only a minimal increase in the O_2 content of the blood because of the flat oxyhemoglobin dissociation curve in that range of partial pressures. Hence, these areas are unable to compensate for regions with low $\dot{V}_A/\dot{Q}$ values. CO_2 elimination is also impaired by $\dot{V}_A/\dot{Q}$ mismatching, but the elevated CO_2 stimulates ventilation. Because the CO_2 dissociation curve is nearly linear in the physiologic range, this increased ventilation is able to compensate for low $\dot{V}_A/\dot{Q}$ areas and maintain CO_2 near normal concen-

trations. With severe $\dot{V}_A/\dot{Q}$ mismatch or impaired ability to increase ventilation, this compensation is inadequate to avoid an increase in CO_2.

3. Physiologic consequences of hypoxemia. Foremost among the clinical manifestations of hypoxemia is cyanosis, which marks the presence of a significant amount of desaturated hemoglobin (usually more than 5 g/100 ml). Although rather subjective, cyanosis usually is observed with hemoglobin saturations less than 85%. This is usually associated with a PaO_2 of 45 to 50 mm Hg in the adult; in the infant, because of the leftward shift of the oxyhemoglobin dissociation curve, it may correspond to a PaO_2 of 35 to 40 mm Hg. Cyanosis may be apparent without actual hypoxemia, as in methemoglobinemia and sulfhemoglobinemia, and, conversely, may not be apparent in the presence of anemia or intense peripheral vasoconstriction. Thus the diagnosis of hypoxemia is established with certainty only when O_2 saturation or PaO_2 is measured.

Hypoxemia is associated with an increased minute ventilation, largely through an increased respiratory rate. The brisk response to low PaO_2 resides in the carotid bodies and is very sensitive to the depressive effects of the volatile anesthetics. These anesthetics exert a similar blunting effect on the circulatory responses to hypoxia. The latter responses also appear to be mediated via the carotid bodies. The circulatory compensation to hypoxia acts to redistribute blood flow and maintain arterial pressure. The aim is to increase the quantity of O_2 carried to important tissues and consists largely of an increased heart rate and cardiac output with vasodilation in brain and heart while the muscle beds and splanchnic circulation undergo constriction.

Ultimately, the consequences of hypoxia manifest themselves by a disruption of the function of all major organ systems. The cerebral cortex, which begins to cease function after about 30 seconds of hypoxia, may suffer irreversible damage after 5 minutes. Cardiac function takes about 5 minutes to cease functioning and experiences tissue death after about 10 minutes.

II. IMPAIRED GAS EXCHANGE ASSOCIATED WITH ANESTHESIA

The abnormal pulmonary gas exchange associated with general anesthesia is manifested by an increased alveolar-arterial O_2 tension difference and an increase in arterial –end-tidal CO_2 tension gradient. The impaired oxygenation and, to some extent, the CO_2 elimination appear to reflect an increased $\dot{V}_A/\dot{Q}$ mismatch, right-to-left intrapulmonary shunting, and an increase in alveolar dead space. All of these changes tend to be increased substantially in the presence of preexisting lung disease. A number of theories have been proposed to account for these changes, many based on the changes in respiratory mechanics associated with general anesthesia. Foremost among these are the reduction in FRC and alterations in the distribution of ventilation.

A. Alterations in respiratory mechanics

General anesthesia affects the static (pressure-volume) and dynamic (pressure-flow) behavior of the respiratory system. These mechanical effects have interested clinicians and investigators because of their potential contribution to the impaired gas exchange so characteristic in anesthetized patients. Perhaps no facet of respiratory system behavior has received as much attention as the change in FRC. A decrease in FRC with induction of general anesthesia was first noted by Bergman.[9] Subsequent observations in supine anesthetized humans indicate that FRC is reduced an average of about 500 ml or 15% to 20% of the awake value.[10] The decreased volume is similar in magnitude to that observed when subjects go from erect to recumbent position. The magnitude of FRC reduction appears to be related to age and body habitus (i.e., weight to height ratio). In fact, morbidly obese patients demonstrate a much larger decrease in FRC, to about 50% of their preanesthetic values.[11] These volumes approach near to the residual volume.

The changes in FRC occur within a minute after induction of anesthesia,[12] do not appear to progress with time, and are not further affected by addition of muscle paralysis.[13] A number of factors may contribute to the FRC reduction, but the underlying mechanisms are complex and as yet not totally clear. Some of these possibilities include atelectasis, increased expiratory muscle activity, trapping of gas in distal airways, cephalad displacement of the diaphragm, decreased outward chest wall recoil, increased lung recoil, and increases in thoracic blood volume. These are discussed in detail elsewhere.[10]

In supine subjects, the induction of general anesthesia reduces FRC such that end-expiratory volume decreases close to residual volume. This FRC may lie below the closing capacity, that is, the volume associated with dependent airway closure or, more precisely, dynamic flow limitation.[14] Early observations with halothane anesthesia suggested a correlation between the degree of impaired oxygenation and the reduction in FRC[15] and led to the hypothesis that airway closure and atelectasis were the consequences of a reduced FRC.

One important aspect of the theory of airway closure lies in the assumption that closing capacity (CC) remains the same in anesthetized and awake states. The decrease in lung compliance in the anesthetized state reflects an increased elastic recoil. As a result, one might expect a decrease in closing capacity (i.e., an increase in airway closure) with general anesthesia. Many early reports suggested no difference in closing capacity between awake and anesthetized states. However, subsequent work provided evidence that both FRC and CC are proportionately reduced with anesthesia.[16] These authors used the foreign gas bolus technique rather than the resident gas (N_2) technique used in the previous study and suggested that the latter might not adequately measure CC when lung volumes are restricted. However, an additional study found no difference when the two techniques were compared.[17] Therefore the issue of whether awake control CC values are the same as those in anesthetized subjects is not resolved.

The degree of intrapulmonary shunting does appear to correlate with the reduction in FRC[18] and with the degree of atelectasis that develops in dependent lung regions.[19] It is thus tempting to attribute such atelectasis simply to the reduced FRC. However, a study in awake supine subjects with thoracoabdominal restriction argues against this simple mechanism.[20] The restriction in these subjects reduced lung volume and altered pulmonary mechanics in a fashion similar to that seen with general anesthesia. The FRC decreased by more than 20% and was matched by a reduction of CC as measured by the resident gas (N_2) technique. No atelectasis was noted with computed tomography scanning and $\dot{V}_A/\dot{Q}$ distribution, and arterial blood gases were unchanged from the control state. Thus gas exchange in these awake subjects with chest restriction differed from that in anesthetized subjects, although they both had some relative decrement in FRC. The authors concluded that the development of compression atelectasis in the anesthetized patients cannot be ascribed solely to a decrease in FRC, nor can the changes in pulmonary mechanics with restriction be attributed solely to the development of atelectasis.

The reductions in FRC with general anesthesia have been accompanied by prompt development of densities in dependent lung regions. These have been interpreted as atelectatic areas. These areas of atelectasis have been reduced in size by phrenic nerve stimulation to increase diaphragmatic tone[21] and by the application of positive end-expiratory pressure (PEEP). Although PEEP diminished the extent of atelectasis, gas exchange was not consistently improved.[22]

On the other hand, recruitment maneuvers consisting of sustained inflation to 40 cm H_2O for 10 seconds virtually eliminated all atelectatic areas.[23] These areas remain expanded for as long as 40 minutes if the lungs are ventilated with a gas mixture containing sufficient amounts of nitrogen (more than 50%).[24] This suggests that resorption of gas plays some role both in the development and recurrences of the atelectatic lung.

B. Alterations in intrapulmonary gas distribution

Ventilation is not normally uniform throughout the lung. The effects of gravity on the lung and the forces that allow it to confirm to the shape of the thorax result in a vertical gradient of pleural pressure. The pleural pressure acting on the upper (nondependent) areas of the lung is more subatmospheric (negative) than that acting on the lower (dependent) portions. As a result, the nondependent areas are more inflated than the dependent ones (Fig. 10-3). The gradient of pleural pressure up and down the lung changes about 0.25 cm H_2O per each centimeter of height. Thus in a lung 30 cm high, a 7.5-cm H_2O pressure difference exists from apex to base. In the supine position, the dorsal areas become dependent. The height of the lungs is reduced by nearly one third; thus the gravitational effect is diminished somewhat.

Although the nondependent lung areas are more distended at FRC, a transpulmonary pressure of 5 cm generated during a normal breath produces a greater volume change or ventilation to the dependent areas (see Fig. 10-3). This is because of the sigmoid shape of the pressure-volume curve. The larger nondependent areas have a lower regional compliance; that is, they lie on a less steep portion of the pressure-volume curve.

These regional differences in ventilation are important in matching ventilation to perfusion. The dependent or basal areas tend to be better perfused because of gravitational ef-

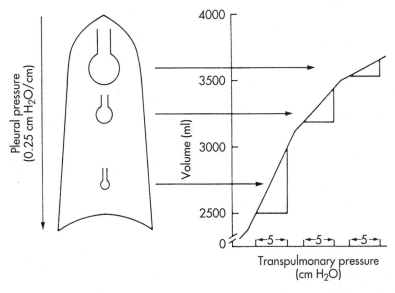

Fig. 10-3. Pleural pressure gradient increases down the lung such that the dependent alveoli are small and nondependent ones are large. A change in transpulmonary pressure of 5 cm H_2O produces a greater change in volume (or ventilation) of the small dependent air spaces because they lie on a steeper portion of the compliance or pressure-volume curve. The large nondependent alveoli lie on a flatter portion of the curve and thus undergo less volume change. (From Benumof JL: Respiration physiology and respiratory function during anesthesia. In Miller RD, ed: *Anesthesia,* ed 3, New York, 1990, Churchill Livingstone.)

Awake

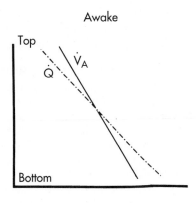

Anesthesia/paralysis

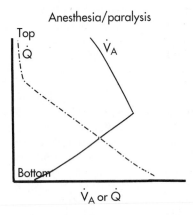

Fig. 10-4. Diagrammatic representation of the distribution of ventilation $(\dot{V}_A)$ and perfusion $(\dot{Q})$ between nondependent *(top)* lung areas and dependent *(bottom)* areas. Note that $\dot{V}_A$ tends to be distributed more uniformly from top to bottom in the anesthetized paralyzed state. (From Gal TJ: Respiratory physiology during anesthesia. In Kaplan JA, ed: *Thoracic anesthesia*, ed 2, New York, 1990, Churchill Livingstone.)

fects. Because the bases are also better ventilated, there is good matching of ventilation and perfusion (Fig. 10-4); that is, both higher ventilation and blood flow are delivered to the bases. In supine anesthetized paralyzed humans, the ventilation or distribution of inspired gas becomes more uniform from top to bottom lung areas (see Fig. 10-4), largely because basal lung units undergo further reduction in size to a point that reduces their regional compliance. Anesthetics, meanwhile, produce a decrease in pulmonary artery pressure that impedes perfusion of nondependent lung regions. Increased alveolar pressures with mechanical ventilation further interfere with perfusion of nondependent areas. Thus dependent lung areas are well perfused but poorly ventilated. In contrast, nondependent areas receive more ventilation but considerably less perfusion.

In addition to changes in static lung mechanics, the overall $\dot{V}_A/\dot{Q}$ in homogeneity may also be increased during anesthesia because of changes in dynamics (i.e., the pressure-flow relationship in the airways). The smooth muscle relaxation associated with anesthetics may be use-

ful in preventing the increased bronchial tone associated with bronchospasm. However, the reductions in normal bronchomotor tone may interfere with the normal $\dot{V}_A/\dot{Q}$ matching and thus impair gas exchange.[25]

In addition, local decreases in alveolar CO_2 tension improve the normal $\dot{V}_A/\dot{Q}$ matching by producing local increases in bronchomotor tone. In a sense, this hypocapnic bronchoconstriction is analogous to HPV. Whether the inhaled anesthetics as a group block this bronchoconstriction induced by hypocapnia is not known. Thus far, only halothane has been shown to reduce this bronchoconstrictive effect of hypocapnia.[26,27]

1. Further alterations in the intrapulmonary distribution of ventilation in the lateral position. Subjects lying in the lateral decubitus position exhibit a greater blood flow to the dependent lung, largely because of gravitational effects. In the awake state, the normal vertical gradient of pleural pressure also allows for greater ventilation of the same dependent lung and maintenance of normal $\dot{V}_A/\dot{Q}$ distribution. This is more true in the case of the larger right lung, which is not subject to compression by an enlarged heart. In fact, in normal persons with unilateral lung disease, respiratory gas exchange is optimal if the good lung is dependent.[28,29] Exceptions appear to occur in infants with chronic obstructive pulmonary disease. In these groups, the nondependent lung appears to be better ventilated.[30,31]

Radiographic and bronchospirometric studies show that the dependent lung normally receives a greater ventilation and has a higher O_2 uptake in the lateral position. Although its FRC is lower than that of the nondependent lung, N_2 washout is also more rapid.[32] When patients are anesthetized in the lateral position, as for thoracic surgery, distribution of the pulmonary blood flow is similar to that of the awake state; that is, the dependent lung receives greater perfusion. However, the greater portion of ventilation is switched from the dependent lung to the nondependent lung. In a sense, the ventilation is more uniform, and this is reflected in more equal N_2 clearance for each lung.[32] This shift in distribution of ventilation results from a loss of lung volume (decreased FRC), which is shared but unequally by both lungs. The dependent lung that undergoes a greater decrease in FRC moves to a less steep portion near the bottom of the pressure-volume curve (see Fig. 10-3). While the nondependent lung moves from a flat portion to a steeper one, the abdominal contents, as well as the mediastinum, also impede dependent lung expansion. Thus the anesthetized patient in the lateral position has a nondependent lung that is well ventilated but poorly perfused. In contrast, the well-perfused dependent lung is poorly ventilated. Opening the chest may only increase the overventilation of the nondependent lung.

In summary, the increased $\dot{V}_A/\dot{Q}$ mismatching that accompanies anesthesia and paralysis, whether in the supine or lateral positions, seems to be largely a result of altered distribution of ventilation with a relative failure of intrapulmonary perfusion to adjust.[33] Although some of this failure of blood flow to adjust for the altered ventilation may relate to inhibition of HPV by the inhaled

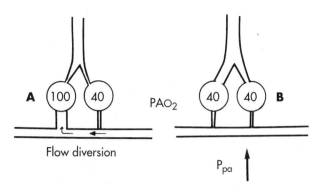

PAO_2

Flow diversion

P_{pa}

Fig. 10-5. Changes in pulmonary artery pressure *(P_{pa})* and diversion of blood flow are depicted for localized hypoxia **(A)** and for diffuse or generalized hypoxia **(B)**. (From Gal TJ: *Respiratory physiology in anesthetic practice,* Baltimore, 1991, Williams & Wilkins.)

anesthetics, the altered pattern of expansion of the lung with anesthesia and paralysis may also affect the distribution of blood flow along with ventilation.

C. Inhibition of hypoxic pulmonary vasoconstriction

In the systemic vascular beds, hypoxia produces vasodilation in order to aid oxygen delivery and carbon dioxide removal. The pulmonary vessels, on the other hand, respond to acute hypoxia by constriction. This unique behavior in response to hypoxia is called hypoxic pulmonary vasoconstriction (HPV). This response is an important compensatory mechanism that diverts flow away from hypoxic alveoli. Blood flow shifts from poorly ventilated alveoli to better ventilated ones in order to match ventilation and perfusion and minimize hypoxemia.

The physiologic manifestations of HPV depend heavily on the size of the lung area that is hypoxic. If the segment of hypoxic lung is small, HPV will result in diversion of flow away from the hypoxic area and little or no change in pulmonary artery pressure (Fig. 10-5, *A*). If the hypoxic area is very large or if the alveolar hypoxia is diffuse and generalized, flow cannot be diverted and the vasoconstriction results in an increased pulmonary artery pressure (Fig. 10-5, *B*). Thus for flow diversion to occur the hypoxic segment must comprise a small fraction of the total lung; that is, flow diversion is inversely related to the size of the hypoxic segment. The increases in pulmonary artery pressure therefore are directly related to the fraction of total lung that is hypoxic. Thus the proportion of flow changes to pressure change decreases as the size of the hypoxic lung segment increases. This distinction between localized and the more generalized or diffuse hypoxia is essential to understanding the nature of HPV.

The major segment of the vascular system at which HPV occurs appears to be at the level of the precapillary arterioles (30 to 35 μm in diameter).[34] These small muscular vessels are closely related to alveoli and are in an ideal position to respond to changes in alveolar oxygen concentration. Indeed, the most important stimulus to HPV appears to be the alveolar oxygen tension (PAO_2). Constriction occurs as PAO_2 decreases below normal, and the response reaches a maximum at about 30 mm Hg. The oxygen tension in the mixed venous blood (PvO_2) also plays a role in the HPV response. The PvO_2 becomes increasingly important at very low PAO_2 values and in an atelectatic lung may be the only stimulus for HPV. At alveolar oxygen tension above 60 mm Hg, PvO_2 appears to have only a minor effect.[35]

The HPV response is attenuated in a number of diverse clinical situations and by many classes of drugs, foremost of which are the anesthetic drugs. Intravenous drugs of most classes used in anesthesia (opioids, barbiturates, benzodiazepine, ketamine) do not appear to have a detectable effect on the HPV response. In vitro and in vivo experiments have shown that the pulmonary vasoconstrictive response to hypoxia is maintained at blood concentrations of these drugs sufficient to produce analgesia and anesthesia.[36,37]

In vitro experiments using isolated perfused lungs generally show that the current halogenated inhalational agents halothane, enflurane, and isoflurane all inhibit HPV in a dosage-related manner. In vitro observation with nitrous oxide suggests that it produces little or no effect on HPV.[38] However, studies in intact animals suggest that 70% nitrous oxide moderately diminishes the HPV response.[37,38] The halogenated anesthetics also appear to antagonize the HPV response in intact animals and humans, but widely divergent results have been reported in contrast to the in vitro experiments. Marshall and Marshall[39] have provided a unifying concept for these findings based on the proportion of the lung that is made hypoxic. They suggest that the differences in most studies arise from the size of the lung segment used. The larger the hypoxic segment studies, the less effective will be the vasoconstriction and flow diversion away from the hypoxic site. They have also suggested that the antagonism of HPV by inhaled anesthetics may be obscured by other hemodynamic effects. The anesthetics depress myocardial function and produce a decrease in cardiac output. The latter is associated with decreased PvO_2 and pulmonary artery pressures, both of which tend to intensify HPV. Thus unless such effects are considered, the anesthetic actions of HPV may be subtle or misinterpreted.

The hypothesis that antagonism of HPV by inhaled anesthetics is important in the etiology of abnormal gas exchange during anesthesia is indeed attractive. However, blunting of the HPV response does not appear to sufficiently account for the impaired oxygenation observed. Inappropriately low PaO_2 values are often seen in patients breathing hyperoxic mixtures that would be expected to provide all open alveolar units in an oxygen tension far above that at which HPV comes into play. Therefore other factors such as altered lung mechanics may play a more significant role in the gas exchange.

D. Alterations in the control of breathing

Although the analysis of the system that controls breathing can be subdivided into chemical and neural elements, clinical appraisal of the neural control system is much more difficult and hazardous. The chemical control system, which is profoundly affected by anesthesia, has been studied extensively and responds to three basic physiologic stimuli: increases in the partial pressure of CO_2, increases in hydrogen ion concentration (decreased blood pH), and decreases in arterial P_{O_2}.

1. Carbon dioxide sensitivity. Metabolically produced CO_2 relies on ventilation for its removal. If ventilation is reduced, Pa_{CO_2} rises. Similarly, if ventilation is voluntarily or reflexly increased, Pa_{CO_2} decreases. The reciprocal relationship between ventilation and CO_2 is described by a rectangular hyperbola. For CO_2 excretion (see Fig. 10-1) it is apparent from the diagram that a doubling of alveolar ventilation (V_A) results in halving of CO_2 tension and CO_2 tension doubles if ventilation is halved. An average normal man has an alveolar ventilation of about 4 L/min and a resting Pa_{CO_2} near 40 mm Hg, shown in the figure as the set point.

In the same normal man, inhalation of CO_2 increases ventilation, which rises in nearly linear fashion with changes in Pa_{CO_2}. Stimulation to breath depends on the hydrogen ion concentration in the extracellular fluid surrounding the CNS chemoreceptors near the ventral-lateral surface of the medulla. The changes in hydrogen ion concentration as a result of inhaled CO_2 depend somewhat on the concentration of bicarbonate in the extracellular fluid. Alterations of bicarbonate concentrations in blood or cerebrospinal fluid from metabolic disturbances can therefore modify the ventilatory response to CO_2. The central chemoreceptors account for about 80% of the total increase in ventilation during inhalation of CO_2. The remaining 20% increase seems to arise from stimulation of peripheral chemoreceptors in the carotid body.

2. Sensitivity to hypoxia. The ventilatory response to decreases in inspired oxygen tension tends to be hyperbolic (Fig. 10-6) such that decreases in oxygen tension exert a greater effect on ventilation when hypoxemia is severe, as opposed to mild reductions in oxygen supply. This curvilinear relationship can be conveniently converted to a straight line by plotting ventilation against the reciprocal of arterial oxygen tension ($1/Pa_{O_2}$) or, as is more common, against arterial O_2 saturation. The nice linear relationship with O_2 saturation suggests that ventilation may be influenced primarily by oxygen content. However, most studies point to oxygen tension or partial pressure (Pa_{O_2}) rather than O_2 saturation as the stimulus to the peripheral chemoreceptors. This is underscored by the effect of inhaling carbon monoxide, which markedly affects O_2 content but has little or no effect on ventilation because Pa_{O_2} is not affected.

The hypoxic ventilatory response is mediated by the peripheral chemoreceptors in the carotid body. In their absence, the hypoxic ventilatory drive is lost, and hypoxia may exert a depressant action on the central chemoreceptors. The carotid bodies exert only a subtle influence on resting ventilation when Pa_{O_2} is greater than 60 mm Hg. Below this, ventilation increases dramatically in hyperbolic fashion, whereas at a Pa_{O_2} of 200 mm Hg or more the carotid body discharge diminishes to a minimal level.

An important interaction occurs between the two major ventilatory stimulants of hypoxia and hypercapnia. The presence of hypoxia enhances the ventilatory response of CO_2. Similarly, an increase in CO_2 results in a greater sensitivity to hypoxia. These interactive effects require an intact central as well as peripheral chemoreceptor function.

3. Response to acidosis. A decrease in arterial pH from metabolic acidosis with normal Pa_{O_2} and Pa_{CO_2} stimulates ventilation primarily by the effect of the acidemia on the peripheral chemoreceptors (carotid bodies). This arises from the concept that neither hydrogen nor bicarbonate ions readily cross the blood-brain barrier and is supported by observations in animals that carotid body denervation attenuates and delays the response. Biscoe, Purves, and Sampson[40] demonstrated in cats that a change of 0.20 pH units (7.45 to 7.25) increased carotid body neural output two to three times. This doubling of ventilation is roughly equivalent to that seen when Pa_{O_2} decreases from normal to about 40 to 50 mm Hg.

In normal volunteers, Knill and Clement[41] noted approximately a doubling of ventilation in normoxic normocarbic volunteers as the hydrogen ion concentration was increased about 13 nmol/L^{-1} (about 0.12 units pH decrease). This response was attenuated by hyperoxia and enhanced by hypoxia, again attesting to the interaction of these stimuli at the peripheral chemoreceptor.

All in all, for the same degree of acidemia or pH change, the addition of CO_2 evokes a larger increment in ventilation than does the addition of fixed acid. The initial response to acute metabolic acidosis is weak because as Pa_{CO_2} decreases from carotid body stimulation, CO_2 tension in the cerebrospinal fluid decreases and pH increases. Thus the strong peripheral stimulation of the hydrogen ion is offset by a central alkalosis and reduced stimulus to the medullary chemoreceptors. Gradually, after several hours, bicarbonate concentrations decrease and permit cerebrospinal fluid pH to decrease back to-

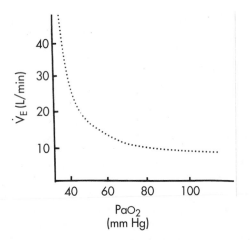

Fig. 10-6. Effects of decreasing arterial oxygen tension (*Pa_{O_2}*) on minute ventilation (V_E). The hyperbolic plot can be linearized by plotting V_E against the reciprocal of Pa_{O_2} or against O_2 saturation. (From Gal TJ: Respiratory physiology during anesthesia. In Kaplan JA, ed: *Thoracic anesthesia*, ed 2, New York, 1990, Churchill Livingstone.)

ward its normal value, and thus restore central chemoreceptor activity to normal.

4. Ventilatory indices of chemosensitivity

a. Carbon dioxide response. The two basic variables of ventilatory control (i.e., resting ventilation and $Paco_2$) may be highly variable and only slightly affected when the ventilatory control system is significantly altered. Nevertheless, they still have been advocated as indices of ventilatory control.

Conventional means of expressing CO_2 sensitivity use a plot of the CO_2 load or stimulus on the abscissa and ventilation on the ordinate. The latter values are obtained from actual data points with steady-state techniques, whereas least-squares linear regression determines the plot with rebreathing data. The carbon dioxide stimulus on the abscissa has included inspired CO_2 concentration, but end-tidal tension is most often used. However, arterial tension ($Paco_2$) may be the most accurate reflection of the CO_2 stimulus, particularly if pulmonary disease is present. The ordinate on the CO_2 ventilation plot is provided by respiratory minute volume ($\dot{V}_E$). The hyperoxic carbon dioxide sensitivity is expressed as the increment in $\dot{V}_E$ per increment in $Paco_2$. This can be quantitated by the equation:

$$\dot{V}_E = S(Paco_2 - B)$$

where S is the slope of the relationship between $\dot{V}_E/Paco_2$, and B is the intercept on the x-axis. The steeper the slope, the more vigorous the response to CO_2 (Fig. 10-7). Thus it provides a measure of the gain of the control system.

In most normal young adults, the slope of the CO_2 response ranged from 1.5 to 5 L/min/mm Hg.[42] Much of the interindividual difference in the response relates to the tidal volume response during rebreathing. In gen-

eral, the lowest ventilatory responses tend to occur in patients whose tidal volumes are small.

Changes in CO_2 sensitivity can be indicated by slope changes in the response. However, factors such as pharmacologic intervention may alter CO_2 sensitivity without changing slope. In this case, the shift of the CO_2 response can be characterized by displacement (see Fig. 10-7). This is the shift across the x-axis (in mm Hg CO_2) at a constant ordinate ($\dot{V}_E$) value, usually 20 or 30 L/min. Another expression for the shift of the CO_2 response curve uses a change in ordinate ($\dot{V}_E$) at a constant CO_2 value (see Fig. 10-7). Often 60 mm Hg is used and the ordinate referred to as the $\dot{V}_E60$. Another interesting term represents an extrapolation of the CO_2 response curve to zero ventilation on the CO_2 axis (see Fig. 10-7). This apneic threshold represents the CO_2 concentration at which apnea should occur from hyperventilation. This value is not easily obtainable in awake subjects and may not provide any more information than the resting CO_2.

b. Hypoxic response. Ideally the hypoxic ventilatory response should be expressed as a change in ventilation for a change in the stimulus (decreased O_2). However, the curvilinear nature of the relationship renders it complex and not easily characterized by a single index. One early index compared the ratio of the slopes of two CO_2 response curves, one performed in the presence of hypoxia ($PAo_2 = 40$ mm Hg) and the other normoxia ($PAo_2 = 150$ mm Hg). This dimensionless ratio has little physiologic meaning and is highly dependent on the hypercapnic response.

Severinghaus et al[43] introduced an index called ΔV_{40}, expressed in liters per minute. This represented the increase in minute ventilation that occurred as oxygen tension was reduced from above 200 mm Hg to 40 mm Hg with normocapnia. At an oxygen tension of 40 mm Hg, the ventilatory response is rather steep (Fig. 10-8). Thus the potential for error exists in establishing the actual ventilation value because small decreases in PO_2 are associated with rather large increases in ventilation. The ΔV_{40} can also be estimated from the two CO_2 response curves, one performed with normoxia and the other at hypoxic level ($Pao_2 = 40$ mm Hg). Ventilations measured at an isocapnic point ($Paco_2 = 40$ mm Hg) can thus be compared.

The ventilatory response to hypoxia can be linearized by plotting the reciprocal of ventilation against PO_2 or more conveniently by relating the change in ventilation to arterial oxyhemoglobin saturation (see Fig. 10-8). Thus the hypoxic response can be quantitated as $\Delta V/\%$ desaturation. Although the latter index is the simplest means of quantitating the hypoxic response, a more complex description of the hyperbolic relationship between ventilation ($\dot{V}_E$) and oxygen tension ($Paco_2$) is equally popular. Parameter A is used to characterize the shape of the curve, which is expressed mathematically by the equation:

$$\dot{V}_E = \dot{V}_O + \frac{A}{Pao_2 - 32}$$

where $\dot{V}_O$ is the asymptote for ventilation, and 32 is the asymptote for Pao_2 at which ventilation is assumed to be infinite. The magnitude of A is related to the briskness of the response.

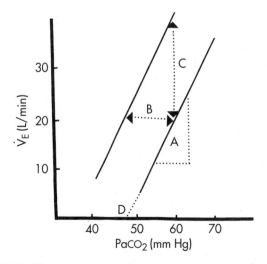

Fig. 10-7. Hypercapneic ventilatory response expressed as increase in minute ventilation *($\dot{V}_E$)* as a function of increased arterial CO_2 tension *($Paco_2$)*. A, Slope of the response; B, displacement of the response (i.e., a change in the abscissa at a constant ordinate value); C, change in ordinate at a constant abscissal value; D, apneic threshold. (From Gal TJ: Respiratory physiology during anesthesia. In Kaplan JA, ed: *Thoracic anesthesia*, ed 2, New York, 1990, Churchill Livingstone.)

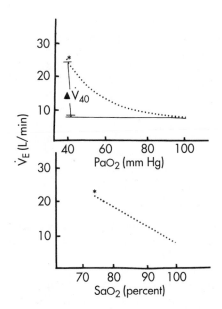

Fig. 10-8. The hyperbolic response to hypoxia can be quantitated as ΔV_{40}, the increase in ventilation ($\dot{V}_E$) at a hypoxic level ($PaO_2 = 40$ mm Hg) compared to normoxia. Note that the increased $\dot{V}_E$ is linearly related to arterial O_2 saturation (SaO_2 percent). At $PaO_2 = 40$ the blood is roughly 25% desaturated ($SaO_2 = 75$). Thus ventilation at this point and at $PaO_2 = 40$ are nearly identical (*). (From Gal TJ: Respiratory physiology during anesthesia. In Kaplan JA, ed: *Thoracic anesthesia*, ed 2, New York, 1990, Churchill Livingstone.)

In normal subjects the ventilatory response to hypoxia appears to be more variable than the hypercapnic response. For example, whereas the mean value for parameter A was 186, the range of values was from 69 to 410.[44] In terms of desaturation, hypoxic sensitivity ranged from 0.16 to 1.35 L/min per 1% desaturation (mean = 0.16 L/min)[45] whereas ΔV_{40} values ranged from 5.4 to 64.8 L/min.[46] Certain mathematical interrelationships can be constructed for the three indices. For example, because normal blood undergoes a 25% desaturation at a PaO_2 of 40 mm Hg, the $\Delta V/1\%$ desaturation and ΔV_{40} are related by a factor of 25 to 1 such that $\Delta V_{40}/25 = \Delta V1\%$ desaturation. Also, if $PaO_2 = 40$ mm Hg is substituted into the equation containing parameter A, the following relationship results:

$$A = \Delta V_{40} \times 8$$

5. Effects of anesthetics on respiratory control. The vast majority of drugs used in the practice of anesthesiology, including the intravenous and volatile anesthetic agents, have as their principal side effect an alteration of respiratory control. This is manifest as a depressed desire to breathe, which assumes great clinical relevance because these drug effects may seriously impair ventilation and thus gas exchange in the perioperative period.

a. Inhaled anesthetics

(1) CARBON DIOXIDE RESPONSES. Present-day halogenated inhaled agents (halothane, enflurane, isoflurane, sevoflurane, and desflurane) produce profound respiratory depression in a dosage-related manner. This respiratory depression is far greater than that associated with outmoded agents (cyclopropane or fluroxene). At concentrations that produce loss of consciousness and surgical anesthesia, tidal volume is reduced. Although respiratory rate increases, minute ventilation decreases, and an elevation of CO_2 occurs in proportion to the depth of anesthesia as a function of the minimum alveolar concentration (MAC). The extent of the hypoventilation and CO_2 retention varies with each agent. At 1.0 MAC, halothane produces a modest increase in CO_2 to about 45 mm Hg. By comparison, the same concentration of isoflurane increases CO_2 to about 50 mm Hg and enflurane produces even more marked hypercapnia (above 60 mm Hg). The effects of sevoflurane and desflurane are similar to those of halothane at 1.0 MAC, but at values above this the ventilatory depression and CO_2 rise are more like those of enflurane.[47,48] Although the effects of surgical stimulation tend to counteract this rise in CO_2, the hypercapnia tends to worsen in patients with COPD in proportion to their degree of airway obstruction.[49] In the face of the added mechanical load, such patients are unable to achieve adequate gas exchange with the rapid shallow breathing pattern associated with halothane.

The normal increase in ventilation with increasing CO_2 (i.e., the slope of the response) is blunted by the halogenated anesthetics in a dose-dependent manner. Whereas sedating halothane doses (0.1 MAC) produce little or no change in the slope of the response, anesthetizing doses (more than 1.0 MAC) produce significant decreases in slope. The observations of Tusiewicz, Bryan, and Froese[50] suggest that much of this ventilatory depression is caused by a reduction of rib cage recruitment that occurs at higher levels of ventilation in the awake state. The latter may also help to explain the effects of surgical stimulation, which produces a decrease in resting CO_2 but no change in the slope of the CO_2 response.[51]

The absence of wakefulness with the inhaled anesthetics results in a complete dependence on the chemical regulation of ventilation. Thus passive hyperventilation that removes the CO_2 stimulus results in apnea. Such apnea is difficult if not impossible to elicit in conscious subjects but easy to achieve during anesthesia. The apneic CO_2 concentration, which is 5 to 9 mm Hg below the normal awake resting value or resting CO_2 tension while anesthetized, is called the apneic threshold. The apneic threshold can be estimated by linear extrapolation of the CO_2 response curve to zero ventilation (see Fig. 10-7).

(2) RESPONSE TO HYPOXIA. Traditional views of the peripheral chemoreceptors considered them the body's last defense and resistant to drug depression. However, present knowledge recognizes that these structures are profoundly depressed in humans by even sedating levels of anesthesia. The initial studies in dogs by Weiskopf, Raymond, and Severinghaus[52] demonstrated blunting of the hypoxic response with 1.1% halothane. Knill and Gelb[53] noted that the response in humans was even more profound. Similar effects were seen with enflurane[54] and isoflurane.[55] Noteworthy is the profound depression of

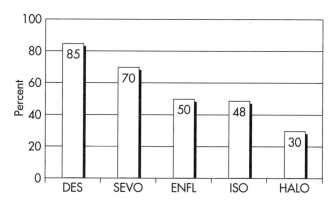

Fig. 10-9. Ventilatory responses to acute hypoxia with sedative concentrations (0.1 MAC) of the five available inhaled anesthetics: desflurane *(DES)*, sevoflurane *(SEVO)*, enflurane *(ENFL)*, Isoflurane *(ISO)* and Halothane *(HALO)*. Mean values are expressed as a percentage of control values, and are estimated from data compiled in Reference 60.

the response in contrast to the hypercapnic response. At levels that minimally affect the CO_2 response, the hypoxic response is nearly abolished. This also appears to be true for nitrous oxide, which at concentrations of 30% to 50% has no effect on the CO_2 response and depresses the ventilatory response to hypoxia.[56] Furthermore, it has been shown in humans that the normal synergistic interaction between hypoxia and hypercapnia is eliminated.[54] Rather than acting to increase ventilation, the two stimuli act to depress ventilation in anesthetized subjects.

Like the response to hypoxia, the response to added (H^+) metabolic acidemia is mediated via peripheral chemoreceptors. Knill and Clement[57] have shown that halothane sedation and anesthesia in humans markedly attenuate the response to acidemia and its attendant interaction with hypoxemia. Thus any patient compensation for these derangements must arise from measures instituted by the physician.

The surprising observations of Temp, Henson, and Ward[58] recently questioned the magnitude of the depression of hypoxic responses. They noted that 0.1 MAC isoflurane did not seem to appreciably affect the hypoxic responses whether hypoxia was induced abruptly (step test) or gradually (ramp test). Later it was noted that depressions of hypoxic responses were mild and variable in the presence of extraneous audio-visual stimuli as used by Temp, and depressant effects of subanesthetic concentrations were demonstrated only when external stimuli were absent.[59] The relative influence of subanesthetic (0.1 MAC) concentrations of the various anesthetics is depicted in Fig. 10-9. The effects of 0.1 MAC are important clinically because they reflect concentrations common during early recovery from general anesthesia. Desflurane has the least effect, followed by sevoflurane. The latter produces depression of the hypoxic response that is not restored by arousal with acute pain.[60]

b. Intravenous agents

(1) Barbiturates. Among the various CNS depressants used to achieve sedation, the barbiturates do not appear to have a significant effect on resting ventilation when used at dosages that produce sedation or drowsiness. Intramuscular pentobarbital (2 mg/kg) reduced the ventilatory response to hypoxia in 5 out of 10 healthy volunteers for a period of about 90 minutes.[61] Sedative dosages of thiopental did not significantly affect resting ventilation or the response to isocapnic hypoxia and hyperoxic hypercapnia.[62] However, hypnotic or anesthetic concentrations of thiopental depressed both hypoxic and hypercapnic responses to nearly the same extent (35% to 45% of control). In this respect, the barbiturates differ from inhaled anesthetics because the latter agents depress hypoxic response far beyond their effects on hypercapnic responses.

(2) Opioids. The prototype of the pure opioid agonists, morphine depresses ventilation at the usual analgesic dosage (10 to 20 mg). This effect is manifest by a decrease in respiratory frequency, small decrease in tidal volume, and a resultant increase in resting CO_2. The CO_2 response to such dosages is altered primarily by a rightward displacement with little or no change in slope (Fig. 10-10). Larger doses of morphine (0.5 mg/kg) begin to depress the slope of the CO_2 response curve in addition to the rightward shift depression in the state of consciousness. Indeed, sleep has been shown to enhance the ventilatory depression of morphine.[63] Other opioids consistently demonstrate the same pattern and degree of respiratory depression when given in equianalgesic doses. Much of the depression is mediated by depression of the contribution of the rib cage to ventilation.[64] This phenomenon is similar but less marked than that observed with halothane anesthesia.[50] However, the decrease in respiratory rate, in contrast to the tachypnea noted with halothane, results in a disproportionate decrease in minute ventilation.

The hypoxic response, much like that with the inhaled anesthetics, was originally felt to be unaffected by opioids. However, depressed hypoxic responses have been demonstrated following morphine (7.5 mg subcutaneously)[65] and meperidine (1.2 mg/kg orally).[66] As with the benzodiazepines and barbiturates, but not the inhaled anesthetics, the magnitude of depression with opioids is approximately the same for both hypoxic and hypercapnic responses.

The safety of parenteral opioids is limited by the risk of severe ventilatory depression with increasing dosages. Intrathecal and epidural administration of opioids was initially thought to be free of such risks because small dosages are required to achieve high concentrations at the dorsal spinal roots, thereby obviating systemic toxicity. However, there is evidence that epidural morphine produces respiratory depression of slightly greater magnitude than the same dosage of drug administered parenterally.[67] The ventilatory depression is delayed and prolonged with the epidural administration and has been attributed to rostral spread of the drug along the neuraxis. With fentanyl the respiratory effects were also greater with epidural administration.[68] Because plasma fentanyl concentrations were lower in the epidural group, the authors also ascribed the effects to rostral spread despite the highly lipid-soluble character of fentanyl. In contrast, observations with another more lipid-soluble opioid, sufentanil, suggest that an important part of the anal-

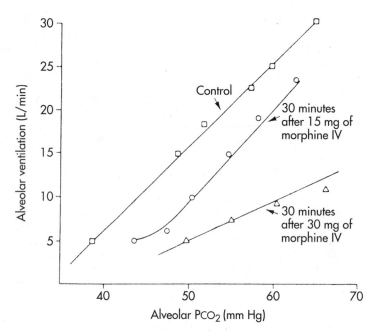

Fig. 10-10. Effects of morphine on the ventilatory response to CO_2. A typical premedicant dose (15 mg) is compared with a larger, more sedating dose (30 mg) likely to be associated with greater decrease in the level of consciousness. (From Bailey PL, Stanley TH: Pharmacology of intravenous narcotic anesthetics. In Miller RD, ed: *Anesthesia,* ed 3, New York, 1990, Churchill Livingstone.)

gesic and respiratory effects of that drug are also mediated centrally, but only after systemic absorption occurs.[69]

(3) BENZODIAZEPINES. The benzodiazepines have become increasingly popular as sedating agents and have virtually replaced barbiturates as preoperative medications, amnestic agents, and adjuvants to opioids. Intravenous dosages of diazepam (0.1 to 0.4 mg/kg) have been shown to depress the slope of the CO_2 response.[70] This respiratory depression does not appear to be consistent in a number of other studies. Gross, Smith, and Smith[71] have clarified the transient nature of the response and have demonstrated that the depressant effect peaks in about 3 minutes and lasts for 30 minutes. More importantly, they showed that the ventilatory depression correlated with the subject's state of consciousness. The effects of another benzodiazepine, midazolam, were qualitatively similar to diazepam's, with perhaps a slightly briefer duration of effects.[72]

The ventilatory response to hypoxia appears to be blunted by diazepam in a transient fashion and to a similar extent as the hypercapnic response. Lakshminarayan et al[73] observed a decrease in parameter A to about one half of control values in eight healthy volunteers. The effect was consistently demonstrated for 30 minutes after 10 mg intravenous diazepam.

(4) KETAMINE. The dissociative anesthetic ketamine appears to have minimal depressant actions on respiratory control. Early observations suggested that intravenous dosages of 2.2 mg/kg did not affect resting ventilation or the response to CO_2 challenge. In a study of dogs anesthetized with ketamine, the hypercapnic response appeared to be increased,[74] and this led to speculation that ketamine may be a respiratory stimulant by virtue of the increased sympathetic nervous system activity. However, another more precisely controlled study in dogs demonstrated that ketamine produces slight but significant depression of both hypoxic and hypercapnic responses.[75] In healthy human volunteers, 3 mg/kg intravenous ketamine appears to produce respiratory depression similar to that observed with premedicant doses of morphine (0.2 mg/kg).[76] In children, an intravenous bolus dose of ketamine produced nearly a 40% decrease in the CO_2 response slope.[77] This transient response disappeared in 30 minutes, whereas the result of a continuous infusion period was similar to that observed in adults, namely, a rightward shift of the CO_2 response curve but no change in slope. These changes are characteristic of premedicant doses of morphine (see Fig. 10-10).

(5) LIDOCAINE. This amide local anesthetic has been widely used to control arrhythmias, produce regional anesthesia, and as an adjunct in combination with other general anesthetics. Lidocaine administered as an intravenous bolus (2.5 mg/kg^{-1}) caused a transient 50% decrease in the slope of the CO_2 ventilatory response.[78] In the same subjects lidocaine infusion increased the slope. Serum lidocaine concentrations during the infusion was about 3 µg/ml^{-1}. This is similar to a concentration that produced up to a 28% reduction in anesthetic requirement.[79] These same steady-state lidocaine concentrations produced depression of the hypoxic ventilatory response manifest by a 20% reduction in parameter A.[80]

(6) ETOMIDATE. This imidazole-based hypnotic agent provides one of the several alternatives to ultra–short-acting barbiturates for inducing general anesthesia.

Many of the early studies with this drug suggest that it may cause less respiratory depression. However, these observations were often subjective and clouded by concomitant administration of drugs such as narcotics. Choi et al[81] noted that etomidate (0.3 mg/kg^{-1}) produced a depression of CO_2 response slope that was comparable to equipotent doses of methohexital (1.5 mg/kg^{-1}). At resting CO_2 tension, however, etomidate appeared to stimulate ventilation slightly. The latter observation suggests that etomidate may be more suitable for induction with maintenance of spontaneous ventilation. However, the frequent development of myoclonus appears to negate this theoretical benefit.

(7) PROPOFOL. This compound, a diisopropyl phenol, is another alternative to barbiturate induction of general anesthesia. Much like with barbiturates, induction of anesthesia with propofol (2.25 mg/kg^{-1}) is often associated with apnea of a minute or more in duration. Studies of CO_2 responsiveness indicate a depression of slope that lasted longer than that produced by thiopental.[82] Interestingly, this ventilatory depression seemed to persist beyond the apparent return of consciousness. Whether patients are at risk for significant ventilatory depression on this basis remains to be seen. During conscious sedation, 1 mg/kg^{-1} propofol significantly decreases the ventilatory response to hypoxia in the presence of hypercapnia.[83] The depressed response appears to return to normal 30 minutes after the propofol infusion is discontinued.

III. OTHER CONTRIBUTING CAUSES OF IMPAIRED GAS EXCHANGE
A. Pulmonary edema

By far the most common cause of pulmonary edema is one in which the forces that drive fluid across the vessel wall are increased. Such increased intravascular pressures are the hallmark of cardiogenic pulmonary edema (i.e., that associated with congestive heart failure). Early in the development of pulmonary edema, well in advance of fluid accumulation in the airspace, interstitial fluid begins to accumulate around arterioles and bronchioles. This cuffing action increases both airway and pulmonary vascular resistance at the lung bases. Both ventilation and perfusion are distributed away from these lower lung zones to more apical areas, and an imbalance in the $\dot{V}_A/\dot{Q}$ relationship results. The immediate consequence of $\dot{V}_A/\dot{Q}$ mismatch is arterial hypoxemia, with PaO_2 values of 50 to 55 mm Hg commonly observed. Hypercapnia is not considered as a usual consequence of pulmonary edema, but elevated $PaCO_2$ values may occur. The mechanism for hypercapnia is not entirely clear but may be related to the severity of the ventilation-perfusion imbalance. Normally hyperventilation can compensate for hypercapnia because the CO_2 dissociation curve is linear. However, if work of breathing is significantly increased, as in the congested stiff lung with increased airway resistance, ventilation may not be able to increase sufficiently to restore $PaCO_2$ to normal. Furthermore, with extremely high work of breathing, the metabolic load of CO_2 by the increased ventilation may offset the exhaled CO_2 and worsen hypercapnia.

Other noncardiac varieties of pulmonary edema consist of conditions in which fluid movement out of vessels is increased because of increased permeability, usually from loss of integrity of the vessel wall. This group includes such states as the adult respiratory distress syndrome, neurogenic pulmonary edema, and the pulmonary edema associated with heroin overdose or exposure to high altitude. The major abnormality of gas exchange in such patients results from large degrees of intrapulmonary shunting. The arterial hypoxemia in these states is also highly influenced by factors that lower PvO_2, particularly cardiac output.

One other variant of pulmonary edema with transient failure of gas exchange in the form of an increased difference between alveolar and arterial O_2 is that associated with the development and relief of acute upper airway obstruction. Many factors play a role in the pathogenesis of such pulmonary edema. However, the fact that it is often called negative pressure pulmonary edema simplistically implies that a marked negative inspiratory pressure is the predominant or only cause. Lloyd et al[84] demonstrated that negative inspiratory pressures associated with breathing through inspiratory resistances promoted lung lymph formation in sheep in a fashion similar to that resulting from elevated intravascular pressures. On the other hand, Hansen, Gest, and Landers[85] were unable to show any effect of inspiratory obstruction on steady-state lung lymph flow. Because they used supplemental O_2, they postulated that a key to development of edema is the presence of alveolar hypoxia, which mediates pulmonary vasoconstriction and may cause capillary leak. This is an attractive explanation because patients with upper airway obstruction may not be receiving O_2 and are likely to experience severe alveolar hypoxia. Other interesting evidence that casts some doubt on the dominant role of negative pressure in the genesis of pulmonary edema is the abundance of studies in which animals[86] and human subjects[87] have breathed against severe extrinsic inspiratory obstructions and developed inspiratory pressures more than 10 times those of quiet breathing and yet have not developed pulmonary edema.

B. Pulmonary embolism

Abnormal gas exchange inevitably accompanies pulmonary embolism. Abnormalities are influenced by the size and extent of the vascular occlusion, the presence of underlying cardiovascular disease, and the time since the acute embolism. Arterial hypoxemia is often but not universally found. However, the patients in whom significant arterial hypoxemia does not develop with ambient air do exhibit an increased alveolar to arterial oxygen gradient. The failure of these patients to develop hypoxemia results from the hyperventilation that usually accompanies the embolism. In most of these patients the increased ventilation is associated with some hypocapnia.

The other significant consequence of the embolism is an increased alveolar dead space because the occlusion is associated with absent flow to distal lung areas. The occlusion may not be total, so regions of high $\dot{V}_A/\dot{Q}$ ratios may prevail. These zones of lung with vascular obstruction develop pneumoconstriction, which may be the result of airway hypocapnia and the release of bronchoconstrictive amines.

This pneumoconstriction teleologically reduces the extent of the alveolar dead space and high $\dot{V}_A/\dot{Q}$ areas but may contribute to development of low $\dot{V}_A/\dot{Q}$ zones. Such zones may preexist in many patients. They can increase acutely from hypoperfusion of the vascular bed in unaffected areas and from the development of atelectasis distal to areas of vascular obstruction.

Another important contributor to the abnormal oxygenation is a reduction in cardiac output because of right ventricular failure. This generally requires massive vascular obstruction (more than 50%). As cardiac output falls, PvO_2 also decreases and amplifies the effect of right-to-left shunting and low $\dot{V}_A/\dot{Q}$ areas in impairing oxygenation.

C. Bronchospasm

Episodes of bronchoconstriction in asthmatics, whether spontaneous or induced by bronchial provocation testing, are associated not only with increased airflow resistance but also with changes in gas exchange. The most prominent manifestation is hypoxemia, and the most current evidence points to $\dot{V}_A/\dot{Q}$ abnormalities as the major cause. There appears to be a marked broadening of $\dot{V}_A/\dot{Q}$ relationships with a preponderance for very low but finite $\dot{V}_A/\dot{Q}$ ratios, but no absolute shunt.[88]

Inhalation of aerosolized β-adrenergic drugs is associated with worsening of hypoxemia and $\dot{V}_A/\dot{Q}$ inequality, presumably from an increased perfusion of lung units with low $\dot{V}_A/\dot{Q}$ ratios. There appears to be a decrease in pulmonary vascular resistance and increased perfusion of low $\dot{V}_A/\dot{Q}$ areas, which suggests that the drugs may be inhibiting HPV. However, because breathing pure oxygen does not seem to increase flow to these low $\dot{V}_A/\dot{Q}$ areas,[88] the phenomenon may simply reflect increased blood flow as a result of increased cardiac output.

Patients with severe acute asthma requiring mechanical ventilation exhibit qualitatively the same pattern of $\dot{V}_A/\dot{Q}$ abnormalities seen in less severe disease. However, they have a high degree of preexisting HPV, which responds to pure oxygen breathing with a significant increase in the amount of shunt.[89]

D. Pulmonary aspiration of gastric contents

The initial response to aspiration of acidic gastric contents is one of intense bronchoconstriction. This irritative reaction is rapidly followed by transudation of large amounts of fluid from the respiratory epithelium into the airspaces. The result is profound arterial hypoxemia (PaO_2 less than 50 mm Hg), as seen in severe cardiogenic pulmonary edema. Increased FIO_2 will offset the hypoxemia, but a large difference in alveolar and arterial O_2 persists as a reflection of the severe ventilation-perfusion mismatch. As in cardiogenic pulmonary edema, this mismatch may be severe enough, given the increased work of breathing, to also impair CO_2 removal. The degree of respiratory acidosis depends on the ability to produce adequate alveolar ventilation, while some metabolic acidosis may result from concomitant tissue hypoxia.

The aspiration of gastric contents in the perioperative period has always been a great concern of anesthesiologists because of the potential for postoperative pulmonary morbidity. The report of Warner, Warner, and Weber[90] suggests that patients who have aspirated gastric contents are unlikely to develop significant respiratory sequelae if they do not develop respiratory symptoms within 2 hours of the aspiration event or end of the anesthetic. The symptoms consist of coughing, wheezing, decreased arterial saturation (more than 10%), or radiographic findings suggesting aspiration.

E. Pneumothorax

The clinical presentation of pneumothorax may be dramatic. The spontaneously breathing patient immediately becomes short of breath, with an abrupt increase in pulse and respiratory rate, while blood pressure decreases. In the patients receiving mechanical ventilation, peak airway pressures may also rise. The latter may lead to some confusion with bronchospasm and lung hyperinflation, especially in patients with COPD. In patients with COPD, it is important to select ventilator settings and patterns that avoid problems of excessive inflation of the lungs. One of the confusing and dangerous aspects of lung hyperinflation is that it may mimic tension pneumothorax. Thus unless circulatory stability is achieved quickly by decreasing lung inflation, the insertion of chest tubes must be considered. Such hyperinflation can be easily identified by interrupting ventilation and disconnecting the circuit to allow lung volume to decrease during the period of apnea.

The prompt diagnosis of pneumothorax in patients with COPD is important because it is more common in such patients and has more dramatic effects in worsening hemodynamics and gas exchange. Progressive expansion of the pneumothorax compresses lung parenchyma and creates more and more areas with low $\dot{V}_A/\dot{Q}$ ratios, and thus hypoxemia. The limited ability to increase ventilation and the cardiac depression may be associated with hypercapnia as well.

F. Influence of chronic disease states on gas exchange

1. Cardiac disease. Cardiac function has its most obvious effect on gas exchange via its effect on the oxygen content of mixed venous blood. If cardiac function is inadequate to match demands of peripheral O_2 delivery, differences in arterial and venous O_2 increase and have an eventual effect on PaO_2. Mild degrees of cardiac failure, in contrast to the effects of pulmonary edema already discussed, are associated with minimal effects on gas exchange and little or no alteration in $\dot{V}_A/\dot{Q}$ distributions.

2. Renal disease. Patients with renal disease often exhibit hypocapnia as a result of attempts to compensate for systemic acidosis by hyperventilation. Coexistent lung disease or cardiac failure may result in hypoxia. Arterial hypoxemia is also observed during and after hemodialysis. Both the acetate and bicarbonate dialysates are associated with hypoxemia while the patient is breathing room air. This appears to be related to a transient hypoventilation.[91] The acetate removes some of the CO_2 load presented, whereas with bicarbonate dialysis respiratory drive appears to be suppressed by a gain in bicarbonate. Ventilation-perfusion abnormalities appear to contribute somewhat to this postdialysis hypoxemia, which is similar in patients with and without lung disease.[92] Another contributing factor may be the reduction in intravascular volume and cardiac output that so commonly occurs with dialysis. However, the principal cause of the reduced arterial O_2 tension appears to be a decrease in alveolar O_2 tension (PAO_2) because of hypoventilation. Thus the $P(A-a)O_2$ does not change and PaO_2 is reduced concomitantly with PAO_2. This is somewhat analogous to the hypoxia that results from hypoventilation following general anesthesia. In either case, the increased alveolar CO_2 is accompanied by a reduction in alveolar oxygen tension, which can be readily corrected by increasing inspired oxygen concentration.

3. Hepatic disease. In patients with liver disease and hepatic cirrhosis, arterial hypoxemia is a common finding and may result from a variety of causes. First of all, because many of these patients smoke, obstructive airway disease may be responsible for $\dot{V}_A/\dot{Q}$ mismatch and the abnormal gas exchange. This problem may be compounded further by repeated episodes of pneumonia. Finally, ascites and sometimes pleural effusions can interfere with gas exchange by restricting ventilation.

Cirrhotic patients tend to hyperventilate. This tends to lessen the decreases in alveolar and arterial O_2 tensions as alveolar CO_2 tension is lowered. Oxygenation is often lower in the upright position than in the recumbent (orthodeoxia). Dyspnea also is worse in the upright position and is relieved by recumbency (platypnea). This is most likely a result of decreased pulmonary vascular tone, which creates a more gravity-dependent flow in the pulmonary vascular bed. Many patients with cirrhosis are believed to have a blunted pulmonary vasoconstriction response to hypoxia. This contributes to an increased perfusion of poorly ventilated lung units, which disproportionately lowers their $\dot{V}_A/\dot{Q}$ ratios and results in hypoxia. An increased cardiac output also contributes to diminishing hypoxic vasoconstriction, and it is reasonable to speculate that the high cardiac output shortens transit times through pulmonary capillaries. The latter may interfere with equilibration of alveolar and capillary oxygen tensions and explains why low carbon monoxide diffusion capacities are often seen in cirrhotic patients.[93]

4. Obesity. The reduced respiratory system compliance and other mechanical ventilatory consequences of obesity would predict that abnormal gas exchange is likely. Indeed, hypoxemia usually unaccompanied by hypercapnia is present.

The hypoxemia largely reflects the presence of low $\dot{V}_A/\dot{Q}$ areas, a consequence of the mass loading on the respiratory system with resultant reduction in lung volumes. This derangement of lung function is intensified by changes in posture from upright to recumbent, to the extent that obese patients often demonstrate significant hypoxemia while supine. Much of this occurs because of

a dramatic reduction in FRC. Following induction of general anesthesia, the reduction in FRC is intensified such that many obese patients reach an FRC close to residual volume. Such large-scale airway closure rapidly results in $\dot{V}_A/\dot{Q}$ mismatch and hypoxemia.

5. Pulmonary disease
a. Restrictive disease. The common element in the many forms of restrictive lung disease is a loss of volume. This is a result of alteration in one of the major structural components of the thorax: skeletal, neuromuscular, pleural, and lung parenchyma (interstitial and alveolar). The reduction in lung volume is associated with a decreased lung compliance, the major consequences of which are increased work of breathing and maldistribution of ventilation. This maldistribution produces low $\dot{V}_A/\dot{Q}$ areas whose major impact on arterial blood gases is a pattern of hypoxemia, hypocapnia, and an increase in $P(A-a)O_2$. The hypocapnia indicates that hyperventilation is effective in maintaining CO_2 excretion. If hypercapnia occurs, it usually indicates advanced terminal disease in restrictive disorders.

b. Obstructive disease. Chronic obstructive disease spans the spectrum between airflow obstruction (bronchitis) and overinflation or air trapping (emphysema). The maldistribution of ventilation that impairs gas exchange results from abnormally long time constants, which essentially describe how rapidly lung areas fill and empty. The time constant *(T)* can simply be thought of as the product of resistance *(R)* times compliance *(C):* T = R × C. In the case of bronchitis, ventilation is impaired by an increased *R*, whereas in emphysema *C* is increased. Many emphysematous patients are called pink puffers because they exhibit only mild hypoxia and are usually normocapnic because of high levels of resting ventilation. In these patients, areas with a high $\dot{V}_A/\dot{Q}$ ratio are common. These are often called dead space areas, but in essence they are areas of wasted ventilation.

In contrast, the more bronchitic types (blue bloaters) characteristically exhibit more low $\dot{V}_A/\dot{Q}$ areas and present with moderate to severe hypoxemia (PaO_2 less than 50 mm Hg) and significant hypercapnia ($PaCO_2$ more than 50 mm Hg). These patients have adopted the economical breathing strategy (described earlier), which lessens the sense of effort and breathlessness at the expense of optimal gas exchange.

REFERENCES

1. Askanazi J, Weissman C, Rosenbaum SH, et al: Nutrition and the respiratory system, *Crit Care Med* 10:163, 1982.
2. Kaplan JA, Bush GL, Lecky JH, et al: Sodium bicarbonate and systemic hemodynamics in volunteers anesthetized with halothane, *Anesthesiology* 42:550, 1975.
3. Shephard RH, Campbell EJM, Martin HB, et al: Factors affecting the pulmonary dead space as determined by single breath analysis, *J Appl Physiol* 11:241, 1975.
4. Gal TJ: Respiratory mechanics and ventilatory failure in patients with chronic obstructive pulmonary disease, *Curr Opin Anaesth* 5:839, 1992.
5. Figueras J, Stein L, Diez V, et al: Relationships between pulmonary hemodynamics and arterial pH and carbon dioxide tension in critically ill patients, *Chest* 70:460, 1976.
6. Juan G, Calverley PK, Talamo C, et al: Effect of carbon dioxide on diaphragmatic function in human beings, *N Engl J Med* 310:874, 1984.

7. Edwards R, Winnie AP, Ramamurthy S: Acute hypocapnic hypokalemia: an iatrogenic anesthetic complication, *Anesth Analg* 56:786, 1977.

8. Cutillo A, Omboni E, Perondi R, et al: Effect of hypocapnia on pulmonary mechanics in normal subjects and in patients with chronic obstructive pulmonary disease, *Am Rev Respir Dis* 110:25, 1974.

9. Bergman NA: Distribution of inspired gas during anesthesia and artificial ventilation, *J Appl Physiol* 18:1085, 1963.

10. Rehder K, Marsh HM: Respiratory mechanics during anesthesia and mechanical ventilation. In Macklem PT, Mead J, eds: *Handbook of physiology. The respiratory system. Mechanics of breathing*, Bethesda, Md, 1986, American Physiological Society.

11. Damia G, Mascheroni D, Croci M, et al: Perioperative changes in functional residual capacity in morbidly obese patients, *Br J Anaesth* 60:574, 1988.

12. Bergman NA: Reduction in resting end-expiratory position of the respiratory system with induction of anesthesia and neuromuscular paralysis, *Anesthesiology* 57:14, 1982.

13. Westbrook PR, Stubbs SE, Sessler AD, et al: Effects of anesthesia and muscle paralysis on respiratory mechanics in normal man, *J Appl Physiol* 34:81, 1973.

14. Rehder K, Marsh HM, Rodarte JR, et al: Airway closure, *Anesthesiology* 47:40, 1977.

15. Hickey RF, Visick WD, Fairley HB, et al: Effects of halothane anesthesia on functional residual capacity and alveolar-arterial oxygen tension difference, *Anesthesiology* 38:20, 1973.

16. Juno P, Marsh HM, Knopp TJ, et al: Closing capacity in awake and anesthetized paralyzed man, *J Appl Physiol* 44:238, 1978.

17. Hedenstierna G, Santesson J: Airway closure during anesthesia: a comparison between resident gas and argon bolus techniques, *J Appl Physiol* 47:874, 1979.

18. Dueck R, Prutow RJ, Davies NJH, et al: The lung volume at which shunting occurs with inhalation anesthesia, *Anesthesiology* 69:854, 1988.

19. Hedenstierna G, Tokics L, Strandberg A, et al: Correlation of gas exchange impairment to development of atelectasis during anesthesia and muscle paralysis, *Acta Anaesthesiol Scand* 30:183, 1986.

20. Tokics L, Hedenstierna G, Brismar BO, et al: Thoracoabdominal restriction in supine men: CT and lung function measurements, *J Appl Physiol* 64:599, 1988.

21. Hedenstierna G, Tokics L, Lundquist H, et al: Phrenic nerve stimulation during anesthesia: effects on atelectasis, *Anesthesiology* 80:751, 1994.

22. Tokics L, Hedenstierna G, Strandberg A, et al: Lung collapse and gas exchange during muscle paralysis and positive end-expiratory pressure, *Anesthesiology* 66:157, 1987.

23. Rothen HU, Sporre B, Engberg G, et al: Reexpansion of atelectasis during general anesthesia: a computed tomography study, *Br J Anaesth* 71:788, 1993.

24. Rothen HU, Sporre B, Engberg G, et al: Influence of gas composition on recurrence of atelectasis after a re-expansion maneuver during general anesthesia, *Anesthesiology* 82:832, 1995.

25. Crawford ABH, Makowska M, Engel LA: Effect of bronchomotor tone on static mechanical properties of lung and ventilation distribution, *J Appl Physiol* 63:2278, 1987.

26. McAslan C, Mima M, Norden I, et al: Effects of halothane and methoxyflurane on pulmonary resistance of gas flow during lung bypass, *Scand J Thorac Cardiovasc Surg* 5:193, 1971.

27. Coon RL, Kampine JP: Hypocapnic bronchoconstriction and inhalation anesthetics, *Anesthesiology* 43:635, 1975.

28. Remolina C, Kahn AU, Santiago TV, et al: Positional hypoxemia in unilateral lung disease, *N Engl J Med* 304:523, 1981.

29. Fishman AF: Down with the good lung, *N Engl J Med* 304:537, 1981.

30. Davies H, Kitchman R, Gordon I, et al: Regional ventilation in infancy: reversal of adult pattern, *N Engl J Med* 313:1626, 1985.

31. Shim C, Chun K, Williams MH, et al: Positional effects on distribution of ventilation in chronic obstructive pulmonary disease, *Ann Intern Med* 105:346, 1986.

32. Rehder K, Hatch DJ, Sessler AD, et al: The function of each lung of anesthetized and paralyzed man during mechanical ventilation, *Anesthesiology* 37:16, 1972.

33. Landmark SJ, Knopp TJ, Rehder K, et al: Regional pulmonary perfusion and V/Q in awake and anesthetized paralyzed man, *J Appl Physiol* 43:993, 1977.

34. Nagasaka Y, Bhattacharya J, Nanjo S, et al: Micro puncture measurements of lung microvascular pressure profile during hypoxia in cats, *Circ Res* 54:90, 1984.

35. Marshall C, Marshall B: Influence of perfusate PO_2 on hypoxic pulmonary vasoconstriction in rats, *Circ Res* 52:691, 1983.

36. Bjertnes LJ: Hypoxia-induced vasoconstriction in isolated perfused lungs exposed to injectable or intravenous anesthetics, *Acta Anesthesiol Scand* 21:133, 1977.

37. Benumof JL, Wahrenbrock EA: Local effects of anesthetics on regional hypoxic pulmonary vasoconstriction, *Anesthesiology* 43:525, 1975.

38. Mathers J, Benumof JL, Wahrenbrock EA: General anesthetics and regional hypoxic pulmonary vasoconstriction, *Anesthesiology* 46:111, 1977.

39. Marshall BE, Marshall C: Continuity of response to hypoxic pulmonary vasoconstriction, *J Appl Physiol* 49:189, 1980.

40. Biscoe TJ, Purves MJ, Sampson SR: The frequency of nerve impulses in single carotid body chemoreceptor afferent fibers recorded in vivo with intact circulation, *J Physiol (Lond)* 208:121, 1970.

41. Knill RL, Clement JL: Ventilatory responses to acute metabolic acidemia in humans awake, sedated, and anesthetized with halothane, *Anesthesiology* 62:745, 1985.

42. Ersigler GB: Carbon dioxide response lines in young adults: the limits of normal response, *Am Rev Respir Dis* 114:529, 1976.

43. Severinghaus J, Bainton CR, Carcelen A: Respiratory insensitivity to hypoxia in chronically hypoxic man, *Respir Physiol* 1:308, 1966.

44. Hirshman CA, McCullough RE, Weil JV: Normal values for hypoxic and hypercapnic ventilatory drives in man, *J Appl Physiol* 38:1095, 1975.

45. Rebuck AS, Woodley WE: Ventilatory effects of hypoxia and their dependence on P_{CO_2}, *J Appl Physiol* 38:16, 1975.

46. Kronenberg RS, Hamilton RN, Gabel R, et al: Comparison of three methods of quantitating respiratory response to hypoxia, *Respir Physiol* 16:109, 1972.

47. Doi M, Ikeda K: Respiratory effects of sevoflurane, *Anesth Analg* 66:241, 1987.

48. Lockhart SH, Rampil IJ, Vasuda N, et al: Depression of ventilation by desflurane in humans, *Anesthesiology* 74:484, 1991.

49. Pietak S, Weenig CS, Hickey RF, et al: Anesthetic effects on ventilation in patients with chronic obstructive pulmonary disease, *Anesthesiology* 42:160, 1975.

50. Tusiewicz K, Bryan AC, Froese AB: Contributions of changing rib cage–diaphragm interactions to the ventilatory depression of halothane anesthesia, *Anesthesiology* 47:327, 1977.

51. Lam AM, Clement JL, Knill RL: Surgical stimulation does not enhance ventilatory chemoreflexes during enflurane anesthesia in man, *Can Anaesth Soc J* 27:22, 1980.

52. Weiskopf RB, Raymond LW, Severinghaus JW: Effects of halothane on canine respiratory responses to hypoxia with and without hypercarbia, *Anesthesiology* 41:350, 1974.

53. Knill RL, Gelb AW: Ventilatory responses to hypoxia and hypercapnia during halothane sedation and anesthesia in man, *Anesthesiology* 49:244, 1978.

54. Knill RL, Manninen PH, Clement JL: Ventilation and chemoreflexes during enflurane sedation and anaesthesia in man, *Can Anaesth Soc J* 26:353, 1979.

55. Kniff RL, Kieraszewicz HT, Dodgson BG: Chemical regulation of ventilation during isoflurane sedation and anaesthesia in humans, *Can Anaesth Soc J* 30:607, 1983.

56. Yacoub O, Doell D, Kryger MH, et al: Depression of hypoxic ventilatory response by nitrous oxide, *Anesthesiology* 45:385, 1976.

57. Knill RL, Clement JL: Ventilatory responses to acute metabolic acidemia in humans awake, sedated, and anesthetized with halothane, *Anesthesiology* 62:745, 1985.

58. Temp JA, Henson LC, Ward DS: Effect of a subanesthetic minimum alveolar concentration of isoflurane on two tests of the hypoxic response, *Anesthesiology* 80:739, 1994.

59. Maarten JL, Vanden Elsen MD, Dahan A, et al: Does subanesthetic isoflurane effect a ventilatory response to isocapnic hypoxia and healthy volunteers, *Anesthesiology* 81:860, 1994.

60. Sarton E, Dahan A, Teppema C, et al: Acute pain and central nervous system arousal do not restore impaired hypoxic ventilatory response during sevoflurane sedation, *Anesthesiology* 85:295, 1996.
61. Hirshman CA, McCullough RE, Cowen PJ, et al: Effect of pentobarbitone on hypoxic ventilatory drive in man, *Br J Anaesth* 47:963, 1975.
62. Knill RL, Bright S, Manninen P: Hypoxic ventilatory responses during thiopentone sedation and anesthesia in man, *Can Anaesth Soc J* 25:366, 1978.
63. Forrest WH Jr, Belleville JW: The effect of sleep plus morphine on the respiratory response to carbon dioxide, *Anesthesiology* 25:137, 1964.
64. Rigg JRA, Rondi P: Changes in rib cage and diaphragm contribution to ventilation after morphine, *Anesthesiology* 55:507, 1981.
65. Weil JV, McCullough RE, Kline JS, et al: Diminished ventilatory response to hypoxia and hypercapnia after morphine in normal man, *N Engl J Med* 292:1103, 1975.
66. Kryger MH, Yacoub O, Dosman J, et al: Effect of meperidine on occlusion pressure responses to hypercapnia and hypoxia with and without external inspiratory resistance, *Am Rev Respir Dis* 114:333, 1976.
67. Knill RL, Clement JL, Thompson WR: Epidural morphine causes delayed and prolonged ventilatory depression, *Can Anaesth Soc J* 28:537, 1981.
68. Negre I, Gueneron J-P, Ecoffey C, et al: Ventilatory response to carbon dioxide after intramuscular and epidural fentanyl, *Anesth Analg* 66:707, 1987.
69. Koren G, Sandler AN, Klein J, et al: Relationship between the pharmacokinetics and the analgesic and respiratory pharmacodynamics of epidural sufentanil, *Clin Pharmacol Ther* 46:458, 1989.
70. Forster A, Gardaz J-P, Suter PM, et al: Respiratory depression by midazolam and diazepam, *Anesthesiology* 53:494, 1980.
71. Gross JB, Smith L, Smith TC: Time course of ventilatory response to carbon dioxide after intravenous diazepam, *Anesthesiology* 57:18, 1982.
72. Gross JB, Zebrowski ME, Carel WD, et al: Time course of ventilatory depression after thiopental and midazolam in normal subjects and in patients with chronic obstructive pulmonary disease, *Anesthesiology* 58:540, 1983.
73. Lakshminarayan S, Sahn SA, Hudson LD, et al: Effect of diazepam on ventilatory responses, *Clin Pharmacol Ther* 20:178, 1976.
74. Soliman MG, Brindle GF, Kuster G: Response to hypercapnia under ketamine anesthesia, *Can Anaesth Soc J* 22:486, 1975.
75. Hirshman CA, McCullough RE, Cohen PJ, et al: Hypoxic ventilatory drive in dogs during thiopental, ketamine, or pentobarbital anesthesia, *Anesthesiology* 43:628, 1975.
76. Bourke DL, Malit LA, Smith TC: Respiratory interactions of ketamine and morphine, *Anesthesiology* 66:156, 1987.
77. Hamza J, Ecoffey C, Gross JB: Ventilatory response to CO₂ following intravenous ketamine in children, *Anesthesiology* 70:422, 1989.
78. Gross JB, Caldwell CB, Shaw LM, et al: The effect of lidocaine on the ventilatory response to carbon dioxide, *Anesthesiology* 59:521, 1983.
79. Himes RS, DiFazio CA, Burney RG: Effects of lidocaine on the anesthetic requirements for nitrous oxide and halothane, *Anesthesiology* 47:437, 1977.
80. Gross JB, Caldwell CB, Shaw LM, et al: The effect of lidocaine infusion on the ventilatory response to hypoxia, *Anesthesiology* 61:662, 1984.
81. Choi SD, Spaulding BC, Gross JB, et al: Comparison of the ventilatory effects of etomidate and methohexital, *Anesthesiology* 62:442, 1985.
82. Blouin RT, Conard PF, Gross JB: Time course of ventilatory depression following induction doses of propofol or thiopental, *Anesthesiology* 75:940, 1991.
83. Blouin RT, Seifert HA, Babenco HD, et al: Propofol depresses the hypoxic ventilatory response during conscious sedation and isohypercapnia, *Anesthesiology* 79:1177, 1993.
84. Lloyd JE, Nolop KB, Parker RE, et al: Effects of inspiratory resistance loading on lung fluid balance in awake sheep, *J Appl Physiol* 60:198, 1986.
85. Hansen TN, Gest AL, Landers S: Inspiratory airway obstruction does not affect lung fluid balance in lambs, *J Appl Physiol* 58:1314, 1985.
86. Bazzy AR, Haddad GG: Diaphragmatic fatigue in unanesthetized adult sheep, *J Appl Physiol* 57:182, 1984.
87. Roussos CS, Macklem PT: Diaphragmatic fatigue in man, *J Appl Physiol* 43:189, 1977.
88. Wagner PD, Dantzker DR, Iacovoni VE, et al: Ventilation-perfusion inequality in asymptomatic asthma, *Am Rev Respir Dis* 118:511, 1978.
89. Rodriguez-Roisin R, Ballester E, Roca J, et al: Mechanisms of hypoxemia in patients with status asthmaticus requiring mechanical ventilation, *Am Rev Respir Dis* 139:732, 1989.
90. Warner MA, Warner ME, Weber JG: Clinical significance of pulmonary aspiration during the perioperative period, *Anesthesiology* 78:56, 1993.
91. Hunt JM, Chappel TR, Henrich WL, et al: Gas exchange during dialysis, *Am J Med* 77:255, 1984.
92. Pitcher WD, Diamond SM, Henrich WL: Pulmonary gas exchange during dialysis in patients with obstructive lung disease, *Chest* 96:1136, 1989.
93. Hourani JM, Bellamy PE, Taskin DP, et al: Pulmonary dysfunction in advanced liver disease. Frequent occurrence of abnormal diffusing capacity, *Am J Med* 90:693, 1991.

Chapter 11

Causes and Consequences of Arrhythmias

Roger L. Royster

I. **Incidence of Arrhythmias**
  A. Healthy, Unanesthetized Persons
  B. Anesthetized Patients
II. **Arrhythmic Effects of Anesthetic Agents**
  A. Mechanisms of Arrhythmia Generation
    1. Normal automaticity
    2. Abnormal automaticity
    3. Triggered automaticity (activity)
      a. Early afterdepolarizations
      b. Delayed afterdepolarizations
    4. Reentry
    5. Reflection
    6. Parasystole
  B. Inhaled Anesthetics (Halothane, Enflurane, Isoflurane, Desflurane, Sevoflurane)
  C. Intravenous Anesthetics
    1. Thiopental
    2. Ketamine
    3. Propofol
  D. Local Anesthetics
    1. Bupivacaine
    2. Ropivacaine
  E. Opioids
  F. Neuromuscular Relaxants
    1. Succinylcholine
    2. Pancuronium
    3. Vecuronium
    4. Rocuronium
    5. Mivacurium and cisatracurium
  G. Reversal Agents
    1. Naloxone
    2. Muscle relaxant reversal
  H. Arrhythmias Induced by Anesthetics and Surgical Procedures

III. **Patients with Arrhythmias Presenting for Anesthesia and Surgery**
  A. Preoperative Evaluation
  B. Causes and Consequences of Supraventricular Arrhythmias
    1. Premature atrial contractions
    2. Paroxysmal supraventricular tachycardia
      a. Sinus node reentry
      b. Atrial tachycardias
      c. Atrioventricular node reentry
      d. Accessory atrioventricular pathways
    3. Atrial fibrillation
    4. Atrial flutter
    5. Multifocal atrial tachycardia
  C. Causes and Consequences of Ventricular Arrhythmias
    1. Benign ventricular arrhythmias
    2. Potentially malignant ventricular arrhythmias
    3. Malignant ventricular arrhythmias
  D. Complications of Antiarrhythmic Therapy
    1. Myocardial depression
    2. Pulmonary toxicity
    3. Hepatic toxicity
    4. Proarrhythmias
    5. Drug interactions
IV. **Patients with Miscellaneous Disease States Associated with Arrhythmias**
  A. Mitral Valve Prolapse
  B. Prolonged QT Syndromes
    1. Congenital
    2. Acquired
  C. Central Nervous System Disease
  D. Valvular Heart Disease
  E. Arrhythmias in Children
  F. Electrolyte Abnormalities

The routine monitoring of cardiac rate and rhythm in patients during anesthesia and surgery is a standard of care in the United States. A retrospective study indicates that electrocardiographic monitoring may be lifesaving in 1 of 3500 cases and through a risk-benefit analysis suggests that electrocardiographic monitoring is indicated in all patients.[1] Thus abnormalities of cardiac rate and rhythm are important indicators of primary changes in cardiac function or secondary physiologic abnormalities or drug effects during the operative period.

For most patients, the continuous monitoring of cardiac rate and rhythm first occurs during anesthesia and postanesthesia care. Anesthesiologists must be aware of the normal baseline variability in cardiac rate and rhythm in healthy unanesthetized people to understand and recognize significant rate and rhythm changes that occur during anesthesia. Moreover, these changes (in cardiac rate and rhythm) may occur during anesthesia secondary to changes in the depth of anesthesia and oxygen delivery to various organ systems; to changes in autonomic balance and catecholamine release; to direct effects of anesthetics, analgesics, muscle relaxants, reversal agents, and other drugs; and to mechanical stimulation secondary to invasive procedures and surgical manipulation.

Often, patients with a history of cardiac arrhythmias require anesthesia and surgery. The number of patients

Table 11-1. Incidence of premature atrial and ventricular contractions in healthy, unanesthetized patients

Study	Year	Number (sex)	Age range (yr)	Monitoring (hr)	PACs (%)	PVCs (%)
Scott et al[2]	1980	131 (M)	10-13	48	13	26
Romhilt et al[3]	1984	200 (F)	20-59	24	28	34
Sobotka et al[4]	1981	50 (F)	22-28	24	64	54
Hinkle et al[5]	1969	301 (M)	55 (median) 6	76	62	
Brodsky et al[6]	1977	50 (M)	23-27	24	56	50
Pilcher et al[7]	1983	80 (MF)	31 (mean)	24	41	50
Kantelip et al[8]	1986	50 (MF)	80-100	24	100	96
Kostis et al[9]	1981	101 (MF)	16-68	24	—	39
Poblete et al[10]	1978	30 (?)	47 (mean)	24	—	40

PACs, Premature atrial contractions; *PVCs,* premature ventricular contractions.

with a history of arrhythmia presenting for surgery is increasing because of a multitude of factors: the general population is aging, survival after myocardial infarction has increased, improved emergency medical services have increased the out-of-hospital survival of sudden death, technologic advances provide surgical procedures for older and sicker patients, and improved monitoring techniques allow physicians greater ability to recognize and diagnose rhythm disturbances. Management during the preoperative, intraoperative, and postoperative periods requires basic knowledge of arrhythmia electrophysiology and antiarrhythmic pharmacology. Awareness of toxic side effects of antiarrhythmic therapy is of tremendous importance and may affect anesthetic management. Potential cofactors involved in arrhythmogenesis during anesthesia include electrolyte abnormalities, acid-base disturbances, hemodynamic alterations, and myocardial ischemia.

This chapter discusses the incidence of cardiac arrhythmias during the unanesthetized and anesthetized states, the effects of anesthetic agents on arrhythmia generation, and the treatment of patients with a history of preoperative arrhythmias during the perioperative period.

I. INCIDENCE OF ARRHYTHMIAS
A. Healthy, unanesthetized persons
Arrhythmias are common in normal, unanesthetized patients (Table 11-1). They occur often in healthy children,[2] women,[3,4] and men.[5,6] A study of 50 male medical students with 24-hour Holter monitoring during various activities revealed a 56% incidence of premature atrial contractions (PACs) and 50% incidence of premature ventricular contractions (PVCs), with 12% having multifocal PVCs and 2% having ventricular tachycardia.[6] In a study of 80 healthy runners all under 40 years of age, 24-hour Holter monitoring revealed PVCs in 41 (50%) and PACs in 33 (41%).[7] There were two episodes of paired PVCs and one episode of nonsustained ventricular tachycardia (five beats). There was no relationship between distances run and incidence of arrhythmias. Kantelip et al[8] found in subjects over 80 years of age without cardiac disease that at least one PAC per hour occurred in 76% and at least one PVC per hour occurred in 72%. The number of PVCs exceeded 10 per hour in 32% and

were multifocal in 18% of subjects. The frequency of arrhythmias in these older subjects surpassed the frequency found in other studies of younger subjects. Others have shown that PVCs increase with age,[3,9] with risk factors for coronary artery disease,[5] and with underlying myocardial disease.[5,10] The long-term prognosis of asymptomatic healthy subjects with frequent complex ventricular ectopy is similar to that of the general healthy population.[11]

B. Anesthetized patients
Arrhythmias are common during anesthesia and surgery (Table 11-2). Publications as early as 1911 reported cardiac irregularities occurring during chloroform anesthesia.[12] Other studies during the 1920s and 1930s documented cardiac arrhythmias during anesthesia and surgery.[13-15] More recent studies using visual inspection of continuous electrocardiographic monitoring (the most common type of clinical monitoring) have documented a high incidence of arrhythmias during anesthesia.[16,17] Vanik and Davis[16] report that 901 of 5013 patients (18%) developed an arrhythmia. There was an increased incidence of arrhythmias with increasing age, intubation of the trachea, cyclopropane anesthesia, preoperative digitalis therapy, and anesthetic induction. Only 47 (1%) specific arrhythmias were considered serious. Dodd et al[17] report an incidence of arrhythmias of 29.9% in 569 patients. The incidence of arrhythmias was greater in patients with preexisting heart disease and intraabdominal surgery.

In studies of patients monitored with continuous electrocardiographic recordings (Holter monitoring) during anesthesia (see Table 11-2), the incidence of arrhythmias is greater, between 60% and 80%. Kuner et al[18] found an incidence of arrhythmias of 61.7% in 154 patients. Arrhythmias were more common in neurologic, thoracic, and head and neck procedures lasting 3 hours or longer. This analysis included any abnormality of cardiac rhythm, including minor abnormalities such as PACs, wandering atrial pacemaker, sinus bradycardia, and atrioventricular (AV) dissociation, and more severe arrhythmias, such as PVCs, atrial fibrillation, and ventricular tachycardia. However, the incidence of clinically significant cardiac arrhythmias was small. In their study of 100

Table 11-2. Incidence of arrhythmias during anesthesia and surgery

Study	Year (%)	Number	Arrhythmia (%)	Monitoring	Highest incidence related to
Dodd et al[17]	1962	569	29.9	Intermittent	Heart disease
Vanik and Davis[16]	1968	5013	17.9	Intermittent	Intraabdominal surgery Age Intubation Heart disease
Kuner et al[18]	1967	154	61.7	Holter	Neurologic, head and 　neck, thoracic surgery Intubation Surgery >3 hr
Bertrand et al[19]	1971	100	84.0	Holter	Intubation Extubation Heart disease

patients, Bertrand et al[19] found that 84 patients had either a supraventricular or a ventricular arrhythmia. Arrhythmias were more common at the time of intubation and extubation, and ventricular arrhythmias were more common in patients with cardiac disease.

In summary, clinical studies have shown a greater incidence of cardiac arrhythmias in anesthetized patients who are tracheally intubated, breathing spontaneously, or treated with digitalis; who have a history of heart disease or preexisting arrhythmias; or whose surgery lasts longer than 3 hours. The incidence of clinically significant arrhythmias in these studies was less than 5%. However, the recognition and evaluation of patients with preexisting arrhythmia and organic heart disease, the knowledge of precipitating and aggravating factors for arrhythmias during anesthesia and surgery, and the necessity of initiating antiarrhythmic therapy are important components of the perioperative anesthetic plan.

II. ARRHYTHMIC EFFECTS OF ANESTHETIC AGENTS
A. Mechanisms of arrhythmia generation*

The specific mechanisms involved in the generation of cardiac rhythm disturbances are fundamental to the development of specific antiarrhythmic therapy (Box 11-1). Scientists have gained greater knowledge in understanding mechanisms of cardiac rhythm disturbances over the past several years, especially in the areas of abnormal automaticity and triggered activity.[20] Determination of the mechanism is helpful in the treatment of supraventricular arrhythmias. For example, sinus node and AV node reentry are responsive to calcium-channel blockers, whereas automatic rhythms from the atrium and AV node are not so responsive to calcium-channel blockers. Moreover, definite electrocardiographic clues help the anesthesiologist differentiate supraventricular reentry from automaticity. Determination of the mechanism in ventricular arrhythmias is difficult clinically, and therapy remains largely empirical. However, knowledge of likely

---

Box 11-1　Classification of mechanisms of ectopic beat formation

Impulse generation
Normal automaticity
Abnormal automaticity
Triggered activity
　Early afterdepolarizations
　Delayed afterdepolarizations

Impulse conduction
Reentry
Reflection

Simultaneous abnormalities of impulse generation and conduction
Parasystole

Modified from Royster RL, Robertie PR: *Anesthesiol Clin North Am* 7:315, 1989.

---

clinical settings that correspond to certain mechanisms may lead to proper therapy for that mechanism. For the more serious student of arrhythmias, Atlee and Bosnjak[21] published a comprehensive review of the probable mechanisms of arrhythmias during anesthesia and surgery.

1. Normal automaticity. Normal automaticity with inherent diastolic depolarization is a property of the sinus node, atrial conduction fibers, areas of the AV nodal complex, and the His-Purkinje system. The rate of automatic depolarization decreases from the sinus node to the Purkinje system; thus all lower automatic cells are generally suppressed and are usually not responsible for ectopic beats but for escape rhythms. However, at lower heart rates and with enhanced intrinsic or extrinsic sympathetic stimulation, it is possible for a normal automatic cell to depolarize before overdrive suppression by a higher automatic focus, resulting in an ectopic complex. An extremely anxious or maximally sympathetically stimulated patient receiving a high-dose opioid anesthetic that resulted in bradycardia would fulfill these criteria for normal automaticity–induced ectopic beats.

---

*Adapted from Royster RL, Robertie PG: Recognition and treatment of ectopic beats. In Thomas S, ed: Diagnosis and management of intraoperative arrhythmias, *Anesthesiol Clin North Am* 7:315, 1989.

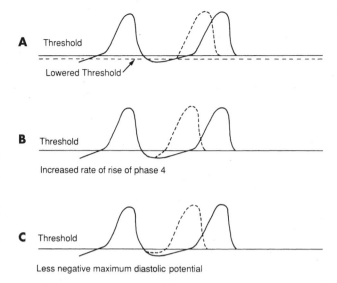

Fig. 11-1. Basic changes in normal electrophysiology of cardiac conducting cells. **A,** Lowered threshold potential. **B,** Increased rate of rise of phase 4 of the action potential. **C,** A less negative resting membrane potential. These changes may result in the generation of an ectopic impulse. (From Royster RL, Robertie PG: *Anesthesiol Clin North Am* 7:315, 1989.)

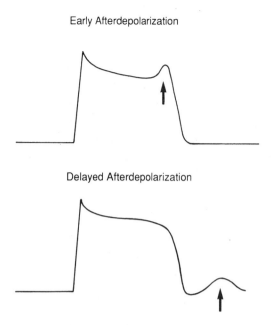

Fig. 11-2. Triggered activity. The top action potential shows an abnormal stimulus *(arrow)* during phase 3 of repolarization. This depolarizing stimulus is called an early afterdepolarization. The bottom action potential demonstrates a depolarizing current *(arrow)* after repolarization is complete, a late afterdepolarization. Causes of these afterdepolarizations are discussed in the text. (From Royster RL, Robertie PG: *Anesthesiol Clin North Am* 7:315, 1989.)

2. Abnormal automaticity. The characteristics of the action potential can be changed by cardiac disease, drug effect, or electrolyte effects. Theoretically, reducing the threshold potential to a more negative value, increasing the rate of rise of phase 4 (spontaneous diastolic depolarization), and increasing the maximum diastolic potential (resting membrane potential) to a less negative value may lead to enhanced automaticity[22] (Fig. 11-1). It appears that a less negative resting membrane potential may be the most important of these effects. Less negative membrane potentials have been found in atrial cells, in patients with rheumatic and congenital heart disease, and in ventricular cells in areas of ischemia and infarction.[22] When the membrane potential reaches -60 mV, spontaneous depolarization may occur in atrial or ventricular fibers or Purkinje cells, probably through activation of the slow Ca^{++} channels.

3. Triggered automaticity (activity). A triggered ectopic beat differs from a truly automatic beat by requiring a preceding action potential for its generation.[23] This activity, occurring after depolarization is complete, may occur during phase 3 of repolarization and is called an early afterdepolarization, or it may occur after repolarization is complete during phase 4, when it is called a delayed afterdepolarization (Fig. 11-2).

a. Early afterdepolarizations. Early afterdepolarizations are believed to occur because of a change in K^+ movement out of the cell during repolarization or to a permeability change to Na^+ or Ca^{++} movement into the cell. These action potential changes have been induced under a variety of conditions, including hypokalemia, high concentrations of catecholamines, acidosis, hypoxia, and drugs that prolong repolarization, such as quinidine and procainamide.[24] Early afterdepolarizations also appear to be more likely during slow heart rates and are probably responsible for ventricular arrhythmias in the prolonged QT syndrome.[25]

b. Delayed afterdepolarizations. Delayed afterdepolarizations appear to be mediated primarily by increases in intracellular Ca^{++}.[23] These can result from inhibition of the Na^+-K^+ pump[26] (digitalis and hypomagnesemia), an increased serum Ca^{++} concentration,[27] stimulation of receptor-operated channels[28] (catecholamines), and failure to pump Ca^{++} out of the cell (ischemia).[29] Delayed afterdepolarizations have been demonstrated in normal canine coronary sinus tissue[30] and in atrial tissue and ventricular specialized conducting tissue from normal and diseased hearts exposed to toxic concentrations of digitalis.[31]

4. Reentry. Reentry is the classic mechanism of ectopic beat formation. Prerequisites for reentry are an available circuit, a difference in refractory periods of two limbs of the circuit, and conduction somewhere in the circuit sufficiently slow to allow the remainder of the circuit to recover responsiveness.[32]

Normally, the conducting impulse of the heart driven by sinus rhythm dies out after sequential activation of the atria and ventricles because it is surrounded by refractory tissue that it has recently excited. But in disease states, differences in refractoriness of tissue and slow conduction may be present, setting up a perfect substrate for reentry formation. This is especially true in Purkinje fibers because of their arborization in the distal conducting system of the ventricle, which sets up a suitable anatomic network for reentry.[32]

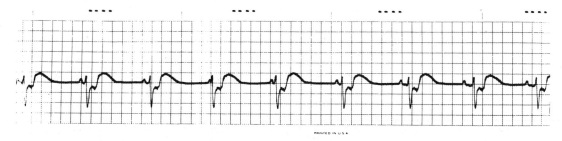

Fig. 11-3. Isorhythmic AV dissociation. This arrhythmia often occurs during inhalational anesthesia and is attributable to an autonomic imbalance, resulting in similar intrinsic rates of the sinus rhythm and an AV escape nodal rhythm. Although usually benign, this arrhythmia may result in hemodynamic compromise in patients with reduced ventricular compliance. Modes of therapy include reduction of the inhaled anesthetic, atropine, succinylcholine (10 to 20 mg), and small doses of β-adrenergic receptor blockers.

Larger anatomic circuits may exist in the sinus node, AV node, accessory pathways, venae cavae, and ventricular aneurysms and may lead to reentry. The prototypical example of reentry is in patients with preexcitation syndromes, using atrial muscle, the AV node, ventricular muscle, and the accessory pathway for the reentry circuit. The AV node also demonstrates dual pathways with different refractory periods and conduction velocities, which may lead to AV nodal reentry arrhythmias.[33]

5. Reflection. Reflection is a form of reentry that occurs in a single fiber and does not require a distinct, circuitous loop, as in classic reentry.[34] Reflection may occur because of abnormal refractoriness of adjacent areas in an individual Purkinje fiber. This process, called longitudinal dissociation, essentially isolates areas of conducting tissue with different refractoriness, potentially allowing recovered tissue to reexcite.[34] Reflection is also believed to occur in areas of ischemic and possibly infarcted conducting tissue, which can transmit depolarizing current (functioning as a passive conduit) without depolarizing.[35] When excitable tissue is reached, depolarization may again occur, with a return of the depolarizing current across this inexcitable segment to reexcite the conducting tissue that originated the depolarizing current.[35]

6. Parasystole. A parasystole is usually a ventricular automatic focus possibly caused by normal automaticity, abnormal automaticity, or triggered activity.[36] This ectopic focus resists overdrive suppression from higher pacemaker cells with faster intrinsic rates. This requires some form of protection surrounding the parasystolic focus, possibly caused by a unidirectional entrance block but not exit block.[37] This allows the parasystole to exit and depolarize the ventricles without allowing depolarization currents to enter and suppress it. Occasionally there may be forms of exit block that cause the parasystole to be intermittent.[38] Therefore a parasystole represents both abnormal impulse generation and abnormal conduction.

B. Inhaled anesthetics (halothane, enflurane, isoflurane, desflurane, sevoflurane)

All inhaled anesthetics have significant electrophysiologic effects. Although the presently used inhaled agents generally decrease sinus rate in awake and anesthetized animals,[39] the effect in humans may be altered by autonomic reflexes. In patients at minimum alveolar concentration (MAC), isoflurane, desflurane, and enflurane generally increase the sinus rate, whereas halothane and sevoflurane cause no change or mild depression of the sinus rate. In animals, halothane and enflurane significantly prolong AV nodal conduction, with minimal prolongation, if any, by isoflurane.[40] Also in this study, His-Purkinje conduction with all three agents was minimally prolonged but statistically significant. Scheffer et al[41] reported the first study of the basic electrophysiologic effects of halothane in humans. In patients breathing twice the MAC of halothane and oxygen, the sinus rate decreased, AV nodal conduction times were prolonged, and the His-Purkinje conduction time did not change.

A very common rhythm disturbance with these agents is isorhythmic AV dissociation (Fig. 11-3), which occurs when an AV nodal pacemaker assumes control of the heart rhythm at a slightly faster rate than the sinus node.[42] This probably occurs because of a greater autonomic effect (vagal) on the sinus node by the inhaled agents as catecholamine stimulation increases the automatic rate of the latent pacemaker in the AV node. Isorhythmic AV dissociation is generally a benign rhythm disturbance, but in patients with noncompliant hypertrophied ventricles who are more dependent on atrial contraction for ventricular filling, this rhythm can cause severe hemodynamic compromise.[43] Reduction of the level of anesthesia or administration of atropine,[43] small doses of succinylcholine,[44] or small doses of β-adrenergic receptor blockers[45,46] are reported to convert AV dissociation back to sinus rhythm.

Many clinical events and pharmacologic agents may interact with inhaled agents to produce arrhythmias (Box 11-2). The inhaled agents themselves are probably not arrhythmogenic, but when they are combined with increased catecholamine stimulation (from hypercapnia,[47] hypoxia,[48] hypertension and tachycardia,[49] light anesthesia, and so forth) or the administration of exogenous catecholamines[50,51] or aminophylline,[52,53] arrhythmias, especially PVCs, may result. In a frequently quoted study, Johnston et al[54] found that the submucosal dose

Box 11-2 Precipitating events and agents associated with halothane-induced arrhythmias

Clinical events

Hypoxia
Hypercapnia
Fasting
Tachycardia
Hypertension

Agents

Thiopental
Ketamine
Succinylcholine
Atropine
Pancuronium and tricyclics
Cocaine
Exogenous catecholamines and vasopressors
Aminophylline
Nitrous oxide

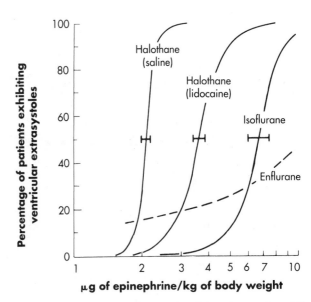

Fig. 11-4. Inhaled anesthetic-epinephrine interaction. The number of patients having PVCs versus the submucosal epinephrine dose during inhalational anesthesia. The submucosal dose of epinephrine required to elicit three or more PVCs in 50% of patients was 2.1 μg/kg for halothane, 6.7 g/kg for isoflurane, and 10.9 μg/kg for enflurane. When lidocaine was added to the epinephrine, the arrhythmic dose was greater in halothane-anesthetized patients. It is suggested that the safe dose of epinephrine during inhalational anesthesia is 1 μg/kg; it may be higher in children. (From Johnston RR, Eger EI II, Wilson C: *Anesth Analg* 55:709, 1976.)

of epinephrine needed to produce ventricular arrhythmias in 50% of adult patients was 2.1 μg/kg with halothane, 3.7 μg/kg with halothane and lidocaine, 6.7 μg/kg with isoflurane, and 10.9 μg/kg with enflurane (Fig. 11-4). Children may be more resistant to catecholamine-induced arrhythmias[55] and may tolerate 10 μg/kg epinephrine subcutaneously during halothane anesthesia without arrhythmias. Sevoflurane[56] and desflurane[57] have similar catecholamine-induced arrhythmia responses as compared to equipotent anesthetic concentrations of isoflurane.

C. Intravenous anesthetics

1. Thiopental. Thiopental may result in no change or slight reduction in the heart rate because it does not completely suppress baroreceptor reflexes.[58] Thiopental potentiates epinephrine-induced arrhythmias with halothane, enflurane, and isoflurane in animal studies.[59,60] However, thiopental does not appear to produce clinically significant arrhythmias in humans.

2. Ketamine. Ketamine may increase the heart rate based on its sympathomimetic effects. Ketamine also potentiates epinephrine-induced arrhythmias during halothane administration in animal studies[61] but makes digitalis-toxic arrhythmias less likely in animals.[62] Ketamine, like thiopental, does not produce clinically significant arrhythmias in humans.

3. Propofol. Propofol may result in little change or, in some patients, a reduction in heart rate.[63] The arrhythmogenic effects of intravenous anesthetic agents, such as etomidate, the benzodiazepines, and propofol, also appear to be clinically insignificant. Propofol prolongs AV node conduction time and effective refractory periods in isolated, perfused guinea pig hearts.[64]

D. Local anesthetics

1. Bupivacaine. Although most local anesthetics have antiarrhythmic activity because of sodium-channel blocking effects, bupivacaine and etidocaine at toxic doses have apparent clinical ventricular arrhythmogenic activity.[65] Animal studies demonstrate multiple arrhythmic effects, including PR and QT interval prolongation, QRS widening, AV block, and ventricular tachycardia and fibrillation[66] (Fig. 11-5). The cause of bupivacaine-induced ventricular arrhythmias is unclear. The recovery time of blocked sodium channels with bupivacaine is almost 10 times that of lidocaine.[67] This prolongation of repolarization may lead to a long QT interval syndrome; torsade de pointes is reported in animals given toxic doses of bupivacaine.[66] Bupivacaine causes a 50% prolongation of the QT interval at a lower concentration than any other local anesthetic.[68] Successful resuscitation with CPR, epinephrine, and lidocaine for arrhythmia control in humans has been reported.[69,70] Animal studies suggest that bretylium may be more effective than lidocaine and may raise the ventricular tachycardia threshold lowered by bupivacaine.[71] Magnesium sulfate suppressed bupivacaine-induced cardiac arrhythmias in an animal study.[72] Acidosis and hypoxia enhance the arrhythmogenic effects and increase the mortality of sheep given intravenous bupivacaine[73] and should be especially avoided in patients likely to have a high serum concentration of bupivacaine.

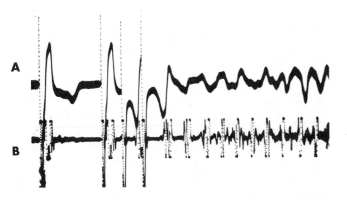

Fig. 11-5. Bupivacaine-induced ventricular fibrillation. **A,** Surface ECG. **B,** Intraaortic electrogram during programmed stimulation of PVCs in the dog. Programmed stimulation did not produce ventricular fibrillation in seven dogs before bupivacaine but did produce ventricular fibrillation in four dogs after 2 mg/kg bupivacaine was given intravenously.

2. Ropivacaine. Animal studies have demonstrated that ropivacaine is less cardiotoxic and is much less likely to produce arrhythmias than bupivacaine. At anesthetically equipotent doses in pigs, ropivacaine produced less QRS prolongation than bupivacaine, but significantly more QRS prolongation than lidocaine.[74]

E. Opioids

All the opioids slow the heart rate by central vagal stimulation[75,76] or suppression of sympathetic activity,[77] except for meperidine,[78] which has anticholinergic effects. Fentanyl, besides slowing the rate of sinus node discharge, also prolongs AV nodal conduction and AV nodal and ventricular refractoriness.[79] There are case reports of AV nodal block and asystole with fentanyl and sufentanil.[80,81] This generalized depression of the conducting system is supported by a canine study that revealed that the incidence of ventricular tachyarrhythmias in fentanyl-anesthetized dogs was less than that in dogs anesthetized with inhaled agents.[82] Additionally, fentanyl increases the ventricular fibrillation threshold in dogs by sympathetic inhibition rather than by vagotonic effects.[83] On the other hand, morphine significantly raises ventricular fibrillation thresholds by increased vagal activity.[76] Suppression of PACs elicited by programmed stimulation by fentanyl has also been reported.[84] Besides decreasing heart rate, there is little information on the effects of remifentanil and cardiac arrhythmias. All these studies suggest that opioid-based anesthesia may be advantageous in patients with significant cardiac arrhythmias.

F. Neuromuscular relaxants

1. Succinylcholine. Most muscle relaxants, except succinylcholine and pancuronium, have little effect on cardiac rhythm. Succinylcholine causes a bradycardia secondary to vagotonic effects probably induced by succinylmonocholine,[85] especially after repeated doses in children. It can precipitate ventricular fibrillation (Box 11-3) secondary to increases in serum K⁺ in burn pa-

---

Box 11-3 Succinylcholine-associated arrhythmias

Sinus bradycardia (repeated doses)
Atrioventricular dissociation
Atrioventricular block and asystole (combined with intravenous induction agents and narcotics)
Ventricular arrhythmias (acute hyperkalemia)
  Burns
  Multiple trauma
  Quadriplegia, paraplegia (spinal cord injury)
  Muscular dystrophy
  Hemiparesis (stroke)
  Closed head injury
  Multiple sclerosis
  Prolonged bed confinement? (muscle disuse, such as Guillain-Barré syndrome, critically ill patients)

---

tients, neurologically injured patients, denervated patients, and patients with multiple trauma.[86] Also, succinylcholine has been reported to cause many other rhythm disturbances, including AV dissociation.[87] Succinylcholine reportedly decreases the threshold of catecholamine-induced ventricular arrhythmias. Several cases of AV nodal block and asystole have also been reported with combinations of sufentanil and alfentanil with succinylcholine.[80,88] However, all these case reports involved the addition of barbiturates or benzodiazepines to the anesthetic induction sequence. Others have shown that rapid-sequence techniques with only sufentanil and succinylcholine result in no change or in increased heart rate.[89]

2. Pancuronium. Pancuronium increases heart rate and shortens AV nodal conduction time[90] because of vagolysis[91] and possible catecholamine release.[92] Pancuronium in combination with halothane and tricyclic antidepressants has been reported to cause PACs and severe ventricular arrhythmias.[93] In an important study stimulated by two patients with severe tachyarrhythmias, pancuronium and halothane in dogs given tricyclics caused worse tachycardia and ventricular arrhythmias than in other dogs receiving pancuronium, enflurane, and tricyclics[93] (Fig. 11-6). In the animals that developed arrhythmias, there was a pronounced increase in the serum norepinephrine concentration. The pancuronium-halothane combination should be avoided in patients receiving these antidepressant drugs. The mechanism of pancuronium-associated arrhythmias was addressed by Jacobs et al,[94] who demonstrated delayed afterdepolarizations and abnormal automaticity in isolated papillary muscle fibers exposed to concentrations of pancuronium and epinephrine.

3. Vecuronium. Vecuronium has been reported to cause bradycardia requiring treatment when combined with a large dose of opioids.[95] Other cases of transient asystole[96] and even cardiac arrest[97,98] after vecuronium administration have been reported when vecuronium was combined with pharmacologic agents or intraoperative reflexes that increase vagal tone.

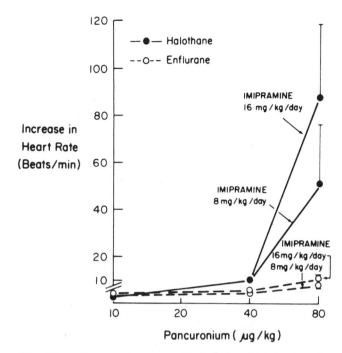

Fig. 11-6. Pancuronium, tricyclic, halothane interaction. In animals fed imipramine (a tricyclic antidepressant compound), extreme increases in heart rate occurred during halothane anesthesia (*closed circles*) after 0.08 µg/kg pancuronium, compared to minimal changes in heart rate during enflurane anesthesia (*open circles*) and pancuronium. (From Edwards RP, Miller RD, Roizen MF, et al: *Anesthesiology* 50:421, 1979.)

Table 11-3. Incidence of arrhythmias after muscle relaxant reversal with atropine-edrophonium in fentanyl-based (group 1) or isoflurane-based (group 2) anesthesia

Arrhythmias	Group 1	Group 2
None	8*	19
Severe	8*	3
Second- and third-degree AV block	6*	
Ventricular arrhythmia	1	1
Heart rate <40 beats/min	1	1
Moderate	7	4
Sinus bradycardia	4	3
First-degree AV block	3	1
Mild	3	3
Junctional rhythm	2	3
P-wave change	1	0

Modified from Urquhart ML, Ramsey FM, Royster RL, et al: *Anesthesiology* 67:561, 1987.
*$p < 0.01$ between group 1 and group 2.

4. Rocuronium. Rocuronium generally causes a 5% to 10% increase in heart rate in human studies, which is smaller than that caused by pancuronium but greater than that caused by vecuronium.[99]

5. Mivacurium and cisatracurium. Mivacurium causes no change or a small decrease in heart rate,[100] whereas cisatracurium causes little change in heart rate.[101] The arrhythmogenic potentials of these drugs are unknown and probably have little clinical significance.

G. Reversal agents

1. Naloxone. Naloxone has caused ventricular tachycardia and fibrillation,[102] in addition to myocardial ischemia, tachycardia, hypertension, and pulmonary edema, during reversal of nonoverdose, opioid-induced sedation and respiratory depression. A sudden increase in sympathomimetic stimulation after opioid withdrawal is hypothesized as the cause. If naloxone is required, very small doses (1 µg/kg intravenously) should be titrated to effect to avoid the surge in sympathetic tone that may cause the arrhythmias.

2. Muscle relaxant reversal. Arrhythmias with atropine-edrophonium reversal of neuromuscular blockade are reported to occur in 36% to 57% of patients.[103,104] Atropine-glycopyrrolate reversal induced arrhythmias in 53% of patients.[103] In a study of 55 patients after atropine-edrophonium reversal in either fentanyl-based or isoflurane-based anesthesia, there was a significantly greater incidence of arrhythmias in the fentanyl group (mainly transient AV

nodal block).[105] Five patients required therapy. However, all types of atrial, nodal, and ventricular arrhythmias occurred, but none were of clinical consequence (Table 11-3).

Cholinesterase inhibitors without anticholinergics cause slowing of sinoatrial (SA) node and AV node conduction and may result in sinus arrest and AV nodal block.[106] Small doses of edrophonium have been used in treatment of sinus tachycardia and paroxysmal supraventricular tachycardia (PSVT). Physostigmine administration has reportedly caused atrial fibrillation in a patient recovering from general anesthesia.[107] Small and large doses of atropine have caused AV dissociation.[108] Ventricular arrhythmias with atropine administration have occurred during inhalational anesthesia.[109]

H. Arrhythmias induced by anesthetics and surgical procedures

Cardiac arrest may occur during spinal anesthesia. Caplan et al[109] reported that in 14 healthy patients who sustained cardiac arrest, central nervous system (CNS) depression and cyanosis resulting in respiratory compromise was the likely cause of cardiac arrest, not cardiac arrhythmias. High spinal anesthesia may also block sympathetic input to the heart and result in bradycardia. Asystole has been reported during spinal anesthesia in a patient with sick sinus syndrome.[110]

As previously mentioned, tracheal intubation is associated with arrhythmias because of reflex sympathetic stimulation.[111] One report found PVCs in 18% of patients[112] during tracheal intubation. Very anxious patients with a high catecholamine concentration who present for anesthetic induction may be especially sensitive to the stimulus of intubation. Intravenous opioids, lidocaine, or β-adrenergic receptor blockers blunt the cardiovascular responses to intubation and may decrease the incidence of arrhythmias.

Insertion of central vascular catheters may also cause arrhythmias. The process of gaining venous access for central venous catheter insertion with the use of an intravenous guidewire may cause arrhythmias[113] if the guidewire is inserted too far into the heart. Furthermore, pulmonary artery catheter insertion often causes atrial and ventricular arrhythmias.[114] These mechanically stimulated ectopic beats generally are not suppressed with antiarrhythmics.[115] Manipulation of the catheter to prevent coiling in a cardiac chamber and repositioning is the proper response. The sudden onset of arrhythmias at any time after insertion should also arouse one's suspicions of a malpositioned catheter.[116]

Numerous surgically induced reflexes and manipulations may cause cardiac arrhythmias. An intrathoracic noncardiac procedure with manual cardiac irritation by the surgeon may lead to arrhythmias. Peritoneal traction, tracheal traction, brainstem compression, and compression of the eye (oculocardiac reflex) may result in either sympathetic-mediated or parasympathetic-mediated arrhythmias. The proper response is to alert the surgeon to discontinue the surgical manipulation, which usually controls the arrhythmia.

III. PATIENTS WITH ARRHYTHMIAS PRESENTING FOR ANESTHESIA AND SURGERY

A. Preoperative evaluation

Patients with a preoperative history of cardiac arrhythmias require a thorough cardiac preoperative evaluation, including specific discussion of the arrhythmia history and the type of antiarrhythmic medication. Precipitating or aggravating factors should be discussed. Relief or lack of relief of symptoms such as palpitations, dizziness, or syncope may be a sign of successful therapy or failure of therapy. Other cardiac symptoms such as dyspnea, angina, or syncope may indicate worsening of associated cardiac disease. Goldman et al[117] have demonstrated that any cardiac rhythm other than sinus rhythms, PACs, and more than five PVCs per minute on preoperative evaluation are directly related to perioperative cardiac morbidity. Arrhythmias are often a marker of associated cardiac disease (ischemic, valvular, cardiomyopathic, and so forth) and treatment of decompensated cardiac disease preoperatively often aids in arrhythmia control in the perioperative period.

All patients with a history of arrhythmia should have an electrocardiogram with rhythm strip before surgery. The electrocardiogram can yield information about worsening ischemic disease (ST segment analysis, new Q waves), possible electrolyte abnormalities, and QT interval changes secondary to antiarrhythmic therapy (proarrhythmic effects). A prolonged rhythm strip will give some baseline information on arrhythmia frequency before surgery. Occasionally, preoperative 24-hour Holter monitoring is indicated, especially if symptoms worsen, to allow one to assess adequacy of therapy and stabilization of arrhythmic events. For example, if a patient has previously controlled bursts of nonsustained ventricular tachycardia every 2 minutes before surgery, this is a sign of electrical instability that may warrant further antiarrhythmic therapy or additional therapy of underlying cardiac disease. Another electrographic technique developed for patients with arrhythmias is signal-averaged electrocar-

diography.[118] This is a computer-based process that eliminates nonrepeating random noise and averages multiple samples of repetitive waveforms to demonstrate periods of late depolarization occurring through slowly conducting tissue at the terminal end of the QRS complex.[119] These late potentials have been demonstrated in patients with ventricular tachycardia, and the elimination of late potentials correlates with successful antiarrhythmic therapy.[119] Last, lack of arrhythmia control and electrical instability preoperatively may require electrophysiologic testing with intravenous drug trials and programmed stimulation. Most of these questions can be addressed by a cardiology consultation with arrhythmia specialists.

Other preoperative laboratory evaluations should include measurement of serum K^+ and Mg^{++} concentrations, antiarrhythmic drug concentration if available, and a chest roentgenogram when structural cardiac disease is present. Many patients with arrhythmias and congestive heart failure require diuretics and digitalis preparations. Diuretic-induced hypokalemia and hypomagnesemia are common.[120] Diuretic therapy in hypertensive disease is associated with a greater mortality secondary to diuretic-induced electrolyte disturbances and arrhythmias.[120] However, because K^+ and Mg^{++} are the two most abundant intracellular ions, normal serum concentrations may not correlate with total body or tissue concentrations of these ions.[121] Digitalis-induced arrhythmias are also more likely in the presence of hypokalemia and hypomagnesemia.[121] Measuring the digitalis concentration before surgery may help to prevent digitalis-toxic arrhythmias and symptoms in the postoperative period. Digitalis toxicity is common in hospitalized patients.[122] Other drug concentrations of antiarrhythmics such as procainamide and its active metabolite (N-acetyl procainamide) are helpful in the assessment of adequate therapeutic or toxic concentrations before surgery.

The continuation of all cardiac antiarrhythmic medication until the time of surgery is important for perioperative arrhythmia control. An increase in arrhythmia frequency and difficulties in arrhythmia control because of the stress of the perioperative period caused by release of catecholamines should be anticipated. Thus adequate preoperative anxiety control with or without sedative-hypnotic agents as indicated is of utmost importance, as with any preoperative preparation.

B. Causes and consequences of supraventricular arrhythmias

1. Premature atrial contractions. The causes of PACs during anesthesia and surgery may include any of the mechanisms previously discussed involving any of the supraventricular structures (SA node, atrial tissue, AV node). However, atrial tissue ectopic activity itself accounts for most premature supraventricular beats. Clinical causes of PACs include ischemic heart disease, congestive heart failure from ischemic or valvular heart disease increasing left atrial dimensions, electrolyte abnormalities, acid-base problems, hypoxemia, drug effects, autonomic imbalance, stress primarily from catecholamine stimulation, surgical manipulations, and central venous catheter insertion. In patients with AV

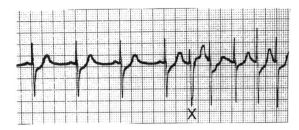

Fig. 11-7. PAC resulting in atrial fibrillation. Notice the changes in T-wave morphology from the normal T waves before and after QRS X, representing PACs in the T waves. The premature QRS *(X)* has a different morphology from the normal QRS complexes, illustrating aberrant ventricular conduction. (From Royster RL, Robertie PG: *Anesthesiol Clin North Am* 7:315, 1989.)

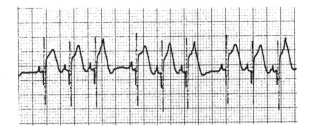

Fig. 11-8. Blocked PACs. Notice the peaked T-wave configuration before the pauses compared to the preceding T-wave morphology. PACs are blocked at the AV node because of their severe prematurity, causing depolarization to enter the AV node during its effective refractory period.

nodal reentry and accessory pathways connecting atrial to ventricular nodes, premature atrial depolarization may occur secondary to retrograde conduction depolarizing the atria from an AV nodal to SA nodal direction, which creates an inverted P wave on the electrocardiogram.[123] This may precipitate sustained PSVT. The PAC is the primary stimulus for most supraventricular arrhythmias such as PSVT, atrial fibrillation, atrial flutter, and multifocal atrial tachycardia (MAT)[123] (Fig. 11-7). Thus preventing the PAC from occurring provides preventive therapy for supraventricular arrhythmias.

The key to diagnosis of PACs is locating the P wave.[124] Lead II or V_1 is usually best for P-wave determination. Depending on the degree of prematurity of the atrial contraction, the P wave may occasionally be located within the T wave, slightly altering the basic T wave morphology (see Fig. 11-7). The shape of the P wave is usually different from that of the sinus P wave, being almost identical when the premature focus is near the sinus node or inverted when the focus is near the atrioventricular groove. The origin of PACs may be either right or left atrial tissue, and because the spread of atrial depolarization proceeds in all directions, the sinus node is usually depolarized prematurely and reset to the intrinsic sinus rate. Therefore the interval after the PAC is equal to the intrinsic PP interval of the sinus rhythm.

The QRS complex with PACs usually appears normal; however, as the degree of prematurity of a PAC increases, the pathway taken through the intraventricular conduction system may become abnormal or aberrant[125] because areas of the distal conducting system have yet to repolarize. The most proximal portion of the right bundle branch is usually the last part of the ventricular conduction system to repolarize; therefore the conduction proceeds down the left bundle, yielding a QRS complex resembling a right bundle-branch block. Aberrantly conducted PACs are also common in atrial fibrillation. It is important to distinguish aberrancy from the wide QRS complex of PVCs. Table 11-4 lists some distinguishing features of aberrantly conducted premature supraventricular complexes and PVCs. Very premature atrial contractions may block at the level of the AV node and fail to conduct to the ventricle, creating a pause in the QRS cycle (Fig. 11-8).

Table 11-4. Differences in morphology of aberrantly conducted premature atrial QRS complexes and premature ventricular QRS complexes

Aberrant conduction (PACs)	PVCs
Preceding P waves	P waves absent
RBBB pattern common	RBBB pattern uncommon
Initial deflection of QRS may be identical to normal QRS	Initial QRS deflection may differ from normal QRS
QRS width >0.12 sec	QRS width >0.14 sec
Noncompensatory pause	Compensatory pause
In atrial fibrillation, varying coupling intervals	In atrial fibrillation, constant coupling intervals

Modified from Royster RL, Robertie PR: *Anesthesiol Clin North Am* 7:315, 1989.
RBBB, Right bundle-branch block.

The class IA antiarrhythmics have atrial electrophysiologic properties suitable for the treatment of premature supraventricular beats. Intravenous procainamide is suitable for the perioperative period to suppress ectopic atrial foci. Additionally, procainamide is effective in converting atrial fibrillation to sinus rhythm, further supporting its antiarrhythmic properties on atrial tissue.[126] Digitalis has been classically used in suppressing atrial arrhythmias; however, its major benefit is slowing AV node conduction and fast ventricular response after supraventricular tachyarrhythmias arise.[127] β-Adrenergic receptor blockers also may aid in the therapy of premature atrial beats associated with high autonomic states or an increased catecholamine concentration.[128] Verapamil may be especially helpful in preventing premature nodal beats that result from AV nodal reentry because verapamil is effective in converting AV nodal reentry supraventricular tachycardias to sinus rhythm.[129]

2. Paroxysmal supraventricular tachycardia. PSVTs originate suddenly in the anatomic structures of the supraventricular area: the sinus node, atrial muscle, AV node, and accessory AV connection.[123] Sinus node, AV node, and accessory AV connection tachycardias are usually attributable to a reentry mechanism, whereas primary atrial tachycardias may be either reentry or some form of automaticity.[123] The QRS complexes may be narrow or wide, and wide complex supraventricular tachycardia must be differentiated from ventricular tachycardia.[130] A basic approach to diagnosis of supraventricular tachy-arrhythmias is shown in Box 11-4. An adequate 12-lead electrocardiogram with an accompanying rhythm strip compared to preceding electrocardiograms is essential for diagnosis of supraventricular arrhythmias. An esophageal lead or intracardiac electrogram may give additional valuable information for diagnosing supraventricular arrhythmias. See Box 11-5 for the most common intravenous drugs for treatment of supraventricular arrhythmias.

Box 11-4 Basic approach to diagnosis of tachyarrhythmias

What is the rate?

1. Ventricular rates of 150 beats/min often represent atrial flutter with 2:1 AV block.
2. Any ventricular rate greater than 200 beats/min in an adult patient suggests an accessory AV connection.

Rhythm: regular or irregular?

1. An irregular ventricular response is highly suggestive of atrial fibrillation.
2. Atrial flutter with variable AV conduction or atrial tachycardias with variable AV block also cause an irregular rhythm (such as multifocal atrial tachycardia).

P waves: present or absent?

1. The presence of P waves indicates a supraventricular tachycardia.
2. P-wave morphology is compared to sinus P-wave morphology (see Box 11-5).
3. The absence of P waves is consistent with a supraventricular tachycardia or ventricular tachycardia.
4. If P waves are not visible on a rhythm strip, then an esophageal lead, saline bridge, or intracardiac electrogram may give further information on atrial activity.

QRS complex: narrow or wide?

1. A narrow QRS complex (<0.12 sec) indicates a supraventricular tachyarrhythmia.
2. A wide QRS (>0.12 sec) complex indicates a supraventricular or a ventricular tachycardia.
3. Wide QRS complexes occur with a supraventricular tachycardia when a preexisting bundle-branch block, aberrant ventricular conduction, or accessory AV connection resulting in preexcitation of the ventricle is present.
4. Ventricular tachycardia is suggested by a QRS complex duration >0.14 sec.

QRS axis: normal or abnormal?

1. A severe left-axis deviation (−60° to −120°) during the tachycardia suggests a ventricular origin.
2. Supraventricular tachycardias usually maintain a normal axis. Ventricular tachycardia is distinguished from supraventricular tachycardia by the following criteria: a QRS duration >0.14 sec, left-axis deviation, a monophasic positive QRS complex in lead V_1, and AV dissociation.

Box 11-5 Intravenous supraventricular antiarrhythmic therapy

Class I

Procainamide (IA) converts acute atrial fibrillation, suppresses PACs and precipitation of atrial fibrillation/flutter, converts accessory pathway SVT. 100 mg IV loading dose every 5 minutes until arrhythmia subsides or total dose of 15 mg/kg (rarely needed) with continuous infusion of 2 to 6 mg/min.

Class II

Esmolol converts or maintains slow ventricular response in acute atrial fibrillation. 0.5 to 1 mg/kg loading dose with each 50 µg/kg/min increase in infusion, with infusions of 50 to 300 µg/kg/min. Hypotension and bradycardia are limiting factors.

Class III

Ibutilide converts atrial flutter, not as good in the conversion of atrial fibrillation. 1 mg given initially, may repeat with another 1 mg if not successful. For patients weighing <60 kg, give 10 µg/kg over 10 minutes, may repeat if unsuccessful. Beware patients with prolonged QT intervals.

Class IV

Verapamil slows ventricular response in acute atrial fibrillation, converts AV node reentry SVT (75 to 150 µg/kg IV bolus).

Diltiazem slows ventricular response in acute atrial fibrillation, converts AV node reentry SVT (250 µg/kg bolus, then 100 to 300 µg/kg/hr infusion).

Others

Adenosine converts AV node reentry SVT and accessory pathway SVT. Aids in diagnosis of atrial fibrillation and flutter.
  Adults: 3 to 6 mg IV bolus, repeat with 6 to 12 mg bolus.
  Children: 100 µg/kg bolus, repeat with 200 µg/kg bolus.
  Increased dosage required with methylxanthines, decreased dosage required with dipyridamole.

Digoxin maintenance intravenous therapy for atrial fibrillation and flutter slows ventricular response.
  Adults: 0.25 mg IV bolus followed by 0.125 mg each 1 to 2 hours until rate controlled, not to exceed 10 µg/kg in 24 hours.
  Children (<10 yr): 10 to 30 µg/kg load given in divided doses over 24 hours. Maintenance: 25% of loading dose.

a. Sinus node reentry. Sinus node reentry is an uncommon form of PSVT, occurring in less than 2% of patients.[123,124] P-wave morphology is identical to sinus P-wave morphology (Box 11-6), with the important differential factor being the sudden onset of tachycardia. Carotid sinus massage may terminate the tachycardia because the sinus node is under vagal innervation. In addition, sinus node depolarization is primarily calcium dependent; verapamil (75 μg/kg given slowly) or β-blockers may be effective in conversion (Fig. 11-9). Sinus node reentry occurs primarily in patients with ischemic heart disease.

b. Atrial tachycardias. Atrial tachycardias, comprising approximately 8% of PSVTs, result from either an ectopic automatic focus or a reentry pathway.[123,124] Atrial tachycardias have a P-wave morphology different from that of the P wave in sinus rhythm (see Box 11-6). This arrhythmia is true paroxysmal atrial tachycardia, which previously was the common term to describe all PSVTs. Atrial tachycardias can be very difficult to treat. Carotid sinus massage and verapamil may slow the ventricular response and cause AV nodal block, but conversion is rare. Therapy is aimed at the underlying process, such as myocardial ischemia, congestive heart failure, chronic obstructive pulmonary disease with hypoxemia and hypercapnia, or electrolyte disturbances. Electrical cardioversion may be required for termination. Type IA antiarrhythmics (quinidine, procainamide, and disopyramide) are beneficial in preventing the recurrence of the premature atrial focus. Intravenous procainamide is preferable in critically ill patients.

c. Atrioventricular node reentry. AV node reentry is the most common PSVT, occurring in 60% of patients.[129] Reentry may occur in the AV node because of dual AV nodal pathways. These AV nodal pathways have different conduction velocities and refractory periods, which present an ideal substrate for the development of a reentrant arrhythmia. Most commonly, P waves are not present on the electrocardiogram because of almost simultaneous retrograde activation of the atria and antegrade activation of the ventricle from the AV nodal focus (Fig. 11-10). Occasionally, inverted P waves in leads II, III, and aV$_F$ may occur either before or after the QRS complex (see Box 11-6). Carotid sinus massage may convert AV nodal reentry, and adenosine (6 mg, repeated in several minutes if no effect is seen) is the drug of choice and is very effective in conversion to sinus rhythm[131] (Fig. 11-11). Verapamil is also effective, and hypotension can be avoided with slow administration. The main advantage of adenosine is an extremely short half-life of a few seconds, which avoids side effects. However, transient AV nodal block and ventricular escape beats may occur before reestablishing sinus rhythm.

d. Accessory atrioventricular pathways. Electrophysiologic studies have demonstrated that the second most common cause (approximately 30%) of PSVT is accessory AV pathways.[123,124] These pathways, along with the AV node, form a reentry pathway between atria and ventricle that can sustain a PSVT. These tachycardias most often have a narrow QRS complex; however, in patients with the preexcitation syndrome (that is, Wolff-Parkinson-White [WPW]) the QRS complex may be wide.[132] This early depolarization of the ventricle creates a slurred upstroke (delta wave) of the QRS complex and a short PR interval, both classic manifestations of WPW

> **Box 11-6** P-wave analysis and cause of paroxysmal supraventricular tachycardias
>
> 1. P waves are absent (usually within QRS) AV node reentry.
> 2. P waves are positive, inferior leads, preceding the QRS.
>   a. Identical morphology to sinus node P waves: SA node reentry
>   b. Morphology different from that of sinus P waves: intraatrial reentry or automaticity
> 3. P waves are inverted before or after the QRS AV node reentry or AV accessory pathway.

PSVT   HR = 153

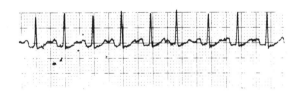

Post Esmolol   100 mg IV, HR = 110

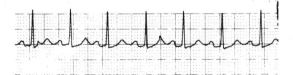

Fig. 11-9. SA node reentry tachycardia. The sudden onset of a paroxysmal supraventricular tachyarrhythmia *(PSVT)* at a heart rate *(HR)* of 153 beats/min that suddenly converted to an HR of 110 after intravenous administration of 100 mg esmolol. P-wave analysis reveals similar P morphology during the tachycardia and sinus rhythm, indicating SA node reentry as the most likely cause.

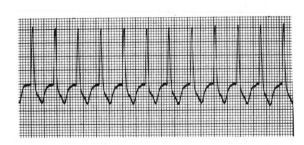

Fig. 11-10. AV nodal reentry. A narrow complex tachycardia at a heart rate of approximately 160 beats/min without evidence of atrial activity is strongly suggestive of atrioventricular nodal reentry.

PSVT

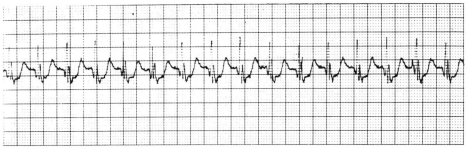

Post 2.5 mg VP

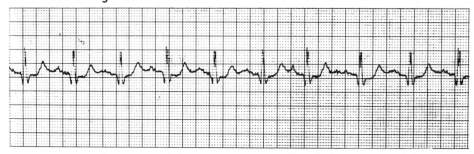

Fig. 11-11. Conversion of AV nodal reentry (paroxysmal supraventricular tachyarrhythmia, *PSVT*) with verapamil *(VP)* 2.5 mg intravenously. Notice the absence of atrial activity on the surface electrocardiogram.

Fig. 11-12. PSVT with retrograde P waves. Inverted P waves following the narrow QRS (rate = 140 beats/min) complex occur with either AV nodal reentry or accessory AV connections.

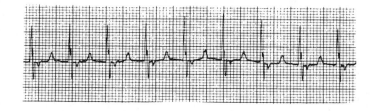

syndrome. During the tachycardia, P waves are often inverted after the QRS complex, an indication of retrograde activation of the atria (Fig. 11-12).

Approximately 50% of patients with the electrocardiographic manifestations of preexcitation have no symptoms, whereas 50% have symptoms of palpitations, dizziness, and syncope, indicating an arrhythmia problem. The most common arrhythmia associated with WPW syndrome is PSVT,[132] occurring in about 80% of patients, whereas atrial fibrillation and atrial flutter occur in the remainder of patients. Because of the potential fast conduction velocity and short refractory period of the accessory pathway, atrial fibrillation or atrial flutter may result in extremely fast ventricular rates (more than 300 beats/min), which can lead to sudden death (Fig. 11-13). These patients conducting at fast ventricular rates should have catheter or surgical ablation of their accessory pathways. In patients with slower ventricular rates, with atrial flutter, fibrillation, or PSVT, pharmacologic therapy is usually beneficial.

If the QRS complex is wide, demonstrating preexcitation, intravenous adenosine[131] or intravenous procainamide[133] (100 mg intravenously every 5 minutes until conversion) is the drug of choice (Figs. 11-14 and 11-15). Intravenous lidocaine[134] is also successful; however, one report demonstrated that an increased heart rate could occur in some patients.[135] Continuous infusions are usually not necessary or beneficial if loading doses fail. Intravenous verapamil[136] and digoxin[137] have been shown to increase the tachycardia rate in atrial fibrillation with wide QRS complexes and therefore are relatively contraindicated in WPW syndrome. However, electrophysiologic studies may demonstrate that verapamil or digoxin is suitable for treatment in some patients. Most anesthetic agents have little effect on accessory pathway function, except droperidol,[138] which has been shown to slow conduction across the pathway. Chronic oral therapy includes the type IA antiarrhythmics or oral agents such as amiodarone or sotalol. The treatment of a PSVT with a narrow QRS complex with

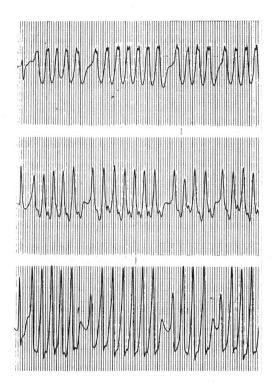

Fig. 11-13. Atrial fibrillation with an accessory pathway. Three different leads show the extremely fast rate (300 beats/min), irregular rhythm, and wide QRS complexes exhibiting preexcitation. These are classic findings of atrial fibrillation in adult patients with accessory pathways (see Figs. 11-14 and 11-15).

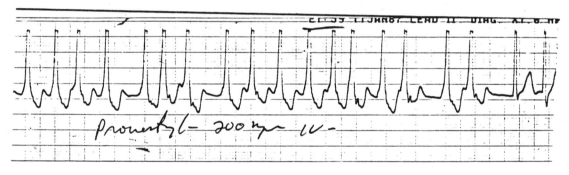

Fig. 11-14. Procainamide slowing of atrial fibrillation in patient with accessory pathway in Fig. 11-13. The patient converted to sinus rhythm after 200 mg procainamide was administered intravenously (see Fig. 11-15).

the reentry pathway proceeding down the AV node across ventricular muscle and conducting retrograde up the accessory pathway to the atria is identical to treatment for most AV nodal reentry supraventricular tachycardias: carotid sinus massage, adenosine, or verapamil.

3. Atrial fibrillation. Atrial fibrillation is an oscillating baseline on the electrocardiogram, best seen in lead II, with conducted ventricular complexes having a totally irregular rhythm. This irregularity is from the constant bombardment of the AV node by impulses that traverse the AV node in a competing and variable fashion, creating periods of physiologic block. The ventricular rate in untreated patients may vary between 120 and 200 beats/min and often results in decreases in cardiac output that are detrimental to the anesthetized or critically ill patient. Occasionally, untreated patients may present for surgery in atrial fibrillation with an intrinsically slow ventricular response because of underlying conducting system disease. These patients do not need preoperative therapy; however, the anesthesiologist should be prepared to treat increases in the ventricular response should they occur during the stress of surgery. Cardiac problems predisposing to atrial fibrillation include congestive heart failure, rheumatic heart disease, coronary artery disease, and pericarditis. Noncardiac conditions include thyrotoxicosis, pulmonary embolus, chronic obstructive lung disease, consumption of alcohol or caffeine, and electrolyte disturbances. Paroxysmal atrial fibrillation may occur intermittently in patients without any associated underlying disease. Anesthesiologists should

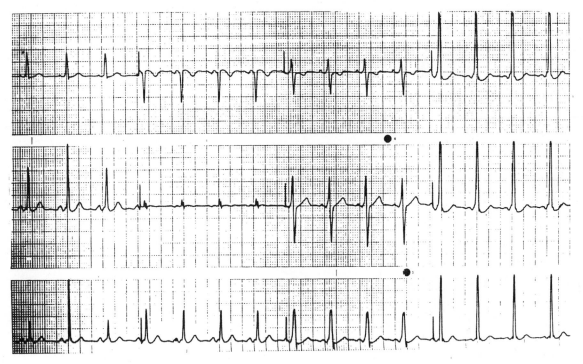

Fig. 11-15. Twelve-lead electrocardiogram after conversion of atrial fibrillation, demonstrating short PR interval and delta waves in most leads of the patient with an accessory pathway (see Figs. 11-13 and 11-14).

assume that the patient with intermittent atrial fibrillation will probably have the arrhythmia occur during his or her anesthetic period.

Verapamil (75 μg/kg) is usually very effective in reducing the ventricular rate in atrial fibrillation within several minutes, but conversion to sinus rhythm is rare.[139] An intravenous bolus of verapamil may result in hypotension, which may be prevented by the slow administration of verapamil (1 mg/min) or by pretreatment with an intravenous dose of calcium.[140] Calcium therapy reverses the hemodynamic effects of verapamil but does not reverse the electrophysiologic effects. A 30% reduction in the ventricular rate can be expected with the initial dose of verapamil, but maximal clinical effects last only 30 to 45 minutes. To maintain heart rate reduction, intravenous digoxin is given after successful rate reduction with verapamil. However, digoxin is as effective as verapamil in rate control during the stress of exercise and may lack effectiveness in rate control during the stress of the perioperative period.[141] Esmolol (0.5 to 1 mg/kg loading dose with a 50 μg/kg/min infusion with repeat loading doses before 50 μg/kg/min increments in infusion up to 250 μg/kg/min) is effective in slowing the ventricular response in atrial fibrillation and also in conversion to sinus rhythm[142] (Fig. 11-16). This short-acting, cardioselective β-blocker may prove effective in rate control during the stress of the perioperative period. Ibutilide (1 to 2 mg) has proven somewhat beneficial in conversion of atrial fibrillation but is more effective in atrial flutter. Amiodarone (5 mg/kg intravenously) is used commonly outside the

United States for conversion of atrial fibrillation, but studies in this country have not shown it to be as successful in conversion of atrial fibrillation as other available drugs.

If the conversion of atrial fibrillation is not accomplished with pharmacologic therapy or treatment of the underlying disease, cardioversion may be necessary. Anesthesiologists are often asked to provide anesthesia for electrical cardioversion of atrial fibrillation and flutter. Patients who are successfully cardioverted usually have atrial fibrillation of less than 1 year's duration, have a left atrial dimension of less than 45 mm by echocardiography, have no ventricular enlargement, and have successful treatment of the precipitating cardiac or noncardiac factors. Anticoagulation for several weeks is considered before elective cardioversion in patients with atrial fibrillation longer than 4 to 5 days and is maintained for several weeks after establishment of sinus rhythm to prevent systemic embolization.[143]

4. Atrial flutter. Atrial flutter is much less common than atrial fibrillation but shares the same predisposing factors. Atrial flutter is categorized into two types[144] (Fig. 11-17). Type I, or classic, atrial flutter usually occurs at a rate of 300 beats/min with a ventricular rate of 150 beats/min. The flutter waves are of a typical sawtooth or biphasic appearance in the inferior leads, and type I flutter may be converted by rapid atrial pacing. Type II atrial flutter exhibits a flat baseline with a positive flutter wave in the inferior leads, with a rate usually greater than 350 beats/min. Type II atrial flutter often cannot be converted by rapid atrial pacing. Electrophysiologic studies

Atrial Fibrillation   HR = 160   2 hrs post-CABG

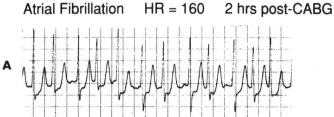

Post Digoxin and Verapamil

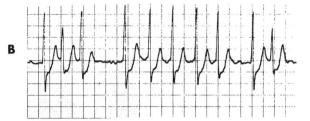

1 hr later, post Esmolol

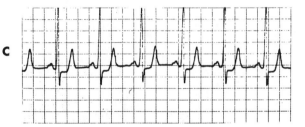

Fig. 11-16. Conversion of atrial fibrillation with esmolol after coronary artery bypass grafting *(CABG)*. **A,** Acute atrial fibrillation. **B,** Digoxin and verapamil slowed the ventricular response, but the rate remained unacceptably fast. **C,** After 1 hour to allow verapamil concentrations to decrease, esmolol (0.5 mg/kg × 2, followed by a 100 μg/kg/min infusion) converted the patient to sinus rhythm).

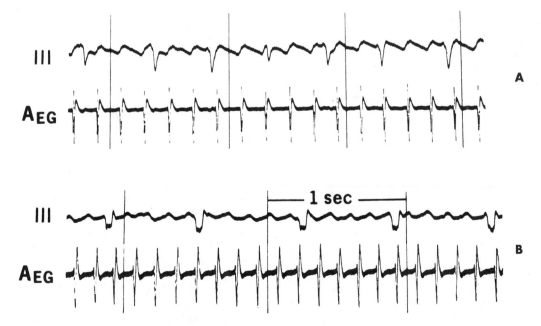

Fig. 11-17. Atrial flutter subtypes. **A,** Type I atrial flutter with the classic sawtooth pattern in lead III and an atrial rate of 300 beats/min on an atrial electrogram (A_{EG}). **B,** Type II flutter with positive flutter waves in lead III and an atrial rate of 400 beats/min. (From Wells JL, MacLean WA, James TN, et al: *Circulation* 60:665, 1979.)

have demonstrated flutter and fibrillation existing in the atria at the same time.

Atrial flutter is usually more difficult to treat than fibrillation. However, rapid atrial pacing in type I atrial flutter is effective.[145] Rapid atrial pacing involves pacing the atria with an atrial pacemaker at a rate approximately 20% faster than the flutter rate (360 for type I) from a site high in the right atrium.[145] In the operating room this can be accomplished with atrial electrodes placed during cardiac surgery, through an atrial electrode inserted through a paceport pulmonary artery catheter, by insertion of a temporary transvenous pacing electrode, or by an esophageal atrial pacing probe. During rapid atrial pacing, a change in the morphology of the flutter pattern is a sign of overdrive suppression. In addition, there is a critical duration of rapid atrial pacing required to convert atrial flutter.[145] After interruption of atrial flutter, pacing should proceed for approximately 30 seconds; pacing for shorter amounts of time may not be successful. Because atrial thresholds are usually higher in atrial flutter[146] than sinus rhythm and determination of capture is difficult, maximal current (usually 20 mA) should be used on all temporary pacemakers for overdrive suppression. If suppression does not occur in type I flutter, it is usually because of inadequate rate, pacing time, or current.

Ibutilide (1 to 2 mg intravenously) is very effective in the conversion of atrial flutter if pharmacologic therapy is required. The QT interval should not be prolonged because a small percentage of patients may develop polymorphic ventricular tachycardia (torsade) after ibutilide.

5. Multifocal atrial tachycardia. The arrhythmia MAT usually occurs in the seriously ill, elderly patient, often in the setting of decompensated chronic obstructive lung disease.[147] However, coronary artery disease, congestive heart failure, and the postoperative state may be associated with this arrhythmia.[148] MAT is diagnosed with the following criteria: three or more P waves with varying morphology and varying P-P cycle lengths, an atrial rate usually between 100 and 200 beats/min with irregular RR intervals, and varying PR intervals with varying degrees of AV block.[147] In most cases of MAT, the ventricular rate is between 100 and 150 beats/min. The ectopic P waves are often large and peaked and resemble the P waves seen in chronic pulmonary disease. Aberrant ventricular conduction may also occur, and this arrhythmia is often misdiagnosed as atrial fibrillation.

The classic treatment for MAT has been the improvement of the underlying chronic lung disease. Correction of hypoxemia, acidemia, and electrolyte disturbances will aid in management. Digoxin and many other antiarrhythmics, including cardioversion, are ineffective.[147] Several reports suggest that the theophylline drugs are highly associated with the development of this arrhythmia[149] and that discontinuation of theophylline agents should result in return to sinus rhythm (Fig. 11-18). Both verapamil[150] and metoprolol[151] decrease the atrial and ventricular rates and convert the arrhythmia to sinus rhythm in some patients.

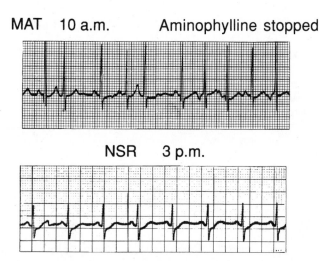

Fig. 11-18. Multifocal atrial tachycardia *(MAT)*. This arrhythmia occurred in a patient with decompensated chronic lung disease and converted to normal sinus rhythm *(NSR)* with discontinuation of an aminophylline infusion.

C. Causes and consequences of ventricular arrhythmias

Treatment of premature ventricular depolarizations requires the anesthesiologist to have an adequate knowledge of arrhythmia history, underlying organic heart disease, and prior antiarrhythmic therapy, as discussed in the preoperative evaluation. Patients with ventricular arrhythmias can be divided into three classes based on their associated risk of sudden death.[152] Most of these patients, especially those with malignant ventricular arrhythmias, need preoperative cardiology consultation. Appropriate questions to ask include "What are the risks of the patient developing ventricular arrhythmia during the increased sympathetic stress of the perioperative period?" and "What antiarrhythmic or other therapy do you recommend if the patient develops ventricular arrhythmia during surgery?"

1. Benign ventricular arrhythmias. Benign ventricular arrhythmias occur in patients without structural heart disease, whose risk of sudden death is minimal.[152] These patients usually have no hemodynamic symptoms and often are not treated; although if palpitations and dizziness are bothersome to the person, therapy may be elected. These patients may or may not have a history of ventricular arrhythmias. As previously discussed, ventricular arrhythmias are common in the normal general population and increase with age.[5,6] During surgery the anesthesiologist may be the first physician to monitor the patient for any prolonged length of time and may uncover these common benign arrhythmias. Therapy is usually not indicated; however, the prudent anesthesiologist should use these cardiac electrical problems as a warning that a noncardiac cause may exist, including myocardial ischemia, hypoxemia, hypercarbia, acidemia, light anesthesia, sympathetic stimulation, electrolyte abnormalities, or drug effects. If intraoperative problems arise associated with ventricular arrhythmias, antiarrhythmic therapy may be justified until the cause of these problems can be determined.

2. Potentially malignant ventricular arrhythmias. Potentially malignant ventricular arrhythmias occur in patients with structural heart disease,[152] with severe coronary artery disease and history of myocardial infarction, and with congestive or hypertrophic cardiomyopathy. All these patients have a higher risk of sudden death than patients with no known heart disease and ventricular arrhythmias. These patients usually are receiving antiarrhythmic therapy before their anesthetic, and if arrhythmias arise during anesthesia and surgery, they should be treated. Once again, after noncardiac causes are ruled out, therapy is based on the patient's organic heart disease and any previous antiarrhythmic therapy. Any patient with ischemic heart disease with new ventricular arrhythmias must have ischemia ruled out. Intravenous nitroglycerin may eliminate premature ventricular depolarizations without antiarrhythmic therapy.[153] Patients with congestive heart failure or congestive cardiomyopathy may have worsening failure with a dilated heart, which should be managed appropriately. Worsening obstruction in hypertrophic cardiomyopathy may require volume loading, pure vasopressors such as phenylephrine (Neo-Synephrine), β-blockade, or calcium-entry blockade to help relieve the obstruction.

3. Malignant ventricular arrhythmias. The final classification, malignant ventricular arrhythmias, is associated with severe structural heart disease with associated hemodynamic abnormalities.[152] These patients have symptoms of dizziness and syncope and may have a history of cardiac arrest. Some of these patients may have automatic implantable cardioverter defibrillator units or have had invasive or noninvasive ablative therapy for their arrhythmia. The treatment of patients with malignant ventricular arrhythmias is basically the same as for potentially malignant ventricular arrhythmias, except that the anesthesiologist and cardiologist must be more aggressive in documenting adequate therapy and considering prophylactic therapy. When a patient with potentially malignant ventricular arrhythmia is receiving antiarrhythmic therapy before surgery, the patient should be questioned to see whether any symptoms have been relieved. Drug concentrations, if available, should be obtained to verify adequate therapeutic concentrations. Most of these patients benefit from intravenous antiarrhythmic therapy during the stress of the perioperative period. The cardiologist should be asked what intravenous antiarrhythmic agent is appropriate for each patient if ventricular arrhythmias occur in the operating room. The most commonly used intravenous agents for control of ventricular arrhythmias are shown in Box 11-7.

Intravenous antiarrhythmic therapy begins with lidocaine, which remains a very effective agent against PVCs with minimal side effects.[154] If lidocaine is not effective, the substitution or addition of intravenous procainamide may prove effective.[154,155] Procainamide is also an excellent antiarrhythmic for PVCs, with efficacy similar to lidocaine; when combined with lidocaine (class IA and IB), it may be more effective than with single-drug ther-

---

Box 11-7 Intravenous ventricular antiarrhythmic therapy[*]

Class I

Procainamide (IA), 100 mg IV loading dose every 5 minutes until arrhythmia subsides or total dose of 15 mg/kg (rarely needed), with continuous infusion of 2 to 6 mg/min.

Lidocaine (IB), 1.5 mg/kg in divided doses given twice over 20 minutes, with continuous intravenous infusion of 1 to 4 mg/min.

Class II

Propranolol, 0.5 to 1 mg given slowly up to a total β-blocking dose of 0.1 mg/kg. Repeat bolus as needed.

Metoprolol, 2.5 mg given slowly up to a total β-blocking dose of 0.2 mg/kg. Repeat bolus as needed.

Esmolol, 0.5 to 1 mg/kg loading dose with each 50 μg/kg/min increase in infusion, with infusions of 50 to 300 μg/kg/min. Hypotension and bradycardia are limiting factors.

Class III

Bretylium, 5 mg/kg loading dose given slowly with a continuous infusion of 1 to 5 mg/min. Hypotension may be a limiting factor with infusion.

Amiodarone, 150 mg intravenously over 10 minutes, followed by 1 mg/min infusion over 6 hours and 0.5 mg/min thereafter.

*Overdrive pacing is effective in conversion of ventricular tachycardia. The procedure is the same as that for atrial flutter: Set rate at 20% faster than ventricular rate, set current at 20 mA, pace for 30 seconds, slowly decrease rate.

---

apy.[156] Theoretically, combination therapy with drugs with different electrophysiologic effects (from different classes) may be successful in patients with refractory ventricular arrhythmias when a single agent fails.[156] For refractory PVCs during the perioperative period, β-adrenergic receptor blockers (class II) are useful because they antagonize the increased catecholamine concentrations that occur during stress and cause PVCs.[128] Intravenous lidocaine, bretylium, and amiodarone (class IB and III) also are a potentially beneficial combination for therapy of PVCs in the perioperative period.[156]

The most common organic heart problem in patients with malignant ventricular arrhythmias is coronary artery disease, and ischemia is a likely precipitating cause. Ischemia during the perioperative period secondary to increases in myocardial demands or decreases in oxygen supply, including coronary vasospasm, may result in atrial or ventricular arrhythmias. Therapy with antiischemic drugs may eliminate the ischemic arrhythmic event. Maseri et al[153] showed that in patients with ventricular arrhythmias secondary to coronary vasospasm, antiischemic therapy was more effective in arrhythmia management than antiarrhythmics. In animal studies, nitroglycerin reverses the decrease in ventricular fibrillation thresholds caused by ischemia and prolongs ventricular refractoriness that was shortened by ischemia.[157] Prophy-

---

Box 11-8 Classification of antiarrhythmic agents with associated significant side effects

Class I

These drugs have local anesthetic or Na$^+$-channel blocking properties and are subdivided into categories A, B, and C.

IA drugs slow conduction velocity and prolong repolarization.

    Quinidine: Hepatic toxicity, prolongs QT interval

    Procainamide: Negative inotropy

    Disopyramide: Significant negative inotropy

    Moricizine: Mild negative inotropy

IB drugs slow conduction velocity and shorten repolarization.

    Lidocaine: Seizures

    Mexiletine: Hepatic toxicity

    Tocainide: Negative inotropy, pulmonary fibrosis, hepatitis

    Phenytoin: Drug interactions

IC drugs slow conduction velocity and have variable effects on repolarization. Recent studies show increased mortality after myocardial infarction.

    Flecainide: Negative inotropy, proarrhythmia

    Propafenone: Negative inotropy

Class II

These drugs block β-adrenergic receptors.

    Propanolol, esmolol, metoprolol: Negative inotropy and hypotension

Class III

These drugs prolong the action potential duration and effective refractory period.

    Bretylium: Hypotension

    Amiodarone: Negative inotropy, pulmonary fibrosis, others

    Sotalol: Negative inotropy, hypotension, proarrhythmia

    Ibutilide: Prolongs QT interval, may induce polymorphic ventricular tachycardia

Class IV

These drugs block calcium entry into the cells.

    Verapamil: Hypotension, contraindicated in wide QRS tachycardia (if ventricular tachycardia, ventricular fibrillation may result) and in neonates (apnea, hypotension, asystole)

    Diltiazem: Negative inotropy, conduction system slowing

---

lactic nitroglycerin with intravenous antiarrhythmic therapy and β-blockade with the usual precautions for anesthetic induction and maintenance in these patients are entirely appropriate.

D. Complications of antiarrhythmic therapy

The important complications of pharmacologic therapy for arrhythmias are best understood by a discussion of the classification of antiarrhythmic agents by Vaughan-Williams (Box 11-8). The most important toxic effects of each drug are also listed. Preoperative assessment of the toxicity of the appropriate organ system is of obvious importance to the anesthesiologist. Patients receiving negative inotrope antiarrhythmics may require a less myocardium-depressant anesthetic. Agents that cause pulmonary toxicity may require more definitive preoperative pulmonary tests and anticipated problems with gas exchange during anesthesia and surgery. The more conservative anesthesiologist may want to avoid inhaled agents in patients who receive potentially hepatotoxic antiarrhythmics. Drug interactions are important because of altered serum concentrations of various pharmacologic agents and of altered hemodynamic responses during anesthesia.

1. Myocardial depression. Negative inotropic effects of the antiarrhythmics are common, with disopyramide (Norpace) having the most significant effect. Acute pulmonary edema may occur with intravenous therapy. One study demonstrated new or worse congestive failure in 50% of patients with a history of congestive failure receiving disopyramide.[158] Anticholinergic effects of acute urinary retention, blurred vision, and dry mouth are other common side effects of disopyramide, with severe hypoglycemia rarely reported. Amiodarone may also cause clinically significant

myocardial depression during anesthesia.[159] Thyroid dysfunction, corneal microdeposits, and bluish skin discoloration are other side effects associated with amiodarone.

2. Pulmonary toxicity. Adverse pulmonary effects, including pulmonary infiltrates and pulmonary fibrosis, have been reported with amiodarone[160] and tocainide.[161] However, the pulmonary complications with amiodarone may occur in as many as 5% to 15% of patients, and autopsy studies indicate that this complication may be underdiagnosed.[162] Although unproven, there may also be an increased risk of adult respiratory distress syndrome if amiodarone is used perioperatively in patients undergoing cardiac surgery. Propafenone and other antiarrhythmics with β-blocking effects may precipitate bronchospasm.

3. Hepatic toxicity. Many antiarrhythmics may induce mild elevations in liver enzymes; however, quinidine[163] may cause a hypersensitivity reaction involving the liver, and tocainide may cause hepatitis. Most antiarrhythmics are hepatically metabolized, and reduced drug administration may be required in patients with hepatic disease. Serum concentrations of antiarrhythmic agents are helpful preoperatively.

4. Proarrhythmias. All antiarrhythmics have the potential to increase the frequency of arrhythmias and cause clinically significant worsening of arrhythmias (proarrhythmic effect). The class IC drugs (flecainide and encainide) are especially likely to cause proarrhythmic events.[164] Verapamil quickly slows the ventricular response in atrial fibrillation but may cause delayed conversion of atrial fibrillation to sinus rhythm. Verapamil is also contraindicated in wide complex tachycardias because it may convert ventricular tachycardia to ventricular fibrillation and cardiac arrest. Ibutilide may cause polymorphic ventricular tachycardia in patients with a prolonged QT interval. Emergency equipment should be available when using this drug.

5. Drug interactions. Other adverse reactions of particular importance to anesthesiologists are drug interactions. Amiodarone,[165] quinidine,[165] propafenone,[166] and verapamil[167] may increase the digitalis concentration. Phenytoin (Dilantin), by inducing liver microsomal enzymes, may reduce the serum concentration of quinidine,[168] disopyramide,[169] and mexiletine.[166] Amiodarone also increases warfarin, quinidine, procainamide, and phenytoin concentrations.[170] Immediate therapy with intravenous β-blockers after intravenous verapamil may result in second- or third-degree AV block. Bretylium (α), amiodarone (α, β), and propafenone (α, β) and other antiarrhythmics with antiadrenergic effects of α- or β-receptor blocking properties may alter hemodynamic responses during anesthesia.

IV. PATIENTS WITH MISCELLANEOUS DISEASE STATES ASSOCIATED WITH ARRHYTHMIAS

A. Mitral valve prolapse

The mitral valve prolapse syndrome is estimated to occur in 5% of the general population and in 10% to 20% of young, healthy females[171] and is accompanied by anxiety, tachycardia, neurasthenia, arrhythmias, and chest pain. More serious complications include acute mitral regurgitation from chordae tendineae rupture, infective endocarditis, stroke, and sudden death.[172] Mitral valve prolapse is associated with autonomic dysfunction, with high serum concentrations of catecholamines present in many patients.[173] Myxomatous degeneration of one or both mitral leaflets has been reported, with atrial muscle–like muscle fibers occasionally seen on pathologic analysis.[172] Atrial and ventricular arrhythmias may occur and are more common in patients with resting ST-segment and T-wave abnormalities.[174] PSVT is the most common tachyarrhythmia[175] caused by AV nodal reentry or accessory AV connections (more common with mitral valve prolapse). QT interval prolongation is also associated with mitral valve prolapse.[176]

Adequate preoperative preparation that provides anxiety relief and antibiotic prophylaxis for infective endocarditis is important. Hemodynamic alterations during anesthesia may make the prolapsing worse. Vasodilation, hypovolemia, or head-up position reduces the size of the left ventricle and allows the leaflets of the mitral valve to prolapse more into the left atrium.[177,178] Maintaining adequate volume and using phenylephrine (Neo-Synephrine) for hypotension may prevent or treat arrhythmias initiated by the prolapse.[178] One study of patients with adrenergic hypersensitivity in mitral valve prolapse showed greater increases in heart rate in response to catecholamine stimulation than in control patients.[173] β-Blockers are often effective antiarrhythmics,[179] although other antiarrhythmic agents may be needed for suppression of refractory atrial and ventricular arrhythmias.

B. Prolonged QT syndromes

1. Congenital. Patients presenting for anesthesia and surgery with a prolonged QT interval have either a congenitally prolonged QT interval or an acquired long QT interval secondary to electrolyte disturbances, drug therapy, or cardiac disease.[180] The congenital syndrome is important to anesthesiologists because of the numerous case reports of ventricular tachyarrhythmias occurring during anesthesia and surgery.[181,182] An imbalance or increase in left sympathetic cardiac input through the sympathetic chain is a possible cause of the congenitally prolonged QT interval.[183] Children with refractory arrhythmias may present for left stellate sympathectomy, which often corrects the prolonged QT interval.[184] Sympathetic stimulation caused by the stress of the perioperative period is a precipitating factor in these patients.[180] β-Blockers shorten the congenital long QT syndrome,[185] and this therapy should be maintained during the perioperative period[181] (Fig. 11-19). Adequate premedication, deep levels of anesthesia during induction and extubation, and postoperative pain relief are important features of the anesthetic plan.[180] Although no specific type of anesthetic has been proved in controlled studies to be beneficial, isoflurane in several case reports appears not to cause worsening of the QT interval.[181,186] Drugs with sympathomimetic effects, such as pancuronium and ketamine, should be avoided.[187]

2. Acquired. In the acquired long QT interval, polymorphic ventricular tachycardia (torsade de pointes) may result[188] (Fig. 11-20). Treatment of hypokalemia, hypomagnesemia, myocardial ischemia, or discontinuation of drugs prolonging the QT interval should be performed before surgery.[180,189] In contrast to therapy for the congenital syndrome, β-receptor stimulation is beneficial in the acquired syndrome.[190,191] Increasing the heart rate with isoproterenol or overdrive pacing prevents the early afterdepolarizations[190,191] that occur during the prolonged period of repolarization. Bradycardia should be avoided. No anesthetic technique appears to have any advantages over others, although inhaled agents that prolong His-Purkinje conduction theoretically may prolong repolarization and the QT interval. However, an abstract comparing isoflurane anesthesia with opioid anesthesia found no difference between the two techniques and the ultimate effect on the QT interval.[192] Some antiarrhythmic agents that prolong refractoriness and the QT interval are associated with torsade de pointes (quinidine),[193] and some are not (amiodarone).[194] Drugs prolonging the QT interval not associated with torsade de pointes have Ca^{++}-antagonistic properties,[195] as the inhaled anesthetic agents do. This finding indicates, but does not prove, that the inhaled agents may be safe to use in the acquired syndrome, as supported by the case reports. As previously mentioned, ibutilide may cause polymorphic ventricular tachycardia in these patients.

C. Central nervous system disease

Cardiac arrhythmias have been known for years to be associated with various CNS diseases. Both supraventricu-

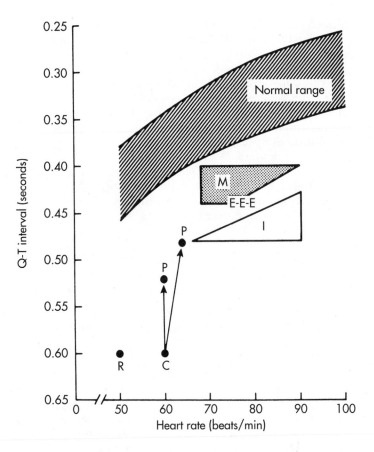

Fig. 11-19. Changes in QT interval during anesthesia with isoflurane in a patient who had an arrest during a previous anesthetic without propranolol pretreatment. The control (C) QT shortens after propranolol (P). The QT intervals during anesthesia are intubation (I), maintenance (M), and emergence (E). The return (R) point QT interval after surgery is similar to the control QT interval. β-adrenergic receptor blockers are indicated in all patients perioperatively with the congenitally long QT interval. (From Medak R, Benumof JL: *Br J Anaesth* 55:361, 1983.)

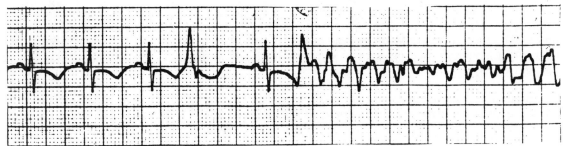

Fig. 11-20. Ventricular tachycardia (torsade de pointes) occurring in a patient with an acquired long QT interval secondary to quinidine toxicity. Notice the second premature ventricular contraction occurring on the inverted T wave, precipitating the ventricular arrhythmia.

lar and ventricular arrhythmias secondary to closed head injury, subarachnoid hemorrhage, and stroke are reported in the literature.[196-198] But few prospective studies of arrhythmias and CNS disease were performed until recently. Di Pasquale et al[199] found arrhythmias in 90% of 107 patients with subarachnoid hemorrhage, with a high incidence of PVCs, PACs, and sinus arrhythmia. Nine patients had atrial fibrillation (Fig. 11-21) or PSVT, and six had ventricular tachycardia or fibrillation. Of these six, four patients had torsade de pointes associated with a long QT interval, which is known to occur with subarachnoid hemorrhage.[200] Other human and animal studies have demonstrated that acutely increased intracranial pressure, brainstem compression, blood injected into the subarachnoid space, and blood irritating

the brainstem or other intracranial structures may precipitate cardiac arrhythmias.[201-204] The neuroanesthesiologist must be aware of this relationship and be prepared to treat associated arrhythmias.

D. Valvular heart disease

There is a high incidence of ventricular arrhythmias occurring in aortic stenosis. Von Olshausen et al[205] found 84% of patients with aortic valve disease to have PVCs, with 73% having multifocal PVCs, couplets, or longer runs of ventricular tachycardia. There appears to be a relationship between left ventricular wall stress, increased pressure gradients, lower ejection fractions, and the more complex ventricular arrhythmias.[205] Some studies have shown a reduction in these complex ventricular ar-

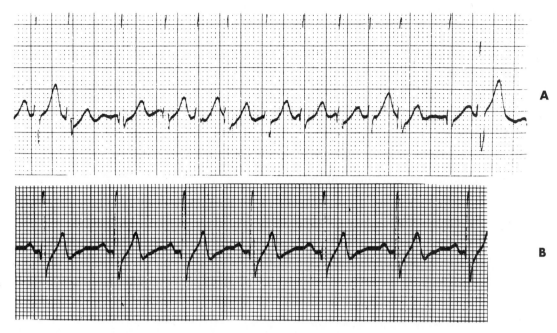

Fig. 11-21. Atrial fibrillation in a 50-year-old man after craniotomy for arteriovenous malformation repair (**A**) and after therapy with esmolol (**B**), which converted the atrial fibrillation to sinus rhythm. Esmolol 500 μg/kg × 4 and a 200 μg/kg/min infusion was required.

rhythmias after valve replacement, and some have not.[206,207] Considering the reduction of ventricular fibrillation thresholds after ischemic periods of cardiac surgery and this high incidence of ventricular arrhythmias, one should give serious consideration to instituting ventricular antiarrhythmic therapy in patients having aortic valve replacement.

Loss of atrial contraction in atrial fibrillation or junctional rhythm may cause severe hemodynamic problems in aortic stenosis because of the increased importance of atrial contraction on ventricular filling. Atrial fibrillation may occur during intravenous guidewire insertion, pulmonary artery catheterization, or venous cannulation before cardiopulmonary bypass. Electrical cardioversion is necessary if hemodynamic collapse occurs. If time and hemodynamics permit, esmolol is very efficacious in converting atrial fibrillation to sinus rhythm. Avoiding inhaled anesthetics in aortic stenosis is wise because junctional rhythms causing AV dissociation commonly occur with these agents.

Tachycardia worsens mitral stenosis by decreasing diastolic filling time, decreasing blood flow across the valve, and increasing the transvalvular gradient. Tachycardia in atrial fibrillation worsens symptoms in patients with mitral stenosis and not the fibrillation itself.[208] Atrial fibrillation does not affect mitral regurgitation as significantly because increased heart rate does not usually increase the left atrial pressure, and atrial contraction is not effective because of the usually giant atrial size.

E. Arrhythmias in children

Junctional ectopic tachycardia (JET) is one of the most dangerous arrhythmias encountered in children, and mortalities are extremely high.[209] There are two forms of junctional ectopic tachycardia: congenital and postsurgical. Anesthesiologists see children with this arrhythmia who have congenital heart disease after cardiac or noncardiac surgery. JET is caused by an enhanced automatic mechanism of the distal conducting system in the area of the His bundle.[210] This arrhythmia may generate ventricular rates as high as 300 beats/min, and a cardiomyopathy with congestive heart failure may develop.[209] Postoperative JET occurs most commonly in infants who have congenital cardiac defects repaired.[211] Most infants have low cardiac output, their lungs are mechanically ventilated, and they are receiving drugs such as meperidine, barbiturates, and pancuronium bromide. Inotropic agents are often required, and many children are mildly acidemic.[211] Thus the cause is multifactorial. Therapy is aimed at reducing adrenergic tone, increasing vagal tone, and maintaining hemodynamic and normal metabolic function.[211] Mild hypothermia also is suggested to be helpful in reducing the tachycardia.[212]

Medical therapy with digoxin or β-blockers, or both, is rarely successful.[209,213] Verapamil, as in other supraventricular tachycardias in infants, should not be given because of reports of apnea, bradycardia, severe hypotension, and death.[214] Overdrive pacing and electrical cardioversion are not effective.[209] Villain et al[215] reported amiodarone to restore the heart rate to below 150 beats/min in 8 of 14 patients with congenital JET. Flecainide, encainide, phenytoin, and propafenone have been reported to be successful in this arrhythmia.[216,217] Because mortality may approach 35%,[215] catheter and surgical ablative therapy should be considered in refractory cases.[209]

F. Electrolyte abnormalities

All physicians are aware of the arrhythmogenic effects of hypokalemia, which increases the automaticity and excitability of the myocardial cell membrane.[218] Controversy exists in the relationship of PVCs to hypokalemia in clinical studies.[218,219] However, there are clear data indicating that hypokalemia is associated with the development of ventricular tachycardia and fibrillation, especially during stressful situations with increased catecholamine concentrations and acute myocardial ischemia.[220]

Patients presenting for anesthesia and surgery who are receiving diuretics are prone to hypokalemia and potassium depletion.[221] In patients with arrhythmias, serum K^+ concentrations should be maintained greater than 4.0 mEq/L before surgery.[217] Further K^+ decreases may occur during surgery because of hyperventilation, which shifts K^+ into cells, and stress-induced epinephrine secretion, which stimulates β_2-adrenergic receptors, promoting an uptake of potassium into cells.[222] The arrhythmogenic electrophysiologic effects of hypokalemia may oppose the antiarrhythmic effects of antiarrhythmic medication.[223]

In contrast to the well-known electrophysiologic effects of hypokalemia, the electrophysiologic effects of hypomagnesemia are less clear.[224] Watanabe and Dreifus[225] demonstrated in perfused rabbit hearts that the effects on transmembrane potentials of hypomagnesemia were entirely dependent on extracellular potassium, with minor changes occurring when extracellular potassium was normal. Magnesium is required as a cofactor for the Na^+-K^+ pump and Ca^{++}-ATPase pump, which maintains low intracellular calcium concentrations. A low serum magnesium concentration reduce Na^+-K^+ pump activity, which increases Na^+-Ca^{++} exchange, increases intracellular Ca^{++}, and reduces intracellular K^+ concentrations.[226] Reduced intracellular Mg^+ also decreases Ca^{++} extrusion via the Ca^{++}-ATPase pump, resulting in increased intracellular Ca^{++} currents, which are arrhythmogenic in triggered automaticity models.[227]

Well-controlled clinical studies have not proved a relationship between hypomagnesemia and PVCs.[228,229] In many of the clinical studies suggesting that hypomagnesemia is arrhythmogenic, concurrent hypokalemia was present.[230-232] However, hypomagnesemia has definite electrophysiologic effects in humans of prolonging SA and AV node recovery times and increasing atrial-His intervals,[233] and such prolongation supports magnesium's effectiveness in treating supraventricular arrhythmias.[234,235] Magnesium is also beneficial in digitalis-toxic arrhythmias,[236] in torsade de pointes,[237] and in managing refractory ventricular arrhythmias.[238]

Chronic Mg^{++} depletion occurs in diuretic usage, aminoglycoside therapy, alcohol abuse, secondary aldosteronism, and malabsorption syndromes.[239] Serum Mg^{++} concentrations do not reflect intracellular Mg^{++} levels, especially in chronic depletion,[240] and treatment is indicated despite normal serum concentrations. Iseri[241] recommends 2 g $MgSO_4$ intravenously given over 2 to 3 minutes when ventricular arrhythmias are refractory to lidocaine and procainamide. A continuous infusion is begun, with 10 g given over 5 hours and, especially if arrhythmias subside, a second 10 g given over 10 hours to restore the intracellular magnesium concentration. Hypotension is a side effect that can be reversed easily with small doses of calcium. Serum K^+ and Mg^{++} concentrations are monitored during Mg^{++} therapy.

REFERENCES

1. Hur D, Gravenstein JS: Is ECG monitoring in the operating room cost effective? *Biotelemetry Patient Monitoring* 6:200, 1979.
2. Scott O, Williams GJ, Fiddler GI: Results of 24 hour ambulatory monitoring of electrocardiogram in 131 healthy boys aged 10 to 13 years, *Br Heart J* 44:304, 1980.
3. Romhilt DW, Chaffin C, Choi SC, et al: Arrhythmias on ambulatory electrocardiographic monitoring in women without apparent heart disease, *Am J Cardiol* 54:582, 1984.
4. Sobotka PA, Mayer JH, Bauernfeind RA, et al: Arrhythmias documented by 24-hour continuous ambulatory electrocardiographic monitoring in young women without apparent heart disease, *Am Heart J* 101:753, 1981.
5. Hinkle LE Jr, Carver ST, Stevens M: The frequency of asymptomatic disturbances of cardiac rhythm and conduction in middle-aged men, *Am J Cardiol* 24:629, 1969.
6. Brodsky M, Wu D, Denes P, et al: Arrhythmias documented by 24 hour continuous electrocardiographic monitoring in 50 male medical students without apparent heart disease, *Am J Cardiol* 39:390, 1977.
7. Pilcher GF, Cook AJ, Johnston BL, et al: Twenty-four-hour continuous electrocardiography during exercise and free activity in 80 apparently healthy runners, *Am J Cardiol* 52:859, 1983.
8. Kantelip J-P, Sage E, Duchene-Marullaz P: Findings on ambulatory electrocardiographic monitoring in subjects older than 80 years, *Am J Cardiol* 57:398, 1986.
9. Kostis JB, McCrone K, Moreyra AE, et al: Premature ventricular complexes in the absence of identifiable heart disease, *Circulation* 63:1351, 1981.
10. Poblete PF, Kennedy HL, Caralis DG: Detection of ventricular ectopy in patients with coronary heart disease and normal subjects by exercise testing and ambulatory electrocardiography, *Chest* 74:402, 1978.
11. Kennedy HL, Whitlock JA, Sprague MK, et al: Long-term follow-up of asymptomatic healthy subjects with frequent and complex ventricular ectopy, *N Engl J Med* 312:193, 1985.
12. Levy AG, Lewis T: Heart irregularities resulting from the inhalation of low percentages of chloroform vapor and their relationship to ventricular fibrillation, *Heart* 3:99, 1911-1912.
13. Lennox WG, Graves RC, Levine SA: An electrocardiographic study of fifty patients during operation, *Arch Intern Med* 30:57, 1922.
14. Marvin HM, Paston RB: The electrocardiogram and blood pressure during operation and convalescence, *Arch Intern Med* 35:768, 1925.
15. Kurtz CM, Bennett JH, Shapiro H: Electrocardiographic studies during surgical anesthesia, *JAMA* 106:434, 1936.
16. Vanik PE, Davis HS: Cardiac arrhythmias during halothane anesthesia, *Anesth Analg* 47:299, 1968.
17. Dodd RB, Sims MA, Bone DJ: Cardiac arrhythmias observed during anesthesia and surgery, *Surgery* 51:440, 1962.
18. Kuner J, Enescu V, Utsu F, et al: Cardiac arrhythmias during anesthesia, *Dis Chest* 52:580, 1967.
19. Bertrand CA, Steiner NV, Jameson AG, et al: Disturbances of cardiac rhythm during anesthesia and surgery, *JAMA* 216:1615, 1971.
20. Wit AL, Rosen MR: Pathophysiologic mechanisms of cardiac arrhythmias, *Am Heart J* 106:798, 1983.
21. Atlee JL, Bosnjak ZJ: Mechanisms for cardiac dysrhythmias during anesthesia, *Anesthesiology* 72:347, 1990.
22. Hoffman BF, Rosen MR: Cellular mechanisms for cardiac arrhythmias, *Circ Res* 49:1, 1981.
23. Cranefield PF: Action potentials, afterpotentials and arrhythmias, *Circ Res* 41:415, 1977.

24. Damiano BP, Rosen MR: Effects of pacing on triggered activity induced by early afterdepolarizations, *Circulation* 69:1013, 1984.
25. Sasyniuk BI, Valois M, Toy W: Recent advances in understanding the mechanisms of drug-induced torsades de pointes arrhythmias, *Am J Cardiol* 64:29J, 1989.
26. Ferrier GR: The effects of tension on acetylstrophanthidin-induced transient depolarizations and after contractions in canine myocardial and Purkinje tissue, *Circ Res* 38:156, 1976.
27. Cranefield PF, Aronson RS: Initiation of sustained rhythmic activity by single propagated action potentials in canine cardiac Purkinje fibers exposed to sodium-free solution or to ouabain, *Circ Res* 34:477, 1974.
28. Hewett KW, Rosen MR: Alpha and beta adrenergic interactions with ouabain-induced delayed after depolarizations, *J Pharmacol Exp Ther* 229:188, 1984.
29. Ferrier GR, Moffat MP, Lukas A: Possible mechanisms of ventricular arrhythmias elicited by ischemia followed by reperfusion, *Circ Res* 56:184, 1985.
30. Wit AL, Cranefield PT: Triggered and automatic activity in the canine coronary sinus, *Circ Res* 44:435, 1977.
31. Ferrier GR: Digitalis arrhythmias: role of oscillatory after potentials, *Prog Cardiovasc Dis* 19:459, 1977.
32. Rosen MR: Mechanisms for arrhythmias, *Am J Cardiol* 61:2A, 1988.
33. Wu D: Supraventricular tachycardias, *JAMA* 249(24):3357, 1983.
34. Wit AL, Hoffman BF, Cranefield PF: Slow conduction and reentry in the ventricular conducting system. I. Return extrasystole in canine Purkinje fibers, *Circ Res* 30:1, 1972.
35. Antzelevitch C, Jalife J, Moe GK: Characteristics of reflection as a mechanism of reentrant arrhythmias and its relationship to parasystole, *Circulation* 61:182, 1980.
36. Kinoshita S: Mechanisms of ventricular parasystole, *Circulation* 58:715, 1978.
37. Scherf D, Choi KY, Bahadori A, et al: Parasystole, *Am J Cardiol* 12:527, 1963.
38. Cohen H, Langendorf R, Pick A: Intermittent parasystole: mechanism of protection, *Circulation* 48:761, 1973.
39. Bosnjak ZJ, Kampine JP: Effects of halothane, enflurane and isoflurane on the SA node, *Anesthesiology* 58:314, 1983.
40. Atlee JL III, Brownlee SW, Burstrom RE: Conscious-state comparisons of the effects of inhalation anesthetics on specialized atrioventricular conduction times in dogs, *Anesthesiology* 64:703, 1986.
41. Scheffer GJ, Jonges R, Holley HS, et al: Effects of halothane on the conduction system of the heart in humans, *Anesth Analg* 69:721, 1989.
42. Sethna DH, Deboer GE, Millar RA: Observations on "junctional rhythms" during anaesthesia, *Br J Anaesth* 56:924, 1984 (letter).
43. Boba A: Significant effects on the blood pressure of an apparently trivial atrial dysrhythmia, *Anesthesiology* 48:282, 1978.
44. Galindo A, Wyte SR, Wetherhold JW: Junctional rhythm induced by halothane anesthesia: treatment with succinylcholine, *Anesthesiology* 37:261, 1972.
45. Breslow MJ, Evers AS, Lebowitz P: Successful treatment of accelerated junctional rhythm with propranolol: possible role of sympathetic stimulation in the genesis of this rhythm disturbance, *Anesthesiology* 62:180, 1985.
46. Hill RF: Treatment of isorhythmic A-V dissociation during general anesthesia with propranolol, *Anesthesiology* 70:141, 1989.
47. Black GW, Linde HW, Dripps RD, et al: Circulatory changes accompanying respiratory acidosis during halothane (Fluothane) anesthesia in man, *Br J Anaesth* 31:238, 1959.
48. Downing SE, Mitchell JH, Wallace AG: Cardiovascular responses to ischemia, hypoxia and hypercapnia of the central nervous system, *Am J Physiol* 204:881, 1963.
49. Zink J, Sasyniuk BI, Dresel PE: Halothane-epinephrine-ninduced cardiac arrhythmias and the role of heart rate, *Anesthesiology* 43:548, 1975.
50. Katz RL, Katz GJ: Surgical infiltration of pressor drugs and their interaction with volatile anaesthetics, *Br J Anaesth* 38:712, 1966.
51. Catenacci AJ, DiPalma JR, Anderson JD, et al: Serious arrhythmias with vasopressors during halothane anesthesia in man, *JAMA* 183:662, 1963.
52. Stirt JA, Berger JM, Ricker SM, et al: Arrhythmogenic effects of aminophylline during halothane anesthesia in experimental animals, *Anesth Analg* 59:410, 1980.
53. Roizen MF, Stevens WC: Multiform ventricular tachycardia due to the interaction of aminophylline and halothane, *Anesth Analg* 57:738, 1978.
54. Johnston RR, Eger EI II, Wilson C: A comparative interaction of epinephrine with enflurane, isoflurane and halothane in man, *Anesth Analg* 55:709, 1976.
55. Karl HW, Swedlow DB, Lee KW, et al: Epinephrine-halothane interactions in children, *Anesthesiology* 58:142, 1983.
56. Navarro R, Weiskopf RB, Moore MA, et al: Humans anesthetized with sevoflurane or isoflurane have similar arrhythmic response to epinephrine, *Anesthesiology* 80:545, 1994.
57. Weiskopf RB, Eger EI II, Holmes MA, et al: Epinephrine-induced premature ventricular contractions and changes in arterial blood pressure and heart rate during I-653, isoflurane, and halothane anesthesia in swine, *Anesthesiology* 70:293, 1989.
58. Bristow JD, Prys-Roberts C, Fisher A, et al: Effects of anesthesia on baroreflex control of heart rate in man, *Anesthesiology* 31:422, 1969.
59. Atlee JL III, Malkinson CE: Potentiation by thiopental of halothane-epinephrine–induced arrhythmias in dogs, *Anesthesiology* 57:285, 1982.
60. Atlee JL, Flaherty MP: Thiopental and epinephrine arrhythmias with enflurane and isoflurane in dogs, *Anesthesiology* 59:A84, 1983 (abstract).
61. Roberts FL, Burstrom RE, Atlee JL: Effects of ketamine and etomidate on epinephrine-induced ventricular dysrhythmias in dogs anesthetized with halothane, *Anesthesiology* 61:A36, 1984 (abstract).
62. Ivankovich AD, El-Etr AA, Janeczko GF, et al: The effects of ketamine and Innovar anesthesia on digitalis tolerance in dogs, *Anesth Analg* 54:106, 1975.
63. Thomson SJ, Yate PM: Bradycardia after propofol infusion, *Anaesthesia* 42:430, 1987.
64. Alphin RS, Martens JR, Dennis DM: Frequency-dependent effects of propofol on atrioventricular nodal conduction in guinea pig isolated heart: mechanism and potential antidysrhythmic properties, *Anesthesiology* 83:382, 1995.
65. Albright GA: Cardiac arrest following regional anesthesia with etidocaine or bupivacaine, *Anesthesiology* 51:285, 1979 (editorial).
66. Kasten GW: High serum bupivacaine concentrations produce rhythm disturbances similar to torsades de pointes in anesthetized dogs, *Reg Anaesth* 11:20, 1986.
67. Clarkson C, Hondeghem L: Mechanism for bupivacaine depression of cardiac conduction: fast block of sodium channels during the action potential with slow recovery from block during diastole, *Anesthesiology* 62:396, 1985.
68. Block A, Covino BG: Effect of local anesthetic agents on cardiac conduction and contractility, *Reg Anaesth* 6:55, 1981.
69. Conklin KA, Ziadlou-Rad F: Bupivacaine cardiotoxicity in a pregnant patient with mitral valve prolapse, *Anesthesiology* 58:596, 1983 (letter).
70. Davis NL, de Jong RH: Successful resuscitation following massive bupivacaine overdose, *Anesth Analg* 61:62, 1982.
71. Kasten GW, Martin ST: Bupivacaine cardiovascular toxicity: comparison of treatment with bretylium and lidocaine, *Anesth Analg* 64:911, 1985.
72. Soloman D, Buneqin L, Albin M: The effect of magnesium sulfate administration on cerebral and cardiac toxicity of bupivacaine in dogs, *Anesthesiology* 72:341, 1990.
73. Rosen M, Thigpen J, Shnider S, et al: Bupivacaine-induced cardiotoxicity in hypoxic and acidotic sheep, *Anesth Analg* 64:1089, 1985.
74. Reiz S, Haggmark S, Johansson G, et al: Cardiotoxicity of ropivacaine: a new amide local anesthetic agents, *Acta Anaesthesiol Scand* 33:93, 1989.
75. Loeb JM, Lichtenthal PR, de Tarnowsky JM: Parasympathomimetic effects of fentanyl on the canine sinus node, *J Auton Nerv Syst* 11:91, 1984.

76. de Silva RA, Verrier RL, Lown B: Protective effect of the vagotonic action of morphine sulphate on ventricular vulnerability, *Cardiovasc Res* 12:167, 1978.

77. Daskalopoulos NT, Laubie M, Schmitt H: Localization of the central sympatho-inhibitory effect of a narcotic analgesic agent, fentanyl, in cats, *Eur J Pharmacol* 33:91, 1975.

78. Tammisto T, Takki S, Toikka P: A comparison of the circulatory effects in man of the analgesics fentanyl, pentazocine, and pethidine, *Br J Anaesth* 42:317, 1970.

79. Royster RL, Keeler KD, Haisty WK, et al: Cardiac electrophysiologic effects of fentanyl and combinations of fentanyl and neuromuscular relaxants in pentobarbital anesthetized dogs, *Anesth Analg* 67:15, 1988.

80. Sherman EP, Lebowitz PW, Street WC: Bradycardia following sufentanil-succinylcholine, *Anesthesiology* 66:106, 1987 (letter).

81. Latson TW, Lappas DG: Use of a pacing catheter to control heart rate in a patient with aortic insufficiency and coronary artery disease, *Anesthesiology* 63:712, 1985.

82. Puerto BA, Wong KC, Puerto AX, et al: Epinephrine-induced dysrhythmias: comparison during anaesthesia with narcotics and halogenated inhalational agents in dogs, *Can Anaesth Soc J* 26:263, 1979.

83. Saini V, Carr DB, Hagestad EL: Antifibrillatory action of the narcotic agonist fentanyl, *Am Heart J* 115:598, 1988 (review).

84. Royster RL, Keeler DK, Prough DS, et al: Fentanyl attenuates stimulation of atrial premature depolarizations and prolongs atrioventricular and ventricular refractoriness in dogs, *Anesthesiology* 63(suppl 3A):A77, 1985 (abstract).

85. Yasuda I, Hirano T, Amaha K, et al: Chronotropic effects of succinylcholine and succinyl monocholine on the sinoatrial node, *Anesthesiology* 57:289, 1982.

86. Cooperman LH: Succinylcholine-induced hyperkalemia in neuromuscular disease, *JAMA* 213:1867, 1970.

87. Stoelting RK, Peterson C: Heart-rate slowing and junctional rhythm following intravenous succinylcholine with and without intramuscular atropine preanesthetic medication, *Anesth Analg* 54:705, 1975.

88. Maryniak JK, Bishop VA: Sinus arrest after alfentanil, *Br J Anaesth* 59:390, 1987.

89. Butterworth JF, Bean VE, Royster RL: Premedication determines the circulatory responses to rapid sequence induction with sufentanil for cardiac surgery, *Br J Anaesth* 63:351, 1989.

90. Geha DG, Rozelle BC, Raessler KL, et al: Pancuronium bromide enhances atrioventricular conduction in halothane-anesthetized dogs, *Anesthesiology* 46:342, 1977.

91. Son SL, Wand BE: Potencies of neuromuscular blocking agents at the receptors of the atrial pacemaker and the motor endplate of the guinea pig, *Anesthesiology* 47:34, 1977.

92. Domenech JS, Garcia RC, Sastain JMR, et al: Pancuronium bromide: an indirect sympathomimetic agent, *Br J Anaesth* 48:1143, 1976.

93. Edwards RP, Miller RD, Roizen MF, et al: Cardiac responses to imipramine and pancuronium during anesthesia with halothane or enflurane, *Anesthesiology* 50:421, 1979.

94. Jacobs HK, Lim S, Salem MR, et al: Cardiac electrophysiologic effects of pancuronium, *Anesth Analg* 64:693, 1985.

95. Gravlee GP, Ramsey FM, Roy RC, et al: Rapid administration of a narcotic and neuromuscular blocker: a hemodynamic comparison of fentanyl, sufentanil, pancuronium, and vecuronium, *Anesth Analg* 67:39, 1988.

96. Starr NJ, Sethna PH, Estafanous FG: Bradycardia and asystole following the rapid administration of sufentanil with vecuronium, *Anesthesiology* 64:521, 1986.

97. Pollok AJP: Cardiac arrest immediately after vecuronium, *Br J Anaesth* 58:936, 1986 (letter).

98. Milligan KR, Beers HT: Vecuronium-associated cardiac arrest, *Anaesthesia* 40:385, 1985 (letter).

99. Cornet JP, Abiad M, Coriate P, et al: Evaluation of the effects of rocuronium bromide on haemodynamics and left ventricular function in patients undergoing abdominal aortic surgery, *Eur J Anaesthesiol Suppl* 9:78, 1994.

100. Kim SY, Cho MH: Neuromuscular and cardiovascular advantages of combinations of mivacurium and rocuronium over either drug alone, *Anaesthesia* 51:929, 1996.

101. Konstadt SN, Reich DL, Stanley TE III, et al: A two-center comparison of the cardiovascular effects of cisatracurium (Nimbex) and vecuronium in patients with coronary artery disease, *Anesth Analg* 81:1010, 1995.

102. Andree RA: Sudden death following naloxone administration, *Anesth Analg* 59:782, 1980.

103. Azar I, Pham AN, Karambelkar DJ, et al: The heart rate following edrophonium-atropine and edrophonium-glycopyrrolate mixtures, *Anesthesiology* 59:139, 1983.

104. Cronnelly R, Morris RB, Miller RO: Edrophonium: duration of action and atropine requirement in humans during halothane anesthesia, *Anesthesiology* 57:261, 1982.

105. Urquhart ML, Ramsey FM, Royster RL, et al: Heart rate and rhythm following an edrophonium/atropine mixture for antagonism of neuromuscular blockade during fentanyl/N$_2$O/O$_2$ or isoflurane/N$_2$O/O$_2$ anesthesia, *Anesthesiology* 67:561, 1987.

106. Sprague DH: Severe bradycardia after neostigmine in a patient taking propranolol to control paroxysmal atrial tachycardia, *Anesthesiology* 42:208, 1975.

107. Maister AH: Atrial fibrillation following physostigmine, *Can Anaesth Soc J* 30:419, 1983.

108. Dauchot P, Gravenstein JS: Effects of atropine on the electrocardiogram in different age groups, *Clin Pharmacol Ther* 12:274, 1971.

109. Caplan RA, Ward RJ, Posner K, et al: Unexpected cardiac arrest during spinal anesthesia: a closed claims analysis of predisposing factors, *Anesthesiology* 68:5, 1988.

110. Cohen LI: Asystole during spinal anesthesia in a patient with sick sinus syndrome, *Anesthesiology* 68:787, 1988.

111. King BD, Harris LC Jr, Greifenstein FE, et al: Reflex circulatory responses to direct laryngoscopy and tracheal intubation performed during general anesthesia, *Anesthesiology* 12:556, 1951.

112. Saanivaara L, Kentala E: Comparison of electrocardiographic changes during microlaryngoscopy under halothane anaesthesia induced by Althesin or thiopentone, *Acta Anaesthesiol Scand* 21:71, 1977.

113. Royster RL, Johnston WE, Gravlee GP, et al: Arrhythmias during venous cannulation prior to pulmonary artery catheter insertion, *Anesth Analg* 64:1214, 1985.

114. Damen J, Bolton D: A prospective analysis of 1400 pulmonary artery catheterizations in patients undergoing cardiac surgery, *Acta Anaesthesiol Scand* 30:386, 1986.

115. Salmenperä M, Peltola K, Rosenberg P: Does prophylactic lidocaine control cardiac arrhythmias associated with pulmonary artery catheterization? *Anesthesiology* 56:210, 1982.

116. Kasten GW, Owens E, Kennedy D: Ventricular tachycardia resulting from central venous catheter tip migration due to arm position changes: report of two cases, *Anesthesiology* 62:185, 1985.

117. Goldman L, Caldera DL, Southwick FS, et al: Cardiac risk factors and complications in non-cardiac surgery, *Medicine* (Baltimore) 57:357, 1978.

118. Berbari EJ, Lazzara R: An introduction to high-resolution ECG recordings of cardiac late potentials, *Arch Intern Med* 148:1859, 1988.

119. Cain ME, Ambros D, Witkowski FX, et al: Fast-Fourier transform analysis of signal-averaged electrocardiograms for identification of patients prone to sustained ventricular tachycardia, *Circulation* 69:711, 1984.

120. Hollifield JW: Electrolyte disarray and cardiovascular disease, *Am J Cardiol* 63:21B, 1989 (review).

121. Cohen L, Kitzes R: Magnesium sulfate and digitalis-toxic arrhythmias, *JAMA* 249:2808, 1983.

122. Shapiro S, Slone D, Lewis PG, et al: The epidemiology of digoxin: a study of three Boston hospitals, *J Chronic Dis* 22:361, 1979.

123. Josephson ME, Kastor JA: Supraventricular tachycardia: mechanisms and management, *Ann Intern Med* 87:346, 1977 (review).

124. Wu D: Supraventricular tachycardias, *JAMA* 249:3357, 1983.

125. Singer DH, Ten Eick RE: Aberrancy: electrophysiologic aspects, *Am J Cardiol* 28:381, 1971.

126. Fenster PE, Comess KA, Marsh R, et al: Conversion of atrial fibrillation to sinus rhythm by acute intravenous procainamide infusion, *Am Heart J* 106:501, 1983.

127. Watanabe AM: Digitalis and the autonomic nervous system, *J Am Coll Cardiol* 5(suppl A):35A, 1985 (review).

128. Venditti FJ Jr, Garan H, Ruskin JN: Electrophysiologic effects of beta blockers in ventricular arrhythmias, *Am J Cardiol* 60:3D, 1987.

129. Littman L, Tenczer J, Fenyvesi T: Atrioventricular nodal reentrant paroxysmal supraventricular tachycardia, *Arch Intern Med* 144:129, 1984.

130. Wellens HJ, Bar FW, Lie KI: The value of the electrocardiogram in the differential diagnosis of a tachycardia with a widened QRS complex, *Am J Med* 64:27, 1978.

131. Garratt C, Linker N, Griffith M, et al: Comparison of adenosine and verapamil for termination of paroxysmal junctional tachycardia, *Am J Cardiol* 64:1310, 1989.

132. Richardson JM: Ventricular preexcitation: practical considerations, *Arch Intern Med* 143:760, 1983.

133. Mandel WJ, Laks MM, Obayashi K, et al: The Wolff-Parkinson-White syndrome: pharmacologic effects of procaine amide, *Am Heart J* 90:744, 1975.

134. Josephson ME, Kastor JA, Kitchen JG III: Lidocaine in Wolff-Parkinson-White syndrome with atrial fibrillation, *Ann Intern Med* 84:44, 1976.

135. Akhtar M, Gilbert CJ, Shenasa M: Effect of lidocaine on atrioventricular response via the accessory pathway in patients with Wolff-Parkinson-White syndrome, *Circulation* 63:435, 1981.

136. McGovern B, Garan H, Ruskin JN: Precipitation of cardiac arrest by verapamil in patients with Wolff-Parkinson-White syndrome, *Ann Intern Med* 104:791, 1986.

137. Sellers TB Jr, Bashore TM, Gallagher JJ: Digitalis in the preexcitation syndrome: analysis during atrial fibrillation, *Circulation* 56:260, 1977.

138. Gómez-Arnau J, Márquez-Montes J, Avello F: Fentanyl and droperidol effects on the refractoriness of the accessory pathway in the Wolff-Parkinson-White syndrome, *Anesthesiology* 58:307, 1983.

139. Rinkenberger RL, Prystowsky EN, Heger JJ, et al: Effects of intravenous and chronic oral verapamil administration in patients with supraventricular tachyarrhythmias, *Circulation* 62:996, 1980.

140. Haft JI, Habbab MA: Treatment of atrial arrhythmias: effectiveness of verapamil when preceded by calcium infusion, *Arch Intern Med* 146:1085, 1986.

141. Goldman S, Probst P, Selzer A, et al: Inefficacy of "therapeutic" serum levels of digoxin in controlling the ventricular rate in atrial fibrillation, *Am J Cardiol* 35:651, 1975.

142. Platia EV, Michelson EL, Porterfield JK, et al: Esmolol versus verapamil in the acute treatment of atrial fibrillation or atrial flutter, *Am J Cardiol* 63:925, 1989.

143. Dunn M, Alexander J, de Silva R, et al: Antithrombotic therapy in atrial fibrillation, *Chest* 89:68S, 1986 (review).

144. Wells JL Jr, Maclean WA, James TN, et al: Characterization of atrial flutter: studies in man after open heart surgery using fixed atrial electrodes, *Circulation* 50:665, 1979.

145. Waldo AL, Wells JL Jr, Cooper TB, et al: Temporary cardiac pacing: applications and techniques in the treatment of cardiac arrhythmias, *Prog Cardiovasc Dis* 23:451, 1981 (review).

146. Plumb VJ, Karp RB, James TN, et al: Atrial excitability and conduction during rapid atrial pacing, *Circulation* 63:1140, 1981.

147. Shine KI, Kastor JA, Yurchak PM: Multifocal atrial tachycardia: clinical and electrocardiographic features in 32 patients, *N Engl J Med* 279:344, 1968.

148. Scher DL, Arsura EL: Multifocal atrial tachycardia: mechanisms, clinical correlates, and treatment, *Am Heart J* 118:574, 1989 (review).

149. Levine JL, Michael JR, Guarnieri T: Multifocal atrial tachycardia: a toxic effect of theophylline, *Lancet* 1:12, 1985.

150. Levine JH, Michael JR, Guarnieri T: Treatment of multifocal atrial tachycardia with verapamil, *N Engl J Med* 312:21, 1985.

151. Hazard PB, Burnett CR: Treatment of multifocal atrial tachycardia with metoprolol, *Crit Care Med* 15:20, 1987.

152. Bigger JT Jr: Identification of patients at high risk for sudden cardiac death, *Am J Cardiol* 54:3D, 1984.

153. Maseri A, L'Abbate A, Chierchia S, et al: Significance of spasm in the pathogenesis of ischemic heart disease, *Am J Cardiol* 44:788, 1979 (review).

154. Bigger JT Jr, Giardina EGV: The pharmacology and clinical use of lidocaine and procainamide, *Med Coll Virginia Q* 9:65, 1973.

155. Giardina EGV, Heissenbuttel RH, Bigger JT Jr: Intermittent intravenous procaine amide to treat ventricular arrhythmias: correlation of plasma concentration with effect on arrhythmia, electrocardiogram, and blood pressure, *Ann Intern Med* 78:183, 1973.

156. Levy S: Combination therapy for cardiac arrhythmias, *Am J Cardiol* 61:95A, 1988 (review).

157. Levites R, Bodenheimer MM, Helfant RH: Electrophysiologic effects of nitroglycerin during experimental coronary occlusion, *Circulation* 52:1050, 1975.

158. Podrid PJ, Schoeneberger A, Lown B: Congestive heart failure caused by oral disopyramide, *N Engl J Med* 302:614, 1980.

159. Gallagher JD, Lieberman RW, Meranze J, et al: Amiodarone-induced complications during coronary artery surgery, *Anesthesiology* 55:186, 1981.

160. Marchlinski FE, Gansler TS, Waxman HL, et al: Amiodarone pulmonary toxicity, *Ann Intern Med* 97:839, 1982.

161. Perlow GM, Jain BP, Pauker SG, et al: Tocainide-associated interstitial pneumonitis, *Ann Intern Med* 94:489, 1981.

162. Dunn M, Glassroth J: Pulmonary complications of amiodarone toxicity, *Prog Cardiovasc Dis* 31:447, 1989 (review).

163. Koch MJ, Seef LB, Crumley CE, et al: Quinidine hepatotoxicity: a report of a case and review of the literature, *Gastroenterology* 70:1136, 1976.

164. Falk RH: Flecainide-induced ventricular tachycardia and fibrillation in patients treated for atrial fibrillation, *Ann Intern Med* 111:107, 1989.

165. Hager WD, Fenster P, Mayersohn M, et al: Digoxin-quinidine interaction: pharmacokinetic evaluation, *N Engl J Med* 300:1238, 1979.

166. Bigger JT Jr: The interaction of mexiletine with other cardiovascular drugs, *Am Heart J* 107:1079, 1984.

167. Klein HO, Lang R, Weiss E, et al: The influence of verapamil on serum digoxin concentration, *Circulation* 65:998, 1982.

168. Data JL, Wilkinson GR, Nies AS: Interaction of quinidine with anticonvulsant drugs, *N Engl J Med* 294:699, 1976.

169. Aitio ML, Mansury L, Tala E, et al: The effect of enzyme induction on the metabolism of disopyramide in man, *Br J Clin Pharmacol* 11:279, 1981.

170. Vrobel TR, Miller PE, Mostow ND, et al: A general overview of amiodarone toxicity: its prevention, detection, and management, *Prog Cardiovasc Dis* 31:393, 1989 (review).

171. Procacci PM, Savran SV, Schreiter SL, et al: Prevalence of clinical mitral-valve prolapse in 1,169 young women, *N Engl J Med* 294:1086, 1976.

172. Mills P, Rose J, Hollingsworth BA, et al: Long-term prognosis of mitral-valve prolapse, *N Engl J Med* 297:13, 1977.

173. Boudoulas H, Reynolds JC, Mazzaferri E, et al: Mitral valve prolapse syndrome: the effect of adrenergic stimulation, *J Am Coll Cardiol* 2:638, 1983.

174. Savage DD, Devereux RB, Garrison RJ, et al: Mitral valve prolapse in the general population. I. Epidemiologic features: the Framingham Study, *Am Heart J* 106:571, 1983.

175. Kramer HM, Kligfield P, Devereux RB, et al: Arrhythmias in mitral valve prolapse: effect of selection bias, *Arch Intern Med* 144:2360, 1984.

176. Puddu PE, Pasternac A, Tubau JF, et al: QT interval prolongation and increased plasma catecholamine levels in patients with mitral valve prolapse, *Am Heart J* 105:422, 1983.

177. Thiagarajah S, Frost EA: Anaesthetic considerations in patients with mitral valve prolapse, *Anaesthesia* 38:560, 1983.

178. Krantz EM, Viljoen JF, Schermer R, et al: Mitral valve prolapse, *Anesth Analg* 59:379, 1980.

179. Barlow JB, Pocock WA: The mitral valve prolapse enigma: two decades later, *Mod Concepts Cardiovasc Dis* 53:13, 1984.

180. Galloway PA, Glass PSA: Anesthetic implications of prolonged QT interval syndromes, *Anesth Analg* 64:612, 1985 (review).

181. Medak R, Benumof JL: Perioperative management of the prolonged QT interval syndrome, *Br J Anaesth* 55:361, 1983.

182. Wig J, Bali IM, Singh RG, et al: Prolonged QT interval syndrome: sudden cardiac arrest during anaesthesia, *Anaesthesia* 34:37, 1979.

183. Yanowitz F, Preston JB, Abildskov JA: Functional distribution of right and left stellate innervation to the ventricles: production of neurogenic electrocardiographic changes by unilateral alteration of sympathetic tone, *Circ Res* 18:416, 1966.

184. Moss AJ, McDonald J: Unilateral cervicothoracic sympathetic ganglionectomy for the treatment of the long QT syndromes, *N Engl J Med* 285:903, 1971.

185. Schwartz PJ, Periti M, Malliani A: The long QT-syndrome, *Am Heart J* 89:378, 1975.

186. Carlock FJ, Brown M, Brown EM: Isoflurane anaesthesia for a patient with long QT syndrome, *Can Anaesth Soc J* 31:83, 1984.

187. Ponte J, Lund J: Prolongation of the QT interval (Romano-Ward syndrome): anaesthetic management, *Br J Anaesth* 53:1347, 1981.

188. Bardy GH, Ungerleider RM, Smith WM, et al: A mechanism of torsades de pointes in a canine model, *Circulation* 67:52, 1983.

189. Tzivoni D, Banai S, Schuger C, et al: Treatment of torsade de pointes with magnesium sulfate, *Circulation* 77:392, 1988.

190. Milne JR, Ward DE, Spurrell AJ, et al: The long QT syndrome: effects of drugs and left stellate ganglion block, *Am Heart J* 104:194, 1982.

191. Kahn MM, Logan KR, McComb JM, et al: Management of recurrent ventricular tachyarrhythmias associated with QT prolongation, *Am J Cardiol* 47:1301, 1981.

192. Roizen MF, Lampe GH, Benefiel DJ, et al: Change in QT interval with anesthesia: should it determine whether to use a narcotic or inhalational agent? *Anesthesiology* 69(3A):A53, 1988 (abstract).

193. Roden DM, Woosley RL, Primm PK: Incidence and clinical features of the quinidine-associated long QT syndrome: implications for patient care, *Am Heart J* 111:1038, 1986.

194. Singh BN, Vaughan-Williams EM: The effect of amiodarone, a new anti-anginal drug, on cardiac muscle, *Br J Pharmacol* 39:357, 1970.

195. Singh BN: When is QT prolongation antiarrhythmic and when is it proarrhythmic? *Am J Cardiol* 63:867, 1989 (editorial).

196. Rotem M, Constantini S, Shir Y, et al: Life-threatening torsade de pointes arrhythmia associated with head injury, *Neurosurgery* 23:89, 1988.

197. Marion DW, Segal R, Thompson ME: Subarachnoid hemorrhage and the heart, *Neurosurgery* 18:101, 1986.

198. Mikolich JR, Jacobs WC, Fletcher GF: Cardiac arrhythmias in patients with acute cerebrovascular accidents, *JAMA* 246:1314, 1981.

199. Di Pasquale G, Pinelli G, Andreoli A, et al: Holter detection of cardiac arrhythmias in intracranial subarachnoid hemorrhage, *Am J Cardiol* 59:596, 1987.

200. Hust MH, Nitsche K, Hohnloser S, et al: Q-T prolongation and torsades de pointes in a patient with subarachnoid hemorrhage, *Clin Cardiol* 7:44, 1984.

201. Stober T, Sen S, Anstatt T, et al: Correlation of cardiac arrhythmias with brainstem compression in patients with intracerebral hemorrhage, *Stroke* 19:688, 1988.

202. Smith M, Ray CT: Cardiac arrhythmias, increased intracranial pressure, and the autonomic nervous system, *Chest* 61(suppl):125, 1972.

203. Estanol BV, Loyo MV, Mateos JH, et al: Cardiac arrhythmias in experimental subarachnoid hemorrhage, *Stroke* 8:440, 1977.

204. Lacy PS, Earle AM: A small animal model for electrocardiographic abnormalities observed after an experimental subarachnoid hemorrhage, *Stroke* 14:371, 1983.

205. von Olshausen K, Amann E, Hofmann M, et al: Ventricular arrhythmias before and late after aortic valve replacement, *Am J Cardiol* 54:142, 1984.

206. von Olshausen K, Schwarz F, Apfelbach J, et al: Determinants of the incidence and severity of ventricular arrhythmias in aortic valve disease, *Am J Cardiol* 51:1103, 1983.

207. Schilling G, Finkbeiner T, Elberskirch P, et al: Incidence of ventricular arrhythmias in patients with aortic valve replacement, *Am J Cardiol* 49:894, 1982 (abstract).

208. Parris TM, Mintz GS, Ross J, et al: Importance of atrial contraction to left ventricular filling in mitral stenosis, *Am J Cardiol* 61:1135, 1988.

209. Gillette PC: Evolving concepts in the management of congenital junctional ectopic tachycardia, *Circulation* 81:1713, 1990 (editorial).

210. Garson A Jr, Gillette PC: Junctional ectopic tachycardia in children: electrocardiography, electrophysiology and pharmacologic response, *Am J Cardiol* 44:298, 1979.

211. Gillette PC: Diagnosis and management of postoperative junctional ectopic tachycardia, *Am Heart J* 118:192, 1989 (editorial).

212. Bash SE, Shah JJ, Albers WH, et al: Hypothermia for the treatment of post-surgical greatly accelerated junctional ectopic tachycardia, *J Am Coll Cardiol* 10:1095, 1987.

213. Grant JW, Serwer GA, Armstrong BE, et al: Junctional tachycardia in infants and children after open heart surgery for congenital heart disease, *Am J Cardiol* 59:1216, 1987.

214. Porter CJ, Gillette PC, Garson A Jr, et al: Effects of verapamil on supraventricular tachycardia in children, *Am J Cardiol* 48:487, 1981.

215. Villain E, Vetter VL, Garcia JM, et al: Evolving concepts in the management of congenital junctional ectopic tachycardia: a multicenter study, *Circulation* 81:1544, 1990 (review).

216. Kunze KP, Kuck KH, Schluter M, et al: Effect of encainide and flecainide on chronic ectopic atrial tachycardia, *J Am Coll Cardiol* 7:1121, 1986.

217. Garson A Jr, Moak JP, Smith RT Jr, et al: Usefulness of intravenous propafenone for control of postoperative junctional ectopic tachycardia, *Am J Cardiol* 59:1422, 1987.

218. Podrid PJ: Potassium and ventricular arrhythmias, *Am J Cardiol* 65:33E, 1990.

219. Papademetriou V, Fletcher R, Khatri IM, et al: Diuretic-induced hypokalemia in uncomplicated systemic hypertension: effect of plasma potassium correction on cardiac arrhythmias, *Am J Cardiol* 52:1017, 1983.

220. Hulting J: In hospital ventricular fibrillation and its relation to serum potassium, *Acta Med Scand* 647(suppl):109, 1981.

221. Hollifield JW: Thiazide treatment of hypertension: effects of thiazide diuretics on serum potassium, magnesium, and ventricular ectopy, *Am J Med* 80(suppl 4A):8, 1986.

222. Struthers AD, Reid JL, Whitesmith R, et al: Effect of intravenous adrenaline on electrocardiogram, blood pressure and serum potassium, *Br Heart J* 49:90, 1983.

223. Watanabe Y, Dreifus LS, Likoff W: Electrophysiologic antagonism and synergism of potassium and antiarrhythmic agents, *Am J Cardiol* 12:702, 1963.

224. Surawicz B: Is hypomagnesemia or magnesium deficiency arrhythmogenic? *J Am Coll Cardiol* 14:1093, 1989.

225. Watanabe Y, Dreifus LS: Electrophysiological effects of magnesium and its interactions with potassium, *Cardiovasc Res* 6:79, 1972.

226. Skou JC: The influence of some actions on an ATPase from peripheral nerves, *Biochim Biophys Acta* 23:394, 1957.

227. January CT, Fozzard HA: Delayed afterdepolarizations in heart muscle: mechanisms and relevance, *Pharmacol Rev* 40:219, 1988.

228. Abraham AS, Rosenman D, Meshulam Z, et al: Serum, lymphocyte, and erythrocyte potassium, magnesium, and calcium concentrations and their relation to tachyarrhythmias in patients with acute myocardial infarction, *Am J Med* 81:983, 1986.

229. Bunton RW: Value of serum magnesium estimation in diagnosing myocardial infarction and predicting dysrhythmias after coronary artery bypass grafting, *Thorax* 38:946, 1983.

230. Ragnarsson J, Hardarson T, Snorrason SP: Ventricular dysrhythmias in middle-aged hypertensive men treated either with a diuretic agent or α-blocker, *Acta Med Scand* 221:143, 1987.

231. Hollifield JW, Slaton PE: Thiazide diuretics, hypokalemia and cardiac arrhythmias, *Acta Med Scand*, suppl 647:67, 1981.

232. Dyckner T: Serum magnesium in acute myocardial infarction: reaction to arrhythmias, *Acta Med Scand* 207:59, 1980.

233. DiCarlo LA Jr, Morady F, de Buitleir M, et al: Effects of magnesium sulfate on cardiac conduction and refractoriness in humans, *J Am Coll Cardiol* 7:1356, 1986.

234. Rasmussen HS, McNair P, Norregard P, et al: Intravenous magnesium in acute myocardial infarction, *Lancet* 1:234, 1986.

235. Boyd LJ, Scherf D: Magnesium sulfate in paroxysmal tachycardia, *Am J Med Sci* 206:43, 1943.
236. French JH, Thomas RG, Siskind AP, et al: Magnesium therapy in massive digoxin intoxication, *Ann Emerg Med* 13:562, 1984.
237. Tzivoni D, Banai S, Schuger C, et al: Treatment of torsade de pointes with magnesium sulfate, *Circulation* 77:392, 1988.
238. Iseri LT, Chung P, Tobis J: Magnesium therapy for intractable ventricular tachyarrhythmias in hormomagnesemic patients, *West J Med* 138:823, 1983.

239. Wester PO: Magnesium, *Am J Clin Nutr* 45:1305, 1987.
240. Reinhart RA: Magnesium metabolism: a review with special reference to the relationship between intracellular content and serum levels, *Arch Intern Med* 148:2415, 1988 (review).
241. Iseri LT: Role of magnesium in cardiac tachyarrhythmias, *Am J Cardiol* 65:47K, 1990.

Chapter 12

Hypotension, Hypertension, Perioperative Myocardial Ischemia, and Infarction

Stephen N. Harris

A continuous supply of oxygenated blood is an absolute necessity for normal human existence. The kinetic and potential energy generated, stored, and distributed by the cardiovascular system provides the vital forces that ensure the constant delivery of nutrient-laden blood. The cardiovascular system is endowed with considerable compensatory capabilities, allowing adaptations to variability in normal human activities as well as compensations for pathophysiologic states. Although they are remarkably efficient within their limits, these compensatory mechanisms can be overwhelmed by the ravages of disease. The administration of anesthesia can also cause complications that are deleterious to both function and structure. In this chapter we focus on hypotension, hypertension, perioperative myocardial ischemia, and perioperative myocardial infarction (MI), listing the major causes of these abnormalities and suggesting appropriate treatment.

I. PERIOPERATIVE HYPOTENSION

Hypotension is probably the most commonly observed and feared complication during anesthesia. The widespread use of continuous arterial manometry and the more recent introduction of automated cuff blood pressure methods have further focused our attention on hypotension.

Generically defined, the term *hypotension* means abnormally low blood pressure. Blood pressure can be low in the systemic circuit or in the pulmonary circuit and can involve systolic or diastolic values. However, in common usage the word *hypotension* refers to an abnormally low systemic systolic blood pressure. Although the systemic systolic blood pressure is certainly not the only pressure affecting critical blood flow, lowering of the systolic pressure serves as a red flag for critical examination of the cardiovascular system.

The dynamics of systolic blood pressure generation and detection are beyond the scope of this chapter. However, any factor that seriously lowers cardiac output or peripheral vascular resistance can significantly lower systolic blood pressure and mean arterial blood pressure. A generalized classification of the causes of systemic arterial hypotension mirrors the classifications of shock, including hypovolemic shock, cardiogenic shock, neurogenic shock, and septic shock. Each of these abnormalities is considered separately.

A. Hypovolemic hypotension

The term *hypovolemia* refers to a reduction in the intravascular blood volume. Hypovolemia may result from losses of whole blood, reductions in red cell volume, reductions in plasma volume, or reductions in free water.

Hypovolemic hypotension during anesthesia can result from decreases in plasma volume. Preoperative and intraoperative use of potent diuretics is a common cause of intraoperative hypovolemic hypotension. Decreases in plasma volume can occur intraoperatively secondary to handling of bowel and mesentery. Even more extensive losses can occur during the retroperitoneal operative dissections done during abdominal aortic aneurysm repair or pancreaticoduodenectomy.[1]

Hemorrhage is often an obvious cause of hypotension because the anesthesiologist may easily detect massive bleeding. However, it can be difficult to observe pelvic bleeding or bleeding into the chest cavity during thoracic surgery. In trauma cases one must keep in mind that bleeding into an unsuspected area of injury remote from the operative site can occur. Likewise, hemorrhage can be hidden, as in the large retroperitoneal hematomas seen with pelvic fractures or the large blood loss into the thigh that can accompany hip or femur fractures.

Early diagnosis of hemorrhagic hypotension is extremely important in minimizing morbidity and mortality, especially in patients with compromised cardiovascular systems. The classic signs of hemorrhagic hypotension are often enumerated as tachycardia, vasoconstriction, low systolic blood pressure, and sometimes low urinary output. To the novice in anesthesia these are the signs of hypovolemic hypotension. However, seasoned clinicians recognize that these abnormalities are not the first signs of hemorrhagic hypotension. Long before these signs occur the astute clinician will notice that blood is suctioned from the operative field much more often and that the demeanor of the surgeons changes. The most competent surgeons faced with acute hemorrhage often become quiet, serious, and directed toward an organized plan. The emotional outbursts of the less competent are easy to detect.

The specific treatment of hypovolemic hypotension is to restore adequate circulating intravascular volume. This can be done with whole blood, packed red blood cells, albumin or hetastarch, or a balanced electrolyte solution such as lactated Ringer's solution. The resistance to fluid flow through an intravenous cannula is directly proportional to cannula length and inversely proportional to the diameter of the cannula. Consequently, if rapid fluid administration is necessary, short, large-bore cannulas (14 or 16 gauge) are very desirable. However, even with optimal intravenous cannulas and pressure-infusion devices, rapid volume repletion is sometimes too slow in restoring systemic blood pressure. The judicious use of a vasoconstrictor such as phenylephrine or a mixed-action drug such as epinephrine allows restoration of improved arterial blood pressure while volume deficits are replaced.

Adjunctive supportive measures are often necessary during the treatment of severe hypovolemic hypotension. Administration of 100% oxygen promotes optimal peripheral oxygen delivery. Volatile anesthetic agents often must be discontinued and muscle relaxants used to immobilize the patient. In this setting, intraanesthetic recall can occur easily unless one administers an amnesic agent with minimal circulatory effects. We have found intravenous scopolamine, 0.2 to 0.4 mg, to be especially useful. Acute renal failure can develop during or after hypotension. Clinicians have commonly administered potent intravenous diuretics such as furosemide in an attempt to minimize renal damage. However, at least two studies indicate that diuretics do not decrease renal damage resulting from hypotension.[2,3]

B. Cardiogenic hypotension

Many different conditions can cause the left ventricle to pump inadequate volumes of blood. When this occurs, the peripheral circulation may attempt to compensate by vasoconstriction, but if impairment of left ventricular ejection is severe enough, hypotension results. This is called cardiogenic hypotension and can be caused by several conditions, which are considered separately.

1. Pharmacologic causes. All modern inhalation agents and many intravenous agents can depress myocardial contractility.[4-8] The cardiogenic hypotension seen with inhalation anesthetics can result from frank overdoses of the agents but more commonly arises when clinically acceptable dosages are given. Previous deficiencies in myocardial contractility or the presence of relative hypovolemia may accentuate cardiogenic hypotension. In the majority of cases, one can treat cardiogenic hypotension associated with volatile agents by decreasing or perhaps temporarily discontinuing the administration of the agent while administering 250 to 500 ml fluid. Patients with healthy cardiovascular systems tolerate such maneuvers very well, but those with preexisting severe cardiovascular disease may require estimation of left ventricular filling pressures using a pulmonary artery catheter. However, it must be recognized that changes in pulmonary capillary wedge pressure (PCWP) do not necessarily correlate well with changes in left ventricular end-diastolic volume (LVEDV), which is the true index of adequate preload.[9,10] Two-dimensional transesophageal echocardiography (TEE) provides a method for estimation of LVEDV, through visual means or through an automated border detection determination of end-diastolic area. It is possible that this method will be more common in the future. At present, however, TEE equipment is expensive and requires significant training before the anesthesiologist or cardiologist can make consistent and accurate diagnoses using this method.

2. Extrinsic cardiac compression. Mechanical compression of the heart or the great veins can impair diastolic filling of the right and left ventricles, resulting in inadequate stroke volume and systemic hypotension. Pericardial tamponade is a classic cause. Trauma, cardiac surgery, and intracardiac catheterization all may lead to pericardial tamponade. The condition can be life-threatening, requiring pericardiocentesis using an 18-gauge spinal needle. If this fails, emergency subxiphoid thoracostomy is indicated.[11] Mechanical displacement of the heart during cardiac surgery and during esophagogastrectomy can also cause hypotension. Tension pneumothorax shifts the mediastinum and kinks the great veins as they enter the thorax. This leads to severe hypotension, which may require emergency decompression using a 16-gauge needle followed by chest tube placement.[11] In supine obstetric patients the gravid uterus may compress the inferior vena cava, leading to impaired venous return, decreased stroke volume, and severe hypotension. This condition can be treated using intravenous fluids, left uterine displacement, and intravenous ephedrine.[12]

3. Impaired myocardial function. Systemic arterial hypotension can result when left ventricular muscle cannot contract adequately. Very severe myocardial contusion can result in transmural MI with attendant hypotension.[13] This condition can also cause severe ventricular arrhythmias. Both antiarrhythmic and inotropic agents may be required for effective treatment.

Stunned myocardium refers to the cardiac response to a brief episode of severe ischemia, followed by prolonged myocardial dysfunction and gradual return of contractile activity.[14,15] Stunned myocardium may be encountered immediately after cardiopulmonary bypass and in other cases in which severe hypotension has persisted for at least 15 to 20 minutes. Likely causes of stunned myocardium are a transient calcium overload of cardiac myocytes immediately after reperfusion, excitation-contraction uncoupling caused by ischemia-induced dysfunction of the sarcoplasmic reticulum, and generation of oxygen free radicals. The resultant left ventricular dysfunction may be clinically significant. Ischemia causes poor cardiac contraction, incomplete ventricular emptying (systolic dysfunction), and impaired ventricular relaxation (diastolic dysfunction). Fortunately, stunned myocardium can be stimulated by infusion of sympathomimetics, which can buy time until the biochemical abnormalities are reversed.[16,17]

Intraoperative MI can cause hypotension. This is especially true of transmural infarction involving a large amount of myocardium. Intraoperative infarcts can be silent, but if a significant amount of myocardium is ischemic, there will be systolic failure with decreased stroke volume, low cardiac output, and systemic arterial hypotension. Failure of ventricular relaxation leads to elevated left ventricular end-diastolic pressures (LVEDPs). The seven-lead ECG may help to establish the diagnosis, particularly if the standard leads are diagnostic as in an inferior infarct. Concentrations of the MB fraction of creatinine phosphokinase (MB-CPK) are not helpful in diagnosing most intraoperative infarcts because the enzyme concentrations may not become elevated until 12 to 24 hours after the infarct.[18] Recent advances in diagnosing MI rely on determination of serum cardiac-specific troponins. Cardiac troponin T (TnT) may be capable of detecting myocardial necrosis below the detection limit of MB-CPK assays.[19]

Most patients who sustain an intraoperative MI who develop hypotension refractory to volume loading may benefit from radial artery and pulmonary artery blood pressure monitoring. Careful titration of fluids and hemodynamic management is important. The use of inotropic and vasoactive drugs may be necessary to support systemic blood pressure. An intraaortic balloon can be helpful in cases with severe circulatory compromise. Thrombolytic therapy could benefit patients with intraoperative infarcts, especially those occurring during operations with minimal bleeding potential. However, today this is conjecture. MI is considered in greater depth later in this chapter.

C. Hypotension secondary to decreased peripheral resistance

The contractile state of smooth muscles in small arterioles determines peripheral vascular resistance. Even small changes in arteriolar diameter can have profound effects on peripheral vascular resistance because it is inversely related to the fourth power of the vessel radius.

1. Premedication. Preoperative hypotension may occasionally be caused by an overdose or relative overdose of premedicant drugs such as barbiturates, narcotics, and benzodiazepine derivatives. This is most likely to occur in patients who are relatively hypovolemic. Often a small bolus, 250 to 500 ml, of lactated Ringer's solution will restore satisfactory blood pressure. If a serious circulatory derangement such as myocardial ischemia or pulmonary embolus can be ruled out, anesthesia can often be induced after the fluid administration.

2. Inhalational agents. All modern inhalation agents cause some decrease in peripheral resistance, which may be partly responsible for intraoperative hypotension. Reduction in the inhaled concentration of the agent, a small bolus of fluids, and judicious use of inotropes or vasoconstrictors can resolve this type of hypotension rapidly.

3. Spinal and epidural anesthesia. Administration of spinal or epidural anesthesia can cause blockade of the sympathetic nervous system, followed by decreased peripheral vascular resistance and severe hypotension. Severe hypotension is most likely to occur in patients with a high sensory level or a diminished intravascular volume. Bradycardia secondary to blockade of the cardioaccelerator fibers (T1-T4) further accentuates the hypotension. Usually, hypotension is easily detected after spinal or epidural anesthesia and can be treated with fluid infusion, oxygen administration, and appropriate dosages of the sympathomimetic ephedrine or vasoconstrictor such as phenylephrine. In very high levels of spinal or epidural anesthesia, ventilation may be inadequate because of loss of intercostal muscle function. The clinician must consider establishment of effective ventilation, which may require endotracheal intubation.

4. Vasodilator adjuncts. Intravenous vasodilators are widely used during anesthetic care. Administration of sodium nitroprusside (SNP), trimethaphan (Arfonad), nitroglycerin, and prostaglandins is often associated with the development of severe hypotension. Hypotension secondary to these agents should be anticipated and can be treated by discontinuing the agent and administering a fluid bolus. If the hypotension is very severe or prolonged, the careful titration of an α_1-adrenergic agent such as phenylephrine may be required. Hypotension secondary to SNP is especially common in hypovolemic patients. Anticipation of hypotension by adequate fluid administration before administration of SNP often allows smooth and predictable control of blood pressure.

5. Antibiotic hypotension. Intravenously administered vancomycin can produce life-threatening hypotension. The predominant mechanism is peripheral vascular dilation, which led to its description as the red man syndrome. The administration of vancomycin may cause an erythematous rash over the face, neck, upper trunk, and upper arms. This is often accompanied by pruritus (in awake patients) and angioedema.[20] The incidence of vancomycin hypotension has been shown to be related to the rate of administration.[21,22] Profound hypotension has been reported when 1000 mg of the drug is given over 30 minutes or less.[23] Rapid infusion has been shown to cause increased plasma histamine concentrations, and it has been suggested that the hypotension is mediated through a histaminergic response. Dogs pretreated with methapyrilene (an antihistamine) do not have hypotension after rapid administration of vancomycin.

Prevention is the best cure for vancomycin hypotension. Administering the drug slowly over 45 minutes definitely minimizes the incidence of hypotension. However, hypotensive episodes have been reported even at very slow rates.[24] Severe vancomycin hypotension can be life-threatening, and we have seen one case in which the systolic arterial pressure decreased to 38 mm Hg. The return toward normal was extremely slow and was accomplished after several minutes of infusion of epinephrine up to 0.15 µg/kg/min. The use of a mixed-action drug such as epinephrine may be rational because Cohen et al[25] showed that cardiac depression is part of the syndrome. Administration of large volumes of crystalloid may also be helpful. If the syndrome does not respond to epinephrine and fluids, the addition of bolus doses of phenylephrine may be appropriate.

6. Methylmethacrylate hypotension. Severe hypotension, hypoxemia, and cardiac arrest have been reported after the introduction of the bone cement methylmethacrylate into the marrow cavities of long bones, especially the femoral shaft. Investigations have shown that methylmethacrylate monomer does not produce hypotension.[26,27] It seems probable that the reaction is caused by fat and gas embolization resulting when high pressure is generated in the marrow cavity during implantation of a prosthesis. Venting the femoral shaft appears to reduce the amount of embolization.[28] The use of high oxygen tensions during implantation may minimize hypoxemia, and careful attention to the pulse oximeter may allow one to identify the reaction early. Effective bone venting should prevent the majority of these reactions, but occasionally a severe reaction requiring pharmacologic support with catecholamines may still be encountered.

7. Carcinoid syndrome. Severe hypotension can occur during the anesthetic care of patients with carcinoid tumors. These tumors, which often occur in the jejunum or ileum, arise from enterochromaffin tissues and may release vasoactive substances, including histamine, prostaglandins, kallikreins, and serotonin. Approximately 5% of patients with carcinoid tumors develop carcinoid syndrome.[29] Carcinoid tumors may metastasize to heart valves, causing tricuspid regurgitation or pulmonary stenosis. Severe bronchospasm can result in air trapping and increased intrathoracic pressures, which may impair venous return and further accentuate hypotension.

The best treatment for hypotension of the carcinoid syndrome is to make every effort to prevent it. H_1 and

H_2 receptor blockers may minimize the effects of histamine. Preoperative administration of cyproheptadine (Periactin) may also block the effects of intraoperative histamine release and can also block the effects of serotonin.[30] Morphine, d-tubocurarine, atracurium, metocurine, and succinylcholine should probably be avoided because they can release histamine. Many different anesthetic techniques have been used in patients with carcinoids, and none has been proved to be superior. However, a general anesthetic consisting of nitrous oxide, short-acting opioids, and pancuronium appears to be a reasonable choice.[31] Monitoring both central venous pressure and pulmonary artery pressures to allow assessment of cardiovascular status is recommended. If hypotension develops, catecholamines should be avoided because they activate kallikreins. Rather, one should give intravascular fluids and be guided by central venous and pulmonary artery pressures. Angiotensin 1.5 mg/kg may also reverse the hypotension.[32]

8. Protamine hypotension. Protamine sulfate given to reverse heparin anticoagulation can produce ominous hypotension secondary to its profound vasodilating properties.[33,34] The noticeable decrease in peripheral vascular resistance is most apparent in patients with poor ventricular function who can compensate only partially for the decreased peripheral resistance.[35] Temporary discontinuation of protamine infusion, increasing intravascular volume, and calcium chloride 1 to 2 g usually reverse this type of protamine hypotension. Occasionally, in the highest-risk patients, inotropic support with epinephrine or vasoconstriction using phenylephrine may be necessary.

Far more serious are anaphylactic reactions to protamine. Several groups of patients, including those taking protamine zinc insulin, vasectomized men, and patients allergic to finned fish may be especially prone to anaphylactic reactions, although good controlled studies are lacking. Lowenstein et al[36] describe catastrophic pulmonary vasoconstriction occurring during protamine reversal of heparin. Pulmonary arterial hypertension, right ventricular dilation, decreased left ventricular filling pressure, and systemic hypotension characterize this serious reaction, which has been reported after only 10 mg protamine. In a later study by the same group, Morel et al[37] describe the mediator profile of patients with catastrophic postprotamine pulmonary reactions. Protamine was injected into the right atrium at a dose of 20 mg for patients undergoing mitral valve repair and 100 mg for patients undergoing coronary artery bypass graft. Of the 48 patients studied, 3 sustained pulmonary vasoconstrictive reactions. The first sign was an increase in peak airway pressure, followed immediately by an acute increase in pulmonary artery pressure and subsequent systemic hypotension requiring treatment with calcium chloride and phenylephrine. Thromboxane B_2 (TXB_2) increased greatly after protamine in all pulmonary reactors but remained normal in the nonreactors. Plasma C5a concentrations also increased greatly in the pulmonary reactors. Acute leukopenia and a significant decrease in the platelet count in systemic blood also occurred in patients who received 100 mg protamine. Morel et al conclude that in the patients who developed catastrophic pulmonary increases in C5a, anaphylatoxin led to thromboxane generation, which in turn caused the pulmonary vasoconstriction and bronchoconstriction. It is important to remember that this reaction involves bronchoconstriction and that an increase in peak airway pressure was the very first sign.

Protamine-induced hypotension can result from other complex mechanisms and can range in severity from mild hypotension to total cardiovascular collapse. In an excellent review article, Horrow[38] classifies the adverse responses to protamine into three types. Type 1 is hypotension related to rapid administration, type 2 includes anaphylactoid responses, and type 3 is catastrophic pulmonary vasoconstriction.

The best treatment for protamine reactions is prospective planning to prevent them whenever possible. However, it can be difficult to predict which patients will develop protamine hypotension. Patients who have a history of having developed severe hypotension in the cardiac catheterization laboratory after receiving protamine should certainly be suspect. Any patient who has had cardiac surgery and reports difficulty after protamine should be treated with a special care. Patients with finned fish (not shellfish) allergies should be suspect. Occasionally, patients who have received neutral protamine Hagedorn insulin may have severe reactions, but we simply cannot predict this reaction with accuracy. Consequently, our approach is as follows: Protamine is always considered to be potentially dangerous. It is diluted to a concentration of 4 mg/ml and administered in low dead-space lines to preclude inadvertent bolus injection. A test dose of 4 to 8 mg protamine is administered slowly with an automated cassette infusion device. The infusion is then stopped, and during the next 1 to 2 minutes we closely follow peak airway pressure, systemic arterial pressure, and pulmonary artery diastolic pressure. If no change occurs in any of these, the calculated protamine dose is slowly administered over 10 minutes by the automatic infusion pump.

If a pronounced increase in airway pressure and pulmonary hypertension occurs after the test dose, we may elect not to administer the drug. At any rate, if a frank catastrophic pulmonary vasoconstrictive reaction occurs, pulmonary artery diastolic pressure will increase greatly. At this point, one might be tempted to administer intravenous nitroglycerin to lower the pulmonary artery diastolic pressure before continuing with the infusion of protamine. However, the right ventricle depends on an increased preload to pump against the elevated pulmonary vascular resistance. Lowering right ventricular preload at this time will cause significant decrease in right ventricular stroke volume. Our plan of action is to first stop the protamine infusion. Second, support the heart and circulation with an appropriate drug, such as epinephrine or milrinone, to increase right ventricular contractility and mediate pulmonary vasodilation. Third, place the patient on 100% oxygen and attempt to decrease CO_2 by hyperventilation, to facilitate further lowering of pulmonary vascular resistance. Once the blood pressure has been restored, careful titration of nitroglycerin may be helpful if pulmonary artery pressures remain elevated.

9. Vascular graft material. Dacron vascular graft material has generally been assumed to be inert. However, Roizen et al[39] recently reported five cases in which severe vasodilation and disseminated intravascular coagulation developed shortly after blood flow began through aortic grafts. Blood samples from two of the patients demonstrated activation of complement and of the kinin system. The graft was urgently replaced in three patients. Two of those made a full recovery and one died. Both patients in whom the graft was not replaced died. Roizen et al postulate that plasticizers in the grafts caused the abnormalities. Although this problem has not been widely recognized, it is worth considering if severe vasodilation and a bleeding diathesis develop shortly after an aortic graft is placed. Definitive therapy appears to be replacement of the Dacron graft with a graft made of a different material.

D. Septic hypotension

Hypotension occurring in a patient with known or suspected infection should always raise suspicion of septic shock. Sepsis-associated hypotension is a complex and very serious condition with a mortality somewhere between 50% and 90%.[40] Septic shock has been recognized since 1831, when Laennec published his early report.[41] The anesthesiologist may encounter septic hypotension in association with a wide variety of surgical conditions (Box 12-1).

A recent consensus conference proposed the term *systemic inflammatory response syndrome* (SIRS) to unify all causes of systemic endothelial inflammation.[42] This was done to create a standardized terminology for describing a hypermetabolic state that includes trauma, burns, pancreatitis, shock, ischemia, and sepsis. Sepsis is the systemic inflammatory response to infection. Severe sepsis includes organ dysfunction, and septic shock includes the sepsis syndrome with hypotension. Sepsis syndrome without shock has been reported to have a mortality of 13%, sepsis syndrome with shock 28%, and shock developing after the onset of sepsis syndrome 43%.[43] The hemodynamic and metabolic abnormalities occurring during septic shock are caused by the activation of the

mediators of inflammation rather than the result of infection per se. Many patients in septic shock develop hypotension and tachycardia, which necessitate hemodynamic monitoring and pharmacologic intervention.[44]

Rational management of the cardiovascular alterations occurring during septic shock necessitate assessment of ventricular filling pressures, cardiac outputs, and peripheral vascular resistance.[45] Myocardial contractility is depressed, as evidenced by an increased end-systolic volume. Causes of decreased myocardial contractility include tumor necrosis factor (TNF), down-regulation of β-adrenergic receptors, lipopolysaccharide, nitric oxide, and relative coronary hypoperfusion. Institution of inotropic therapy improves ventricular performance and end organ perfusion in septic shock. Dopamine has limited efficacy because of β-adrenergic down-regulation and may be effective only in the early stages of sepsis.[46] The combination of norepinephrine and dobutamine results in similar increases in cardiac output (CO) and mean arterial pressure (MAP) as epinephrine, but they increase splanchnic oxygen consumption and blood flow to a much greater extent. This combination therapy results in less lactic acidosis and a higher gastric mucosal pH than epinephrine alone.

In septic shock there is a loss of correlation between LVEDP and LVEDV. This loss of ventricular compliance means that PCWP will not correlate with LVEDP. Volume administration should be monitored following the changes in cardiac output until the plateau of the Starling curve is reached. Each patient has an individual response curve, and it is unusual to push the PCWP higher than 10 to 14 mm Hg in septic shock.[47] Use of a pulmonary artery catheter and radial artery blood pressure measurement is critical in diagnosis and guidance of therapy.

Septic shock also alters the relationship between oxygen delivery (DO_2) and oxygen consumption (VO_2). In patients in septic shock and lactic acidosis, therapy should be aimed at increasing DO_2 by increasing preload and contractility, until a plateau VO_2 occurs. Pearl[48] recommends a treatment algorithm for treatment of septic shock. All patients are initially started with low-dose dopamine (2 to 5 μg/kg/min). If an adequate CO is present (cardiac index [CI] more than 4.5, lactate less than 2 mmol/L) and MAP is less than 70 mm Hg, then treatment with norepinephrine is indicated. If the CO is inadequate (CI less than 4.5, lactate more than 2 mmol/L), the preload should be optimized until the plateau on the Starling curve is reached. If MAP is less than 70, consider starting dobutamine plus norepinephrine. If MAP is greater than 70, then start dobutamine. Pearl stresses that the hemodynamic status is constantly changing, so that therapy must be constantly reevaluated to fit the appropriate hemodynamic state. If the patient remains hypotensive despite this therapy, the prognosis is extremely poor.[49] Steroid therapy is no longer advocated because prospective controlled studies have shown that they offer no benefit.[50-52]

Septic shock is a complex disease. Specific treatment necessitates surgical drainage of the infected area, if identified, and administration of antibiotics. However, one must also deal with the toxic aspects of the disease. These

---

Box 12-1 Surgical conditions that may be associated with septic shock

Urinary tract infections
Pelvic abscess
Intraperitoneal abscess
Necrotizing fasciitis
Respiratory tract infection (particularly in patients with a tracheostomy)
Ascending cholangitis
Infected burns
Septic abortions
Postpartum infections
Subphrenic abscess

are particularly apparent in gram-negative shock. In the future, it is possible that specific monoclonal antibodies can be used to eradicate endotoxins. However, at present no trial involved with attacking specific mediators of SIRS has demonstrated statistically significant reductions in mortality.

II. PERIOPERATIVE HYPERTENSION

Hypertension can be a significant complication in the preoperative, intraoperative, and postoperative care of surgical patients. The term *hypertension* denotes an elevated systemic systolic arterial pressure. Abnormally high systolic arterial pressure is often accompanied by increases in the diastolic and mean arterial pressure.

Hypertension commonly exists in elderly patients and can represent a substantial anesthetic risk. Known complications of severe perioperative hypertension include cerebrovascular accident, cerebral changes of malignant hypertension, myocardial ischemia, left ventricular failure, malignant cardiac arrhythmias, and rupture of preexisting aneurysms or atherosclerotic vessels.

A. Preoperative hypertension

Preoperative hypertension can be associated with a wide variety of clinical conditions. Essential hypertension is probably the most common cause. In the early phases of essential hypertension, blood pressure may be normal during nonstressed conditions but may rise abnormally in response to stresses such as preoperative pain or preoperative anxiety. These conditions can be treated with opioids and anxiolytics. In chronic hypertension the blood pressure is consistently above 140/90 and requires treatment. Although antihypertensive therapy is usually continued until the time of operation, the clinician may occasionally encounter a patient whose antihypertensive medications have been discontinued in preparation for operation. This can be seen in patients receiving many different types of drugs, including clonidine.[53] Less common causes of preoperative hypertension are pheochromocytoma, Conn's syndrome, coarctation of the aorta, renal artery stenosis, and increased intracranial pressure. Occasionally, preoperative hypertension may be seen in a trauma patient who has received excessive fluid during resuscitation.

B. Intraoperative hypertension

1. Verifying hypertension. Severe intraoperative hypertension is a substantial risk to the patient. On the other hand, treatment with potent vasodilators also carries substantial risks, making it necessary to eliminate errors in diagnosis. If systemic hypertension is diagnosed from an arterial line, it is important to establish that the zero point and the calibration are both accurate. This can be done very rapidly. Another method for verifying arterial blood pressure is to inflate a blood pressure cuff on the catheterized arm until the arterial tracing disappears. The cuff is slowly deflated. The systemic arterial pressure is roughly equivalent to the point at which arterial pulsations reappear.[54] It is also axiomatic that the anesthesiologist must examine the arterial pressure wave-

form before accepting the digital readout. This is important because detection of spikes at peak arterial pressure indicate systolic overshoot, an error in measurement attributable to resonance in the system.[47]

Once the diagnosis of intraoperative hypertension has been firmly established, the cause must be pursued. Hypertension can be caused by many different factors during anesthesia, which are considered separately.

2. Intubation hypertension. Laryngoscopy and endotracheal intubation are known causes of hypertension during anesthesia. Intubation hypertension is most likely to occur during administration of a general anesthetic induced with a hypnotic such as pentothal, followed rapidly by the administration of a muscle relaxant for intubation. The reaction does not occur often in patients who have received a high-dose fentanyl or sufentanil induction. Intubation hypertension is most severe when laryngoscopy is prolonged and can be minimized by preadministration of lidocaine 1.5 mg/kg or SNP.[55] In healthy patients intubation hypertension is usually not harmful, but during anesthesia for aneurysm surgery or in patients with myocardial ischemia or left ventricular failure it can be very significant.

3. Inadequate anesthesia. Surgical stimulation during an inadequate depth of anesthesia results in sympathetic nervous system activation and subsequent increases in arterial pressure. Recent advances in anesthesia monitoring, such as the bispectral index (BIS), may make it possible to monitor the depth of anesthesia in a straightforward fashion during surgery. The electroencephalogram-based BIS uses four frontal leads to monitor central nervous system (CNS) electrical activity during anesthesia. This technology will enable the anesthesiologist to anticipate situations of intense surgical stimulus and titrate anesthetic doses appropriately. However, without the use of such monitoring, the anesthesiologist must rely on increases in heart rate and systemic arterial pressure after surgical incision, exploration of the peritoneum, scraping of periosteal surfaces of bone, or other significant surgical stimuli to deduce that the anesthesia is too light. Correlative findings include tachycardia, sweating, grimacing, tearing, or movement on the operative table. The doses of each agent given must be reviewed and compared to usual amounts. Individual factors such as alcoholism or narcotic addiction may increase anesthetic requirements and must be considered. Occasionally, hypertension arising during a primarily inhalation anesthetic may result when vaporizers are empty or deliver a concentration of agent lower than that selected. Proper vigilance toward monitoring of end-tidal concentrations of inspired gases and carbon dioxide through the use of mass spectrometry or infrared technology can be very useful in assessing ventilation and detecting the appropriate administration of a particular volatile agent.

4. Hypercapnia. Intraoperative hypercapnia causes sympathetic stimulation and may result in hypertension.[56-59] During anesthesia intraoperative hypercapnia can result from inadequate tidal volume, inadequate minute volume, depleted soda lime, malfunctioning valves within the anesthetic circle, disconnection of the inner hose of a Bain circuit, inadequate fresh gas flow to a Bain circuit, or increased production caused by malignant hyperthermia or thyrotoxicosis. Exogenous administration of CO_2 during laparoscopic procedures may similarly increase total CO_2 load on the circulatory system. Elevated end-tidal CO_2 concentrations detected by infrared capnography or by a mass spectrometer are highly suggestive of hypercapnia. However, the conclusive diagnosis is established by arterial blood gases. Proper treatment depends on which of these factors is causing hypercapnia.

5. Hypoxemia. Severe hypoxemia increases cardiac output to almost every organ. In the early phases of hypoxemia, systolic arterial pressure may be affected little. But in very severe hypoxemia, and provided the depth of anesthesia is only moderate, the systolic arterial pressure is greatly elevated. It must be emphasized that systolic hypertension is a very late sign in hypoxemia and is often the harbinger of complete circulatory collapse.[60]

6. Pharmacologic adjuncts. Administration of inotropic and vasoconstrictor agents is an obvious cause of intraoperative hypertension. Bolus doses of phenylephrine or epinephrine given in urgent situations can often cause severe hypertension. Medication errors resulting from failure to identify ampoules or labeled syringes may produce severe hypertension. Another cause is flushing an intravenous line that contains a vasopressor or inotropic drug. Hypertension can occur during regional anesthetic blocks if an epinephrine-containing local anesthetic solution is injected intravenously. During ophthalmic surgery, 10% phenylephrine drops may be instilled in the eye to produce mydriasis. Significant amounts of this drug can pass through the nasolacrimal duct to the nasal mucosa, where rapid absorption results in hypertension. These reactions can be minimized by limiting the concentration of phenylephrine to 5%[61] and applying pressure over the medial canthus to occlude the nasolacrimal duct.[62]

7. Pheochromocytoma. Massive amounts of epinephrine and norepinephrine can rapidly enter the circulation in patients with pheochromocytomas. If the diagnosis is known before operation, intraoperative hypertension is easily explained. However, in the case of occult pheochromocytomas, the cause of severe hypertension may be less obvious. Pheochromocytoma must always be considered in the differential diagnosis of unexplained intraoperative hypertension. In such cases, it is usually impossible to establish the definitive diagnosis until a postoperative workup has been done. Fortunately, the intraoperative control of blood pressure and tachycardia in these patients is nonspecific and involves vasodilators, β-adrenergic receptor blockers, and perhaps calcium-channel blockers.

8. Distention of urinary bladder. Distention of the urinary bladder causes increased sympathetic activity, leading to hypertension. This is often diagnosed in the recovery room.[63]

9. Aortic cross-clamping. Cross-clamping the aorta at any of several locations may be required during vascular surgery procedures. Hypertension from this cause is most commonly seen during abdominal aortic aneurysm surgery. It may also be seen during repair of coarctation of the aorta and during operations for thoracic aortic aneurysms. Hypertension from cross-clamping is usually obvious, occurring almost immediately after placement of an aortic clamp. The patient who presents with aortic lesions that have had time to develop collateral circulation (i.e., aortic occlusive disease and coarctation) may develop minimal hemodynamic changes when the aorta is cross-clamped. Good communication between surgical and anesthetic teams is essential in minimizing cross-clamping hypertension and preventing hypertensive crises.

10. Aortic valve replacement. Patients with long-standing aortic stenosis develop concentric left ventricle hypertrophy. This hypertrophied ventricle is capable of generating very high systolic pressures. During aortic valve replacement the stenotic area in the left ventricular outflow tract is removed, allowing the full peak systolic left ventricular pressure to be transmitted to the vascular tree. This can result in severe hypertension. This cause is obvious and well known to most cardiac anesthesiologists.

11. Hypertension after carotid endarterectomy. Baroreceptor dysfunction is a common cause of hypertension after carotid endarterectomy.[64] Surgical dissection renders the carotid sinus less sensitive to increases in blood pressure, thereby permitting development of significant arterial hypertension. Knowledge of this fact will prevent an unnecessary search for the cause of hypertension in these patients. Treatment usually includes antihypertensive agents.

12. Hypertension after extubation. Removal of an endotracheal tube may cause significant sympathetic stimulation, with resultant hypertension. Usually extubation hypertension is short lived. However, if prevention is necessary, a bolus dose of lidocaine given several minutes before extubation can minimize extubation hypertension.[65]

13. Postpartum hypertension. A vasoconstrictor administered before delivery can lead to severe postpartum hypertension. After delivery, the normal uterine autotransfusion causes an increased cardiac output. If this increased output faces an increased afterload because of the administration of a vasoconstrictor, severe hypertension occurs. This should be a rare event in obstetrics because potent vasoconstrictors such as methoxamine and phenylephrine decrease uterine blood flow and are usually avoided in modern obstetric anesthesia.

III. PERIOPERATIVE MYOCARDIAL ISCHEMIA
A. Definition of myocardial ischemia

Myocardial ischemia is a dual state composed of inadequate myocardial oxygenation and accumulation of anaerobic metabolites. It occurs when myocardial oxygen demand exceeds myocardial oxygen supply. A thorough grasp of this complication depends on an understanding of the dynamics of normal coronary blood flow and the deranged flow that occurs in disease.

B. Dynamics of normal myocardial oxygenation

The coronary circulation is far more complex than the circulation to other organs. Large epicardial arteries originate at the aorta and travel across the epicardial surface of the heart. These vessels branch into smaller penetrating vessels that arise approximately at right angles to the surface epicardial coronary arteries. The penetrating or intramural arteries course downward between muscle fibers of the cardiac syncytium. Anastomotic connections without an intervening capillary bed exist between portions of the same coronary artery and between different coronary arteries. Under normal circumstances these collaterals are almost invisible; they become apparent only when a major coronary artery is occluded. After passing through a dense capillary bed, cardiac venous blood travels either through the coronary sinus to the right atrium or into the left ventricle. Coronary perfusion pressure is the pressure in a coronary artery minus the right atrial or left ventricular end-diastolic pressure, depending on whether the blood drains into the coronary sinus or the left ventricle.

Flow in the proximal coronary arteries meets significant resistance in the penetrating or intramural arteries. These intramural arteries have both an intrinsic and an extrinsic resistance. Intrinsic coronary resistance is the resistance that originates within the substance of the intramural vessels themselves and is influenced by many factors. The coronary arteries contain sympathetic and parasympathetic nerves. Stimulation of the sympathetic nerves causes coronary vasoconstriction. Stimulation of the parasympathetic nerves results in coronary vasodilation. Myogenic factors refer to the tendency of vascular smooth muscle to contract when perfusion pressure increases. This mechanism is called the Bayliss effect.[66] Metabolic factors also exert a pronounced effect on intrinsic coronary resistance. When a region of myocardium is hypoperfused, vasodilator metabolites accumulate and dilate the coronary vasculature. Adenosine is an especially powerful coronary vasodilator[67] that blocks a receptor on the surface of vascular smooth muscle cells and prevents entry of calcium into muscle cells.[66] Although adenosine is probably the major metabolic coronary vasodilator, prostaglandins such as PGI_2 and PGE_2 can cause coronary vasodilation. Several other substances such as acetylcholine, adenosine triphosphate, adenosine diphosphate, bradykinin, and histamine are capable of dilating coronary arteries but must act through an intact endothelium. The endothelium of muscular arteries may have receptors for these vasodilators. When vasodilators bind to these receptors, they cause the endothelial cells to release a substance that causes relaxation of vascular smooth muscle. This substance has been called endothelium-derived relaxing factor (EDRF). EDRF is a labile compound that activates guanylate cyclase in vascular smooth muscle, resulting in an increase in intracellular cyclic guanosine monophosphate, causing vascular relaxation.[68-71] Damage to the coronary vascular endothelium can impair this relaxation response.[72]

Extrinsic coronary vascular resistance of the intramural arteries is the factor that clearly distinguishes the coronary circulation. The intramural coronary arteries and arterioles are virtually surrounded by the cardiac muscle syncytium. During systole, contraction of cardiac muscle squeezes coronary arteries and at end-systole coronary blood flow ceases.[73] As the diastolic period begins, cardiac muscle relaxes, the extrinsic squeezing of the coronary arteries is relieved, and the cardiac muscle receives a rush of blood. The diastolic portion of the cardiac cycle is extremely important for adequate coronary perfusion[73] because approximately 85% of coronary blood flow occurs during diastole in the normal person. Tachycardia decreases diastolic time and thereby decreases coronary flow.

Increases in myocardial oxygen demand occur frequently during exercise and intense emotion. People with normal coronary arteries can accommodate increased oxygen demands because their total coronary blood flow can increase five times over the resting level. In addition, regional increases in myocardial blood flow can occur through adenosine-induced decreases in intrinsic coronary vascular tone called autoregulation.[74]

C. Major conditions predisposing to myocardial ischemia

The two most common conditions that predispose to myocardial ischemia are coronary artery disease and left ventricular hypertrophy.

1. Coronary artery disease. The fixed and dynamic obstructions encountered in coronary artery disease severely limit myocardial blood flow. Autoregulation is faulty because the poststenotic coronary vascular bed may be maximally vasodilated in the resting state and cannot dilate further during exercise or stress. Left ventricular dilation secondary to heart failure may increase ventricular wall tension, particularly in the subendocardial area, leading to poor subendocardial flow and resultant ischemia. A tachycardia may severely limit the time for coronary blood flow.

2. Left ventricular hypertrophy. Left ventricular hypertrophy predisposes to myocardial ischemia because the increased oxygen requirements of the thickened myocardium can easily exceed oxygen supply. Impairment of oxygen supply occurs because abnormal diastolic relaxation increases impedance to coronary flow. Left ventricular hypertrophy leading to myocardial ischemia is most commonly seen in patients with chronic hypertension.

D. Types of myocardial ischemia

Myocardial ischemia may be either symptomatic or silent.

1. Symptomatic. Symptomatic myocardial ischemia usually is ischemia that causes cardiac pain. The presence of typical cardiac pain may lead to thorough preoperative evaluation and treatment and specialized plans for intraanesthetic and postanesthetic monitoring and treatment. Treatment of patients with symptomatic ischemia can be challenging but at least one can be prepared for it.

2. Silent. Silent myocardial ischemia is especially dangerous because of its concealed nature. Two major types of problems can arise from silent ischemia. The first is that a patient with advanced coronary disease and active ischemia may come to anesthesia without the caregivers realizing that the patient is prone to ischemia. Indeed, some 2% to 4% of middle-aged men have asymptomatic coronary artery disease with silent ischemia.[75] Because the anesthesiologist has no reason to suspect coronary disease, provision for ECG ischemia monitoring may not be made. Repeated and prolonged ischemic episodes may go unrecognized. This can lead to MI[76,77] and intraoperative or postoperative death. In this setting, it is very likely that the infarction or death would be attributed to substandard anesthetic care. It is obviously important to obtain a postmortem examination in such cases because the demonstration of fresh coronary thrombosis or plaque rupture may exonerate the anesthesiologist. The second major problem posed by silent ischemia is that episodes of myocardial ischemia in patients with known coronary artery disease may be missed. This is a real problem because approximately 70% of ischemic episodes in patients with stable angina are silent.[75] Bouts of silent ischemia are most likely to be missed when the patient is not monitored for ischemia. Most elective surgical patients with coronary disease do not have constant ECG ischemia monitoring in the hours immediately preceding their operations. Ischemia monitoring during transport to and from the operating room is not often done. And ischemia monitoring in many recovery rooms is certainly not optimal. Thus it is very likely that ischemic events can be easily missed in coronary artery disease patients with silent ischemia.

E. Myocardial ischemia without hemodynamic alterations

The fact that hemodynamic alterations can be valuable in predicting, detecting, and treating myocardial ischemia is discussed in the following paragraphs. However, it must be emphasized that studies done in coronary bypass patients indicate that the majority of perioperative ischemic episodes are not accompanied by hemodynamic changes.[78] Likewise, Cheng et al[79] report that good control of blood pressure and pulse rate does not necessarily prevent myocardial ischemia. This perplexing and frustrating observation is explained by the contention that most episodes of preoperative myocardial ischemia are associated with distal coronary vasospasm or reversible platelet aggregation. Neither of these conditions can be detected directly by our current monitoring.

F. Myocardial ischemia associated with hemodynamic alterations

1. Tachycardia. Perioperative myocardial ischemia may follow the onset of adverse hemodynamic changes. The occurrence of tachycardia is particularly dangerous because it increases oxygen demand and simultaneously decreases myocardial oxygen supply. The decrease in supply is particularly severe because the time available for coronary flow is drastically and disproportionly reduced. For example, at a heart rate of approximately 60 beats/min, the total diastolic time is approximately 800 ms. Increasing the heart rate to 90 beats/min decreases

coronary flow time to only 200 ms.[80] It is important to emphasize that increases in heart rate that would ordinarily be within the normal range can be a serious threat to the patient with coronary vascular disease.

Perioperative tachycardia can result from many causes, including light anesthesia, endotracheal intubation, hypovolemia, fever, anemia, congestive heart failure, and postoperative pain. Treating the underlying cause is obviously the sensible thing to do. However, in practicality, if myocardial ischemia clearly accompanies tachycardia, damage to the myocardium may be time dependent, so it may be appropriate to use esmolol to decrease the heart rate while the causal condition is treated. For example, a patient with severe coronary vascular disease who has a temperature of 103° F (39.3° C) may develop tachycardia and myocardial ischemia. In principle, treating the elevated temperature would remove the cause and result in cardiac slowing. However, the process of cooling is so slow that severe myocardial damage could occur while the temperature is being lowered. Alternatively, if tachycardia is caused by an ectopic supraventricular pacemaker, the administration of esmolol, metoprolol, verapamil, or adenosine may be important in the differentiation and treatment of the dysrhythmia.

2. Tachycardia and hypotension. The combination of tachycardia and hypotension is especially likely to precipitate myocardial ischemia because two supply factors are simultaneously decreased. Hypotension reduces the driving force across the coronary bed, and tachycardia reduces the time available for coronary blood flow. These two hemodynamic derangements are commonly encountered in hypovolemia. Treating the basic cause is always rational, but when evidence of ischemia accompanies these two changes, the time required for appropriate volume replacement may result in prolonged ischemia and possible evolution into MI. This is particularly true if the placement of a pulmonary artery catheter or central venous pressure catheter is required before volume replacement. Consequently, in severe hypotension and tachycardia it may be necessary to buy time by increasing coronary perfusion pressure with a potent α-adrenergic agent such as phenylephrine. This drug may also decrease cardiac rate via a baroreceptor response.

3. Hypervolemia. Iatrogenic hypervolemia can cause myocardial ischemia. Overzealous fluid administration can easily result in an abnormally large LVEDV. As left ventricular volume increases, the LVEDP and the mean myocardial wall tension both increase, leading to an increase in myocardial oxygen consumption. If the coronary vessels are unable to increase flow to match this increased demand, myocardial ischemia can result. Detection of hypervolemia using a single measurement can be difficult. Central venous pressure monitoring often fails to detect changes in LVEDV. An abnormally high PCWP can correlate with a large LVEDV if compliance of the left ventricle is normal. However, it is possible that direct estimation of LVEDV obtained with the use of a transesophageal two-dimensional echocardiogram (2-D TEE) may be more accurate. This method also has limitations because TEE provides a measurement of left ventricular end-diastolic area, not a direct measurement of LVEDV or LVEDP. Accurate diagnosis of hypervolemia can be difficult and may require consideration of changes in several measurements, including PCWP, cardiac output, arterial oxygen tension, and heart size on chest roentgenograms.

4. Postpartum hypervolemia. Hypervolemia-induced myocardial ischemia may also occur in obstetric patients. Palmer et al[81] found ST segment or T-wave changes in 44 of 93 otherwise healthy women giving birth through cesarean section under regional anesthesia. Fifteen of these patients developed chest pain, pressure, or dyspnea. No patient without ECG changes developed chest symptoms. The authors speculate that the ECG changes were caused by myocardial ischemia related to sudden hypervolemia resulting from fluid loading and autotransfusion during delivery. Mathew et al[82] report a 25% incidence of ST segment depression in women undergoing cesarean delivery. This occurred most commonly in the 30 minutes following delivery. Transthoracic echocardiography was unable to detect regional wall motion abnormalities (RWMAs) during the ST segment depression but did reveal significant decreases in ejection fraction area during these episodes. Despite the incidence of ST segment changes in these two studies, clinically significant myocardial impairment during cesarean delivery probably does not occur. However, significant ST segment depression may not be an artifact of parturition.

The treatment of myocardial ischemia secondary to hypervolemia involves preload reduction, diuretics, and occasionally phlebotomy. Endotracheal intubation, controlled ventilation, and oxygen supplementation are often required to maintain adequate arterial oxygenation.

5. Hypertension. Hypertension is another adverse condition in patients with coronary artery disease. Systemic arterial hypertension increases myocardial oxygen consumption. In the presence of coronary artery disease, the increased myocardial oxygen consumption may exceed myocardial oxygen supply, resulting in acute ischemia. This is particularly true if tachycardia coexists with hypertension. Although the role of hypertension as a predictor for the onset of ischemia has been questioned,[75,83] some studies suggest that acute hypertensive episodes precede as many as 50% of intraoperative ischemic episodes.[84,85]

G. Myocardial ischemia associated with other conditions

1. Coronary spasm (Prinzmetal's angina). Coronary artery spasm can produce severe transmural myocardial ischemia. Coronary spasm that accompanies Prinzmetal's (variant) angina occurs at rest, is usually not precipitated by physical or emotional exertion, and is accompanied by ST segment elevations on the ECG.[86] This type of myocardial ischemia results from a transient abrupt decrease in the diameter of an epicardial or large septal coronary artery. The spasm can be demonstrated clearly by coronary arteriography.[87] Prinzmetal's angina may be associated with MI, serious cardiac dysrhythmias, including ventricular tachycardia and fibrillation, and

even sudden death.[88] Ganz and Alexander[89] suggest that the abnormality in Prinzmetal's angina is a hypercontractility of the arterial wall related to the atherosclerotic process. Others suggest that endothelial damage reverses the dilator response associated with EDRF.[90] Unless a history of Prinzmetal's angina is known, its occurrence under anesthesia, including the pronounced ST segment elevation, can mimic an acute MI.

2. Handling the heart. Direct handling of the heart may cause ischemia, particularly in patients with coronary artery disease. Lifting, twisting, and compressing the heart all may kink atherosclerotic coronary arteries, which may predispose to spasm, plaque rupture, and even thrombosis and occlusion. Hyduke et al[91] report severe intraoperative myocardial ischemia after manipulation of the heart in a patient undergoing esophagogastrectomy. It may be impossible to avoid cardiac manipulation completely during certain surgical procedures. Lifting or displacement of the heart may impair venous return to the heart. This would decrease preload and thus stroke volume. The drop in blood pressure following manipulation may decrease perfusion pressure across stenotic coronary lesions and lead to myocardial ischemia. The incidence of attendant myocardial ischemia may be lessened by handling the heart gently and minimizing the degree and duration of cardiac displacement.

3. Carbon monoxide exposure. Carbon monoxide exposure may predispose the patient with coronary artery disease to myocardial ischemia. Allred et al[92] found that during incremental exercise testing, patients with coronary artery disease who were exposed to carbon monoxide had a reduction in the time to a threshold ischemic ST segment change. The stressed surgical patient might have a similar response. For example, burned patients who have suffered smoke inhalation may be particularly prone to myocardial ischemia. Likewise, a period of heavy cigarette smoking before surgery in an ambulatory setting might predispose the patient with coronary disease to myocardial ischemia.

4. Cocaine abuse. It is widely accepted that cocaine use can precipitate myocardial ischemia and chest pain is the most common cocaine-related medical problem. The possibility of cocaine-induced myocardial ischemia may not be suspected during nasal surgery.[93] However, combinations of topical cocaine and injected lidocaine with epinephrine (1:100,000) may precipitate ischemia. Recommended doses in the range of 3 to 4 mg/kg have been advocated.

The effects of cocaine are mediated through a sympathomimetic response, inhibiting the reuptake of both norepinephrine and epinephrine while stimulating the presynaptic release of norepinephrine. The increases in norepinephrine at postsynaptic α-receptors account for the drug's stimulatory effects. Its central effects lead to increased neuronal firing and, combined with inhibited reuptake, contribute to an exaggerated sympathetic response. Further CNS activity leads to hyperthermia and seizure activity.

Cocaine produces myocardial ischemia through a combination of factors. Cocaine is a coronary vasoconstrictor and its presence increases α-adrenergic–mediated platelet aggregability. Cocaine also stimulates thrombus formation in situ and predisposes to premature development of coronary atherosclerosis. Cocaine-induced coronary vasoconstriction can be reversed by phentolamine and exacerbated by propanolol. Most cocaine users are cigarette smokers, and the combination of nicotine and cocaine has synergistic effects on development of coronary vasoconstriction.[94] It is well known that cocaine elevates blood pressure and heart rate and increases myocardial oxygen consumption. Knowing these facts, it is not surprising that cocaine is an ideal drug for precipitating myocardial ischemia.

Treatment of cocaine-induced myocardial ischemia should be based on the understanding of cocaine's central and peripheral mechanisms of action. Hollander[95] recommends initial treatment of suspected cocaine-induced myocardial ischemia with benzodiazepines, relying not only on their anxiolytic effects but also their ability to decrease blood pressure and heart rate. Aspirin, or suitable antiplatelet therapy, should be administered to reduce the formation of thrombi. Nitroglycerin relieves cocaine-induced coronary vasoconstriction and should be administered with a goal of decreasing mean arterial pressure of 10% to 15%. Oxygen should be administered. Phentolamine, 1 mg, and verapamil may be useful second-line drugs. β-Blockers and labetalol may worsen coronary vasoconstriction through unopposed α-adrenergic stimulation.[96] In the absence of risk for subarachnoid hemorrhage, thrombolytic therapy may be indicated if ST segments do not resolve. Cocaine withdrawal may lead to asymptomatic episodes of ST segment changes. This has been demonstrated by Holter monitoring of a group of known cocaine addicts.[97]

H. Diagnosing myocardial ischemia

With the onset of myocardial ischemia, a series of events occur that can have diagnostic implications. Ischemia may result in cardiac pain, myocardial lactate production, RWMAs, decreased myocardial contractility, decreased ejection fraction, increased LVEDP, and ST segment abnormalities. Although each of these sequelae can accompany myocardial ischemia, some of these abnormalities are highly useful in the state-of-the-art diagnosis in the late 1990s. Others hold promise for the future and some, such as lactate production, require sampling methods, which are simply impractical for day-to-day use. Although innovative methods such as TEE present exciting possibilities for the future, it is important to understand how to use our current state-of-the-art monitoring.

1. New cardiac pain. The onset of new cardiac pain can be extremely important when one is diagnosing myocardial ischemia preoperatively, during surgery under local or regional anesthesia, and postoperatively in the recovery room. One should certainly be aware that chest pressure, chest pain, and a sense of chest constriction are symptoms of myocardial ischemia. Cardiac pain may also be referred to either arm, the neck, the jaws, the teeth, and even the posterior scapular areas. The onset of any of these symptoms should not be ignored. Cardiac pain is extremely useful as a diagnostic aid when it occurs. However, it is important to remember that the absence of cardiac pain does not rule out myocardial ischemia.[98] Diabetic patients may have myocardial ischemia without perceiving pain because pain pathways may be impaired by diabetic neuropathy.[99] Silent myocardial ischemia can also occur in nondiabetic patients. In fact, many authorities agree that approximately 70% of ischemic episodes in patients with symptomatic coronary artery disease are not associated with angina.[100] Because 70% of myocardial ischemic episodes in fully awake humans are asymptomatic, it is sobering to consider that the elderly, sedated patient receiving regional anesthesia probably will have no symptoms even if he or she develops myocardial ischemia.

2. Electrocardiography: anachronism or standard? Contemporary literature contains many reports emphasizing the limitations of electrocardiography compared to futuristic monitors such as echocardiography and cardiokymography. However, electrocardiography is an extremely important method for detecting myocardial ischemia. It can be used preoperatively, intraoperatively, and postoperatively. It can be used in patients undergoing regional anesthesia and with general anesthesia with or without endotracheal intubation. ECG leads can be applied to the patient without pain and at minimal cost. Deviations in the ST segment can be recognized, recorded, and measured easily. The proper frequency bandwidth for diagnostic electrocardiography and the criteria for proper voltage standardization have been established. Postoperative ECGs can be compared easily to preoperative tracings. The ST segment can be analyzed by computer, recorded, and trended both during and after anesthesia. Because of its practicality, the ECG remains the standard for the diagnosis of myocardial ischemia in the late 1990s.

The value of electrocardiography depends on its proper use. The ECG must be calibrated to give a pen deflection of 10 mm for 1 mV potential. This is extremely important because excessive gain can produce false ST segment depression and inadequate gain can mask such depression. The proper frequency bandwidth must be used. Most modern operating room ECG monitors contain both a diagnostic and a monitor mode. The monitoring mode is designed to filter out electrical interference. However, ischemia monitoring using the monitor mode may produce false T-wave and ST segment changes. Proper diagnosis of ischemia from the ECG depends on the use of the diagnostic mode, which brackets a frequency bandwidth of 0.05 to 100 Hz.

The standard ECG consists of 12 leads. Inclusion of all 12 leads gives the best overall assessment and can be used preoperatively and postoperatively. However, during anesthesia, monitoring is usually limited to seven leads. Selection of the best leads is important. Blackburn and Katigbak[101] demonstrated that 89% of significant ST segment depression after exercise was found in precordial lead V_5. They also demonstrated that 100% of ST segment changes can be detected by recording leads V_3-V_6 and leads II and aVF.[102] The seven-lead system allows the standard leads and lead V_5 to be monitored. Any of these seven leads can be recorded when necessary. In routine practice, leads II and V_5 are continuously monitored, giving views of the inferior and lateral myocardium. Continuous scanning of several leads seems to improve the detection of myocardial ischemia. Kotrly et al[103] described the use of a modified microcomputer-based ECG that continuously monitors leads I, II, and V_5 and gives a summation of ST segment deviations. Many commercial monitors are available with computer analysis and automatic ST segment trending.

Whether one uses computerized ST segment trending, it is still important to have a working knowledge of critical ST segment analysis. In the normal ECG, the ST segment is isoelectric. Elevations or depressions are fairly easy to recognize. Depressions of 1 mm or more are usually indicative of subendocardial ischemia, and upsloping depression of this magnitude may be the first sign of myocardial ischemia. Horizontal or downsloping ST segment depression of 1 mm or more indicates significant subendocardial ischemia. ST segment elevation greater than 1 mm indicates severe transmural ischemia.[104] ST segment depression is usually measured 80 milliseconds after the J-point, which is the junction of the S-wave and the ST segment. However, the ST segment may be distorted by the preoperative presence of a left bundle-branch block (LBBB), left ventricular hypertrophy, digitalis effect, and ventricular pacing. These conditions make the ECG diagnosis of ischemia extremely difficult.

3. Pulmonary artery catheter measurements during ischemia. With the onset of myocardial ischemia, myocardial compliance decreases, leading to a stiff heart. Theoretically this stiffness should result in an increased PCWP. Kaplan and Wells[105] report that increases in PCWP could be used to diagnose early myocardial ischemia. Other studies indicate an increase in PCWP during ischemia induced by cardiac pacing[106-108] and during coronary angioplasty.[109-111] However, these observations do not necessarily mean that increases in PCWP can be used as an early and reliable indicator of myocardial ischemia during anesthesia. In order to examine the value of increases in PCWP as an early indicator of myocardial ischemia detected by electrocardiography and echocardiography, van Daele et al[112] studied 100 patients undergoing coronary artery bypass grafting. Increases in wedge pressure often did not occur during ischemia. From these results it appears that increases in PCWP are not a sensitive or specific indicator of the onset of myocardial ischemia during anesthesia.

4. Echocardiography: futuristic or current standard? During normal cardiac systole the myocardium thickens. Within seconds after total interruption of circulation to a region, systolic thickening decreases and other aspects of wall motion are impaired. Both systolic thickening and wall motion can be monitored by use of 2-D TEE. The TEE probe is a modified gastroscope that can be inserted easily after endotracheal intubation. Studies done during coronary angioplasty have shown that echocardiography is more sensitive than electrocardiography in the detection of myocardial ischemia.[111] Other experimental data and clinical studies suggest that RWMAs are more sensitive than ST segment changes for the early detection of myocardial ischemia.[113-116] Continuous online images provide the anesthesiologist with beat-to-beat observations of the heart. The recent introduction of quad-screen technology allows the anesthesiologist to freeze previous cardiac images for comparison with the online measurements. Color flow Doppler technology gives the potential for detection of acute mitral regurgitation secondary to ischemic papillary muscle dysfunction. Left ventricular end-diastolic area can be measured and recorded during rapid volume infusion, which may help in the early detection of overdistention of the left ventricle. Complications associated with the use of the TEE probe are rare. Ultrasound has no known medical complications.

All these facts and prominent exposure at national anesthesia meetings have contributed to enthusiasm for the use of TEE as an extremely sensitive monitor of myocardial ischemia. However, its value must be viewed in perspective. The studies were done by investigators who had extensive training and experience in TEE. In their hands, TEE may indeed be a more sensitive indicator of myocardial ischemia than the ECG. The use of TEE by an untrained person may result in an incorrect diagnosis caused by lack of training and experience. Preinduction imaging would require preoperative passage of the probe or use of a transthoracic probe for cardiac imaging. Transesophageal echocardiography cannot be used easily in the awake patient undergoing regional anesthesia. Its use as an ischemia detector in the recovery room is limited unless the patient is still sedated and intubated. When one is monitoring for myocardial ischemia, the most commonly used view is a transgastric midpapillary view of the left ventricle. Ischemia confined to the right ventricle or to the base or apex of the left ventricle may be missed. Rotation or translation of the entire heart can make segmental contraction difficult to evaluate. Discoordinated contraction may not be attributable to ischemia if a patient has a preexisting bundle-branch block or is undergoing ventricular pacing. Other wall motion abnormalities may represent stunned, or hibernating, myocardium instead of acutely ischemic myocardium. Quantitative methods for wall-thickening analysis are tedious and often limited by inadequate visualization of the epicardium.[117] Finally, because of biologic differences, not all normal hearts contract normally and not all parts of the same heart contract to the same degree.[118] However, TEE has even more serious limitations. London et al[119] compared echocardiography to electrocardiography as an ischemia monitor. They report that many ischemic episodes detected by electrocardiography were missed by echocardiography. The authors conclude that "the discordant relation between TEE and ECG changes observed here necessitates careful monitoring of the ECG when TEE is used clinically." Development of multiplane TEE gives the practitioner an electronically controlled rotating array to allow the rapid, consistent acquisition of standard and off-axis views from a single transducer position. Apical and basal segments are easily viewed using the multiplane TEE. This modality should facilitate interrogation of greater areas of the heart for ischemia detection, as compared to the transgastric midpapillary view of the left ventricle commonly acquired with monoplane TEE. Edge detection software and real-time determination of ejection fraction area further assist the anesthesiologist in determination of RWMAs. In summary, if the anesthesiologist has the training, experience, and equipment to perform TEE, it can be invaluable in the early detection of myocardial ischemia.

I. Treatment of perioperative myocardial ischemia

1. Prevention of myocardial ischemia. The best treatment for perioperative myocardial ischemia is prevention. This can be a very difficult task because many factors are simply not under the control of the anesthesiologist. Careful preoperative histories and appropriate preoperative workup will do much to identify susceptible patients. However, these conscientious efforts will not result in identification of all patients at risk. Some patients have silent myocardial ischemia. Others simply deny serious cardiac symptoms. However, suspicion of coronary artery disease in the elderly, patients with noticeable truncal obesity, heavy smokers, and those with a family history of coronary artery disease will help in preoperative identification.

Careful attention to prevention of tachycardia during anesthesia is extremely important, and it must be remembered that seemingly normal heart rates (such as 80 beats/min) may precipitate myocardial ischemia in patients with coronary artery disease. Careful titration of appropriate levels of anesthesia, particularly if it includes fentanyl, will do much to prevent tachycardia. Judicious use of ultra–short-acting β-blockers can also be very beneficial in preventing tachycardia. In perspective, the perceived dangers of β-blockers are probably more imaginary than real. Although β-blockers do have serious side effects, the majority of cardiac side effects can be reversed very rapidly using common drugs such as atropine or calcium chloride.

Coriat et al[120] demonstrated that the prophylactic administration of intravenous nitroglycerin 1 μg/kg/min will significantly decrease the incidence of intraoperative myocardial ischemia in patients with coronary artery disease. Seitelberger et al[121] showed that the intravenous infusion of nifedipine after coronary artery bypass grafting decreases the incidence of myocardial ischemia. Although nifedipine is not available as an intravenous preparation in the United States, other calcium-channel blockers might have similar prophylactic effects.

Despite our best preventive efforts, perioperative myocardial ischemia may still occur. Because myocardial ischemia may be secondary to complex and interrelated causes, the specifics of treatment in any given case depend on the details of that case. However, it is possible to make some useful generalizations.

2. Establishment of temporal relationships. Myocardial ischemia can occur with or without significant hemodynamic aberrations. If hemodynamic aberrations are associated with myocardial ischemia, they may precede and be the cause of the ischemia. On the other hand, ischemia may precede and may cause the hemodynamic aberrations. Close monitoring and establishment of a temporal relationship may be extremely important. For example, if an anesthetized patient has normal ST segments and then develops tachycardia followed by ST segment depression, it is reasonable to assume that tachycardia caused the ischemia, so efforts should be directed at reducing the pulse rate. If hypovolemic hypotension precedes the onset of ST segment depression, perhaps the hypotension and decrease in myocardial oxygen supply may be the cause. Details of treatment in any given case also depend on the urgency of the situation and whether appropriate monitoring lines are in place when ischemia occurs.

3. Ischemia without hemodynamic alterations. In susceptible patients, myocardial ischemia manifested by ST segment depression often occurs without attendant hemodynamic aberrations. In these cases the administration of nitroglycerin can be extremely helpful. Nitroglycerin decreases preload and wall tension, dilates epicardial coronary arteries, and increases subendocardial blood flow. Intravenous administration is preferred in acute situations. However, if the intravenous preparation is not immediately available, a 0.4-mg tablet can be placed sublingually or be dissolved in 1 ml saline solution and administered intranasally.[122] Because intranasal administration of 0.4 mg of dissolved nitroglycerin can occasionally produce hypotension, we recommend an initial dose of 0.2 mg. However, even with careful dose selection, intranasal administration is less predictable than intravenous administration.

4. Ischemia accompanied by tachycardia and hypertension. A combination of tachycardia and hypertension can lead to a hyperdynamic state precipitating myocardial ischemia. Hypertension increases myocardial oxygen demand and tachycardia decreases oxygen supply. After satisfactory ventilation, oxygenation, and anesthetic administration have been quickly verified, intervention with a β-adrenergic receptor blocking drug is recommended. These types of drugs should be administered if there is no evidence of congestive heart failure or bronchospasm. Despite the $β_1$-receptor selectivity of esmolol and metoprolol, these drugs should be titrated carefully in the setting of a patient with severe chronic obstructive pulmonary disease or reactive airway disease. In many cases this hyperdynamic state subsides as the pulse rate slows. If hypertension and ECG evidence of ischemia continue after the pulse rate is decreased to approximately 70 beats/min, nitroglycerin is recommended in small titrated doses guided by blood pressure monitoring.

5. Ischemia: hypotension and tachycardia. The combination of hypotension and tachycardia is particularly likely to produce myocardial ischemia because both derangements can drastically reduce myocardial oxygen supply. A common cause of this combination is hypovolemia. Treatment of hypovolemia as the first priority appears to be logical. However, in the face of hypotension and myocardial ischemia, volume replacement as the only treatment may be too slow. Certainly we would begin volume replacement as rapidly as possible, but in the interim it is critical to restore coronary perfusion pressure and slow the pulse rate. Phenylephrine is extremely useful in this situation. In critical cases we would administer phenylephrine using a 1-ml syringe. A small syringe facilitates the accurate administration of a reasonable first dose of 0.020 to 0.050 mg. The response can be assessed rapidly and more drug can be given easily if necessary. Slow titration of phenylephrine may buy time while intravascular volume is restored.

6. Coronary spasm and ischemia. Coronary spasm may produce acute, severe transmural myocardial ischemia manifested by ST segment elevation. Prinzmetal's variant angina was first described in 1959 and is characterized as cardiac pain secondary to myocardial ischemia that occurs exclusively at rest, not precipitated by physical exertion or emotional stress, and is associated with ECG ST segment elevations. This syndrome commonly occurs in younger patients rather than those affected by chronic stable or unstable angina. They are without significant coronary artery disease risk factors except that they are often heavy cigarette smokers. This condition might easily be confused with the early stages of a transmural MI. However, with a history of variant angina, one may treat this condition effectively. Sublingual or intravenous nitrates will abolish coronary spasm by directly vasodilating the spastic coronary artery. When combined with calcium-channel blocking drugs, the nitrates may have an additive effect. Diltiazem, verapamil, and nifedipine all have exhibited similar efficacy rates when administered in this clinical scenario. These two types of drugs are mainstays of treatment for this condition. β-Adrenergic blocking drugs have variable efficacy in this syndrome.

7. Ectopic supraventricular tachycardia. The sudden onset of a supraventricular tachycardia may precipitate myocardial ischemia. In this case, slowing the pulse rate is extremely important and drugs such as esmolol, propranolol, verapamil, and adenosine[123] should be considered. One may rapidly terminate the myocardial ischemia by restoring normal sinus rhythm at a slow rate.

8. Severe resistant myocardial ischemia. Occasionally the anesthesiologist will encounter severe myocardial ischemia resistant to reasonable doses of all antianginal drugs. In this setting, the intraaortic balloon can be invaluable. Counterpulsation provided by an intraaortic balloon acutely decreases myocardial oxygen requirements and may increase myocardial oxygen supply. The balloon can be quickly inserted percutaneously by a cardiac surgeon or an invasive cardiologist. It is important that a radial artery line also be inserted to establish the correct timing of the balloon and to ensure that it is not advanced into the arch of the aorta.

IV. PERIOPERATIVE MYOCARDIAL INFARCTION
A. Significance of infarction

MI occurring before, during, or after anesthesia and operation is a major complication with significant morbidity and mortality. This is especially true in patients who have suffered an MI in the 6 months immediately preceding an operation. Older data indicated that 27% to 37% of these patients will sustain a perioperative reinfarction and of these approximately 50% will die before leaving the hospital.[124-126] Although inconclusive, newer studies suggest that the use of aggressive invasive hemodynamic monitoring and prompt treatment of hemodynamic abnormalities can greatly decrease the reinfarction and mortality rates.[127,128] Despite these apparent improvements, perioperative MI still occurs and can lead to major problems such as pulmonary edema, low cardiac output, severe intractable cardiac arrhythmias, cerebral and renal damage, and death.

B. Factors associated with infarction

The overwhelming majority of perioperative infarctions occur in patients with significant preexisting coronary vascular disease. However, hypertensive patients with left ventricular hypertrophy and patients with left ventricular hypertrophy secondary to aortic valve disease are also very susceptible to perioperative MI.

Perioperative MI can occur after many pathophysiologic processes. Sloghoff and Keats[129,130] demonstrated that myocardial ischemia occurring during coronary artery bypass operations leads to an increased incidence of postoperative MI. Although this relationship has been established in patients undergoing coronary artery bypass grafting, conclusive studies establishing the relationship during other operations have not been done. However, it is the authors' firm opinion that significant myocardial ischemia during many different types of operations leads to an increased incidence of postoperative MI, especially if the ischemic episode is severe and prolonged.

Coronary atherosclerotic plaques may undergo sudden changes, resulting in perioperative MI. It must be emphasized that these changes can occur without apparent precipitating factors and at any time. When a sudden MI occurs, surgeons and anesthesiologists are likely to ask, "Why did this happen now?" This cannot always be answered easily. It has been shown that the majority of MIs in unanesthetized patients follow a circadian variation, with an increase beginning about 7 AM and reaching its peak at approximately 8 AM. This is the time when anesthesia is being induced in many patients. There is also an evening peak beginning around 6 PM and reaching the zenith at about 10 PM.[131] The cause of these peaks is unknown. We do know that sudden acute MI can result from plaque rupture leading to an occlusive intimal flap. Hemorrhage into an existing plaque is another mechanism. The development of a fissure in an atherosclerotic plaque can expose platelets to collagen, which leads to thrombus formation. Prolonged or repetitive coronary artery spasm may also lead to coronary thrombosis.[132] Withdrawing cocaine addicts may develop coronary spasm with silent myocardial ischemia demonstrated by Holter monitoring. These episodes occur spontaneously and may not be associated with stress.[133] Chronic cocaine addicts have accelerated coronary atherogenesis, making it especially likely that a withdrawing addict could develop a perioperative infarction.

Box 12-2 Myocardial infarction not associated with coronary atherosclerosis

Congenital coronary anomalies
Coronary artery aneurysms
Left coronary artery arising from anterior sinus of Valsalva
Coronary arteriovenous fistulas
Origin of left coronary artery from pulmonary artery

Hematologic
Thrombocytosis
Hypercoagulability
Disseminated intravascular coagulation
Thrombocytopenic purpura
Polycythemia vera

Coronary artery emboli
Left atrial or ventricular mural thrombus
Prolapse of mitral valve
Prosthetic valve emboli
Papillary fibroelastoma of the aortic valve
Cardiac myxoma
Paradoxic emboli

Arteritis
Ankylosing spondylitis
Rheumatoid arthritis
Disseminated lupus erythematosus
Kawasaki's syndrome
Takayasu's disease
Polyarteritis nodosa
Luetic aortitis

Miscellaneous
Carbon monoxide poisoning
Thyrotoxicosis
Aortic insufficiency
Mucopolysaccharidosis
Fabry's disease
Amyloidosis
Pseudoxanthoma elasticum

It has recently been demonstrated that cocaine use can lead to acute coronary spasm, making it probable that cocaine abusers arriving for surgery may develop perioperative coronary artery spasm and infarction.[97] Chest injury can also lead to trauma of coronary arteries, with laceration and thrombosis. Other numerous conditions not involving coronary atherosclerosis can be associated with acute MI (Box 12-2).

C. Diagnosing perioperative myocardial infarction

1. Preoperative diagnosis. All MIs occurring in the 3 months immediately before an operation must be considered present perioperative MIs because they can lead to major present perioperative morbidity and mortality. In some cases a preoperative infarct is associated with a discrete event characterized by hospitalization, a thorough workup, and a complete description of therapy and complications. Perusal of hospital records will substantiate the diagnosis and document the severity of the infarct. In other cases, a patient may come to the preoperative holding area and experience crushing substernal chest pain radiating to the left arm and appear dyspneic and cyanotic. Acute MI is clearly the most likely cause. But pain does not always accompany MI, particularly in diabetic or elderly patients.[134] Studies indicate that 20% to 60% of nonfatal MIs are completely unrecognized by the patient and are discovered on subsequent ECG or postmortem examinations.[135] Other patients have clear-cut cardiac symptoms for which they seek medical advice, but they subsequently deny them. Preoperative MIs may be detected occasionally by the new appearance of Q-waves on the preoperative ECG or by the appearance of a new LBBB. The new onset of atrial fibrillation may be another marker for preoperative infarction, particularly in the elderly patient. The very early stage of an acute MI may be indicated by tall, narrow T-waves, a phenomenon called peaked or hyperacute T-waves. The new appearance of tall R-waves in lead V_1 may indicate a true posterior MI, particularly if there is ST segment depression in lead I.[136] It may be tedious to consider all these alternatives preoperatively, but the benefits in minimizing morbidity and mortality and promoting good risk management will repay the anesthesiologist a hundredfold for the effort.

2. Intraoperative diagnosis. Diagnosing an MI that occurs during the administration of an anesthetic can be difficult for several reasons. Many intraoperative infarcts are subendocardial and do not cause hypotension or arrhythmias. Complete electrocardiographic tracings usually cannot be done during an operation, and evolutionary electrocardiographic changes often occur after the operation is completed. Diagnostic increases in cardiac enzyme concentrations usually peak postoperatively. Because of these diagnostic limitations, it is important for the anesthesiologist to maximally use the information he or she does have. The criteria for diagnosis of an acute MI includes at least two of three conditions: a history of ischemic-type chest discomfort, evolutionary changes on serially obtained ECG tracings, and a rise and fall in serum cardiac markers.

Intraoperative MI is probably easier to diagnose in patients undergoing local or regional anesthetics than it is in patients undergoing general anesthesia. Although the onset of cardiac pain does not always accompany MI, when it does occur it can be extremely useful. The astute clinician will not only consider chest pain or chest pressure, but will also carefully consider the new onset of pain in the right or left arm, the neck, jaws, teeth, or posterior scapular regions. The most obvious infarcts are glaringly apparent, and occasionally a patient dies soon after experiencing cardiac pain.

In less severe infarcts, findings from a seven-lead intraoperative ECG may be helpful. The seven-lead ECG includes leads II, III, and aVF, which allow a good look at the inferior surface of the heart, and lead V_5, which gives a good view of the lateral aspect of the heart. T-wave inversions, ST segment depressions, or ST segment elevations in any of these leads may indicate a developing MI. Infarcts associated with extensive myocardial damage are probably associated with hypotension and cardiac arrhythmias.

Patients receiving general anesthetics obviously will not complain of pain but may have hypotension, arrhythmias, signs of congestive heart failure, and ECG changes of subendocardial or transmural ischemia. The sudden appearance of severe wall motion abnormalities in patients being monitored with transesophageal echocardiography may also indicate MI, although the differential diagnosis between acute ischemia, evolving infarction, stunned myocardium, and hibernating myocardium may be difficult to distinguish using echocardiographic findings.[137] Increased concentrations of the MB-CPK are not useful intraoperatively because the leakage of these enzymes into the circulation can occur 8 to 24 hours after an MI. Indeed, some investigators have indicated that peak MB-CPK concentrations occur at highly variable times after an infarct, with a range of 12 to 24 hours.[18] Although the MB-CPK concentration cannot be expected to increase in the first few hours after an infarct, if an infarct is suspected it may be useful to draw blood for levels to establish a baseline value. Serial MB-CPK concentrations in the postoperative period for up to 24 hours after the first signs and symptoms of the infarct will obviously assist in the diagnosis.

Because of inherent diagnostic limitations of MB-CPK concentrations, MI may be best detected with cardiac TnT concentrations. Recent advances in diagnosing MI rely on determination of serum cardiac-specific troponins. TnT binds to tropomyosin, troponin C binds to Ca^{++}, and troponin I (TnI) binds to actin and inhibits actin-myosin interactions. These three subunits regulate the calcium-mediated contractile process of striated muscle. Specific antibodies to these isoforms are available, so sensitive immunoassays are currently used to detect serum concentrations.[19] Under normal conditions, MB-CPK concentrations may be detected in the peripheral circulation while specific cardiac forms of TnT and TnI are not present. MB-CPK concentrations may rise only 10 to 20 times normal during infarction and return to normal range within 72 hours. In contrast, TnT and TnI levels may rise more than 20 times above the reference range within 3 hours after the onset of chest pain and may persist for up to 10 to 14 days. This may assist in late diagnosis of infarction.[138] Cardiac TnT may be capable of detecting myocardial necrosis below the detection limit of MB-CPK assays, possibly identifying patients who have sustained minor myocardial damage.[139]

Serial postoperative ECGs play a major role in documenting a probable intraoperative or early postoperative MI. The initial 12-lead ECG is often nondiagnostic.

Therefore a series of ECGs is necessary to determine whether evolution of the ECG changes of infarction has occurred. The earliest ECG changes in MI involve T-wave peaking followed by symmetric inversion of the T-waves. Later, ST segment elevation is seen, and finally new Q-waves appear. It is important to distinguish true pathologic Q-waves from the normal Q-waves caused by septal depolarization. Pathologic Q-waves are greater than 0.04 second in duration, and the depth of the Q-wave must be at least one third of the height of the R-wave in the same QRS complex. (An exception to this rule applies to lead aV_R, which normally has a very deep Q-wave.) New pathologic Q-waves appear within hours to days after an onset of an MI, and in most patients they persist throughout life.[140]

In most cases, the diagnosis of intraoperative or postoperative MI is established by clinical signs and symptoms, elevation of cardiac isoenzymes, and evolutionary ECG changes. However, a small number of infarcts may be missed by these methods. Infarct-avid technetium pyrophosphate scanning using single-photon emission computed tomography may be helpful in diagnosing elusive postoperative MIs.[79] However, this type of scanning may overestimate the incidence and size of postoperative MIs because technetium pyrophosphate is known to bind not only to infarcted tissue but also to severely damaged but nonetheless viable myocardium.

Magnetic resonance imaging can be used to detect, localize, and establish the size of an acute MI. It can also assess perfusion of infarcted and noninfarcted tissues and can help identify areas of jeopardized but viable myocardium. Magnetic resonance imaging can also reveal myocardial edema, myocardial fibrosis, wall thinning, and hypertrophy.[141] Although magnetic resonance appears to have many advantages in diagnosing MIs, the need to move the patient to the magnetic resonance scanner places a practical limitation on its widespread use in this disease.

D. Treatment of perioperative myocardial infarction

Treatment of patients who have sustained an acute preoperative or postoperative MI is usually done by cardiologists or surgeons. However, the anesthesiologist has a major intraoperative role in caring for patients who develop MI during anesthesia. In addition, the anesthesiologist may initiate and direct care in the postanesthesia care unit (PACU) following an episode of intraoperative ischemia or new onset of ischemia during anesthetic recovery. The specific treatment plan for any patient depends on the details of the case.

If the diagnosis of MI seems probable, it is obviously important to monitor the patient closely. Attention to the pulse oximeter allows very early detection of hypoxemia and may give early warning of significant decreases in pulse volume. If blood pressures have been determined using the Riva-Rocci method, a rapid change to an automated blood pressure cuff will provide more frequent blood pressures. An automated method of blood pressure determination may seriously underestimate systemic arterial pressure in patients with intense vasoconstriction; therefore in appropriate patients a radial arterial line should be inserted as soon as possible in the contralateral arm.

Hypotension should be treated rapidly in order to restore coronary perfusion pressure and perhaps to open up collateral vessels. In the patient anesthetized with potent volatile anesthetic agents, hypotension should be treated by decreasing or discontinuing these agents. Administration of 100% oxygen should always be instituted. Moderate hypotension in the patient experiencing an acute MI often responds to volume expansion consisting of a 300- to 500-ml rapid infusion of crystalloid. If systolic pressures of 60 to 80 mm Hg persist after conservative volume expansion, vasoactive or inotropic drugs should be given to elevate coronary perfusion pressure. Although it is true that vasoactive or inotropic agents increase myocardial oxygen consumption, it is also true that a critical coronary perfusion pressure must exist or the patient will certainly die. Use of inotropes maximizes the contractile power of myocardium unaffected by the infarct. Administration of these agents may be necessary for a brief duration, for they may support the patient through a tenuous period.

The use of invasive hemodynamic monitoring should be based on a number of findings. If difficulty arises in interpreting the clinical findings of pulmonary congestion (rales and radiographic findings), one may underestimate elevations in left ventricular filling pressures. A patient who is experiencing arterial hypotension unresponsive to volume loading or markedly diminished ventricular compliance requiring careful titration of fluids may similarly benefit from such monitoring.[142]

Patients will benefit from pulmonary artery catheterization during an acute MI if there is hypotension refractory to fluid administration, hypotension in the presence of congestive heart failure, or hemodynamic deterioration severe enough to require vasopressors, vasodilators, or an intraaortic balloon pump (IABP). Additionally, a high clinical suspicion of pericardial tamponade, ventricular septal defect, or rupture of a papillary muscle may demand central monitoring.[142]

This procedure can be done in both awake and asleep patients from several peripheral sites. The internal jugular route is the preferred route of access in the anesthetized patient. If operative considerations preclude this, the left medial basilic vein is another alternative, as is the femoral vein. Because of the possibility of pneumothorax and laceration of major vessels, the subclavian route is the least favorable option. If pulmonary artery wedge pressures are 12 mm Hg or less, volume expansion with a crystalloid should continue if hematocrit concentrations allow moderate hemodilution without impairing arterial oxygen content. If pulmonary wedge pressures are high, use of an inotropic agent such as dopamine 3 to 5 µg/kg/min or dobutamine 2.5 to 20 µg/kg/min should be considered. However, if severe hypotension persists after 5 µg/kg/min dopamine or dobutamine 10-15 µg/kg/min, one should consider the addition of epinephrine or milrinone.

Milrinone is a noncatecholamine, class III cyclic adenosine monophosphate phosphodiesterase inhibitor that may be useful if additional inotropic support is needed during intraoperative MI. Milrinone is 10 times as potent as amrinone, with a shorter half-life and less potential for thrombocytopenia. Its actions are to increase cardiac contractility through increasing availability of intracellular calcium and acting as a peripheral vasodilator.[143] After a bolus dose of 25 to 50 µg/kg and initiation of maintenance infusion of 0.375 to 0.75 µg/kg/min, cardiac output and blood pressure often increase within a few minutes. Although it is not a first-line drug, it may be useful in selected patients in need of an inodilator. Dosage must be adjusted in patients with impaired creatinine clearance.

Some patients with intraoperative MI do not respond adequately to pharmacologic and volume expansion. In some of these patients the use of an intraaortic balloon can be lifesaving. The balloon can be inserted percutaneously and can almost immediately decrease myocardial oxygen requirements and may possibly increase myocardial oxygen supply. Early use of the balloon in severe intraoperative infarctions may help to decrease the size of the resultant infarct.

Metabolic acidosis may result from low cardiac output. This can lead to a vicious cycle in which the acidosis further depresses cardiac function and limits the effectiveness of inotropic drugs. Early treatment of metabolic acidosis may help to restore cardiac function in a patient with an intraoperative infarct. Hypoxemia also often follows acute myocardial infarction. Measures to increase arterial oxygen tension may help to limit the size of an intraoperative infarct.

A wide variety of cardiac dysrhythmias can accompany acute MI. Sinus bradycardia occurs commonly in inferior and posterior infarctions.[144-146] Sinus tachycardia may be the result of pain, anxiety, or congestive heart failure. Atrial fibrillation can occur especially in patients with cardiac failure and increased left atrial pressure. Ventricular arrhythmias ranging from premature ventricular beats to ventricular fibrillation are also seen in acute infarctions. Unifocal or multifocal premature ventricular contractions can usually be controlled with intravenous lidocaine. However, an occasional patient may require procainamide or propranolol. Ventricular fibrillation necessitate electrical defibrillation.

Some patients with severe bradycardia require cardiac pacing. Noninvasive temporary ventricular pacing can be done using the Zoll external pacer.[147] This requires the application of large conductive pregelled pacing electrodes to the front and back of the left chest. Transcutaneous pacing may be uncomfortable for the awake patient. Discomfort from external pacing is not a consideration under general anesthesia. Emergency intraoperative cardiac pacing can be achieved by passing a straight pacer wire through a 7.5-French introducer in the internal jugular vein. One may also accomplish pacing by using the pace-port pulmonary artery catheter. This is a modification of a standard pulmonary artery catheter that has a right ventricular port through which a small pacing wire can be passed.[148]

After acute hemodynamic aberrations have been treated, we should consider myocardial salvage to minimize the damage caused by an intraoperative infarct. Intravenous thrombolysis using tissue thromboplastic activator (t-PA) or streptokinase has revolutionized care of patients with acute MI. To be effective the drugs must be given within 4 hours of onset of symptoms. The major limitation of thrombolysis in surgical patients is a predisposition for excessive bleeding. It is therefore contraindicated in patients with fresh surgical wounds. However thrombolysis may be valuable in selected patients. For example, the patient who has sustained an MI during a cystoscopy or diagnostic laryngoscopy may be a very good candidate for thrombolysis. If radial and pulmonary artery monitoring appear to be necessary, the catheters should be inserted before thrombolytic drugs are administered. Patients who receive t-PA should also be given a sustained infusion of heparin.[149]

In addition to thrombolysis, medical therapy with β-blockers and antithrombotic and antiplatelet drugs can also be important components of maximum myocardial salvage. Use of β-blockers in the setting of acute MI has been shown to limit infarct size when given in the early phases (within 4 hours after onset of pain) of an acute MI.[150] There is also a decrease the incidence of nonfatal reinfarction and cardiac arrest as well as a decrease in mortality at 7 days.[151] Calcium-channel blockers have not been shown to be beneficial in the acute phase of MI and have been implicated in an increased risk of mortality when administered to such a population.[152]

Antithrombotic and antiplatelet therapies are critical areas of therapy in the development and treatment of an acute MI, considering the role of platelets in the development of coronary thrombosis.[153] Significant reductions in mortality, nonfatal reduction of recurrent infarction, and nonfatal stroke are all realized with antiplatelet therapy. If no thrombolytic therapy is planned to be given to the patient, then heparin should be considered strongly. Heparin has been shown to reduce mortality and morbidity from reinfarction and thromboembolism. An activated partial thromboplastin time of 1.5 to 2 times normal should be the target range.[154] During the perioperative period, it may be difficult to administer such agents, especially when bleeding may be a problem. Aspirin may be administered per rectum if possible, and orally when the patient is admitted to the PACU. Open discussion with the surgeon, weighing the immediate benefits of prompt antiplatelet and antithrombotic therapy against the risks of bleeding in a patient who is currently being operated on, is vital to the prompt treatment of a perioperative MI.

V. SUMMARY

In everyday practice, the paradigm of hemodynamic stability is challenged constantly. Occasionally, severe hemodynamic disturbances may occur and may lead to un-

toward events in the perioperative period. It would be unrealistic to propose that such hemodynamic changes can be eliminated completely. Rather, the anesthesiologist should anticipate and prevent these complications whenever possible. Early recognition and prompt treatment are essential. We hope that the material presented in this chapter will assist in management when these situations arise.

REFERENCES

1. Proctor HJ: Fluid and electrolyte management. In Hardy JD, ed: *Hardy's textbook of surgery,* Philadelphia, 1983, JB Lippincott.
2. Kleinknecht D, Ganeval D, Gonzalez-Duque LA, et al: Furosemide in acute oliguric renal failure: a controlled trial, *Nephron* 17:51, 1976.
3. Brown CB, Ogg CS, Cameron JS: High dose furosemide in acute renal failure: a controlled trial, *Clin Nephrol* 15:90, 1981.
4. Johnstone M: Human cardiovascular response to Fluothane anesthesia, *Br J Anaesth* 28:392, 1954.
5. Stevens WC, Eger EI II: Comparative evaluation of new inhalation anesthetics, *Anesthesiology* 35:125, 1971.
6. Dobkin AB, Nisioka K, Gengaje DB, et al: Ethrane (compound 347) anesthesia: a clinical and laboratory review of 700 cases, *Anesth Analg* 48:477, 1969.
7. Stevens WC, Cromwell TH, Halsey MJ, et al: The cardiovascular effects of a new inhalation anesthetic, Forane, in human volunteers at constant arterial carbon dioxide tension, *Anesthesiology* 35:8, 1971.
8. Calverley RK, Smith NT, Jones CW, et al: Ventilatory and cardiovascular effects of enflurane during spontaneous ventilation in man, *Anesth Analg* 57:610, 1978.
9. Beaupre PN, Cahalan MK, Kremer PF, et al: Does pulmonary artery occlusion pressure adequately reflect left ventricular filling during anesthesia and surgery? *Anesthesiology* 59:A3, 1983.
10. Ellis RJ, Mangano DT, VanDyke DC: Relationship of wedge pressure to end-diastolic volume in patients undergoing myocardial revascularization, *J Thorac Cardiovasc Surg* 78:605, 1979.
11. Trunkey DD, Holcroft JW: Trauma: general survey in synopsis of management of specific injuries. In Hardy JD, ed: *Hardy's textbook of surgery,* Philadelphia, 1983, JB Lippincott.
12. Pregnant patients. In Stoelting RK, Dierdorf SF, McCammon RL, eds: *Anesthesia and co-existing disease,* ed 2, Edinburgh, 1988, Churchill Livingstone.
13. Jones FL Jr: Transmural myocardial necrosis after nonpenetrating cardiac trauma, *Am J Cardiol* 26:419, 1970.
14. Braunwald E, Kloner RA: The stunned myocardium: prolonged post-ischemic ventricular dysfunction, *Circulation* 66:1146, 1982.
15. Vatner SF, Heyndrickx GR, Fallon JT: Effects of brief periods of myocardial ischemia on regional myocardial function and creatine kinase release in conscious dogs and baboons, *Can J Cardiol,* Suppl A:19, July 1986.
16. Arnold JM, Braumwald E, Sandor T, et al: Inotropic stimulation of reperfused myocardium with dopamine: effects on infarct size and myocardial function, *J Am Coll Cardiol* 6:1026, 1985.
17. Ellis G, Wynne J, Braunwald E, et al: Response of reperfused-salvaged stunned myocardium to inotropic stimulation, *Am Heart J* 107:13, 1984.
18. Lee T, Goldman L: Serum enzyme assays in the diagnosis of acute myocardial infarction: recommendations based on a quantitative analysis, *Ann Intern Med* 102:221, 1986.
19. Katus H, Scheffold T, Remppis A, et al: Proteins of the troponin complex, *Lab Med* 32:311, 1992.
20. Rothenberg HJ: Anaphylactoid reaction to vancomycin, *JAMA* 171:1101, 1959.
21. Schaad UB, McCraken GH Jr, Nelson JD: Clinical pharmacology and efficacy of vancomycin in pediatric patients, *J Pediatr* 96:119, 1980.
22. Wold JS, Turnipseed SA: Toxicology of vancomycin in laboratory animals, *Rev Infect Dis* 3(suppl):224, 1981.

23. Southorn PA, Plevak EJ, Wright AAJ, et al: Adverse effects of vancomycin administered in the perioperative period, *Mayo Clin Proc* 61:721, 1986.

24. Pau AK, Kahakoo R: "Red-neck syndrome" with slow infusion of vancomycin, *N Engl J Med* 313:576, 1985.

25. Cohen LS, Wechsler AS, Mitchell JH, et al: Depression of cardiac function by streptomycin and other antimicrobial agents, *Am J Cardiol* 26:505, 1970.

26. Modig J, Busch C, Waernbaum G: Effect of graded infusions of monomethylmethacrylate on coagulation, blood lipids, respiration and circulation, *Clin Orthop* 113:187, 1975.

27. Modig J, Busch C, Olerud S, et al: Arterial hypotension and hypoxemia during total hip replacement: the importance of thromboplastic products, fat embolism and acrylic monomers, *Acta Anaesthesiol Scand* 19:28, 1975.

28. Kallos T: Impaired arterial oxygenation associated with use of bone cement in the femoral shaft, *Anesthesiology* 42:210, 1975.

29. Weidner FA, Zieter FMH: Carcinoid tumors of the gastrointestinal tract, *JAMA* 245:1153, 1981.

30. Stone CA, Wenger HC, Ludden CT, et al: Antiserotonin-antihistamine properties of cyproheptadine, *J Pharmacol Exp Ther* 131:73, 1961.

31. Stoelting RK, Dierdorf SF, McCammon RL: *Anesthesia and co-existing disease,* ed 2, New York, 1988, Churchill Livingstone.

32. Barash PG, Cullen BF, Stoelting RK: *Clinical anesthesia,* Philadelphia, 1992, JB Lippincott.

33. Houghie C: Anticoagulant action of protamine sulfate, *Proc Soc Exp Biol Med* 98:130, 1958.

34. Fadali MA, Ledbetter M, Papacostas CA, et al: Mechanism responsible for the cardiovascular depression effect of protamine sulfate, *Ann Surg* 180:232, 1974.

35. Michaels I, Barash PG: Hemodynamic changes during protamine administration, *Anesth Analg* 62:831, 1983.

36. Lowenstein E, Johnston WE, Lappas DG, et al: Catastrophic pulmonary vasoconstriction associated with protamine reversal of heparin, *Anesthesiology* 59:470, 1983.

37. Morel DR, Zapol WM, Thomas SJ, et al: C5a and thromboxane generation associated with pulmonary vaso and broncho constriction during protamine reversal of heparin, *Anesthesiology* 66:597, 1987.

38. Horrow JC: Protamine: a review of its toxicity, *Anesth Analg* 64:348, 1985.

39. Roizen MF, Rodgers GM, Valone FJ, et al: Anaphylactoid reactions to vascular graft material presenting with vasodilatation and subsequent disseminated intravascular coagulation, *Anesthesiology* 71:331, 1989.

40. Shoemaker WC, Ayres S, Grenvik A, et al: *Textbook of critical care,* ed 2, Philadelphia, 1989, WB Saunders.

41. Laennec RTH: *Traite de l'auscultation mediate et des maladies des poumons et du coeur,* Paris, 1831, JS Chaude.

42. Bone RC, Balk RA, Cerra FB, et al: Definitions for sepsis and organ failure and guidelines for the use of innovative therapies in sepsis, *Chest* 101:1644, 1992.

43. Bone RC: Pathogenesis of sepsis, *Ann Int Med* 115:457, 1991.

44. Snell RJ, Parrillo JE: Cardiovascular dysfunction in septic shock, *Chest* 99:1000, 1991.

45. Ognibene FP: Pathogenesis and innovative treatment of septic shock, *Adv Int Med* 42:313, 1997.

46. Martin C, Papazian L, Perrin G, et al: Norepinephrine or dopamine for the treatment of hyperdynamic septic shock? *Chest* 103:1826, 1993.

47. Thompson JS, Pearl RG: Sepsis, Part II: Medical management of septic shock, *Semin Anesth* 13:195, 1994.

48. Pearl RG: Treatment of shock: 1998, *Anesth Analg Suppl, IARS Rev Lectures* 86:75, 1998.

49. Shoemaker WC, Ayres S, Grenvik A, et al: *Textbook of critical care,* ed 2, Philadelphia, 1989, WB Saunders.

50. Bone RG, Fisher CJ, Clemmer TP, et al: A controlled clinical trial of high-dose methylprednisolone in the treatment of severe sepsis and septic shock, *N Engl J Med* 317:653, 1987.

51. Veterans Administration Systemic Sepsis Cooperative Study Group: Effects of high-dose glucocorticoid therapy on mortality in patients with clinical signs of systemic sepsis, *N Engl J Med* 317:659, 1987.

52. Parrillo JE: High dose glucocorticoid therapy: two prospective randomized, controlled trials find no efficacy: update, *Crit Care Med* 2:1, 1987.

53. Brodsky JB, Brabo JJ: Acute postoperative clonidine withdrawal syndrome, *Anesthesiology* 44:519, 1976.

54. Bruner JMR: *Handbook of blood pressure monitoring,* Littleton, Mass, 1978, PSG.

55. Stoelting RK: Attenuation of blood pressure response to laryngoscopy and tracheal intubation with sodium nitroprusside, *Anesth Analg* 58:116, 1979.

56. Cullen BF, Eger EI II, Smith NT, et al: The circulatory response to hypercapnia during fluroxene anesthesia in man, *Anesthesiology* 34:415, 1971.

57. Hornbein TF, Martin WE, Bonica JJ, et al: Nitrous oxide effect on the circulatory and ventilatory responses to halothane, *Anesthesiology* 31:250, 1969.

58. Marshall BE, Cohen PJ, Klingenmaier CH, et al: Some pulmonary and cardiovascular effects of enflurane (Ethrane) anesthesia with varying $PaCO_2$ in man, *Br J Anaesth* 43:996, 1971.

59. Cromwell TH, Stevens WC, Eger EI II, et al: The cardiovascular effects of compound 469 (Forane) during spontaneous ventilation and carbon dioxide challenge in man, *Anesthesiology* 35:17, 1971.

60. Collins VJ: *Principles of anesthesiology,* ed 2, Philadelphia, 1976, Lea & Febiger.

61. Haddad NJ, Moyer NJ, Riley FC: Mydriatic effects of phenylephrine hydrochloride, *Am J Ophthalmol* 70:729, 1970.

62. Zimmerman J, Konner AS, Kandarakis AS, et al: Improving the therapeutic index of topically applied ocular drugs, *Arch Ophthalmol* 102:551, 1984.

63. Barash PG, Cullen BF, Stoelting RK: *Clinical anesthesia,* Philadelphia, 1992, JB Lippincott.

64. Bove EL, Fry WJ, Gross WS, et al: Hypotension and hypertension as consequences of baroreceptor dysfunction following carotid endarterectomy, *Surgery* 85:633, 1979.

65. Bidwai AV, Bidwai VA, Rogers CA: Blood pressure and pulse rate responses to endotracheal extubation with and without prior injection of lidocaine, *Anesthesiology* 51:171, 1971.

66. Berne RM, Rubio R: Coronary circulation. In Burne RM, Sperelakis N, Geiger SR, eds: *Handbook of physiology,* Bethesda, Md, 1979, American Physiological Society.

67. Rubio R, Berne RM: Release of adenosine by the normal myocardium and its relationship to the regulation of coronary resistance, *Circ Res* 25:407, 1969.

68. Furchgott RF, Zawadski JB: The obligatory role of endothelial cells in the relaxation of arterial smooth muscle by acetylcholine, *Nature* 288:373, 1980.

69. Deboer LWV, Rude RE, Davis RF, et al: Extension of myocardial necrosis into normal epicardium following hypotension during experimental coronary occlusion, *Cardiovasc Res* 16:423, 1982.

70. Peach MJ, Loeb AL, Singer HA: Endothelium-derived vascular relaxing factor, *Hypertension* 7(suppl 1):94, 1985.

71. Peach MJ, Singer HA, Izzo NJ Jr, et al: Role of calcium in endothelium-dependent relaxation of arterial smooth muscle, *Am J Cardiol* 59:35A, 1987.

72. Freiman PC, Mitchell GG, Heistad DD, et al: Atherosclerosis impairs endothelium-dependent vascular relaxation to acetylcholine and thrombin in primates, *Circ Res* 58:783, 1986.

73. Braunwald E: *Heart disease: a textbook of cardiovascular medicine,* ed 5, Philadelphia, 1997, WB Saunders.

74. Parmley WW: Prevalence and clinical significance of silent myocardial ischemia, *Circulation* 80(6, suppl IV):66, 1989.

76. Geft IL, Fishbein MC, Ninomiya K, et al: Intermittent brief periods of ischemia have a cumulative effect and may cause myocardial necrosis, *Circulation* 66:1150, 1982.

77. Cohn PF: Total ischemic burden: pathophysiology and prognosis, *Am J Cardiol* 59:3C, 1987.

78. Knight AA, Hollenberg M, London MJ: Perioperative myocardial ischemia: importance of the preoperative ischemic pattern, *Anesthesiology* 68:681, 1988.

79. Cheng DC, Chung F, Burns RJ, et al: Postoperative myocardial infarction documented by technetium pyrophosphate scan using single photon emission computed tomography: significance of intraoperative myocardial ischemia and hemodynamic control, *Anesthesiology* 71:818, 1989.

80. Boudoulas H, Lewis RP, Rittgers SE, et al: Increased diastolic time: a possible important factor in the beneficial effect of propranolol in patients with coronary artery disease, *J Cardiovasc Pharmacol* 1:503, 1979.

81. Palmer CM, Norris MC, Giudici MC, et al: Incidence of electrocardiographic changes during caesarean delivery under regional anesthesia, *Anesth Analg* 70:36, 1990.

82. Mathew JP, Fleisher LA, Rinehouse JA, et al: ST segment depression during labor and delivery, *Anesthesiology* 77:635, 1992.

83. Mangano DT: Perioperative cardiac morbidity, *Anesthesiology* 72:153, 1990.

84. Roy WL, Edelist G, Gilbert B: Myocardial ischemia during noncardiac surgical procedures in patients with coronary artery disease, *Anesthesiology* 51:393, 1979.

85. Coriat P, Harari A, Daloz M, et al: Clinical predictors of intraoperative myocardial ischemia in patients with coronary artery disease undergoing non-cardiac surgery, *Acta Anaesthesiol Scand* 26:287, 1982.

86. Prinzmetal M, Kennamer R, Merliss R, et al: A variant form of angina pectoris, *Am J Med* 27:375, 1959.

87. Oliva PB, Potts DE, Pluss RG: Coronary arterial spasm in Prinzmetal angina: documentation by coronary arteriography, *N Engl J Med* 288:745, 1973.

88. Braunwald E: *Heart disease: a textbook of cardiovascular medicine,* ed 5, Philadelphia, 1997, WB Saunders.

89. Ganz P, Alexander RW: New insights into the cellular mechanisms of vasospasms, *Am J Cardiol* 56:11E, 1985.

90. Ludmer PL, Celwyn AP, Shook TL, et al: Paradoxical vasoconstriction induced by acetylcholine in atherosclerotic coronary arteries, *N Engl J Med* 315:1046, 1986.

91. Hyduke JF, Pineda JJ, Smith CE, et al: Severe intraoperative myocardial ischemia following manipulation of the heart in a patient undergoing esophagogastrectomy, *Anesthesiology* 71:154, 1989.

92. Allred EN, Bleecker ER, Chaitman DR, et al: Short-term effects of carbon monoxide exposure on the exercise performance of subjects with coronary artery disease, *N Engl J Med* 321:1426, 1989.

93. Lange RA, Cigarroa RG, Yancy CW, et al: Cocaine induced coronary artery vasoconstriction, *N Engl J Med* 321:1557, 1989.

94. Moliterno DJ, Willard JE, Lange RA, et al: Coronary artery vasoconstriction induced by cocaine, cigarette smoking, or both, *N Engl J Med* 330:454, 1994.

95. Hollander JE: The management of cocaine induced myocardial ischemia, *N Engl J Med* 333:1267, 1995.

96. Lange RA, Cigarroa RG, Yancy CV Jr, et al: Potentiation of cocaine-induced coronary vasoconstriction by beta-adrenergic blockade, *Ann Intern Med* 112:897, 1990.

97. Nademanee K, Gorelick DA, Josephson MA, et al: Myocardial ischemia during cocaine withdrawal, *Ann Intern Med* 111:876, 1989.

98. Parmley WW: Prevalence and clinical significance of silent myocardial ischemia, *Circulation* 80(6, suppl IV):S68, 1989.

99. Margolis JR, Kannel WS, Feinleib M, et al: Clinical features of unrecognized myocardial infarction, silent and symptomatic: eighteen year follow-up: the Framingham Study, *Am J Cardiol* 32:1, 1973.

100. Epstein SE, Quyyumi AA, Bonow R: Myocardial ischemia: silent or asymptomatic, *N Engl J Med* 318:1038, 1988.

101. Blackburn H, Katigbak R: What electrocardiographic leads to take after exercise? *Am Heart J* 67:184, 1964.

102. Blackburn H, Taylor HL, Okamato N, et al: Standardization of the exercise electrocardiogram: a systematic comparison of chest lead configurations employed for monitoring during exercise. In Karoonen MJ, Barry AJ, eds: *Physical activity and the heart,* Springfield, Ill, 1967, Charles C Thomas.

103. Kotrly KJ, Kotter GS, Mortara D, et al: Intraoperative detection of myocardial ischemia with an ST-segment trend monitoring system, *Anesth Analg* 63:343, 1984.

104. Kaplan JA: Electrocardiographic monitoring. In Kaplan JA, ed: *Cardiac anesthesia,* New York, 1979, Grune & Stratton.

105. Kaplan JA, Wells PH: Early diagnosis of myocardial ischemia using the pulmonary arterial catheter, *Anesth Analg* 60:789, 1981.

106. Aroesty JM, McKay RG, Heller GB, et al: Simultaneous assessment of left ventricular systolic and diastolic dysfunction during pacing-induced ischemia, *Circulation* 71:889, 1985.

107. Iskandrian AS, Bemis CE, Hakki AH, et al: Ventricular systolic and diastolic impairment during pacing-induced myocardial ischemia in coronary artery disease: simultaneous hemodynamic electrocardiographic and radionuclide angiographic evaluation, *Am Heart J* 112:382, 1986.

108. Bourdillon PD, Lorell BH, Mirsky I, et al: Increased regional myocardial stiffness of the left ventricle during pacing-induced angina in man, *Circulation* 67:316, 1983.

109. Wyns W, Serruys PW, Slager C, et al: Effects of coronary occlusion during percutaneous transluminal angioplasty in humans on left ventricular chamber stiffness and regional diastolic pressure–radius relations, *J Am Coll Cardiol* 7:455, 1986.

110. Serruys PW, van den Brand M, Wijns W, et al: Systolic and diastolic left ventricular function during transluminal acute occlusion, *Circulation* 68(suppl III):237, 1983.

111. Bowman LK, Cleman MW, Cabin HS, et al: Dynamics of early and late left ventricular filling determined by Doppler 2-dimensional echocardiography during percutaneous transluminal coronary angioplasty, *Am J Cardiol* 61:541, 1988.

112. van Daele M, Sutherland GR, Mitchell MM, et al: Do changes in pulmonary capillary wedge pressure adequately reflect myocardial ischemia during anesthesia? A correlative preoperative hemodynamic, electrocardiographic, and transesophageal echocardiographic study, *Circulation* 81:865, 1990.

113. Smith JS, Cahalan MK, Benefiel CJ, et al: Intraoperative detection of myocardial ischemia in high-risk patients: electrocardiography versus 2-dimensional transesophageal echocardiography, *Circulation* 72:1015, 1985.

114. Hauser AM, Gangadharn V, Ramos RG, et al: Sequence of mechanical electrocardiographic and clinical effects of repeated coronary artery occlusion in human beings: echocardiographic observations during coronary angioplasty, *J Am Coll Cardiol* 5:193, 1985.

115. Wohlgelerter D, Cleman M, Higman HA, et al: Regional myocardial dysfunction during coronary angioplasty: evaluation by 2-dimensional echocardiography and 12-lead electrocardiography, *J Am Coll Cardiol* 7:1245, 1986.

116. Leung J, O'Kelly MB, Mangano DT: Relationship of regional wall motion abnormalities to hemodynamic indices of myocardial oxygen supply and demand in patients undergoing CABG surgery, *Anesthesiology* 73:802, 1990.

117. Cahalan MK: Intraoperative evaluation of left ventricular function with transesophageal echocardiography: problems and pitfalls, Monograph of 1990 Workshops "Update on Intraoperative Echo," Orlando, Fla, 1990, Society of Cardiovascular Anesthesiologists (Richmond, Va), 12th annual meeting, p 142.

118. Pandian NG, Skorton DJ, Collins SM, et al: Heterogenicity of left ventricular segmental wall motion thickening and excursion in 2-dimensional echocardiograms of normal human subjects, *Am J Cardiol* 51:1667, 1983.

119. London MJ, Tubau TF, Wong MG, et al: The "natural history" of segmental wall motion abnormalities in patients undergoing non-cardiac surgery, *Anesthesiology* 73:644, 1990.

120. Coriat P, Daloz M, Bousseau D, et al: Prevention of intraoperative myocardial ischemia during noncardiac surgery with intravenous nitroglycerin, *Anesthesiology* 61:193, 1984.

121. Seitelberger R, Zwolfer W, Binder TM, et al: Infusion of nifedipine after coronary artery bypass grafting decreases the incidence of early postoperative myocardial ischemia, *Ann Thorac Surg* 49:61, 1990.

122. Hill AB, Bowley CJ, and Nahrwold ML: Intranasal administration of nitroglycerin, *Anesthesiology* 51:567, 1979.

123. DiMarco JP, Miles W, Akhtar M, et al: Adenosine for paroxysmal supraventricular tachycardia: dose ranging and comparison with verapamil, *Ann Intern Med* 113:104, 1990.

124. Arkins R, Smessaert AA, Hicks RG: Mortality and morbidity in surgical patients with coronary artery disease, *JAMA* 190:93, 1964.

125. Steen PA, Tinker JH, Tarhan S: Myocardial reinfarction after anesthesia and surgery, *JAMA* 239:2566, 1968.

126. Topkins MJ, Artusio JF: Myocardial infarction and surgery, a five year study, *Anesth Analg* 43:716, 1964.

127. Wells PH, Kaplan JA: Optimal management of patients with ischemic heart disease for non-cardiac surgery by complementary anesthesiologist and cardiologist interaction, *Am Heart J* 102:102, 1981.

128. Rao TLK, Jacobs KH, El-Etr AA: Reinfarction following anesthesia in patients with myocardial infarction, *Anesthesiology* 59:499, 1983.

129. Sloghoff S, Keats AS: Does perioperative myocardial ischemia lead to postoperative myocardial infarction? *Anesthesiology* 62:107, 1985.

130. Sloghoff S, Keats AS: Further observations on perioperative myocardial ischemia, *Anesthesiology* 65:539, 1986.

131. Muller JE, Stone PH, Turi ZG, et al: Circadian variation in the frequency of onset of acute myocardial infarction, *N Engl J Med* 313:1315, 1985.

132. Dressler FA, Malekzadeh S, Roberts WC: Quantitative analysis of amounts of coronary arterial narrowing in cocaine addicts, *Am J Cardiol* 65:303, 1990.

133. Benacerraf A, Scholl JM, Achard F, et al: Coronary spasm and thrombosis associated with myocardial infarction in a patient with nearly normal coronary arteries, *Circulation* 67:1147, 1983.

134. Norris RM: *Myocardial infarction,* Edinburgh, 1982, Churchill Livingstone.

135. Roseman MD: Painless myocardial infarction: a review of the literature and analysis of 220 cases, *Ann Intern Med* 41:1, 1954.

136. Thaler MS: *The only EKG book you'll ever need,* Philadelphia, 1988, JB Lippincott.

137. Braunwald E, Kloner RA: The stunned myocardium: prolonged post-ischemic ventricular dysfunction, *Circulation* 66:1146, 1982.

138. Adams JE, Schectman KB, Landt Y, et al: Comparable detection of acute myocardial infarction by creatine kinase MB isozyme and cardiac troponin I, *Clin Chem* 40:1291,1994.

139. Newby LK, Gibler WB, Ohman WM, et al: Biochemical markers in suspected acute myocardial infarction: the need for early assessment, *Clin Chem* 41:1263, 1995.

140. Thaler MS: *The only EKG book you'll ever need,* Philadelphia, 1988, JB Lippincott.

141. Braunwald E: *Heart disease: a textbook of cardiovascular medicine,* ed 5, Philadelphia, 1997, WB Saunders.

142. Antman EM, Braunwald E. Acute myocardial infarction. In *Heart disease,* ed 5, Philadelphia, 1997, WB Saunders.

143. Kikura M, Levy JH: New cardiac drugs, *Int Anesthesiol Clin* 33:21, 1995.

144. Adgey AAJ, Alley JD, Geddes JS, et al: Acute phase of myocardial infarction, *Lancet* 2:501, 1971.

145. Graner LE, Gershen BJ, Orlando MM, et al: Bradycardia and its complications in pre-hospital phase of acute myocardial infarction, *Am J Cardiol* 32:607, 1973.

146. Zipes DP: The clinical significance of bradycardic rhythms in acute myocardial infarction, *Am J Cardiol* 24:814, 1969.

147. Zoll PM, Zoll RH, Falx RH, et al: External non-invasive temporary cardiac pacing: clinical trials, *Circulation* 71:937, 1985.

148. Product information from Baxter Healthcare Corp, Santa Ana, Calif 92711-1150.

149. Braunwald E: *Heart disease: a textbook of cardiovascular medicine,* ed 5, Philadelphia, 1997, WB Saunders.

150. Chamberlain D: β-Blockers and calcium antagonists. In: Julian D, Braunwald E, eds: *Management of acute myocardial infarction,* London, 1993, WB Saunders.

151. Yusuf S: The use of beta-blockers in the acute phase of myocardial infarction. In Califf RM, Wagner CS, eds: *Acute coronary care,* Boston, 1986, Martinus Nijhoff.

152. Yusuf S, Held P, Furberg C: Update of effects of calcium antagonists in myocardial infarction or angina in light of the second Danish Verapamil Infarction Trial (DAVIT-I) and other recent studies, *Am J Cardiol* 67:1295, 1991.

153. Patrono C: Aspirin as an antiplatelet drug, *N Engl J Med* 330:1287, 1994.

154. Granger CB, Hirsch J, Califf RM, et al: Activated partial thromboplastin time and outcome after thrombolytic therapy for acute myocardial infarction: results from the GUSTO-I trial, *Circulation* 93:870, 1996.

Chapter 13

Complications Related to Cardiopulmonary Bypass

Anne T. Rogers

John C. Lundell

Sylvia Y. Dolinsky

I. INTRODUCTION

A. Definition of cardiopulmonary bypass

During cardiopulmonary bypass (CPB), venous blood returning to the right heart from the systemic circulation is allowed to drain into an external reservoir under the influence of gravity. A mechanical pump then moves the blood from the reservoir, through an oxygenator, and back into the circulation, usually via a cannula placed in the ascending aorta. The CPB apparatus effectively takes over the pumping function of the heart and the oxygenation and ventilation functions of the lungs. The heart is emptied of blood and brought to an electrical and mechanical standstill to provide optimal surgical conditions while the patient's vital organs are perfused with oxygenated blood.

B. Historical background

In the early 1950s experimental models of CPB showed promise, but initial human trials were disappointing. In that era the preoperative diagnosis, based on history, physical examination, chest radiography, cardiac fluoroscopy, and electrocardiography, did not always match the intraoperative diagnosis because cardiac catheterization was not yet available. Compounding the clinical challenge, the surgical field was usually obscured by blood because of the perceived need to maintain high perfusion flow rates in the range of 100 to 165 ml/kg/min. During this same time, John F. Lewis and others were successful in closing atrial septal defects of the ostium secundum type using systemic hypothermia, temporary vena caval occlusion (also called inflow stasis), and rapid surgical repair (5.5 minutes) with sutures.[1] But this technique was unsatisfactory for more complex lesions. Attempts to bypass only the heart using the patients' native lungs to oxygenate blood were abandoned because bronchopulmonary collateral blood flow continuously flooded the surgical field. Pulmonary edema caused by higher flow rates or by displaced or kinked cannulas at lower flow rates was also a persistent problem.

In the midst of this discouragement, surgeons at the University of Minnesota working with dogs made two major advances. First, they found that flow rates in the range of 8 to 14 ml/kg/min were "sufficient to sustain perfusion safely in every animal for a minimum of 30 minutes at normothermia."[2] This modification greatly improved the surgical view by reducing considerably the amount of blood that would have to be removed from the surgical field. Second, by using one dog to perfuse another dog, they performed procedures with fewer deaths and recovery was faster using controlled cross-circulation than it was in dogs undergoing conventional CPB.[3] This observation implied that serious physiologic disturbances occurred during CPB, probably caused by blood contact with foreign surfaces and the mechanical limitations of the pumps and oxygenators at that time.

On March 26, 1954, a team of surgeons at the University of Minnesota, including Cohen, Warden, and Lillehei, closed a ventricular septal defect (VSD) in a 1-year-old child using the patient's father's circulatory system to pump and oxygenate the baby's blood. This team of surgeons went on to perform 45 open-heart operations in 1954-1955, including VSD closure and correction of other defects with remarkable results. This success heralded a rapid expansion of cardiac surgical services while the technology required for safe CPB was still being developed.[4]

Simultaneously progress was being made in the development of oxygenators. Surgeons at the Mayo Clinic experimented with the Gibbon-Mayo film oxygenator, but it proved too complex and expensive and required a large priming volume. In contrast, the bubble oxygenator, introduced by Lillehei in 1955, was readily assembled from available equipment and could be primed with a smaller volume. At first the bubble oxygenator was widely criticized, but it was demonstrated to be a safe and effective way to oxygenate blood without causing obvious nervous system complications. Despite a long and reasonably safe track record, American practitioners remained reluctant to introduce oxygen bubbles deliberately into the circulation. Once the membrane oxygenator was developed, it became the clinical standard. However, the bubble oxygenator is still used in less developed countries because of its lower costs.

In just 40 years CPB has progressed from a risky laboratory experiment to an event occurring many times daily throughout the world. In the United States alone, more than 450,000 procedures involving CPB are performed each year. Coronary artery bypass grafting (CABG) accounts for approximately 75% to 80% of these, cardiac valve repair or replacement accounts for around 20% to 25%, and repair of congenital defects accounts for less than 1%.[5] Accumulated experience and technologic advances now enable surgery to be performed in patients who would have been considered inoperable even a decade ago. This is particularly true for neonates and infants with serious congenital heart disease, in whom early correction is now favored over palliation for many defects. Now it is not unusual for octogenarians, and even nonagenarians, to undergo CABG or valve repair or replacement. Recently, the circulation in patients with cardiogenic shock and undergoing high-risk angioplasty has been supported with partial CPB in the interventional cardiology laboratory.[6]

II. CARDIOPULMONARY BYPASS: A PATHOPHYSIOLOGIC STATE
A. Vascular breach

CPB entails breaching the vascular system, extracorporeal transit of blood, loss of pulsatile flow, hemodilution, and hypothermia. Each of these steps has deleterious consequences and makes CPB a pathophysiologic state. Typically venous blood is drained from the circulation either through a single two-stage cannula with ports in the right atrium and inferior vena cava, through two separate cannulas passed into the superior vena cava and inferior vena cava via the right atrium, or through a femoral venous cannula. Under the influence of gravity, the venous blood flows through the venous cannula into the venous reservoir. From here it is pumped mechanically through a heat exchanger and an oxygenator before passing through a filter into the arterial limb of the CPB circuit. Oxygenated blood enters the ascending aorta through an arterial cannula and perfuses the body under pressure from the mechanical pump. Some procedures, such as repair of a thoracic aneurysm, require only left heart bypass, in which case blood is drained from the left atrium to the venous reservoir. For other procedures, such as repair of the aortic arch, the arterial inflow cannula is placed in the descending aorta or the femoral artery. Blood that appears in the surgical field is suctioned actively and collected in a cardiotomy reservoir. Then it passes through a filter before draining into the main venous reservoir. Three other cannulas are also typically used: an anterograde cardioplegia cannula inserted into the aortic root, a retrograde cardioplegia cannula inserted into the coronary sinus via the right atrium, and a left ventricular vent inserted either through the apex of the left ventricle or into the left ventricle via a superior pulmonary vein, left atrium, and mitral valve.

B. Cardiovascular trauma associated with CPB

Clearly establishing extracorporeal circulation carries the risk of unintended injury to the heart and great vessels. The structures at particular risk depend on preoperative patient factors and the type of surgery. Mitral valve repair requires selective cannulation of both the superior and inferior vena cavae. Repairing a tear in the inferior vena cava where it penetrates the diaphragm is a considerable surgical challenge. Inserting a catheter into the coronary sinus may tear the posterior atrioventricular ring. In a patient with calcific mitral valve disease, or in a patient with pericardial adhesions undergoing reoperation for coronary artery bypass, this injury is potentially fatal, even in the best hands.

An important source of vascular trauma is the intraaortic balloon counterpulsation pump (IABP). Usually inserted into the femoral artery, the IABP is threaded retrograde into the descending aorta until the inflatable balloon lies between the renal arteries and the left subclavian artery. A tear or dissection of the aortic wall can occur during insertion or later.[7] This injury is usually fatal even with attempted surgical repair, but fortunately, it is rare. In some dissections endovascular stenting may be successful.[8] Most IABP complications are ischemic. A renal artery can become occluded by the balloon if the cannula is improperly positioned. The ipsilateral lower extremity can become ischemic if insufficient blood passes through the femoral artery whose lumen is occupied by the cannula. The contralateral lower extremity can become ischemic during removal of the balloon cannula if a thrombus adhering to it becomes dislodged and embolizes. Data from 472 patients who had the IABP inserted were reviewed retrospectively by Busch et al.[9] The overall mortality rate was 28%, and was greater for patients with ischemic limb complications, who made up one third of the total. Forty-two percent of the ischemic limbs were treated with thromboembolectomy, and amputation was necessary in 3%. Diabetes mellitus and peripheral vascular disease were predictive of ipsilateral limb ischemia when an IABP was needed.

C. Systemic embolism

The appearance of emboli in the circulation is almost unavoidable during CPB. The challenge is to minimize this risk.

1. Massive air emboli. Most incidents of massive air embolism involve human error by the perfusionist or surgeon.[10] Entrainment of air into the venous outflow cannula causes an airlock, with cessation of venous flow and an abrupt decrease in the blood level in the venous reservoir. Kinking the venous outflow cannula has the same effect. In both instances the pump flow rate must be decreased or stopped by the perfusionist within seconds to prevent the pumping of air from an empty venous reservoir through the arterial cannula into the systemic circulation. If the perfusionist stops the pump in time, management depends on the stage of surgery. If the patient is normothermic and has a normal electrical cardiac rhythm, the heart may be able to support the circulation. If the patient is cold and the heart asystolic, the CPB circuit and tubing must be rapidly de-aired or replaced during brief circulatory arrest. The hypothermia may protect the brain until circulation is restored. The risk of massive air embolism has been addressed by im-

provements in CPB circuit design such as the incorporation of an alarm that is activated if the volume in the venous reservoir decreases below a certain level. This device may be coupled with another that automatically reduces pump flow rate. But the best protection still remains the vigilance of an experienced perfusionist. Massive air embolism results from pumping of air not only through the arterial cannula but also through the blood cardioplegia cannula.[11]

If a significant quantity of air is injected into the systemic circulation, a potentially fatal cascade of events is launched, affecting the brain and other organs. Organ blood flow is diminished because air is compressible. Inflammatory mediators are released that cause serious and extensive vascular and interstitial changes. No therapeutic regimen has been studied in appropriate clinical trials. Although systemic air is distributed to all vital organs, most reports focus on the brain because the neurologic consequences are so devastating. Using a computer model, Dexter and Hindman[12] calculated that if air emboli are large enough to be seen on a computed tomography (CT) scan, clearance will take 15 hours with a fractional inspired oxygen concentration of 40%, or longer if cerebral blood flow is depressed by the previously mentioned factors. If air bubbles are seen on an emergency postoperative CT scan, some recommend that the patient be transferred to a hyperbaric facility, even if this facility is several hours away. Successful treatment has been documented.[13]

2. Smaller air emboli. Lesser degrees of gas embolism may be clinically undetectable, or bubbles may be seen in the left ventricular vent. Doppler instruments placed over the carotid and middle cerebral arteries reveal emboli at some time during cardiac surgery in virtually all adult and pediatric patients.[14,15] Although a few emboli are particulate matter, most are air bubbles loculated in endocardial trabeculations. Currently available instruments do not differentiate large from small emboli, merely the presence or absence of reflected signals. The count varies from a few emboli to several thousand during the course of a procedure. Open chamber surgery, such as valve replacement or repair of septal defects, is associated with more emboli than coronary artery bypass surgery. Some Doppler signals coincide with specific maneuvers, such as removal of the aortic cross-clamp. Other emboli appear to become manifest throughout CPB in a random fashion. Transesophageal echocardiographic (TEE) imaging may aid in detecting the source of air entry into the heart (e.g., the vent site) and direct the surgeon to tighten the sutures around the cannula or close the hole.

3. Particulate emboli. Particulate material may enter the circulation from the CPB apparatus itself or from the surgical field. Although emboli are distributed to all vital organs, frank stroke is the most dreaded complication. Historically, patients with valvular calcifications or vegetations, left ventricular thrombi, and atherosclerotic plaques in the aorta were known to be at high risk for major brain injury.[16,17] Once brain imaging became available, clinical correlation and diagnosis were greatly enhanced. Angiography and TEE have established preexisting vascular disease as a risk factor in particulate embolism. Some patients have post-CBP complications compatible with a discrete area of tissue infarction because of one or more large emboli. Others present with a syndrome caused by intravascular showers of cholesterol crystals or atherothrombotic debris, with occlusion of small vessels.[18] Mortality can be as high as 70%, with the scope of injury ranging from a cyanotic toe to multiorgan failure.

4. Histologic studies. In 1990 Moody and colleagues reported brain autopsy studies of dogs and patients who had recently undergone CPB. Alkaline phosphatase staining revealed focal dilations in terminal arterioles and capillaries. Called small capillary and arterial dilations (SCADs), these lesions were acellular lipid deposits 10 to 70 µm in length.[19] Associated histologic changes, such as focal vacuolation, neuron loss, and gliosis, are signs of tissue injury. Finding no differences in the SCAD count when CABG and valve repair are compared suggests that they are a function of the CPB circuit rather than patient or surgical factors.[20] Brain SCADs decrease in number with elapsed time after CPB. Most are cleared by 1 week after operation. Challa et al[21] used laser microprobe mass spectrometry on brain sections from patients who died after CPB to detect higher concentrations of aluminum and silicone in the SCADs than in nearby brain tissue. This observation suggests that the modern CPB circuit is still a source of contamination. Brooker et al[22] determined that dogs undergoing CPB with cardiotomy suction and reinfusion of shed blood had a greater density of SCADs than those in which shed blood was not reinfused. The authors interpret this as evidence of lipid microembolization.

5. Aortic atherosclerosis. Tuman et al[23] found a stroke rate of 9% in patients undergoing CABG at 75 years of age or older, 4% in patients between 65 and 75 years, and 1% in patients less than 65 years. The link is the severity of aortic atherosclerosis. Significant aortic atherosclerotic lesions increase the risk of cerebral embolism in both medical and surgical patients.[24] Retrospective studies demonstrate a strong association between large lesions, 4 to 5 mm plaque thickness, and previous embolic disease. Prospective studies have shown that patients with large lesions have a 12% to 33% incidence of stroke and peripheral events within 14 months.[25] Using TEE, Barbut et al[26] determined the severity of atheroma in the ascending aorta, the aortic arch, and the descending aorta in 84 patients undergoing CABG. The incidence of stroke was 33% among those with mobile plaque of the arch and 2.7% among those with nonmobile plaque.

Until the mid-1980s cardiac surgeons palpated the ascending aorta to feel for plaques at the intended site of aortic cannulation. However, friable, pedunculated material is not felt through the exterior aortic wall. TEE yields better images of the anterior aortic wall than does epiaortic scanning. But part of the ascending aorta is obscured by the left mainstem bronchus during TEE, making epiaortic scanning advisable if severe atherosclerotic disease is detected in the descending aorta.[27,28] Surgical teams now modify their approach to patients with severe aortic disease, using intraoperative TEE to select the arterial cannulation site, a single cross-clamping of the aorta during the surgery, or even opting for deep hypothermic circulatory arrest to avoid cross-clamping completely. Data are now accumulating that show the benefit of such modifications in reducing stroke.[29]

D. Prothrombotic and inflammatory response to CPB

Endothelial cells are the only nonthrombogenic cells in the body. When the great vessels are cannulated, blood comes in contact with nonendothelial cells. Once CPB is initiated, blood flows across nonbiologic surfaces, predominantly composed of polyvinyl chloride. Without heparin, an antithrombin III inhibitor, the clotting cascade would be activated and the result would be lethal diffuse intravascular coagulation. To avoid this scenario, it is important to document a heparin effect before initiating CPB. An intense inflammatory response begins. Both cellular (neutrophils and nonendothelial cells) and humoral mediators (contact activation cascades, the complement system, and cytokines) are involved. Activated neutrophils emigrate to the interstitium, where they become cytotoxic. Interstitial edema, subclinical thrombi, and microemboli cause small vessel obstruction with cellular ischemia. The resulting tissue dysfunction can be permanent if CPB is prolonged or the preoperative reserve is low. This state is called postperfusion syndrome. Paradoxically, restoring blood flow can worsen injury. For example, following the release of the aortic cross-clamp during CABG, hypoxic coronary endothelial cells are reoxygenated, endothelial edema worsens, neutrophil and platelet plugging occurs, and thrombosis and spasm of small coronary arteries cause myocardial ischemia. Thus myocardial dysfunction secondary to preoperative stunning or infarction is exacerbated initially by reperfusion, despite patent bypass grafts. Both the prothrombotic and inflammatory aspects of this response can be moderated by the physical, chemical, and rheologic properties of the CPB apparatus. Other measures that inhibit the process reversibly include heparin bonding of circuits, leukocyte depletion filters, plasma ultrafiltration, and administration of steroids, aprotinin, and antioxidants.[30]

1. Heparin-bonded CPB circuits. Heparin has both anticoagulant and antiinflammatory properties. Heparin-bonded CPB circuits have been shown to reduce the need for blood transfusion in cardiac surgical patients.[31] Indicators of inflammation (e.g., cytokine concentrations, elastase, and complement components) are lower with heparin-bonded circuits than with conventional bypass circuits.[32] It is not clear whether these observations translate into a clinical benefit in routine adult CPB cases. Children are particularly prone to proinflammatory reactions on CPB because of the large surface area of the circuit relative to their body surface areas. A recent study in children using a heparin-bonded oxygenator, which is 80% of the circuit, showed lower concentrations of inflammatory mediators and shorter duration of mechanical ventilation than with conventional CPB.[33]

2. Neutrophil filtration. Filtration of activated neutrophils reduces the severity of postperfusion syndrome in animals. The major effect is improved gas exchange, with fewer white cells sequestered in the pulmonary circulation. The clinical utility is less apparent because pulmonary indices are not always improved. In some studies benefits are small, transient, and of no significance to major outcome markers. Despite these reservations, their use is increasing in clinical practice.[34,35]

3. Plasma ultrafiltration. During CPB the venous reservoir volume may be large because of preexisting congestive heart failure, oliguria, or high cardioplegia volumes. An ultrafiltration coil added to the circuit enables the removal of isotonic fluid devoid of plasma proteins. Inflammatory mediators are also removed, with corresponding reductions in postoperative complications. Because the severity of the inflammatory response depends in part on the ratio of body surface area to CPB circuit area, neonates and infants are more likely to benefit from ultrafiltration than adults.[36,37]

4. Aprotinin. Aprotinin is a serum protease inhibitor that reduces the appearance of prothrombin fragments, thrombin-antithrombin III complexes, fibrinopeptide A, and fibrin monomers in the circulation. Not only does it appear to reduce blood loss in high-risk patients undergoing CPB, but it may also moderate the inflammatory cascade.[38] Widespread clinical use of aprotinin has been limited by two factors: cost and safety. The expense is considered prohibitive by some, but it must be balanced against the cost of blood component administration. Infusion also sensitizes patients to aprotinin so that its use may be precluded for future procedures. The package insert recommends a 1-ml initial dose in all patients to test for prior sensitization.

E. Hemodilution

Early CPB circuits required large volumes of blood to prime the circuit, sometimes more than 8 units. These volumes placed a strain on blood-banking resources and exposed recipients to bloodborne pathogens. As clinical experience increased, more cases of pump lung and homologous blood syndrome were seen postoperatively. When bubble oxygenators were introduced, these complications decreased in incidence and severity, apparently because of the smaller priming volume. By 1960 experience with moderate hemodilution in animals and clinical emergencies was considerable. Priming the CPB circuit with nonblood solutions, both colloid and crystalloid, became the standard of practice, and the need for blood products decreased.

The hematocrit preferred during CPB varies from institution to institution and from surgeon to surgeon. A general rule is 25% to 30% at systemic temperatures of 30° to 35° C and 20% to 25% for core temperatures less than 25° C. In patients with myocardial ischemia or a history of cerebrovascular disease, it seems prudent to maintain a hematocrit greater than 25%.[39] In a computer model of focal stroke, Dexter and Hindman[40] calculated

oxygen balance in the ischemic penumbra surrounding a cerebral infarct. They concluded that a hematocrit of 33% was a rational transfusion trigger for the acutely anemic normothermic stroke victim. Although these data were derived in a non-CPB model, the underlying principle seems applicable to patients with neurologic complications of cardiac surgery. Thus there is evidence favoring a higher hematocrit in patients after surgery requiring CPB.

However, maintaining a higher hematocrit means an increased risk of viral transmission from blood products. Some patients preparing for elective cardiac surgery opt to have several units of autologous blood withdrawn preoperatively and stored for use intraoperatively or postoperatively. The number of units that can be drawn is limited by the patient's blood volume and initial hematocrit, the time necessary for the body to restore red cell mass, and the risk of exacerbating cardiac failure or myocardial ischemia. If an adult presents for cardiac surgery with a normal or high hematocrit, some clinicians choose to withdraw one or more units of fresh whole blood into a heparinized, citrated solution immediately before CPB is initiated. The blood is clearly labeled and stored at room temperature for reinfusion after heparin reversal. The rationale is that fresh whole blood, including platelets, will be spared the trauma of CPB, will contribute to hemostasis after CPB, and will carry more oxygen than older units of bank blood. If this course is adopted, care must be taken to calculate the expected hematocrit during CPB and contingencies prepared in case of acute blood loss, unexpectedly profound anemia, or myocardial ischemia. Because less blood is now being salvaged from the surgical field in some centers than in previous years (e.g., blood recovered from the cardiotomy suction, because of its emboli content),[22] patients are more likely to have lower hematocrits and thus be considered candidates for red cell transfusions.

F. Hypothermia

The basis of the protective effect of hypothermia is metabolic suppression and decreased tissue oxygen consumption. Lower perfusion flow rates are required, which means less trauma to formed elements of blood and perhaps fewer microemboli. Lower perfusion rates also reduce bronchopulmonary collateral flow, improve surgical visualization, and prevent myocardial ischemia. Because CPB is such an invasive procedure, with the ever-present threat of mechanical or electrical failure, hypothermia provides a margin of safety should a clinical catastrophe occur. After the aorta is cross-clamped and cold cardioplegia is infused, myocardial temperature is generally colder than core body temperature, 12° C versus 28° C at moderate hypothermia.

G. Other factors affecting outcome

1. Age. At any institution, the 30-day mortality rate increases with advancing age. Similarly, postoperative morbidity also increases with advancing age. Major complications occur in 25% of patients older than 70 years. The result is an increase in the length of stay and cost of care. However, 19% were discharged by the fifth postoperative day, compared with 48% of younger patients. Cardiovascular morbidity has decreased steadily in the geriatric age group, but the stroke rate increases with advancing age.[23,41,42]

2. Reoperation. In general, perioperative mortality and morbidity are higher for the second cardiac surgery than for the first cardiac operation a patient requires. In describing 622 redo CABG procedures, He et al[43] report an operative mortality of 11%, compared with 4% in first-time operations. Patients presenting for a second cardiac operation are more likely to have a New York Heart Association functional class of III or IV and a lower ejection fraction than first-time patients. The technical challenges are greater because of mediastinal adhesions, longer surgery, increased likelihood of coagulopathy, and greater need for transfusion. Even so, Awad et al[44] report only a 7% operative mortality in 111 patients older than 70 years, one third of them in the emergent or urgent category.

3. Emergency reexploration. Hemorrhage requiring reexploration after CABG increases both mortality and morbidity. Dacey et al[45] describe a series of 8586 patients undergoing isolated CABG between 1992 and 1995 at five centers. A total of 305 patients (3.6%) underwent reexploration for bleeding. The in-hospital mortality rate was nearly three times as high (9.5% versus 3.3%) and average length of stay from surgery to discharge was significantly longer (14.5 days versus 8.6 days) than in other cardiac patients who did not have bleeding problems. Risk factors include older age, preoperative renal insufficiency, operation other than CABG, and prolonged bypass time. Interestingly the preoperative use of aspirin, heparin, or thrombolytic agents and the bleeding time were not identified as predictors of reexploration.

III. CARDIAC COMPLICATIONS RELATED TO CPB

A. Reperfusion injury

Ironically, surgery designed to improve cardiac function causes a degree of myocardial injury that may be transient or permanent. While studying biochemical markers of cell death, Eikvar et al[46] noticed that most CPB patients without demonstrable myocardial infarction had an increased concentration of cardiospecific troponin at day 4, suggesting irreversible damage. The cause of this injury is felt to be primarily the ischemia of myocardial cells during aortic cross-clamping. On release of the aortic cross-clamp, hypoxic endothelial cells in the coronary circulation initiate an inflammatory reaction that may intensify tissue injury for several hours.[47] This phenomenon, known as reperfusion injury, is not limited to the coronary circulation. It can affect any organ after interruption of blood flow. Blocking the inflammatory response provides significant improvements in left ventricular function and myocardial blood flow, with a 40% to 50% reduction in myocardial necrosis in experimental models. Other causes of myocardial ischemia include mechanical interference with coronary blood flow, incomplete revascularization, and coronary embolism.

B. Cardioplegia

Over the last 25 years a vast amount of research has been done on myocardial protection.[48,49] Ischemic injury is avoided by reducing myocardial oxygen demand by causing immediate cardiac arrest and cooling the heart to approximately 10° C. The perfusion solutions used to facilitate this process are potassium enriched (40 mEq/L) to induce electrical asystole. These cardioplegia solutions are also intermittently infused to reoxygenate the myocardium, maintain hypothermia, and wash out accumulated metabolites. Reperfusion injury may be reduced if the cardioplegia solutions are made hyperosmotic and include oxygen free radical scavengers or inhibitors to reduce membrane lipid peroxidation and myocellular and endothelial damage.

If the aortic valve is competent, cardioplegia solution injected via a small-bore catheter (e.g., 16 gauge) into the aortic root enters the coronary ostia and the coronary vascular tree. Antegrade infusions are distributed selectively to areas with less severe coronary stenosis and not to the areas where there is significant disease. A technique for retrograde infusion of cardioplegia into the coronary sinus veins, venules, and capillaries was developed that provided more even distribution of the cardioplegia solution and did not require the surgeon to interrupt what he or she was doing to infuse more, as was necessary with antegrade cardioplegia. Administration of retrograde cardioplegia also does not require a competent aortic valve. Many surgeons combine both approaches to ensure optimal protection, especially for resuscitation of an acutely ischemic heart.

C. Perioperative myocardial infarction

Perioperative myocardial infarction is detected in a number of ways. Historically, the reference standard was the appearance of new Q waves on the electrocardiogram (ECG) or new left bundle-branch block combined with significant elevation of myocardium-specific serum creatine kinase (CK-MB). Using these criteria, Slogoff et al[16] reported that perioperative myocardial infarction occurred in 4% of 1023 patients who underwent elective CABG. More recent studies question the significance and predictive value of Q-wave changes. Svedjeholm et al[50] studied 302 CABG patients. New Q waves were noted in 8% of patients, whereas only 1% had the combination of new Q waves and CK-MB concentrations of 70 μg/L or more. One fourth of all patients with new Q waves had a serum cardiac troponin concentration less than the detection limit of the laboratory, (i.e., 0.2 μg/L), suggesting no myocardial necrosis. Furthermore, new Q waves, in contrast to biochemical markers, did not correlate with short-term clinical outcome. In another study of patients undergoing CPB, the plasma troponin concentrations were less than 15 μg/L and suggested that no significant myocardial necrosis had occurred.[51] Echocardiographic regional wall motion abnormalities (RWMA) during CABG have been compared to ECG criteria for myocardial ischemia and perioperative myocardial infarction. Changes in both ECG and RWMA were sensitive indicators of myocardial ischemia (RWMA more so than ECG).

However, both modalities lacked a high degree of specificity. Again, changes may be noted in the absence of cellular ischemia or necrosis.[52,53] Communale et al[54] studied 351 CABG patients with TEE and Holter monitoring of ST segments. Sixty-two (18%) had perioperative myocardial infarction (new Q wave, CK-MB more than 100 ng/dL, or both), half of whom had intraoperative ischemia. Of those with intraoperative ischemia, 28 (88%) were identified by TEE and 13 (41%) were identified by ECG. Prediction of myocardial infarction was greater for TEE than for ECG. Clinically, myocardial infarction may be silent or present as atrial fibrillation,[55] ventricular arrhythmias, low cardiac output,[56] failure to separate from CPB, or cardiac arrest.[57]

D. Low cardiac output

After CPB, myocardial dysfunction may indicate myocardial stunning caused by tissue hypoxia and reperfusion injury rather than a perioperative myocardial infarction.[58] Recognition of myocardial stunning is important because this form of contractile dysfunction can be compensated for with inotropic therapy.[56] Normal preoperative left ventricular function does not preclude dysfunction after CPB, but patients with a preoperative ejection fraction less than 55% tend to be more severely depressed and to take longer to recover (e.g., more than 24 hours rather than 6 to 12 hours). The combination of preoperative left ventricular dysfunction and reperfusion-induced myocardial stunning may require combinations of inotropic agents such as β-receptor agonists and phosphodiesterase inhibitors.[59]

E. Perioperative arrhythmia

1. Atrial fibrillation. Atrial fibrillation affects one third of postoperative cardiac patients and is the most common reason for readmission to the intensive care unit in patients after CABG.[55,60] It tends to occur in paroxysms between the second and fifth postoperative day. Several causes have been proposed, including pericarditis, changes in autonomic tone, cardioplegia, myocardial damage, and fluid shifts. Preoperative patient characteristics associated with a higher incidence of atrial fibrillation include older age, chronic lung disease, digoxin use, hypertension, and left atrial enlargement. Intraoperative techniques associated with a greater incidence include right superior pulmonary vein venting, mitral valve surgery, no topical ice slush, and the use of inotropic drugs. The mortality and morbidity rate, including perioperative myocardial infarction, is twice that of patients without atrial fibrillation. Prophylactic regimens that include combinations of β-antagonists and amiodarone have been reported to decrease the incidence.[61]

2. Ventricular premature beats. Ventricular premature beats are common and usually of little consequence after CPB. However, 2% of patients have episodes of sustained ventricular tachycardia or fibrillation requiring treatment. The first priority is to diagnose and treat myocardial ischemia. Supportive therapy includes potassium and magnesium supplementation.[62]

3. Temporary pacing. Transient minor conduction disturbances are common after CPB and may necessitate temporary pacing. Most cardiac centers routinely apply temporary epicardial pacing leads in all patients. In some patients persistent atrioventricular block and sinus node dysfunction develop, in which case a permanent pacemaker may be required.

IV. NEUROLOGIC COMPLICATIONS
A. Clinical evidence

1. Neurologic dysfunction. The reported incidence of clinical neurologic dysfunction after CPB varies considerably. Prospective studies identify a greater incidence of new deficits than do retrospective studies. In most retrospective studies a brief screening examination is performed on admission to the hospital and a Glasgow coma scale or equivalent measure is used in the postoperative intensive care unit. In most prospective studies the neurologic examination is more comprehensive and includes mental status; cranial nerve function; motor, sensory, and cerebellar function; deep tendon reflexes; plantar reflexes; and neurovascular status. Many patients presenting for CABG have neurologic findings on comprehensive examination, even though their histories are negative for cerebral events. This observation emphasizes the importance of comparing preoperative and postoperative findings in assessing the impact of CPB.[63]

The clinical term *stroke* describes profound damage to a brain region of major social significance in that it impairs speech, movement, or vision. One to five percent of CPB patients suffer frank strokes.[23,64-66] A greater proportion experience more subtle neurologic deterioration (e.g., disturbances of consciousness, gait, reflexes, and vibration sense). Because more than 450,000 adult CPB procedures are performed each year in the United States, up to 22,500 strokes occur annually during or after surgery. One-third of stroke patients die during their hospitalization for cardiac surgery. Of the survivors, one third recover substantially and two thirds experience major morbidity.[23] Although stroke is uncommon after CPB, it constitutes a significant public health problem.

2. Neuropsychologic dysfunction. The neurologic examination leaves portions of the brain function untested. Neuropsychologic testing detects other functional change that may appear subtle to the clinician but can be critical for the patient because it may affect memory, the ability to focus attention, and hand-eye coordination.[15,66,67] As in the neurologic examination, it is important to focus on changes from the preoperative to the postoperative interval. To be broadly applicable in the perioperative setting, the neuropsychologic battery of tests must be concise.[68] This is different from the comprehensive and exhaustive approach used in other situations. In defining a neuropsychologic deficit, the most popular method requires a 20% decrement in individual performance from the preoperative interval on two or more neuropsychologic tests. Because of the expected effect of learning with repeat performance, any deterioration constitutes an abnormality. The 20% cutoff is considered reflective of a disorder rather than intertest variability. For comparison, the nondominant hand consistently performs at a level 10% poorer than the dominant hand. One week after CPB, 50% of patients have a neuropsychologic defect.

The clinical expression of post-CPB dysfunction (i.e., stroke, lesser neurologic findings, and neuropsychologic deficits) depends on the specific location and severity of the ischemic insult. For example, necrosis of a tiny brain region in the dominant hemisphere might have devastating consequences. A comparable lesion in the nondominant hemisphere, or a large infarct in either frontal lobe, might appear clinically minor. In turn, the impact of a given pathologic lesion on a patient's quality of life is affected by many interrelated factors, such as geographic location, socioeconomic status, education level, prior expectations, availability of caregivers, mood, and the ability to adapt. It should not be assumed that neuropsychologic deficits reflect brain injury of a lesser severity than more conventional neurologic findings because they may lead to considerable disability.

B. Radiologic evidence

Magnetic resonance imaging studies in patients before and after CABG and valve replacement have demonstrated that 48% to 95% of preoperative scans are abnormal, with cortical infarcts, lacunae, and white matter hyperintensity consistent with preexisting cerebrovascular disease.[20,69] New postoperative findings are seen in 0% to 58% of scans 1 week after CPB.[69] Harris and colleagues reported on magnetic resonance imaging performed in patients 1 hour after coronary artery surgery using both hypothermic and normothermic CPB.[70,71] All patients had marked cerebral edema with obliteration of cortical sulci; the edema had resolved on the 1-week follow-up imaging study.

C. Biochemical evidence

More than 50% of CPB patients have an increase in brain-specific enzymes such as adenylate kinase, neuron-specific enolase, and protein S-100, whereas no increase occurs in noncardiac surgery patients.[69,72,73]

D. Etiology

Although emboli were known to be a problem associated with cardiac surgery and CPB, early circumstantial evidence favored global brain hypoperfusion as the primary culprit. First, post-CPB stroke was more common in the elderly, perhaps because of a greater incidence of extracranial and intracranial cerebrovascular disease. Second, hypotension was common during CPB at a time when the understanding of the physiology of cerebral autoregulation was incompletely understood.[74] Third, when cerebral blood flow was measured by xenon-133 washout, the cerebral blood flow was found to be low in comparison to that of awake humans.[75] In the 1980s Slogoff et al[16] reported that patients undergoing cardiac valve replacement had twice the incidence of neuropsychologic sequelae as patients undergoing CABG. Thus attention was focused on cerebral embolization. For the next 10 years, the working model assumed that brain in-

jury stemmed from global hypoperfusion in a few patients (e.g., after deep hypothermic circulatory arrest), whereas most patients experienced embolic insults. More recent thinking emphasizes that hypoperfusion and embolism coexist and interact within the cerebral microvasculature. Low cerebral blood flow in patients with preexisting cerebrovascular disease hinders washout of emboli and contributes to downstream ischemia because of poor collateral flow.[76] The number of cerebral emboli detected by Doppler techniques correlates with post-CPB neurologic and neuropsychologic dysfunction.[15,77] Cerebral embolic events occur particularly during manipulation of the aorta (i.e., during cannulation, clamping, declamping, and decannulation), during resumption of left ventricular ejection, and during separation from CPB. Modification of surgical technique may reduce the number of emboli considerably.[66]

E. Risk factors

Advanced age, history of neurologic disease, diabetes mellitus, history of vascular disease, previous CABG, unstable angina, and history of pulmonary disease are predictors of stroke in patients undergoing coronary revascularization. Preexisting cerebrovascular disease, such as stroke and carotid artery stenosis, carries a particularly high perioperative stroke risk.[78,79] Recent reports support the recommendation that combined carotid endarterectomy and CABG is appropriate for patients who have coronary artery disease and a significant carotid artery lesion, defined as unilateral stenosis of more than 70%, unilateral stenosis of more than 50% with ulcerated plaque, bilateral stenoses of more than 50%, or unilateral carotid occlusion.[80-82]

F. Hypothermia and the brain during cardiac surgery

Historically, brain protection inherent in hypothermia was taken for granted. With the advent of normothermic CABG surgery with retrograde cardioplegia, questions arose as to the cerebral impact of warmer brain temperatures.[83] Because most embolic cerebral injury occurs at the time of aortic cannulation, rewarming, and separation from CPB, when the brain temperature is closer to normothermia than to the target temperature for hypothermic CPB, the brain may not have been as well protected as previously assumed. But confusion has also been fueled by the misnomer "warm" or "normothermic" CPB, when in fact most "warm CPB" involves mild hypothermia (32° to 35° C), which confers significant brain protection in animal models.[84] Martin et al[85] studied 1001 patients in two groups, core temperature higher than 35° C and core temperature lower than 28° C, and found a neurologic complication rate of 4.5% in warm CPB and 1.4% in cold CPB. In contrast, the Warm Heart Investigators[83] studied 1732 patients and found no difference in stroke rates (1.5% for both groups) for mild versus moderate hypothermic CPB. A crucial methodologic distinction between the two studies is that in the study by Martin et al, active rewarming kept core temperature at 37° C, whereas in the study by the Warm

Heart Investigators core temperature was allowed to drift to approximately 34° C. Cook et al[86] found that 54% of patients undergoing normothermic CPB with core temperature of 37° C experienced desaturation of cerebral (jugular bulb) venous blood (SjvO$_2$ less than 50%), and Croughwell et al[87] reported that only 20% of patients experience desaturation of cerebral venous blood during rewarming after moderately hypothermic CPB. An SjvO$_2$ less than 50% correlates with greater risk of neuropsychologic deterioration. To complicate the picture McClean et al,[88] in a subgroup of patients in the Warm Heart study, were unable to demonstrate a neuroprotective role for moderate versus mild hypothermia using neuropsychologic measures of outcomes. In summary, unanswered questions include the following: What is the ideal core temperature during CPB? How should this core temperature be attained? How can actual brain temperature be best approximated?[89]

G. Pharmacologic protection

To date, thiopental is the only agent demonstrated to protect the brain during CPB, and then only in specific circumstances of surgery requiring an open ventricle during normothermic CPB with no arterial line filter.[17] Thiopental has not become the standard of practice in CPB because of lingering questions about study design and interpretation, lack of efficacy in CABG, and side effects, which include prolonged intubation, prolonged intensive care unit stay, and increased need for inotropic drugs.[90] In other settings, thiopental is used empirically in situations for which its efficacy has not been demonstrated (e.g., for adults or children undergoing deep hypothermic circulatory arrest).[91] If electroencephalographic monitoring is used to ensure the adequacy of brain cooling, it is important to understand that thiopental will induce a burst-suppression pattern at doses of 15 to 18 mg/kg at normothermia.[17]

H. Blood pressure during CPB

1. Adults. In adults undergoing CPB with moderate hypothermia, brain autoregulation is preserved with α-stat blood gas management during fentanyl-based anesthesia (50 to 100 µg/kg). Mean arterial pressures as low as 30 mm Hg were associated with cerebral blood flows similar to those observed at higher perfusion pressures.[74,92] Throughout the 1980s and 1990s, studies of mean arterial pressure and neurologic outcome showed little correlation. More recently, Gold et al[93] conducted a clinical trial in which 248 CABG patients were randomized into two groups, one with mean arterial pressure maintained at 50 to 60 mm Hg and one with mean arterial pressure maintained at 70 to 80 mm Hg. The overall incidence of combined cardiac and neurologic complications was significantly less in the high-pressure group (4.8%) than in the low-pressure group 12.9%). At 6 months the mortality rate was 1.6% in the high-pressure group and 4.0% in the low-pressure group; the stroke rate was 2.4% versus 7.2%, and the cardiac complication rate was 2.4% versus 4.8%. Cognitive and functional status did not differ between groups. The differ-

ence from earlier studies may be attributable to the older age of CABG patients in the Gold study, a greater proportion of patients with preexisting cerebrovascular disease, a higher prevalence of diabetes mellitus, warmer temperatures during CPB, and lower doses of opioids. In patients known to be at risk for stroke, the data suggest maintaining their mean arterial pressure in the 70 to 80 mm Hg range.

2. Children. In children, cerebral vascular autoregulation persists at moderate hypothermia but is lost progressively as the patient's temperature approaches deep hypothermia, even if α-stat blood gas management is used.[94] Based on clinical trials, most pediatric cardiac anesthesiologists use pH-stat management to increase cerebral blood flow, hasten brain cooling, and maximize brain oxygenation before deep hypothermic circulatory arrest.[95]

V. HEPATIC AND GASTROINTESTINAL COMPLICATIONS

Gastrointestinal (GI) complications, although uncommon, worsen clinical outcomes after CPB. In the post-CPB setting the symptoms of GI problems may be vague, atypical, or absent, with few positive clinical findings. In the face of unexplained sepsis, lactic acidosis, or hemodynamic instability, abdominal ultrasonography and a CT scan should be considered.[96-99] Orlando and Crowell[100] report the use of video-laparoscopy in 26 surgical intensive care unit patients, 19 of whom had undergone CPB. The endoscopic examination was performed at the bedside in 8 patients. The examination was positive in 19 patients. Of these, a laparoscopic cholecystectomy was performed in 4 patients. In the remaining 15, open surgical procedures were performed in the operating room. The preoperative diagnoses were perforation of a viscus, mesenteric infarction, and acute cholecystitis.

Peptic ulceration is the most common GI complication seen in the post-CPB period, even when reasonable prophylaxis with histamine-2 antagonists occurs. Patients who develop peptic ulcers are generally older and more likely to have a history of peptic ulcer disease. If upper GI bleeding or free perforation supervenes, the mortality rate is 15% despite operative intervention.[98] Mesenteric infarction, probably caused by embolism, is fatal in 85% of cases.[99] Even acalculous cholecystitis after CPB is potentially lethal.[97] In a study of 6393 patients who had undergone cardiac surgery, 22 were diagnosed with cholecystitis. Only 15 of the 22 survived, a mortality rate of 32% despite emergent cholecystectomy or biliary drainage. In a prospective study of 300 patients undergoing CPB, biochemical evidence of pancreatic injury was detected in 80, of whom 23 had signs or symptoms and 3 had severe pancreatitis, 2 with pancreatic abscess and 1 with necrotizing hemorrhagic pancreatitis.[101] Moderate to severe pancreatitis carries a mortality rate greater than 50%.[102] Risk factors for development of pancreatitis include prolonged duration of CPB, prolonged hypotension, low cardiac output, and perioperative administration of calcium.

Hepatic injury during and after CPB can result from trauma from the inadvertent placement of thoracostomy tubes or vascular tears associated with the inferior vena caval cannula. Either of these situations can lead to occult bleeding into the abdominal cavity, which manifests as unexplained hypovolemia. Postpump jaundice is more common in patients undergoing multiple valve procedures, either because of higher transfusion requirements, longer bypass times, or high right atrial pressures with subsequent hepatic congestion. Hepatitis from cytomegalovirus, hepatitis A, B, or C antigens, human immunodeficiency virus, and other infectious agents still occurs but with less frequency than in the past because of effective screening of blood. In a study of 3041 patients with normal preoperative liver function, 96 (3.2%) developed jaundice.[103] Determinants of hepatic dysfunction include New York Heart Association class, valve versus coronary bypass surgery, duration of surgery, low cardiac output syndrome requiring administration of inotropic agents or insertion of an IABP, cardiac arrest, and number of blood transfusions. Patients with hepatic dysfunction required prolonged mechanical ventilation, stayed longer in the intensive care unit, and experienced an 11.4% mortality rate.

VI. RENAL COMPLICATIONS

Renal function can improve after cardiac surgery if the surgery corrects defects associated with heart failure or low cardiac output. The hemodilution that occurs during and after CPB also tends to be protective, especially if hypothermia is used or there is considerable breakdown of blood cells during long bypass runs or with considerable cardiotomy suction. However, some degree of renal failure occurs in 1% to 10% of patients after CPB.[104,105] There is a strong correlation between the severity of renal failure and mortality. Renal failure is seen more often with bubble oxygenators than with membrane oxygenators and more often with valve surgery than with coronary artery surgery. The previous two observations suggest that microembolism is the primary mechanism of injury. Interestingly, hemodilution leads to an increased renal blood flow, which makes the kidney more vulnerable to embolic injury. Other causes include the use of vasopressors before bypass, perioperative myocardial infarction, the use of an IABP, high transfusion volumes, emergency surgery, and preoperative renal insufficiency. Interventions that have been shown to help protect the kidneys include administration of furosemide and low-dose dopamine.[106]

VII. PULMONARY COMPLICATIONS

At least five major mechanisms of pulmonary dysfunction are associated with CPB: atelectasis, microembolism, elevated pulmonary artery pressures, noncardiogenic pulmonary edema, and bronchospasm.[107] Atelectasis occurs in about 70% of patients after heart surgery. During CPB the lungs are allowed to collapse. Subsequent reexpansion and ventilation rarely eliminate all atelectasis. Atelectasis leads to a decrease in functional residual capacity and lung compliance, which in turn leads to an increase in the alveolar arterial oxygen gradient and possible hypoxemia. The classic picture of pump

lung is caused by microembolism of solid particulate matter such as aggregated protein, leukocyte and platelet aggregates, damaged blood cells, fat globules, and foreign materials from the bypass circuit. Activated leukocytes and platelets intensify the problem by promoting an acute inflammatory response. Use of membrane oxygenators and arterial filters has reduced this problem. In most situations, increased pulmonary artery pressures are avoided by decompressing the left ventricle with vents. But when pulmonary hypertension is a problem, inhalation of nitric oxide has been used with success. Noncardiogenic pulmonary edema most often occurs with the administration of blood products and fresh frozen plasma after CPB.[108] Finally, bronchospasm can occur during CPB even in patients without a history of asthma. The most likely cause is activation of human C5a anaphylatoxin by the extracorporeal circuit. Aprotinin, a serine protease inhibitor that is administered to reduce blood loss by preventing platelet aggregation and inhibiting fibrinolysis, also prevents the activation of kininogen and formation of bradykinin. Its role in the prevention of acute lung injury in cardiac surgery is unclear, however.

VIII. INFECTIOUS COMPLICATIONS

Patients undergoing cardiac surgery are at high risk for infectious complications.[109] Nosocomial pneumonia, surgical wound infections, and vascular access–related bacteremia have caused the most illness and death.[110] In any patient who has been hospitalized, bacterial colonization with nosocomial organisms may occur. Pseudomonads, staphylococci, and *Escherichia coli* are called the troika of nosocomial infections. Coexistent illness, such as diabetes mellitus or chronic renal failure, depresses the immune system and increases susceptibility to infection. Likewise, various intrinsic features of CPB, such as systemic hypothermia and leukocyte activation,[111] also impair the immune response. To make things worse, these patients must be cared for in intensive care units, which are the epicenters of antibiotic resistance. Vancomycin-resistant *Staphylococcus aureus* is the pathogen of greatest concern because vancomycin is the antibiotic of last choice. Methicillin-resistant *S. aureus* and gentamicin-resistant *E. coli* are now being encountered more often. In some centers, this problem has forced the closure of intensive care units. Established bacterial infection can lead to severe illness with multiorgan failure.[112,113]

Because CPB entails extracorporeal blood flow through foreign materials with innumerable portals for infectious agents, prophylactic antibiotic administration remains a standard of care. A history of penicillin allergy should be reviewed carefully with patients to avoid using vancomycin frivolously. In a review of published reports and postmarketing data from pharmaceutical companies, Anne and Reisman[114] concluded that second- and third-generation cephalosporins can be used safely in patients with penicillin allergy. Penicillin skin tests are not predictive of cross-allergenicity.

Sternal wound infection must be treated with early surgical exploration, evacuation of pus, and excision of necrotic tissue. Once established, mediastinitis carries a grave prognosis because of sternal instability, respiratory failure, pericarditis, and septicemia. Even patients with minimal drainage can become gravely ill in just a few hours. If primary closure of the wound is not possible, plastic repair of the sternal region may prove necessary once the infection is treated. Reconstructive methods include omental, rectus abdominis, or pectoralis major flaps. Jones et al[115] reported 20 years experience with 409 sternal wound infections. In 1975 the diagnosis carried a mortality rate greater than 50%. Today the mortality rate is less than 10% because of early diagnosis and aggressive surgical treatment. Postoperatively, a period of controlled mechanical ventilation may be necessary until bacteremia has resolved and the patient can resume the mechanical and metabolic work of breathing.

IX. CONCLUSION

If all possible complications of CPB were spelled out fully in a preoperative consent form, few patients would agree to cardiac surgery. An experienced cardiac surgeon describes how meticulous each member of the health care team must be when taking care of these patients: "We must always remind ourselves that we are surrounded by assassins and saboteurs." Knowing what can go wrong only makes the success of cardiac surgery all the more impressive. Huge demands are placed on everyone involved. However, most cardiac anesthesiologists, cardiac surgeons, perfusionists, operating room and intensive care nurses, and intensivists enjoy the challenge, the camaraderie, and the success.

REFERENCES

1. Lewis FJ, Taufic M: Closure of atrial septal defects with the aid of hypothermia: experimental accomplishments and the report of one successful case, *Surgery* 33:52, 1953.
2. Cohen M, Lillehei CW: A quantitative study of the "azygos factor" during vena caval occlusion in the dog, *Surg Gynecol Obstet* 98:225, 1954.
3. Warden HE, Cohen M, DeWall RA, et al: Experimental closure of intraventricular septal defects and further physiologic studies on controlled cross circulation, *Surg Forum* 5:22, 1954.
4. Lillehei CW, Varco RL, Ferlic RM, et al: Results in the first 2,500 patients undergoing open-heart surgery at the University of Minnesota Medical Center, *Surgery* 62:819, 1967.
5. Roach GW, Kanchuger M, Mangano CM, et al: Adverse cerebral outcomes after coronary artery bypass surgery. Multicenter study of Perioperative Ischemia Research Group and the Ischemia Research and Education Foundation Investigators, *N Engl J Med* 335:1857, 1996.
6. Shawl FA, Baxley WA: Role of percutaneous cardiopulmonary bypass and other support devices in interventional cardiology, *Cardiol Clin* 12:543, 1994.
7. Wolff T, Stulz P: Successful surgery for perforation of the thoracic aorta caused by the tip of an intra-aortic balloon pump, *Eur J Cardiothorac Surg* 11:1176, 1997.
8. Johnson MS, Lalka SG: Successful treatment of an iatrogenic infrarenal aortic dissection with serial wall stents, *Ann Vasc Surg* 11:295, 1997.
9. Busch T, Sirbu H, Zenker D, et al: Vascular complications related to intra-aortic balloon counterpulsation: an analysis of ten years experience, *Thorac Cardiovasc Surg* 45:55, 1997.
10. Tovar EA, Del Campo C, Borsari A, et al: Postoperative management of cerebral air embolism: gas physiology for surgeons, *Ann Thorac Surg* 60:1138, 1995.
11. Jones NC, Howell CW: Massive arterial air embolism during cardiopulmonary bypass: antegrade blood cardioplegia delivered by the pump: an accident waiting to happen, *Perfusion* 11:157, 1996.
12. Dexter F, Hindman BJ: Recommendations for hyperbaric oxygen therapy based on a mathematical model of bubble absorption, *Anesth Analg* 84:1203, 1997.
13. Lin WL, Liu CL, Li WR. Massive arterial air embolism during cardiac operation: successful treatment in hyperbaric chamber under 3 ATA, *J Thorac Cardiovasc Surg* 100:928, 1990.
14. O'Brien JJ, Butterworth J, Hammon JW, et al: Cerebral emboli during cardiac surgery in children, *Anesthesiology* 87:1063, 1997.
15. Stump DA, Kon ND, Rogers AT, et al: Emboli and neuropsychological outcome following cardiopulmonary bypass, *Echocardiography* 13:555, 1996.
16. Slogoff S, Girgis KZ, Keats AS: Etiologic factors in neuropsychiatric complications associated with cardiopulmonary bypass, *Anesth Analg* 61:903, 1982.
17. Nussmeier NA, Arlund C, Slogoff S: Neuropsychiatric complications after cardiopulmonary bypass: cerebral protection by a barbiturate, *Anesthesiology* 64:165, 1986.
18. Applebaum RM, Kronzon I: Evaluation and management of cholesterol embolization and the blue toe syndrome, *Curr Opin Cardiol* 11:533, 1996.
19. Moody DM, Bell MA, Challa VR, et al: Brain microemboli during cardiac surgery or aortography, *Ann Neurol* 28:477, 1990.
20. Moody DM, Brown WR, Challa VR, et al: Brain microemboli associated with cardiopulmonary bypass: a histologic and magnetic resonance imaging study, *Ann Thorac Surg* 59:1304, 1995.
21. Challa VR, Lovell MA, Moody DM, et al: Laser microprobe mass spectrometric study of aluminum and silicon in brain emboli related to cardiac surgery, *J Neuropathol Exp Neurol* 57:140, 1998.
22. Brooker RF, Brown WR, Moody DM, et al: Cardiotomy suction: a major source of brain lipid emboli during cardiopulmonary bypass, *Ann Thorac Surg* 65:1651, 1998.
23. Tuman KJ, McCarthy RJ, Najafi H, et al: Differential effects of advanced age on neurologic and cardiac risks of coronary artery operations, *J Thorac Cardiovasc Surg* 104:1510, 1992.
24. Amarenco P, Cohen A, Tzourio C, et al: Atherosclerotic disease of the aortic arch and the risk of ischemic stroke, *N Engl J Med* 331:1474, 1994.
25. Kronzon I, Tunick PA: Atheromatous disease of the thoracic aorta: pathologic and clinical implications, *Ann Intern Med* 126:629, 1997.
26. Barbut D, Lo YW, Hartman GS, et al: Aortic atheroma is related to outcome but not numbers of emboli during coronary bypass, *Ann Thorac Surg* 64:454, 1997.
27. Konstadt SN, Reich DL, Quintana C, et al: The ascending aorta: how much does transesophageal echocardiography see? *Anesth Analg* 78:240, 1994.
28. Barbut D, Hinton RB, Szatrowski TP, et al: Cerebral emboli detected during bypass surgery are associated with clamp removal, *Stroke* 25:2398, 1994.
29. Trehan N, Mishra M, Dhole S, et al: Significantly reduced incidence of stroke during coronary artery bypass grafting using transesophageal echocardiography, *Eur J Cardiothorac Surg* 11:234, 1997.
30. Janvier G, Baquey C, Roth C, et al: Extracorporeal circulation, hemocompatability, and biomaterials, *Ann Thorac Surg* 62:1926, 1996.
31. Aldea GS, O'Gara P, Shapira OM, et al: Effect of anticoagulation protocol on outcome in patients undergoing CABG with heparin-bonded cardiopulmonary bypass circuits, *Ann Thorac Surg* 65:425, 1998.
32. Levy M, Hartman AR: Heparin-coated bypass circuits in cardiopulmonary bypass: improved biocompatibility or not? *Int J Cardiol* 53:S81, 1996.
33. Ashraf S, Tian Y, Cowan D, et al: Release of proinflammatory cytokines during pediatric cardiopulmonary bypass: heparin-bonded versus nonbonded oxygenators, *Ann Thorac Surg* 64:1790, 1997.
34. Mihaljevic T, Tonz M, von Segesser KL, et al: The influence of leukocyte filtration during cardiopulmonary bypass on postoperative lung function: a clinical study, *J Thorac Cardiovasc Surg* 109:1138, 1995.

35. Johnson D, Thomson D, Mycyk T, et al: Depletion of neutrophils by filter during aortocoronary bypass surgery transiently improves postoperative cardiorespiratory status, *Chest* 107:1253, 1995.

36. Journois D, Pouard P, Greeley WJ, et al: Hemofiltration during cardiopulmonary bypass in pediatric cardiac surgery: effects on hemostasis, cytokines, and complement components, *Anesthesiology* 81:1181, 1994.

37. Ungerleider RM: Effects of cardiopulmonary bypass and use of modified ultrafiltration, *Ann Thorac Surg* 65:S35, 1998.

38. Murkin JM: Cardiopulmonary bypass and the inflammatory response: a role for serine protease inhibitors? *J Cardiothorac Vasc Anesth* 11:19, 1997.

39. Spahn DR, Leone BJ, Reves JG, et al: Cardiovascular and coronary physiology of acute isovolemic hemodilution: a review of non–oxygen-carrying and oxygen-carrying solutions, *Anesth Analg* 78:1000, 1994.

40. Dexter F, Hindman BJ: Effect of haemoglobin concentration on brain oxygenation in focal stroke: a mathematical modeling study, *Br J Anaesth* 79:346, 1997.

41. He GW, Acuff TE, Ryan WH, et al: Determinants of operative mortality in elderly patients undergoing bypass grafting: emphasis on the influence of internal mammary artery grafting on mortality and morbidity, *J Thorac Cardiovasc Surg* 108:73, 1994.

42. Rady MY, Ryan T, Starr NJU: Perioperative determinants of morbidity and mortality in elderly patients undergoing cardiac surgery, *Crit Care Med* 26:225, 1998.

43. He GW, Acuff TE, Ryan WH, et al: Determinants of operative mortality in reoperative coronary artery bypass grafting, *J Thorac Cardiovasc Surg* 110:971, 1995.

44. Awad WI, De Souza AC, Magee PG, et al: Re-do cardiac surgery in patients over 70 years old, *Eur J Cardiothorac Surg* 12:40, 1997.

45. Dacey LJ, Munoz JJ, Baribeau YR, et al: Reexploration for hemorrhage following coronary artery bypass grafting: incidence and risk factors, *Arch Surg* 133:442, 1998.

46. Eikvar L, Pillgram-Larsen J, Skjaeggestad O, et al: Serum cardiospecific troponin T after open heart surgery in patients with and without perioperative myocardial infarction, *Scand J Clin Lab Invest* 54:329, 1994.

47. Appleyard RF, Cohn LH: Myocardial stunning and reperfusion injury in cardiac surgery, *J Card Surg* 8:316, 1993.

48. Damiano RJ Jr: The electrophysiology of ischemia and cardioplegia: implications for myocardial protection, *J Card Surg* 10:445, 1995.

49. Guyton RA, Gott JP, Brown WM, et al: Cold and warm myocardial protection techniques, *Adv Card Surg* 7:1, 1996.

50. Svedjeholm R, Dahlin LG, Lundberg C, et al: Are electrocardiographic Q-wave criteria reliable for diagnosis of perioperative myocardial infarction after coronary artery surgery? *Eur J Cardiothorac Surg* 13:655, 1998.

51. Alyanakian MA, Dehoux M, Chatelo D, et al: Cardiac troponin I in diagnosis of perioperative myocardial infarction after cardiac surgery, *J Cardiothorac Vasc Anesth* 12:288, 1998.

52. Smith JS, Cahalan MK, Benefiel DJ, et al: Intraoperative detection of myocardial ischemia in high-risk patients: electrocardiography versus two-dimensional transesophageal echocardiography, *Circulation* 72:1015, 1985.

53. Koide Y, Keehn L, Nomura T, et al: Relationship of regional wall motion abnormalities detected by biplane transesophageal echocardiography and electrocardiographic changes in patients undergoing coronary artery bypass graft surgery, *J Cardiothorac Vasc Anesth* 10:719, 1996.

54. Communale ME, Body SC, Ley C, et al: The concordance of intraoperative left ventricular wall-motion abnormalities and electrocardiographic S-T segment changes: association with outcome after coronary revascularization, *Anesthesiology* 88:945, 1998.

55. Almassi GH, Schowalter T, Nicolosi AC, et al: Atrial fibrillation after cardiac surgery: a major morbid event? *Ann Surg* 226:501, 1997.

56. Butterworth JF IV, Legault C, Royster RL, et al: Factors that predict the use of positive inotropic drug support after cardiac valve surgery, *Anesth Analg* 86:461, 1998.

57. Anthi A, Tzelepis GE, Alivizatos P, et al: Unexpected cardiac arrest after cardiac surgery: incidence, predisposing causes, and outcome of open chest cardiopulmonary resuscitation, *Chest* 113:15, 1998.

58. Bolli R: Basic and clinical aspects of myocardial stunning, *Prog Cardiovasc Dis* 40:477, 1998.

59. Royster RL: Myocardial dysfunction following cardiopulmonary bypass: recovery patterns, predictors of inotropic need, theoretical concepts of inotropic administration, *J Cardiothorac Vasc Anesth* 7(suppl 2):19, 1993.

60. Asher CR, Miller DP, Grimm RA, et al: Analysis of risk factors for development of atrial fibrillation early after cardiac valve surgery, *Am J Cardiol* 82:892, 1998.

61. Daoud EG, Strickberger SA, Man KC, et al: Preoperative amiodarone as prophylaxis against atrial fibrillation after heart surgery, *N Engl J Med* 337:1785, 1997.

62. Pires LA, Wagshal AB, Lancey R, et al: Arrhythmias and conduction disturbances after coronary artery bypass graft surgery: epidemiology, management, and prognosis, *Am Heart J* 129:799, 1995.

63. Baird DL, Murkin JM, Lee DL: Neurologic findings in coronary artery bypass patients: perioperative or preexisting? *J Cardiothorac Vasc Anesth* 11:694, 1997.

64. Kuroda Y, Uchimoto R, Kaieda R, et al: Central nervous system complications after cardiac surgery: a comparison between coronary bypass grafting and valve surgery, *Anesth Analg* 76:222, 1993.

65. Ahlgren E, Aren C: Cerebral complications after coronary artery bypass and heart valve surgery: risk factors and onset of symptoms, *J Cardiothorac Vasc Anesth* 12:270, 1998.

66. Hammon JW, Stump DA, Kon ND, et al: Risk factors and solutions for the development of neurobehavioral changes after coronary artery bypass grafting, *Ann Thorac Surg* 63:1613, 1997.

67. Bruggermans EF, van de Vijver FJ, Huysmans HA: Assessment of cognitive deterioration in individual patients following cardiac surgery: correcting for measurement error and practice effects, *J Clin Exp Neuropsychol* 19:543, 1997.

68. Murkin JM, Newman SP, Stump DA, et al: Statement of consensus on assessment of neurobehavioral outcomes after cardiac surgery, *Ann Thorac Surg* 59:1289, 1995.

69. Steinberg GK, de LaPaz R, Mitchell RS, et al: Magnetic resonance imaging and CSF enzymes as sensitive indicators of subclinical cerebral injury following open-heart valve replacement surgery, *Stroke* 23:161, 1992.

70. Harris DN, Bailey SM, Smith PL, et al: Brain swelling in first hour after coronary artery bypass surgery, *Lancet* 342:586, 1993.

71. Harris DN, Oatridge A, Dob D, et al: Cerebral swelling after normothermic cardiopulmonary bypass, *Anesthesiology* 88:340, 1998.

72. Johnsson P, Lundqvist C, Lindgren A, et al: Cerebral complications after cardiac surgery assessed by S-100 and NSE levels in blood, *J Cardiothorac Vasc Anesth* 9:694, 1995.

73. Blomquist S, Johnsson P, Luhrs C, et al: The appearance of S-100 protein in serum during and immediately after cardiopulmonary bypass surgery: a possible marker for cerebral injury, *J Cardiothorac Vasc Anesth* 11:699, 1997.

74. Rogers AT, Stump DA, Gravlee GP, et al: Response of cerebral blood flow to phenylephrine infusion during hypothermic cardiopulmonary bypass: influence of $PaCO_2$ management, *Anesthesiology* 69:547, 1988.

75. Prough DS, Stump DA, Roy RC, et al: Response of cerebral blood flow to changes in carbon dioxide tension during hypothermic cardiopulmonary bypass, *Anesthesiology* 64:576, 1986.

76. Caplan LR, Hennerici M: Impaired clearance of emboli (washout) is an important link between hypoperfusion, embolism, and ischemic stroke, *Arch Neurol* 55:1475, 1998.

77. Pugsley W, Klinger L, Paschalis C, et al: The impact of microemboli during cardiopulmonary bypass on neuropsychological functioning, *Stroke* 25:1393, 1994.

78. Mills SA: Risk factors for cerebral injury and cardiac surgery, *Ann Thorac Surg* 59:1296, 1995.

79. Redmond JM, Greene PS, Goldsborough MA, et al: Neurologic injury in cardiac surgical patients with a history of stroke, *Ann Thorac Surg* 61:42, 1996.

80. Akins CW: Combined carotid endarterectomy and coronary revascularization operation, *Ann Thorac Surg* 66:1483, 1998.

81. Donatelli F, Pelenghi S, Pocar M, et al: Combined carotid and cardiac procedures: improved results and surgical approach, *Cardiovasc Surg* 6:506, 1998.

82. Darling RC III, Dylewski M, Chang BB, et al: Combined carotid endarterectomy and coronary artery bypass grafting does not increase the risk of perioperative stroke, *Cardiovasc Surg* 6:448, 1998.

83. The Warm Heart Investigators: Randomized trial of normothermic versus hypothermic coronary artery bypass surgery, *Lancet* 343:559, 1994.

84. Ginsberg MD, Sternau LL, Globus MYT, et al: Therapeutic modulation of brain temperature: relevance to ischemic brain injury, *Cerebrovasc Brain Metab Rev* 4:189, 1992.

85. Martin TD, Craver JM, Gott JP, et al: Prospective, randomized trial of retrograde warm blood cardioplegia: myocardial benefit and neurologic threat, *Ann Thorac Surg* 57:298, 1994.

86. Cook DJ, Oliver WC Jr, Orszulak TA, et al: A prospective, randomized comparison of cerebral venous oxygen saturation during normothermic and hypothermic cardiopulmonary bypass, *J Thorac Cardiovasc Surg* 107:1020, 1994.

87. Croughwell ND, Newman MF, Blumenthal JA, et al: Jugular bulb saturation and cognitive dysfunction after cardiopulmonary bypass, *Ann Thorac* 58:1702, 1994.

88. McLean RF, Wong BI, Naylor CD, et al: Cardiopulmonary bypass, temperature, and central nervous system dysfunction, *Circulation* 90(2):250, 1994.

89. Stone JG, Young WL, Smith CR, et al: Do standard monitoring sites reflect true brain temperature when profound hypothermia is rapidly induced and reversed? *Anesthesiology* 82:344, 1995.

90. Todd M: Barbiturate protection and cardiac surgery: a different result, *Anesthesiology* 74:402, 1991.

91. Mossad EB: Thiopental should not be used before deep hypothermic circulatory arrest in pediatric patients, *J Cardiothorac Vasc Anesth* 12:595, 1998.

92. Murkin JM, Farrar JF, Tweed WA, et al: Cerebral autoregulation and flow/metabolism coupling during cardiopulmonary bypass: the influence of $PaCO_2$, *Anesth Analg* 66:825, 1987.

93. Gold JP, Charlson ME, Williams-Russo P, et al: Improvement of outcomes after coronary artery bypass: a randomized trial comparing intraoperative high versus low mean arterial pressure, *J Thorac Cardiovasc Surg* 110:1302, 1995.

94. Greely WJ, Kern FH, Meliones JN, et al: Effect of deep hypothermia and circulatory arrest on cerebral blood flow and metabolism, *Ann Thorac Surg* 56:1464, 1993.

95. Kern FH, Ungerleider RM, Schulman SR, et al: Comparing two strategies of cardiopulmonary bypass cooling on jugular venous oxygen saturation in neonates and infants, *Ann Thorac Surg* 60:1198, 1995.

96. Eustace S, Connolly B, Egleston C, et al: Imaging of abdominal complications following cardiac surgery, *Abdom Imaging* 19:405, 1994.

97. Sessions SC, Scoma RS, Sheikh FA, et al: Acute acalculous cholecystitis following open heart surgery, *Am Surg* 59:74, 1993.

98. Johnston G, Vitikainen K, Knight R, et al: Changing perspectives on gastrointestinal complications in patients undergoing cardiac surgery, *Am J Surg* 163:525, 1992.

99. Yilmaz AT, Arslan M, Demirkilc U, et al: Gastrointestinal complications after cardiac surgery, *Eur J Cardiothorac Surg* 10:763, 1996.

100. Orlando R III, Crowell KL: Laparoscopy in the critically ill, *Surg Endosc* 11:1072, 1997.

101. Fernandez-del Castillo C, Harringer W, Warshaw AL, et al: Risk factors for pancreatic cellular injury after cardiopulmonary bypass, *N Engl J Med* 325:382, 1991.

102. Lefor AT, Vuocolo P, Parker FB Jr, et al: Pancreatic complications following cardiopulmonary bypass: factors influencing mortality, *Arch Surg* 127:1225, 1992.

103. Michaelopoulos A, Alivizatos P, Geroulanos S: Hepatic dysfunction following cardiac surgery: determinants and consequences, *Hepatogastroenterology* 44:779, 1997.

104. Chertow GM, Levy EM, Hammermeister KE, et al: Independent association between acute renal failure and mortality following cardiac surgery, *Am J Med* 104:343, 1998.

105. Zanardo G, Michielon P, Paccagnella A, et al: Acute renal failure in the patient undergoing cardiac operation: prevalence, mortality rate, and main risk factors, *J Thorac Cardiovasc Surg* 107:1489, 1994.

106. Kron IL, Joob AW, Meter CV: Acute renal failure in the cardiovascular surgical patient, *Ann Thorac Surg* 39:590, 1985.

107. Sladen RN, Berkowitz DE: Cardiopulmonary bypass and the lung. In Gravlee GP, Davis RF, Utley JR, eds: *Cardiopulmonary bypass: principles and practice*, Baltimore, 1993, Williams & Wilkins.

108. Roy RC, Stafford MA, Hudspeth AS, et al: Failure of prophylaxis with fresh frozen plasma after cardiopulmonary bypass, *Anesthesiology* 69:254, 1988.

109. Lutwick LI, Vaghjimal A, Connolly MW: Postcardiac surgery infections, *Crit Care Clin* 14:221, 1998.

110. Weinstein RA: Nosocomial infection update, *Emerg Infect Dis* 4:416, 1998.

111. van de Watering LM, Hermans J, Houbiers JG, et al: Beneficial effects of leukocyte depletion of transfused blood on postoperative complications in patients undergoing cardiac surgery: a randomized clinical trial, *Circulation* 97:562, 1998.

112. Ryan T, McCarthy JF, Rady MY, et al: Early bloodstream infection after cardiopulmonary bypass: frequency rate, risk factors, and implications, *Crit Care Med* 25:2009, 1997.

113. Michalopoulos A, Stavridis G, Geroulanos S: Severe sepsis in cardiac surgical patients, *Eur J Surg* 164:217, 1998.

114. Anne S, Reisman RE: Risk of administering cephalosporin antibiotics to patients with histories of penicillin allergy, *Ann Allergy Asthma Immunol* 74:167, 1995.

115. Jones G, Jurkiewicz MJ, Bostwick J, et al: Management of the infected median sternotomy wound with muscle flaps: the Emory 20-year experience, *Ann Surg* 225:766, 1997.

Chapter 14

Anesthetic Complications Related to Endocrine Disease

Richard A. Wiklund
Stanley H. Rosenbaum

The endocrine system is a complex but integrated system of first- and second-messenger chemical compounds, hormones, that act as ligands at receptor binding sites to produce homeostasis in response to stress. Abnormal endocrine function can result from excess or insufficient production, release, or availability of these hormones. Alternatively, abnormal endocrine function can result from acquired or induced abnormalities of the ligand-specific receptor proteins, G-proteins related to transmission of receptor-ligand signal or disrupted intracellular cascade of metabolic activity, often protein kinase–mediated phosphorylation of functional proteins. Thus many endocrine hormones have been called first messengers and their intracellular partners, cyclic nucleotides, second messengers.[1] Their physiologic effect is rapid in onset and short-lived. The thyroid, adrenal cortical, and pancreatic islet cell hormones are exceptions to this rule because their homeostatic effect is not mediated by cyclic nucleotides, it is not rapid in onset, and their ef-

fects are long-lived. These hormones cause transduction that leads to increased expression of the genes that control the transcription of messenger RNA, which, in turn, controls intracellular protein synthesis. Permutations of enhanced, limited, or absent control mechanisms in a number of endocrine organs could lead to a disjointed discussion of postoperative endocrine complications. In this chapter we discuss complications related to preoperative hyperactivity and hypoactivity as well as physical complications related to surgery involving specific endocrine glands. We limit our review to the glands and endocrinopathies commonly encountered by anesthesiologists: neurohypophysis-pituitary (anterior and posterior), thyroid, parathyroid, and adrenal glands and the pancreatic islet cells. Many other interesting hormone systems are beyond the scope of this chapter. Included are the hormones that control sexual function, obesity, response to starvation, prostaglandins, intestinal vasopeptides, and many others.

I. NEUROHYPOPHYSIS-PITUITARY AXIS

The pituitary gland is a source of messenger hormones whose release from the pituitary is controlled by other messenger hormones from the paraventricular nuclei in the hypothalamus. Pituitary hormones are ligands for specific receptors in a number of other endocrine glands. Control of the release of pituitary hormones is exerted primarily through closed-loop feedback inhibition, but the tropostat for hormone release is influenced by numerous factors from the internal milieu (e.g., stress, emotion, temperature, metabolic balance, osmolarity) as well as the external environment. Therefore many postoperative complications not directly related to the endocrine system exert secondary influences on pituitary function, with either increased or decreased secretion of its messenger hormones.

A. Hypophysis

Release of the six trophic hormones (adrenocorticotropic hormone [ACTH], thyroid-stimulating hormone [TSH], luteinizing hormone [LH], growth hormone [GH], follicle-stimulating hormone [FSH], and prolactin) of the anterior pituitary is controlled by corresponding releasing hormones secreted in the adenohypophysis and transported to the pituitary by a portal system of capillaries transcending the pituitary stalk. Secretion of posterior pituitary hormones (antidiuretic hormone [ADH] and vasopressin) is controlled by active transport of precursors (neurophysins) in the neurohypophysis down the neurons of the pituitary stalk. Hypothalamic activity and a variety of ligands and their antagonists influence the release of releasing hormones. Important inhibitors of adenohypophysis and neurohypophysis include γ-aminobutyric acid (GABA), opioid peptides, dopaminergic compounds, and α- and β-adrenergic blocking compounds. Central nervous system trauma, ischemia, infection, tumors, elevated cerebrospinal fluid pressure, hyperthermia or hypothermia, and centrally acting pharmacologic agents can lead to disruption of hypothalamic and hypophyseal function in the postoperative period.

B. Anterior pituitary gland

The anterior pituitary gland secretes six trophic hormones from five types of cells that are now called tropocytes.[2] These include corticotropes (ACTH), thyrotropes (TSH), lactotropes (prolactin), somatotropes (GH), and gonadotropes (FSH and LH). Perioperative complications may result from disturbed hypothalamic control, ablation of the tropocytes, or excess secretion associated with hyperplasia or neoplasia of the pituitary gland. When global central nervous system injury occurs (e.g., trauma, infection, or inflammation), all of the anterior pituitary tropocytes are destroyed and the patient is at risk of developing panhypopituitarism.

Pituitary hyperplasia usually results from long-standing trophic stimulation by trophocyte-specific releasing hormones. This is one cause of acromegaly (growth hormone–releasing factor [GHRF] and GH) and Cushing's disease (corticotropin-releasing factor [CRF] and ACTH). Thyrotrope hyperplasia may result from long-standing hypothyroidism with elevated concentrations of thyrotropic hormone–releasing factor (THRF) and TSH. Accordingly, these endocrinopathies may present in the postoperative period of patients undergoing pituitary surgery for hyperplasia. Neoplasia of the pituitary is a clonal disease, so excess secretion of trophic hormones is specific to the tropocyte from which the adenoma arose.[3] Functioning adenomas may develop from mutations of tumor suppression genes (multiple endocrine neoplasia [MEN-1], Rb, p53, and other oncogenes). The most common functioning adenomas arise from gonadotropes (FSH and LH) and somatotropes (GH) and lead to hypogonadism, galactorrhea, and acromegaly, respectively. ACTH-secreting adenomas may lead to Cushing's disease or may occur after bilateral adrenalectomy (Nelson's syndrome). Following resection of secreting pituitary adenomas, postoperative complications may result from the anatomic features of acromegaly or from acute withdrawal of ACTH stimulation of adrenal secretion. TSH-secreting adenomas are rare but are a cause of hyperthyroidism.

Acromegaly is an endocrinopathy of particular concern to the anesthesiologist because of the somatic expression of the disease. It results from the unrestrained secretion of GH caused in many cases by a genetic abnormality of the G-protein that couples GHRF receptor occupancy to activation of adenylate cyclase in the pituitary gonadotrope. The clinical picture of acromegaly may be influenced by polymorphous secretion of other trophic hormones along with GH (e.g., TSH or prolactin). Furthermore, acromegaly may be seen as part of a syndrome of multiple endocrine neoplasia (MEN-1 syndrome; Table 14-1).

GH-secreting adenomas may cause severe headache from local expansion of the tumor, acute systemic metabolic effects (diabetes mellitus), and the long-term structural features of acromegaly. GH causes insulin resistance, and excess secretion can aggravate diabetes mellitus. After hypophysectomy, blood glucose concentrations must be

Table 14-1. Clinical presentation of the multiple endocrine neoplasia (MEN) syndromes

	MEN-1	MEN-2A	MEN-2B
Adrenal	Hyperplasia, neoplasia	Pheochromocytoma	Pheochromocytoma
Thyroid	Hyperplasia, neoplasia	Medullary carcinoma	Medullary carcinoma
Parathyroid	Hyperplasia, neoplasia	Hyperplasia	Not involved
Pituitary	Hyperplasia, neoplasia	Not involved	Not involved
Pancreas	Islet adenoma	Not involved	Not involved
Ganglia	Not involved	Not involved	Marfanoid habitus
Other diseases	Carcinoid syndrome	None	None

monitored closely and increased insulin sensitivity should be anticipated. The somatic features of acromegaly include enlargement of the bones and thickening of the tissues of the airway. Thickening of the tissues can lead to nerve entrapment syndromes, including paresis of the recurrent laryngeal nerve. Tissue thickening can involve the tongue and glottis, making endotracheal intubation and extubation more difficult. Therefore postoperative airway surveillance should include the expectation of partial or complete airway obstruction and the need for prolonged intubation and possibly tracheostomy.

Virtually all pituitary adenomas can be treated surgically by transsphenoidal hypophysectomy.[4] Only 1% or less require a transcranial approach for tumor extending well beyond the sella turcica. The morbidity and mortality rates are very low, and transphenoidal hypophysectomy is feasible even in patients who would be considered high-risk patients for craniotomy.

C. Posterior pituitary gland

The posterior portion of the pituitary gland secretes two hormones, vasopressin or ADH and oxytocin. Vasopressin-secreting cells are much more abundant than those that secrete oxytocin. Few, if any, postoperative complications are related to inadequate or excess secretion of oxytocin. This is not the case with vasopressin, a nonapeptide that enables the reabsorption of water in the distal or collecting tubules of the kidney. In the absence of vasopressin, the renal tubules are impermeable to water and a large volume of dilute urine is excreted. Vasopressin is the ligand for renal tubular receptors (V2), which open permeability channels for water through a G-protein–cyclic adenosine monophosphate (cAMP) mediated mechanism. The stimulus for secretion of vasopressin by the posterior pituitary is complex and may be altered by physiologic, physical, and pharmacologic forces associated with anesthesia and surgery. The two primary mechanisms that control vasopressin release in the undisturbed, resting state are plasma osmolarity sensed by osmoreceptor neurons in the central nervous system and the hydrostatic pressure sensed by baroreceptors in the cardiovascular system. Abnormal increases or decreases in activity of either mechanism can cause postoperative complications (oliguria or polyuria) related to vasopressin secretion. Postoperative complications may also occur secondary to disruption of the osmotic gradient in the renal medulla, which impairs the reabsorption of water in response to increased secretion of vasopressin.

Osmoreceptors in the central nervous system are exquisitely sensitive to changes in plasma osmolarity, which is established primarily by the concentration of plasma sodium and its associated anions. Hyponatremia suppresses the secretion of vasopressin and increases urinary excretion of water in the distal tubules, whereas sodium is reabsorbed in the proximal tubules. Hypernatremia leads to hyperosmolarity. The set point for markedly increased vasopressin secretion is approximately 275 to 290 mOsm in plasma.[5] Hyperosmolarity increases vasopressin secretion and causes rapid renal tubular reab-

sorption of water, decreased urine volume, and increased urine osmolarity. Thirst plays a major role in stimulation of vasopressin release, and the effect of thirst is independent of baroreceptor mechanisms of blood pressure and volume. A patient experiences thirst when he or she is hyperosmolar, regardless of whether blood pressure and extracellular fluid volume are increased or decreased.

The plasma osmolarity set point of 275 to 290 mOsm can be inhibited by agents used to control postoperative nausea and vomiting, specifically dopaminergic antagonists such as fluphenazine, haloperidol, droperidol, and promethazine.[6] Glucocorticoids also inhibit the release of vasopressin. Vasopressin secretion is stimulated by a variety of stimuli, including some pharmacologic drugs, apomorphine, and high-dose morphine. Nausea, a common postoperative problem, causes a marked increase in vasopressin secretion, 100 to 1000 times basal secretion. These effects must be mediated through the chemoreceptor trigger zone because these drugs do not alter vasopressin secretion in response to hyperosmolarity or changes in intravascular volume (baroreceptor mechanisms).

Sodium is not the only solute that produces hyperosmolarity and increased secretion of vasopressin. The increase in vasopressin secretion caused by hyperosmolarity secondary to mannitol administration is equal to that caused by hypernatremia.[7] Urea is less potent but can cause increased vasopressin secretion. Increased secretion of vasopressin in response to hyperosmolarity caused by glucose depends on the presence of elevated blood concentrations of insulin. If insulin is deficient, hyperglycemia does not increase vasopressin secretion. If increased concentrations of insulin are present, glucose increases secretion of vasopressin. This suggests that hyperglycemia must lead to increased intracellular concentrations of glucose before osmoreceptor neurons secrete vasopressin.

The administration of mannitol can have secondary effects on vasopressin physiology in the postoperative period. By increasing renal blood flow, mannitol may eliminate the hypertonic gradient in the renal medulla. Vasopressin-mediated reabsorption of water is passive, and while cAMP-gated channels are opened in response to vasopressin, significant water reabsorption does not occur if the hypertonic gradient is not present.

Use of a vasopressin antagonist in humans has been described.[8] To be useful for treatment of the antidiuretic effect of vasopressin, as opposed to the pressor effect, antagonists have to be specific for the V2 (renal tubular) rather than the V1 (cardiovascular) vasopressin receptor. Intravenous vasopressin is a potent vasoconstrictor. It reduces mesenteric and portal blood flow, a benefit in patients with portal hypertension, but its usefulness is limited by myocardial ischemia secondary to coronary artery vasoconstriction.

Vasopressin secretion is controlled by baroreceptor mechanisms that stimulate V1 receptors in response to hypotension or hypovolemia. These are located at numerous sites outside the central nervous system (heart and larger arteries), with afferent transmission via the vagus and glossopharyngeal nerves. This mechanism is not as sensitive as the osmoreceptor mechanism in the central nervous system. Although the two mechanisms are cooperative, baroreceptor-influenced vasopressin secretion (increased or decreased) does not interfere with osmoreceptor control of osmolarity.

Virtually any mechanism or pharmacologic agent that increases or decreases blood pressure or effective blood volume will decrease or increase vasopressin secretion. These certainly include the vasopressors used intraoperatively and postoperatively, the stress of surgery, controlled ventilation, controlled vasodilation, and administration of narcotics and antiemetics. The effects of these interventions on other baroreceptor mechanisms is probably more important, especially baroreceptor control of heart rate.

D. Diabetes insipidus

Diabetes insipidus more properly should be called polyuria. The three well-known types of diabetes insipidus are neurogenic, nephrogenic, and dipsogenic. Neurogenic or hypothalamic diabetes insipidus results from lack of secretion of vasopressin in response to osmotic stimulation of central osmoreceptors. Nephrogenic diabetes insipidus results from renal tubular insensitivity to normal or elevated blood concentrations of vasopressin. The third form, dipsogenic, results from excess intake of water and is usually psychogenic in origin, but it is important to keep in mind when trying to sort out the other forms of diabetes insipidus.

Neurogenic diabetes insipidus is probably the most common form of diabetes insipidus presenting as a postoperative complication, and it is most likely to be caused by head trauma or neurosurgery in the area of the hypothalamus or pituitary gland. Other causes in the postoperative setting may include Sheehan's syndrome, intracranial aneurysm, a variety of intracranial tumors, and infections. Idiopathic neurogenic diabetes insipidus may be an immune disease or an immune reaction in which pitressin is the antigen. Tumors (craniopharyngioma, glioma, and germinoma) are the cause of diabetes insipidus in 13% of cases.[9]

Anterior pituitary tumors can lead to a combination of neurogenic and nephrogenic diabetes insipidus in the postoperative period by an unusual mechanism. Glucocorticoids are essential for vasopressin-induced distal renal tubular permeability to water. Inadequate ACTH secretion after anterior pituitary surgery or inadequate glucocorticoid secretion after adrenal surgery may cause renal tubular insensitivity to vasopressin with polyuria.

The most common causes of nephrogenic diabetes insipidus in the postoperative period are serum electrolyte abnormalities, particularly hypercalcemia and hypokalemia. The former should be considered in patients with hyperparathyroidism. Nephrogenic diabetes insipidus induced by drugs (lithium, demeclocycline) is not commonly encountered postoperatively.

Neurogenic diabetes insipidus is diagnosed by determining plasma and urine osmolarity and vasopressin concentrations in response to osmotic stimulation (fluid restriction or hypertonic saline administration). Patients with nephrogenic diabetes insipidus have high vasopressin concentrations and hyposmolar urine.

Neurogenic diabetes insipidus can be treated with intravenous or intranasal administration of arginine vasopressin. However, this peptide is a nonspecific ligand that binds to both V1 and V2 receptors and may lead to hypertension and myocardial ischemia in patients with coronary artery disease. Desmopressin, a safer alternative, is specific for the V2 receptor and may be given intranasally or intravenously.[10] Although desmopressin will not cause hypertension, dilutional hyponatremia can occur if a postoperative patient being treated with desmopressin has free access to water. Nephrogenic diabetes insipidus is more difficult to treat unless it was caused by an adverse drug reaction, in which case withdrawal of the drug may cause spontaneous reversal.

E. Central pontine myelosis

Central pontine myelosis is a potentially fatal complication of rapid correction of chronic hypernatremia regardless of the cause of the electrolyte imbalance.[11] It can be a significant problem in the operative and postoperative anesthesia care of patients with refractory ascites, particularly those undergoing orthotopic liver transplantation or portal decompression procedures associated with large amounts of blood loss. The duration of hyponatremia is important in the postoperative approach to correction of hyponatremia. Acute hyponatremia (less than 48 hours) is a significant risk for neurologic harm, and rapid correction to a sodium concentration at which neurologic symptoms disappear is not associated with cerebral demyelination.[12] Chronic hyponatremia, on the other hand, usually is not associated with neurologic symptoms, but rapid correction will cause demyelination. If a patient with refractory ascites and hyponatremia requires alkali therapy for correction of severe acidosis associated with blood volume replacement, the serum sodium concentration must be monitored closely to prevent pontine myelosis. Postoperative pontine myelosis can be prevented if preoperative preparation includes gradual correction of hyponatremia. Maximum recommended rates of correction of hyponatremia range from 0.5 to 2.0 mEq/L per hour, not to exceed 12 mEq/L in a 12- to 24-hour period or 25 mEq/L in a 48-hour period.[13] Within those guidelines, end points for correction include reversal of neurologic symptoms or achievement of a serum sodium concentration greater than 120 mEq/L.

F. Syndrome of inappropriate ADH secretion

This syndrome is the cause of hyposmolarity in 30% to 40% of all hyposmolar patients. Criteria for the syndrome of inappropriate ADH secretion (SIADH) were described in 1967 by Barter and Schwartz.[14] They include plasma osmolarity less than 275 mOsm, urine osmolarity greater than 100 mOsm, normal renal function, normovolemia, elevated urinary sodium concentration with normal salt and water intake, no history of recent diuretic use, and the absence of other endocrinopathies (Addison's disease or hypothyroidism). It can be confirmed by direct measurement of the plasma concentration of vasopressin in conjunction with measurement of plasma and urinary osmolarity. In the postoperative period, positive pressure ventilation is the most likely cause of SIADH, although a number of tumors, central nervous system disorders, drugs, and pulmonary disorders should also be considered. Overall, tumors are the most common cause and the leading offender is oat cell or small cell carcinoma of the lung. There is no common thread in the long list of central nervous system causes of SIADH. Chlorpropamide (Diabinese) has been the leading cause of drug-induced SIADH, but its use in the treatment of diabetes mellitus has diminished considerably.[15] Pulmonary disease as a cause of SIADH is almost always associated with early, severe respiratory failure and most often with mechanical ventilation or positive end-expiratory pressure therapy.[16] It resolves with improvement of the respiratory disease and resumption of spontaneous ventilation.

Treatment of SIADH is determined by an estimation of extracellular fluid volume. If the patient is hypervolemic, diuretics will cause a hyposmolar diuresis with partial correction of hyponatremia. If the patient is hypovolemic or diuretic therapy is the cause of SIADH, intravenous saline with potassium supplementation should be given. If the patient is normovolemic, solute depletion (extracellular sodium) is likely and intravenous saline should be given. In these patients, corticosteroids may be indicated because of the possibility of primary or secondary corticosteroid insufficiency.

G. Pituitary apoplexy

Necrosis of the pituitary gland can result from hemorrhagic infarction secondary to an enlarging adenoma, trauma, or severe hypotension secondary to systemic hemorrhage. When this occurs in the peripartum period it is called Sheehan's syndrome and may result from acute arterial vasospasm of vessels supplying the anterior pituitary gland.[17] The pituitary may be at increased risk because of the physiologic enlargement of the gland that occurs during pregnancy. Features of Sheehan's syndrome include hypotension that does not respond to appropriate fluid volume replacement, hypoglycemia, failure to lactate, and low blood concentrations of ACTH. Treatment consists of administration of glucocorticoids and appropriate intravenous fluids. Following recovery, imaging of the pituitary may show an empty sella turcica, a classic radiologic finding. In some cases, not all of the anterior pituitary is lost and the need for long-term hormone replacement is determined by blood hormone assay.

When pituitary apoplexy results from trauma or hemorrhage of a pituitary adenoma, presenting signs may include meningismus, visual disturbances, headache, and coma. In severe cases, craniotomy may be necessary to decompress the area of hemorrhage. Again, diagnosis can be made by radiologic imaging.

H. Pituitary surgery

Pituitary surgery can lead to postoperative endocrinopathies including acute adrenal insufficiency, hypothyroidism, and neurogenic diabetes insipidus. These problems are easily anticipated, and suspicions are raised by appropriate monitoring of hemodynamic variables, urinary output, and serum electrolytes. Despite the less invasive nature of transphenoidal surgery, inappropriate behavior, unstable vital signs, and visual difficulties are indications for neurologic examination and diagnostic imaging to rule out postoperative hemorrhage and the need for decompression.

II. THYROID GLAND

The thyroid gland has been the subject of medical scrutiny and surgical ablation for more than a century. Disorders of thyroid function, including myxedema and cretinism, were characterized in the mid- to late-1800s. Hypothyroidism is the most commonly diagnosed endocrinopathy, found in up to 2% of the population.[18] Surgery for thyroid disease is highly effective, commonly performed, and nearly free of complications when performed by competent surgeons. Similarly, postoperative complications are exceedingly rare because of the routine nature of preoperative medical preparation of patients with thyroid dysfunction, well-described surgical technique, and modern standards of monitoring during and after anesthesia. We review the recognition and management of intraoperative and postoperative thyroid dysfunction, myxedema, and thyroid storm at the extremes, but these are extremely rare postoperative complications. The most common complications result from inadvertent or unavoidable surgical trauma to surrounding tissues.

A. Hyperthyroidism

Hyperthyroidism results from excess stimulation of thyroid follicles by thyrotropin or by autoantibodies to thyroidal peroxidase (TPO) that bind to thyrotropin binding sites and cause Graves' disease. The natural history of the disease is not consistent and, indeed, it may remit after an unpredictable period of antithyroid therapy. Patients treated with radioactive iodine isotopes usually develop overt hypothyroidism at some point in their lives. Other causes of hyperthyroidism include excess pituitary secretion of thyrotropin, solitary autonomous thyroid nodules, toxic multinodular goiter, thyroid tumors, excess iodine in patients with underlying thyroid disease, and the spectrum of thyroiditis.

Postoperative complications of hyperthyroidism are best treated by preoperative preparation aimed at controlling thyroid function. This includes administration of inhibitors of thyroid hormone synthesis, propylthiouracil or methimazole, and the administration of iodides to decrease thyroid secretion and decrease thyroid gland vascularity. β-Adrenergic inhibitors may be needed to control tachycardia and hypertension, the clinical manifestations of hyperthyroidism. Lithium carbonate may also inhibit the release of thyroid hormones, but its clinical use is limited by systemic toxicity. Radioactive iodine therapy with ^{131}I is effective and provides long-term control of hyperthyroidism. Although it has not been shown to lead to thyroid cancer or to produce gonadal abnormalities, it is not routinely used in women of childbearing age but is used more often in older patients.

Thyroid storm is an exaggerated expression of hyperthyroidism. Presenting signs and symptoms include tachycardia, hypertension, high-output congestive heart failure, fever, anxiety, nausea, vomiting, and diarrhea.[19] It occurs in patients with untreated or suboptimally treated hyperthyroidism in patients undergoing surgery, both thyroidal and nonthyroidal. It also occurs during or after obstetric delivery, in patients with sepsis (particularly pharyngeal or pulmonary infections), or following trauma. Thyroid storm has been reported even after minor trauma.[20] It may also occur in patients with hyperthyroidism who have received iodine or iodide treatment preoperatively for either diagnostic or therapeutic reasons (^{131}I, supersaturated potassium iodide [SSKI] or Lugol's solution, iodide containing contrast media, or amiodarone). Amiodarone-induced thyrotoxicosis may not respond to conventional therapy, including antithyroid drugs, corticosteroids, and plasmapheresis.[21]

Thyroid storm leads to a hypermetabolic crisis similar to malignant hyperpyrexia with hypertension, tachycardia, fever, and metabolic acidosis. Untreated patients will develop coma and die. This syndrome is exceptionally rare, more so than malignant hyperthermia, and is never seen by most anesthesiologists. Because of the improved outcome with dantrolene therapy for malignant hyperpyrexia, dantrolene should be considered in all patients with the signs of a hypermetabolic crisis. Nonspecific treatment of hypermetabolic crisis induced by thyroid storm includes administration of β-adrenergic inhibitors (esmolol, propranolol, labetalol), systemic vasodilators (nitroprusside, labetalol, nitroglycerin), corticosteroids, iodides preceded by antithyroid drugs (propylthiouracil or methimazole) several hours beforehand, surface cooling, and acetaminophen. Benzodiazepines may be needed for the hyperactive, uncontrollable patient with near coma. If inotropic support is needed for congestive heart failure, phosphodiesterase inhibitors may offer the advantage of enhanced contractility without increasing heart rate. Plasma exchange has been used in a patient to control a thyrotoxic crisis.[22] Dialysis and charcoal hemofiltration may accomplish the same goals, presumably by sequestering active thyroid hormone from the circulating blood volume. When thyroid storm results from acute surgical problems, adequate blood concentrations of antithyroid drugs, including propylthiouracil and iodide, can be achieved by rectal administration, even in the presence of gastrointestinal dysfunction.[23] Metastatic lesions from follicular thyroid adenocarcinoma can be the source of hormone production leading to thyroid storm. Naito et al[24] report the prolonged course of thyroid storm seen in a patient with extensive burns following a suicide attempt that proved to be successful after an 80-day hospitalization. Despite aggressive therapy with thyroid blocking agents, β-adrenergic blocking drugs, and steroids, the patient developed all the complications associated with thyroid storm, including uncontrolled atrial fibrillation and congestive heart failure. The effects of free thyroid hormones were enhanced by marked hypoproteinemia.

B. Graves' disease

Graves' disease is the most common cause of hyperthyroidism, but the distinction between Graves' disease and other autoimmune thyroid disorders that cause hyperthyroidism is not as clear as previously thought.[25] Autoantibodies to the thyrotropin receptor or thyroidal peroxidase of follicular cells cause unregulated activation

of G-protein–regulated intracellular production of thyroid hormones. With long-term antithyroid therapy, Graves' disease may remit and 55% of patients may not need ongoing therapy.[26] Therefore thyroid function tests must be repeated periodically in patients on antithyroid therapy. [131]I therapy may be titrated to achieve normal thyroid function, but the majority of patients treated with ^{131}I therapy eventually become hypothyroid and require hormone supplementation. Thus to prevent intraoperative or postoperative hyperthyroidism or hypothyroidism, preoperative assessment should include at least the determination of blood T_4 and TSH concentrations. Elective surgery should be delayed if studies suggest inadequate treatment of hyperthyroidism.

Ironically, patients with hyperthyroidism may have impaired hemodynamic ability to respond to stress. In one study, patients with Graves' disease had higher resting heart rates and ejection fractions than controls but had limited ability to increase those parameters with exercise beyond the anaerobic threshold.[27] Paroxysmal atrial fibrillation is reported to occur in as many as 25% of patients with hyperthyroidism. In fact, hyperthyroidism is the cause of atrial fibrillation in 15% of patients presenting with the arrhythmia. The signal-averaged P-wave duration may be able to predict which patients with hyperthyroidism are at risk of developing atrial fibrillation.[28] β-Adrenergic blocking therapy would be the logical choice for control of atrial fibrillation occurring as a complication of surgical stress.

C. Jodbasedow phenomenon

Transient hyperthyroidism may occur in patients with autonomously active thyroid nodules who move from an endemic area of iodide deficiency to an area with excess iodide in the diet.[29] Hyperthyroidism may occur anywhere from 6 months to 3 years after relocation and may not return to baseline for several years. Of more concern in the United States, where there are no areas of iodide deficiency, is a similar syndrome of hyperthyroidism that may occur following administration of iodinated antiinfective agents, SSKI, iodinated oral or intravenous contrast agents, or amiodarone as an antiarrhythmic.[30] The risk of this phenomenon is low and probably requires the presence of a goiter with loss of controlled production of thyroid hormones.

D. Thyroiditis

Thyroiditis is often a self-limited inflammatory disease with autoantibodies that stimulate the thyrotropin receptor. Hashimoto's thyroiditis is an advanced form of thyroiditis that eventually results in replacement of thyroid follicles by a lymphocytic infiltrate. Postpartum thyroiditis occurs in up to 10% of women during the first year after delivery. It tends to reoccur with subsequent pregnancies and may progress to clinical hyperthyroidism or hypothyroidism. Again, postoperative complications can be prevented by baseline blood testing of thyroid function.

E. Hyperthyroidism in pregnancy

Perioperative complications secondary to hyperthyroidism occur in both the mother and the neonate when the endocrinopathy is not controlled with antithyroid drugs during pregnancy. The prevalence of hyperthyroidism in pregnancy is 0.2%, and the usual cause is Graves' disease. Thyroid storm, toxemia, premature delivery, placenta abruptio, congestive heart failure, and thyroid crisis are common in patients whose hyperthyroidism has not been controlled throughout pregnancy.[31] Neonatal mortality is increased, as are prematurity and neonatal growth abnormalities. If administration of maternal antithyroid medication has been excessive, neonates may have goiter at the time of delivery.[32] In one series of 32 patients, even among those with hyperthyroidism known and treated before conception, the incidence of maternal and fetal complications was high: preterm labor 25%, pregnancy-induced hypertension 22%, thyroid crisis 9%, and intrauterine growth retardation 13%. One maternal death occurred because of thyroid storm. One neonate developed thyrotoxicosis, and two were hypothyroid.[31]

F. Thyroid adenoma

Thyroid adenomas may function independently, that is, without the need for TSH stimulation. When trophic hormone control is lost, T_4 secretion is not regulated and hyperthyroidism results. On scan, these adenomas present as hot nodules and hyperthyroidism can be controlled by thyroid lobectomy.

G. Factitious hyperthyroidism

Thyroid hormone supplements, most commonly levothyroxine, are commonly prescribed medications; as with other medications, poor compliance with the prescription may include surreptitious or inadvertent overdose leading to untreated clinical hyperthyroidism. In one case, a patient with an evolving myocardial infarction developed severe thyrotoxicosis that required β-adrenergic blocker therapy to control heart rate and fever.[33] Myocardial contractility was compromised by esmolol but improved with amrinone.

H. Hypothyroidism

Hypothyroidism is the most common endocrinopathy, and its most common cause is long-standing Hashimoto's thyroiditis. Another common cause is ^{131}I therapy for hyperthyroidism. It is found in approximately 2% of the population and is more common in women over the age of 40.[18] Unfortunately, it is often overdiagnosed, and long-term therapy with levothyroxine may be overprescribed.

Patients with hypothyroidism can be divided into two groups based on outcomes following anesthesia and surgery. First, patients with subclinical or clinical hypothyroidism may have suggestive findings on history and physical examination with decreased T_4 and increased TSH blood concentrations; second, patients with advanced myxedema have clear-cut findings on examination, cold and exercise intolerance, abnormal metabolism, and markedly low T_4 and increased TSH blood concentrations. Because of frequently cited case reports of adverse outcome following anesthesia and surgery in patients with hypothyroidism, there has been unnecessary delay before elective surgery in many patients whose thyroid function tests are minimally abnormal.[34,35] Case-controlled studies of a large number of patients with clinical hypothyroidism show no significant difference in outcome between patients with hypothyroidism and matched controls.[36,37] Patients with clinical hypothyroidism do not have increased sensitivity to anesthetic agents, hemodynamic instability, or unusual need for vasopressors. They are not at greater risk of developing hypothermia or metabolic acidosis postoperatively.

If a patient has been diagnosed as having clinical or subclinical hypothyroidism, improvement in symptoms may occur within a few days of initiation of levothyroxine therapy, but optimal improvement may not occur for several weeks. It is unnecessary to delay elective surgery until optimal hormone effect has been achieved.[38] It has been suggested that patients with clinical hypothyroidism may have difficulty with separation from cardiopulmonary bypass following cardiac surgery. However, a review of controlled studies failed to show significant decreases in cardiac output, increased need for vasopressor support, or prolonged length of stay.[39] Klemperer et al[40] showed that levothyroxine therapy during and after cardiopulmonary bypass increased cardiac index, but control patients had no significant difference in the need for inotropic support and there was no difference in outcome between the two groups. Preoperative thyroxine therapy is not without risk in patients scheduled for coronary artery bypass surgery. Increases in heart rate and myocardial contractility following levothyroxine therapy may exacerbate myocardial ischemia and lead to increased risk of infarction.[41]

Myxedema has been recognized since the late 1800s, when it was described as a cretinoid state. Patients with severe hypothyroidism can survive without difficulty until faced with a complicating medical condition, which may precipitate myxedema coma. Until the advent of intensive care, myxedema coma was often fatal. Levothyroxine, 400 to 500 mg intravenously, combined with adrenocorticosteroids is effective in resuscitating the patient with myxedema coma as long as the precipitating systemic disease is controlled.[42] Treatment should also include reversal of hypothermia, cardiovascular support, and support of ventilation.

I. Euthyroid sick syndrome

During periods of critical illness, high-risk patients may appear to have an inadequate hemodynamic response to stress, become hypothermic, and appear to have clinical hypothyroidism.[43] The blood concentration of levothyroxine is low and that of thyrotropin is normal. Secondary hypothyroidism from pituitary dysfunction can be ruled out by measuring the response to ACTH. Mortality is increased in patients with euthyroid sick syndrome and is not improved by treatment with levothyroxine. The syndrome may represent impaired receptor sensitivity or down-regulation of the thyrotropin receptor.

III. SURGERY INVOLVING THE THYROID GLAND

Thyroid surgery has been well described and performed since the 1860s. Despite the clearly defined technique, the same complications continue to occur. The more common complications include injury to the recurrent laryngeal nerve, inadvertent removal or devascularization injury to the parathyroid glands, and postoperative hematoma formation. Thyroid storm may result from manipulation of the thyroid when thyroidectomy is being performed for hyperthyroidism, thyroid adenoma, multinodular goiter, or functioning follicular thyroid carcinoma. Rarer complications may occur when extensive lymph node dissection is performed. These include venous air embolism and injury to major vessels, nerves other than the recurrent laryngeal, the thoracic duct, the trachea, and the esophagus. With very large suprasternal or substernal goiters or thyroid tumors, removal may unmask instability of the anterior tracheal rings with tracheomalacia and postoperative respiratory distress.

A. Vocal cord injury

Risk of vocal cord injury is related to the skill and experience of the surgeon and the extent of the surgery, but most reports estimate the risk at 2% or less.[44] Injury may be unilateral, particularly with subtotal thyroidectomy, or bilateral with more extensive surgery. Injury does not require transection of the nerves. Excessive traction or devascularization can result in temporary or permanent paresis of the abductor muscles of the larynx. When unilateral, the patient is left with hoarseness; when bilateral, aphonia and near total airway obstruction may occur. The cords lie in the median position at rest and are tightly opposed with activation of the adductor muscles. Respiratory distress may require reintubation and elective, long-term tracheostomy followed by vocal cord stenting procedures.

It is often forgotten that dissection of the superior pole of the thyroid gland and division of its blood supply can lead to injury of the superior laryngeal nerve with loss of forceful phonation. With this injury, the vocal cords may be tightly abducted by unopposed recurrent laryngeal nerve innervation of the abductor muscles, leaving the patient at risk of aspiration.

Traditionally, it is taught that the laryngeal nerves are best protected by gentle identification throughout their course, but many filmy slips of areolar tissue can be mistaken for these nerves. Preoperative endoscopy with phonation establishes the integrity of the laryngeal nerves before surgical dissection. Invasive tumors can destroy these nerves and cause vocal cord paresis. With identification of intact laryngeal nerves, most anesthesiologists do not perform direct laryngoscopy at extubation. However, if the status of the nerves is in doubt, if the surgery has been extensive, or if the patient has abnormal phonation or signs of airway obstruction, direct laryngoscopy should be carried out to determine whether reintubation and tracheostomy is needed. At the conclusion of surgery, inspection of the vocal cords can be performed with extubation under direct vision with a rigid laryngoscope or with removal of the endotracheal tube over a fiberoptic laryngoscope.

In a unique approach, the vocal cords can be observed directly during dissection and stimulation of the recurrent laryngeal nerve.[45] General anesthesia is maintained by use of a laryngeal mask airway, and a fiberoptic endoscope is positioned just proximal to the glottis. Adduction of the cords can be seen when they are stimulated with a nerve stimulator at the conclusion of the thyroidectomy.

B. Acute hypoparathyroidism

The risk of iatrogenic hypoparathyroidism after thyroidectomy is directly related to the extent of thyroid surgery. It is greater with total thyroidectomy than with subtotal thyroidectomy and greatest if radical lymphadenectomy has been performed in addition to thyroidectomy. Injury of the vascular supply to the parathyroid glands may be as effective as inadvertent parathyroidectomy in causing acute postoperative hypoparathyroidism. Estimates of incidence range from 0.9% to 20%.[46] Acute hypoparathyroidism can be recognized by classic symptoms of severe hypocalcemia: anxiety, circumoral numbness, and signs of skeletal muscle hyperreactivity (Chvostek's sign). Significant adverse cardiovascular effects of severe hypocalcemia can be prevented by heightened awareness of the potential problem and frequent testing of blood calcium concentrations after thyroid surgery.

If radical excision of a thyroid tumor is performed and parathyroids are identified, they can be transplanted into the sternocleidomastoid muscle.[47] As noted later in this chapter, in patients with hyperparathyroidism secondary to chronic renal failure, total parathyroidectomy can be performed and a solitary gland transplanted to the subcutaneous tissue of the forearm.

If a patient develops significant hypocalcemia after thyroid or parathyroid surgery, calcium should be administered as an intravenous bolus for control of acute symptoms and should be followed by a continuous calcium infusion because of the short half-life of the initial bolus. Intravenous calcium should be continued until the patient is able to take oral calcium supplements along with vitamin D.

C. Thyroid goiter

Goiter is a nonspecific diagnosis describing a thyroid gland that is twice or more its normal size. Goiter can result from a variety of causes, including iodine-deficient diet, excessive iodine intake, drug reaction, chronic inflammatory reaction, long-term TSH stimulation, or autonomous thyroid function. Goiter may present in the neck or it may extend into the substernal area (Fig. 14-1). The enlarged thyroid may be associated with apparently normal thyroid function (euthyroid) or with hyperthyroidism or hypothyroidism.

Goiters are usually nontoxic, and the major complaint is the patient's concern about a mass in the neck, with worry about malignancy or disfigurement. The sudden onset of pain and enlargement of the goiter may result from hemorrhage in the substance of the gland. Hashimoto's thyroiditis with goiter may lead to neck tenderness. Otherwise, goiters usually are not painful. Distortion of the normal neck anatomy may cause neuropraxia of the recurrent laryngeal nerve, with hoarseness. Venous engorgement can result from thoracic outlet obstruction from very large or malignant goiters. Goiters usually do not respond to TSH suppression with levothyroxine or to ^{131}I irradiation preoperatively and require surgical removal if the patient is symptomatic.

Thyroid goiters may distort the normal anatomy of the upper airway. At the subglottic level, goiters may displace the glottis and lead to difficulty with bag-mask ventilation or tracheal intubation. At the substernal level,

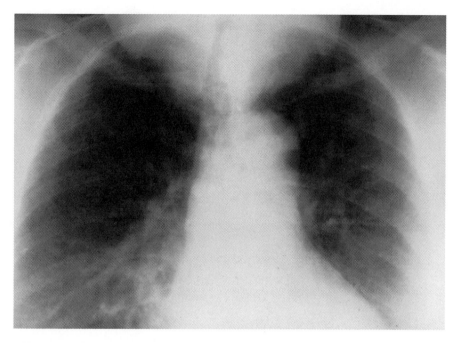

Fig. 14-1. Goiter may present in the neck or it may extend into the substernal area.

goiters may compress the trachea with a narrow tracheal lumen or they may produce tracheomalacia by compression of tracheal rings. Tracheomalacia usually is not a problem until tracheal extubation is attempted following removal of the substernal goiter. At that point, the tracheal lumen can be seen to collapse with voluntary inspiration because of the lack of extraluminal support. This phenomenon is best observed by fiberoptic bronchoscopy through the endotracheal tube at the time of extubation. If the airway is seen to "fish-mouth," the bronchoscope is left in place and the endotracheal tube is immediately reinserted. Then ventilation is supported with positive pressure and either controlled or spontaneous ventilation. Positive-pressure support may be required for a period of days before the surrounding mediastinal tissues are able to support the tracheal wall during inspiration, with subatmospheric pressure applied during inspiration. Preoperative posteroanterior chest radiograph and computed tomography (CT) scan of the neck are particularly helpful in predicting difficulty with endotracheal intubation and collapse of the trachea postoperatively. The flow-volume loop on pulmonary function testing may show findings typical of intrathoracic or extrathoracic obstruction with goiters (Fig. 14-2).

D. Expanding hematoma

Expanding hematoma in the neck following thyroidectomy can be a life-threatening complication because of acute airway obstruction. The most likely cause is dislodging a surgical ligature from a thyroidal artery or vein. The risk of this complication argues in favor of a minimal surgical dressing following neck surgery. Bulky dressings, wrapped towels, and neck collars will obscure an expanding hematoma until airway compression occurs.

Treatment consists of immediate opening of the surgical incision to allow decompression of the hematoma. If there has been significant blood loss and the patient is hypotensive from bleeding from a large neck vein, he or she may be at increased risk of air entrainment and venous air embolism if the hematoma is drained with the patient breathing spontaneously in the sitting position.

E. Thyroid tumors

Patients with thyroid tumors often require subtotal or total thyroidectomy, often with lymph node sampling or extensive lymph node dissection, depending on the nature of the thyroid tumor.[48] Preoperative or intraoperative histologic diagnosis based on fine needle aspiration or frozen section examination will determine the extent of surgical resection and the likelihood of postoperative complications. Mechanical complications (hematoma, nerve injury, iatrogenic parathyroidectomy, thoracic duct injury, phrenic or cranial nerve injury) are more common in these patients.

F. Parathyroid glands

The average person has four parathyroid glands symmetrically located, two located superiorly in the neck and two inferiorly. However, the number of glands may vary from one to twelve and the variability of their location may be a challenge to the surgeon. The parathyroid glands secrete parathyroid hormone (PTH) in response to a low serum concentration of ionized calcium. However, PTH is only one of three hormones that respond to hypocalcemia; the others are calcitonin secreted from C-cells in the thyroid gland and 1,25-dihydroxyvitamin D (1,25[OH$_2$]D) produced in the proximal tubules of the kidney. Parathyroid gland cells sense a decreased ionized calcium blood concentration and secrete PTH.

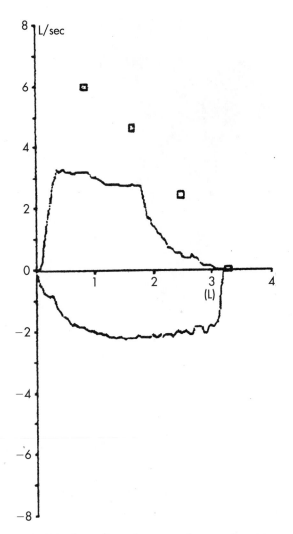

Fig. 14-2. The flow-volume loop on pulmonary function testing may show findings typical of intrathoracic or extrathoracic obstruction with goiters with diminished peak expiratory flow.

PTH increases renal excretion of phosphate, increases reabsorption of calcium, and stimulates the production of $1,25(OH_2)D$. The $1,25(OH_2)D$ increases absorption of calcium and phosphorus from the intestine. PTH and $1,25(OH_2)D$ increase the release of calcium from bone. An increasing plasma concentration of ionized calcium inhibits the secretion of PTH and closes the loop of negative feedback inhibition. PTH, like so many other endocrine hormones, is a first messenger, which is a ligand for G-protein–associated receptors that increase adenylate cyclase and phospholipase C activity. cAMP-mediated phosphorylation controls calcium-activated mechanisms that produce the primary messenger hormone effect.

Calcitonin is an enigma. It is not clear how its release from the thyroid is controlled, nor is its role in controlling the plasma concentration of ionized understood. It promotes the excretion of calcium in the urine and seems to protect bone from excessive reabsorption of calcium.

G. Hyperparathyroidism

Hyperparathyroidism results from parathyroid hyperplasia with a normal set point for response to plasma calcium concentrations but with a simple excess of parathyroid cells. Parathyroid adenoma is the second cause of hyperparathyroidism and usually involves a single gland functioning autonomously. Benign adenomas have a large number of PTH-secreting cells with an excessively high set point for inhibition of release of PTH. These tumors probably result from the abnormal expression of a monoclonal gene, either the PTH or the PRAD1 oncogene.[49] Parathyroid carcinoma is present in less than 0.5% of patients with hypercalcemia but should be suspected when there is marked hypercalcemia (more than 16 mg/dl), a palpable mass in the neck, and recent onset of hoarseness.[50]

Excess PTH in hyperparathyroidism causes hypercalcemia, renal lithiasis, proximal muscle atrophy, and osteitis fibrosa cystica. Pancreatitis, peptic ulceration, and systemic hypertension are other manifestations of hyperparathyroidism. Hypercalcemia produces a shortened QT interval on ECG. Indications for surgery include a serum calcium concentration greater than 12 mg/dl, marked hypercalcuria, overt manifestations of the disease, markedly reduced bone density, impaired renal function without other cause, and age less than 50 years.[51] The majority of patients are asymptomatic and are diagnosed on routine measurement of serum calcium concentration. Medical treatment of hyperparathyroidism has few options, although oral phosphates, 1 to 2 g/day, may reduce the serum calcium concentration 0.5 to 1 mg/dl.

The risk of postoperative complications is directly related to the number of parathyroid glands removed because of their appearance, hyperplastic or adenomatous. The highest risk is when all four glands are removed because of hyperplasia. Subtotal parathyroidectomy results in recurrent hyperparathyroidism in up to 16% of patients with nonfamilial hyperplasia. In this group, permanent hypoparathyroidism occurs in 4% to 5% of patients.[52] The incidence of recurrent disease is greater (26% to 36% at 5 years) in patients with MEN-1 syndrome, a familial form of the disease.[53] Postoperative hypoparathyroidism leads to severe hypocalcemia and must be treated with a continuous intravenous infusion of calcium.

Recurrent hyperparathyroidism results from inadequate resection of parathyroid tissue at the time of initial surgery, and reexploration of the neck looking for additional parathyroid tissue can be difficult. Alternatives for further control include repeated resection and autotransplantation of a reduced-size gland to an area, such as the forearm, where repeated resection can be performed easily under local anesthesia.

H. Hypoparathyroidism

Hypoparathyroidism is most often a surgical complication of thyroid surgery or excessive removal of parathyroid tissue. Nonsurgical causes are rare but their presentation includes hypocalcemia, usually with skeletal defects. It may be part of a polyendocrinopathy associated with hypoadrenalism and mucocutaneous candidiasis (HAM syndrome). Pseudohypoparathyroidism leads to hypocalcemia in the presence of elevated blood concentrations of PTH because of the absence of PTH receptors in the renal tubules. This may result in musculoskeletal abnormalities in children and adults that require surgery and may manifest significant hypocalcemia in the postoperative period.

IV. ADRENAL GLANDS

Much like the pituitary gland, the adrenal glands are functionally two glands in one, with distinctly different hormones secreted from the medullary and cortical portion. In fact, the two portions of the gland have separate arterial supplies, with a conjoined venous drainage.[54] The adrenal cortex is a typical endocrine gland, with a closed-loop negative feedback mechanism of corticotropin-releasing hormone (CRH) and ACTH secretion controlling its activity.[55] The adrenocortical hormones affect most tissues in the body and have a prolonged onset time compared to the medullary hormones; their half-life is controlled by hepatic metabolism and renal excretion. The medullary portions of the adrenal glands are part of the neuroendocrine system, with control exhibited from the vasomotor centers in the central nervous system via the efferent autonomic nervous system. The effects of medullary hormones are terminated primarily by uptake with high affinity at preganglionic sympathetic nerve terminals (uptake 1) and by low affinity into muscle tissue (uptake 2). Metabolism occurs in both neuronal and nonneuronal tissue and involves monamine oxidase and catechol-o-methyl transferase, respectively. The neuroendocrine function of the adrenal medulla does not have the distinct closed-loop negative feedback control seen in the adrenal cortex, pituitary, and thyroid glands. Both the adrenal cortical and adrenal medullary hormones have direct physiologic effects on virtually all tissues in the body, especially the cardiovascular systems. Thus these endocrine glands are an important consideration in understanding the nature of postoperative complications.

A. Adrenal cortical hormones

The adrenal cortical hormones include a number of compounds derived from substitutions on the basic steroid nucleus. By common name they include aldosterone, corticosterone, cortisol (hydrocortisone), cortisone, dehydroepiandrosterone, deoxycorticosterone, deoxycortisol, estradiol, progesterone, and testosterone. Postoperative complications seldom involve the last three, and we do not address postoperative reproductive function in this chapter. The others are conveniently divided into mineralocorticoids (primarily aldosterone) and glucocorticoids (primarily cortisol). Corticosterone shares both glucocorticoid and mineralocorticoid activity and is a synthetic precursor of both.

Cortisol secretion is controlled by ACTH that, like TSH, is a specific ligand for a G-protein–linked receptor that activates adenylate cyclase and produces cAMP. As discussed earlier, pituitary adenomas arising from corticotropic cells secrete excessive ACTH and produce Cushing's disease with hyperadrenocorticalism. Panhypopituitarism leads to chronic adrenal suppression and is one cause of adrenal insufficiency. Aldosterone secretion is controlled by the kidney, not the pituitary. The ligand for the adrenal receptor, again G-protein linked to adenylate cyclase, that controls aldosterone secretion is angiotensin II.[56] The angiotensin-converting enzyme (ACE) controls production of angiotensin II from angiotensin I. Angiotensin I secretion is stimulated by renin in response to decreases in renal vascular pressure and changes in potassium concentration. To a limited extent, aldosterone secretion also is stimulated by ACTH.[57] This simplified outline of the control of adrenal hormone secretion will be helpful in understanding the mechanisms involved in a variety of postoperative complications.

B. Cushing's syndrome

Cushing's disease is adrenal hyperplasia in response to excess ACTH production. Cushing's syndrome is adrenal hyperplasia with excess production of cortisol from endogenous or exogenous sources. Endogenous causes of hypercortisolism depend on ACTH production (usually pituitary or hypothalamic; rarely ectopic production of CRH) or are independent of ACTH (adrenal hyperplasia, adenoma, carcinoma). Exogenous causes include prednisone or cortisone therapy for inflammatory or autoimmune disease or immunosuppression or may result from illicit steroid (androgen) ingestion.

Cushing's syndrome is diagnosed on the results of blood hormone assays performed in patients with hypertension and classic physical findings of the syndrome. The more florid features of the syndrome usually result from ACTH-dependent causes, whereas functioning adrenal adenomas present only with signs and symptoms of increased protein catabolism. These are diagnosed on CT scans obtained for evaluation of abdominal complaints. Alternatives for treatment include surgery (transphenoidal hypophysectomy or adrenalectomy), pituitary irradiation with cobalt-60, or administration of competitive inhibitors of ligands or noncompetitive antagonists of ligand synthesis. In one series of 79 consecutive patients with Cushing's syndrome, there were 3 early postoperative deaths following bilateral adrenalectomy.[58]

Of the inhibitors, etomidate is uniquely important to the anesthesiologist because it is an inhibitor of adrenal 11-β-hydroxylase, an enzyme important to the synthesis of both aldosterone and cortisol.[59] Although it is used often in patients with hemodynamic concerns, it should be remembered that adrenal suppression may last 5 to 8 hours after a single induction dose of etomidate.[60] Etomidate has been used in large doses for cerebral protection during aneurysm surgery, and it may be used in procedures in which it is important to monitor evoked somatosensory potentials. In these settings, resulting postoperative adrenal insufficiency may be important and necessitate supplemental corticosteroid therapy. Etomidate has been shown to increase mortality secondary to adrenal suppression when used for long-term sedation. It is not used for therapy of hypercortisolism because of its anesthetic effect.

Pituitary surgery for an ACTH-secreting microadenoma or macroadenoma is minimally invasive and highly successful in controlling Cushing's disease. Complete resection of an adenoma can usually be achieved without producing adrenal suppression secondary to ACTH deficiency. However, postoperative cardiovascular instability might be secondary to adrenal insufficiency and warrants intravenous administration of glucocorticoids.

Adrenal surgery for a functioning adenoma may cause adrenal insufficiency because of the long-standing negative feedback inhibition of ACTH secretion. This surgery produces temporary adrenal insufficiency of the second adrenal gland, and the patient may need cortisol replacement for over a year before the remaining adrenal gland returns to normal function.

Adrenal hyperplasia independent of ACTH stimulation requires bilateral adrenalectomy with life-long corticosteroid replacement therapy. Nelson's syndrome is a complication of bilateral adrenalectomy. In the absence of negative feedback inhibition of ACTH secretion, pituitary corticotrope hyperplasia or adenoma develops and excess secretion of ACTH results in hyperpigmentation.

Carcinoma of the adrenal gland is a highly malignant disease. Excess hormone production may be controlled temporarily by surgery or antagonist therapy but recurrence is common and is associated with hypercortisolism.

C. Hyperaldosteronism (Conn syndrome)

The renin-angiotensin-aldosterone system regulates extracellular fluid volume and its sodium and potassium concentrations. Excess aldosterone secretion results in hypertension, expanded extracellular fluid volume, sodium retention, and potassium loss. Primary hyperaldosteronism results from the uncontrolled production of aldosterone in the adrenal gland and is responsible for approximately 2% of cases of hypertension.[61] Primary hyperaldosteronism may be caused by a unilateral adrenal adenoma or by bilateral adrenal hyperplasia, with the cause determining surgical or combined medical-surgical therapy. Adrenalectomy does not cure hypertension in patients with idiopathic hyperaldosteronism, and they should be treated with calcium-channel blockers, ACE inhibitors, or angiotensin IIB inhibitors. If spironolactone administration controls hypertension, adrenalectomy may be indicated. In one form of primary hyperaldosteronism, dexamethasone suppresses ACTH and aldosterone secretion. Unfortunately, this is associated with overall adrenal suppression. The important findings in primary hyperaldosteronism include hypertension and hypokalemia, a clue to the cause of postoperative hypertension.

D. Hypoaldosteronism

Isolated hypoaldosteronism results from a number of causes but is distinguished from adrenal insufficiency by the presence of normal cortisol production. Isolated hypoaldosteronism leads to hyperkalemia, with muscle weakness and cardiac arrhythmias. It can result from inherited metabolic defects that prevent the synthesis of aldosterone, or it can evolve from autoimmune adrenalitis with early selective involvement of the portion of the gland that produces aldosterone. This may be part of the multiple autoimmune endocrinopathy described earlier.

Plasma renin activity is high, aldosterone may be not detectable, and adrenal antibodies can be demonstrated. Serum electrolytes may show metabolic acidosis and hyponatremia. Hypoaldosteronism may also occur in critically ill patients such as those with septic or cardiogenic shock. A stress-evoked chronically increased ACTH concentration may inhibit the enzymes involved in aldosterone production. Atrial natruretic hormone is markedly increased in chronic illness and is a natural inhibitor of aldosterone production. Other mediators associated with critical illness that inhibit production of aldosterone include interleukin-1 and tumor necrosis factor. Competitive inhibitors of the renin-angiotensin system, such as valsartan, may cause hypoaldosteronism, but these are seldom significant causes of clinically important hypoaldosteronism. However, they must be avoided when patients may have hypoaldosteronism from other causes.

Chronic renal disease is a common cause of secondary hypoaldosteronism. These patients have low plasma renin activity. Electrolyte abnormalities include hyperkalemia in all patients as well as hyponatremia and hyperchloremic metabolic acidosis in many. This syndrome, hyporeninemic hypoaldosteronism (SHH), may be seen in many forms of chronic renal disease, including diabetic nephrosclerosis, interstitial nephritis, anatomic urinary tract abnormalities, analgesic abuse, and human immunodeficiency virus nephropathy.[62] Drug therapy can also produce hypoaldosteronism in the postoperative period. Responsible agents include cyclosporine, long-term heparin therapy, β-adrenergic blockers, and prostaglandin synthetase inhibitors. ACE inhibitors and dopaminergic antagonists also may reduce aldosterone secretion.

Pseudohypoaldosteronism is known to occur in two forms, one in children (type I) and the other in adults (type II or Gordon's syndrome). Severe salt wasting occurs in children but not in adults. A low aldosterone concentration is associated with decreased renin production and electrolyte abnormalities, mainly hyperchloremic acidosis.

E. Adrenal insufficiency (Addison's disease)

Adrenal insufficiency may be primary or secondary. We have already alluded to causes of secondary adrenal insufficiency, those caused by hypothalamic or pituitary dysfunction with loss of corticotrophin-releasing factor or ACTH. Other secondary causes include exogenous glucocorticoids or ACTH and cures used for Cushing's syndrome.

Primary adrenal insufficiency can be caused by autoimmune adrenalitis or tuberculosis. Adrenalitis is recognized as the more common of the two and is responsible for approximately 70% of cases of primary adrenal insufficiency.[63] One form of the syndrome is seen in children, and another occurs in adults. Autoimmune adrenalitis may be part of a multiple endocrine autoimmune disease in which adrenal insufficiency occurs along with hypothyroidism, hypoparathyroidism, mucocutaneous candidiasis, ovarian failure, type I diabetes mellitus, pernicious anemia, or other autoimmune syndromes. Antibodies to adrenal enzymes, 21-hydroxylase in adults and

Table 14-2. Intravenous glucocorticoid recommendations for urgent treatment of suspected adrenocortical insufficiency

Corticoid	Proprietary name	Intravenous bolus dose (mg)	Time to onset	HPA suppression duration (hr)	20-mg cortisol equivalent (mg)
Methylprednisolone	Solumedrol	10-250	Immediate	12-36	4
Dexamethasone	Decadron	0.5-25	Rapid	36-54	0.75
Hydrocortisone	Solucortef	20-300	Immediate	30-36	25

HPA, Hypophyseal-pituitary-adrenal.

17-hydroxylase in children, can be identified in two thirds of patients with primary adrenal insufficiency.

For the detection and management of postoperative complications, the most important other cause of acute adrenal insufficiency is adrenal hemorrhage associated with septic shock such as that seen with severe meningococcemia (Waterhouse-Friderichsen syndrome). Adrenal hemorrhage should be suspected in the patient with postoperative sepsis when hypotension does not respond to fluid volume replacement and vasopressor support. If these patients develop a cortisol concentration less than 20 mg/dl, they should be treated with intravenous glucocorticoids. Often, the blood cortisol concentration may be nearly unmeasurable. Again, acute adrenal insufficiency should be suspected in any critically ill patient whose hypotension does not respond appropriately to standard therapy.

Secondary adrenal insufficiency may be seen in patients who have abused steroids or have received long-term prednisone or cortisone therapy. Adrenal suppression usually does not occur with short-term (less than 1 week) steroid therapy (equivalent to 20 to 30 mg of prednisone per day).[64] For patients who have received larger dosages or for longer periods of time, an ACTH stimulation test can determine whether they have persistent adrenal suppression. If this test has not been done, it is prudent to suspect adrenal suppression for a year after termination of steroid therapy. Replacement or stress-dosage steroid therapy for adults typically has included hydrocortisone, 100 mg every 12 hours (Table 14-2). This dosage is probably excessive based on the estimation of normal daily production of cortisol in adults. Dexamethasone is the most potent of the available corticosteroids for replacement therapy. It has the longest half-life as well. Cortisone acetate and prednisone depend on hepatic metabolism before becoming bioactive. They have the shortest half-lives. Corticosteroids used for replacement therapy may aggravate systemic hypertension, a consideration to be kept in mind in patients with increased intracranial pressure or myocardial ischemia.

F. Adrenal medullary hormones

The adrenal medulla functions as a postganglionic neuron in the sympathetic nervous system. It is capable of secreting three humoral neurotransmitters: dopamine, norepinephrine, and epinephrine. Because of the redundancy of the autonomic nervous system, adrenal secretion of catecholamines is not essential for normal well-being. Therefore bilateral adrenalectomy does not lead to catecholamine deficiency.

G. Pheochromocytoma

Pheochromocytoma is the important endocrinopathy related to the adrenal medulla. It may be benign or malignant, unilateral or bilateral, familial or nonfamilial. The "rule of 10s" applies: 10% are bilateral, 10% are familial, 10% are malignant.

Norepinephrine is the principal hormone secreted in the majority of pheochromocytomas, with epinephrine and dopamine being secreted in lesser amounts. Epinephrine may be the principal catecholamine secreted when the pheochromocytoma arises from adrenal or extraadrenal chromaffin cells containing phenylethanolamine *N*-methyl transferase, the enzyme that converts norepinephrine to epinephrine. These sites include the brain, lung, urinary bladder, and the organ of Zuckerkandl. Other extraadrenal sites where these tumors can grow include the carotid body, aortic chemoreceptors, and sympathetic ganglia.

The treatment of patients with pheochromocytoma is well described in all anesthesiology texts. Standard treatment includes the use of α-adrenergic blocking agents to control hypertension and, when necessary, β-adrenergic blocking agents to control reflex tachycardia. Phenoxybenzamine therapy has given way to prazosin therapy as managed care practitioners have prescribed outpatient preparation for surgery. α-Adrenergic blocking agents are given as needed to control hypertension, perhaps to the point of orthostatic hypotension. Secondary correction of extracellular fluid volume expansion occurs and is monitored by progressive lowering of the hematocrit. Intraoperatively, sodium nitroprusside and either esmolol or labetalol are used to control hypertension and tachycardia during excision of the tumor. Magnesium sulfate has been used for additional control of hemodynamics during tumor removal.[65]

Postoperative complications are more appropriately considered management of the persistent effects of adrenergic blocking agents following removal of the source of excess catecholamine secretion. In addition, catecholamine-induced cardiomyopathy may be a significant cause of hypotension and decreased cardiac output after removal of a pheochromocytoma. Invasive hemodynamic monitoring should guide postoperative fluid volume expansion and hemodynamic support with vasopressors, usually phenylephrine. If bilateral adrenalectomy has been performed or if the patient has had long-standing hypertension from a pheochromocytoma, concurrent adrenocortical suppression may be present and the patient may need intravenous glucocorticoids for refractory hypotension.

Acute and chronic adrenal insufficiency will occur following bilateral adrenalectomy for bilateral pheochromocytoma in patients with MEN syndrome. This will require short-term parenteral glucocorticoid replacement and long-term oral steroid therapy. This postoperative problem can be prevented by cortical-sparing adrenalectomy. In one series, cortical sparing was possible in 14 of 15 patients who had bilateral adrenalectomy for benign bilateral pheochromocytomas.[66] Thirteen of the 14 patients had a normal blood cortisol concentration postoperatively. However, three patients developed late (average 17 years) recurrence of pheochromocytoma. Two patients died of metastatic medullary thyroid carcinoma.

Like many other abdominal procedures, adrenalectomy, even bilateral, can be performed successfully in most patients with minimal blood loss and shortened length of stay, without the discomfort and morbidity associated with an extensive laparotomy or bilateral flank incision.[67]

H. Multiple endocrinopathy

Pheochromocytoma occurs in patients with MEN type IIA and IIB. Pheochromocytoma is seen in 50% of patients with MEN type IIA.[68] All patients with pheochromocytoma should have determinations of serum calcium and calcitonin for the diagnosis of coexisting hyperparathyroidism and medullary carcinoma of the thyroid gland. These measurements must be repeated indefinitely if there is evidence of familial transmission. When coexisting endocrinopathy exists, removal of the pheochromocytoma takes precedence over treatment of hyperparathyroidism and medullary carcinoma. Therefore magnesium therapy may be needed to control postoperative hypercalcemia in a patient with MEN II syndrome.

V. PANCREATIC ISLET CELLS

The pancreas is one of the glands of the digestive system that has the unique property of having both endocrine and exocrine function, and the endocrine function involves more than one hormone. However, for this chapter we limit our discussion to the postoperative complications related to the secretion of insulin.

A. Diabetes mellitus

It is the function of the pancreas to moderate the various factors that determine glucose homeostasis. In the perioperative period the usual determinants of glucose production by the liver and glucose use by the tissues (including insulin-independent tissues such as kidney and brain) are complicated by exogenous glucose loading and an amplified and variable stress response. This pancreatic control comes from the insulin-producing β-cells and the glucagon-producing α-cells. Insulin, which functions as the primary hormone in this process, has many effects, generally acting via receptors on cell surfaces. It activates cellular transport of glucose, has important anabolic properties, and opposes the catabolic breakdown of glycogen, proteins, and fats.

The normal pancreas in a basal, unstressed state produces approximately 1 unit of insulin per hour. This free insulin has a plasma half-life on the order of 5 minutes, being cleared by hepatic, renal, and muscle pathways. In the kidney, insulin is filtered and then reabsorbed and degraded by the tubules. Insulin taken up by the muscles and adipose tissues has the important effect of stimulating glucose uptake into these tissues.

In diabetes mellitus, glucose control by insulin goes awry and many other tissues are also affected. In a rough classification, with considerable overlap, diabetes mellitus is divided into two groups. In type I diabetes mellitus, often called juvenile-onset or insulin-dependent diabetes mellitus, there is an earlier, more rapid onset, with a greater tendency to ketosis and the absolute need for exogenous insulin for metabolic control. In type II diabetes mellitus, often called adult-onset or non–insulin-dependent diabetes mellitus, the onset is later in life, more gradual, and often associated with obesity; insulin therapy is not universally needed for treatment. Of course, there is much overlap in this classification, and it is not rare for diabetic adults to develop insulin dependence.

The classic pathologic abnormality of diabetes mellitus is an impairment of glucose tolerance. This means that the patient does not clear blood glucose appropriately (i.e., does not transport the glucose efficiently into the tissues) and has abnormally high blood concentrations of glucose. In typical type I diabetes, the cause of this is abnormally low to practically absent concentrations of circulating insulin. Many type II diabetic patients have normal or even somewhat elevated concentrations of insulin, but because of resistance to insulin effect at the tissue level, they still have inadequate insulin effect.

Along with the hyperglycemia induced by insufficient insulin is the stimulation of lipolysis in fatty tissues, producing free fatty acids. These are broken down in the liver to ketone bodies. The ketone bodies, mostly acetoacetate and β-hydroxybutyrate, are important sources of fuel to the brain during starvation. When diabetes mellitus is markedly out of control, the concentrations of circulating ketones can become quite high, producing severe metabolic acidosis.

Glucagon and the stress-induced counterregulatory hormones oppose the glucose-lowering effect of insulin. Glucagon stimulates gluconeogenesis and glycogenolysis. The counterregulatory hormones epinephrine, cortisol, and GH all produce a tendency to hyperglycemia. Under medical stress, particularly infection or surgery, normal patients often are slightly hyperglycemic and diabetic patients may have major instabilities in glucose homeostasis.

The postoperative treatment of patients with diabetes mellitus must reflect the need for caloric intake to be met by glucose administration and the need for supplemental potassium replacement.[69] The method of insulin administration is determined by the scope of the surgical procedure and the ability of the patient to resume a normal diet. If surgery has been extensive and it is anticipated that the patient will not be able to resume a normal diet for a prolonged period of time, insulin should be administered as a continuous intravenous infusion, or by sliding scale, along with glucose and potassium. Hirsch et al[70] have provided guidelines for the perioperative treatment of diabetic patients (Table 14-3).[70]

Table 14-3. Algorithm for administration of intravenous insulin

Blood glucose concentration	Insulin infusion
<80 mg/dl	Discontinue; give 1.0 g dextrose; recheck.
80-120 mg/dl	Decrease by 0.3 units/hr.
120-180 mg/dl	Start infusion at 0.5-1.0 units/hr.
180-240 mg/dl	Increase by 0.3 units/hr.
>240 mg/dl	Increase by 0.5 units/hr.

Modified from Hirsch IB, McGill JB, Cryer PE, et al: *Anesthesiology* 74:346, 1991.

B. Hyperglycemia

Decreased glucose clearance from the blood combined with increased glucose production by gluconeogenesis leads to hyperglycemia. This condition can be exacerbated by metabolic stress stimulating the counterregulatory hormones. Although the nondiabetic patient can vary insulin production to maintain fairly tight control of blood glucose, even patients with type II diabetes do not have optimum control of the glucose concentration. Therefore all diabetics are subject to hyperglycemia.

The acute complications of hyperglycemia result mostly from the effects of hyperosmolarity and fluid and electrolyte imbalances. The hyperglycemia generally induces an osmotic diuresis, leading to hypovolemia and washout of electrolytes, especially potassium ion. In the setting of ketoacidosis, the plasma potassium concentration may be increased, even if cellular potassium stores are depleted, by the effect of acidosis stimulating the extracellular transport of potassium.

It is important to recognize that small amounts of circulating insulin may be enough to prevent major ketosis without being sufficient to control hyperglycemia. Therefore it is common for patients to have an increased glucose concentration before or without ketoacidosis. In some patients, hypovolemia may become very pronounced, with extreme hyperglycemia (greater than 1000 mg/dl) without ketoacidosis. This syndrome, called hyperosmolar hyperglycemic nonketotic coma, often responds nicely to rehydration with only minimal insulin supplementation.

In the hospitalized patient, particularly in the perioperative period, vigorous intravenous fluid loading is common. If glucose-containing fluids are used for this, enormous amounts of glucose can be given in a short period of time. In this setting, even normal patients may become hyperglycemic; the diabetic patient is especially vulnerable to pronounced iatrogenic hyperglycemia. This is commonly associated with hypokalemia from both the induced glycosuric diuresis and the intracellular shift of potassium stimulated by the increased concentration of glucose in the presence of even marginal amounts of insulin.

In addition to the acute effects of diabetic hyperglycemia, the diabetic patient is subject to multiple end-organ prob-

lems, each of which has its own array of potential acute complications. The chronic effects of diabetes mellitus have multiple causes and generally are not the direct results of hyperglycemia. However, it is generally accepted that long-term close control of blood glucose minimizes these end-organ effects.[71] Because of the chronic nature of the disease, it is not correct to generalize from the fact that close control of blood glucose is important in the long term to the conclusion that very tight control is necessary in the setting of acute illness or surgery. Indeed, because of the varying metabolic demands and the acute stimulation of counterregulatory systems, close control in the acute setting may be very difficult and may induce untoward hypoglycemia.

The multiple effects of chronic diabetes mellitus are often very relevant in the treatment of patients with critical illness and surgical disease. Chronic renal impairment, peripheral vascular disease, premature coronary artery disease, and cerebrovascular disease are all potentially life threatening.

C. Autonomic dysfunction

In the perioperative setting the autonomic dysfunction associated with long-standing diabetes mellitus may lead to subtle yet disabling complications. Gastric atony, with slow emptying before surgery and a delayed return of function after a postoperative ileus, predisposes the patient to vomiting and pulmonary aspiration of stomach contents.[72] Similarly, poor bladder emptying may lead to a prolonged requirement for an indwelling catheter and the concomitant discomfort and risk of infection. Autonomic cardiovascular instability may complicate the postoperative assessment of hemodynamic status and the management of fluid replacement.

D. Hyperglycemia and the brain

Hyperglycemia exacerbates the effect of ischemia on the brain. It is likely that an increased supply of glucose to the brain during ischemia leads to increased intracellular glycolysis and lactic acid production. Because glucose transport in the brain is not dependent on insulin, even if the patient is insulin deficient, hyperglycemia will result in increased brain intracellular glucose. Because mild cerebral ischemia is a potential risk for all anesthetics, and a common risk during neurosurgery or cardiopulmonary bypass, careful glucose control during anesthesia is desirable. During neurosurgery and cardiac procedures, tight glucose control is standard practice, maintaining plasma glucose in the 150 to 200 mg/dl range.[73]

E. Diabetic ketoacidosis

The diabetic patient with a severe deficiency of insulin plus stimulation of the counterregulatory hormones is at great risk for developing diabetic ketoacidosis (DKA). This is characterized by an increased concentration of ketone bodies, leading to metabolic acidosis. Hyperglycemia is almost always present but may not be very extreme; the blood glucose concentration is generally less than 500 mg/dl, and may even be as low as 250 mg/dl. Patients with DKA are generally hypovolemic, weak, and confused, with polyuria and often abdominal pain. The acidosis may be very marked, and the compensatory hyperventilation may be profound. This deep and rapid breathing, called Kussmaul respiration, may itself be a compromising factor in the perioperative or critically ill patient. It is possible for patients with DKA to develop arterial blood pH in the range of 7.0 and arterial PCO_2 down to 10 mm Hg. This condition is generally regarded as a critical situation for which expert consultation is often necessary. Therapy includes insulin and careful replacement of fluids, potassium, and bicarbonate. Once severe hyperglycemia is reversed, intravenous glucose is generally necessary to end the production of ketones. A good guide is to provide glucose with the insulin once the blood glucose concentration is less than 300 mg/dl; 10 g of glucose hourly is a reasonable dosage for an adult. Potassium changes, reflecting depleted stores and rapid alteration of cellular fluxes in responses to changes in pH, may be rapid and dangerous. Once oliguria and hyperkalemia are excluded, potassium replacement is usually a standard part of therapy. Very close monitoring of blood values and therapy is generally the best way to monitor the patient in DKA; flow sheets with hourly recordings are quite helpful.

F. Hypoglycemia

The brain uses glucose as its principal metabolic substrate. In periods of starvation or carbohydrate depletion, the brain is able to use ketone bodies as an partial alternative. However, hypoglycemia seriously interferes with cerebral function. Mild hypoglycemia may cause somnolence and confusion. Marked hypoglycemia can cause coma, seizure, and even permanent brain damage. The precise concentration at which symptoms develop is variable. Patients with a chronically increased blood glucose concentration may need a higher concentration to avoid symptoms than do normal patients. In normal patients, a plasma glucose concentration less than 50 mg/dl may be sufficient to induce symptoms.

Patients with hypoglycemia generally demonstrate a stimulation of the counterregulatory system, marked by sympathetic hyperactivity. Often the first signs are tachycardia and diaphoresis. Under anesthesia, the signs of hypoglycemia may be entirely masked or suppressed; sympathetic hyperactivity is also a classic marker of light anesthesia.

Under anesthesia, hypoglycemia may be a very subtle diagnosis, and the cerebral effects of hypoglycemia, especially if prolonged, may be very deleterious; therefore it seems essential to control diabetic patients under anesthesia so as to maintain a safe but abnormal degree of perioperative hyperglycemia. Indeed, it is a common practice to maintain perioperative plasma glucose near 200 mg/dl.

VI. CONCLUSION

In this chapter we have tried to provide the background information concerning the common endocrinopathies. Often they are coincidental medical problems in patients requiring surgery for other problems. More often, however, the surgical procedure aims to correct the underlying endocrinopathy. Postoperative complications may result from either situation. The basic pathophysiology we have presented should provide a framework for understanding the evolution of potential problems in the postoperative period.

REFERENCES

1. Sutherland EW: Nobel prize in physiology or medicine 1971: the action of hormones outlined, *Lakartidningen* 68:4991, 1971.
2. Thapar K, Kovacs K, Horvath E: Morphology of the pituitary in health and disease. In Becker KL, ed: *Principles and practice of endocrinology and metabolism*, ed 2, Philadelphia, 1995, JB Lippincott.
3. Herman V, Fagan J, Gonsky R, et al: Clonal origin of pituitary adenomas, *J Clin Endocrinol Metab* 71:1427, 1990.
4. Wilson CB: Role of surgery in the management of pituitary tumors, *Neurosurg Clin North Am* 1:139, 1990.
5. Robertson GL: Thirst and vasopressin function in normal and disordered states of water balance, *J Lab Clin Med* 101:351, 1983.
6. Robertson GL, Bwerl T: Water metabolism. In Brenner BM, Rector FC, eds: *The kidney*, ed 3, Philadelphia, 1986, WB Saunders.
7. Robertson GL: Disorders of the posterior pituitary. In Stein JH, ed: *Internal medicine*, Boston, 1983, Little, Brown.
8. Ohnishi A, Orita Y, Okahara R, et al: Potent aquaretic agent: a novel nonpeptide selective vasopressin 2 antagonist (OPC-31260) in men, *J Clin Invest* 92:2653, 1993.
9. Moses AM, Notman DD: Diabetes insipidus and syndrome of inappropriate antidiuretic hormone secretion (SIADH), *Adv Intern Med* 27:73, 1982.
10. Cobb WE, Spare S, Reichlin S: Neurogenic diabetes insipidus: management with DDAVP (1-desamino-8-D-arginine vasopressin), *Ann Intern Med* 88:183, 1978.
11. Sterns RH, Riggs JE, Schochet SS Jr: Osmotic demyelination syndrome following correction of hyponatremia, *N Engl J Med* 314:1535, 1986.
12. Cheng JC, Zikos D, Skopicki HA, et al: Long-term neurologic outcome in psychogenic water drinkers with severe symptomatic hyponatremia: the effect of rapid correction, *Am J Med* 88:561, 1990.
13. Ayus JC, Krothapalli RK, Arieff AI: Treatment of symptomatic hyponatremia and its relation to brain damage: a prospective study, *N Engl J Med* 317:1190, 1987.
14. Bartter FC, Schwartz WB: The syndrome of inappropriate secretion of antidiuretic hormone, *Am J Med* 42:790, 1967.
15. Miller M, Moses AM: Drug-induced states of impaired water excretion, *Kidney Int* 10:96, 1976.
16. Farber MO, Roberts LR, Weinberger MH, et al: Abnormalities of sodium and H_2O handling in chronic obstructive lung disease, *Arch Intern Med* 142:1326, 1982.
17. Sheehan HL: The recognition of chronic hypopituitarism resulting from postpartum pituitary necrosis, *Am J Obstet Gynecol* 111:852, 1971.
18. Helfand M, Crapo LM: Screening for thyroid disease, *Ann Intern Med* 112:840, 1990.
19. Dillman WH: Thyroid storm, *Curr Ther Endocrinol Metab* 6:81, 1997.
20. Yoshida D: Thyroid storm precipitated by trauma, *J Emerg Med* 14:697, 1996.
21. Samaras K, Marel GM: Failure of plasmapheresis, corticosteroids and thionamines to ameliorate a case of protracted amiodarone-induced thyroiditis, *Clin Endocrinol* 45:365, 1996.
22. Tajiri J, Katsuya H, Kiyokawa T, et al: Successful treatment of thyrotoxic crisis with plasma exchange, *Crit Care Med* 12:536, 1984.
23. Yeung SC, Go R, Balasubramanyam A: Rectal administration of iodide and propylthiouracil in the treatment of thyroid storm, *Thyroid* 5:403, 1995.
24. Naito Y, Sone T, Kataoka K, et al: Thyroid storm due to functioning metastatic thyroid carcinoma in a burn patient, *Anesthesiology* 87:433, 1997.
25. Paschke R, Ludgate M: The thyrotropin receptor in thyroid disease, *N Engl J Med* 337:1675, 1997.
26. Wartofsky L: Treatment options for hyperthyroidism, *Hosp Pract* 31:69, 1996.
27. Kahaly G, Hellermann J, Mohr-Kahaly S, et al: Impaired cardiopulmonary exercise capacity in patients with hyperthyroidism, *Chest* 109:57, 1996.

28. Montereggi A, Masrconi P, Olivotto I, et al: Signal-averaged P-wave duration and risk of paroxysmal atrial fibrillation in hyperthyroidism, *Am J Cardiol* 77:266, 1996.

29. Vagenakis AG, Wang C, Burger A, et al: Iodide-induced thyrotoxicosis in Boston, *N Engl J Med* 287:523, 1972.

30. Martino E, Aghini-Lombardi F, Mariotti S, et al: Amiodarone: a common source of iodine induced thyrotoxicosis, *Horm Res* 26:158, 1987.

31. Kriplani A, Buckshee K, Bhargava VL, et al: Maternal and perinatal outcome in thyrotoxicosis complicating pregnancy, *Eur J Obstet Gynecol Reprod Biol* 54:159, 1994.

32. Mestman JH: Hyperthyroidism in pregnancy, *Clin Obstet Gynecol* 40:45, 1997.

33. Redahan C, Karski JM: Thyrotoxicosis factitia in a post-aortocoronary bypass patient, *Can J Anaesth* 41:969, 1994.

34. Abbott TR: Anaesthesia in untreated myxoedema: report of two cases, *Br J Anaesth* 39:510, 1967.

35. Kim JM, Hackman L: Anesthesia for untreated hypothyroidism: report of three cases, *Anesth Analg* 56:299, 1977.

36. Weinberg AD, Brennan AD, Gorman CA, et al: Outcome of anesthesia and surgery in hypothyroid patients, *Arch Intern Med* 143:893, 1983.

37. Ladenson PW, Levin AA, Ridgway EC, et al: Complications of surgery in hypothyroid patients, *Am J Med* 77:261, 1984.

38. Weinberg AD, Ehrenwerth J: Anesthetic considerations and perioperative management of patients with hypothyroidism, *Adv Anesthesiol* 4:185, 1987.

39. Becker C: Hypothyroidism and atherosclerotic heart disease: pathogenesis, medical management, and the role of coronary artery bypass surgery, *Endocr Rev* 6:432, 1985.

40. Klemperer JD, Klein I, Gomez M, et al: Thyroid hormone treatment after coronary-artery bypass surgery, *N Engl J Med* 333:1552, 1995.

41. Toft AD: Thyroxine therapy, *N Engl J Med* 331:174, 1994.

42. McConahey WM: Diagnosing and treating myxedema and myxedema coma, *Geriatrics* 33:61, 1978.

43. Slag MF, Morley JE, Elson MK, et al: Hypothyroxinemia in critically ill patients as a predictor of high mortality, *JAMA* 245:43, 1981.

44. Jatzko GR, Lisborg PH, Muller MG, et al: Recurrent nerve palsy after thyroid operations: principal nerve identification and a literature review, *Surgery* 115:139, 1994.

45. Rosenblatt W. Personal communication, 1998.

46. Mazzaferri EL: Papillary and follicular cancer: a selective approach to diagnosis and treatment, *Annu Rev Med* 32:73, 1981.

47. Olson JA Jr, DeBenedetti MK, Baumann DS, et al: Parathyroid autotransplantation during thyroidectomy: results of long-term follow-up, *Ann Surg* 223:472, 1996.

48. Schlumberger MJ: Medical progress: papillary and follicular thyroid carcinoma, *N Engl J Med* 338:297, 1998.

49. Arnold A: Genetic basis of endocrine disease: molecular genetics of parathyroid gland neoplasia, *J Clin Endocrinol Metab* 77:1108, 1993.

50. Schantz A, Castleman B: Parathyroid carcinoma: a study of 70 cases, *Cancer* 31:600, 1973.

51. Anonymous: Proceedings of the NIH Consensus Development Conference Statement on diagnosis and management of symptomatic primary hyperparathyroidism, *J Bone Miner Res* 6(suppl 2):S1, 1991.

52. Rudberg C, Akerstrom G, Palmer M, et al: Late results of operation for primary hyperparathyroidism in 441 patients, *Surgery* 99:643, 1986.

53. Rizzoli R, Green J, Marx SJ: Primary hyperparathyroidism in familial multiple endocrine neoplasia type I: long-term follow-up of serum calcium levels after parathyroidectomy, *Am J Med* 78:467, 1985.

54. Breslow MJ: Regulation of adrenal medullary and cortical blood flow, *Am J Physiol* 262:H1317, 1992.

55. Waterman MR, Simpson ER: Regulation of steroid hydroxylase gene expression is multifactorial in nature, *Recent Prog Horm Res* 45:533, 1989.

56. Hsueh WA: Components of the renin-angiotensin system: an update, *Am J Nephrol* 3:109, 1983.

57. Williams GH, Dluhy RG: Aldosterone biosynthesis: interrelationship of regulatory factors, *Am J Med* 53:595, 1972.

58. Welbourn RB: Survival and cause of death after an adrenalectomy for Cushing's disease, *Surgery* 97:16, 1985.

59. Wagner RL, White PF, Kan PB, et al: Inhibition of adrenal steroidogenesis by the anesthetic etomidate, *N Engl J Med* 310:1415, 1984.

60. Wagner RL, White PF: Etomidate inhibits adrenocortical function in surgical patients, *Anesthesiology* 61:647, 1984.

61. Irony I, Kater CE, Biglieri EG, et al: Correctable subsets of primary aldosteronism, primary adrenal hyperplasia and renin responsive adenoma, *Am J Hypertens* 3:576, 1990.

62. Schambelan M, Sebastian A, Biglieri EG: Prevalence, pathogenesis and functional significance of aldosterone deficiency in hyperkalemic patients with chronic renal insufficiency, *Kidney Int* 17:89, 1980.

63. Neufeld M, MacLaren N, Blizzard R: Autoimmune polyglandular syndromes, *Pediatr Ann* 9:154, 1980.

64. Axelrod L: Glucocorticoid therapy, *Medicine* 55:39, 1976.

65. James MFM: Clinical use of magnesium infusions in anesthesia, *Anesth Analg* 74:129, 1992.

66. Lee JE, Curley SA, Gagel RF, et al: Cortical-sparing adrenalectomy for patients with bilateral pheochromocytoma, *Surgery* 120:1064, 1996.

67. De Canniere L, Michel L, Hamoir E, et al: Videoendoscopic adrenalectomy: multicentric study from the Belgian Group for Endoscopic Surgery (BGES), *Int Surg* 81:6, 1996.

68. Neumann HP, Berger DP, Sigmund G, et al: Pheochromocytomas, multiple endocrine neoplasia type 2, and von Hippel–Lindau disease, *N Engl J Med* 329:1531, 1993.

69. Peters A, Kerner W: Perioperative management of the diabetic patient, *Exp Clin Endocrinol Diabetes* 103:213, 1995.

70. Hirsch IB, McGill JB, Cryuer PE, et al: Perioperative management of surgical patients with diabetes mellitus, *Anesthesiology* 74:346, 1991.

71. The Diabetes Control and Complications Trial Research Group: The effect of intensive treatment of diabetes on the development and progression of long-term complication in insulin-dependent diabetes mellitus, *N Engl J Med* 329:977, 1993.

72. Ishihara H, Singh H, Giesecke AH: Relationship between diabetic autonomic neuropathy and gastric contents, *Anesth Analg* 78:943, 1994.

73. Sieber FE: The neurologic implications of diabetic hyperglycemia during surgical procedures at increased risk for brain ischemia, *J Clin Anesth* 9:334, 1997.

Chapter 15

Causes and Consequences of Hypothermia and Hyperthermia

Henry Rosenberg
Steven M. Frank

I. HEAT BALANCE PHYSIOLOGY

A. Heat and temperature

Heat, which is energy in the form of molecular motion, differs from temperature, which is a measure of the concentration of heat energy. When a substance is divided into two equal parts, each half contains half as much heat as the original but the same temperature. Heat, like other forms of energy, follows conservation laws. Heat transfer, however, depends on the existence of a temperature gradient. By analogy, gas contents (mass) are conserved, whereas gas transfer occurs with differences in partial pressure.

Heat and temperature are related by the ability of a substance to contain heat, called specific heat. The specific heat of water and thus of body tissues defines the unit of heat energy, the calorie: the addition of 1 calorie to 1 g water results in a 1° C increase in temperature.

B. Heat production

Basal metabolic energy appears as heat at the rate of 1 kcal/kg^{-1}/hr^{-1}, or 44 W/m^{-2}. Were all this heat retained, body temperature would increase at the rate of 1° C/hr^{-1}. The liver, heart, and skeletal muscle serve as major heat generators, whereas skin and respiratory mucosal surfaces provide opportunities for heat dissipation. Muscle tension alone, in the absence of shivering, generates additional heat. In hypothyroidism, a depressed basal metabolic rate results in decreased heat production.

Likewise, impaired catecholamine excretion or inhibition of catecholamine peripheral action decreases heat generation and may lead to symptoms and heat-conserving behaviors. Furthermore, thyroid hormone potentiates the calorigenic effects of epinephrine.[1]

C. Heat loss

Approximately 3000 kcal of heat are lost per day by the average adult male. Ninety-five percent of those 3000 kcal dissipate through the skin and respiratory mucosa. Warming of inspired air (3%) and elimination of urine and feces (2%) account for the remainder. The four mechanisms of heat loss are convection, evaporation, conduction, and radiation. Convective transfer, accounting for 15% of total heat loss, occurs by moving air. The loss increases with the square of air speed, up to 60 miles/hr.

Conductive heat loss occurs by direct contact with a cooler material, such as the cold mattress of a stretcher, or by intravenous infusion of cold solution. (Strictly speaking, because the fluid becomes part of the body, the total heat content remains constant even though temperature decreases.) Normally there is little conductive heat loss.

Conversion of 1 ml water from a liquid to a vapor state (that is, evaporation) from the skin or respiratory tract permits dissipation of 0.58 kcal of energy. Evaporation is facilitated by low ambient humidity and hindered in damp atmospheres. Nearly 1 oz of water is lost each hour from the skin (two thirds) and lungs (one third) at room temperature, accounting for 17 kcal of energy.

Radiation of heat through the skin constitutes the major mechanism of heat loss, reaching 50% of the total, or about 50 kcal/hr^{-1}, when a person is naked. Radiant heat transfer occurs by infrared electromagnetic waves traveling from a hotter object to a cooler one. Radiant heat loss increases with the temperature differential and with the amount of exposed surface. By increasing skin temperature, vasodilation promotes heat loss.

D. Thermoregulation

The anterior hypothalamus is the center of thermoregulatory control.[2] There are three general components to the thermoregulatory system: the afferent input of thermal information, central processing of this information, and the efferent responses that control heat loss and production (Fig. 15-1).[3] Afferent information is taken from thermoreceptors in the hypothalamus itself, other parts of the brain and spinal cord, deep visceral tissues, and the skin surface. The relative contribution of thermal information to the central thermoregulatory system is 80% from the core and deep body tissues and 20% from the skin surface.[4] In the hypothalamus this information is compared to an internal set point temperature, which is analogous to the setting on a thermostat. When body temperature is above or below this set point, the first response to correct the body's temperature is a behavioral one that involves changing the ambient temperature to which the person is exposed or altering one's clothing to optimize heat balance. When behavioral thermoregulation is inadequate and temperature exceeds the set point, vasodilation and sweating are triggered to release heat to

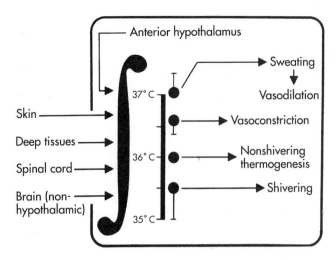

Fig. 15-1. A model of thermoregulatory control. Afferent input of thermal information is derived from tissues throughout the body, including the brain, skin surface, spinal cord, and deep tissues. A mean body temperature below the set point initiates cold responses (vasoconstriction, shivering, and nonshivering thermogenesis). A mean body temperature above the set point triggers the warm responses (vasodilation and sweating). (From Sessler DI: *N Engl J Med* 336:1730, 1997.)

the atmosphere. When temperature is below the set point, vasoconstriction is triggered to conserve heat, and shivering and nonshivering thermogenesis are triggered to produce heat. Nonshivering thermogenesis is not thought to occur in adult humans, but contributes significantly to heat production in neonates.

The efferent thermoregulatory responses are characterized by three concepts known as threshold, gain, and maximum intensity.[5] Threshold is the core temperature at which the response is triggered. The interthreshold range is the range of core temperatures over which no thermoregulatory responses occur. This range is normally 0.2° C in adult humans between the sweating and the vasoconstriction thresholds.[6] Gain is the change in response intensity for a given change in body temperature. For example, shivering is quantitatively assessed by measuring total body oxygen consumption. The gain for shivering is determined by plotting O_2 consumption against core temperature and using the slope of the regression line to represent gain. Maximum intensity of a response is the highest value that occurs under maximal thermal stress. The maximum intensity of shivering, for example, is a threefold to fourfold increase in oxygen consumption above baseline levels.[7] The threshold, gain, and maximum intensities of the various thermoregulatory responses are important concepts because they are used to quantitatively assess the degree of thermoregulatory impairment with the various anesthetics as well as the differences in thermoregulation between young and old and between men and women.

E. Body temperature monitoring

As DuBois[8] described, there are "many different temperatures of the human body and its parts." In the simplest model, the body is divided into two thermal compart-

Fig. 15-2. Body temperature monitoring in a patient on full cardiopulmonary bypass. The relative ability of each monitoring site to reflect core temperature is shown. Arterial blood temperature coming from the bypass pump into the ascending aorta is shown along with various sites used to monitor core temperature. The fastest temperatures to show change during cooling and warming are those measured at the nasopharynx, tympanic membrane, and esophagus. Temperatures in the urinary bladder and rectum are slower to change and are considered intermediate temperatures rather than core temperatures. These sites are helpful in assessing the completeness of cooling and warming during cardiac surgery.

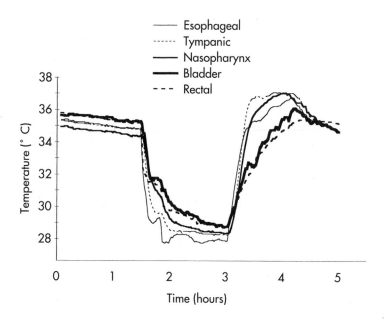

ments: the core and the periphery. The core has a fairly constant internal temperature that is protected by the insulation from the peripheral compartment. The chest, abdomen, pelvis, and head make up the core compartment. The extremities and skin surface make up the peripheral compartment. Mean body temperature lies somewhere between the two and is defined as 0.66 (core temperature) + 0.34 (mean skin surface temperature).[9]

For the purposes of temperature monitoring during anesthesia and surgery, the best monitoring sites are those that are closest to blood temperature, which is considered to be the true core temperature. These sites are as follows, in order of greatest to least correlation with core temperature: pulmonary artery, esophagus (distal one third), tympanic membrane, nasopharynx, oral/sublingual cavity, urinary bladder, rectum, and skin surface.[10] When body temperature is constant, all these sites (except skin surface) are good estimates of core temperature. The skin surface is usually 2° to 3° C lower than core temperature, but the core-to-skin gradient depends on ambient temperature and vasomotor tone. For this reason, liquid crystal thermometers on the forehead skin surface give a reasonable estimate of core temperature. In one study, skin surface temperature was within 0.5° C of core temperature in two thirds of patients and rarely did skin surface temperature differ from core temperature by more than 1° C.[11] When body temperature is changing (i.e., during anesthesia and surgery), bladder and rectal temperatures are the slowest to change and are likely to underestimate the magnitude of alteration in body temperature.[12] In some clinical situations (e.g., cardiac surgery) these sites are deliberately monitored because the slow change is helpful in assessing the completeness of cooling and warming on cardiopulmonary bypass. Besides blood temperature in the pulmonary artery, nasopharyngeal and esophageal temperatures are

the most accurate estimates of core temperature. However, esophageal measurements must be taken from the lower third of the esophagus.[13,14] If the probe is placed in the upper or middle third, the respiratory gases will heat or cool the temperature probe. The distal third can be reached by going 10 cm beyond the point of maximum heart sounds with an esophageal stethoscope. Tympanic measurements are an excellent representation of core temperature because the internal carotid artery passes near the tympanic membrane.[15] A special flexible tympanic probe with a cotton tip is used. This probe is commercially available and has been used extensively without complications. The relative changes in body temperature from various monitoring sites are shown during cooling and rewarming on cardiopulmonary bypass in Fig. 15-2.

The definition of normal core temperature varies because there is a circadian rhythm of 1° C or more, with a nadir in the morning and a peak in the afternoon. There is also a monthly variation in menstruating women of 0.5° C. When these changes are taken into account along with the differences among measurement sites, it is difficult to define a normal core temperature, but 36.5° to 37.5° C is within the normal range.

II. HYPOTHERMIA
A. Effect of anesthetics on heat balance

Drugs can modify heat balance by altering one or more of the three components of the thermoregulatory system: the afferent pathway, the central control mechanism, or the efferent paths. Atropine, for example, may result in hyperthermia by blocking the efferent sympathetic diaphoresis response to warm environments. General anesthetics impair all three components, and regional anesthesia (major conduction blockade) impairs the afferent and efferent pathways but not the central

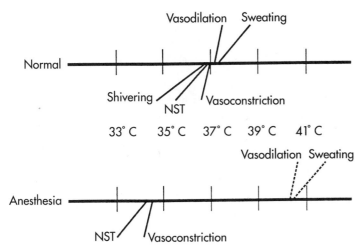

Fig. 15-3. A schematic illustrating thresholds and gains for thermoregulatory responses in awake and anesthetized humans. The *x*-axis represents mean body temperature. For each individual thermoregulatory response the threshold is indicated by the intersection with the *x*-axis and the gain is represented by the slope of the line that intersects. The interthreshold range is shown as the range of temperatures that do not trigger a response. This range (between sweating and vasoconstriction) is expanded approximately tenfold by anesthesia. This effect of anesthesia renders patients poikilothermic, and body temperature drifts toward environmental temperature. (From Sessler DI: Temperature monitoring. In Miller RD, ed: *Anesthesia*, ed 3, New York, 1990, Churchill Livingstone.)

pathway. Over the past decade, numerous studies have characterized the effects of different anesthetic drugs and techniques on thermoregulatory function. The results of these studies show that virtually all anesthetics (regional and general) impair thermoregulation, rendering patients poikilothermic during surgery.[3,5] The overall effects of anesthesia on thermoregulation are illustrated in Fig. 15-3. Considering the cold operating room environment, hypothermia occurs in approximately 50% of patients when defined as a core temperature less than 36° C, and in 33% of patients when defined as a core temperature less than 35° C.[16,17]

1. Sedatives. Direct cerebral application of barbiturates induces an increase in skin blood flow, with resultant radiant heat loss to the environment.[18] Benzodiazepines lower the thresholds for sweating, vasoconstriction, and shivering, but only minimally compared to other anesthetic drugs.[19] Propofol has little effect on sweating but significantly inhibits responses to cold (vasoconstriction and shivering) in a dose-dependent fashion, thus predisposing to hypothermia.[20]

2. Opioids. Intracerebral morphine decreases body heat production.[21] All opioids in large doses given systemically cause hypothermia.[22] Meperidine is most effective in treating postoperative shivering when compared to fentanyl and morphine, an effect related to the κ-receptor agonist properties of the drug.[23] Alfentanil (a μ-agonist) causes a linear dose-dependent inhibition of vasoconstriction and shivering but has little effect on sweating.[24] In general, opioids predispose patients to hypothermia by significantly impairing thermoregulation.

3. Inhaled anesthetics. The volatile anesthetics and nitrous oxide inhibit all thermoregulatory responses in a dose-dependent fashion.[5] There is a sudden redistribution of heat within the body after induction of general anesthesia, which is characterized by a 1° C decrease in core temperature in the first 30 to 60 minutes of general anesthesia.[3] This represents heat flow from the core to the peripheral thermal compartment from vasodilation.[25] At a typical dose of volatile anesthetic, the interthreshold range is expanded tenfold and vasoconstriction is not

triggered until core temperature is near 34° C. Thus core temperature continues to decrease over the first 2 to 3 hours of general anesthesia. At this time the core temperature often plateaus because of activation of vasoconstriction. Upon emergence, active vasoconstriction and shivering are often observed as the anesthetic is discontinued in the hypothermic patient.[26,27]

4. Regional anesthesia. Unlike general anesthetics, epidural and spinal anesthesia do not modify central thermoregulatory activity. However, major conduction blockade is associated with approximately the same magnitude of hypothermia as occurs during general anesthesia when all other factors are the same.[16] In a controlled randomized trial comparing epidural and general anesthesia in patients undergoing radical prostatectomy, mean core temperature was identical at the end of the surgical procedure.[16] Thus when all factors are taken into consideration, the risks of hypothermia appear to be similar with regional and general anesthetics.

The effects of regional anesthesia on afferent thermal signals are such that the hypothalamus is fooled by apparent warm signals from the lower body as the dominant cold signals are blocked.[28] The efferent responses are also blocked because vasoconstriction and shivering cannot occur below the level of the block and heat loss continues without the plateau phase, as with general anesthesia. There is some evidence that a higher block level predisposes to more hypothermia.[29] It also may be that core temperature is slower to recover in the postoperative period with regional than with general anesthesia because of residual sympathectomy and the resultant heat loss.[30] Shivering occurs, but with less heat production because only the upper body contributes.

Despite the risks and consequences of hypothermia, body temperature is largely ignored during regional anesthesia, and hypothermia often is not recognized, prevented, or treated.[30a] Body temperature monitoring sites typically used during general anesthesia (nasopharynx, esophagus, and oropharynx) are not tolerated in awake or sedated patients, so some clinicians think it is not convenient to monitor temperature during regional anesthesia. Historically, temperature monitoring became popular in the early 1960s, when malignant hyperthermia (MH) was first described. Because regional anesthesia is not associated with MH, temperature monitoring was initially not thought to be important. We now recognize that hypothermia is common during regional anesthesia and that temperature should be monitored and controlled.

5. Combined regional and general anesthesia. Vasoconstriction thresholds are reduced and core cooling rates are higher in patients receiving combined regional and general anesthesia than in those receiving only general anesthesia.[31] This difference appears to be related to lower-extremity heat loss in the complete absence of vasomotor tone during regional anesthesia, in addition to the central thermoregulatory inhibition from general anesthesia. For this reason core temperature should be carefully monitored and active warming used to maintain body temperature when combined regional and general anesthesia is used.

B. Benefits of hypothermia

1. Brain protection. The benefits of hypothermia are well recognized during surgical procedures that put the brain at risk for ischemic injury. These procedures include cerebral aneurysm clipping, carotid endarterectomy, and cardiac surgery. Hypothermia reduces oxygen consumption by 5% to 7% for each 1° C of cooling, and this reduction is linear.[32] Thus at typical hypothermic cardiopulmonary bypass temperature (28° C), brain metabolism is 50% lower than normal. Several animal studies suggest that even mild hypothermia (34° C) provides significant cerebral protection,[33,34] perhaps not only by reducing brain oxygen consumption but also by decreasing the release of excitatory amino acids.[35] Conversely, mild hyperthermia (39° C) can increase injury during ischemia.[33] For this reason, it is optimal to use slow, gradual rewarming during cardiopulmonary bypass to avoid overheating the brain in patients undergoing cardiac surgery.

Human studies on temperature and perioperative cerebral outcomes are difficult to perform because of the low incidence of cerebral injury and the resulting large sample size required to show an effect on outcome. Results from a randomized trial on thermal management and cerebral injury during coronary bypass surgery demonstrate that active warming to maintain normothermia (37° C) during cardiopulmonary bypass was associated with a higher incidence of neurologic deficit than was traditional hypothermic bypass (28° C).[36] Other studies have shown similar rates of neurologic injury with mild hypothermia (34° C) and moderate hypothermia (28° C). In summary, mild hypothermia provides significant cerebral protection but moderate hypothermia does not provide much additional benefit. Although hypothermia is beneficial for most procedures in which the brain is at risk, carotid surgery may be an exception because these procedures are often short in duration, not allowing time for cooling and rewarming. In addition, patients undergoing carotid surgery are at significant risk for perioperative myocardial infarction, and residual hypothermia in the postoperative period is associated with increased myocardial ischemia[37] and cardiac morbidity.[38]

2. Spinal cord protection. Paraplegia is a well recognized complication of aortic surgical procedures, especially when aortic cross-clamps are placed high on the aorta. The incidence of paraplegia is as great as 20% to 40% in some series in which aortic cross-clamping is prolonged or the aneurysm is dissecting.[39] In a series of patients cooled to 30° C on partial cardiopulmonary bypass, we found no neurologic deficits in 20 patients.[40] Certainly, many variables contribute to spinal cord injury, but mild to moderate hypothermia appears to be protective. Animal studies show that the duration of aortic cross-clamping required to produce paraplegia is twice as long at 35° C as at 37° C,[34] thus supporting the findings in brain studies of the benefits of mild hypothermia for neurologic protection.

C. Consequences of hypothermia

1. Shivering and metabolism. One of the most commonly recognized effects of hypothermia is postoperative shivering. Despite earlier suggestions that inhaled anesthetics cause shivering by disassociation of spinal reflexes from cortical centers in the brain, it is now believed that virtually all perioperative shivering (with general or regional anesthesia) is thermoregulatory in origin.[5]

Based on studies from 20 to 30 years ago with very small numbers of patients and questionable methods, the myth has been perpetuated that shivering dramatically increases total body oxygen consumption by 400% or more above baseline. In these earlier studies, single patients reportedly increased their metabolic rates by more than 400%,[41,42] but the methods used to measure oxygen consumption were inferior and the average increase with shivering was about 100%. In general, these were young patients receiving little or no opioid analgesia. Recent more carefully conducted studies have shown that shivering increases oxygen consumption, but the average increase is 40%, with a maximum increase of 100%.[26] Other predictors of increased oxygen consumption were male gender and increased core temperature (Fig. 15-4). Although shivering is uncomfortable for most patients, it is unlikely that this small increase in total body oxygen consumption in the average shivering patient is associated with perioperative morbidity.

It is common for patients to complain that their worst memory from the recovery room is the intense cold sensation and uncontrollable shivering. Shivering can be attenuated by small doses of opioids. Although all opioids reduce shivering, meperidine (12.5 to 25 mg) is most effective.[42,43] Other drugs that are effective in the treatment of shivering include clonidine, neostigmine, and ketanserin (a serotonin antagonist). Thermal comfort is significantly improved and shivering can be virtually eliminated with the use of cutaneous warming during or following surgery with forced-air heaters.[44] For every 1° C of core hypothermia, approximately 4° C of skin surface warming is required to attenuate the shivering response.[4]

2. Respiratory. Whole-body CO_2 production decreases with hypothermia. The magnitude of this de-

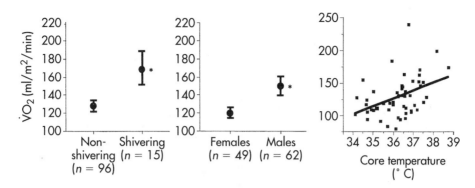

Fig. 15-4. Total body oxygen consumption in the early postoperative period and the effects of shivering, gender, and core temperature. Oxygen consumption is higher in shivering patients than in nonshivering patients, but the magnitude of difference was only 40%. Males had a 25% greater metabolic response than females because of a greater lean body mass. Core temperature was directly proportional to oxygen consumption. These findings indicate that even when shivering is accounted for, hypothermia is associated with a decrease in metabolism, not the increase that one would expect if all hypothermic patients shivered and all shivering were associated with a large increase in metabolism. *$p < 0.05$. (Modified from Frank SM, Fleisher LA, Olson KF, et al: *Anesthesiology* 83:241, 1995.)

crease reflects the behavior of most enzyme-controlled biologic phenomena, that is, a halving of activity with fall in temperature of 10° C. This halving is formally expressed as a Q_{10}, or the quotient of measured activities at two temperatures 10° C apart. Initially, cooling increases respiratory rate by central stimulation; ventilatory depression supervenes. Decreases in both tidal volume and respiratory rate contribute to the decreased minute ventilation. Body CO_2 content remains constant at hypothermia. One might expect the magnitude of decrease in minute ventilation to parallel that of CO_2 production. However, ventilatory dead space increases with hypothermia, thus blunting the decrease in minute ventilation.[45]

As with other gases, CO_2 solubility increases with cooling. Because content is the product of solubility and partial pressure, preservation of CO_2 blood content in the face of increased solubility yields a decreased $PaCO_2$ with hypothermia. Solubility changes are not enzymatically mediated and thus do not follow a "Q_{10} one-half" rule; $PaCO_2$ changes only about 4.5%/1° C. Fortunately, one may apply a convenient guideline to the relationship of $PaCO_2$ to temperature: Normocapnia occurs when the temperature-corrected $PaCO_2$ (mm Hg) numerically equals the temperature (degrees Celsius). Thus a patient at 33° C should have a blood temperature-corrected $PaCO_2$ of 33 mm Hg. Blood pH increases by 0.015 units/1° C, in parallel with the elevation of the pH of water with cold.

Hypothermia blunts the ventilatory response to CO_2. The slope of the CO_2 response curve decreases from 0.38 L/min^{-1}/mm^{-1} Hg at 37° C to 0.10 L/min^{-1}/mm^{-1} Hg at 28° C.[46] The respiratory quotient, or ratio of CO_2 production to oxygen use, does not change with hypothermia. Thus oxygen use decreases at the same rate as CO_2 production. Like CO_2 content, oxygen content does not change. An increase of oxygen solubility in blood compounds an

overall 7.5% per 1° C increase in oxygen affinity of hemoglobin. Thus PaO_2 decreases with cooling. Even mild hypothermia induces pulmonary vasoconstriction, which interferes with hypoxic pulmonary vasoconstriction.[47]

3. Adrenergic. The adrenergic response to hypothermia is significant. Although this response is not manifested during anesthesia, norepinephrine concentrations are significantly increased postoperatively in mildly hypothermic patients. A core temperature of less than 35.5° C following surgery triggers a twofold increase in norepinephrine, vasoconstriction, and increased arterial blood pressure.[27] When human volunteers are cooled to a core temperature of 35.2° C, a 700% increase in norepinephrine is induced, along with vasoconstriction and increased arterial blood pressure. This response appears to result primarily from the peripheral sympathetic nervous system, with little or no adrenal response, because epinephrine and cortisol are unchanged with core hypothermia (Fig. 15-5).[7] The adrenergic response is greater in younger patients, which may explain the decreased ability for the elderly to protect their core temperatures during cold challenge.

4. Cardiovascular. It is well known that cold stress adversely affects the cardiovascular system by triggering myocardial ischemia. For more than 50 years a seasonal variation in death rate from myocardial infarction has been recognized, with increased morbidity during the winter.[48,49] This effect appears to be temperature related and independent of snowfall or other climatic changes. The classic model of cold stress that is used to precipitate myocardial ischemia is the cold pressor test. The test was described over 50 years ago and involves a brief period of immersion of the hand and forearm into a cold ice bath.[50] The stimulus triggers a significant increase in both norepinephrine and epinephrine along with α-adrenergically mediated coronary vasoconstriction in the coronary vascular

Fig. 15-5. The adrenergic response to core cooling. Mild core hypothermia (35° to 35.5° C) was induced by infusion of high- or low-dose cold intravenous fluid. Norepinephrine increased 700%, whereas epinephrine and cortisol were unchanged. Thus a peripheral sympathetic response is activated by core hypothermia but the adrenal response is absent. The norepinephrine response is associated with increased vasomotor tone and increased arterial blood pressure. *$p < 0.05$ vs. preinfusion baseline, #$p < 0.05$ vs. 30 ml/kg group. (Modified from Frank SM, Higgins MS, Fleisher LA, et al: *Am J Physiol* 272:R557, 1997.)

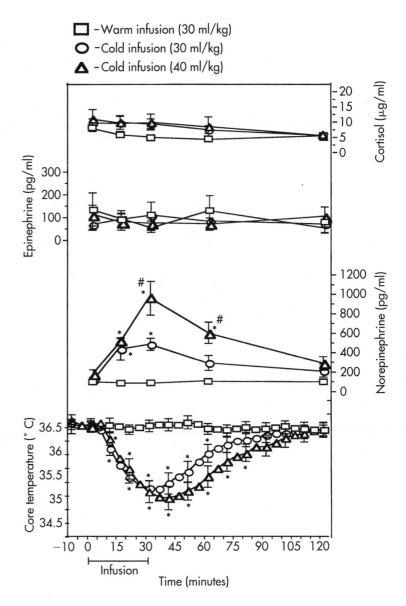

bed.[51] In high-risk patients (those undergoing peripheral vascular surgery), a core temperature less than 35° C is associated with a twofold to threefold increase in the incidence of early postoperative myocardial ischemia.[37] This cold-induced myocardial ischemia is independent of anesthetic technique (regional or general) and age (median age was 65 years). In a recently completed randomized trial, we demonstrated a 55% reduction of the relative risk for early postoperative cardiac morbidity in patients who were aggressively warmed during surgery.[38] The incidence of postoperative ventricular tachycardia and morbid cardiac events was lower in the normothermic group (36.7° C) than in the hypothermic group (35.3° C) (Fig. 15-6). Intraoperatively, cardiac outcomes occurred with similar frequency in the two groups. This suggests that cold-induced perioperative cardiovascular morbidity is likely to be mediated by the adrenergic response because the effect of temperature on outcome is significant in the postoperative pe-

riod after emergence, not during anesthesia, when the adrenergic response to hypothermia is attenuated.

Conduction velocity decreases throughout the hypothermic heart, yielding prolonged PR and QT intervals as well as a widening of the QRS complex on the electrocardiogram. Both J-point elevation, called Osborne waves, and T-wave flattening or inversions occur with hypothermia. Atrial fibrillation is common when core temperature approaches 30° C, especially when the atrium has been traumatized by cannulation for cardiopulmonary bypass. Between 24° C and 28° C, ventricular fibrillation develops. Hypothermia-induced ventricular fibrillation is refractory to pharmacologic therapy.

5. Coagulation and bleeding. The coagulation system is significantly influenced by hypothermia through three different mechanisms: platelet function, the coagulation cascade, and fibrinolysis. The function of platelets

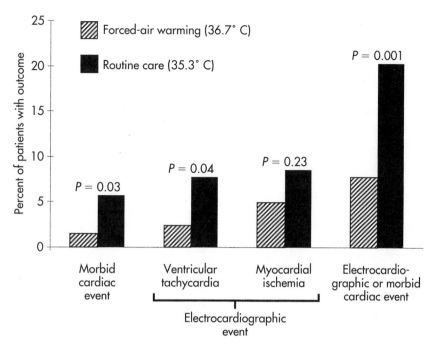

Fig. 15-6. Cardiac morbidity increases during the early postoperative period in patients who are mildly hypothermic (35.3° C) following surgery. Three hundred patients having vascular, thoracic, or major abdominal surgery with documented coronary artery disease (CAD) or risk factors for CAD were randomly assigned to receive forced-air warming or routine thermal care during surgery. Morbid cardiac events included cardiac arrest, myocardial infarction, and unstable angina or ischemia. Ventricular tachycardia was defined as five or more consecutive beats detected by Holter monitor. (Modified from Frank SM, Fleisher LA, Breslow MJ, et al: *JAMA* 277:1127, 1997.)

is impaired by hypothermia because of reduced concentrations of thromboxane B_2 at the site of tissue injury.[52,53] There is also reduced activity of coagulation factors in the coagulation cascade because the enzymes involved in the cascade, like all enzymes, are temperature dependent.[54] Because the prothrombin and partial thromboplastin time tests are routinely performed at a temperature of 37° C in most laboratories, it is likely that most temperature-related coagulopathies are missed in the clinical setting.[54] Fibrinolysis is enhanced with hypothermia, which destabilizes clot and predisposes to increased bleeding.[55] Platelet sequestration is also thought to contribute to hypothermia-related coagulopathy. However, sequestration has been shown only in severely hypothermic dogs (20° C)[56] and is unlikely to be significant in the perioperative setting. A recently completed study in patients undergoing total hip arthroplasty showed a significantly lower blood loss and lower requirements for allogeneic blood transfusion in patients maintained normothermic than in those with mild hypothermia (35° C).[57]

6. Wound healing and infection. There is evidence that wound healing is impaired and that patients are more susceptible to wound infection when hypothermia (core temperature lower than 35° C) occurs during surgery.[58] The incidence of wound infection was more than three times as high in mild hypothermia (34.7° C) than in normothermic patients (36.6° C) undergoing

colon surgery (19% vs. 6%). This effect is thought to be related to impaired macrophage function and reduced tissue oxygen tension secondary to thermoregulatory vasoconstriction. Collagen deposition in the wound has also been shown to be impaired with hypothermia. Increased susceptibility to infection with hypothermia at the time of introduction of bacteria into the skin has also been shown in animal models.[59] The window of opportunity for infection to become established is reportedly in the first 3 hours following inoculation. If hypothermia occurs at this critical time, then infection occurs more often.

7. Altered pharmacokinetics and pharmacodynamics. The minimum alveolar concentration (MAC) for potent inhaled anesthetics decreases by 5% for each 1° C reduction in body temperature.[60] In addition, the blood gas solubility for inhaled anesthetics increases with hypothermia. In combination, these effects contribute to the slow emergence from general anesthesia in hypothermic patients. In a recently completed blinded randomized trial, the duration of time needed in the postanesthesia care unit (PACU) needed before discharge was an average of 40 minutes longer in hypothermic (34.8° C) than in normothermic (36.7° C) patients.[61] These findings suggest that substantial cost savings can be achieved by maintaining normothermia and expediting recovery from general anesthesia.

Mild hypothermia increases the duration of action of nondepolarizing neuromuscular blockers. At 34° C the duration of vecuronium is doubled.[62] This effect is thought to be pharmacokinetic, not pharmacodynamic. Atracurium is also prolonged, but somewhat less; a 60% increase in duration occurs at 34° C.[63] When added to the changes in MAC and solubility for inhaled anesthetics, this prolongation of neuromuscular blockade can delay or prevent emergence from general anesthesia, especially in the elderly, who already have a reduced MAC and are especially susceptible to hypothermia.

D. Methods of controlling body temperature

1. Ambient temperature. Anesthesia induces poikilothermia, whereby patients tend to equilibrate body temperature with ambient temperature. At the turn of the century, heat stroke during surgery was reported in anesthetized patients in hot operating rooms before the use of air conditioning.[64] Operating rooms are now maintained at temperatures between 65° and 70° F, primarily for the comfort of the staff. At these temperatures, patients are subject to hypothermia, especially with the high rate of air exchange, which creates a windchill effect. When ambient temperature is greater than 23° C (73° F), unintentional hypothermia occurs less often during surgery,[16,65] but this warm environment is not well tolerated by the surgical staff because surgical gowns are now impermeable to fluids and very uncomfortable to wear. It is therefore preferable to warm the patient rather than the entire operating room and the surgical staff therein.

2. Airway heating and humidification. Active heating and humidification of the inspired gases have little or no effect on core temperature except in neonates, in whom this method may help in maintaining normothermia.[66] Less than 10% of total heat loss during surgery occurs from the respiratory tract in adult patients, but this fraction is higher in small children. Earlier studies showing a significant effect on core temperature may have been flawed because core temperature was measured in the esophagus, where direct heating of the temperature probe occurs when airway gases are warmed. Passive humidification with heat-moisture exchangers (HMEs) increases humidity in the airway but has no effect on the patient's core temperature. Current recommendations are to use an HME for any patient who would benefit from added moisture. This includes patients with chronic obstructive pulmonary disease, asthma, or significant pulmonary conditions in which secretions are not well cleared. Active heating and humidification of the respiratory gases are not necessary unless other methods of warming small children (forced-air warming) are unavailable. The approximate cost of an HME is $1, whereas the cost of an active heated humidifier system is $14. Active heater and humidifier systems have been associated with inadvertent disconnects in the breathing circuit and overheating of the inspired gases.

3. Intravenous fluid warming. Fluid warming can be used to help reduce the magnitude of hypothermia during surgery but cannot be used to warm patients because fluids cannot be delivered at temperatures significantly greater than 37° C. For minor procedures requiring minimal fluids (less than 2 L), it is unnecessary to warm the intravenous fluids. For procedures in which fluids are given at higher flow rates or volumes, it becomes necessary to warm the fluids in order to maintain normothermia. Prewarmed fluids can be given or an in-line fluid or blood warmer may be used. When transfusion is likely, a fluid or blood warmer should be used because blood is stored at 4° C. When a unit of cold blood or room-temperature crystalloid is given to the patient, mean body temperature decreases by 0.25° C.[3] When this decrease is added to ongoing heat loss from the skin surface, the problem with unwarmed fluids is compounded.

When fluid warmers are used, two factors must be considered in determining the temperature at which the fluid is delivered to the patient: flow rate and length of intravenous (IV) tubing (Fig. 15-7).[67] At low flow rates, the fluid returns to ambient room temperature after it leaves the warmer and before it reaches the patient. This

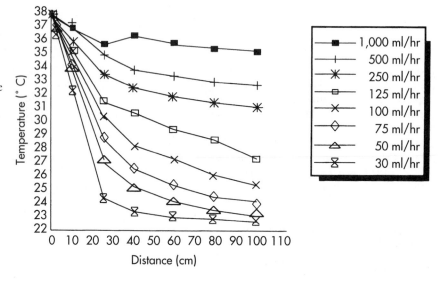

Fig. 15-7. Temperature measurements of normal saline in intravenous tubing at various distances from the fluid warmer at various flow rates. Fluid started at ambient room temperature and was warmed to 37° C by an in-line fluid warmer. Both distance and flow rate have a significant effect on the temperature at which the fluid is delivered. (From Faries G, Johnston C, Pruitt KM, et al: *Ann Emerg Med* 20:1198, 1991.)

Legend:
- 1,000 ml/hr
- 500 ml/hr
- 250 ml/hr
- 125 ml/hr
- 100 ml/hr
- 75 ml/hr
- 50 ml/hr
- 30 ml/hr

Temperature (° C) vs Distance (cm)

heat loss can be eliminated by a warmed fluid-filled jacket around the IV tubing, but heat loss from low-flow fluid administration is not significant except in pediatric patients.[68] At high flows, fluids pass through the warmer so quickly that the fluids cannot be warmed sufficiently. Newer warmers are designed for delivery of warm fluids even at high flow rates. The cost of the average fluid warmer setup is $10 to $15, but some high-capacity warmers cost $60 or even $300 to set up, depending on the device.

4. Passive insulation. A layer of passive insulation reduces heat loss from the skin surface by 30%. The type of insulator is unimportant because there is little difference between materials (plastic, cotton, paper, or reflective space blankets).[69] The layer of air between the insulation cover and the patient's skin provides the insulation, independent of the material itself. Prewarmed cotton blankets are commonly used in the operating room. Patients feel immediate warmth and comfort, but actual heat flux through the skin is virtually identical with both warmed and unwarmed cotton blankets.

5. Active warming. Although passive insulation and intravenous fluid warming can reduce heat loss from the patient, these therapies cannot be used to transfer heat into the patient. Therefore active warming is required to maintain normothermia during the intraoperative period. Of the available warming systems, the most effective is forced air (Fig. 15-8).[70] This type of warming became available in the late 1980s and its use has increased dramatically over the last decade. Forced air was initially used to actively warm hypothermic patients in the postoperative period, but it was quickly recognized that preventing hypothermia was more desirable than treating hypothermia. The forced-air system consists of two components: the forced-air generator and the blanket. The generator blows air at various flow rates and delivery temperatures into the attached blanket through a hose that inserts into the blanket. The blankets are baffled to fill with warm air, with small holes for the air to exit onto the patient's skin surface. They are designed for covering the upper body, lower body, or full body, and the appro-

priate design is chosen based on the location of the surgical field. Child-size blankets are available. Heat transfer with these systems is 60 to 100 W,[71] which makes this therapy more efficient than other warming systems, such as circulating water mattresses or radiant heaters.

Circulating water mattresses are also designed to actively warm patients during surgery. These mattresses are placed underneath the patient and are connected to a warm water source that circulates flow through the mattress. Heat transfer with this device is limited because cutaneous blood flow to the patient's back is limited by pressure on the capillary beds from the body's weight. Heat flux through the skin surface over the back of a patient is 7 W, compared to 3 W with the standard foam mattress used on operating room tables.[72] Water mattresses have been shown to be most effective in transferring heat when used over the ventral surface of the patient, which is sometimes an option in the postoperative period but is impractical during surgery.

Radiant heat is another type of active warming system. These systems are often used during the intraoperative period and are incorporated into the beds used for neonates. Radiant heaters should be used with a skin surface thermistor that provides thermostatic feedback to the warmer and reduces the risk of burning. Radiant heaters have also been used in the recovery room for adult patients. Shivering is immediately attenuated with radiant warming.[73] The effectiveness of radiant heating has not been compared with that of other active warming methods with regard to core rewarming of hypothermic patients.

A relatively new technology has been introduced to clinical practice that combines subatmospheric pressure and cutaneous warming in the upper extremity. The concept is to increase cutaneous blood flow using a vacuum chamber that surrounds the arm, which allows the rapid transfer of cutaneous heat into the central circulation. The new device (Thermo-STAT) is being used for postoperative warming therapy[73a] because other methods of surface warming can be ineffective in hypothermic vasoconstricted patients with limited cutaneous blood flow.

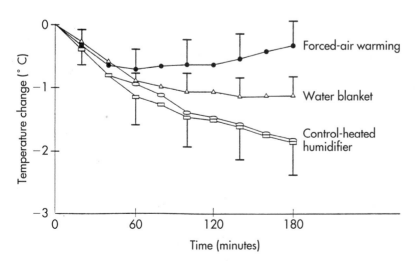

Fig. 15-8. Core temperature was compared in patients receiving four different warming methods during renal transplant surgery. Core temperature decreased 1° C in the first hour in all patients because of redistribution of heat. In the next 2 hours, heated humidification did not maintain core temperature better than control, circulating water mattresses prevented further hypothermia, but only forced-air warming increased core temperature back to baseline values. (Modified from Hynson JM, Sessler DI: *J Clin Anesth* 4:194, 1992.)

III. HYPERTHERMIA
A. Causes of hyperthermia

Body temperature depends on an intricate interplay between environmental temperature and mechanisms of heat gain and heat loss controlled by the central thermoregulatory centers. Hyperthermia may therefore be a result of an inadequate or inappropriate response to increased environmental temperature, an alteration of the internal set point of the "thermostat" located in the hypothalamus, or overwhelming peripheral heat production.

There are numerous causes of hyperthermia. Fever is one of the most common reasons for seeking medical attention. Bacteremia, viremia, and infectious diseases are perhaps the most common causes of fever. Fever in such situations results from a change in thermostatic set point from pyrogens and cytokines of various causes directly resulting from the organism, or from the release of such substances from macrophages and white cells.[73b]

Other causes of hyperthermia include inability to vasodilate or perspire because of drugs or disease.[74] Examples include Parkinson's disease, anticholinergic medications, and failure to adapt to high environmental temperatures, as may occur in elderly or psychiatrically impaired patients during periods of increased temperature. Hyperthermia is common during strenuous exercise in those not well adapted to heat or in whom fluid intake has been inadequate.[75]

1. Iatrogenic causes. The preceding generalizations about hyperthermia apply also to the anesthetized patient. Environmental temperatures in the operating room usually produce hypothermia. However, the microenvironment of the patient may be elevated by the use of convective warming devices. During anesthesia, iatrogenic hyperthermia results from active warming of patients (particularly pediatric patients), as may occur during application of warming devices applied to the patient's skin or unintentional overuse of heated airway humidifiers. Hyperthermia, usually mild, may occur during long procedures when the patient is covered with nonpermeable drapes and the operative area is small (e.g., eye surgery). Less common reasons have been reported. Application of tourniquets to upper or lower extremities for prolonged periods of time, especially in children, induces hyperthermia secondary to constraint of body heat to the core and reduction of body surface area.[76] For reasons still poorly understood, the injection of arteriovenous malformations with sclerosing solution may increase body temperature.[77] Induced hyperthermia for patients undergoing treatment for malignancy is another iatrogenic cause of hyperthermia.[78] This modality of treatment is no longer commonly used.

In days before temperature control of the operating room and air conditioning, heat stroke during anesthesia was a common problem. As already mentioned, this results from failure of physiologic processes to dissipate heat effectively during anesthesia.[64] In addition to the increased temperature and humidity, increased catecholamine release (as occurs with the then-common agents ether and cyclopropane), especially in the face of hypercapnia, was also responsible for the hyperthermia.

Recent studies by Sessler's group clearly show that the normal vasoconstriction response to cold is depressed during all forms of general anesthesia.[79] Vasodilation and sweating, which normally occur in response to increased body temperature, are also affected by general anesthetics; instead of occurring when body temperature exceeds 37.5° C central temperature, vasodilation and sweating may not occur until the body temperature exceeds 38° C or 39° C.[5] Therefore in some situations general anesthesia may promote hyperthermia.

2. Hyperthermia secondary to diseases
a. Pheochromocytoma. An increased plasma concentration of norepinephrine causes vasoconstriction in the periphery, inhibiting heat dissipation and hence increasing body temperature. Pheochromocytoma results in a profound increase in circulating catecholamines. Cases of mild to significant hyperthermia have been reported during or in the absence of anesthesia in patients with a pheochromocytoma.[80]

Because of the associated tachycardia and hypertension, MH may be suspected.

b. Thyrotoxicosis and thyroid storm. Thyrotoxicosis and thyroid storm may also cause intraoperative hyperthermia.[81] (See also Chapter 14.) Thyroid storm, an uncommon diagnosis in this era, presents with hypertension, hyperthermia, and tachycardia. Unlike in MH, however, muscle rigidity does not occur and acidosis is unusual. Clinical observation indicates that thyroid gland surgery causes mild hyperthermia, perhaps because of release of thyroid hormone with manipulation of the gland. Alternatively, the increased temperature may be unrelated to thyroid surgery itself but related to inadequate heat dissipation from the small surgical site in a completely draped patient. The hypermetabolism of thyroid-induced hyperthermia is sodium–potassium adenosine triphosphatase (ATPase) mediated,[82] unlike that of MH, in which intracellular calcium is elevated.[83]

c. Riley-Day syndrome. Increased body temperature also complicates Riley-Day syndrome, a deficiency of dopamine β-hydroxylase.[84] Patients so affected exhibit pronounced instability of the autonomic nervous system, with wide variation in blood pressure, heart rate, and temperature, apparently unrelated to external stimuli.

d. Osteogenesis imperfecta. Hyperthermia occurs during anesthesia in patients with osteogenesis imperfecta,[85] a metabolic bone disease characterized by easy and frequent bone fractures and blue scleras. Although a few episodes of true MH have been reported with osteogenesis imperfecta, in many cases clinical and laboratory testing revealed that MH was mistakenly diagnosed.

e. Central nervous system dysfunction. Central nervous system (CNS) dysfunction may induce hyperthermia.[87] In status epilepticus, fever may occur, presumably secondary to the intense muscle activity. However, any major CNS catastrophe may also lead to hyperthermia: Patients who experience hypoxic encephalopathy characteristically develop hyperthermia. After resuscitation from cardiac arrest, hyperthermia may accompany loss of consciousness, seizures, and increased muscle tone manifested by abnormal posturing. If cardiac arrest has occurred under anesthesia, the combination of autonomic imbalance associated with hypoxic encephalopathy, hyperthermia, and muscle rigidity render the distinction from MH problematic.

f. Infectious agents. Bacteremia, viremia, and a host of infectious agents produce sepsis and fever. Body temperature usually decreases when febrile patients are anesthetized. However, hyperthermia recurs after surgery, characterized by rigors and intense peripheral vasoconstriction. Sepsis, bacteremia, and hyperthermia may be induced by surgical manipulation, leading to postoperative and occasionally intraoperative hyperthermia. Appendectomy is a common scenario for this occurrence, with fever engendered by release of pyrogens with handling of the septic organ. Fever may occur during surgery for head trauma, particularly with disruption of the oral cavity. In this case, the bountiful oral bacteria can readily enter the bloodstream. Prolonged surgery on the urinary tract (e.g., nephrolithotomy) may lead to gram-negative sepsis and shock.

3. Drug-induced hyperthermia. A wide variety of drugs have been associated with fever.[87] We concentrate here on drug fevers in the perioperative period or related to conditions that may call for the attention of the anesthesiologist. The two most important pathophysiologic states causing hyperthermia from drug administration are MH[88] and the neuroleptic malignant syndrome (NMS).[89]

The anesthesiologist may be asked to treat patients suffering from hyperthermia caused by ingestion of sympathetic stimulants, such as cocaine, or methylenedioxyamphetamine (MDMA) activators such as Ecstasy or Eve.[90]

a. Malignant hyperthermia. MH occurs in genetically predisposed patients anesthetized with certain potent inhaled agents or succinylcholine. The incidence of MH ranges approximately from 1 in 15 to 1 in 200,000 anesthetics, with most authorities claiming an incidence of 1 in 50,000 anesthetics. The incidence depends on the gene pool for MH and the frequency of use of triggering anesthetic agents. Anesthesiologists who never use triggering agents will not see MH, whereas those who use such drugs regularly will see a higher frequency of MH. Also, elderly patients seem resistant to MH triggers, so anesthesiologists caring primarily for elderly patients will see MH infrequently. The largest gene pools for MH in North America may be found in Wisconsin, Michigan, and southeastern Canada.[91] The precise cause of MH remains elusive. However, increased intracellular calcium ion concentration in skeletal muscle cells clearly is one of the final pathophysiologic steps. Controversy exists as to whether animals or patients who are MH susceptible have increased intracellular calcium concentration before exposure to triggering anesthetics and whether increased intracellular calcium ion concentration occurs in cells other than skeletal muscle cells.[92] In swine, intracellular calcium ion concentration increases before the induction of MH and then increases dramatically during an MH episode. However, in vitro studies using different measurement techniques document normal resting calcium concentrations in skeletal muscle that increase only upon exposure to MH trigger agents.[83]

What leads to the increased intracellular calcium ion concentrations? Perhaps an alteration in excitation-contraction coupling in skeletal muscle of MH susceptible patients permits excessive release of calcium from sar-

coplasmic reticulum (SR) upon exposure to triggering agents.[93] Perhaps mitochondrial oxidative phosphorylation and calcium uptake are altered.[94] Perhaps elevated intracellular calcium results from elevation of certain free fatty acids within the cell, which in turn leads to calcium ion release from the SR.[95,96] The consequences of increased intracellular calcium are clear: activation of ATPases with ensuing depletion of adenosine triphosphate (ATP), actin-myosin interaction causing muscle contraction or increased muscle tone, breakdown of glucose and glycogen, and generation of heat. With sufficient ATP depletion, compromise of membrane integrity occurs, leading to increased cellular permeability and release of intracellular potassium, myoglobin, creatine kinase (CK), and tissue thromboplastin. The clinical consequences include hyperkalemia, myoglobinemia, rhabdomyolysis, and disseminated intravascular coagulation (DIC).

The molecular genetics of MH have been the subject of many studies in recent years.[97-99] It is clear that MH is a heterogenetic disorder; several genes on different chromosomes may lead to the syndrome. In many human families, and in virtually all pigs studied to date, MH is associated with a defect in the gene that elaborates a calcium channel in muscle (the ryanodine receptor) that mediates excitation-contraction coupling and release of cellular calcium. This gene is very large, so the potential for mutation within the gene is great. The ryanodine receptor gene is located on chromosome 19 in humans and chromosome 6 in pigs.

Other genes implicated in the cause of MH include the gene responsible for the dihydropyridine receptor (another protein involved in excitation-contraction coupling)[100] and the gene responsible for the elaboration of the sodium channel.[101]

Two unusual myopathies have been associated with MH: central core disease and King Denborough syndrome. Central core disease is a slowly progressive myopathy that is inherited in an autosomal dominant fashion. There also may be an association with a rare variant of myotonia, myotonia fluctuans.

Patients with Duchenne muscular dystrophy (DMD) and the similar but far rarer Becker's muscular dystrophy develop hyperkalemia, rhabdomyolysis, fever, and mild rigidity on exposure to succinylcholine and MH trigger drugs.[102] Therefore these patients are felt to be at risk for MH. In reality, the pathophysiology is probably different. Hyperkalemia is life-threatening in this situation and calls for immediate treatment.[103]

The gene for DMD is located on the X chromosome, so the disorder is limited to males. It is believed that chronically elevated intracellular calcium produces progressive muscle destruction in DMD.[104] Because inhaled agents normally cause calcium release from the SR,[105] in DMD the normal response of intracellular calcium to inhaled agents against a background of intracellular hypercalcemia may lead to an MH-like syndrome. Unlike MH, where the first line of treatment should be dantrolene, in DMD states, calcium, bicarbonate, insulin, and hyperventilation should be used first in order to abort the elevated hyperkalemia.

The clinical presentation of MH requires both a susceptible patient and exposure to specific drugs. The trigger drugs are the potent inhaled agents, including halothane, isoflurane, sevoflurane enflurane, cyclopropane, ether, and methoxyflurane, and the depolarizing neuromuscular relaxant succinylcholine. Local anesthetics, both amides and esters, do not trigger MH,[106] nor do intravenous induction agents, including propofol, barbiturates, ketamine, and benzodiazepines. Other drugs that do not trigger MH include digitalis, calcium, parasympatholytics, anticholinesterases, and nondepolarizing muscle relaxants. However, hyperkalemia may trigger MH or may retrigger an episode of MH.[107] We believe that catecholamines do not trigger MH, although others state that they should not be used during MH episodes.

MH may occur in pigs without drug intervention. Case reports indicate that MH-susceptible patients may be at increased risk of heat stroke[108]; likewise, in pigs high environmental temperatures and stress may induce an episode of MH. However, in humans there is no direct evidence that full-blown MH may occur without being induced by drugs.

An intriguing case report suggests that chronic exposure to low levels of hydrocarbons with a structure similar to that of anesthetics may lead to a hyperthermic reaction. The patient developed hyperthermia, muscle aches, and malaise; symptoms resolved after removal of the compound from the environment.[109]

b. Neuroleptic malignant syndrome. Psychiatrists have noted a syndrome characterized by hyperthermia, muscle rigidity, rhabdomyolysis, arrhythmia, acidosis, and death. It is precipitated by haloperidol alone or in combination with phenothiazines, or occasionally with antidepressant medications. Indeed, all antipsychotic agents have been known to cause this syndrome. Fortunately, the syndrome is not common (less than 1% of patients taking such medications). NMS should not be confused with hyperthermia and arrhythmias induced by overdose of monoamine oxidase (MAO) inhibitors or by combination of an MAO inhibitor and meperidine[110]; they originate from a different mechanism.

Despite the clinical similarity to MH, the cause of NMS is probably different from that of MH. Most believe that NMS results from blockade of dopamine receptors in the CNS. The dopamine agonist bromocriptine is one of the drugs effective in treating NMS.

Is the patient who has experienced NMS also at risk for MH? Probably not.[111] For example, succinylcholine, if preceded by barbiturate, as may occur for electroconvulsive therapy,[112] does not precipitate MH syndrome in the patient with NMS. However, there is little experience with general anesthesia in patients who have experienced NMS. Retrospective surveys have failed to link an increased incidence of NMS in MH families or an increased risk of MH in families where NMS has occurred. In addition, NMS is not genetically linked.

c. Other drug-induced hyperthermias. Cocaine toxicity, particularly in association with alcohol abuse, leads to hyperthermia, increased muscle tone, arrhythmias, and ventricular fibrillation.[113] This toxic effect of the drug is not related to MH.

Sympathetic stimulants such as amphetamines and the MDMA drug Ecstasy also lead to hyperthermia. The usual setting for the latter drug is in association with vigorous dancing ("rave parties"). Acidosis, rhabdomyolysis, and death often accompany some cases. Although dantrolene has been used in such life-threatening situations, it is felt to be a nonspecific treatment.[90]

B. Consequences of hyperthermia

Hyperthermia itself increases metabolic rate and oxygen consumption. Increased cardiac output, heart rate, and stroke volume ensue. Patients unable to increase cardiac output may develop significant acidemia and myocardial ischemia. Hyperthermic patients may perspire during anesthesia, but usually do not until body temperature exceeds 38° C or 39° C. Children may exhibit seizures. Coma, brain damage, and DIC occur with pronounced (greater than 42° C) hyperthermia. Seizures increase the metabolic demand for oxygen even further. Despite temperatures greater than 41° C, vigorous treatment of hyperthermia may reverse CNS dysfunction.[114] Although documentation is poor, case reports before air conditioning record death during anesthesia from hyperthermia, presumably because of acidosis and DIC.

1. Clinical diagnosis of malignant hyperthermia. The signs and symptoms of MH may be classified as specific or nonspecific. Nonspecific responses in MH include tachycardia, tachypnea, and diaphoresis. Increased concentrations of catecholamines secondary to sympathetic stimulation may lead to peripheral vasoconstriction, represented by mottled cyanosis in some cases. Temperature elevation is a nonspecific, late sign of MH that follows the increase in oxygen consumption.

More specific signs of MH include skeletal muscle rigidity (sometimes involving only the masseter muscles), muscle destruction with increased concentrations of CK, myoglobinuria and myoglobinemia, hyperkalemia, and hypercalcemia. Respiratory and metabolic acidosis often accompany MH. Acidemia is mild when cardiac output and oxygen delivery to the periphery are maintained. In more dramatic cases, however, acidosis and hyperkalemia produce arrhythmias, myocardial depression, and cardiac arrest. DIC occurs in severe MH. DIC has been the usual cause of death in MH in recent years.

Masseter muscle rigidity (MMR) presages MH.[115] MMR occurs in pediatric patients after halothane and succinylcholine induction in up to 1 in 100 cases.[116,117] Fifty percent of those patients, when biopsied and tested with the halothane-caffeine contracture test, demonstrate MH susceptibility. Clinically, however, a much smaller number of those experiencing MMR go on to develop MH. This discrepancy may arise from a high false positive rate of diagnostic muscle biopsy, or because subclinical MH susceptibility occurs more often in the population than otherwise suspected. The association of MH with generalized rigidity is much higher than with isolated MMR.

MH may begin in an explosive manner with tachycardia, marked elevation of end-tidal carbon dioxide, and muscle rigidity, or in a slower, more insidious form. In recent years, with the diminishing use of succinylcholine, slowly (over 20 to 30 minutes) increasing concentrations of carbon dioxide and increasing ventilatory requirements may be the earliest sign of MH.[118] MH may occur at any point during anesthesia or even in the PACU. Hyperthermia per se is a late sign of MH and, in the absence of other metabolic changes, a poor predictor of MH.

2. Clinical diagnosis of neuroleptic malignant syndrome. Despite its presumed CNS cause (dopamine receptor alteration), NMS displays manifestations that imply direct involvement of skeletal muscle, such as rhabdomyolysis, rigidity, and release of CK. In contrast to MH, however, nondepolarizing muscle relaxants block the muscle rigidity of NMS. Fever, autonomic imbalance, and acidosis are consequences of the hyperthermia.

C. Prevention of hyperthermia

A thorough history, familiarity with the patient's preoperative condition, and careful attention to application of heating devices are essential in the prevention of intraoperative hyperthermia. Screening for the disorders mentioned previously and for evidence of myopathy should be routine. Osteogenesis imperfecta should be suspected in a patient with multiple fractures and blue scleras. A family or personal history of an adverse response to anesthesia should arouse suspicions of MH. MH is not the most common cause of intraoperative morbidity and mortality, however. Not all cases of unexplained death in the perioperative period should be ascribed to MH. A history of sudden, unexpected cardiac arrest in the perioperative period should raise the suspicion of an inherited myopathy. Where available, old records should be consulted.

Intraoperative monitoring plays a key role in the early diagnosis of MH. Unexplained elevation in end-tidal carbon dioxide constitutes the earliest, most sensitive sign of MH.[117] A doubling or tripling of end-tidal carbon dioxide may occur in less than 5 minutes. However, a more insidious onset may occur in which the end-tidal carbon dioxide rises slowly and is maintained within normal limits by increasing minute ventilation. In such a scenario, MH or other causes of hypermetabolism should be considered.[118] Hemoglobin oxygen saturation usually does not decrease during acute episodes of MH, depending on the degree of peripheral vasoconstriction, inspired oxygen concentration, and delivery of oxygen to the periphery.

Although simple and readily available, body temperature is not always monitored during anesthesia in clinical practice. We believe that temperature is a vital sign that should be recorded in all patients undergoing general anesthesia lasting for more than 20 minutes and during major conduction anesthesia. Despite being a late sign of MH, temperature elevation may nevertheless be a determining clinical indicator of MH.

Most authorities agree that esophageal, pulmonary artery, and tympanic membrane measurement sites provide the greatest accuracy and reliability. Less accurate indicators of central temperature include rectal and urinary catheter temperature.[119] How skin temperature changes during MH in humans has not been studied. In pigs, skin temperature lags significantly behind core temperature.[120] Theoretically, vasoconstriction from catecholamine release during MH

might render skin temperature monitoring inaccurate. However, if the heat load is sufficient, peripheral vasodilation to transfer heat to the skin may occur, overcoming the vasoconstriction. Recently it has been shown that forehead skin temperature is a reasonably good representative of core temperature during routine surgery.[11] The American Society of Anesthesiologists standards indicate that temperature monitoring should be used wherever temperature changes are anticipated. We contend that temperature changes should be anticipated with every general anesthetic.

Dantrolene, a hydantoin derivative, inhibits the release of calcium from SR and may enhance reuptake of calcium into the SR as well. Prophylaxis against MH is by dantrolene administration before surgery at a dose of 2 to 2.5 mg/kg^{-1} intravenously. The same blood concentrations may be achieved with 5 mg/kg^{-1} orally over 24 hours.[121] Dantrolene may exacerbate preexisting muscle weakness and elicit nausea and vomiting. Routine prophylaxis with dantrolene for patients who have a history of MH is no longer recommended. Some would use dantrolene prophylactically in a patient who has experienced a life-threatening episode of MH. Dantrolene should be available in all facilities where general anesthesia is administered.

For the MH-susceptible patient requiring general anesthesia, the anesthesia vaporizers should be disabled by removal, drainage, or taping the control mechanism temporarily. Flowing oxygen at 10 L/min for 20 minutes combined with changing CO_2 absorbant is sufficient to reduce the concentrations of inhaled agent so that they will not trigger MH.[122] Of course, succinylcholine and potent inhaled agents should be avoided.

D. Treatment of hyperthermia

1. Nonspecific. The management of intraoperative hyperthermia not attributable to MH consists of removal of warming devices such as heating blankets, heated humidifiers, and coverings. Iced or cooled intravenous solutions are also of help. Where possible, blowing cool air with a fan over the patient and cooling the room provide additional means of heat dissipation. In hyperthermia not related to MH, these simple surface-cooling maneuvers should be sufficient to restore normothermia. With more pronounced hyperthermia, ice packs should be placed along the superficial sites of major blood vessels such as the neck, groin, axilla, and scalp.

Iced-solution lavage of the stomach, rectum, and wound provides internal cooling, as does infusion of iced intravenous fluid. Peritoneal lavage, in cases where the abdomen is not open, has also been reported to be effective.[123] A recent report has shown that total body immersion in an ice-water bath is the most rapid means of cooling.[124] However, the technique is very impractical. Those experienced in managing heat stroke advise application of tepid water by spray and blowing cool air over the patient as an effective cooling technique.[125] In extreme cases, cardiopulmonary bypass rapidly cools patients. This highly invasive step is reserved for the most desperate situations. Only when heart rate exceeds 160 beats/min with compromise of cardiac output or signs of myocardial ischemia should β-blocker administration occur.

Box 15-1 Suggested treatment of malignant hyperthermia

1. Stop potent inhaled agents and succinylcholine.
2. Increase minute ventilation to lower end-tidal CO_2
3. Get help.
4. Prepare and administer dantrolene 2.5 mg/kg initial dose. Titrate dantrolene to tachycardia and hypercarbia. Ten mg/kg is suggested as the upper limit, but more may be given as needed.
5. Begin cooling measures, if hyperthermic (iced solutions, ice packs in groin, axilla, and neck). Perform nasogastric lavage with iced solution. Use more aggressive measures as needed. Stop cooling measures at 38.5° C.
6. Treat arrhythmias as needed. Do not use calcium-channel blockers.
7. Secure blood gases, electrolytes, CK, blood, and urine for myoglobin, coagulation profile. Check values every 6 to 12 hours. Treat hyperkalemia with hyperventilation, glucose, and insulin as needed.
8. Continue dantrolene at 1 mg/kg every 4 to 8 hours for 24 to 48 hours.
9. Ensure urine output of 2 ml/kg/hr with mannitol, furosemide, and fluids as needed.
10. Evaluate need for invasive monitoring and continued mechanical ventilation.
11. Observe patient in ICU for at least 36 hours.
12. Refer patient to the Malignant Hyperthermia Association of the United States for information and counseling. Complete form for enrollment in the North American MH registry.
13. Refer to biopsy center for biopsy.

Box 15-2 Malignant Hyperthermia Association of the United States and the North American MH Registry

Address
P.O. Box 1069
Sherburne, New York 13460

Web site: www.mhaus.org

MHAUS general number: 1-800-98-MHAUS

MHAUS hotline: 1-800-MHHYPER

Fax: 607-674-7910

2. *Specific for malignant hyperthermia.* Upon diagnosing MH, the anesthesiologist should discontinue inhaled anesthetics and institute hyperventilation at two to three times the predicted minute ventilation (Box 15-1). Hypotension or other cardiovascular compromise indicates use of sodium bicarbonate 1 to 2 mg/kg^{-1} IV. However, rapid conversion of bicarbonate to carbon dioxide requires that minute ventilation be increased further.

Dantrolene, the specific drug treatment for MH, is prepared as a lyophilized solution of 20 mg per vial. Because it must be reconstituted with 60 ml distilled water or 5% glucose solution, additional help should be sought to mix and solubilize the drug. Once it is mixed, 2.5 mg/kg^{-1} of the drug should be given intravenously, titrated to heart rate, body temperature, and muscle rigidity. Despite the recommended upper dosage limit of 10 mg/kg^{-1}, more may be administered if needed to establish control. This is rarely necessary. Once MH is under control, dantrolene should be continued for at a least 48 hours, with use of an empiric dose of 1 to 2 mg/kg^{-1} IV every 4 to 6 hours. Total amounts of greater than 10 mg/kg^{-1} may be necessary with recrudescence or persistence of the syndrome. Dantrolene's half-life is approximately 12 hours.[126] Once the patient has responded to treatment and is awake, orally administered dantrolene is appropriate.

Upon diagnosing MH, one should measure arterial blood gases, activated PTT, platelet count, plasma fibrinogen, fibrinogen degradation products (if available), and calcium and phosphate ion concentrations. Baseline CK and myoglobin concentrations in the blood and urine should be obtained. Because CK peaks 24 hours after an MH episode, it should not be elevated initially. Myoglobinuria may occur at the time of first diagnosis of MH. Liver enzymes are also elevated in many patients.

Use of dantrolene, hyperventilation, and cooling measures usually prevent arrhythmias. Lidocaine may be used in the management of arrhythmias as necessary. Amide local anesthetics do not exacerbate MH episodes in swine, and lidocaine has allowed successful management of arrhythmias during MH.[127]

The use of calcium-channel blockers should be avoided. The combination of dantrolene, hyperkalemia, and hypotension complicates the use of calcium-channel blockers in MH.[128] Similarly, coagulation abnormalities and DIC often revert with control of the underlying disorder. MH does not modify the customary treatment of acute DIC; many clinicians will want to enlist the aid of a hematologist to treat DIC.

Once resuscitated, the patient should undergo observation in an intensive care unit for at least 24 hours. Up to 25% of treated MH episodes may recur within that period of time, and dantrolene should be administered for at least 48 hours. Serial CK concentrations serve to detect ongoing muscle destruction. Muscle weakness and myalgias are common after an episode of MH because a massive amount of muscle destruction may occur.

3. *Management of masseter muscle spasm.* The specific management of MMR is controversial.[129] We and others advocate that trismus is an indication to stop an anesthetic for elective surgery. Because it is not clear whether MH may supervene and because myoglobinuria is expected after MMR whether or not MH supervenes, others prefer converting to nontriggering anesthetics. A third group contends that MMR is insignificant; they would continue a triggering anesthetic. This approach is risky. Serum CK should be measured at 6, 12, and 24 hours after MMR. Myoglobinuria and hyperkalemia may occur. Because myoglobinuria carries particular risk of renal morbidity, we recommend 1 to 2 mg/kg^{-1} dantrolene after an episode of MMR, even in the absence of other signs of MH.

After an episode of MH or MMR, patients should receive follow-up counseling for MH susceptibility through organizations such as the Malignant Hyperthermia Association of the United States (MHAUS; Box 15-2). Relatives of these patients should also consider being tested for MH.

At present, the only agreed-upon diagnostic test for MH is the halothane-caffeine contracture test. Performed in over 40 centers worldwide, the test involves removal of 1 to 2 g muscle with testing for a contracture response to halothane and caffeine. Muscle from MH patients displays a contracture to halothane and a left-shifted dose-response curve to caffeine. The sensitivity of the test is 100% and the specificity is approximately 90%.[130] No patient with a negative biopsy has subsequently developed MH, even when challenged.[131] A variety of other diagnostic tests have been found to be of no value, including the calcium uptake test, the calcium ATPase test, the platelet ATP depletion test, and a test of released calcium from lymphocytes. Serum CK concentrations are not an appropriate screening test for MH. Recent identification of the gene for MH on chromosome 19 in some families holds prospect for a DNA-based test that could be performed on white cells. However, it is also clear that not all MH susceptibles share a similar genetic defect.

Measurements of intracellular high-energy phosphates using magnetic resonance imaging of arm muscles reveal a depletion of CK in MH-susceptible patients.[132,133] Because reduced concentrations of CK in muscle are also found in patients with a variety of other muscle disorders, this test may prove useful for screening family members once MH has been otherwise diagnosed.

4. Neuroleptic malignant syndrome. The management of NMS consists of discontinuing the offending psychotropic drug, administration of dantrolene and bromocriptine, and supportive treatment. We would also avoid triggering anesthetics. Dantrolene's effectiveness in NMS may be related to a nonspecific reduction of muscle tone and thus heat production or to blocking of a specific pathophysiologic process of heat production related to calcium release from the SR in muscle.

An organization now exists to provide information about NMS and its treatment. The Neuroleptic Malignant Syndrome Information Service (NMSIS) supports a Web site (www.nmsis.org). The NMSIS is a subsidiary of MHAUS; its phone number is 888-776-6747.

5. Other syndromes. Treatment of patients who have fevers unrelated to MH and NMS includes the administration of salicylates and antipyretic agents along with the nonspecific measures mentioned earlier in this chapter. Of course, specific treatment for pheochromocytoma, hyperthyroidism, and status epilepticus should be instituted when these are the precipitating causes of hyperthermia.

IV. SUMMARY

Alteration in body temperature is common during anesthesia. In the unanesthetized patient, body temperature is maintained within a very narrow range by way of af-ferent sensing, central processing, and efferent thermoregulatory responses. All these components of the thermoregulatory system are impaired by anesthesia, thus creating a state of poikilothermia in which body temperature tends to equilibrate with ambient temperature. Although MH is rarely encountered, the potential morbidity associated with MH is significant and the syndrome must be recognized and treated expeditiously. The role of the anesthesiologist is to maintain physiologic homeostasis during the perioperative period, a time during which anesthesia and surgery create an abnormal physiologic state. Body temperature should be managed in a similar fashion to the other vital signs, and efforts should be made to maintain normothermia.

ACKNOWLEDGMENT

The authors wish to acknowledge the assistance of Dr. Jan Horrow, Professor of Anesthesiology, MCP-Hahnemann, for assistance with the preparation of this information for the first edition of this book.

REFERENCES

1. Ring GC: The importance of thyroid hormone in maintaining an adequate production of heat during exposure to cold, *Am J Physiol* 137:582, 1942.
2. Benzinger TH: Heat regulation: homeostasis of central temperature in men, *Physiol Rev* 49:671, 1969.
3. Sessler DI: Mild perioperative hypothermia, *N Engl J Med* 336:1730, 1997.
4. Cheng C, Matsukawa T, Sessler DI, et al: Increasing mean skin temperature linearly reduces the core-temperature thresholds for vasoconstriction and shivering in humans, *Anesthesiology* 82:1160, 1995.
5. Sessler DI: Perianesthetic thermoregulation and heat balance in humans, *FASEB J* 7:638, 1993.
6. Lopez M, Sessler DI, Walter K, et al: Rate and gender dependence of the sweating, vasoconstriction, and shivering thresholds in humans, *Anesthesiology* 80:780, 1994.
7. Frank SM, Higgins MS, Fleisher LA, et al: The adrenergic, respiratory, and cardiovascular effects of core cooling in humans, *Am J Physiol* 272:R557, 1997.
8. DuBois EF: The many different temperatures of the human body and its parts, *West J Surg Obstet Gynecol* 59:476, 1951.
9. Colin J, Timbal J, Houdas Y, et al: Computation of mean body temperature from rectal and skin temperatures, *J Appl Physiol* 31:484, 1971.
10. Cork RC, Vaughan RW, Humphrey LS: Precision and accuracy of intraoperative temperature monitoring, *Anesth Analg* 62:211, 1983.
11. Ikeda T, Sessler DI, Marder D, et al: The influence of thermoregulatory vasomotion and ambient temperature variation on the accuracy of core-temperature estimates by cutaneous liquid-crystal thermometers, *Anesthesiology* 86:603, 1997.
12. Frank SM: Body temperature monitoring. In Levitt R, ed: *Anesthesiology clinics of North America*, Philadelphia, 1994, WB Saunders, p 387.
13. Cranston WI: Oral, rectal and oesophageal temperatures and some factors affecting them in man, *J Physiol* 126:347, 1954.
14. Whitby JD, Dunkin LJ: Temperature differences in the oesophagus, *Br J Anaesth* 40:991, 1968.
15. Benzinger M: Tympanic thermometry in surgery and anesthesia, *JAMA* 209:1207, 1969.
16. Frank SM, Beattie C, Christopherson R, et al: Epidural versus general anesthesia, ambient operating room temperature, and patient age as predictors of inadvertent hypothermia, *Anesthesiology* 77:252, 1992.
17. Vaughan MS, Vaughan RW, Cork RC: Postoperative hypothermia in adults: relationship of age, anesthesia, and shivering in rewarming, *Anesth Analg* 60:746, 1981.

18. Lomax P: The hypothermic effect of pentobarbital in the rat: sites and mechanisms of action, *Brain Res* 1:296, 1966.

19. Kurz A, Sessler DI, Annadata R, et al: Midazolam minimally impairs thermoregulatory control, *Anesth Analg* 81:393, 1995.

20. Leslie K, Sessler DI, Bjorksten AR, et al: Propofol causes a dose-dependent decrease in the thermoregulatory threshold for vasoconstriction but has little effect on sweating, *Anesthesiology* 81:353, 1994.

21. Lotti VJ, Lomax P, George R: Temperature responses in the rat following intracerebral microinjection of morphine, *J Pharmacol Exp Ther* 150:135, 1965.

22. Rosow CE, Miller JM, Pelikan EW, et al: Opiates and thermoregulation in mice. I. Agonists, *J Pharmacol Exp Ther* 213:273, 1980.

23. Pauca AL, Savage RT, Simpson S, et al: Effect of pethidine, fentanyl, and morphine on postoperative shivering in man, *Acta Anaesthesiol Scand* 28:138, 1984.

24. Kurz A, Go JC, Sessler DI, et al: Alfentanil slightly increases the sweating threshold and markedly reduces the vasoconstriction and shivering thresholds, *Anesthesiology* 82:293, 1995.

25. Matsukawa T, Sessler DI, Sessler AM, et al: Heat flow and distribution during induction of general anesthesia, *Anesthesiology* 82:662, 1995.

26. Frank SM, Fleisher LA, Olson KF, et al: Multivariate determinants of early postoperative oxygen consumption: the effects of shivering, core temperature, and gender, *Anesthesiology* 83:241, 1995.

27. Frank SM, Higgins MS, Breslow MJ, et al: The catecholamine, cortisol, and hemodynamic responses to mild perioperative hypothermia: a randomized clinical trial, *Anesthesiology* 82:83, 1995.

28. Emerick TH, Ozaki M, Sessler DI, et al: Epidural anesthesia increases apparent leg temperature and decreases the shivering threshold, *Anesthesiology* 81:289, 1994.

29. Leslie K, Sessler DI: Reduction in the shivering threshold is proportional to spinal block height, *Anesthesiology* 84:1327, 1996.

30. Frank SM, Shir Y, Raja SN, et al: Core hypothermia and skin-surface temperature gradients: epidural vs. general anesthesia and the effects of age, *Anesthesiology* 80:502, 1994.

30a. Frank SM, Nguyen JM, Garcia CM, et al: Temperature monitoring practices during regional anesthesia, *Anesth Analg* 88:373, 1999.

31. Joris J, Ozaki M, Sessler DI, et al: Epidural anesthesia impairs both central and peripheral thermoregulatory control during general anesthesia, *Anesthesiology* 80:268, 1994.

32. Michenfelder JD, Uihlen A, Saw EF, et al:: Moderate hypothermia in man: hemodynamic and metabolic effects, *Br J Anaesth* 37:738, 1965.

33. Busto R, Dietrich WD, Globus MY, et al: Small differences in intraischemic brain temperature critically determine the extent of ischemic neuronal injury, *J Cereb Blood Flow Metab* 7:729, 1987.

34. Vacanti FX, Ames AA: Mild hypothermia and Mg++ protect against irreversible damage during CNS ischemia, *Stroke* 15:695, 1983.

35. Todd MM, Warner DS: A comfortable hypothesis reevaluated: cerebral metabolic depression and brain protection during ischemia, *Anesthesiology* 76:161, 1992 (editorial).

36. Mora CT, Henson MB, Weintraub WS, et al: The effects of temperature management during cardiopulmonary bypass on neurologic and neuropsychologic outcomes in patients undergoing coronary revascularization, *J Thorac Cardiovasc Surg* 112:514, 1996.

37. Frank SM, Beattie C, Christopherson R, et al: Unintentional hypothermia is associated with postoperative myocardial ischemia, *Anesthesiology* 78:468, 1993.

38. Frank SM, Fleisher LA, Breslow MJ, et al: Perioperative maintenance of normothermia reduces the incidence of morbid cardiac events: a randomized trial, *JAMA* 277:1127, 1997.

39. Crawford SE, Crawford JL, Safi HJ, et al: Thoracoabdominal aortic aneurysms: preoperative and intraoperative factors determining immediate and long term results of operations in 605 patients, *J Vasc Surg* 3:389, 1986.

40. Frank SM, Parker SD, Rock P, et al: Moderate hypothermia with partial bypass and segmental sequential repair for thoracoabdominal aortic aneurysm, *J Vasc Surg* 19:687, 1994.

41. Bay J, Nunn JF, Prys-Roberts C: Factors influencing arterial PO_2 during recovery from anaesthesia, *Br J Anaesth* 17:398, 1968.

42. MacIntyre PE, Pavlin EG, Dwersteg JF: Effect of meperidine on oxygen consumption, carbon dioxide production, and respiratory gas exchange in postanesthetic shivering, *Anesth Analg* 66:751, 1987.

43. Kurz M, Belani K, Sessler DI, et al: Naloxone, meperidine, and shivering, *Anesthesiology* 79:1193, 1993.

44. Krenzischeck DA, Frank SM, Kelly S: Forced-air skin-surface warming vs. routine thermal care and core temperature monitoring sites, *J Postanesth Nurs* 10:69, 1995.

45. Severinghaus JW, Stupfel M: Respiratory dead space increase following atropine in man, and atropine, vagal or ganglionic blockade and hypothermia in dogs, *J Appl Physiol* 8:81, 1955.

46. Regan MJ, Eger EI: Ventilatory responses to hypercapnia and hypoxia at normothermia and moderate hypothermia during constant-depth halothane anesthesia, *Anesthesiology* 27:624, 1966.

47. Benumof JL, Wahrenbrock EA: Dependency of hypoxic pulmonary vasoconstriction on temperature, *J Appl Physiol* 42:56, 1977.

48. Bainton D, Moore F, Sweetnam P: Temperature and deaths from ischemic heart disease, *Br J Prev Soc Med* 31:49, 1977.

49. Rose G: Cold weather and ischaemic heart disease, *Br J Prev Soc Med* 20:97, 1966.

50. Hines EA, Brown GE: The cold pressor test for measuring the reactibility of the blood pressure: data concerning 571 normal and hypertensive subjects, *Am Heart J* 11:1, 1936.

51. Mudge GH, Grossman W, Mills RM, et al: Reflex increase in coronary vascular resistance in patients with ischemic heart disease, *N Engl J Med* 295:1333, 1976.

52. Kattlove HE, Alexander B: The effect of cold on platelets. I. Cold-induced platelet aggregation, *Blood* 38:39, 1971.

53. Valeri CR, Feingold H, Cassidy G, et al: Hypothermia-induced reversible platelet dysfunction, *Ann Surg* 205:175, 1987.

54. Rohrer MJ, Natale AM: Effect of hypothermia on the coagulation cascade, *Crit Care Med* 20:1402, 1992.

55. Yoshihara H, Yamamoto T, Mihara H: Changes in coagulation and fibrinolysis occurring in dogs during hypothermia, *Thromb Res* 37:503, 1985.

56. Hessel EA, Schmer G, Dillard DH: Platelet kinetics during deep hypothermia, *J Surg Res* 28:23, 1980.

57. Schmied H, Kurz A, Sessler DI, et al: Mild hypothermia increases blood loss and transfusion requirements during total hip arthroplasty, *Lancet* 347:289, 1996.

58. Kurz A, Sessler DI, Lenhardt R, et al: Perioperative normothermia to reduce the incidence of surgical-wound infection and shorten hospitalization, *N Engl J Med* 334:1209, 1996.

59. Sheffield CW, Sessler DI, Hunt TK: Mild hypothermia impairs resistance to *E. coli* infection in guinea pigs, *Acta Anesthesiol Scand* 38:201, 1994.

60. Vitez TS, White PF, Eger EI: Effects of hypothermia of halothane MAC and isoflurane MAC in the rat, *Anesthesiology* 41:80, 1974.

61. Lenhardt R, Marker E, Goll V, et al: Mild intraoperative hypothermia prolongs postanesthetic recovery, *Anesthesiology* 87:1318, 1997.

62. Heier T, Caldwell JE, Sessler DI, et al: Mild intraoperative hypothermia increases duration of action and spontaneous recovery of vecuronium blockade during nitrous oxide-isoflurane anesthesia in humans, *Anesthesiology* 74:815, 1991.

63. Leslie K, Sessler DI, Bjorksten AR, et al: Mild hypothermia prolongs the duration of action of atracurium, *Anesth Analg* 80:1007, 1995.

64. Moschcowitz AV: Post-operative heat stroke, *Surg Gynecol Obstet* 23:443, 1916.

65. Morris RH: Operating room temperature and the anesthetized paralyzed patient, *Arch Surg* 103:95, 1971.

66. Bissonnette B, Sessler DI: Passive or active inspired gas humidification increases thermal steady-state temperatures in anesthetized infants, *Anesth Analg* 69:783, 1989.

67. Faries G, Johnston C, Pruitt KM, et al: Temperature relationship to distance and flow rate of warmed IV fluids, *Ann Emerg Med* 20:1198, 1991.

68. Presson RGJ, Bezruczko AP, Hillier SC, et al: Evaluation of a new fluid warmer effective at low to moderate flow rates, *Anesthesiology* 78:974, 1993.

69. Sessler DI, McGuire J, Sessler AM: Perioperative thermal insulation, *Anesthesiology* 74:875, 1991.

70. Hynson JM, Sessler DI: Intraoperative warming therapies: a comparison of three devices, *J Clin Anesth* 4:194, 1992.

71. Giesbrecht GG, Ducharme MB, McGuire JP: Comparison of forced-air patient warming systems for perioperative use, *Anesthesiology* 80:671, 1994.

72. Sessler DI, Moayeri A: Skin-surface warming: heat flux and central temperature, *Anesthesiology* 73:218, 1990.

73. Sharkey A, Lipton JM, Murphy MT, et al: Inhibition of postanesthetic shivering with radiant heat, *Anesthesiology* 66:249, 1987.

73a. Tran K, Frank SM, El-Rahmany H, et al: Thermal and hemodynamic effects of subatmospheric postoperative rewarming, *J Therm Biol* (in press).

73b. Bernheim HA, Block LH, Atkins E: Fever: pathogenesis, pathophysiology, and purpose, *Ann Intern Med* 91:261, 1979.

74. Clark WG, Lipton JM: Drug-related heatstroke, *Pharmacol Ther* 26:345, 1984.

75. Kim RC, Collins G, Cho C, et al: Heat stroke: report of three fatal cases with emphasis on findings in skeletal muscle, *Arch Pathol Lab Med* 104:345, 1980.

76. Bloch EC: Hyperthermia resulting from tourniquet application in children, *Ann R Coll Surg Engl* 68:193, 1986.

77. Gomes AS, Busuttil RW, Baker JD, et al: Congenital arteriovenous malformations, *Arch Surg* 118:817, 1983.

78. Henderson MA, Pettigrew RT: Induction of controlled hyperthermia in the treatment of cancer, *Lancet* 1:1275, 1971.

79. Stoen R, Sessler DI: The thermoregulatory threshold is inversely proportional to isoflurane concentration, *Anesthesiology* 72:822, 1990.

80. Crowley KJ, Cunningham AJ, Conroy D, et al: Phaeochromocytoma: a presentation mimicking malignant hyperthermia, *Anaesthesia* 43:1031, 1988.

81. Bennett MH, Wainwright AP: Acute thyroid crisis on induction of anaesthesia, *Anaesthesia* 44:28, 1989.

82. Ismail-Beigi F, Edelman IS: The mechanism of the calorigenic action of thyroid hormone, *J Gen Physiol* 57:710, 1971.

83. Iaizzo PA, Klein W, Lehmann Horn F: Fura-2 detected myoplasmic calcium and its correlation with contracture force in skeletal muscle from normal and malignant hyperthermia susceptible pigs, *Pflugers Arch* 411:648, 1988.

84. Axelrod FB, Donenfeld R, Denziger F, et al: Anesthesia in familial dysautonomia, *Anesthesiology* 68:631, 1988.

85. Rampton AJ, Kelly DA, Shanahan EC, et al: Occurrence of malignant hyperpyrexia in a patient with osteogenesis imperfecta, *Br J Anaesth* 56:1443, 1984.

86. Plum F, Posner JB, Hain RF: Delayed neurological deterioration after anoxia, *Arch Intern Med* 110:18, 1962.

87. Chan TC, Evans SD, Clark RF: Drug induced hyperthermia. In Carlson RW, Geheb MA, eds: *Critical care clinics,* Philadelphia, 1997, WB Saunders, p 785.

88. Rosenberg H, Fletcher JE, Seitman D: Pharmacogenetics. In Barash P, Cullen B, Stoelting RK, eds: *Clinical anesthesia,* ed 3, Philadelphia, 1996, Lippincott-Raven, p 489.

89. Lazarus A, Mann SC, Caroff SN: *The neuroleptic malignant syndrome and related conditions,* Washington, DC, 1989, American Psychiatric Press.

90. Hall AP: "Ecstasy" and the anesthetist, *Br J Anaesth* 79:697, 1997.

91. Bachand M, Vachon N, Boisvert M, et al: Clinical reassessment of malignant hyperthermia in Abitibi-Temiscamingue, *Can J Anaesth* 44:696, 1997.

92. Lopez JR, Allen PD, Alamo L, et al: Myoplasmic free Ca^{+2} during a malignant hyperthermia episode in swine, *Muscle Nerve* 11:82, 1988.

93. Mickelson JR, Gallant EM, Litterer LA, et al: Abnormal sarcoplasmic reticulum ryanodine receptor in malignant hyperthermia, *J Biol Chem* 263:9310, 1988.

94. Cheah KS: Skeletal-muscle mitochondria and phospholipase A_2 in malignant hyperthermia, *Biochem Soc Trans* 12:358, 1984.

95. Fletcher JE, Rosenberg H, Michaux K, et al: Triglycerides, not phospholipids, are the source of elevated free fatty acids in muscle from patients susceptible to malignant hyperthermia, *Eur J Anaesthesiol* 6(5):355, 1989.

96. Pessah IN, Lynch C, Gronert GA: Complex pharmacology of malignant hyperthermia, *Anesthesiology* 84:1275, 1996.

97. MacLennon DH, Phillips MS: Malignant hyperthermia, *Science* 256:789, 1992.

98. Levitt RC, Olckers A, Meyers S, et al: Evidence for the localization of a malignant hyperthermia susceptibility locus (MHS2) to human chromosome 17q, *Genomics* 14:562, 1992.

99. McCarthy TV: Localization of the malignant hyperthermia susceptibility locus to human chromosome 19q12-13.2, *Nature* 343(6258):562, 1990.

100. Monnier N, Procaccio V, Stieglitz P, et al: Malignant hyperthermia susceptibility is associated with a mutation of the alpha 1 subunit of the human dihydropyridine-sensitive L-type voltage dependent calcium-channel receptor in skeletal muscle, *Am J Hum Genet* 60:1316, 1997.

101. Fletcher JE, Wieland SJ, Karan SM, et al: Sodium channel in malignant hyperthermia, *Anesthesiology* 86:1023, 1997.

102. Brownell AK, Paasuke RT, Elash A, et al: Malignant hyperthermia in Duchenne muscular dystrophy, *Anesthesiology* 58:180, 1983.

103. Larach MG, Rosenberg H, Gronert GA, et al: Hyperkalemic cardiac arrest during anesthetics in infants and children with occult myopathies, *Clin Pediatr* 36:9, 1997.

104. Bertorini TE, Bhattacharya SK, Palmieri GM, et al: Muscle calcium and magnesium content in Duchenne muscular dystrophy, *Neurology* 32:1088, 1982.

105. Masayuki K: Volatile anesthetics decrease calcium content of isolated myocytes, *Anesthesiology* 70:954, 1989.

106. Minasian A, Yagiela JA: The use of amide local anesthetics in patients susceptible to malignant hyperthermia, *Oral Surg Oral Med Oral Pathol* 66:405, 1988.

107. Gronert GA, Ahern CP, Milde JH, et al: Effect of CO_2, calcium, digoxin, and potassium on cardiac and skeletal muscle metabolism in malignant hyperthermia susceptible swine, *Anesthesiology* 64:24, 1986.

108. Nagarajan K, Fishbein NN, Muldoon SM, et al: Calcium uptake in frozen muscle biopsy sections compared with other predictors of malignant hyperthermia susceptibility, *Anesthesiology* 66:680, 1987.

109. Denborough MA, Hopkinson KC, Banney DG: Firefighting and malignant hyperthermia, *Br Med J Clin Res* 296(6634):1442, 1988.

110. Mirchandani H, Reich LE: Fatal malignant hyperthermia as a result of ingestion of tranylcypromine (Parnate) combined with white wine and cheese, *J Forensic Sci* 30:217, 1985.

111. Krivosic Horber R, Adnet P, Guevart E, et al: Neuroleptic malignant syndrome and malignant hyperthermia: in vitro comparison with halothane and caffeine contracture tests, *Br J Anaesth* 59:1554, 1987.

112. Geiduschek J, Cohen SA, Kahn A, et al: Repeated anesthesia for a patient with neuroleptic malignant syndrome, *Anesthesiology* 68:134, 1988.

113. Loghmanee F, Tobak M: Fatal malignant hyperthermia associated with recreational cocaine and ethanol abuse, *Am J Forensic Med Pathol* 7:246, 1986.

114. Cabral R, Prior PF, Scott D, et al: Reversible profound depression of cerebral electrical activity in hyperthermia, *Electroencephalogr Clin Neurophysiol* 42:697, 1977.

115. Rosenberg H, Fletcher JE: Masseter muscle rigidity and malignant hyperthermia susceptibility, *Anesth Analg* 65:161, 1986.

116. Schwartz L, Rockoff MA, Koka BV: Masseter spasm with anesthesia: incidence and implications, *Anesthesiology* 61:772, 1984.

117. Lazell VA, Carr AS, Lerman J, et al: The incidence of masseter muscle rigidity after succinylcholine in infants and children, *Can J Anaesth* 41:475, 1994.

118. Karan Sm, Crowl F, Muldoon SM: Malignant hyperthermia masked by capnographic monitoring, *Anesth Analg* 78:590, 1994.

119. Horrow JC, Rosenberg H: Does urinary catheter temperature reflect core temperature during cardiac surgery? *Anesthesiology* 69:986, 1988.
120. Iaizzo PA, Kehler CH, Zink RS, et al: Thermal response in acute porcine malignant hyperthermia, *Anesth Analg* 82:803, 1996.
121. Allen GC, Cattran CB, Peterson RG, et al: Plasma levels of dantrolene following oral administration in malignant hyperthermia–susceptible patients, *Anesthesiology* 69:900, 1988.
122. Beebe JJ, Sessler DI: Preparation of anesthesia machines for patients susceptible to malignant hyperthermia, *Anesthesiology* 69:395, 1988.
123. Horowitz BZ: The golden hour in heat stroke: use of iced peritoneal lavage, *Am J Emerg Med* 7:616, 1989.
124. Plattner O, Kurz A, Sessler DI, et al: Efficacy of intraoperative cooling methods, *Anesthesiology* 87:1089, 1997.
125. Khogali M, Mustafa MKE, Gumma K: Management of heatstroke, *Lancet* 2:1225, 1982.
126. Ward A, Chaffman MO, Sorkin EM: Dantrolene: a review of its pharmacodynamic and pharmacokinetic properties and therapeutic use in malignant hyperthermia, the neuroleptic malignant syndrome and an update of its use in muscle spasticity, *Drugs* 32:130, 1986.
127. Katz D: Recurrent malignant hyperthermia during anesthesia, *Anesth Analg* 49:225, 1975.
128. Rubin AS, Zablocki AD: Hyperkalemia, verapamil, and dantrolene, *Anesthesiology* 66:246, 1987.
129. Rosenberg H: Trismus is not trivial, *Anesthesiology* 67:453, 1987 (editorial).
130. Allen GC, Larach MG, Kunselman AR, et al: The sensitivity and specificity of the caffeine halothane contracture test: a report from the North American Malignant Hyperthermia Registry, *Anesthesiology,* 88:579, 1998.
131. Allen GC, Rosenberg H, Fletcher JE: Safety of general anesthesia in patients previously tested negative for malignant hyperthermia susceptibility, *Anesthesiology* 72:619, 1990.
132. Olgin J, Argov Z, Rosenberg H, et al: Non-invasive evaluation of malignant hyperthermia susceptibility with phosphorus nuclear magnetic resonance spectroscopy, *Anesthesiology* 68:507, 1988.
133. Payan JF, Bosson JL, Bourdon L, et al: Improved noninvasive diagnostic testing for malignant hyperthermia susceptibility from a combination of metabolites determined in vivo with ^{31}P-magnetic resonance spectroscopy, *Anesthesiology* 78:848, 1993.

Chapter 16

Impaired Central Nervous System Function

Deborah J. Culley
Gregory Crosby

General anesthesia, by definition, is central nervous system (CNS) dysfunction. Hence, some degree of postoperative CNS impairment, at least in the immediate postanesthetic period, is a natural and unavoidable consequence of general anesthesia. The problem is that general anesthesia can contribute to and complicate diagnosis of serious CNS events that occur infrequently in anesthetized patients, thereby making the assessment of abnormal emergence difficult. Accordingly, this chapter focuses on the causes, diagnosis, and prevention of perioperative CNS complications associated with general anesthesia and on surgical procedures in which the risk of an adverse neurologic event is high.

The first section considers four topics: normal cognitive and psychologic consequences of anesthesia, delirium, new neurologic deficits in the perioperative period, and evaluation of delayed or abnormal emergence. The second section of the chapter examines the risk of adverse neurologic outcome associated with carotid endarterectomy, cardiac surgery, and thoracoabdominal aortic surgery. This chapter does not deal with the neurologic complications of spinal, epidural, or regional anesthesia or with injury to the peripheral nervous system because these are covered in Chapters 3, 4, and 8, respectively.

Most data on CNS dysfunction in the perioperative period are limited because they are based almost entirely on associations between a particular adverse event and certain patient characteristics, medications, physiologic changes, procedures, and so on. Rarely have cause-and-effect relationships been established directly. Likewise, evidence that anesthetic management influences neurologic outcome in the clinical setting is sparse. With these caveats, our aim is to help the clinician develop a rational and realistic approach to anticipating, avoiding, identifying, and managing CNS dysfunction in the perioperative period.

I. CNS DYSFUNCTION AFTER NON-CNS, NONCARDIAC SURGERY

A. Postanesthetic cognitive and psychomotor dysfunction

All agents used for premedication, induction, and maintenance of anesthesia have lingering CNS effects. Thus it is accurate to say that every general anesthetic produces some postanesthetic impairment of cognitive and psychomotor performance. There are numerous examples of this. Diazepam and meperidine impair reaction time and coordination for as long as 5 to 12 hours in healthy volunteers[1] and an antiemetic dose of droperidol leaves 25% of patients with feelings of anxiety and restlessness for 24 to 36 hours.[2] Even short-acting drugs can produce long-lasting CNS dysfunction. Memory is impaired for up to 5 hours after sedative doses of midazolam[3] and residual effects of methohexital are evident on psychomotor testing 12 hours after a single dose.[4] Psychomotor performance is diminished in volunteers for 5 hours following 7 mg/kg of thiopental, whereas after an induction dose of propofol, recovery of cognitive and psychomotor performance occurs within an hour.[5] Inhaled anesthetics also have prolonged effects on mental function. Psychomotor performance is impaired for 5 hours after inhalation induction and maintenance of anesthesia for only 3.5 minutes with halothane or enflurane in normal volunteers.[6] In volunteers, somatic and behavioral symptoms persist for 6 to 8 days after 7 hours of halothane or isoflurane (with or without nitrous oxide) anesthesia,[7] and perceptual-motor and intellectual function take 2 days to return to normal after 10 to 14 hours of halothane or enflurane anesthesia.[8] The newer agents desflurane and sevoflurane, with low blood/gas partition coefficients, are an improvement in this regard.[9] Short- and intermediate-term cognitive and psychomotor recovery occurs more quickly than with the older inhaled agents,[10,11] but long-term recovery of psychomotor performance has not been assessed thoroughly. In humans, the only nonbehavioral measure of persistent dysfunction that has been evaluated carefully is natural sleep.

Electrophysiologic data indicate that natural patterns of rapid-eye-movement and slow-wave sleep in humans are disrupted for 24 hours after a brief anesthetic and remain abnormal for several days after anesthesia and surgery.[12] Although these types of cognitive and psychomotor impairments are rarely noticed by clinicians, patients will almost certainly notice. In fact, some combinations of sedatives and analgesics used commonly in anesthesia produce transient impairment similar to or greater than that produced by large doses of alcohol.[13]

There has been special concern that general anesthesia produces prolonged or permanent changes in memory and cognitive ability in the elderly.[14,15] Several studies using neuropsychologic testing before and from 1 to several months after anesthesia and surgery fail to support that notion, however.[14,16,17] Two recent studies[18,19] are notable and provocative exceptions. The first was a prospective, randomized trial of general versus epidural anesthesia with sedation for total knee replacement in patients older than 70 years of age.[18] The results show that cognitive performance was worse than the preoperative baseline in 4% to 6% of patients 6 months after anesthesia and surgery. Interestingly, there was no difference between the general and epidural anesthesia groups.[18] This is consistent with previous work indicating that cognitive performance after regional anesthesia in the elderly is typically no better than after general anesthesia, particularly if intravenous sedation is used to supplement a regional technique.[16,17,20,21] However, one limitation of the study[18] was that it lacked a control group for the effects of time or hospitalization alone. Therefore the extent to which the natural aging process or factors associated with hospitalization and surgery (e.g., postoperative sedatives and analgesics, immobility, social isolation, loss of independence) contribute cannot be determined. This issue was addressed recently by another study that was both prospective and controlled.[19] Moller et al[19] studied the incidence of long-term postoperative cognitive dysfunction

in the elderly (Table 16-1). In this international study, neuropsychologic tests were performed before and 1 week and 3 months after anesthesia and surgery in elderly patients (mean age 68 years; 1218 enrolled and 947 completed the study) undergoing general anesthesia for orthopedic, major abdominal, or noncardiac thoracic surgery. Controls consisted of 176 volunteers from the United Kingdom and 145 nationals. The study demonstrated a 9.9% incidence of deterioration on psychomotor tests of cognitive performance in elderly patients 3 months after general anesthesia for a variety of surgical procedures, whereas performance worsened in only 2.8% of nonhospitalized controls. The relationship of this deterioration to functional impairment (i.e., activities of daily living) was not examined. Risk factors, other than age, are not obvious; for example, deterioration did not correlate with episodes of arterial hemoglobin desaturation or hypotension. Although these data clearly implicate some aspect of anesthesia and surgery in cognitive deterioration in elderly patients, the anesthetic technique and agents were not specified, so the contribution of anesthesia itself remains unclear. In any case, these results are both interesting and sobering. Long-lasting cognitive deterioration may be a heretofore unrecognized risk of anesthesia and surgery in the elderly.

Why does anesthesia have lingering effects on cognitive and psychomotor function? The most obvious explanation is that some anesthetic agent remains in the brain even when gross clinical recovery is complete.[22] This has been demonstrated in animals; using magnetic resonance, 15% to 20% of the signal for halothane and isoflurane is still detectable in the brain 90 minutes after a 60- to 90-minute anesthetic.[22,23] Moreover, at the time of gross clinical recovery, cerebral metabolic rate is still 20% less than that of the awake state.[24] Newer agents (e.g., remifentanil, desflurane) with rapid and predictable redistribution and clearance are an improvement in this regard. However, to the extent that complex brain functions are exquisitely sensitive to drug effects, even trace amounts of anesthetics may disrupt normal function.[25,26] Another problem is that anesthetic requirements are determined clinically by crude indices of anesthetic depth (e.g., movement, blood pressure, and heart rate) that may have little direct relationship to the state of higher brain function or consciousness. For instance, the minimum alveolar concentration (MAC), a traditional measure of anesthetic depth, is heavily influenced by anesthetic action at the spinal level and is independent of forebrain structures.[27] Newer approaches to determining anesthetic depth, such as bispectral analysis of the electroencephalogram (EEG), may facilitate immediate recovery,[28] but whether these devices can also reduce the magnitude and duration of longer-term postanesthetic cognitive impairment is unknown. A third possibility is that anesthesia produces lasting changes in brain function. Evidence for this hypothesis is limited to a preliminary report of brain atrophy in rats[29] 6 months after uncomplicated general anesthesia and the observation that in patients with severe depression, isoflurane-induced burst suppression is as effective as electroconvulsive therapy[30] (indicating that isoflurane, burst suppression, or

Table 16-1. Long-term postoperative cognitive dysfunction in the elderly

	Control	Anesthesia and surgery
1 Week	3.4%	25.8%
3 Months	2.8%	9.9%

From Moller JT, Cluitmans P, Rasmussen LS, *Lancet* 351:857, 1998.

both can produce permanent alterations in brain function).[31] Whatever the reason, awakening and recovery from anesthesia are normally associated with cerebral metabolic, neurophysiologic, behavioral, and cognitive changes that persist for hours to days from the time of exposure. These changes are fundamentally benign and self-limited and are best considered side effects rather than complications of anesthesia. Clearly more worrisome is the observation that routine anesthesia and surgery may produce lasting decrements in cognitive performance in the elderly.

B. Delirium

Delirium is a common clinical entity associated with significant morbidity and mortality[32-34] Characteristic features include abnormalities in cognition, memory, perception, and thinking. The differential diagnosis is extensive and of more than academic interest because postoperative delirium can be a warning of serious but treatable underlying disease.[35] Preexisting organic cerebral pathology, endocrine and metabolic abnormalities, cognitive impairment, male gender, polypharmacy, advanced age, poor functional status, alcohol abuse, and the type of surgery (aortic aneurysm,[36] noncardiac thoracic,[36] cardiac,[37] and orthopedic[38,39]) have all been associated with an increased risk of postoperative delirium. It has also been proposed that delirium may be a manifestation of awareness during anesthesia.[40] Interestingly, most studies indicate that the incidence of postoperative delirium is similar regardless of whether regional or general anesthesia is used.[16,18]

Clinically, it is important to identify the potentially treatable causes of postoperative delirium. In particular, conditions that unbalance the normally close relationship between cerebral oxygen supply and demand are the most ominous and important to recognize. Thus cerebral hypoxia, regardless of cause, must be considered immediately in any patient who is delirious in the perioperative period.[41] Only after the possibility of cerebral hypoxia has been excluded should one consider other treatable causes of delirium such as endocrine or ionic imbalances, postoperative pain, sepsis, bowel or bladder distention, language difficulties, the porphyrias (acute intermittent and variegate), and medications.

A delirious patient's medication history is important.[33] High-dose steroids may produce an acute psychotic reaction[42] and delirium may also occur during withdrawal from drugs of abuse such as alcohol, opioids, and hallucinogens. Several anesthetic agents and adjuvants have been implicated in postoperative confusional states. Ketamine, a derivative of phencyclidine (PCP), has hallucinogenic and convulsive properties; emergence delirium and vivid, unpleasant dreams, perceptual distortion, disorientation, agitation, and nightmares can also occur.[43] The incidence of psychologic disturbances associated with ketamine is lowest among the elderly and children and can be reduced by the intravenous administration of benzodiazepines before awakening.[43,44] Anticholinergic medications such as atropine and scopolamine are another classic pharmacologic cause of postoperative confusion, particularly in the elderly.[38,45,46] This is not surprising because a deficiency of central cholinergic activity

is thought to account partially for the memory impairment that occurs with aging and some neurodegenerative diseases.[47] Other medications often used in the perioperative period that are associated with postoperative delirium or hallucinations include H_2 blockers,[48] droperidol,[49] and propofol.[50] Although medications can and do cause postanesthetic delirium, the key point is that delirium should not mistakenly be attributed to a drug effect when cerebral hypoxia or some other correctable disturbance is actually the cause. On rare occasions, circumstances may require a pharmacologic solution. If the delirious patient endangers himself or others, administration of haldol[51] is usually effective.

C. Neurologic complications after routine surgery

Major neurologic complications after nonneurologic, noncardiac surgery are rare but devastating. In a large prospective, randomized study of outcome after anesthesia,[52] the incidence of perioperative stroke was 0.04%. In the ambulatory surgical setting, the risk of a central nervous system event is less than 0.02%.[53] Seizures and hypoxic brain injury also occur perioperatively, but both are probably less common than stroke. For example, a large retrospective review of insurance claims made on just over 1 million anesthetics administered at nine teaching hospitals reported eight claims for severe hypoxia-induced CNS injury usually related to catastrophes of airway management.[54] From a clinical perspective, the central questions are what precipitates perioperative neurologic events, whether they can be prevented, and how one distinguishes between cerebral disease and "normal" CNS dysfunction in the patient recovering from anesthesia.

1. Perioperative stroke. The incidence of perioperative stroke after noncardiac, nonvascular, nonneurologic surgery is 0.02% to 0.07%.[52,53,55] The incidence is about 10 times greater in the elderly[56] and those having peripheral vascular surgical procedures,[57,58] presumably because of coexisting cerebral or carotid vascular disease. Although development of a new focal neurologic deficit during the perioperative period is uncommon and unpredictable, it may not be random. In one report,[59] for example, 12 strokes occurred in a general surgical population, whereas demographic data concerning the yearly incidence of stroke in age-matched nonhospitalized persons predicted only one such event. Another study[60] found three cases of perioperative stroke when only 0.1 was predicted from demographic data. Thus the risk of stroke is apparently increased perioperatively, but the conditions that predispose surgical patients to stroke are not obvious.

The potential roles of preexisting cerebrovascular disease and hypotension have been explored in some studies, but the data are limited and often inconsistent. There is strong agreement that an asymptomatic carotid bruit, present in about 14% of surgical patients over age 55 and 20% of vascular surgical patients, is not itself a risk factor for perioperative stroke.[55,61] Surgery need not be delayed in such patients, but they should be referred for further evaluation because recent evidence suggests that carotid endarterectomy may benefit asymptomatic patients with high-grade carotid stenosis.[62,63] The relationship between symptomatic cerebrovascular disease and perioperative stroke is controversial. There is disagreement as to whether reversible ischemic neurologic deficits (RINDs) or amaurosis fugax are associated with a higher incidence of perioperative stroke,[57,58] but the risk of perioperative cerebral reinfarction may be as much as 10 times greater in patients with a recent stroke.[64] The reasons for this greater vulnerability are unknown but may relate to a prolonged period of altered cerebrovascular reactivity after stroke.[65] There is no proven benefit of delaying elective surgery in this situation, although it is often recommended. Hypotension is another potential cause of perioperative stroke. There is no question that hypotension can produce cerebral ischemia and infarction.[66] Nevertheless, studies indicate that most patients who suffer a postoperative stroke experienced and survived intraoperative hypotension without neurologic sequelae.[58,59] The only direct investigation of the role of hypotension as a cause of stroke in humans comes from a study[67] of 37 patients with RINDs deliberately exposed to nearly a 60% decrease in systolic blood pressure. Such profound hypotension, albeit for a brief period, recreated a true transient ischemic attack (TIA) or RIND in only one person; others developed unrelated focal signs, and 17 had no focal findings at all before developing signs of global cerebral ischemia. Similarly, an autopsy study[68] of the brains of 135 patients who survived at least 1 day after a cardiac arrest (by definition, a hypotensive episode) found a relationship between the severity of cerebral atherosclerosis and brain infarction in only seven patients. This is not to suggest that transient intraoperative hypotension is benign, but rather that its role in precipitating perioperative stroke is not well established.

Thrombotic and embolic events appear to be responsible for most perioperative strokes. Dissection and thrombosis of the carotid or vertebral arteries have been reported perioperatively, ostensibly in conjunction with malpositioning of the neck.[69,70] Such patients are typically intact upon emergence but acutely develop severe neurologic symptoms and massive cerebral infarction hours or days later. Although neck hyperextension and rotation have been implicated, such dissections also occur spontaneously in association with common activities such as sneezing and coughing.[71] With respect to embolic events, cardiogenic embolism accounted for 5 of 12 perioperative strokes in a retrospective review[59] (only 1 was attributed to hypotension) and all but 2 occurred postoperatively. An antecedent myocardial infarction was present in 17% of the patients, and 33% were in atrial fibrillation at the time of the stroke.[59] Similarly, in a retrospective study of nearly 59,000 cases, 2 of 3 cases of new focal neurologic deficits detected upon emergence from anesthesia were attributed to embolism (one cardiogenic, the other paradoxic embolization of CO_2) and one was caused by a cerebral hemorrhage.[60] Indeed, the potential for hemorrhagic stroke exists but it appears to be extremely rare during uncomplicated anesthesia and surgery.[72] Because of the apparent prevalence of embolic sources for perioperative stroke, a thorough cardiac examination should not be neglected when evaluating a patient afflicted with a new postoperative focal deficit.

2. Perioperative seizures. Perioperative seizures may be idiopathic or related to hypoxia, metabolic disorders such as hypocalcemia and hypoglycemia, fever, or occult concomitant CNS diseases (e.g., cerebrovascular disease, brain tumor).[73] Anesthetic agents can also produce seizures, but evidence that anesthetic agents precipitate postoperative convulsions is weak. For example, enflurane produces epileptiform EEG activity in both normal and epileptic patients that is influenced by the depth of anesthesia and the PCO_2. At a given enflurane concentration, hyperventilation increases seizure activity and hypoventilation decreases it such that the minimum epileptogenic concentration is approximately 1% less at a $PaCO_2$ of 20 mm Hg and 1% greater at a $PaCO_2$ of 60 mm Hg than it is at 40 mm Hg.[74,75] Although seizures have been reported hours to days after enflurane anesthesia in nonepileptic patients,[76,77] EEG documentation of postoperative seizure activity is rare.[76-78] In volunteers followed for 6 to 30 days with surface EEG recordings after receiving enflurane, only nonepileptiform changes were observed even though one half had clinical and EEG evidence of seizures during anesthesia.[75] Halothane, isoflurane, and nitrous oxide have also been the subject of case reports of seizurelike activity during exposure, but none are believed to cause postoperative seizures.[79] Evidence that the newer inhaled anesthetics produce postoperative seizures is also mostly anecdotal. Desflurane appears not to cause seizure activity,[80] whereas there are a few case reports of seizures upon emergence from anesthesia with sevoflurane.[81]

Seizure activity has also been associated with certain intravenous anesthetics. Methohexital, well known to produce excitatory phenomena such as tremor and muscle movements,[82] does not precipitate clinical or EEG-demonstrated seizures in patients with generalized convulsive disorders but is epileptogenic in patients with psychomotor epilepsy.[83] Etomidate produces involuntary myoclonic movements during induction of anesthesia that occasionally persist into the recovery period.[82,84] This myoclonic activity is occasionally associated with EEG spikes in nonepileptic patients, but these do not progress to seizures.[82,85] In contrast, seizures occur in a large percentage of epileptic patients anesthetized with etomidate[86] and appear in 20% of nonepileptic patients undergoing open-heart surgery under etomidate anesthesia.[87] Ketamine is another agent that activates epileptogenic foci and may increase seizure frequency in patients with a seizure disorder[88,89] but does not produce electroencephalographic seizures in nonepileptic patients.[83] Propofol has been associated with excitatory activity such as movement, myoclonus, and muscle tremors during the induction of anesthesia[82] but evidently does not precipitate epileptiform activity in patients without preexisting CNS pathology.[82,90] However, it may activate preexisting seizure foci and has been associated with seizure activity in patients with CNS pathology.[91] In epileptic patients undergoing seizure surgery, these effects of propofol may be dose-dependent[92]; depression of EEG activity is seen at high dosages,[93-95] whereas increases in spike activity occur at sedative doses.[96] In terms of postoperative seizures, there are isolated case reports of EEG-documented seizures in epileptic[97] and nonepileptic patients following propofol administration.[98]

Opioid analgesics can also produce seizures. Meperidine (or, more accurately, its metabolite normeperidine) may produce tremulousness, myoclonus, and seizures.[99] Because normeperidine has a long half-life (14 to 21 hours), this effect may persist into the postoperative period, particularly in patients with reduced clearance because of renal failure or in those receiving very large doses of meperidine for chronic pain.[100-102] Morphine, on the other hand, has no seizure activity in humans at clinically relevant dosages.[79] Reports of grand mal seizure–like behavior after administration of fentanyl, sufentanil, and alfentanil lack EEG confirmation.[34,79,103-106] Indeed, with the exception of a few studies[107,108] that reported isolated sharp waves, abnormal EEG patterns have not been documented in normal patients treated with fentanyl or its analogs.[108-110] However, fentanyl[111] and alfentanyl[112] may induce electrocorticographic seizures in patients with preexisting epilepsy.

Although selected inhaled and intravenous anesthetics may produce abnormal EEG activity in nonepileptic patients and activate seizure foci in epileptic patients, it is uncertain whether these electrophysiologic events are neurologically meaningful, require treatment, or respond appropriately to it. Traditional seizure therapy with diazepam[76] or low-dose thiopental,[113] for example, may actually intensify enflurane-induced seizures. This issue is further complicated by the fact that most anesthetics have anticonvulsant properties.[114,115] Many reduce seizure duration during electroconvulsive therapy, and most have been used successfully to treat status epilepticus.[115-119] In summary, although many anesthetics and anesthetic adjuncts may precipitate intraoperative EEG changes, evidence that such changes increase the risk of postoperative seizures, even in seizure-prone patients, is weak.

3. Miscellaneous types of perioperative neurologic injury. In addition to hypoxia, stroke, and seizures, other types of central neurologic injury can develop perioperatively. Postoperative blindness is one such complication. Reports of blindness after otherwise uncomplicated general anesthesia are rare, and causes are difficult to define.[120,121] Blindness can be the result of injury to the eye itself (retina or optic nerve) or to the visual cortex (also see Chapter 17). Proposed mechanisms, based exclusively on anecdotal reports, include direct compression of the globe as well as hypoxia, hypotension, and anemia, either alone or in combination.[120, 121] Paraplegia is another rare perioperative complication that, like blindness, is described only in case reports.[122, 123] Here again the mechanism is unclear, but spinal cord compression caused by extreme flexion or extension, perhaps combined with hypotension, has been implicated.[122,123] Another cause of multiple neurologic signs and symptoms in the postanesthetic period is nitrous oxide–induced subacute combined degeneration of the spinal cord.[124,125] This syndrome is unique in that it presents 3 to 5 weeks after anesthesia and surgery with weakness and spasticity of the legs, ataxia, paresthesias, personality changes, cognitive impairment, and bowel and bladder dysfunc-

---

Box 16-1 Causes of delayed or abnormal awakening

Pharmacologic
  Excessive anesthesia
  Preoperative self-medication (drug abuse)
Metabolic derangements
  Ventilatory: hypoxia, hypercarbia
  Systemic: hyponatremia, hyperglycemia or hypoglycemia, uremia, liver failure, extremes of body temperature
Neurologic
  Ischemic or hemorrhagic stroke
  Occult intracranial mass lesion
Fictitious (hysteria)

---

tion.[124,125] The cause is a nitrous oxide–induced oxidation of cobalamin, which inactivates vitamin B_{12}. Patients with normal vitamin B_{12} concentrations are not at risk, but in those with pernicious anemia the disease can occur after administration of nitrous oxide for as little as 1.5 hours. Because of the delayed onset, an anesthetic cause may not be considered.[124,125] Prompt treatment with vitamin B_{12} is simple and usually effective, but symptoms may not resolve completely in all cases.[124,125]

D. Clinical evaluation of CNS dysfunction upon emergence

Emergence from anesthesia may be unsatisfactory from a neurologic standpoint because of prolonged drowsiness, delirium, an obvious focal neurologic deficit, or even true coma. The most important diagnostic issue in such a situation is whether the problem is attributable to an exaggerated but reversible anesthetic effect or a potentially permanent neurologic event (Box 16-1).

Other than personal experience, there is little guidance in what constitutes prolonged emergence under actual clinical circumstances. In a study of more than 17,000 patients randomized to receive one of four anesthetic agents (enflurane, halothane, isoflurane, and fentanyl), 6% and 3% were scored as not recovered at 60 and 90 minutes after anesthesia, respectively.[52] Because the incidence of stroke and other major CNS events in this population was only 0.04%, one can safely assume that non-CNS problems (such as protracted vomiting, pain, hemodynamic or respiratory instability) accounted for low recovery scores in most cases. Data specifically concerning neurologic recovery after anesthesia are surprisingly few. Gross clinical recovery (response to commands, eye opening, orientation) typically occurs within 10 to 15 minutes of discontinuing nitrous oxide, but some neurologically intact patients remain unarousable for significantly longer periods.[126] This illustrates two features of postanesthesia neurologic recovery: Most patients awaken promptly after anesthesia, but the variability is large, and delayed arousal is much more commonly attributable to drug effects than to neurologic events.

The first step in evaluating a patient whose emergence from anesthesia is abnormal or delayed is to perform a neurologic examination. Surprisingly, however, formal study of the neurology of emergence from anesthesia has been rare, so the definition of *normal* is not well characterized. Moreover, one of the most important parts of the neurologic examination, namely, evaluation of consciousness and orientation, is difficult to interpret because, by design, it is altered by general anesthesia. Often, therefore, one must rely on an abbreviated evaluation of cognition, motor function, pupillary signs, and reflexes. In this context, several factors should be considered. First, a simple explanation (such as dilated pupils caused by mydriatics or eye trauma) may account for an otherwise alarming finding. Second, even neurologically normal patients awakening from anesthesia often have abnormal eye signs and "pathologic" reflexes.[127] For instance, 40% to 100% of neurologically normal patients have an absent pupillary response to light 20 minutes after anesthesia, and in 10% the pupillary and lid responses can be depressed for 40 minutes.[127] Biceps and quadriceps hyperreflexia, sustained and unsustained ankle clonus, and a plantar (Babinski) reflex occur in a large percentage of neurologically intact patients recovering from anesthesia, and in many cases abnormalities are present even when patients are awake and responsive.[127] The age of the patients and anesthetic agents used influence the incidence of such transient neurologic abnormalities; hyperreflexia is more common in younger patients, and the incidence is greater after enflurane or halothane than nitrous oxide–opioid anesthesia.[127,128] Surprisingly, according to a preliminary report, transient neurologic abnormalities that occur in normal patients emerging from general anesthesia are not always bilateral.[128] Thus unilateral reflex changes, which are always a worrisome finding but are particularly so in a unresponsive patient, can occur in the course of normal neurologic recovery from anesthesia. In most cases, however, these drug-induced changes resolve shortly after anesthesia is discontinued. Therefore persistence of these neurologic abnormalities, particularly if the patient's level of consciousness remains depressed, is most worrisome. Also reported are opisthotonus[129] and difficulty with eye opening[130] after propofol anesthesia, extrapyramidal reactions with droperidol,[131] seizures with several agents,[79,83] and ophthalmoplegia, which may signal thrombosis of the basilar artery. Furthermore, certain anesthetic agents can unmask or exacerbate an underlying focal neurologic deficit.[132,133] This is best demonstrated for fentanyl and midazolam but is likely to occur with many anesthetics. Clinically, this means that even small doses of CNS depressants may make a minor or fully compensated preexisting focal deficit seem worse when, in fact, there has been no further damage to the nervous system (Fig. 16-1). Although this possibility should be considered in the patient with a seemingly new postoperative focal deficit, evaluation should not be delayed because such drug-induced exacerbation of an old deficit is transient and cannot explain persistent findings. When recovery does not occur promptly or normally, the most likely explanation is an exaggerated or prolonged drug effect. Though clearly undesirable and anxiety pro-

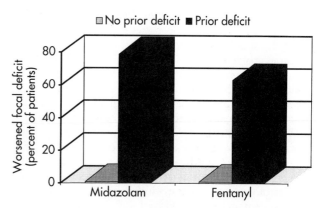

Fig. 16-1. Exacerbation or unmasking of neurologic deficits by midazolam or fentanyl. The study was conducted in patients about to undergo carotid endarterectomy or supratentorial brain tumor resection. After a baseline neurologic examination, patients received a small dose of fentanyl or midazolam and the examination was repeated. Transient worsening of the neurologic examination was detected in most of the patients who had recently recovered from a focal deficit or had a focal deficit at baseline, whereas no focal findings developed in patients without a preexisting focal deficit. (From Thal GD, Szabo MD, Lopez-Bresnahan M, et al: *Anesthesiology* 85:21, 1996.)

voking, this effect is not life threatening as long as the problem is recognized and supportive management (such as airway protection and ventilation) appropriate. Nevertheless, it is the clinician's responsibility to rule out the possibility that abnormal emergence is caused by a serious, and potentially treatable, neurologic event.

Because an individual patient may have received several drugs capable of obtunding consciousness, identifying a pharmacologic cause may not be easy. A relative opioid overdosage might be suspected clinically in a patient with slow, deep inspirations and pinpoint pupils, whereas midposition pupils and rapid, shallow breathing might suggest lingering inhaled agent. The possibility of continuing neuromuscular blockade, which might limit patient cooperation but does not explain drowsiness or unconsciousness, can be evaluated by hand-grasp strength, ability to sustain a head lift, or train-of-four testing. More often than not, a combination of drugs, rather than a single agent, is the cause of delayed emergence, and determining whether anesthetics are responsible is further complicated by the fact that only a few anesthetic agents and adjuvants have pharmacologic antagonists. In this context, antagonists such as naloxone, physostigmine, and flumazenil should be viewed as diagnostic aids, not therapy. Given the limited selection of antagonists and the multiplicity of drugs a patient may have received, one must be pragmatic: If in doubt, reverse what can be reversed. The goal of this approach is to permit a brief period of arousal during which clinical neurologic evaluation can be performed.[134,135]

Residual drug-induced paralysis is usually easily corrected with an anticholinesterase and antimuscarinic agent such as atropine or glycopyrrolate. If an opioid has been administered, a very small dose of naloxone (40 to 80 μg intravenously) typically reverses respiratory depression and awakens the patient transiently without intensifying incisional pain or producing nausea and vomiting.[134] Some caution should be exercised when one is using naloxone, however, because even small dosages rarely may produce severe hypertension, arrhythmias, and pulmonary edema.[136,137] An attempt to reverse the CNS effects of an inhaled agent with a nonspecific analeptic such as physostigmine should be considered,[135] but the clinical arousal obtained is unreliable and short lived. Physostigmine is a specific antagonist for the CNS depression or agitation caused by scopalamine or atropine[138] and may produce improvement in postoperative somnolence caused by benzodiazepines.[139] Flumazenil produces prompt recovery from benzodiazepine sedation with minimal side effects and is useful when emergence is believed to be delayed by lingering effects of diazepam or midazolam.[140] The premise underlying this approach is that if a patient is arousable (even if only transiently) by pharmacologic means and is neurologically intact, no further evaluation is necessary. Recovery from anesthesia can proceed naturally, with judgments as to the need for continued support such as intubation and mechanical ventilation made according to the usual criteria.

Failure of time and active attempts to reverse components of the anesthetic is worrisome and requires an active search for nonanesthetic causes of abnormal awakening or coma. Reviewing the history for prior TIAs, subarachnoid hemorrhage, seizures, or medical conditions that are associated with coma (such as diabetes[141] and porphyria[142]) is essential. Hypothermia may delay awakening,[143,144] particularly in the elderly, but CNS changes probably do not occur unless body temperature is 28° to 30° C.[145] Chronically administered medications, such as cimetidine,[146] may slow metabolism or elimination of anesthetic drugs and adjuvants. Severe hyperglycemia,[141] hyperosmolarity, and illicit drug usage should also be considered at this stage. An active seizure focus can depress consciousness, but in the absence of gross tonic-clonic movements the diagnosis requires EEG documentation. An unrecognized preexisting intracranial mass lesion such as a meningioma or new intracerebral hemorrhage may delay emergence from anesthesia,[72,147] but focal neurologic findings would be expected. The diagnosis should be confirmed by computed tomography (CT) or magnetic resonance (MR) scan. Finally, hysteria has been mistaken for an abnormal state of consciousness or a neurologic injury in the perianesthetic period.[148]

If a new and persistent focal neurologic deficit is identified, both additional diagnostic procedures and neurologic consultation are required. The history should be reviewed carefully for cardiac conditions such as arrhythmias, recent myocardial infarction, and intracardiac shunts that could predispose to emboli.[59,60] A thorough auscultatory examination of the heart should be performed with the same objective in mind. In view of the high incidence of embolic stroke,[59,60] an echocardiogram can be diagnostically helpful and is essential whenever the history or physical examination is suggestive of an intracardiac source for emboli. A pre-

cordial echocardiogram is not reliable for detecting a patent foramen ovale, however, so a negative study does not eliminate the possibility of a paradoxic embolism.[149] A CT scan is required to identify an intracranial mass lesion such as tumor or hemorrhage and, if contrast is used, may help identify a vascular anomaly (such as arteriovenous malformation) as well. Until recently, ischemic areas were not identifiable radiographically for hours to days following the event. However, newer diagnostic modalities such as perfusion-weighted MR imaging[150] and perfusion imaging[151] permit the detection of ischemic zones within the brain in as little as 3 hours following the onset of neurologic symptoms.

Early detection becomes important as promising new therapeutic modalities to reverse or minimize the permanent consequences of injury are tested.[152] In most cases, however, results are conflicting. A prospective, randomized, placebo-controlled, double-blind study of the calcium-channel antagonist nimodipine[153] indicated that it improved neurologic outcome and reduced mortality in patients suffering an acute ischemic stroke, but a more recent study[154] failed to confirm these results. Likewise, investigations are ongoing to evaluate the use of low-molecular-weight heparins and intraarterial thrombolytics such as tissue plasminogen activator in the setting of acute stroke, but results are again mixed.[155-162] Moreover, the safety of thrombolytics and heparin in the treatment of the surgical patient with acute stroke has not been established and the risk of hemorrhage remains a concern. Nevertheless, it is important to make the diagnosis expediently because for the first time, there is real potential for effective treatment of stroke, and promptness of treatment is an important factor. Finally, it may be important to recognize the potential for a variety of commonly used drugs to adversely affect neurologic outcome from stroke. A recent retrospective review[163] identified a direct correlation between poor outcome and the use of benzodiazepines, dopamine antagonists, α_2 agonists, α_1 antagonists, and phenytoin or phenobarbital in the first 28 days following stroke. This is particularly germane to the perioperative setting because it suggests that common drugs can have unanticipated neurologic consequences in patients with cerebral ischemia. Hence, pharmacotherapy should be judicious if acute stroke is suspected.

II. NEUROLOGIC PROBLEMS ASSOCIATED WITH SPECIFIC SURGICAL PROCEDURES
A. Carotid endarterectomy

Although various neurologic complications have been attributed to carotid endarterectomy (CEA), the most serious is stroke. This is not surprising because CEA is the clinical prototype of transient focal cerebral ischemia with reperfusion. Several large prospective studies indicate that in experienced hands the combined risk of stroke and death after CEA is about 3% to 6%, but the risk of cardiac or neurologic morbidity approaches 10% if the patient is neurologically unstable preoperatively.[164-166] If combined morbidity and mortality is within this range, long-term neurologic outcome is improved by surgery in symptomatic[167-169] patients with high-grade stenosis. Data concerning the efficacy of CEA in asymptomatic patients are less clear.[170] Because of these data, combined with aging of the population, the annual number of CEAs performed has nearly doubled.[170]

Causes of stroke in the perioperative period include hypoperfusion, emboli, and reperfusion cerebral hyperemia.[171-174] Causation is difficult to establish in individual cases, however, and studies often disagree as to the most common pathophysiology. Generally speaking, fewer than a quarter of perioperative strokes appear to be caused by hypoperfusion,[171,173] and some studies suggest that cerebral hyperemia after carotid reconstruction is a more likely culprit.[174] There is no question that emboli play a role. Cerebral emboli can be detected in virtually all patients during CEA, but the volume and frequency of emboli are evidently insufficient to produce frank stroke in all but a few patients.[171,175,176] With respect to pathophysiology and potential prevention, it is important to recognize that strokes associated with CEA commonly occur postoperatively[174,176,177] and may be related to surgical technique.[174,175] Although it may be difficult to imagine how intraoperative anesthetic management could directly precipitate or prevent such postoperative complications, one should recognize that intraoperative neurologic deterioration is associated with an increased incidence of postoperative neurologic instability[176] and stroke.[178]

The goals of perioperative management are to prevent ischemia by maintaining an acceptable balance between cerebral metabolic demand and blood supply and to minimize the consequences of unavoidable cerebral ischemia before it becomes severe enough to produce permanent CNS injury. In practice, there are many approaches to this problem. Surgeons attempt to preserve adequate cerebral blood flow (CBF) during CEA by limiting cross-clamp time or inserting a shunt. Routine shunt insertion is controversial, however, because the shunt itself may cause cerebral emboli and increase neurologic morbidity,[179] so many surgeons shunt selectively. In the patient under general anesthesia, some surgeons neither shunt nor monitor,[180] others shunt routinely without monitoring,[181] and some shunt selectively on the basis of EEG,[182,183] somatosensory evoked potentials (SSEPs),[184,185] or transcranial Doppler (TCD).[173,174,186-188] Alternatively, some prefer selective shunting based on neurologic status in the awake patient under cervical plexus block.[189,190] Each approach has proponents, but whether one or any combination leads to improved neurologic outcome remains controversial.[191]

The basis for EEG monitoring is that EEG changes occur when CBF falls below a critical level.[192] As CBF decreases, it reaches a level that is inadequate to support neuronal activity but is still sufficient to prevent neuronal death.[193] This hypothetical zone has been called the penumbra and is characterized by electrically and functionally silent but viable neurons.[169,194] Therefore EEG changes are not necessarily indicative of irreversible neuronal injury because neurons become electrically silent before their structural integrity is threatened.[193,194] In

practice, however, during CEA performed under local anesthesia, direct comparison of EEG and the neurologic examination indicates that agreement between the two is usually good, even though both false-positive and false-negative EEGs can occur.[195] Nevertheless, whether EEG monitoring positively influences neurologic outcome remains a matter of speculation because no prospective, controlled studies have been performed. The possibility that intraoperative interventions to normalize the EEG are effective in preventing stroke is suggested by clinical studies that monitored the EEG (one simultaneously monitored SSEPs)[196] and noted that major, untreated, cross-clamp–associated EEG changes are predictive of stroke in some patients.[196-198]

The basis for SSEP monitoring is the same as that of EEG monitoring except that, whereas EEG is primarily a cortical signal, SSEPs can evaluate the integrity of subcortical pathways.[184,196] Therefore during carotid cross-clamping, SSEPs may provide sensitivity and specificity similar to that of EEG monitoring,[184,185,199] but proof of efficacy in this setting awaits large prospective randomized studies. Stump pressure measurements lack both sensitivity and specificity in measuring the adequacy of cerebral perfusion during CEA,[200,201] whereas TCD can detect cerebral hypoperfusion as well as cerebral hyperemia and thromboembolic events.[171,173,174,186,188] In fact, there appears to be an association between embolic load detected by TCD both intraoperatively and postoperatively and the incidence of stroke.[173,202,203] The challenge, therefore, is to use TCD monitoring to guide surgery and decrease the embolic load. Finally, near-infrared spectroscopy (NIRS), which measures cerebral oxygenation noninvasively, has been used during CEA. However, this is a new device and its role in CEA and other procedures is still being defined.[204,205]

Apart from monitoring issues, the main focus of anesthetic management is on maintaining normal cerebral physiology. Chiefly, this means attention to blood pressure, arterial carbon dioxide (Pa_{CO_2}), and metabolic considerations such as the plasma glucose concentration. Vessels distal to a carotid stenosis have impaired autoregulation and carbon dioxide reactivity.[206] Hence, a decrease in arterial pressure may reduce CBF, whereas moderate induced hypertension may improve flow to marginal regions.[207] Accordingly, moderate induced hypertension is used occasionally during the period of carotid cross-clamping in an attempt to improve CBF.[174,176,187] Theoretical considerations concerning intracerebral steal[208] or inverse steal phenomena[209] notwithstanding, the role of hypocapnia or hypercapnia in intraoperative stroke during CEA is not well studied.[210] Indeed, hypocapnia is of no therapeutic benefit in acute ischemic stroke.[211] It seems unlikely, therefore, that either hypocapnia or hypercapnia has a significant impact on the likelihood of stroke during CEA, but normocapnia is usually recommended. The plasma glucose concentration is another important physiologic consideration in CEA patients at risk for cerebral ischemia. Studies in animals[212,213] demonstrate that hyperglycemia may worsen neurologic outcome from focal ischemic brain injury. An association between hyperglycemia and poor neurologic outcome after traumatic or ischemic brain injury has also been demonstrated in humans.[213,214] Although there is general agreement that hyperglycemia can be deleterious in the setting of cerebral ischemia, the critical plasma glucose concentration is not well defined and hypoglycemia has its own risks. Accordingly, opinions vary as to the acceptable plasma glucose concentration. Because of the risk of cerebral ischemia, it is prudent to avoid administering glucose-containing solutions to a nondiabetic patient undergoing CEA and to maintain plasma glucose concentration within broadly normal limits (i.e., 80 to 150 mg/dl in nondiabetic patients and 100 to 200 mg/dl in a patient with diabetes). However, one should recognize that such guidelines are not firmly established.[212,213]

Because of their profound effects on cerebral physiology, anesthetic agents may improve the tolerance of the brain to low-flow states.[215-218] However, few agents have been studied in the context of CEA. In a retrospective review of over 2000 CEA patients, intraoperative cerebral ischemia as determined by EEG criteria was significantly less common during anesthesia with isoflurane than either enflurane or halothane,[219] but there was no difference in neurologic outcome. The critical rCBF (that is, the regional CBF below which ischemic EEG changes are likely) is also lower with isoflurane (approximately 10 ml/100 g/min) than with either halothane or enflurane anesthesia (about 18 ml/100 g/min).[192,220] However, animal work challenges the idea that isoflurane can provide meaningful protection in this setting.[217,221] Interestingly, recent data indicate the critical rCBF of sevoflurane is probably similar to that of isoflurane.[222] Barbiturates have also been advocated for brain protection during CEA,[223,224] but prospective, randomized studies with a concurrent control group are lacking. Furthermore, despite evidence that low-dose barbiturates offer protection in rats,[225] issues related to timing, dose, and duration of therapy must be addressed before such therapy can confidently be considered protective during CEA. Few other anesthetics have been subjected to even this level of clinical investigation, so no particular anesthetic agent or technique can be recommended as superior to another at present. Indeed, because regional anesthesia appears to be associated with the same incidence of adverse neurologic events after CEA as general anesthesia,[189] one must question the role of general anesthetics as neuroprotective agents in this setting. Lastly, though not protective strategies, alternative procedures such as angioplasty and vascular stents are being evaluated in an attempt to treat carotid stenosis while avoiding the neurologic complications associated with CEA.[226] However, the place of such new treatments in the treatment of carotid disease remains to be proven.

Despite meticulous intraoperative management, some patients awaken from CEA with a neurologic deficit. In this situation, the first step is to rule out anesthetic-induced neurologic dysfunction. Of particular interest is the fact that mild preexisting focal neurologic deficits may be worsened transiently by sedative medications in CEA patients.[132] Because the only surgically remediable cause of stroke after CEA is carotid occlusion,[176] the pa-

tient awakening from CEA with a dense hemiplegia or other major focal deficit should be evaluated promptly with carotid noninvasive studies or angiography once nonsurgical causes of the problem have been excluded. Assuming that no correctable reason for stroke exists, another strategy to consider in order to minimize the permanent consequences of the injury is use of intraarterial thrombolytics. These agents have shown promise when used early after acute ischemic stroke, but experience in the perioperative setting is limited and the risks of precipitating incisional and intracerebral hemorrhage mandate a cautious approach.[227,228]

B. Cardiac surgery and cardiopulmonary bypass

Despite numerous technical advances, neurologic and neuropsychologic dysfunction continue to be significant and undeniable risks of cardiac surgery. (Also see Chapter 13.) A recent, large, multicenter study[229] of coronary bypass surgery patients determined predictors of adverse CNS outcomes after coronary artery bypass grafting (CABG) with a reported cumulative incidence of 6.1% (Table 16-2). Focal neurologic injury, stupor, or coma (Type I) accounted for about half of these complications; the remainder were caused by deterioration in intellectual function or seizures (Type II). However, this study, which did not use psychometric testing or other sensitive forms of neurologic evaluation, probably underestimates the true incidence of these complications. For example, cerebral swelling occurs after both hypothermic and normothermic bypass,[230] and a large percentage of patients have cerebrospinal fluid evidence of subclinical brain injury after bypass.[231] After open-chamber cardiac procedures, nearly 60% of patients have new ischemic lesions on MR scan but only 25% have an associated focal neurologic deficit.[232] Similarly, when cognitive performance is assessed with psychometric tests before and after hypothermic bypass, 25% to 79% of patients demonstrate deterioration and in about a quarter of these the deterioration is moderate or severe.[233,234] The natural history of the intellectual deterioration is that it resolves in most patients over a few months,[234,235] but 10% to 30% remain neuropsychologically impaired for 12 months or more.[234,236] To the extent that these complications of bypass are associated with a higher mortality rate and

Table 16-2. Predictors of adverse CNS outcome after CABG

Type I	Type II
Age	Age
Pulmonary disease	Pulmonary disease
Hypertension	Hypertension
Aortic atheroma	Excessive alcohol consumption
Prior neurologic abnormality	Postoperative arrhythmia
	Prior CABG
Diabetes	Peripheral vascular disease

From Roach GW, Kanchuger M, Mangano LM: *N Engl J Med* 335:1857, 1996.
CABG, Coronary artery bypass graft; *CNS*, central nervous system.

greater consumption of medical resources,[229] they obviously represent a major public health issue.

Apart from rare cases of equipment malfunction or human error, the causes of this neurologic morbidity include emboli, hypoperfusion,[237] or some combination of the two. Macroemboli from the aortic root or valves are a likely cause of stroke. The fact that proximal aortic atherosclerosis is the strongest predictor of an adverse neurologic event supports this contention.[229,238] Microembolism of air and other debris is also very common throughout bypass, but particularly around the time of aortic manipulation.[239] Evidence of a relationship between these microemboli and subsequent neurologic or cognitive deterioration is strong but mainly circumstantial. In patients undergoing bypass, microemboli have been documented in the retina,[237] the left ventricle,[240] and the cerebral vasculature.[241] The observation that arterial filtration reduces the incidence of both cerebral microembolization and CNS dysfunction[241] provides additional support for the microemboli theory. Hypoperfusion is often considered secondary to emboli as a cause of perioperative neurologic and cognitive deterioration after routine bypass,[242,243] perhaps because CBF is adequate at a perfusion pressure as low as 30 mm Hg during hypothermic bypass.[244] However, recent data suggest that a higher perfusion pressure (mean arterial pressure 80 to 100 mm Hg) during cardiopulmonary bypass (CPB) may help reduce the risk of stroke in patients with severe proximal atherosclerosis[238] and cognitive decline in the elderly.[238,245] In this regard, it is important to note that most studies examining the role of perfusion pressure have been conducted during hypothermic bypass. There is no reason to assume that similar results will be obtained under normothermic conditions.

Both nonmodifiable and modifiable factors contribute to the risk of an adverse cerebral outcome from cardiac surgery (Box 16-2).[246] Among the former, older age, proximal aortic atherosclerosis, and preexisting cerebrovascular disease are particularly important. Age greater than 70 years is associated with at least a 15% risk of an adverse cerebral event,[229] perhaps because such patients have altered cerebral autoregulation and more severe aortic atheroma. The extent and severity of aortic atherosclerosis are an independent predictor of the risk of stroke after cardiopulmonary bypass.[229,238,247] A history of stroke also increases the risk of stroke after CPB severalfold,[248] but asymptomatic carotid artery disease has no effect on either the likelihood of stroke or neuropsychologic dysfunction.[57,249] If a patient is a candidate for CEA, however, this may best be performed in conjunction with the cardiac procedure.[166] This is because the risk of stroke appears to be greater if the cardiac procedure precedes CEA, whereas cardiac complications appear to be more common if CEA precedes CABG. Thus combined carotid-CABG surgery, though still quite controversial, seems reasonable and may lower the aggregate risk of cardiac and cerebral morbidity.[166] Another nonmodifiable factor is the type of surgery. Some studies indicate that open-cardiac procedures, such as valve replacement, are associated with a higher incidence of

---

Box 16-2 Neurologic injury and cardiopulmonary bypass

Nonmodifiable factors
Age
Prior cerebrovascular disease
Aortic atheroma
Genetic predisposition (Apo E4)

Modifiable factors
Surgical technique
  Bypass duration
  Embolic load
Bypass technique
  Oxygenator type
  Filters
  Pulsatile versus nonpulsatile
Physiologic management
  Perfusion pressure
  Alpha versus pH stat
  Glucose
  Temperature

---

postoperative neurologic or neuropsychologic deficits than CABG surgery.[231,246] Newer comparative studies[234,250] show no difference, however, and in some series involving only open procedures[251,252] the incidence of gross neurologic deficits (4% to 8%) is comparable to that reported for CABG. Finally, there may be a genetic predisposition for cognitive deterioration after bypass. Specifically, possession of the ε4 allele of the apolipoprotein E gene, which influences susceptibility to several other neurologic insults and diseases, appears to be a predictor of cognitive decline after CPB.[253]

The list of modifiable factors that may improve cerebral outcome from CPB is lengthy. A short bypass duration is preferable to a long period on pump,[246] and membrane oxygenators are associated with fewer clinical and subclinical deficits than bubble oxygenators.[254] The issue of optimal perfusion pressure has already been discussed, but it is important to reiterate that most work in this area has been performed during hypothermic, nonpulsatile bypass. Clinical trials of pulsatile bypass have been few. In animal work, there is little or no difference in CBF or metabolism between perfusion techniques.[255,256] In human trials, no differences in neurologic or cognitive outcome have been identified as a result of perfusion techniques, but the studies are small.[257,258] Interest in the ability of arterial filters to reduce the cerebral risks of bypass follows from evidence that microemboli are likely to be a major cause of adverse neurologic and cognitive outcomes.[241] Filters clearly reduce cerebral embolization[259] and at least one study confirms an associated improvement in neuropsychologic outcome.[241] Another way to reduce cerebral embolization is with careful selection of the site of aortic cannulation. Because palpation of the aorta is not particularly sensitive, transesophageal echocardiography (TEE) has become a popular method of directing placement of the cannula.[260] There appears to be an association between the severity of TEE-identified aortic atherosclerosis and stroke risk,[238] so modification of practice based on such monitoring may reduce the risk of neurologic morbidity. There has long been uncertainty about how to best manage CO_2 during hypothermic CPB. This uncertainty is based on a debate over what constitutes normocapnia in hypothermic patients[261] and concern that hypercapnia could increase CBF, thereby predisposing to cerebral microembolism, whereas hypocapnia might produce cerebral hypoperfusion.[262] In practical terms, pH-stat management corrects the values measured in the blood gas machine for body temperature, increases $PaCO_2$ approximately 50% at a body temperature of 28° C, and produces "luxury perfusion" and impaired autoregulation during CPB.[263,264] α-Stat management aims for normal pH and $PaCO_2$ values as measured in the blood gas machine at 37° C, and is associated with maintained CO_2 responsiveness and intact autoregulation but a lower CBF.[262,264] Several studies have examined this issue and, with few exceptions, show that α-stat management is no worse than pH-stat management and may be better in terms of the neurologic and neuropsychologic morbidity of CPB.[236,250,257] However, pH-stat management could have advantages in some circumstances. Because it produces higher CBF, use of pH-stat management during circulatory arrest may produce better, more homogeneous cooling of the brain and more rapid recovery of flow patterns upon rewarming from deep hypothermia.[265,266]

Another approach to improving cerebral outcome during cardiac surgery is to use drugs or techniques that might protect the brain. Barbiturates have been used for this purpose, with mixed results. In a prospective, controlled study[267] of patients undergoing open-ventricle procedures during normothermic CPB, thiopental administered to produce burst suppression before aortic cannulation reduced the frequency of persistent neuropsychiatric deficits. Subsequently, however, no protection was found when a similar dose of thiopental was used in patients undergoing CABG.[268,269] Given these inconsistent results, the disadvantages of high-dose thiopental treatment (i.e., longer postoperative intubation, more inotropic support),[267] and a trend toward fast-track cardiac surgery,[270] use of thiopental for this purpose is not widespread. Propofol-induced burst suppression has proven ineffective in mitigating adverse cerebral outcomes of cardiac valve surgery. This suggests that neither cerebral metabolic depression nor cerebral blood flow reduction (which should reduce the embolic load) reliably protect the brain during open heart surgery.[270a] Nimodipine, a calcium-channel antagonist with protective effects in models of focal cerebral ischemia, has also been tested in cardiac surgical patients. Although initial results were promising,[271] a prospective, randomized trial was terminated early because of excessive surgical bleeding in the nimodipine group.[272]

By far, the most commonly used form of cerebral protection during CPB is hypothermia. Hypothermia has a number of effects that can contribute to its protective action, including the ability to decrease neuronal activity and metabolic demands associated with maintenance of cellular integrity[273] and to reduce release of excitotoxic metabolites such as glutamate that can initiate and exacerbate neuronal injury.[274] Even mild hypothermia (2° to 5° C decrease), which has only a modest effect on cerebral metabolic rate, is profoundly protective in animal models of cerebral ischemia.[275] Because of consistently positive animal data and abundant clinical experience, the protective efficacy of hypothermia in cardiac surgery has not been subjected to prospective, randomized clinical trials until recently. The impetus for such studies was the recent trend toward normothermic bypass. Normothermia has advantages in terms of cardiac outcomes, but if hypothermia is protective, normothermia could worsen neurologic outcome. One large study reported no worsening of neurologic outcomes with normothermia,[276] whereas others reported fewer neurologic events in patients undergoing hypothermic bypass.[277,278] None of these studies are optimal, however, because they were either uncontrolled or used historic controls or did not use formal neurologic or neuropsychologic assessments. The only available well-controlled, randomized, prospective, single-blind study demonstrates no difference in the incidence of a neuropsychologic or focal neurologic deficit between normothermic and hypothermic bypass for CABG but is limited by a very small sample size.[279] Thus present evidence suggests that normothermic bypass is not associated with a worse neurologic outcome than hypothermic bypass, but the issue is likely to be debated for years. There are several possible explanations for this counterintuitive result. First, during "normothermic" bypass, patients are typically cooled a few degrees and thus may still benefit from mild hypothermia. Second, CNS injury may occur before or after hypothermia is instituted or, in the case of embolic occlusion of a cerebral vessel, persist beyond the hypothermic interval. Finally, just as small decreases in brain temperature are protective, mild cerebral hyperthermia (38° C) worsens outcome from focal cerebral ischemia.[280] In this context, it has been shown that cerebral hyperthermia and desaturation occur during rapid rewarming from hypothermic bypass,[281,282] possibly negating any advantage of hypothermia during the bypass run. Therefore until the role of hypothermia is resolved, it seems prudent at least to avoid cerebral hyperthermia by rewarming slowly after a hypothermic bypass run.

Treatment of a patient with a post-CPB neurologic deficit is primarily supportive, with the aim of preventing a secondary neurologic insult because of hypoxia, hypoventilation, or hypoperfusion. However, one rare cause of post-CPB CNS injury, namely, cerebral embolization of large amounts of air, lends itself to an unusual and specific form of treatment. Hyperbaric therapy capitalizes on the fact that a gas-filled space will decrease in size as pressure surrounding it increases. Thus hyperbaric therapy is believed to reduce the size of cerebral air emboli and speed reabsorption. Few patients have been treated this way,[283] probably reflecting the limited number of such chambers and the practical difficulties encountered in caring for critically ill patients in such a de-

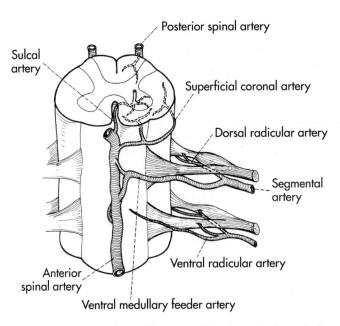

Fig. 16-2. Cross-section of the spinal cord illustrating blood supply through the anterior and posterior spinal arteries. The flow through the anterior spinal artery is supplemented at various levels by segmental arteries arising from the aorta. The anterior spinal artery provides flow to the ventral two thirds of the spinal cord, whereas the posterior spinal artery supplies the dorsal one third.

vice. Results have nonetheless been encouraging, even when treatment is begun hours after the embolic event.

C. Thoracoabdominal aortic surgery

Despite recent developments, paraplegia is still a common complication of surgery on the thoracoabdominal aorta (TAA). The incidence of paraplegia varies between 0% and 15% for elective surgery, and the risk is greater still for emergency surgical resections of acute dissection or aortic rupture.[284,285] The largest series reported to date involved 1509 patients undergoing TAA surgery and found proximal resections, long cross-clamp time, advanced age, extensive lesions, or a history of renal dysfunction to be strong predictors of paraplegia or paraparesis.[286,287]

Thoracoabdominal aneurysm surgery subjects the spinal cord to potential ischemia as well as reperfusion injury.[288] The cord is vulnerable to ischemia because of the pecularities of spinal vascular anatomy (Fig. 16-2). The spinal cord has essentially separate anterior and posterior circulations.[289] A single anterior spinal artery provides flow to the ventral two thirds of the spinal cord, including motor neurons in the anterior horn and the corticospinal tracts. Paired posterior spinal arteries form a plexuslike arrangement on the dorsal surface of the cord and supply the dorsal third of the spinal cord parenchyma, including the posterior columns. The anterior spinal artery travels the entire length of the spinal cord but may be narrow or occluded in some areas,[289] rendering these regions of the spinal cord heavily dependent on collateral flow from segmental vessels arising from the aorta. Of 62 segmental vessels present at birth, only a small fraction remain into adult life.[290] These are

typically unpaired, arising on the left from intercostal or lumbar arteries.[285,289] One segmental vessel of note is the artery of Adamkiewicz (or great radicular artery), which arises from the aorta, usually between the seventh thoracic and fourth lumbar nerve roots.[289] This vessel is a significant contributor to the blood supply of the spinal cord, and its location relative to the site of aortic cross-clamping and resection can be a decisive factor for the risk of ischemic spinal cord injury. The clinical problem is that the extent to which the spinal cord depends on flow through aortic collaterals is quite variable, and it is often impossible to identify patients at greatest risk for spinal ischemia preoperatively. Thus TAA surgery can interfere with spinal cord blood supply directly by sacrificing a critical segmental vessel during the repair or by producing hypoperfusion through segmental vessels distal to the aortic cross-clamp. In addition, spinal cord perfusion can be further compromised by an aortic cross-clamp–induced increase in cerebrospinal fluid pressure (CSFP).[291,292] Finally, when the cross-clamp is removed, spinal cord hyperemia probably occurs. This suggests that biochemically mediated reperfusion injury may play a role in the development of postoperative paraplegia.[288] The fact that some patients develop paraplegia 24 to 48 hours postoperatively is consistent with such a mechanism.

Accordingly, strategies to reduce the incidence of paraplegia following thoracoabdominal aortic surgery address the general problems of spinal cord hypoperfusion and subsequent reperfusion injury. These range from efforts to identify patients at greatest risk to the administration of putatively protective agents directly into the subarachnoid space. Direct approaches to reducing the incidence of neurologic complications during aortic surgery include reducing the duration of ischemia by decreasing cross-clamp time, improving distal perfusion during cross-clamping using induced hypertension[293] and bypass procedures or shunts,[284] or reimplantation of critical intercostal arteries.[294] None of these procedures is without controversy, however, and the surgical community is divided. For example, some workers[295,296] claim that maintaining distal aortic pressure above 60 mm Hg with some form of bypass or shunt in some patients is beneficial,[294,297] whereas others assert that shunting or bypass is of no benefit.[298,299] Monitoring the spinal cord for evidence of ischemia to allow selective interventions is another strategy. Techniques such as SSEPs[300,301] and motor evoked potential monitoring,[302,303] which evaluate neuronal conduction in the posterior and anterior spinal cord, respectively, as well as qualitative hydrogen clearance measurements of spinal cord perfusion,[304] are popular in this regard. However, their utility is limited by the frequency of false positives and negatives and the extent to which anesthetics and anesthetic adjuncts affect the measured variables.[301,305] Though promising, none of these techniques has been rigorously investigated, and their efficacy in improving neurologic outcome from surgery on the TAA remain unresolved.

With respect to perioperative physiologic and anesthetic management, interest has focused on CSF drainage, blood pressure management, and spinal cord protection. Multiple studies have investigated ways to attenuate or prevent the increase in CSFP that occurs with aortic cross-clamping, but such work is hampered by the fact that the mechanism underlying the increase is unknown. In animal models, reducing CSFP with either osmotic diuretics or withdrawal of CSF has produced mixed results in terms of neurologic outcome, and most show that if spinal cord blood flow increases at all with such interventions, it still remains well below normal.[306-309] Most human series examining CSF drainage have not been randomized and often used multiple treatment modalities simultaneously. The one exception, a prospective randomized clinical study, failed to demonstrate a benefit of CSF drainage during thoracoabdominal aneurysm surgery, but sample sizes were small and CSF drainage was limited to 50 ml.[310] CSF drainage has also been used in the postoperative period[293] to attenuate the risk of delayed neurologic injury. However, except for case studies, there is no evidence of its efficacy in this regard. Management of the arterial hypertension that develops proximal to the aortic clamp can also influence CSFP. Sodium nitroprusside can increase CSFP and, in an animal model of aortic cross-clamping, compromises spinal cord blood flow,[311] whereas β-blockers and trimethaphan[312] have no such effect.

Numerous pharmacologic strategies have been evaluated for their ability to protect the spinal cord, but only a few have been investigated thoroughly enough to warrant attention. Glucose management deserves serious consideration because studies in both animals and humans[212] show convincingly that small increases in plasma glucose have an adverse effect on neurologic outcome.[212,213] Thus it is reasonable to avoid exogenous glucose in patients at

risk for spinal cord ischemia during TAA surgery and to normalize plasma glucose in the hyperglycemic patient. Although the concentration of glucose that exacerbates neurologic injury is debated, maintenance of plasma glucose less than 200 mg/dl in diabetic patients and 150 mg/dl in nondiabetic patients is advocated by some.[213] Some anesthetics[313] and neuroanesthetic adjuncts (e.g., hyperventilation, mannitol)[314] improve tolerance of the spinal cord to ischemia in animals, as do magnesium,[315,316] nimodipine,[317] oxygen free radical scavengers,[318] and excitatory amino acid antagonists.[319] However, none of these have been studied thoroughly in humans. In fact, in terms of human investigation, interest has focused on use of steroids, gangliosides, and hypothermia in the setting of spinal cord trauma rather than ischemia. Massive dosages of steroids, but not naloxone, produce modest improvements in the outcome of spinal cord trauma,[320] and the ganglioside GM1 has shown promise.[321] Gangliosides are particularly interesting because they may be effective when administered many hours after injury. Neither drug has been studied in TAA surgery, however. The ability to administer drugs or solutions into the epidural or subarachnoid space has also been exploited. For example, CSF drainage combined with intrathecal papaverine, which improves thoracic spinal cord blood flow in animals during aortic cross-clamping,[322,323] reduced the incidence of paraparesis or paraplegia in one study,[323,324] but there were only 11 patients in the papaverine group. These approaches notwithstanding, hypothermia is perhaps the modality that has generated the most recent interest. In patients undergoing TAA surgery, there have been various approaches to both systemic[325] and regional hypothermia.[308,326] These include using bypass or shunts to cool the whole body or just the cord and irrigation of the epidural space with iced saline to produce local hypothermia.[327] Unfortunately, most reports are case series rather than controlled studies, so efficacy remains to be determined.

Ultimately, the best way to reduce the risk of neurologic morbidity associated with thoracic aneurysm repair may be with alternative surgical procedures. Along these lines, percutaneous, intravascular stenting obviates TAA surgery and shows encouraging preliminary results.[328] The procedure does not eliminate neurologic morbidity,[329] however, and the long-term effectiveness and safety of this new procedure compared to open repair must await larger trials.

REFERENCES

1. Korttila K, Linnoila M: Psychomotor skills related to driving after intramuscular administration of diazepam and meperidine, *Anesthesiology* 42:685, 1975.
2. Melnick B, Sawyer R, Karambelkar D, et al: Delayed side effects of droperidol after ambulatory general anesthesia, *Anesth Analg* 69:748, 1989.
3. Skelly AM, Boscoe MJ, Dawling S, et al: A comparison of diazepam and midazolam as sedatives for minor oral surgery, *Eur J Anaesthesiol* 1:253, 1984.
4. Korttila K, Linnoila M, Ertama P, et al: Recovery and simulated driving after intravenous anesthesia with thiopental, methohexital, propanidid, or alphadione, *Anesthesiology* 43, 291, 1975.

5. Korttila K, Nuotto EJ, Lichtor JL, et al: Clinical recovery and psychomotor function after brief anesthesia with propofol or thiopental, *Anesthesiology* 76:676, 1992.
6. Kortilla K, Tammisto T, Ertama P, et al: Recovery, psychomotor skills, and simulated driving after brief inhalational anesthesia with halothane or enflurane combined with nitrous oxide and oxygen, *Anesthesiology* 46:20, 1977.
7. Davison LA, Steinhelber JC, Eger EI, et al: Psychological effects of halothane and isoflurane anesthesia, *Anesthesiology* 43:313, 1975.
8. Storms LH, Stark AH, Calverley RK, et al: Psychological functioning after halothane or enflurane anesthesia, *Anesth Analg* 59:245, 1980.
9. Nathanson MH, Fredman B, Smith I, et al: Sevoflurane versus desflurane for outpatient anesthesia: a comparison of maintenance and recovery profiles, *Anesth Analg* 81:1186, 1995.
10. Philip BK, Kallar SK, Bogetz MS, et al: A multicenter comparison of maintenance and recovery with sevoflurane or isoflurane for adult ambulatory anesthesia. The Sevoflurane Multicenter Ambulatory Group, *Anesth Analg* 83:314, 1996.
11. Fletcher JE, Sebel PS, Murphy MR, et al: Psychomotor performance after desflurane anesthesia: a comparison with isoflurane, *Anesth Analg* 73:260, 1991.
12. Knill RL, Moote CA, Skinner MI, et al: Anesthesia with abdominal surgery leads to intense REM sleep during the first postoperative week, *Anesthesiology* 73:52, 1990.
13. Thapar P, Zacny JP, Thompson W, et al: Using alcohol as a standard to assess the degree of impairment induced by sedative and analgesic drugs used in ambulatory surgery, *Anesthesiology* 82:53, 1995.
14. Chung F, Seyone C, Dyck B, et al: Age-related cognitive recovery after general anesthesia, *Anesth Analg* 71:217, 1990.
15. Smith RJ, Roberts NM, Rodgers RJ, et al: Adverse cognitive effects of general anaesthesia in young and elderly patients. *Int Clin Psychopharmacol* 1:253, 1986.
16. Chung FF, Chung A, Meier RH, et al: Comparison of perioperative mental function after general anaesthesia and spinal anaesthesia with intravenous sedation, *Can J Anaesth* 36:382, 1989.
17. Ghoneim MM, Hinrichs JV, O'Hara MW, et al: Comparison of psychologic and cognitive functions after general or regional anesthesia, *Anesthesiology* 69:507, 1988.
18. Williams-Russo P, Sharrock NE, Mattis S, et al: Cognitive effects after epidural vs general anesthesia in older adults. A randomized trial, *JAMA* 274:44, 1995.
19. Moller JT, Cluitmans P, Rasmussen LS, et al: Long-term postoperative cognitive dysfunction in the elderly ISPOCD1 study. International Study of Post-Operative Cognitive Dysfunction, *Lancet* 351:857, 1998.
20. Riis J, Lomholt B, Haxholdt O, et al: Immediate and long-term mental recovery from general versus epidural anesthesia in elderly patients, *Acta Anaesthesiol Scand* 27:44, 1983.
21. Chung F, Meier R, Lautenschlager E, et al: General or spinal anesthesia: which is better in the elderly? *Anesthesiology* 67:422, 1987.
22. Wyrwicz AM, Pszenny MH, Schofield JC, et al: Noninvasive observations of fluorinated anesthetics in rabbit brain by fluorine-19 nuclear magnetic resonance, *Science* 222:428, 1983.
23. Litt L, González-Méndez R, James TL, et al: An *in vivo* study of halothane uptake and elimination in the rat brain with fluorine nuclear magnetic resonance spectroscopy, *Anesthesiology* 67:161, 1987.
24. Albrecht RF, Miletich DJ, Rosenberg R, et al: Cerebral blood flow and metabolic changes from induction to onset of anesthesia with halothane or pentobarbital, *Anesthesiology* 47:252, 1977.
25. Bruce DL, Bach MJ, Arbit J: Trace anesthetic effects on perceptual, cognitive, and motor skills, *Anesthesiology* 40:453, 1974.
26. Galinkin JL, Janiszewski D, Young CJ, et al: Subjective, psychomotor, cognitive, and analgesic effects of subanesthetic concentrations of sevoflurane and nitrous oxide, *Anesthesiology* 87:1082, 1997.
27. Rampil IJ, Mason P, Singh H: Anesthetic potency (MAC) is independent of forebrain structures in the rat, *Anesthesiology* 78:707, 1993.
28. Gan TJ, Glass PS, Windsor A, et al: Bispectral index monitoring allows faster emergence and improved recovery from propofol, alfentanil, and nitrous oxide anesthesia. BIS Utility Study Group, *Anesthesiology* 87:808, 1997.
29. Davies, K, Hans FJ, Livingstone D, Wei L, et al: Accelerated cerebral atrophy following general anesthesia and surgery, *Anesthesiology* 85:A698, 1996.
30. Engelhardt W, Carl G, Hartung E: Intra-individual open comparison of burst-suppression-isoflurane anaesthesia versus electroconvulsive therapy in the treatment of severe depression, *Eur J Anaesthesiol* 10:113, 1993.
31. Langer G, Karazman R, Neumark J, et al: Isoflurane narcotherapy in depressive patients refractory to conventional antidepressant drug treatment. A double-blind comparison with electroconvulsive treatment, *Neuropsychobiology* 31:182, 1995.
32. Eckenhoff JE, Kneale DH, Dripps RD: The incidence and etiology of post-anesthetic excitement, *Anesthesiology* 22:667, 1961.
33. Parikh SS, Chung F: Postoperative delirium in the elderly, *Anesth Analg* 80:1223, 1995.
34. Marcantonio ER, Juarez G, Goldman L, et al: The relationship of postoperative delirium with psychoactive medications, *JAMA* 272:1518, 1994.
35. Lipowski ZJ: Delirium in the elderly patient, *N Engl J Med* 320:578, 1989.
36. Marcantonio ER, Goldman L, Mangione CM, et al: A clinical prediction rule for delirium after elective noncardiac surgery, *JAMA* 271:134, 1994.
37. Heller SS, Frank KA, Kornfeld DS, et al: Psychological outcome following open-heart surgery, *Arch Intern Med* 134:908, 1974.
38. Berggren D, Gustafson Y, Eriksson B, et al: Postoperative confusion after anesthesia in elderly patients with femoral neck fractures, *Anesth Analg* 66:497, 1987.
39. Williams-Russo P, Urquhart BL, Sharrock NE, et al: Post-operative delirium: predictors and prognosis in elderly orthopedic patients, *J Am Geriatr Soc* 40:759, 1992.
40. Hutchinson R: Awareness during surgery: a study of its incidence, *Br J Anaesth* 33:463, 1960.
41. Aakerlund LP, Rosenberg J: Postoperative delirium: treatment of supplementary oxygen, *Br J Anaesth* 72:286, 1994.
42. Lewis DA, Smith RE: Steroid-induced psychiatric syndromes. A report of 14 cases and a review of the literature, *J Affect Disord* 5:319, 1983.
43. White PF, Way WL, Trevor AJ: Ketamine: its pharmacology and therapeutic uses, *Anesthesiology* 56:119, 1982.
44. Sussman DR: A comparative evaluation of ketamine anesthesia in children and adults, *Anesthesiology* 40:459, 1974.
45. Simpson KH, Smith RJ, Davies LF: Comparison of the effects of atropine and glycopyrrolate on cognitive function following general anaesthesia, *Br J Anaesth* 59:966, 1987.
46. Tune L, Carr S, Cooper T, et al: Association of anticholinergic activity of prescribed medications with postoperative delirium. *J Neuropsychiatry Clin Neurosci* 5:208, 1993.
47. Parnetti L, Senin U, Mecocci P: Cognitive enhancement therapy for Alzheimer's disease: the way forward, *Drugs* 53:752, 1997.
48. Cantu TG, Korek JS: Central nervous system reactions to histamine-2 receptor blockers, *Ann Intern Med* 114:1027, 1991.
49. Lee CM, Yeakel AE: Patient refusal of surgery following Innovar premedication, *Anesth Analg* 54:224, 1975.
50. Gadalla F, Spencer J: Prolonged delirium after propofol, *Can J Anaesth* 43:877, 1996.
51. Trzepacz PT: Delirium: advances in diagnosis, pathophysiology, and treatment, *Psychiatr Clin North Am* 19:429, 1996.
52. Forrest JB, Cahalan MK, Rehder K, et al: Multicenter study of general anesthesia. II. Results, *Anesthesiology* 72:262, 1990.
53. Warner MA, Shields SE, Chute CG: Major morbidity and mortality within 1 month of ambulatory surgery and anesthesia, *JAMA* 270:1437, 1993.
54. Eichhorn JH: Prevention of intraoperative anesthesia accidents and related severe injury through safety monitoring, *Anesthesiology* 70:572, 1989.
55. Ropper AH, Wechsler LR, Wilson LS: Carotid bruit and the risk of stroke in elective surgery, *N Engl J Med* 307:1388, 1982.
56. Wilder AJ, Fishbein RH. Operative experiences with patients over 80 years of age, *Surg Gynecol Obstet* 113:205, 1961.

57. Turnipseed WD, Berkoff HA, Belzer FO: Postoperative stroke in cardiac and peripheral vascular disease, *Ann Surg* 192:365, 1980.
58. Barnes RW, Liebman PR, Marszalek PB, et al: The natural history of asymptomatic carotid disease in patients undergoing cardiovascular surgery, *Surgery* 90:1075, 1981.
59. Hart R, Hindman B: Mechanisms of perioperative cerebral infarction, *Stroke* 13:766, 1982.
60. Oliver SB, Cucchiara RF, Warner MA, et al: Unexpected focal neurologic deficit on emergence from anesthesia: a report of three cases, *Anesthesiology* 67:823, 1987.
61. Van Ruiswyk J, Noble H, Sigmann P: The natural history of carotid bruits in elderly persons. *Ann Intern Med* 112:340, 1990.
62. Mayberg MR, Winn HR: Endarterectomy for asymptomatic carotid artery stenosis: resolving the controversy, *JAMA* 273:1459, 1995.
63. Executive Committee for the Asymptomatic Carotid Atherosclerosis Study: Endarterectomy for asymptomatic carotid artery stenosis, *JAMA* 273:1421, 1995.
64. Landercasper J, Merz BJ, Cogbill TH, et al: Perioperative stroke risk in 173 consecutive patients with a past history of stroke, *Arch Surg* 125:986, 1990.
65. Widder B, Kleiser B, Krapf H: Course of cerebrovascular reactivity in patients with carotid artery occlusions, *Stroke* 25:1963, 1994.
66. Bladein CF, Chambers BR: Frequency and pathogenesis of hemodynamic stroke, *Stroke* 25:2179, 1994.
67. Kendell RE, Marshall J: Role of hypotension in the genesis of transient focal cerebral ischaemic attacks, *BMJ* 344, 1963.
68. Torvik A, Skullerud K: How often are brain infarcts caused by hypotensive episodes? *Stroke* 7:255, 1976.
69. Sherman DG, Hart RG, Easton JD: Abrupt change in head position and cerebral infarction, *Stroke* 12:2, 1981.
70. Tettenborn B, Caplan LR, Sloan MA, et al: Postoperative brainstem and cerebellar infarcts, *Neurology* 43:471, 1993.
71. Nwokolo N, Bateman DE: Stroke after a visit to the hairdresser, *Lancet* 350:866, 1997.
72. Black S, Enneking FK, Cucchiara RF: Failure to awaken after general anesthesia due to cerebrovascular events, *J Neurosurg Anesthesiol* 10:10, 1998.
73. Manners JM, Wills A: Post-operative convulsions: a review based on a case report, *Anaesthesia* 26:66, 1971.
74. Lebowitz MH, Blitt CD, Dillon JB: Enflurane-induced central nervous system excitation and its relation to carbon dioxide tension, *Anesth Analg* 51:355, 1972.
75. Burchiel KJ, Stockard JJ, Calverley RK, et al: Relationship of pre- and postanesthetic EEG abnormalities to enflurane-induced seizure activity, *Anesth Analg* 56:509, 1977.
76. Kruczek M, Albin MS, Wolf S, et al: Postoperative seizure activity following enflurane anesthesia, *Anesthesiology* 53:175, 1980.
77. Ohm WW, Cullen BF, Amory DW, et al: Delayed seizure activity following enflurane anesthesia, *Anesthesiology* 42:367, 1975.
78. Fariello RG: Epileptogenic properties of enflurane and their clinical interpretation, *Electroencephalogr Clin Neurophysiol* 48:595, 1980.
79. Modica PA, Tempelhoff R, White PF: Pro- and anticonvulsant effects of anesthetics (part I), *Anesth Analg* 70:303, 1990.
80. Rampil IJ, Lockhart SH, Eger EI, et al: The electroencephalographic effects of desflurane in humans, *Anesthesiology* 74:434, 1991.
81. Komatsu H, Taie S, Endo S, et al: Electrical seizures during sevoflurane anesthesia in two pediatric patients with epilepsy, *Anesthesiology* 81:1535, 1994.
82. Reddy RV, Moorthy SS, Dierdorf SF, et al: Excitatory effects and electroencephalographic correlation of etomidate, thiopental, methohexital, and propofol, *Anesth Analg* 77:1008, 1993.
83. Modica PA, Tempelhoff R, White PF: Pro- and anticonvulsant effects of anesthetics (part II), *Anesth Analg* 70:433, 1990.
84. Laughlin TP, Newberg LA: Prolonged myoclonus after etomidate anesthesia, *Anesth Analg* 64:80, 1985.
85. Ghoneim MM, Yamada T: Etomidate: a clinical and electroencephalographic comparison with thiopental, *Anesth Analg* 56:479, 1977.
86. Ebrahim ZY, DeBoer GE, Luders H, et al: Effect of etomidate on the electroencephalogram of patients with epilepsy, *Anesth Analg* 65:1004, 1986.
87. Krieger W, Copperman J, Laxer KD: Seizures with etomidate anesthesia, *Anesth Analg* 64:1226, 1985.
88. Ferrer-Allado T, Brechner VL, Dymond A, et al: Ketamine-induced electroconvulsive phenomena in the human limbic and thalamic regions, *Anesthesiology* 38:333, 1973.
89. Bennett DR, Madsen JA, Jordan WS, et al: Ketamine anesthesia in brain-damaged epileptics. Electroencephalographic and clinical observations, *Neurology* 23:449, 1973.
90. Borgeat A, Dessibourg C, Popovic V, et al: Propofol and spontaneous movements: an EEG study, *Anesthesiology* 74:24, 1991.
91. Cochran D, Price W, Gwinnutt CL: Unilateral convulsion after induction of anaesthesia with propofol, *Br J Anaesth* 76:570, 1996.
92. Wang B, Bai Q, Jiao X, et al: Effect of sedative and hypnotic doses of propofol on the EEG activity of patients with or without a history of seizure disorders, *J Neurosurg Anesthesiol* 9:335, 1997.
93. Samra SK, Sneyd JR, Ross DA, et al: Effects of propofol sedation on seizures and intracranially recorded epileptiform activity in patients with partial epilepsy, *Anesthesiology* 82:843, 1995.
94. Cheng MA, Tempelhoff R, Silbergeld DL, et al: Large-dose propofol alone in adult epileptic patients: electrocorticographic results, *Anesth Analg* 83:169, 1996.
95. Ebrahim ZY, Schubert A, Van Ness P, et al: The effect of propofol on the electroencephalogram of patients with epilepsy, *Anesth Analg* 78:275, 1994.
96. Smith M, Smith SJ, Scott CA, et al: Activation of the electrocorticogram by propofol during surgery for epilepsy, *Br J Anaesth* 76:499, 1996.
97. Makela JP, Iivanainen M, Pieninkeroinen IP, et al: Seizures associated with propofol anesthesia, *Epilepsia* 34:832, 1993.
98. Nowack WJ, Jordan R: Propofol, seizures and generalized paroxysmal fast activity in the EEG, *Clin Electroencephalogr* 25:110, 1994.
99. Goetting MG, Thirman MJ: Neurotoxicity of meperidine, *Ann Emerg Med* 14:1007, 1985.
100. Szeto HH, Inturrisi CE, Houde R, et al: Accumulation of normeperidine, an active metabolite of meperidine, in patients with renal failure of cancer, *Ann Intern Med* 86:738, 1977.
101. Kaiko RF, Foley KM, Grabinski PY, et al: Central nervous system excitatory effects of meperidine in cancer patients, *Ann Neurol* 13:180, 1983.
102. Marinella MA: Meperidine-induced generalized seizures with normal renal function, *South Med J* 90:556, 1997.
103. Rao TLK, Mummaneni N, El-Etr AA: Convulsions: an unusual response to intravenous fentanyl administration, *Anesth Analg* 61:1020, 1982.
104. Molbegott LP, Flashburg MH, Karasic HL, et al: Probable seizures after sufentanil, *Anesth Analg* 66:91, 1987.
105. Strong WE, Matson M: Probable seizure after alfentanil, *Anesth Analg* 68:692, 1989.
106. Safwat AM, Daniel D: Grand mal seizure after fentanyl administration, *Anesthesiology* 59:78, 1983.
107. Sebel PS, Bovill JG, Wauquier A, et al: Effects of high-dose fentanyl anesthesia on the electroencephalogram, *Anesthesiology* 55:203, 1981.
108. Wauquier A, Bovill JG, Sebel PS: Electroencephalographic effects of fentanyl, sufentanil and alfentanil anaesthesia in man, *Neuropsychobiology* 11:203, 1984.
109. Bovill JG, Sebel PS, Wauquier A, et al: Influence of high-dose alfentanil anaesthesia on the electroencephalogram: correlation with plasma concentrations, *Br J Anaesth* 55(suppl 2):199S, 1983.
110. Kearse LAJ, Koski G, Husain MV, et al: Epileptiform activity during opioid anesthesia, *Electroencephalogr Clin Neurophysiol* 87:374, 1993.
111. Tempelhoff R, Modica PA, Bernardo KL, et al: Fentanyl-induced electrocorticographic seizures in patients with complex partial epilepsy, *J Neurosurg* 77:201, 1992.

112. Keene DL, Roberts D, Splinter WM, et al: Alfentanil mediated activation of epileptiform activity in the electrocorticogram during resection of epileptogenic foci, *Can J Neurol Sci* 24:37, 1997.

113. Furgang FA, Sohn JJ: The effect of thiopentone on enflurane-induced cortical seizures, *Br J Anaesth* 49:127, 1977.

114. Kofke WA, Tempelhoff R, Dasheiff RM: Anesthetic implications of epilepsy, status epilepticus, and epilepsy surgery, *J Neurosurg Anesthesiol* 9:349, 1997.

115. Opitz A, Marschall M, Degen R, et al: General anesthesia in patients with epilepsy and status epilepticus. *Adv Neurol* 34:531, 1983.

116. Gallagher TJ, Galindo A, Richey ET: Inhibition of seizure activity during enflurance anesthesia, *Anesth Analg* 57:130, 1978.

117. Yeoman P, Hutchinson A, Byrne A, et al: Etomidate infusions for the control of refractory status epilepticus, *Intensive Care Med* 15:255, 1989.

118. Simpson KH, Halsall PJ, Carr CM, et al: Propofol reduces seizure duration in patients having anaesthesia for electroconvulsive therapy, *Br J Anaesth* 61:343, 1988.

119. Mackenzie SJ, Kapadia F, Grant IS: Propofol infusion for control of status epilepticus, *Anaesthesia* 45:1043, 1990.

120. Brown RH, Schauble JF, Miller NR: Anemia and hypotension as contributors to perioperative loss of vision, *Anesthesiology* 80:222, 1994.

121. Roth S, Thisted RA, Erickson JP, et al: Eye injuries after nonocular surgery. A study of 60, 965 anesthetics from 1988 to 1992, *Anesthesiology* 85:1020, 1996.

122. Condon HA: Deliberate hypotension in ENT surgery, *Clin Otolaryngol* 4:241, 1979.

123. Wilkes LL: Paraplegia from operating position and spinal stenosis in non-spinal surgery: a case report, *Clin Orthop* 148, 1980.

124. Flippo TS, Holder WDJ: Neurologic degeneration associated with nitrous oxide anesthesia in patients with vitamin B_{12} deficiency, *Arch Surg* 128:1391, 1993.

125. Hadzic A, Glab K, Sanborn KV, et al: Severe neurologic deficit after nitrous oxide anesthesia, *Anesthesiology* 83:863, 1995.

126. Zelcer J, Wells DG: Anaesthetic-related recovery room complications, *Anaesth Intens Care* 15:168, 1987.

127. Rosenberg H, Clofine R, Bialik O: Neurologic changes during awakening from anesthesia, *Anesthesiology* 54:125, 1981.

128. Thal GD, Szabo MD, Lopez-Bresnahan M, et al: Neurologic changes during emergence from general anesthesia in neurologically normal patients, *Anesthesiology* 79:A192, 1993.

129. Laycock GJ: Opisthotonos and propofol: a possible association, *Anaesthesia* 43:257, 1988.

130. Marsch SC, Schaefer HG: Problems with eye opening after propofol anesthesia, *Anesth Analg* 70:127, 1990.

131. Melnick BM: Extrapyramidal reactions to low-dose droperidol, *Anesthesiology* 69:424, 1988.

132. Thal GD, Szabo MD, Lopez-Bresnahan M, et al: Exacerbation or unmasking of focal neurologic deficits by sedatives, *Anesthesiology* 85:21, 1996.

133. Cucchiara RF: Differential awakening, *Anesth Analg* 75:467, 1992.

134. Finck AD, Salcman M, Balis E: Alleviation of prolonged postoperative central nervous system depression after treament with naloxone, *Anesthesiology* 47:392, 1977.

135. Artru AA, Hui GS: Physostigmine reversal of general anesthesia for intraoperative neurological testing: associated EEG changes, *Anesth Analg* 65:1059, 1986.

136. Prough DS, Roy R, Bumgarner J, et al: Acute pulmonary edema in healthy teenagers following conservative doses of intravenous naloxone, *Anesthesiology* 60:485, 1984.

137. Azar I, Turndorf H: Severe hypertension and multiple atrial premature contractions following naloxone administration, *Anesth Analg* 58:524, 1979.

138. Holzgrafe RE, Vondrell JJ, Mintz SM: Reversal of postoperative reactions to scopolamine with physostigmine, *Anesth Analg* 52:921, 1973.

139. Bidwai AV, Stanley TH, Rogers C, et al: Reversal of diazepam-induced postanesthetic somnolence with physostigmine, *Anesthesiology* 51:256, 1979.

140. Hoffman EJ, Warren EW: Flumazenil: a benzodiazepine antagonist, *Clin Pharmacol* 12:641, 1993.

141. Toker P: Hyperosmolar hyperglycemic nonketotic coma, a cause of delayed recovery from anesthesia, *Anesthesiology* 41:284, 1974.

142. Mustajoki P, Heinonen J: General anesthesia in "inducible" porphyrias, *Anesthesiology* 53:15, 1980.

143. Johnston KR, Vaughan RS: Delayed recovery from general anaesthesia, *Anaesthesia* 43:1024, 1988.

144. Regan MJ, Eger EI: Effect of hypothermia in dogs on anesthetizing and apneic doses of inhalation agents. Determination of the anesthetic index (Apnea/MAC), *Anesthesiology* 28:689, 1967.

145. Granberg PO: Human physiology under cold exposure, *Arctic Med Res* 50(suppl 6):23, 1991.

146. Lam AM, Parkin JA: Cimetidine and prolonged post-operative somnolence, *Can Anaesth Soc J* 28:450, 1981.

147. Schubert A, Mascha EJ, Bloomfield EL, et al: Effect of cranial surgery and brain tumor size on emergence from anesthesia, *Anesthesiology* 85:513, 1996.

148. Adams AP, Goroszeniuk T: Hysteria. A cause of failure to recover after anaesthesia, *Anaesthesia* 46:932, 1991.

149. Black S, Muzzi DA, Nishimura RA, et al: Preoperative and intraoperative echocardiography to detect right-to-left shunt in patients undergoing neurosurgical procedures in the sitting position, *Anesthesiology* 72:436, 1990.

150. Warach S, Gaa J, Siewert B, et al: Acute human stroke studied by whole brain echo planar diffusion-weighted magnetic resonance imaging, *Ann Neurol* 37:231, 1995.

151. Fisher M, Prichard JW, Warach S: New magnetic resonance techniques for acute ischemic stroke, *JAMA* 274:908, 1995.

152. Rothman SM, Olney JW: Glutamate and the pathophysiology of hypoxic-ischemic brain damage, *Ann Neurol* 19:105, 1986.

153. Gelmers HJ, Gorter K, De Weerdt CJ, et al: A controlled trial of nimodipine in acute ischemic stroke, *N Engl J Med* 318:203, 1988.

154. Kaste M, Fogelholm R, Erila T, et al: A randomized, double-blind, placebo-controlled trial of nimodipine in acute ischemic hemispheric stroke, *Stroke* 25:1348, 1994.

155. Barnwell SL, Clark WM, Nguyen TT, et al: Safety and efficacy of delayed intraarterial urokinase therapy with mechanical clot disruption of thromboembolic stroke, *AJNR Am J Neuroradiol* 15:1817, 1994.

156. Ferguson RD, Ferguson JG: Cerebral intraarterial fibrinolysis at the crossroads: is a phase III trial advisable at this time? *AJNR Am J Neuroradiol* 15:1201, 1994.

157. Hacke W, Kaste M, Fieschi C, et al: Intravenous thrombolysis with recombinant tissue plasminogen activator for acute hemispheric stroke. The European Cooperative Acute Stroke Study (ECASS), *JAMA* 274:1017, 1995.

158. The National Institute of Neurological Disorders and Stroke rt-PA Stroke Study Group: Tissue plasminogen activator for acute ischemic stroke, *N Engl J Med* 333:1581, 1995.

159. Kay R, Wong KS, Yu YL, et al: Low-molecular-weight heparin for the treatment of acute ischemic stroke, *N Engl J Med* 333:1588, 1995.

160. The Publications Committee for the Trial of ORG 10172 in Acute Stroke Treatment (TOAST) Investigators: Low molecular weight heparinoid, ORG 10172 (Danaparoid), and outcome after acute ischemic stroke, *JAMA* 279:1265, 1998.

161. Schriger DL, Kalafut M, Starkman S, et al: Cranial computed tomography interpretation in acute stroke, *JAMA* 279:1293, 1998.

162. Fisher M, Bogousslavsky J: Further evolution toward effective therapy for acute ischemic stroke, *JAMA* 279:1298, 1998.

163. Goldstein LB: Common drugs may influence motor recovery after stroke. The Sygen in Acute Stroke Study Investigators, *Neurology* 45:865, 1995.

164. Rothwell PM, Slattery J, Warlow CP: A systematic comparison of the risks of stroke and death due to carotid endarterectomy for symptomatic and asymptomatic stenosis, *Stroke* 27:266, 1996.

165. Rothwell PM, Slattery J, Warlow CP: A systematic review of the risks of stroke and death due to endarterectomy for symptomatic carotid stenosis, *Stroke* 27:260, 1996.

166. Moore WS, Barnett HJ, Beebe HG, et al: Guidelines for carotid endarterectomy. A multidisciplinary consensus statement from the ad hoc Committee, American Heart Association, *Stroke* 26:188, 1995.

167. MRC European Carotid Surgery Trial: Interim results for symptomatic patients with severe (70-99%) or with mild (0-29%) carotid stenosis. European Carotid Surgery Trialists' Collaborative Group, *Lancet* 337:1235, 1991.
168. North American Symptomatic Carotid Endarterectomy Trial Collaborators: Beneficial effect of carotid endarterectomy in symptomatic patients with high-grade carotid stenosis, *N Engl J Med* 325:445, 1991.
169. Mayberg MR, Wilson SE, Yatsu F, et al: Carotid endarterectomy and prevention of cerebral ischemia in symptomatic carotid stenosis. Veterans Affairs Cooperative Studies Program 309 Trialist Group, *JAMA* 266:3289, 1991.
170. Wennberg DE, Lucas L, Birkmeyer JD, et al: Variation in carotid endarterectomy mortality in the medicare population, *JAMA* 279:1278, 1998.
171. Gaunt ME, Naylor AR, Bell PR: Preventing strokes associated with carotid endarterectomy: detection of embolisation by transcranial Doppler monitoring, *Eur J Vasc Endovasc Surg* 14:1, 1997.
172. Penn AA, Schomer DF, Steinberg GK: Imaging studies of cerebral hyperperfusion after carotid endarterectomy. Case report, *J Neurosurg* 83:133, 1995.
173. Ghali R, Palazzo EG, Rodriguez DI, et al: Transcranial Doppler intraoperative monitoring during carotid endarterectomy: experience with regional or general anesthesia, with and without shunting, *Ann Vasc Surg* 11:9, 1997.
174. Spencer MP: Transcranial Doppler monitoring and causes of stroke from carotid endarterectomy, *Stroke* 28:685, 1997.
175. Gavrilescu T, Babikian VL, Cantelmo NL, et al: Cerebral microembolism during carotid endarterectomy, *Am J Surg* 170:159, 1995.
176. Walleck P, Becquemin JP, Desgranges P, et al: Are neurologic events occurring during carotid artery surgery predictive of postoperative neurologic complications? *Acta Anaesthesiol Scand* 40:167, 1996.
177. Riles TS, Imparato AM, Jacobowitz GR, et al: The cause of perioperative stroke after carotid endarterectomy, *J Vasc Surg* 19:206, 1994.
178. Davies MJ, Mooney PH, Scott DA, et al: Neurologic changes during carotid endarterectomy under cervical block predict a high risk of postoperative stroke, *Anesthesiology* 78:829, 1993.
179. Prioleau WH Jr, Aiken AF, Hairston P: Carotid endarterectomy: neurologic complications as related to surgical techniques, *Ann Surg* 185:678, 1977.
180. Whitney EG, Brophy CM, Kahn EM, et al: Inadequate cerebral perfusion is an unlikely cause of perioperative stroke, *Ann Vasc Surg* 11:109, 1997.
181. Schiro J, Mertz GH, Cannon JA, et al: Routine use of a shunt for carotid endarterectomy, *Am J Surg* 142:735, 1981.
182. Cho I, Smullens SN, Streletz LJ, et al: The value of intraoperative EEG monitoring during carotid endarterectomy, *Ann Neurol* 20:508, 1986.
183. Plestis KA, Loubser P, Mizrahi EM, et al: Continuous electroencephalographic monitoring and selective shunting reduces neurologic morbidity rates in carotid endarterectomy, *J Vasc Surg* 25:620, 1997.
184. Fiori L, Parenti G: Electrophysiological monitoring for selective shunting during carotid endarterectomy, *J Neurosurg Anesthesiol* 7:168, 1995.
185. Prokop A, Meyer GP, Walter M, et al: Validity of SEP monitoring in carotid surgery. Review and own results, *J Cardiovasc Surg* 37:337, 1996.
186. Jansen C, Vriens EM, Eikelboom BC, et al: Carotid endarterectomy with transcranial Doppler and electroencephalographic monitoring: a prospective study in 130 operations, *Stroke* 24:665, 1993.
187. Giannoni MF, Sbarigia E, Panico MA, et al: Intraoperative transcranial Doppler sonography monitoring during carotid surgery under locoregional anaesthesia, *Eur J Vasc Endovasc Surg* 12:407, 1996.
188. Jansen C, Ramos LMP, van Heesewijk JPM, et al: Impact of microembolism and hemodynamic changes in the brain during carotid endarterectomy, *Stroke* 25:992, 1994.
189. Allen BT, Anderson CB, Rubin BG, et al: The influence of anesthetic technique on perioperative complications after carotid endarterectomy, *J Vasc Surg* 19:834, 1994.
190. Benjamin ME, Silva MBJ, Watt C, et al: Awake patient monitoring to determine the need for shunting during carotid endarterectomy, *Surgery* 114:673, 1993.
191. Arnold M, Sturzenegger M, Schaffler L, et al: Continuous intraoperative monitoring of middle cerebral artery blood flow velocities and electroencephalography during carotid endarterectomy: a comparison of the two methods to detect cerebral ischemia, *Stroke* 28:1345, 1997.
192. Sharbrough FW, Messick JM Jr, Sundt TM Jr: Correlation of continuous electroencephalograms with cerebral blood flow measurements during carotid endarterectomy, *Stroke* 4:674, 1973.
193. Astrup J, Siesjo BK, Symon L: Thresholds in cerebral ischemia: the ischemic penumbra, *Stroke* 12:723, 1981.
194. Heiss WD: Flow thresholds of functional and morphological damage of brain tissue, *Stroke* 14:329, 1983.
195. Evans WE, Hayes JP, Waltke EA, et al: Optimal cerebral monitoring during carotid endarterectomy: neurologic response under local anesthesia, *J Vasc Surg* 2:775, 1985.
196. Lam AM, Manninen PH, Ferguson GG, et al: Monitoring electrophysiologic function during carotid endarterectomy: a comparison of somatosensory evoked potentials and conventional electroencephalogram, *Anesthesiology* 75:15, 1991.
197. Chiappa KH, Burke SR, Young RR: Results of electroencephalographic monitoring during 367 carotid endarterectomies: use of a dedicated minicomputer, *Stroke* 10:381, 1979.
198. Blume WT, Ferguson GG, McNeill DK: Significance of EEG changes at carotid endarterectomy, *Stroke* 17:891, 1986.
199. Krul JMJ, van Gijn J, Ackerstaff RGA, et al: Site and pathogenesis of infarcts associated with carotid endarterectomy, *Stroke* 20:324, 1989.
200. Kalra M, al-Khaffaf H, Farrell A, et al: Comparison of measurement of stump pressure and transcranial measurement of flow velocity in the middle cerebral artery in carotid surgery, *Ann Vasc Surg* 8:225, 1994.
201. Harada RN, Comerota AJ, Good GM, et al: Stump pressure, electroencephalographic changes, and the contralateral carotid artery: another look at selective shunting, *Am J Surg* 170:148, 1995.
202. van Zuilen EV, Moll FL, Vermeulen FE, et al: Detection of cerebral microemboli by means of transcranial Doppler monitoring before and after carotid endarterectomy, *Stroke* 26:210, 1995.
203. Levi CR, O'Malley HM, Fell G, et al: Transcranial Doppler detected cerebral microembolism following carotid endarterectomy: high microembolic signal loads predict postoperative cerebral ischaemia, *Brain* 120:621, 1997.
204. Kuroda S, Houkin K, Abe H, et al: Near-infrared monitoring of cerebral oxygenation state during carotid endarterectomy, *Surg Neurol* 45:450, 1996.
205. Samra SK, Dorje P, Zelenock GB, et al: Cerebral oximetry in patients undergoing carotid endarterectomy under regional anesthesia, *Stroke* 27:49, 1996.
206. White RP, Markus HS: Impaired dynamic cerebral autoregulation in carotid artery stenosis, *Stroke* 28:1340, 1997.
207. Drummond JC, Oh YS, Cole DJ, et al: Phenylephrine-induced hypertension reduces ischemia following middle cerebral artery occlusion in rats, *Stroke* 20:1538, 1989.
208. Boysen G, Ladegaard-Pedersen HJ, Henriksen H, et al: The effects of $PaCO_2$ on regional cerebral blood flow and internal carotid arterial pressure during carotid clamping, *Anesthesiology* 35:286, 1971.
209. Mohr LL, Smith LL, Hinshaw DB: Blood gas and carotid pressure: factors in stroke risk, *Ann Surg* 184:723, 1976.
210. Baker WH, Rodman JA, Barnes RW, et al: An evaluation of hypocarbia and hypercarbia during carotid endarterectomy, *Stroke* 7:451, 1976.
211. Christensen MS, Paulson OB, Olesen J, et al: Cerebral apoplexy (stroke) treated with or without prolonged artificial hyperventilation. I. Cerebral circulation, clinical course, and cause of death, *Stroke* 4:568, 1973.

212. Sieber FE, Traystman RJ: Special issues: glucose and the brain, *Crit Care Med* 20:104, 1991.

213. Wass CT, Lanier WL: Glucose modulation of ischemic brain injury: review and clinical recommendations, *Mayo Clin Proc* 71:801, 1996.

214. Lam AM, Winn HR, Cullen BF, et al: Hyperglycemia and neurological outcome in patients with head injury, *J Neurosurg* 75:545, 1991.

215. Verhaegen MJ, Todd MM, Warner DS: A comparison of cerebral ischemic flow thresholds during halothane/N$_2$O and isoflurane/N$_2$O anesthesia in rats, *Anesthesiology* 76:743, 1992.

216. Young Y, Menon DK, Tisavipat N, et al: Propofol neuroprotection in a rat model of ischaemia reperfusion injury, *Eur J Anaesthesiol* 14:320, 1997.

217. Drummond JC, Cole DJ, Patel PM, et al: Focal cerebral ischemia during anesthesia with etomidate, isoflurane, or thiopental: a comparison of the extent of cerebral injury, *Neurosurgery* 37:742, 1995.

218. Messick JM Jr, Newberg LA, Nugent M, et al: Principles of neuroanesthesia for the nonneurosurgical patient with CNS pathophysiology, *Anesth Analg* 64:143, 1985.

219. Michenfelder JD, Sundt TM, Fode N, et al: Isoflurane when compared to enflurane and halothane decreases the frequency of cerebral ischemia during carotid endarterectomy, *Anesthesiology* 67:336, 1987.

220. Messick JM Jr, Casement B, Sharbrough FW, et al: Correlation of regional cerebral blood flow (rCBF) with EEG changes during isoflurane anesthesia for carotid endarterectomy: critical rCBF, *Anesthesiology* 66:344, 1987.

221. Todd MM, Warner DS: A comfortable hypothesis reevaluated: cerebral metabolic depression and brain protection during ischemia, *Anesthesiology* 76:161, 1992.

222. Grady RE, Weglinski MR, Sharbrough FW, et al: Correlation of regional cerebral blood flow with ischemic electroencephalographic changes during sevoflurane–nitrous oxide anesthesia for carotid endarterectomy, *Anesthesiology* 88:892, 1998.

223. Frawley JE, Hicks RG, Horton DA, et al: Thiopental sodium cerebral protection during carotid endarterectomy: perioperative disease and death, *J Vasc Surg* 19:732, 1994.

224. Spetzler RF, Martin N, Hadley MN, et al: Microsurgical endarterectomy under barbiturate protection: a prospective study, *J Neurosurg* 65:63, 1986.

225. Warner DS, Takaoka S, Wu B, et al: Electroencephalographic burst suppression is not required to elicit maximal neuroprotection from pentobarbital in a rat model of focal cerebral ischemia, *Anesthesiology* 84:1475, 1996.

226. Jordan WDJ, Schroeder PT, Fisher WS, et al: A comparison of angioplasty with stenting versus endarterectomy for the treatment of carotid artery stenosis, *Ann Vasc Surg* 11:2, 1997.

227. Comerota AJ, Eze AR: Intraoperative high-dose regional urokinase infusion for cerebrovascular occlusion after carotid endarterectomy, *J Vasc Surg* 24:1008, 1996.

228. Barr JD, Horowitz MB, Mathis JM, et al: Intraoperative urokinase infusion for embolic stroke during carotid endarterectomy, *Neurosurgery* 36:606, 1995.

229. Roach GW, Kanchuger M, Mangano CM, et al: Adverse cerebral outcomes after coronary bypass surgery. Multicenter Study of Perioperative Ischemia Research Group and the Ischemia Research and Education Foundation Investigators, *N Engl J Med* 335:1857, 1996.

230. Harris DN, Oatridge A, Dob D, et al: Cerebral swelling after normothermic cardiopulmonary bypass, *Anesthesiology* 88:340, 1998.

231. Aberg T, Ronquist G, Tydén H, et al: Adverse effects on the brain in cardiac operations as assessed by biochemical, psychometric, and radiologic methods, *J Thorac Cardiovasc Surg* 87:99, 1984.

232. Steinberg GK, De La Paz R, Mitchell RS, et al: MR and cerebrospinal fluid enzymes as sensitive indicators of subclinical cerebral injury after open-heart valve replacement surgery, *AJNR Am J Neuroradiol* 17:205, 1996.

233. Shaw PJ, Bates D, Cartlidge NEF, et al: Neurologic and neuropsychological morbidity following major surgery: comparison of coronary artery bypass and peripheral vascular surgery, *Stroke* 18:700, 1987.

234. Townes BD, Bashein G, Hornbein TF, et al: Neurobehavioral outcomes in cardiac operations: a prospective controlled study, *J Thorac Cardiovasc Surg* 98:774, 1989.

235. Klonoff H, Clark C, Kavanagh-Gray D, et al: Two-year follow-up study of coronary bypass surgery: psychologic status, employment status, and quality of life, *J Thorac Cardiovasc Surg* 97:78, 1989.

236. Venn GE, Patel RL, Chambers DJ: Cardiopulmonary bypass: perioperative cerebral blood flow and postoperative cognitive deficit, *Ann Thorac Surg* 59:1331, 1995.

237. Blauth CI: Macroemboli and microemboli during cardiopulmonary bypass, *Ann Thorac Surg* 59:1300, 1995.

238. Hartman GS, Yao FS, Bruefach M, et al: Severity of aortic atheromatous disease diagnosed by transesophageal echocardiography predicts stroke and other outcomes associated with coronary artery surgery: a prospective study, *Anesth Analg* 83:701, 1996.

239. Barbut D, Hinton RB, Szatrowski TP, et al: Cerebral emboli detected during bypass surgery are associated with clamp removal, *Stroke* 25:2398, 1994.

240. Rodigas PC, Meyer FJ, Haasler GB, et al: Intraoperative 2-dimensional echocardiography: ejection of microbubbles from the left ventricle after cardiac surgery, *Am J Cardiol* 50:1130, 1982.

241. Pugsley W, Klinger L, Paschalis C, et al: The impact of microemboli during cardiopulmonary bypass on neuropsychological functioning, *Stroke* 25:1393, 1994.

242. Ellis RJ, Wisniewski A, Potts R, et al: Reduction of flow rate and arterial pressure at moderate hypothermia does not result in cerebral dysfunction, *J Thorac Cardiovasc Surg* 79:173, 1980.

243. Kolkka R, Hilberman M: Neurologic dysfunction following cardiac operation with low-flow, low-pressure cardiopulmonary bypass, *J Thorac Cardiovasc Surg* 79:432, 1980.

244. Schell RM, Kern FH, Greeley WJ, et al: Cerebral blood flow and metabolism during cardiopulmonary bypass, *Anesth Analg* 76:849, 1993.

245. Gold JP, Charlson ME, Williams-Russo P, et al: Improvement of outcomes after coronary artery bypass. A randomized trial comparing intraoperative high versus low mean arterial pressure, *J Thorac Cardiovasc Surg* 110:1302, 1995.

246. Slogoff S, Girgis KZ, Keats AS: Etiologic factors in neuropsychiatric complications associated with cardiopulmonary bypass, *Anesth Analg* 61:903, 1982.

247. Katz ES, Tunick PA, Rusinek H, et al: Protruding aortic atheromas predict stroke in elderly patients undergoing cardiopulmonary bypass: experience with intraoperative transesophageal echocardiography, *J Am Coll Cardiol* 20:70, 1992.

248. Redmond JM, Greene PS, Goldsborough MA, et al: Neurologic injury in cardiac surgical patients with a history of stroke, *Ann Thorac Surg* 61:42, 1996.

249. Harrison MJG, Schneidau A, Ho R, et al: Cerebrovascular disease and functional outcome after coronary artery bypass surgery, *Stroke* 20:235, 1989.

250. Bashein G, Townes BD, Nessly ML, et al: A randomized study of carbon dioxide management during hypothermic cardiopulmonary bypass, *Anesthesiology* 72:7, 1990.

251. Michenfelder JD: A valid demonstration of barbiturate-induced brain protection in man—at last, *Anesthesiology* 64:140, 1986.

252. Nussmeier NA, Fish KJ: Neuropsychological dysfunction after cardiopulmonary bypass: a comparison of two institutions, *J Cardiothorac Vasc Anesth* 5:584, 1991.

253. Tardiff BE, Newman MF, Saunders AM, et al: Preliminary report of a genetic basis for cognitive decline after cardiac operations: the Neurologic Outcome Research Group of the Duke Heart Center, *Ann Thorac Surg* 64:715, 1997.

254. Blauth CI, Smith PL, Arnold JV, et al: Influence of oxygenator type on the prevalence and extent of microembolic retinal ischemia during cardiopulmonary bypass. Assessment by digital image analysis, *J Thorac Cardiovasc Surg* 99:61, 1990.

255. Hindman BJ, Dexter F, Smith T, et al: Pulsatile versus nonpulsatile flow. No difference in cerebral blood flow or metabolism during normothermic cardiopulmonary bypass in rabbits, *Anesthesiology* 82:241, 1995.

256. Hindman B: Cerebral physiology during cardiopulmonary bypass: pulsatile versus nonpulsatile flow, *Adv Pharmacol* 31:607, 1994.

257. Murkin JM, Martzke JS, Buchan AM, et al: A randomized study of the influence of perfusion technique and pH management strategy in 316 patients undergoing coronary artery bypass surgery. II. Neurologic and cognitive outcomes, *J Thorac Cardiovasc Surg* 110:349, 1995.

258. Henze T, Stephan H, Sonntag H: Cerebral dysfunction following extracorporeal circulation for aortocoronary bypass surgery: no differences in neuropsychological outcome after pulsatile versus nonpulsatile flow, *Thorac Cardiovasc Surg* 38:65, 1990.

259. Padayachee TS, Parsons S, Theobold R, et al: The effect of arterial filtration on reduction of gaseous microemboli in the middle cerebral artery during cardiopulmonary bypass, *Ann Thorac Surg* 45:647, 1988.

260. Konstadt SN, Reich DL, Kahn R, et al: Transesophageal echocardiography can be used to screen for ascending aortic atherosclerosis, *Anesth Analg* 81:225, 1995.

261. Swain JA: Hypothermia and blood pH. A review, *Arch Intern Med* 148:1643, 1988.

262. Prough DS, Stump DA, Troost BT: $PaCO_2$ management during cardiopulmonary bypass: intriguing physiologic rationale, convincing clinical date, evolving hypothesis? *Anesthesiology* 72:3, 1990.

263. Rogers AT, Stump DA, Gravlee GP, et al: Response of cerebral blood flow to phenylephrine infusion during hypothermic cardiopulmonary bypass: influence of $PaCO_2$ management, *Anesthesiology* 69:547, 1988.

264. Murkin JM, Farrar JK, Tweed WA, et al: Cerebral autoregulation and flow/metabolism coupling during cardiopulmonary bypass: influence of $PaCO_2$, *Anesth Analg* 66:825, 1987.

265. Hindman BJ, Dexter F, Cutkomp J, et al: pH-stat management reduces the cerebral metabolic rate for oxygen during profound hypothermia (17° C). A study during cardiopulmonary bypass in rabbits, *Anesthesiology* 82:983, 1995.

266. Kirshbom PM, Skaryak LR, DiBernardo LR, et al: pH-stat cooling improves cerebral metabolic recovery after circulatory arrest in a piglet model of aortopulmonary collaterals, *J Thorac Cardiovac Surg* 111:147, 1996.

267. Nussmeier NA, Arlund C, Slogoff S: Neuropsychiatric complications after cardiopulmonary bypass: cerebral protection by a barbiturate, *Anesthesiology* 64:165, 1986.

268. Prough DS, Mills SA: Should thiopental sodium administration be a standard of care for open cardiac procedures? *J Clin Anesth* 2:221, 1990.

269. Zaidan JR, Klochany A, Martin WM, et al: Effect of thiopental on neurologic outcome following coronary artery bypass grafting, *Anesthesiology* 74:406, 1991.

270. Engelman RM, Rousou JA, Flack JE, et al: Fast-track recovery of the coronary bypass patient, *Ann Thorac Surg* 58:1742, 1994.

270a. Roach GW, Newman MF, Murkin JM, et al: Ineffectiveness of burst suppression therapy in mitigating perioperative cerebrovascular dysfunction, *Anesthesiology* 90:1255, 1999.

271. Forsman M, Olsnes BT, Semb G, et al: Effects of nimodipine on cerebral blood flow and neuropsychological outcome after cardiac surgery, *Br J Anaesth* 65:514, 1990.

272. Legault C, Furberg CD, Wagenknecht LE, et al: Nimodipine neuroprotection in cardiac valve replacement: report of an early terminated trial, *Stroke* 27:593, 1996.

273. Michenfelder JD, Theye RA: Hypothermia: effect on canine brain and whole-body metabolism, *Anesthesiology* 29:1107, 1968.

274. Conroy BP, Lin CY, Jenkins LW, et al: Hypothermic modulation of cerebral ischemic injury during cardiopulmonary bypass in pigs, *Anesthesiology* 88:390, 1998.

275. Busto R, Dietrich WD, Globus MY, et al: Small differences in intraischemic brain temperature critically determine the extent of ischemic neuronal injury, *J Cereb Blood Flow Metab* 7:729, 1987.

276. Warm Heart Investigators: Randomized trial of normothermic versus hypothermic coronary bypass surgery, *Lancet* 343:559, 1994.

277. Craver JM, Bufkin BL, Weintraub WS, et al: Neurologic events after coronary bypass grafting: further observations with warm cardioplegia, *Ann Thorac Surg* 59:1429, 1995.

278. Martin TD, Craver JM, Gott JP, et al: Prospective, randomized trial of retrograde warm blood cardioplegia: myocardial benefit and neurologic threat, *Ann Thorac Surg* 57:298, 1994.

279. McLean RF, Wong BI, Naylor CD, et al: Cardiopulmonary bypass, temperature, and central nervous system dysfunction, *Circulation* 90(2):250, 1994.

280. Wass CT, Lanier WL, Hofer RE, et al: Temperature changes of > or = 1° C alter functional neurologic outcome and histopathology in a canine model of complete cerebral ischemia, *Anesthesiology* 83:325, 1995.

281. Croughwell ND, Frasco P, Blumenthal JA, et al: Warming during cardiopulmonary bypass is associated with jugular bulb desaturation, *Ann Thorac Surg* 53:827, 1992.

282. Croughwell ND, Newman MF, Blumenthal JA, et al: Jugular bulb saturation and cognitive dysfunction after cardiopulmonary bypass, *Ann Thorac Surg* 58:1702, 1994.

283. Winter PM, Alvis HJ, Gage AA: Hyperbaric treatment of cerebral air embolism during cardiopulmonary bypass, *JAMA* 215:1786, 1971.

284. Verdant A, Cossette R, Page A, et al: Aneurysms of the descending thoracic aorta: three hundred sixty-six consecutive cases resected without paraplegia, *J Vasc Surg* 21:385, 1995.

285. Mauney MC, Blackbourne LH, Langenburg SE, et al: Prevention of spinal cord injury after repair of the thoracic or thoracoabdominal aorta, *Ann Thorac Surg* 59:245, 1995.

286. Svensson LG, Crawford ES, Hess KR, et al: Experience with 1509 patients undergoing thoracoabdominal aortic operations, *J Vasc Surg* 17:357, 1993.

287. Coselli JS, LeMaire SA, de Figueiredo LP, et al: Paraplegia after thoracoabdominal aortic aneurysm repair: is dissection a risk factor? *Ann Thorac Surg* 63:28, 1997.

288. Svensson LG: New and future approaches for spinal cord protection, *Semin Thorac Cardiovasc Surg* 9:206, 1997.

289. Ross RT: Spinal cord infarction in disease and surgery of the aorta, *Can J Neurol Sci* 12:289, 1985.

290. Adams HD VGH: Neurologic complications of aortic surgery, *Ann Surg* 144:574, 1956.

291. Drenger B, Parker SD, Frank SM, et al: Changes in cerebrospinal fluid pressure and lactate concentrations during thoracoabdominal aortic aneurysm surgery, *Anesthesiology* 86:41, 1997.

292. Berendes JN, Bredée JJ, Schipperheyn JJ, et al: Mechanisms of spinal cord injury after cross-clamping of the descending thoracic aorta, *Circulation* 66:I112, 1982.

293. Hollier LH, Money SR, Naslund TC, et al: Risk of spinal cord dysfunction in patients undergoing thoracoabdominal aortic replacement, *Am J Surg* 164:210, 1992.

294. Svensson LG, Hess KR, Coselli JS, et al: Influence of segmental arteries, extent, and atriofemoral bypass on postoperative paraplegia after thoracoabdominal aortic operations, *J Vasc Surg* 20:255, 1994.

295. Cunningham JN Jr, Laschinger JC, Spencer FC: Monitoring of somatosensory evoked potentials during surgical procedures on the thoracoabdominal aorta: IV. Clinical observations and data, *J Thorac Cardiovasc Surg* 94:275, 1987.

296. Matsui Y, Goh K, Shiiya N, et al: Clinical application of evoked spinal cord potentials elicited by direct stimulation of the cord during temporary occlusion of the thoracic aorta, *J Thorac Cardiovasc Surg* 107:1519, 1994.

297. Svensson LG, Crawford ES, Hess KR, et al: Variables predictive of outcome in 832 patients undergoing repairs of the descending thoracic aorta, *Chest* 104:1248, 1993.

298. DeBakey ME, McCollum CH, Crawford ES, et al: Dissection and dissecting aneurysms of the aorta: twenty-year follow-up of five hundred twenty-seven patients treated surgically, *Surgery* 92:1118, 1982.

299. Livesay JJ, Cooley DA, Ventemiglia RA, et al: Surgical experience in descending thoracic aneurysmectomy with and without adjuncts to avoid ischemia, *Ann Thorac Surg* 39:37, 1985.

300. Griepp RB, Ergin MA, Galla JD, et al: Looking for the artery of Adamkiewicz: a quest to minimize paraplegia after operations for aneurysms of the descending thoracic and thoracoabdominal aorta, *J Thorac Cardiovasc Surg* 112:1202, 1996.

301. Galla JD, Ergin MA, Sadeghi AM, et al: A new technique using somatosensory evoked potential guidance during descending and thoracoabdominal aortic repairs, *J Card Surg* 9:662, 1994.

302. de Haan P, Kalkman CJ, de Mol BA, et al: Efficacy of transcranial motor-evoked myogenic potentials to detect spinal cord ischemia during operations for thoracoabdominal aneurysms, *J Thorac Cardiovasc Surg* 113:87, 1997.

303. Drenger B, Parker SD, McPherson RW, et al: Spinal cord stimulation evoked potentials during thoracoabdominal aortic aneurysm surgery, *Anesthesiology* 76:689, 1992.

304. Svensson LG: Intraoperative identification of spinal cord blood supply during repairs of descending aorta and thoracoabdominal aorta, *J Thorac Cardiovasc Surg* 112:1455, 1996.

305. Koht A, Schutz W, Schmidt G, et al: Effects of etomidate, midazolam, and thiopental on median nerve somatosensory evoked potentials and the additive effects of fentanyl and nitrous oxide, *Anesth Analg* 67:435, 1988.

306. Blaisdell FW, Cooley DA: The mechanism of paraplegia after temporary thoracic aortic occlusion and its relationship to spinal fluid pressure, *Surgery* 51:351, 1962.

307. Bower TC, Murray MJ, Gloviczki P, et al: Effects of thoracic aortic occlusion and cerebrospinal fluid drainage on regional spinal cord blood flow in dogs: correlation with neurologic outcome, *J Vasc Surg* 9:135, 1988.

308. Wisselink W, Becker MO, Nguyen JH, et al: Protecting the ischemic spinal cord during aortic clamping: the influence of selective hypothermia and spinal cord perfusion pressure, *J Vasc Surg* 19:788, 1994.

309. Kazama S, Masaki Y, Maruyama S, et al: Effect of altering cerebrospinal fluid pressure on spinal cord blood flow, *Ann Thorac Surg* 58:112, 1994.

310. Crawford ES, Svensson LG, Hess KR, et al: A prospective randomized study of cerebrospinal fluid drainage to prevent paraplegia after high-risk surgery on the thoracoabdominal aorta, *J Vasc Surg* 13:36, 1990.

311. Ryan T, Mannion D, O'Brien W, et al: Spinal cord perfusion pressure in dogs after control of proximal aortic hypertension during thoracic aortic cross-clamping with esmolol or sodium nitroprusside, *Anesthesiology* 78:317, 1993.

312. Simpson JI, Eide TR, Newman SB, et al: Trimethaphan versus sodium nitroprusside for the control of proximal hypertension during thoracic aortic cross-clamping: the effects on spinal cord ischemia, *Anesth Analg* 82:68, 1996.

313. Cole DJ, Shapiro HM, Drummond JC, et al: Halothane, fentanyl/nitrous oxide, and spinal lidocaine protect against spinal cord injury in the rat, *Anesthesiology* 70:967, 1989.

314. Mutch WAC, Graham MR, Halliday WC, et al: Use of neuroanesthesia adjuncts (hyperventilation and mannitol administration) improves neurological outcome after thoracic aortic cross-clamping in dogs, *Stroke* 24:1204, 1993.

315. Robertson CS, Foltz R, Grossman RG, et al: Protection against experimental ischemic spinal cord injury, *J Neurosurg* 64:633, 1986.

316. Simpson JI, Eide TR, Schiff GA, et al: Intrathecal magnesium sulfate protects the spinal cord from ischemic injury during thoracic aortic cross-clamping, *Anesthesiology* 81:1493, 1994.

317. Schittek A, Bennink GBWE, Cooley DA, et al: Spinal cord protection with intravenous nimodipine: a functional and morphologic evaluation, *J Thorac Cardiovasc Surg* 104:1100, 1992.

318. Qayumi AK, Janusz MT, Jamieson WRE, et al: Pharmacologic interventions for prevention of spinal cord injury caused by aortic cross-clamping, *J Thorac Cardiovasc Surg* 104:256, 1992.

319. Madden KP, Clark WM, Kochhar A, et al: Efficacy of LY233053, a competitive glutamate antagonist, in experimental central nervous system ischemia, *J Neurosurg* 76:106, 1992.

320. Bracken MB, Shepard MJ, Holford TR, et al: Administration of methylprednisolone for 24 or 48 hours or tirilazad mesylate for 48 hours in the treatment of acute spinal cord injury. Results of the Third National Acute Spinal Cord Injury Randomized Controlled Trial. National Acute Spinal Cord Injury Study, *JAMA* 277:1597, 1997.

321. Geisler FH, Dorsey FC, Coleman WP: Recovery of motor function after spinal-cord injury: a randomized, placebo-controlled trial with GM-1 ganglioside, *N Engl J Med* 324:1829, 1991.

322. Svensson LG, Rickards E, Coull A, et al: Relationship of spinal cord blood flow to vascular anatomy during thoracic aortic cross-clamping and shunting, *J Thorac Cardiovasc Surg* 91:71, 1986.

323. Svensson LG, Grum DF, Bednarski M, et al: Appraisal of cerebrospinal fluid alterations during aortic surgery with intrathecal papaverine administration and cerebrospinal fluid drainage, *J Vasc Surg* 11:423, 1990.

324. Svensson LG, Stewart RW, Cosgrove DMI, et al: Intrathecal papaverine for the prevention of paraplegia after operation on the thoracic or thoracoabdominal aorta, *J Thorac Cardiovasc Surg* 96:823, 1988.

325. Kwun BD, Vacanti FX: Mild hypothermia protects against irreversible damage during prolonged spinal cord ischemia, *J Surg Res* 59:780, 1995.

326. Allen BT, Davis CG, Osborne D, et al: Spinal cord ischemia and reperfusion metabolism: the effect of hypothermia, *J Vasc Surg* 19:332, 1994.

327. Cambria RP, Davison JK, Zannetti S, et al: Clinical experience with epidural cooling for spinal cord protection during thoracic and thoracoabdominal aneurysm repair, *J Vasc Surg* 25:234, 1997.

328. Dake MD, Miller DC, Semba CP, et al: Transluminal placement of endovascular stent-grafts for the treatment of descending thoracic aortic aneurysms, *N Engl J Med* 331:1729, 1994.

329. Mitchell RS, Dake MD, Sembra CP, et al: Endovascular stent-graft repair of thoracic aortic aneurysms, *J Thorac Cardiovasc Surg* 111:1054, 1996.

Chapter 17

Injuries to the Visual System and Other Sense Organs

Steven Roth

Inger Gillesberg

The number of eye injuries associated with nonocular surgery and anesthesia is low, and most discussions of eye injuries appear in case reports, of which only a few are found in the anesthetic literature. Only one large study has appeared in the anesthesia literature. In 60,965 patients in our hospital undergoing nonocular surgery over a 4.5-year period,[1] the incidence of eye injury was 0.056% (34 patients). The true incidence may be greater because of underreporting of incidents for fear of legal action. In the American Society of Anesthesiologists (ASA) Closed Claims Study, which analyzed only cases in which litigation was involved, eye injuries accounted for just 3% of all claims, yet were responsible for large monetary awards,[2] reflecting the serious nature of some of these injuries.

Although uncommon, eye injuries result in discomfort and occasionally permanent visual impairment. Symptoms and signs of eye injury may be subtle and, generally, are not familiar to most anesthesiologists. Moreover, excepting the extensive consideration of the impact of anesthetic agents on intraocular pressure, there are few data on the influence of anesthesia on visual function. Accordingly, this chapter will familiarize anesthesiologists with the incidence, risk factors, diagnosis, and treatment of eye injuries that may be encountered in the perioperative period. The discussion is confined to injuries that follow nonocular surgery because eye damage after ocular surgery is well considered in the ophthalmology literature. Injuries to both the anterior segment of the eye (cornea, iris, and lens) and posterior segment (vitreous, retina, and optic nerve [ON]), as well as the visual connections to the brain, are considered. Because injuries to the posterior segment are far more likely to result in permanent or severe visual loss, the causes, detection, and prevention of these serious events are analyzed in more detail.

Even more rarely reported after anesthesia are injuries that affect other senses, such as hearing, taste, and smell. Following extensive discussion of the more common and generally more serious visual system injuries, we briefly mention these other types of complications that may affect other senses.

I. ANATOMY OF THE VISUAL PATHWAY

The anatomy of the eye and visual pathway are overviewed briefly. The visual system is divided into the anterior segment, consisting of the portions of the eye anterior to the vitreous, and the posterior segment (the vitreous, retina, ON, and intracranial visual pathways).

A. Overall structure and organization of the eye

The refractive system is formed by the cornea and lens, which focuses light on the retina; the jellylike vitreous fills the space between the lens and the retina. The iris controls the amount of light reaching the retina by regulating pupillary size.[3] The eye has three chambers: the anterior chamber extending from the cornea to the iris, the posterior chamber extending from the iris and ciliary body to the vitreous, and the vitreous chamber containing the jellylike vitreous. The ciliary body constantly produces aqueous humor that flows through the posterior chamber via the pupil to the anterior chamber and drains to the venous system via the canal of Schlemm in the angle between the iris and cornea. Another important function of the ciliary body is accommodation. Vitreous humor is not produced in the mature eye, but it may be replaced by saline after extraction. Except for the cornea, the eye is coated by the outer avascular sclera, the vascular intermediate choroid, and the inner pigmented retina. Anteriorly, the sclera is covered by conjunctiva.[4]

B. The retina

The retina is the sensory part of the eye consisting of an outer avascular region of pigmented epithelium in close contact with the photoreceptor cells (rods and cones), which transmit visual information to cells in the inner retina (bipolar, ganglion, Müller, horizontal, and amacrine cells) (Fig. 17-1). The photoreceptor layer contains 6 to 7 million cones, which provide central reading and color vision. Rod cells, which number 120 million, provide night vision and detect motion. The inner two thirds of the retina contains the retinal vessels and various cell bodies: the bipolar cells that transmit impulses from the photoreceptors and the ganglion cells, whose axons transmit visual information to the ON and then to the brain. The visual axis extends through the fovea centralis, which is avascular and contains 650,000 cones, concentrated in that region for central vision.[3]

C. The optic nerve and visual pathway

Axons of the ON arise from retinal ganglion cells and merge toward the optic disc in a well-defined manner. Those from the nasal part of the retina merge straight to the optic disc, axons from the fovea form the papillomacular bundle and enter the temporal part of the optic disc, and axons from the remaining parts of retina merge to the superior and inferior poles of the optic disc.[5] Arrangement of the ON axons is important in the differential diagnosis of visual field disturbances (i.e., when differentiating between ON disease and visual loss caused by glaucoma or cerebral insults).[6]

The optic disc comprises the intraocular part of the ON and is further divided into intraorbital, intracanalicular (within the optic canal), and intracranial portions. The two ONs merge into the optic chiasm, where axons derived from the nasal portion of the retina cross over. From the chiasm, each ON tract carries the axons from the nasal retina of the contralateral eye and the temporal retina of the ipsilateral eye to the lateral geniculate nucleus (LGN) in the midbrain for the first synapse of the retinal ganglion cells. Some axons continue through the LGN and terminate in the superior colliculus (for control of eye movement), other axons terminate in the pretectal region (for control of the pupillary light reflex), and some continue directly to the peristriate and parastriate areas in the occipital cortex, next to the primary visual cortex (same as striate cortex).

From the LGN, postsynaptic axons form the optic radiation projecting the neurons to the visual cortex. Neu-

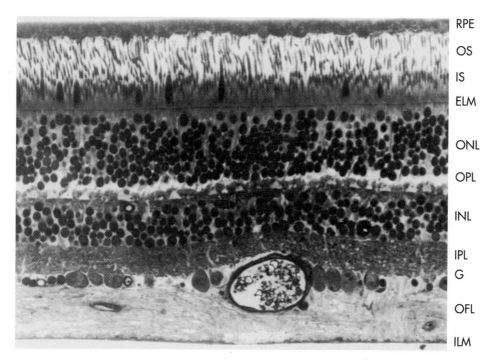

RPE
OS
IS
ELM
ONL
OPL
INL
IPL
G
OFL
ILM

Fig. 17-1. Section of the human retina demonstrating its organization into layers. The outer retina contains the photoreceptors, and the inner retina contains neurons responsible for the transmission of visual information to the brain. *RPE,* Retinal pigment epithelium; *OS,* photoreceptor outer segments; *IS,* photoreceptor inner segments; *ELM,* external limiting membrane; *ONL,* outer nuclear layer (contains cell bodies of rods and cones); *OPL,* outer plexiform layer (contains synapses between rods and cones and second-order neurons); *INL,* inner nuclear layer (contains cell bodies of horizontal, amacrine, bipolar, interplexiform, and Müller cells); *IPL,* inner plexiform layer (synapses of third-order neurons); *G,* ganglion cell layer (contains cell bodies of ganglion cells); *OFL,* optic fiber layer (axons of ganglion cells); *ILM,* internal limiting membrane. (From Cohen AI: The retina. In Hart WM Jr, ed: *Adler's physiology of the eye,* ed 9, St Louis, 1992, Mosby.)

rons carrying information from the inferior half of the retina pass in a loop (Meyer's loop) through the temporal lobe, whereas impulses from the upper half of the retina take a more direct course through the parietooccipital cortex to the visual cortex. The visual cortex connects to areas in the occipital and parietotemporal lobes for more complicated visual perception.[7]

D. Anatomy and physiology of the ocular circulation

Ocular blood supply arises from the ophthalmic artery (OA), which is the first intracranial branch of the internal carotid artery. Supplying the retina is the central retinal artery (CRA), a branch of the OA. Other important branches of the OA are two long posterior ciliary arteries (PCAs) supplying the ciliary body; anterior long ciliary arteries supplying the ciliary body, iris, and choroid; and 10 to 15 short PCAs penetrating the sclera (lamina cribrosa) to supply the anterior portion of the ON and the choroid.[8] The anterior portion of the ON is proximal to the lamina cribrosa, an elastic, collagenous tissue through which the ON, CRA, and central retinal vein pass as they enter the optic disc. The long PCAs are end arteries with-

out anastomoses, and there is a watershed zone in the ON, varying between individuals, that may be found anywhere between the fovea and the nasal border of the optic disc.[9,10] The retrolaminar, posterior portion of the ON is supplied by perforating branches of pial arteries and, in some patients, branches of the CRA (Fig. 17-2).[11]

Individually varying anastomoses exist between the internal carotid system from which the OA arises and the external carotid artery. The lacrimal artery, arising from the OA, anastomoses to the middle meningeal artery, and in the eyelids and nose, distal branches of the OA and distal branches of the external carotid artery anastomose.[12] Although these connections may not be significant in the ocular blood supply under normal circumstances, they may be of pathophysiologic importance as potential pathways for iatrogenic particle embolization after intraarterial injections into the external carotid system.[13]

The choroid is drained by four vortex veins located in each posterior quadrant of the eye. Blood from the retina is almost exclusively drained by the central retinal vein to the cavernous sinus.[8,14]

The visual cortex is supplied by the posterior cerebral arteries, whereas the ON radiation is supplied by the

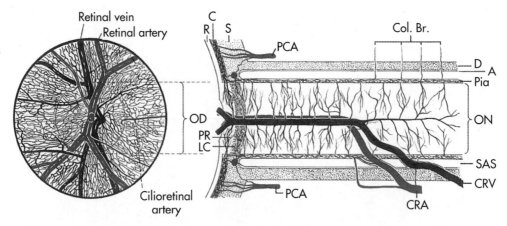

Fig. 17-2. The blood supply to the optic nerve *(ON)*. The anterior portion of the ON is located to the left, and the posterior portion (closer to the brain) is on the right. The anterior portion of the nerve derives its blood supply from the posterior ciliary arteries *(PCA)* and the choroid *(C)*, whereas the posterior ON derives its blood supply from penetrating pial arteries *(Col. Br.)* and branches of the central retinal artery *(CRA)*. *A,* Arachnoid; *CRV,* central retinal vein; *D,* dura; *LC,* long ciliary artery; *OD,* optic disc; *PR,* short ciliary artery, *R,* retina; *S,* sclera; *SAS,* subarachnoid space.(Courtesy Dr. SS Hayreh, Department of Ophthalmology, the University of Iowa Hospitals and Clinics, Iowa City).

middle cerebral arteries in the parietotemporal lobes. Occlusion of both posterior cerebral arteries does not necessarily produce blindness because there is collateral circulation via the circle of Willis.[15] Infarction in the visual cortex is believed to be embolic in origin, or the result of a bilateral watershed incident caused by hypotension in the distal branches of the posterior cerebral arteries.[15-18]

Two distinct vascular systems, the retinal and the choroidal vessels, supply blood to the retina. The choroid, also known as the choriocapillaris, provides oxygen to the outer layers of the retina (where the photoreceptors are located) via diffusion. Blood flow in the choroid is the highest in the body (about 2000 ml/min^{-1}/100 g^{-1}) and oxygen extraction is low (3%) under normal conditions.[19] About 60% to 80% of the retinal oxygen supply comes from the choroid.[8] Although it was previously thought that the choroid was a passive circulation, not significant for retinal homeostasis, its importance in maintenance of retinal health, especially that of the photoreceptors, is becoming increasingly recognized.[20] The choroid has adrenergic innervation and shows vasoactive responses to changes in arterial blood pressure, oxygen, or carbon dioxide tension.[21,22] Recent studies in healthy human volunteers using laser Doppler flowmetry indicate a capacity for autoregulation in the choroid in response to changes in perfusion pressure.[23] The retinal vessels nourish the inner two thirds of the retina; these vessels display autoregulation in response to changes in arterial O_2 or CO_2 content or to changes in perfusion pressure similar to those observed in the cerebral vasculature. Compared to the choroid, retinal O_2 extraction is high (38%) and blood flow is low (about 40 to 100 ml/min^{-1}/100 g^{-1}).[8]

Retinal or choroidal blood flow may be altered by clinically relevant phenomena encountered during anesthesia and surgery. Inhalation of 7% CO_2, resulting in an increase of arterial P_{CO_2} to 80 mm Hg, increases retinal

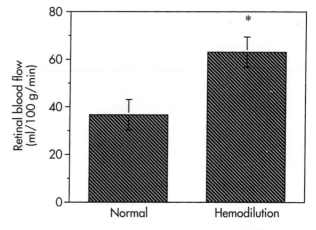

Fig. 17-3. Hemodilution increases retinal blood flow in cats. Blood flow was measured using radioactively labeled microspheres (see Reference 27). Hematocrit was decreased from 36 ± 1 to 20 ± 1%. *$p < 0.05$ compared to normal conditions.

blood flow by 300% to 400%. Likewise, inhalation of 4% to 6% CO_2 increases choroidal blood flow.[8] Inhalation of hypercarbic gas mixtures has been used empirically in humans after retinal arterial occlusion or spasm as a means of increasing retinal blood flow.[24]

A decrease in mean arterial blood pressure diminishes the ocular perfusion pressure (difference between mean arterial and retinal venous pressures).[8] In nearly all studies, the intraocular pressure (IOP) has been taken as equivalent to retinal venous pressure. Although not strictly valid,[25] this equivalency does not change the interpretation of the effects of decreased perfusion pressure on ocular blood flow. Increases in IOP decrease retinal and choroidal blood flow.[21,22] Under conditions of extremely high IOP in cats (i.e., IOP more than 40 mm Hg above systolic blood pressure), ocular blood flow virtually ceases.[26] Under these con-

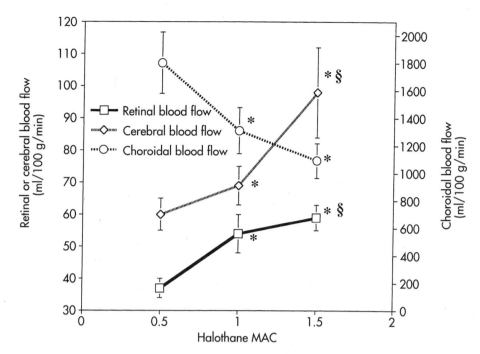

Fig. 17-4. Halothane alters retinal and choroidal blood flow in cats. Note that the changes in retinal blood flow parallel those in the cerebral cortex. *MAC,* Minimum alveolar concentration; *p < 0.0167 versus 0.5 MAC; §p < 0.0167 versus 1.0 MAC. (Adapted from Roth S: *Anesthesiology* 76:455, 1992.)

ditions, choroidal blood flow was reduced to 6% and retinal blood flow to 0.6% of baseline. Also, changes in hematocrit may alter ocular blood flow. Hemodilution (hematocrit changed from 36% ± 1% to 20% ± 1%) increased retinal blood flow by 71% and preserved retinal oxygen delivery while producing a non–statistically significant 19% decrease in choroidal blood flow[27] (Fig. 17-3). Accordingly, hemodilution has been used in humans to treat central retinal vein occlusion, in which increased blood viscosity may contribute to decreased retinal blood flow.[28]

Anesthetics alter ocular blood flow (Fig. 17-4). Both halothane and enflurane produce dose-related increases in retinal and decreases in choroidal blood flow. In cats, retinal blood flow measured 75 ± 13, 90 ± 9, and 88 ± 11 ml/min^{-1}/100 g^{-1} (mean ± SEM) at 0.5, 1, and 1.5 minimum alveolar concentration (MAC) enflurane, respectively. Corresponding values for choroidal blood flow were 1275 ± 124, 876 ± 106, and 843 ± 102 ml/min^{-1}/100 g^{-1}. For halothane, retinal blood flow was 37 ± 3, 54 ± 6, and 59 ± 4 ml/min^{-1}/100 g^{-1} at 0.5, 1, and 1.5 MAC, and choroidal blood flow measured 1801 ± 222, 1309 ± 167, and 1091 ± 126 ml/100 g^{-1}/min^{-1}.[19,29] Decreases in choroidal blood flow parallel decreases in perfusion pressure. The clinical significance of these findings is not yet known.

Most studies of ocular blood flow have been performed in animals such as rabbits and cats; however, in nonprimates the retina and ON are supplied by the PCAs and there is no CRA. Primates (e.g., the monkey) have an ocular circulation similar to that of humans and are a better model for the study of ocular blood flow, particularly that of the ON. In primates, blood flow in the ON head is au-

toregulated within a range of perfusion pressures similar to that of the brain.[30] In atherosclerotic monkeys, however, autoregulation was defective.[31] Recent data obtained in human volunteers indicate that blood flow in the ON head measured by laser Doppler flowmetry is constant until ocular pressure reaches 40 mm Hg. However, 2 of 10 healthy young volunteers failed to demonstrate autoregulation.[32] This finding seems to support speculation that watershed areas in the distribution of the PCAs predispose some patients to infarction of the anterior portion of the ON when perfusion pressure is decreased as a result of either decreased systemic blood pressure or elevated IOP. At present, however, there is no clinically proven, cost-effective technique for reliable detection of such patients.

II. CLINICAL STUDIES OF EYE INJURIES AND ANESTHESIA
A. Incidence

Table 17-1 summarizes studies of visual damage after anesthesia for nonocular surgery. The incidence varies considerably with the type of study (retrospective or prospective) and the types of surgery. Nearly all of these studies have included specific subsets of patients, the most common being those who have had open heart operations. The vast majority of studies are retrospective. Incidence data may be biased by the selected nature of the patient populations. In some instances (e.g., the study by Silverstein and Krieger[33]), eye injuries were noted incidentally in the course of an evaluation for neurologic damage after surgery.

The only studies reported in the anesthesia literature to date that specifically examine the incidence of eye injuries are those of Roth et al[1] and Cucchiara and Black.[34]

Table 17-1. Incidence of eye damage

Reference	Type of study	No. of operations	No. of eye complications	Operative setting	Period	Incidence %	Type of injury (no. of cases)
Little (1955)	Retrospective multicenter questionnaire	27,930	130	Controlled hypotensive anesthesia	NI	0.47	Retinal emboli (3), blurred vision (127)
Silverstein (1960)	Prospective*	55	2	Open heart and great vessel surgery	1958	3.64	CB (homonymous hemianopia) (2)
Gutman and Zegarra (1971)	Prospective	100	17	CABG surgery	NI	17.00	Subconjunctival hemorrhage (13), retinal hemorrhage (2), retinal cholesterol emboli (1), retinal infarcts and homonymous hemianopia (1)
Williams (1971)	Prospective, preliminary	7	7	Heart valve surgery	NI	100	White retinal emboli (4), bright embolic plaques in retinal vessels (3)†
Taugher (1976)	Cases per number of surgeries	808	10	CABG surgery	1974	1.24	Cortical blindness
Plate and Asboe (1981)	Cases per number of surgeries	20,000	3	Nasal surgery	10 yr	0.02	RH (1), CRAO/BRAO (2)
Sweeney et al (1982)	Cases per number of surgeries	7685	7	CABG surgery	36 mo	0.09	AION
Meyendorf (1982)	Retrospective	150	15	Cardiac	1972-1973	10.00	Spontaneous complaint of visual disturbance
Meyendorf (1982)	Prospective	120	30	Cardiac	1977-1978	25.00	Visual disturbance
Breuer et al (1983)	Prospective	421	7	CABG surgery	1980	1.66	Retinal infarction (5), ION (2)
Fazio et al (1985)	Retrospective	913	9	Spinal or general anesthesia	1955-1980	0.99	Acute angle closure glaucoma
Shaw et al (1987)	Prospective	312	78	CABG surgery	1983-1984	25.00	Retinal infarction, retinal emboli, visual field defect, reduced visual acuity
Blauth et al (1988)	Prospective	21	21	CABG surgery	—	100.00	Retinal microemboli
Cucchiara and Black (1988)	Prospective	4652	8	Neurosurgery	1986-1987	0.17	Corneal abrasion
Shahian and Speert (1989)	Cases per number of surgeries	700	4	Open heart surgery	NI	0.57	Retinal emboli, AION, occipital lobe infarcts (2)
Stein et al (1992)	Retrospective	46	4	Liver transplantation	1984-1988	8.70	Hallucinations (2), cortical blindness (3)
Quinlan and Salmon (1993)	Cases per number of surgeries	133	1	Heart transplantation	1967-1991	0.75	Occipital lobe infarction
Pugsley et al (1994)	Prospective	105	0	CABG surgery	NI	0.00	
Roth (1995)	Retrospective	60,965	34	Nonocular surgery	1988-1992	0.06	AION (1), corneal abrasion (21), red eye (7), other injury in anterior segment (3)
Shapira et al (1996)	Retrospective	602	8	CABG and heart valve surgery	1990-1992	1.30	AION
Myers et al (1997)	Retrospective survey of spine surgeons	—	37	Lumbar spinal fusion	NI	—	AION (8), PION (14), CRAO (9), cortical blindness (3), other (3)

*Focus on neurologic complications.

†1 patient with visual defects, 2 deaths.

NI, Not indicated; CB, cortical blindness; CABG, coronary artery bypass grafting; AION, anterior ischemic optic neuropathy; CRAO, central retinal artery occlusion; BRAO, branch retinal artery occlusion; ION, ischemic optic neuropathy; PION, posterior ischemic optic neuropathy; RH, retrobulbar hemorrhage.

These studies differ in their methods and in the types of patients studied. Although both studies have their limitations, they provide incidence data and some indications of risk factors for eye injuries after anesthesia. Cucchiara and Black[34] prospectively examined the incidence of a specific ocular injury, corneal abrasion, after 4692 neurosurgical operations in their hospital. Although prospective, this study examined only a small number of patients and only in a carefully selected group of patients. They report corneal abrasion in 0.17% of patients. The study of Roth et al[1] used retrospective and prospective data collection methods, primarily of quality improvement data, to examine 60,965 unselected anesthetics in patients older than 6 years of age for nonocular surgery in a busy academic anesthesia practice. Although it included nearly all types of surgery, with large amounts of data for each patient, the limitation of this study was the possibility of missing some injuries, especially in outpatients (constituting 23% of the patient population). The overall incidence of eye injury in this study was 0.056%; of the 34 patients found to have an eye injury, 21 of these incidents involved a corneal abrasion.

The most seriously affected patient in our study sustained ischemic optic neuropathy (ION). We have described in more detail this and another similarly affected patient from our institution.[35] Both of these patients had undergone complex lumbar spine operations while positioned prone with a head-down table tilt, accompanied by considerable blood loss, mild deliberate hypotension, and transfusion of large quantities of fluid and blood to maintain intravascular volume. Similar cases have been reported by others.[36-38]

But the incidence of ION or other retinal and ON abnormalities is apparently greater in selected groups such as patients undergoing coronary artery bypass grafting (CABG). Sweeney et al[39] found an incidence of postoperative blindness of 0.091% in a study of 7685 CABG patients. Shaw et al[40] prospectively searched for neurologic abnormalities in 312 CABG patients and found ophthalmologic abnormalities in 25%: retinal infarctions in 17.3%, retinal emboli in 2.6%, visual field defects in 2.6%, and a reduction in visual acuity in 4.5%. Breuer et al[41] found an incidence of ON damage of 1.67%. In a retrospective study, Shahian and Speert[42] found 4 cases of irreversible visual loss among 700 patients after open heart operations (including CABG surgery and valvular heart procedures). The same group, in a subsequent study, has found no significant change in incidence in this patient population.[43]

From these studies, it is apparent that the incidence of visual problems after CABG is difficult to estimate precisely. This problem is clearly significant, considering the rapidly increasing number of CABG operations in the United States; in 1991 there were 407,000 procedures,[44] compared to 360,000 in 1989.[45] Extrapolation from these studies suggests a possible incidence of visual deficits after CABG surgery of 37,000 to 102,000 per year in the United States. Although many of these visual changes are transient, such a projected incidence seems worrisome. Larger studies are needed to determine the true incidence and risk factors for eye injuries in this patient population.

B. Risk factors

An association between ION and atherosclerosis has been suggested by studies in nonhuman primates. In monkeys fed an atherogenic diet for 12.5 years, in which IOP was increased, resulting in decreased ocular perfusion pressure, there was evidence of impaired oxygen supply and anaerobic glycolysis in the inner and outer retina and the ON.[31] The results suggest that autoregulation of blood flow in the retina and ON may be impaired by atherosclerosis in the ocular circulation. These results cannot be extrapolated to humans, but they do provide evidence that long-standing atherosclerosis could be a risk factor for ON injury when perfusion pressure is reduced. In a prospective study of 15 patients with nonarteritic anterior ION, the frequency of carotid artery atherosclerosis was not greater than in 30 age-matched asymptomatic controls with atrial fibrillation. However, the authors note that the study population was too small for generalization of the results to conclude that anterior ischemic optic neuropathy (AION) and atherosclerosis are not associated.[46] On the other hand, in patients who underwent CABG, peripheral vascular disease, increasing age, preexisting cerebrovascular disease, and hypertension were risk factors in patients who developed neurologic deficits after cardiopulmonary bypass.[40,47] As mentioned earlier, this is the patient population from which most reports of ION in the perioperative period have emerged. Thus it seems logical to attempt to preserve systemic perfusion pressure in patients who may be at risk.

Although uncommon, preexisting eye conditions not previously diagnosed may be precipitated or recognized initially in the perioperative period. A case of Fuchs's epithelial dystrophy, a chronic and slowly developing degeneration of the cornea, was first recognized after an iliac lymph node resection followed by perfusion of one leg with the cytostatic agent melphalan. Various factors were thought to cause the acute changes in the cornea found postoperatively, which were accompanied in this case by frontal headache, nausea, blurred vision, pain in the eyes, and lacrimation. Systemic uptake of a small dose of melphalan was documented.[48]

Various chronic medical therapies, such as chronic immunosuppressive therapy after heart transplantation,[49] may predispose for complications; lens changes, cytomegalovirus retinitis, and vascular events including AION, central retinal vein occlusion, and bilateral occipital lobe infarction have been described. These more serious vascular complications all occurred months after heart transplantation. It is important to recognize that the effect of immunosuppressive therapy is a possible risk factor for any patient after surgery.

C. The role of general anesthesia, patient positioning, and site of surgery

In an earlier report, we used logistic regression with univariate and multivariate analysis to identify the importance of possible risk factors for eye injuries after nonocular surgery.[1] The most common injury among the 34 patients detected by our survey was corneal abrasion (21 cases).

Other injuries we found included conjunctivitis, blurry vision, red eye, chemical injury, direct trauma to the eye, and blindness. Independent factors associated with a greater relative risk of eye injury were long surgical procedures (odds ratio 1.16 per hour of anesthetic care, confidence interval [CI] = 1.1 to 1.3), lateral positioning during surgery (odds ratio 4.7, CI = 2 to 11), operation on the head or neck (odds ratio 4.4, CI = 2.2 to 9), general anesthesia (odds ratio 3, CI = 2.2 to 38), and surgery on a Monday (odds ratio 2.7, CI = 1.4 to 5.3). Risk of eye injury increased with patient age, but age was not an independent risk factor. The elderly patient tends to undergo lengthier procedures, more often with general anesthesia, and more procedures on the head and neck or while in the lateral position.

Our study did not allow for conclusions about the cause of most of these injuries because we could identify a specific mechanism of injury in only 21% of cases. This finding is in agreement with that of the ASA Closed Claims Study of eye injuries.[2] Perhaps tear production is affected by lengthy surgery or decreased in elderly patients. These factors could increase the risk of corneal abrasion. Operations on the head or neck could increase risk because of the greater chance of unintentional contact with the eye by the surgeon or the greater chance of irritating or toxic liquids such as prep solutions contacting the eye. It is not clear why lateral positioning is a risk factor, especially because in our study there was no association between the occurrence of eye injury and the position of the eye affected (i.e., dependent or nondependent eye). General anesthesia may be a risk factor because of potential alterations in tear production or unintentional contact with the eye by the surgeon or anesthesiologist. The increased risk in patients operated upon on Monday was a surprising finding, and it is not clear whether that result is due to some unknown patient factor or perhaps to some difference in the reporting of these injuries. Overall, these data from a large patient population are helpful in identifying patterns of risk and injury that will be useful in future studies.

III. INJURIES TO THE ANTERIOR SEGMENT
A. Anatomy and physiology

The cornea is a clear, avascular tissue anterior to the iris and pupil through which light rays pass to enter the eye en route to the retina. The cornea is 1 mm thick at the periphery and 0.8 mm thick at the center; it inserts at the limbus, in a circular depression called the scleral sulcus. The cornea consists of five layers: epithelium, Bowman's membrane, stroma, Descemet's membrane, and endothelium. Nutrients are supplied by tears, aqueous humor, and blood vessels at the limbus, which receive oxygen at the superficial cornea from the atmosphere. Sensory innervation comes from the first (ophthalmic) division of the fifth cranial nerve; rich innervation for pain sensation makes the cornea exquisitely sensitive to even minor abrasions of the epithelial layer.[4]

B. Diagnosis and treatment of injury

By far, the most common problem encountered perioperatively is corneal abrasion. Pain, tearing, and photophobia are the predominant symptoms and signs. The patient may complain of a foreign body sensation. Pain is worsened by blinking and eye movement and is temporarily relieved by manually holding the eyelids wide apart. The initial symptoms are frequently reported as the patient awakens from the anesthetic, but recognition may be delayed in patients who remain asleep for a prolonged period postoperatively. Many corneal abrasions heal spontaneously and completely after 12 to 24 hours. Treatment consists of patching the affected eye shut. Antibiotic drops or ointments are not usually indicated, but are used by some.

Although corneal abrasions almost always heal quickly and with complete resolution, even within hours, recurrent epithelial erosions can occur and are treated with patching or a bandage contact lens. Primary perioperative concerns include appropriate diagnosis (ruling out infections, for example) and enhancing patient comfort and assuring the patient of the expected speedy recovery.

Serious or permanent corneal damage has been caused by contact with chlorhexidine gluconate and Hibiclens, agents commonly used to prepare the skin for facial surgery.[50,51] Therefore precautions to prevent eye contact with these solutions are essential. In an animal study, various commonly used presurgical skin preparations were tested for corneal toxicity. Tincture of iodine (iodine, sodium iodine, and alcohol), Hibiclens, pHisoHex (a combination of octyphenoxypolyethoxyethanol ether and hexachlorophene), 70% alcohol, 7.5% povidone iodine scrub with detergent, and 10% povidone iodine solution without detergent were tested in rabbits. All agents caused corneal epithelial edema progressing to corneal deepithelialization and chemosis within 3 hours after application.[52] In the event of accidental contact in patients, eyes should be irrigated copiously with balanced saline solution.

There are two reports of injury caused by insufficient rinsing of anesthesia masks. Obviously, increasing use of disposable masks should eliminate this problem. In one instance, glutaraldehyde was retained in the pneumatic cushion of the anesthesia mask, causing a moderate chemical conjunctivitis.[53] Another patient developed a chemical burn of sclera when Cidex spilled onto the eye from the incompletely rinsed reusable anesthetic mask.[1]

Though unlikely in the postoperative setting, the painful red eye may be caused by acute glaucoma; when this condition is suspected, immediate ophthalmology consultation should be obtained.

C. Pathophysiology of injury

An intact corneal epithelium prevents the development of corneal ulceration. The eye's response to acute corneal injury consists of hyperemia, pupillary changes, and increases in IOP. These effects are mediated by prostaglandins.[54] Chemical injuries, especially by alkaline liquids, damage cell membranes, leading to cell disruption and death.[55] Following corneal injury, recovery depends on centripetal movement of the most proximal viable epithelium. Persistent inflammation may slow this process. Because collagen constitutes over 80% of the corneal stromal components, its synthesis by keratocytes is critical for recovery. Infiltration by white blood cells is more prominent after chemical injury and requires more prolonged recovery.[56]

D. Role of anesthesia

Multiple factors are likely to contribute to formation of corneal abrasion in the perioperative period: general anesthesia reduces tear production,[57] predisposing to a dry eye; normal corneal reflexes and the perception of pain and ability to communicate and to adjust one's position are all absent during and for a brief period after general anesthesia.[1] The cornea may be abraded subtly by the anesthesia mask, surgical drapes, or other items, including the wrist watch or identification tag of the person performing intubation[58] or listening devices and pens carried in the anesthetist's pocket.[34] Improper taping or closure of the eyes could lead to exposure keratopathy; then desquamation of the epithelial layer of the cornea results in an abrasion typically located in the inferior third of the cornea.[59]

Retrospective analysis failed to determine the cause of postoperative corneal abrasions in more than 80% of cases.[2] It is possible that many corneal injuries actually occur in the postoperative period. They may be caused by patients rubbing their eyes with the pulse oximeter finger probe. Even without the probe, patients are uncoordinated upon initial awakening, and while rubbing their eyes, as commonly occurs immediately upon awakening, they may accidentally produce a corneal abrasion.

Measures used to prevent corneal abrasion intraoperatively include taping the eyes shut, applying protective goggles, and instilling protective ointments or liquids into the eyes. Each of these techniques has some disadvantages. Ointments are flammable and in some instances may trigger allergic reactions or cause blurred vision in the postoperative period. Blurred vision may stimulate the patient to rub the eyes, possibly causing corneal abrasions by the placement of clumsy fingers or equipment such as pulse oximeter probes in the eye.

The use of ointment did not reduce the incidence of perioperative corneal abrasion.[60] Simply closing the eyes with tape appears adequately protective, although if the eye opens under the tape, contact with the tape itself could induce corneal abrasion. Suturing the eyelids closed is another possible protective option that is sometimes used in plastic surgical procedures performed in the immediate vicinity of the eyes. Taping the eyes closed immediately after induction and during laryngoscopy or ventilation via mask may be prudent, especially when working with trainees or during anticipated prolonged intubation attempts. During ventilation via mask, dry anesthetic breathing gas may be accidentally blown beneath the patient's eyelids and could dry the cornea. For surgical procedures involving the face, it may not be possible to tape eyes shut, and many clinicians choose to apply eye ointment. It may be best to restrict ointments to high-risk patients (e.g., patients with paresis of the facial nerve) and high-risk surgery (e.g., prone position surgery or prolonged surgery).[61]

Certain medical problems are associated with corneal damage secondary to drying: Graves's ophthalmopathy, Bell's palsy, and exophthalmus. Careful attention during mask ventilation and appropriate mask selection may prevent abrasions in these patients.

E. Acute glaucoma

Acute angle-closure glaucoma rarely has been described following general anesthesia. The disease usually occurs spontaneously and is of multifactorial origin, with an increased risk in patients with a genetic predisposition, shallow anterior chamber, and increased thickness of the lens; it is more common in women and the elderly.[62] It is believed to be associated with emotional stress, and it is thus somewhat surprising that it is not seen more often in the perioperative period. Three patient series have been reported. Gartner and Billet[63] describe acute angle-closure glaucoma in 4 of 3437 patients (0.1%) who received either general or spinal anesthesia. One of these 4 had spinal anesthesia. Subsequently, Wang et al[64] reported 5 cases in 25,000 surgical patients, an incidence of 0.02%. The most recent series, which reports the highest incidence, was that of Fazio et al.[65] These authors reviewed 913 patients who received general or spinal anesthesia. There were nine cases, two of which were bilateral (1%). It is not clear why these authors found a higher risk than in previous reports. None of these studies found an association between acute glaucoma and a particular anesthetic technique or drug.

Acute angle-closure glaucoma occurs when the passage of aqueous humor from the posterior to the anterior chamber is obstructed by apposition of the iris to the anterior surface of the lens. The pupil is middilated, with associated pupillary block. If uncorrected, increased IOP may result in ON damage. The diagnosis should be suspected in patients presenting with a painful, red eye, cloudy or blurred vision, possibly accompanied by headache, nausea, and vomiting. Symptoms may not appear for hours to days after a surgical procedure. Acute glaucoma is an emergency, and ophthalmologic consultation should be obtained immediately. Patients are treated with intravenous acetazolamide to acutely decrease IOP, and with pilocarpine 4% applied topically to the eye. Systemic analgesic agents are given as needed. A peripheral iridectomy should be performed later to form a permanent opening between the anterior and posterior chambers.[62]

IV. INJURIES TO THE POSTERIOR SEGMENT: GENERAL CONSIDERATIONS

Perioperative damage to the retina or visual pathway may result in blindness. These are therefore the most serious ocular injuries that can follow anesthesia and surgery. Because of the small incidence of this complication, few clinical studies address the problem and the vast majority of incidents are published as case reports. Accurate incidence data are not available, nor is it known what percentage of complications actually are reported. Nonetheless, the large number of case reports over a lengthy period of time affords considerable information on the nature of these visual abnormalities.

Case reports were obtained by performing a Medline search. The search criteria included ION, retinal vascular occlusion, cortical blindness (CB), and anesthesia and

Table 17-2. Summary of case reports on visual disturbance in the posterior segment

	AION	RH	PION	CB	CRAO/BRAO
No. of cases	34	20	19	40	29
References	Chisholm (1969)	Griffiths (1971)	Milner (1960)	Hollenhorst (1950)	Givner (1950)
	Sweeney (1982)	Plate (1981)	Mazzia (1962)	Wortham (1952)	Gillan (1953)
	Jaben (1983)	Maniglia (1981)	Chutkow (1973)	Gillan (1953)	Hollenhorst (1954)
	Alpert (1987)	Sacks (1988)	Johnson (1987)	Alfano (1957)	Torti (1964)
	Hayreh (1987)	Maniglia (1989)	Rizzo (1987)	Gutman (1971)	Gutman (1971)
	Larkin (1987)	Buus (1990)	Wessels (1987)	Taugher (1976)	Whiteman (1980)
	Shahian (1989)	Vanden Abeele (1994)	Kirkall (1990)	Fennel (1977)	Plate (1981)
	Savino (1990)		Marks (1990)	Ross-Russell (1978)	Bradish (1987)
	Wilson (1991)		Savino (1990)	Aldrich (1987)	Cheney (1987)
	Sharma (1993)		Buus (1990)	Shahian (1989)	Rettinger (1990)
	Brown (1994)		Nawa (1992)	Stein (1989)	Savino (1990)
	Katz (1994)		Brown (1994)	Weissman (1989)	Wolfe (1992)
	Lund (1994)		Katz (1994)	Stiller (1990)	Wisotsky (1993)
	Roth (1995)		Schobel (1995)	Wong (1991)	Bekar (1996)
	Strome (1997)		Roth (1997)		
	Dilger (1998)				
Surgery					
CABG	53%	0	11%	55%	7%
Other thoracovascular	12%	0	0%	23%	0%
Neck	6%	0	37%	5%	4%
Nasal/sinus	3%	100%	11%	0%	29%
Spinal	15%	0	16%	0%	28%
Other	11%	0	25%	18%	32%
Patient demography and symptoms					
% Males	74%	65%	58%	73%	61%
Age median	55	45	51	50	37
Age interval	[16;74]	[19;76]	[13;81]	[0;67]	[12;71]
% Bilateral	56%	15%	68%	98%	7%
Blind	13%	95%	63%	35%	45%
Perioperative risk factors					
% Prone position	15%	0%	21%	0%	31% (+7% sitting)
Hypotension	50%	0%	68%	45%	45%
Anemia and hemodilution	38%	0%	42%	23%	11%
Blood loss ≥2 L	29%	0%	58%	0%	10%
Nasal injection	3%	5%	7%	0%	28%
None	18%	0%	0%	8%	0%
RH	0%	100%	0%	0%	0%
Pressure from mask or head rest	0%	0%	0%	0%	52%
Patient risk factors					
CAD	56%	0%	11%	55%	7%
HTN	26%	0%	26%	5%	4%
Chronic anemia	9%	0%	5%	0%	0%
DM	21%	5%	5%	0%	4%
Carotid disease or previous stroke	6%	0%	0%	8%	4%
Ocular disease	3%	0%	16%	3%	0%
Other	21%	45%	20%	43%	44% (20% low nasal bridge)
None	9%	50%	20%	0%	4%
Time of symptoms					
NI	3%	45%	7%	48%	7%
Awakening	12%	25%	26%	25%	32%
On or before postop day 1	12%	30%	32%	8%	93%
After postop day 1	59%	0%	37%	20%	0%
Ocular findings					
Pupillary reaction NI	32%	80%	5%	18%	31%
Afferent pupillary defect	62%	5%	68%	0%	17%
No pupillary reaction	3%	15%	32%	0%	45%
Funduscopy NI	29%	80%	11%	23%	3%
Normal disc	3%	10%	58%	73%	7%
Optic disc edema	62%	5%	11%	0%	4%
Flame-shaped hemorrhage	15%	0%	0%	0%	0%
Disc pallor	44%	10%	16%	3%	0%
Cherry-red macula	3%	0%	0%	0%	59%
Retinal edema or pale retina	3%	5%	0%	3%	75%
Visual defect					
NI	6%	5%	0%	33%	10%
Altitudinal defect	66%	0%	11%	3%	7%
Central scotoma	12%	0%	21%	8%	7%
Blind in one or both eyes	9%	95%	63%	33%	71%
Hemianopia	0%	0%	0%	28%	0%
Outcome					
NI	26%	0%	32%	23%	10%
Improvement in visual defect	16%	5%	5%	65%	14%
No improvement	53%	95%	63%	13%	69%
Other objective findings					
NI	15%	50%	21%	5%	21%
Paresis, limbs or abnormal reflexes	9%	0%	5%	38%	3%
Paresis, face or ocular region	3%	30%	5%	0%	7%
Proptosis, facial edema or bruises	3%	35%	33%	0%	32%
Confusion	0%	0%	0%	25%	3%
None	63%	0%	42%	20%	41%

AION, Anterior ischemic optic neuropathy; *RH,* retrobulbar hemorrhage; *PION,* posterior ischemic optic neuropathy; *CB,* cortical blindness; *CRAO,* central retinal artery occlusion; *BRAO,* branch retinal artery occlusion; *CABG,* coronary artery bypass grafting; *CAD,* coronary artery disease; *HTN,* hypertension; *DM,* diabetes mellitus; *NI,* not indicated.

Table 17-3. Differential diagnosis: eye examination in posterior segment injury

	AION	PION	CB	CRAO	BRAO
Optic disc	Pale swelling Peripapillary flame-shaped hemorrhages	Normal (initially)	Normal	Normal	Normal
Retina	Opacification	Opacification	Normal	Cherry-red macula* Pallor and edema Narrowed retinal arteries	Emboli may be seen† Partial retinal whitening and edema
Light reflex	Absent or RAPD	Absent or RAPD	Normal	Absent or RAPD	Normal or RAPD
Fixation and accommodation reflexes	Normal	Normal	Impaired	Normal	Normal
Response to visual threat	Yes	Yes	No response	Yes	Yes
Opticokinetic nystagmus	Normal	Normal	Absent	Normal	Normal
Tracking objects	Normal	Normal	Absent	Normal	Normal
Ocular muscle function	Normal	Normal	Normal	Sometimes impaired	Normal
Perimetry (gross)	Altitudinal defect	Altitudinal defect or blind eye	Often hemianopia (depends on anatomy of lesion) Periphery usually affected	Affected eye blind	Scotoma Peripheral vision usually intact

*Because of lack of overlying inner retinal cells in the fovea, the intact choroidal circulation is visible as a cherry-red spot.
†Cholesterol, platelet-fibrin emboli, calcified atheromatous material.
AION, Anterior ischemic optic neuropathy; *PION,* posterior ischemic optic neuropathy; *CB,* cortical blindness; *CRAO,* central retinal arterial occlusion; *BRAO,* branch retinal arterial occlusion; *RAPD,* relative afferent pupillary defect.

surgery. Only English-language publications were included. From review of these case reports, data on posterior segment damage were divided into vascular damage to the retina and ON and CB. After presenting estimates of incidence (see Table 17-1) and data from case reports (Table 17-2), risk factors and differential diagnosis are discussed (Table 17-3). These first sections will be useful for the reader who is interested only in an overview. In the next section, the specific mechanisms responsible for retinal and ON injury are explained in detail.

A. Spectrum of injuries

Retinal damage may result from central retinal arterial occlusion (CRAO) or branch retinal arterial occlusion (BRAO). Damage to the circulatory supply of the ON produces anterior or posterior ischemic optic neuropathy (AION or PION). Brain injury rostral to the ON may cause CB. Case reports of visual damage, with special emphasis on ION and apparently associated with different types of surgical procedures and a possible mechanism of occurrence, have been summarized recently by Williams et al.[66] Visual disturbance related to retinal and ON damage (see Table 17-2) has been reported after a wide range of surgical procedures. These include abdominal surgery (exploratory laparotomy, cholecystectomy, gastroduodenectomy, liver transplantation, partial gastrectomy),[37,67-70] cardiovascular surgery (CABG, pedi-

atric cardiac and adult heart valve surgery, aortocoronary and aortobifemoral bypass, and heart transplantation),* thoracic surgery (pulmonectomy, thoracoplasty),[70,82] neurosurgery (spinal surgery, ganglionectomy),† orthopedic surgery (removal of hip prosthesis),[76] head and neck surgery (nasal or sinus surgery, cancer surgery of the neck, parathyroidectomy, tonsillectomy),[71,73,85-105] obstetric surgery (induced abortion, partum and repair of vaginal tear, cesarean section),[93,106-110] and catheterization of the subclavian artery.[111]

B. Case reports

Table 17-2 presents 142 cases of lesions of the posterior segment that presented after surgery and anesthesia. Patients with visual disturbances following hemodialysis, brain operations, or bleeding not related to surgical procedures who were included in these reports were excluded from this summary, as was one case report with insufficient data. Sixty-four journal articles are represented, spanning a period of 47 years. Two recent small retrospective series concentrating primarily on postoperative AION, one in CABG patients[43] and the other in patients undergoing instrumented spinal fusion,[36] were ex-

---

*References 16, 18, 33, 37, 39, 49, 70-81.
†References 1, 35, 37, 38, 83, 84.

cluded from this analysis because individual patient data were not provided and in the latter some patient data are taken from other studies. The results from these two important studies are discussed in the AION section that follows. Summaries of demographic data, the most common speculated risk factors, and objective findings and outcomes are presented from the case reports. In the next section, the specific mechanisms, diagnosis, treatment, and prevention of each of these disorders are discussed in detail.

Age of the patients ranged from 0 to 81 years, with a median age of 49 years. There was a strong tendency for male predominance, with two out of three cases occurring in men. Operative duration has been excluded from the analysis because in 79% of the cases these times were not reported. The type of surgery, perioperative risk factors, and patient risk factors are grouped after the most commonly reported complications. Factors such as hypotension or anemia could not be delimited precisely because in many instances these factors were not defined specifically by the authors. Moreover, the duration of decreased blood pressure or hemoglobin concentration was not provided consistently. However, as important speculated risk factors, hypotension and anemia were listed as present when mentioned by the authors.

1. Anterior ischemic optic neuropathy. Fifty-three percent of AION cases followed CABG surgery; the next largest surgical category was spinal surgery (12%). Males outnumbered females 4 to 1. Bilateral lesions were present in 56%, but only 13% of patients claimed to be blind at the time of initial onset of symptoms, with blurry or decreased vision being far more common presenting symptoms. The main speculated perioperative risk factors were hypotension (50%), anemia or hemodilution (38%), and blood loss exceeding 2 L (38%). There was a large incidence of preexisting cardiovascular disease, including coronary artery disease (56%), hypertension (26%), and diabetes mellitus (21%). In 59% of the patients, symptoms were not noted until the first postoperative day or later. The typical objective findings were altitudinal visual defects (66%), optic disc edema (62%) or pallor (44%), and an afferent pupillary defect (62%). Other neurologic deficits or facial abnormalities were not present. One patient had a cherry-red macula, indicating simultaneous occlusion of the CRA. Two had visible retinal emboli. In more than half of the patients, there was no improvement in visual dysfunction. From these reports, perioperative AION appears to be a multifactorial disease typically occurring in patients with predisposing cardiovascular disease and perioperative hypotension or anemia, all of which may lead to impaired oxygen delivery to the ON head. As pointed out later in this chapter, other factors such as impaired venous return and aberrant vascular anatomy in the ON may also be responsible. CABG, other thoracovascular operations, and spinal surgery accounted for the majority of the cases. Unfortunately, the lesion is usually permanent.

2. Retrobulbar hemorrhage. Retrobulbar hemorrhage (RH) was reported only after nasal and sinus surgery. This category is listed separately because the exact cause of visual loss was not always described. Not surprisingly, RH resulted in visual loss that was usually unilateral, and all but one patient complained of total blindness of the affected eyes. Intense pain in the ocular region as the hematoma develops in the orbit is a classic symptom of RH, but in these case reports only one author noted this symptom. Perhaps this is because it is considered obvious to the readers of otorhinolaryngology journals in which the reports were published. Patient factors noted to predispose for RH were chronic sinusitis and the presence of a neoplasm in sinus structures, leading perhaps to vulnerable sinus bone that may be damaged surgically. For half of the cases, the time of symptom onset was not described; for the other half symptoms were noted intraoperatively (for operation under local anesthesia alone), upon awakening from general anesthesia, or within the first 24 hours of recovery. Common objective findings besides blindness were proptosis, paresis of ocular muscles, and edema in the eye region. The blindness was permanent in nearly every case (95%). In summary, blindness after RH is most probably the result of surgical damage to orbital walls and vessels in a patient undergoing nasal or sinus surgery that may be predisposed to weak bone by infection or neoplasm.

3. Posterior ischemic optic neuropathy. In contrast to AION, nearly half (48%) of the cases of PION were reported after surgery involving the neck, nose, or sinuses, 16% followed spinal surgery, and only 11% were reported after CABG. As in AION, males outnumbered women 4 to 1. Sixty-three percent of the patients complained of blindness and 58% noted symptoms within the first 24 hours after their operations. However, in some patients the onset of symptoms was delayed by several days. In as many as 68% of the cases hypotension was reported; anemia or hemodilution was present in 42% and blood loss of more than 2 L in 58% of the patients. In 16%, there was evidence of preexisting eye disease or an abnormal ocular blood supply (glaucoma, temporal arteritis, or verified 50% stenosis of ophthalmic arteries), 11% had coronary artery disease, 26% systemic hypertension, and 5% diabetes mellitus. In 20% of the patients no predisposing systemic factors could be found. Typical objective findings were afferent pupillary defect (68%) or nonreactive pupil (32%). In one case optic disc edema was reported; the diagnosis of PION may be disputed in this case because disc edema is a feature of AION. A normal optic disc was generally reported (58%), consistent with the anatomic defect in PION, which involves the retroorbital portion of the ON. In 33% of patients, proptosis, facial edema, or ptosis (and one case of venous dilation at funduscopy) were found, as opposed to no extraocular symptoms in 27%. Sixty percent showed no improvement in vision. In conclusion, perioperative PION appears to be less related to the presence of preexisting cardiovascular disease than does AION and may be the result of a local vascular disturbance of the distal ON, a region supplied by penetrating pial arterial branches. Compromise of arterial supply or venous drainage or embolic phenomena may be involved.

4. Cortical blindness. CB accounted for the largest number of patients described in case reports (40). Fifty-five percent of the cases were reported after CABG surgery and 23% after other thoracovascular surgery. This was the only category in which cases were found in children. In 45% of the cases, hypotension was considered a risk factor and in 23% anemia or hemodilution was present. Over half of the patients had coronary artery disease, but the group of other possible disposing patient factors was very large; it included congenital heart disease, liver failure, postpartum pulmonary embolism, and hypercholesterolemia. Unfortunately, the time of onset of symptoms was not reported in half of the cases, but for the remaining 50%, two thirds complained within the first postoperative day and one third did so later. As would be expected, funduscopy, where findings were indicated, was normal in virtually all patients except one, in whom AION occurred in combination with CB. Visual defects were bilateral in all but one patient, who presented with a lesion near the LGN. As expected, the incidence of other objective neurologic findings was high (38%). Confusion was present in 25%. In direct contrast to all the other diagnosis groups, the majority (65%) of the patients experienced improvement in visual outcome. In summary, patients of any age may present with CB that is usually bilateral and improvement may generally be expected. Embolic or other low-flow conditions that could occur during cardiac and other thoracovascular surgery appear to be involved.

5. Central retinal arterial occlusion and branch retinal arterial occlusion. In this group, 75% of the reported cases followed spinal, nasal, or sinus surgery. Half of the cases share characteristic similarities; these reports are from the 1950s, and pressure from the headrest in the prone position or anesthesia mask in supine patients probably is responsible in part for the visual symptoms. As a group these were healthy patients, and they were considerably younger (median age 37) than those in the other diagnostic categories. Twenty percent were thought to have low nasal bridges, which may have predisposed for damage from external pressure on the eye. The perioperative risk factors were somewhat different from those of the other diagnosis groups; there was a lower incidence of hypotension and anemia, and one third of the cases followed intraarterial injections of corticosteroids or local anesthetics in branches of the external carotid artery, with possible retrograde embolization to the ocular blood supply. Of the remaining cases, one had signs of external pressure (abrasion), two followed CABG surgery and had visible retinal emboli, eight occurred after spinal surgery, and one followed neck surgery; in these cases hypotension was also reported. One case occurred after induced abortion in a patient in whom patent foramen ovale was diagnosed by transesophageal echocardiography on follow-up. Symptoms occurred within the first postoperative day for all patients and were severe, with 71% blind or with vision reduced

to light perception. Patients with CRAO, but none with BRAO, had accompanying symptoms such as eye muscle paresis, periorbital edema, bruises, or proptosis. In patients with CRAO, no improvement was found (except in one patient); following BRAO some improvement was usually found. In conclusion, preventing external pressure by careful positioning has proven important for reduction in incidence of perioperative CRAO and BRAO. Embolization is possible after intraarterial injection near the ocular region, during CABG surgery, or in patients with patent foramen ovale, and whether these injuries are preventable has not been established. Neck and spinal surgery may present a risk of CRAO by a combination of systemic hypotension and compromised venous drainage.

6. Overall impression. There does not seem to be any age limitation to symptoms from perioperative injury to the posterior segment. Any complaint about visual disturbances should be taken seriously. Because the symptoms are caused by ischemia of the retina, ON, or brain, diagnosis should be made as early as possible to allow an attempt to shorten ischemic time. AION and CB are significant concerns in patients undergoing CABG, and systemic disease is often present. At least for CB, some improvement may be expected. In PION, RH, and CRAO or BRAO the patients are generally healthier preoperatively, yet more than half of the patients are blind in the affected eyes and remain so.

V. INJURIES TO THE POSTERIOR SEGMENT: SPECIFIC MECHANISMS

Differential diagnosis is presented first. For each clinical entity we then discuss clinical significance, pathophysiology, risk factors, prognosis, treatment, and prevention.

A. Differential diagnosis

1. Symptoms. Typical patient complaints are blurry vision, progressive visual loss, or blindness. ION and vascular damage to the retina both present as acute visual loss that is usually painless. AION may present as complete or partial loss of light perception. A visual field deficit is present, generally in the inferior visual field. Central visual loss may be present. Retinal arterial occlusion also results in visual field loss. In contrast, RH and narrow-angle glaucoma produce intense pain in the periorbital region.

Visual loss in all of these conditions is generally recognized within the first postoperative day, typically when the patient awakens from the anesthesia. However, the onset of ON edema may proceed at a slow pace, and symptoms may not appear for several days. In some patients, the diagnosis may be delayed even after early onset because of slow awakening from anesthesia. Visual symptoms could be misdiagnosed as delirium upon awakening from anesthesia. The presence of accompanying focal neurologic complaints such as unilateral weakness suggests a concomitant stroke, a common feature with CB.

Complete or incomplete CB is visual impairment caused by damage of the visual pathway beyond the LGN or the visual cortex in the occipital lobe. As reviewed in Table 17-3, the optic disc and pupillary responses are normal, but the patients do not react to visual threat or they show loss of optokinetic nystagmus with normal eye motility.

2. Eye examination. The patient's chart should be checked for preexisting abnormalities such as glaucoma, cataract, or retinopathy. Initial examination of the visual pathway includes pupillary, fixation, and accommodation reflexes, digital examination of IOP, eye movements by tracking a finger, rough visual field examination, and ophthalmoscopy. More sophisticated studies include formal visual field testing, fluorescein angiography, electroretinography, visual evoked potentials (VEPs), computed tomography (CT), and magnetic resonance imaging (MRI) scanning.

Table 17-3 reviews reflexes and findings of eye examination. An impaired direct pupillary light reflex indicates an ipsilateral ON lesion. The abnormality in ION is known as an afferent pupillary defect. Retinal arterial occlusion may also result in a similarly abnormal light reflex. A preserved consensual light reflex indicates that the optic chiasma and the pretectal region are intact. Impaired accommodation and fixation reflexes indicate loss of connection between the visual cortex, pretectal region, and superior colliculus. Absence of optokinetic nystagmus also indicates cortical damage, as does indifference to visual threats. Typical findings in CB are preserved pupillary reflexes, regaining of most of the visual field within days, and impairment of spatial perception and sense of relationship between sizes and distances. Restricted visual attention and inability to notice images formed on all parts of the retina at one time are also features. These factors can lead to inability to read. Denial sometimes accompanies CB.

Pupil signs in the postoperative period are easily overlooked or misdiagnosed, particularly after narcotic-based anesthetic techniques or with the use of postoperative parenterally administered analgesia. Except in cases of bilateral visual dysfunction, a clue that visual damage may have occurred is the presence of a unilateral pupillary defect.

CRAO and BRAO may be accompanied by extraocular muscle dysfunction. Facial or periorbital edema may be present if venous obstruction is associated.

3. Ophthalmoscopy. Ophthalmoscopy is critical in differential diagnosis. Pupils must first be dilated pharmacologically. The examination is normal in cortical damage. In retinal or ON damage, characteristic temporal changes can be seen; within the first hour of ischemia mild pallor of the optic disc and opacification or whitening of the ischemic retina with narrowing of retinal arterioles may be visible.[10,112] In BRAO, bright yellowish, glistening cholesterol emboli or calcific (white, nonglistening) or migrant pale emboli of platelet fibrin (dull, dirty white) may be seen. A cherry-red macula with a white ground-glass appearance of the retina and attenuated arterioles signify CRAO with a preserved choriocapillaris (Fig. 17-5). The red appearance is caused by pallor in the ischemic, overlying retina, which allows the intact choroidal circulation to reflect light.

A cherry-red macula is not seen in ION. In the acute

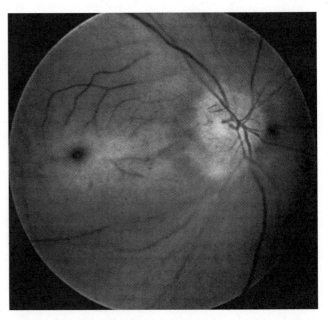

Fig. 17-5. The funduscopic appearance of retinal vascular occlusion. The retinal vessels are severely attenuated. Note the pallor of the retina and the cherry-red spot, the clinical hallmark of retinal arterial occlusion, visible in the fovea near the center of the picture. The ischemic retina loses its normal transparency, and because the fovea is thinner than the surrounding retina, the underlying choroid is visible as the cherry-red spot. (From Ryan: *Retina,* ed 2, St Louis, 1995, Mosby.)

stage (first day), AION is signified by pale swelling of the optic disc and flame-shaped peripapillary hemorrhages, whereas the disc is normal in PION. Within days white optic atrophy appears in AION and PION (Fig. 17-6); these changes may include only a section of the ON and disc.[10]

4. Perimetry. Perimetry is used for precise evaluation of the visual field. This test requires a fully cooperative patient and obviously would usually not be useful in the immediate postoperative period. In AION, the typical lesion is altitudinal (i.e., affecting the superior or inferior part of the visual field), combined with a circumferential constriction of the visual field, whereas the overall visual acuity may be unaffected. This restriction in vision reflects a watershed infarction in PCAs combined with edema of the ON in the region of lamina cribrosa. Any edema in this region would result in damage to the axons in the peripheral diameter of the ON, as described earlier in this chapter.[6,10,46] In CRAO, the eye is usually blind initially. In BRAO, the visual loss is sectorial, corresponding to the area supplied by the occluded arterial segment. In patients undergoing CABG surgery, multiple calcific emboli in branches of the CRA are not unusual,[10] and may produce visual field deficits of varying size and location.

5. Computed tomography. CT and MRI are important in determining the extent of infarction of the brain associated with CB. Occipital lesions are usually bilateral; symptoms and CT findings indicate posterior cerebral artery throm-

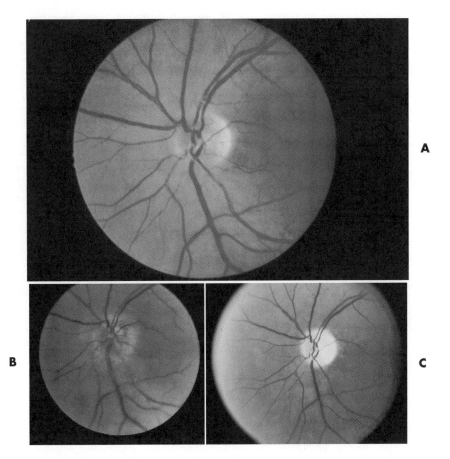

Fig. 17-6. Funduscopic images showing the time course of changes in AION. **A,** Normal fundus. **B,** In AION, initial optic disc edema. **C,** In the late stages, optic atrophy. (Courtesy Dr. SS Hayreh, Department of Ophthalmology, the University of Iowa Hospitals and Clinics, Iowa City).

bosis, basilar artery occlusion, posterior cerebral artery branch occlusion, or watershed infarctions.[71] Lesions after CABG often include the parietooccipital regions.[16,18,71] CT is helpful in distinguishing ischemic brain damage from psychogenic visual loss or in the presence of preexisting pupillary abnormalities that raise the possibility of ON lesions.[71]

MRI or CT may also be helpful in diagnosis of ION, where the typical finding is enlargement of the ONs by ischemic edema.[68] ON atrophy is likewise visible using MRI.[113] MRI is normal in CRAO and BRAO. In recent studies, MRI has shown an increased incidence of white matter lesions in the brains of patients with ION. The significance of this finding is not yet clear.

6. Electroretinogram and visual evoked potentials. Electroretinogram (ERG) and VEPs are useful diagnostic tests. The full-field flash ERG is the most widely used.[114] A contact lens electrode is placed on the cornea and a reference electrode on the conjunctiva or the skin. The characteristic response is a small, early negative a-wave and a larger, immediately following positive b-wave. This mass response is a sensitive indicator for the presence of retinal injury, but it may not be able to localize precisely the retinal cell layers affected. ERG may be used for differential

diagnosis between AION and retinal ischemia following CRAO or BRAO because the ERG is normal in AION, whereas the b-wave is depressed after CRAO with irreversible ischemic damage (Fig. 17-7). ION would not result in an abnormal ERG recording unless there was damage to the retinal ganglion cells or choroidal ischemia.[115]

The VEP records the response to flash or checkerboard pattern stimuli presented in front of the eye and is recorded with electrodes over the occipital cortex. Abnormal VEP responses suggest pathology distal to the orbit (i.e., the ON and its projections to the brain, or occipital cortex). In a study of neurologically normal young children with acute onset of CB, a normal flash visually evoked potential (FVEP) was found to be a highly specific and reliable prognostic factor for the recovery of vision. The children recovering usually suffered CB caused by hypotension during cardiac surgery, rather than traumatic damage.[116] In a study of children with preexisting neurologic deficits, FVEP was found to be nonspecific.[78] In adults, the role of FVEP as a diagnostic tool is inconclusive.[71]

7. Fluorescein angiography. In fluorescein angiography, 5 ml sodium fluorescein dye is injected into an antecubital vein. Within 3 to 5 minutes, the fluorescein is

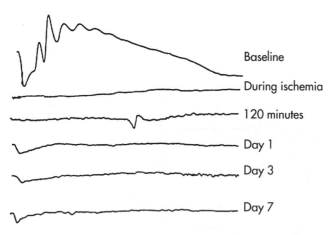

Fig. 17-7. The electroretinogram (ERG) in central retinal arterial occlusion. The ERG is shown before, during, and after ischemia, up to 7 days later. (From Roth S, Li B, Rosenbaum PS, et al: *Invest Ophthalmol Vis Sci* 39:777, 1998.)

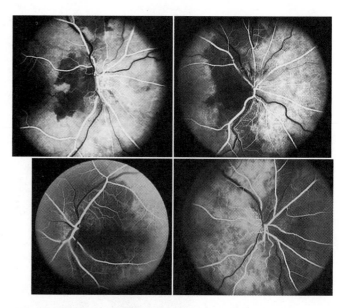

Fig. 17-8. Fluorescein angiography in AION, with the dark areas corresponding to absence of filling of the choroid and optic disc with fluorescein dye. (Courtesy Dr. SS Hayreh, Department of Ophthalmology, the University of Iowa Hospitals and Clinics, Iowa City).

distributed throughout the body. The fluorescein is excited by light at certain frequencies, and the emitted light after excitation can be visualized in the eye using high-speed fundus photography. In recent years, digital video imaging has been used to enhance analysis.[117] The retinal and choroidal circulation are separated by the pigment epithelium and can be visualized simultaneously and distinguished by three-dimensional stereo images. Also, there is a distinct temporal perfusion pattern because the choroid fills before the retina.[115] In AION, there is a delay in the onset and completion of optic disc filling (Fig. 17-8).[118] CRAO and BRAO produce characteristic perfusion deficits in the retinal circulation. But the follow-up angiography has little prognostic value.[112]

8. Ultrasound. Ultrasound uses a high-frequency (7.5 MHz) transducer held over the eye. Two-dimensional (B-mode) imaging is useful for visualization of gross ocular anatomy, whereas one-dimensional (A-mode) gives more detailed information on the thickness and reflectivity of ocular structures.[115] In a preliminary study, it was found that combining the A- and B-modes may enable evaluation of fluid in the ON sheath (e.g., in AION).[119] Using color Doppler ultrasonography, visualization of flow patterns of the ocular blood vessels is possible.[120] Analysis of flow patterns in the posterior ciliary circulation may assist in the diagnosis of ION.

To summarize, CRAO, BRAO, and ION produce abnormal pupillary responses, whereas CB does not. CRAO, BRAO, and ION can be distinguished generally by the findings on ophthalmoscopy. CRAO and BRAO may produce retinal pallor and a cherry-red spot, whereas ION is characterized by optic disc edema initially and optic atrophy later in the most severe cases. CT and MRI are most useful for delineating the area of cerebral cortex damaged in CB. Other diagnostic tests are

highly useful for quantitating the extent and location of injury and the prognosis and results of treatment.

B. Retinal ischemia: BRAO and CRAO

1. Clinical significance. There are several possible causes of retinal ischemia, including increased ocular venous pressure (caused by impaired venous drainage or increased IOP, for example), reduction in arterial supply (e.g., caused by emboli or systemic hypotension), and combinations of these. Impaired venous drainage by surgical damage (in radical neck or cancer surgery), external pressure (e.g., from a headrest), and internal pressure resulting from RH are causes of perioperative retinal ischemia. Cardiac surgery could be accompanied by emboli that lodge in the retinal arterial supply; in fact, an incidence of retinal microemboli of up to 100% diagnosed by fluorescein retinal angiography has been documented in prospective studies.[121,122] In contrast, the incidence of retinal ischemia after hypotensive anesthesia is low (3 cases out of 27,930 hypotensive anesthetics in a multicenter questionnaire).[123] The degree of injury depends on the extent of retinal arterial occlusion; CRAO results in decreased blood supply to the entire retina, and BRAO results in a localized injury that affects only a portion of the retina.

2. Pathophysiology. Retinal ischemia is a common mechanism of injury resulting in blindness or severe visual disability in vascular diseases such as retinal vascular occlusion, retinopathy of prematurity, and diabetes.[124] This mechanism is significant because most severe visual loss in the United States is caused by diseases that ultimately result in retinal ischemia. Increases in extracellular glutamate concentration during retinal ischemia[125] and attenuation of ischemic injury in vitro and in vivo by glutamate receptor antagonists[126-128] support a role for excitotoxicity in the retina. It is believed that increased intracellular Ca^{+2} concentration, as a result of enhanced glutamate release, ultimately initiates mechanisms that result in cellular destruction.

In addition to ischemia-related chemical alterations, two distinct flow patterns follow a period of ischemia. In cats, we showed that retinal and choroidal blood flow increase dramatically (hyperemia) immediately following the end of ischemia.[26] Adenosine and nitric oxide are responsible for this hyperemia.[129-131] Hyperemia is of clinical relevance when reperfusion occurs after a period of ischemia; increased flow at a time when vessels or the blood-retinal barrier are damaged might lead to macular edema.[132] Alternatively, hyperemia may represent a necessary physiologic adjustment to a previous profound disturbance in blood flow. Hypoperfusion represents the other extreme in blood flow derangement. Delayed retinal hypoperfusion 1 to 4 hours after the end of a period of ischemia has been shown in adult rats,[133] results resembling the low-flow state found in other models after global cerebral ischemia.[134,135] The mechanism of these changes in blood flow has not been clearly established; although depletion of vasodilators such as adenosine or nitric oxide may be responsible, a predominance of vasoconstrictors such as endothelins cannot be excluded.[136]

Altered gene expression may also play a pathologic role. For example, increased activity of the tyrosine kinase pathway was found in the rat retina after ischemia and reperfusion. Activation of signal proteins could lead to ischemia-induced cellular proliferation.[137] mRNA for vascular endothelial growth factor was increased in retinal capillary endothelial cells and pericytes exposed to hypoxia, suggesting a pathogenic mechanism for vasoproliferative diseases.[137-139] Recently, we documented the existence of a powerful endogenous mechanism that completely protects the retina against injury from ischemia.[140,141] This phenomenon, known as ischemic preconditioning, requires de novo protein synthesis.[141] How these exciting findings will translate into clinical practice remains to be determined.

In humans, the retinal blood supply consists of contributions from the retinal vessels and the choroidal vessels.[8,142] Occlusion of both circulations would be extremely unusual in humans. Therefore following a retinal vascular occlusion, some oxygen may still be supplied from the choroid. This and a supply of available glucose in the vitreous may account for the lengthy survival time of the retina following ischemia.[143] Moreover, cells of the inner retina such as ganglion cells are more susceptible to ischemic damage than the photoreceptor cells of the outer retina, even in animals in which both the retinal and choroidal blood supplies are occluded.[132,141,144] The implication is that there may be a relative selectivity to ischemic damage in the retina. But in humans, this finding may also result in part from the choroidal circulation supplying primarily the photoreceptors in the outer retina. Whatever the mechanism, the retina differs from the cerebral cortex in that longer periods of ischemia can be tolerated, and the retina may therefore be amenable to more delayed treatment following ischemia. By implication, a patient presenting with retinal ischemia in the postoperative period should be treated aggressively in an attempt to salvage vision.

3. Patient risk factors

a. CRAO. Various causes of CRAO have been proposed by Wray[10] and by Rettinger et al.[92] These mechanisms include emboli, atheromatous disease in vessels with superimposed thrombosis or hemorrhage, inflammation (e.g., giant cell arteritis), vasospasm, and arterial occlusion caused by high IOP or low retinal perfusion pressure.

Some patients with altered facial anatomy may be predisposed to damage from external pressure by anesthesia masks or headrests when patients are prone. Osteogenesis imperfecta is associated with blue sclerae. Fibrous coats of the eye are thin and immature because of a deficiency of collagen fibers, persistent reticulin fibers, and increased mucopolysaccharide ground substance. Sclerae and corneas are unusually thin, and exophthalmos caused by bony facial abnormalities is common. All of these factors render the eye more vulnerable to damage from external pressure. A greater incidence of CRAO among those of Asian descent, caused by lower nasal bridges, has been suggested.[83] Low nasal bridge and other facial and ocular abnormalities were also speculated to be an additional risk factor in a case of a 12-year-old girl suffering from osteogenesis imperfecta who developed CRAO after spinal surgery.[83] If the nasal bridge is low, pressure from an anesthesia mask or from a headrest in the prone position is more easily transmitted to the globe, perhaps resulting in increased IOP.

Improper positioning even in patients with normal anatomy may compress the ocular and periorbital contents, occluding retinal blood flow.[84,145,146] In old reports of verified external pressure on the eye during mask anesthesia and hypovolemic shock (abdominal surgery and ureterostomy), CRAO was found in combination with corneal abrasion. Upon induction of anesthesia, the patient complained of pressure from the anesthesia mask on the eye, and edema of eyelids and conjunctiva was found postoperatively.[147,148] The risk of direct compression of the eye is particularly of concern during surgery performed in the prone position.[145,149] Adding to the risk during such procedures would be the use of deliberate hypotension and a steep head-down position because both factors could further reduce ocular perfusion pressure. However, whether the presence of the latter two factors alone could lead to retinal arterial or venous occlusion has never been documented.

One case of retinal venous hemorrhage has been described in an otherwise healthy young woman who immediately upon awakening complained of seeing red. No other symptoms were found. By the end of surgery the patient had frequent premature ventricular contractions that disappeared with hyperventilation. Funduscopy revealed a venous retinal hemorrhage involving the macula. The patient recovered fully and the tentative diagnosis was Valsalva hemorrhagic retinopathy. This is a rare entity in which activities physiologically similar to the Valsalva maneuver, such as vomiting, "stormy" emergence from anesthesia, or blowing up air mattresses are thought to cause retinal venous hemorrhage. The postulated mechanism in this case was a combination of retinal vasodilation and increased intracranial pressure (ICP) caused by hypoxemia and hypercarbia, and obstructed retinal venous return by the Valsalva maneuver.[150] However, this mechanism does not result in permanent visual loss.

Neck and nasal or sinus surgery account for the majority of reported cases of CRAO postoperatively (see Table 17-2). During nasal or sinus surgery, direct damage to the vascular system of the eye may result in thrombosis or spasm in arteries, or the CRA may be compressed by retrobulbar hematoma that may follow iatrogenic fracture of the lamina papyracea.[151] Indirect damage of the CRAO by intraarterial injections of 1% lidocaine with epinephrine[86,94] or lidocaine mixed with vasopressin[92] has also been described; the mechanism of action is speculated to be arterial spasm or embolism.[94] Embolization of cerebral cortical vessels may also occur; one case was associated with transient confusion and left-sided weakness.[86]

CRAO after spinal surgery and radical neck dissection was accompanied by periorbital edema or chemosis and ocular muscle dysfunction, suggesting decreased venous drainage from the region.[99,149] Perhaps this condition was caused by extraocular pressure in the prone position or bilateral surgical removal of external jugular veins, respectively. In any event, such facial signs and symptoms are useful in differentiating CRAO or BRAO from ION. It should be noted that intraoperative hypotension was hypothesized to have played a role in these cases.

b. BRAO. BRAO usually leads to permanent ischemic retinal damage with partial visual field loss. Unlike in CRAO, some visual preservation would be expected because the entire retinal blood supply has not been compromised. Symptoms may not be noticed by the patient immediately when there is only a peripheral visual field loss or a small scotoma. BRAO is primarily the result of emboli of various origin, but vasospasm has been described in a few cases. Most case reports describe embolization of material from intravascular injections and circulating embolic material from the surgical field or bypass equipment in cardiac surgery.

Microemboli to the retina during cardiopulmonary bypass have been shown by retinal fluorescein angiography. The occurrence and extent of perfusion defects were related to oxygenator type; when a bubble oxygenator was used, all patients had perfusion defects indicative of microemboli, whereas retinal perfusion defects were found in only half of the patients when a membrane oxygenator was used and the degree of perfusion defect was significantly smaller. Unfortunately, the study did not present neurologic outcome.[122] Also, a preliminary study in seven patients during heart valve surgery showed retinal emboli, some temporarily in all seven patients. None of these resulted in visual defects in surviving patients, but one patient had findings of concomitant CB.[79]

There are case reports describing sudden irreversible blindness with BRAO in patients after injection of various drugs in the head and neck region. Several authors reported nearly instant loss of vision when injecting steroids in the nasal mucosa.[97,152-154] In approximately half of the reported cases, crystalline emboli could be seen at funduscopy and in one incident vasospasm appeared to be present. This injury appears to be preventable. In 1981 Mabry[154] summarized 100,000 injections without neurologic or ophthalmologic injury and pointed out that knowledge of the anastomosis (as described earlier) between terminal branches of the OA and the external carotid system should prompt a refined technique for reducing the risk of intraarterial injections and embolization to the ophthalmic system. To produce retrograde flow into the OA branches, the injection needle must be located intraarterially and the perfusion pressure must be overcome during injection. Consequently, topical nasal vasoconstrictors should be applied to reduce the size of the vascular bed and a small (25-gauge) needle on a low-volume syringe should be used to minimize injection pressure.

Two case reports describe visual loss after injections of combinations of corticosteroids, penicillin, and lidocaine into the tonsillar fossae and steroid, lidocaine, and epinephrine into the pterygopalatine fissure to relieve trigeminal neuralgia. Bilateral multiple retinal emboli were seen, and one patient had symptoms of multiple cerebral emboli with confusion, hypotension, and tachycardia.[155] It is thought that mixing of steroids with other drugs may enhance formation of drug crystals and should be discouraged.

Local infiltration anesthesia with lidocaine or bupivacaine in combination with epinephrine (ratio 1:100,000 or 1:200,000) for nasal septal surgery has also been reported to cause partial or total visual field defects postoperatively, presumed to be caused by BRAO.[91,94] No emboli were visible at funduscopy in these cases. It was speculated that the cause of BRAO might have been accidental intraarterial retrograde injection into branches of the external carotid artery with epinephrine or the combination of lidocaine and epinephrine causing vasospasm. Another possible contributing factor might have been epinephrine-induced platelet aggregation with retrograde embolization.[94] Although all are speculated mechanisms, this latter possibility is supported by a case report of verified platelet hypersensitivity to epinephrine. This patient used a sympathomimetic spray (oxymetazoline) chronically as a nasal decongestant. After an acute incident of decreased visual acuity, funduscopy revealed a fibrin platelet embolus in a retinal artery branch.[156]

An animal study has been performed to examine these mechanisms. In a canine model, intracarotid injections of lidocaine, epinephrine, and corticosteroid were administered. Injection of 2 ml lidocaine showed no visible funduscopic change. Injection of 2 ml 1:100,000 epinephrine alone or with lidocaine produced transient vasospasm. An injection of partly dissolved steroid (with particles) and 1:100,000 epinephrine or epinephrine/lidocaine caused permanent retinal ischemic damage. The authors concluded that injection of particulate matter was necessary to produce permanent damage.[157] Yet this may not be the entire explanation in humans, where platelet-induced hypercoagulability appears to play a role as well.[156] Also, the human ocular circulation differs from that of the canine; in humans a single CRA supplies the retina, whereas in dogs the retinal circulation derives from multiple branches of the posterior ciliary circulation. Accordingly, the canine retinal circulation may be somewhat more protected from the deleterious effects of arterial embolism and occlusion than human circulation.

One unusual case described BRAO following elective termination of pregnancy in the first trimester. The next day the patient noted decreased vision in one eye, and retinal findings suggestive of BRAO combined with no indications of pregnancy-induced hypercoagulability led to further evaluation and a diagnosis of patent foramen ovale and a tentative diagnosis of amnionic fluid emboli in a cilioretinal artery.[110]

4. Prognosis. Perioperative retinal arterial occlusion resulted in permanent loss of vision in all of the reported cases, and in general the prognosis is very poor, with only one of five eyes recovering useful vision.[10] This may be because of the limited therapeutic time interval available in retinal ischemia. The time delay is of particular importance in the postoperative patient. The diagnosis is not ordinarily sought in the absence of patient symptoms. Slow awakening from anesthesia generally delays the recognition of symptoms. Hayreh and Weingast[143] found in studies in monkeys that the critical time limit of irreversible retinal damage is approximately 100 minutes. CRAO of 105 minutes' duration produced irreversible damage, whereas recovery was seen if ischemic time was limited to 97 minutes. Shorter periods of retinal ischemia have been associated with varying degrees of recovery in animal studies.[141,144,158] The recovery pattern after BRAO would be expected to be similar, but there is more likely to be some remaining visual function.

5. Treatment. The currently available methods of treatment are not satisfactory. Some initial treatment could be instituted by the anesthesiologist. It consists of ocular massage to lower IOP (contraindicated if glaucoma cannot be ruled out) and thereby dislodge an embolus to more peripheral arterial branches.[10] Intravenous acetazolamide should be administered to increase retinal blood flow,[159] and the patient may inhale 5% CO_2 in oxygen to enhance dilation of and increase oxygen delivery from retinal and choroidal vessels.[8] Further treatment should be prescribed by the ophthalmologist and may in the future include thrombolysis, although this may be contraindicated following certain surgical procedures. A recent preliminary clinical study showed that early fibrinolysis (within 6 to 8 hours) through a catheter in the OA was associated with improved visual outcome.[160] Localized application of hypothermia to the affected eye is a simple technique that has been shown to decrease injury in animal studies following ischemia,[161] and is probably reasonable to institute in humans because of its minimal risk.

6. Prevention. The most important principle would be the avoidance of accidental application of external pressure to the eye. Pressure on the eye from anesthetic masks should be easily avoidable. If a strap is used to hold the anesthetic mask in place, it should not be placed tightly on the eye. If surgery is occurring near the face, the surgeon's arm must not be allowed to rest on the patient's eye. In patients positioned prone for surgery, a padded headrest should be used. For neurosurgical or orthopedic procedures involving the cervical spine, the head is often placed on a headrest. The eyes must be in the opening of this headrest. Because the headrest is not supported from below, the anesthesiologist can intermittently examine the eyes for pressure. Intermittent examination is advisable, but the appropriate time interval has not been established. If the patient's head does not fit the headrest adequately (e.g., it is too large), it may be preferable to secure the head with a pin head-holder. For most other procedures in which the patient is prone, we recommend a square foam headrest. The head is positioned straight down in the neutral position. The eyes and nose are then located in the open portion of the headrest, and the anesthesiologist can easily reach underneath to check for pressure intermittently. It is also important, and simply accomplished, to ensure that the endotracheal tube, esophageal stethoscope, temperature probe, and wires (such as those connected to ECG leads) are positioned so as to produce no contact with the eyes.

In some patients, especially during lumbar spine procedures, the prone position may be used in combination with a steep Trendelenburg (head-down) orientation to improve surgical exposure and decrease venous bleeding at the operative site. This position could predispose to an increased venous pressure in the head and theoretically decrease retinal perfusion pressure. However, it is not known to what extent IOP is altered under these conditions. But when this type of patient positioning is combined with deliberate hypotension and administration of large quantities of fluid, the risk of further compromise of ocular circulation is present.[35] Therefore it may be prudent to limit the extent of these interventions as much as possible.

In nasal and sinus surgery, the most important principle is the avoidance of accidental injections into or compromise of the ocular circulation, as explained previously. Embolization during cardiopulmonary bypass remains a cause of retinal vascular occlusion. Better means of detecting this complication are needed. However, there are surgical maneuvers that may lower the incidence of arterial emboli.[162]

C. Anterior ischemic optic neuropathy

1. Clinical significance. ION is the leading cause of sudden visual loss in patients 50 years of age or older. AION is divided into two types: arteritic AION and nonarteritic AION. Arteritic AION is the most serious type and is caused by temporal arteritis. This systemic disease usually occurs in patients aged 60 and older and has a female predominance. About three fourths of these patients feel ill and have flulike symptoms. Arteritic AION is an emergency and will lead to permanent blindness if untreated.

Nonarteritic AION is much more common and is not accompanied by or related to inflammation of the arteries. Generally seen in older patients, it may also occur in young patients with diabetes, malignant hypertension, eclampsia, migraine, systemic lupus, and a number of other systemic vascular diseases. About one quarter of patients with AION have both eyes involved within 3 years, and about half are so affected within 10 years. The incidence of nonarteritic ION is estimated to be 2.30 per 100,000 inhabitants per year in the United States.[163] These estimates are similar to those in surgical patients. In nonocular surgery, an incidence of about 1 per 60,000 patients more than 6 years of age was found at the University of Chicago Hospitals,[1,35] and at Johns Hopkins Hospital six patients were found with the diagnosis of postoperative AION in a 10-year period, or about 1 in 30,000 patients.[37] As indicated in Table 17-2, AION has been found following a wide variety of surgical procedures, with the majority after cardiothoracic operations.[39,42,43] However, recently there has been heightened awareness of its occurrence following complex instrumented spinal fusion operations.[1,35,36]

2. Pathophysiology. The arteritic form is caused by giant cell arteritis, whereas postoperative ION is nonarteritic. Findings in the arteritic form have been documented histologically and by fluorescein angiography.[164-166] The lesion appears to be the result of occlusion by embolus or thrombus of the PCAs in a watershed zone, resulting in regional loss of perfusion to the ON. On the other hand, the pathology has not been completely elucidated for nonarteritic AION, but is thought to be caused by temporary hypoperfusion or nonperfusion of the vessels supplying the anterior portion of the ON.[118,165]

Delayed onset and filling of the prelaminar optic disc, demonstrated by fluorescein angiography, suggests an impaired perfusion within the microcirculation of the ON head. However, intraaxonal swelling could produce the same effect. This edema could be a contributor to or a result of decreased flow. Deprivation of blood flow to the ON sets in motion a complex set of biochemical changes in the neurons. A series of cytoplasmic and membrane events culminates in axonal destruction. Adenosine triphosphate depletion caused by decreased oxygen delivery leads to membrane depolarization, influx of Na^+ and Ca^{2+} via specific voltage-gated channels and reversed operation of the Na^+/Ca^{2+} exchange pump. Ca^{2+} overload results in direct cellular damage from activation of proteolytic and other enzymes.[167] Recent data suggest that ION may lead to neuronal injury via apoptotic or programmed cell death, which may be stimulated by a reduction in oxygen delivery.[168]

Reduced perfusion pressure in the region of paraoptic branches of the short PCAs results in optic disc hypoperfusion.[9] The ON head derives its blood supply from the choriocapillaries and branches of the PCAs. The PCAs are end arteries, which display autoregulation similar to that in the cerebral cortex. Variations in the circulatory supply of the ON in some patients may predispose them to the development of AION,[32] especially under conditions such as increased IOP or decreased systemic arterial blood pressure. These variations in blood supply could result in underperfused or watershed areas, similar to the circulatory mechanisms involved in hypo-perfusion of regions of the cerebral cortex.[11,164]

The most commonly noted factors by authors of case reports are massive bleeding, anemia, and hypotension. Hayreh[69] reviewed 600 cases of posthemorrhagic blindness since the seventeenth century and summarized the clinical features: The hemorrhage is massive and recurrent, but blindness after a single hemorrhage cannot be excluded, especially not in iatrogenic bleeding during operations. The most common site of bleeding in non–surgically related blindness is the gastrointestinal tract, followed by uterine bleeding. Visual loss from ION is exceedingly rare in children. The visual loss is usually bilateral and ranges from blurred vision to blindness in one or both eyes.

Onset of AION is sudden and painless and may progress over several hours, but there is typically a time lag between the bleeding and onset of visual symptoms; lags of 10 days to 3 weeks have been described. Symptoms commonly occur upon awakening in the morning, and this effect is thought to result from the superimposed influence of nocturnal hypotension in a susceptible patient. Visual field defects are typically an inferior altitudinal hemianopic defect with or without constriction of the visual field, or superior altitudinal defect, nasal hemoptic defect, or central scotoma. Bedside ophthalmologic findings are summarized in Table 17-3.

Based on a review of the literature, Hayreh[69,169] hypothesized that AION following hemorrhage could be caused by a combination of three factors. First, recurrent hemorrhage increases peripheral vascular resistance with the release of systemic endogenous vasoconstrictors such as angiotensin, epinephrine, and vasopressin, all of which freely enter the choroidal interstitial fluid and result in vasoconstriction in the ON head vessels and the peripapillary choroidal arteries. Second, a decrease in systemic blood pressure from bleeding and superimposed sleep leads to decreased perfusion of the ON head. Third, autoregulatory failure of the ON blood supply also diminishes perfusion.

Prospective studies in humans have shown that AION is a multifactorial disease characterized by hypoperfusion and ischemic changes in the anterior part of the ON.[169] Systemic disease, particularly cardiovascular, is often found in patients with AION. The prevalence of systemic disease in 406 patients ages 11 to 91 years with AION was compared to that in a race-, gender-, and age-matched group in the general population.[170] Criteria for AION included a history of sudden visual loss with documented optic disc edema that resolved spontaneously within 2 to 3 months and left residual optic disc–related visual defects. For all ages there was a significantly higher prevalence of arterial hypertension, diabetes mellitus, and gastrointestinal ulcer in patients with AION. For patients older than 45 years, a significantly higher prevalence of ischemic heart disease and thyroid disease was found. Furthermore, middle-aged patients also had a significantly higher prevalence of chronic obstructive pulmonary disease (COPD) and cerebrovascular disease. If the patient had diabetes mellitus and arterial hypertension, a significantly higher incidence of cerebrovascular disease was present.

Perioperative AION is a multifactorial disease for which the risk factors have not been precisely delineated. Apart from systemic patient risk factors just cited, some operations are more likely to be associated with AION, especially CABG surgery, other thoracovascular surgery, and spinal surgery (see Table 17-2). Intraoperative hypotension has been cited as an important risk factor by several authors[37,38,171] but is not always present, suggesting that other factors may be more important. For example, in a recent retrospective study of patients undergoing spinal fusion, hypotension and anemia were equally prevalent in patients who developed ION and in those who did not.[36] This study was a retrospective survey of spine surgeons throughout the United States. Although there may be design flaws, it is the largest attempt to date to analyze the causes of AION after spinal surgery. Similarly, in a recent retrospective study of 602 patients undergoing open heart surgery at one institution during a 2-year period, eight cases of AION were found. Lowest perfusion pressure intraoperatively was no different between affected and normal patients.[43] These authors found that the principal distinguishing factors between affected and normal patients were a longer cardiopulmonary bypass time and a greater weight gain postoperatively. Even if hypotension is important, it is difficult to define precisely the degree of hypotension that is harmful because actual preoperative and intraoperative blood pressures were not available in many of the reported cases in the literature. Nonetheless, when reported, hypotension was generally significant and lasted for at least 1 hour.

Disturbed autoregulation in the circulation of the ON head in patients without other preexisting systemic disease may be important in the pathogenesis of AION perioperatively.[32] Using laser Doppler flowmetry, these authors showed that about 20% of normal volunteers have nonperfused regions of the ON. These patients could theoretically be susceptible to ON damage watershed areas under conditions of increased IOP or decreased blood pressure, but this speculation has not been tested rigorously. At this time, there is no clinically available test to determine which patients are so susceptible.

Possible factors involved in the cause of perioperative ION are emboli, decreased systemic blood pressure, blood loss, increased intraocular or orbital venous pressure, or localized compression of the ON blood supply. More than one of these may be required in a particular patient (e.g., hypotension plus increased venous pressure). Emboli may directly obstruct flow and are most likely to occur during cardiac surgery[162,172] as particulate matter enters the arterial circulation directly. Profound hypotension or large increases in IOP could theoretically decrease ON blood flow, but only when autoregulatory limits are exceeded. From the currently available data, the degree of hypotension or the duration of decreases in blood pressure that may lead to AION have not been established.

Increases in IOP (e.g., caused by extrinsic compression of the eye) are likely to decrease retinal blood flow and thereby produce retinal and ON damage.[173] Localized compression of the ON with or without increased IOP could result from large fluid transfusion when the patient's head is dependent (e.g., during spinal surgery with the operating table in Trendelenburg position). These patients may demonstrate significant periorbital edema postoperatively.[35,174] Large fluid transfusions with the patient's head in a dependent position could increase venous pressure in the orbital venous plexus that drains blood from the eye and the ON, resulting in a decreased

perfusion pressure gradient (the difference between inflow and outflow pressure) in the ON head. There is one case report of a patient undergoing lumbar spinal fusion in whom ION developed despite the maintenance of normotension. The patient's head and face were notably edematous after the completion of a lengthy operation.[174]

A recent study has identified possible risk factors in cardiac surgical patients.[43] During cardiac surgery, there may be transient increases in IOP during cardiopulmonary bypass that could decrease ocular perfusion pressure. This change in IOP appears to correlate with the degree of hemodilution and the use of crystalloid priming solution. Interestingly, patients with AION were more likely to develop significant weight gain 24 hours after open heart surgery, again suggesting a possible role for increases in ocular venous pressure. A similar but more sustained mechanism could explain reports of ION after radical neck dissection with compression or ligation of the internal jugular vein.[175,176] In cardiac surgical patients, other identified risk factors included longer cardiopulmonary bypass time and the use of vasoactive agents such as epinephrine and amrinone.[43] The latter fits in well with Hayreh's theory that AION is related to excessive secretion of vasoconstrictors, which could lower ON perfusion to dangerously low levels.[69,169]

Another related explanation for decreased ON perfusion is an increase in ICP. The ON is surrounded by the dura, and increased ICP could lead to significant declines in pressure in the OA. Therefore changes in venous pressure could have an important influence on blood supply to the ON.

With intraoperative blood loss, intravascular volume could be maintained by infusion of colloid or crystalloid solution, resulting in hemodilution. Although it is cited as a risk factor by some authors,[37,38,171] the supposition that isovolemic hemodilution and AION are linked is not well supported by available data. Hemodilution with preserved circulating volume is not likely to be detrimental to the ON because it results in preservation of choroidal oxygen delivery,[27] and the choroid is the origin of the PCAs that supply the anterior portion of the ON. Moreover, very deep levels of hemodilution (hemoglobin 50 g/L) are well tolerated in healthy patients, producing no disturbance in systemic oxygen delivery.[177] In the eye, isovolemic hemodilution in cats increased retinal tissue oxygen tension.[178] Combined hemodilution and hypotension may alter ON oxygen delivery, but this hypothesis has not been tested. This technique is commonly used in patients undergoing spinal surgery. In animal studies, combined hemodilution and hypotension did not appear to alter tissue oxygen delivery.[179] Even if O_2 delivery were altered, this would not necessarily imply that hemodilution is detrimental without knowledge of tissue O_2 consumption. Definitive data on the effects of hemodilution and hypotension on ON function are not likely to be obtained in humans, and we must await the results of animal experiments before coming to definite conclusions.

In summary, the pathogenesis of perioperative AION is not yet completely understood and requires further study.

Such studies should probably be undertaken in higher-risk patients, such as those undergoing cardiac surgery or spinal fusion operations. A complex interaction of factors such as altered ocular venous pressure, systemic hypotension and hemodilution, release of endogenous vasoconstrictors, and individual risk factors such as atherosclerosis and aberrant ON circulation may be responsible.

3. Distinction between nonarteritic and arteritic AION. It is very important to differentiate arteritic AION from nonarteritic AION because the arteritic form responds to steroid treatment, which must be instituted rapidly. Arteritic AION may also progress to bilateral blindness if untreated. Several symptoms and findings aid in distinguishing between the two conditions. In arteritic AION the patient is typically 60 years of age or older. Symptoms such as a vague feeling of sickness, fever of unknown origin, flulike symptoms, scalp tenderness, and usually palpable, hard, nodular changes in the temporal arteries are often present. Also, there are biochemical findings indicating inflammation. The erythrocyte sedimentation rate is greater than 80 mm, although it may be normal. Likewise, the C-reactive protein concentration may be markedly elevated.[165]

In 50% of patients the optic disc swelling typically appears chalky-white and is strongly suggestive of arteritic AION. The finding of cilioretinal artery occlusion and matching retinal infarction by funduscopy is diagnostic of arteritic AION. This finding is a consequence of underlying PCA occlusion, so fundus angiography will show nonfilling of the choroid in the corresponding area. Temporal artery biopsy must be performed to confirm this diagnosis.[165]

4. Prognosis and treatment. Unfortunately, there is no recognized specific treatment of AION. As reviewed by Williams et al,[66] many treatments have been tested. Acetazolamide lowers IOP and may improve flow to the ON head and retina.[159,180] Diuretics such as mannitol and Lasix could be useful for reducing edema. Corticosteroids in the acute phase may reduce axonal swelling, but corticosteroids in the postoperative period may increase the risk of wound infection. Because steroids are of unproven benefit, their use must be weighed carefully. Restoration of normal ocular perfusion or of hemoglobin concentration may be called for when AION occurs in conjunction with significant decreases in blood pressure and hemoglobin concentration. Maintaining head-up position could be valuable if increased ocular venous pressure is suspected. Similarly, IOP should be lowered if an increased IOP is documented. ON decompression is a recently developed operative procedure that could restore circulation in the ON, but in a multicenter trial sponsored by the National Eye Institute, this operation was found to be ineffective and possibly harmful.[181] This finding resulted in premature conclusion of the study before patient randomization was complete, although these patients are being followed to acquire further data on the pathogenesis of this disease. There is no proven method for preventing ION of the unaffected eye.

The recently completed multicenter trial demonstrated that 6 months after onset of symptoms, 43% of patients improved their vision by three or more lines.[181] This improvement was much greater than in previous studies, in which the spontaneous improvement rate was approximately 10% or less. The reason for this discrepancy is not clear, nor is it known whether postoperatively related ION has a different prognosis from that occurring in nonsurgical patients.

5. Prevention. It is difficult at this time to recommend specific preventive strategies. The major difficulties are that the status of patients' ON circulation is not known preoperatively, and there is no effective or practical method for monitoring ON function intraoperatively. However, some general recommendations could be made. In patients with preexisting cardiovascular disease, long-standing or poorly controlled hypertension, end-organ damage, or known visual disorders such as glaucoma, it seems prudent to maintain systemic blood pressure as close to baseline values as possible and to avoid prolonged decreases in ocular perfusion pressure. Obviously, external pressure on the eyes must be avoided. Whether hematocrit should be maintained at baseline value is controversial and must be weighed against any possible risks of blood transfusion. It may be advisable to minimize prolonged periods of dependency of the head during prolonged surgery in the prone position, if possible and consistent with surgical requirements. Similarly, it is controversial whether patients should be warned about the possibility of ION during the process of informed consent, especially those undergoing apparently higher-risk operations such as CABG and complex instrumented spinal fusion surgery.[173] Despite the devastating nature of this injury, our limited understanding of the pathogenesis of this disorder does not yet enable us to make rational recommendations that are likely to prevent its occurrence completely.

D. Posterior ischemic optic neuropathy

1. Clinical significance. PION is less common and hence has not been described as extensively as AION. As seen in Table 17-2, PION occurs postoperatively after an equally diverse set of operative procedures, but unlike AION, it is not common after CABG. Head and neck and spinal surgery are more often associated with PION than AION. Nonsurgical settings in which PION is found include cardiac arrest, treatment for malignant hypertension, severe anemia, and direct trauma to the eye.

2. Pathophysiology. Whereas AION is the result of interruption of the blood supply to the anterior portion of the ON, PION is produced by decreased oxygen delivery to the more posterior, retrolaminar portion of the nerve. Blood supply to the retrolaminar portion of the ON is derived from the peripheral centripetal vascular system, which is formed by the pial vessels. These are supplied by small collateral arteries arising from the OA, and this blood supply is derived developmentally from a source other than the blood supply to the optic disc.[11] Most probably, compression of these vessels or embolic phenomena result in ischemia.[182] However, a low flow state from systemic hypoperfusion or venous stasis could also play a role.

The development of ischemic damage generally proceeds at a slower pace in PION than in AION. Autopsy studies in postoperative PION have shown edema and enlargement of the ON, with central retrolaminar hemorrhagic infarction of the ON.[68,76,100,103] CT in the immediate postoperative period may reveal enlargement of the intraorbital portion of the ON.[68] However, a symptom-free period is usually present initially, with minimal or no abnormalities found on ophthalmoscopic examination. An initially normal optic disc and no perfusion abnormalities on fluorescein angiography distinguish AION from PION. Mild disc edema occurs over a period of days. Later (within 5 to 6 weeks) the optic disc is pale and atrophied. The sudden onset of visual disturbance may not affect visual acuity. There will be an ON-related visual field defect, and systemic (vascular) disease is often present.

As is the case in AION, PION also seems to reflect a multifactorial disease, although with a higher frequency of bilateral postoperative blindness than in AION. Bilateral blindness indicates involvement of the optic chiasm or a disease process affecting both ONs simultaneously. Severe hypotension and anemia appear to be risk factors. In Table 17-2 it is shown that 63% of the cases lead to blindness, and no improvement in vision is found in cases where data were provided. An important feature may be concomitant disease of the eye or ocular blood supply because in 20% of the cases, glaucoma, arteritis temporalis, or verified stenosis of the ophthalmic arteries was found.

3. Prognosis and treatment. In most cases, there is improvement. No treatment has proven efficient for PION. Steroids may be considered for reduction of ON swelling.[182]

4. Prevention. The same principles apply as described earlier for AION.

5. Retrobulbar hemorrhage and ION. An additional consideration is the association of retrobulbar hemorrhage and ION. Because of the close anatomic relationship of the sphenoid sinus and ethmoidal cells to the orbit and ON, surgery of the nose and paranasal sinuses poses a special risk of damage to the visual pathway. Furthermore, the bone is very fragile in this area and there is anatomic variation because pneumatization depends on the individual pattern of growth developmentally. In a CT study of the relationship of the ON to the paranasal sinuses (in which half of the patients had suspected disease of the ON) it was found that in 48% of the patients the posterior ethmoid cells were separated from the ON by only the thin wall of the optic canal, and in 90% the sphenoid sinus contacted the nerve; in 10% this contact was found bilaterally. In 26% there was projection of the ON into the sinuses. The close anatomic relationship of these structures to the ON may predispose to compression-type damage from direct surgical trauma or bleeding.[183]

Ophthalmic complications of nasal or sinus surgery are uncommon but well recognized, and when they occur they may result in significant morbidity. They occur especially with an intranasal approach because the surgical field is small, the arteries are not well visualized, and the operations are technically difficult. The blood supply is rich, and bleeding from the nasal and sinus mucosa is common. RH may occur following surgical damage to the fragile

lateral wall of the ethmoidal cells, the lamina papyracea. Sinus endoscopy has improved visualization of structures in the surgical field significantly, but with this technique, blindness has occasionally been reported.[85,96,184] Direct surgical lesion of the ON may occur,[89] but indirect ON lesion by compression from retrobulbar hematoma leading to ION has been reported more often (see Table 17-2). Most authors do not describe findings at funduscopy, so the cases cannot be classified as AION or PION but rather ION caused by RH. Paresis of eye muscles (mostly the medial rectus muscle), including ptosis, is often seen.[87,90,91] The outcome is poor; in only one case is temporary blindness reported,[95] whereas all other reported cases of retrobulbar hematoma resulted in permanent blindness (see Table 17-2 for references).

Less severe cases of surgical damage to the orbital walls may cause herniation of the eye muscles, leading to strabismus and permanent double vision in parts of the visual field. Damage to the superior oblique, the inferior rectus, and the medial rectus has been described.[89,185-187]

E. Cortical blindness

1. Clinical significance. Complete CB is defined as bilateral visual loss and loss of optokinetic nystagmus, absent lid reflex response to threat, a normal pupillary response, normal eye motility, and a normal retina and ON. Interestingly, patients often fail to recognize the blindness themselves, known as Anton's syndrome.[188] Each visual cortex receives data from the contralateral visual field and connects to nearby areas in the occipital and parietotemporal cortex for more advanced visual functions such as analysis of movement, color vision, and three-dimensional form. The primary visual cortex processes retinal information to give a sense of orientation and binocular vision for depth perception. Complete blindness implies damage to both the left and right occipital cortex. A more localized injury would produce homonymous hemianopia.

Total blindness caused by bilateral occipital infarction is rare. Because the visual pathway travels through the parietotemporal lobes, a perioperative cerebrovascular accident related to the internal carotid, middle cerebral, basilar, or posterior cerebral arteries is the more common scenario that produces CB. Yet because of collateral circulation, the degree of visual damage is actually difficult to predict.[7] About 80% of cases of CB reported postoperatively have followed cardiac or other thoracic surgery. Depending on the neuropsychologic testing profile used, these patients may show evidence of postoperative neurologic sequelae.[189]

Initially, total CB is usually accompanied by cortical sensory symptoms as signs of stroke in the parietooccipital region. The patient may suffer agnosia, an inability to interpret sensory stimuli. Usually vision improves over time, leaving incomplete lesions in the visual field combined with visual disorientation. Typical findings are preserved pupillary reflexes and regaining of most of the visual field within days, but impairment of spatial perception and sense of relationship between sizes and distances may remain. Restricted visual attention and an inability to notice images formed on all parts of the retina at one time are also features. These factors can lead to inability to read. Denial sometimes accompanies CB.

Delay in the recognition of blindness is a particular problem with CB. Examining 50 cases of CB, Aldrich et al[71] found five factors contributing to a delay in diagnosis: preexisting pupillary abnormalities, macular sparing, variation of visual perception over time, disproportion between visual complaints and measured visual field loss, and CB as the only symptom. Denial or unawareness may also confuse and delay the diagnosis of CB.[71,190,191]

The incidence of CB after cardiac surgery has been studied. CB was present in 10 out of 808 CABG surgeries in one hospital, with brain scans in 5 of them demonstrating occipital infarcts.[16] In a retrospective series of 700 CABG and valve replacement operations performed by a single surgeon, 2 had unilateral occipital cortical infarcts.[42] Shaw et al[40] prospectively studied 312 patients undergoing CABG. They found an overall incidence of CB of 5%. At least 50% of these patients had other associated neurologic deficits. In another study, the onset of visual deficits was shown to follow a similar time course to that of neurologic damage postoperatively (see Table 17-2).[192] One of the largest, most recent studies of neurologic dysfunction after cardiac surgery was that of Roach et al.[193] A total of 2108 CABG patients from 24 different hospitals were studied prospectively. There was a 6% incidence of neurologic complications. Risk factors included aortic atherosclerosis, old age, prior neurologic dysfunction, hypertension, pulmonary disease, and alcohol consumption. Unfortunately, the incidence of visual disorders was not reported.

Angiography often is performed in the preoperative period in patients presenting for cardiac and vascular surgical operations. Transient (and in one case permanent[71]) CB has been reported following intraarterial injection of iodinated contrast material. The possibility that CB is associated with such procedures should be considered. An incidence of CB of 1 in 12,367 coronary angiographies[194] and of 10 in 619 patients after vertebral angiography has been reported.[195] CB has been seen after angiography of the coronary[196-199] and cerebral arteries.[200,201] It is believed that vasospasm, emboli, or damage to the blood-brain barrier, as a result of lipid solubility or the high osmolality of the contrast material, is responsible.[191,201]

2. Pathophysiology. Many different causes could result in diminished oxygen delivery to the visual pathway between the ON and the occipital cortex. Among these are global ischemia, cardiac arrest, hypoxemia, intracranial hypertension, exsanguinating hemorrhage, focal ischemia, vascular occlusion, thrombosis, intracranial hemorrhage, vasospasm, and emboli. If blood and oxygen deprivation persist long enough, the cellular energy supply ceases and a series of biochemical events is initiated that ultimately leads to cell death. The pathways responsible for neuronal injury in the cerebral cortex have been reviewed extensively.[202]

CABG is the most common operation associated with CB. The pathophysiology of CB after CABG is incompletely understood. The major source of brain and visual

damage is controversial but is believed to be the result of macroembolism from the surgical field, such as fat and atheroma, or microemboli of lipid and fibrin-platelet aggregates.[71,81] Indeed, a high incidence of emboli in the retinal circulation in patients undergoing CABG has been documented.[172] Patients with aortic atherosclerosis appear to be at particular risk.[193] Edema could also be responsible for CB,[203,204] but a pilot study of early MRI of the brain after CABG showed cortical swelling present within 20 to 40 minutes that was not found on follow-up 1 to 3 weeks later, leading to a question about its pathogenic role.[205] This edema may somehow contribute to the vague visual disturbances found in up to 25% of patients after CABG (see Table 17-1).[206] Transient embolization is an alternative explanation for the often temporary nature of CB. In addition to emboli, transient decreases in blood flow to border zones of perfusion between the middle and posterior cerebral arteries, especially in patients with preexisting cerebrovascular disease, probably is another responsible factor.[18]

3. Prognosis, treatment, and prevention. Visual recovery from CB may be prolonged, but in previously healthy patients, it may be considerable. Therefore when CB is accompanied by focal neurologic signs, treatment should be directed at preventing progression of stroke.

The optimal strategy to prevent neurologic injury during cardiac surgery remains controversial. Because of heightened awareness of the risk of embolism from an atherosclerotic aorta,[207,208] several different techniques have been advocated to decrease intraoperative manipulation of the aorta.[42,162,209] Adequate removal of air and particulate matter from the heart during valvular operations may decrease the risk of embolism. In patients less than 70 years old without evidence of cerebrovascular disease, the use of an arterial line filter during cardiopulmonary bypass reduces significantly the number of microemboli detectable by transcranial Doppler ultrasonography. The frequency of subtle neuropsychologic and neurologic changes (including nystagmus) is also reduced. There were no visual defects in the study patients.[210] Maintenance of adequate systemic perfusion pressure may prevent episodes of hypoperfusion in patients with cerebrovascular disease. Better development of transcranial Doppler techniques may enhance detection of embolic events. There are as yet no proven neuroprotective agents for these patients.[211]

VI. ANESTHETICS AND TRANSIENT VISUAL IMPAIRMENT

Intravenous anesthetic agents commonly produce transient visual changes. Nystagmus, blurry vision, double vision, and visual illusions at emergence from ketamine anesthesia are well-known phenomena,[212] but transient blindness is rare. Three cases of transient blindness accompanied by normal pupillary reflexes, lasting 25 minutes, have been reported.[213] The exact mechanism is not known. While ketamine has been shown to depress glucose use in auditory brain structures in rats, a nonsignificant rise in visual cortex glucose use was seen with unaltered metabolism in LGN and the superior colliculus.[214,215] However, the distribution of activity in the visual cortex was altered.[214] A speculated mechanism of action of ketamine is that it produces misperception or misinterpretation of visual stimuli in the cortex.[216]

In a double-blind study comparing recovery after short-acting anesthetics, propofol was associated with a significantly longer time to eye opening on command: 7 minutes as compared to 6 minutes for thiopental and 5.3 minutes for etomidate. After case reports of external ophthalmoplegia following propofol anesthesia,[217,218] Marsch[219] examined the effect of total intravenous anesthesia with propofol on eye opening and eye movements. One hundred ten patients were examined immediately after extubation, and after they were able to lift their heads and follow commands. There were 21 patients with total gaze paresis and 30 with various degrees of impaired eye opening or eye movements; after 20 minutes normal eye opening and movements had reappeared in a symmetric manner. From the study, the underlying mechanisms could not be discerned, but the authors suggested that propofol probably produces these alterations by action at a midbrain or pontine level. The effect of propofol on eye opening seems to be of such a limited duration that it may not even be noticed following anesthesia in daily practice.[219,220] However, the possibility that transient alterations in eye movements could be caused by propofol should be kept in mind in the differential diagnosis of impaired eye movement in the postoperative period.

VII. EPIDURAL INJECTION AND VISUAL IMPAIRMENT

Retinal venous hemorrhage has been reported after injections of local anesthetic, steroids, or saline into the lumbar epidural space. These cases have been reported in both the anesthetic and ophthalmologic literature and have been recently summarized by Purdy and Ajimal.[221] In all patients affected, at least 40 ml was injected into the epidural space. They subsequently developed blurry vision or headaches, in some cases with onset 12 hours or more later. Retinal hemorrhage was consistently present on funduscopic examination. Of the 9 patients reported, all but one had complete recovery. It is believed that the hemorrhage is the result of acute increases in intracranial pressure, resulting in a transient elevation of retinal venous pressure. There may be other risk factors that are additive, such as hypertension, pseudotumor cerebri, and retinal vascular diseases such as diabetic retinopathy. This complication can probably be avoided by minimizing the volume and speed of injection into the epidural space.

VIII. VISUAL CHANGES AFTER TRANSURETHRAL RESECTION OF THE PROSTATE
A. Clinical significance

The possibility of visual changes occurring during or after transurethral resection of the prostate (TURP) has been recognized for nearly 40 years.[222-231] Visual changes may occur alone or as part of a syndrome involving excessive absorption of irrigating fluid, resulting in hyponatremia, cerebral edema, seizures, coma, and cardiac failure from fluid overload.[226] TURP is one of the most commonly performed surgical procedures in the United States. By the late 1940s, the transurethral approach was preferred in North America because of its demonstrated low mortality and morbidity compared to open procedures.[232,233]

Successful completion of TURP requires copious irrigation of the bladder to remove clots and debris, keeping the surgeon's view of the field clear. Despite aspiration of the irrigant, 1 L or more of it may be absorbed by the patient[234] at a rate of approximately 10 to 30 ml/min,[235] and rates as high as 200 ml/min have been reported.[236] Absorption of the irrigant is the major source of non–surgically related complications. The determinants of the amount of irrigant absorbed are somewhat controversial. Duration of the resection, extent of opening of the prostatic venous sinuses, hydrostatic pressure of the irrigation fluid, and venous pressure at the irrigant-blood interface are proposed factors.[233] However, Stewart et al[237] dispute the role of operative time; they found that a longer resection time did not result in increased absorption, suggesting that the veins and capsule of the smaller prostate may be exposed earlier in the resection, so that a greater absorption during a quick resection leads to the same amount of irrigant absorption as a slower absorption during a long resection. Nonetheless, significant amounts may be absorbed even if the surgeon believes no venous sinuses are open, and the operator thus cannot predict or estimate the amounts.[238] The absorption of irrigating fluid may continue postoperatively through the retroperitoneal and perivesical spaces.[239] Vigilance and a high index of suspicion for development of the syndrome are important components of the anesthetic plan. The possibility of earlier detection of central nervous system (CNS) signs and symptoms of TURP syndrome accounts for the preference by many anesthesiologists for regional anesthesia for these procedures.

B. Presenting signs and symptoms

Visual deficits may present during the resection, several hours after, or, rarely, on the second postoperative day as the patient awakens from a TURP-related coma.[231] The range of presenting signs and symptoms is wide, from complete loss of light perception to more subtle defects. The initial complaint may be visual halos and a blue visual hue.[225] Dilated pupils that are unreactive to light, a normal IOP, normal extraocular muscle movement, and normal fundus examination without evidence of papilledema are the objective findings in these cases.[225] These visual changes may resolve over a few hours or persist for up to 80 hours.[231] There are no reports of permanent visual loss.

C. Role of irrigating fluid

The choice of irrigant is very important in explaining the mechanisms of cerebral and visual dysfunction associated with TURP. A desirable irrigant fluid is clear (for better visualization), nonionized, nontoxic, inexpensive, and easily sterilized. Unfortunately, the best visualization occurs with use of hemolytic fluids (such as water) that dissolve red cells, dispelling any cloudiness in the operative field. Solutes used to make irrigation fluid safe must be effective osmoles to prevent hemolysis and cerebral edema. Ionized solvents cause dispersal and weakening of the current from the cautery, making cutting and coagulation ineffective.[240]

Glycine 1.5% is probably the most extensively used solution. It is slightly hypoosmolar, but it does not cause clinically significant hemolysis.[241] A 1.5% solution of glycine has an osmolarity of 200 mOsm/kg.[231] The half-life of infused glycine in plasma is reported to be between 26 and 245 minutes, depending on the dose administered.[242] Glycine is metabolized to serine and ammonia, both of which are associated with CNS complications after TURP.[243] Other important metabolites include glyoxylic acid, an inhibitor of oxidative phosphorylation, and methylene tetrahydrofolate, an inhibitor of presynaptic glutamate uptake.[244]

D. Mechanisms of visual dysfunction

The precise mechanisms leading to visual dysfunction probably are multifactorial. Proposed mechanisms of the visual changes include cerebral edema,[224] hyponatremia,[223] glycine toxicity to the retina and cerebral cortex,[225] ammonia toxicity,[243,245] increased IOP caused by water absorption,[246] and cranial nerve dysfunction caused by spinal anesthesia. Each of these is reviewed briefly.

1. Glycine toxicity. This mechanism has been the most widely studied and is probably the most important. Glycine is the smallest amino acid. It enters cells primarily through a carrier-mediated process, but its rate of transport is slow. As long as glycine remains in the extracellular space, it acts as an effective osmole. The glycine solution usually used, with an osmolarity of 200 mOsm/L, contains 300 ml/L free water, and two thirds of it will enter cells while one third enters the extracellular fluid.[231]

Glycine easily crosses the blood-brain barrier, and in the CNS it functions as an inhibitory neurotransmitter. Glycine depresses the spontaneous and evoked activity of retinal neurons and hyperpolarizes cells via blockade of chloride channels.[247,248] The highest glycine concentration is present in the amacrine cells, inner plexiform, and ganglion cell layers of the retina.[225] When injected into the vitreous in rabbits, glycine has an inhibitory action on the ERG, which reverses spontaneously within 24 hours. Similar effects were seen in the ERG of patients with TURP syndrome and glycine toxicity.[227] Because of a profound effect on oscillatory potentials of the ERG, the predominant site of action may be amacrine cells,[249] although other inner retinal cells probably are involved as well. Moreover, glycine altered visual evoked potentials in dogs and in humans, suggesting an effect on neural transmission in the ON as well.[250,251] The threshold for visual symptoms is a plasma glycine concentration greater than 4000 μmol/L.[250] Glycine concentration does not correlate well with the presence of visual symptoms, suggesting that perhaps its metabolites (e.g., serine)[252] play an important role in causing visual changes. A GABA-like antianxiety effect of the transmitter may account for the inappropriate calmness reported with visual changes in patients with TURP syndrome.

Metabolism of glycine may produce ammonia, serine, glucose, proteins, creatinine, hippurate, and glyoxylate. Hyperammonemia with toxicity caused by glycine absorp-

tion during TURP has been reported.[243,245] Ammonia concentrationss are increased in many but not all patients after glycine administration. Correlation between CNS changes and ammonia concentrations has been lacking, however. Preexisting liver disease has been suggested as a risk factor for development of significant hyperammonemia during glycine administration[253] Serine, a major metabolite, has inhibitory effects on the retina similar to those of glycine.[254] These metabolites may also play a role, via unknown mechanisms, in visual dysfunction after TURP.[229,252]

2. Cerebral edema. It is suggested that hyponatremia or hypoosmolality occurring during TURP produces occipital cortical edema. This effect has never been confirmed. Perhaps segmental vascular disease in the blood supply to the occipital cortex placed that portion of the brain more at risk for swelling.[226]

3. Hyponatremia. Hyponatremia indicates that hypoosmolality is present. Absorption of irrigant fluid by damaged blood vessels or leakage into the retroperitoneal space is the cause of symptoms from hypoosmolality.[255] Hyponatremia syndrome is dominated by CNS dysfunction secondary to hypoosmolality. The osmolal gradient causes water to move into the brain. The amount of CNS dysfunction is related to the rapidity as well as the degree of decline in sodium concentration.[256] Symptoms include hallucinations, psychosis, seizures, and focal neurologic signs. Hyponatremia and glycine toxicity may occur independently.

4. Increased intraocular pressure. Ocular hypertension causes enlarged blind spots and paracentral scotoma. In the presence of water overload, it seemed logical that an increase in IOP could be involved in TURP syndrome. However, in a prospective study of 22 patients undergoing TURP, Peters et al[246] found no change in IOP in the affected patients.

5. Spinal anesthesia. Spinal anesthesia is often used for TURP. Cranial nerve palsies, particularly of the sixth nerve, have been reported as a complication of spinal anesthesia, theoretically caused by a reduction in intracranial pressure from loss of CSF. These palsies occur several hours after the procedure along with postdural puncture headache. However, a cranial nerve dysfunction does not explain complete blindness. In addition, the visual disturbance seen with TURP has occurred after general anesthesia as well, and regional techniques are unlikely to be causative.

Visual changes following TURP are transient and often associated with TURP syndrome. The most important means of prevention is to maintain high vigilance to avoid excessive absorption of irrigating solution.

IX. OCULAR LIGHT DAMAGE

The eye is extremely sensitive to photic injury and may be permanently damaged by direct or reflected light beams. Light in the 280- to 400-nm range (UV-A and UV-B) is absorbed by the anterior segment of the lens and cornea.[257] Laser light (400 to 1400 nm) is a particular hazard to the retina; even very brief exposure could result in profound damage.[258] Prolonged exposure to blue and UV light is capable of producing retinal damage in patients. This damage could result from lengthy use of the operating microscope during eye surgery.[259]

Laser light, which is commonly used in the operating room, poses a hazard to patients undergoing laser surgery as well as to operating room personnel. The extent of damage is a function of the laser irradiance, duration of exposure, and the size of the beam.[260] Most of these injuries are painless. They may result in subretinal and vitreous hemorrhage and macular hole formation. When the injury is located outside of the fovea, chances of recovery are improved. The Q-switched neodymium–yttrium aluminum garnet (Nd:YAG) laser is especially hazardous because the beam is invisible and the retina lacks sensory innervation. Photoacoustic retinal damage may produce an audible pop at the time of exposure.[261]

The major means of prevention of laser injuries is the use of proper eye protection in both laser users and in patients exposed to laser light during surgery. Laser operators must be trained properly; most institutions have specific guidelines governing laser use in the operating room. Determination of the correct protective goggles for operating room personnel has been reviewed elsewhere.[262] The eyes of patients undergoing laser surgery must be protected correctly as well. Appropriate minigoggles are available, but care must be taken not to expose the straps to laser light because they are combustible. For use of laser light near the eyes, stainless steel or lead eye shields are available. These are positioned on the corneal surface with the use of topical anesthetic.

Photic injury to the retina after prolonged exposure to the operating microscope has been well described.[259,263] Of particular interest to the anesthesiologist is the need to minimize inspired oxygen concentration in patients undergoing eye surgery with the operating microscope under general anesthesia. Jaffe et al[264] showed in monkeys that exposure to 99% O_2 produced retinal lesions three times as large as those in monkeys exposed to 21% O_2 when the operating microscope was used for 1.5 to 20 minutes per exposure.

X. RETINOPATHY OF PREMATURITY

Retinopathy of prematurity (ROP) is a well-described but complex phenomenon that occurs in premature infants.[265] ROP was initially believed to be caused by exposure to oxygen; recent studies have called this theory into question.[266] Exposure to bright lights and vitamin E deficiency are other factors that have been implicated.[267] Nonetheless, some cases might still be explainable as a result of hyperoxia. When caring for a premature baby requiring general anesthesia, it is prudent to avoid hyperoxia and to maintain arterial oxygen saturation between 93% and 95%, or a PaO_2 between 60 and 100 mm Hg.[268]

XI. HEARING

The loss of hearing secondary to barotrauma has been described after anesthesia and surgery involving the middle ear. The pathogenesis of this problem is related to increases in middle ear pressure secondary to the administration of nitrous oxide. Nitrous oxide enters the ear cavities at a rate greater than that at which nitrogen can leave. Normally, increases in pressure within the inner ear are vented through the eustachian tube, but surgical trauma may attenuate this avenue for the relief of increased pressure. Moreover, a negative pressure within the ear may develop after nitrous oxide has been discontinued. Such pressure changes may result in rupture of the tympanic membrane, transient decreases in middle ear function, nausea, and vomiting. Impairment of eustachian tube patency (e.g., caused by previous ear surgery, chronic otitis media, upper respiratory tract infection, and abnormalities of the nasopharynx) increases the risk of this complication. Discontinuing nitrous oxide at least 15 minutes before the closure of the middle ear and limiting its concentration to 50% are recommended steps to diminish the risk of middle ear damage.[269]

XII. TASTE AND SMELL

There are reports of vaguely defined changes in taste and smell following anesthesia and surgery not involving the oral cavity, nasopharynx, or the olfactory lobes of the cerebral cortex. Diminished smell and taste in a 47-year-old woman followed a cystoscopy performed under general anesthesia with propofol, lidocaine, succinylcholine, and isoflurane.[270] Loss of taste, flavor sensation, or smell; dysgeusia (bad taste); and dysosmia (bad smell) were described in 59 patients evaluated at a taste and smell disorders clinic at varying times following anesthesia and surgery.[271] Although they were found after a variety of procedures, including abdominal, genitourinary, and cardiac bypass, all of which were remote from the mouth and nose, the risk factors and causes of these conditions are unknown. These alterations have also been described after tonsillectomy, middle ear surgery, and intracranial procedures, but these latter cases are more likely to be related to surgical trauma than to an effect of anesthesia. In any event, further research is necessary to ascertain whether there is any role of anesthesia in the occurrence of these changes in taste and smell.

XIII. CONCLUSIONS

Complications to the sense organs range from vague symptoms of altered taste and smell to the more serious permanent loss of vision. Although some of these complications, such as corneal abrasions and those caused by pressure on the eyes, can be but are not always avoidable, the cause of some of the more serious complications still remains enigmatic. Heightened awareness by the anesthesiologist of the risk of these complications may lead to improved means of detection and prevention of these injuries.

ACKNOWLEDGMENTS
Dr Roth's research on this topic is supported by National Institutes of Health Grant EY10343.

REFERENCES
1. Roth S, Thisted RA, Erickson JP, et al: Eye injuries after nonocular surgery: a study of 60,965 anesthetics from 1988-1992, *Anesthesiology* 85:1020, 1996.

2. Gild WA, Posner KL, Caplan RA, et al: Eye injuries associated with anesthesia, *Anesthesiology* 76:204, 1992.

3. Heimer L: Visual system. In *The human brain and spinal cord. Functional neuroanatomy and dissection guide,* New York, 1983, Springer Verlag.

4. Goldberg S: *Ophthalmology made ridiculously simple,* Miami, Fla, 1982, Medmaster.

5. Anderson DR: The optic nerve. In Moses A, Hart C, eds: *Adler's physiology of the eye,* ed 8, St Louis, 1987, Mosby.

6. Quigley HA, Miller NR, Green WR: The pattern of optic nerve fiber loss in anterior ischemic optic neuropathy, *Am J Ophthalmol* 100:769, 1985.

7. Heimer L: Cerebral cortex. In *The human brain and spinal cord. Functional neuroanatomy and dissection guide.* New York, 1983, Springer-Verlag.

8. Alm A, Bill A: Ocular circulation. In Moses A, Hart C, eds: *Adler's physiology of the eye,* ed 8, St Louis, 1987, Mosby.

9. Olver JM, Spalton DJ, McCartney ACE: Microvascular study of the retrolaminar optic nerve in man. The possible significance in anterior ischaemic optic neuropathy, *Eye* 4:7, 1990.

10. Wray SH: The management of acute visual failure, *J Neurol Neurosurg Psychiatry* 56:234, 1993.

11. Isayama Y, Hiramatsu K, Asakura S, et al: Posterior ischemic optic neuropathy. I. Blood supply of the optic nerve, *Ophthalmology* 186:197, 1983.

12. Feneis H: *Anatomisk billedordbog,* ed 2, Copenhagen, 1983, Munksgaard.

13. Mames RN, McCoy LS, Guy J: Central retinal and posterior ciliate artery occlusion after particle embolization of the external carotid artery system, *Ophthalmology* 98:527, 1991.

14. Lieberman MF, Maumenee E, Green WR: Histologic studies of the vasculature of the anterior optic nerve, *Am J Ophthalmol* 82:405, 1976.

15. Symonds C, Mackenzie I: Bilateral loss of vision from cerebral infarction, *Brain* 80:415, 1957.

16. Taugher PJ: Visual loss after cardiopulmonary bypass, *Am J Ophthalmol* 81:280, 1976.

17. Hoyt HS, Goebel JL, Lee HI, et al: Types of shock-like reaction during transurethral resection and relation to acute renal failure, *J Urol* 79:500, 1958.

18. Ross-Russell RW, Bharucha N: The recognition and prevention of border zone cerebral ischaemia during cardiac surgery, *QJM* 187:303, 1978.

19. Roth S: The effects of halothane on retinal and choroidal blood flow in cats, *Anesthesiology* 76:455, 1992.

20. Spraul CW, Lang GE, Grossniklaus HE: Morphometric analysis of the choroid, Bruch's membrane, and retinal pigment epithelium in eyes with age-related macular degeneration, *Invest Ophthalmol Vis Sci* 37:2724, 1997.

21. Kiel JW, van Heuven WA: Ocular perfusion pressure and choroidal blood flow in the rabbit, *Invest Ophthalmol Vis Sci* 36:579, 1995.

22. Kiel JW, Lovell MD: Adrenergic modulation of choroidal blood flow in the rabbit, *Invest Ophthalmol Vis Sci* 37:673, 1996.

23. Riva CE, Titze P, Hero M, et al: Effect of acute decreases of perfusion pressure on choroidal blood flow in humans, *Invest Ophthalmol Vis Sci* 38:1752, 1997.

24. Schmetterer L, Lexer F, Findl O, et al: The effect of inhalation of different mixtures of O_2 and CO_2 on ocular fundus pulsations, *Exp Eye Res* 14:351, 1996.

25. Attariwala R, Giebs CP, Glucksberg MR: The influence of elevated intraocular pressure on vascular pressures in the cat retina, *Invest Ophthalmol Vis Sci* 35:1019, 1996.

26. Roth S, Pietrzyk Z: Blood flow after retinal ischemia in cats, *Invest Ophthalmol Vis Sci* 35:3209, 1994.

27. Roth S: The effects of isovolumic hemodilution on ocular blood flow, *Exp Eye Res* 55:59, 1992.

28. Wiek J, Schade M, Wiederholt M, et al: Haemorheological changes in patients with retinal vein occlusion after isovolemic hemodilution, *Br J Ophthalmol* 74:665, 1990.

29. Roth S, Pietrzyk Z, Crittenden AP: The effects of enflurane on ocular flow, *J Ocul Pharmacol* 9:251, 1993.

30. Sperber GO, Bill A: Blood flow and glucose consumption in the optic nerve, retina and the brain: effects of high intraocular pressure, *Exp Eye Res* 41:639, 1985.

31. Hayreh SS, Bill A, Sperber GO: Effects of high intraocular pressure on the glucose metabolism in the retina and the optic nerve in atheroschlerotic monkeys, *Graefe's Arch Clin Exp Ophthalmol* 232:745, 1994.

32. Pillunat LE, Anderson DR, Knighton RW, et al: Autoregulation of human optic nerve head circulation in response to increased intraocular pressure, *Exp Eye Res* 64:737, 1997.

33. Silverstein A, Krieger HP: Neurologic complications of cardiac surgery, *Trans Am Neurol Assoc* 85:151, 1960.

34. Cucchiara RF, Black S: Corneal abrasion during anesthesia and surgery, *Anesthesiology* 69:978, 1988.

35. Roth S, Nunez R, Schreider BD: Visual loss after lumbar spine fusion, *J Neurosurg Anesthesiol* 9:346, 1997.

36. Myers MA, Hamilton SR, Bogosian AJ, et al: Visual loss as a complication of spinal surgery, *Spine* 22:1325, 1997.

37. Brown RH, Schauble JF, Miller NR: Anemia and hypotension as contributors to perioperative loss of vision, *Anesthesiology* 80:222, 1994.

38. Katz DM, Trobe JD, Cornblath WT, et al: Ischemic optic neuropathy after lumbar spine surgery, *Arch Ophthalmol* 112:925, 1994.

39. Sweeney PJ, Breuer AC, Selhorst JB, et al: Ischemic optic neuropathy: a complication of cardiopulmonary bypass surgery, *Neurology* 32:560, 1982.

40. Shaw PJ, Bates D, Cartlidge NEF, et al: Neurologic and neuropsychologic morbidity following major surgery: comparison of coronary artery bypass and peripheral vascular surgery, *Stroke* 18:700, 1987.

41. Breuer AC, Furlan AJ, Hanson MR, et al: Central nervous system complications of coronary artery bypass surgery. Prospective analysis of 421 patients, *Stroke* 14:682, 1983.

42. Shahian DM, Speert PK: Symptomatic visual deficits after open heart operations, *Ann Thorac Surg* 48:275, 1989.

43. Shapira OM, Kimmel WA, Lindsey PS, et al: Anterior ischemic optic neuropathy after open heart operations, *Ann Thorac Surg* 61:660, 1996.

44. Graves EJ: Detailed diagnoses and procedures, National Hospital Discharge Survey, 1991, *Vital Health Stat 13* 115:1, 1994.

45. Graves EJ: National hospital discharge survey: annual summary 1989, *Vital Health Stat 13* 199:4, 1991.

46. Fry CL, Carter JE, Kanter MC, et al: Anterior ischemic optic neuropathy is not associated with carotid artery atherosclerosis, *Stroke* 24:539, 1993.

47. Kuroda Y, Uchimoto R, Kaieda R, et al: Central nervous system complications after cardiac surgery: a comparison between coronary artery bypass grafting and valve surgery, *Anesth Analg* 76:222, 1993.

48. Richardson RB, McBride CM, Berkeley RG, et al: An unusual ocular complication after anesthesia, *Anesthesiology* 43:357, 1975.

49. Quinlan MF, Salmon JF: Ophthalmic complications after heart transplantation, *J Heart Lung Transplant* 12:252, 1993.

50. Hamed LM, Ellis D, Boudreault G, et al: Hibiclens keratitis, *Am J Ophthalmol* 104:50, 1987.

51. Tabor E, Bostwick B, Evans C: Corneal damage due to eye contact with chlorhexidine gluconate, *JAMA* 261:557, 1984.

52. MacRae SM, Brown B, Edelhausser H: The corneal toxicity of presurgical skin antiseptics, *Am J Ophthalmol* 97:221, 1984.

53. Murray WJ, Ruddy MP: Toxic eye injury during induction of anesthesia, *South Med J* 78:1012, 1985.

54. Jampol LM, Neufeld AH, Sears ML: Pathways for the response of the eye to injury, *Invest Ophthalmol* 14:184, 1975.

55. Shingleton BJ: Eye injuries, *N Engl J Med* 325:408, 1991.

56. Waggoner MD: Chemical injuries of the eye: current concepts in pathophysiology and therapy, *Surv Ophthalmol* 41:275, 1997.

57. Krupin T, Cross DA, Becker B: Decreased basal tear production associated with general anesthesia, *Arch Ophthalmol* 95:107, 1977.

58. Watson WJ, Moran RL: Corneal abrasion during induction, *Anesthesiology* 66:440, 1987 (letter).

59. Rosenberg M: Ocular injuries during general anesthesia, *J Oral Surg* 39:945, 1981.
60. Schmidt P, Boggild-Madsen NB: Protection of the eyes with ophthalmic ointments during general anesthesia, *Acta Ophthalmologica* 59:422, 1981.
61. Siffring PA, Poulton TJ: Prevention of ophthalmic complications during general anesthesia, *Anesthesiology* 66:569, 1987.
62. Vaughan DG, Asbury T, Riordan-Eva P: *General ophthalmology*, Norwalk, Conn, 1995, Appleton & Lange.
63. Gartner S, Billet E: Acute glaucoma: as a complication of general surgery, *Am J Ophthalmol* 45:668, 1958.
64. Wang BC, Tannenbaum CS, Robertazzi RW: Acute glaucoma after general surgery, *JAMA* 177:108, 1961.
65. Fazio DT, Bateman JB, Christensen RE: Acute angle-closure glaucoma associated with surgical anesthesia, *Arch Ophthalmol* 103:360, 1985.
66. Williams EL, Hart WA, Tempelhoff R: Postoperative ischemic optic neuropathy, *Anesth Analg* 80:1018, 1995.
67. Stein DP, Lederman RJ, Vogt DP, et al: Neurological complications following liver transplantation, *Ann Neurol* 31:644, 1992.
68. Johnson MW, Kincaid MC, Trobe JD: Bilateral retrobulbar optic nerve infarctions after blood loss and hypotension, *Ophthalmology* 94:1577, 1987.
69. Hayreh SS: Anterior ischemic optic neuropathy. VIII. Clinical features and pathogenesis of post-hemorrhagic amaurosis, *Ophthalmology* 94:1488, 1987.
70. Chisholm IA: Optic neuropathy of recurrent blood loss, *Br J Ophthalmol* 53:289, 1969.
71. Aldrich MS, Alessi AG, Beck RW, et al: Cortical blindness: etiology, diagnosis, and prognosis, *Ann Neurol* 21:149, 1987.
72. Alpert JN, Pena Y, Leachman DR: Anterior ischemic optic neuropathy after coronary bypass surgery, *Texas Med* 83:45, 1987.
73. Jaben SL, Glaser JS, Daily M: Ischemic optic neuropathy following general surgical procedures, *J Clin Neuro-ophthalmol* 3:239, 1983.
74. Larkin DFP, Connolly P, Magner JB, et al: Intraocular pressure during cardiopulmonary bypass, *Br J Ophthalmol* 71:177, 1987.
75. Lund PE, Madsen K: Bilateral blindness after cardiopulmonary bypass, *J Cardiothorac Vasc Anesth* 8:448, 1994.
76. Rizzo III JF, Lessel S: Posterior ischemic optic neuropathy during general surgery, *Am J Ophthalmol* 103:808, 1987.
77. Wessels IF: Posterior ischemic optic neuropathy during general surgery, *Am J Ophthalmol* 104:555, 1987.
78. Wong V: Cortical blindness in children: a study of etiology and prognosis, *Pediatr Neurol* 7:178, 1991.
79. Williams IM: Intravascular changes in the retina during open-heart surgery, *Lancet* 2:688, 1971.
80. Alfano JE, Fabritius RE, Garland MA: Visual loss following mitral commisurotomy for mitral stenosis, *Am J Ophthalmol* 44:213, 1957.
81. Gutman FA, Zegarra H: Ocular complications in cardiac surgery, *Surg Clin North Am* 51:1095, 1971.
82. Wortham E, Levin G, Wick HW: Altitudinal anopsia following thoracoplasty, *Arch Ophthalmol* 47:248, 1952.
83. Bradish CF, Flowers M: Central retinal artery occlusion in association with osteogenesis imperfecta, *Spine* 12:193, 1987.
84. Hollenhorst RW, Svien HJ, Benoit CF: Unilateral blindness occuring during anesthesia for neurosurgical operations, *Arch Ophthalmol* 52:819, 1954.
85. Buus DR, Tse DT, Farris BK: Ophthalmic complications of sinus surgery, *Ophthalmology* 97:612, 1990.
86. Cheney ML, Blair BA: Blindness as a complication of rhinoplasty, *Arch Otolaryngol Head Neck Surg* 113:768, 1987.
87. Griffith JD, Smith B: Optic atrophy following Caldwell-Luc procedure, *Arch Ophthalmol* 86:15, 1971.
88. Hollenhorst RW, Wagener HP: Loss of vision after distant hemorrhage, *Am J Med Sci* 219:209, 1950.
89. Maniglia AJ, Chandler JR, Goodwin WJ, et al: Rare complications following ethmoidectomies: a report of eleven cases, *Laryngoscope* 91:1234, 1981.
90. Maniglia AJ: Fatal and major complications secondary to nasal and sinus surgery, *Laryngoscope* 99:276, 1989.
91. Plate S, Asboe S: Blindness as a complication of rhinosurgery, *J Laryngol Otololaryngol* 95:17, 1981.
92. Rettinger G, Christ P, Meythaler FH: Erblindung durch Zentralarterienverschluβ nach Septumkorrektur, *HNO* 38:105, 1990.
93. Sachs SH, Edelstein D, Green RP: Surgical treatment of blindness secondary to intraorbital hemorrhage, *Arch Otolaryngol Head Neck Surg* 114:801, 1988.
94. Savino PJ, Burde RM, Mills RP: Visual loss following intranasal anesthetic injection, *J Clin Neuroophthalmol* 10:140, 1990.
95. Stankiewicz JA. Complications of endoscopic intranasal ethmoidectomy, *Laryngoscope* 97:1270, 1987.
96. Vanden Abeele D, Clemens A, Tassignon M-J, et al: Blindheid ten gevolge van electrocoagulatie na FESS, *Acta Otorhinolaryngol Belg* 48:11, 1994.
97. Whiteman DW, Rosen DA, Pinkerton RMH: Retinal and choroidal microvascular embolism after intranasal corticosteroid injection, *Am J Ophthalmol* 89:851, 1980.
98. Wilson JF, Freeman SB, Breene DP: Anterior ischemic optic neuropathy causing blindness in the head and neck surgery patient, *Arch Otolaryngol Head Neck Surg* 117:1304, 1991.
99. Torti RA, Ballantyne AJ, Houston RG: Sudden blindness after simultaneous bilateral radical neck dissection, *Arch Surg* 88:271, 1964.
100. Nawa Y, Jaques JD, Miller NR, et al: Bilateral posterior optic neuropathy after bilateral radical neck dissection and hypotension, *Graefes Arch Clin Exp Ophthalmol* 230:301, 1992.
101. Milner GAW. A case of blindness after bilateral neck dissection, *J Laryngol* 74:880, 1960.
102. Mazzia VDB, Mark LC, Schrier RI, et al: Blindness after hemorrhage, *N Y State J Med* 62:2549, 1962.
103. Marks SC, Jaques DA, Hirata RM, et al: Blindness following bilateral radical neck dissection, *Head Neck* 12:342, 1990.
104. Kirkali P, Kansu T: A case of unilateral posterior ischemic optic neuropathy after radical neck dissection, *Ann Ophthalmol* 22:297, 1990.
105. Chutkow JG, Sharbrough FW, Riley FC: Blindness following simultaneous bilateral neck dissection, *Mayo Clin Proc* 48:713, 1973.
106. Sharma R, Desai S: Postpartum hemorrhage producing acute ischemic optic neuropathy, *Asia-Oceania J Obstet Gynaecol* 19:249, 1993.
107. Stein LB, Roberts RI, Marx J, et al: Transient cortical blindness following an acute hypotensive event in the postpartum period, *N Y State J Med* 89:682, 1989.
108. Stiller RJ: Postpartum pulmonary embolus as an unusual cause of cortical blindness, *Am J Obstet Gynecol* 162:696, 1990.
109. Weissman A, Peretz BA, Michaelson M, et al: Air embolism following intra-uterine hypertonic saline instillation: treatment in a high-pressure chamber; a case report, *Eur J Obstet Gynecol Reprod Biol* 33:271, 1989.
110. Wisotsky BJ, Engel HM: Transesophageal echocardiography in the diagnosis of branch retinal artery obstruction, *Am J Ophthalmol* 115:653, 1993.
111. Fennell SJ: Cortical blindness following unintended catheterization of the subclavan artery, *J Pediatr* 90:491, 1977.
112. Hayreh SS, Kolder HE, Weingeist TA: Central retinal artery occlusion and retinal tolerance time, *Ophthalmology* 87:75, 1980.
113. Oshitari K, Mashima Y, Imamura Y, et al: T2-weighted fast-spin echo MR imaging of the optic nerve and subarachnoid space around the optic nerve, *Invest Ophthalmol Vis Sci* 36:S677, 1995.
114. Fishman GA, Sokol S: Electrophysiological testing in disorders of the retina, optic nerve, and visual pathway, San Francisco, American Academy of Ophthalmology, 1990 Ophthalmology Monographs.
115. Federman JL, Gouras P, Schubert H, et al: Retina and vitreous. In Podos SM, Yanoff M, eds, *Textbook of ophthalmology*, vol 9, St Louis, 1994, Mosby.
116. Taylor MJ, McCulloch DL: Prognostic value of VEPs in young children with acute onset of cortical blindness, *Pediatr Neurol* 7:111, 1991.

117. Cavallerano RA: Ophthalmic fluorescein angiography, *Optom Clin* 5:1, 1996.

118. Arnold AC, Hepler RS: Fluorescein angiography in acute nonarteritic anterior optic neuropathy, *Am J Ophthalmol* 117:222, 1994.

119. Samadani EE, Rizzuto PR, Tinoosh F, et al: Detection and evaluation of optic nerve sheath fluid with ultrasonography: correlation between 30 degree A scan test and B scan ultrasonography, *Invest Ophthalmol Vis Sci* 36:S677, 1995.

120. Baxter GM, Williamson TH, McKillop G, et al: Color Doppler ultrasound of orbital and optic nerve blood flow: effects of posture and timolol 0.5%, *Invest Ophthalmol Vis Sci* 33:604, 1992.

121. Blauth CI, Arnold JV, Schulenberg WE, et al: Cerebral microembolism during cardiopulmonary bypass, *J Thorac Cardiovasc Surg* 95:668, 1988.

122. Blauth CI, Smith PL, Arnold JV, et al: Influence of oxygenator type on the prevalence and extent of microembolic retinal ischemia during cardiopulmonary bypass, *J Thorac Cardiovasc Surg* 99:61, 1990.

123. Little D: Induced hypotension during anaesthesia and surgery, *Anesthesiology* 16:320, 1955.

124. Aiello LP: Vascular endothelial growth factor: 20th-century mechanisms, 21st-century therapies, *Invest Ophthalmol Vis Sci* 38:1647, 1997.

125. Louzada-Junior P, Dias JJ, Santos WF, et al: Glutamate release in experimental ischaemia of the retina: an approach using microdialysis, *J Neurochem* 59:358, 1992.

126. Mosinger JL, Price MT, Bai HY, et al: Blockade of both NMDA and non-NMDA receptors is required for optimal protection against ischemic neuronal degeneration in the in vivo adult mammalian retina, *Exp Neurol* 113:10, 1991.

127. Zeevalk GD, Nicklas WJ: Chemically induced hypoglycemia and anoxia: relationship to glutamate receptor–mediated toxicity in retina, *J Pharmacol Exp Ther* 253:1285, 1990.

128. Yoon Y, Marmor M: Dextromethorphan protects retina against ischemic injury in vivo, *Arch Ophthalmol* 107:409, 1989.

129. Ostwald P, Goldstein IM, Pachnanda A, et al: Effect of nitric oxide synthase inhibition on blood flow after retinal ischemia in cats, *Invest Ophthalmol Vis Sci* 36:2396, 1995.

130. Ostwald P, Park SS, Toledano AY, et al: Adenosine receptor blockade and nitric oxide synthase inhibition: impact upon blood flow and the electroretinogram following retinal ischemia, *Vision Res* 37:3453, 1997.

131. Roth S: Post-ischemic hyperemia in the retina: the effects of adenosine receptor blockade, *Curr Eye Res* 14:323, 1995.

132. Hughes WF: Quantitation of ischemic damage in the rat retina, *Exp Eye Res* 53:573, 1991.

133. Lin J, Roth S: Retinal hypoperfusion following ischemia in rats depends upon the duration of ischemia, *Invest Ophthalmol Vis Sci* 1999 (in press).

134. Kato H, Araki T, Kogure K, et al: Sequential cerebral blood flow changes in short-term cerebral ischemia in gerbils, *Stroke* 21:1346, 1990.

135. Leffler CW, Busija DW, Mirro R, et al: Effects of ischemia on brain blood flow and oxygen consumption of newborn pigs, *Am J Physiol* 257:H1917, 1989.

136. Samdami AF, Dawson TM, Dawson VL: Nitric oxide synthase in models of focal ischemia, *Stroke* 28:1283, 1997.

137. Hayashi A, Koroma BM, Imai K Jr, et al: Increase of protein tyrosine phosphorylation in rat retina after ischemia-reperfusion injury, *Invest Ophthalmol Vis Sci* 37:2146, 1996.

138. Takagi H, King GL, Robinson GS, et al: Adenosine mediates hypoxic induction of vascular endothelial growth factor in retinal pericytes and endothelial cells, *Invest Ophthalmol Vis Sci* 37:2165, 1996.

139. Takagi H, King GL, Ferrara N, et al: Hypoxia regulates vascular endothelial growth factor receptor KDR/Flk gene expression through adenosine A2 receptors in retinal capillary endothelial cells, *Invest Ophthalmol Vis Sci* 37:1311, 1996.

140. Li B, Roth S: Retinal ischemic preconditioning in the rat: requirement for adenosine and repetitive induction, *Invest Ophthalmol Vis Sci* 40:1200, 1999.

141. Roth S, Li B, Rosenbaum PS, et al: Preconditioning provides complete protection against retinal ischemic injury in rats, *Invest Ophthalmol Vis Sci* 39:775, 1998.

142. Alm A, Bill A: The oxygen supply to the retina. II. Effects of high intraocular pressure and of increased arterial carbon dioxide tension on uveal and retinal blood flow in cats. A study with radioactively labelled microspheres including flow determinations in brain and some tissues, *Acta Physiol Scand* 84:306, 1972.

143. Hayreh SS, Weingast TA: Experimental occlusion of the central retinal artery of the retina. IV. Retinal tolerance time to acute ischaemia, *Br J Ophthalmol* 64:818, 1980.

144. Selles-Navarro I, Villegras-Perez MP, Salvador-Silva M, et al: Retinal ganglion cell death after different transient periods of pressure-induced ischemia and survival intervals, *Invest Ophthalmol Vis Sci* 37:2002, 1996.

145. Grossman W, Ward WT: Central retinal artery occlusion after scoliosis surgery with a horseshoe headrest, *Spine* 18:1226, 1993.

146. Bekar A, Tureyen K, Aksoy K: Unilateral blindness due to patient positioning during cervical syringomyelia surgery: unilateral blindness after prone position, *J Neurosurg Anesthesiol* 8:227, 1996.

147. Gillan JG: Two cases of unilateral blindness following anesthesia with vascular hypotension, *Can Med Assoc J* 69:294, 1953.

148. Givner I, Jaffe N: Occlusion of the central retinal artery following anesthesia, *Arch Ophthalmol* 43:197, 1950.

149. Wolfe SW, Lospinuso MF, Burke SW: Unilateral blindness as a complication of patient positioning for spinal surgery, *Spine* 17:600, 1992.

150. Bolder PM, Norton ML: Retinal hemorrhage following anesthesia, *Anesthesiology* 61:595, 1984.

151. Hepler RS, Sugimura GI, Straatsma BR: On the occurrence of blindness in association with blepharoplasty, *Plast Reconstr Surg* 57:233, 1976.

152. Byers B: Blindness secondary to steroid injections into the nasal turbinates, *Arch Ophthalmol* 97:79, 1979.

153. Evans DE, Zahorchak JA, Kennerdell JS: Visual loss as a result of primary optic nerve neuropathy after intranasal corticosteroid injection, *Am J Ophthalmol* 90:641, 1980.

154. Mabry RL: Visual loss after intranasal corticosteroid injection, *Arch Otolaryngol* 107:484, 1981.

155. McGrew RN, Wilson RS, Havener WH: Sudden blindness secondary to injections of common drugs in the head and neck: I. Clinical experiences, *Otolaryngology* 86:147, 1978.

156. Magargal LE, Sanborn GE, Donoso LA, et al: Branch retinal artery occlusion after excessive use of nasal spray, *Ann Ophthalmol* 17:500, 1985.

157. McGrew RN, Wilson RS, Havener WH: Sudden blindness secondary to injections of common drugs in the head and neck: II. Animal studies, *Otolaryngology* 86:152, 1978.

158. Rosenbaum DM, Rosenbaum PS, Gupta H, et al: An electrophysiological and histopathological comparison of two models to produce ischemia in the intact *in vivo* rat retina, *Invest Ophthalmol Vis Sci* 37(suppl):S676, 1996.

159. Rassam SM, Patel V, Kohner EM: The effect of acetazolamide on the retinal circulation, *Eye* 7:697, 1993.

160. Schumacher M, Schmidt D, Wakhloo AK: Intra-arterial fibrinolytic therapy in central retinal artery occlusion, *Neuroradiology* 35:600, 1993.

161. Faberowski N, Stefansson E, Davidson RC: Local hypothermia protects the retina from ischemia. A quantitative study in the rat, *Invest Ophthalmol Vis Sci* 30:2309, 1989.

162. Wareing TH, Davila-Roman VG, Barzilai B, et al: Management of the severely atherosclerotic ascending aorta during cardiac operations. A strategy for detection and treatment, *J Thorac Cardiovasc Surg* 103:453, 1992.

163. Johnson LJ, Arnold AC: Incidence of nonarteritic and arteritic anterior ischemic optic neuropathy. A population-based study in the state of Missouri and Los Angeles County, California, *J Clin Neuro-ophthalmol* 14:38, 1994.

164. Hayreh SS: In vivo choroidal circulation and its watershed zones, *Eye* 4:273, 1990.

165. Hayreh SS: Anterior ischaemic optic neuropathy. Differentiation of arteritic from nonarteritic type and its management, *Eye* 4:25, 1990.

166. Siatkowski RM, Gass JDM, Glaser JS, et al: Fluorescein angiography in the diagnosis of giant cell arteritis, *Am J Ophthalmol* 115:57, 1993.

167. Potarazu SV: Ischemic optic neuropathy: models for mechanism of disease, *Clin Neurosci* 4:264, 1997.

168. Levin LA, Louhab A: Apoptosis of retinal ganglion cells in anterior ischemic optic neuropathy, *Arch Ophthalmol* 114:488, 1996.

169. Hayreh SS, Zimmerman MB, Podhajsky P, et al: Nocturnal arterial hypotension and its role in optic nerve head and ocular ischemic disorders, *Am J Ophthalmol* 117:603, 1994.

170. Hayreh SS, Joos KM, Podhajsky PA, et al: Systemic disease associated with nonarteritic anterior ischemic optic neuropathy, *Am J Ophthalmol* 118:766, 1994.

171. Lee AG: Ischemic optic neuropathy following lumbar spine surgery, *J Neurosurg* 83:348, 1995.

172. Blauth CI, Cosgrove DM, Webb BW, et al: Atheroembolism from the ascending aorta. An emerging problem in cardiac surgery, *J Thorac Cardiovasc Surg* 103:1104, 1992.

173. Roth S, Roizen MF: Ischemic optic neuropathy: role of the anesthesiologist? *Anesth Analg* 82:435, 1996 (letter).

174. Dilger JA, Tetzlaff JE, Bell GR, et al: Ischaemic optic neuropathy after spinal fusion, *Can J Anaesth* 45:63, 1998.

175. Schobel GA, Schmidbauer M, Millesi W, et al: Posterior ischemic optic neuropathy following bilateral radical neck dissection, *Int J Oral Maxillofac Surg* 24:283, 1995.

176. Strome SE, Hill JS, Burnstine MA, et al: Anterior ischemic optic neuropathy following neck dissection, *Head Neck* 19:148, 1997.

177. Weiskopf RB, Viele MV, Feiner J, et al: Human cardiovascular and metabolic response to acute, severe isovolemic anemia, *JAMA* 279:217, 1998.

178. Neely KA, Ernest JT, Goldstick TK, et al: Isovolemic hemodilution increases retinal oxygen tension, *Graefes Archiv Clin Exp Ophthalmol* 234:688, 1996.

179. Crystal GJ: Myocardial oxygen supply-demand relations during isovolemic hemodilution, *Adv Pharmacol* 31:285, 1994.

180. Hayreh SS: Anterior ischaemic optic neuropathy. III. Treatment, prophylaxis, and differential diagnosis, *Br J Ophthalmol* 58:981, 1974.

181. The Ischemic Optic Neuropathy Decompression Trial Research Group: Optic nerve decompression surgery is not effective and may be harmful, *JAMA* 273:625, 1995.

182. Hayreh SS: Posterior ischemic optic neuropathy, *Ophthalmologica* 182:29, 1981.

183. Bansberg SF: Harner SG, Forbes G: Relationship of the optic nerve to paranasal sinuses, *Otolaryngol Head Neck Surg* 96:331, 1987.

184. Stankiewicz JA: Complications in endoscopic intranasal ethmoidectomy: an update, *Laryngoscope* 99:686, 1989.

185. Flynn JT, Mitchell KB, Fuller DG, et al: Ocular motility complications following intranasal surgery, *Arch Ophthalmol* 97:453, 1979.

186. Mark LE, Kennerdell JS: Medial rectus injury from intranasal surgery, *Arch Ophthalmol* 97:459, 1979.

187. Rosenbaum AL, Astle WF: Superior oblique and inferior rectus muscle injury following frontal and intranasal sinus surgery, *J Pediatr Ophthalmol Strabismus* 22:194, 1985.

188. Hoyt WF, Walsh FB: Cortical blindness with partial recovery following acute cerebral anoxia from cardiac arrest, *Arch Ophthalmol* 60:1061, 1958.

189. McKhann GM, Goldsborough MA, Borowicz LM, et al: Cognitive outcome after coronary artery bypass: a one-year prospective study, *Ann Thorac Surg* 63:510, 1997.

190. Horwitz NH, Wener L: Temporary cortical blindness following angiography, *J Neurosurg* 40:583, 1974.

191. Studdard WE, David DO, Young SW: Cortical blindness after cerebral angiography, *J Neurosurg* 54:240, 1981.

192. Tettenborn B, Caplan LR, Sloan MA, et al: Postoperative brainstem and cerebellar infarcts, *Neurology* 43:471, 1993.

193. Roach GW, Kanchuger M, Mangano CM, et al: Adverse cerebral outcomes after coronary bypass surgery, *N Engl J Med* 335:1857, 1996.

194. Fischer-Williams M, Gottschalk PG: Transient cortical blindness. An unusual complication of coronary aniography, *Neurology* 20:353, 1970.

195. Jørgensen J, Sigurdsson J, Ovesen N: Complications of vertebral arteriography by the Seldinger technique. A survey of 619 cases, *Dan Med Bull* 17:132, 1970.

196. Rama BN, Pagano TV, DelCore M, et al: Cortical blindness after cardiac catheterization: effect of rechallenge with dye, *Cathet Cardiovasc Diagn* 28:149, 1993.

197. Parry R, Russell Rees J, Wilde P: Transient cortical blindness after coronary angiography, *Br Heart J* 70:563, 1993.

198. Silverman SM, Bergman PS, Bender MB: The dynamics of transient cerebral blindness. Report of nine episodes following vertebral angiography, *Arch Neurol* 4:333, 1961.

199. Demirtas M: Transient cortical blindness after second coronary angiography: is an immunological mechanism possible? *Cathet Cardiovasc Diagn* 31:161, 1994.

200. Shyn PB, Bell KA: Transient cortical blindness following cerebral angiography, *J Louisiana State Med Soc* 141:35, 1989.

201. Kermode AG, Chakera T, Mastaglia FL: Low osmolar and nonionic x-ray contrast media and cortical blindness, *Clin Exp Neurol* 29:272, 1992.

202. Siesjö BK: Pathophysiology and treatment of focal cerebral ischemia. II: mechanisms of damage and treatment, *J Neurosurg* 77:337, 1992.

203. Marra TR, Shah M, Mikus MA: Transient cortical blindness due to hypertensive encephalopathy. Magnetic resonance imaging correlation, *J Clin Neuroophthalmol* 13:35, 1993.

204. Makino A, Soga T, Obayashi M, et al: Cortical blindness caused by acute general cerebral swelling, *Surg Neurol* 29:393, 1988.

205. Harris DNF, Bailey SM, Smith PLC, et al: Brain swelling in first hour after coronary artery bypass surgery, *Lancet* 342:586, 1993.

206. Meyendorf R: Psychopatho-ophthalmology, gnostic disorders, and psychosis in cardiac surgery. Visual disturbances after open heart surgery, *Arch Psychiatr Nervenkr* 232:119, 1982.

207. Goto T, Yoshitake A, Baba T, et al: Cerebral ischemic disorders and cerebral oxygen balance during cardiopulmonary bypass surgery: preoperative evaluation using magnetic resonance imaging and angiography, *Anesth Analg* 84:5, 1997.

208. Hartman GS, Yao FS, Bruefach M, et al: Severity of aortic atheromatous disease diagnosed by transesophageal echocardiography predicts stroke and other outcomes associated with coronary artery surgery: a prospective study, *Anesth Analg* 83:701, 1996.

209. Kouchoukos NT, Wareing TH, Daily BB, et al: Management of the severely atherosclerotic aorta during cardiac operations, *J Card Surg* 9:490, 1994.

210. Pugsley W, Klinger L, Paschalis C, et al: The impact of microemboli during cardiopulmonary bypass on neuropsychological functioning, *Stroke* 25:1393, 1994.

211. Nussmeier MA: Adverse neurologic events: risks of intracardiac versus extracardiac surgery, *J Cardiothorac Vasc Anesth* 10:31, 1996.

212. Garfield JM, Garfield FB, Stone JB, et al: A comparison of psychologic responses to ketamine and thiopental–nitrous oxide–halothane anesthesia, *Anesthesiology* 36:329, 1972.

213. Fine J, Weissman J, Finestone SC: Side effects after ketamine anesthesia: transient blindness, *Anesth Analg* 53:72, 1974.

214. Crosby G, Crane AM, Sokoloff L: Local changes in cerebral glucose utilization during ketamine anesthesia, *Anesthesiology* 56:437, 1982.

215. Nelson SR, Howard RB, Cross RS, et al: Ketamine-induced changes in regional glucose utilization in the rat brain, *Anesthesiology* 52:330, 1980.

216. White PF, Way WL, Trevor AJ: Ketamine: its pharmacology and therapeutic uses, *Anesthesiology* 56:119, 1980.

217. Marsch SCU, Schaefer HG: Problems with eye opening after propofol anesthesia, *Anesth Analg* 70:127, 1990.

218. Schaefer HG, Marsch SCU: Am I blind? The fear of a 4-year old boy after total intravenous anaesthesia with propofol, *Paediatr Anaesth* 1:53, 1991.

219. Marsch SCU: External ophthalmoplegia after total intravenous anaesthesia, *Anaesthesia* 49:525, 1994.

220. Boysen K, Sanchez R, Krintel JJ, et al: Induction and recovery characteristics of propofol, thiopental and etomidate, *Acta Anaesthesiol Scand* 33:689, 1989.

221. Purdy EP, Ajimal GS: Vision loss after lumbar epidural steroid injection, *Anesth Analg* 86:119, 1998.

222. Ceccarelli FE, Smith PC: Studies on fluid and electrolyte alterations during transurethral prostatectomy: II, *J Urol* 86:434, 1961.

223. Harrison RH III, Boren JS, Robison JR: Dilutional hyponatriemic shock: another concept of the transurethral prostatic resection reaction, *J Urol* 75:95, 1956.

224. Defalque RJ, Miller DW: Visual disturbances during transurethral resection of the prostate, *Can Anaesth Soc J* 22:620, 1975.

225. Ovassapian A, Joshi CW, Brunner EA: Visual disturbances: an unusual symptom of transurethral prostatic resection reaction, *Anesthesiology* 57:332, 1982.

226. Appelt GL, Benson GS, Corriere JN Jr: Transient blindness: unusual initial symptom of transurethral prostatic resection reaction, *Urology* 13:402, 1979.

227. Creel DJ, Wang JM, Wong KC: Transient blindness associated with transsurethral resection of the prostate, *Arch Ophthalmol* 105:1537, 1987.

228. Kaiser R, Adragna MG, Weis FR, et al: Transient blindness following transurethral resection of the prostate in an achondroplastic dwarf, *J Urol* 133:685, 1985.

229. Mizutani AR, Parker J, Katz J, et al: Visual disturbances, serum glycine levels and transurethral resection of the prostate, *J Urol* 144:697, 1990.

230. Russell D: Painless loss of vision after transurethral resection of the prostate, *Anaesthesia* 45:218, 1990.

231. Agarwal R, Emmett M: The post-transurethral resection of prostate syndrome: therapeutic proposals, *Am J Kidney Dis* 24:108, 1994.

232. Creevy CD: The mortality of transurethral prostatic resection, *J Urol* 65:876, 1951.

233. Hatch PD: Surgical and anaestetic considerations in transurethral resection of the prostate, *Anaesth Intensive Care* 15:203, 1987.

234. Rao PN: Fluid absorption during urological endoscopy, *Br J Urol* 60:93, 1987.

235. Hagstrom RS: Studies on fluid absorption during transurethral prostatic resection, *J Urol* 73:852, 1955.

236. Hahn RG, Ekengren JC: Patterns of irrigating fluid absorption during transurethral resection of the prostate as indicated by ethanol, *J Urol* 149:502, 1993.

237. Stewart PA, Hamilton PA, Barlow IM: Metabolic effects of prostatectomy, *J R Soc Med* 82:725, 1989.

238. Taylor RO, Maxson ES, Carter FH, et al: Volumetric, gravimetric and radioisotopic determination of fluid transfer in transurethral prostatectomy, *J Urol* 79:490, 1958.

239. Gravenstein D: Transurethral resection of the prostate (TURP) syndrome: a review of the pathophysiology and management, *Anesth Analg* 84:438, 1997.

240. Creevy CD, Webb EA: A fatal hemolytic reaction following transurethral resection of the prostate gland, *Surgery* 21:56, 1947.

241. Nesbit RM, Glickman SI: The use of glycine solution as an irrigating medium during transurethral resection, *J Urol* 59:1212, 1948.

242. Hahn RG: Dose-dependent half-life of glycine, *Urol Res* 21:289, 1993.

243. Hoekstra PT, Kahnoski R, McCamish MA, et al: Transurethral prostatic resection syndrome—a new perspective: encephalopathy with associated hyperammonemia, *J Urol* 130:704, 1983.

244. Zucker JR, Bull AP: Independent plasma levels of sodium and glycine during transurethral resection of the prostate, *Can Anaesth Soc J* 31:307, 1984.

245. Roesch RP, Stoelting RK, Lingeman JE, et al: Ammonia toxicity resulting from glycine absorption during a transurethral resection of the prostate, *Anesthesiology* 58:577, 1983.

246. Peters KR, Muir J, Wingard DW: Intraocular pressure after transurethral prostatic surgery, *Anesthesiology* 55:327, 1981.

247. Gilbertson TA, Borges S, Wilson M: The effects of glycine and GABA on isolated horizontal cells from the salamander retina, *J Neurophysiol* 66:2002, 1991.

248. Schneider SP, Fyffe REW: Involvement of GABA and glycine in recurrent inhibition of spinal motoneurons, *J Neurophysiol* 68:397, 1992.

249. Korol S, Leuenberger PM, Englert U, et al: In vivo effects of glycine on retinal ultrastructure and averaged electroretinogram, *Brain Res* 97:235, 1975.

250. Wang JML, Creel DJ, Wong KC: Transurethral resection of the prostate, serum glycine levels, and ocular evoked potentials, *Anesthesiology* 70:36, 1989.

251. Wang JM, Wong KC, Creel DJ, et al: Effects of glycine on hemodynamic responses and visual evoked potentials in the dog, *Anesth Analg* 64:1071, 1985.

252. Mantha S, Rao SM, Singh AK, et al: Visual evoked potentials and visual acuity after transurethral resection of the prostate, *Anaesthesia* 46:491, 1991.

253. Frink EJ, DiGiovanni DA, Davis JR, et al: Serum ammonia levels in response to glycine infusion in normal and cirrhotic rats, *Anesth Analg* 69:776, 1989.

254. Slaughter MM, Miller RF: Characterization of serine inhibitory action on neurons in the mudpuppy retina, *Neuroscience* 41:817, 1991.

255. Sunderrajan S, Bauer JH, Vopat RL, et al: Posttransurethral prostatic resection hyponatremic syndrome: case report and review of the literature, *Am J Kidney Dis* 4:80, 1984.

256. Arieff AI, Llach F, Massry SG: Neurological manifestations and morbidity of hyponatremia: correlation with brain water and electrolytes, *Medicine* 55:121, 1976.

257. Zigman S: Ocular light damage, *Photochem Photobiol* 57:1060, 1993.

258. Anonymous: Laser energy and its dangers to eyes, *Health Devices* 22:159, 1993.

259. Cowan CL: Light hazards in the operating room, *J Natl Med Assoc* 84:425, 1992.

260. Sliney DH: Laser safety, *Lasers Surg Med,* 16:215, 1995.

261. Lam TT, Tso MM: Retinal injury by neodymium: YAG laser, *Retina* 16:42, 1996.

262. Occupational Safety and Health Administration, US Dept of Labor: *Guidelines for laser safety and hazard assessment.* #8-1.7 O.I.P. 1991.

263. Michels M, Sternberg P: Operating microscope-induced retinal phototoxicity: pathophysiology, clinical manifestations and prevention, *Surv Ophthalmol* 34:237, 1990.

264. Jaffe GJ, Irvine AR, Wood IS, et al: Retinal phototoxicity from the operating microscope: the role of inspired oxygen, *Ophthalmology* 95:1130, 1988.

265. Flynn JT, Sola A, Good WV, et al: Screening for retinopathy of prematurity: a problem solved? *Pediatrics* 95:755, 1995.

266. Jacobson RM, Feinstein AR: Oxygen as a cause of blindness in premature infants: "autopsy" of a decade of errors in clinical epidemiologic research, *J Clin Epidemiol* 65:1265, 1992.

267. Robinson J, Fielder AR: Light and the immature visual system, *Eye* 6:166, 1992.

268. Bucher HU, Fanconi S, Baeckert P: Hyperoxemia in newborn infants: detection by pulse oximetry, *Pediatrics* 84:226, 1989.

269. Donlon JV: Anesthesia for eye, ear, nose and throat surgery. In Miller RD, ed: *Anesthesia,* ed 4, vol 2, New York, 1994, Churchill Livingstone.

270. Adelman BT: Altered taste and smell after anesthesia: cause and effect? *Anesthesiology* 83:647, 1995 (letter).

271. Henkin RI: Altered taste and smell after anesthesia: cause and effect? *Anesthesiology* 83:648, 1995 (reply).

Chapter 18

Immunologic Complications

Jerrold H. Levy
Mette Veien
Michael E. Weiss

Among the many adverse events that can occur in the perioperative period, immunologic complications are important causes of morbidity and mortality. Anaphylaxis is the most life-threatening of these complications and requires immediate intervention. In 1902, Portier and Richet coined the word *anaphylaxis* when they noted that a second sublethal injection of a sea anemone extract, which had produced minimal effects after first injection, caused dogs to die of profound shock. Thus the term was initially used to describe a phenomenon in which repeated exposure to a foreign protein produced an adverse reaction rather than the intended immunization or prophylaxis (i.e., *ana*, "against," *phylaxis*, "protection").

The different terms used to describe immunologic mechanisms can be confusing. Allergic reactions or hypersensitivity reactions are best defined as untoward physiologic events triggered by immune processes.[1]

When we speak of an immunologic reaction, we mean the interaction of a foreign antigen with an immunospecific antibody or sensitized lymphocyte. When the antigen bridges cell surface immunoglobulin E (IgE) antibodies, the antibodies undergo conformational changes resulting in mediator release that may produce inflammation in the host.[1] This inflammation produces pathophysiologic changes in the cardiopulmonary, vascular, cutaneous, and gastrointestinal systems.[1] It should be emphasized that these inappropriate reactions are the same as those produced as part of normal host defense immunosurveillance.

More than 80 years after the original description, we now understand that classic anaphylaxis is a clinical syndrome produced by an IgE antibody–mediated reaction, resulting in immediate, severe alterations in the cutaneous (urticaria or angioedema), respiratory (bronchospasm, laryngeal edema, increased secretions), gastrointestinal (nausea, vomiting, abdominal pain, diarrhea), or cardiovascular (vasodilation, tachycardia, cardiovascular collapse) systems.[1] The same clinical manifestations may occur consequent to non–IgE-mediated, direct drug–mediated, or complement-mediated reactions and have previously been called anaphylactoid reactions.[1]

I. CLASSIFICATION OF ALLERGIC REACTIONS

Gell and Coombs[2] classified four types of immunopathologic reactions, to which can be added a fifth: idiopathic type. Types I, II, and III depend on different classes of antibodies and are immediate reactions, whereas type IV depends on T-lymphocytes and is known as a delayed hypersensitivity reaction. It should be noted that some pharmacologic agents, such as penicillin, can cause all the reactions described here (Table 18-1).

A. Type I reactions: immediate hypersensitivity

Type I reactions result from the interaction of antigens with preformed antigen-specific IgE antibodies from previous exposure that are bound to tissue mast cells or circulating basophils by high-affinity IgE receptors. Cross-linking two or more IgE receptors by antigen liberates both preformed and newly generated mediators, resulting in constriction of the bronchioles and bronchi, contraction of smooth muscle, and dilation of capillaries, which produce urticaria, laryngeal edema, and bronchospasm with or without cardiovascular collapse. Examples of type I reactions are atopic allergies, classic penicillin allergy, and bee sting (Hymenoptera) reactions.

B. Type II reactions: cytotoxic antibodies

Type II reactions result when IgG or IgM antibody reacts with a cell-bound antigen (that is, blood group antigens, penicillin determinants bound to red blood cells). The antigen-antibody interaction activates the complement system, resulting in cell lysis. Type II reactions may also be complement independent. IgG or IgM antibody may bind to cell membrane–bound antigen. Neutrophils or macrophages may then attach to the antibody through their Fc receptors, and this opsonization can result in injury to the antigen-laden cell. Examples of type II reactions include ABO-incompatible transfusion reactions, drug-induced autoimmune hemolytic anemia or thrombocytopenia, Rh disease of the newborn, and Goodpasture syndrome.

C. Type III reactions: immune complexes (Arthus reaction)

Type III reactions are similar to type II, but the antigens are not cell-bound. Instead, circulating complexes are formed between antigens and antigen-specific IgG and IgM antibodies. The complexes lodge in tissue sites, fix complement, and attract polymorphonuclear leukocytes, which attempt to phagocytize the immune complexes. The release of proteolytic enzymes from the phagocytic cells results in tissue damage. Immune complex reactions typically appear 7 to 14 days after continual exposure to antigen, such as a persistent infection, autoimmunity to self-components, or repeated exposure to environmental agents. Examples include serum sickness glomerulonephritis, farmer's lung, and possibly drug fever.

D. Type IV reactions: cell-mediated hypersensitivity

Type IV reactions are not mediated by an antibody but rather by T-lymphocytes that are specifically sensitized to recognize a particular antigen. After being modified by antigen-processing cells (i.e., macrophages or Langerhans cells), the modified antigen is presented, in association with major histocompatibility (MHC) class II molecules, to the T-lymphocyte. The sensitized T-lymphocyte recognizes the processed antigen through an antigen-specific T-cell receptor. This triggers the T-cell to release substances, known as cytokines, that orchestrate the immune response by recruiting and stimulating proliferation of other lymphocytes and mononuclear cells, which ultimately cause tissue inflammation and in-

Table 18-1. Characterization of immune mechanisms

	Type I	Type II	Type III	Type IV
Mechanisms	Immediate IgE-mediated hypersensitivity	Cytotoxic IgG or IgM antibody	Circulating IgG or IgM antibody antigen complexes	T-lymphocyte–mediated delayed hypersensitivity
	Antigens bind to specific IgE antibodies on sensitized mast cells, resulting in mediator release	Antibody reacts with a cell-bound antigen, resulting in cell lysis	Circulating antibody-antigen complexes are deposited in tissue, resulting in cellular destruction	Sensitized T-lymphocytes release cytokines, resulting in cellular damage
Time course	Minutes	Hours	Hours to days	Days
Examples	Atopic allergies Systemic allergies	ABO-incompatible transfusion reactions Rh disease of the newborn	Glomerulonephritis Farmer's lung	Tuberculin skin testing Graft versus host disease
Penicillin reactions	Urticaria Systemic anaphylaxis	Hemolytic anemia	Serum sickness	Contact dermatitis

jury. Examples of cell-mediated immune reactions are tuberculin skin testing, contact dermatitis (as from poison ivy), and graft versus host disease.

E. Idiopathic reactions

The immunologic pathogenesis of some reactions is unclear and they are considered to be idiopathic. Examples include eosinophilia, Stevens-Johnson syndrome, exfoliative dermatitis, and maculopapular eruptions.

II. MEDIATOR RELEASE

Anaphylaxis is produced by mast cell or basophil release of vasoactive mediators, and represents the most important clinical example of an allergic reaction because of its potential for sudden onset with catastrophic outcome. Tissue mast cells or circulating basophils may be triggered to release their mediators by both IgE anaphylactic reactions and non-IgE mechanisms (anaphylactoid reactions). The various mechanisms inducing mediator release are considered next.

A. IgE-mediated anaphylaxis (type I reaction)

Foreign molecules capable of stimulating IgE antibody production may cause IgE-mediated anaphylaxis on re-

exposure. Some drugs or macromolecules are complete antigens and can stimulate an immune response by themselves (e.g., protamine), whereas other low-molecular-weight substances called haptens (e.g., penicillin) must form a stable bond to serum proteins to become complete antigens capable of stimulating antibody production.[3] IgE antibodies, once produced, become fixed to tissue mast cells or circulating basophils, both of which contain high-affinity IgE receptors.[4] This attachment takes place at the Fc region of the IgE molecule, which allows the antigen binding (Fab) region of the IgE antibody to bind antigen. Reexposure to antigens or haptens that are functionally multivalent (have two or more antigenic sites) is required to cross-link IgE antibodies bound to mast cells or basophils. Cross-linking of IgE antibodies causes the direct bridging of IgE receptor molecules on mast cell and basophil cell membranes, which induces activation of membrane-associated enzymes, causing complex biochemical cascades that lead to an influx of extracellular calcium and a mobilization of intracellular calcium, with subsequent release of preformed granule-associated mediators and the generation of new mediators from cell membrane phospholipids[5,6] (Fig. 18-1). Examples of IgE antibody–mediated allergic

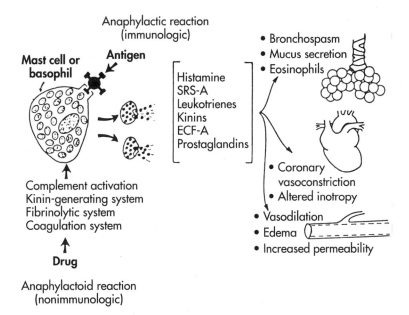

Fig. 18-1. Summary of the pathophysiologic changes producing anaphylactic and anaphylactoid reactions. Anaphylactic reactions *(upper left):* The allergen enters the body and combines with allergen-specific IgE antibodies on the surface of mast cells and basophils. This interaction causes mast cell and basophil activation, releasing vasoactive mediators (histamine, leukotrienes, kinins, eosinophilic chemotactic factor of anaphylaxis [ECF-A], prostaglandins, and others). The release of these substances may cause the signs and symptoms of anaphylaxis, that is, bronchospasm; pharyngeal, glottic, and pulmonary edema; vasodilation; hypotension; alterations in cardiac contractility and arrhythmias; subcutaneous edema; and urticaria. Anaphylactoid reactions *(lower left):* The offending agent enters the body and works by nonimmunologically activating systems that cause degranulation of mast cells and basophils or activation of other humoral amplification systems. The systems that can be activated to cause release of mediators from basophils and mast cells include the complement system, the coagulation and fibrinolytic system, and the kinin-generating system. Activation of these systems can result in the release of the same mediators from basophils and mast cells and can result in a syndrome that is clinically indistinguishable from anaphylaxis. (From Levy JH, Roizen MF, Morris JM: *Spine* 11:282, 1986.)

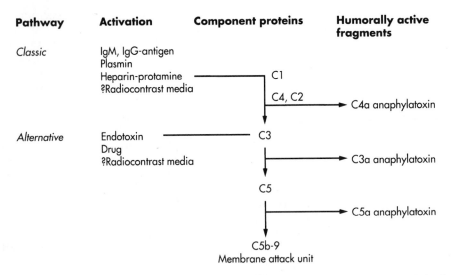

Pathway	Activation	Component proteins	Humorally active fragments

Classic   IgM, IgG-antigen
Plasmin
Heparin-protamine ——————— C1
?Radiocontrast media

    C4, C2 ————→ C4a anaphylatoxin

Alternative   Endotoxin ——————— C3
Drug
?Radiocontrast media

    C3 ————→ C3a anaphylatoxin

    C5

    C5 ————→ C5a anaphylatoxin

    C5b-9
    Membrane attack unit

Fig. 18-2. Complement activation pathways, the involved component proteins, and the humorally active fragments. (Modified from Levy JH: *Anaphylactic reactions in anesthesia and intensive care,* ed 2, Stoneham, Mass, 1992, Butterworth-Heinemann.)

reactions include those induced by insulin, chymopapain, muscle relaxants, and penicillin (hapten).

B. Anaphylactoid reactions

1. Complement-mediated reactions. Activation of the complement system results in generation of a membrane attack unit and the liberation of low-molecular-weight peptides C3a, C4a, and C5a, known as the anaphylatoxins[7] (Fig. 18-2). The anaphylatoxins are capable of causing mast cell and basophil mediator release, directly increasing vascular permeability, contracting smooth muscles, aggregating platelets, and stimulating macrophages to produce thromboxane[7,8] (see Fig. 18-1). The complement cascade may be activated through the classical pathway or the alternative pathway. Complement activation through the classical pathway can be initiated through IgG or IgM antibody binding to antigens, as in hemolytic ABO-incompatible blood transfusion reactions. Heparin-protamine complexes have also been shown in vitro[9] and in vivo[10,11] to activate complement by the classical pathway. Injection of preformed immune complexes or IgG aggregates can activate complement and mimic clinical anaphylaxis.[12] Patients lacking IgA antibody may develop IgG anti-IgA antibodies after receiving multiple transfusions, which may result in complement activation and anaphylactic reactions.[13] Complement activation by the alternative pathway may be stimulated by cell membranes from gram-negative or gram-positive bacteria (endotoxin or exotoxin),[14] cell wall products from fungi (zymosan),[14] Althesin,[15] radiocontrast media,[16] and membranes used for cardiopulmonary bypass and dialysis.[17]

2. Pharmacologic (nonimmunologic) mast cell activators. A variety of unrelated molecules and endogenous neuropeptides can release histamine by a non-immunologic mechanism (see Fig. 18-1). The pathophysiology of nonimmunologic mediator release is not well understood, but does not require previous exposure to the drug, is dose dependent, and can be produced by certain molecular structures. Drugs that induce nonimmunologic release include the opiates (morphine, meperidine, codeine),[18,19] benzylisoquinoline-derived neuromuscular blocking agents (*d*-tubocurarine, metocurine, atracurium),[20] and vancomycin. Although less common, true allergic reactions to the neuromuscular blocking agents can also release multiple mast cell mediators by means of IgE antibodies directed against quaternary or tertiary ammonium ion epitopes characteristic of all muscle relaxants.[21-23]

C. Mediators from mast cells or basophils

Mast cell or basophil activation releases both preformed mediators that are stored in the granules and newly generated mediators after immunologic activation. The released mediators cause various pathophysiologic responses that may result in life-threatening clinical manifestations. The various preformed and newly generated mediators released by mast cells or basophils and their biologic actions and physiologic manifestations are complex (Table 18-2). However, nonimmunologic activation results only in release of preformed mediators.

III. CLINICAL MANIFESTATIONS OF ANAPHYLAXIS

The time of onset and manifestations of anaphylaxis can vary. The clinical manifestations can range from minimal changes in blood pressure to life-threatening cardiopulmonary collapse. Usually signs and symptoms begin within minutes after parenteral injection of the causative agent, but they may be delayed for up to 2 hours after oral administration. The primary targets of anaphylaxis in humans are the cutaneous, gastrointestinal, respiratory, and cardiovascular systems and the signs and symptoms are described here and in Table 18-3.

Table 18.2. Biologic actions and clinical manifestations of mast cell or basophil mediators, both preformed and newly synthesized

Mediators	Biologic actions	Clinical manifestations
Preformed		
Histamine	Smooth muscle relaxation	Vasodilation, hypotension
	Smooth muscle contraction	Bronchospasm, coronary spasm, increased gastrointestinal motility
	Increases capillary permeability	Angioedema, urticaria, influx of inflammatory cells
	Positive inotropic	Increased contractility
	Positive chronotropic	Tachycardia
Eosinophilic chemotactic factor of anaphylaxis	Eosinophil chemotaxis	Inflammation
Neutrophilic chemotactic factor	Neutrophil chemotaxis	Inflammation
Neutral proteases	Proteolysis	Inflammation
Heparin	Anticoagulant	Coagulopathy
Newly synthesized		
Prostaglandin D_2	Smooth muscle relaxation	Vasodilation, hypotension
	Smooth muscle contraction	Bronchospasm, coronary spasm, increased gastrointestinal motility
	Stimulates mucus secretion	Bronchorrhea, rhinorrhea
	Enhances basophil mediator release	Potentiates reactions
	Inhibits platelet aggregation	
Leukotrienes (C_4, D_4, E_4)	Smooth muscle relaxation	Vasodilation, hypotension
	Smooth muscle contraction	Bronchospasm, coronary spasm, increased gastrointestinal motility
	Increases capillary permeability	Angioedema, urticaria, influx of inflammatory cells
	Stimulates mucus secretion	Bronchorrhea, rhinorrhea
	Negative inotropic	Myocardial depression, hypotension
Platelet activating factor	Smooth muscle relaxation	Vasodilation, hypotension
	Smooth muscle contraction	Bronchospasm, coronary spasm, increased gastrointestinal motility
	Increases capillary permeability	Angioedema, urticaria, influx of inflammatory cells
	Neutrophil aggregation	Neutrophil activation
	Platelet aggregation	Platelet activation

Table 18-3. Recognition of anaphylaxis during anesthesia

Systems	Symptoms	Signs
Respiratory	Dyspnea, chest discomfort	Coughing, wheezing, sneezing, laryngeal edema, decreased pulmonary compliance, fulminant pulmonary edema, acute respiratory distress
Cardiovascular	Dizziness, malaise, retrosternal oppression	Disorientation, diaphoresis, loss of consciousness, hypotension, tachycardia, or arrhythmias, decreased systemic vascular resistance, cardiac arrest, pulmonary hypertension
Cutaneous	Itching, burning	Urticaria (hives), flushing, periorbital edema, perioral edema

From Levy JH: *Anaphylactic reactions in anesthesia and intensive care,* Stoneham, Mass, 1992, Butterworth-Heinemann.

A. Cardiovascular manifestations

Cardiovascular complications include varying degrees of hypotension to cardiovascular collapse, atrial and ventricular arrhythmias, myocardial ischemia and infarction, and right ventricular dysfunction. Symptoms include light-headedness, faintness, and a sense of impending doom.

B. Respiratory manifestations

Upper respiratory tract involvement may include laryngeal edema, which may progress to asphyxia. Early symptoms of laryngeal edema include hoarseness, dysphonia, stridor, or sensations of a "lump in the throat." Lower respiratory tract involvement is often indicated by chest tightness, shortness of breath, cough, or wheezing.

C. Cutaneous manifestations

Initial signs and symptoms may include erythema, flushing, and pruritus (especially of the palms, soles, and groin), which often progress to urticaria and angioedema. Angioedema refers to edema in serosal, mucosal, and other vascular-rich tissues that can produce obstruction of the glottis and larynx.

D. Gastrointestinal manifestations

Gastrointestinal findings include nausea, cramping, abdominal pain, vomiting, and severe diarrhea, which may be bloody.

Other signs and symptoms reported in anaphylaxis include nasal, ocular, and palatal pruritus, sneezing, diaphoresis, disorientation, and incontinence. Some patients redevelop manifestations of anaphylaxis 8 to 24 hours after successful resuscitation (late-phase responses). In a large study of numerous fatal anaphylactic reactions caused by bee stings, 70% of the deaths were ascribed to respiratory complications and 24% to cardiovascular complications.[24] However, cardiovascular collapse accounted for 80% of anaphylactic reactions to perioperative anesthetic agents.

E. Intraoperative and perioperative anaphylaxis

The diagnosis and treatment of patients who develop anaphylaxis in the operating room is difficult, even for the experienced physician. In the perioperative period, multiple medications are often given either simultaneously or in rapid succession, making temporal relationships more difficult to interpret. In addition, patients often are unconscious and draped, potentially masking early signs and symptoms of anaphylaxis.[25] Anesthetics themselves have been shown in vitro to alter mediator release, possibly delaying early recognition of the syndrome.[26] Often the only observable manifestation of anaphylaxis occurring during anesthesia is cardiovascular collapse,[27] a late event in the syndrome. In suspected anaphylactic reactions in patients undergoing hemodynamic monitoring, cardiovascular changes were characterized by decreases in systolic, diastolic, and mean arterial pressure.[27] Systemic vascular resistance also decreased, and cardiac output and stroke volume increased.[27] Sudden decreases in pulmonary compliance

and increases in airway resistance may be manifested by an increase in airway pressures during positive-pressure ventilation. Cardiovascular collapse accounts for 80% of anaphylactic reactions to perioperative anesthetic agents.

F. Differential diagnosis

In the awake patient, anaphylaxis is most easily confused with a vasovagal reaction, which may occur after an injection or the onset of intense pain. In vasovagal reactions, the patient looks pale and complains of nausea before syncope. Respiratory difficulty does not occur, and symptoms are almost immediately relieved once the patient is supine. The syndrome is usually accompanied by profuse diaphoresis and bradycardia, without flushing, urticaria, angioedema, pruritus, or wheezing. A differential diagnosis of sudden collapse perioperatively may also include arrhythmia, myocardial infarction, and pulmonary or air embolism.

In the presence of laryngeal edema, especially when accompanied by abdominal pain, the diagnosis of hereditary angioedema should be considered. When respiratory symptoms are present, globus hystericus and fictitious asthma are included in the differential diagnosis.

Other conditions that can mimic anaphylaxis include sedation from analgesics, overdose of vasodilators, or inadvertent discontinuation of vasopressors, cold urticaria (especially if generalized), idiopathic urticaria, carcinoid tumors, and systemic mastocytosis.

IV. SPECIFIC ALLERGIC REACTIONS SEEN BY THE ANESTHESIOLOGIST

Almost any drug may produce an anaphylactic reaction.[28-126] However, some drugs have been implicated more often than others or have been investigated in greater detail. We consider the drugs most often suspected of causing life-threatening anaphylactic reactions and discuss their pathophysiology.

A. Antibiotics

1. Penicillins. Of all the medications capable of causing allergic drug reactions, penicillin antibiotics are the most frequent offenders. Various studies report an incidence of 0.7% to 0.8% of allergic reactions to penicillin.[67] Anaphylaxis occurs in 0.004% to 0.015% of penicillin treatment cases.[67] Fatality from penicillin anaphylaxis occurs about once in every 50,000 to 100,000 treatment cases,[67] causing approximately 400 to 800 deaths per year.[68] Penicillin can produce all four types of immunopathologic reaction described by Gell and Coombs,[2] including anaphylaxis (type I), penicillin-induced hemolysis (type II), serum sickness (type III), and contact dermatitis (type IV). Some reactions to penicillin have an obscure pathogenesis and have been labeled idiopathic. Among these are the common maculopapular rash, eosinophilia, Stevens-Johnson syndrome, exfoliative dermatitis, and toxic epidermal necrolysis. For unknown reasons, ampicillin induces rashes with much greater frequency than penicillin does.[34,69] Pseudoanaphylactic reactions have been observed after intramuscular or inadvertent intravenous injection of procaine penicillin, most likely because of a combination of toxic and embolic phenomena from the procaine.[70]

Penicillin has a low molecular weight (356 Da) and must first covalently combine with tissue macromolecules (presumably serum albumin) to produce multivalent hapten-protein complexes, which are required for both sensitization (with production of immunospecific antibodies) and elicitation of an allergic reaction.[71] Levine[72] showed that the β-lactam ring in penicillins spontaneously opens under certain physiologic conditions, forming the penicilloyl group. Recent evidence indicates that this reaction may be facilitated by low-molecular-weight molecules in serum.[73] The penicilloyl group has been designated the major determinant because about 95% of the penicillin molecules irreversibly combine with proteins from penicilloyl groups.[3] This reaction occurs with the prototype benzylpenicillin and with virtually all semisynthetic penicillins. Benzylpenicillin can also be degraded by other metabolic pathways to form additional antigenic determinants.[74] These derivatives are formed in small quantities and stimulate a variable immune response and thus have been called the minor determinants. Therefore IgE antibodies can be produced against several haptenic derivatives of the major and minor determinants to penicillin and other β-lactams. Anaphylactic reactions to penicillin are usually mediated by IgE antibodies directed against minor determinants, although some anaphylactic reactions have occurred in patients with only penicilloyl-specific IgE antibodies.[3,74,75,84] Accelerated and late urticarial reactions are generally mediated by penicilloyl-specific IgE antibody (major determinant).[3]

Parenteral administration of penicillin produces more allergic reactions than oral administration of penicillin does.[63] Recent evidence indicates that this difference may be more related to dose than to route of administration. When equivalent doses of penicillin are given orally, the incidence of allergic reactions is comparable to that of intramuscularly administered procaine penicillin.[76] Patients with a history of penicillin reactions have a fourfold to sixfold higher risk of subsequent reactions to penicillin than those without such histories.[77] However, most serious and fatal allergic reactions to penicillin and β-lactam antibiotics occur in patients who have never had an allergic reaction to these drugs. Sensitization of these patients may have occurred from a previous therapeutic course of penicillin.

Approximately 10% to 20% of hospitalized patients claim a history of penicillin allergy. However, studies have shown that many of these patients have been incorrectly labeled as allergic to penicillin or have lost their sensitivity to it. The most useful piece of information in the assessment of a person's potential for an immediate IgE-mediated reaction is the skin test response to major and minor penicillin determinants.[121] Radioallergosorbent tests (RASTs) have been developed to detect IgE antibodies to the penicilloyl determinant.[55] At present, there is no in vitro RAST for minor determinant antibodies. Therefore RASTs and other in vitro analogs have limited clinical utility.

2. Cephalosporins. Cephalosporins have a β-lactam ring like penicillins, but the five-membered thiazolidine ring of penicillin is replaced by the six-membered dihydrothiazine ring of cephalosporins. Shortly after the cephalosporins came into clinical use, allergic reactions, including anaphylaxis, were reported, and the question of cross-reactivity between cephalosporins and penicillins was raised.[78] Studies in both animals and humans have clearly demonstrated cross-reactivity between penicillins and cephalosporins using immunoassays and bioassays to evaluate IgG, IgM, and IgE antibodies.[79-81] Primary cephalosporin allergy in non–penicillin-allergic patients has been reported, but the exact incidence is not clear.[82,83] Studies have been limited because the haptenic determinants involved in cephalosporin allergy are unknown. The exact incidence of clinically relevant cross-reactivity between the penicillins and the cephalosporins is unknown and probably small, but anaphylactic cross-reactivity has occurred.[84]

3. Vancomycin. Hypotension is the most serious adverse effect associated with intravenous vancomycin. Non–immunologically mediated histamine release[20,88] has been reported recently as the mechanism of vancomycin-induced hypotension. Hypotension occurs when the drug is infused rapidly or when it is administered in a concentrated solution.[20,87] Vancomycin can produce the red-neck syndrome, or red-man's syndrome, characterized by pruritus and an intense erythematous discoloration of the upper trunk, arms, and neck. To minimize the risk of histamine release, vancomycin should be infused over a period of at least 60 minutes and in a dilute solution (500 mg/dl). Hypotension should be treated by discontinuance of the vancomycin infusion and by volume and vasopressor administration.

B. Muscle relaxants

The benzylisoquinoline-derived muscle relaxants, such as *d*-tubocurarine, metocurine, atracurium, doxacurium, and mivacurium, produce nonimmunologic histamine release.[27] However, Vervloet et al[23,48] and Baldo and colleagues[21,22] have also demonstrated IgE-mediated anaphylactic reactions to muscle relaxants. Evidence supporting an IgE-mediated mechanism includes positive passive transfer tests, basophil histamine release studies, inhibition of basophil histamine release after desensitization to anti-IgE, and the demonstration of drug-specific IgE antibodies in sera from patients who have had adverse reactions to muscle relaxants.[21-23,48] It appears that IgE antibodies are directed against the quaternary or tertiary ammonium ions present in muscle relaxants.[21] Extensive in vitro cross-reactivity has been reported between the muscle relaxants and other compounds that contain quaternary and tertiary ammonium ions.[21] These compounds occur widely in drugs, foods, cosmetics, disinfectants, and industrial materials. The clinical significance of this in vitro cross-reactivity is unclear, although it has been postulated that patients may become sensitized through environmental contact with these various compounds.[21] Because the muscle relaxants contain two ammonium ions, they appear to be functionally divalent, capable of cross-linking cell surface IgE and initiating mediator release from mast cells and basophils without haptenating to carrier molecules.[48] Molecules with ammonium ions 0.4 nm apart or closer appear incapable of inducing histamine release, whereas the optimal length for cross-linking cell-surface IgE appears to be 0.6 nm or more.[89] Muscle relaxants with a rigid backbone between the two ammonium ions (i.e., pancuronium and vecuronium) appear to be less likely than flexible molecules (i.e., atracurium, succinylcholine) in initiating mediator release.[89]

Atopy does not appear to be a risk factor for the occurrence of anaphylactic reactions to muscle relaxants.[90] It is of interest that 90% to 95% of anaphylactic reactions to muscle relaxants occur in females.[91] The reason for this is unclear. However, sensitization to ammonium ion epitopes in cosmetics has been postulated to explain the predominance of reactions in women.[21]

Skin testing and RAST can be used to evaluate the presence of IgE antibody directed against muscle relaxants.[21,35,66] However, more studies are needed to determine the predictive value of these tests.

C. Barbiturates

Anaphylaxis has been reported after thiobarbiturate administration, most often associated with thiopental.[27] Proposed mechanisms for thiobarbiturate reactions include non–immunologically induced mediator release and IgE-mediated reactions.[27] Positive skin tests to thiopental have been reported in patients who have had anaphylactic reactions after induction of general anesthesia.[35,92] Recently a thiopental RAST has been reported,[56] but the value of skin testing and RAST in predicting reactions to thiopental is uncertain at present.

D. Local anesthetics

Despite the fact that patients commonly report adverse reactions to local anesthetics and are advised that they are "allergic" to these agents, true allergic reactions to injected local anesthetics are rare. Reactions to local anesthetics are often the result of vasovagal changes, toxic reactions (probably because of inadvertent intravenous injection), side effects from epinephrine, or psychomotor responses, including hyperventilation. Toxic symptoms often involve the central nervous and cardiovascular systems and may produce slurred speech, euphoria, dizziness, excitement, nausea, emesis, disorientation, or convulsions.[93] Vasovagal reactions are usually associated with bradycardia, sweating, pallor, and rapid improvement in symptoms when the patient is supine. Sympathetic stimulation, either from epinephrine or anxiety, may result in tremor, diaphoresis, tachycardia, or hypertension. Rarely, symptoms of reaction to local anesthetics are consistent with IgE-mediated reactions such as urticaria, bronchospasm, and anaphylactic shock. However, acceptable documentation of IgE-mediated reactivity against local anesthetics in such patients is almost totally lacking.[94] IgE-mediated sensitivity has also been reported, though rarely, for methylparaben, which is a preservative used in local anesthetics.[95] Local anes-

thetics are divided into two chemical groups: group I comprises chemicals containing benzoate esters, which may cross-react with each other but not with group II drugs, and group II agents include mostly amides, which do not cross-react substantially with each other.

Evaluation of a patient with a history of adverse reaction to local anesthetics should include a complete history of the episode and skin testing, along with incremental drug challenge.[93,94] The local anesthetic tested should be one that is appropriate for the proposed procedure and that would not be expected to cross-react with the drug implicated in the previous reaction. If the previous drug is unknown, a group II anesthetic (probably lidocaine) should be chosen. In a patient with a history suggestive of methylparaben sensitivity, preparations without paraben should be used for testing, challenge, and treatment. Preparations without epinephrine should be used for skin testing because epinephrine may mask a positive skin test[96] and may induce toxic effects.

E. Opioids

Morphine, meperidine, and codeine are the cause of non-immunologically mediated histamine release from cutaneous mast cells.[18] In vitro studies indicate that the cutaneous mast cell is uniquely sensitive to opioids and that neither the gastrointestinal nor the lung mast cell nor the circulating basophil releases histamine when exposed to these agents.[97] Most histamine-induced reactions are self-limiting reactions, restricted to hives and pruritus, or hypotension treated by fluid administration. However, anaphylaxis induced by meperidine, fentanyl, and morphine has been documented.[98-100] IgE antibodies can be induced, which bind epitopes contained in opiates.[98-100]

F. Radiocontrast media

The incidence of reactions induced by radiocontrast media injections is between 5% and 8%.[16] Vasomotor reactions (nausea, vomiting, flushing, or warmth) occur in 5% to 8% of patients.[16] Anaphylactoid reactions (urticaria, angioedema, wheezing, dyspnea, hypotension, or death) occur in 2% to 3% of patients receiving intravenous or interarterial infusions.[65] Most reactions occur 1 to 3 minutes after intravascular administration. Fatal reactions after radiocontrast media administration occur in about 1:50,000 intravenous procedures,[65] and it has been estimated that as many as 500 deaths per year are attributable to reactions to radiocontrast media. The cause or causes of adverse reactions to radiocontrast media are unknown at present, but different mechanisms have been considered. Histamine liberation appears to be a feature of some reactions,[16] although elevations in plasma histamine have occurred without hemodynamic changes or anaphylactic reactions.[16] Activation of serum complement occurs after the intravascular injection of radiocontrast media[16] and may occur by the classical or alternative pathway. Therefore it has been suggested that production of anaphylatoxins, with subsequent mast cell and basophil mediator release, is the cause of radiocontrast media reactions. Yet radiocontrast media is capable of inducing nonimmunologic histamine release from mast cells and basophils in the absence of complement activation.[16] It has been suggested that the hypertonicity of radiocontrast media results in nonimmunologic mediator release from mast cells and basophils.[16] Although it appears clear that the vasomotor reactions (pain, nausea, vomiting, and warmth) as well as histamine release in vitro are caused by hyperosmolarity, it is unclear whether hyperosmolarity is the cause of all radiocontrast media reactions in humans. There is no evidence that IgE-mediated mechanisms play a role in radiocontrast media reactions.

A patient who requires radiocontrast media administration and who has had a previous anaphylactoid reaction to it has an increased (35% to 60%) risk for a reaction on reexposure.[16] Pretreatment of these high-risk patients with prednisone (50 mg) 13 hours, 7 hours, and 1 hour before radiocontrast media administration, along with diphenhydramine (50 mg) 1 hour before radiocontrast media administration, reduces the risk of reactions to 9%.[101] Almost all reactions in pretreated patients are so mild as to be of no clinical importance (that is, mild urticaria).[16] The addition of ephedrine (25 mg) 1 hour before radiocontrast media administration (in patients without angina, arrhythmia, or other contraindications for ephedrine) resulted in a reaction rate of 3.1%.[16] It might be expected that the addition of an H_2-receptor antagonist, such as cimetidine or ranitidine, would further decrease the incidence of radiocontrast media reactions, but no study has shown a benefit from the addition of H_2-receptor antagonists to radiocontrast media pretreatment regimens. A recent study showed that steroid pretreatment before the administration of hyperosmolar radiocontrast media is as effective as and much less expensive than the use of recent nonhyperosmolar radiocontrast media.[102]

G. Protamine

Protamine sulfate is a polycationic, strongly basic small protein with a molecular weight of 4000 to 5000 Da. Protamine is extracted from salmon sperm in a protein purification process and is used medicinally to reverse heparin anticoagulation and to retard the absorption of certain insulins, namely, neutral protamine Hagedorn (NPH) and protamine zinc insulin. The use of intravenous protamine has increased in the last decade with the advent of cardiopulmonary bypass technology, cardiac catheterization, and hemodialysis. This increase in intravenous protamine use has resulted in more frequent reports of adverse reactions.

A spectrum of adverse reactions to intravenous protamine administration has been described, including rash, urticaria, bronchospasm, pulmonary vasoconstriction, and systemic hypotension leading at times to cardiovascular collapse and death.[103-105] Diabetic patients receiving daily subcutaneous injections of insulin containing protamine have a thirtyfold to fiftyfold greater risk for life-threatening reactions when given protamine intravenously.[103-105] The actual risk for anaphylactic reactions in NPH insulin-dependent diabetics is 0.6% to 2%.[104,105] Another group putatively at increased risk for protamine

reactions is men who have undergone vasectomies. With disruption of the blood-testis barrier, studies have shown that 20% to 33% of such men develop hemagglutinating autoantibodies against protamine-like compounds.[106] It has been postulated that these autoantibodies may cross-react with medicinal protamine, causing adverse reactions.[107] Although protamine reactions in vasectomized men have been reported,[108] Levy et al[105] did not observe any clinical reactions in a prospective evaluation of 16 vasectomized patients undergoing cardiac surgery with protamine reversal of heparin. Fish-allergic patients may also be at potential risk for protamine reactions. Because protamine is produced from the matured testis of salmon or a related species of fish belonging to the family Salmonidae or Clupeidae, it has been suggested that patients allergic to fish may have serum antibodies directed against protamine. On the other hand, commercial protamine preparations may be contaminated with fish proteins that fish-allergic patients may react to. Evidence supporting the increased risk of protamine reactions in fish-allergic patients is lacking and is limited to case reports.[108] Levy et al[105] did not observe any clinical reactions to protamine in six patients with a history of fish allergy after cardiac surgery. Finally, previous exposure to intravenous protamine given for reversal of heparin anticoagulation may increase the risk of a reaction on subsequent protamine administration.[116]

The exact mechanisms by which acute protamine reactions occur are incompletely understood. Protamine may be able to cause direct, nonimmunologic release of histamine in mast cells in vitro.[122] Protamine is also 70% arginine by weight, and may increase the formation of nitric oxide by providing substrate 6 or vascular endothelium.[123] Some protamine reactions may be associated with complement activation, either through protamine-heparin complexes[9-11,111] or through protamine and complement fixing, and antiprotamine IgG antibody interaction.[112] These reactions may lead to increased pulmonary artery pressure and have been associated with the generation of thromboxane, a pulmonary vasoconstrictor.[113,114] Recent evidence indicates that protamine may inhibit the action of plasma carboxypeptidase N, which cleaves the C-terminal arginine residue from the anaphylatoxins and bradykinin, converting them to their less active *des arg* metabolites.[115]

Lakin et al[112] provided evidence that protamine-specific IgG antibodies could cause protamine reactions by activating complement, whereas others[116,117] have also reported the presence of protamine-specific IgE antibodies in small numbers of protamine reactors. Weiss et al,[58] in a case control study, showed that in diabetic patients who had received previous protamine insulin injections, the presence of antiprotamine IgE antibody was a significant risk factor for acute protamine reactions, as was the presence of antiprotamine. In patients without prior exposure to protamine insulin injections, antiprotamine IgG antibody was also a risk factor for protamine reactions.[58] It appears that in protamine insulin–dependent diabetic patients, antibody-mediated mechanisms are the likely cause for the increased risk of protamine reactions seen in this group. Prescreening high-risk patients (protamine insulin–dependent diabetics) for the presence of antiprotamine antibodies before elective procedures that would involve the administration of intravenous protamine might be worthwhile. If such antibodies are present, special precautions could be taken or alternative heparin antagonists, such as hexadimethrine, could be substituted.[118]

Skin testing with protamine does not appear to be useful in discriminating between subjects with significant serum antiprotamine IgE antibody and control subjects.[124,125] It has been suggested that protamine may be an incomplete or univalent antigen that first must combine with a tissue macromolecule, or possibly heparin, to become a complete, multivalent antigen capable of eliciting mediator release. Thus it appears likely that more than one mechanism may be responsible for the adverse reactions associated with protamine.[126]

H. Chymopapain

Chymopapain is injected intradiskally for chemonucleolysis of herniated lumbar intervertebral disks. The incidence of anaphylaxis to chymopapain is about 1%, whereas the incidence of fatal anaphylaxis appears to be about 0.14%.[37] Women appear to be three times more likely to develop anaphylaxis than men.[106] Chymopapain is obtained from a crude fraction, called papain, that is extracted from the papaya tree and may be found in meat tenderizers, cosmetics, beer, and soft contact lenses.[17] Evidence indicates that chymopapain reactions may be IgE mediated.[37,65] Both in vivo skin tests and in vitro immunoassays have been used to detect antichymopapain IgE antibody,[37] but more studies are required to determine the predictive value of these tests.

I. Mannitol

The administration of mannitol or other hyperosmotic agents may cause direct, nonimmunologic histamine release from circulating basophils and mast cells.[27] There is no evidence that mannitol causes immunologically mediated reactions. It is believed that slow infusion helps to avoid this problem.

J. Methylmethacrylate

Methylmethacrylate (bone cement) is used during orthopedic surgery to attach a prosthetic joint to raw bone. Cardiopulmonary complications from the use of methylmethacrylate include hypotension, hypoxemia, noncariogenic pulmonary edema, and cardiac arrest. Many reasons have been postulated for these physiologic manifestations, none of which implicate mechanisms that are allergic in nature.[1]

K. Latex

For the anesthesiologist, certain environmental agents typical of hospital settings (i.e., latex) are also important causes of anaphylaxis, and health care workers, children with spina bifida, and urogenital abnormalities have also been recognized as having increased risk for anaphylaxis to latex.[26-28] Because latex is such a ubiquitous environmental antigen, avoidance of latex can be difficult. During operations, surgical gloves are in repeated and intense contact with mucous membranes and open wounds. Tissue barriers are destroyed, and blood and secretions provide an environment in which latex may be eluted from the gloves and absorbed. This may explain why some patients develop localized cutaneous reactions when wearing rubber gloves but react with severe anaphylaxis during surgical, gynecologic, or dental procedures. The relative rarity of anaphylaxis to latex despite the presence of rubber products in daily life suggests that long-standing and repeated contact is necessary for sensitization to occur. Latex allergy should be suspected if unexpected anaphylactic reactions occur after the start of surgical procedures without obvious temporal relationships to drug or blood product administration. Because of the increasing awareness of latex allergy and growing numbers of patients reported to have reactions, it is extremely important that latex sensitivity be included in the preoperative evaluation in all health care workers and in rescue and support personnel (e.g., firefighters, police officers). The important symptoms of itching, hives or rashes, or difficulty breathing (i.e., wheezing) after wearing latex gloves, inflating toy balloons, or other exposure to latex may be important. The most important preventive therapy is to avoid antigen exposure.

V. TREATMENT OF ANAPHYLAXIS

Anaphylactic reactions must be recognized immediately because death may occur within minutes.[1] The longer initial therapy is delayed, the greater is the incidence of death.[24] Because anaphylactic reactions are associated primarily with acute cardiovascular and respiratory dysfunction, close monitoring of hemodynamics, including heart rate and blood pressure, as well as airway patency and ventilation, is most important in assessing the severity of the reaction and the response to therapy. Treatment of anaphylactic reactions can be divided into initial and secondary therapies and is discussed here. Therapy must be titrated to clinical effect (Box 18-1).

A. Initial therapy

First, steps should be taken to interrupt further drug administration, when possible, and decrease absorption of the offending agent. Intravenous infusions of suspected allergens should be stopped immediately. If the antigen has been given subcutaneously (that is, insulin or immunotherapy), a venous tourniquet should be placed proximally to the site and 0.01 ml/kg aqueous epinephrine 1:1000 (maximal dose 0.3 to 0.5 ml) should be injected directly into the antigen source to reduce the local circulation and systemic absorption of antigen.

Second, maintain the airway and administer 100% oxygen; adequate oxygenation should be monitored using pulse oximetry or arterial blood gases. If the patient is not already intubated and there is any suggestion of airway compromise secondary to laryngeal edema, the patient should be intubated immediately. If laryngospasm or laryngeal edema is present, epinephrine, either aerosolized (three inhalations of 0.16 to 0.20 mg

---

Box 18-1 Management of anaphylaxis

Initial therapy
1. Stop administration of antigen.
2. Maintain airway with 100% oxygen.
3. Discontinue all anesthetic agents.
4. Start intravascular volume expansion (2 to 4 L crystalloid with hypotension).
5. Give epinephrine (5 to 10 μg IV bolus with hypotension, titrate as needed; 0.1 to 0.5 mg IV with cardiovascular collapse).

Secondary treatment
1. Administer antihistamines (0.5 to 1 mg/kg diphenhydramine).
2. Administer catecholamine infusions (starting doses: epinephrine 5 to 10 μg/min, norepinephrine 5 to 10 μg/min, as an infusion, titrated to desired effect).
3. Administer aminophylline (5 to 6 mg/kg over 20 minutes for persistent bronchospasm).
4. Administer corticosteroids (0.25 to 1 g hydrocortisone or 1 to 2 mg/kg methylprednisolone; methylprednisolone may be the drug of choice if one suspects that the reaction is mediated by complement).
5. Administer sodium bicarbonate (0.5 to 1 mEq/kg with persistent hypotension or acidosis).
6. Evaluate airway (before extubation).

From Levy JH: *Anaphylactic reactions in anesthesia and intensive care,* Stoneham, Mass, 1992, Butterworth-Heinemann.

---

epinephrine per inhalation) or nebulized (8 to 15 drops 2.25% epinephrine in 2 ml normal saline) may be useful. If laryngospasm or laryngeal edema is refractory to these measures or is progressing too rapidly, a catheter cricothyrotomy or emergency surgical cricothyrotomy may be necessary.

Third, discontinue all anesthetic agents because they have negative inotropic properties and may interfere with the reflex compensatory response to shock. Halothane also sensitizes the heart to catecholamines, which may be required for resuscitation.

Fourth, rapid intravenous volume administration of 25 to 50 ml/kg (2 to 4 L in an adult) of isotonic crystalloid (lactated Ringer's or normal saline) or colloidal solutions is important in the initial shock therapy. Military antishock trousers (MAST suit) can be useful in patients suffering hypotension secondary to anaphylaxis.[29,30] The MAST suit provides perfusion to vital organs and may be helpful in obtaining peripheral venous access in the upper extremities.[30]

Fifth, epinephrine is the mainstay of initial treatment and should be given intravenously. The α-adrenergic effects constrict vascular capacitance and arterial resistance vessels, the β$_1$-adrenergic effects increase contractility, and the β$_2$-adrenergic effects function as bronchodilators and may attenuate mast cell activation. The exact dose depends on the clinical condition and common sense. In cases of severe hypotension, an initial dose of 0.05 to 0.1

ml 1:10,000 epinephrine (100 μg/ml) should be given intravenously and increased until blood pressure improves. Depending on the patient's condition, a higher dose may be needed, especially in the patient who is partially sympathectomized after spinal or epidural anesthesia.[31] If an intravenous line is not in place, 0.5 ml 1:1000 epinephrine can be given intramuscularly or 10 ml 1:10,000 epinephrine can be administered through the endotracheal tube. However, in a patient in shock, the absorption of intramuscular or subcutaneous epinephrine is unreliable.

B. Secondary treatment

Once a patient's condition has begun to stabilize, administration of other pharmacologic agents may be warranted. First, an antihistamine, such as diphenhydramine (1 mg/kg, up to 50 mg), given either intravenously or intramuscularly, is helpful for symptomatic relief of itching. Although there is no evidence demonstrating the effectiveness of H$_2$-receptor antagonists in the treatment of anaphylaxis, ranitidine (1 mg/kg intravenously) may be useful in combination with an H$_1$-receptor antagonist when hypotension is persistent because peripheral vasodilation may be exacerbated by the effects of histamine on endothelial H$_2$-receptors.

Second, for persistent hypotension, catecholamine infusions may be used. Epinephrine may be useful if both hypotension and bronchospasm persist. Suggested starting doses of epinephrine are 0.05 to 0.1 μg/kg/min (5 to 10 μg/min), which should be titrated to increase blood pressure. If high doses are required, tachycardia may be a significant side effect, in which case norepinephrine may be a more effective alternative. Suggested starting dose for norepinephrine is 0.05 to 0.1 μg/kg/min (5 to 10 μg/min), titrated to maintain systemic perfusion pressure.

Third, if bronchospasm persists, inhaled β$_2$-catecholamine administration, with terbutaline or isoetharine, should be given. Aminophylline 5 to 6 mg/kg administered over 20 minutes may be useful, but has a complex series of effects.

Fourth, glucocorticoids may be useful in preventing potential late-phase reactions but will have no immediate effect. Hydrocortisone 5 mg/kg (up to a 200-mg initial dose) and then 2.5 mg/kg every 6 hours, or methylprednisolone 1 mg/kg initially and every 6 hours for the first 24 hours, may be given. If the reaction is suspected of being complement mediated, higher doses of methylprednisolone may be given.

Fifth, if acidosis is suspected, sodium bicarbonate (0.5 to 1 mg/kg) should be administered initially. Acid-base status must be monitored by use of arterial blood gas concentrations to guide further therapeutic interventions.

Sixth, before extubation the airway should be evaluated for patency, especially if the patient has developed angioedema.

Despite all the preceding measures, some patients may be refractory to therapy. In one study in which the efficacy of immunotherapy for insect sting allergy was assessed by deliberate sting challenge, investigators found that even when they were totally prepared to treat anaphylaxis in an intensive care unit setting, severe persistent hypotension occurred that was difficult to treat despite repeated doses of intravenously administered epinephrine.[32] During spinal or epidural anesthesia, patients may be partially sympathectomized and require larger doses of epinephrine. Treatment of anaphylaxis may also be complicated by the increased use of β-adrenergic receptor blocking agents.[33] Treatment of the patient with persistent bronchospasm, pulmonary hypertension, or right ventricular failure can be complex and require additional therapeutic interventions with appropriate hemodynamic monitoring. In patients with refractory shock, transesophageal echocardiography is an important tool to help evaluate the cause of the hypotension.

VI. DETERMINING THE CAUSE OF ALLERGIC REACTIONS

Patients who have had anaphylactic reactions to drugs administered in the operating room require evaluation to identify the causal agents and to guide selection and use of future medications.

A. Detailed history

Evaluation should start with a detailed history, including any concurrent illness or prior allergic or anesthetic encounters.[120] The patient's reaction should be reviewed carefully to determine the temporal relationship between the clinical manifestations of the reaction and the medications received, including indications, when initiated, dosage, and duration of therapy. Equally important information is previous exposure to the same or structurally related medications, effect of drug discontinuation, response to treatment, and any prior diagnostic testing or rechallenge. Medications should be considered with regard to their known propensity for causing anaphylaxis. The proximity of drug administration to the onset of acute reactions should also be documented. In general, agents that have been used for long, continuous periods of time before the onset of an acute reaction are less likely to be implicated than agents recently introduced or reintroduced. However, in the perioperative period, it is common for patients to receive many medications in temporal proximity, making a diagnosis more difficult by history alone.

B. Immunodiagnostic tests

1. *Skin testing for immediate hypersensitivity reactions.* Skin testing is a standardized procedure commonly used by allergists to diagnose immediate hypersensitivity to pollens and bee stings. However, evaluating anesthetic drug allergy is complicated by the unavailability of relevant drug metabolites or appropriate multivalent testing reagents. Intradermal skin tests are still the most readily available and generally useful diagnostic tests for drug allergy. Skin testing has an established role in the evaluation of IgE-mediated penicillin allergy,[34] and it is also useful in the evaluation of allergy to muscle relaxants,[23,35] barbiturates,[35,36] chymopapain,[37] streptokinase,[38] insulin,[39] and miscellaneous other drugs. Specific

protocols for skin testing are well documented[40,41] but are not discussed in detail here.

For safety, a scratch or puncture (epicutaneous) test should be performed before the more definitive intradermal test.[41] When one is skin testing with drugs or reagents that have not been well validated previously, all positive skin test responses should be confirmed by skin testing of five normal subjects with the same drug concentration as an appropriate control for irritative, false positive skin responses. Appropriate skin test concentrations of medications commonly used in anesthesia practice have been published.[23,42] It is prudent to discount negative skin test results unless prior studies have established their reliability. Skin testing must be done in the absence of medications that will affect the skin test response (especially H_1-antihistamines, tricyclic antidepressants, and sympathomimetic agents). Appropriate positive (histamine or morphine) and negative (diluent) controls should be used.

2. *In vitro tests*

a. *Total serum IgE concentrations.* Although increased total serum IgE concentrations have been reported after allergic reactions,[43] the concentration of total IgE is rarely if ever helpful in establishing the diagnosis of an allergic drug reaction.

b. *Complement activation.* Assays to measure complement activation include measuring decreases in complement components (that is, C4, C3, or total hemolytic complement [CH50]) and assays to measure the generation of products of complement activation (C3a, C4a, C5a, and so forth). If positive, these assays may implicate complement activation in specific reactions.

c. *Release of histamine and other mediators by basophils and mast cells.* Washed leukocytes comprising 1% to 2% basophils with IgE antibody on their cell surfaces degranulate and release histamine and other mediators when incubated with relevant antigens.[44] In general, results appear to correlate with the results of the direct immediate skin test.[45,46] Although the in vitro basophil histamine release assay avoids exposing a patient to a drug, the assay is time-consuming and requires whole blood drawn immediately before the test, and its availability is limited. Leukocyte histamine release has been used to demonstrate sensitivity to thiopental,[47] muscle relaxants,[23,48] and penicillins.[49]

d. *Measurements of tryptase and other mediators.* During or shortly after allergic reactions, blood may be obtained and analyzed for the release of various mediators such as histamine, prostaglandin D_2 (PGD_2), or high-molecular-weight neutrophil chemotactic factor.[32,50] Urine may also be analyzed for metabolites of histamine or PGD_2. Plasma histamine and PGD_2 concentrations remain elevated only briefly, limiting their clinical utility. Tryptase (a protease released specifically from mast cells) is important in the clinical assessment of mast cell–mediated allergic reactions.[51] Serum tryptase has a half life of 2 hours in serum, is considered to be a specific mast cell marker, and is useful in determining the causes of unexplained shock.

e. *Radioallergosorbent testing.* A solid-phase radioimmunoassay, called the radioallergosorbent test (RAST), was first introduced in 1967. The RAST measures circulating allergen-specific IgE antibody, and its basic principle is quite simple. Allergen is attached to a solid phase (carbohydrate particle, paper disk, or the wall of a polystyrene test tubes or plastic microtiter wells) and incubated with serum under study, during which time specific antibody of all immunoglobulin classes is bound. The particles are then washed, and a second incubation is undertaken with a radiolabeled, highly specific anti-IgE antibody. After washes, the bound radioactivity is directly related to the allergen-specific IgE antibody content in the original serum. Results from the serum under study are compared to a positive reference serum and a negative control serum. When appropriately done, RAST correlates well with skin test end-point titration, basophil histamine release, and provocation tests.[45,52-54] Application of the RAST to the diagnosis of a drug hypersensitivity attributable to IgE antibody has been limited because of insufficient knowledge of the drug metabolite acting as antigen or hapten. In 1971, a RAST was developed to measure IgE antibody to the major determinant of penicillin,[55] and more recently RASTs have been developed to measure IgE antibody to insulin,[39] chymopapain,[37] muscle relaxants,[21,22] thiopental,[56] trimethoprim,[57] and protamine.[58] False positive test results may occur because of large nonspecific binding, high total serum IgE concentrations, or poor technique.[59] False negative results may occur because of interference of high concentrations of IgG blocking antibodies or inability to maximize assay sensitivity.[60]

In recent years, the commercialization of the RAST has led to abuses. Some commercial laboratories have offered RAST for testing numerous substances not known to cause IgE-mediated allergic disease (that is, local anesthetics and radiocontrast media). Relying on misleading information from such inappropriate RASTs should be discouraged.

f. Measurement of specific IgG or IgM antibodies. Except for drug-induced (i.e., heparin-induced) thrombocytopenia, hemolytic anemia, and agranulocytosis, there often is little correlation between the presence of antigen-specific IgG and IgM antibodies and the occurrence of an allergic drug reaction. Recent evidence indicates that certain protamine reactions are mediated through protamine-specific IgG antibody.[58]

VII. TREATMENT OF THE ALLERGIC PATIENT

If a patient has a history of an allergic reaction to a specific medication but requires its use again, the physician must weigh the risks and benefits of using that medication. If an equally effective, non–cross-reacting alternative is available, it should be used. If alternative drugs are unavailable, induce unacceptable side effects, or are clearly less effective, cautious administration of the offending drug, with use of a premedication regimen or a desensitization protocol, may be considered.

Premedication regimens have been tested, validated, and used primarily in patients who have had previous reactions to ionic radiocontrast agents and who again require procedures using radiocontrast.[16] However, there is little evidence supporting the use of premedication regimens to prevent IgE-mediated anaphylaxis, and premedication with antihistamines or steroids is not recommended for reactions mediated by IgE antibodies.[61,62] Desensitization protocols have been developed and used in patients with acute allergic reactions to penicillin,[63,64] insulin,[65] sulfonamides,[66] and heterologous antisera.[65] In general, desensitization protocols use the initial administration of low doses (usually 1:10,000 of a conventional dose) of the suspect drug. Oral or parenteral doses are usually doubled every 15 to 30 minutes, and full doses are usually achieved within 4 to 8 hours, although longer intervals often are needed for aspirin desensitization. Desensitization should be performed only by an appropriately trained physician in an intensive care setting. Desensitization usually is not practical for the anesthesiologist.

VIII. EFFECTS OF ANESTHESIA ON IMMUNE RESPONSES

Patients undergoing both anesthesia and surgery develop depressions of both T-cell–mediated and B-cell–mediated lymphocyte responsiveness as well as depression of nonspecific host resistance mechanisms, including phagocytosis.[119] A spectrum of anesthetic drugs have been shown in vitro to decrease immune responses; however, the effects are short lived and may be modified by multiple other factors such as increases in stress responses that occur perioperatively.[119] Immune competence during surgery can be affected by direct and hormonal effects of anesthetic drugs, immunologic consequences of other drugs used, type of surgery, and coincidence infections. Although multiple studies demonstrate in vitro alterations of immune function, no studies have ever demonstrated the actual clinical significance or actual importance.[119] Furthermore, they are likely to be of minor importance when compared with the general systemic hormonal aspects of stress responses and their abilities to depress immune function transiently.

REFERENCES

1. Levy JH: *Anaphylactic reactions in anesthesia and intensive care,* ed 2, Stoneham, Mass, 1992, Butterworth-Heinemann.
2. Gell PGH, Coombs RRA: Classification of allergic reactions responsible for clinical hypersensitivity and disease. In Gell PGH, Coombs RRA, Hachmann PJ, eds: *Clinical aspects of immunology,* Oxford, 1975, Blackwell Scientific.
3. Levine BB: Immunologic mechanisms of penicillin allergy: a haptenic model system for the study of allergic diseases of man, *N Engl J Med* 275:1115, 1966.
4. Metzger H, Alcaraz G, Hohman R, et al: The receptor with high affinity for immunoglobulin E, *Ann Rev Immunol* 4:419, 1986.
5. Ishizaka T: Mechanisms of IgE-mediated hypersensitivity. In Middleton E Jr, Reed CE, Ellis EF, et al, eds: *Allergy: principles and practice,* ed 3, St Louis, 1988, Mosby.
6. Siraganian RP: Histamine secretion from mast cells and basophils, *Trends Pharmacol Sci* 4:432, 1983.
7. Ghebrehiwet B: The complement system: mechanisms of activation, regulation, and biological functions. In Kaplan AP, ed: *Allergy,* New York, 1985, Churchill Livingstone.

8. Yancey KB, Hammer CH, Harvath L, et al: Studies of human C5a as a mediator of inflammation in normal human skin, *J Clin Invest* 75:486, 1985.
9. Rent R, Ertel N, Eisenstein R, et al: Complement activation by interaction of polyanions and polycations. I. Heparin-protamine induced consumption of complement, *J Immunol* 114:120, 1975.
10. Kirklin JK, Chenoweth DE, Naftel DC, et al: Effects of protamine administration after cardiopulmonary bypass on complement, blood elements, and the hemodynamic state, *Ann Thorac Surg* 41:193, 1986.
11. Best N, Sinosich MJ, Teisner B, et al: Complement activation during cardiopulmonary bypass by heparin-protamine interaction, *Br J Anaesth* 56:339, 1984.
12. Wasserman SI, Marquardt DL: Anaphylaxis. In Middleton E Jr, Reed CE, Ellis EF, et al, eds: *Allergy: principles and practice*, ed 3, St Louis, 1988, Mosby.
13. Vyas GN, Perkins HA, Fundenberg HH: Anaphylactoid transfusion reactions associated with anti-IgA, *Lancet* 2:312, 1968.
14. Frank MM: Complement: a brief review, *J Allergy Clin Immunol* 84:411, 1988.
15. Watkins J, Clark A, Appleyard TN, et al: Immune mediated reactions to althesin (alphaxalone), *Br J Anaesth* 55:231, 1976.
16. Greenberger PA: Contrast media reactions, *J Allergy Clin Immunol* 74:600, 1984.
17. Craddock PR, Fehr J, Brigham KL, et al: Complement and leukocyte-mediated pulmonary dysfunction in hemodialysis, *N Engl J Med* 296:769, 1977.
18. Levy JH, Brister NW, Shearin A, et al: Wheal and flare responses to opioids in humans, *Anesthesiology* 70:756, 1989.
19. North FC, Kettlekamp N, Hirshman CA: Comparison of cutaneous and in vitro histamine release by muscle relaxants, *Anesthesiology* 66:543, 1987.
20. Levy JH, Kettlekamp N, Goertz P, et al: Histamine release by vancomycin: a mechanism for hypotension in man, *Anesthesiology* 67:122, 1987.
21. Baldo BA, Fisher MM: Substituted ammonium ions as allergenic determinants in drug allergy, *Nature* 306:262, 1983.
22. Harle DG, Baldo BA, Fisher MM: Detection of IgE antibodies to suxamethonium after anaphylactoid reactions during anaesthesia, *Lancet* 1:930, 1984.
23. Vervloet D, Nizankowska E, Arnaud A, et al: Adverse reactions to suxamethonium and other muscle relaxants under general anesthesia, *J Allergy Clin Immunol* 71:552, 1983.
24. Barnard JH: Studies of 400 Hymenoptera sting deaths in the United States, *J Allergy Clin Immunol* 52:259, 1973.
25. Laxenaire MC, Moneret-Vautrin DA, Boileau S, et al: Adverse reactions to intravenous agents in anaesthesia in France, *Klin Wochenschr* 60:1006, 1982.
26. Moneret-Vautrin DA, Laxenaire MC, Bavoux F: Allergic shock to latex and ethylene oxide during surgery for spina bifida, *Anesthesiology* 73:556, 1990.
27. Gold M, Swartz JS, Braude BM, et al: Intraoperative anaphylaxis: an association with latex sensitivity, *J Allergy Clin Immunol* 87:662, 1991.
28. Holzman RS: Latex allergy: an emerging operating room problem, *Anesth Analg* 76: 635, 1993.
29. Bickell WH, Dice WH: Military antishock trousers in a patient with adrenergic-resistant anaphylaxis, *Ann Emerg Med* 13:189, 1984.
30. Loehr MM: Suit up against anaphylaxis, *Emerg Med* April 1985, p 127.
31. Levy JH: Cardiovascular changes during anaphylactic/anaphylactoid reactions in man, *J Clin Anesth* 1:426, 1989.
32. Smith PL, Kagey-Sobotka A, Bleecker ER, et al: Physiologic manifestations of human anaphylaxis, *J Clin Invest* 66:1072, 1980.
33. Jacobs RL, Geoffrey WR Jr, Fournier DC, et al: Potentiated anaphylaxis in patients with drug-induced beta-adrenergic blockade, *J Allergy Clin Immunol* 68:125, 1981.
34. Weiss ME, Adkinson NF Jr: Immediate hypersensitivity reactions to penicillin and related antibiotics, *Clin Allergy* 18:515, 1988.
35. Fisher MM: Intradermal testing in the diagnosis of acute anaphylaxis during anaesthesia: results of five years' experience, *Anaesth Intensive Care* 7:58, 1979.
36. Moscicki RA, Sockin SM, Corsello BF, et al: Anaphylaxis during induction of general anesthesia: subsequent evaluation and management, *J Allergy Clin Immunol* 86:325, 1990.
37. Grammer LC, Patterson R: Proteins: chymopapain and insulin, *J Allergy Clin Immunol* 74:635, 1984.
38. Dykewicz MS, McGrath KG, Davison R, et al: Identification of patients at risk for anaphylaxis due to streptokinase, *Arch Intern Med* 146:305, 1986.
39. Hamilton RG, Rendell M, Adkinson NF Jr: Serological analysis of human IgG and IgE anti-insulin antibodies by solid-phase radioimmunoassays, *J Lab Clin Med* 96:1022, 1980.
40. Norman PS: Skin testing. In Rose NR, Friedman H, Fahey JL, eds: *Manual of clinical laboratory immunology*, ed 3, Washington, DC, 1986, American Society for Microbiology.
41. Adkinson NF Jr: Tests for immunological drug reactions. In Rose NF, Friedman H, Fahey JL, eds: *Manual of clinical immunology*, ed 3, Washington, DC, 1986, American Society for Microbiology.
42. Fisher M: Intradermal testing after anaphylactoid reaction to anaesthetic drugs: practical aspects of performance and interpretation, *Anaesth Intensive Care* 12:115, 1984.
43. Etter MS, Helrich M, Mackenzie CF: Immunoglobulin E fluctuation in thiopental anaphylaxis, *Anesthesiology* 52:181, 1980.
44. Lichtenstein LM, Osler AG: Studies on the mechanisms of hypersensitivity phenomena. IX. Histamine release from leukocytes by ragweed pollen antigen, *J Exp Med* 120:507, 1964.
45. Norman PS, Lichtenstein LM, Ishizaka K: Diagnostic tests in ragweed hay fever: a comparison of direct skin tests, IgE antibody measurements, and basophil histamine release, *J Allergy Clin Immunol* 52:210, 1973.
46. Bruce CA, Rosenthal RR, Lichtenstein LM, et al: Diagnostic tests in ragweed-allergic asthma: a comparison of direct skin tests, leukocyte histamine release, and quantitative bronchial challenge, *J Allergy Clin Immunol* 53:230, 1974.
47. Hirshman CA, Peters J, Cartwright-Lee I: Leukocyte histamine release to thiopental, *Anesthesiology* 56:64, 1982.
48. Vervloet D, Arnaud A, Senft M, et al: Leukocyte histamine release to suxamethonium in patients with adverse reactions to muscle relaxants, *J Allergy Clin Immunol* 75:338, 1985.
49. Pienkowski MM, Kazmier WJ, Adkinson NF Jr: Basophil histamine release remains unaffected by clinical desensitization to penicillin, *J Allergy Clin Immunol* 82:171, 1988.
50. Atkins PC, Norman M, Weiner H, et al: Release of neutrophil chemotactic activity during immediate hypersensitivity reactions in humans, *Ann Intern Med* 86:415, 1977.
51. Schwartz LB, Metcalfe DD, Miller JS, et al: Tryptase levels as an indicator of mast-cell activation in systemic anaphylaxis and mastocytosis, *N Engl J Med* 316:1622, 1987.
52. Council on Scientific Affairs: In vitro testing for allergy. Report II of the Allergy Panel, *JAMA* 258:1639, 1987.
53. Plaut M, Lichtenstein LM, Henney CS: Properties of a subpopulation of T cells bearing histamine receptors, *J Clin Invest* 55:856, 1975.
54. Santrach PJ, Parker JL, Jones RT, et al: Diagnostic and therapeutic applications of a modified radioallergosorbent test and comparison with the conventional radioallergosorbent test, *J Allergy Clin Immunol* 67:97, 1981.
55. Wide L, Juhlin L: Detection of penicillin allergy of the immediate type by radioimmunoassay of reagins (IgE) to penicilloyl conjugates, *Clin Allergy* 1:171, 1971.
56. Harle DG, Baldo BA, Smal MA, et al: Detection of thiopentone-reactive IgE antibodies following anaphylactoid reactions during anaesthesia, *Clin Allergy* 16:493, 1986.
57. Harle DG, Baldo BA, Smal SA, et al: An immunoassay for the detection of IgE antibodies to trimethoprim in the sera of allergic patients, *Clin Allergy* 17:209, 1987.
58. Weiss ME, Nyhan D, Zhikang P, et al: Association of protamine IgE and IgG antibodies with life-threatening reactions to intravenous protamine, *N Engl J Med* 320:886, 1989.
59. Hamilton RG, Adkinson NF Jr: Serological methods in the diagnosis and management of human allergic disease, *CRC Crit Rev Clin Lab Sci* 21:1, 1984.

60. Zeiss CR, Grammer LC, Levitz D: Comparison of the radioallergosorbent test and a quantitative solid-phase radioimmunoassay for the detection of ragweed-specific immunoglobulin E antibody in patients undergoing immunotherapy, *J Allergy Clin Immunol* 67:105, 1981.

61. Mathews KP, Hemphill FM, Lovell RG, et al: A controlled study on the use of parenteral and oral antihistamines in preventing penicillin reactions, *J Allergy* 27:1, 1956.

62. Sciple GW, Knox JM, Montgomery CH: Incidence of penicillin reactions after an antihistaminic simultaneously administered parenterally, *N Engl J Med* 261:1123, 1959.

63. Sullivan TJ, Yecies LD, Shatz GS, et al: Desensitization of patients allergic to penicillin using orally administered beta-lactam antibiotics, *J Allergy Clin Immunol* 69:275, 1982.

64. Adkinson NF Jr: Penicillin allergy. In Lichtenstein LM, Fauci A, eds: *Current therapy in allergy, immunology and rheumatology,* Burlington, Ontario, 1983, BC Decker.

65. Patterson R, DeSwarte RD, Greenberger PA, et al: Drug allergy and protocols for management of drug allergies, *N Engl Reg Allergy Proc* 4:325, 1986.

66. Smith RM, Iwamoto GK, Richerson HB, et al: Trimethoprim-sulfamethoxazole desensitization in the acquired immunodeficiency syndrome, *Ann Intern Med* 106:335, 1987.

67. Idsoe O, Guthe T, Willcox RR, et al: Nature and extent of penicillin side-reactions, with particular reference to fatalities from anaphylactic shock, *Bull World Health Organ* 38:159, 1968.

68. Sheffer AL: Anaphylaxis, *J Allergy Clin Immunol* 75:227, 1985.

69. Shapiro S, Siskind V, Slone D, et al: Drug rash with ampicillin and other penicillins, *Lancet* 2:969, 1969.

70. Galpin JE, Chow AW, Yoshikawa TT, et al: "Pseudoanaphylactic" reactions from inadvertent infusion of procaine penicillin G, *Ann Intern Med* 81:358, 1974.

71. Eisen HN: Hypersensitivity to simple chemicals. In Lawrence HS, ed: *Cellular and humoral aspects of the hypersensitive states,* New York, 1959, PB Hoeber.

72. Levine BB: Immunochemical mechanisms involved in penicillin hypersensitivity in experimental animals and in human beings, *Fed Proc* 24:45, 1965.

73. Sullivan TJ: Facilitated haptenation of human proteins by penicillin, *J Allergy Clin Immunol* 83:255, 1989 (abstract).

74. Levine BB, Redmond AP: Minor haptenic determinant-specific reagins of penicillin hypersensitivity in man, *Int Arch Allergy* 35:445, 1969.

75. Levine BB, Redmond AP, Fellner MJ, et al: Penicillin allergy and the heterogeneous immune responses of man to benzylpenicillin, *J Clin Invest* 45:1895, 1966.

76. Adkinson NF Jr, Wheeler B: Risk factors for IgE-dependent reactions to penicillin. In Kerr JW, Ganderton MA, eds: *XI International Congress of Allergology and Clinical Immunology,* London, 1983, Macmillan, p 55.

77. Sogn DD: Prevention of allergic reactions to penicillin, *J Allergy Clin Immunol* 78:1051, 1987.

78. Grieco MH: Cross-allergenicity of the penicillins and the cephalosporins, *Arch Intern Med* 119:141, 1967.

79. Petz L: Immunologic cross-reactivity between penicillins and cephalosporins: a review, *J Infect Dis* 137:S74, 1978.

80. Shibata K, Atsumi T, Horiuchi Y, et al: Immunological cross-reactivities of cephalothin and its related compounds with benzylpenicillin (penicillin G), *Nature* 212:419, 1966.

81. Abraham GN, Petz LD, Fudenberg HH: Immunohaematological cross-allergenicity between penicillin and cephalothin in humans, *Clin Exp Immunol* 3:343, 1968.

82. Abraham GN, Petz LD, Fudenberg HH: Cephalothin hypersensitivity associated with anti-cephalothin antibodies, *Int Arch Allergy* 34:65, 1968.

83. Ong R, Sullivan T: Detection and characterization of human IgE to cephalosporin determinants, *J Allergy Clin Immunol* 81:222, 1988.

84. Saxon A, Beall GN, Rohr AS, et al: Immediate hypersensitivity reactions to beta-lactam antibiotics, *Ann Intern Med* 107:204, 1987.

85. Adkinson NF Jr, Swabb EA, Sugerman AA: Immunology of the monobactam aztreonam, *Antimicrob Agents Chemother* 25:93, 1984.

86. Adkinson NF Jr, Wheeler B, Swabb EA: Clinical tolerance of the monobactam aztreonam in penicillin allergic subjects. Abstract (WS-26-4) presented at the 14th International Congress of Chemotherapy, June 23-28, Kyoto, Japan, 1984.

87. Southorn PA, Plevak DJ, Wright AJ, et al: Adverse effects of vancomycin administered in the perioperative period, *Mayo Clin Proc* 61:721, 1986.

88. Verburg KM, Bowsher RR, Israel KS, et al: Histamine release by vancomycin in humans, *Fed Proc* 44:1247, 1985.

89. Didier A, Cador D, Bongrand P, et al: Role of the quaternary ammonium ion determinants in allergy to muscle relaxants, *J Allergy Clin Immunol* 79:578, 1987.

90. Charpin D, Benzarti M, Hemon Y, et al: Atopy and anaphylactic reactions to suxamethonium, *J Allergy Clin Immunol* 82:356, 1988.

91. Youngman PR, Taylor KM, Wilson JD: Anaphylactoid reactions to neuromuscular blocking agents, *Lancet* 2:597, 1983.

92. Dolovich J, Evans S, Rosenbloom D, et al: Anaphylaxis due to thiopental sodium anesthesia, *Can Med Assoc J* 123:292, 1980.

93. Schatz M: Skin testing and incremental challenge in the evaluation of adverse reactions to local anesthetics, *J Allergy Clin Immunol* 606:616, 1989.

94. deShazo RD, Nelson HS: An approach to the patient with a history of local anesthetic hypersensitivity: experience with 90 patients, *J Allergy Clin Immunol* 63:387, 1989.

95. Nagel JE, Fuscaldo JT, Fireman PL: Paraben allergy, *JAMA* 237:1594, 1977.

96. DeSwarte RD: Drug allergy. In Patterson R, ed: *Allergic diseases: diagnosis and management,* ed 3, Philadelphia, 1989, JB Lippincott.

97. Lawrence ID, Warner JA, Cohan VL, et al: Purification and characterization of human skin mast cells: evidence for human mast cell heterogeneity, *J Immunol* 139:3062, 1987.

98. Harle DG, Baldo BA, Coroneos NJ, et al: Anaphylaxis following administration of papaveretum: case report: implication of IgE antibodies that react with morphine and codeine, and identification of an allergenic determinant, *Anesthesiology* 71:489, 1989.

99. Zucker-Pinchoff B, Ramanathan S: Anaphylactic reaction to epidural fentanyl, *Anesthesiology* 71:599, 1989.

100. Levy JH. Rockoff MR: Anaphylaxis to meperidine, *Anesth Analg* 61:301, 1982.

101. Kelly JF, Patterson R, Lieberman P, et al: Radiographic contrast media studies in high risk patients, *J Allergy Clin Immunol* 62:181, 1978.

102. Lasser EC, Berry CC, Talner LB, et al: Pretreatment with corticosteroids to alleviate reactions to intravenous contrast material, *N Engl J Med* 317:845, 1987.

103. Sharath MD, Metzger WJ, Richerson HB, et al: Protamine-induced fatal anaphylaxis, *J Thorac Cardiovasc Surg* 90:86, 1985.

104. Levy JH, Zaidan JR, Faraj BA: Prospective evaluation of risk of protamine reactions in NPH insulin–dependent diabetics, *Anesth Analg* 65:739, 1986.

105. Levy JH, Schwieger IM, Zaidan JR, et al: Evaluation of patients at risk for protamine reactions, *J Thorac Cardiovasc Surg* 98:200, 1989.

106. Samuel T: Antibodies reacting with salmon in human protamines in sera from infertile men and from vasectomized men and monkeys, *Clin Exp Immunol* 30:181, 1977.

107. Watson RA, Ansbacher R, Barry M, et al: Allergic reaction to protamine: a late complication of elective vasectomy? *Urology* 22:493, 1983.

108. Knape JTA, Schuller JL, De Haan P, et al: An anaphylactic reaction to protamine in a patient allergic to fish, *Anesthesiology* 55:324, 1981.

109. Keller R: Interrelations between different types of cells, *Int Arch Allergy* 34:139, 1968.

110. Levy JH, Faraj BA, Zaidan JR, et al: Effects of protamine on histamine release from human lung, *Agents Actions* 28:70, 1989.

111. Cavarocchi NG, Schaff HV, Orszulak TA, et al: Evidence for complement activation by protamine-heparin interaction after cardiopulmonary bypass, *Surgery* 98:525, 1985.

112. Lakin JD, Blocker TJ, Strong DM, et al: Anaphylaxis to protamine sulfate mediated by a complement-dependent IgG antibody, *J Allergy Clin Immunol* 61:102, 1977.

113. Degges RD, Foster ME, Dang AQ, et al: Pulmonary hypertensive effect of heparin and protamine interaction: evidence for thromboxane B$_2$ release from the lung, *Am J Surg* 154:696, 1987.
114. Morel DR, Zapol WM, Thomas SJ, et al: C5a and thromboxane generation associated with pulmonary-, vaso- and broncho-constriction during protamine reversal of heparin, *Anesthesiology* 66:597, 1987.
115. Skidgel RA, Tan F, Jackman H, et al: Protamine inhibits plasma carboxypeptidase N (CPN), the inactivator of anaphylatoxins and kinins, *Fed Proc* 2:A1382, 1988 (abstract).
116. Grant JA, Cooper JR, Albyn KC, et al: Anaphylactic reactions to protamine in insulin-dependent diabetics after cardiovascular procedures, *J Allergy Clin Immunol* 73:180, 1984 (abstract).
117. Gottschlich GM, Georgitis JW: Protamine-specific antibodies in protamine anaphylaxis, *Ann Allergy* 60:249, 1988 (abstract).
118. Doolan L, McKenzie I, Krafchek J, et al: Protamine sulphate hypersensitivity, *Anaesth Intensive Care* 9:147, 1981.
119. Stevenson GW, Hall SC, Rodnick S, et al: The effect of anesthetic agents on the human immune response, *Anesthesiology* 72:542, 1990.
120. Weiss ME, Adkinson NF Jr, Hirshman CA: Evaluation of allergic drug reactions in the perioperative period, *Anesthesiology* 71:483, 1989.
121. Weiss ME, Adkinson NF Jr: Immediate hypersensitivity reactions to penicillin and related antibiotics, *Clin Allergy* 18:515, 1988.
122. North FC, Kettelkamp N, Hirshman CA: Comparison of cutaneous and in vitro histamine release by muscle relaxants, *Anesthesiology* 66:543, 1987.
123. Foreman JC, Lichtenstein LM: Induction of histamine secretion by polycations, *Biochim Biophys Acta* 629:587, 1980.
124. Weiler JM, Gelhaus MA, Carter JG, et al: A prospective study of the risk of an immediate adverse reaction to protamine sulfate during cardiopulmonary bypass surgery, *J Allergy Clin Immunol* 85:713, 1990.
125. Weiss ME, Chatham F, Kagey-Sobotka A, et al: Serial immunological investigations in a patient who had a life-threatening reaction to intravenous protamine, *Clin Exp Allergy* 20:713, 1990.
126. Cormack JG, Levy JH: Adverse reactions to protamine, *Coron Artery Dis* 4:420, 1993.

Chapter 19

Postoperative Nausea and Vomiting

John B. Rose

Mehernoor F. Watcha

The decrease in the incidence of life-threatening anesthetic-related complications has led clinicians to focus on the more common distressing symptoms following surgery: pain and postoperative nausea and vomiting (PONV). Although much effort rightly has been placed on providing adequate pain relief after surgery, many physicians continue to view PONV as a minor complication that poses little threat to the patient. In contrast, some patients view PONV as being more debilitating than the operation itself.[1] This complication is not only unpleasant and aesthetically displeasing to patients and their caregivers, but, when severe, may also be associated with stress on suture lines, wound dehiscence, bleeding, electrolyte disturbances, dehydration, and, on rare occasions, pulmonary aspiration of gastric contents.[2] More commonly, PONV delays discharge from the ambulatory surgery center and results in an increased use of resources such as intravenous fluids, drugs, supplies, and physician and nursing attention, all of which have finan-

cial implications. Yet this complication has been called the "big, little problem."[3] This chapter reviews the physiology of vomiting, factors associated with PONV, and therapeutic measures available today for the management and prevention of PONV.

I. DEFINITIONS AND INCIDENCE

The terms *nausea, vomiting,* and *retching* are not synonymous. Nausea is an unpleasant sensation in the epigastrium and throat associated with the urge to vomit, whereas vomiting is the forceful expulsion of gastric contents from the mouth. Retching is the rhythmic, labored contractions of the respiratory muscles, including the diaphragm and abdominal muscles, without expulsion of gastric contents.[2]

The incidence of PONV is remarkably constant at 18% to 30% in many large series from around the world, but varies between institutions and even between anesthesiologists within each hospital.[4,5] This is a dramatic improvement over the 75% to 80% incidence during the days of ether and cyclopropane.[6] However, the incidence of severe vomiting has remained remarkably constant at 0.1% to 0.6%.[4,6] Some subsets of patients are at high risk for PONV.

II. PHYSIOLOGY OF VOMITING

Vomiting evolved as an important physiologic mechanism for protecting animals and humans from the ingestion of harmful materials.[7] The emetic center, located in the lateral reticular formation of the medulla, mediates the vomiting response via efferent impulses through the vagus and phrenic nerves and the spinal nerves of the abdominal muscles. Electrical stimulation of this center (or the tractus solitarius) results in immediate vomiting, and ablation eliminates vomiting.[7,8] At present no drugs are known to act directly on the emetic center (Fig. 19-1). However, the emetic center does receive input from several areas, including higher cortical centers, somatic structures (gastrointestinal [GI] tract, pharynx, heart, mediastinum, testes), and optic, olfactory, vagal, glossopharyngeal, and trigeminal nerves. An important source of input to the vomiting center comes from the chemoreceptor trigger zone (CTZ), which is located in the area postrema, a highly vascularized area where no effective blood-brain barrier exists. The CTZ can be activated by direct chemical stimulation via blood or cerebrospinal fluid, but not by direct electrical stimulation.

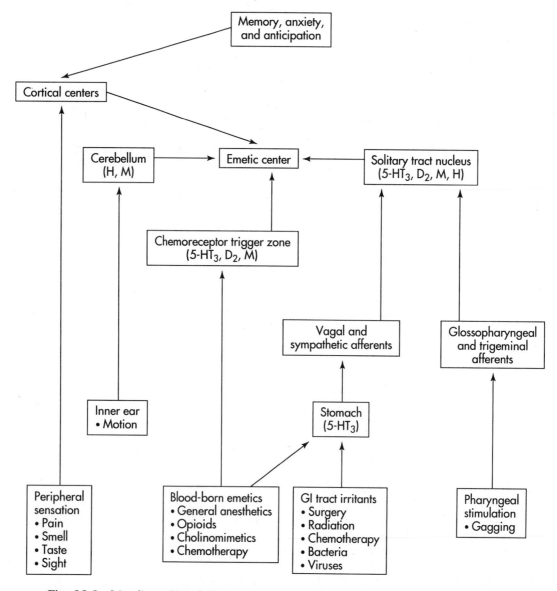

Fig. 19-1. Stimuli capable of eliciting the emetic response. (Modified from Brunton LL: Agents affecting gastrointestinal water flux and motility, emesis, bile acids, and pancreatic enzymes. In Hardman JG, Limbird LE, eds: *Goodman and Gilman's pharmacologic basis of therapeutics,* ed 9, New York, 1996, McGraw-Hill.)

However, ablation of the CTZ prevents vomiting in response to apomorphine but not in response to GI or vestibular stimulation. The central structures involved in the vomiting response are rich in dopaminergic, muscarinic, serotoninergic, histaminic, and opioid receptors, and antiemetic medications exert their effects by interacting with these receptors and blocking neurotransmitter access.[9]

III. NONANESTHETIC FACTORS ASSOCIATED WITH PONV

Given the diverse nature of stimuli capable of eliciting the vomiting response, it is not surprising that myriad nonanesthetic as well as anesthetic factors can contribute to the occurrence of postoperative nausea, retching, and vomiting (Box 19-1).

A. Patient factors

Patient factors associated with an increased risk for PONV include age, gender, increased body mass index (obesity), gastroparesis, a previous history of PONV or motion sickness, and anxiety.

1. Age. Children have a greater incidence of PONV than adults.[2] Within the pediatric age group the risk increases from 5% in infants less than 12 months old, to 20% in children 1 to 5 years old, to 34% in children 6 to 10 years old, and plateaus in children older than 11 years old at a rate of 32%.[10] Some investigators have reported

---

Box 19-1 Factors associated with PONV

Nonanesthetic

Patient factors
  Age
  Gender
  Obesity
  Motion sickness
  History of PONV
  Anxiety
  Gastroparesis
Surgical factors
  Operative procedure
  Duration of surgery

Anesthetic

Preoperative
  Premedication
Intraoperative
  Agents
  Techniques
  Airway management
  Regional anesthesia
  Monitored anesthesia care
Postoperative
  Pain and pain management
  Dizziness
  Ambulation
  Oral intake
  Hydration status

---

that PONV decreases with increasing age in adults[4,11] but this was not confirmed in women undergoing laparotomy or abdominal hysterectomy.

2. Gender. Patient gender has a greater influence on PONV than age in adult patients, with males having less PONV than females, including postmenopausal women less than 60 years old.[2,4,11] Variations in serum gonadotropins or other hormones may be responsible for the greater incidence of PONV in women, as suggested by the observation that gender has no influence on emetic symptoms in prepubertal children or in adults beyond the eighth decade of life. This speculation is supported by reports of variations in the incidence of PONV during the preovulatory and perimenstrual phases of the menstrual cycle.[12-14]

3. Obesity. Obesity, defined by a body mass index greater than 30 kg/m² (weight divided by height squared), is associated with increased PONV.[15,16] This association may be secondary to associated GI diseases (gastroesophageal reflux, hiatal hernia, liver diseases), gastric insufflation during the management of the usually more difficult airway in the obese, and the large reserves for fat-soluble anesthetic agents.[15,16]

4. Motion sickness or prior PONV. Patients with a history of motion sickness or PONV after previous surgery are at greater risk for PONV, perhaps because they have a well-developed vomiting reflex arc.[17-19]

5. Anxiety. Anxiety from anticipation, memory, or fear of unpleasant or unknown perioperative events and experiences decreases gastric pH and increases gastric fluid volume, and thus may increase the risk of PONV.[2,20] Although some investigators did not correlate gastric volumes and pH with preoperative anxiety,[21] others have shown decreased PONV when hypnosis or relaxation techniques were used to reduce perioperative anxiety during plastic surgery operations performed under monitored anesthesia care.[22]

6. Gastroparesis. Altered gastric motility and delayed gastric emptying (ileus) may be related to surgical interventions (i.e., vagotomy, partial gastrectomy) and gastric outlet obstruction, but more commonly accompany the use of anesthetic and opioid analgesics. Gastric hypomotility can accompany scleroderma, amyloidosis, familial visceral myopathy, dysautonomia, muscular dystrophies, and diabetes mellitus.[23]

B. Surgical factors

1. Operative procedure. Nausea, vomiting, and retching are more apt to occur after certain types of surgical procedures than others, regardless of the anesthetic agents used.[24] Gynecologic, general abdominal, head and neck, pediatric, dental, laparoscopic, and some orthopedic surgeries are often cited as procedures with a greater risk for PONV. Pediatric patients undergoing strabismus repair, adenotonsillectomy, orchiopexy, middle ear surgery, and laparotomy are also at increased risk.[2,25]

2. Duration. The incidence of PONV increases with the duration of an operative procedure, perhaps because there is greater exposure to emetogenic anesthetic agents.[2,5,26]

IV. ANESTHETIC FACTORS ASSOCIATED WITH PONV

Nausea and vomiting can occur after general, spinal, epidural, and regional anesthesia as well as after local anesthesia with conscious sedation. Although anesthesiologists cannot control the patient and surgical factors just described, other factors can be influenced by the anesthesiologist's actions, and these anesthetic-related factors are reviewed here.

Many of these factors have been defined in clinical trials, but the quality of such trials varies considerably. It is therefore appropriate to consider the elements of the ideal study design in order to ensure that the observed differences in PONV rates are related to a specific anesthetic intervention. The ideal study will be a randomized, double-blind controlled trial of patients undergoing a standardized surgical procedure with a standardized anesthetic, where the only variation is the administration of one of the study drugs. The number of patients enrolled should be determined by a priori power analysis with a predetermined α and β. If the study compares the efficacy of two or more drugs, the power analysis should be based on differences in PONV rates between the study groups, not the difference between a treated group and a placebo group. The groups should be similar in all demographic factors that affect PONV.

The primary efficacy end point should be the number of patients free from both nausea and vomiting. The data should be analyzed separately for early, late, and total PONV rates and differentiate between nausea and emesis. The criteria for use of rescue antiemetics must be enforced rigorously so that the number of patients requiring rescue antiemetics for recurrent or intractable PONV reflects patient-evaluated severity of symptoms and not variability in the threshold of postanesthesia care unit (PACU) nursing in administering rescue drugs. An estimate should be made of the number of patients in each group with severe emesis, which may be arbitrarily defined as three or more episodes in 24 hours. The time and frequency of emetic episodes and the number of patients who required unanticipated admission to hospital for control of PONV are easy to determine. However, it is more difficult to assess the severity of nausea because this symptom waxes and wanes. Serial visual analog scales of nausea are a sensitive measure of the degree of nausea.

Traditionally, the statistical analysis for PONV studies is based on a chi-square analysis of the patients with PONV in each group. In addition to the p values, the authors should provide the 95% confidence limits in their reports. The investigators should also use the numbers-needed-to-treat method so that readers can determine the clinical importance of the proposed strategy and not just the statistical significance.[27] In addition, the authors should include a Kaplan-Meier survival curve of the time to failure to compare the duration of antiemetic efficacy. The numbers of patients with PONV in each treatment group are surrogate end points for the more important end points of duration of stay in the PACU and the rate of unexpected admission for control of PONV. These data should be provided along with an estimate of patient satisfaction with the regimen and the relative costs of the strategies used.[28]

A. Preoperative

1. Premedication. Anesthesiologists often administer drugs before induction with the aim of reducing anxiety; providing analgesia, amnesia, and vagolysis; drying oral secretions; raising gastric pH; and promoting gastric emptying. The benzodiazepines have become popular because they reduce anxiety, produce amnesia, and are associated with decreased PONV,[29-31] although they do not appear to reduce gastric volume and pH.[21] Similarly, the preoperative use of the α_2 agonist clonidine for sedation is associated with decreased PONV, perhaps as the need for anesthetic agents is reduced.[32] The preoperative use of atropine and glycopyrrolate as antisialagogues and vagolytics is a common practice. In one study, glycopyrrolate was associated with a greater incidence of early postoperative nausea and antiemetic rescue was required three times more often than in patients who received atropine.[33]

Before the advent of benzodiazepines, it was traditional to use opioids for preanesthetic sedation, but this practice is associated with increased PONV.[34-36] The concomitant use of atropine or scopolamine would ameliorate the increased PONV, but the use of glycopyrrolate, which does not cross the blood-brain barrier, would not alter the incidence of opioid-induced emetic symptoms.[2] Fentanyl has recently become available in a candy matrix for transmucosal administration (Fentanyl Oralet). Though useful in children undergoing painful procedures outside the operating room, the transmucosal preparation has not become popular for routine anesthetic premedication in pediatric patients because it increases preinduction emesis.[37,38] It should be emphasized that opioid premedication can be given under some circumstances without increasing the incidence of PONV and that avoidance of opioids when pain exists may result in an increased incidence of emetic symptoms.[2]

B. Intraoperative

1. General anesthetic agents
a. Nitrous oxide. Although early reviews questioned the clinical effect of nitrous oxide on PONV, three independent meta-analyses of existing studies concluded that omission of nitrous oxide reduces the incidence of PONV.[39-41] Perhaps the earlier confusion was based on different effects of nitrous oxide on emesis and on nausea. A number of physiologic mechanisms have been invoked to explain how nitrous oxide could increase the incidence of PONV, including its ability to diffuse into closed spaces (i.e., bowel and middle ear), resulting in bowel distention or stimulation of the vestibular apparatus, to activate the medullary dopaminergic system, and to increase cerebrospinal opioids. However, omission of nitrous oxide results in a significant increase in intraoperative awareness and therefore may not be warranted on the grounds of preventing PONV.[41]

b. Potent inhaled agents. Ether and cyclopropane are associated with a very high incidence of postoperative emetic sequelae, probably secondary to the release of endogenous catecholamines.[2,42] Few studies exist comparing halothane, enflurane, isoflurane, desflurane, and sevoflurane with respect to their incidence of PONV, but the lack of consistent results suggests there is probably little difference in associated PONV. There are some suggestions that sevoflurane is associated with decreased PONV,[43,44] but these results need confirmation by other authors.[45,46] Perhaps the variations in results indicate that there is an interaction between sevoflurane and antiemetic therapy.[46a]

c. Intravenous anesthetics

(1) PROPOFOL. Propofol is a new intravenous drug used initially for anesthetic induction, but now also used for maintenance of general anesthesia and for sedation.[47,48] Numerous clinical investigations have demonstrated that anesthetic induction or maintenance with propofol is associated with lower postoperative emetic sequelae than a variety of other techniques.[47,49-51] A single induction dose of propofol may not be effective in preventing PONV, particularly for long cases, but when used as an infusion for both induction and maintenance of anesthesia the antiemetic benefit of propofol appears to be greatest.[2,51] Some investigators have demonstrated that subhypnotic doses of propofol can be used to treat nausea and vomiting associated with a variety of emetogenic stimuli, including surgery, anesthesia, intrathecal morphine, and cancer chemotherapy.[52-54] The short duration of this effect makes it unlikely that subhypnotic doses of propofol will be practical for the management of established PONV.[55]

The mechanism of the antiemetic effect of propofol is not clear. It does not appear to be related to anxiolysis or sedation because the antiemetic effect of propofol outlasts its effect on consciousness and because subhypnotic doses of propofol appear to have antiemetic properties. Some authors speculate that propofol has direct interactions with receptor sites in subcortical regions known to be involved in the emetic response.[48] However, Appadu et al[56] report that propofol does not interact with D_2 dopamine receptors. Whereas one investigation reports that propofol produces a functional block of 5-HT$_3$ receptors, an important mechanism for antiemesis, other intravenous anesthetics not known to have antiemetic properties (thiopental and etomidate) also produce this block.[56,57] Furthermore, other investigators have demonstrated that propofol exerts little direct effect on 5-HT$_3$ receptors in a cultured neuroblastoma cell model.[58]

(2) ETOMIDATE. Etomidate is a useful sedative-hypnotic agent for anesthetic induction and endotracheal intubation in patients with limited cardiovascular reserve as well as compromised cerebral perfusion. However, it is associated with a greater incidence of PONV than propofol for total intravenous anesthesia (TIVA) in women undergoing gynecologic procedures.[59,60]

(3) KETAMINE. Ketamine, a dissociative anesthetic with profound analgesic properties, has been used for both induction and maintenance of anesthesia, but is associated with a greater incidence of PONV than barbiturates, etomidate, or propofol.[2] It has been suggested that

the increase in emetic sequelae after ketamine is related to its release of endogenous catecholamines.[2] Under some circumstances ketamine may have a beneficial effect on postoperative pain control and therefore reduce narcotic consumption and emetic symptoms.[61]

(4) BARBITURATES. Barbiturates, including sodium thiopental, methohexital, and sodium thiamylal, have long been used to induce general anesthesia. Because other agents are often needed to maintain anesthesia, few studies address the emetogenicity of barbiturates. However, in a number of studies, TIVA with barbiturates (thiamylal, methohexital, or pentothal) was associated with more frequent PONV than propofol.[62-64] Eltanolone, a new steroid-based hypnotic agent, resulted in a similar rate of PONV when compared with sodium thiopental for induction and maintenance of general anesthesia supplemented with nitrous oxide for termination of pregnancy.[65]

2. Nondepolarizing muscle relaxants. Nondepolarizing muscle relaxants are an important component of many general anesthetics. The use of cholinesterase inhibitors to antagonize significant residual neuromuscular blockade (NMB) is a common anesthetic practice and may increase PONV. However, with the introduction of short- and intermediate-acting muscle relaxants, the routine use of antagonists has been questioned, and some suggest that spontaneous recovery of NMB is preferable in order to minimize the incidence of PONV secondary to reversal agents. There are conflicting reports regarding the effect of neostigmine on PONV, with no significant differences noted in adult patients who received low-dose neostigmine (1.5 mg IV) with atropine (0.5 mg IV) and those who were allowed to recover neuromuscular function spontaneously.[66] In another investigation, neostigmine (0.02 mg/kg IV) provided adequate antagonism of NMB with mivacurium in adults without increasing the incidence of PONV.[67] Yet other investigators have demonstrated an antiemetic benefit to patients who recovered neuromuscular function without NMB antagonists.[68] Perhaps these differences relate to the concomitant use of atropine. In one study, children who received neostigmine (0.07 mg/kg^{-1} IV) and glycopyrrolate (0.01 mg/kg^{-1}) following mivacurium infusions had more vomiting in the PACU than children who received placebo or edrophonium (1 mg/kg^{-1} IV) and atropine (0.01 mg/kg^{-1} IV).[68] Recently, neostigmine has been administered in the intrathecal space to provide postoperative analgesia, but it is associated with increased PONV.[69]

3. Techniques. A variety of techniques including inhaled anesthesia (potent inhaled agent with or without nitrous oxide), balanced anesthesia (a combination of inhaled agents and opioid analgesics), and TIVA produce general anesthesia. When antiemetic drugs have not been administered prophylactically, the incidence of PONV has traditionally been reported as greatest with balanced anesthesia, intermediate with inhaled anesthesia, and least with propofol-based TIVA.[2,49,70,71] Propofol may have a greater effect on the control of nausea than of emesis in low-risk patients. In a study comparing TIVA with propofol and isoflurane anesthesia for major abdominal surgery, only nausea during the first 2 post-operative hours was decreased in the TIVA group.[72] In a recent systematic review of randomized controlled trials of propofol, Tramer et al[51] conclude that propofol has a clinically relevant effect on PONV, but only in the short term, when given as a continuous infusion, and if the control rate for emesis was greater than 20%. These authors state that propofol may have statistically significant benefits in other situations but the clinical relevance is unclear.[51]

4. Airway management and gastric distention. Intraoperative gastric distention occurs during controlled ventilation if there is partial airway obstruction and inexperienced personnel.[73] However, the routine placement of orogastric tubes and suctioning of gastric contents just before the conclusion of general anesthesia have been shown to have no effect or to increase the incidence of PONV.[74,75]

5. Regional anesthesia. Regional anesthesia often is associated with a lower incidence of PONV than is general anesthesia.[2,76] However, regional anesthesia may take longer to perform than general anesthesia, may result in other complications such as dural puncture, headache or hypotension, and may not always work, necessitating general anesthesia.[76] Nausea and vomiting during spinal or epidural anesthesia is greater than during peripheral nerve blocks. This may be related to a postural hypotension, light-headedness, hypoxemia of the vomiting center, or vagal stimulation associated with a sympathetic nerve block and can be reduced by pretreatment with crystalloid infusions, atropine, and administration of 100% oxygen.[2,77]

6. Monitored anesthesia care. Local anesthesia with conscious sedation under the supervision of an anesthesiologist (monitored anesthesia care [MAC]) is becoming increasingly popular for many types of surgical, diagnostic, and therapeutic procedures, including plastic surgery, cataract extractions, breast biopsies, endoscopy, vascular access catheter or shunt placement, lumbar puncture, bone marrow aspiration, and dental surgery.[2] In many instances, studies have demonstrated a lower incidence of nausea and vomiting after procedures done under MAC than under general anesthesia, particularly if propofol has been used.[78] However, some patients do develop PONV after MAC, depending on the drugs (opioids in particular) and doses used.[31,79] Nonsteroidal antiinflammatory drugs may reduce opioid requirements and consequently reduce PONV.[79]

C. Postoperative factors

The incidence of nausea and vomiting after surgery may be influenced by several postoperative factors, including pain, pain management, dizziness, ambulation, oral intake, and hydration status.

1. Pain and pain management. Pain has long been recognized as a causative factor in PONV.[2] The quality of postoperative analgesia has improved greatly over the last 20 years with the introduction of patient-controlled analgesia, neuraxial opioids, and continuous epidural analgesia.[80-82] However, opioid analgesics used in pain management can also increase PONV by direct stimulation of the CTZ and the vestibular apparatus, decreased gastric emptying, and atony of the small and large intestine.[41] Some patients prefer to experience pain rather than tolerate PONV associated with opioids.[83] When administered in equianalgesic doses, all opioids are capable of eliciting emetic symptoms.[84] Nevertheless, the emetogenic effects of individual opioids available today vary tremendously from one patient to another. Therefore in patients with severe opioid-related nausea and emesis, selecting a different opioid analgesic may have significant antiemetic benefit.[2]

Multimodal analgesia relies on combinations of regional anesthesia, nonsteroidal antiinflammatory agents, and other medications such as clonidine in order to potentiate the analgesic effects and reduce the incidence and severity of PONV and other opioid-related side effects.[85]

2. Dizziness. PONV can be exacerbated by light-headedness or dizziness caused by opioids or lingering anesthetic effects, hypovolemia, postural hypotension, increased vagal tone, hypoxemia, or anemia.[2] Treatment should be directed at the underlying cause.

3. Ambulation. Motion during the recovery from anesthesia including a change in posture, transport on a stretcher or wheelchair or in an automobile, and ambulation can precipitate nausea and vomiting, particularly in patients who have received opioid analgesics. The vestibular apparatus may become sensitized by general anesthetics such as nitrous oxide (by diffusion into the middle ear) or opioids and result in activation of the emetic response.[42,86] For this reason, many anesthesiologists recommend that patients with PONV restrict their activities until their need for opioid analgesics is over.

4. Oral intake. The first oral intake after surgery may precipitate emesis. Van Der Berg et al[87] report that restricting fluids during the first 8 hours after ophthalmic surgery did not decrease the incidence of PONV. But they demonstrated that half of the patients who do vomit during this recovery period do so immediately after taking their first drinks. Pediatric ambulatory surgery patients required to drink without vomiting before discharge have been shown to have a greater incidence of PONV and longer hospitalization than those who were not required to drink in the early postoperative period.[88]

5. Hydration status. It is a common ambulatory anesthesia practice to administer intravenous fluids in excess of maintenance fluids during the surgical procedure, despite the fact that with liberalized preoperative non per os guidelines, few patients have large fluid deficits. The reason given for this practice is to prevent PONV that may result from hypovolemia, orthostatic hypotension, and dizziness and to prevent dehydration in the event patients are unable to tolerate oral liquids in the early postoperative period. In a study of women undergoing minor gynecologic surgery, the intraoperative intravenous administration of 1000 ml crystalloid decreased dizziness but had no effect on PONV during the first 6 hours of recovery when compared to women who did not receive the fluid bolus.[89]

V. PREVENTION AND TREATMENT

Routine antiemetic prophylaxis is not warranted for all surgical patients because the overall incidence of PONV is less than 36%[2,10,24,55] and most patients with PONV have one or two emetic episodes and minimal nausea.[2,5,10] Furthermore, commonly used antiemetics can produce side effects, which require further pharmacologic interventions and may result in a prolonged hospitalization (Table 19-1). These side effects include sedation, dysphoria, extrapyramidal symptoms, dry mouth, blurred vision, and headache. Although the serotonin antagonists have fewer side effects, their high costs limit their availability in many hospitals and ambulatory surgery facilities. However, many anesthesiologists believe patients at high risk for PONV should routinely receive prophylactic antiemetics because intractable PONV may otherwise occur in up to 1% of surgical patients. These patients require repeated doses of rescue antiemetic therapy, and unanticipated hospitalization may be necessary in up to 1 in 3000.[90] In this section, the various antiemetic agents available for prophylaxis are considered along with nonpharmacologic interventions. The question of which patients should receive prophylactic antiemetics also is considered. Finally, the evaluation and treatment of patients with established PONV are presented.

A. Pharmacologic

As described earlier in this chapter, the emetic response is complex and may be elicited by a wide variety of stimuli. Dopaminergic, muscarinic, histaminic, serotonergic, and opioid receptors may be involved in the myriad

Table 19-1. Antiemetics, site of action, and side effects

Class	Site of action	Drugs	Side effects
Phenothiazines	Central D_2	Promethazine (Phenergan) Adult: 12.5-25 mg PO, PR, IM Pediatric: 0.25-1 mg/kg PR Prochlorperazine (Compazine) Adult: 5-10 mg IM, 5-25 mg PR Pediatric: 0.1 mg/kg PR Chlorpromazine (Thorazine) Adult: 12.5-50 mg IM Pediatric: 1 mg/kg PR	Extrapyramidal signs, sedation, confusion, excitation
Butyrophenones	Central D_2	Droperidol (Inapsine) Adult: 0.625-2.5 mg IV Pediatric: 25-75 μg/kg IV	Sedation, lethargy, agitation, extrapyramidal signs
Antihistamines	H_1	Diphenhydramine (Benadryl) Adult: 10-50 mg IV, IM, PO Pediatric: 1 mg/kg IV, PO Hydroxyzine (Atarax, Vistaril) Adult: 25-100 mg IM Pediatric: 1 mg/kg IV, IM Cyclizine (Marezine) Adult: 50 mg IM Pediatric: 1 mg/kg IM (max 25 mg)	Sedation
Anticholinergics	M, H_1	Scopolamine Adult: 0.3-0.65 mg IM, IV Pediatric: 6 μg/kg IV, IM, SC	Dry mouth, sedation, dysphoria, confusion, disorientation, hallucinations, visual disturbance
Benzamides	D_2, 5-HT$_3$	Metoclopramide Adult: 10-20 mg PO, IM, IV Pediatric: 0.1-0.25 mg/kg PO, IM, IV Trimethobenzamide Adult: 200-250 mg PO, PR, IV Pediatric: <15 kg, 100 mg PR, PO >15 kg, 200 mg PR, PO	Extrapyramidal signs, dystonia
Serotonin antagonists	5-HT$_3$	Ondansetron Adult: 4 mg IV or 8 mg PO Pediatric: 50-100 μg/kg IV or 150 μg/kg PO Granisetron Adult: 1-3 mg IV Pediatric: 40 μg/kg IV	Headache, light-headedness, dizziness, flushing at IV site, constipation

neural pathways connecting peripheral, visceral, and central structures sensitive to emetogenic stimuli to the emetic center. Although antiemetic medications may exert their effects by antagonism of one or more of these receptors, no single drug antagonizes all receptors or exerts an antiemetic effect directly on the emetic center. Thus none of the antiemetic drugs available today are capable of eliminating nausea and vomiting associated with all emetogenic stimuli.

1. Phenothiazines. The phenothiazines are tricyclic compounds characterized by two benzene rings joined by a sulfur and nitrogen atom at positions 5 and 10, respectively, to form the third ring. Individual drugs of this class are further defined by the substitutions on the nitrogen atom and the carbon atom at position 2. Chlorpromazine, promethazine, perphenazine, and dixyrazine are phenothiazines that have been used in the prevention and treatment of PONV.[2] Their antiemetic effects are believed to be related primarily to an interaction with central dopaminergic receptors of the CTZ. They are most effective in preventing opioid-related nausea and emesis. Although their antiemetic effects are achieved at low doses, all phenothiazines are capable of producing significant toxicity, including extrapyramidal effects and sedation. Thus the phenothiazine drugs may complicate postoperative care and result in prolonged hospitalization. Nevertheless, in a recent study comparing the antiemetic efficacy of preoperative perphenazine (5 mg IV), with placebo, ondansetron (4 mg IV), droperidol (1.25 mg IV), and metoclopramide (10 mg IV) in 360 women undergoing transabdominal hysterectomy, perphenazine was the only agent free of side effects.[91] Furthermore, it was as effective as ondansetron and droperidol in preventing severe postoperative emesis. Similarly, prochlorperazine (0.2 mg intramuscularly) was more effective than placebo and just as effective as ondansetron (0.06 mg/kg IV) in reducing posttympanoplasty nausea and vomiting.[92] Dixyrazine reduced nausea after general surgery and orthopedic surgery but did not result in an increase in sedation postoperatively.[93]

2. Butyrophenones. Like phenothiazines, butyrophenones are heterocyclic neuroleptic compounds with significant antiemetic effects from competitive antagonism of dopamine at central D_2 receptors. Droperidol is the only drug in this class in common use today by anesthesiologists for the treatment or prevention of PONV. Droperidol in adults (2.5 mg IV) as well as children (0.075 mg/kg IV) is associated with excessive sedation, lethargy, agitation, and extrapyramidal effects.[2,94-96] Despite these findings, many investigators have found droperidol to be an effective antiemetic in postoperative patients of all ages, with few serious side effects. In a meta-analytic study of antiemetics used to prevent vomiting in children after strabismus repair, droperidol (0.075 mg/kg IV) had the best documented antiemetic effect and was associated with few adverse events.[27] Droperidol in a dose as low as 0.02 mg/kg intravenously may be effective in preventing PONV after pediatric day surgery and was not associated with any adverse side effects in one recent investigation.[97] In healthy women undergoing outpatient gynecologic surgery, droperidol (0.625 mg IV) was as effective as ondansetron (4 mg IV) in preventing PONV, without producing untoward effects or delaying discharge, and it was more cost-effective.[28]

3. Antihistamines. H_1 antagonists such as diphenhydramine, dimenhydrinate, hydroxyzine, and cyclizine may be useful in the control of emesis resulting from vestibular stimulation, as occurs in patients with motion sickness or following middle ear surgery. However, these drugs are weakly antiemetic in most chemotherapy, radiation therapy, and postoperative settings. They are used often in drug regimens to combat chemotherapy-induced emesis because they counteract the extrapyramidal symptoms that can occur with the more efficacious dopamine receptor antagonists. Promethazine is a phenothiazine with an ethylamine moiety (like many H_1 antagonists) attached to the nitrogen atom and has significant antiemetic and sedative properties. The antiemetic effects of promethazine may be related to antagonism of dopaminergic, histaminergic, or muscarinic receptors.[2] The sedative and hypnotic effects of this group of drugs make them less suitable for use in postoperative patients. Nevertheless, because these drugs are inexpensive, there is some interest in their use as antiemetics. Cyclizine has been shown to be an effective postoperative antiemetic and may have fewer side effects than other drugs in this class.[2] However, in one recent study of metoclopramide (10 mg IV), ondansetron (4 mg IV), or cyclizine (50 mg IV) in women undergoing laparoscopic gynecologic surgery, cyclizine was no better than a regimen of no antiemetic in reducing PONV.[98] In children undergoing strabismus surgery, dimenhydrinate (0.5 mg/kg IV) significantly reduced the incidence of in-hospital and 24-hour vomiting when compared to placebo.[99]

4. Anticholinergics. The vestibular apparatus and the nucleus of the tractus solitarius are rich in muscarinic and histaminic receptors. Muscarinic receptor antagonists, like antihistamines, are effective in the prevention of motion sickness and the treatment of postoperative vomiting related to vestibular stimulation. However, in a randomized, placebo-controlled, double-blinded study, neither atropine nor glycopyrrolate reduced the incidence of emesis after strabismus repair in children.[100] Scopolamine and atropine are often added to opioid premedication to reduce PONV but may have disturbing postoperative side effects, including dry mouth, sedation, dysphoria, confusion, disorientation, hallucinations, and visual disturbances.[2] Kamath et al[101] did not observe a lower incidence of PONV in general surgical or orthopedic patients premedicated with morphine-scopolamine than in those receiving placebo. Doyle et al[102] demonstrated a reduction in PONV for 48 hours with transdermal scopolamine in children using patient-controlled morphine analgesia. But the children also had a significant increase in sedation and dry mouth. Similarly, Reinhart et al[103] observed a reduction in nausea and vertigo in adults after outpatient ear surgery but an increase in dry mouth associated with transdermal scopolamine. However, Honkavaara et al[104] report that transdermal scopolamine reduced PONV without producing significant side effects after middle ear surgery.

5. Benzamides. The benzamides and benzimidazole derivatives metoclopramide, trimethobenzamide, cisapride, and domperidone all have prokinetic and antiemetic effects. Metoclopramide is the most effective antiemetic of this class of compounds. Although it is structurally related to procainamide, it does not have any antiarrhythmic or local anesthetic activity.[105] The primary mechanism of antiemetic action of metoclopramide is believed to be a result of central D_2 receptor antagonism, but at large doses antagonism of serotonin (5-HT_3) receptors also occurs. In the GI tract metoclopramide has significant dopaminergic and cholinergic actions, and it increases motility from the distal esophagus to the ileocecal valve, perhaps by increasing acetylcholine release from the myenteric neurons. Furthermore, antimuscarinic drugs such as atropine antagonize the prokinetic effects of benzamides.

Large doses of metoclopramide are well tolerated in adults but often are associated with dystonic reactions in children. For this reason, metoclopramide often is combined with diphenhydramine or lorazepam when used to prevent chemotherapy-induced emesis in children. Fortunately, smaller doses of metoclopramide are effective in preventing and treating PONV. Cisapride is primarily a prokinetic agent and devoid of central dopamine antagonism. Domperidone is a dopamine antagonist but because it does not penetrate the central nervous system significantly, its effects are limited to peripheral GI sites; like cisapride, it is used for its prokinetic effects. Cardiovascular side effects led to the abandonment of this drug.

Several investigations have confirmed earlier studies that metoclopramide has a statistically significant antiemetic efficacy in a variety of settings.[2,98,106] Ali-Melkkila et al[107] observed that metoclopramide (0.25 mg/kg IV) but not tropisetron (0.1 mg/kg IV) provided effective prophylaxis against PONV in patients undergoing elective ophthalmic surgery. Similarly, Pugh et al[108] found that metoclopramide (10 mg IV) had greater antiemetic efficacy than ondansetron (8 mg IV) in adults undergoing major neurosurgical procedures. However, other recent studies show metoclopramide to be of no or limited value when compared to other antiemetics.[55,109] In a comparison with three serotonin antagonists (ondansetron, tropisetron, and granisetron), metoclopramide (10 mg IV) was no more effective than placebo in preventing PONV in adults undergoing laparoscopic cholecystectomy.[109] In contrast, antiemetic prophylaxis with ondansetron (4 mg IV) was the most efficacious treatment. In a study comparing the antiemetic efficacy of ondansetron (8 mg PO), metoclopramide (10 mg PO), or placebo before major orthopedic surgery in adults, ondansetron but not metoclopramide reduced PONV when compared to placebo.[110] When given as an intravenous bolus followed by administration with morphine during patient-controlled analgesia, metoclopramide was only marginally effective in reducing PONV, unlike droperidol given in a similar fashion or tropisetron given as a single intravenous dose.[111] Both

Lacroix et al[55] and Polati et al[112] found metoclopramide to have moderate antiemetic efficacy in the treatment of established PONV. However, metoclopramide was not as effective as droperidol in the former study or ondansetron in the latter study.[55] The earlier popularity of metoclopramide was based on its lack of sedative side effects compared to other antiemetics available at that time. However, with the introduction of antiserotonin agents that have a greater efficacy with a similar lack of sedative side effects, metoclopramide is not used as often as before.[112]

6. Serotonin antagonists. Serotonin or 5-hydroxytryptamine (5-HT) antagonists were discovered fortuitously when compounds structurally related to metoclopramide were found to have significant antiemetic effects but were devoid of any affinity for dopamine receptors, while having antagonistic effects at the 5-hydroxytryptamine (type 3) receptor site.[113] Ondansetron was the first drug of this class to become available for clinical use in 1991. Since that time granisetron, tropisetron, and dolasetron have also been introduced. After studies demonstrated that ondansetron was more effective than metoclopramide and droperidol in preventing chemotherapy-induced nausea and vomiting, numerous clinical investigations of its use in the perioperative period were conducted. Ondansetron is a 5-hydroxytryptamine type 3 receptor antagonist, and so does not have the side effects of dopamine receptor antagonists (e.g., chlorpromazine, droperidol, metoclopramide), muscarinic receptor antagonists (e.g., scopolamine, atropine), or histamine receptor antagonists (e.g., diphenhydramine, promethazine). These side effects include sedation, dysphoria, dystonia, visual disturbances, dry mouth, and urinary retention. Psychomotor function is unaffected by ondansetron.[114] Rapid intravenous infusion of ondansetron in adults is not associated with changes in heart rate, blood pressure, or respiratory rate.[115] Asymptomatic, brief prolongation of the QRS and PR intervals has been documented after intravenous infusion of 5-HT_3 receptor antagonists. Ondansetron does not potentiate respiratory depression induced by alfentanil. Although colonic transit time is reduced and constipation is a known side effect of ondansetron, gastric emptying and small bowel transit are not affected by ondansetron. Headache, light-headedness, dizziness, flushing at the infusion site, and a warm epigastric sensation are reported side effects of the serotonin antagonists.[116] The most serious side effects of ondansetron appear to be rare hypersensitivity reactions and transient increases in liver enzymes. Liver enzyme increases have been reported only in patients receiving antineoplastic drugs at the same time, and it is unclear whether this complication is a result of the chemotherapy or ondansetron.

Prophylactic ondansetron (0.05 to 0.20 mg/kg intravenously or orally) reduces the incidence of PONV in adults and children at increased risk for these complications.[115-120] Although the antiemetic effects of ondansetron appear to be superior to those of other prophylactic antiemetics in many studies, more recent data suggest that a small dose of droperidol (0.625 to 1.25 mg) may be equally effective. In a comparison of costs and efficacy of prophylactic ondansetron with those of droperidol in adults having elective gynecologic surgery, Tang et al[28] concluded that droperidol (0.625 mg IV) was more cost-effective than ondansetron (4 mg IV) and was not associated with any adverse effects, including prolonged length of stay.[28] In a similar study of prophylactic ondansetron versus droperidol for gynecologic procedures, Sniadach et al[117] conclude that droperidol was as effective as ondansetron in preventing PONV and that significant cost savings can be realized if droperidol is used rather than ondansetron in this setting. Jellish et al also conclude that prophylactic ondansetron (4 mg IV) was no more effective than droperidol (25 µg/kg IV) in preventing PONV in adults after middle ear surgery, and ondansetron did not result in any cost advantage as measured by lower use of rescue antiemetics or shorter PACU times. Prophylactic ondansetron (0.1 mg/kg IV) decreased PONV compared to placebo and droperidol (75 µg/kg IV) and reduced hospital length of stay compared to droperidol (75 µg/kg IV) in pediatric ambulatory surgery patients.[95,119] In these patients the administration of ondansetron (0.1 mg/kg IV) before pediatric ambulatory surgery resulted in a 30-minute reduction in time to meet home-readiness when compared to placebo-treated patients.[119] In other studies, ondansetron-treated patients required fewer and shorter nursing interventions postoperatively and ondansetron-treated patients consumed fewer resources for the management of PONV.[118]

The numerous clinical trials of ondansetron have recently been subjected to a systematic review to test whether there is evidence of antiemetic efficacy with ondansetron, assess the dose-response relationship for ondansetron, and determine whether the differences in efficacy between doses have any clinical relevance.[120] The authors found that ondansetron could prevent further PONV in one of four patients who would otherwise continued to have these symptoms. The investigators found no evidence for a dose-response effect between 4 and 8 mg of ondansetron. A disturbing finding of this meta-analysis was that a false impression of the ability of ondansetron to control nausea and vomiting may have resulted from duplication of roughly 25% of reports. Tramer et al[120] also claimed that ondansetron did not differ from metoclopramide or droperidol in controlling further emetic symptoms when administered to patients with established PONV, but other studies have shown ondansetron to provide better and longer-lasting control than metoclopramide.[112]

Granisetron in doses of 5 to 60 µg/kg IV is very effective in decreasing emetic symptoms in adult and pediatric patients at increased risk for PONV, including patients with motion sickness and in women throughout their menstrual cycles.[19,121] In comparative studies of granisetron and other antiemetics, granisetron was superior to metoclopramide and droperidol.[19,121] Although granisetron is an effective antiemetic, Cieslak et al[122] estimate the cost of treating pediatric ambulatory surgery patients at increased risk for PONV to be $101.00 per patient (including the cost of nursing labor). Further studies on the cost-effectiveness of this and other antiemetics are required before routine prophylactic therapy with granisetron can be advocated.[123]

Tropisetron is another 5-HT$_3$ antagonist available for clinical use today. In a dose-response investigation, Capouet[124] reported that tropisetron (2 mg IV) was the least effective dose in terms of 24-hour incidence of nausea and vomiting and need for rescue antiemetic therapy in women during gynecologic procedures. In another study, tropisetron (but not droperidol 1.25 mg IV) reduced the incidence of emesis and number of emetic episodes per patient observed when compared to placebo-treated patients.[109] In addition, the investigators observed a greater level of postoperative anxiety in droperidol-treated patients. Whether tropisetron offers any advantages over other 5-HT$_3$ receptor antagonists or other antiemetics remains to be determined.

Dolasetron, a pseudopelletierine-derived 5-HT$_3$ receptor antagonist, is the latest member of this class of antiemetics to be introduced into clinical practice. After intravenous administration, it is rapidly converted into hydrodolasetron, which is responsible for much of the parent compound's pharmacologic properties. Hydrodolasetron has a half-life of about 8 hours, giving dolasetron a potential advantage over the other serotonin antagonists. Like the other serotonin antagonists, dolasetron was initially used clinically for the management of chemotherapy and radiation therapy–induced nausea and vomiting. Dolasetron (1.8 mg/kg IV or 200 mg PO) resulted in a complete response (no nausea or vomiting) in 50% of patients receiving highly emetogenic chemotherapy.[125] Although granisetron (3 mg IV) and ondansetron (32 mg IV) have equivalent antiemetic efficacy as dolasetron (1.8 mg/kg IV) in patients receiving highly emetogenic chemotherapy, dolasetron appears to be superior to metoclopramide in this setting. Initial studies of the effects of dolasetron (12.5 mg to 100 mg IV or 25 mg to 200 mg PO) in women before gynecologic surgery show that it is significantly better than placebo in preventing PONV.[125]

Dolasetron is well tolerated in large doses, but dizziness, headache, light-headedness, and increased appetite occurred more often in dolasetron-treated patients than in placebo-treated patients.[126] Other investigators report that adverse events occurred in 3% of patients, regardless of whether they received placebo or dolasetron. In this study, three different doses of dolasetron (12.5 mg, 25 mg, and 50 mg IV) were compared with placebo to test the antiemetic efficacy of prophylactic dolasetron in 635 women undergoing laparoscopic gynecologic procedures. All three doses were effective in reducing nausea scores and increasing the number of patients who experienced a complete response (no nausea or vomiting during the first 24 postoperative hours) compared to the placebo group, but there were no differences between the three dolasetron-treated groups. In other studies, dolasetron was shown to be effective in the treatment of PONV. Of 1557 patients enrolled in the study before ambulatory surgery under general anesthesia, 620 patients were eligible for treatment postoperatively and received either placebo or one of four different doses of dolasetron (12.5 mg, 25 mg, 50 mg, and 100 mg). Complete response rates during the 24 hours after study drug administration were better for each dose of dolasetron (35%, 28%, 29%, and 29%, respectively) than for placebo (11%).[125] Of interest is the finding that the dose-response relationship of dolasetron differs if it is given at the end of the operation (when 12.5 mg is an effective dose) than at the start of the procedure (when 50 mg is effective). The preliminary studies of dolasetron are very encouraging, and in one study dolasetron was shown to be as effective as ondansetron (4 mg IV). Further studies evaluating cost-effectiveness of dolasetron in comparison with other antiemetics are required.

7. Other drugs: steroids, cannabinoids. A variety of medications from diverse classes of pharmacologic agents, including corticosteroids, benzodiazepines, α_2 agonists (clonidine), and cannabinoids, are also known to have antiemetic actions, although their mechanisms of action are not completely understood and may be indirect rather than direct effects. For example, the benzodiazepines primarily reduce anxiety and induce sedation. Their antiemetic benefits appear to be secondary to anxiolysis and sedation, and are particularly useful in patients with anticipatory emesis during multiple chemotherapeutic and other procedures.[127] Similarly, clonidine is an anxiolytic and sedative medication but also has analgesic properties useful in anesthetic practice. Clonidine reduces general anesthetic and opioid requirements and thus may have an effect on PONV by reducing patient exposure to emetogenic substances.[32] Ephedrine, an indirect-acting sympathomimetic agent, has been used to treat motion sickness and prevent PONV.[2] Its antiemetic benefit may be secondary to its ability to prevent hypotension, especially that secondary to spinal or epidural anesthesia.

Dexamethasone has significant, prolonged antiemetic effects both in the perioperative period and when administered before chemotherapy. It is not clear how dexamethasone reduces PONV. However, dexamethasone is known to have multiple central nervous system effects, including effects on mood and sense of well-being. The antiemetic effect of dexamethasone is present when dexamethasone is used as the sole antiemetic.[127] However, it is more commonly used in combination with other antiemetics and is discussed further in the following section.

The cannabinoids have been used to reduce nausea and vomiting associated with moderately emetogenic chemotherapy.[2] Yet their use in postoperative patients is limited because of a low efficacy and a high frequency of undesirable side effects including vertigo, ataxia, postural hypotension, visual disturbances, and confusion. Furthermore, in a recent study of women undergoing general anesthesia for total abdominal hysterectomy, the antiemetic effect was limited at best. Rates of postoperative nausea and vomiting after preoperative tetrahydrocannabinol (2 mg PO) were high (73% and 54%, respec-

tively) and no different from the rates observed for women who received metoclopramide (70% and 67%, respectively).

8. Combination antiemetic therapy. The combination of antiemetics from different pharmacologic classes to enhance antiemetic efficacy and reduce the incidence of side effects has been well studied and documented in chemotherapy patients. Over the last 5 years, interest has developed in this approach to PONV, and studies have confirmed that combinations of antiemetics are more efficacious than the medications given alone.[128] Dexamethasone in combination with a serotonin antagonist improves antiemetic efficacy in studies of adults and children after a variety of surgical procedures.[128] However, in one study of women undergoing major gynecologic surgery, it was observed that the addition of dexamethasone to a combination of propofol and ondansetron did not result in lower rates of PONV than did propofol and ondansetron alone.[129] In another study of the same patient population, dexamethasone did not enhance the antiemetic effects of droperidol or metoclopramide, but did improve the control of nausea and vomiting with granisetron.

Other combinations of antiemetics have been examined for the prevention of PONV. The combination of a central dopamine antagonist (droperidol) with a 5-HT$_3$ antagonist (ondansetron) resulted in a significantly higher number of patients with a complete response (no PONV in 24 hours), longer time to first emetic episode, fewer emetic episodes, and less nausea after tubal banding when compared to patients who received droperidol alone.[130] Similarly, during patient-controlled analgesia with morphine, the addition of both droperidol and ondansetron to the morphine solutions provided better control of emetic symptoms than either drug alone.[131] In another study, freedom from PONV during the first 48 hours after general anesthesia for elective abdominal surgery was significantly higher (92%) with ondansetron combined with droperidol than with ondansetron alone (56%), droperidol alone (60%), and placebo (28%).[132]

Other combinations of antiemetics may provide superior control over nausea and vomiting postoperatively. In one study, promethazine (10 mg PO) combined with transdermal scopolamine (1.5 mg) was more effective in reducing the number of patients who vomited and the number of emetic episodes following spinal anesthesia with bupivacaine and intrathecal morphine for arthroscopic surgery of the lower extremity than was promethazine alone or diazepam.[53] Also of interest is the finding that the combination of the inexpensive antiemetics metoclopramide (10 mg IV) and droperidol (0.625 mg) was associated with a greater reduction in PONV than ondansetron (4 mg IV) administered before laparoscopic cholecystectomy.[133]

In conclusion, it appears that as in cancer chemotherapy patients, some combinations of antiemetics provide superior control of nausea and vomiting in some postoperative patients. It remains to be seen whether this technique can result in lower costs of antiemesis and a lower incidence of undesirable side effects.

B. Nonpharmacologic

Strategies to prevent or treat PONV most commonly involve pharmacologic interventions, including the use of antiemetic medications discussed in this chapter or the selection of certain anesthetic agents and techniques over those known to be more emetogenic. However, several nonpharmacologic techniques may have antiemetic benefits. Furthermore, concern over the costs of newer antiemetic agents and side effects of the older agents has resulted in an increased interest in some of these techniques.[134]

1. Acupuncture and acupressure. Early studies of the antiemetic efficacy of acupuncture, acupressure, and electrical stimulation of the P6 or Neiguan point (located on the anterior surface of the wrist approximately three fingerbreadths above the distal skin crease of the wrist joint and between the tendons of the flexor carpi radialis and palmaris longus muscles) in postoperative patients have yielded mixed results and have been reviewed.[2] Recently, Yentis and Bisonette[135] reported that 5 minutes of intraoperative acupuncture treatment was ineffective in preventing postoperative vomiting in children undergoing strabismus repair, even when combined with droperidol (0.075 mg IV). However, in a randomized, prospective, controlled study of women undergoing outpatient laparoscopic surgery, bilateral P6 acupuncture treatment (beginning after the induction of anesthesia but before surgery or morphine administration) lasting the entire duration of the procedure resulted in a significant reduction in predischarge and postdischarge vomiting. In another randomized, controlled study of women following hysterectomy, electrical stimulation of the P6 point with a transcutaneous electrical nerve stimulation (TENS) unit for 6 hours resulted in a significant reduction in the incidence of vomiting during therapy. However, this effect disappeared 2 hours after discontinuation of P6 TENS therapy.[136] The use of an elastic wrist band with an embedded plastic bead (Sea Band) to exert pressure (acupressure) on the P6 point has also been used successfully to reduce vomiting associated with brief surgical procedures in adults.[137] Acupressure at the P6 point or metoclopramide (10 mg IV) reduced the incidence of nausea and vomiting during spinal anesthesia for cesarean section.[106] Although it appears from these studies that acupressure, acupuncture, and TENS at the P6 point provide reliable antiemetic benefits in certain circumstances, antiemetic efficacy may depend on the timing and duration of treatment and on the location of the surgery. At least part of the antiemetic effect of these nonpharmacologic interventions may be related to placebo effect. The extent to which these interventions will be used for the prevention and treatment of PONV is unclear.

2. Environmental factors. Control of environmental factors can be important in reducing the incidence and severity of PONV. Noise, activity, motion, and light can aggravate symptoms of nausea and emesis. In patients who have a history of PONV or motion sickness, or in patients with established PONV, ensuring that they rest in a quiet, darkened room, with little activity around them can reduce vestibular stimuli and emetic sequelae. In a recent study of women after elective gynecologic surgery, movement was identified as a significant factor associated with and causing nausea.[101]

3. Diet. Over the last decade, the approach to postoperative diet has been reviewed extensively. During the early postoperative period, nausea and vomiting may be precipitated by oral intake of any kind. In fact, half the patients who vomited after ophthalmic surgery in one study did so after drinking for the first time.[88] Insisting that patients drink without vomiting before discharge following ambulatory surgery is no longer routine. However, it is essential to ensure that patients are well hydrated before discharge in order to eliminate the need for them to take fluids immediately. Once patients do experience thirst, they should take clear liquids in small quantities or sips. If they tolerate sips without experiencing nausea or vomiting, it is reasonable to advance their diets gradually to normal solids. In a study of short-stay orthopedic surgery patients, 84% of patients received a normal diet during their first meal after surgery, but because of adverse abdominal symptoms, about half of the patients were not able to eat anything.[88] However, 40% of patients reported that they ate everything provided. After the second postoperative meal, there were many fewer complaints of adverse symptoms. It was concluded that although patients vary considerably in postoperative symptoms, meal tolerance, and meal preferences, recovery after general anesthesia was quick in the majority of patients. After tonsillectomy in children, dietary restrictions to soft foods only during the first 12 hours did not reduce emesis or pain when compared to an unrestricted diet, and parents perceived a more successful recovery in the unrestricted diet group.[114] In another study of the effect of diet on recovery after tonsillectomy in children, there were no differences between soft diet, rough diet, or the no dietary advice groups with respect to healing or analgesia after 2 weeks of follow-up. The authors concluded that no specific dietary advice was required other than to encourage regular eating.[138]

VI. PHARMACOECONOMICS

With the recent change in the methods of payment for health care in the United States from an indemnity basis to a managed care basis, physicians are under increasing pressure to reduce the costs of interventions. As this change occurred, many newer anesthetic drugs have been introduced. These newer drugs are shorter-acting and easier to use, and have fewer side effects than currently used drugs, but they are more expensive. Administrators have begun questioning the wisdom of using these newer drugs and asking physicians whether they can obtain acceptable results with the use of cheaper, older drugs. The unfortunate practice of concentrating solely on the acquisition price of drugs is short-sighted because the major costs of medical care relate to labor costs. In this setting it is up to the anesthesiologist to be the patient advocate and demonstrate that there are benefits to the patient, society, and the health care institution from the use of these drugs. It is a good principle to limit the replacement of older drugs with newer ones only when the new drug has been shown to be more effective, is associated with fewer side effects, or is cheaper.[139]

Some investigators have tried to use cost accounting principles to examine the cost-effectiveness of their strategies. One question that is often asked is the justification of routine antiemetic prophylaxis versus a strategy of waiting for a patient to develop symptoms and then treating only those with symptoms. Both approaches have associated costs beyond the acquisition of antiemetic drugs. There are nursing labor costs associated with the management of problems arising from the withholding of a drug until symptoms appear and costs from the side effects of drugs. Using a decision analysis model, Watcha and Smith[140] have shown that the cost-effectiveness of routine antiemetic prophylaxis depends on the costs of the drug used, the incidence of PONV symptoms, and side effects from the prophylactic use of drugs. They note that it was cost-effective to use ondansetron for the prophylaxis of PONV only if the incidence of predischarge emesis was greater than 30%. These authors also showed that in their model ondansetron was less cost-effective than droperidol but more cost-effective than metoclopramide. The same model was used in studies of the cost-effectiveness of granisetron and droperidol.[28]

These studies assume a linear relationship between labor costs and the time taken to provide drugs. However, unless there is a direct reduction in the number of nurses required for patient care, faster emergence and reduced emesis will not result in true nursing labor cost savings. Dexter and Tinker[141] used computer simulations to show that the total elimination of emesis would have a modest impact on nursing costs and that the peak number of patients arriving in the PACU has a greater impact on PACU economics.

As mentioned earlier, it is our duty as patient advocates to provide sufficient data to demonstrate greater patient satisfaction with reduced emesis. With such data we can be more effective in justifying the use of the more expensive drugs. Unfortunately, these data often are not obtained during drug studies.

VII. EVALUATION OF THE PATIENT WITH INTRACTABLE PONV

Anesthesiologists may be called upon to evaluate and treat patients with PONV in a variety of settings, including the PACU, day surgery unit, general surgical ward, and increasingly the home after discharge from day surgery. These latter patients pose the greatest challenge because they are not immediately available for examination or follow-up and do not have intravenous lines in place. Before a patient with established PONV is treated, age, medical history, surgical procedure, hydration status, and the severity and frequency of symptoms as well as any precipitating factors (i.e., car ride home, severe pain, analgesics, forced oral intake) should be ascertained. The dose, route, and time of any antiemetics already received should also be noted in order to avoid side effects resulting from further antiemetic therapy and

in order to select an antiemetic that may be more effective than one taken previously. When symptoms are related to dietary or environmental factors such as a long car ride home from the hospital in stop-and-go traffic, therapy may consist of only conservative nonpharmacologic environmental or dietary instructions. When symptoms persist despite adherence to these instructions, antiemetic medications may be required. If intractable PONV or dehydration exists or may potentially develop, the patient must return to the hospital for further evaluation. In these instances, intravenous fluid and electrolyte therapy may be required in addition to therapy to control the symptoms of nausea and vomiting.

From time to time an anesthesiologist is faced with the problem of managing a patient with a history of severe postoperative emesis after a previous operation. In this setting, the anesthesiologist should examine the previous anesthetic records carefully. The anesthetic plan should aim at reducing these risks by the use of premedication to reduce perioperative anxiety and the preferential use of regional anesthetic techniques. If general anesthesia is essential, the anesthesiologist should use techniques known to reduce the risk of PONV. These include the use of propofol for both induction and maintenance of anesthesia; the avoidance of nitrous oxide, opioids, and neuromuscular antagonists; the use of nonsteroidal anti-inflammatory drugs; and the administration of a combination of dexamethasone, a $5-HT_3$ antagonist, and an antiemetic of a different class (e.g., low-dose droperidol). In the postoperative period the patient should not be moved suddenly from one position to another. Adequate intravenous fluids should be provided and the patient not forced to drink before discharge. Nonpharmacologic approaches such as perioperative suggestion and acupressure should also be considered as part of the overall plan. When such a multimodal approach is taken, the overall experience for the patient should be better than on previous occasions.

VIII. SUMMARY

PONV has been considered to be as inevitable as postoperative pain. Although recent improvements in therapy have reduced the incidence of PONV, it still remains high. We should continue to investigate better methods of reducing this debilitating complication and improving the patient's perioperative experience. It should be our aim to make nausea and vomiting as unacceptable as pain in the postoperative period.

REFERENCES

1. Lee PJ, Pandit SK, Green CR: Postanesthetic side effects in the outpatient: which are the most important? *Anesth Analg* 79:S271, 1995.
2. Watcha MF, White PF: Postoperative nausea and vomiting: its etiology, treatment and prevention, *Anesthesiology* 77:162, 1992.
3. Kapur PA: The big "little problem," *Anesth Analg* 73:243, 1991.
4. Forrest JB, Cahalan MK, Rehder K, et al: Multicenter study of general anesthesia. II. Results, *Anesthesiology* 72:262, 1990.
5. Cohen MM, Duncan PG, Tweed WA: The postoperative interview: assessing risk factors for nausea and vomiting, *Anesth Analg* 78:7, 1994.

6. Burtles R, Peckett BW: Postoperative vomiting, *Br J Anaesth* 29:114, 1955.
7. Andrews PLR, David CJ, Binham S: The abdominal visceral innervation and the emetic reflex: pathways, pharmacology and plasticity, *Can J Physiol Pharmacol* 68:325, 1990.
8. Borison HL: Area postrema: chemoreceptor circumventricular organ of the medulla oblongata, *Prog Neurobiol* 32:351, 1989.
9. Peroutka SJ, Snyder SH: Neurotransmitter receptor binding predicts therapeutic action, *Lancet* 1:658, 1982.
10. Cohen M, Cameron CB, Duncan PG: Pediatric anesthesia morbidity and mortality in the perioperative period, *Anesth Analg* 70:160, 1990.
11. Palazzo MGA, Strunin L: Anaesthesia and emesis. I. Etiology, *Can Anaesth Soc J* 31:178, 1984.
12. Beattie WS, Lindblad T, Buckley DN, et al: Menstruation increases the risk of nausea and vomiting after laparoscopy: a prospective and randomized study, *Anesthesiology* 78:272, 1993.
13. Honkavaara P, Pekko I, Rutanen EM: Increased incidence of retching and vomiting during the preovulatory phase after middle ear surgery, *Can J Anaesth* 43:1108, 1996.
14. Beattie WS, Lindblad T, Buckley DN, et al: The incidence of postoperative nausea and vomiting in women undergoing laparoscopy is influenced by the day of the menstrual cycle, *Can J Anaesth* 37:298, 1991.
15. Shankman Z, Shin Y, Brodsky JB: Perioperative management of the obese patient, *Br J Anaesth* 70:349, 1993.
16. Palazzo M, Evans R: Logistic regression analysis of fixed patient factors for postoperative sickness: a model for risk assessment, *Br J Anaesth* 75:301, 1995.
17. Watcha MF, Simeon RM, White PF, et al: Effect of propofol on the incidence of postoperative vomiting after strabismus surgery in pediatric outpatients, *Br J Anaesth* 75:204, 1991.
18. Toner CC, Bromhead CJ, Littlejohn IH, et al: Prediction of postoperative nausea and vomiting using a logistic regression model, *Br J Anaesth* 76:347, 1996.
19. Fujii, Y, Tanaka H, Toyooka H: Granisetron reduces postoperative nausea and vomiting throughout menstrual cycle, *Can J Anaesth* 44:489, 1997.
20. Kallar SK, Everett LL: Potential risks and preventative measures for pulmonary aspiration: new concepts in preoperative fasting guidelines, *Anesth Analg* 77:171, 1993.
21. Haavik PE, Soreide E, Hofstad B, et al: Does preoperative anxiety influence gastric fluid volume and acidity? *Anesth Analg* 75:91, 1992.
22. Faymonville ME, Fissette J, Mambourg PH, et al: Hypnosis as an adjunct in conscious sedation for plastic surgery, *Reg Anesth* 20:145, 1995.
23. Read NW, Houghton LA: Physiology of gastric emptying and the pathophysiology of gastroparesis, *Gastroenterol Clin North Am* 18:359, 1989.
24. Haigh CG, Kaplan LA, Dunham JM, et al: Nausea and vomiting after gynaecological surgery: a meta-analysis of factors affecting their incidence, *Br J Anaesth* 71:517, 1993.
25. Patel RI, Hannallah RS: Anesthetic complications following pediatric ambulatory surgery, *Anesthesiology* 69:1009, 1988.
26. Larsson S, Lundberg D: A prospective survey of postoperative nausea and vomiting with special regard to incidence and relations to patient characteristics, anesthetic routines and surgical procedures, *Acta Anaesthesiol Scand* 39:539, 1995.
27. Tramer M, Moore A, McQuay H: Prevention of vomiting after paediatric strabismus repair: a systematic review using the numbers-needed-to-treat method, *Br J Anaesth* 75:556, 1995.
28. Tang J, Watcha MF, White PF: A comparison of costs and efficacy of ondansetron and droperidol as prophylactic antiemetic therapy for elective outpatient gynecologic procedures, *Anesth Analg* 83:304, 1996.
29. Khalil SN, Berry JM, Howard G, et al: The antiemetic effect of lorazepam after outpatient strabismus surgery in children, *Anesthesiology* 77:915, 1992.
30. Splinter WM, MacNeill HB, Menard EA, et al: Midazolam reduces vomiting after tonsillectomy in children, *Can J Anaesth* 42:201, 1995.
31. Avramov MN, Smith I, White PF: Interactions between midazolam and remifentanil during monitored anesthesia care, *Anesthesiology* 85:1283, 1996.
32. Mikawa K, Nishina K, Maekawa N, et al: Oral clonidine reduces vomiting after strabismus surgery, *Can J Anaesth* 42:977, 1995.
33. Salmenpera M, Kuoppamaki R, Salmonpera A: Do anticholinergic agents affect the occurrence of postanaesthetic nausea? *Acta Anaesthesiol Scand* 36:445, 1992.
34. Pandit SK, Kothary SP: Intravenous narcotics for premedication in outpatient anaesthesia, *Acta Anaesthesiol Scand* 33:353, 1989.
35. Zedie N, Amory DW, Wagner BK, et al: Intravenous narcotics for premedication in outpatient anaesthesia, *Clin Pharmacol Ther* 59:341, 1996.
36. White PF, Shafer A: Nausea and vomiting: causes and prophylaxis, *Semin Anesth* 6:300, 1998.
37. Schecter NL, Weisman SJ, Rosenblum M, et al: The use of oral transmucosal fentanyl citrate for painful procedures in children, *Pediatrics* 95:335, 1995.
38. Epstein RH, Mendel HG, Witkowski TA, et al: The safety and efficacy of oral transmucosal fentanyl citrate for preoperative sedation in young children, *Anesth Analg* 83:1200, 1996.
39. Hartung J: Twenty-four of twenty-seven studies show a greater incidence of emesis with nitrous oxide than with alternative anesthetics, *Anesth Analg* 83:114, 1996.
40. Divatia JV, Vaidya JS, Badwe RA, et al: Omission of nitrous oxide during anesthesia reduces the incidence of postoperative nausea and vomiting: a meta-analysis, *Anesthesiology* 85:1055, 1996.
41. Tramer M, Moore A, McQuay H: Omitting nitrous oxide in general anesthesia: metaanalysis of intraoperative awareness and postoperative emesis in randomized controlled trials, *Br J Anaesth* 76:86, 1996.
42. Kenny GN: Risk factors for postoperative nausea and vomiting, *Anaesthesia* 49(suppl):6, 1994.
43. Johannesson GP, Floren M, Lindahl SG: Sevoflurane for ENT-surgery in children, *Acta Anaesthesiol Scand* 39:546, 1995.
44. Hobbhahn J, Funk W: Sevoflurane in pediatric anesthesia, *Anaesthesia* 45:22, 1998.
45. Fredman B, Nathanson MH, Smith I, et al: Sevoflurane for outpatient anesthesia: a comparison with propofol, *Anesth Analg* 81:823, 1995.
46. Jellish WS, Lein CA, Fontenot HJ: The comparative effects of sevoflurane versus propofol in the induction and maintenance of anesthesia in adult patients, *Anesth Analg* 82:479, 1996.
46a. P. White: Personal communication, 1998.
47. Sebel PS, Lowdon JD: Propofol: a new intravenous anesthetic, *Anesthesiology* 71:260, 1989.
48. Biebuyck J, Gouldson R, Nathanson M, et al: Propofol: an update on its clinical use, *Anesthesiology* 81:1005, 1994.
49. Raftery S, Sherry E: Total intravenous anesthesia with propofol and alfentanil protects against nausea and vomiting, *Can J Anaesth* 39:37, 1992.
50. Gan TJ, Ginsberg B, Grant APS, et al: Double-blind, randomized, comparison of ondansetron and intraoperative propofol to prevent postoperative nausea and vomiting, *Anesthesiology* 85:1036, 1996.
51. Tramer M, Moore A, McQuay H: Propofol anaesthesia and postoperative nausea and vomiting: quantitative systematic review of randomized controlled studies, *Br J Anaesth* 78:247, 1997.
52. Borgeat A, Wilder-Smith OHG, Forni M, et al: Adjuvant propofol enables better control of nausea and emesis secondary to chemotherapy for breast cancer, *Can J Anaesth* 41:1117, 1994.
53. Torn K, Tuominen, Tarkkila P, et al: Effects of sub-hypnotic doses of propofol on the side-effects of intrathecal morphine, *Br J Anaesth* 73:411, 1994.
54. Scher CS, Amar D, McDowell RH, et al: Use of propofol for the prevention of chemotherapy induced nausea and emesis, *Can J Anaesth* 39:170, 1992.
55. Lacroix G, Lessard MR, Trepanier CA: Treatment of postoperative nausea and vomiting: comparison of propofol, droperidol, and metoclopramide, *Can J Anaesth* 43:115, 1996.
56. Appadu BL, Strange PG, Lambert DG: Does propofol interact with D2 dopamine receptors? *Anesth Analg* 79:1191, 1994.

57. Barann M, Gothert M, Fink K, et al: Inhibition by anesthetics of 14-C-quanidium flux through the voltage-gated sodium channel and the cation channel of the 5-HT₃ receptor of N1E-115 neuroblastoma cells, *Naunyn Schmiedebergs Arch Pharmacol* 347:125, 1993.

58. Appadu B, Lambert DG: Interaction of IV anesthetic agent with 5-HT₃ receptors, *Br J Anaesth* 76:271, 1996.

59. Fruergaard K, Jenstrup M, Schierbeck J, et al: Total intravenous anesthesia with propofol or etomidate, *Eur J Anaesthesiol* 8:385, 1991.

60. Kestin IG, Dorje P: Anaesthesia for the evacuation of retained products of conception: comparison between alfentanil plus etomidate and fentanyl plus thiopentone, *Br J Anaesth* 59:364, 1987.

61. Javery KB, Ussery TW, Steger HG, et al: Comparison of morphine and morphine with ketamine for postoperative analgesia, *Can J Anaesth* 43:212, 1996.

62. Sampson IH, Plosker H, Cohen M, et al: Comparison of propofol and thiamylal for induction and maintenance of anesthesia for outpatient surgery, *Br J Anaesth* 61:707, 1988.

63. Best N, Traugott F: Comparative evaluation of propofol and methohexitone as the sole anesthetic agent for microlaryngeal surgery, *Anaesth Intensive Care* 19:50: 1991.

64. Chittleborough MC, Osborne GA, Rudkin GE, et al: Double blind comparison of patient recovery after induction with propofol or thiopentone for day case relaxant general anaesthesia, *Anaesth Intensive Care* 20:169, 1992.

65. Eriksson H, Hassio J, Korttila K: Comparison of eltanolone and thiopental in anaesthesia for termination of pregnancy, *Acta Anaesthesiol Scand* 39:479, 1995.

66. Boeke AJ, de Lange JJ, van Druenen, et al: Effect of antagonizing residual neuromuscular block by neostigmine and atropine on postoperative vomiting, *Br J Anaesth* 72:654, 1994.

67. Lessard MR, Trepanier CA, Rouillard JF: Neostigmine requirements for reversal of neuromuscular blockade following an infusion of mivacurium, *Can J Anaesth* 44:836, 1997.

68. Ding Y, Fredman B, White PF: Use of mivacurium during laparoscopic surgery: effect of reversal drugs on postoperative recovery, *Anesth Analg* 78:450, 1994.

69. Lauretti GR, Mattos AL, Reis MP, et al: Intrathecal neostigmine for postoperative analgesia after orthopedic surgery, *J Clin Anesth* 9:473, 1997.

70. Jellish WS, Leonetti JP, Murdoch JR, et al: Propofol-based anesthesia as compared with standard anesthetic techniques for middle ear surgery, *J Clin Anesth* 7:292, 1995.

71. Lim BL, Low TC: Total intravenous anaesthesia versus inhalational anaesthesia for dental day surgery, *Anaesth Intensive Care* 20:475, 1992.

72. Phillips AS, Mirakhur RK, Glen JB, et al: Total intravenous anesthesia with propofol or inhalational anaesthesia with isoflurane for major abdominal surgery: recovery characteristics and postoperative oxygenation—an international multicentre study, *Anaesthesia* 51:1055, 1996.

73. Hovorka J, Korttila K, Erkola O: The experience of the person ventilating the lungs does influence postoperative nausea and vomiting, *Acta Anaesthesiol Scand* 34:203, 1990.

74. Hovorka J, Korttila K, Erkola O: Gastric aspiration at the end of anaesthesia does not decrease postoperative nausea and vomiting, *Anaesth Intensive Care* 18:58, 1990.

75. Trepanier CA, Isabel LI: Perioperative gastric aspiration increases postoperative nausea and vomiting in outpatients, *Can J Anaesth* 40:325, 1993.

76. Mulroy MF: Regional anesthesia techniques, *Int Anesthesiol Clin* 32:81, 1994.

77. Carpenter RL, Caplan RA, Brown DL, et al: Incidence and risk factors for side effects of spinal anesthesia, *Anesthesiology* 76:906, 1992.

78. Bokesch PM, Huffnagle FT, Macauley C: Local versus general anesthesia for lumbar percutaneous discectomy, *J Neurosurg Anesthesiol* 5:81, 1993.

79. Ramirez-Ruiz M, Smith I, White PF: Use of analgesics during propofol sedation: a comparison of ketorolac, dezocine, and fentanyl, *J Clin Anesth* 7:481, 1995.

80. Moote CA: Postoperative pain management: back to the basics, *Can J Anaesth* 42:453, 1995.

81. Rapp SE, Egan KJ, Ross BK, et al: A multidimensional comparison of morphine and hydromorphone patient-controlled analgesia, *Anesth Analg* 82:1043, 1996.

82. Doyle E, Robinson D, Morton NS: Comparison of patient-controlled analgesia with and without a background infusion after lower abdominal surgery in children, *Br J Anaesth* 71:670, 1993.

83. Orkin F: What do patients want? Preferences for immediate postoperative recovery, *Anesth Analg* 74:S225, 1992 (abstract).

84. Reisine T, Pasternak G: Opioid analgesics and antagonists. In Hardman JG, Limbird LE, eds: *Goodman & Gilman's pharmacological basis of therapeutics*, ed 9, New York, 1996, McGraw-Hill, p 531.

85. White PF: Practical issues in outpatient anaesthesia: management of postoperative pain and emesis, *Can J Anaesth* 42:1053, 1995.

86. Comroe JH, Dripps RD: Reactions to morphine in ambulatory patients, *Surg Gynecol Obstet* 87:221, 1948.

87. Van Der Berg AA, Lambourne A, Yazji NS, et al: Vomiting after ophthalmic surgery: effects of intra-operative anti-emetics and postoperative oral fluid restriction, *Anaesthesia* 42:270, 1987.

88. Schreiner MS, Nicolson SC, Martin T, et al: Should children drink before discharge from day surgery? *Anesthesiology* 76:528, 1992.

89. Spencer EM: Intravenous fluids in minor gynecological surgery: their effect on postoperative morbidity, *Anesthesiology* 43:1050, 1988.

90. Gold BS, Kitz DS, Lecky JH, et al: Unanticipated hospital admission following ambulatory surgery, *JAMA* 262:3008, 1989.

91. Desilva PH, Darvish AH, McDonald S, et al: The efficacy of prophylactic ondansetron, droperidol, perphenazine, and metoclopramide in the prevention of nausea and vomiting after major gynecologic surgery, *Anesth Analg* 81:139, 1995.

92. Van Den Berg AA: A comparison of ondansetron and prochlorperazine for the prevention of nausea and vomiting after tympanoplasty, *Anesth Analg* 43:939, 1996.

93. Larsson S, Hagerdal M, Lundberg D: A controlled double-blind comparison with morphine-scopolamine and placebo, *Acta Anaesthesiol Scand* 32:131, 1988.

94. Grond S, Lynch J, Diefenbach C, et al: Comparison of ondansetron and droperidol in the prevention of nausea and vomiting after inpatient minor gynecologic surgery, *Anesth Analg* 81:603, 1995.

95. Davis PJ, McGowan FX, Landsmann I, et al: Effect of antiemetic therapy on recovery and hospital discharge time: a double-blind assessment of ondansetron, droperidol and placebo in pediatric patients undergoing ambulatory surgery, *Anesthesiology* 83:956, 1995.

96. Foster PN, Stickle BR, Dale M, et al: Akathisia after low-dose droperidol, *Anesthesiology* 74:477, 1995.

97. Lunn DV, Lauder GR, Williams AR, et al: Low-dose droperidol reduces postoperative vomiting in paediatric day surgery, *Br J Anaesth* 74:509, 1995.

98. Watts SA: A randomized double-blinded comparison of metoclopramide, ondansetron and cyclizine in daycase laparoscopy, *Anaesth Intensive Care* 24:546, 1996.

99. Vener DF, Carr AS, Bissonette B, et al: Dimenhydrinate decreases vomiting after strabismus surgery in children, *Anesth Analg* 82:728, 1996.

100. Chisakuta AM, Mirakhur RK: Anticholinergic prophylaxis does not prevent emesis following strabismus surgery in children, *Paediatr Anaesth* 5:97, 1995.

101. Kamath B, Curran J, Hawkey C, et al: Anesthesia movement and emesis, *Br J Anaesth* 64:728, 1990.

102. Doyle E, Byers G, McNicol LR, et al: Prevention of postoperative nausea and vomiting with transdermal hyoscine in children using patient-controlled analgesia, *Br J Anaesth* 72:72, 1994.

103. Reinhart DJ, Klein KW, Schroff E: Transdermal scopolamine for the reduction of postoperative nausea in outpatient ear surgery: a double-blind, randomized study, *Anesth Analg* 79:281, 1994.

104. Honkavaara P, Saarnivaara L, Klenola UM: Prevention of nausea and vomiting with transdermal hyoscine in adults after middle ear surgery, *Br J Anaesth* 73:763, 1994.

105. Naylor RJ, Inall FC: The physiology and pharmacology of postoperative nausea and vomiting, *Anaesthesia* 49(suppl):2, 1994.

106. Stein DJ, Birnbach DJ, Danzer BI, et al: Acupressure versus intravenous metoclopramide to prevent nausea and vomiting during spinal anesthesia for caesarean section, *Anesth Analg* 84:342, 1997.

107. Ali-Melkkila T, Kanto J, Katevou R: Tropisetron and metoclopramide in the prevention of postoperative nausea and vomiting: a comparative, placebo-controlled study in patients undergoing opthalmic surgery, *Anaesthesia* 51:232, 1996.

108. Pugh SC, Jones NC, Barsoum LZ: A comparison of prophylactic ondansetron and metoclopramide administration in patients undergoing major neurosurgical procedures, *Anaesthesia* 51:1162, 1996.

109. Naguib M, el Bakry AK, Khoshim MH, et al: Prophylactic antiemetic therapy with ondansetron, tropisetron, granisetron and metoclopramide in patients undergoing laparoscopic cholecystectomy, *Can J Anaesth* 43:226, 1996.

110. Alexander R, Fennelly M: Comparison of ondansetron, metoclopramide and placebo as premedicants to reduce nausea and vomiting after major surgery, *Anaesthesia* 52:695, 1997.

111. Kaufman MA, Rosow C, Schnieper P, et al: Prophylactic antiemetic therapy with patient-controlled analgesia: a double-blind, placebo-controlled comparison of droperidol, metoclopramide and tropisetron, *Anesth Analg* 78:988, 1997.

112. Polati E, Verlato G, Finco G, et al: Ondansetron versus metoclopramide in the treatment of postoperative nausea and vomiting, *Anesth Analg* 85:395, 1997.

113. Hesketh PJ, Gandara DR: Serotonin antagonists: a new class of antiemetic agents, *J Natl Cancer Inst* 83:613, 1991.

114. Hall MD, Brodsky L: The effect of post-operative diet on recovery in the first 12 hours after tonsillectomy, *Int J Pediatr Otorhinolaryngol* 31:215, 1995.

115. Pearman MH: Single dose intravenous ondansetron in the prevention of postoperative nausea and vomiting, *Anaesthesia* 49:11, 1994.

116. Russell D, Kenny GNC: 5-HT$_3$ antagonists in postoperative nausea and vomiting, *Br J Anaesth* 69(suppl):63S, 1992.

117. Sniadach MS, Alberts MS: A comparison of the prophylactic antiemetic effect of ondansetron and droperidol on patients undergoing gynecologic laparoscopy, *Anesth Analg* 85:797, 1997.

118. Markham A, Sorkin EM: Ondansetron: an update of its therapeutic use in chemotherapy-induced and postoperative nausea and vomiting, *Drugs* 45:931, 1993.

119. Patel RI, Davis PJ, Orr RJ, et al: Single-dose ondansetron prevents postoperative vomiting in pediatric outpatients, *Anesth Analg* 85:538, 1997.

120. Tramer MR, Moore RA, Reynolds DJ, et al: A quantitative systematic review of ondansetron in treatment of established postoperative nausea and vomiting, *BMJ* 314:1088, 1997.

121. Fujii Y, Toyooka H, Tanaka H: Antiemetic effects of granisetron on postoperative nausea and vomiting in patients with and without motion sickness, *Can J Anaesth* 43:110, 1996.

122. Cieslak GD, Watcha MF, Phillips MB, et al: The dose-response relation and cost-effectiveness of granisetron for the prophylaxis of pediatric postoperative emesis, *Anesthesiology* 85:1076, 1996.

123. White PF, Watcha MF: Are new drugs cost-effective for patients undergoing ambulatory surgery? *Anesthesiology* 78:2, 1998.

124. Capouet V, De PC, Vernet B, et al: Single dose I.V. tropisetron in the prevention of postoperative nausea and vomiting after gynaecological surgery, *Br J Anaesth* 76:54, 1996.

125. Balfour JA, Goa KL: Dolasetron: a review of its pharmacology and therapeutic potential in the management of nausea and vomiting induced by chemotherapy, radiotherapy or surgery, *Drugs* 54:273, 1997.

126. Dixon RM, Cramer M, Shah AK, et al: Single-dose, placebo-controlled, phase I study of oral dolasetron, *Pharmacotherapy* 16:245, 1996.

127. Splinter WM, Roberts DJ: Dexamethasone decreases vomiting by children after tonsillectomy, *Anesth Analg* 83:913, 1996.

128. Lopez-Olaondo L, Carrascosa F, Pueyo FJ, et al: Combination of ondansetron and dexamethasone in the prophylaxis of postoperative nausea and vomiting, *Br J Anaesth* 76:835, 1996.

129. Mckenzie R, Tantisira B, Karambelkar DJ, et al: Comparison of ondansetron with ondansetron plus dexamethasone in the prevention of postoperative nausea and vomiting, *Anesth Analg* 79:961, 1994.

130. McKenzie R, Uy NT, Riley TJ, et al: Droperidol/ondansetron combination controls nausea and vomiting after tubal banding, *Anesth Analg* 83:1218, 1996.

131. Wrench IJ, Ward JE, Walder AD, et al: The prevention of postoperative nausea and vomiting using a combination of ondansetron and droperidol, *Anaesthesia* 51:776, 1996.

132. Pueyo FJ, Carrascosa F, Lopez L, et al: Combination of ondansetron and droperidol in the prevention of postoperative nausea and vomiting, *Anesth Analg* 83:117, 1996.

133. Steinbrook RA, Freiberger D, Gosnell JL, et al: Prophylactic antiemetics for laparoscopic cholecystectomy: ondansetron versus droperidol plus metoclopramide, *Anesth Analg* 83:1081, 1996.

134. White PF: Are nonpharmacologic techniques useful alternatives to antiemetic drugs for the prevention of nausea and vomiting? *Anesth Analg* 84:712, 1987.

135. Yentis SM, Bisonette B: Ineffectiveness of acupressure and droperidol in preventing vomiting following strabismus repair in children, *Can J Anaesth* 39:173, 1992.

136. al-Sadi M, Newman B, Julious SA: Acupuncture in the prevention of postoperative nausea and vomiting, *Anaesthesia* 52:658, 1997.

137. Fan CF, Tanhui E, Joshi S, et al: Acupressure treatment for the prevention of postoperative nausea and vomiting, *Anesth Analg* 84:821, 1997.

138. Cook JA, Murrant NJ, Evans KL, et al: A randomized comparison of three post-tonsillectomy diets, *Clin Otolaryngol* 17:28, 1992.

139. Watcha MF, White PF: Postoperative nausea and vomiting: do they matter? *Eur J Anaesthesiol* 12(suppl 10):18, 1995.

140. Watcha MF, Smith I: Cost-effectiveness analysis of antiemetic therapy for ambulatory surgery, *J Clin Anesth* 6:370, 1994.

141. Dexter F, Tinker JH: Analysis of strategies to decrease postanesthesia care unit costs, *Anesthesiology* 82:94, 1995.

Chapter 20
Liver Dysfunction After Anesthesia

Phillip S. Mushlin
Simon Gelman

Although postoperative liver dysfunction (POLD) can be a direct consequence of anesthesia or surgery, it may also reflect the progression of a preexisting liver disorder that is unaffected, or perhaps exacerbated, by perioperative events. Thus a careful preoperative patient evaluation is of great importance in the differential diagnosis of POLD. The evaluation should be thorough enough to detect subtle presentations of liver disease and to identify risk factors for POLD, such as ethanol abuse, prior blood transfusions, infection with hepatitis virus, or previous episodes of unexplained postoperative jaundice.

Nonetheless, there are times when the analysis of preoperative factors and intraoperative events will fail to suggest the cause of POLD. In such cases, the anesthetic is a prime suspect.

The diagnosis of anesthesia-induced liver disease (AILD) is typically based on circumstantial evidence and predicated on an exclusion of other possible causes of POLD. There are no distinct diagnostic criteria for AILD and no pathognomonic features. It is therefore inappropriate to implicate the anesthetic before duly considering the multifarious causes of POLD, such as viruses, medications, perioperative circulatory disturbances, and surgical trauma. Probing the diagnostic possibilities, which include analyses of an abundance of clinical, laboratory, and histopathologic data, clearly requires an understanding of liver disease. Such an understanding is imperative for those of us who seek to critically evaluate a diagnosis of AILD and to optimally treat patients at risk for developing severe POLD.

I. PRESENTATIONS OF POSTOPERATIVE LIVER DYSFUNCTION

POLD is common, and its presentation ranges from asymptomatic injury to overt liver failure. Mild, transient increases in serum concentrations of hepatic enzymes are often detectable within hours of surgery but do not usually persist for more than 2 days. Such subclinical hepatocellular injury occurs in as many as 20% of patients who receive enflurane anesthesia and in nearly 50% of those receiving halothane.[1,2] Jaundice rarely occurs in healthy patients following minor operations but appears in up to 20% of patients after major surgical procedures.[3] Jaundice is typically the earliest sign of serious hepatic or hepatobiliary dysfunction and therefore requires prompt medical attention. Marked increases of serum aminotransferase activities are an ominous finding, reflecting extensive hepatocellular necrosis.

Some cases of severe POLD are apparent hours after surgery (e.g., with hypoxic injury), whereas other cases are delayed in onset for days to weeks (e.g., with anesthesia-induced hepatitis [AIH]). With severe POLD, residual liver function may fall below a critical threshold, leading to the development of hepatic encephalopathy. If encephalopathy occurs within 2 weeks of the onset of jaundice or within 8 weeks of the initial manifestation of hepatic disease, the disorder is defined as fulminant hepatic failure (FHF).[4] FHF has a wide variety of causes (Table 20-1). The mortality rate from FHF correlates with the severity of encephalopathy. The shorter the time interval between the appearance of jaundice and presentation of encephalopathy, the worse the prognosis.

To effectively treat patients with FHF, the clinician must be able to make prompt and accurate predictions about the outcome of the disease. Through proper recognition of reversible disease, unnecessary orthotopic liver transplantation (OLT) is avoided. Cases of FHF that are destined to be irreversible must be identified without delay (Box 20-1). Otherwise, the severe complications of FHF that develop may render patients unacceptable candidates for OLT.

II. ASSESSMENT OF HEPATIC FUNCTION

A broad array of laboratory and clinical tests are available for the assessment of hepatic function (Box 20-2).[5] The majority of the "liver function tests" (LFTs) do not actually measure functions of the liver (e.g., serum aminotransferase activity, alkaline phosphatase [AP] activity); they mainly reflect the presence of hepatobiliary injury and may suggest a general category of disease, such as hepatitis, biliary obstruction, or steatosis. Although LFTs often provide the earliest indication of a subclinical injury, they rarely indicate the specific cause of the problem or the current status of a patient's hepatic function.[5]

The extent of hepatocellular injury can often be inferred from the degree of increase of serum aspartate aminotransferase activity (AST, formerly called SGOT) or alanine aminotransferase activity (ALT, formerly called SGPT). ALT and AST are elevated in almost all

---

Box 20-1 Criteria for liver transplantation*

PT > 100 seconds (INR > 7.7) (irrespective of grade of encephalopathy)
or any three of the following:
  Age < 10 or > 40
  Bad etiology (non-A/non-B hepatitis, halothane, idiosyncratic drug reaction, Wilson's disease)
  Period of jaundice to encephalopathy > 7 days
  PT > 50 seconds (INR > 3.85)
  Serum bilirubin > 300 μmol/L (17 mg/dl)

Modified from Sussman N: Fulminant hepatic failure. In Zakim D, Boyer T, eds: *Hepatology: a textbook of liver disease,* Philadelphia, 1996, WB Saunders.
*Criteria for liver transplantation for causes other than acetaminophen; likelihood of survival considered <20%.
PT, Prothrombin time (British units); *INR,* International Normalization Ratio.

Table 20-1. Four etiologic categories of fulminant hepatic failure

Infections	Drugs, toxins, and other chemicals	Cardiovascular	Metabolic
Viral hepatitis	Acetaminophen	Portal vein thrombosis	Acute fatty liver of pregnancy
Type A	Halothane	Budd-Chiari syndrome	Wilson's disease
Type B	Isoniazid	Right ventricular failure	Reye's syndrome
Type C	Sodium valproate	Cardiac tamponade	Galactosemia
Type D	Tetracycline	Circulatory shock	Hereditary fructose intolerance
Type E	NSAIDs	Metastatic tumor	Hereditary tyrosinemia
	Pirprofen	Heat stroke	
Yellow fever	*Amanita phalloides*		
Q fever	Yellow phosphorus		
Other viruses	Ketoconazole		

From Sussman N: Fulminant hepatic failure. In Zakim D, Boyer T: *Hepatology: a textbook of liver disease,* Philadelphia, 1996, WB Saunders.

types of hepatic disease. A small increase (less than three-fold) typically occurs with fatty liver disease or chronic viral hepatitis, whereas a larger increase (three- to twentyfold) is suggestive of acute hepatitis or exacerbations of chronic hepatitis (alcoholic hepatitis). The largest increases (greater than twentyfold) are indicative of massive hepatocellular necrosis and usually result from the effects of drugs (including anesthetics), toxins, circulatory shock, or severe viral hepatitis.

It is important to realize that changes in ALT or AST do not invariably reflect the severity or even the presence of hepatocellular injury. For example, in patients with severe hepatitis, decreases of ALT or AST may indicate that the liver is either recovering from the disease or being destroyed by it, with few remaining hepatocytes to release these enzymes into the circulation. Moreover, increases of AST or ALT may occur in the absence of liver disease, reflecting diseases of other tissues such as heart or skeletal muscle. In this regard, ALT, which is localized primarily in the liver, is a more specific marker of hepatic injury than AST; AST is present in a variety of tissues including liver, heart, skeletal muscle, kidney, and brain.

In addition to ALT and AST, lactate dehydrogenase (LDH) activity is often measured as a test for hepatic injury. A marked increase of LDH may be indicative of hepatocellular necrosis, shock liver, or hemolysis combined with liver disease. However, LDH can be increased in many nonhepatic diseases and is therefore of little value as a diagnostic test for liver disease.

Measurement of hepatic isoenzymes of glutathione S-transferase (GST) has been purported to be a highly sensitive and specific method for detection of drug-induced hepatocellular damage.[2] Because GSTs are rapidly released into the circulation following hepatic injury and have a short plasma half-life (90 minutes), the monitoring of GST can provide detailed information about the time course of the injury, from onset to resolution. Unlike the aminotransferases, which have a periportal (zone 1) localization, GST concentrations are greater in centrilobular (zone 3) hepatocytes than in midzonal or periportal hepatocytes.[6] Thus agents such as anesthetics, which can selectively injure centrilobular hepatocytes, may cause a disproportionately greater increase of GST than of serum aminotransferases.

AP is a highly sensitive test for assessing the integrity of intrahepatic and extrahepatic bile ducts. However, AP must be used in conjunction with other LFTs for the diagnosis of hepatobiliary disease because isozymes of alkaline phosphatase are present in liver, intestine, bone, placenta, kidney, and leukocytes. Indeed, on routine laboratory testing, transient, mild increases of AP are observed in up to one third of patients in the absence of hepatobiliary disease. During pregnancy, AP nearly doubles just from placental release of the enzyme. Although various diseases increase AP, the increases are greatest in the presence of cholestatic disorders. It is noteworthy that a relatively low AP in the presence of an increased serum bilirubin concentration (AP to bilirubin ratio) is generally associated with a poor prognosis in patients with FHF.

Measurement of 5'-nucleotidase activity in blood (5'NT) is a highly specific method for detecting hepatobiliary dysfunction. (5'NT has largely replaced measurement of serum γ-glutamyl transpeptidases [GGT], which is the most sensitive test for biliary tract disease, but too nonspecific to be useful). Although these nucleotidases are present in liver, brain, intestine, heart, blood vessels, and endocrine pancreas, only hepatobiliary tissue can release the enzymes into the circulation, because the release of 5'NT may require the detergent action of bile salts on plasma membranes. Perhaps the greatest utility of measuring 5'NT is for confirming or rejecting assumptions about the hepatic origin of an increased AP. 5'NT is useful in this regard because it closely correlates with AP in patients with liver disease.

Measurement of serum bilirubin (an endogenous organic anion derived primarily from the breakdown of hemoglobin) plays a central role in the evaluation of hepatobiliary disease. Hyperbilirubinemia has a wide range of causes, and is classified as either unconjugated (indirect) or conjugated (direct reacting bilirubin) on the basis of the predominant form of bilirubin in the systemic circulation (Box 20-3). Unconjugated hyperbilirubinemia, with a serum concentration between 17 and 70 μmol/L (1 mg/dl to 4 mg/dl), generally results from any or a combination of the following disorders: excessive bilirubin production, impaired transport of bilirubin into hepatocytes, or defective bilirubin conjugation by hepatocytes. The total serum bilirubin concentration rarely exceeds 70 μmol/L when hepatic function is normal, even in cases of severe hemolysis. Thus hepatic disease can be inferred when the total bilirubin concentration either exceeds 70 μmol/L or ranges between 17 and 70 μmol/L in the presence of other abnormal LFTs. Hepatobiliary disease is characterized by conjugated hyper-

---

Box 20-2 Classification of liver function tests

Tests that reflect injury to hepatocytes (serum aminotransferase activities) or bile ducts (alkaline phosphatase activity)

Tests that measure the liver's capacity to transport organic ions and clear both endogenous and exogenous substances from the circulation (serum bilirubin concentration, bile acid concentration)

Tests that measure hepatic blood flow or the metabolic capacity of the liver (indocyanine green, bromsulfophthalein, galactose, lidocaine clearance)

Tests that reflect hepatic synthetic function (serum albumin concentration, concentration of coagulation factors)

Miscellaneous tests that facilitate accurate diagnosis of hepatic disease but do not necessarily assess liver function (titers of immunoglobulin-specific autoantibody and serologic tests for viral hepatitis)

From Friedman L, Martin P, Munoz S: Liver function tests and the objective evaluation of the patient with liver disease. In Zakim D, Boyer T, eds: *Hepatology: a textbook of liver disease,* Philadelphia, 1996, WB Saunders.

> **Box 20-3** Causes of hyperbilirubinemia
>
> **Unconjugated (indirect)**
> Excessive bilirubin production (hemolysis)
> Immaturity of enzyme systems
>   Physiologic jaundice of newborn
>   Jaundice of prematurity
> Inherited defects
>   Gilbert's syndrome
>   Crigler-Najjar syndrome
> Drug effects
>
> **Conjugated (direct)**
> Hepatocellular disease (hepatitis, cirrhosis, drugs)
> Intrahepatic cholestasis (drugs, pregnancy)
> Benign postoperative jaundice, sepsis
> Congenital conjugated hyperbilirubinemia
>   Dubin-Johnson syndrome
>   Rotor's syndrome
> Obstructive jaundice
>   Extrahepatic (calculus, stricture, neoplasm)
>   Intrahepatic (sclerosing cholangitis, neoplasm, primary biliary cirrhosis)

From Friedman L, Martin P, Munoz S: Liver function tests and the objective evaluation of the patient with liver disease. In Zakim D, Boyer T, eds: *Hepatology: a textbook of liver disease,* Philadelphia, 1996, WB Saunders.

bilirubinemia. With complete bile duct obstruction, serum bilirubin may reach 500 μmol/L (35 mg/dl), but it rarely exceeds this concentration because of continued urinary excretion of conjugated bilirubin. Thus a bilirubin concentration of greater than 500 μmol/L is indicative of severe hepatocellular disease accompanied by hemolysis or renal failure.

Blood concentrations of albumin, coagulation factors, and lipoproteins are often useful to detect severe impairments of hepatic synthetic function. To be meaningful, these tests, which lack sensitivity and specificity for liver disease, must be interpreted in the context of the clinical presentation and the other laboratory findings. For example, a low serum albumin concentration in the presence of chronic liver disease is highly suggestive of severe disease, provided that other causes of hypoalbuminemia (poor nutritional status, hormonal imbalance, nephropathy, and derangements of osmotic pressure) have been excluded. In acute liver failure, however, the long plasma half-life of albumin (nearly 20 days) renders it an insensitive and unreliable index of hepatic synthetic function. By contrast, assessment of coagulation function can provide useful information about the severity of both acute and chronic liver disease. Because the liver synthesizes quantities of coagulation factors (I, II, V, VII, IX, and X) that are far greater than what is needed for normal coagulation, abnormalities of clotting do not result from liver disease alone unless it is severe. Thus the appearance of a coagulopathy in a patient with liver disease may be ominous. In acute hepatocellular disease, a prothrombin time (PT) that is markedly prolonged and progressively worsening often signals the development of FHF. Of course, the prolongation of PT may be totally unrelated

to liver disease, resulting instead from congenital deficiencies of coagulation factors or acquired conditions, such as consumptive coagulopathy, vitamin K deficiency, or ingestion of drugs that antagonize the prothrombin complex (coumarin).

Less common in the evaluation of hepatic dysfunction are tests that measure hepatic blood flow and the capacity of the liver to metabolize drugs. Studies comparing effects of anesthetics on hepatic blood flow often use the indocyanine green method (ICG). ICG is a nontoxic dye that binds avidly to plasma proteins and is highly extracted by the liver following an intravenous injection; the hepatic extraction ratio of ICG (70% to 90%) exceeds that of bromsulfophthalein (BSP 50% to 80%). Although ICG is unaltered by hepatic biotransformation processes and is excreted unchanged in bile, it also undergoes extrahepatic clearance. Therefore measurements of hepatic blood flow by ICG clearance may be inaccurate without measurements of ICG concentrations in hepatic venous blood. Tests that measure the capacity of the liver to metabolize drugs include antipyrine clearance from plasma (C14 aminopyrine breath test), caffeine clearance, galactose elimination, maximum rate of urea synthesis, and the rate of formation of lidocaine metabolites. In general, the agents used to evaluate the liver's metabolic capacity have low intrinsic clearances and are selectively metabolized by hepatic microsomal enzymes. Thus the elimination of these agents depends on the functional mass of the liver and is independent of hepatic blood flow.

Another category of laboratory tests provides information that is critically important for accurate diagnosis of liver disease but offers no specific information about hepatic function. Included in this category are serologic profiles for viral hepatitis and measurements of plasma immunoglobulins, which may reveal autoantibodies or antibodies to anesthetic-induced neoantigens.

Liver biopsy continues to have a central role in the evaluation of patients with suspected liver disease because it provides the only means of determining the precise nature of hepatic damage (necrosis, inflammation, or fibrosis). It is often used in the evaluation of unexplained abnormalities of LFTs. Postoperatively, liver biopsy can be invaluable for resolving diagnostic dilemmas because it may reveal the type and extent of various chronic hepatic injuries, identity and location of intrahepatic viral antigens, and patterns of acute hepatic injury that are characteristic of hepatotoxic drugs. Liver biopsy is also helpful for evaluating the effectiveness of therapies for liver disease. However, it is contraindicated in the presence of coagulopathy (e.g., PT more than 3 seconds greater than control, platelet count less than 60,000/mm³).

III. HALOGENATED INHALED ANESTHETICS AND POSTOPERATIVE LIVER DYSFUNCTION
A. Comparison of hepatotoxic potentials of halogenated agents: an overview

Of the many drugs that can produce or contribute to POLD, none have caused greater concern than the halogenated inhaled anesthetics. Indeed, the recognition of

Table 20-2. Relationship between metabolism of volatile halogenated agents and anesthetic-induced hepatitis

Agent	Year introduced into clinical practice in the United States	No. of cases of hepatitis	Percentage of agent taken up that is metabolized	Metabolites fluororacetylate and hepatic proteins
Halothane	1958	More than 500[7]	20-46[15,16]	Yes
Enflurane	1972	Approximately 50[7-9]	2.5-8.5[16,17]	Yes
Isoflurane	1981	6[7,10]	0.2-2[16,19]	Yes
Desflurane	1993	1[14]	0.02[20]	Yes
Sevoflurane	1995	3[11,12,13]	2-5[131]	No

halothane's potential to cause significant hepatotoxicity has prompted a dramatic decrease in its use in adult patients in the United States and has paved the way for the use of newer agents: enflurane (1972), isoflurane (1981), desflurane (1993), and sevoflurane (1995).

Table 20-2 shows a comparison of the halogenated agents in clinical use and the number of cases in which hepatitis was attributed to the anesthetic. Several hundred cases of halothane hepatitis have been reported since the introduction of halothane into clinical practice in the 1950s.[7] This is many times more than the total number of cases attributed to all the other inhaled agents combined. Thus far, enflurane has been implicated as a cause of severe hepatic injury in approximately 50 cases[7-9] and isoflurane may have been responsible for another six cases.[7,10] Three cases of hepatitis have been attributed to sevoflurane use,[11-13] and there is only a single report that implicates desflurane as a possible cause of hepatitis.[14] The very low incidence of hepatitis with desflurane and sevoflurane is probably a reason for optimism, but such optimism should be tempered by recognition of the limited clinical experience with these new agents.

The potential of halogenated inhaled agents to cause severe liver dysfunction appears to be associated with the extent of their metabolism. Of the halothane taken up during anesthesia, 20% to 46% is metabolized,[15,16] compared to 2.5% to 8.5% for enflurane,[16,17] 2% to 5% for sevoflurane,[18,131] 0.2% to 2% for isoflurane,[16,19] and 0.02% for desflurane[20] (see Table 20-2). Each of these anesthetics, with the exception of sevoflurane, is oxidized via cytochrome P-450 2E1 to produce highly reactive intermediates that bind covalently (acylation) to a variety of hepatocellular macromolecules (Fig. 20-1). In susceptible people, these altered hepatic proteins may trigger an immunologic response that causes massive hepatic necrosis[7] (discussed later).

B. Halothane

Halothane produces both mild and severe forms of postoperative hepatic dysfunction.[21] Mild hepatic injury is detectable in 20% to 50% of adult patients after halothane anesthesia.[1,2,22-25] The injury is almost invariably asymptomatic and manifested only by minor abnormalities of LFTs.[1,2,25] The severe form, called halothane hepatitis, is a rare, unpredictable disorder with an estimated incidence between 1 in 3000 and 1 in 30,000 halothane anesthetics.[26-29] This disorder is characterized by massive hepatocellular necrosis, marked increases of

serum aminotransferases, and jaundice, and it may progress to FHF and death.[1,26,30]

1. Mild hepatic injury. AST and ALT are the most commonly used clinical tests for assessing the presence or absence of hepatocellular injury. Mild increases of serum aminotransferases (ALT or AST) occur postoperatively in approximately 25% of patients anesthetized with halothane,[25] and the increases may persist for up to 2 weeks after anesthesia.[22-24,31] As mentioned earlier, GST is even more sensitive than aminotransferases for detecting anesthetic-induced hepatic injury.[1,2,32] Postoperative increases in plasma GST may be seen in up to half of the patients having halothane anesthesia for minor operative procedures.[2] Under similar conditions, GST is increased in about 20% of those receiving enflurane anesthesia, and no increase occurs after isoflurane anesthesia.[2]

There is evidence that nitrous oxide can increase the hepatotoxicity of halothane. For example, in urologic patients anesthetized with either halothane plus 70% nitrous oxide (30% O_2), halothane alone (100% O_2), or isoflurane plus 70% nitrous oxide (30% O_2),[1] postoperative increases of GST occurred only in the two halothane groups and were seen more often in patients who had received nitrous oxide. These small but significant increases in GST appeared 3 to 6 hours after halothane in one third of the patients receiving nitrous oxide and in one fourth of those whose anesthetic did not include nitrous oxide. A second peak in GST activity at 24 hours has been observed with both halothane[1] and enflurane anesthesia.[2] The exact mechanism of the increased GST is unknown, but it seems plausible that early increases reflect effects of hepatic hypoxia from anesthesia-induced decreases of hepatic blood flow, whereas the delayed increases result from the production of toxic metabolites of halothane and enflurane.

A single halothane anesthetic administered to adults often causes transient hepatic injury. Children are much less likely than adults to experience hepatic injury following halothane anesthesia.[33-35] In a prospective study of 25 children who received at least 10 halothane anesthetics in a single year, the only evidence of POLD was a minimal increase of hepatic enzymes, which occurred in 5% to 11% of the children.[36] Similarly, repeated halothane anesthetics at intervals of less than 28 days did not produce overt POLD; only minor elevations of hepatic enzymes occurred, with an incidence of about 3%. Just as children are much less susceptible than adults to halothane-induced subclinical hepatic injury, they are

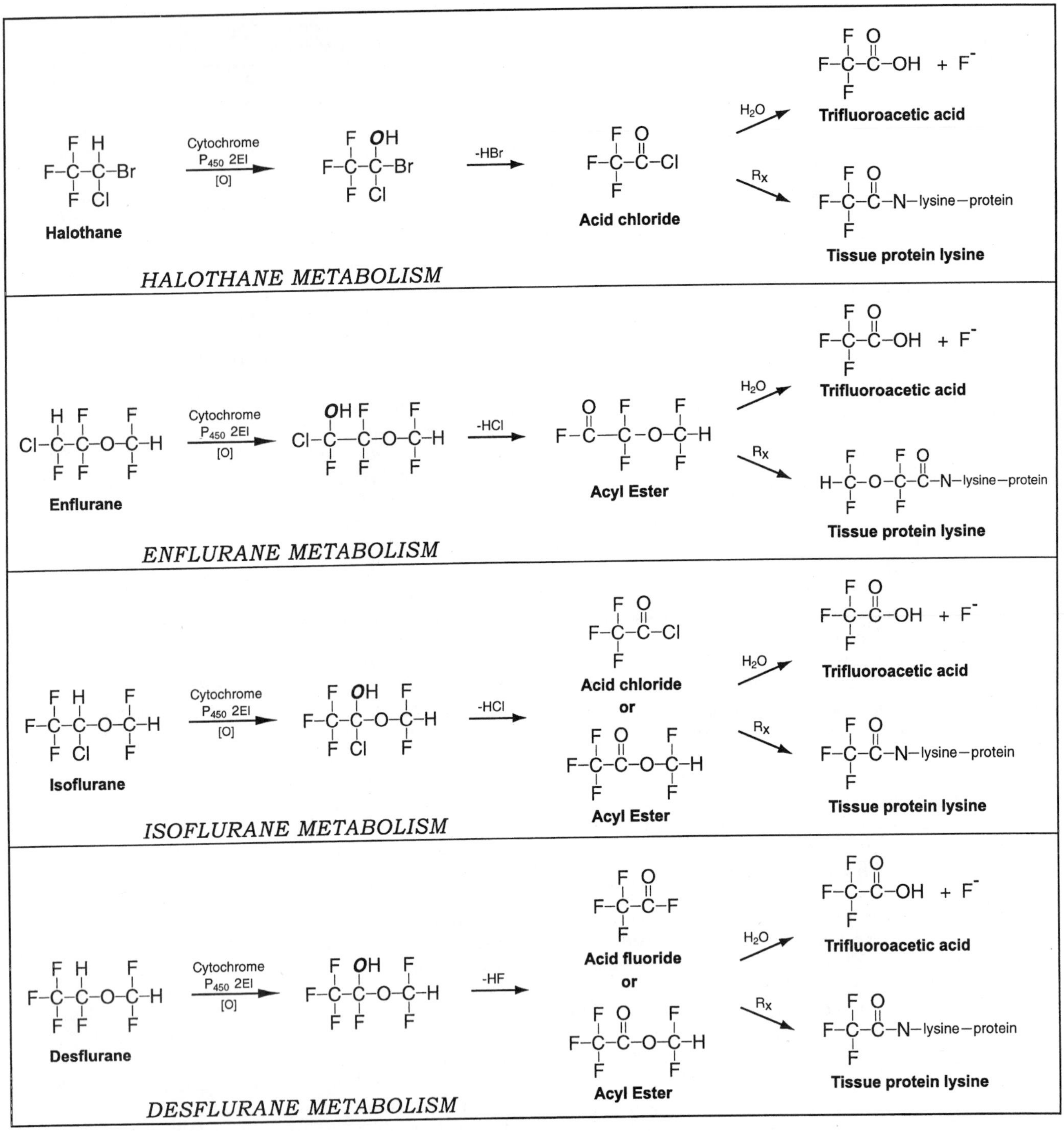

Fig. 20-1. Proposed pathways of cytochrome P-450 2E1 catalyzed metabolism of halothane, enflurane, isoflurane, and desflurane to produce highly reactive intermediates that acylate hepatic proteins. The acylated liver proteins appear to function as haptens to elicit an immune response. There is no evidence that sevoflurane produces an acylating intermediate, so it is not included in this figure (see Fig. 20-6). (Modified from Frink EJ Jr: *Anesth Analg* 81[suppl 6]:S46, 1995; Kenna JG, Jones RM: *Anesth Analg* 81[suppl 6]:S51, 1995; Njoku D, Laster MJ, Gong DH, et al: *Anesth Analg* 84:173, 1997.)

also considerably more resistant to the development of halothane hepatitis. However, it is unclear whether the reversible, mild forms of halothane toxicity are related to or in any way predispose to halothane hepatitis.

2. Halothane hepatitis

a. The National Halothane Study. Several years after the clinical introduction of halothane in 1955, an association was noted between halothane anesthesia and severe postoperative liver damage. Concerned that halothane could cause fulminant hepatitis, the Committee on Anesthesia of the National Academy of Sciences/National Research Council launched one of the largest epidemiologic studies ever completed: the National Halothane Study.[37] This retrospective review of anesthetics performed over a 4-year period, from 1959 to 1962, was designed to determine the incidence of massive hepatic necrosis after anesthesia. Based on a review of 856,600 surgical anesthetics, the study concluded that fatal, postoperative massive hepatic necrosis was very rare and usually explainable on a nonanesthetic basis, and that halothane, when compared with other anesthetics, was associated with an overall lower anesthetic mortality rate.

To understand the conclusions of the National Halothane Study, one must be aware of its major limitations, including significant problems with experimental design. Initially, the study included 54 centers, but only 38 were able to comply with the protocol's restrictions, and only 35 contributed data. Among these 35 institutions, marked differences existed in patterns of anesthetic use (halothane use varied from 6.2% to 62.7%), and overall anesthesia death rates varied widely (0.27% to 6.41%). Because the study required that necropsy be performed (15,722 deaths; autopsy rate was 65%), 35% of the deaths were excluded from the data analysis. Moreover, most cases believed to involve massive necrosis were excluded because postmortem autolysis made it impossible to assess hepatic morphology (724 excluded out of 946 cases). Of the 222 cases that revealed hepatic necrosis, all but 82 were eliminated by the reviewing pathologists as demonstrating less than "massive" necrosis, neglecting the fact that submassive necrosis can also be fatal. Of the remaining 82 cases, only 9 were attributed to anesthetic toxicity and only 7 of those patients had received halothane. In short, although the study reported an incidence of fulminant hepatic necrosis of approximately 1 per 35,000 anesthetics, the true incidence of halothane hepatitis cannot be ascertained from the study.[38] This is because the study was designed to look only at cases in which massive hepatic necrosis terminated in death and did not address the incidence of lesser degrees of hepatic injury. Based on more recent studies, the incidence of halothane hepatitis is probably somewhere between 1 in 3000 and 1 in 30,000.[26-29]

b. Clinical presentation and risk factors for halothane hepatitis. Halothane hepatitis often develops after minor, uneventful procedures of brief duration (less than 30 minutes). The disease does not become clinically apparent for several days after the halothane anesthetic (Table 20-3).[38] The classic presentation includes fever, anorexia, nausea, chills, myalgias, and a rash, followed by the appearance of jaundice 3 to 6 days later. Overt jaundice signals severe disease and portends a mortality rate that may be as great as 40%. Indicators of poor prognosis include a short latency period between the halothane anesthetic and the appearance of clinical symptoms, age greater than 40 years, obesity, a PT greater than 20 seconds, and a bilirubin concentration greater than 10 mg/dl (see Table 20-3).[38]

Several risk factors for the development of halothane hepatitis have been identified (Box 20-4). The most important is prior exposure to halothane.[39] Clinical studies indicate that between 71% and 95% of patients who develop jaundice after halothane have had at least one prior exposure to this agent.[28,38,40-44] Severe, idiosyncratic reactions to halothane occur about 10 times more often in patients who have had multiple halothane anesthetics than in those having their first-ever halothane anesthetic.[25] The shorter the interval between the two most recent exposures, the more rapid is the onset of jaundice and the more serious the disease. The risk of halothane hepatitis is greater for women than men. Women who

Table 20-3. Clinical and prognostic features of halothane hepatitis

Effects of frequency of exposure on latency period

Single exposure	6 days to first symptom	11 days to jaundice
Multiple exposures	3 days to first symptom	6 days to jaundice

Clinical presentation

Signs and symptoms	Percentage of cases
Fever	75
Anorexia, nausea	50
Chills	30
Myalgias	20
Rash	10

Indicators of poor prognosis

Short latency period
Age >40 years
Obesity
Prothrombin time >20 seconds (nearly 100% mortality)
Bilirubin >10 mg/dl (approximately 60% mortality)

From Touloukian J, Kaplowitz N: *Semin Liver Dis* 1:134, 1981.

Box 20-4 Risk factors for halothane hepatitis

Multiple exposures
Frequent exposures, especially with short intervals between anesthetics
Middle age (40 to 65 years)
Obesity
Female gender
Hispanic ethnicity

Modified from Brown BR, ed: *Anesthesia in hepatic and biliary tract disease*, Philadelphia, 1988, FA Davis.

develop the disease outnumber men 1.8 to 1, although men have a greater mortality rate from FHF. Obese women[45] seem to be more likely to develop halothane hepatitis than their nonobese counterparts. An increased susceptibility could result from obesity-related increases in the metabolism of halothane[46] as well as the prolonged postoperative exposure to halothane and its metabolites (increased sequestration by, and subsequent release from, adipose tissue) that occurs in obese patients. Some ethnic groups (Mexican-American) appear to be at greater risk,[47] and the disease may have a genetic basis.[48] Chromosomal differences have been noted between patients who recovered from halothane hepatitis and halothane-treated patients who did not develop the disease.[49]

Age is a significant risk factor for halothane hepatitis. Approximately half of the cases of halothane-associated FHF occur in patients older than 50.[25] Children are highly resistant to the development of halothane hepatitis[33-35] for reasons that are not yet clear. The rare cases that have been documented in children have involved multiple exposures to halothane.[50] Table 20-4 shows clinical details and results of biochemical tests in seven children who developed halothane hepatitis. It is unclear whether fetal exposure to halothane (transplacental) can sensitize very young children to the drug and thereby place them at increased risk for halothane hepatitis after postnatal anesthetics with halothane.

There is no evidence that preexisting liver disease increases the risk of halothane hepatitis.[51,52] In addition, there is no compelling evidence that concomitant administration of medications increases the risk of halothane hepatitis.

c. Diagnosis of halothane hepatitis. The differential diagnosis of POLD following halothane anesthesia can be quite challenging; it includes halothane hepatitis, viral hepatitis, benign postoperative jaundice, circulatory disturbances, and biliary injury (Table 20-5). Important clues as to the cause of the dysfunction often are found in the clinical presentation (presence or absence of fever, latency between the end of surgery and the onset of liver dysfunction), in results of laboratory tests (ALT and AP), or on liver biopsy (centrilobular necrosis). Nonetheless, because halothane hepatitis has no pathognomonic features, in certain cases it may be indistinguishable from other types of hepatitis. Thus unexplained hepatitis following a halothane anesthetic is often labeled as halothane hepatitis unless another cause is clearly identified.

A carefully performed preoperative evaluation will often contain invaluable diagnostic clues relating to POLD, such as a history of unexplained fever or jaundice

Table 20-4. Clinical details and results of biochemical tests in seven children with halothane hepatitis

Case no.	Age (yr)	Sex	Last operation	No. halothane exposures	Bilirubin (mg/dl)	Serum AST (IU/L)	Halothane antibody	Outcome
1	13	F	Ureterocele	3	37.2	3755	+	Alive
2	1½	F	Scar removal	3	Not assessed	>1500	+	Alive
3	1	M	Fistula repair	6	21.4	5080	+	Alive
4	14	F	Ortho repair	3	30.1	4000	+	Alive
5	15	F	Ortho manipulation	2	21.5	1005	+	Alive
6	3½	M	Hypospadias	3	86.1	960	+	Died
7	4	M	Ortho repair	2	9.3	3120	+	Alive

From Kenna JG, Jones RM: *Anesth Analg* 81:S51, 1995.
AST, Aspartate aminotransferase.

Table 20-5. Differential diagnosis of postoperative liver dysfunction

Disorder	Type of surgery	Fever	Time to onset	ALT (IU/L)	AP
Halothane hepatitis	No relationship	Common	2-15 days	>500	Slight ↑
Viral hepatitis	No relationship	Uncommon	>3 weeks	>500	Slight ↑
Benign postoperative jaundice	Major surgery with sepsis	Common	<7 days	Slight ↑	↑↑
Shock	No relationship (cardiac disease)	Uncommon	1-4 days	>500	Slight ↑ (high LDH)
Bile duct injury	Biliary tract and stomach	Common	Days-weeks	200-300	↑↑

From Boyer T: Preoperative and postoperative hepatic dysfunction. In Zakim D, Boyer T, eds: *Hepatology: a textbook of liver disease,* Philadelphia, 1996, WB Saunders.
ALT, Alanine aminotransferase; *AP,* alkaline phosphatase; *LDH,* lactate dehydrogenase.

following a previous general anesthetic or the presence of risk factors for non–anesthesia-related hepatic diseases. Severe POLD in a previously healthy patient is more likely to result from some preexisting liver disease than from halothane. Clinical studies have indicated that approximately 1 out of every 700 healthy-appearing preoperative patients (ASA Physical Status I) has undetected liver disease, and about 1 of 2500 ASA Physical Status I patients develops jaundice within days of a preoperative visit, solely on the basis of preoperative liver disease.[53,54] Thus it is difficult to know how often fulminant hepatitis that develops in the days that follow an anesthetic is erroneously attributed to the anesthetic agent. For example, Douglas et al[55] describe a case of hepatitis following enflurane anesthesia in which herpes virus was eventually isolated and identified as the cause of liver failure. In another case, laparotomy for suspected extrahepatic biliary obstruction was followed by acute hepatic deterioration; the cause of the deterioration was ultimately identified as viral hepatitis.[56]

Indeed, the clinical presentation and laboratory abnormalities seen in viral hepatitis can be indistinguishable from AIH. Even liver biopsy may not be helpful in the differential diagnosis because both conditions can produce centrilobular necrosis (as evidence of direct cytotoxicity) rather than cholestatic injury.[37] Thus serologic markers for infections with either hepatotropic viruses (A, B, C, D, E, G) or other viruses (cytomegalovirus [CMV], herpes) are important in the differential diagnosis. However, patients with recently acquired viral infections may have undetectable, low blood concentrations of viral antigen and nonexistent antibody titers. In such cases, the potential for misdiagnosing the cause of postoperative hepatic injury is clear. At least initially, the diagnosis may rest on circumstantial evidence, including demographic information (patients with fulminant viral hepatitis are typically much younger than those with halothane-associated FHF[25]; median age 30 versus 57 years old) and an analysis of the risk factors associated with viral versus other forms of hepatitis.

d. Mechanisms of halothane hepatitis. The mechanisms of hepatic dysfunction following halothane anesthesia remain unclear. The reported cases of halothane hepatitis do not form a homogeneous group, and it seems unlikely that a single mechanism will explain the different types of halothane hepatotoxicity.[57] Animal studies indicate that effects of halothane on hepatic blood flow and oxygen demand can cause hypoxic injury and that halothane metabolites can exert direct hepatotoxic effects. However, for reasons discussed later in this chapter, these mechanisms are either unimportant or unrelated to the development of halothane hepatitis in humans. The preponderance of evidence indicates that halothane hepatitis is an immunologically mediated disease. The pathogenesis appears to involve the generation of highly reactive intermediates that covalently bind to, and thereby modify, hepatic macromolecules. The immune theory posits that hepatocytes containing these modified macromolecules become targets for immune destruction in susceptible patients.

(1) BIOTRANSFORMATION. Halothane can be metabolized extensively via reductive pathways (O_2 less than 50 μmol/L) or oxidative pathways (O_2 greater than 50 μmol/L) (Fig. 20-2), and it also reacts with soda lime to form 2-chloro-2 bromo-1,1,difluoroethylene (CBDFE). CBDFE does not appear to be a clinically important hepatotoxin, nor do the stable end products of either reductive metabolism (2-chloro-1,1,1-trifluoroethane [CTE] and 2-chloro-1,1-difluoroethylene [CDE]) or oxidative metabolism (trifluoroacetic acid [TFA]); these compounds are chemically stable and lack hepatotoxicity. However, the intermediates of halothane metabolism, which are highly reactive species, can bind covalently to various hepatocellular molecules: CTE radical (reductive intermediate) forms adducts with hepatocellular phospholipids, whereas trifluoro (TF)-acetyl chloride (oxidative intermediate) forms TF-acetyl adducts with macromolecular nucleophiles in hepatocytes (e.g., with amino or sulfhydryl groups of proteins). It seems likely that such reactions injure the liver directly by impairing hepatocellular homeostasis or indirectly by generating neoantigens or autoantigens that ultimately trigger immunologically mediated hepatocellular necrosis.

The role of reductive or oxidative pathways in the genesis of halothane-mediated liver injury will depend on the O_2 tension in hepatocytes as well as on the activity of the cytochrome P-450 system (Figs. 20-2 and 20-3).[58] In some experimental models, halothane toxicity is mediated via oxidative pathways (guinea pig, isoniazid-pretreated rats, rat hepatocyte suspensions),[59] whereas in others it is related to reductive metabolism (various rat models) (Table 20-6). In fact, the mechanism of halothane hepatotoxicity in an animal model is merely a reflection of the paradigm used and may therefore be either germane or irrelevant to the clinical toxicity of halothane. The earliest paradigms of halothane hepatotoxicity were developed under the assumption that reductive metabolism is clinically relevant. Both phenobarbital pretreatment and hypoxia are used to promote reductive metabolism, which is accompanied by free radical generation, lipid peroxidation, and hepatocellular injury.[60] For example, halothane administration to phenobarbital-pretreated rats under normoxic conditions (21% O_2) causes a fivefold increase in liver F(2)-isoprostane concentrations (measure of lipid peroxidation in vivo); no lipid peroxidation occurs in the absence of phenobarbital pretreatment or following enflurane or desflurane anesthesia. Under hypoxic conditions (14% O_2), halothane produces a twentyfold increase in lipid peroxidation in phenobarbital-pretreated rats and an elevenfold increase in the absence of pretreatment.[60] Thus halothane anesthesia delivered under hypoxic conditions is sufficient to cause hepatocellular injury (increases in ALT) in this rat model.

(2) HYPOXIA AND ISCHEMIA. An inverse correlation exists between hepatic injury and hepatic oxygen supply, regardless of the intervention used to decrease the oxygen supply, be it halothane, isoflurane, or hemorrhage.[61] Experimental conditions that lower hepatic oxygen consumption, such as hypothermia or pretreatment with

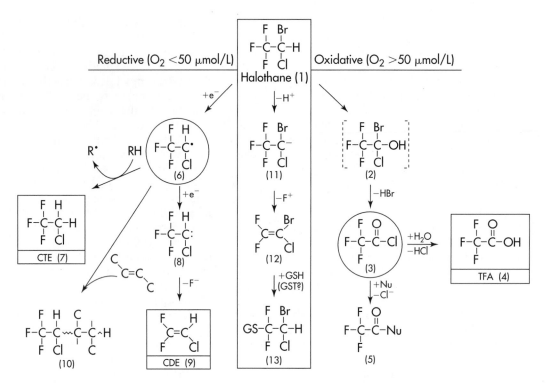

Fig. 20-2. Pathways of oxidative and reductive metabolism of halothane: *1*, halothane; *2*, unstable halohydrin; *3*, trifluoroacetyl chloride; *4*, trifluoroacetic acid (TFA); *5*, trifluoroacetyl adduct with nucleophile; *6*, 2-chloro-1,1,1-trifluoroethyl radical; *7*, 2-chloro-1,1,1-trifluoroethane; *8*, carbanion derivative of compound (6); *9*, 2-chloro-1,1-difluoroethylene; *10*, phospholipid adduct of compound (6); *11*, 2-bromo-2-chloro-1,1-difluoroethyl anion; *12*, 2-bromo-2-chloro-1,1-difluoroethylene; *13*, glutathione adduct of compound (12). Circled intermediates are highly reactive species that may bind covalently to hepatic molecules. Stable end products of halothane metabolism are shown in boxes. (Modified from Bass N, Ockner R: Drug-induced liver disease. In Zakim D, Boyer T, eds: *Hepatology: a textbook of liver disease,* Philadelphia, 1996, WB Saunders.)

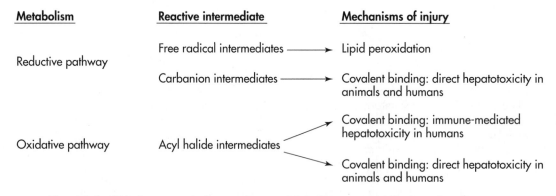

Fig. 20-3. Halothane metabolism and potential mechanism of halothane hepatotoxicity. (Modified from Bass N, Ockner R: Drug-induced liver disease. In Zakim D, Boyer T, eds: *Hepatology: a textbook of liver disease,* Philadelphia, 1996, WB Saunders.)

cimetidine or metyrapone, provide protection against hepatic injury.[62] Indeed, the high susceptibility of the liver to hypoxic injury confounds correlations between the reductive metabolism and hepatotoxity of halothane because the conditions required to stimulate reductive metabolism also increase the oxygen demand of the liver (see Table 20-6). Thus it is difficult to know

whether necrosis in the rat model is caused by halothane metabolism per se or by hypoxia or some combination of the two. However, no special conditions are needed to produce halothane hepatotoxicity in guinea pigs; the toxicity occurs without enzyme inducers (no phenobarbital pretreatment) and without hypoxic gas mixtures. The exquisite sensitivity of guinea pigs to halothane is

Table 20-6. Animal models of halothane hepatotoxicity*

Species	Special conditions required	Mechanism of toxicity
Rat	Pretreatment with polychlorinated biphenyls Mild hypoxia (14% O_2)	Reductive metabolites and hypoxia
Rat	Pretreatment with phenobarbitone Mild hypoxia (14% O_2)	Reductive metabolites and hypoxia
Rat	Pretreatment with triiodothyronine	Hypoxia
Rat	Pretreatment with phenobarbital Severe hypoxia (8%-12% O_2)	Hypoxia
Rat	Pretreatment with isoniazid	Oxidative metabolites
Guinea pig	None	Oxidative metabolites

From Kenna JG, Jones RM: *Anesth Analg* 81:S51, 1995.
*Note: no model for halothane hepatitis.

probably related to the very low hepatic arterial blood flow in these animals (2% to 3% of total hepatic blood flow versus 20% to 35% in other species). Guinea pigs are also highly susceptible to hepatic injury from surgical stress, hemorrhage, and anesthetic agents that are characteristically nontoxic (isoflurane, nitrous oxide). Of the inhaled anesthetics, halothane causes the most pronounced cardiovascular and respiratory depression (greatest hepatic oxygen deprivation) and also causes the most severe liver dysfunction in the guinea pig model. Thus in the setting of an unfavorable oxygen supply-to-demand ratio, halothane can produce, or exacerbate, hepatic ischemia or hypoxia.

The histopathologic lesions (primarily centrolobular necrosis) that result from an ischemic insult are remarkably similar to those associated with halothane anesthesia. This finding may be more than coincidental because anesthetics not only decrease hepatic blood flow but also may inhibit oxidative phosphorylation at the step of nicotinamide adenine dinucleotide (NAD) formation. Such inhibition has been reported to occur at low concentrations of halothane, enflurane, and isoflurane and could contribute to depletion of high-energy phosphates.[63] In the absence of hypoxemia, however, anesthesia with halothane, enflurane, or isoflurane does not decrease hepatic concentrations of high-energy phosphates in rats undergoing laparotomy and liver biopsy.[64] In vitro studies indicate that hypoxic conditions promote the covalent binding of halothane metabolites to hepatocytes (see Figs. 20-2 and 20-3). Thus hepatic oxygen deprivation may somehow contribute to halothane-induced liver dysfunction; however, its contribution to halothane hepatitis, if any, remains unknown.

(3) IMMUNE INJURY. Although halothane can produce direct hepatotoxic effects and hepatic necrosis in a variety of experimental models, such findings are of questionable relevance to the pathogenesis of halothane hepatitis in humans. The characteristic features of halothane hepatitis are highly suggestive of an injurious process that is immunologically mediated rather than a disorder caused by direct cytotoxicity or hypoxia. For example, halothane hepatitis is an idiosyncratic disease: it is unrelated to the dose of halothane used and occurs in only a

very small minority of those who receive the drug. Its development typically requires multiple prior halothane anesthetics, rather than a single exposure to halothane. The disease has a delayed onset, not becoming manifest for at least several days after halothane anesthesia, and the clinical presentation is often associated with findings of a hypersensitivity reaction, such as peripheral eosinophilia,[65] circulating immune complexes, and organ nonspecific autoantibodies.[66]

Occupational exposure to subanesthetic concentrations of halothane is sufficient to cause liver injury in highly susceptible individuals. In one case, an anesthesiologist suspected of having halothane-induced liver disease was given subanesthetic doses of halothane in a controlled setting; after each administration, he developed clinical, laboratory, and histopathologic manifestations of halothane hepatotoxicity.[67] Clinical hepatitis also developed in a laboratory investigator who conducted animal experiments with halothane during a 3-year period; the hepatitis promptly resolved after the exposure to halothane was terminated.[68] Similarly, hepatic injury occurred in two surgeons who were chronically exposed to subanesthetic doses of halothane; both surgeons were ultimately found to have a circulating antibody that reacted specifically with halothane-altered hepatocyte membrane components.[69]

The potential for halothane to produce immune injury appears to be related to its ability to stimulate the formation of hepatic antigens (Table 20-7). Many halothane-induced antigens (neoantigens) result from the production of TF-acetyl chloride (oxidative intermediate of halothane metabolism) and its covalent binding to various hepatic macromolecules[70-74]; the TF-acetyl moiety acts as a hapten and enhances the immune recognition of the carrier protein. Many of the neoantigens identified via immunoblot technology are modified endoplasmic reticulum (site of halothane oxidation by CYP2E1) proteins. Neoantigens detected via enzyme-linked immunosorbent assays (ELISA) (Box 20-5) but absent on immunoblot are TF-acetylated integral membrane proteins (unknown identity) whose immunogenicity probably depends on their conformation. A variety of autoantigens that lack TF-acetyl adducts also arise following halothane anesthesia. Which, if any, of these neoantigens or autoantigens is important in the pathogenesis of halothane hepatitis remains to be determined.

The humeral immune response is a characteristic feature of halothane hepatitis. Most patients with halothane hepatitis have antibodies in their blood that bind to specific antigens isolated from halothane-treated animals (rabbits); 70% of patients have antibodies that recognize TF-acetyl–modified epitopes, whereas 90% have antibodies that recognize non–TF-acetyl–modified epitopes (Box 20-6). Thus testing for the presence of halothane antibodies may be a useful approach for identifying pa-

tients at risk for the development of halothane hepatitis, as well as for determining whether cases of unexplained hepatitis after halothane anesthesia were likely to have been caused by halothane. However, at present no test is totally sensitive or specific for the detection of halothane hepatitis. The ELISA method of antibody detection has been reported to have a sensitivity of about 75% and a specificity of 88%.[72]

Although the evidence supporting the TF-acetyl–hapten theory appears to be strong, it is still conceivable that the antigen-antibody responses associated with halothane hepatitis are a result of the hepatic injury, not its cause. Proponents of the hapten theory still need to explain how most (if not all) patients anesthetized with halothane form the same set of TF-acetylated liver proteins but so few develop halothane hepatitis. Potential explanations include the possibilities that only a few of the TF-acetyl proteins are actually immunogenic or that a critical threshold of TF-acetyl liver proteins is needed to stimulate the immune response (antigenic threshold theory) (Box 20-7).

3. Clinical use of halothane. Guidelines for the clinical use of halothane should take into consideration the following issues and concerns[58]: Halothane has very low potential to produce liver damage in children, even with repeated exposures; severe halothane-related liver damage is uncommon after a single exposure to halothane; repeated exposures in adults, especially obese, middle-aged women, over a brief period of time (less than 6 weeks) increase the risk of halothane hepatitis; and no totally reliable test exists for the detection of patients susceptible to halothane hepatitis.

4. Conclusions. Clearly the greatest concern with halothane anesthesia is development of FHF, but there are many other germane concerns: Halothane markedly decreases blood flow and oxygen supply to the liver; it often causes mild, transient liver injury; and its use has

Table 20-7. Halothane-induced hepatic antigens that are recognized by antibodies from patients with halothane hepatitis

Protein carrier	Subunit molecular mass (kDa)
Endoplasmin/Erp99/GRP94	100
BiP/GRP94	82
Erp72	80
Calreticulin	63
Microsomal carboxylase	59
Unknown function	58
Protein disulfide isomerase	57
Unknown, not purified	54

Modified from Kenna JG, Jones RM: *Anesth Analg* 81:S51, 1995.

Box 20-5 Liver antigens in patients with halothane hepatitis*

Neoantigens detected by immunoblot

Peripheral membrane proteins (54-100 kDa) that are abundant and normally reside within the lumen of the endoplasmic reticulum.
Not involved themselves in halothane metabolism.
TF-acetyl covalently bound to ϵ-amino groups of lysine.
Related to oxidative metabolism of halothane (probably CYP2E1).

Neoantigens detected by ELISA but not immunoblot

Integral membrane proteins.
Proteins are TF-acetylated.
Identity of antigens is unknown.
Probably stimulate autoantibody formation.
Conformation important to immunogenicity (therefore not detected on immunoblot).
Likely to be important targets in halothane hepatitis.
Recognition by antibodies presumably results from loss of T-cell tolerance.

From Kenna JG, Jones RM: The organ toxicity of inhaled anesthetics, *Anesth Analg* 81(suppl 6):S51, 1995.
*Harsh conditions during immunoblotting may destroy conformational components of halothane-induced epitopes. Refer to Box 20-6 for information about antibodies in patients with halothane hepatitis.

Box 20-6 Types of antibodies identified in patients with halothane hepatitis*

70% of patients have specific antibodies that recognize at least one of the halothane-induced antigens that are detectable by immunoblotting.
  These antibodies recognize epitopes in which the TF-acetyl is linked to the essential features of the protein carriers.
90% of patients have antibodies that recognize at least one of the halothane-induced antigens that are detectable by ELISA but not by immunoblotting.
  Antibodies recognize the essential structural features of the protein carriers; this recognition does not require the presence of TF-acetyl moieties.
  These appear to be autoantibodies and probably are involved in the immune injury caused by halothane.

From Kenna JG, Jones RM: *Anesth Analg* 81(suppl 6):S51, 1995.
*Refer to Box 20-5 for information about liver antigens to which these antibodies may be directed.

medicolegal implications, which may plague anesthesiologists whenever unexplained hepatic dysfunction develops in the postoperative period. So why use halothane at all? The main advantage of halothane over other agents would appear to be its low cost. However, when medicolegal costs are factored in, the cost-benefit analysis might actually favor the elimination of halothane from anesthesia practice.[75] To illustrate, let us consider the following hypothetic example. The average cost of an isoflurane anesthetic is $5 greater than that of a halothane anesthetic, the incidence of halothane hepatitis is 1 in 20,000 halothane anesthetics, and the average malpractice claim per case of halothane hepatitis results in a $500,000 loss. In this hypothetical example, because of the medicolegal cost of a halothane anesthetic ($25 per halothane anesthetic, or $500,000/20,0000 cases), the average halothane anesthetic would cost $20 more than the average isoflurane anesthetic (medicolegal cost − agent cost = $25 − $5). Based only on such considerations, the financially prudent decision would be to replace halothane with another comparable agent, even if its direct cost is $25 more per anesthetic than halothane. It is our opinion that halothane's place in modern anesthesia practice will continue to diminish as the advantages of using this agent are contrasted with its disadvantages and risks.

C. Enflurane

About a decade after the clinical introduction of enflurane in 1972, Lewis et al[8] published a case-control study involving 24 cases of suspected enflurane hepatitis. The clinical, biochemical, and histopathologic profiles were similar to those seen in halothane-induced hepatitis. Fever was the most common presenting feature (79%); jaundice eventually appeared in 79% of the patients after a latent period (from anesthetic exposure to onset of symptoms or jaundice) of 8 days; a shorter latent period occurred in patients who had had prior anesthetics with either enflurane or halothane. Liver biopsy characteristically showed centrilobular necrosis, and 20% of the patients died from FHF.

Eger et al[9] reevaluated the data from Lewis et al's study by creating a syndrome score for each patient, based on a composite of 12 variables, including presence of fever, chills, nausea, rash, eosinophilia, death, and hepatic histopathology. Finding no differences between the syndrome scores of patients identified by Lewis et al as having "probable postanesthetic enflurane hepatitis" and those with postoperative hepatitis from other causes (such as sepsis or shock), these investigators concluded that there was still no proof of the existence of enflurane hepatitis. This conclusion notwithstanding, the many unexplained cases of massive or submassive necrosis that have followed enflurane anesthesia[76-78] provide presumptive evidence that the disorder exists. In addition, results of experimental studies and clinical investigations indicate that enflurane, like halothane, can produce both mild and severe forms of liver disease.

1. Mechanisms of enflurane hepatotoxicity. Many of the same mechanisms that have been proposed to explain the hepatotoxicity of halothane also merit consideration as possible mechanisms of enflurane hepatotoxicity. Enflurane-induced liver injury may result from direct cytotoxic effects of metabolites of enflurane; hepatic hypoxia caused by effects of enflurane on liver blood flow and oxygen demand; and immune reactions triggered by neoantigens that arise from covalent binding of enflurane metabolites to hepatic macromolecules.

The lower hepatotoxic potential of enflurane relative to halothane may be a direct result of differences in the metabolism of these two agents: enflurane is much less extensively metabolized than halothane (2.5% to 8.5% of the enflurane taken up into the body is metabolized).[16,17] Although both are oxidized via cytochrome P-450 (isoform CYP2E1)[79,80] to highly reactive intermediates (TF-acetyl chloride for halothane, difluoromethoxydifluoroacetyl fluoride for enflurane) that bind covalently to hepatic macromolecules, the binding is quite extensive with halothane anesthesia but only minimal with enflurane (Fig. 20-4).

A wide range of drugs and physiologic factors can modify enflurane metabolism, which could conceivably alter the hepatotoxic potential of enflurane. For example, the ratio of dietary fat to carbohydrate affects P-450 activity, and the metabolism of enflurane can be doubled by a diet that is high in fat.[81] Acute ethanol ingestion produces a tenfold increase in enflurane metabolism in pair-fed rats.[82] Chronic ethanol consumption similarly enhances enflurane metabolism.[83]

Alterations in enflurane metabolism are not necessarily coupled to changes in microsomal content of cytochrome P-450. For example, the ethanol-induced increases occur in the absence of an increase in P-450 content, whereas phenobarbital treatment increases P-450 content but not enflurane defluoridation (86% of con-

---

Box 20-7 Immune basis for halothane hepatitis

Unresolved issue

All patients exposed to halothane appear to form the same set of TF-acetyl liver proteins, but halothane hepatitis occurs only rarely.

Possible explanations

Only a few of these proteins may be immunogenic: Antibody populations from patients with halothane hepatitis recognize one or more, but not all, TF-acetyl–labeled hepatic proteins from rats or humans. Such selective recognition may result from differential presentations of TF-acetyl liver proteins to the immune system.

A critical threshold of TF-acetyl liver proteins may be needed to stimulate the immune response (antigenic threshold theory).

From Kenna JG, Jones RM: The organ toxicity of inhaled anesthetics, *Anesth Analg* 81(suppl 6):S51, 1995.

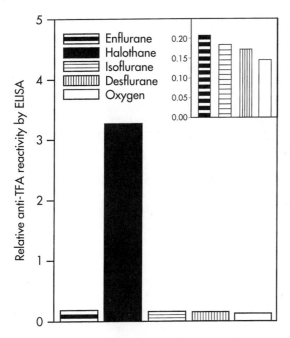

Fig. 20-4. Detection of anti-TF-acetyl (anti-TFA) reactivity in rat liver microsomes by enzyme-linked immunoabsorbent assay *(ELISA)* after inhalation exposure to halothane, enflurane, isoflurane, desflurane, or oxygen. The response to halothane was more than 50 times greater than to enflurane or the other agents (response = reactivity for anesthetic − reactivity for oxygen). Inset compares incremental difference in anti-TFA reactivity for all agents except halothane. (From Njoku D, Laster MJ, Gong DH, et al: *Anesth Analg* 84:173, 1997.)

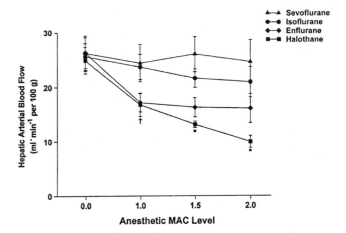

Fig. 20-5. Dose-dependent effect of inhaled anesthetics on hepatic arterial blood flow in chronically instrumented dogs in the absence of surgical stress. Sevoflurane and isoflurane preserve hepatic arterial blood flow even at higher minimum alveolar anesthetic concentration *(MAC)* levels. *Differs from sevoflurane and isoflurane at same MAC values ($p < 0.05$). †Differs from sevoflurane at same MAC value ($p < 0.05$). (From Frink EJ Jr: *Anesth Analg* 81[suppl 6]:S46, 1995.)

trol). The implication of the aforementioned metabolic alterations on the hepatotoxicity of enflurane remains to be determined.

2. Hypoxia and ischemia. Enflurane produces greater reductions of hepatic blood flow and splanchnic perfusion than any of the clinically used halogenated inhaled agents (isoflurane, sevoflurane, or desflurane), with the exception of halothane. Studies in dogs indicate that enflurane causes a dose-related reduction in portal venous blood flow[85,86] and either decreases (Fig. 20-5)[85] or does not change hepatic artery blood flow.[86] Enflurane-induced decreases in mean arterial pressure (MAP) and cardiac output in patients are associated with decreases in splanchnic perfusion.[87] Enflurane also decreases hepatic venous SvO_2, reflecting increases in splanchnic O_2 extraction.[87]

Although hypoxia itself can produce liver injury, hypoxic conditions may actually decrease the hepatotoxic potential of enflurane by decreasing its metabolism (oxidative).[90] In contrast, halothane metabolism (reductive rather than oxidative) continues to occur under hypoxic conditions, spewing out toxic free radical intermediates that can exacerbate the liver injury produced by hypoxia. Thus enflurane would be expected to have a lesser toxic potential than halothane in settings where hepatic blood flow is critically limited and the adequacy of the balance between O_2 supply and demand is in question. In such

settings, isoflurane or sevoflurane may be even better agents than enflurane because of their more favorable effects on hepatic blood flow.

3. Cytotoxic effects. Enflurane is considerably less cytotoxic than halothane in experimental models of halothane hepatotoxicity. Studies in guinea pig liver slices indicate that the viability of hepatic tissue is better maintained in the presence of enflurane than with either halothane or isoflurane.[88,89] Enflurane causes less of a decrease in protein synthesis than either isoflurane or halothane, and it actually increases protein secretion, in contrast to halothane, which causes a pronounced decrease.

4. Immune mechanisms. The pathogenesis of enflurane- and halothane-induced liver injury may be similar or the same. Both anesthetics are biotransformed to highly reactive intermediates that acylate hepatic macromolecules, thereby creating neoantigens that appear to trigger immunologically mediated liver injury. Although the acyl haptens produced by oxidative metabolism of enflurane (difluoromethoxydifluoroacetyl halide) and halothane (TF-acetyl halide) are chemically distinct, liver protein adducts containing these haptens are sufficiently similar to be recognizable by serum antibodies from patients with halothane hepatitis. In one study, the enflurane metabolites generated in the rat were found to react immunologically with sera of patients who had recovered from halothane hepatitis.[91] In another study, administration of enflurane to rats and guinea pigs stimulated the production of neoantigens (fluorinated adducts) that were detected by halothane-induced antibodies. These neoantigens were located in the centrilobular region of the liver, appeared in both microsomal and cytosolic fractions of liver homogenates,[92] and were up to 20 times more abundant in guinea pigs than in rats.

Proposed pathways for the formation of acylating intermediates from the oxidative metabolism of several inhaled agents are shown in Fig. 20-1. The use of enflurane anesthesia has preceded cases of unexplained hepatic injury following anesthesia with other inhaled agents, including halothane,[93] isoflurane,[94] and sevoflurane.[12] Whether such an association is merely coincidental or represents true immune crossover sensitivity between enflurane and other halogenated inhaled agents remains to be determined.

5. Conclusions. The consensus at present is that enflurane, via its oxidative metabolites, can cause serious liver dysfunction.[26,95] However, this disorder is extremely rare. Even if all unexplained cases of hepatitis that have followed enflurane anesthetics were considered enflurane-induced, the incidence of enflurane hepatitis would be only 0.36 cases per million, about $\frac{1}{200}$ that associated with halothane. The risk of enflurane-induced liver injury appears to be increased by the same factors that increase the risk of halothane hepatitis.

D. Isoflurane

This agent has a very low hepatotoxic potential as compared to halothane or even enflurane. Isoflurane undergoes minimal biodegradation[16,19] (see Table 20-2), preserves hepatic oxygen delivery even during laparotomy,[96] and does not undergo reductive metabolism. It has been found to protect the liver from carbon tetrachloride (CCl_4) toxicity, probably by inhibiting the cytochrome P-450 isozyme that metabolizes CCl_4 and possibly by dismutating haloperoxyl radicals.[97] In addition, isoflurane has no adverse effects on hepatic function of rats with CCl_4-induced cirrhosis.[98]

1. Isoflurane metabolism and the immune theory of anesthesia-induced hepatitis. Isoflurane causes centrilobular necrosis under certain experimental conditions,[99] and there is a theoretical basis for suspecting that it may cause hepatitis in humans. Like halothane, enflurane, and desflurane, isoflurane undergoes oxidative metabolism by P-450 2E1, yielding highly reactive intermediates (TF-acetyl chloride; acyl ester) that bind covalently to hepatic macromolecules (see Fig. 20-1). These altered macromolecules (both neoantigens and autoantigens) are apparently recognized as nonself and attacked by the immune system, leading to extensive hepatocellular necrosis.[92] Although this theory of isoflurane hepatotoxicity seems plausible, the likelihood of isoflurane hepatitis occurring via this mechanism is extremely low; only about 0.2% of the isoflurane taken up into the body is actually metabolized, and only trace amounts of isoflurane metabolites are bound to hepatocellular macromolecules following treatment with isoflurane. Also, according to this theory, a prior exposure to any of the halogenated agents that are metabolized to fluoroacyl intermediates could predispose to the development of isoflurane-induced hepatitis.

2. Conclusions. It is plausible that isoflurane, on very rare occasions, produces clinically significant liver disease. Numerous reports have described severe, unexplained hepatic dysfunction following isoflurane anesthe-

sia.[10,94,100-103] Many of the cases involved patients who had had prior exposure to halogenated agents (e.g., halothane,[103] enflurane,[94] or isoflurane[104]), as might be predicted from the immune theory. A recent review in the *American Journal of Gastroenterology* concluded that ample direct evidence exists to implicate isoflurane as a hepatotoxin and that isoflurane should be considered a potential cause of postoperative increases of serum aminotransferases.[102] This opinion notwithstanding, the vast majority of cases of unexplained hepatitis following isoflurane anesthesia are not caused by isoflurane, as attested to by a subcommittee report from the Anesthetic and Life Support Advisory Committee of the Food and Drug Administration (FDA).[100] The subcommittee carefully reviewed 47 cases of suspected isoflurane-induced hepatic injury reported to the FDA from 1981 through 1984. In most instances, a potential cause other than isoflurane was identified, including sepsis, hypoxia, biliary obstruction, nutritional deficiency, circulatory shock, viral hepatitis (including herpesvirus), and antibiotic therapy (erythromycin estolate). In fact, the committee concluded that there was no compelling evidence of a causal relationship between use of isoflurane and the occurrence of postoperative hepatic dysfunction.[100]

E. Desflurane

To date, only one case of hepatitis has been attributed to desflurane anesthesia.[14] The case involved a healthy 65-year-old woman who developed pruritus, malaise, nausea, and polyarthralgias 12 days after a minor operation under desflurane anesthesia. Four days later she had a macular rash, dermal jaundice, epigastric pain, and laboratory evidence of significant hepatic dysfunction (serum ALT was 1886 IU, total bilirubin was 27 mg/dl, and PT was 27 seconds, with negative serologies). She was readmitted to the hospital, and there was concern about the need for an OLT, but her condition gradually improved on conservative therapy. A blood sample collected on postoperative day 48 contained antibodies that reacted with TF-acylated liver microsomal proteins, providing circumstantial evidence that the liver injury was immunologically mediated. In this regard, it is noteworthy that the patient had received two halothane anesthetics more than a decade before the desflurane anesthetic. Could the prior exposures to halothane have sensitized this patient to desflurane hepatitis, or could this actually be a case of halothane hepatitis, triggered by traces of halothane that had been retained in the anesthesia machine during recent anesthetics?[105] It is unclear whether desflurane itself can actually cause postoperative hepatitis.

1. Desflurane metabolism and the immune theory of anesthesia-induced hepatitis. With desflurane, as with the other halogenated agents, metabolism can theoretically lead to hepatotoxicity. However, only 0.02% to 0.2% of the desflurane taken up by the body is metabolized (1/1000 that of halothane). Desflurane does not undergo reductive metabolism; it is oxidized via cytochrome P-450 2E1[106] to yield fluorinated acyl compounds, inorganic fluoride, and TFA (see Fig. 20-1).[20,107]

Metabolites are usually undetectable in plasma unless there has been prolonged exposure to desflurane. Data from patients and volunteers indicate that TFA concentrations in serum and urine after desflurane anesthesia are approximately 1/10 that of concentrations after a similar exposure to isoflurane.[20]

Because desflurane is biotransformed to trifluroacyl metabolites, it is theoretically possible for desflurane to cause immunologically mediated hepatic injury via the generation of neoantigens through trifluoroacylation of hepatic macromolecules (see Fig. 20-1). With desflurane anesthesia, however, there appears to be little or no acylation of hepatic tissue. For example, in rats pretreated with isoniazid (induces P-450 2E1 in rats) the extent of acylation of hepatic proteins (via immunochemical analysis or ELISA) after 8 hours of inhaled anesthesia (1.25 minimum alveolar concentration [MAC]) was as follows: halothane >> enflurane > isoflurane > desflurane = oxygen.[7] Moreover, sera taken from patients with a clinical diagnosis of halothane hepatitis exhibited no antibody reactivity against hepatic proteins isolated from desflurane- or isoflurane-treated rats, whereas significant reactivity occurred with the proteins isolated from rats exposed to halothane or enflurane.[7] Thus the potential for desflurane or isoflurane to produce immune-mediated hepatic injury appears to be considerably lower than that of either halothane or enflurane.

Desflurane, like the other inhaled agents, might conceivably cause hepatic injury by adversely affecting the oxygen supply-to-demand relationship in the liver. Desflurane anesthesia decreases hepatic blood flow in both experimental and clinical settings.[108] Administration of 1 MAC desflurane to patients before skin incision causes about a 30% reduction of hepatic blood flow (measured by ICG), which is similar to the reduction produced by 1 MAC of halothane or isoflurane.[108] Desflurane anesthesia in domestic pigs[109] produces dose-dependent reductions of mean arterial blood pressure, cardiac output, and total hepatic blood flow; at 0.5 MAC, portal venous and superior mesenteric arterial blood flows are decreased, and at 1 MAC, hepatic arterial blood flow is also decreased. Despite a marked reduction in O_2 delivery to the liver and small intestine, O_2 uptake is maintained, and there are no adverse effects on the metabolic function of the liver or small intestine. Nevertheless, desflurane decreases the O_2 reserve capacity of the liver and small intestine.

The effects of desflurane on the hepatic microcirculation (sinusoidal diameters or the sinusoidal blood flow) of mechanically ventilated rats, as assessed by intravital fluorescence microscopy,[110] are similar to those of isoflurane or pentobarbital. Additional studies in both the normoxic[60] and hypoxic rat models (enzyme induction plus hypoxia) indicate that desflurane neither causes hypoxic liver injury nor increases the potential of hypoxia to cause hepatocellular necrosis.[111]

In the setting of marginal hepatic oxygenation, it is theoretically possible for carbon monoxide, generated via degradation of desflurane in the CO_2 absorber of the anesthesia machine, to contribute to hypoxic liver injury

and POLD. Although other anesthetics can also be degraded to carbon monoxide, desflurane and enflurane are the most problematic in this regard (desflurane ≥ enflurane > isoflurane >> halothane = sevoflurane).[112,113]

2. Conclusions. Desflurane is less hepatotoxic than halothane or enflurane, and may produce even less POLD than isoflurane. The very low hepatotoxic potential of desflurane is presumably related to the very limited metabolism of this agent. Nonetheless, there is at least a theoretical basis for desflurane to cause immunologically mediated hepatic injury because it is biotransformed, albeit in small amounts, to highly reactive intermediates that can acylate hepatic proteins and thereby create hepatic neoantigens. In addition, desflurane anesthesia can decrease hepatic blood flow and O_2 delivery to the liver, which may contribute to POLD in settings of marginal hepatic oxygenation.

F. Sevoflurane

Although sevoflurane was synthesized in the late 1960s, its commercial development was delayed because of concerns about the potential toxicity of its metabolites and breakdown products. Such concerns were mitigated by the apparent safety of sevoflurane in clinical trials, conducted initially in Japan and later throughout the world.[114] Sevoflurane was approved for clinical use in Japan in 1990. By 1995, when it became clinically available in the United States, more than 2 million Japanese patients had already received sevoflurane. To date, three cases of severe POLD have been attributed to sevoflurane anesthesia; all occurred in Japanese patients in the early 1990s.[11,12,13]

None of the cases resemble the classic presentation of halothane hepatitis. Two cases involved infants: an 11-month-old, who developed POLD (maximum serum AST of 836 IU/L) 2 weeks after receiving sevoflurane anesthesia for foot surgery[13] and a 1-month-old who developed increases of serum aminotransferases and LDH that peaked 12 to 16 days after administration of sevoflurane for an inguinal herniorrhaphy.[11] The 1-month-old presented with frequent vomiting, anorexia, and fever on the second postoperative day, and the disorder did not fully resolve for 2 months. The only case involving an adult occurred in a 63-year-old man who had had an enflurane anesthetic for cerebral aneurysm clipping approximately 7 weeks before he received sevoflurane for a cranioplasty. Postoperative hepatic injury was characterized by an increase in ALT (700 IU/L), AST (800 IU/L), and bilirubin (15 mg/dl); there was no encephalopathy and the test results improved on conservative therapy.[12] These cases suggest that sevoflurane may be capable on rare occasions of producing clinically significant hepatic injury. Because the presentations of hepatitis associated with sevoflurane have been different from those typically associated with halothane or enflurane, the mechanisms of the hepatic injury may well have been different.

1. Experimental evaluation of the hepatotoxic potential of sevoflurane. Many studies have been conducted to provide a better understanding of the hepatotoxic potential of sevoflurane. Most of the studies suggest that sevoflurane anesthesia can produce mild and transient hepatic dysfunction in animals and humans. The administration of sevoflurane or isoflurane (total gas flow rate of 1 L/min) to surgical patients ($n = 100$) undergoing minor operative procedures is associated with a similar postoperative increase of hepatic enzymes.[116] Based on other clinical investigations, the use of sevoflurane anesthesia for major intraabdominal operations did not produce significant POLD.[117,118] In beagles, sevoflurane (1.8 MAC) causes only mild, transient increases in blood concentrations of hepatic enzymes, which are comparable to those caused by enflurane or halothane.[119] Even with repeated administrations of sevoflurane (closed-circle absorption with soda lime), no toxicologically significant changes occurred during a 2-week study in dogs and rats.[120] Similarly, multiple, prolonged sevoflurane anesthetics (up to 2 MAC, for 3 hr/day, 3 days/week) did not cause significant POLD in monkeys. Although increases in aminotransferases and LDH were observed within the first weeks of sevoflurane administration, they were no longer present at the end of the 8-week study. Moreover, sevoflurane did not cause any gross pathologic, histopathologic, or ultrastructural abnormalities of the liver.[121]

Sevoflurane also has minimal toxicity in a variety of in vitro systems. For example, in guinea pig liver slices, sevoflurane treatment maintains tissue viability for up to 24 hours,[122] in contrast to treatments with enflurane, isoflurane, or halothane, which cause dose- and time-related decreases of hepatocellular viability (decreases in intracellular slice K^+).[89] In isolated liver preparations, sevoflurane produces less inhibition of protein synthesis and secretion than halothane, and similar inhibition to that produced by enflurane or isoflurane.

2. Sevoflurane hepatotoxicity and hepatic blood flow.
Sevoflurane does not appear to produce liver damage by causing hepatic hypoxia or by exacerbating the injurious effects of hypoxia on the liver. Sevoflurane (1 or 2 MAC) maintains hepatic blood flow (ICG clearance) at awake, preanesthetic levels in patients having elective operations, despite significant reductions in mean arterial blood pressure. Similar results are obtained with isoflurane anesthesia (1 or 2 MAC), whereas halothane anesthesia (2 MAC) causes a significant reduction of hepatic blood flow.[123]

Data from animal studies also indicate that sevoflurane anesthesia generally preserves hepatic blood flow. Administration of sevoflurane (1.66 vol%) to mechanically ventilated rats does not reduce total hepatic blood flow (microsphere technique) despite significant reductions in mean arterial blood pressure.[124] Sevoflurane produces dose-dependent increases of hepatic arterial blood flow (HABF) and dose-dependent decreases of portal venous blood flow (PVBF) in chronically instrumented dogs.[125] At 2 MAC, sevoflurane increases HABF by 33% and decreases PVBF by 33%, and these effects are accompanied by significant decreases of MAP (37%) and CO (21%). By comparison, HABF is minimally decreased by 2 MAC isoflurane,[125] moderately decreased (about 30%)

by 1 MAC doses of either halothane or enflurane, and markedly decreased by larger doses of halothane (1.5 or 2 MAC) (see Fig. 20-5). Sevoflurane at 1.5 MAC reduces PVBF to the same degree as isoflurane. At 2 MAC, sevoflurane produces a greater reduction of PVBF than isoflurane, but less of a reduction than enflurane and much less of a reduction than halothane.[85]

Under a condition of marginal hepatic oxygen supply (hepatic artery ligation in beagles), sevoflurane and halothane produce greater reductions of portal blood flow (electromagnetic flow meter) and hepatic oxygen supply than isoflurane. In addition, hepatic O_2 uptake is greater with sevoflurane than halothane anesthesia (3.7 ml/min versus 2.7 ml/min per 100 g of liver) possibly because halothane causes greater decreases of hepatic metabolism and oxygen requirements than sevoflurane. Thus the hepatic O_2 supply/uptake ratio is actually lower with sevoflurane than with halothane anesthesia. Nonetheless, hepatic function seems to be better preserved during sevoflurane anesthesia than during halothane anesthesia (via ICG clearance; 40 ml/min versus 31 ml/min),[126] even in the presence of hypoxia. In the enzyme-induced hypoxic rat model, 1 MAC sevoflurane produces the same degree of hepatic injury as 1 MAC isoflurane, and less injury than 1 MAC halothane.[127]

3. Sevoflurane degradation, metabolism, and hepatotoxicity.
Nephrotoxicity rather than hepatotoxicity has been the greater concern with sevoflurane. Animal studies indicate that the nephrotoxicity is caused by a degradation product of sevoflurane known as compound A ($CF_2 = C[CF_3]OCH_2F$; fluoromethyl-2,2-difluoro-1-[trifluoromethyl] vinyl ether). Compound A results from the extraction of hydrogen fluoride by CO_2 absorbents at low fresh gas flows (Fig. 20-6). Although controversy exists about the nephrotoxic potential of compound A in humans,[128] there is no evidence that compound A itself causes hepatotoxicity.[127] In rats, the combination of acetaminophen (up to 1000 mg/kg) and compound A (100 ppm) causes greater hepatotoxicity (hepatocyte hyperchromicity, centrilobular pallor, and early vacuolization) than either agent alone.[129] However, the exceedingly large doses of acetaminophen and compound A that are needed to produce hepatotoxicity in this rat model raise questions about the clinical applicability of this study.

The extent of the metabolism of sevoflurane is less than that of halothane and enflurane: only 2% to 5% of the sevoflurane taken up by the body is metabolized.[130,131] The metabolism is rapid (1.5 to 2 times faster than enflurane), and the major metabolites, fluoride and hexafluoroisopropanol (HPIF), appear in the plasma within minutes of the start of sevoflurane administration. HPIF is rapidly conjugated in the liver and released into the systemic circulation as the HPIF-glucuronide (more than 85%). Plasma concentrations of fluoride generally peak within the first hour following sevoflurane administration and then begin to decline. Metabolism of sevoflurane is decreased nearly fivefold in patients taking disulfiram, an effective inhibitor of cy-

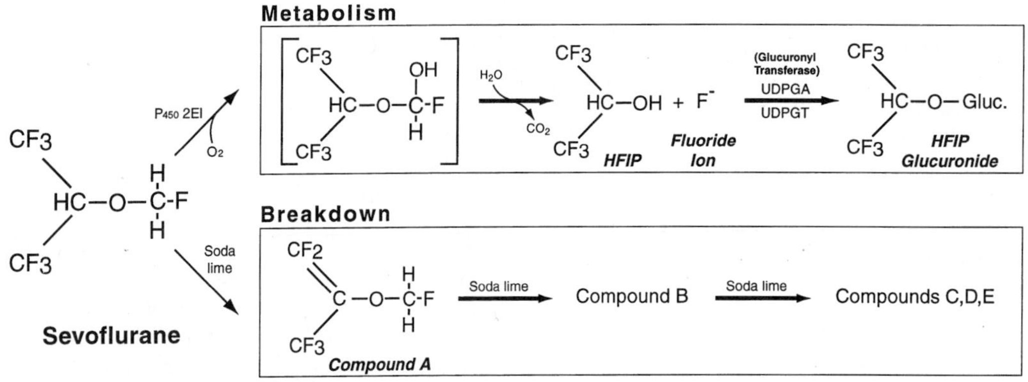

Fig. 20-6. Cytochrome P-450 2E1–catalyzed biotransformation of sevoflurane, producing inorganic fluoride and hexafluoroisopropanol *(HFIP)*, which is rapidly metabolized to HFIP-glucuronide. Sevoflurane undergoes breakdown in soda lime to produce compound A, which in animals may predispose to hepatotoxicity. (Modified from Frink EJ Jr: The hepatic effects of sevoflurane, *Anesth Analg* 81[6 suppl]:S46, 1995; Njoku D, Laster MJ, Gong DH, et al: *Anesth Analg* 84:173, 1997.)

tochrome P-450 2E1.[18] This finding suggests that P-450 2E1 is the major isoform responsible for sevoflurane metabolism in humans[18] and that drugs or pathophysiologic factors that alter its activity will also alter sevoflurane metabolism.

Although the apparent lack of severe hepatic dysfunction following sevoflurane anesthesia may simply reflect the limited clinical experience with this agent, it may also relate to differences in the metabolism of sevoflurane versus the other inhaled anesthetics.[107] In contrast to halothane, enflurane, isoflurane, and desflurane, sevoflurane has no reactive (fluoroacyl) metabolites and does not give rise to the fluoroacetylated liver proteins (see Fig. 20-4) that appear to play a critical role in immune-mediated hepatic injury.[131] Experience to date does not suggest a causal link between sevoflurane biotransformation and hepatic toxicity.[107]

4. Conclusions. Animal and human studies that have evaluated the hepatotoxic potential of sevoflurane indicate that it is less toxic than either halothane or enflurane, and no more toxic than either desflurane or isoflurane. Sevoflurane is less extensively metabolized than halothane or enflurane, and its metabolic products are less reactive, and therefore probably less injurious, than those resulting from halothane, enflurane (Box 20-8), isoflurane, or even desflurane.[132] Moreover, sevoflurane better preserves hepatic blood flow than halothane, enflurane, or desflurane; its effects on hepatic perfusion and metabolic function are similar to those of isoflurane. At present, it seems unlikely that sevoflurane will emerge as a clinically important cause of severe POLD.

IV. AGENTS USED DURING ANESTHESIA OTHER THAN POTENT HALOGENATED VAPORS

A. Nitrous oxide

Nitrous oxide administered by itself has little effect on hepatic function,[21,133] although it has been shown to enhance the hepatotoxicity of halothane in hypoxic rats.[134] Fifty percent nitrous oxide inhibits the enzyme methio-

---

Box 20-8 Sevoflurane differs from other clinically used fluorinated vapors

It is not metabolized to reactive acyl halide intermediates.
Its metabolites do not covalently bind to liver proteins.
Its primary, and perhaps only, organic metabolite, hexafluoroisopropanol, does not appear to be reactive.

From Kenna JG, Jones RM: The organ toxicity of inhaled anesthetics, *Anesth Analg* 81(suppl 6):S51, 1995.

---

nine synthetase, which can cause derangements of folate and methionine metabolism.[135] Cohen et al[136] reported that the incidence of liver disease in dentists who are chronically exposed to N_2O is approximately seven times greater than in other professionals without similar exposure. By contrast, in patients with mild alcoholic hepatitis, a nitrous oxide–opioid anesthetic administered for peripheral surgery has no adverse effects on postoperative liver function. Other studies similarly indicate that N_2O by itself lacks hepatotoxicity.[137]

B. Nonopioid sedative-hypnotic agents

Intravenous agents commonly used in the induction of anesthesia do not appear to produce serious hepatotoxicity.[138] The usual clinical doses of thiopental have little effect on liver function, although very large doses (greater than 750 mg) have been associated with hepatic dysfunction.[139,140] Ketamine has been reported to produce dose-dependent alterations of postoperative liver function.[141] Fourteen of 34 patients (41%) anesthetized with ketamine plus oxygen for intermediate procedures developed significant increases in hepatic enzyme concentrations postoperatively, compared to 7 of 34 (21%) who received a "control" anesthetic. It is unclear from such studies whether the observed changes in liver enzymes relate to direct hepatotoxic effects of ketamine, effects of ketamine on hepatic metabolism, or ketamine-induced increases of serum catecholamines, which lead to decreases in hepatic blood flow and oxygen delivery to the liver. Other intravenous anesthetic agents, such as etomidate, midazolam, propofol, and althesin, have not been shown to significantly alter hepatic function in patients undergoing minor operative procedures.[142] In the final analysis, it is highly unlikely that a standard dose of any of the clinically used intravenous hypnotic agents will cause more than minimal alterations of commonly used LFTs.[143]

C. Opioids

Opioids can increase the tone of the common bile duct and sphincter of Oddi, leading to increased intrabiliary pressures. As a result, patients may develop severe epigastric or abdominal pain, radiographic abnormalities on studies of the biliary system, and increased concentrations of serum lipase and amylase, which may persist for up to 24 hours after a dose of a μ-agonist. Equianalgesic doses of fentanyl and morphine have been reported to cause larger increases in biliary pressure than meperidine or pentazocine[144]; butorphanol and nalbuphine do not cause biliary spasm. Studies in volunteers indicate that morphine causes a greater increase in tone of the sphincter of Oddi than meperidine. Opioid-induced increases in biliary pressure can be antagonized by nitroglycerin, atropine, glucagon, and naloxone, as well as by volatile anesthetics.

Opioids have been found in mice to cause fatty infiltration of the liver and up to a tenfold increase in AST after a single intraperitoneal injection. These changes could be blocked by naloxone, reserpine, or propranolol administration, suggesting that the fatty changes may result from sympathetic nervous system activation and subsequent decreases in hepatic blood flow. It is unlikely that these data are relevant to humans undergoing major surgery, but they could possibly be of relevance to the management of opioid abusers with liver failure.[145]

D. Nonopioid analgesics

1. Acetaminophen. Acetaminophen is widely prescribed for the treatment of postoperative pain, being used alone (Tylenol) or in combination with opioid analgesics, such as oxycodone (Percocet) and hydrocodone (Vicodin). Although acetaminophen has enjoyed a reputation for being a tremendously safe analgesic, it is well recognized that extremely large doses (suicide attempts) produce extensive hepatocellular necrosis. In fact, acetaminophen has been the most common cause of FHF in the United Kingdom.[4] Recent evidence indicates that daily doses in the range of 3 to 8 g can produce chronic hepatotoxicity. Thus iatrogenic overdosing of acetaminophen is a germane concern if patients are instructed to take two tablets every 4 to 6 hours, as needed, for pain relief (combination analgesic products may contain 500 to 750 mg acetaminophen per tablet).

Some individuals are highly susceptible to acetaminophen toxicity. Recognized determinants of increased susceptibility include chronic use of ethanol,

therapeutic use of other inducers of hepatic microsomal drug metabolism, and poor nutritional status.

The differential diagnosis of acute acetaminophen hepatotoxicity includes all other causes of acute hepatic necrosis, such as viral hepatitis, ethanol-induced and other forms of drug-induced liver injury, and acute exacerbation of preexisting chronic liver disease. When acetaminophen hepatotoxicity seems probable, specific treatment (*N*-acetyl cysteine) should be instituted without undue delay because it is highly effective with minimal risk to the patient.

2. Nonsteroidal antiinflammatory drugs, including aspirin. Aspirin is a well-documented cause of a dose-related, reversible form of hepatotoxicity. This disorder can develop in days to weeks after initiation of high-dose aspirin therapy and has been commonly seen in patients with chronic rheumatic diseases or acute rheumatic fever. Usually, patients are asymptomatic, with mild to moderate increases of serum aminotransferases activity. Jaundice is uncommon, and severe clinical hepatitis is rare.

The Arthritis Advising Committee of the Food and Drug Administration concluded in 1992 that hepatotoxicity is "class characteristic" of nonsteroidal antiinflammatory drugs (NSAIDs). Major offenders in this regard have been diclofenac, sulindac, and phenylbutazone. Other offenders include piroxicam, ibuprofen, naproxen, and fenoprofen. The basis of hepatotoxicity from NSAIDs appears to be largely but not entirely idiosyncratic; cross-sensitivity between different NSAID classes may occur.

V. NONPHARMACOLOGIC CAUSES OF POSTOPERATIVE LIVER DYSFUNCTION
A. Systemic or regional circulatory derangements

Passive congestion of the liver per se, even when caused by congestive heart failure, rarely produces more than minor hepatic injury. By contrast, extreme liver injury is not uncommon in patients with prolonged shock or sepsis; total infarction of a lobe or of the entire liver may occur in the absence of portal or hepatic arterial occlusion.[147] Lesser degrees of hypotension can produce a hepatitis-like illness (ischemic hepatitis). Patients develop jaundice, systemic symptoms, and pronounced increases of serum transaminases; liver biopsy shows centrilobular necrosis with little or no inflammatory response.[148]

The hepatic dysfunction that follows a period of documented ischemia is usually mild, and prognosis depends on the underlying cardiac or systemic illness. Abnormal LFTs secondary to ischemia usually persist for 3 to 11 days. Clinical and biochemical criteria alone are usually sufficient to allow differentiation of ischemic and viral hepatitis. With ischemic hepatitis, patients have a probable history of inadequate systemic perfusion, accompanied by increases in liver enzyme concentrations, which are often greater than those associated with viral hepatitis. The mechanism of ischemic hepatitis remains to be fully elucidated, but may involve free radical production because hepatocytes contain very high concentrations of xanthine oxidase. (Ischemia and reperfusion increase xanthine oxidase activity; this enzyme catalyzes the oxidation of purines to uric acid and the associated reduction of O_2 to superoxide anion, which initiates toxic free radical reactions.)

B. Hemolysis and transfusion

Reabsorption of large surgical hematomas and blood transfusions are the major causes of jaundice in the absence of overt hepatocellular dysfunction. At least 10% of transfused erythrocytes hemolyze in the initial 24 hours following a blood transfusion (bilirubin load of approximately 250 mg per unit transfused). The normal liver readily clears the bilirubin loads that result from mild hemolysis. With severe hemolysis, the bilirubin loads are excessive, leading to unconjugated hyperbilirubinemia that persists until the liver conjugates and excretes the excess bilirubin.

In addition to massive blood transfusions, excessive bilirubin loads can result from severe hemolytic disorders such as sickle cell disease (hemoglobinopathies) or glucose-6-phosphate dehydrogenase (G6PD) deficiency (derangements of erythrocyte metabolism). Thus unconjugated hyperbilirubinemia may be seen in the perioperative period as a result of exacerbations of sickle cell disease (via hypovolemia, hypoxia, hypothermia, stress) or G6PD deficiency (via sulfonamides, chloramphenicol, nitrofurantoin). Significant hemolysis can also be associated with prosthetic cardiac valves and various other causes.

C. Surgically induced liver hypoxia or hepatobiliary injury

Minor operations do not produce POLD in healthy patients. Similarly, patients with marginal hepatic function usually tolerate peripheral procedures, even those performed under halothane anesthesia, without postoperative hepatic complications.[137] A randomized study in patients with mild alcoholic hepatitis compared spinal anesthesia and general anesthesia (enflurane plus N_2O versus N_2O plus opioid) and found no anesthesia-related differences in values of LFTs following peripheral or superficial surgery.[133]

Major surgery (especially laparotomy) is often associated with elevated blood concentration of enzymes putatively released from the liver. The magnitude of such increases depends more on the type of operation than on a particular anesthetic technique.[137,150] Nonetheless, the hepatic dysfunction produced by major operations is rarely of concern in healthy patients. In patients with advanced hepatic disease (marginal hepatic function), however, laparotomy is often associated with extremely high postoperative morbidity and mortality.[151,152] These patients are probably unable to tolerate the decreased hepatic oxygen supply caused by surgical stress.

1. Laparotomy. Early clinical studies reported very high postoperative mortality rates in patients with active hepatitis. The deaths typically occurred after laparotomy performed to identify the cause of liver failure. It now seems that the high susceptibility of patients with active hepatitis to laparotomy-induced decreases in hepatic blood flow and oxygen delivery may have played a major role in the development of hepatic failure in these pa-

tients. Fortunately, because of improved diagnostic methods (serologic tests, transhepatic cholangiography, endoscopic retrograde cholangiography, and percutaneous needle biopsy), laparotomy is rarely needed anymore to find the cause of liver failure.

Anesthetic techniques might be expected to modify the effects of laparotomy on POLD because some anesthetics (halothane or enflurane) produce much greater decreases of hepatic blood flow and oxygen supply than others (isoflurane or sevoflurane).[96,153-155] Support for this idea comes from experiments conducted in phenobarbital-pretreated rats (microsomal enzyme induction) that were anesthetized with either thiamylal, halothane, enflurane, or isoflurane for various operative interventions, including hepatic artery ligation.[156] Centrilobular necrosis occurred only in the rats anesthetized with halothane; the severity of the injury was related to both duration of anesthesia and the operative location. The hepatic damage associated with upper abdominal (sham for hepatic artery ligation) and lower abdominal operations was comparable and exceeded that occurring after peripheral surgery. Thus mesenteric vasoconstriction and reductions of hepatic and intestinal blood flow probably play an important role in the hepatic injury that accompanies laparotomy. These vascular changes may be mediated by neuroendocrine stress responses to major operations because they can be abolished in animals via hypophysectomy.[157]

2. Hepatobiliary procedures. Postoperative jaundice may result from intraoperative cholestasis or from extrahepatic biliary obstruction caused by stones in the bilary duct, iatrogenic strictures, or pancreatitis. Benign postoperative intrahepatic cholestasis is a syndrome that often follows severe shock, hypoxemia, major surgical procedures, and blood transfusion. Bilirubin concentrations may exceed 40 mg/dl, but hepatocellular function is well preserved. Mortality is uncommon unless the surgical procedure fails or a concurrent disease, such as sepsis, cardiac failure, or renal failure, is severe.[158]

3. Procedures requiring cardiopulmonary bypass. Cardiac failure itself does not usually lead to significant hepatic dysfunction, but jaundice and hepatocellular necrosis may occur in patients who experience severe hypotension.[159] Cardiopulmonary bypass with low-flow states and nonpulsatile perfusion can probably aggravate preexisting hepatic dysfunction. If catecholamine administration is necessary to improve cardiac performance, either before or after bypass, hepatic oxygen delivery may be compromised. Hypothermia during cardiopulmonary bypass probably limits the hepatic damage created by the abnormal hemodynamics, thus limiting the development of POLD.

VI. PREEXISTING LIVER DISEASE AND POSTOPERATIVE LIVER DYSFUNCTION
A. Preexisting asymptomatic or mild liver disease

Although postoperative liver disease is occasionally produced or exacerbated by anesthetic or surgical interventions, POLD is often unrelated to perioperative factors, arising instead from preexisting liver disease that escaped detection preoperatively. A study by Schemel[53] provides some insight into the prevalence of asymptomatic liver disease in a healthy-appearing surgical population. During a 1-year period, multiple laboratory screening tests were performed in 7620 patients (ASA Physical Status I) scheduled to have elective surgical procedures. In 11 of the patients (approximately 1 of 700), abnormal increases of AST (SGOT), ALT (SGPT), and LDH were detected and the proposed surgeries were canceled. All 11 proved to have overt hepatic disorders (infectious mononucleosis, viral hepatitis, cirrhosis, or alcoholic hepatitis), and three later became clinically jaundiced (overall incidence of jaundice of 1:2540). If any of these three patients had actually received general anesthesia with halogenated vapors and overt hepatic disease had appeared between the sixth and fourteenth postoperative days, their disease may well have been diagnosed erroneously as AIH. Of the 7609 patients who actually underwent anesthesia and surgery, none had laboratory evidence of preexisting hepatic disease and none developed unexplained postsurgical jaundice. Another clinical study[54] has documented a prevalence of unsuspected preoperative hepatic dysfunction similar to that reported by Schemel. Thus it appears that approximately 1 out of every 2500 healthy patients who undergo anesthesia and surgery will develop clinically significant POLD that is totally unrelated to surgery or anesthesia.

Because preexisting conditions are more likely than anesthetics to contribute to or cause severe POLD, preoperative evaluation of the patient should address preexisting risk factors for POLD. These risk factors include use of potentially hepatotoxic medications or illicit drugs (cocaine), use of ethanol, prior episodes of jaundice or history of viral hepatitis, congenital disorders (e.g., Gilbert's disease), and systemic diseases or conditions associated with hepatic pathology (e.g., preeclampsia). Exposure to environmental and occupational hepatotoxins should also be considered as a possible cause of liver disease of unknown origin.[160] Hepatotoxins, like the other major causes of hepatic disease, can produce a broad spectrum of hepatic dysfunction, including abnormal LFTs in asymptomatic patients, steatosis, acute or chronic hepatitis, fulminant hepatic necrosis, cirrhosis, venoocclusive disease, and hepatic neoplasia.

1. Pharmacologically induced. Use of prescription and over-the-counter medications is ubiquitous. Polypharmacy is the rule rather than the exception in patients who are elderly, debilitated, or undergoing major operations. Thus the ability of pharmacologic agents to cause liver injury is an important perioperative concern. Some 500 to 1000 therapeutic agents have been implicated in a broad spectrum of liver diseases.[161] These diseases may be classified in accordance with whether the drug produces primarily direct cell toxicity (necrosis), cholestasis (cessation of bile flow), or steatosis (fatty liver). Most forms of drug-induced liver disease are benign and of little consequence (estrogen-induced cholestasis), producing only transient alterations of LFTs. Severe drug toxicities, which are typically dose-related (acetaminophen) or idiosyncratic (halothane), are responsible for 15% to 30% of the cases of FHF and 20% to 50% of the cases of chronic hepatitis (nonviral). Moreover, when drug reactions produce hepatocellular necrosis, the estimated case fatality rate approaches 50%.

Drugs that can produce hepatocellular injury and centrilobular necrosis include acetaminophen, isoniazid, and methyldopa. Other cytotoxic drugs include oxyphenisatin, rifampin, papaverine, phenytoin,[162] indomethacin, monoamine oxidase inhibitors, and amitriptyline.[163] The use of dantrolene for treatment of muscle spastic disorders has been linked to the development of hepatic failure in patients receiving the drug for more than 60 days. Cholestatic reactions can result from drugs such as chlorpromazine, phenylbutazone, and androgenic and anabolic steroids. Erythromycin (ethylsuccinate form) has caused hepatic failure that was initially attributed to halothane administration.

The potential of a drug to cause hepatotoxicity can be markedly enhanced by pharmacologic (other drugs) or pathophysiologic (hepatitis) conditions. For example, the combination of trimethoprim-sulfamethoxazole is nearly five times more frequently associated with hepatotoxicity than sulfamethoxazole alone. Drugs that induce hepatic microsomal drug-metabolizing systems can markedly increase the toxic potential of other drugs by altering their metabolism, favoring the production of highly reactive intermediates or toxic metabolites. Phenobarbital can increase halothane-induced liver dysfunction[164] as well as the hepatotoxic potential of other drugs such as chemotherapeutic agents (methotrexate) and antibiotics (tetracycline).[165]

2. Ethanol-induced. Postoperative hepatic dysfunction should raise the question of preoperative alcohol excess. Chronic alcoholism, an important cause of POLD, can produce a wide spectrum of liver disease, including steatosis (fatty liver), alcoholic hepatitis, and cirrhosis. However, this condition is notoriously difficult to detect by a brief patient history and physical examination, and laboratory values can be misleading. Moreover, there is a poor correlation between clinical presentation and hepatic histopathology because patients with extensive liver disease may be remarkably well compensated clinically.[166]

Although elective surgery is not contraindicated in patients with steatosis, the mortality from acute alcoholic hepatitis, even without surgery, is significant. Animal studies indicate that alcohol ingestion increases the likelihood that centrilobular necrosis will develop after halothane anesthesia, which may relate to the ability of ethanol to increase hepatic hypoxia. Thus if alcoholic hepatitis is suspected, further examination of liver function is warranted.

3. Viral hepatitis. Viral hepatitides are important causes of postoperative hepatic dysfunction; they can elude preoperative detection, especially during the incubation period, when the disease is asymptomatic. The viruses that most commonly cause hepatic dysfunction are called heterotropic viruses, and include hepatitis A virus (HAV, infectious hepatitis), hepatitis B virus (HBV, serum hepatitis), hepatitis C virus (HCV, previously lumped with non-A, non-B viruses), hepatitis D virus

(HDV, delta), hepatitis E virus (HEV), and non-A, non-B/C virus. HDV is a defective but pathogenic agent that requires HBV or a similar hepadnavirus for its replication. Table 20-8 compares hepatitis types A, B, C, D, and E with respect to taxonomy, clinical presentation, laboratory data, outcomes, and modes of transmission.

Other important but much less common causes of viral hepatitis include CMV, Epstein-Barr virus (EBV), herpes simplex virus, rubella virus, varicella zoster virus, measles virus, Coxsackie viruses, and echoviruses (Box 20-9). Although these viruses typically produce benign, anicteric disease, which escapes detection by surgical and anesthesia teams,[55,167] in rare circumstances, particularly in immunocompromised patients, they can cause acute hepatitis, FHF, and death.

The differential diagnosis of viral hepatitis and AIH can be quite difficult; the clinical presentations may be similar, laboratory findings may be inconclusive, and liver biopsy results may fail to provide a basis for etiologic differentiation. A diagnosis of viral hepatitis is based on a constellation of findings suggestive of viral infection coupled with hepatocellular necrosis.[168] In general, the clinical presentation of viral hepatitis includes the following four phases: (1) an early prodromal phase, which typically begins 2 to 3 weeks before jaundice develops, and resembles serum sickness, with fever, arthral-

Table 20-8. Comparison of hepatitis types A, B, C, D, and E

Item	A	B	C	D	E
Taxonomy					
Family	Picornaviridae	Hepadnaviridae	Flaviviridae	Delta viridae	Caliciviridae
Nucleic acid	RNA	DNA	RNA	RNA	RNA
Clinical presentation					
Age group	Primarily young	All ages	? All ages	? All ages	Mostly adults
Onset	Abrupt	Insidious	Insidious	Abrupt insidious	Abrupt
Inoculation period					
Range (days)	15-50	28-160	14-160	Varies	15-45
Mean (days)	±30	±80	±50	Varies	±40
Symptoms					
Arthralgias, rash	Uncommon	Common	Uncommon	Uncommon	Common
Fever	Common	Uncommon	Uncommon	Common	Common
Nausea, vomiting	Common	Common	Common	Common	Common
Jaundice	Uncommon in children	Less common than in hepatitis A	Uncommon	Common	Common
Laboratory data					
Duration of enzymes	Short	Prolonged	Prolonged	Variable	Short
Location of virus					
Blood	Transient	Prolonged	Prolonged	Prolonged	Prolonged
Stool	Yes	No	No	No	Yes
Outcomes					
Acute disease	Mild	Moderate	Mild	Can be severe	Severe in pregnant women
Mortality	Low	Low	Low	High	As above
Chronic hepatitis	No	Yes	Yes	Yes	No
Transmission					
Oral	+	±	−	−	+
Percutaneous	Rare	+	+	+	−
Sexual	+	+	?	++	−
Perinatal	−	+	?	−−	−
Homologous immunity	Yes	Yes	Can have second bouts	Yes	?

From Seeff L: Diagnosis, therapy, and prognosis of viral hepatitis. In Zakim D, Boyer T: *Hepatology: a textbook of liver disease,* Philadelphia, 1996, WB Saunders.
+, *Yes;* −, *no;* ±, *unknown.*

gias, arthritis, rash, and angioneurotic edema; (2) a pre-icteric phase, characterized by nonspecific constitutional symptoms including malaise, unusual fatigue, myalgias, anorexia, nausea, vomiting, occasional midepigastric or right upper quadrant pain, and diarrhea; (3) an icteric phase, marked by onset of jaundice, a decrease in fever, and lessening of constitutional symptoms; and (4) a convalescent phase, wherein jaundice begins to subside, constitutional symptoms disappear, and a sense of well-being returns to the patient.

HAV infection is not associated with blood transfusion. The viremia is short lived, and the incubation period is only 3 to 4 weeks long. There are no chronic carriers, and chronic liver disease is not a feature of HAV infection. FHF is rarely caused by HAV (0.14% to 2%) in the absence of preexisting liver disease. Although most patients with hepatitis B who acquire an HAV infection have an uncomplicated clinical course, an HAV superinfection of patients with chronic hepatitis C has been reported to produce fulminant hepatitis in 41% of patients, with a fatality rate of 35%. In these cases, propensity to develop liver failure was unrelated to the severity of preexisting liver disease.[169] The potential for HBV to cause FHF is markedly increased by an HDV superinfection. Unlike HCV, which by itself is not very pathogenic, HDV infections are almost invariably associated with active liver disease, either acute or chronic.

Posttransfusion hepatitis is caused primarily by non-A non-B hepatitis viruses (either HCV or other non-A non-B viruses), and there is now strong evidence that HCV has been the major cause of transfusion-related hepatitis for decades. For example, reports from the 1960s indicated that the type of hepatitis that followed transfusions did not become clinically manifest for approximately 7 weeks after the transfusion; this incubation period is the same as described for HCV (discovered in 1989) and is distinctly different from the incubation periods of infections with HAV (3 to 4 weeks) or HBV (12 weeks). Thus even in the years that preceded the screening of donor blood for hepatitis surface antigen (HBsAg), it was not HBV but rather HCV that was usually responsible for posttransfusion hepatitis. From an epidemiologic perspective, this is of concern because infections with HCV more often progress to chronic liver disease than those of other hepatitis viruses. Fortunately, a serologic test for HCV now exists, and because of its use in screening donated blood, the incidence of transfusion-related hepatitis from HCV is lower than that from HBV (1 case per 100,000 versus 1 case per 60,000 units transfused) (Fig 20-7).

Serologic tests have been the mainstay in the diagnosis of viral hepatitis. For example, an acute infection with HAV is documented by serum immunoglobulin M (IgM) antibody to the HAV capsid, as well as HAV RNA in stool; recovery is associated with IgG anti-HAV. HBV infections are indicated by either HBsAg or antibody (IgM) to core antigen (HBV core), hepatitis B e antigen (HBeAg), antibody to HBeAg (anti-HBe), antibody to HBsAg (anti-HBs), or HBV DNA measured by the polymerase chain reaction (PCR). An infection with HDV, which requires a coexisting HBV infection, is documented by IgM and total antibody to HDV. HCV can be detected by anti-HCV or the presence of HCV RNA. Assay for viral genomes are also used in the detection of hepatitis G virus (HGV).

Autoantibodies are often seen in both HBV and HCV infections, especially anti–smooth-muscle antibodies and antinuclear antibodies, the latter of which are associated with an HLA phenotype of A1,B8,DR3. Anti–asialoglycoprotein-receptor antibodies often are found in HAV infections, as well as autoimmune hepatitis, and are almost undetectable in HCV infections. It has been suggested that HAV may trigger autoimmune mechanisms (partially primed by HCV) in susceptible patients, leading to massive hepatocellular necrosis. These same types of antibodies have been identified in patients with HCV infections. HLA phenotype of A1,B8,DR3 may be a marker for susceptibility to fulminant viral hepatitis.

One should keep in mind that the serologic tests used in the diagnosis of viral hepatitis have their limitations; they are neither 100% sensitive nor 100% specific. For example, screening tests for HBsAg are negative during the incubation period of HBV infections (approximately 12 weeks). In addition, blood may contain HDV in the absence of detectable HBsAg, and serologic tests may be negative despite chronic liver disease, presumed to be caused by HBV, as suggested by the identification of hepatitis B viral DNA in such cases.[170] In addition, acute infections with HAV can cause previously detected HBV RNA or HCV RNA to become undetectable until recovery from HAV infection, and HDV infections suppress HBV replication. Moreover, viral hepatitis may be caused by a non-A, non-B/C virus that is undetectable by present assays.

4. Congenital disorders. The most common cause of jaundice in the United States is a benign metabolic dis-

---

Box 20-9 Nonhepatotropic viruses that may involve the human liver

RNA viruses

Picornaviruses (enteroviruses): coxsackie viruses, echoviruses
Togaviruses: rubella virus, yellow fever virus
Arenaviruses: Junin virus, Machupo virus, Lassa virus, Rift Valley fever virus
Rhabdoviruses: Marburg virus, Ebola virus
Paramyxoviruses: measles virus

DNA viruses

Herpes viruses: cytomegalovirus, Epstein-Barr virus, herpes simplex virus, varicella zoster virus

Unclassified viruses (agents causing infectious hepatitis thought to be viral)

Non-A, non-B, non-C hepatitis virus

From Robinson W: Biology of human hepatitis viruses. In Zakim D, Boyer T, eds: *Hepatology: a textbook of liver disease,* Philadelphia, 1996, WB Saunders.

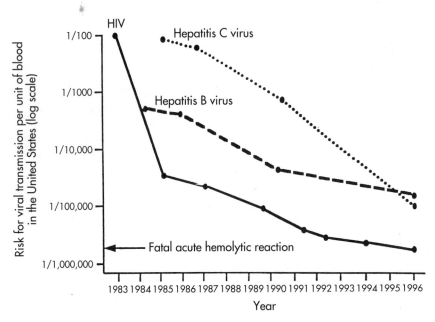

Fig. 20-7. Decrease in per-unit risk for transmission of hepatitis B virus *(broken line)*, hepatitis C virus *(dotted line)*, and human immunodeficiency virus *(solid line)* by blood transfusion in the United States. The arrow shows the current risk for death from acute hemolysis for comparison.

order known as Gilbert's syndrome (familial unconjugated hyperbilirubinemia). In this syndrome, bilirubin uptake by the liver is impaired and bilirubin glucuronyl transferase activity is decreased. Patients often do not manifest their disease until the second decade of life. This condition can be exacerbated by stress, fasting, fever, and infection. Diagnosis is suggested by clinical (jaundice without dark urine) and laboratory (unconjugated hyperbilirubinemia) abnormalities.

A less common metabolic disorder, the Crigler-Najjar syndrome (type II), is also associated with unconjugated hyperbilirubinemia; surgical and anesthetic-related problems are apparently minimal. Dubin-Johnson syndrome can be exacerbated after surgery.

5. Pregnancy-related. Well-known disorders of pregnancy that cause FHF during the third trimester or in the immediate postpartum period include acute fatty liver of pregnancy (AFLP) and the HELLP syndrome (hemolysis, elevated liver enzymes, and low platelet count). In addition, parturients are unusually susceptible to morbidity and mortality from hepatitis E infection.[171] It is unclear how the natural courses of these diseases are affected by the analgesic or anesthetic techniques used for vaginal or abdominal deliveries.

AFLP is a rare disease that occurs in the late stage of pregnancy. It is probably caused by an abnormality of lipid metabolism that remains to be fully characterized. Jaundice, encephalopathy, hypoglycemia, and preeclampsia are common, but hypertension is rare (incidence of 1 in 13,000 births) with advanced liver failure. Liver biopsy shows infiltration of centrilobular hepatocytes with microvesicular fat, producing a histopathologic picture that is strikingly similar to that seen in disorders

called hepatic microvesicular steatosis (includes Reye syndrome and injury produced by valproic acid or tetracycline). Serum aminotransferases typically do not exceed 1000 IU/L because hepatocellular necrosis is not a major feature of this disease. When the diagnosis of AFLP is made, delivery of the fetus is expedited, usually by induction of labor or, occasionally, cesarean section. Some patients continue to decline clinically after delivery, but most begin to recover by the third day postpartum. On rare occasions, liver transplantation has been necessary. Recurrence of AFLP with future pregnancy is rare.

HELLP syndrome, defined by Louis Weinstein in 1982, is much more common and generally occurs earlier in pregnancy than AFLP. This syndrome appears to represent a severe manifestation of preeclampsia, and affects about 10% of all preeclamptic women. In some cases, pregnancy-induced hypertension (in the absence of preeclampsia) appears to adversely affect hepatic function, presumably on the basis of marginal hepatic perfusion secondary to profound peripheral vasoconstriction accompanied by hypovolemia and starvation.[172]

On liver biopsy, preeclampsia has three characteristic histopathologic features: diffuse fibrin deposition along the sinusoids, periportal and portal tract hemorrhage, and ischemic necrosis that is usually focal but occasionally confluent. Because hepatocellular necrosis is present in all patients with HELLP, serum aminotransferases are almost invariably increased; mean values of AST and ALT are 434 IU/L and 239 IU/L, respectively. At times, the degree to which laboratory abnormalities reflect hepatic dysfunction is difficult to assess. For example, hyperbilirubinemia, which is present in 42% of cases of HELLP, probably results from a combination of hemolysis and liver dysfunction.

Hepatic hemorrhage or rupture is probably caused by confluent hepatocellular necrosis from preeclampsia and may occur in up to 2% of women with preeclampsia, based on abdominal computed tomography scans in women with few symptoms other than right upper quadrant abdominal pain. The most important factors in ensuring maternal survival following hepatic rupture are prompt identification of this disorder before irreversible shock occurs, vigorous hemodynamic support, and, if rupture of Glisson's capsule has occurred, an emergency laparotomy.

B. Preexisting moderate to severe liver disease (hepatitis, cirrhosis)

Large surveys indicate that the risk of postoperative hepatic complications is greatly increased in patients with preexisting liver disease, especially following emergency operations.[173] Cirrhosis is associated with an increased risk of operative and postoperative complications, with the risk being greater for abdominal than nonabdominal procedures. Child's classification of hepatic dysfunction (A, 10%; B, 31%; C, 76%) has been found to correlate with the incidence of both postoperative complications (liver failure, bleeding, infection, sepsis, renal failure, pulmonary failure, and ascites)[174,175] and operative mortality. Fortunately, clinically significant liver disease is not difficult to recognize with a careful history and physical examination, and LFTs.[152]

VII. PREVENTION AND TREATMENT OF ANESTHESIA-RELATED POSTOPERATIVE LIVER DYSFUNCTION

It seems likely that perioperative physicians can decrease the incidence of severe POLD by performing careful preoperative evaluations of patients to detect preexisting liver diseases and identify important risk factors for anesthesia-induced disease. When liver dysfunction is recognized preoperatively, it is prudent to defer elective procedures until the course of the disease can be determined. Fever or unexplained jaundice after a previous halothane anesthetic is a contraindication to another halothane anesthetic. A history of AIH may also be reason to avoid the use of other inhaled anesthetics, given the theoretical potential for immune crossover between the agents and the possibility that trace amounts of anesthetic retained in the anesthesia apparatus might trigger an allergic response. Even though halothane has an impressive record of safety in pediatric patients, it is difficult to justify its use in children at risk for halothane hepatitis. In the final analysis, avoiding the use of halothane is the single most effective way to decrease the frequency of AIH.

Which anesthetic technique best preserves hepatic function? For peripheral or minor surgery (operations that do not affect splanchnic blood flow), choice of anesthetic is usually an insignificant issue. However, the selection of anesthetics has important implications for those at increased risk for developing POLD, such as pa-

tients with preexisting liver disease or those undergoing major abdominal operations.

In the absence of liver disease, hepatic hypoperfusion is usually well tolerated; conversely, patients recovering from infectious hepatitis or chronic alcoholics may be highly susceptible to hepatic ischemia because of critically compromised liver blood flow and impaired autoregulation. Invasive monitoring of the circulation is indicated in patients with liver disease who undergo major operations, so that acute hypovolemia can be rapidly detected and effectively treated. Spinal anesthesia has been used successfully in patients at increased risk for POLD. A rational approach to general anesthesia would include the use of agents (e.g., isoflurane and fentanyl or remifentanil) that preserve cardiac output and do not adversely affect the hepatic oxygen supply-and-demand relationships.

Although the mainstay of therapy for postoperative hepatic injury is supportive, a thorough search must be made for any reversible cause of the injury. All medications should be examined for hepatotoxic potential and withdrawn if suspect. Sources of sepsis should be sought and treated. Extrahepatic biliary obstruction, which should be considered in the differential diagnosis, may require surgical intervention when present. In some cases, percutaneous liver biopsy may be needed to identify the pathogen or at least document the type of liver injury that is present. Judicious use of biochemical tests and imaging studies, which can help delineate hepatocellular from cholestatic dysfunction, will usually shorten the list of diagnostic possibilities and provide useful prognostic information. If liver function is rapidly deteriorating, the clinician must be able to predict without undue delay whether the hepatic injury will be reversible or irreversible. Accurate prognostications about reversible disease prevent unnecessary OLTs; prompt recognition of irreversible disease allows OLT to be performed expeditiously, before the complications of FHF render the patient an unacceptable candidate for this operation.

VIII. SUMMARY AND CONCLUSIONS

Manifestations of POLD can range from subclinical abnormalities of LFTs to FHF and death. The incidence and severity of POLD are influenced by a variety of patient factors (preexisting liver diseases, poor general health), surgical variables (extent of operation, operative site), and anesthetic techniques. Minor hepatic damage may occur in nearly 20% of patients who receive enflurane anesthesia, and in almost half of those having halothane anesthesia for peripheral or superficial surgery. Most major operative procedures (particularly those involving, or in close proximity to, the liver) are complicated by mild or moderate POLD, regardless of the anesthetic technique used. Up to 20% of patients undergoing such procedures develop postoperative jaundice, which usually reflects a benign condition but may indicate biliary tract obstruction or serious liver disease. Fortunately, severe POLD is an infrequent occurrence. It can result from a variety of perioperative interventions or events or from conditions that are totally independent of anesthesia and surgery.

Severe POLD is rarely caused by anesthetic agents. Much more commonly, this disorder develops in patients who appeared healthy preoperatively but had a preexisting liver disease that was not diagnosed during the preoperative assessment. A thorough preoperative history and physical examination will often reveal important clues in the diagnosis of POLD. A failure to identify patients who abuse alcohol or intravenous drugs or who have been exposed to environmental hepatotoxins (phenols, polycyclic compounds) will result in cases of unexplained POLD. Because medications can cause hepatobiliary dysfunction, anesthesiologists should familiarize themselves with those that have been associated with hepatocellular damage, cholestatic disease, or steatosis. Viral hepatitides are another important cause of POLD; these infections may have been contracted from a needlestick or a preoperative blood transfusion and remained asymptomatic (e.g., 8-week incubation period for HCV) until in the postoperative period. Incubating viral hepatitis may be responsible for 1 case of POLD per 2500 operations, whereas halothane accounts for fewer than 1 case of severe POLD per 10,000 anesthetics, and the newer volatile agents (enflurane, isoflurane, sevoflurane, desflurane) account for fewer than 1 case per million anesthetics.

It is important to realize that anesthetic-induced POLD is a diagnosis of exclusion. There are neither pathognomonic features nor highly specific tests for this disorder, and the clinical presentation provides the key to the diagnosis. More cases of AIH have been attributed to halothane (500 cases) than to all the other anesthetics combined (enflurane, 50 cases; isoflurane, 10 cases; sevoflurane, 3 cases; desflurane, 1 case). Accordingly, much more is known about halothane hepatitis than the hepatitides that have been attributed to the other inhaled anesthetics. Halothane hepatitis typically affects middle-aged patients, especially obese women, and very rarely occurs in children. It most often occurs after brief, minor surgical procedures in patients who have had prior halothane anesthetics. It usually presents 3 to 14 days after the halothane anesthetic, with fever or jaundice as the initial manifestation in about 70% of cases. The most predictive of the risk factors for halothane hepatitis is a recent (within 28 days) exposure to halothane, which has been noted in 80% of patients who subsequently developed the disease.

The mechanisms of AILD are complex and have not been fully elucidated. Mild hepatic injuries that follow anesthesia (especially with halothane or enflurane) and surgery probably result from anesthesia-induced derangements of hepatic circulation and oxygen-supply demand ratios or cytotoxic effects associated with anesthetic metabolism. All the volatile agents decrease portal blood flow as cardiac output decreases, and although some produce increases in hepatic arterial flow (isoflurane or sevoflurane), the net result is usually a lowering of total hepatic blood flow during anesthesia. Such effects are likely to increase the potential of major operations (especially laparotomy) or perioperative stresses to cause liver injury. Nonetheless, the effects of anesthetics on hepatic circulation and oxygen supply-to-demand ratios are not responsible for the development of AIH.

The cytochrome P-450 2E1 catalyzed oxidation of anesthetics appears to play a major role in the pathogenesis of AIH. Highly reactive oxidative intermediates (trifluoroacyl derivative, TF-acyl) of halothane, and perhaps enflurane, bind covalently to a variety of hepatic macromolecules, thereby creating both neoantigens (TF-acyl moieties act as haptens) and autoantigens. In susceptible individuals, these antigens apparently trigger an immunologic response directed at the affected hepatocytes (centrilobular area of liver), causing massive hepatic necrosis. Isoflurane and desflurane can theoretically cause hepatitis via a similar mechanism, although these agents are much less extensively metabolized than halothane or enflurane. Thus an exposure to any of these agents could conceivably sensitize patients to the other volatile agents (immune crossover).

Antibodies isolated from patients with halothane hepatitis are able to recognize antigens induced by enflurane anesthesia or from exposure to isoflurane or desflurane. The phenomenon of immune crossover could underlie the association between prior halothane or enflurane anesthetics and the many cases of hepatitis attributable to the newer anesthetics. Thus anesthesia with halothane, and perhaps enflurane, might endanger patients in a subtle way, predisposing them to hepatitis from agents (isoflurane or desflurane) that otherwise would be safe. This concern may not pertain to sevoflurane because its metabolism is unique; neither trifluoroacylated hepatic macromolecules nor neoantigens have been detected following sevoflurane administration. If the pathogenesis of AIH truly requires trifluorolacylation of hepatic proteins, sevoflurane would not be expected to cause hepatitis. Of the various mechanisms proposed as explanations for the development of severe AIH, the immune theory is the most compelling to date. But like any useful theory, it has generated a multitude of provocative questions, the answers to which will either challenge or support its validity.

REFERENCES

1. Allan LG, Hussey AJ, Howie J, et al: Hepatic glutathione S-transferase release after halothane anaesthesia: open randomised comparison with isoflurane, *Lancet* 1:771, 1987.
2. Hussey AJ, Aldridge LM, Paul D, et al: Plasma glutathione S-transferase concentration as a measure of hepatocellular integrity following a single general anaesthetic with halothane, enflurane or isoflurane, *Br J Anaesth* 60:130, 1988.
3. Evans C, Evans M, Pollock AV: The incidence and causes of postoperative jaundice: a prospective study, *Br J Anaesth* 46:520, 1974.
4. Sussman N: Fulminant hepatic failure. In Zakim D, Boyer T, eds: *Hepatology: a textbook of liver disease*, Philadelphia, 1996, WB Saunders, p 618.
5. Friedman L, Martin P, Munoz S: Liver function tests and the objective evaluation of the patient with liver disease. In Zakim D, Boyer T, eds: *Hepatology: a textbook of liver disease*, Philadelphia, 1996, WB Saunders, p 791.

6. Redick JA, Jakoby WB, Baron J: Immunohistochemical localization of glutathione S-transferases in livers of untreated rats, *J Biol Chem* 257:15200, 1982.
7. Njoku D, Laster MJ, Gong DH, et al: Biotransformation of halothane, enflurane, isoflurane, and desflurane to trifluoroacetylated liver proteins: association between protein acylation and hepatic injury, *Anesth Analg* 84:173, 1997.
8. Lewis JH, Zimmermann HJ, Ishak KG, et al: Enflurane hepatotoxicity: a clinicopathologic study of 24 cases, *Ann Intern Med* 98:984, 1983.
9. Eger EI, Smuckler EA, Ferrell LD, et al: Is enflurane hepatotoxic? *Anesth Analg* 65:21, 1986.
10. Carrigan TW, Straughen WJ: A report of hepatic necrosis and death following isoflurane anesthesia, *Anesthesiology* 67:581, 1987.
11. Watanabe K, Hatakenaka S, Ikemune K, et al: A case of suspected liver dysfunction induced by sevoflurane anesthesia, *Masui* 42:902, 1993.
12. Shichinohe Y, Masuda Y, Takahashi H, et al: A case of postoperative hepatic injury after sevoflurane anesthesia, *Masui* 41:1802, 1992.
13. Ogawa M, Doi K, Mitsufuji T, et al: Drug-induced hepatitis following sevoflurane anesthesia in a child, *Masui* 40:1542, 1991.
14. Martin JL, Plevak DJ, Flannery KD, et al: Hepatotoxicity after desflurane anesthesia, *Anesthesiology* 83:1125, 1995.
15. Cohen EN, Trudell JR, Edmunds HN, et al: Urinary metabolites of halothane in man, *Anesthesiology* 43:392, 1975.
16. Carpenter RL, Eger EI, Johnson BH, et al: The extent of metabolism of inhaled anesthetics in humans, *Anesthesiology* 65:201, 1986.
17. Chase RE, Holaday DA, Fiserova-Bergerova V, et al: The biotransformation of ethrane in man, *Anesthesiology* 35:262, 1971.
18. Kharasch ED, Armstrong AS, Gunn K, et al: Clinical sevoflurane metabolism and disposition. II. The role of cytochrome P450 2E1 in fluoride and hexafluoroisopropanol formation, *Anesthesiology* 82:1379, 1995.
19. Holaday DA, Fiserova-Bergerova V, Latto IP, et al: Resistance of isoflurane to biotransformation in man, *Anesthesiology* 43:325, 1975.
20. Sutton TS, Koblin DD, Gruenke LD, et al: Fluoride metabolites after prolonged exposure of volunteers and patients to desflurane, *Anesth Analg* 73:180, 1991.
21. Ray DC, Drummond GB: Halothane hepatitis, *Br J Anaesth* 67:84, 1991.
22. Trowell J, Peto R, Campton-Smith A: Controlled trial of repeated halothane hepatitis in patients of the uterine cervix treated with radium, *Lancet* 1:824, 1975.
23. Fee JP, Black GW, Dundee JW, et al: A prospective study of liver enzyme and other changes following repeat administration of halothane and enflurane, *Br J Anaesth* 51:1133, 1979.
24. Wright R, Eade OE, Chisholm M, et al: Controlled prospective study of the effect on liver function of multiple exposures to halothane, *Lancet* 1:817, 1975.
25. Neuberger J, Williams R: Halothane anaesthesia and liver damage, *BMJ* 289:1136, 1984.
26. Kenna JG, Jones RM: The organ toxicity of inhaled anesthetics, *Anesth Analg* 81(suppl 6):S51, 1995.
27. Eger E: Anesthetic-induced hepatitis, International Anesthesia Research Society Review Course Lectures, Cleveland, Ohio, 1986, p 116.
28. Inman WH, Mushin WW: Jaundice after repeated exposure to halothane: an analysis of Reports to the Committee on Safety of Medicines, *BMJ* 1:5, 1974.
29. Bottiger L, Dalen E, Hallen B: Halothane-induced liver damage: an analysis of the material reported to the Swedish Adverse Drug Reaction Committee 1966-1973, *Acta Anaesthesiol Scand* 20:40, 1976.
30. Elliott RH, Strunin L: Hepatotoxicity of volatile anaesthetics, *Br J Anaesth* 70:339, 1993.
31. Neuberger J: Halothane hepatitis, *ISI Atlas of Science & Pharmacology* vol 2, no 4, 1988, p 303.
32. Hussey AJ, Howie J, Allan LG, et al: Impaired hepatocellular integrity during general anaesthesia, as assessed by measurement of plasma glutathione S-transferase, *Clin Chim Acta* 161:19, 1986.
33. Kenna JG, Neuberger J, Mieli-Vergani G, et al: Halothane hepatitis in children, *BMJ* 294:1209, 1987.
34. Warner LO, Beach TP, Garvin JP, et al: Halothane and children: the first quarter century, *Anesth Analg* 63:838, 1984.
35. Hassall E, Israel DM, Gunasekaran T, et al: Halothane hepatitis in children, *J Pediatr Gastroenterol Nutr* 11:553, 1990.
36. Wark H, O'Halloran M, Overton J: Prospective study of liver function in children following multiple halothane anaesthetics at short intervals, *Br J Anaesth* 58:1224, 1986.
37. Anonymous: Summary of National Halothane Study: possible association between halothane anesthesia and postoperative hepatic necrosis, *JAMA* 197:775, 1966.
38. Touloukian J, Kaplowitz N: Halothane-induced hepatic disease, *Semin Liver Dis* 1:134, 1981.
39. Anonymous: Halothane-associated liver damage, *Lancet* 1:1251, 1986 (editorial).
40. Bottiger LE, Dalen E, Hallen B: Halothane-induced liver damage: an analysis of the material reported to the Swedish Adverse Drug Reaction Committee, 1966-1973, *Acta Anaesthesiol Scand* 20:40, 1976.
41. Moult PJ, Sherlock S: Halothane-related hepatitis: a clinical study of twenty-six cases, *Q J Med* 44:99, 1975.
42. Walton B, Simpson BR, Strunin L, et al: Unexplained hepatitis following halothane, *BMJ* 1:1171, 1976.
43. Peters RL, Edmondson HA, Reynolds TB, et al: Hepatic necrosis associated with halothane anaesthesia, *Am J Med* 47:748, 1969.
44. Klion FM, Schaffner F, Popper H: Hepatitis after exposure to halothane, *Ann Intern Med* 71:467, 1969.
45. Mushin W, Rosen M, Jones E: Post-halothane jaundice in relation to previous administration of halothane, *BMJ* 3:18, 1971.
46. Biermann J, Rice SA, Fish KJ, et al: Metabolism of halothane in obese Fischer 344 rats, *Anesthesiology* 71:431, 1989.
47. Brown BJ, Gandolfi A: Adverse effects of volatile anaesthetics, *Br J Anaesth* 59:14, 1987.
48. Hoft R, Bunker JP, Goodman HI, et al: Halothane hepatitis in three pairs of closely related women, *N Engl J Med* 304:1023, 1981.
49. Otsuka S, Yamamoto M, Kasuya S, et al: HLA antigens in patients with unexplained hepatitis following halothane anesthesia, *Acta Anaesthesiol Scand* 29:497, 1985.
50. Kenna J: Halothane hepatitis in children, *BMJ* 294:1209, 1987.
51. Brown BJ: General anesthetics and hepatic toxicity, *Ariz Med* 34:5, 1977.
52. Nomura F, Hitoshi H, Iida S, et al: Halothane hepatotoxicity and reductive metabolism of halothane in acute experimental liver injury in rats, *Anesth Analg* 67:448, 1988.
53. Schemel WH: Unexpected hepatic dysfunction found by multiple laboratory screening, *Anesth Analg* 55:810, 1976.
54. Wataneeyawech M, Kelly K: Hepatic diseases—unsuspected before surgery, *N Y State J Med* 75:1278, 1975.
55. Douglas HJ, Eger EI, Biava CG, et al: Hepatic necrosis associated with viral infection after enflurane anesthesia, *N Engl J Med* 296:553, 1977.
56. Morley TS: "Halothane hepatitis," *JAMA* 225(13):1659, 1973.
57. Cousins MJ, Plummer JL, Hall PD: Toxicity of volatile anaesthetic agents, *Can Anaesth Soc J* 32(3 pt 2):S52, 1985.
58. Stock JG, Strunin L: Unexplained hepatitis following halothane, *Anesthesiology* 63:424, 1985.
59. DiRenzo AB, Gandolfi AJ, Brooks SD, et al: Toxicity and biotransformation of volatile halogenated anesthetics in rat hepatocyte suspensions, *Drug Chem Toxicol* 8:207, 1985.
60. Awad JA, Horn JL, Roberts LJ, et al: Demonstration of halothane-induced hepatic lipid peroxidation in rats by quantification of F2-isoprostanes, *Anesthesiology* 84:910, 1996.
61. Gelman S: General anesthesia and hepatic circulation, *Can J Physiol Pharmacol* 65:1762, 1987.
62. Gelman S, Van Dyke R: Mechanism of halothane-induced hepatotoxicity: another step on a long path, *Anesthesiology* 68:479, 1988.

63. Van Dyke R, Madson T: Stimulation of phosphorylase activity by volatile anesthetics in isolated rat hepatocytes, *Fed Proc* 45:699, 1986.

64. Mets B, Janicki PK, James MF, et al: Hepatic energy charge and adenine nucleotide status in rats anesthetized with halothane, isoflurane or enflurane, *Acta Anaesthesiol Scand* 41:252, 1997.

65. Fujiwara M, Watanabe A, Sato Y, et al: Clinical significance of eosinophilia in the diagnosis of halothane-induced liver injury, *Acta Med Okayama* 38:35, 1984.

66. Hubbard AK, Roth TP, Gandolfi AJ, et al: Halothane hepatitis patients generate an antibody response toward a covalently bound metabolite of halothane, *Anesthesiology* 68:791, 1988.

67. Klatskin G, Kimberg DV: Recurrent hepatitis attributable to halothane sensitization in an anesthetist, *N Engl J Med* 280:515, 1969.

68. Sutherland DE, Smith WA: Chemical heptitis associated with occupational exposure to halothane in a research laboratory, *Vet Hum Toxicol* 34:423, 1992.

69. Neuberger J, Vergani D, Mieli-Vergani G, et al: Hepatic damage after exposure to halothane in medical personnel, *Br J Anaesth* 53:1173, 1981.

70. Callis AH, Brooks SD, Roth TP, et al: Characterization of a halothane-induced humoral immune response in rabbits, *Clin Exp Immunol* 67:343, 1987.

71. Hals J, Dodgson MS, Skulberg A, et al: Halothane-associated liver damage and renal failure in a young child, *Acta Anaesthesiol Scand* 30:651, 1986.

72. Martin JL, Kenna JG, Pohl LR: Antibody assays for the detection of patients sensitized to halothane, *Anesth Analg* 70:154, 1990.

73. Neuberger J, Gimson AE, Davis M, et al: Specific serological markers in the diagnosis of fulminant hepatic failure associated with halothane anaesthesia, *Br J Anaesth* 55:15, 1983.

74. Kenna JG, Neuberger J, Williams R: Specific antibodies to halothane-induced liver antigens in halothane-associated hepatitis, *Br J Anaesth* 59:1286, 1987.

75. Taylor M, Lack J: Letter to the editor, *BMJ* 293:335, 1986.

76. Schneider M: Fatal hepatic necrosis following cardiac surgery and enflurane anaesthesia, *Anaesth Intensive Care* 23:225, 1995.

77. Hausmann R, Schmidt B, Schellmann B, et al: Differential diagnosis of postoperative liver failure in a 12-year-old child, *Int J Legal Med* 109:210, 1996.

78. Reeves M: Acute hepatitis following enflurane anaesthesia, *Anaesth Intensive Care* 25:80, 1997.

79. Kharasch ED, Thummel KE, Mautz D, et al: Clinical enflurane metabolism by cytochrome P450 2E1, *Clin Pharmacol Ther* 55:434, 1994.

80. Garton KJ, Yuen P, Meinwald J, et al: Stereoselective metabolism of enflurane by human liver cytochrome P450 2E1, *Drug Metab Dispos* 23:1426, 1995.

81. Yoo JS, Ning SM, Pantuck CB, et al: Regulation of hepatic microsomal cytochrome P450IIE1 level by dietary lipids and carbohydrates in rats, *J Nutr* 121:959, 1991.

82. Pantuck EJ, Pantuck CB, Ryan DE, et al: Inhibition and stimulation of enflurane metabolism in the rat following a single dose or chronic administration of ethanol, *Anesthesiology* 62:255, 1985.

83. Rice SA, Dooley JR, Mazze RI: Metabolism by rat hepatic microsomes of fluorinated ether anesthetics following ethanol consumption, *Anesthesiology* 58:237, 1983.

84. Reference deleted in pages.

85. Frink EJ Jr, Morgan SE, Coetzee A, et al: The effects of sevoflurane, halothane, enflurane, and isoflurane on hepatic blood flow and oxygenation in chronically instrumented greyhound dogs, *Anesthesiology* 76:85, 1992.

86. Bernard JM, Doursout MF, Wouters P, et al: Effects of enflurane and isoflurane on hepatic and renal circulations in chronically instrumented dogs, *Anesthesiology* 74:298, 1991.

87. Berendes E, Lippert G, Loick HM, et al: Effects of enflurane and isoflurane on splanchnic oxygenation in humans, *J Clin Anesth* 8:456, 1996.

88. Ghantous H, Fernando J, Gandolfi AJ, et al: Inhibition of protein synthesis and secretion by volatile anesthetics in guinea pig liver slices, *Adv Exp Med Biol* 283:725, 1991.

89. Ghantous HN, Fernando J, Gandolfi AJ, et al: Toxicity of halothane in guinea pig liver slices, *Toxicology* 62:59, 1990.

90. Lind RC, Gandolfi AJ, Sipes IG, et al: Comparison of the requirements for hepatic injury with halothane and enflurane in rats, *Anesth Analg* 64:955, 1985.

91. Christ DD, Kenna JG, Kammerer W, et al: Enflurane metabolism produces covalently bound liver adducts recognized by antibodies from patients with halothane hepatitis, *Anesthesiology* 69:833, 1988.

92. Clarke JB, Thomas C, Chen M, et al: Halogenated anesthetics form liver adducts and antigens that cross-react with halothane-induced antibodies, *Int Arch Allergy Immunol* 108:24, 1995.

93. Gogus FY, Toker K, Baykan N: Hepatitis following use of two different fluorinated anesthetic agents, *Isr J Med Sci* 27:156, 1991.

94. Weitz J, Kienle P, Bohrer H, et al: Fatal hepatic necrosis after isoflurane anaesthesia, *Anaesthesia* 52:892, 1997.

95. Boyer T: Preoperative and postoperative hepatic dysfunction. In Zakim D, Boyer T, eds: *Hepatology: a textbook of liver disease*, Philadelphia, 1996, WB Saunders, p 1912.

96. Gelman S, Dillard E, Bradley EL Jr: Hepatic circulation during surgical stress and anesthesia with halothane, isoflurane, or fentanyl, *Anesth Analg* 66:936, 1987.

97. Gil F, Fiserova-Bergerova V, Altman NH: Hepatic protection from chemical injury by isoflurane, *Anesth Analg* 67:860, 1988.

98. Baden JM: Hepatotoxicity and metabolism of isoflurane in rats with cirrhosis, *Anesth Analg* 68:214, 1989.

99. Van Dyke RA: Hepatic centrilobular necrosis in rats after exposure to halothane, enflurane, or isoflurane, *Anesth Analg* 61:812, 1982.

100. Stoelting RK, Blitt CD, Cohen PJ, et al: Hepatic dysfunction after isoflurane anesthesia, *Anesth Analg* 66:147, 1987.

101. Shiraishi N, Saito H, Shiraishi H, et al: A case of liver dysfunction after isoflurane anesthesia, *Masui* 42:910, 1993.

102. Sinha A, Clatch RJ, Stuck G, et al: Isoflurane hepatotoxicity: a case report and review of the literature, *Am J Gastroenterol* 91:2406, 1996.

103. Gunaratnam NT, Benson J, Gandolfi AJ, et al: Suspected isoflurane hepatitis in an obese patient with a history of halothane hepatitis, *Anesthesiology* 83:1361, 1995.

104. Gelven PL, Cina SJ, Lee JD, et al: Massive hepatic necrosis and death following repeated isoflurane exposure: case report and review of the literature, *Am J Forensic Med Pathol* 17:61, 1996.

105. Varma RR, Whitesell RC, Iskandarani MM: Halothane hepatitis without halothane: role of inapparent circuit contamination of its prevention, *Hepatology* 5:1159, 1985.

106. Kharasch ED, Thummel KE: Identification of cytochrome P450 2E1 as the predominant enzyme catalyzing human liver microsomal defluorination of sevoflurane, isoflurane, and methoxyflurane, *Anesthesiology* 79:795, 1993.

107. Kharasch ED: Metabolism and toxicity of the new anesthetic agents, *Acta Anaesthesiol Belg* 47:7, 1996.

108. Schindler E, Muller M, Zickmann B, et al: Blood supply to the liver in the human after 1 MAC desflurane in comparison with isoflurane and halothane, *Anasthesiol Intensivmed Notfallmed Schmerzther* 31:344, 1996.

109. Armbruster K, Noldge-Schomburg GF, Dressler IM, et al: The effects of desflurane on splanchnic hemodynamics and oxygenation in the anesthetized pig, *Anesth Analg* 84:271, 1997.

110. Bauer C, Sattel C, Grundmann U, et al: Effects of desflurane on liver microcirculation in comparison with isoflurane and pentobarbital: an intravital microscopy study in the rat, *Anasthesiol Intensivmed Notfallmed Schmerzther* 30:226, 1995.

111. Eger EI, Johnson BH, Strum DP, et al: Studies of the toxicity of I-653, halothane, and isoflurane in enzyme-induced, hypoxic rats, *Anesth Analg* 66:1227, 1987.

112. Fang ZX, Eger EI, Laster MJ, et al: Carbon monoxide production from degradation of desflurane, enflurane, isoflurane, halothane, and sevoflurane by soda lime and Baralyme, *Anesth Analg* 80:1187, 1995.

113. Baxter PJ, Kharasch ED: Rehydration of desiccated Baralyme prevents carbon monoxide formation from desflurane in an anesthesia machine, *Anesthesiology* 86:1061, 1997.

114. Brown B Jr: Sevoflurane: introduction and overview, *Anesth Analg* 81(6 suppl):S1, 1995.

115. Reference deleted in pages.

116. Bito H, Ikeda K: Renal and hepatic function in surgical patients after low-flow sevoflurane or isoflurane anesthesia, *Anesth Analg* 82:173, 1996.

117. Newman PJ, Quinn AC, Hall GM, et al: Circulating fluoride changes and hepatorenal function following sevoflurane anaesthesia, *Anaesthesia* 49:936, 1994.

118. Quinn AC, Newman PJ, Hall GM, et al: Sevoflurane anaesthesia for major intra-abdominal surgery, *Anaesthesia* 49:567, 1994.

119. Nagata R, Sameshima H, Komaki T, et al: The effect of inhalation of sevoflurane for an hour on the liver of beagles, *Masui* 40:887, 1991.

120. Wallin RF, Regan BM, Napoli MD, et al: Sevoflurane: a new inhalational anesthetic agent, *Anesth Analg* 54:758, 1975.

121. Soma LR, Tierney WJ, Hogan GK, et al: The effects of multiple administrations of sevoflurane to cynomolgus monkeys: clinical pathologic, hematologic, and pathologic study, *Anesth Analg* 81:347, 1995.

122. Ghantous HN, Fernando J, Gandolfi AJ, et al: Sevoflurane is biotransformed by guinea pig liver slices but causes minimal cytotoxicity, *Anesth Analg* 75:436, 1992.

123. Kanaya N, Nakayama M, Fujita S, et al: Comparison of the effects of sevoflurane, isoflurane and halothane on indocyanine green clearance, *Br J Anaesth* 74:164, 1995.

124. Conzen PF, Vollmar B, Habazettl H, et al: Systemic and regional hemodynamics of isoflurane and sevoflurane in rats, *Anesth Analg* 74:79, 1992.

125. Bernard JM, Doursout MF, Wouters P, et al: Effects of sevoflurane and isoflurane on hepatic circulation in the chronically instrumented dog, *Anesthesiology* 77:541, 1992.

126. Fujita Y, Kimura K, Hamada H, et al: Comparative effects of halothane, isoflurane, and sevoflurane on the liver with hepatic artery ligation in the beagle, *Anesthesiology* 75:313, 1991.

127. Strum DP, Eger EI, Johnson BH, et al: Toxicity of sevoflurane in rats, *Anesth Analg* 66:769, 1987.

128. Kharasch ED, Frink EJ Jr, Zager R, et al: Assessment of low-flow sevoflurane and isoflurane effects on renal function using sensitive markers of tubular toxicity, *Anesthesiology* 86:1238, 1997.

129. Laster MJ, Gong D, Kerschmann RL, et al: Acetaminophen predisposes to renal and hepatic injury from compound A in the fasting rat, *Anesth Analg* 84:169, 1997.

130. Shiraishi Y, Ikeda K: Uptake and biotransformation of sevoflurane in humans: a comparative study of sevoflurane with halothane, enflurane, and isoflurane, *J Clin Anesth* 2:381, 1990.

131. Kharasch ED: Biotransformation of sevoflurane, *Anesth Analg* 81(suppl 6):S27, 1995.

132. Frink EJ Jr: The hepatic effects of sevoflurane, *Anesth Analg* 81(suppl 6):S46, 1995.

133. Zinn SE, Fairley HB, Glenn JD: Liver function in patients with mild alcoholic hepatitis, after enflurane, nitrous oxide narcotic, and spinal anesthesia, *Anesth Analg* 64:487, 1985.

134. Ross JA, Monk SJ, Duffy SW: Effect of nitrous oxide on halothane-induced hepatotoxicity in hypoxic, enzyme-induced rats, *Br J Anaesth* 56:527, 1984.

135. Lumb M, Deacon R, Perry J, et al: The effect of nitrous oxide inactivation of vitamin B$_{12}$ on rat hepatic folate: implications for the methylfolate-trap hypothesis, *Biochem J* 186:933, 1980.

136. Cohen EN, Gift HC, Brown BW, et al: Occupational disease in dentistry and chronic exposure to trace anesthetic gases, *J Am Dent Assoc* 101:21, 1980.

137. Clarke RS, Doggart JR, Lavery T: Changes in liver function after different types of surgery, *Br J Anaesth* 48:119, 1976.

138. Tiainen P, Lindgren L, Rosenberg PH: Disturbance of hepatocellular integrity associated with propofol anaesthesia in surgical patients, *Acta Anaesthesiol Scand* 39:840, 1995.

139. Clarke R, Kirwan MJ, Dundee JW, et al: Clinical studies of induction agents. XIII. Liver function after propanidid and thiopentone anaesthesia, *Br J Anaesth* 37:415, 1965.

140. Dundee J: Thiopentone as a factor in the production of liver dysfunction, *Br J Anaesth* 27:14, 1955.

141. Dundee JW, Fee JP, Moore J, et al: Changes in serum enzyme levels following ketamine infusions, *Anaesthesia* 35:12, 1980.

142. Gelman S: Anesthesia and the liver. In Barash P, Cullen B, Stoelting R, eds: *Clinical anesthesia*, Philadelphia, 1989, JB Lippincott.

143. Sear JW: Toxicity of IV anaesthetics, *Br J Anaesth* 59:24, 1987.

144. Arguelles JE, Franatovic Y, Romo-Salas F, et al: Intrabiliary pressure changes produced by narcotic drugs and inhalation anesthetics in guinea pigs, *Anesth Analg* 58:120, 1979.

145. Needham WP, Shuster L, Kanel GC, et al: Liver damage from narcotics in mice, *Toxicol Appl Pharmacol* 58:157, 1981.

146. Neuberger J: Halothane and the liver: the present situation, *J Clin Pharm Ther* 12:269, 1987 (editorial).

147. Bynum TE, Boitnott JK, Maddrey WC: Ischemic hepatitis, *Dig Dis Sci* 24:129, 1979.

148. Gibson PR, Dudley FJ: Ischemic hepatitis: clinical features, diagnosis and prognosis, *Aust N Z J Med* 14:822, 1984.

149. Berman ML, Kuhnert L, Phythyon JM, et al: Isoflurane and enflurane-induced hepatic necrosis in triiodothyronine-pretreated rats, *Anesthesiology* 58:1, 1983.

150. Viegas O, Stoelting RK: LDH5 changes after cholecystectomy or hysterectomy in patients receiving halothane, enflurane, or fentanyl, *Anesthesiology* 51:556, 1979.

151. Aranha GV, Greenlee HB: Intra-abdominal surgery in patients with advanced cirrhosis, *Arch Surg* 121:275, 1986.

152. Powell-Jackson P, Greenway B, Williams R: Adverse effects of exploratory laparotomy in patients with unsuspected liver disease, *Br J Surg* 69:449, 1982.

153. Gelman S, Rimerman V, Fowler KC, et al: The effect of halothane, isoflurane, and blood loss on hepatotoxicity and hepatic oxygen availability in phenobarbital-pretreated hypoxic rats, *Anesth Analg* 63:965, 1984.

154. Gelman S, Fowler KC, Smith LR: Regional blood flow during isoflurane and halothane anesthesia, *Anesth Analg* 63:557, 1984.

155. Gelman S, Fowler KC, Smith LR: Liver circulation and function during isoflurane and halothane anesthesia, *Anesthesiology* 61:726, 1984.

156. Harper MH, Collins P, Johnson BH, et al: Postanesthetic hepatic injury in rats: influence of alterations in hepatic blood flow, surgery, and anesthesia time, *Anesth Analg* 61:79, 1982.

157. McNeill JR, Pang CC: Effect of pentobarbital anesthesia and surgery on the control of arterial pressure and mesenteric resistance in cats: role of vasopressin and angiotensin, *Can J Physiol Pharmacol* 60:363, 1982.

158. Schmid M, Hefti M, Gattiker R, et al: A benign postoperative intrahepatic cholestasis, *N Engl J Med* 272:545, 1965.

159. Maze M, Baden J: Anesthesia for patients with liver disease. In Miller R, ed: *Anesthesia*, New York, 1986, Churchill Livingstone.

160. Gitlin N: Clinical aspects of liver disease caused by industrial and environmental toxins. In Zakim D, Boyer T, eds: *Hepatology: a textbook of liver disease*, Philadelphia, 1996, WB Saunders, p 1018.

161. Bass N, Ockner R: Drug-induced liver disease. In Zakim D, Boyer T, eds: *Hepatology: a textbook of liver disease*, Philadelphia, 1996, WB Saunders, p 962.

162. Dossing M, Andreasen PB: Drug-induced liver disease in Denmark: an analysis of 572 cases of hepatotoxicity reported to the Danish Board of Adverse Reactions to Drugs, *Scand J Gastroenterol* 17:205, 1982.

163. Brown B: *Anesthesia in hepatic and biliary tract disease*, Philadelphia, 1988, FA Davis.

164. Nomura F, Hatano H, Ohnishi K, et al: Effects of anticonvulsant agents on halothane-induced liver injury in human subjects and experimental animals, *Hepatology* 6:952, 1986.

165. Gilman A: *The pharmacological basis of therapeutics*, New York, 1985, Macmillan.

166. Maddrey W: Alcoholic hepatitis. In Williams R, Maddrey W, eds: *Liver*, London, 1984, Butterworth.

167. Scully R, Mark E, McNeely W, et al: Case records of the Massachusetts General Hospital, *N Engl J Med* 322:318, 1990.

168. Seeff L: Diagnosis, therapy, and prognosis of viral hepatitis. In Zakim D, Boyer T, eds: *Hepatology: a textbook of liver disease.* Philadelphia, 1996, WB Saunders, p 1067.

169. Vento S, Garofano T, Renzini C, et al: Fulminant hepatitis associated with hepatitis A virus superinfection in patients with chronic hepatitis C, *N Engl J Med* 338:286, 1998.

170. Brechot C, Degas F, Lugassy C: Hepatitis B virus DNA in patients with chronic liver disease and negative tests for hepatitis B surface antigen, *N Engl J Med* 312:270, 1985.

171. Van Dyke R: The liver in pregnancy. In Zakim D, Boyer T, eds: *Hepatology: a textbook of liver disease,* Philadelphia, 1996, WB Saunders, p 1734.

172. James F, Wheeler A, Dewan D: *Obstetric anesthesia: the complicated patient,* Philadelphia, 1988, FA Davis.

173. Friedman L, Maddrey W: Surgery in the patient with liver disease, *Med Clin North Am* 71:454, 1987.

174. Bloch RS, Allaben RD, Walt AJ: Cholecystectomy in patients with cirrhosis: a surgical challenge, *Arch Surg* 120:669, 1985.

175. Brown MW, Burk RF: Development of intractable ascites following upper abdominal surgery in patients with cirrhosis, *Am J Med* 80:879, 1986.

Chapter 21

Renal Dysfunction

Robert J. Lowes
Donald S. Prough

ABBREVIATIONS

ACE	Angiotensin-converting enzyme
ADH	Antidiuretic hormone
ANH	Atrial natriuretic hormone
ANP	Atrial natriuretic peptide
ARF	Acute renal failure
ATN	Acute tubular necrosis
BUN	Blood urea nitrogen
CCr	Creatinine clearance
CVVH	Continuous venovenous hemofiltration
CVVHD	Continuous venovenous hemodialysis
DA	Dopaminergic
DO_2	Systemic oxygen delivery
ECF	Extracellular fluid
FE_{NA}	Fractional excretion of sodium
FF	Filtration fraction
GFR	Glomerular filtration rate
ICU	Intensive care unit
K_f	Glomerular filtration coefficient
MAC	Minimum alveolar concentration
mTAL	Medullary thick ascending loop of Henle
NSAIDS	Nonsteroidal antiinflammatory drugs
P_{BC}	Bowman's capsule hydraulic pressure
PCr	Phosphocreatine
PCT	Proximal convoluted tubule
PEEP	Positive end-expiratory pressure
P_{GC}	Glomerular capillary hydraulic pressure
PGE_2	Prostaglandin E_2
PGI_2	Prostaglandin I_2
π_{GC}	Plasma oncotic pressure
RBF	Renal blood flow
SCr	Serum creatinine
Tx	Thromboxane
UCr	Urinary creatinine concentration
U_{Na}	Urinary sodium concentration

I. INCIDENCE OF PERIOPERATIVE RENAL FAILURE

Anesthesia and surgery have long been associated with decrements in renal function.[1,2] Although few of the anesthetic agents in current use are associated with direct renal injury, anesthesia is implicated in perioperative renal dysfunction,[3,4] an association attributed to anesthetic-induced decreases in effective blood volume.[4] Consequently, Klahr and Miller[3] have suggested that general anesthetics be avoided, along with nonsteroidal antiinflammatory drugs (NSAIDs), aminoglycosides, radiographic contrast agents, angiotensin-converting enzyme

(ACE) inhibitors, amphotericin B, and many chemotherapeutic agents, in patients with prerenal oliguria. However, that advice often is not practical.

Discussion of perioperative renal dysfunction is complicated by the lack of a standard definition of acute renal failure (ARF).[4,5] In general, ARF is defined as "the loss of renal function over a period of hours to days, as reflected in the glomerular filtration rate (GFR)."[6] Useful operational definitions include an increase in serum creatinine (SCr) exceeding 0.5 mg/dl, an increase in SCr of more than 50% of the baseline level, or a decrement in renal function sufficient to necessitate dialysis.[4] For purposes of diagnosis and management, ARF is subclassified as prerenal, intrarenal, and postrenal. Of all patients with ARF, about 70% have a prerenal cause; about 25% have intrarenal or parenchymal injury (including acute tubular necrosis [ATN]); and less than 5% have a postrenal cause.[7] Frequently, in the perioperative period, the distinction between prerenal and intrarenal causes of ARF is difficult.

Renal insults present as a spectrum ranging from mild elevations of SCr to ARF requiring renal dialysis. Acute elevations in blood urea nitrogen (BUN) and SCr occur in approximately 5% of all general hospital admissions and in up to 20% of intensive care unit (ICU) patients. After noncardiac surgery, SCr increased significantly in 23% of patients with moderately severe preexisting disease.[8] Although most postoperative patients recover normal, or at least adequate, renal function, a subset of patients are seriously and permanently impaired. Major surgery may, in fact, be secondary only to medically related decreased renal perfusion as a cause of renal insufficiency.[9] In elderly patients, the effects of surgical insults are compounded by the loss of functional reserve and reduced ability to withstand acute insults associated with aging.[4,10]

The incidence of ARF after high-risk procedures involving interruption of aortic flow varies from 2.6% to 28%.[11-16] Cardiac procedures requiring cardiopulmonary bypass are associated with a 0.9% to 7.5% incidence of ARF.[17-19] In a series of more than 40,000 patients undergoing coronary artery bypass grafting with or without other procedures, the factors most strongly associated with postoperative ARF were valvular surgery, creatinine clearance less than 80 ml/min, previous heart surgery, New York Heart Association Class IV, and systolic blood pressure greater than 160 mm Hg.[20] Preexisting renal insufficiency, defined as a GFR of 25 to 50 ml/min, is an important contributing factor in ARF after either cardiac or noncardiac surgery; a preoperative SCr exceeding 2 mg/dl is a highly significant predictor of postoperative ARF after cardiac surgery.[21]

The most severe renal dysfunction, ARF, represents an abrupt reduction of renal function, resulting in retention of nitrogenous waste products and inability to maintain fluid and electrolyte homeostasis. Perioperative ARF, which accounts for the majority of patients who require acute dialysis,[22] is associated with a mortality rate exceeding 50%.[9,23] The mortality associated with ARF has changed little[24-28] over the past several decades and has possibly increased,[23] owing to immediate survival from injuries that previously were lethal. Mortality approaches 100% when ominous variables, such as multiple organ failure, cardiac failure, sepsis, and a requirement for multiple transfusions, accompany ARF.[25,26] Such patients are vulnerable to repeated insults in the presence of altered renal function.[27,28] The high mortality rate of ARF, 42% to 88% in recent series,[29] previously had been attributed to comorbid conditions, but a recent case-control study isolated ARF as a cause of increased mortality, independent of coexisting diseases.[30]

ARF also occurs frequently in patients undergoing certain gastrointestinal procedures,[31] in patients with hepatic insufficiency,[9] and in patients with sepsis or volume depletion. McMurray et al[32] reported that gastrointestinal surgery was responsible for 32% of postoperative ARF. Postoperative ARF developed in 6.8% of 103 jaundiced patients compared with 0.1% of 2353 emergency gastric surgical procedures, despite an equal or greater incidence and severity of hypotension.[9] Overall, volume depletion may account for at least 17% of cases of hospital-acquired ARF in surgical and medical patients.[9]

Traumatic causes of ARF include direct renal trauma, hemorrhagic shock, abdominal tamponade, and multiple organ dysfunction. Of 72,757 admissions to nine regional trauma centers, only 78 patients, an incidence of 0.01%, developed dialysis-dependent ARF.[33] Approximately one third developed "early" ARF within 1 week, presumably directly related to an ischemic insult; two thirds developed "late" ARF, associated with multiorgan system failure, at an average interval of 3 weeks after injury.

The significance of ARF lies not only in the high mortality that continues to accompany perioperative ARF but also in the cost to society for renal replacement therapy and lost productivity. Hamel et al[34] quantified the cost-effectiveness of renal replacement therapy in seriously ill hospitalized patients. Of 490 patients prospectively evaluated to determine the cost per quality-adjusted life-year, the cost for the most high-risk patients, with the lowest predicted survival, was $274,100 (Table 21-1).

To reduce the incidence, morbidity, mortality, and cost of perioperative ARF, the surgical team must understand basic renal physiology, be aware of the effects of anesthetic drugs, recognize and monitor threatened renal function,

Table 21-1. Cost of dialysis-dependent acute renal failure as a function of predicted and actual survival

Number of patients (n)	Probability of 6-month survival (%)	Actual 6-month survival (%)	Cost per QALY ($)
103	0-10	7	274,100
114	11-20	18	122,600
83	21-30	27	85,800
96	31-40	33	80,000
94	41-60	46	61,900

Modified from Hamel MB, Phillips RS, Davis RB, et al: *Ann Intern med* 127:195, 1997.
QALY, Quality-adjusted life-years.

attempt to prevent ARF, and for patients who develop ARF, provide adequate renal replacement therapy.

II. RENAL PHYSIOLOGY
A. Renal blood flow and function

The kidney performs three major excretory functions: filtration, reabsorption, and secretion. One unique aspect of the complex renal circulation is that it provides both the filtrate and the oxygen required for the active processes that convert filtrate to urine. Plasma filtration at the glomerulus begins the process of urine formation. The blood supply of the energy-consuming cells of the distal nephrons are in series with, and distal to, the glomerular capillaries. The oxygen supply to these active tubular cells is tightly linked to glomerular flow and therefore to tubular oxygen demand.

The total kidney receives a high blood flow rate and extracts a small percentage of arterial oxygen. The change from a renal arterial PO_2 of 95 mm Hg to a renal venous PO_2 of 70 mm Hg suggests that renal ischemic complications should be unusual. However, especially in the outer medulla in the region of the medullary thick ascending loop of Henle (mTAL), the combination of limited oxygen supply and high oxygen consumption results in tenuous tissue oxygenation.[35] Even before arterial blood arrives in the renal medulla, PO_2 has decreased substantially in the intervening efferent arteriole. Relatively low blood flow containing relatively decreased oxygen content explains much of the paradox of an apparently richly perfused organ that is highly vulnerable to ischemia.

1. Delivery of plasma for filtration. Under normal conditions, total perfusion to the kidneys is luxurious. Renal blood flow equals 20% to 25% of total cardiac output (or 1000 to 1250 ml/min), 10% of which is normally filtered. Therefore normal GFR is ~125 ml/min, and total filtration is ~180 L/day. This high blood flow allows the kidneys to serve as a blood reservoir in times of stress. Sympathetically mediated renal vasoconstriction can reduce the proportion of systemic blood flow perfusing the kidneys and increase the proportion available to other organs. This compensatory mechanism makes estimation of renal blood flow from blood pressure measurement extremely difficult during hypovolemia.[36,37]

2. Delivery of oxygen. Renal blood flow (RBF) has conventionally been considered to be "autoregulated." This concept originated with in vitro studies demonstrating a relatively constant RBF as renal perfusion pressure was varied from 85 to 200 mm Hg (Fig. 21-1).[36,38] However, autoregulation cannot completely compensate for decreases in mean arterial pressure to less than 85 mm Hg and is virtually absent at mean arterial pressures less than 70 mm Hg.[38]

Renal circulatory function undergoes considerable adaptation during episodes of decreased cardiac output and hypovolemia. Both the efferent and afferent arterioles are extensively sympathetically innervated. Renal arterioles constrict in response to increased sympathetic

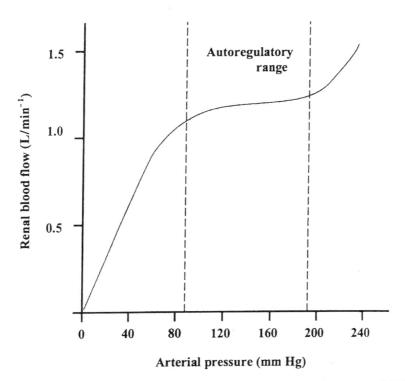

Fig. 21-1. The autoregulation of renal blood flow. In the "autoregulatory range" (90 to 200 mm Hg), a change in the mean renal perfusion pressure has little effect on the blood flow. The graph can be misleading because in vivo, the kidneys do not respond passively to changes in blood pressure but are active components of blood pressure regulation.

tone and increased circulating epinephrine as a consequence of arterial hypotension. Increasing *afferent* arteriolar tone acts to decrease both RBF and glomerular perfusion pressure. Increases in *efferent* arteriolar tone maintain GFR by raising filtration pressure. The opposing forces of sympathetically mediated vasoconstriction and autoregulatory vasodilatation produce a variable effect on total RBF during periods of hemodynamic fluctuation.

Blood enters the glomeruli through the afferent arterioles that arise from the renal arteries via the interlobar,

arcuate, and interlobular arteries. The afferent arterioles supplying deep juxtamedullary glomeruli are noteworthy in that they branch from the interlobular arteries at right angles or even more acutely (Fig. 21-2).[36] Plasma skimming, which occurs because of the sharp angulation, results in hematocrit values of approximately 10% in the corresponding glomeruli. The preglomerular decrease in hematocrit attenuates the increase in viscosity that otherwise would occur as solute is reabsorbed during passage through the hypertonic renal medulla.[36]

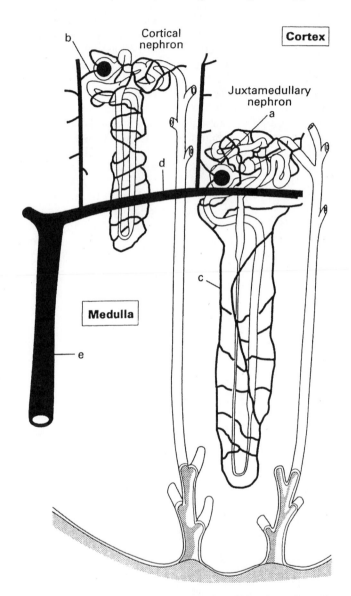

Fig. 21-2. Diagram showing the anatomic arrangement of blood supply to the nephrons. For clarity, venules and veins are omitted. A typical juxtamedullary nephron (15% of the total) and cortical nephron (85% of the total) are shown on the right and left, respectively. Note that the afferent arterioles of the juxtamedullary nephrons *(a)* leave the interlobular artery at a hyperacute angle, whereas the afferent arteriole of the cortical nephron *(b)* leaves at a shallow angle. Thus plasma skimming is more likely in the blood to the juxtamedullary nephron, the efferent arteriole of which supplies the vasa recta *(c)*. Only two nephrons are shown completely. Other afferent arterioles are shown, but not the glomeruli. Other labels: arcuate artery *(d)*, running along corticomedullary boundary. Interlobar artery *(e)*. (From Lote CJ, Harper L, Savage COS: *Br J Anaesth* 77:82, 1996.)

Blood leaves the glomeruli via the efferent arterioles. These arterioles then form the vasa recta, which extend to the papillary tip. Capillaries branching from the descending vasa recta provide the blood supply to the loop of Henle before draining back into the ascending vasa recta (see Fig. 21-2).[36] This structure produces the countercurrent circulation that maintains the high medullary osmotic concentration (a necessity for urinary concentration) and also permits movement of oxygen from the descending to ascending vasa recta. The gradient between cortical and medullary PO_2 produced by this arrangement has been repeatedly demonstrated.[39,40]

The renal medulla is therefore supplied by relatively low blood flow with a relatively low hematocrit, owing to plasma skimming, which is further depleted of oxygen by diffusion before reaching the deep medulla and papillae. Measurements of renal arterial blood flow, even measurements of medullary blood flow, therefore suggest greater medullary oxygen delivery than is actually available.[36]

B. Physiology and pharmacology of urine formation

Filtration and reabsorption ultimately form urine. Normal adult kidneys produce approximately 180 L/day of filtrate, 99% of which is reabsorbed in the tubules and collecting ducts, generating approximately 1 to 2 L/day of urine. The process of urine formation can best be visualized by tracing the course of a single nephron.[41] Afferent arterioles enter the glomeruli, then branch to form the glomerular capillary network before exiting the glomeruli as efferent arterioles (see Fig. 21-2).

The initial quantity of filtrate is governed by the factors that determine movement across all biologic membranes, that is, gradients in hydrostatic pressures, oncotic pressures, and membrane permeability. The relevant variables determining filtration are the glomerular filtration coefficient (K_f), which is the product of glomerular membrane permeability and surface area, the glomerular capillary hydraulic pressure (P_{GC}), the hydraulic pressure in Bowman's capsule (P_{BC}), and the plasma oncotic pressure (π_{GC}), according to the equation[42]:

$$GFR = K_f \times (P_{GC} - P_{BC} - \pi_{GC})$$

Of these variables, P_{GC} is subject to the greatest physiologic variation. P_{GC} and RBF are determined by inflow resistance and outflow resistance. The P_{GC} will decline if the resistance in the afferent arterioles increases or if resistance in the efferent arterioles decreases. Conversely, a decrease in afferent arteriolar resistance or an increase in efferent arteriolar resistance will increase P_{GC}. The renin-angiotensin and prostaglandin systems alter both afferent and efferent resistance. Sympathetic nervous system activation and high levels of circulating catecholamines can induce afferent arteriolar constriction that overrides autoregulatory mechanisms and decreases cortical perfusion and GFR.[43] The volume of glomerular filtrate determines the volume that must be processed through passive and energy-consuming processes in the collecting tubules. The ability to reduce the volume of initial filtrate allows the kidney to reduce medullary oxygen consumption.[35] This ability becomes particularly important during times of reduced perfusion or otherwise limited energy availability (Fig. 21-3).[35]

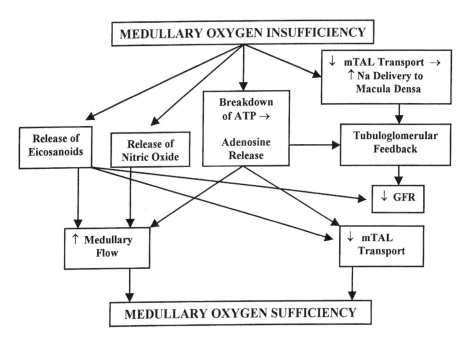

Fig. 21-3. In response to medullary oxygen insufficiency, homeostatic mechanisms act to improve medullary flow and decrease the need for oxygen-consuming processes in the medullary thick ascending loop of Henle *(mTAL)*. The processes acting to decrease oxygen consumption in the mTAL include the reduction of the glomerular filtration rate *(GFR)* through tubuloglomerular feedback. (Modified from Heyman SN, Fuchs S, Brezis M: *New Horiz* 3:597, 1995.)

Reduction of glomerular filtration results in a smaller volume of urine presented to the distal nephron. In fact, oliguria, regarded as an ominous sign in ARF, may be an effective protective mechanism to decrease oxygen demand in response to decreased oxygen supply.[44] Pharmacologic inhibition of active reabsorption by loop diuretics also decreases tubular energy consumption.[45,46]

1. Sodium filtration and reabsorption. The sodium concentration of glomerular filtrate is similar to that in plasma. In the proximal convoluted tubule (PCT), under normovolemic conditions, approximately 65% of filtered sodium is reabsorbed, with water following passively. In hypovolemic states an increased percentage is reabsorbed. Because equal percentages of sodium and water are reabsorbed, the concentration of sodium remains similar throughout the proximal tubule. In addition to sodium reabsorption, glucose, potassium, uric acid, and amino acids also are reabsorbed in the PCT up to tubular threshold limits. Acid-base regulation in the PCT includes almost complete reabsorption of bicarbonate.

The reduced volume of isosmotic tubular fluid proceeds to the loop of Henle, which in some nephrons is short but in others is long and dips deeply into the medulla. Cortical tissue contains the glomeruli, PCT, and distal convoluted tubules, whereas the medulla consists of the loops of Henle, collecting ducts, vasa recta, and interstitium. As the filtrate passes through the ascending limb of Henle's loop, a primary active process reabsorbs an additional 25% of filtered sodium. The remaining 10% of sodium undergoes continued reabsorption in the distal tubules and collecting ducts by means of both aldosterone-dependent and aldosterone-independent processes. Only 1% of the sodium originally filtered by the glomeruli is ultimately excreted in the urine.[38] Also, in the distal convoluted tubule, the remaining bicarbonate continues to be reabsorbed as hydrogen ions are actively secreted.

2. Water reabsorption. As noted previously, 65% of filtered water is reabsorbed in the proximal tubule.[38] In Henle's loop, proportionately less water than sodium is reabsorbed. Although fluid leaving the loop is isosmotic, half of the total osmolar content consists of urea rather than sodium and chloride. The medullary countercurrent multiplier system is a critical component of renal sodium and water conservation. The vasa recta, which are medullary vessels arising from the efferent renal arterioles, preserve the hypertonicity of the medullary interstitium. Either increases or decreases in flow within the vasa recta may diminish the osmotic gradient, as will sodium depletion and malnutrition. In addition, an increased filtrate flow rate through Henle's loop reduces renal concentrating ability; a greatly accelerated flow rate, such as that produced by the infusion of mannitol, may "wash out" the concentrating gradient. Water is reabsorbed to a variable extent in the distal tubules, cortical collecting tubules, and medullary collecting ducts, dependent primarily on the presence of antidiuretic hormone (ADH). A summary of the constituents of glomerular filtrate during the various stages of urine formation and sodium excretion is presented in Table 21-2.

Table 21-2. Sodium, water, and osmolar excretion

	Flow rate (ml/min)	[Na⁺] (mEq/L)	Urea (mg/dl)	Osmolality (mOsm/kg)
Plasma	750	140	10	290
Filtrate	125	140	10	290
Proximal tubule	44	140	50	290
Henle's loop	25	70	50	150
Distal tubule	20	10	50	100
Final urine	2	100	250	100

Reabsorption of sodium chloride in the mTAL generates the medullary osmotic gradient.[35] Chloride is actively transported out of the lumen of the mTAL, resulting in hypotonic tubular fluid passing into the distal convoluted tubule. This active transport represents one of the most important renal energy expenditures. As mentioned earlier, this high-energy requirement occurs in a region of the kidney that is predisposed to hypoxia because of limited oxygen delivery. Therefore one protective strategy for preventing renal ischemia is reduction of tubular reabsorption.[35]

C. Regulation of extracellular fluid volume

Alterations in extracellular fluid (ECF) volume result in parallel changes in plasma volume. Thus the primary monitors of ECF volume are located within the vascular system. The body protects ECF volume by controlling the secretion of sodium and water; however, renal conservation of ECF incurs a renal metabolic expense.

1. Afferent limb. Low-pressure intrathoracic volume receptors are located within the cardiac atria, great veins, cardiac ventricles, and pulmonary capillaries.[47] Because 85% of circulating blood volume resides within the high-compliance venous system, these receptors are of primary importance for detecting decreases in intravascular and ECF volume. Stimulation of atrial stretch receptors by volume expansion results in the release of atrial natriuretic peptide (ANP) and natriuresis.[48,49] High-pressure arterial receptors are found within the carotid sinuses, aortic arch, and intrarenal arterioles. These receptors, relatively insensitive to small changes in intravascular volume, act to preserve perfusion when blood pressure is decreased. Stimulation of these high-pressure arterial receptors by volume overload induces natriuresis.

Intrarenal baroreceptors cause renin release in response to decreased renal perfusion pressure. Renin, released from the juxtaglomerular apparatus in response to reduced arterial volume, catalyzes the conversion of circulating angiotensinogen to angiotensin I, which is transformed in the lungs by ACE inhibitors into angiotensin II, which in turn stimulates the adrenal cortex to release aldosterone. Acting primarily on the distal convoluted tubule, aldosterone influences the reabsorption of about 2% of filtered sodium.[50-54] Overall, the renin-angiotensin system acts to preserve circulating blood volume by causing aldosterone-induced sodium retention during periods of intravascular volume depletion. These hormones increase blood pressure, increase afferent glomerular arteriolar tone (decreasing RBF), and stimulate sodium reabsorption. The renal baroreceptors also stimulate natriuresis in response to increased perfusion pressure.

Secretion of antidiuretic hormone (ADH) increases in response to increases in serum osmolality and to decreases in intravascular volume.[55] Antidiuretic hormone increases water reabsorption in the distal convoluted tubules and collecting ducts, resulting in the formation of small amounts of highly concentrated urine. Urinary volume may vary 100-fold, depending on the ADH concentration.[54]

2. Efferent limb. Adequate circulating blood volume is essential for maintenance of organ perfusion and survival. Afferent signals are converted to efferent signals, which serve to maintain ECF volume and vital organ perfusion.[47] Activation of the sympathetic nervous system, renin-angiotensin-aldosterone axis, secretion of ADH, and suppression of ANP release serve to increase systemic vascular resistance and conserve sodium and water during volume depletion. Thirst and salt craving are activated in an attempt to increase intake. Aldosterone also decreases salt loss in sweat. Insufficiency of these systems or the use of pharmacologic antagonists may aggravate hypovolemic states.

3. Renal response to ECF volume depletion. The kidney has a remarkable ability to maintain homeostasis despite substantial reductions in ECF volume. Renal adaptation to decreases in ECF volume (and cardiac output) occurs through three primary mechanisms: RBF, glomerular filtration, and tubular reabsorption. Initially, RBF is maintained as perfusion pressure decreases (i.e., by autoregulation) by reductions in renal vascular resistance (primarily at the level of the afferent arteriole). Under normal conditions, RBF remains constant (autoregulates) over a considerable range of perfusion pressures (see Fig. 21-1). However, RBF decreases when perfusion pressure decreases below the autoregulatory range. In addition, autoregulation may be diminished or lost during acute hypovolemia.[47,56,57]

During acute hypovolemia, RBF is influenced by secretion of α-adrenergic catecholamines[58] and angiotensin II and by renal sympathetic stimulation. RBF is determined by a balance among opposing factors: intrinsic renal autoregulatory capacity, the vasodilatory capacity of prostaglandins to maintain RBF, and the ability of the renal sympathetic nerves, angiotensin II, and catecholamines to decrease RBF.[59] Because the kidney has few β_2 receptors, both epinephrine and norepinephrine induce renal vasoconstriction. Sympathetically mediated renal cortical vasoconstriction may redistribute blood flow to the relatively hypoxic renal medulla, but at the expense of inducing cortical ischemia.[60] Release of nitric oxide also acts to preserve medullary blood flow during circulatory stress.[35] In addition to changes in total RBF, hypovolemia also changes the intrarenal distribution of

perfusion, redistributing blood flow from outer cortical nephrons to inner cortical nephrons,[47] which have longer loops of Henle and tend to conserve more sodium and thus protect circulating blood volume.

In the setting of volume depletion, GFR may be either maintained or decreased. As noted earlier, GFR depends on glomerular plasma flow, P_{GC}, π_{GC}, and glomerular capillary permeability. During hypovolemia, plasma flow decreases, but filtration pressure tends to increase secondary to increased efferent arteriolar resistance, thereby serving to increase the filtration fraction (FF). The FF normally increases as ECF volume decreases. As RBF decreases, the efferent arterioles constrict, primarily in response to angiotensin II and norepinephrine. The net result is that GFR tends to be preserved despite reduced ECF volume. Stimulation of the sympathetic nervous system and release of ADH and aldosterone increase sodium and water reabsorption.

The kidneys respond to ECF depletion by reabsorbing water and sodium in response to hormonal factors ADH, ANP, and the renal prostaglandins (Fig. 21-4). Diminished water excretion is accomplished by ADH-dependent and ADH-independent mechanisms. ADH secretion from the posterior pituitary responds not only to changing osmolarity but also to changing intravascular volume (Fig. 21-5).[55] A 1% to 2% increase in osmolarity significantly increases ADH secretion, as does decreased stretch of the atrial baroreceptors. However, the ADH response to volume depletion is less sensitive than the response to changes in osmolality. A 10% to 20% decrease in blood volume is necessary to stimulate ADH secretion.[55] Antidiuretic hormone acts primarily on the medullary collecting ducts and to a lesser extent on the cortical collecting tubules to increase water permeability, resulting in greater water reabsorption and the excretion of smaller volumes of more highly concentrated urine. Water excretion is further reduced in volume-depleted patients by impaired delivery of tubular fluid to distal nephron sites and by ADH-independent water reabsorption by the collecting ducts.

In volume-depleted states, sodium conservation results both from decreased filtration of sodium (decreased GFR) and from increased tubular reabsorption of sodium. The major effectors of sodium reabsorption are activation of the renin-angiotensin-aldosterone axis and suppression of ANP secretion. However, increased peritubular capillary oncotic pressure and autonomic nervous system activation also contribute to increased tubular sodium reabsorption. Acting primarily in the distal convoluted tubules, high concentrations of aldosterone may reduce urinary concentrations of sodium nearly to zero, whereas low levels of aldosterone permit excretion of urine high in sodium.

Although the complete physiologic role of ANP has yet to be defined, the hormone clearly causes vasodilation and increases the renal excretion of sodium and water.[48,49,61-65] During volume depletion, ANP secretion is decreased. Many of the physiologic effects of ANP appear to be mediated by hemodynamic effects that increase GFR and thus result in diuresis. Acute sodium loading

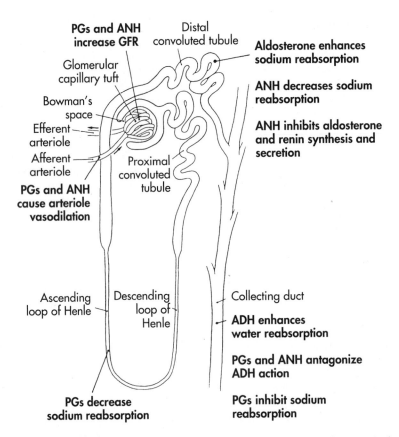

Fig. 21-4. Important neuroendocrine modifiers of glomerular and tubular function include al-dosterone, antidiuretic hormone *(ADH)*, atrial natriuretic hormone *(ANH;* also termed atrial natriuretic peptide), and the renal prostaglandins *(PGs)*. The primary sites of action include the afferent and efferent arterioles, glomerular filtration, loop of Henle, the distal convoluted tubule, and the collecting ducts. *GFR,* Glomerular filtration rate.

significantly increases ANP secretion; in contrast, chronic sodium loading does not change ANP levels.

The kidney also contains large quantities of pros-taglandin metabolites, including PGE_2 and thromboxane A_2 (TxA_2). These products appear to modulate the renal effects of other hormones.[66] For instance, the vasodilator PGE_2 decreases the contraction of glomerular mesangial cells produced by angiotensin II.[67] Vasodilatory prostaglandins are important for maintaining RBF dur-ing states of ECF volume depletion. In contrast, TxA_2 produces mesangial contraction.[67]

Prostaglandins may play a crucial role in protecting the kidney from the effects of systemic vasoconstrictor hormones and for maintaining RBF during hypo-volemia. The protective effect of endogenous renal prostaglandins is emphasized by the many reports of ARF in patients in whom circulatory compromise was superimposed upon treatment with NSAIDs.[68] Arachi-donic acid is converted to the molecular precursor of the vasodilator prostaglandins by cyclooxygenase, an en-zyme that is reversibly inhibited by NSAIDs for 8 to 24 hours. A single dose of aspirin causes irreversible acety-lation of cyclooxygenase, which in the kidney suppresses prostaglandin synthesis for 24 to 48 hours. The renal protective effect of prostaglandins is illustrated by the

fact that NSAIDs (e.g., indomethacin, meclofenamate, ketorolac) cause nephrotoxicity in ischemic but not in normal kidneys. Adverse renal effects of NSAIDs or as-pirin have been demonstrated in animal models of hem-orrhage, endotoxemia, increased venous pressure or low cardiac output, and in patients with congestive heart failure, ascites, mild underlying renal dysfunction, or systemic lupus erythematosus.[69] However, in hospital-ized patients, including surgical patients, parenteral ad-ministration of ketorolac for less than 5 days was not as-sociated with a higher incidence of ARF than was administration of opioids.[70] Experimental administra-tion of the NSAID indomethacin to rats decreased both medullary Po_2 and medullary blood flow (Fig. 21-6).[35] However, in rats exposed to small and large doses of ke-torolac plus a variety of interventions, including dehy-dration and gentamicin, only the combination of ke-torolac and gentamicin produced functional and structural renal damage.[71]

Nitric oxide may play an important role in maintain-ing medullary perfusion during intervals of circulatory compromise. The inducible form of nitric oxide syn-thase, one of the isozymes that generate nitric oxide, is concentrated in the outer medulla of the rat kidney.[72] Inhibition of inducible nitric oxide synthase aggravates

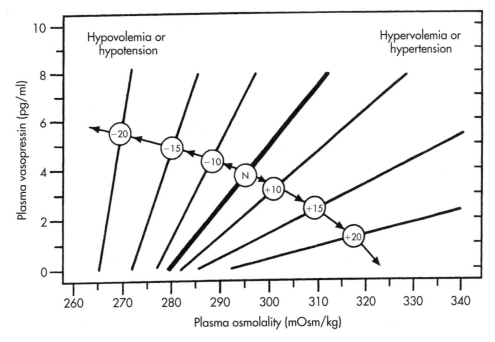

Fig. 21-5. Antidiuretic hormone (also termed *vasopressin*) is released in response to stimulation of the hypothalamic osmoreceptors by increased blood osmolarity and in response to decreased stretch of the atrial baroreceptors. A 1% to 2% change in osmolarity significantly alters vasopressin secretion. However, the response of vasopressin to volume depletion is less sensitive than the response to changes in osmolality. A 10% to 20% decrease in blood volume is necessary to stimulate vasopressin secretion. (From Fried LF, Palevsky PM: Hyponatremia and hypernatremia. In Saklayen MG, ed: *The Medical Clinics of North America: renal disease,* Philadelphia, 1997, WB Saunders.)

medullary hypoxia.[73,74] Heyman et al[35] have speculated, based on experimental evidence,[75-77] that the increased vulnerability of aged, diabetic, or hypertensive patients could be due in part to impaired nitrovasodilation.

The kidneys have a remarkable ability to preserve function during progressive circulatory stress.[59] However, when the limits of renal homeostatic mechanisms are reached, renal decompensation rapidly ensues, resulting in excessive vasoconstriction, decreased RBF, and renal ischemia. The three critical homeostatic functions of the kidneys consist of the ability of intrarenal factors to influence the fraction of cardiac output received by the kidneys, the intrinsic renal regulation of the FF (GFR/glomerular plasma flow), and control of fluid reabsorption.[59] RBF is maintained as cardiac output decreases by afferent arteriolar dilation induced by the myogenic reflex of the renal vasculature and by tubuloglomerular feedback, a process whereby decreases in delivery of solute to the cells of the macula densa result in afferent arteriolar relaxation. In addition, the kidneys adjust to high circulating levels of vasoconstrictors by release of endogenous vasodilatory products of arachidonic acid (e.g., prostaglandin I_2 [PGI_2]).[59] Nitric oxide also may play a role in renal vasodilation in response to circulatory stress.[73,74] The FF is maintained during reduced cardiac output in part through the action of intrarenal angiotensin II on the efferent arteriole, constric-

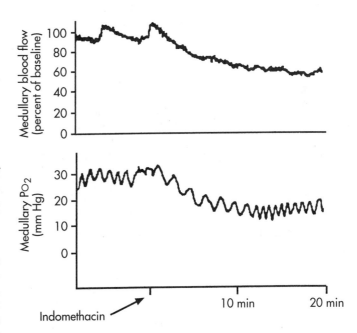

Fig. 21-6. Administration of indomethacin, a cyclooxygenase inhibitor, decreases medullary blood flow and medullary oxygen delivery by reducing the production of vasodilator prostaglandins; however, because tubular energy consumption is relatively unaffected, medullary Po_2 decreases. (From Heyman SN, Fuchs S, Brezis M: *New Horiz* 3:597, 1995.)

tion of which increases glomerular hydrostatic pressure, especially if renal afferent arteriolar resistance is decreased.[59] As described previously, decreased renal perfusion also results in aldosterone-mediated sodium reabsorption in the renal tubules and ADH-mediated water reabsorption.

When the limits of renal compensatory mechanisms are reached, RBF decreases. The kidneys maintain RBF less effectively as perfusion pressure decreases below 80 mm Hg.[59] As circulating levels of vasopressin and catecholamines increase and as renal sympathetic stimulation increases, afferent arteriolar resistance increases, decreasing the fraction of total cardiac output that perfuses the kidneys. Excessively high local levels

of angiotensin II may cause afferent constriction, which, in the presence of maximal efferent constriction, causes a decrease in filtration pressure.[59] To summarize this sequence of initially effective, then failed intrinsic renal homeostatic regulation, Badr and Ichikawa[59] have suggested the term *preprerenal failure* to describe the compensated state preceding prerenal failure (Fig. 21-7).

As further decreases in cardiac output decrease the fraction of cardiac output delivered to kidneys, increases in renal vascular resistance shunt blood away from the kidneys. If sufficiently severe and prolonged, this response may result in renal ischemia and the development of ARF.

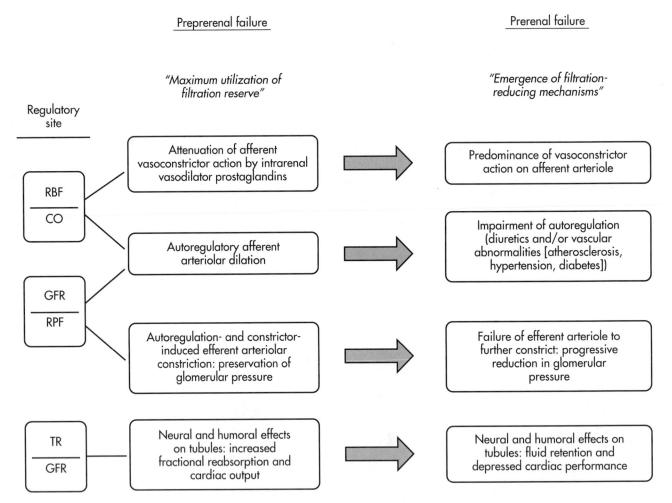

Fig. 21-7. Renal mechanisms involved in preprerenal and prerenal failure. Three important regulatory sites for glomerular filtration are listed on the left of the diagram. As perfusion pressure decreases, filtration reserve is progressively used. Inhibition by intrarenal vasodilator prostaglandins antagonizes afferent vasoconstrictor activity and maintains the fraction of cardiac output *(CO)* that serves as renal blood flow *(RBF)*. Autoregulatory dilation of the afferent arterioles also increases RBF/CO and, by increasing glomerular hydrostatic pressure, increases the filtration fraction, defined as the fraction of renal plasma flow *(RPF)* that is filtered at the glomerulus (glomerular filtration rate *[GFR]*). In addition, neural and humoral effects, such as aldosterone and vasopressin, on the renal tubules increase tubular reabsorption *(TR)* as a fraction of the GFR. During decompensation, the mechanisms are exhausted by the factors in the right column and prerenal failure supervenes. (From Badr KF, Ichikawa I: *N Engl J Med* 319:623, 1988.)

Postischemic ARF is usually multifactorial. Both vascular factors (i.e., renal vasoconstriction, altered glomerular function) and tubular factors (i.e., intraluminal obstruction, back-leak) combine to reduce GFR. Factors that appear to enhance the risk of ARF include volume depletion, sepsis, liver failure, nephrotoxic antibiotics and other drugs, and myoglobinuria. Loop diuretics such as furosemide exert unpredictable effects in patients with threatened ARF. By impairing sodium reabsorption and worsening hypovolemia, furosemide may potentiate renal hypoperfusion; however, by inhibiting tubular reabsorption of sodium, furosemide may improve medullary oxygenation (Fig. 21-8).[35]

III. RENAL RESPONSES TO ANESTHESIA AND SURGERY

The physiologic stress of trauma and surgery is associated with reduced urinary excretion of sodium and water, which occurs in response to changes in intravascular and extracellular volume and to secondary neuroendocrine effects, especially the release of ADH, catecholamines, and aldosterone.[78,79] Although anesthetics may not directly stimulate release of ADH and aldosterone, anesthetic-related changes in hemodynamics function may trigger those neuroendocrine responses. Table 21-3 summarizes the average and maximal effects of surgical stress on urinary flow, urinary sodium, and water excretion.

Table 21-3. Renal responses to surgery or trauma

	Urinary flow rate (ml/min)	U_{Na} (mEq/L)	Urea (mg/dl)	Osmolality (mOsm/kg)
Euvolemic, young adult	2.0	100	250	300
"Average" perioperative patient	0.5	20	500	800
Maximal antidiuretic hormone and aldosterone	0.2	1	1000	1200

U_{Na}, Urinary sodium concentration.

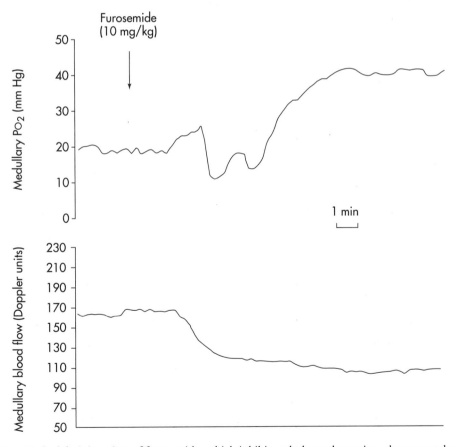

Fig. 21-8. Administration of furosemide, which inhibits tubular reabsorption, decreases tubular energy consumption in addition to medullary blood flow and medullary oxygen delivery; therefore medullary P_{O_2} increases. (From Heyman SN, Fuchs S, Brezis M: *New Horiz* 3:597, 1995.)

Anesthetic drugs may alter RBF, glomerular filtration, or tubular function. Anesthetics may directly alter renal function or exert indirect effects, secondary to changes in cardiovascular function or neuroendocrine activity. Anesthetic drugs and techniques exert diverse effects on myocardial contractility, intravascular volume, regional blood flow, autonomic reflexes, coronary blood flow, vascular tone, and the response to catecholamines.[80] In high concentrations, potent inhaled anesthetics decrease myocardial contractility and reduce cardiac output. Spinal or epidural anesthesia may reduce cardiac output through sympathectomy-induced venodilation. Either an increase or a decrease in peripheral vascular resistance may indirectly reduce RBF.

Because anesthesia interferes with compensatory hemodynamic responses, physiologic insults such as hemorrhage may produce exaggerated hemodynamic effects in comparison to the conscious state.[80] For example, moderate hemorrhage in anesthetized animals results in intense peripheral vasoconstriction of renal, muscular, and mesenteric vascular beds. In conscious animals, renal vasodilation occurs despite vasoconstriction in mesenteric and limb circulations.[80] The coronary vascular response to norepinephrine and dopamine is diminished in anesthetized animals. In addition, the inotropic response to dobutamine and dopamine is increased in anesthetized animals.[80]

Other perioperative interventions also directly and indirectly modify renal function. Mechanical ventilation and positive end-expiratory pressure (PEEP) are associated with reduced urinary output,[81] which improves in response to volume expansion.[82] Ventilation with PEEP reduces both urinary sodium excretion and plasma levels of ANP, an indication of a role of that hormone in the renal response to increased intrathoracic pressure.[83] In contrast, ADH release appears to exert little effect on renal function during ventilation with PEEP.[84]

A. Inhaled anesthetics

1. Methoxyflurane. Now rarely used, methoxyflurane is partially metabolized to inorganic fluoride ion, which produces dose-dependent renal toxicity, including hypoosmotic diuresis, azotemia, hypernatremia, and hyperosmolality. Clinical toxicity correlates with serum inorganic fluoride concentrations and appears consistently at levels exceeding 50 μmol/ml.[85]

2. Enflurane, isoflurane, and halothane. Enflurane decreases GFR and urinary output.[86] Although isoflurane does not reduce RBF, it does reduce GFR and urinary output.[87,88] Enflurane, unlike halothane or isoflurane, releases significant amounts of fluoride ion.[86] After prolonged (about 9 hours) enflurane anesthesia, fluoride concentrations of 30 to 40 μmol/ml, sufficient to decrease urinary concentrating ability, have been reported.[89] Potentially harmful concentrations of fluoride ion (more than 50 μmol/ml) accumulate in obese patients after prolonged exposure to enflurane and in patients who have received isoniazid.[90] Clinical doses of halothane decrease renal vascular resistance but have little effect on RBF.[91] Halothane-induced hypotension

does not reduce RBF until mean arterial pressure is 60 mm Hg or less.[92] Even during acute hemorrhagic hypovolemia in halothane-anesthetized animals, autoregulation remains intact and decreased renal vascular resistance maintains RBF at normal levels.[93]

3. Sevoflurane and desflurane. Although also metabolized to inorganic fluoride, sevoflurane appears to be a less potent nephrotoxin than methoxyflurane, perhaps because sevoflurane is renally metabolized to fluoride ion at a much slower rate than is methoxyflurane.[94] Sevoflurane also is metabolized to another nephrotoxin, compound A, a vinyl chloride, by degradation in soda lime or Baralyme. The suggestion that fresh gas flows be maintained at greater than 2 L/min during prolonged anesthesia is intended to dilute any compound A produced in a circle system. Nevertheless, no significant renal effects were noted with low-flow (1 L/min) sevoflurane anesthesia for long general surgical procedures.[95] In volunteers, administration of sevoflurane at a concentration of 1.25 times the minimum alveolar concentration (MAC) at a fresh gas flow of 1 L/min for 4 hours did not result in any clinically significant changes in sensitive biochemical markers of renal dysfunction.[96] Volunteers tolerated administration of sevoflurane at a concentration of 1.25 times MAC at a fresh gas flow of 2 L/min for 8 hours without any clinically significant changes in biochemical markers of renal or hepatic dysfunction.[97] In contrast, Eger et al[98] reported subtle evidence of transient glomerular and tubular injury after 4 hours of 1.25 MAC sevoflurane.

B. Effects of intravenous agents

1. Thiopental. In humans, low doses of thiopental produce little change in systemic blood pressure, renal vascular resistance, or RBF.[99] Higher doses produce venodilation and decrease cardiac preload and myocardial contractility.[100] During thiopental administration, RBF is preserved by reduced renal vascular resistance.[100]

2. Propofol. In rats, sedation with propofol or thiopental reduced GFR by 20% to 30%.[101] Both propofol and thiopental decreased urinary output (−24% and −48%, respectively); in contrast, midazolam produced sedation without influencing renal function.[101] In septic sheep, propofol reduced RBF to 60% ± 10% of the presptic baseline and to 39% ± 4% of the septic value.[102] In healthy sheep, propofol caused only minor hemodynamic changes.[102] Neither chronic renal failure nor hepatic failure influences the percentage of unbound propofol in serum after intravenous injection. In healthy volunteers, patients with chronic renal failure, and patients with hepatic cirrhosis, only about 1% of propofol was unbound.[103]

3. Opioids. Morphine, even when given in doses that lower blood pressure, does not reduce RBF.[104] Fentanyl decreases urine flow and GFR, but its effects on RBF are less well defined.[105,106]

4. Ketorolac tromethamine. The injectable analgesic ketorolac, an NSAID, blocks production of PGE_2 and PGI_2 and has been associated with episodes of ARF.[107-109] A large retrospective study of medical and surgical pa-

Table 21-4. Adjusted odds ratios for hospitalization from acute renal failure in patients taking NSAIDs*

Risk factor	Odds ratio (95% confidence interval)
Use of any NSAID	
No	1.0 (Reference)
Current	4.1 (1.5-10.8)
Recent	0.8 (0.2-4.1)
Past	1.5 (0.4-5.6)
Daily NSAID dose in current users	
No use	1.0 (Reference)
Low dose	4.0 (1.1-15.2)
High dose	9.8 (3.2-30.5)
Duration of NSAID use	
No use	1.0 (Reference)
≤1 Month	8.5 (2.5-28.6)
>6 Months	2.7 (0.7-9.9)
Age	
15-65 Years	1.0 (Reference)
≥65 Years	3.5 (1.3-9.8)

*Data obtained from Perez Guthann S, Garcia Rodriquez LA, Raiford DS, et al: *Arch Intern Med* 156:2433, 1996.
From Goldfarb S, Henrich WL: *Ann Intern Med* 128:49, 1998.
NSAID, Nonsteroidal antiinflammatory drug.

tients found no difference in the incidence of ARF when treatment with opioids or ketorolac lasted less than 5 days. Treatment longer than 5 days resulted in a risk ratio for ARF of 2.08 in the ketorolac-treated patients.[70] However, chronic administration of NSAIDs increases the odds ratio that patients will require hospitalization for ARF (Table 21-4).[110]

C. Effects of regional anesthesia

The renal and systemic hemodynamic responses to spinal and epidural anesthesia are strongly influenced by preanesthetic intravascular volume. Epidural block performed with epinephrine-free solutions generates little change in systemic hemodynamics and only a small decrease in GFR and RBF.[111] Thoracic levels of epidural block, using epinephrine-containing local anesthetics, moderately reduced RBF and GFR in parallel with the decrease in mean arterial pressure.[112]

IV. MONITORING AND EVALUATION OF RENAL FUNCTION

Prevention of perioperative ARF depends on the recognition of patients who are at increased risk of ARF and the use of appropriate diagnostic techniques and monitoring to evaluate renal function. Unfortunately, no monitors or diagnostic tests are sufficiently sensitive and specific to accurately classify all patients with threatened renal function.[113] Among the tests that are commonly used, those most important to understand include urinary output, SCr, creatinine clearance (CCr), BUN, and measures of tubular reabsorption of sodium and water.

Although renal compromise is often heralded by oliguria, urinary output is not a reliable index of renal func-tion. Anuria suggests mechanical obstruction of the urinary tract or catheter system. Completely reversible oliguria is the normal response to hypovolemia, yet patients with preexisting renal insufficiency and chronic loss of concentrating ability may not become oliguric in response to threatened renal perfusion. As a consequence, oliguria in perioperative patients should be assumed to be hemodynamically mediated and potentially reversible (i.e., prerenal) until otherwise proven, and efforts should be made to enhance cardiac output and RBF (especially blood flow in the mTAL).

Creatinine, an endogenous end-product of creatine phosphate metabolism, is generated from muscle at a uniform rate that is proportional to muscle mass. Creatinine is primarily filtered by the glomerulus, although a small amount is secreted by the renal tubules. A relatively accurate reflection of chronic glomerular function, SCr is unreliable when renal function is rapidly changing. The relationship between phosphocreatine (PCr) and GFR is inverse and exponential; that is, if GFR is halved, SCr will ultimately double. However, if creatinine excretion were to suddenly cease (i.e., GFR of zero), SCr would increase at a rate of only 1 to 3 mg/dl per day. After a transient renal insult, such as that caused by suprarenal aortic cross-clamping, SCr may continue to increase for a few days while GFR is actually recovering.

CCr is defined as the virtual volume of plasma cleared of creatinine per unit time, in millimeters per minute:

$$CCr = (UCr/SCr)V$$

where *UCr* is urinary creatinine concentration and *V* is urinary flow rate in ml/min.

Estimation of CCr provides useful prognostic information. The CCr provides earlier warning of renal dysfunction than the SCr because the creatinine excretion rate (UCr × V) rapidly reflects changes in GFR. Precisely timed and measured urinary collection is more important than the absolute duration of collection.[114] In trauma patients undergoing surgery, Shin, Mackenzie, and Helrich[115] found that a 1-hour CCr of less than 25 ml/min within 6 hours of injury was the most reliable predictor of subsequent renal dysfunction or failure. In postoperative patients, the 2-hour CCr provides a rapid assessment of GFR during intervals of rapidly changing renal function. Two-hour measurements of CCr in catheterized patients with urinary flow rates greater than 15 ml/hr correlated well with values obtained with 12- to 24-hour urinary collections.[114]

In patients in whom renal function is not rapidly changing, GFR can be estimated through the Cockcroft-Gault equation, which incorporates SCr, age, weight (in kg), and sex as follows:

$$GFR\ (male) = (140 - age)(weight)/(SCr)(72)$$

and

$$GFR\ (female) = (140 - age)(weight)(0.85)/(SCr)(72)$$

where 0.85 corrects the equation for the smaller muscle mass of women. However, the Cockcroft-Gault equation is inaccurate if renal function is rapidly changing and overestimates renal function in obese or edematous patients in whom total body weight is much greater than muscle mass.

The time frame in which perioperative oliguria occurs often prevents extensive diagnostic evaluation; that is, the problem must be addressed before diagnostic information would be available from the laboratory. However, tests of renal tubular function may help to differentiate prerenal oliguria from ATN (Table 21-5).[3] Renal hypoperfusion, acting via intrarenal and systemic mechanisms, stimulates the renal tubules to preserve intravascular volume by reabsorbing sodium and water. Therefore a hypovolemic patient should excrete small volumes of concentrated urine with a low sodium. In established ATN, the tubules cannot normally conserve sodium and water, and the urine becomes more dilute and higher in sodium. It is essential to remember that most of the tests of tubular function are valid only in the evaluation of oliguria. Healthy, well-hydrated, sodium-replete persons excrete relatively large volumes of dilute urine with a high sodium concentration. In addition, tests of tubular function do not accurately predict whether the kidneys will respond to improvement of systemic hemodynamics. In hepatorenal syndrome and sepsis, oliguria may occur despite apparently adequate hemodynamic function and may respond poorly to attempts to further enhance intravascular volume. Potent diuretics (e.g., furosemide, mannitol, low-dose dopamine) may increase water and sodium excretion and confound interpretation of tests of tubular function.

Avid reabsorption of water in the collecting ducts increases the UCr-to-SCr ratio, a useful and simply calculated index of tubular function. In prerenal states the ratio may be as high as 100:1 and should be greater than 40:1, but in ATN the ratio declines to less than 20:1. For example, the combination of an SCr of 2 mg/dl and a UCr of 100 mg/dl (UCr/SCr ratio = 50:1) suggests prerenal oliguria; however, if UCr were 20 mg/dl, ATN would be more likely (ratio = 10:1).

Avid tubular reabsorption of sodium is a central feature of the renal response to hypovolemia; therefore in prerenal oliguria, urinary sodium (U_{Na}) should be less than 10 mEq/L and is usually less than 20 mEq/L. In established ATN, the ability to conserve sodium is lost;

therefore U_{Na} should be at least 40 mEq/L and is usually greater than 60 to 80 mEq/L. If diuretics have recently been given, U_{Na} may be high despite normal tubular function. However, U_{Na} may remain low despite low-dose dopamine administration in patients for whom fluid is restricted before surgery.[116] Unfortunately, U_{Na} is an imperfect test of the likelihood that a patient will develop ARF. Table 21-6 summarizes the performance characteristics of urinary sodium as a means of discriminating between prerenal oliguria and ATN.[113]

The fractional excretion of sodium (FE_{Na}) expresses sodium clearance as a percentage of CCr as follows:

$$FE_{Na}(\%) = \left[(U_{Na}/P_{Na})/(U_{Cr}/P_{Cr}) \right](100)$$

where P_{Na} is plasma sodium. Because the FE_{Na} can be calculated from spot samples of blood and urine, less time is required to obtain this calculation than to obtain a CCr, which requires a timed collection of urine.

In oliguria secondary to actual or relative hypovolemia, FE_{Na} decreases to <1%. In contrast, in ARF, FE_{Na} should increase to >3% and usually will be >1%. However, an increased FE_{Na} is a normal response to diuretic therapy and postoperative salt and water mobilization. Sequential increases in FE_{Na} associated with declining CCr more reliably indicate deteriorating renal function than an isolated high FE_{Na}. Table 21-7 describes the performance of the FE_{Na} in evaluating oliguria.[113]

Table 21-5. Characteristic urinary indexes in patients with acute oliguria owing to prerenal or renal (intrinsic) causes

Index	Prerenal causes	Renal causes
Urinary sodium concentration (mmol/L)	<20	>40
Fractional excretion of sodium (%)	<1	>1
Ratio of urinary to plasma creatinine	>40	<20
Ratio of urinary to plasma osmolarity	>1.5	<1.1

From Klahr S, Miller SB: *N Engl J Med* 338:671, 1998.

Table 21-6 Meta-analysis of the performance characteristics of urinary sodium in evaluation of oliguria

Characteristic	Prerenal	ATN
Sensitivity	0.55 (0.39-0.70)	0.50 (0.42-0.58)
Specificity	0.84 (0.73-0.96)	0.90 (0.78-1.00)
LRP	4.58 (2.0-10.47)	3.40 (1.79-6.46)

From Kellen M, Aronson S, Roizen MF, et al: *Anesth Analg* 78:134, 1994.
ATN, Acute tubular necrosis; Sensitivity = N(+test and +disease)/N(+disease), where N = number of patients; Specificity = N(−test and −disease)/N(−disease); likelihood ratio of a positive test *(LRP)* = Sensitivity/(1 − Specificity).

Table 21-7. Meta-analysis of the performance characteristics of fractional excretion of sodium in evaluation of oliguria

Characteristic	Prerenal	ATN
Sensitivity	0.96 (0.89-1.00)	0.95 (0.88-1.00)
Specificity	0.95 (0.88-1.00)	0.96 (0.89-1.00)
LRP	11.18 (8.9-14.04)	12.79 (10.18-16.06)

From Kellen M, Aronson S, Roizen MF, et al: *Anesth Analg* 78:134, 1994.
ATN, Acute tubular necrosis; Sensitivity = N(+test and +disease)/N(+disease) where N = number of patients; Specificity = N(−test and −disease)/N(−disease); likelihood ratio of a positive test *(LRP)* = Sensitivity/(1 − Specificity).

V. ACUTE RENAL DYSFUNCTION

Transient perioperative decreases in urine formation or increases in SCr are common. The majority of these, however, soon return to baseline.[8] Persistent or severe changes, such as ARF, are of greater concern to anesthesiologists. Acute renal dysfunction is conventionally divided into three categories: postrenal, prerenal, and intrinsic renal (Fig. 21-9).[4] The actual causes of ARF are, however, often multifactorial. Because postrenal, prerenal, and intrinsic renal dysfunction may progress to ARF, rapid treatment is essential to restore or maintain urinary flow and prevent the development of ARF.

A. Postrenal dysfunction

Postrenal (obstructive) dysfunction typically presents as anuria or erratically fluctuating urinary output, although oliguria or nonoliguric renal failure may also be the initial finding. Treatment necessitates identification of the site of obstruction, including evaluation of the patency of existing urinary bladder catheters. Prostatic hypertrophy, autonomic dysfunction, and drugs with anticholinergic side effects increase the risk of perioperative urinary retention. Abdominal ultrasonography, computer tomography, cystoscopy, and retrograde pyelography occasionally may be necessary for accurate diagnosis.

B. Prerenal dysfunction

Prerenal dysfunction describes a state in which tubular and glomerular functions remain intact, but clearance of solutes is limited by renal perfusion. This category accounts for most episodes of ARF occurring before hospital admission.[4] Prerenal dysfunction, often but not in-

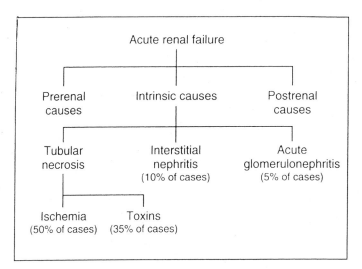

Fig. 21-9. Main categories of acute renal failure. The causes of acute renal failure are conventionally categorized as prerenal, intrinsic, and postrenal. Once prerenal and postrenal causes have been excluded, the remainder are due to intrinsic causes, which are associated with high rates of morbidity and mortality. The percentages listed reflect the experience in one institution[4]; proportions may vary from one institution or country to another. (From Thadhani R, Pascual M, Bonventre JV: *N Engl J Med* 334:1448, 1996.)

variably evidenced by oliguria (urinary output less than $0.5 \, ml \cdot kg^{-1} \cdot hr^{-1}$), is initiated by decreased renal perfusion. In response to circulatory compromise, renin, angiotensin II, aldosterone, and ADH avidly conserve sodium and water. The renal vasodilating prostaglandins, especially PGE_2, act to preserve RBF and GFR. Nitric oxide may also cause afferent arteriolar dilation. Autonomic nervous system activation helps to maintain RBF by increasing renal perfusion pressure.

Renin is released from the juxtaglomerular apparatus in response to decreased afferent arteriolar pressure,[117] to catecholamine secretion, and to increasing tubular concentrations of sodium and chloride delivered to the macula densa.[118] Angiotensin II is generated and constricts both afferent and efferent arterioles, thereby reducing GFR, and releases aldosterone, which leads to increased sodium reabsorption in the distal tubule. Renal hypoperfusion also is associated with reduction of factors that facilitate sodium excretion. Circulating levels of ANP are reduced during hypotensive hemorrhage,[119] and the response to exogenous ANP is reduced.[120] Moderate hypovolemia reduces the stimulation of atrial stretch receptors, thereby initiating ADH release and increasing reabsorption of water from urine in the collecting ducts. Frank hypotension stimulates the vagally innervated aortic arch and carotid sinus baroreceptors, leading to further ADH secretion. Because maximal ADH stimulation can increase urinary osmolality to nearly 1200 mOsm/L, excretion of the normal dietary solute load of 400 to 600 mOsm per day requires the kidneys to produce 300 to 500 ml per day of urine. Therefore the conventional medical definition of oliguria is 400 ml per day. However, because surgical patients or traumatized patients typically cannot achieve maximal urinary concentration, oliguria is defined as urinary output less than $0.5 \, ml \cdot kg^{-1} \cdot hr^{-1}$. Excretion of increased catabolic wastes in hypermetabolic patients may require even greater urinary flow. Failure to remove accumulated waste products indicates prerenal failure.

The renal response to hypovolemia and hypotension depends on the severity of the insult. Ischemic tubular damage is the eventual end point of escalating prerenal azotemia. There are many mechanisms of intrinsic renal damage (Fig. 21-10).[4] Severely reduced renal perfusion depletes high-energy phosphates and initiates a series of biochemical insults that may lead to progressive renal injury,[121] especially if mean arterial pressure declines below the level necessary to preserve renal autoregulation.[37] In experimental models, GFR declines more profoundly if acute hypotension is superimposed on preexisting renal hypoperfusion, such as that produced by acute water deprivation or congestive heart failure.[122]

Although the kidneys are capable of substantial adjustment in response to declining perfusion, at some point decompensation ensues.[43] When renal hypoperfusion precipitates prerenal oliguria, the primary treatment is to improve renal perfusion. Prompt restoration of RBF may increase urinary flow, diminish hormonal responses to circulatory depression, and prevent ARF. Failure to restore RBF may lead to postischemic ARF. Thus there is

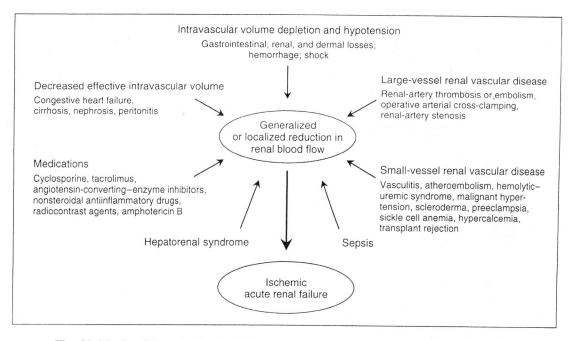

Fig. 21-10. Conditions that lead to ischemic acute renal failure. A wide spectrum of clinical conditions can result in a generalized or localized reduction in renal blood flow, thus increasing the likelihood of ischemic acute renal failure. The most common condition leading to ischemic acute renal failure is severe and sustained prerenal azotemia. Kidney ischemia and acute renal failure are often the result of a combination of factors. (From Thadhani R, Pascual M, Bonventre JV: *N Engl J Med* 334:1448, 1996.)

a continuum between prerenal azotemia and postischemic ARF.

C. Acute renal failure

Postoperative, hemodynamically mediated ARF can be divided into three distinct patterns.[123] In some patients, glomerular filtration abruptly declines at the time of surgery and then promptly recovers (Fig. 21-11, *A*). In such patients, the peak increase in SCr may be reached as the GFR is already returning toward normal. Dialysis is rarely required. The second pattern of ARF is associated with prolonged hemodynamic insufficiency (Fig. 21-11, *B*). As hemodynamic function recovers, GFR will increase and SCr will decline. The third category of ARF is highly lethal, usually developing in association with delayed septic complications, recurrent episodes of hypotension, and failure of other organ systems (Fig. 21-11, *C*). Recurrent episodes of renal ischemia may induce new renal lesions and prevent healing of existing lesions, resulting in permanent loss of renal function. Renal replacement therapy then becomes part of an escalating series of therapeutic interventions in progressively worsening, often terminal illness.

Once ARF is established, improving prerenal or postrenal factors cannot reverse the insult.[124] In prerenal states, improvements in RBF improve GFR, whereas in established ARF, increases in RBF do not increase GFR. Prompt intervention in prerenal states is essential, as is apparent from a brief review of common models of renal failure. Experimental ischemic ATN requires a severe in-

Table 21-8. Mechanisms contributing to the initiation and maintenance of acute renal failure

Initiation	Maintenance
Renal hypoperfusion	Decreased renal blood flow
Nephrotoxins	Decreased glomerular filtration
	Tubular obstruction
	Tubular dysfunction

sult of substantial duration. Perhaps the best established model consists of an infusion of norepinephrine directly into a renal artery in a dose sufficient to produce complete renal ischemia.[125] A 60-minute infusion results in oliguria but not tubular damage. An infusion lasting 60 to 120 minutes causes ischemic tubular damage, analogous to clinical ATN. An infusion persisting more than 120 minutes causes irreversible cortical necrosis. In predicting the probable clinical efficacy of interventions that have been proven effective in this experimental model, it is essential to recognize that virtually no intervention limits renal injury as effectively as shortening the duration of infusion. Therefore in the clinical setting, prompt reversal of prerenal insults before ARF ensues is also likely to be more effective than other therapeutic modalities.

Contributing mechanisms to hemodynamically mediated ARF include factors that initiate and those that maintain ARF (Table 21-8). After initiation by renal hypoperfusion or nephrotoxins (i.e., causes of renal is-

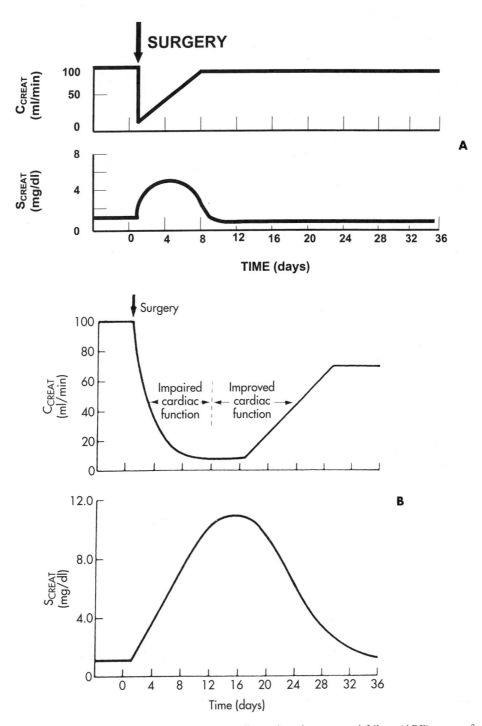

Fig. 21-11. Three patterns of hemodynamically mediated acute renal failure (ARF) occur after major trauma or surgery. **A,** Abbreviated ARF. Acute reduction in creatinine clearance
(C_{Creat}) with prompt recovery. Serum creatinine (S_{Creat}) may be increasing even as C_{Creat} recovers. **B,** Overt ARF. Concurrent, mirror-image decreases in C_{Creat} and increases in S_{Creat}, usually
in association with compromised cardiac function followed by recovery. (From Myers BD,
Moran SM: *N Engl J Med* 314:97, 1986.)

Continued

chemia or direct toxic injury), ARF is maintained by
both reduced RBF and by tubular abnormalities.

The vulnerability of the renal medulla to ischemia explains the magnitude of tubular injury.[126] However, the
renal cortex is also vulnerable to severe insults. When total RBF declines because of ECF volume depletion or
compensatory vasoconstriction, blood flow is redistrib-
uted from cortical to juxtamedullary nephrons.[127] Ischemic dysfunction of renal endothelial cells disrupts
both the synthesis of and response to vasodilator agents.

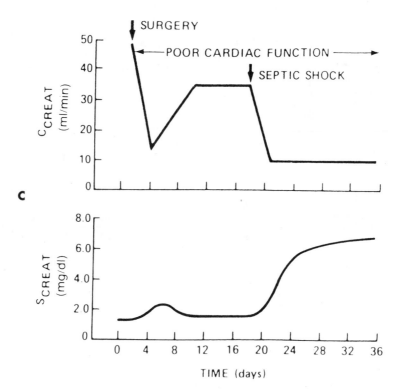

Fig. 21-11, cont'd. C, Protracted ARF. Development as a consequence of prolonged hemodynamic compromise, often complicated by systemic sepsis. (From Myers BD, Moran SM: *N Engl J Med* 314:97, 1986.)

Cortical vasoconstriction is augmented by intrarenal renin, released by increased delivery to the macula densa of sodium and chloride, which are no longer adequately absorbed by ischemic tubular epithelium. In ARF, the kidneys lose the ability to autoregulate and are more dependent on renal arterial pressure for perfusion than are normal kidneys.[128,129] Such kidneys are susceptible to repeated ischemic insults, especially recurrent episodes of hypotension.

In postischemic ARF, GFR declines to a greater degree than RBF, although the glomeruli usually appear structurally normal.[130] Because GFR also remains depressed in ARF despite therapeutic interventions that increase RBF, it is apparent that reduced glomerular permeability or perfusion pressure, owing to a derangement of the balance between afferent and efferent arteriolar tone, contributes to ARF. Angiotensin II acts on receptors on mesangial cells of the glomerular tuft, causing them to contract, thus decreasing glomerular surface area and GFR. After the initial tubular insult, vasoconstrictor responses mediated by tubuloglomerular feedback help to sustain a reduced GFR.

Renal tubular dysfunction appears to consist of two primary components: obstruction and "back-leak." Obstruction of tubular flow by intratubular debris, produced by ischemic desquamation of brush-border microvilli[131] or by pigmented casts, can result in back-pressure that opposes glomerular filtration.[132] Tubular obstruction may maintain but rarely initiates ARF (except that caused by pigmenturia or crystalluria). Disrup-

tion of tubular epithelial integrity permits pathologic back-leak of filtered waste products from the tubular lumen into the peritubular interstitium and peritubular capillaries. Aggravated by tubular obstruction from intraluminal debris, back-leak may prevent excretion of nearly 50% of total filtrate, leading to azotemia and retention of sodium and water.[133]

One puzzling aspect of ARF is the ability of the normal kidney to tolerate hypotension and significant decreases in RBF despite the apparent vulnerability of the medulla. Although the concept that the renal medulla exists on the verge of hypoxia provides an approach for understanding renal ischemia, objective data are somewhat contradictory. Experimentally, extreme decreases in renal perfusion pressure are required to demonstrate changes consistent with ARF.[134,135] Laboratory investigation of ARF has frequently been based on experiments that completely interrupt renal arterial blood flow because the magnitude of hypotension required to initiate ARF consistently is incompatible with survival of experimental animals.[136] The explanation for the resilience of the normal kidney may lie in the effective protective mechanisms. The oxygen demand of the nephron varies with the rate of active reabsorption in the mTAL. Oliguria, which is viewed as an ominous sign, actually represents reduction of GFR and therefore reduction of filtrate that must be processed in the mTAL and reduction of the oxygen required to process the filtrate (see Fig. 21-3).[137,138] Similarly, although loop diuretics reduce medullary blood flow, the accompanying reduction of tubular work may markedly increase medullary P_{O_2} (see Fig. 21-8).[4,139]

1. Contributing factors to acute renal failure. Often, clinical ARF results from a combination of insults, such as hypoperfusion compounded by a nephrotoxin or an agent that interferes with compensation (see Fig. 21-10).[140] Other predisposing factors, including chronic renal insufficiency, diabetes mellitus, hypertension, congestive heart failure, cirrhosis, and even normal aging, may increase the vulnerability of the kidney to acute insults.[35] The specific nature and mechanism of these triggering insults are varied.

Many antibiotics are nephrotoxic. Aminoglycoside-induced nephrotoxicity, occurring in 10% to 26% of patients receiving these drugs, is characterized by enzymuria, reduced glomerular permeability, decreased concentrating ability, and progressively declining GFR.[141,142] Neomycin, the most toxic aminoglycoside, may be absorbed from surgical irrigating fluid. In a prospective, controlled trial,[143] 8% to 10% of patients receiving gentamicin developed nephrotoxicity, in contrast to 18% of those receiving tobramycin. Sustained high blood levels, advanced age, volume depletion, concurrent cephalosporin antibiotics, potent diuretics, acidemia, endotoxemia, and a history of recent exposure to aminoglycosides and NSAIDs increase the risk of aminoglycoside nephrotoxicity. Recent evidence suggests that single daily doses of aminoglycosides are as effective as multiple daily doses and are possibly less nephrotoxic.[144] Amphotericin induces renal vasoconstriction and may also increase oxygen requirements via augmented sodium pump activity.[35] Vancomycin, once considered highly nephrotoxic, appears to have little effect in the absence of extremely high serum trough levels.[145]

Renal toxicity is frequently a dose-limiting feature of antineoplastic agents. Patients receiving chemotherapy may be at increased risk because of hypovolemia, tumor lysis syndrome, or unrelated coexisting diseases.[146] Cisplatin is a potent tubular nephrotoxin, necessitating aggressive volume expansion before dosing.[147] The nitrosoureas, especially streptozocin, produce renal dysfunction in 28% to 73% of patients through an unclear mechanism.[148] Nephrotoxicity with methotrexate was a common feature before recognition of the importance of hydration in treatment protocols.[149] Mithramycin has been linked to significant decreases in creatinine clearance, particularly in patients with preexisting renal insufficiency.[150,151]

Immunomodulating agents that have been associated with ARF include interleukin-2, cyclosporine, and interferon. Interleukin-2, a glycoprotein that may mediate regression of metastatic cancer, has been associated with azotemia.[152] Cyclosporine adversely affects renal function via renal vasoconstriction, in part mediated by endothelin.[153] Interferon has been associated with proteinuria and rarely ARF.[154,155]

As noted earlier, one potent mechanism in the renal cortex that resists the development of ARF involves the vasodilating prostaglandins PGE_2 and PGI_2 (prostacyclin), which modulate renin release and reduce renal vas-

---

Box 21-1 Risk factors contributing to the development of contrast-induced acute renal failure

Definite risk factor
Preexisting renal insufficiency

Probable risk factors
Diabetes mellitus
Dehydration
Large doses of contrast medium
Previous contrast medium–induced acute renal failure
Congestive heart failure
Multiple myeloma

---

cular resistance. By inhibiting the production of vasodilating prostaglandins, NSAIDs increase the risk of ARF.[68,156-158] Although NSAIDs appear to have little effect on renal function in healthy patients, in patients with compromised renal perfusion, the reduced vasodilator synthesis may be critical.[157,158]

The potentially detrimental effects of ACE inhibitors in patients with bilateral renal arterial stenosis or arterial stenosis of a solitary kidney are well documented.[159,160] In contrast, patients with hypertension and chronic renal insufficiency or congestive heart failure may experience some improvement in renal function after therapy with ACE inhibitors.[161]

Nearly all patients undergoing elective or emergent major vascular surgery and many of those requiring surgery after trauma will have undergone radiographic procedures requiring contrast media. The risk of contrast medium–induced ARF is increased by multiple risk factors, most importantly preexisting renal insufficiency (Box 21-1). If SCr is less than 1.5 mg/dl, the risk of contrast medium–induced ARF is 0.6%, increasing to 3% if SCr is 1.5 to 4.5 mg/dl.[162] Other risk factors include diabetes mellitus, dehydration, congestive heart failure, multiple myeloma, liver disease, and vascular disease. The combination of diabetes mellitus and renal insufficiency is associated with an incidence of contrast-induced ARF of nearly 9%.[163] After radiographic contrast studies, renal injury produces evidence of azotemia beginning 24 to 48 hours after exposure; SCr rapidly increases 3 to 5 days after injury and then typically becomes normal within 2 weeks.

Agents that alter the agglutination of red cells (dextran and volume expansion) protect against ARF induced by contrast media. Hydration with 0.9% saline has been shown to be more effective than mannitol or a combination of saline and furosemide in reducing the incidence of renal dysfunction after contrast media.[164] Minimizing the total dose of contrast media also helps to limit injury. The newer radiocontrast agents are minimally toxic in the absence of risk factors.

Rhabdomyolysis releases myoglobin, the oxygen-carrying heme pigment of muscle. If released in sufficient quantities from injured or ischemic skeletal muscle, myoglobinemia causes ARF. Several clinical situations associated with myoglobin-induced ARF include severe hypophosphatemia; nontraumatic myonecrosis; embolic arterial ischemia and rhabdomyolysis; the crush syndrome, which combines muscle injury and hypovolemia; and severe hypokalemia, especially if combined with exercise.[165,166] Rhabdomyolysis also is associated with prolonged immobilization, protracted fever, status epilepticus, myoclonus, and acute alcohol or cocaine intoxication.

Myoglobin is rapidly filtered through the glomerular capillary membrane when the plasma level exceeds 0.03 mg/dl. Predictors of myoglobinemic ARF include a serum myoglobin greater than 400 μg/L, urinary myoglobin greater than 1000 ng/ml, and myoglobin clearance less than 4 ml/min.[167,168] In clinical practice, serial estimations of total creatinine phosphokinase (CPK) are the most useful guide to the severity and progress of rhabdomyolysis and the potential for renal damage.[169]

Myoglobin toxicity is enhanced by dehydration, which decreases tubular flow, and by acidic urine (pH less than 5.6). Urinary alkalinization prevents conversion of myoglobin to ferrihematin, decreases tubular obstruction, and reduces tubular toxicity.[170] Myoglobinemia is associated with a precipitously falling GFR, probably related both to swelling of glomerular epithelial cells and mesangial cells and to tubular obstruction. Mannitol in doses of 25 to 50 g induces diuresis and prevents tubular obstruction by decreasing glomerular edema and maintaining tubular flow. In experimental models, furosemide aggravates myoglobin-induced ARF.

Atheromatous material dislodged by thoracic or abdominal trauma, by cardiac or aortic surgery, or by intraaortic catheters can embolize to the renal circulation and cause ischemia. The clinical diagnosis, often difficult, requires a high index of suspicion and the recognition of evidence of peripheral embolization (such as ischemic injury to fingers and toes). Livedo reticularis, an irregular cutaneous mottling at sites of small vessel occlusion, is strongly suggestive of atheroembolic disease. No specific findings or laboratory values are diagnostic; the only clinical manifestation may be oliguria with increasing hypertension. There is no specific therapy.

A variety of surgical procedures are associated with renal compromise. In cardiac patients, duration of cardiopulmonary bypass has been implicated as a significant determinant of renal impairment. Perioperative alterations in RBF and hemoglobinemia caused by the trauma of the bypass circuit appear to play major roles, rather than any direct effects of cardiopulmonary bypass.[171] Postoperative depression of cardiac function and use of vasopressors are associated with an increased risk of ARF.[17,172]

Major vascular surgery threatens renal perfusion in several ways. First, aortic procedures involve extensive tissue manipulation with substantial loss of plasma volume into the interstitial space. Second, aortic procedures are associated with variable, sometimes massive, hemorrhage. Third, aortic procedures produce frank renal ischemia or disturbed renal hemodynamics because of

temporary occlusion of aortic flow. Significant decreases in RBF may occur even with the placement of the aortic cross-clamp below the renal arteries.[173,174] Finally, manipulation of the aorta in the presence of atheromatous disease may result in renal artery emboli. Patients who develop ARF after vascular surgery have a particularly poor prognosis. In a series of 47 patients who developed ARF after aortic aneurysm surgery, 75% died within 30 days of the procedure; only 20% of patients recovered sufficient renal function to allow withdrawal of hemodialysis.[175]

Although all surgery requiring cross-clamping of the aorta carries some risk of postoperative renal dysfunction, the risk is less when flow is interrupted distal to the renal arteries.[16] The incidence of ARF requiring hemodialysis after surgery on the infrarenal aorta may be 5% or lower.[176] A small retrospective series[177] suggested that mild perioperative renal insufficiency was associated with an acceptable risk of ARF after infrarenal aortic surgery. Only 1 of 16 patients with a baseline SCr between 2 and 4 mg/dl required perioperative hemodialysis. In contrast, 4 of 6 patients who had SCr levels greater than 4 mg/dl but who had not previously undergone hemodialysis required acute perioperative hemodialysis. A retrospective study by Bush et al[178] of patients undergoing infrarenal cross-clamping suggested that adequate volume loading, monitored by either central venous pressure or pulmonary arterial occlusion pressure, could reduce the incidence of postoperative oliguric renal failure.

Emergency operations and those involving the thoracic aorta carry a substantially higher risk of perioperative renal dysfunction. Emergency surgery for ruptured or leaking abdominal aneurysms carries up to a 32% risk of perioperative renal failure.[179,180] Patients who undergo thoracic aortic cross-clamping have an incidence of ARF of 2.6% to 28%.[11-16] The incidence of less severe renal dysfunction can be as high as 51%.[12] A comparison of 39 patients undergoing suprarenal cross-clamping with 166 patients who had infrarenal clamping showed a higher incidence of renal insufficiency in the former (28% versus 10%) but no significant difference in the frequency at which postoperative dialysis was required (3% versus 2%).[16]

Sepsis, a common complication of critical surgical illness, is a significant risk factor for the development of irreversible ARF. The mechanisms postulated involve a complex interplay of bacteria, endotoxins, neutrophil activation, disseminated intravascular coagulation, and cytokines.[181] Renal perfusion is often compromised in both congestive heart failure and advanced liver disease. Compromised arterial filling results in retention of sodium and water by the kidney, which further worsens the oxygen supply and demand relationship.

D. Prevention and treatment of acute renal failure

Renal ischemia must be prevented or limited in duration because of the high mortality associated with the progression from prerenal insults to ARF. Efforts to prevent or attenuate renal ischemia should be particularly emphasized in patients who are at increased risk for ARF, including those who are elderly or have underlying renal disease, hepatic disease, sepsis, or cardiac disease. The fundamental strategy for the prevention of ARF is to limit the magnitude and duration of renal ischemia. In general, effective therapeutic interventions in acute, hemodynamically mediated oliguria should improve the balance between oxygen supply and demand in the mTAL.[29] Theoretically, tubular oxygen supply should be increased by an increase in cardiac output, RBF, or arterial oxygen content, and tubular oxygen consumption should be decreased by reducing the amount of solute that must be reabsorbed. In relatively or absolutely hypovolemic patients, fluid administration suppresses reflex vasoconstriction, increases cardiac output, and, by causing atrial distension, releases endogenous ANP, a renal vasodilator that also increases sodium and water excretion.

1. Maintenance of intravascular volume and oxygen transport. Compromised renal perfusion, upon which additional renal insults are superimposed, usually constitutes the substrate for ARF. Preoperative and intraoperative restoration and maintenance of intravascular volume are essential, especially in patients who are hypovolemic as a consequence of angiography, bowel preparation, or prolonged fasting.[182] Early institution of appropriate monitoring is also essential for effective renal protection and the treatment of oliguria. Bladder catheterization is mandatory for high-risk cases. Pulmonary arterial catheterization is indicated when close monitoring of intravascular volume status is important (preexisting renal dysfunction, respiratory failure, congestive heart failure) and is difficult to interpret by central venous pressure alone. Evidence indicates that optimal volume loading, using information derived from pulmonary arterial catheterization, can reduce renal injury associated with vascular surgery.[178,182] Similarly, maintenance of volume homeostasis has been shown to markedly reduce the risk of contrast nephrotoxicity.[164]

There remain some inconsistencies between clinical and experimental data regarding whether a nonspecific increase in systemic oxygen delivery alters renal outcome. A clinical report from Shoemaker et al[183] suggested that goal-directed hemodynamic therapy (i.e., maintenance of systemic oxygen delivery greater than $600 \ ml \cdot min^{-1} \cdot m^{-2}$) reduced the incidence of ARF in high-risk surgical patients. However, the apparent decrease in the incidence of ARF was identified through a secondary analysis of the data and was not addressed as a primary hypothesis. In septic sheep, decreased renal oxygen delivery did not appear to cause tubular damage,[184] perhaps because the decrease in GFR decreased the tubular oxygen consumption required for sodium reabsorption. Experimental data are unclear regarding the relationship between systemic oxygen delivery and renal outcome. In fluid-loaded septic swine, dobutamine increased systemic oxygen delivery but did not achieve a concomitant increase in renal oxygen delivery.[185]

2. Pharmacologic therapies. The protective or therapeutic value of clinically available adjuvant pharmacologic therapies has been difficult to establish. Many interventions, especially dopamine, mannitol, and furosemide, are applied empirically with limited evidence of probable efficacy. Most clinical approaches to the reduction of perioperative ARF are based on anecdotal experience and inferences from animal models involving complete renal ischemia.[125] In experimental ATN, tubular injury, especially tubular back-leak, is reduced, oliguria does not occur, and recovery is more rapid if the insult is preceded by saline loading, osmotic diuresis with mannitol, or vasodilation with dopamine, furosemide, or PGE_1.[186] Mannitol, dopamine, and furosemide promote urinary flow and reduce the renal damage produced by experimental renal ischemia of fixed magnitude and duration.[125,187-192]

a. Mannitol. Mannitol improves renal cortical blood flow and may exert cellular protective effects, particularly when given before the ischemic insult.[189,193,194] Intravenous mannitol osmotically expands plasma, thereby increasing ventricular preload, cardiac output, RBF, transglomerular hydrostatic pressure, and GFR. Osmotic opposition to water reabsorption increases tubular flow, which in turn diminishes tubular obstruction. Osmotic volume expansion of the atria by mannitol may suppress renin activation by stimulating the release of ANP.[195] Osmotic hemodilution may protect against the "no-reflow" phenomenon, that is, hypoperfusion caused by red cell aggregation and endothelial swelling in the vessels of the inner medulla as a consequence of renal ischemia.[196] Mannitol appears to be a free radical scavenger and also appears to increase the release of vasodilator intrarenal prostaglandins, which may further protect against ischemic injury.[197] Paradoxically, however, mannitol may reduce medullary PO_2 by increasing the amount of solute available for energy-requiring reabsorption.[35]

Osmotic diuresis with mannitol appears to protect against renal injury associated with rhabdomyolysis and obstructive jaundice. To limit the tubular toxicity of myoglobinemia, urinary flow should be maintained at greater than 100 ml/hr using mannitol and intravenous hydration, often with furosemide. Urinary alkalinization, using sodium bicarbonate or acetazolamide, to a pH greater than 5.6 decreases the conversion of myoglobin to acid ferrihematin. In surgical patients with obstructive jaundice, prophylactic intravenous administration of mannitol or oral administration of sodium taurocholate prevented postoperative ARF.[198] Previous series had reported a rate of 4% to 18%, with an associated mortality rate of 76%.[199]

Mannitol does not, however, reverse the profound reduction in GFR and RBF induced by suprarenal aortic cross-clamping for 60 minutes in dogs.[191] In fact, prospective, controlled studies have failed to demonstrate any prophylactic benefits of mannitol in surgical patients,[200,201] with the exception of those undergoing renal transplantation.[193,194] Despite mannitol infusion, infrarenal cross-clamping was associated with a 75% increase in calculated renal vascular resistance, a 38% decrease in RBF, and a 25% decrease in urinary flow.[173] The increased RBF demonstrated after mannitol therapy may even be potentially harmful if the increased filtrate, which requires increased tubular energy for processing, is not accompanied by an increase in medullary blood flow.[202,203]

b. Dopamine. Low-dose dopamine (0.5 to 3 μg · kg^{-1}· min^{-1}) acts as a nonselective agonist at the two types of dopaminergic (DA) receptors,[204] as a β_1 agonist at doses of 3 to 10 μg · kg^{-1} · min^{-1}, and as an α-adrenergic agonist at doses greater than 10 μg · kg^{-1} · min^{-1}. DA$_1$ receptors mediate smooth muscle relaxation in the renal and splanchnic vasculature. Stimulation of DA$_1$ receptors localized on the luminal and basolateral membranes of the proximal tubules activates adenylate cyclase and phospholipase C, thereby inhibiting active sodium reabsorption and resulting in natriuresis and diuresis.[205,206] Stimulation of DA$_2$ receptors, located presynaptically on postganglionic sympathetic nerves that innervate renal vessels, inhibits release of norepinephrine. The effects on urinary output may be secondary to renal vasodilation (DA$_1$, DA$_2$ agonists), tubular saliuresis (DA$_1$ agonist), or increased cardiac output (β_1 agonist). Dopamine induces natriuresis, often increases GFR, and, most consistently, improves urinary flow.[207-209] In healthy volunteers, dopamine at a dose of 3 μg · kg^{-1} · min^{-1} increased effective RBF and reversed the reduction in effective RBF associated with norepinephrine infusion; however, GFR did not change with infusion of either drug alone or with the combination.[210] Potential adverse effects include tachycardia from β_1-adrenergic agonists and renal vasoconstriction secondary to α agonists.

During cardiopulmonary bypass, in 36 patients with mild preoperative renal dysfunction (CCr less than 50 ml/min), placebo, dopamine, or a combination of dopamine and nitroprusside were associated with similar values for CCr, FE$_{Na}$, osmolality and C$_{H2O}$.[211] After cardiac surgery, dopamine and dobutamine in equiinotropic doses exerted similar effects on GFR and renal plasma flow; however, dopamine produced greater urinary flow (2.8 versus 1 ml/min) and FE$_{Na}$ (2.5% versus 0.7%), suggesting that tubular dopaminergic receptors were active.[212] In hemodynamically stable patients with normal renal function, low-dose dopamine (200 μg/min) appeared to have only a diuretic effect, without improving CCr; in contrast, low-dose dobutamine (175 μg/min) consistently improved CCr.[208]

In patients with chronic renal disease, dopaminergic agonists induce natriuresis but do not improve renal perfusion. Dopamine did not significantly increase GFR or RBF in patients in whom baseline GFR was less than 50 ml · min^{-1} · m^{-2}.[213] The response of effective renal plasma flow and filtration fraction to fenoldopam, a dopamine analog and a selective DA$_1$ receptor agonist, was also impaired, but the natriuretic effect was conserved.[214]

Schwartz and Gewertz[207] summarized nine uncontrolled studies that suggested beneficial effect of dopamine infusion (1 to 4 μg · kg^{-1} · min^{-1}) in oliguria. In eight of the nine studies, patients had either failed prior furosemide therapy or were concomitantly given furosemide in doses ranging from 1 to 15 mg · kg^{-1} · day^{-1}. Mean urinary flow increased from 15 to 80 ml/hr.

More recently, Flancbaum, Choban, and Dasta[209] demonstrated that low-dose dopamine increased mean urinary output from 0.3 to 1 ml · kg^{-1} · hr^{-1} without altering systemic hemodynamics in nine surgical ICU patients who had remained oliguric despite fluid resuscitation. Urinary flow decreased when dopamine was stopped and increased when it was restarted.

Like mannitol, dopamine is ineffective in reversing the renal injury produced by aortic cross-clamping.[191,215] In humans, dopamine infusion induced saluresis and reversed the decline in CCr caused by infrarenal aortic cross-clamping.[216] However, the effect of dopamine (or mannitol) on GFR was no greater than that provided by extravascular fluid volume expansion during infrarenal aortic cross-clamping[215] or after elective, major vascular surgery.[217] Although a retrospective study of patients undergoing orthotopic liver transplantation suggested that low-dose dopamine, started before surgery, increased urinary flow and CCr and decreased the incidence of dialysis-dependent ARF from 27% to 9.5%,[218] a controlled, prospective trial demonstrated no benefit.[219] After renal transplantation, dopamine in combination with furosemide not only failed to reduce the incidence of postoperative renal failure but also caused more fluid and electrolyte disturbances and arrhythmias.[220]

Infusion of dopamine to increase urinary output is appropriate in patients who remain oliguric (urinary output less than 0.5 ml · kg^{-1} · hr^{-1}) despite restoration of adequate intravascular volume and stable hemodynamics. However, dopamine used in this situation has not been shown to reduce the incidence of ARF. Relatively few data suggest that prophylactic administration of low-dose dopamine protects the kidney from injury. In 256 patients with ARF (PCr increase greater than 1 mg/dl in the preceding 24 to 48 hours), dopamine did not improve survival or reduce the need for dialysis.[221] There is no evidence that use of low-dose dopamine prevented or altered the course of established ARF[217,221-224] or that it prevented ARF. The prophylactic use of low-dose dopamine also entails the risk of complications. In a Holter monitoring study that documented a high incidence of supraventricular and ventricular arrhythmias after cardiac surgery, dopamine (especially low-dose dopamine) emerged as the only factor directly correlated with the incidence of complex ventricular arrhythmias.[225]

Dopexamine, a potent, synthetic β_2 agonist, has one-third the dopaminergic effect of dopamine but has minimal β_1 agonist and no α-adrenoceptor activity. Dopexamine provides positive inotropy, arterial dilation, and positive chronotropy, usually without generating cardiac arrhythmias. Used in the dose range of 1 to 5 μg · kg^{-1} · min^{-1}, dopexamine reduces left and right ventricular afterload in acute and chronic heart failure, while augmenting RBF through its dopaminergic and β_2-adrenergic effects.[226] In patients undergoing orthotopic liver transplantation, dopexamine was associated with less renal dysfunction.[227]

Fenoldopam, also a dopaminergic agonist, dilates the renal and mesenteric vasculature and increases RBF at doses that do not influence blood pressure; higher doses reduce blood pressure but maintain renal perfusion. Fenoldopam is natriuretic, possibly resulting from a direct effect on DA_1 receptors on the proximal convoluted tubule. Given by intravenous infusion at 0.1 to 0.5 μg · kg^{-1} · min^{-1}, it has a rapid onset and offset of action with an elimination half-life of 10 minutes. In patients with chronic renal insufficiency, oral administration of fenoldopam significantly reduced blood pressure but did not change renal plasma flow, GFR, or FE_{Na}; intravenous infusion of fenoldopam induced natriuresis but did not change renal plasma flow or GFR.[228]

c. Furosemide. Furosemide improves renal perfusion and GFR in experimental models of complete renal ischemia,[188,189] though less effectively than mannitol. One important protective effect of loop diuretics appears to be inhibition in the mTAL of the sodium-potassium-ATPase pump, thereby decreasing active tubular sodium transport and tubular oxygen consumption (see Fig. 21-8).

In established oliguric ARF, furosemide increases urinary output but does not improve outcome or reduce the frequency at which dialysis is required.[45,229,230] Although nonoliguric ARF is associated with lower mortality, there is no evidence that converting oliguric ARF to nonoliguric ARF with the use of diuretics improves outcome. When GFR is low, delivery of furosemide to the renal tubules is impaired, so that high-dose boluses or continuous infusions of furosemide are required to effect diuresis.[231] In patients susceptible to ARF, the greatest risk associated with the administration of diuretics is that chemically induced diuresis, in the absence of adequate volume expansion, may delay effective therapy and further deplete intravascular volume. Furosemide is less controversial in situations in which cellular debris or pigment may cause tubular obstruction and damage. The use of small doses of furosemide (5 to 10 mg intravenously), given in combination with mannitol (see following text), is well established in standard protocols to maintain high urinary flow for the prevention of renal damage in the presence of hemolysis or rhabdomyolysis.

d. Future promising approaches. In addition to the commonly discussed renal protective effects of volume expansion, mannitol, dopamine, and furosemide, a variety of agents have demonstrated efficacy in experimental ARF. The intense investigative activity in this field suggests that improved pharmacologic renal protective therapy will be available within the next few years. Recent reviews address research that may lead to therapeutic progress.[200,232-235] Some of the more promising approaches are summarized.

In the kidney, as in other organs, ischemia causes a potentially toxic increase in intracellular free calcium. Calcium-channel blockers can be either protective or injurious to the kidneys, depending on the experimental or clinical circumstances. Protective effects include the prevention of reflow-induced vasoconstriction after ischemia, inhibition of angiotensin action in the glomerulus, and reduction of circulating interleukin-2 receptors.[236] Pretreatment with calcium-channel blockers limits renal injury produced by experimental complete renal ischemia.[237,238] Diltiazem improved renal function

in patients undergoing cadaveric renal transplantation and conferred important protection against nephrotoxicity induced by cyclosporin A.[239] Nitrendipine conferred renal protection against radiocontrast dye toxicity.[240] In hypertensive patients, including some patients with GFR greater than 80 ml/min, diltiazem and nifedipine produced natriuresis and diuresis; diltiazem actually increased RBF and GFR.[241]

In partial renal ischemia, calcium-channel blockers may produce salutary or deleterious effects, depending on the magnitude of the drug-induced reduction in blood pressure and the cause(s) of renal hypoperfusion.[242-244] In patients with renal insufficiency, nifedipine precipitated nonoliguric renal failure, which improved when the drug was discontinued.[245] Additional clinical evidence is necessary before calcium-channel blockers can be routinely given to patients who must undergo complete renal ischemia.[246]

Renal hypoperfusion reduces the concentration of high-energy phosphates.[247] Infusion of adenine nucleotides in combination with magnesium chloride preserves postischemic renal function.[248,249] Inhibition of 5′-nucleotidase similarly enhances metabolic and functional recovery after renal ischemia.[250] Infusion of fructose-1,6-diphosphate, a high-energy metabolite, also enhanced the ability of the kidney to withstand ischemic injury.[251] Presumably, the renal protective effects of hypothermia also depend on preservation of high-energy phosphates.[252]

Oxygen free radicals, arachidonate metabolites, leukotrienes, and neutrophils have also been implicated in ischemic renal damage. Oxygen free radicals probably are produced in large quantities during and after renal ischemia,[253] an observation that may explain why superoxide dismutase or allopurinol reduce experimental renal ischemic injury when administered before ischemia.[254] Evidence indicates that renal vascular tone is regulated in part by the balance between the synthesis of the vasodilator prostaglandin PGI_2 and the vasoconstrictor TxA_2. Inhibition of TxA_2 synthesis protects against tubular necrosis after experimental ischemia in rats[255] and improves renal function in patients with lupus nephritis.[256] Scavengers of oxygen free radicals also inhibit synthesis of TxA_2 and improve renal outcome in experimental models.[257]

Just as inhibition of the production of vasoconstrictive arachidonate metabolites attenuates experimental renal injury, so too does therapeutic administration of vasodilator prostaglandins such as PGE_2,[256,258] PGE_1,[259,260] and PGI_2.[261]

There is evidence that nitric oxide or, in various forms of ARF, its inhibitors may play a role in prevention or recovery.[262-264] Nitric oxide has been implicated in the prevention of radiocontrast nephrotoxicity in rats.[73] Antbodies to endothelin and intercellular adhesion molecule-1 (ICAM-1) may prove to contribute to prevention of ARF.[262,265,266]

Under specific circumstances, ACE inhibitors exert renal protective effects. As discussed earlier, local release of angiotensin II causes predominantly efferent arteriolar vasoconstriction, which maintains glomerular filtration despite mild to moderate decreases in RBF or perfusion pressure. High levels of angiotensin II cause constriction of the afferent arterioles and the glomerular mesangial cells, which decreases RBF and glomerular surface area, and thereby FF and GFR.[59] By inference, inhibition of the local effects of smaller concentrations of angiotensin II might be harmful, and inhibition of the effects of high circulating levels might ameliorate renal damage. Accordingly, deterioration in renal function with ACE inhibitors has been reported in patients with hypotension, renal insufficiency, or unilateral renal artery stenosis, probably related to the block of compensatory angiotensin-mediated efferent arteriolar constriction.[267] Hyperkalemia can occur in patients with renal insufficiency who receive ACE inhibitors, especially in association with β-blockade. It is wise to avoid ACE inhibitors in patients who are hypovolemic or hypotensive or who have renal vascular occlusive disease or renal insufficiency.

In contrast, Colson et al[268] compared short-term pretreatment with captopril versus placebo in patients without preexisting cardiac or renal failure undergoing coronary revascularization with cardiopulmonary bypass. Renal plasma flow and GFR decreased in the placebo group and remained unaltered in the captopril group. During bypass, urinary excretion of sodium was greater in patients receiving captopril. The authors concluded that additional studies on the protective value of ACE inhibitors are warranted.

Perhaps the most promising category of renal protective agents consists of ANP and its synthetic congeners. In experimental animals, ANP and its congeners ameliorate ischemic or nephrotoxic injury to the kidney, even when administered after insult.[234,269] After 90 minutes of unilateral renal arterial occlusion in dogs, ANP significantly increased CCr, FF, natriuresis, and sodium reabsorption.[270] In nephrotoxic ARF in rats, ANP improved RBF and GFR, induced profound natriuresis, and decreased azotemia and renal histologic damage.[271] Even 2 days after induction of ischemic ARF, a 4-hour infusion of atriopeptin III and dopamine doubled RBF and GFR in comparison to saline controls and decreased SCr to baseline within 2 days after the infusion.[272]

More recent clinical studies have shown an improvement in dialysis-free survival for patients with oliguric, but not nonoliguric, ARF.[272-274] In eight patients who developed ARF after liver transplantation and fulfilled the requirements for hemodialysis, infusion of an ANP congener, urodilatin, resulted in natriuresis and improved electrolyte disturbances, CCr, SCr, and BUN; six patients avoided treatment but two patients still required renal replacement therapy.[275] Allgren et al[274] recently published a multicenter, randomized, double-blind, placebo-controlled clinical trial of anaritide, a 25-amino-acid synthetic form of ANP, in 504 critically ill patients with ATN. All patients received a 24-hour intravenous infusion of either anaritide ($0.2 \ \mu g \cdot kg^{-1} \cdot min^{-1}$) or placebo. In patients with oliguria (urinary output less than 400 ml per day), dialysis-free survival was 8% in the placebo group and 27% in the anaritide group ($p = 0.008$). In patients without oliguria, anaritide appeared to worsen survival (59% in the placebo group versus 48% in the anaritide group). In nonoliguric patients, anaritide induced a greater decrease in blood pressure (which may have reduced renal perfusion) and reduced urinary output, whereas in oliguric patients, blood pressure decreased less and urinary output increased.

3. Prevention and treatment algorithms. Although a variety of agents appear promising, clinical application requires cumbersome testing. Clinical ARF is heterogeneous, frequently involving elderly patients with reduced renal reserve and highly variable degrees of renal ischemia. Fig. 21-12 summarizes three general approaches to the prevention of ARF. The left-hand algorithm, similar to that currently used by many clinicians, emphasizes the essential role of volume expansion, supplemented by hemodynamic monitoring and pharmacologic interventions in patients who fail to respond to volume expansion. The middle algorithm, based on extrapolations from the data of Shoemaker et al,[183] depends on prospective identification of high-risk patients rather than waiting for the development of oliguria; in such patients, support of systemic oxygen delivery (DO_2) to achieve a specific target may be justified. The right-hand algorithm combines aggressive hemodynamic support with preventive pharmacotherapy, based on experimental models in which earlier pharmacologic intervention is more effective.

E. Renal replacement therapy

Renal replacement therapy improves most of the medical complications of ARF, including hypervolemia, metabolic acidosis, electrolyte imbalance, muscle weakness, and hypertension. The artificial kidney was developed in 1944 by Kolff and Berk; by 1960 dialysis medicine was an established area of specialization.[276] Widespread hemodialysis was established in 1973 when Medicare extended coverage to all patients with end-stage renal disease (ESRD). In 1995, 205,000 patients were enrolled in chronic hemodialysis programs in the United States. Approximately 10,000 renal transplants are performed annually in the United States.[277]

The two basic modalities used in renal replacement therapy are dialysis and ultrafiltration.[278] The dialysis principle involves equilibration of circulating blood constituents (e.g., potassium or catabolic products) with dialysate across a semipermeable membrane. The ionic content and tonicity of the dialysate may be altered based on the patient's electrolyte and volume status. Ultrafiltration removes fluid and solutes in bulk, with filtration of solutes dependent on molecular size. The variety of techniques for renal replacement currently provides the ability to select a specific modality based on a patient's clinical condition (Table 21-9). Factors of particular interest in perioperative patients include efficacy in controlling extracellular fluid volume and applicability in patients who are hemodynamically unstable.

Peritoneal dialysis is occasionally used in acute situations but more commonly is used for long-term maintenance of patients with chronic renal failure. The technique requires a peritoneal access catheter and uses the peritoneal lining as the semipermeable membrane, thus

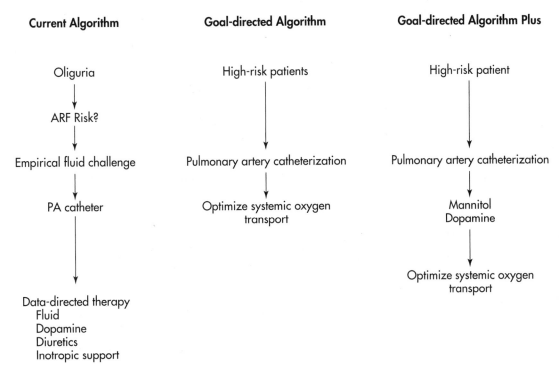

Fig. 21-12. Three possible approaches to prevention of acute renal failure *(ARF)*. The left-hand algorithm is derived from the approach used by many clinicians. Once oliguria is recognized, the diagnostic and therapeutic approach consists of empirical volume expansion, supplemented if necessary by pulmonary artery *(PA)* catheterization, with subsequent data-directed therapy consisting of fluid, dopamine, inotropic support, mannitol, or furosemide. In contrast, the goal-directed algorithm is based on identification of high-risk patients. Such patients would undergo pulmonary artery catheterization with subsequent support of systemic oxygen transport [(cardiac output)(arterial oxygen content)] at levels associated with improved survival in high-risk surgical patients. The right-hand figure combines goal-oriented therapy with early pharmacologic support because of the frequent experimental observation that earlier intervention is more efficacious.

Table 21-9. Types of renal replacement therapy for acute renal failure

Type	Complexity	Efficiency	Cost	Anti-coagulant therapy	Risk of hemorrhage	Risk of infection	ECF volume control	Use in hypo-tension
Peritoneal dialysis	Low	Moderate	Moderate	No	Low	High	Moderate	Yes
Intermittent hemodialysis	Moderate	High	Low	Yes	Moderate	Low	Intermittent	No
Continuous arteriovenous hemofiltration	Moderate	Low and variable	Moderate	Yes	Moderate	Low	Good	No
Continuous arteriovenous hemodialysis with filtration	High	Moderate and variable	High	Yes	Moderate	Low	Good	Variable
Continuous venovenous hemofiltration	Moderate	High	Moderate	Yes	Moderate	Low	Good	Yes
Continuous venovenous hemodialysis with filtration	High	High	High	Yes	Moderate	Low	Good	Yes

From Forni LG, Hilton PJ: *N Engl J Med* 336:1303, 1997.
ECF, Extracellular fluid.

avoiding vascular cannulae and the associated complications. Peritoneal dialysis is less efficient than hemodialysis, so dialysis times are longer. Also, peritonitis is a known complication, and some patients experience abdominal pain during dialysis.

Hemodialysis is more widely used than peritoneal dialysis. The establishment and maintenance of acceptable vascular access frequently require surgery. For acute hemodialysis or continuous techniques (see later text), a double-lumen catheter may be placed into a central vein using standard venous access techniques. For chronic hemodialysis, subcutaneous arteriovenous fistulae have proven to be the best method of access. Approximately 60% of indwelling arteriovenous fistulae will be patent after 1 year.[279] Hemodialysis uses an extracorporeal circuit linked to the patient via an arteriovenous anastomosis. To prevent clotting of the dialysis circuit, heparin is given before dialysis with protamine reversal after dialysis. The patient undergoes dialysis typically for 4 to 5 hours, 3 times per week. During a 5-hour treatment, the dialysate flow rates are about 500 ml/min so that the blood is exposed to 150 L of dialysate fluid. Prospective trials have demonstrated that newer biocompatible dialytic membranes improved recovery from ARF and reduced the mortality rate.[280,281]

Recently, continuous techniques have gained considerable popularity for the management of ARF in critically ill patients. Continuous venovenous hemofiltration (CVVH) uses a pump to generate hydrostatic pressure to remove large quantities of water and solutes across a filter.[278] Because solutes are removed in proportion to their concentration in the plasma ultrafiltrate, the final concentration in blood is then adjusted by infusing fluid in which approximately physiologic concentrations of most constituents are present (Table 21-10). Although the efficiency of CVVH is less than conventional intermittent hemodialysis, those who have extensive experience in using CVVH encounter few if any patients in whom metabolic control cannot be achieved.[278] One of the advantages of CVVH is maintenance of hemodynamic stability during treatment. In trauma patients with the multiple organ dysfunction syndrome, CVVH improved hemodynamic and respiratory variables.[282]

The efficiency of solute removal can be increased by circulating blood through dialysate in a process known as continuous venovenous hemodialysis (CVVHD).[278] Although debate continues about whether this modality is superior to conventional hemodialysis, the ability to remove large quantities of sodium and water while maintaining stable hemodynamics has made CVVH and CVVHD popular with some nephrologists and intensivists. However, the cost of CVVH for a typical episode of ARF is more than double the cost of conventional hemodialysis,[278] a factor that may be acceptable based on preliminary evidence that survival may be better in patients who are treated with CVVH.[283-286]

VI. CONCLUSION

Patients undergoing extensive surgical procedures, especially those involving cardiopulmonary bypass and aortic cross-clamping, are at risk for ARF. The kidneys have substantial ability to maintain renal integrity during intervals of circulatory stress by altering renal vascular resistance in the afferent and efferent arterioles; however, stress of sufficient magnitude and duration will precipitate renal decompensation. The renal medulla, in which oxygen delivery is critically low and metabolic oxygen consumption is relatively high, appears to be the most vulnerable region of the kidney. Although virtually all anesthetic agents and techniques have been associated with a decrease in GFR and urinary output under certain conditions, there is little reason to believe that anesthetic agents play a primary etiologic role in perioperative ARF. Few data describe interactions among the many drugs commonly combined in clinical anesthesia. Specific responses vary with respect to the characteristics of the subjects studied, the control of confounding variables, and the choice of measurement techniques. Surprisingly little is known about the integrity of RBF autoregulation during the administration of various individual anesthetic drugs and combinations of anesthetic drugs and adjuvants.

Prevention of perioperative ARF depends on appropriate monitoring and systemic circulatory support. In the acute, short-term situation, only urinary output is a practical, though certainly imperfect, diagnostic test. Maintenance of adequate circulating blood volume, supplemented when necessary by invasive hemodynamic monitoring, is the approach most likely to avoid ARF. Pharmacologic interventions do not replace, and at present minimally supplement, careful attention to systemic oxygen delivery.

In those patients who nevertheless develop ARF, a variety of renal replacement therapies are available. The continuous forms offer the advantages of providing hemodynamic stability while removing large quantities of water and solutes.

Table 21-10. Typical composition of hemofiltration replacement fluid*

Component	Value (mmol/L)
Sodium	140
Potassium	0
Calcium	1.6
Magnesium	0.75
Chloride	101
Lactate	45
Glucose	11

From Forni LG, Hilton PJ: *N Engl J Med* 336:1303, 1997.
*The values shown are for Gambro Hemofiltrasol 22. Potassium chloride is added to the solution immediately before use in concentrations of up to 4 mmol/L, depending on the serum potassium concentration. To convert the value for calcium to milligrams per deciliter, divide by 0.25; to convert the value for magnesium to milliequivalents per liter, divide by 0.5; and to convert the value for glucose to milligrams per deciliter, divide by 0.05551.

REFERENCES

1. Mazze RI, Schwartz FD, Slocum HC, et al: Renal function during anesthesia and surgery. I. The effects of halothane anesthesia, *Anesthesiology* 24:279, 1963.
2. Deutsch S, Bastron RD, Pierce EC II, et al: The effects of anaesthesia with thiopentone, nitrous oxide, narcotics and neuromuscular blocking drugs on renal function in normal man, *Br J Anaesth* 41:807, 1969.
3. Klahr S, Miller SB: Acute oliguria, *N Engl J Med* 338:671, 1998.
4. Thadhani R, Pascual M, Bonventre JV: Acute renal failure, *N Engl J Med* 334:1448, 1996.
5. Novis BK, Roizen MF, Aronson S, et al: Association of preoperative risk factors with postoperative acute renal failure, *Anesth Analg* 78:143, 1994.
6. Mindell JA, Chertow GM: A practical approach to acute renal failure, *Med Clin North Am* 81:731, 1997.
7. Brady HR, Singer GG: Acute renal failure, *Lancet* 346:1533, 1995.
8. Charlson ME, MacKenzie CR, Gold JP, et al: Postoperative changes in serum creatinine. When do they occur and how much is important? *Ann Surg* 209:328, 1989.
9. Hou SH, Bushinsky DA, Wish JB, et al: Hospital-acquired renal insufficiency: a prospective study, *Am J Med* 74:243, 1983.
10. Pascual J, Liaño F, Ortuño J: The elderly patient with acute renal failure, *J Am Soc Nephrol* 6:144, 1995.
11. Crawford ES, Walker HS III, Salch SA, et al: Graft replacement of aneurysm in descending thoracic aorta: results without bypass or shunting, *Surgery* 89:73, 1981.
12. Carlson DE, Karp RB, Kouchoukos NT: Surgical treatment of aneurysms of the descending thoracic aorta: an analysis of 85 patients, *Ann Thorac Surg* 35:58, 1983.
13. Crawford ES, Crawford JL, Safi HJ, et al: Thoracoabdominal aortic aneurysms: preoperative and intraoperative factors determining immediate and long-term results of operations in 605 patients, *J Vasc Surg* 3:389, 1986.
14. Svensson LG, Coselli JS, Safi HJ, et al: Appraisal of adjuncts to prevent acute renal failure after surgery on the thoracic or thoracoabdominal aorta, *J Vasc Surg* 10:230, 1989.
15. Sturm JT, Billiar TR, Luxenberg MG, et al: Risk factors for the development of renal failure following the surgical treatment of traumatic aortic rupture, *Ann Thorac Surg* 43:425, 1987.
16. Breckwoldt WL, Mackey WC, Belkin M, et al: The effect of suprarenal cross-clamping on abdominal aortic aneurysm repair, *Arch Surg* 127:520, 1992.
17. Koning HM, Koning AJ, Leusink JA: Serious acute renal failure following open heart surgery, *Thorac Cardiovasc Surgeon* 33:283, 1985.
18. Heikkinen L, Harjula A, Merikallio E: Acute renal failure related to open-heart surgery, *Ann Chir Gynaecol* 74:203, 1985.
19. Mangano CM, Diamondstone LS, Ramsay JG, et al: Renal dysfunction after myocardial revascularization: risk factors, adverse outcomes, and hospital resource utilization. The Multicenter Study of Perioperative Ischemia Research Group, *Ann Intern Med* 128:194, 1998.
20. Chertow GM, Lazarus JM, Christiansen CL, et al: Preoperative renal risk stratification, *Circulation* 95:878, 1997.
21. Higgins TL, Estafanous FG, Loop FD, et al: Stratification of morbidity and mortality outcome by preoperative risk factors in coronary artery bypass patients: a clinical severity score, *JAMA* 267:2344, 1992.
22. Kasiske BL, Kjellstrand CM: Perioperative management of patients with chronic renal failure and postoperative acute renal failure, *Urol Clin North Am* 10:35, 1983.
23. Abreo K, Moorthy AV, Osborne M: Changing patterns and outcome of acute renal failure requiring hemodialysis, *Arch Intern Med* 146:1338, 1986.
24. Cameron JS: Acute renal failure in the intensive care unit today, *Intensive Care Med* 12:64, 1986.
25. Cioffi WG, Ashikaga T, Gamelli RL: Probability of surviving postoperative acute renal failure, *Ann Surg* 200:205, 1984.
26. Lohr JW, McFarlane MJ, Grantham JJ: A clinical index to predict survival in acute renal failure patients requiring dialysis, *Am J Kidney Dis* 3:254, 1988.
27. Druml W: Prognosis of acute renal failure 1975-1995, *Nephron* 73:8, 1996.
28. Lameire N, Hoste E, Loo AV, et al: Pathophysiology, causes, and prognosis of acute renal failure in the elderly, *Ren Fail* 18:333, 1996.
29. Gelman S: Preserving renal function during surgery, *Anesth Analg* 74:88, 1992.
30. Levy EM, Viscoli CM, Horwitz RI: The effect of acute renal failure on mortality: a cohort analysis, *JAMA* 275:1489, 1996.
31. Dawson JL: The incidence of postoperative renal failure in obstructive jaundice, *Br J Surg* 52:663, 1965.
32. McMurray SD, Luft FC, Maxwell DR, et al: Prevailing patterns and predictor variables in patients with acute tubular necrosis, *Arch Intern Med* 138:950, 1978.
33. Morris JA Jr, Mucha P Jr, Ross SE, et al: Acute posttraumatic renal failure: a multicenter perspective, *J Trauma* 31:1584, 1991.
34. Hamel MB, Phillips RS, Davis RB, et al: Outcomes and cost-effectiveness of initiating dialysis and continuing aggressive care in seriously ill hospitalized adults, *Ann Intern Med* 127:195, 1997.
35. Heyman SN, Fuchs S, Brezis M: The role of medullary ischemia in acute renal failure, *New Horiz* 3:597, 1995.
36. Lote CJ, Harper L, Savage COS: Mechanisms of acute renal failure, *Br J Anaesth* 77:82, 1996.
37. Hamaji M, Nakamura M, Izukura M, et al: Autoregulation and regional blood flow of the dog during hemorrhagic shock, *Circ Shock* 19:245, 1986.
38. Vander AJ: *Renal physiology,* New York, 1995, McGraw-Hill.
39. Leichtweiss HP, Lübbers DW, Weiss C, et al: The oxygen supply of the rat kidney: measurements of intrarenal Po_2, *Pflugers Arch* 309:328, 1969.
40. Baumgärtl H, Leichtweiss HP, Lübbers DW, et al: The oxygen supply of the dog kidney: measurements of intrarenal Po_2, *Microvasc Res* 4:247, 1972.
41. Anderson S: Relevance of single nephron studies to human glomerular function, *Kidney Int* 45:384, 1994.
42. Arendshorst WJ, Finn WF, Gottschalk CW: Autoregulation of blood flow in the rat kidney, *Am J Physiol* 228:127: 1975.
43. Badr KF, Ichikawa I: Prerenal failure: a deleterious shift from renal compensation to decompensation, *N Engl J Med* 319:623, 1988.
44. Thurau K, Boylan JW: Acute renal success: the unexpected logic of oliguria in acute renal failure, *Am J Med* 61:308, 1976.
45. Shiliday I, Allison MEM: Diuretics in acute renal failure, *Ren Fail* 16:3, 1994.
46. Memoli B, Libetta C, Conte G, et al: Loop diuretics and renal vasolidators in acute renal failure, *Nephrol Dial Transplant* 9(suppl):168, 1994.
47. Stone AM, Stahl WM: Renal effect of hemorrhage in normal man, *Ann Surg* 172:825, 1970.
48. Inagami T: Atrial natriuretic factor as a volume regulator, *J Clin Pharmacol* 34:424, 1994.
49. Ardaillou R, Dussaule JC: Role of atrial natriuretic peptide in the control of sodium balance in chronic renal failure, *Nephron* 66:249, 1994.
50. Kamel KS, Quaggin S, Scheich A, et al: Disorders of potassium homeostasis: an approach based on pathophysiology, *Am J Kidney Dis* 24:597, 1994.
51. Vallotton MB, Rossier MF, Capponi AM: Potassium-angiotensin interplay in the regulation of aldosterone biosynthesis, *Clin Endocrinol* 42:111, 1995.
52. Laragh JH: Renin-angiotensin-aldosterone system for blood pressure and electrolyte homeostasis and its involvement in hypertension, in congestive heart failure and in associated cardiovascular damage (myocardial infarction and stroke), *J Hum Hypertens* 9:385, 1995.
53. Müller J: Aldosterone: the minority hormone of the adrenal cortex, *Steroids* 60:2, 1995.
54. Franci CR: Aspects of neural and hormonal control of water and sodium balance, *Braz J Med Biol Res* 27:885, 1994.
55. Fried LF, Palevsky PM: Hyponatremia and hypernatremia. In Saklayen MG, ed: *The Medical Clinics of North America: renal disease,* Philadelphia, 1997, WB Saunders, p 585.

56. Aukland K, Kirkebo A, Loyning E, et al: Effect of hemorrhagic hypotension on the distribution of renal cortical blood flow in anesthetized dogs, *Acta Physiol Scand* 87:514, 1973.

57. Henrich WL, Pettinger WA, Cronin RE: The influence of circulating catecholamines and prostaglandins on canine renal hemodynamics during hemorrhage, *Circ Res* 48:424, 1981.

58. Henrich WL, Anderson RJ, Berns AS, et al: The role of renal nerves and prostaglandins in control of renal hemodynamics and plasma renin activity during hypotensive hemorrhage in the dog, *J Clin Invest* 61:744, 1978.

59. Badr KF, Ichikawa I: Mechanisms of disease. Prerenal failure: a deleterious shift from renal compensation to decompensation, *N Engl J Med* 319:623, 1988.

60. Brezis M, Rosen S, Epstein F: The pathophysiologic implications of medullary hypoxia, *Am J Kidney Dis* 13:253, 1989.

61. Salazar FJ, Romero JC, Burnett JC Jr: Atrial natriuretic peptide levels during acute and chronic saline loading in conscious dogs, *Am J Physiol* 251:R499, 1986.

62. Needleman P, Greenwald JE: Atriopeptin: a cardiac hormone intimately involved in fluid, electrolyte, and blood-pressure homeostasis, *N Engl J Med* 314:828, 1986.

63. Roy LF, Ogilvie RI, Larochelle P: Cardiac and vascular effects of atrial natriuretic factor and sodium nitroprusside in healthy men, *Circulation* 79:383, 1989.

64. Cernacek P, Maher E, Crawhall JC, et al: Renal dose response and pharmacokinetics of atrial natriuretic factor in dogs, *Am J Physiol* 255:R929, 1988.

65. Shenker Y: Atrial natriuretic hormone effect on renal function and aldosterone secretion in sodium depletion, *Am J Physiol* 255:R867, 1988.

66. Schramek H, Coroneos E, Dunn MJ: Interactions of the vasoconstrictor peptides, angiotensin II and endothelin-1, with vasodilatory prostaglandins, *Semin Nephrol* 15:195, 1995.

67. Scharschmidt LA, Lianos E, Dunn MJ: Arachidonate metabolites and the control of glomerular function, *Fed Proc* 42:3058, 1983.

68. Murray MD, Brater DC: Adverse effect of nonsteroidal anti-inflammatory drugs on renal function, *Ann Intern Med* 112:559, 1990.

69. Clive D, Stoff J: Renal syndromes associated with nonsteroidal antiinflammatory drugs, *N Engl J Med* 310:563, 1984.

70. Feldman HI, Kinman JL, Berlin JA, et al: Parenteral ketorolac: the risk for acute renal failure, *Ann Intern Med* 126:193, 1997.

71. Jaquenod M, Ronnhedh C, Cousins MJ, et al: Factors influencing ketorolac-associated perioperative renal dysfunction, *Anesth Analg* 86:1090, 1998.

72. Morrissey JJ, McCracken R, Kaneto H, et al: Location of an inducible nitric oxide synthase mRNA in the normal kidney, *Kidney Int* 45:998, 1994.

73. Agmon Y, Peleg H, Greenfeld Z, et al: Nitric oxide and prostanoids protect the renal outer medulla from radiocontrast toxicity in the rat, *J Clin Invest* 94:1069, 1994.

74. Brezis M, Heyman SN, Dinour D, et al: Role of nitric oxide in renal medullary oxygenation: studies in isolated and intact rat kidneys, *J Clin Invest* 88:390, 1991.

75. Lerman A, Burnett JC Jr: Intact and altered endothelium in regulation of vasomotion, *Circulation* 86:III12, 1992.

76. Scherrer U, Randin D, Vollenweider P, et al: Nitric oxide release accounts for insulin's vascular effects in humans, *J Clin Invest* 94:2511, 1994.

77. Wang YX, Brooks DP, Edwards RM: Attenuated glomerular cGMP production and renal vasodilation in streptozotocin-induced diabetic rats, *Am J Physiol* 264:R952, 1993.

78. Sladen RN: Effect of anesthesia and surgery on renal function, *Crit Care Clin* 3:373, 1987.

79. Philbin D, Coggins CH: Plasma antidiuretic hormone levels in cardiac surgical patients during morphine and halothane anesthesia, *Anesthesiology* 49:95, 1978.

80. Vatner SF, Braunwald E: Cardiovascular control mechanisms in the conscious state, *N Engl J Med* 293:970, 1975.

81. Marquez JM, Douglas ME, Downs JB, et al: Renal function and cardiovascular responses during positive airway pressure, *Anesthesiology* 50:393, 1979.

82. Priebe H-J, Heimann JC, Hedley-Whyte J: Mechanisms of renal dysfunction during positive end-expiratory pressure ventilation, *J Appl Physiol* 50:643, 1981.

83. Andrivet P, Adnot S, Brun-Buisson C, et al: Involvement of ANF in the acute antidiuresis during PEEP ventilation, *J Appl Physiol* 65:1967, 1988.

84. Payen DM, Farge D, Beloucif S, et al: No involvement of antidiuretic hormone in acute antidiuresis during PEEP ventilation in humans, *Anesthesiology* 66:17, 1987.

85. Cousins MJ, Mazze RI: Methoxyflurane nephrotoxicity: a study of dose response in man, *JAMA* 225:1611, 1973.

86. Cousins MJ, Greenstein LR, Hitt BA, et al: Metabolism and renal effects of enflurane in man, *Anesthesiology* 44:44, 1976.

87. Lundeen G, Manohar M, Parks C: Systemic distribution of blood flow in swine while awake and during 1.0 and 1.5 MAC isoflurane anesthesia with or without 50% nitrous oxide, *Anesth Analg* 62:499, 1983.

88. Gelman S, Fowler KC, Smith LR: Regional blood flow during isoflurane and halothane anesthesia, *Anesth Analg* 63:557, 1984.

89. Mazze RI, Calverley RK, Smith NT: Inorganic fluoride nephrotoxicity: prolonged enflurane and halothane anesthesia in volunteers, *Anesthesiology* 46:265, 1977.

90. Mazze RI, Woodruff RE, Heerdt ME: Isoniazid-induced enflurane defluorination in humans, *Anesthesiology* 57:5, 1982.

91. Theye RA, Maher FT: The effects of halothane on canine renal function and oxygen consumption, *Anesthesiology* 35:54, 1971.

92. Ohmura A, Wong KC, Pace NL, et al: Effects of halothane and sodium nitroprusside on renal function and autoregulation, *Br J Anaesth* 54:103, 1982.

93. Priano LL: Effect of halothane on renal hemodynamics during normovolemia and acute hemorrhagic hypovolemia, *Anesthesiology* 63:357, 1985.

94. Kharasch ED, Hankins DC, Thummel KE: Human kidney methoxyflurane and sevoflurane metabolism: intrarenal fluoride production as a possible mechanism of methoxyflurane nephrotoxicity, *Anesthesiology* 82:689, 1995.

95. Bito H, Ikeuchi Y, Ikeda K: Effect of low-flow sevoflurane anesthesia on renal function, *Anesthesiology* 86:1231, 1997.

96. Ebert TJ, Messana LD, Uhrich TD, et al: Absence of renal and hepatic toxicity after four hours of 1.25 minimum alveolar anesthetic concentration sevoflurane anesthesia in volunteers, *Anesth Analg* 86:662, 1998.

97. Ebert TJ, Fink EJ Jr, Kharasch ED: Absence of biochemical evidence for renal and hepatic dysfunction after 8 hours of 1.25 minimum alveolar concentration sevoflurane anesthesia in volunteers, *Anesthesiology* 88:601, 1998.

98. Eger EI II, Gong D, Koblin DD, et al: Dose-related biochemical markers of renal injury after sevoflurane versus desflurane anesthesia in volunteers, *Anesth Analg* 85:1154, 1997.

99. Lebowitz PW, Cote ME, Daniels AL, et al: Comparative renal effects of midazolam and thiopental in humans, *Anesthesiology* 59:381, 1983.

100. Priano LL: Alteration of renal hemodynamics by thiopental, diazepam, and ketamine in conscious dogs, *Anesth Analg* 61:853, 1982.

101. Petersen JS, Shalmi M, Christensen S, et al: Comparison of the renal effects of six sedating agents in rats, *Physiol Behav* 60:759, 1996.

102. Booke M, Armstrong C, Hinder F, et al: The effects of propofol on hemodynamics and renal blood flow in healthy and in septic sheep, and combined with fentanyl in septic sheep, *Anesth Analg* 82:738, 1996.

103. Costela JL, Jimenez R, Calvo R, et al: Serum protein binding of propofol in patients with renal failure or hepatic cirrhosis, *Acta Anaesthesiol Scand* 40:741, 1996.

104. Bidwai AV, Stanley TH, Bloomer HA, et al: Effects of anesthetic doses of morphine on renal function in the dog, *Anesth Analg* 54:357, 1975.

105. Hunter JM, Jones RS, Utting JE: Effect of anaesthesia with nitrous oxide in oxygen and fentanyl on renal function in the artificially ventilated dog, *Br J Anaesth* 52:343, 1980.

106. Priano LL: Effects of high-dose fentanyl on renal haemodynamics in conscious dogs, *Can Anaesth Soc J* 30:10, 1983.

107. Pearce CJ, Gonzalez FM, Wallin JD: Renal failure and hyperkalemia associated with ketorolac tromethamine, *Arch Intern Med* 153:1000, 1993.
108. Quan DJ, Kayser SR: Ketorolac induced acute renal failure following a single dose, *J Toxicol Clin Toxicol* 32:305,1994.
109. Haragsim L, Dalal R, Bagga H, et al: Ketorolac-induced acute renal failure and hyperkalemia: report of three cases, *Am J Kidney Dis* 24:578, 1994.
110. Goldfarb S, Henrich WL: Update in nephrology, *Ann Intern Med* 128:49, 1998.
111. Sivarajan M, Amory DW, Lindbloom LE: Systemic and regional blood flow during epidural anesthesia without epinephrine in the rhesus monkey, *Anesthesiology* 45:300, 1976.
112. Kennedy WF Jr, Sawyer TK, Gerbershagen HY, et al: Systemic cardiovascular and renal hemodynamic alterations during peridural anesthesia in normal man, *Anesthesiology* 31:414, 1969.
113. Kellen M, Aronson S, Roizen MF, et al: Predictive and diagnostic tests of renal failure: a review, *Anesth Analg* 78:134, 1994.
114. Sladen RN, Endo E, Harrison T: Two-hour versus 22-hour creatinine clearance in critically ill patients, *Anesthesiology* 67:1013, 1987.
115. Shin B, Mackenzie CF, Helrich M: Creatinine clearance for early detection of posttraumatic renal dysfunction, *Anesthesiology* 64:605, 1986.
116. Bryan AG, Bolsin SN, Vianna PTG, et al: Modification of the diuretic and natriuretic effects of a dopamine infusion by fluid loading in preoperative cardiac surgical patients, *J Cardiothorac Vasc Anesth* 9:158, 1995.
117. Vander AJ: Control of renin release, *Physiol Rev* 47:359, 1967.
118. Thurau K, Schnermann J, Nagel W, et al: Composition of tubular fluid in the macula densa segment as a factor regulating the function of the juxtaglomerular apparatus, *Circ Res* 20:79, 1967.
119. Edwards BS, Zimmerman RS, Schwab TR, et al: Role of atrial peptide system in renal and endocrine adaptation to hypotensive hemorrhage, *Am J Physiol* 254:R56, 1988.
120. Habib BR, Hanet C, Van Mechelen H, et al: Effects of atriopeptin III on renal function, regional blood flows and left ventricular function in conscious dogs in presence or absence of hypovolaemia, *Eur J Clin Invest* 16:461, 1986.
121. Burke TJ, Burnier M, Langberg H, et al: Renal response to shock, *Ann Emerg Med* 15:1397, 1986.
122. Yoshioka T, Yared A, Kon V, et al: Impaired preservation of GFR during hypotension in preexistent renal hypoperfusion, *Am J Physiol* 256:F314, 1989.
123. Myers BD, Moran SM: Hemodynamically mediated acute renal failure, *N Engl J Med* 314:97, 1986.
124. Schrier RW: Acute renal failure, *JAMA* 247:2518, 1982.
125. Cronin RE, Erickson AM, de Torrente A, et al: Norepinephrine-induced acute renal failure: a reversible ischemic model of acute renal failure, *Kidney Int* 14:187, 1978.
126. Olsen TS, Hansen HE: Ultrastructure of medullary tubules in ischemic acute tubular necrosis and acute interstitial nephritis in man, *APMIS* 98:1139, 1990.
127. Hollenberg NK, Adams DF, Oken DE: Acute renal failure due to nephrotoxins, *N Engl J Med* 282:1329, 1970.
128. Williams RH, Thomas CE, Navar LG, et al: Hemodynamic and single nephron function during the maintenance phase of ischemic acute renal failure in the dog, *Kidney Int* 19:503, 1981.
129. Conger JD, Robinette JB: Loss of blood flow autoregulation in acute renal failure (ARF), *Kidney Int* 16:850, 1979.
130. Humes HD: Acute renal failure: prevailing challenges and prospects for the future, *Kidney Int* 48:S26, 1995.
131. Donohoe JF, Venkatachalam MA, Bernard DB, et al: Tubular leakage and obstruction after renal ischemia: structural-functional correlations, *Kidney Int* 13:208, 1978.
132. Thurau K: Pathophysiology of the acutely failing kidney, *Clin Exp Dial Apheresis* 7:9, 1983.
133. Moran SM, Myers BD: Pathophysiology of protracted acute renal failure in man, *J Clin Invest* 76:1440, 1985.
134. Zager RA: Partial aortic ligation: a hypoperfusion model of ischemic acute renal failure and a comparison with renal artery occlusion, *J Lab Clin Med* 110:396, 1987.
135. Zager RA: Alterations of intravascular volume: influence on renal susceptibility to ischemic injury, *J Lab Clin Med* 108:60, 1986.
136. Zager RA: Ischemic acute renal failure: a multifactorial disease? In Solez K, Racusen LC, eds: *Acute renal failure: diagnosis, treatment, and prevention*, New York, 1991, Marcel Dekker, p 149.
137. Prough DS, Zaloga G: Hypovolemia and renal dysfunction. In Benumof JL, Saidman LJ, eds: *Anesthesia and perioperative complications*, St Louis, 1992, Mosby, p 434.
138. Brezis M, Heyman SN, Epstein FH: Determinants of intrarenal oxygenation. II. Hemodynamic effects, *Am J Physiol (Renal Fluid Electrolyte Physiol)* 267:F1063, 1994.
139. Brezis M, Agmon Y, Epstein FH: Determinants of intrarenal oxygenation. I. Effects of diuretics, *Am J Physiol (Renal Fluid Electrolyte Physiol)* 267:F1059, 1994.
140. Rasmussen HH, Ibels LS: Acute renal failure: multivariate analysis of causes and risk factors, *Am J Med* 73:211, 1982.
141. Porter GA, Bennett WM: Nephrotoxic acute renal failure due to common drugs, *Am J Physiol* 241:F1, 1981.
142. Moore RD, Smith CR, Lipsky JJ, et al: Risk factors for nephrotoxicity in patients treated with aminoglycosides, *Ann Intern Med* 100:352, 1984.
143. Matzke GR, Lucarotti RL, Shapiro HS: Controlled comparison of gentamicin and tobramycin nephrotoxicity, *Am J Nephrol* 3:11, 1983.
144. Barza M, Ioannidis JP, Cappelleri JC, et al: Single or multiple daily doses of aminoglycosides: a metaanalysis, *BMJ* 312:338, 1996.
145. Cimino MA, Rotstein C, Slaughter RL, et al: Relationship of serum antibiotic concentrations to nephrotoxicity in cancer patients receiving concurrent aminoglycoside and vancomycin therapy, *Am J Med* 83:1091, 1987.
146. Dillon JJ, Finn WF: Acute renal failure caused by antibacterial, antifungal, and antineoplastic agents. In Solez K, Racusen LC, eds: *Acute renal failure: diagnosis, treatment, and prevention*, New York, 1991, Marcel Dekker, p 49.
147. Ozols RF, Corden BJ, Jacob J, et al: High-dose cisplatin in hypertonic saline, *Ann Intern Med* 100:19, 1984.
148. Weiss RB: Streptozocin: a review of its pharmacology, efficacy, and toxicity, *Cancer Treat Rep* 66:427, 1982.
149. Pitman SW, Frei E: Weekly methotrexate-calcium leucovorin rescue: effect of alkalinization on nephrotoxicity: pharmacokinetics in the CNS: and use in non-Hodgkins lymphoma, *Cancer Treat Rep* 61:695, 1977.
150. Kennedy BJ: Metabolic and toxin effects of mithramycin during tumor therapy, *Am J Med* 49:494, 1970.
151. Benedetti RG, Heilman KJI, Gabow PA: Nephrotoxicity following single dose mithramycin therapy, *Am J Nephrol* 3:277, 1983.
152. Belldegrun A, Webb DE, Austin HAI, et al: Effects of interleukin-2 on renal function in patients receiving immunotherapy for advanced cancer, *Ann Intern Med* 106:817, 1987.
153. Perico N, Dadan J, Remuzzi G: Endothelin mediates the renal vasoconstriction induced by cyclosporine in the rat, *J Am Soc Nephrol* 1:76, 1990.
154. Quesada JR, Talpaz M, Rios A, et al: Clinical toxicity of interferons in cancer patients: a review, *J Clin Oncol* 4:234, 1986.
155. Averbuch SD, Austin HAI, Sherwin SA, et al: Acute interstitial nephritis with the nephrotic syndrome following recombinant leukocyte α interferon therapy for mycosis fungoides, *N Engl J Med* 310:32, 1994.
156. Mann JFE, Goerig M, Brune K, et al: Ibuprofen as an over-the-counter drug: is there a risk for renal injury? *Clin Nephrol* 39:1,1993.
157. Palmer BF, Henrich WL: Clinical acute renal failure with nonsteroidal anti-inflammatory drugs, *Semin Nephrol* 15:214, 1995.
158. Bennett WM, Henrich WL, Stoff JS: The renal effects of nonsteroidal anti-inflammatory drugs: summary and recommendations, *Am J Kidney Dis* 28:S56, 1996.
159. Hricik DE, Browning PJ, Kopelman R, et al: Captopril-induced functional renal insufficiency in patients with bilateral renal-artery stenoses or renal-artery stenosis in a solitary kidney, *N Engl J Med* 308:373, 1983.
160. Coulie P, DePlaen JF, van Ypersele de Strihou C: Captopril-induced acute reversible renal failure, *Nephron* 35:108, 1983.
161. Nuyts GD, Rutsaert RJ, DeBroe ME: Primum non nocere, acute renal failure caused by angiotensin-converting enzyme inhibitors. In Solez K, Racusen LC, eds: *Acute renal failure: diagnosis, treatment, and prevention*, New York, 1991, Marcel Dekker, p 473.

162. VanZee BE, Hoy WE, Talley TE, et al: Renal injury associated with intravenous pyelography in nondiabetic and diabetic patients, *Ann Intern Med* 89:51, 1978.

163. Parfrey PS, Griffiths SM, Barrett BJ, et al: Contrast material–induced renal failure in patients with diabetes mellitus, renal insufficiency, or both: a prospective controlled study, *N Engl J Med* 320:143, 1989.

164. Solomon R, Werner C, Mann D, et al: Effects of saline, mannitol, and furosemide on acute decreases in renal function induced by radiocontrast agents, *N Engl J Med* 331:1416, 1994.

165. Knochel JP, Schlein EM: On the mechanism of rhabdomyolysis in potassium depletion, *J Clin Invest* 51:1750, 1972.

166. Dubrow A, Flamenbaum W: Acute renal failure associated with myoglobinuria and hemoglobinuria. In Brenner BM, Lazarus JM, eds: *Acute renal failure,* New York, 1988, Churchill Livingstone.

167. Feinfeld DA, Cheng JT, Beysolow TD, et al: A prospective study of urine and serum myoglobin levels in patients with acute rhabdomyolysis, *Clin Nephrol* 38:193, 1992.

168. Wu AH, Laios I, Green S, et al: Immunoassays for serum and urine myoglobin: myoglobin clearance assessed as a risk factor for acute renal failure, *Clin Chem* 40:796, 1994.

169. Ellinas PA, Rosner F: Rhabdomyolysis: report of eleven cases, *J Natl Med Assoc* 84:617, 1992.

170. Ron D, Taitelman U, Michaelson MD, et al: Prevention of acute renal failure in traumatic rhadomyolysis, *Arch Intern Med* 144:277, 1984.

171. Lema G, Meneses G, Urzua J, et al: Effects of extracorporeal circulation on renal function in coronary surgical patients, *Anesth Analg* 81:446, 1995.

172. Hilberman M, Myers BD, Carrie BJ, et al: Acute renal failure following cardiac surgery, *J Thorac Cardiovasc Surg* 77:880, 1979.

173. Gamulin Z, Forster A, Morel D, et al: Effects of infrarenal aortic cross-clamping on renal hemodynamics in humans, *Anesthesiology* 61:394, 1984.

174. Gamulin Z, Forster A, Simonet F, et al: Effects of renal sympathetic blockade on renal hemodynamics in patients undergoing major aortic abdominal surgery, *Anesthesiology* 65:688, 1986.

175. Gornick CC Jr, Kjellstrand CM: Acute renal failure complicating aortic aneurysm surgery, *Nephron* 35:145, 1983.

176. McCombs PR, Roberts B: Acute renal failure following resection of abdominal aortic aneurysm, *Surg Gynecol Obstet* 48:175, 1979.

177. Cohen JR, Mannick JA, Couch NP, et al: Abdominal aortic aneurysm repair in patients with preoperative renal failure, *J Vasc Surg* 3:867, 1986.

178. Bush HL Jr, Huse JB, Johnson WC, et al: Prevention of renal insufficiency after abdominal aortic aneurysm resection by optimal volume loading, *Arch Surg* 116:1517, 1981.

179. Sinicrope RA, Serra RM, Engle JE, et al: Mortality of acute renal failure after rupture of abdominal aortic aneurysms, *Am J Surg* 141:240, 1981.

180. Chawla SK, Najafi H, Ing TS, et al: Acute renal failure complicating ruptured abdominal aortic aneurysm, *Arch Surg* 110:521, 1975.

181. Johnson JP, Rokaw MD: Sepsis or ischemia in experimental acute renal failure: what have we learned? *New Horiz* 3:608, 1995.

182. Hesdorffer CS, Milne JF, Meyers AM, et al: The value of Swan-Ganz catheterization and volume loading in preventing renal failure in patients undergoing abdominal aneurysmectomy, *Clin Nephrol* 28:272, 1987.

183. Shoemaker WC, Appel PL, Kram HB, et al: Prospective trial of supranormal values of survivors as therapeutic goals in high-risk surgical patients, *Chest* 94:1176, 1988.

184. Weber A, Schwieger IM, Poinsot O, et al: Sequential changes in renal oxygen consumption and sodium transport during hyperdynamic sepsis in sheep, *Am J Physiol* 262:F965, 1992.

185. Haywood GA, Tighe D, Moss R, et al: Goal directed therapy with dobutamine in a porcine model of septic shock: effects on systemic and renal oxygen transport, *Postgrad Med J* 67(suppl 1):36, 1991.

186. Myers B: Pathogenesis of postischemic acute renal failure in man, *Kidney Int* 16:37, 1983.

187. Burke TJ, Cronin RE, Duchin KL, et al: Ischemia and tubule obstruction during acute renal failure in dogs: mannitol in protection, *Am J Physiol* 238:F305, 1980.

188. Patak RV, Fadem SZ, Lifschitz MD, et al: Study of factors which modify the development of norepinephrine-induced acute renal failure in the dog, *Kidney Int* 15:227, 1979.

189. Hanley MJ, Davidson K: Prior mannitol and furosemide infusion in a model of ischemic acute renal failure, *Am J Physiol* 241:F556, 1981.

190. Sinsteden TD, O'Neil TJ, Hill S, et al: The role of high-energy phosphate in norepinephrine-induced acute renal failure in the dog, *Circ Res* 49:93, 1986.

191. Pass LJ, Eberhart RC, Brown JC, et al: The effect of mannitol and dopamine on the renal response to thoracic aortic cross-clamping, *J Thorac Cardiovasc Surg* 95:608, 1988.

192. Lindner A, Cutler RE, Goodman WG: Synergism of dopamine plus furosemide in preventing acute renal failure in the dog, *Kidney Int* 16:158, 1979.

193. Weimar W, Geerlings W, Bijnen AB, et al: A controlled study on the effect of mannitol on immediate renal function after cadaver donor kidney transplantation, *Transplantation* 35:99, 1983.

194. Tiggeler GWL, Berden JHM, Hoitsma AJ, et al: Prevention of acute tubular necrosis in cadaveric kidney transplantation by the combined used of mannitol and moderate hydration, *Ann Surg* 201:246, 1985.

195. Laragh JH. Atrial natriuretic hormone, the renin-aldosterone axis, and blood pressure-electrolyte homeostasis, *N Engl J Med* 313:1330, 1985.

196. Mason J: The pathophysiology of ischaemic acute renal failure: a new hypothesis about the initiation phase, *Renal Physiol* 9:129, 1986.

197. Johnston PA, Bernard DB, Perrin NS, et al: Prostaglandins mediate the vasodilatory effect of mannitol in the hypoperfused rat kidney, *J Clin Invest* 68:127, 1981.

198. Plusa SM, Clark NW: Prevention of postoperative renal dysfunction in patients with obstructive jaundice: a comparison of mannitol-induced diuresis and oral sodium taurocholate, *J R Coll Surg Edinb* 36:303, 1991.

199. Wait RB, Kahng KU: Renal failure complicating obstructive jaundice, *Am J Surg* 157:256, 1989.

200. Conger JD: Interventions in clinical acute renal failure: what are the data? *Am J Kidney Dis* 26:565, 1995.

201. Gubern JM, Sancho JJ, Sitges-Serra A, et al: A randomized trial on the effect of mannitol on postoperative renal function in patients with obstructive jaundice, *Surgery* 39:44:1988.

202. Behnia R, Koushanpour E, Brunner EA: Effects of hyperosmotic mannitol infusion on hemodynamics of dog kidney, *Anesth Analg* 82:902, 1996.

203. Gelman S: Does mannitol save the kidney? *Anesth Analg* 82:899, 1996.

204. Goldberg LI, Rajfer SI: Dopamine receptors: applications in clinical cardiology, *Circulation* 72:245, 1985.

205. Bello-Reuss E, Higashi Y, Kaneda Y: Dopamine decreases fluid reabsorption in straight portions of rabbit proximal tubule, *Am J Physiol* 242:F634, 1982.

206. Lokhandwala MF, Amenta F: Anatomical distribution and function of dopamine receptors in the kidney, *FASEB J* 5:3023, 1991.

207. Schwartz LB, Gewertz BL: The renal response to low dose dopamine, *J Surg Res* 45:574, 1988.

208. Duke GJ, Briedis JH, Weaver RA. Renal support in critically ill patients: low-dose dopamine or low-dose dobutamine? *Crit Care Med* 22:1919, 1994.

209. Flancbaum L, Choban PS, Dasta JF: Quantitative effects of low-dose dopamine in urine output in oliguric surgical intensive care unit patients, *Crit Care Med* 22:61: 1994.

210. Richer M, Robert S, Lebel M: Renal hemodynamics during norepinephrine and low-dose dopamine infusions in man, *Crit Care Med* 24:1150, 1996.

211. Costa P, Ottino GM, Matani A, et al: Low-dose dopamine during cardiopulmonary bypass in patients with renal dysfunction, *J Cardiothorac Anesth* 4:469, 1990.

212. Hilberman M, Maseda J, Stinson EB, et al: The diuretic properties of dopamine in patients after open-heart operation, *Anesthesiology* 61:489, 1984.

213. ter Wee PM, Smit AJ, Rosman JB, et al: Effect of intravenous infusion of low-dose dopamine on renal function in normal individuals and in patients with renal disease, *Am J Nephrol* 6:42, 1986.

214. Smit AJ: Dopamine in chronic renal failure, *Am J Hypertens* 3:75S, 1990.

215. Paul MD, Mazer CD, Byrick RJ, et al: Influence of mannitol and dopamine on renal function during elective infrarenal aortic cross-clamping in man, *Am J Nephrol* 6:427, 1986.

216. Salem MG, Crooke JW, McLoughlin GA, et al: The effect of dopamine on renal function during aortic cross-clamping, *Ann R Coll Surg Engl* 70:9, 1988.

217. Baldwin L, Henderson A, Hickman P: Effect of postoperative low-dose dopamine on renal function after elective major vascular surgery, *Ann Intern Med* 120:744, 1994.

218. Polson RJ, Park GR, Lindop MJ, et al: The prevention of renal impairment in patients undergoing orthotopic liver grafting by infusion of low dose dopamine, *Anaesthesia* 42:15, 1987.

219. Swygert TH, Roberts LC, Valek TR, et al: Effect of intraoperative low-dose dopamine on renal function in liver transplant recipients, *Anesthesiology* 75:571, 1991.

220. De Los Angeles A, Baquero A, Bannett A, et al: Dopamine (D) Furosemide (F) infusion for prevention of posttransplant oliguric renal failure (TORF), *Kidney Int* 27:339, 1985 (abstract).

221. Chertow GM, Sayegh MH, Allgren RL, et al: Is the administration of dopamine associated with adverse or favorable outcomes in acute renal failure? *Am J Med* 101:49, 1996.

222. Cottee DBF: Is renal dose dopamine protective or therapeutic? No, *Crit Care Clin* 12:687, 1996.

223. Denton MD, Chertow GM, Brady HR: "Renal-dose" dopamine for the treatment of acute renal failures: scientific rationale, experimental studies and clinical trials, *Kidney Int* 49:4, 1996.

224. Myles PS, Buckland MR, Schenk NJ, et al: Effect of "renal-dose" dopamine on renal function following cardiac surgery, *Anaesth Intensive Care* 21:56, 1993.

225. Chiolero R, Borgeat A, Fisher A: Postoperative arrhythmias and risk factors after open heart surgery, *Thorac Cardiovasc Surg* 39:81, 1991.

226. Ghosh S, Gray B, Oduro A, et al: Dopexamine hydrochloride: pharmacology and use in low cardiac output states, *J Cardiothorac Vasc Anesth* 5:382, 1991.

227. Burns A, Gray PA, Bodenham AR, et al: Dopexamine: studies in the general intensive care unit and after liver transplantation, *J Auton Pharmacol* 10(suppl 1):S109, 1990.

228. de Fijter CW, Comans EF, de Vries PM, et al: The effect of fenoldopam on renal haemodynamics and natriuresis in chronic renal failure, *Neth J Med* 36:267, 1990.

229. Brown CB, Ogg CS, Cameron JS: High dose furosemide in acute renal failure: a controlled trial, *Clin Nephrol* 15:90, 1981.

230. Kleinknecht D, Ganeval D, Gonzales-Duque LA, et al: Furosemide in acute oliguric renal failure: a controlled trial, *Nephron* 17:51, 1976.

231. Krasna MJ, Scott GE, Scholz PM, et al: Postoperative enhancement of urinary output in patients with acute renal failure using continuous furosemide therapy, *Chest* 89:294, 1986.

232. Fischereder M, Trick W, Nath KA: Therapeutic strategies in the prevention of acute renal failure, *Semin Nephrol* 14:41, 1994.

233. Rodicio JL, Ruilope LM: Assessing renal effects and renal protection, *J Hypertens* 13:S19, 1995.

234. Alkhunaizi AM, Schrier RW: Management of acute renal failure: new perspectives, *Am J Kidney Dis* 28:315, 1996.

235. Bonventre JV: Mediators of ischemic renal injury, *Annu Rev Med* 39:531, 1988.

236. Neumayer HH, Gellert J, Luft FC: Calcium antagonists and renal protection, *Ren Fail* 15:353, 1993.

237. Goldfarb D, Iaina A, Serban I, et al: Beneficial effect of verapamil in ischemic acute renal failure in the rat, *Proc Soc Exp Biol Med* 172:389, 1983.

238. Silverman M, Rose H, Puschett JB: Modification in proximal tubular function induced by nitrendipine in a rat model of acute ischemic renal failure, *J Cardiovasc Pharmacol* 14:799, 1989.

239. Neumayer HH, Kunzendorf U, Schrieber M: Protective effects of calcium antagonists in human renal transplantation, *Kidney Int* 36:87, 1992.

240. Neumayer HH, Junge W, Kufner A, et al: Prevention of radio-contrast-media-induced nephrotoxicity by the calcium channel blocker nitrendipine: a prospective randomised clinical trial, *Nephrol Dial Transplant* 4:1030, 1989.

241. Bauer JH, Sunderrajan S, Reams G: Effects of calcium entry blockers on renin-angiotensin-aldosterone system, renal function and hemodynamics, salt and water excretion and body fluid composition, *Am J Cardiol* 56:62H, 1985.

242. Leahy AL, Galla J, Fitzpatrick JM, et al: The canine kidney in haemorrhagic shock: effect of verapamil, *Eur Urol* 13:401, 1987.

243. Loutzenhiser RD, Epstein M: Renal hemodynamic effects of calcium antagonists, *Am J Med* 82:23, 1987.

244. Diamond JR, Cheung JY, Fang LST: Nifedipine-induced renal dysfunction. Alterations in renal hemodynamics, *Am J Med* 77:905, 1984.

245. Diamond J, Cheung J, Fang L: Nifedipine-induced renal dysfunction, *Am J Med* 77:905, 1984.

246. Russell JD, Churchill DN: Calcium antagonists and acute renal failure, *Am J Med* 87:306, 1989.

247. Ratcliffe PJ, Moonen CTW, Holloway PAH, et al: Acute renal failure in hemorrhagic hypotension: cellular energetics and renal function, *Kidney Int* 30:355, 1986.

248. Hirasawa H, Odaka M, Soeda K, et al: Experimental and clinical study on ATP-MgCl$_2$ administration for postischemic acute renal failure, *Clin Exp Dial Apheresis* 7:37, 1983.

249. Siegel NJ, Glazier WB, Chaudrey IH, et al: Enhanced recovery from acute renal failure by the postischemic infusion of adenine nucleotides and magnesium chloride in rats, *Kidney Int* 17:338, 1980.

250. van Waarde A, Stromski ME, Thulin G, et al: Protection of the kidney against ischemic injury by inhibition of 5'-nucleotidase, *Am J Physiol* 256:F298, 1989.

251. Didlake R, Kirchner KA, Lewin J, et al: Protection from ischemic renal injury by fructose-1, 6-diphosphate infusion in the rat, *Circ Shock* 16:205, 1985.

252. Zager RA, Gmur DJ, Bredl CR, et al: Degree and time sequence of hypothermic protection against experimental ischemic acute renal failure, *Circ Res* 65:1263, 1989.

253. Canavese C, Stratta P, Vercellone A: The case for oxygen free radicals in the pathogenesis of ischemic acute renal failure, *Nephron* 49:9, 1988.

254. Ratych RE, Bulkley GB: Free-radical-mediated postischemic reperfusion injury in the kidney, *J Free Radic Biol Med* 2:311, 1986.

255. Lelcuk S, Alexander F, Kobzik L, et al: Prostacyclin and thromboxane A$_2$ moderate postischemic renal failure, *Surgery* 98:207, 1985.

256. Pierucci A, Simonetti BM, Pecci G, et al: Improvement of renal function with selective thromboxane antagonism in lupus nephritis, *N Engl J Med* 320:421, 1989.

257. Kaufman RP Jr, Klausner JM, Anner H, et al: Inhibition of thromboxane (Tx) synthesis by free radical scavengers, *J Trauma* 28:458, 1988.

258. Mandal AK, Miller J: Protection against ischemic acute renal failure by prostaglandin infusion, *Prostaglandins Leukot Med* 8:361, 1982.

259. Tobimatsu M, Konomi K, Saito S, et al: Protective effect of prostaglandin E1 on ischemia-induced acute renal failure in dogs, *Surgery* 98:45, 1985.

260. Torsello G, Schror K, Szabo Z, et al: Effects of prostaglandin E1 (PGE1) on experimental renal ischaemia, *Eur J Vasc Surg* 3:5, 1989.

261. Lifschitz MD, Barnes JL: Prostaglandin I$_2$ attenuates ischemic acute renal failure in the rat, *Am J Physiol* 247:F714, 1984.

262. Simon EE: Review: new aspects of acute renal failure, *Am J Med Sci* 310:217, 1995.

263. Raij L, Baylis C: Glomerular actions of nitric oxide, *Kidney Int* 48:20, 1995.

264. Peer G, Blum M, Iaina A: Nitric oxide and acute renal failure, *Nephron* 73:375, 1996.

265. Kon V, Yoshioka T, Fogo A, et al: Glomerular actions of endothelin in vivo, *J Clin Invest* 83:1762, 1989.

266. Kelly KJ, Williams WW Jr, Colvin RB, et al: Intercellular adhesion molecule-1-deficient mice are protected against ischemic renal injury, *J Clin Invest* 97:1056, 1996.

267. Bender W, La France N, Walker WG: Mechanism of deterioration in renal function in patients with renovascular hypertension treated with enalapril, *Hypertension* 6:I193, 1984.

268. Colson P, Ribstein J, Mimran A, et al: Effect of angiotensin converting enzyme inhibition on blood pressure and renal function during open heart surgery, *Anesthesiology* 72:23, 1990.

269. Conger JD: Interventions in clinical acute renal failure: what are the data? *Am J Kidney Dis* 26:565, 1995.

270. Atanasova I, Girchev R, Dimitrov D, et al: Atrial natriuretic peptide and dopamine in a dog model of acute renal ischemia, *Acta Physiol Hung* 82:75, 1994.

271. Seki G, Suzuki K, Nonaka T, et al: Effects of atrial natriuretic peptide on glycerol induced acute renal failure in the rat, *Jpn Heart J* 33:383, 1992.

272. Conger JD, Falk SA, Hammond WS: Atrial natriuretic peptide and dopamine in established acute renal failure in the rat, *Kidney Int* 40:21, 1991.

273. Rahman SN, Kim GE, Mathew AS, et al: Effects of atrial natriuretic peptide in clinical acute renal failure, *Kidney Int* 45:1731, 1994.

274. Allgren RL, Marbury TC, Rahman SN, et al: Anaritide in acute tubular necrosis, *N Engl J Med* 336:828, 1997.

275. Cedidi C, Meyer M, Kuse ER, et al: Urodilatin: a new approach for the treatment of therapy-resistant acute renal failure after liver transplantation, *Eur J Clin Invest* 24:632, 1994.

276. Schreiner GE: Acute renal failure. In Black DAK, ed: *Renal disease*, Philadelphia, 1967, FA Davis, p 309.

277. Rettig RA: End-stage renal disease therapy: an American success story, *JAMA* 275:1118, 1996.

278. Forni LG, Hilton PJ: Continuous hemofiltration in the treatment of acute renal failure, *N Engl J Med* 336:1303, 1997.

279. Fan P-Y, Schwab SJ: Hemodialysis vascular access. In Henrich WL, ed: *Principles and practice of dialysis*, Baltimore, 1994, Williams & Wilkins, p 22.

280. Hakim RM, Wingard RL, Parker RA: Effect of the dialysis membrane in the treatment of patients with acute renal failure, *N Engl J Med* 331:1338, 1994.

281. Schiffl H, Lang SM, König A, et al: Biocompatible membranes in acute renal failure: prospective case-controlled study, *Lancet* 344:570, 1994.

282. Sanchez-Izquierdo Riera JA, Alted E, Lozano MJ, et al: Influence of continuous hemofiltration on the hemodynamics of trauma patients, *Surgery* 122:902, 1997.

283. Barton IK, Hilton PJ, Taub NA, et al: Acute renal failure treated by haemofiltration: factors affecting outcome, *Q J Med* 86:81, 1993.

284. Forni LG, Wright DA, Hilton PJ, et al: Prognostic stratification in acute renal failure, *Arch Intern Med* 156:1023, 1996.

285. McDonald BR, Mehta RL: Decreased mortality in patients with acute renal failure undergoing continuous arteriovenous hemodialysis, *Contrib Nephrol* 93:51, 1991.

286. van Bommel EFH, Bouvy ND, So KL, et al: Acute dialytic support for the critically ill: intermittent hemodialysis versus continuous arteriovenous hemodiafiltration, *Am J Nephrol* 15:192, 1995.

Chapter 22

Perioperative Electrolyte and Acid-Base Abnormalities

John L. Ard, Jr.
Donald S. Prough

I. Electrolyte Abnormalities
  A. Sodium
    1. Regulation of water and sodium
    2. Hyponatremia
      a. Pathophysiology
      b. Clinical features
      c. Causes
      d. Diagnosis
      e. Treatment
    3. Hypernatremia
      a. Pathophysiology
      b. Clinical features
      c. Causes
      d. Diagnosis
      e. Treatment
  B. Potassium
    1. Potassium homeostasis
    2. Hypokalemia
      a. Pathophysiology
      b. Clinical features
      c. Diagnosis
      d. Treatment
    3. Hyperkalemia
      a. Pathophysiology
      b. Clinical features
      c. Diagnosis
      d. Treatment
  C. Calcium
    1. Calcium homeostasis
    2. Physiologic actions of calcium
    3. Hypocalcemia
      a. Pathophysiology
      b. Clinical features
      c. Diagnosis
      d. Treatment
    4. Hypercalcemia
      a. Pathophysiology
      b. Clinical features
      c. Treatment
  D. Magnesium
    1. Physiologic considerations
    2. Hypomagnesemia
      a. Pathophysiology
      b. Clinical features
      c. Diagnosis
      d. Treatment
    3. Hypermagnesemia
      a. Pathophysiology
      b. Clinical features
      c. Diagnosis
      d. Treatment
  E. Phosphate
    1. Physiologic considerations
    2. Hypophosphatemia
      a. Pathophysiology
      b. Clinical features
      c. Diagnosis
      d. Treatment
    3. Hyperphosphatemia
      a. Pathophysiology
      b. Clinical features
      c. Diagnosis
      d. Treatment
II. Acid-Base Disorders and Treatment
  A. Overview of Acid-Base Equilibrium
    1. Metabolic alkalosis
    2. Metabolic acidosis
    3. Respiratory alkalosis
    4. Respiratory acidosis
  B. Rapid Bedside Analysis of Acid-Base Status
  C. Example
III. Summary

Disorders of the internal milieu occur commonly in surgical patients. Many patients, because of chronic underlying diseases or previous medical treatment, have preoperative disorders of electrolytes and acid-base status. Others undergo acute physiologic changes in response to acute surgical illness. During surgery, hemorrhage, infusion of intravenous fluids, and substitution of mechanical ventilation for spontaneous ventilation represent additional stresses that may disrupt homeostasis. Surgical patients require replacement of fluid and electrolyte losses secondary to blood loss, wound or burn edema, ascites, and loss of gastrointestinal (GI) secretions.

If sufficiently severe, abnormalities of electrolytes and acid-base status may increase the likelihood of perioperative mortality and morbidity. Consequently, one key responsibility of anesthesiologists is prompt diagnosis and effective treatment of abnormalities in the concentrations of sodium, potassium, calcium, magnesium, phosphate, hydrogen ion, bicarbonate, and $Paco_2$. This chapter reviews the diagnosis, physiologic implications, and treatment of excesses or deficits of these important substances.

I. ELECTROLYTE ABNORMALITIES
A. Sodium

Sodium, the principal extracellular cation, is the main determinant of plasma osmolality. Plasma osmolality (P_{Osm}), which expresses the ratio of solute content to water, is calculated as follows:

$$P_{Osm} = 2([Na^+]) + (P_{glu} \div 18) + (BUN \div 2.8) \quad (22\text{-}1)$$

where:

$[Na^+]$ = sodium concentration
P_{glu} = plasma glucose
BUN = blood urea nitrogen

An increase or decrease in total body sodium tends to increase or decrease extracellular volume and plasma volume. In contrast, changes in $[Na^+]$ primarily reflect changes in total body water. Total body water, which in adults approximates 60% of total body weight, includes intracellular volume (40% of total body weight) and extracellular volume (20% of body weight). Extracellular volume contains most of total body sodium, with equal $[Na^+]$ in the plasma volume (4% of total body weight) and interstitial fluid volume (16% of total body weight). The predominant intracellular cation, potassium, has an intracellular concentration ($[K^+]$) approximating 150 mEq/L.

1. Regulation of water and sodium. Total body water content is regulated by the intake and output of water. Water intake includes ingested liquids plus an average of 750 ml ingested in solid food and 350 ml that is generated metabolically.[1] Insensible losses are normally 1 L/day, and GI losses are 100 to 150 ml/day. Thirst, the primary mechanism of controlling water intake, is triggered by an increase in body fluid tonicity or by a decrease in extracellular volume.[2]

Renal water handling can be conceptualized as having three components: delivery of fluid to the diluting segments of the nephron, separation of solute and water in the diluting segment, and variable reabsorption of water in the collecting ducts.[2] Renal regulation of water output begins as tubular fluid is concentrated in the descending loop of Henle, from which water is reabsorbed while solute is retained to achieve a final osmolality of tubular fluid of approximately 1200 mOsm/kg (Fig. 22-1). This

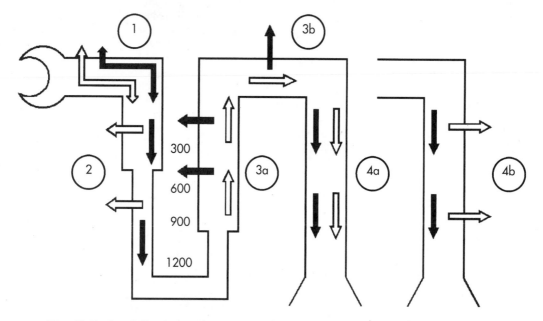

Fig. 22-1. Renal filtration, reabsorption, and excretion of water. Open arrows represent water and solid arrows represent electrolytes. Water and electrolytes are filtered by the glomerulus. In the proximal tubule *(1)*, water and electrolytes are absorbed isotonically. In the descending loop of Henle *(2)*, water is absorbed to achieve osmotic equilibrium with the interstitium while electrolytes are retained. The numbers (300, 600, 900, and 1200) between the descending and ascending limbs represent the osmolality of the interstitium (in mOsm/kg). The delivery of solute and fluid to the distal nephron is a function of proximal tubular reabsorption; as proximal tubular reabsorption increases, delivery of solute to the medullary *(3a)* and cortical *(3b)* diluting sites decreases. In the diluting sites, electrolyte-free water is generated through selective reabsorption of electrolytes while water is retained in the tubular lumen, generating a dilute tubular fluid. In the absence of vasopressin, the collecting duct *(4a)* remains impermeable to water and a dilute urine is excreted. When vasopressin acts on the collecting ducts *(4b)*, water is reabsorbed from these vasopressin-responsive nephron segments, allowing the excretion of a concentrated urine. (From Fried LF, Palevsky PM: Hyponatremia and hypernatremia. In Saklayen MG, ed: *The Medical Clinics of North America: renal disease,* Philadelphia, 1997, WB Saunders.)

concentrated fluid is then diluted by the active reabsorption of electrolytes in the ascending limb of the loop of Henle and in the distal tubule, both of which are largely impermeable to water.[2] As fluid exits the distal tubule and enters the collecting duct, osmolality is approximately 50 mOsm/kg. Within the collecting duct water reabsorption is modulated by antidiuretic hormone (ADH, also called vasopressin). Vasopressin binds to V_2 receptors along the basolateral membrane of the collecting duct cells,[3] then stimulates the synthesis and insertion of the aquaporin-2 water channel into the luminal membrane of collecting duct cells.[3-5]

Plasma hypotonicity suppresses ADH release, resulting in excretion of dilute urine. Hypertonicity stimulates ADH secretion, which increases the permeability of the collecting duct to water and enhances water reabsorption. In response to changing plasma $[Na^+]$, changing secretion of ADH can vary urinary osmolality from 50 to 1200 mOsm/kg and urinary volume from 0.4 to 20 L/day (Fig. 22-2). Other factors that stimulate ADH secretion, though none as powerfully as plasma tonicity, include hypotension, hypovolemia, and nonosmotic stimuli such as nausea, pain, and medications, including opiates.[2]

Two powerful hormonal systems regulate total body sodium. The renin-angiotensin-aldosterone axis defends against sodium depletion and hypovolemia and the natriuretic peptides (atrial natriuretic peptide [ANP], brain natriuretic peptide, and C-type natriuretic peptide) defend against sodium overload.[6] Aldosterone is the final common pathway in a complex response to decreased effective arterial volume, whether decreased effective arterial volume is true or relative (as in edematous states or hypoalbuminemia). In this pathway, decreased stretch in the baroreceptors of the aortic arch and carotid body and stretch receptors in the great veins, pulmonary vasculature, and atria result in increased sympathetic tone. Increased sympathetic tone, in combination with decreased renal perfusion, leads to renin release and formation of angiotensin I from angiotensinogen.[7] Angiotensin-converting enzyme (ACE) converts angiotensin I to angiotensin II, which stimulates the adrenal cortex to synthesize and release aldosterone.[8] Acting primarily in the distal tubules, high concentrations of aldosterone cause sodium reabsorption[8] (Fig. 22-3) and may reduce urinary excretion of sodium nearly to zero.

Released in response to increased atrial stretch (hypervolemia), ANP increases renal excretion of sodium and water to decrease plasma volume.[9] Even in patients with chronic renal insufficiency, infusion of ANP in low, nonhypotensive doses increases sodium excretion and augments urinary losses of retained solutes (Fig. 22-4).[10] Intrarenal physical factors are also important in regulating sodium balance. Sodium loading decreases colloid osmotic pressure, thereby increasing the glomerular filtration rate (GFR), decreasing net sodium reabsorption, and increasing distal sodium delivery, which, in turn, suppresses renin secretion.[8]

2. Hyponatremia

a. Pathophysiology. Hyponatremia ($[Na^+]$ less than 130 mEq/L) indicates that body fluids are diluted by an excess of water relative to total solute. Most hyponatremia results from impaired urinary diluting capacity, although the causes of the impairment are diverse. It is important to recognize that hyponatremia is not equivalent to sodium depletion; in fact, most hospitalized patients with hyponatremia have normal or increased quantities of total body sodium.

b. Clinical features. Hyponatremia is the most common electrolyte disturbance in hospitalized patients.[11] In one series of hyponatremic patients, the postoperative state was the most common association (30% of patients), followed by acute intracranial disease (17%), malignant disease (17%), medications (9%), and pneumonia (5%).[11] Although hyponatremia is associated with a sevenfold to sixtyfold increase in mortality,[11,12] it is unclear whether the increased mortality is a direct effect of hy-

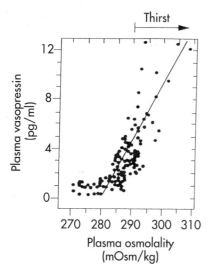

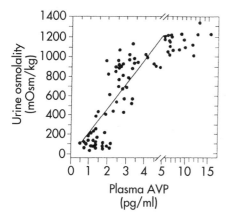

Fig. 22-2. *Top:* Relationship between plasma osmolality and plasma vasopressin (*AVP;* also called ADH). *Bottom:* Relationship between plasma AVP and urinary osmolality. (From Fried LF, Palevsky PM: Hyponatremia and hypernatremia. In Saklayen MG, ed: *The Medical Clinics of North America: renal disease,* Philadelphia, 1997, WB Saunders.)

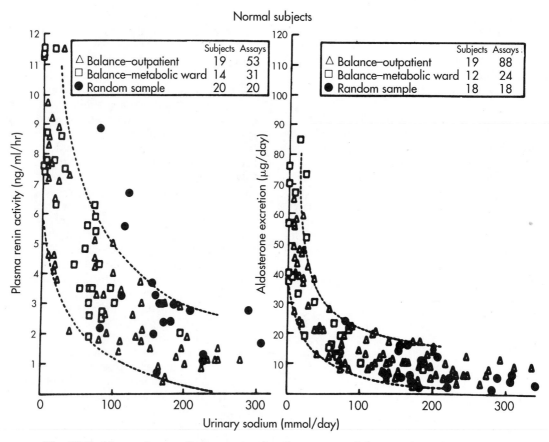

Fig. 22-3. Mean urinary sodium excretion for given ranges of plasma renin activity and urinary aldosterone excretion in humans. Aldosterone exerts a regulatory effect on urinary sodium excretion even at low levels of secretory activity and high levels of sodium excretion. (From Laragh JH: *J Hypertens* 4[suppl 2]:S143, 1986.)

ponatremia or whether hyponatremia simply serves as a secondary marker of severe systemic disease.[2]

Symptoms that can accompany severe hyponatremia ([Na+] less than 120 mEq/L) include loss of appetite, nausea, vomiting, cramps, weakness, altered level of consciousness, coma, and seizures. The severity of signs and symptoms depends on the rapidity and severity of the decrease in [Na+]. The most severe symptoms, typically neurologic, are in part related to cerebral overhydration. Because the blood-brain barrier is poorly permeable to sodium but freely permeable to water, a rapid decrease in [Na+] results in an increase in intracellular and extracellular brain water and may, if sufficiently severe, result in clinically important cerebral edema.

The symptoms of chronic hyponatremia probably relate to depletion of brain electrolytes. In response to a decrease in plasma osmolality, the brain compensatorily loses intracellular electrolytes (Na+, K+, Cl−) as well as other intracellular osmolytes (taurine, phosphocreatine, myoinositol, glutamine, and glutamate).[13,14] Requiring approximately 48 hours to counteract brain overhydration, this adaptive process can be overwhelmed if hyponatremia develops rapidly. After correction of hyponatremia, electrolytes return to brain cells in about 24 hours and osmolytes return over 5 to 7 days.

c. Causes. Hyponatremia may be accompanied by normal plasma osmolality (normotonic hyponatremia), by hyperosmolality, or by plasma hypoosmolality.[2] Hyponatremia with normal or high plasma osmolality can result from the laboratory abnormality called pseudohyponatremia and from retention of nonsodium solutes in plasma.

Extreme hyperproteinemia or hyperlipidemia can generate pseudohyponatremia by holding water in plasma. As the term suggests, pseudohyponatremia is not an electrolyte abnormality but a consequence of the fact that certain techniques used to measure serum sodium are confounded by an increase in nonaqueous components of plasma. Normal human plasma is composed of 93% water and 7% nonaqueous components (i.e., lipids and proteins). Older measurements of [Na+], based on flame emission spectrophotometry, used the total mass of sodium divided by the total volume of plasma or serum. If the nonaqueous components were increased, plasma [Na+] was artifactually depressed. Current methods usually use direct potentiometry, which directly measures [Na+][2] and is uninfluenced by nonaqueous components. Although [Na+] is conveniently reported in terms of mEq/L, true [Na+] is expressed per unit volume of plasma divided by the percentage of plasma made up of water. No treatment is required for pseudohyponatremia.

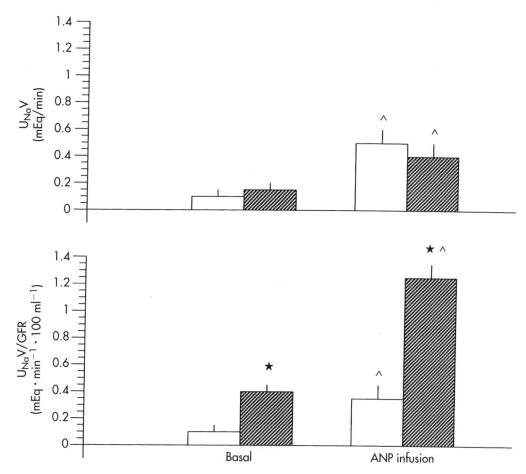

Fig. 22-4. Absolute *(top)* and fractional *(bottom)* urinary excretion of sodium under basal conditions and during 16 ng/kg^{-1}/min^{-1} of atrial natriuretic peptide *(ANP)* infusion in normal subjects *(open bars)* and in glomerulonephritic patients with chronic renal failure *(shaded bars)* kept on a low-sodium diet. $^\wedge p < 0.05$ vs. normal; $^* p < 0.05$ vs. basal. *GFR,* Glomerular filtration rate. (From Conte G, Bellizzi V, Cianciaruso B, et al: *Kidney Int* 51:S28, 1997.)

Hyponatremia with a normal or high serum osmolality can also result from the presence of a nonsodium solute, such as glucose or mannitol, that does not diffuse freely across cell membranes. For instance, plasma [Na$^+$] decreases approximately 1.6 mEq/L for each 100-mg/dl rise in glucose concentration.[15] Postoperative hyponatremia with normal serum osmolality is sometimes seen after transurethral resection of the prostate (TURP), because of absorption of large amounts of sodium-free irrigating solutions containing mannitol, glycine, or sorbitol.[16] These solutes cause a dilutional hyponatremia that is responsible for the clinical features of the TURP syndrome.[17,18] Neurologic symptoms are minimal if mannitol is given because the agent does not cross the blood-brain barrier and is excreted with water in the urine. In contrast, as glycine or sorbitol is metabolized, hypoosmolality gradually develops and cerebral edema may appear as a late complication.[16]

The disorders responsible for hyponatremia with plasma hypoosmolality are distinguished by differences in extracellular volume: hypovolemic, hypervolemic, and normovolemic (Fig. 22-5). Because of the distinct pathogenesis of each disorder, the treatments differ. In hypovolemic patients, ADH is secreted to preserve intravascular volume, even at the expense of hypotonicity. Angiotensin II also decreases free water generation.[2] Increased extracellular volume (in association with decreased effective arterial volume or hypovolemia) is associated with hyponatremia and hypoosmolality in edematous states, such as congestive heart failure,[1] cirrhosis, and renal insufficiency. Euvolemic hyponatremia most commonly is associated with nonosmotic vasopressin (ADH) secretion, such as in glucocorticoid deficiency, hypothyroidism, thiazide-induced hyponatremia, the syndrome of inappropriate antidiuretic hormone (SIADH), and the reset osmostat syndrome.[2] SIADH may be idiopathic but also is associated with diseases of the central nervous system and with pulmonary disease (Box 22-1).

Postoperative hyponatremia has been attributed to intravenous administration of hypotonic fluids and to nonosmotically stimulated secretion of ADH (Box

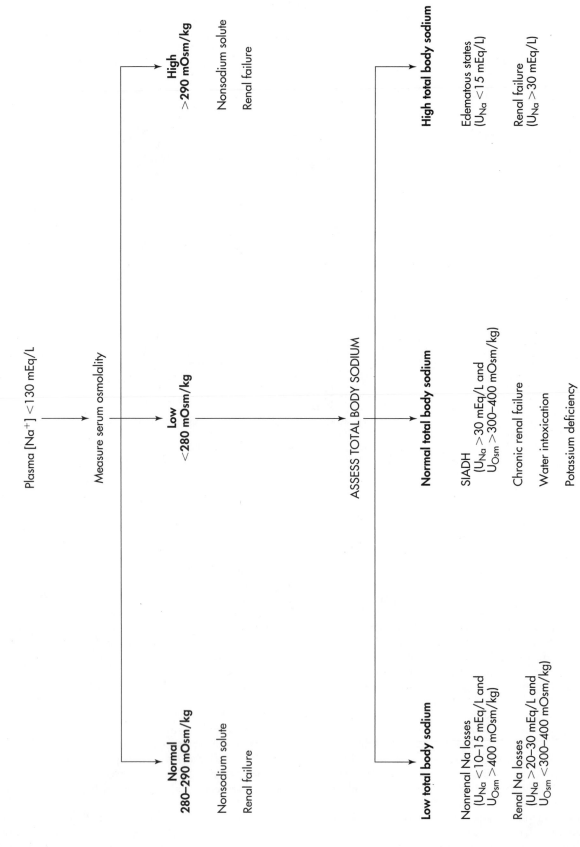

Fig. 22-5. Algorithm for evaluation of hyponatremia. *[Na⁺],* Sodium concentration; *SIADH,* syndrome of inappropriate antidiuretic hormone secretion; *U_Osm,* urinary osmolality.

Hyponatremia: Evaluation

Plasma [Na⁺] <130 mEq/L

Measure serum osmolality

Normal
280–290 mOsm/kg

Nonsodium solute

Renal failure

Low
<280 mOsm/kg

High
>290 mOsm/kg

Nonsodium solute

Renal failure

ASSESS TOTAL BODY SODIUM

Low total body sodium

Nonrenal Na losses
(U_{Na} <10–15 mEq/L and
U_{Osm} >400 mOsm/kg)

Renal Na losses
(U_{Na} >20–30 mEq/L and
U_{Osm} <300–400 mOsm/kg)

Normal total body sodium

SIADH
(U_{Na} >30 mEq/L and
U_{Osm} >300–400 mOsm/kg)

Chronic renal failure

Water intoxication

Potassium deficiency

High total body sodium

Edematous states
(U_{Na} <15 mEq/L)

Renal failure
(U_{Na} >30 mEq/L)

Box 22-1 Causes of the syndrome of inappropriate secretion of antidiuretic hormone

Neoplasms

Bronchogenic
    carcinoma
Pancreatic carcinoma
Carcinoma of the
    duodenum
Prostate carcinoma
Thymoma
Lymphoma
Mesothelioma

**Central nervous
system diseases**

Head trauma
Subdural hematoma
Subarachnoid
    hemorrhage
Cerebrovascular
    accident
Meningitis
Encephalitis
Brain abscess
Hydrocephalus
Brain tumors
Guillain-Barré
Acute intermittent
    porphyria
Delirium tremens

Pulmonary diseases

Tuberculosis
Pneumonia
Bronchiectasis
Aspergillosis
Cystic fibrosis
Positive-pressure
    ventilation

Medications

Opiates
Chlorpropamide
Carbamazepine
Phenothiazines
Tricyclic antidepressants
Clofibrate
Vincristine
Cyclophosphamide
Oxytocin

Miscellaneous

General surgery
Pain
Nausea
Psychosis

From Fried LF, Palevsky PM: Hyponatremia and hypernatremia. In Saklayen MG, ed: *The Medical Clinics of North America: renal disease*, Philadelphia, 1997, WB Saunders.

Box 22-2 Nonosmotically stimulated secretion of antidiuretic hormone

Surgical and traumatic stress
Catecholamines
Angiotensin II
Hypovolemia
Pain
Nausea and vomiting
Opioids
Hypoglycemia
Hypercapnia
Hypoxia

22-2). At least 4% of postoperative patients develop plasma [Na$^+$] less than 130 mEq/L.[19] Patients at particular risk of hyponatremia include children, premenstrual women, and elderly patients.

In an editorial accompanying a report[20] of apparent postoperative SIADH in a 30-kg, 10-year-old girl, Arieff[21] attributed the relationship between surgery in children and hyponatremic brain damage to elevated ADH, excessive sodium-free water in perioperative fluids, and respiratory failure secondary to hyposmolar encephalopathy. He suggested that children receive no sodium-free water perioperatively.

Women may be particularly vulnerable because estrogens stimulate and androgens suppress ADH release.[22,23] In experimental animals, hyponatremia produces greater brain swelling in females than in males.[24] In extreme cases, administration of hypotonic fluids to young, healthy, female surgical patients has resulted in severe neurologic symptoms and death secondary to transtentorial herniation.[25] Steele et al[26] studied 22 women (mean age 42 years) undergoing uncomplicated gynecologic surgery. Twenty-four hours after surgery, plasma [Na$^+$] had decreased in 21 of 22 patients; mean plasma [Na$^+$] had decreased from 140 ± 1 mEq/L to 136 ±

0.5 mEq/L.[26] In two patients, plasma [Na$^+$] decreased to 131 mEq/L. Although the patients retained sodium perioperatively, they retained proportionately more water (an average of 1.1 L of electrolyte-free water). In a subsequent letter to the editor, Ayus and Arieff[27] state that of 158 patients studied because of perioperative hyponatremic encephalopathy, none had received isotonic saline; the authors advise against routine perioperative use of hypotonic fluids.

In elderly patients, unlike younger patients, SIADH often has no discernible precipitating cause.[28] Cornforth[29] reports a 71-year-old woman who developed postoperative seizures in the setting of a plasma [Na$^+$] of 112 mEq/L; she recovered with treatment and had no apparent risk factors other than age. Because of the risk of postoperative hyponatremia, hypotonic fluids are best avoided in both children and adults in the early postoperative period unless such fluids are specifically indicated, patients are closely monitored, and serum electrolytes are determined frequently.[30]

d. Diagnosis (see Fig. 22-5). In the diagnostic evaluation of hyponatremia, the first step, exclusion of pseudohyponatremia and hyponatremia caused by an excess of a nonsodium solute, is accomplished by comparing measured serum osmolality with calculated serum osmolality (see Equation 22-1). If calculated osmolality exceeds measured osmolality by more than 10 mOsm/kg, the likelihood is that the patient has pseudohyponatremia or has accumulated a nonsodium solute. Also useful is calculation of effective osmolality, as follows:

$$\text{Effective osmolality} = 2[\text{Na}^+] + \text{Glucose}/18 \quad \textbf{(22-2)}$$

This calculation provides a more accurate assessment of true hypotonicity by eliminating the influence of urea, which distributes throughout total body water and therefore does not change the distribution of body water.

If both [Na$^+$] and measured osmolality are below the normal range, hyponatremia is further evaluated by first assessing volume status using physical findings and laboratory data. Often, physical findings are equivocal. In hypovolemic patients or edematous patients, urinary volume should be decreased and urinary composition should show signs of water and sodium conservation. The ratio of BUN to serum creatinine (SCr) should be more than

20:1. Urinary [Na^+] is generally less than 15 mEq/L in edematous states and volume depletion and more than 20 mEq/L if hyponatremia is caused by renal salt wasting or renal failure with water retention. One important cause of hypovolemic, hypotonic hyponatremia is the cerebral salt-wasting syndrome, an often severe, symptomatic salt-losing diathesis that appears to be mediated by ANP and is independent of SIADH; patients at risk include those with cerebral lesions caused by trauma, subarachnoid hemorrhage, tumors, and infection.[31-34]

In SIADH, in which normovolemia should minimize stimuli for sodium retention, urinary [Na^+] should be more than 30 mEq/L unless fluids have been restricted. The criteria for the diagnosis of SIADH include hypotonic hyponatremia, urinary osmolality greater than 100 or 150 mmol/kg, absence of extracellular volume depletion, normal thyroid and adrenal function, and normal cardiac, hepatic, and renal function.[2] Arieff[21] argues that the diagnosis of SIADH may be inaccurately applied to postoperative patients because they often are functionally hypovolemic. Therefore ADH secretion, by definition, would be appropriate. The actual relationship of postoperative hyponatremia to ADH secretion remains poorly characterized. ADH is only one of many factors, including drugs, intravenous fluid administration, and renal function, that influence perioperative water balance.[35] However, in most patients who are not postoperative, the various types of normovolemic hyponatremia can be differentiated by careful review of specific features of the history, such as associated diseases, drug therapy, and fluid intake.

e. Treatment. Therapy of hyponatremia depends on the cause and the severity of symptoms (Fig. 22-6). The first steps are to eliminate the cause or stop offending drugs. Hyponatremia with normal or high serum osmolality requires elimination of the increased concentration of the responsible solute. Uremic patients can be treated with free water restriction or dialysis. Treatment of edematous patients necessitates restriction or removal of both sodium and water, ideally by improving cardiac output (effective arterial volume) and renal perfusion and using diuretics to inhibit sodium and water reabsorption. In hypovolemic, hyponatremic patients, infusion of 0.9% saline increases plasma volume and increases plasma [Na^+] as the hypovolemic stimulus for water retention is removed.

The cornerstone of SIADH treatment is free water restriction and elimination of precipitating causes. Water restriction sufficient to decrease total body water by 0.5 to 1 L/day decreases extracellular fluid volume even if excessive ADH secretion continues. The resultant reduction in GFR enhances proximal tubular reabsorption of salt and water, thereby decreasing free water generation, and stimulates aldosterone secretion. As long as free water losses (i.e., renal, skin, GI) exceed free water intake, plasma [Na^+] will increase. During treatment of hyponatremia, increases in plasma [Na^+] are determined not only by the composition of the infused fluid but also, to a major degree, by the rate of renal free water excretion.[36]

In hypervolemic, hyponatremic patients who have severe symptoms, more rapid correction can be achieved by increasing free water excretion with furosemide in combination with replacement of sodium losses with 0.9% or 3% saline. Furosemide usually induces greater urinary water losses than sodium losses, thereby increasing plasma [Na^+] with less risk of excessive extracellular volume expansion.

Hyponatremia with neurologic symptoms is an indication for aggressive therapy with 3% (hypertonic) saline. However, infusion of hypertonic saline, as well as excessively rapid correction of hyponatremia using any treatment, entails the risk of central pontine and extrapontine myelinolysis (the osmotic demyelination syndrome), a neurologic injury in which symptoms range from transient behavioral disturbances or seizures to pseudobulbar palsy and quadriparesis.[13,37] The principal determinants of neurologic injury appear to be the magnitude of hyponatremia, the chronicity of hyponatremia, and the rate of correction. The osmotic demyelination syndrome is more likely when hyponatremia has persisted more than 48 hours.[38] Other risk factors for the development of this lesion include alcoholism, poor nutritional status, liver disease, burns, and hypokalemia.[39] Within 3 to 4 weeks of the clinical onset of the syndrome, areas of demyelination are apparent on magnetic resonance imaging.[40]

Although more rapid correction of hyponatremia clearly increases the risk of the osmotic demyelination syndrome, defining a rate of correction that is completely safe may be impossible.[41,42] A rate of 1 to 2 ml/kg/hr of 3% saline appears to be safe for most patients. Treatment of 25 hyponatremic children in this fashion promptly terminated seizures and resulted in no delayed neurologic sequelae.[43] However, in SIADH, 3% saline may only transiently increase plasma [Na^+] because expansion of extracellular volume results in increased urinary sodium excretion.

To assist in preventing overcorrection of plasma [Na^+], the expected change in plasma [Na^+] resulting from 1 L selected infusate can be estimated using the following equation[44]:

$$\frac{\Delta[Na^+]_s = [Na^+]_{inf} - [Na^+]_s}{TBW + 1} \quad (22\text{-}3)$$

where:

$\Delta[Na^+]_s$ = the change in the patient's serum sodium
$[Na^+]_{inf}$ = sodium concentration of the infusate
$[Na^+]_s$ = the patient's serum sodium concentration
TBW = the patient's estimated total body water in liters
1 = a factor added to take into account the volume of infusate.

Treatment should be interrupted or slowed when symptoms improve. Frequent determinations of [Na^+] are important to prevent correction at a rate faster than 10 mEq/L/24 hr.[38] Once plasma [Na^+] exceeds 120 mEq/L, water restriction alone is usually sufficient to normalize [Na^+].

Demeclocycline and lithium, though potentially toxic, have been used effectively to reverse SIADH in patients in whom the primary disease is irreversible. Although better tolerated than lithium, demeclocycline may induce or worsen renal dysfunction. Hemodialysis is occa-

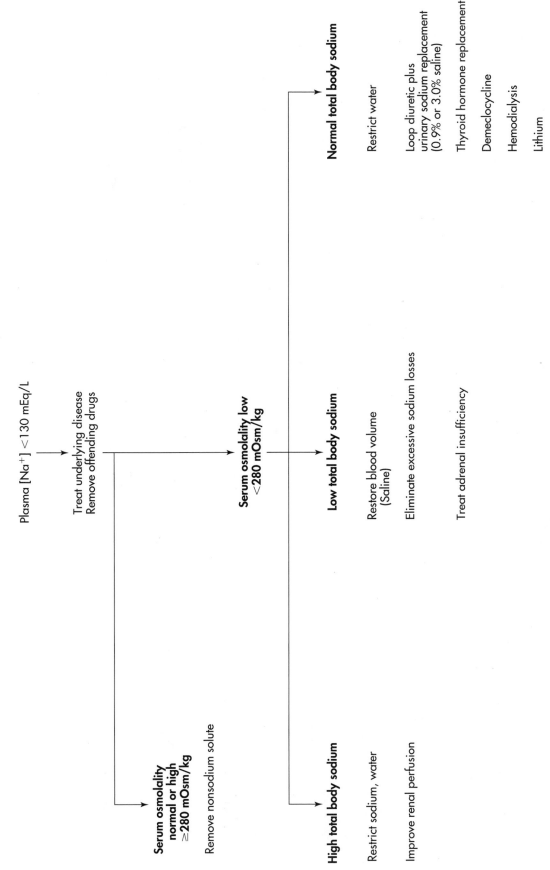

Fig. 22-6. Hyponatremia is treated according to the cause of the disturbance, the level of serum osmolality, and a clinical estimation of total body sodium. *[Na⁺]*, Serum sodium concentration.

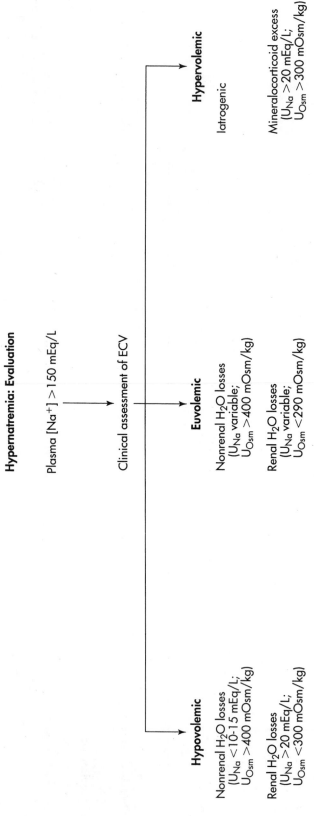

Fig. 22-7. Severe hypernatremia is evaluated by first assessing extracellular volume (*ECV*) to separate patients into hypovolemic, euvolemic, and hypervolemic groups. Next, potential etiologic factors are assessed diagnostically. *[Na⁺]*, Serum sodium concentration; U_{Na}, urinary sodium concentration; U_{Osm}, urinary osmolality.

sionally necessary in severely hyponatremic patients who cannot be treated adequately with more conservative measures. In the future, perhaps aquaporin antagonists will be effective in treating hyponatremia, particularly in patients with SIADH and no correctable primary cause.

3. Hypernatremia

a. Pathophysiology. Hypernatremia ([Na$^+$] greater than 150 mEq/L) indicates an absolute or relative water deficit. Normally, minimal increases in tonicity or sodium stimulate thirst and ADH secretion. This is the first and best line of defense against hypernatremia. Severe, persistent hypernatremia occurs only in patients who cannot respond to thirst by voluntary ingestion of fluid (i.e., obtunded patients, anesthetized patients, and infants).

b. Clinical features. The principal manifestations of hypernatremia are neurologic, including restlessness, irritability, muscle twitching, hyperreflexia, and spasticity. More serious manifestations include stupor, coma, and seizures. Although the mortality of hypernatremia is 40% to 55%, it is unclear whether hypernatremia is the cause or a marker of severe associated disease.[2]

The magnitude of symptoms depends on the severity of hyperosmolality. Neurologic symptoms appear to be caused by acute dehydration of brain cells. Brain shrinkage may damage delicate cerebral vessels, leading to subdural hematoma, parenchymal hemorrhage, subarachnoid hemorrhage, or venous thrombosis. Clinical consequences are most serious at the extremes of age and when hypernatremia develops abruptly.

Surprisingly, moderate acute increases in plasma [Na$^+$] do not appear to precipitate central pontine myelinolysis if plasma [Na$^+$] is initially normal. In clinical trials of prehospital resuscitation from hypovolemic shock using hypertonic saline, acute increases in serum sodium to 155 to 160 mEq/L produced no apparent harm.[45,46] However, larger accidental increases in plasma [Na$^+$] have produced severe consequences in children. In a 12-year-old diabetic child who accidentally received 500 ml of 5% saline during treatment for diabetic ketoacidosis (DKA), plasma [Na$^+$] acutely increased to 172 mEq/L; subsequent cranial computed tomography showed many subcortical hemorrhages, and the child suffered brain death.[47] In experimental animals, acute hypernatremia (acute increase from 146 to 170 mEq/L) caused neuronal damage at 24 hours, suggestive of early central pontine myelinolysis.[48]

c. Causes. The primary defect in hypernatremia is impaired water intake.[2] Hypernatremia can be generated by isolated water loss, as in diabetes insipidus (DI), or by hypotonic fluid loss, as in burns, GI losses, diuretic therapy, or osmotic diuresis. Other causes include renal disease, mineralocorticoid excess or deficiency, and iatrogenic causes (Fig. 22-7). Geriatric patients are at increased risk of hypernatremia because of decreased renal concentrating ability and thirst, although the responsiveness of osmoreceptors to hypernatremia is maintained during normal aging.[49,50] Isolated sodium gain is uncommon but occurs in patients who receive large quantities of sodium, such as treatment of metabolic acidosis with 8.4% sodium bicarbonate, in which [Na$^+$] is approximately 1000

mEq/L, or perioperative or prehospital treatment with hypertonic saline resuscitation solutions.

d. Diagnosis. Diagnosis requires distinction between three groups of patients: hypovolemic, euvolemic, and hypervolemic (see Fig. 22-7). Measurement of urinary sodium and osmolality can help to differentiate the various causes. A urinary osmolality less than 150 mOsm/kg in the setting of hypertonicity and polyuria is diagnostic of DI. Postoperative neurosurgical patients who have undergone pituitary surgery are at particular risk of developing DI secondary to decreased or absent ADH secretion.[51] In traumatic DI, polyuria may be present only transiently after surgery, may be permanent, or may demonstrate a triphasic sequence: early DI, return of urinary concentrating ability, then recurrent DI.

e. Treatment (Box 22-3). The treatment of hypovolemic hypernatremia consists of correcting hypovolemia with 0.9% saline and then cautiously replacing water deficits with oral or intravenous hypotonic fluid. Although 0.9% saline has 154 mEq/L of sodium, the solution is effective in treating the volume deficit and will reduce [Na$^+$] if it exceeds 154 mEq/L. After correcting hypovolemia, the free water deficit can be estimated using the following formula:

$$\text{Free water deficit} = 0.6 \times \text{Body weight (kg)} \times [([Na^+] - 140)/140] \quad (22\text{-}4)$$

where 140 is the middle of the normal range for [Na$^+$]. Common errors in treating hypernatremia include failing to appreciate the magnitude of the water deficit and failing to account for ongoing maintenance requirements and continued fluid losses in planning therapy.

Hypernatremia must be corrected slowly because of the risk of neurologic sequelae such as seizures or cerebral edema.[52] The plasma [Na$^+$] should not decrease more than 2 mEq/L/hr. At the cellular level, restoration

---

Box 22-3 Hypernatremia: acute treatment

Sodium depletion (hypovolemia)
  Hypovolemia correction (0.9% saline)
  Hypernatremia correction (hypotonic fluids)
Sodium overload (hypervolemia)
  Enhance sodium removal (loop diuretics, dialysis)
  Replace water deficit (hypotonic fluids)
Normal total body sodium (euvolemia)
  Replace water deficit (hypotonic fluids)
Control diabetes insipidus
  Central diabetes insipidus
    DDAVP, 10-20 μg intranasally; 2-4 μg SC
    Aqueous vasopressin, 5 U q 2-4 hr IM or SC
  Nephrogenic diabetes insipidus
    Restrict sodium, water intake
    Thiazide diuretics

From Lang JD, Prough DS: Diagnosis and management of electrolyte abnormalities. In Murray MJ, Coursin DB, Pearl RG, et al, eds: *Critical care medicine: perioperative management*, Philadelphia, 1997, Lippincott-Raven.
DDAVP, Desmopressin.

of cell volume occurs remarkably quickly after tonicity is altered; as a consequence, acute treatment of hypertonicity may result in overshooting the original, normotonic cell volume (Fig. 22-8).[53-55] Reversible underlying causes of hypernatremia should be treated. In the sodium-overloaded patient, sodium excretion can be accelerated using a loop diuretic or dialysis.

The management of DI varies according to whether the cause is central or nephrogenic. The two most suitable agents for correcting central DI are desmopressin (1-deamino-[8-D-arginine]-vasopressin; DDAVP) and aqueous vasopressin.[1,56,57] Given subcutaneously in a dose of 1 to 4 μg or intranasally in a dose of 5 to 20 μg every 12 to 24 hours, DDAVP is effective in most patients (Fig. 22-9).[57] Patients with partial central DI often do not require hormone therapy. Chlorpropamide, which potentiates the renal effects of vasopressin, and carbamazepine, which enhances vasopressin secretion, have been used to treat partial central DI, but are associated with clinically important side effects. In nephrogenic DI, urinary water losses can be decreased by using salt and water restriction or thiazide diuretics to induce extracellular volume contraction, thereby enhancing fluid reabsorption in the proximal tubules. If less filtrate passes through into the collecting ducts, less water will be excreted.

B. Potassium

1. Potassium homeostasis. Potassium, the principal intracellular cation, plays an important role in maintaining resting membrane potentials and in generating action potentials in the central nervous system and the heart. Potassium is actively transported into cells by a Na-K adenosine triphosphatase (ATPase) pump. This pump maintains an intracellular potassium concentration $[K^+]$ that is at least 30 times greater than extracellular $[K^+]$ (i.e., the intracellular $[K^+]$ is 150 mEq/L, and the extracellular $[K^+]$ is 3.5 to 5 mEq/L). In a 70-kg person, in whom intracellular fluid volume is 28 L (0.4 × total body weight), total body potassium is approximately 4200 mEq. Of this, only 2% is extracellular.

The usual potassium intake is between 50 and 150 mEq/day. Most is excreted in the urine, with some fecal elimination. Freely filtered at the glomerulus, 85% to 90% of potassium is reabsorbed in the proximal convoluted tubule and loop of Henle. The remaining 10% to 15% reaches the distal convoluted tubule, which is the major site at which potassium excretion is regulated. As long as GFR is greater than 8 ml/min, dietary potassium intake, unless greater than normal, can be excreted. Four factors that favor K^+ excretion are alkalemia, increased aldosterone activity, increased delivery of Na^+ to the distal tubule and collecting duct, and increased urinary flow to these segments. The two most important regulators of potassium secretion are the plasma $[K^+]$ and aldosterone, although there is some evidence to suggest the involvement of an enteric reflex mediated by a potassium-rich meal and of the central nervous system.[58] Within the distal nephron, a magnesium-dependent Na-K ATPase plays a critical role in potassium reabsorp-

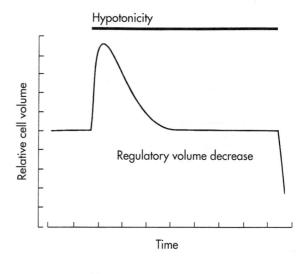

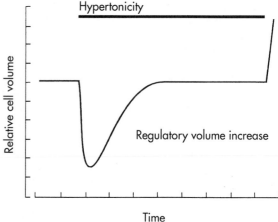

Fig. 22-8. Activation of mechanisms regulating cell volume in response to acute osmotic stress. Regulatory volume decrease and regulatory volume increase are compensatory losses and gains of solutes. Although the course of these regulatory volume decreases and increases varies with the type of cell and experimental conditions, typically the responses occur over a period of minutes. Returning volume-regulated cells to normotonic conditions causes shrinkage or swelling. (From McManus ML, Churchwill KB, Strange K: *N Engl J Med* 333:1260, 1995.)

tion.[59] Magnesium depletion impairs the function of this enzyme, resulting in renal potassium wasting.

The relationship between plasma and intracellular potassium is influenced by the hormones epinephrine (through β_2 receptors) and insulin, which promote movement of potassium into cells, whereas α-adrenergic agonists impair cellular potassium uptake.[60] Metabolic acidosis tends to shift potassium out of cells, whereas metabolic alkalosis favors movement into cells.

2. Hypokalemia

a. Pathophysiology. Uncommon among healthy people, hypokalemia ($[K^+]$ less than 3 mEq/L) is a common complication of treatment with diuretic drugs and occasionally complicates other diseases and treatment regi-

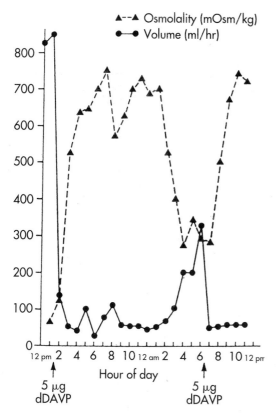

Fig. 22-9. Effect of 5 μg of intranasal desmopressin *(DDAVP)* on volume and osmolality of hourly urine collections in a patient who developed diabetes insipidus after removal of a craniopharyngioma. (From Cobb WE, Spare S, Reichlin S: *Ann Intern Med* 88:183, 1978.)

Box 22-4 Common nonrenal causes of hypokalemia

Gastrointestinal disorders (vomiting, gastric suction, diarrhea)
Trauma
β_2 agonists
Phosphodiesterase inhibitors

Box 22-5 Causes of renal potassium loss

Drugs
  Diuretics
    Thiazide diuretics
    Loop diuretics
    Osmotic diuretics
  Antibiotics
    Penicillin and
      penicillin analogues
    Amphotericin B
  Aminoglycosides
  Hormones
    Aldosterone
    Glucocorticoid excess
      states

Bicarbonaturia
  Distal renal tubular
    acidosis
  Treatment of proximal
    renal tubular acidosis
  Correction phase of
    metabolic alkalosis
Magnesium deficiency
Other less common
  causes
  Cisplatin
  Carbonic anhydrase
    inhibitors
  Leukemia
  Diuretic phase of acute
    tubular necrosis
Intrinsic renal transport
  defects
  Barter's syndrome
  Gitelman's syndrome

Modified from Weiner ID, Wingo CS: *J Am Soc Nephrol* 8:1179, 1997.

---

mens (Boxes 22-4 and 22-5).[60] Because extracellular [K+] is small in relation to intracellular [K+], small variations in extracellular [K+] produce large variations in the intracellular/extracellular ratio. Conversely, only large changes in intracellular [K+] influence the ratio significantly. Plasma [K+] imperfectly reflects total body potassium (i.e., plasma hypokalemia can occur with high, low, or normal total body potassium). As a general rule, however, a chronic decrement of 1 mEq/L in plasma [K+] corresponds to a total body deficit of 200 to 300 mEq.

b. Clinical features. The most prominent features of hypokalemia are neuromuscular. Hypokalemia causes muscle weakness that, when severe, can progress to paralysis and death. Additionally, acute hypokalemia causes hyperpolarization of the cardiac cells and may lead to ventricular escape activity, reentrant phenomena, ectopic tachycardias, and delayed conduction. Hypokalemia can be especially dangerous in patients taking digoxin because hypokalemia increases myocardial binding, pharmacologic effectiveness, and toxicity of cardiac glycosides. Despite the influence of acutely decreased [K+] on cardiac rhythm, chronic hypokalemia ([K+] 2.6 to 3.4 mEq/L) did not increase the incidence of intraoperative arrhythmias in several prospective studies.[61,62] Hypokalemia contributes to systemic hypertension, especially when combined with a high-sodium diet.[63] In

diabetic patients, hypokalemia impairs insulin secretion and end-organ sensitivity to insulin, thereby worsening hyperglycemia.[64] If hypokalemia is sufficiently prolonged, chronic renal interstitial damage can decrease renal concentrating ability.

c. Diagnosis. The diagnosis of hypokalemia requires knowledge of risk factors for excessive potassium excretion or intracellular redistribution, recognition of clinical findings suggestive of hypokalemia, and laboratory confirmation. The most common risk factor precipitating hypokalemia is treatment with diuretics. Thiazides, loop diuretics, and carbonic anhydrase inhibitors increase K+ excretion. Abrupt reduction of dietary K+ intake may result in a potassium deficit because of the delay in the renal potassium-conserving response. Intracellular movement of potassium occurs in response to insulin, β_2 agonists, and to some extent aldosterone. Intrinsic renal diseases that result in increased K+ loss (see Box 22-5) include Bartter's syndrome and renin-secreting tumors. GI disorders in which vomiting, diarrhea, or loss of GI secretions is prominent can lead to hypokalemia. Magnesium deficiency, associated with aminoglycoside and cisplatin therapy, can generate hypokalemia that is resistant to replacement therapy. A majority of trauma pa-

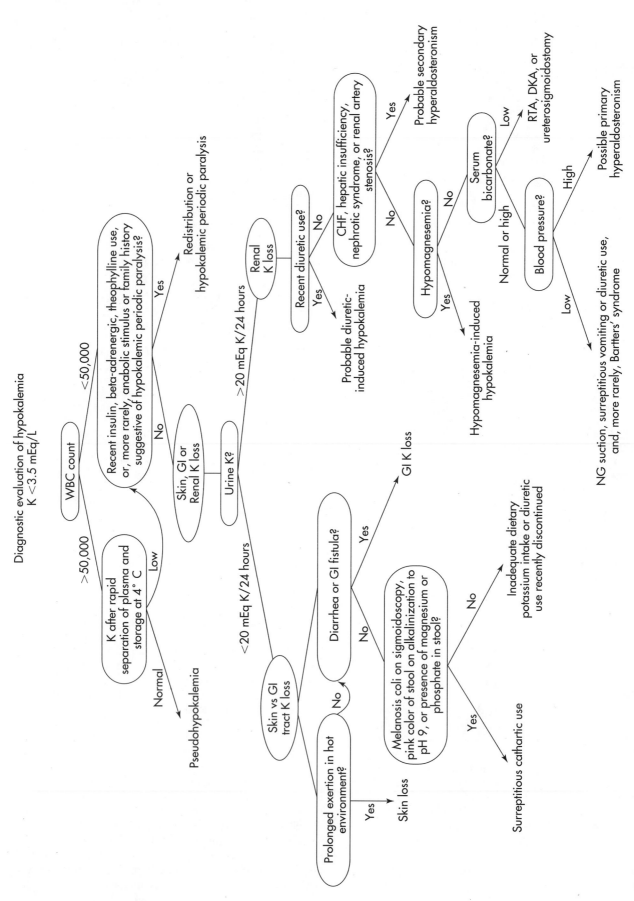

Fig. 22-10. Diagnostic evaluation of hypokalemia. *DKA,* Diabetic ketoacidosis; *GI,* gastrointestinal; *K,* potassium; *WBC,* white blood cell. (From Weiner ID, Wingo CS: *J Am Soc Nephrol* 8:1179, 1997.)

tients develop hypokalemia that returns to normal within 24 hours without specific therapy.[60]

In addition to the nonspecific symptoms of hypokalemia, characteristic electrocardiographic changes include flat or inverted T waves, prominent U waves, and ST segment depression. Laboratory diagnosis is occasionally confounded by pseudohypokalemia, which results from excessive delay before analyzing a leukemic blood sample in which excessive white cell uptake of potassium reduces the plasma [K$^+$].

Initial evaluation of hypokalemia includes a medical history (drug use, vomiting), physical examination, and measurement of other serum electrolytes (e.g., magnesium) (Fig. 22-10). Measurement of 24-hour urinary excretion of potassium and sodium may help to distinguish between renal and extrarenal causes. In selected cases, plasma renin and aldosterone concentrations can help to establish an accurate diagnosis.

d. Treatment. The treatment of hypokalemia consists of potassium repletion, correction of alkalemia, and removal of offending drugs. Potassium replacement may not be necessary in patients with asymptomatic, mild hypokalemia (3 to 3.5 mEq/L). Low potassium secondary to intracellular redistribution alone requires no therapy. If total body potassium is depleted, oral supplementation is more effective than intravenous replacement. Intravenous therapy should be reserved for patients with cardiac arrhythmias, familial periodic paralysis, and severe myopathy. Potassium usually is replaced as the chloride salt because coexisting chloride deficiency may limit the ability of the kidney to conserve potassium.

When required, intravenous potassium replacement should be performed cautiously (rate less than 20 mEq/hr).[60,65] The plasma [K$^+$] and electrocardiogram (ECG) should be monitored to detect inadvertent hyperkalemia. Particular care should be taken in patients with acidemia, type IV renal tubular acidosis, diabetes mellitus, or renal insufficiency, or in patients receiving nonsteroidal antiinflammatory drugs, ACE inhibitors, or β-blockers, all of which delay movement of extracellular potassium into cells or decrease potassium secretion.

Hypokalemia associated with hyperaldosteronemia (i.e., primary hyperaldosteronism, Cushing's disease) usually responds favorably to reduced sodium intake and increased potassium intake. Intercurrent hypomagnesemia also should be treated. In patients with acidemia and hypokalemia, such as those in DKA, potassium administration should precede correction of acidosis to avoid a precipitous drop in plasma [K$^+$] as pH increases.

3. Hyperkalemia

a. Pathophysiology. Hyperkalemia ([K$^+$] greater than 5 mEq/L) can occur with low, normal, or high total body potassium. It is uncommon except in patients with renal insufficiency. Patients with chronic renal insufficiency can maintain a normal plasma [K$^+$] via tubular secretion until GFR falls below 8 ml/min. However, a variety of other clinical situations are occasionally associated with hyperkalemia. Pseudohyperkalemia can occur secondary to extravascular hemolysis of red blood cells, especially if a blood sample is forcibly aspirated through a small-

gauge needle. When hyperkalemia is suspected, a repeat sample should be obtained; if sampling error is confirmed, no treatment is required. Drugs that limit the excretion of potassium and may precipitate hyperkalemia include nonsteroidal antiinflammatory drugs, ACE inhibitors, cyclosporine, and potassium-sparing diuretics, especially in the setting of renal insufficiency, diabetes mellitus, and metabolic acidosis.[66] In patients with denervating injuries, such as traumatic paraplegia or quadriplegia, succinylcholine causes a rapid, severe increase in [K$^+$]. Hyperkalemia always accompanies malignant hyperthermia. A deficiency of aldosterone, as in Addison's disease, will lead to hyperkalemia. In patients with normal total body potassium, hyperkalemia may accompany a sudden shift of potassium from the intracellular to the extracellular volume because of acidemia, increased catabolism, or rhabdomyolysis.

b. Clinical features. The most lethal manifestations of hyperkalemia involve the cardiac conduction system and include arrhythmias, conduction abnormalities, and cardiac arrest. If plasma [K$^+$] is less than 6 mEq/L, cardiac effects are negligible. As [K$^+$] progressively increases, the ECG first shows tall, peaked T waves, especially in the precordial leads, then the PR interval becomes prolonged, followed by a decrease in the amplitude of the P wave. Finally, the QRS complex widens as a prelude to cardiac standstill (Fig. 22-11).[67] Hyperkalemic cardiotoxicity is enhanced by hyponatremia, hypocalcemia, and acidemia. Progression to cardiac standstill is unpredictable and often swift. Ascending muscle weakness appears when plasma [K$^+$] approaches 7 mEq/L and may progress to flaccid paralysis, inability to phonate, and even respiratory arrest.

c. Diagnosis. The most important aspects of diagnosis are a medical history, emphasizing recent drug therapy, and assessment of renal function. The ECG may provide the first suggestion of hyperkalemia in some patients. Despite the familiar effects of hyperkalemia on cardiac conduction and rhythm, the ECG is an insensitive and nonspecific method of detecting hyperkalemia.[68] If hyponatremia is also present, adrenal function should be evaluated.

d. Treatment. The priorities in treatment of severe hyperkalemia are to reverse membrane hyperexcitability, reduce serum [K$^+$], remove potassium from the body, and eliminate the cause of hyperkalemia (Box 22-6). Calcium chloride (1 g over 3 minutes) or calcium gluconate acutely depresses the membrane threshold potential and can be used until more definitive therapy takes effect (see Fig. 22-11). Membrane hyperexcitability also can be antagonized temporarily by moving potassium into cells. Acute alkalinization of plasma using sodium bicarbonate (50 to 100 mEq over 5 to 10 minutes in a 70-kg adult) transiently moves potassium into the intracellular volume. Insulin, which increases the activity of the Na-K ATPase pump, also moves potassium into cells. The recommended dose in an adult is 5 to 10 U of regular insulin with 50 ml of 50% dextrose. Salbutamol, a selective β$_2$ agonist, decreases serum potassium acutely when given by inhalation or intravenously. In 15 pediatric pa-

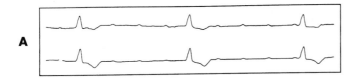

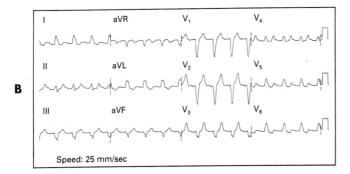

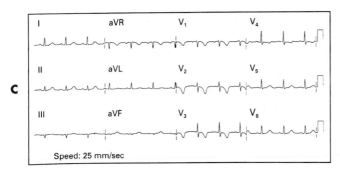

Fig. 22-11. Electrocardiographic changes caused by hyperkalemia occurring in a 42-year-old woman undergoing placement of an arteriovenous fistula for permanent hemodialysis access to treat end-stage renal disease. **A,** During dissection of the brachial artery under local anesthesia, her cardiac rhythm converted from normal sinus rhythm to complete heart block with ventricular escape (approximately 25 beats per minute). **B,** Two ampules of calcium gluconate (9.2 mEq) were administered intravenously. An electrocardiogram revealed sinus tachycardia with profound prolongation of the QRS interval (left bundle-branch morphology), first-degree atrioventricular block, and peaked T waves. The serum potassium concentration was 8.6 mmol/L. After reduction of the serum potassium concentration, the electrocardiogram showed sinus rhythm with normalization of the PR and QRS intervals. **C,** Anteroseptal ST wave and T wave changes were noted on subsequent electrocardiograms. A cardiac exercise imaging study did not show ischemia. (From Kuvin JT: *N Engl J Med* 338:662, 1998.)

tients with baseline serum [K⁺] of 6.6 mEq/L, a single infusion of salbutamol (5 μg/kg over 15 minutes) reduced serum [K⁺] to 5.7 mEq/L after 30 minutes and to 4.9 mEq/L after 120 minutes.[69]

Potassium may be removed from the body by the kidneys (loop diuretic) or the GI tract. Sodium polystyrene resin (Kayexalate), which exchanges sodium for potassium, can be given orally or as a retention enema. Emergency hemodialysis may occasionally be necessary. Mineralocorticoid deficiency can be treated with 9-α-fludrocortisone. Hyperkalemia secondary to digitalis in-

---

Box 22-6 Severe* hyperkalemia: goals of treatment

Reverse membrane effects
    Calcium (10 ml of 10% calcium chloride intravenously over 2-5 minutes)
Transfer extracellular [K⁺] into cells
    Glucose and insulin (D10W + 5-10 U regular insulin per 25-50 g glucose)
    Sodium bicarbonate (50-100 mEq over 5-10 minutes)
    β₂ agonists
Remove potassium from body
    Diuretics, proximal or loop
    Potassium exchange resins (sodium polystyrene sulfonate)
    Hemodialysis
Monitor ECG and serum [K⁺] level

From Lang JD, Prough DS: Diagnosis and management of electrolyte abnormalities. In Murray MJ, Coursin DB, Pearl RG, et al, eds: *Critical care medicine: perioperative management,* Philadelphia, 1997, Lippincott-Raven.
*Potassium concentration *([K⁺])* > 7 mEq/L or electrocardiographic *(ECG)* changes.
D10W, 10% dextrose in water.

---

toxication may be resistant to therapy because attempts to shift potassium intracellularly are often ineffective. In this situation, administration of a digoxin-specific antibody may be lifesaving.

C. Calcium

1. Calcium homeostasis. Calcium is a divalent cation found primarily in the mineral lattice of the bone. Ninety-nine percent of calcium exists in bone, whereas the remaining 1% exists within cells and their surrounding medium. Of this 1%, most is extracellular. The concentration of free calcium in extracellular volume is approximately 1 mmol/L; in the intracellular volume, the free calcium is approximately 100 nmol/L. Therefore the gradient from extracellular to intracellular concentrations is 10,000:1. Circulating calcium includes protein-bound (40%), chelated (10%), and ionized fractions (50%); only the ionized fraction is physiologically active. Because total serum calcium correlates poorly with the concentration of ionized calcium ([Ca²⁺]) in critically ill patients, [Ca²⁺] should be measured whenever possible.[70]

Serum [Ca²⁺] is regulated by multiple factors (Fig. 22-12).[71] The "three hormone, three organ rule" is a simplified statement of the fact that three organs (kidney, bone, and small intestine) and three hormones (parathyroid hormone [PTH], activated vitamin D, and calcitonin) regulate calcium homeostasis.[72] Vitamin D (through its metabolites) and PTH mobilize calcium from bone, increase reabsorption of calcium from renal tubule, and enhance intestinal absorption of calcium. Metabolites of vitamin D exert a major role in long-term control of circulating calcium. Vitamin D, after ingestion or synthesis in the skin, is 25-hydroxylated to calcidiol in the liver and then is 1-hydroxylated in the kidney to calcitriol, the active metabolite. Vitamin D and PTH can

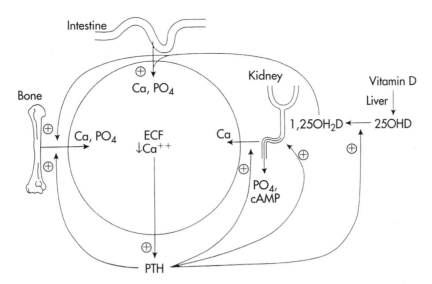

Fig. 22-12. The hormonal control of serum calcium is depicted. *Ca,* Calcium; *cAMP,* cyclic adenosine monophosphate; *ECF,* extracellular fluid; *PO$_4$,* phosphate; *PTH,* parathyroid hormone; *25OHD,* calcidiol; *1,25OH$_2$D,* calcitriol. (From Edelson GW, Kleerekoper M: *Med Clin North Am* 79:79, 1995.)

maintain normal circulating calcium concentrations, even in the absence of dietary calcium, by mobilizing calcium from bone.

2. Physiologic actions of calcium. Calcium is the secondary messenger responsible for stimulus-excitation coupling and transmembrane signal transduction in a wide variety of cells. It is also required for secretion of hormones, release of neurotransmitters, and initiation of coagulation. Additionally, calcium is essential for the generation of electrical impulses in cells of the cardiac conduction system.

3. Hypocalcemia

a. Pathophysiology. As many as 12% of critically ill patients have a decreased [Ca^{2+}]. Because ionized hypocalcemia influences cardiac, respiratory, and neuromuscular function, [Ca^{2+}] should be measured routinely in patients at risk for clinically important hypocalcemia. Hypocalcemia can occur as a result of failure of PTH or calcitriol action (Box 22-7). PTH deficiency can result from parathyroid suppression, surgical damage, or removal. Parathyroid gland suppression may occur during severe hypomagnesemia or hypermagnesemia, extensive burns, sepsis, or pancreatitis. Vitamin D deficiency results from dietary lack or malabsorption in patients who lack sunlight exposure. Extreme hyperventilation and bicarbonate injection can cause an acute decrease in [Ca^{2+}].

Hypocalcemia also can occur secondary to precipitation or chelation. Precipitation occurs with hyperphosphatemia secondary to the formation of CaHPO$_4$ complexes. However, ionized [Ca^{2+}] decreases only approximately 0.019 mmol/L for each 1-mmol/L increase in phosphate concentration.[73] In massive transfusions, citrate may produce transient hypocalcemia by chelating calcium. A healthy, normothermic adult who has intact hepatic and renal function can metabolize the citrate present in 20 units of blood per hour without be-

Box 22-7 Nonparathyroid causes of hypocalcemia

Parathyroid hormone resistance
  Pseudohypoparathyroidism
  Hypomagnesemia
Vitamin D deficiency
  Nutritional
  Renal failure
  Malabsorption
  Anticonvulsant therapy
  Liver disease
1α-Hydroxylase deficiency (vitamin D–dependent rickets, type I)
Vitamin D resistance (vitamin D–dependent rickets, type II)
Medications
  Plicamycin, calcitonin, bisphosphonates, phosphate
  Phenobarbital, dilantin
  Citrated blood, radiographic contrast dyes
  Fluoride
  Foscarnet, pentamidine
Malignancy
  Osteoblastic metastases
  Tumor lysis syndrome
Acute pancreatitis
Toxic shock syndrome
Acute rhabdomyolysis
Prematurity

From Guise TA, Mundy GR: *J Clin Endocrinol Metab* 80:1473, 1995.

coming hypocalcemic.[74] However, when citrate clearance is reduced (e.g., hepatic or renal disease or hypothermia) and when blood transfusion is rapid (more than 0.5 ml/kg/min), hypocalcemia and cardiovascular compromise may occur.

b. Clinical features. The hallmark of hypocalcemia (ionized $[Ca^{2+}]$ less than 4 mg/dl) is increased neuronal membrane irritability and tetany. Early symptoms include sensations of numbness and tingling involving fingers, toes, and the circumoral region. Latent hypocalcemia can be diagnosed by tapping on the facial nerve or inflating a sphygmomanometer to 20 mm Hg above systolic pressure. Tapping on the facial nerve elicits muscle spasms known as Chvostek's sign, and radial and ulnar nerve ischemia elicits carpal spasm known as Trousseau's sign.[75] In frank tetany, tonic contraction of respiratory muscles may lead to laryngospasm, bronchospasm, or respiratory arrest. Smooth muscle contraction can lead to abdominal cramping and urinary frequency. Mental status alterations include irritability, depression, psychosis, and dementia. Hypocalcemia has been associated with heart failure, hypotension, arrhythmias, insensitivity to digitalis, and impaired β-adrenergic action.

c. Diagnosis. Initial evaluation should concentrate on history and physical examination, laboratory evaluation of renal function, and measurement of serum phosphate concentration. The differential diagnosis of hypocalcemia can be approached by addressing four issues: age of the patient, serum phosphate concentration, general clinical status, and duration of hypocalcemia.[76] High phosphate concentrations suggest renal failure or hypoparathyroidism. Low or normal phosphate concentrations imply vitamin D or magnesium deficiency. An otherwise healthy patient with chronic hypocalcemia probably is hypoparathyroid. Chronically ill adults with hypocalcemia often have disorders such as malabsorption, osteomalacia, or osteoblastic metastases.

Table 22-1. Treatment of concomitant hypocalcemia and hyperphosphatemia

Treatment of hyperphosphatemia	Treatment of hypocalcemia
Increased renal excretion	Urgently required if symptomatic
Diuresis	Calcium IV to increase $[Ca^{2+}]$ to the low normal range
Dopamine	Immediate measures to normalize $[PO_4]$
Redistribution	
Dextrose/insulin	
Correct acidosis	
Deposition into bone	
Administer calcium	
Decreased absorption	
Oral phosphate binders	
Direct removal	
Hemodialysis	

From Sutters M, Gaboury CL, Bennett WM: *J Am Soc Nephrol* 7:2055, 1996.
[Ca²⁺], Ionized calcium concentration; *[PO₄],* plasma phosphate concentration.

d. Treatment. In treating hypocalcemia, unnecessary offending drugs should be discontinued. Hypocalcemia resulting from hypomagnesemia or hyperphosphatemia is treated by repletion or removal of magnesium or phosphate, respectively. Treatment of a patient who has tetany and hyperphosphatemia requires coordination of therapy to avoid the consequences of metastatic soft tissue calcification (Table 22-1).[77] Hyperkalemia and hypomagnesemia potentiate hypocalcemia-induced cardiac and neuromuscular irritability. In contrast, hypokalemia protects against hypocalcemic tetany; therefore correction of hypokalemia without correction of hypocalcemia may provoke tetany.

Mild, ionized hypocalcemia should not be overtreated, especially when it is incidentally discovered during perioperative laboratory testing. For instance, in most patients after cardiac surgery, administration of calcium only increases mean arterial pressure and attenuates the β-adrenergic effects of epinephrine.[78] In normocalcemic dogs, the predominant effect of calcium chloride was peripheral vasoconstriction; in hypocalcemic dogs, calcium infusion improved both cardiac contractile performance and blood pressure.[79]

The cornerstone of therapy for confirmed, symptomatic, ionized hypocalcemia ($[Ca^{2+}]$ less than 0.7 mmol) is calcium administration. In patients who have severe or symptomatic hypocalcemia, calcium should be administered intravenously. In emergency situations, in an averaged-sized adult, the "rule of 10s" advises infusion of 10 ml of 10% calcium gluconate (93 mg elemental calcium) over 10 minutes, followed by a continuous infusion of elemental calcium, 0.3 to 2 mg/kg/hr (i.e., 3 to 16 ml/hr of 10% calcium gluconate for a 70-kg adult). Calcium salts should be diluted in 50 to 100 ml dextrose in water (to limit venous irritation and thrombosis), should not be mixed with bicarbonate (to prevent precipitation), and must be given cautiously to patients receiving digoxin because calcium increases the toxicity of digoxin. Continuous ECG monitoring during initial therapy will detect cardiotoxicity (e.g., heart block, ventricular fibrillation). During calcium replacement, the clinician should monitor total serum calcium, magnesium, phosphate, potassium, and creatinine. Once the $[Ca^{2+}]$ is stable in the range of 4 to 5 mg/dl (1 to 1.25 mmol), oral calcium supplements can substitute for parenteral therapy. Urinary calcium should be monitored in an attempt to avoid hypercalciuria (more than 5 mg/kg/24 hr) and associated urinary tract stone formation.

When supplementation fails to maintain serum calcium within the normal range, or if hypercalciuria develops, vitamin D may be added to raise the serum calcium into the low normal range. When rapid changes in dosage are anticipated or an immediate effect is required (e.g., postoperative hypoparathyroidism), shorter-acting calciferols such as dihydrotachysterol may be preferable.

4. Hypercalcemia

a. Pathophysiology. Hypercalcemia occurs when calcium enters the extracellular volume more rapidly than the kidneys can excrete the excess. Clinically, hypercalcemia most commonly results from an excess of bone resorption over bone formation, usually secondary to malignant disease, hyperparathyroidism, thyrotoxicosis, granulomatous diseases, and immobilization.[80] Factors that promote hypercalcemia may be offset by coexisting disorders, such as pancreatitis, sepsis, or hyperphosphatemia, that reduce serum calcium.

b. Clinical features. Although [Ca^{2+}] greater than 1.3 mmol most accurately defines physiologically significant hypercalcemia, the conventional definition is a total serum calcium greater than 10.5 mg/dl. Patients in whom total serum calcium is less than 11.5 mg/dl are usually asymptomatic. Patients with moderate hypercalcemia (total serum calcium 11.5 to 13 mg/dl) may have lethargy, anorexia, nausea, and polyuria. Severe hypercalcemia (total serum calcium greater than 13 mg/dl) is associated with more severe symptoms, including muscle weakness, depression, impaired memory, emotional lability, lethargy, stupor, and coma. The cardiovascular effects of hypercalcemia include hypertension, arrhythmias, heart block, cardiac arrest, and digitalis sensitivity.

Hypercalcemia impairs urinary concentrating ability and the renal excretory capacity for calcium by irreversibly precipitating calcium salts within the renal parenchyma and by reducing renal blood flow and GFR. In response to hypovolemia, renal tubular reabsorption of sodium results in enhanced renal calcium reabsorption. Effective treatment of severe hypercalcemia is necessary to prevent progressive dehydration and renal failure, leading to further increases in total serum calcium. Skeletal disease may occur secondary to direct osteolysis or humoral bone resorption.

c. Treatment. Although definitive treatment of hypercalcemia requires correction of the underlying cause, temporizing therapy may be necessary to avoid complications and relieve symptoms. The decision to treat should be based on the presence and severity of symptoms as well as the actual serum calcium concentration. A total serum calcium greater than 14 mg/dl should be treated in most cases. General supportive measures include hydration, correction of associated electrolyte abnormalities, removal of offending drugs, and increased physical activity. Hypercalcemia invariably leads to sodium and water depletion because hypercalcemia causes anorexia and antagonizes ADH action. Therefore

infusion of 0.9% saline dilutes serum calcium, promotes renal excretion, and reduces total serum calcium by 1.5 to 3 mg/dl. As GFR increases, the sodium ion increases calcium excretion by competing with the calcium ion for reabsorption in the proximal renal tubules and the loop of Henle. Furosemide further enhances calcium excretion by increasing tubular sodium. During saline infusion and forced diuresis, careful monitoring of cardiopulmonary status and electrolytes, especially magnesium and potassium, is required. Intensive diuresis and saline administration can achieve net calcium excretion rates of 2000 to 4000 mg per 24 hours, a rate 8 times greater than that of saline alone but still less than the rate of removal achieved by hemodialysis (i.e., 6000 mg every 8 hours.)

Bone reabsorption, the primary cause of hypercalcemia, can be minimized by physical mobilization and drug therapy (Table 22-2).[71] Bisphosphonates, currently the first-line therapy for acute hypercalcemia, have an inhibitory effect on osteoclast function and viability. Etidronate, the first bisphosphonate to be studied and approved for use in hypercalcemia, lowers serum calcium for up to 2 weeks in many patients with hypercalcemia of malignancy.[81] Pamidronate, an aminobisphosphonate 100 times more potent than etidronate, normalized serum calcium in 70% of patients with malignancy-related hypercalcemia.[82] Other osteoclast-inhibiting agents used to treat hypercalcemia include mithramycin and calcitonin (Fig. 22-13).[83]

Glucocorticoids are effective in treating certain causes of hypercalcemia, including hypercalcemia secondary to lymphatic malignancies, vitamin D and A intoxication, and granulomatous diseases. Although intravenous phosphate can treat acute hypercalcemia effectively, the major drawback to this therapy is the risk of precipitating calcium salts in soft tissue. Therefore intravenous phosphate should be reserved for cases in which all else has failed.

D. Magnesium

1. Physiologic considerations. Magnesium is a divalent cation located primarily intracellularly. Fifty percent is found in bone, 25% in muscle, and less than 1% in serum, in which only the ionized form is metabolically active.

Table 22-2. Drugs currently approved by the Food and Drug Administration that are effective in lowering serum calcium acutely

Generic name	Trade name	Recommended starting dosage
Synthetic human calcitonin	Cibacalcin	0.5 mg SC daily
Synthetic salmon calcitonin	Calcimar Miacalcin	4 IU/kg body weight every 12 hr SC or IM
Etidronate	Didronel	7.5 mg/kg body weight/day for 3 days
Pamidronate	Aredia	60-90 mg IV over 24 hr
Plicamycin	Mithracin	25 μg/kg body weight/day IV for 3-4 days
Gallium nitrate	Ganite	200 mg/m² body surface area/day for 5 days

From Edelson GW, Kleerekoper M: *Med Clin North Am* 79:79, 1995.
SC, Subcutaneously; *IM,* intramuscularly; *IV,* intravenously.

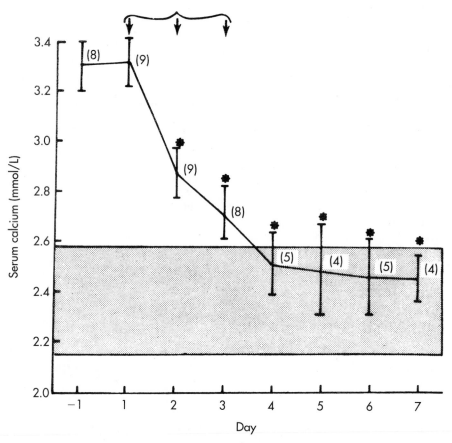

Fig. 22-13. Decrease in the albumin-corrected serum calcium concentration during combined salmon calcitonin and etidronate therapy of nine patients with cancer. Each patient had been hydrated with intravenous saline solution for at least 48 hours before treatment. Each patient received 7.5 mg/kg etidronate intravenously daily and 100 IU salmon calcitonin subcutaneously every 12 hours for 3 days. There was a significant decrease in the serum calcium within 24 hours ($p < 0.001$). The shaded area is the normal range for serum calcium concentration. (From Fatemi S, Singer FR, Rude RK: *Calcif Tissue Int* 50:107, 1992.)

The normal serum concentration is 1.6 to 2.4 mEq/L. Magnesium is widely available in foods and is absorbed through the GI tract.[84] Serum magnesium is regulated primarily by renal mechanisms (Table 22-3),[85] although PTH and vitamin D exert minor influences.

Magnesium is necessary for enzymatic reactions involving DNA and protein synthesis (Box 22-8).[85] As a primary regulator or cofactor in many enzyme systems, magnesium is important for the regulation of the Na-K pump, Ca-ATPase enzymes, adenylate cyclase, proton pumps, and slow calcium channels. Magnesium has been called an endogenous calcium antagonist because its regulation of slow calcium channels contributes to maintenance of normal vascular tone, prevention of vasospasm, and perhaps prevention of calcium overload in many tissues. Because magnesium partially regulates PTH secretion and is important for the maintenance of end-organ sensitivity to both PTH and vitamin D, abnormalities in ionized magnesium concentration ($[Mg^{2+}]$) may result in abnormal calcium metabolism. Magnesium functions in potassium metabolism primarily by regulating sodium-potassium ATPase, an enzyme that controls potassium entry into cells, especially in potassium-depleted states, and controls reabsorption of potassium by the renal tubules. In addition, magnesium functions as a regulator of membrane excitability and serves as a structural component in both cell membranes and the skeleton.

Because magnesium stabilizes axonal membranes, reduction of magnesium concentration decreases the threshold for axonal stimulation and increases nerve conduction velocity. Magnesium also influences the release of neurotransmitters at the neuromuscular junction by competitively inhibiting the entry of calcium into the presynaptic nerve terminals. The concentration of calcium required to trigger calcium release and the rate at which calcium is released from the sarcoplasmic reticulum have been shown to be inversely related to the ambient magnesium concentration.

2. Hypomagnesemia

a. Pathophysiology. Hypomagnesemia, identified in 11% of hospitalized patients[86] and as many as 47% of blood samples collected for determination of other elec-

Box 22-8 Proposed metabolic roles for magnesium

Protein synthesis
DNA synthesis
Glucose phosphorylation
Mitochondrial oxidative metabolism
Adenylate cyclase activity
Peptide hormone modulation

From Whang R, Hampton EM, Whang DD: *Ann Pharmacother* 28:220, 1997.

Table 22-3. Renal magnesium handling

Factors associated with increased magnesium excretion	Factors associated with decreased magnesium excretion
Metabolic	**Metabolic**
Hypermagnesemia	Hypomagnesemia
Hypercalcemia	Hypocalcemia
Fluid overload	Fluid depletion
Phosphate depletion	Hypothyroidism
Metabolic acidosis	Increased parathyroid hormone
Increased carbohydrate intake	
Increased protein intake	
Drug-induced	
Thiazide and thiazide-like diuretics	
Loop diuretics	
Osmotic diuretics	
Alcohol	
Cisplatin	
Cyclosporine	
Ticarcillin	
Gentamicin (aminoglycosides)	
Carbenicillin	

From Whang R, Hampton EM, Whang DD: *Ann Pharmacother* 28:220, 1997.

Box 22-9 Causes of magnesium deficiency

Nutritional and intestinal causes (inadequate intake or malabsorption)
Prolonged parenteral fluid administration
Parenteral nutrition without added magnesium
Chronic alcoholism
Severe prolonged diarrhea, inflammatory bowel disease, laxative abuse, villous adenoma, cancer of the colon
Intestinal malabsorption (short bowel syndrome, gluten enteropathy, tropical sprue)
Starvation with ketosis
Protein calorie malnutrition
Diabetic ketoacidosis

Renal causes
Diuretics
Drug-induced renal tubular injury (amphotericin B, gentamicin, cisplatin)
Renal tubular acidosis
Recovery from acute tubular necrosis
Chronic glomerulonephritis and pyelonephritis (rarely)
Familial and sporadic renal wastage of magnesium

Neonatal and childhood-associated conditions
Infantile convulsions with hypomagnesemia and hypocalcemia
Newborns of diabetic mothers
Genetic (male) hypomagnesemia (specific malabsorption syndrome)
Exchange transfusions (citrate effect)
Congenital hypoparathyroidism
Infant born of mother with hyperparathyroidism

Endocrine and metabolic causes
Primary and secondary aldosteronism
Hyperthyroidism
Hyperparathyroidism
Malacic bone disease
Excessive lactation
Last trimester of pregnancy

From Flink EB: *West J Med* 133:304, 1980.

trolytes,[87] is associated with hypokalemia, hyponatremia, hypophosphatemia, and hypocalcemia. Hypomagnesemia rarely results from inadequate dietary intake. The most common causes of hypomagnesemia are inadequate GI absorption, excessive magnesium losses, or failure of renal magnesium conservation (Box 22-9). Excessive magnesium loss is associated with GI disease, prolonged nasogastric suctioning, GI or biliary fistulas, intestinal drains, and polyuria. Inability of renal tubules to conserve magnesium complicates a variety of systemic and renal diseases, although advanced renal disease with a decreased GFR may lead to magnesium retention. Various drugs and toxins, including aminoglycosides, cisplatin, cardiac glycosides, osmotic diuretics, and alcohol, enhance urinary magnesium excretion. Intracellular shifts of magnesium as a result of thyroid hormone or insulin administration may also decrease serum $[Mg^{2+}]$.

b. Clinical features. The clinical features of hypomagnesemia ($[Mg^{2+}]$ less than 1.7 mg/dl), like those of hypocalcemia, are characterized by increased neuronal irritability and tetany.[88] Hypomagnesemia can aggravate digoxin toxicity and CHF. Although hypomagnesemia is common in critically ill patients, serum $[Mg^{2+}]$ may not reflect intracellular magnesium content.[89] Symptoms are rare when the serum $[Mg^{2+}]$ is 1.5 to 1.7 mg/dl; in most symptomatic patients serum $[Mg^{2+}]$ is less than 1 mg/dl. Patients often complain of weakness, lethargy, muscle spasms, paresthesias, and depression. When severe, hypomagnesemia may induce seizures, confusion, and coma. Cardiovascular abnormalities include coronary artery spasm, cardiac failure, arrhythmias, and hypotension.

c. Diagnosis. Measurement of 24-hour urinary magnesium excretion is useful in separating renal from nonrenal causes of hypomagnesemia. Normal kidneys can reduce magnesium excretion to less than 2 mEq/day in response to magnesium depletion. Hypomagnesemia accompanied by high urinary excretion of magnesium (more than 3 mEq/day) suggests excessive renal losses. Parenteral magnesium tolerance testing is useful in confirming magnesium deficiency in the presence of normal renal function.

d. Treatment. Magnesium deficiency is treated by the administration of magnesium supplements (Box 22-10). One gram of magnesium sulfate provides approximately 4 mmol (8 mEq, or 98 mg) of elemental magnesium. Mild deficiencies can be treated with diet alone. Replacement of deficiencies must be added to daily magnesium requirements (0.3 to 0.4 mEq/kg/day). Symptomatic or severe hypomagnesemia ($[Mg^{2+}]$ less than 1 mg/dl) should be treated with parenteral magnesium: 1 to 2 g (8 to 16 mEq) of magnesium sulfate as an intravenous bolus over the first hour, followed by a continuous infusion of 0.5 to 1 g/hr (4 to 8 mEq/hr). Therapy should be guided subsequently by the serum magnesium concentration. The rate of infusion should not exceed 1 mEq/min, even in emergent situations. Patients receiving rapid infusions should have continuous ECG monitoring to detect cardiotoxicity. Because magnesium antagonizes calcium, blood pressure and cardiac function should be monitored, although clinical effects of acute magnesium administration on myocardial contractility and blood pressure appear to be modest.

Magnesium administration may decrease arrhythmias by directly affecting myocardial membranes, altering cellular potassium and sodium concentrations, inhibiting cellular calcium entry, improving myocardial oxygen supply and demand, prolonging the effective refractory period, depressing conduction, antagonizing catecholamine action on the conducting system, and preventing vasospasm.[89a] Treatment of hypomagnesemia, which often occurs after cardiopulmonary bypass, decreases the incidence of ventricular arrhythmias after heart surgery from 63% to 22%.[90] Several studies have shown a decrease in short-term mortality when intravenous magnesium was administered after acute myocardial infarction.[91] In addition, magnesium may be useful as treatment for torsades de pointes, even in normomagnesemic patients.[92]

Because the sodium-potassium pump is magnesium dependent, hypomagnesemia increases myocardial sensitivity to digitalis preparations and may cause hypokalemia as a result of renal potassium wasting. Attempts to correct potassium deficits with potassium replacement alone may not be successful without simul-

taneous magnesium therapy. Magnesium is important in the regulation of potassium channels. The interrelationships of magnesium and potassium in cardiac tissue have probably the greatest clinical relevance in terms of arrhythmias, digoxin toxicity, and myocardial infarction. Severe hypomagnesemia suppresses PTH secretion and can cause hypocalcemia. Severe hypomagnesemia may also impair end-organ responses to PTH.

During magnesium repletion, the patellar reflexes should be monitored frequently and treatment discontinued if they become suppressed. Patients who have renal insufficiency have a diminished ability to excrete magnesium and require careful monitoring during therapy. Repletion of systemic magnesium stores usually requires 5 to 7 days of therapy, after which daily maintenance doses of magnesium should be provided. Magnesium can be given orally, usually in a dose of 60 to 90 mEq/day of magnesium oxide. Hypocalcemic, hypomagnesemic patients should receive magnesium as the chloride salt because the sulfate ion can chelate calcium and further reduce serum $[Ca^{2+}]$.

3. Hypermagnesemia

a. Pathophysiology. Therapeutic hypermagnesemia is used to treat patients with premature labor, preeclampsia, and eclampsia. Because magnesium blocks the release of catecholamines from adrenergic nerve terminals and the adrenal glands, magnesium has been used to reduce the hypertensive response to tracheal intubation and to reduce the effects of catecholamine excess in patients with tetanus and pheochromocytoma.[93]

b. Clinical features. Most cases of clinically important hypermagnesemia ($[Mg^{2+}]$ greater than 2.5 mg/dl) are iatrogenic in origin, resulting from the administration of magnesium-containing antacids, enemas, and parenteral nutrition formulas, especially to patients with impaired renal function. Hypermagnesemia is less common than hypomagnesemia in hospitalized patients, present in 5.7% to 9.3% of blood samples drawn for electrolyte determinations.[86.87]

c. Diagnosis. Because magnesium antagonizes the release and effect of acetylcholine at the neuromuscular junction, hypermagnesemia depresses skeletal muscle function and induces neuromuscular blockade. Magnesium potentiates the action of nondepolarizing muscle relaxants.

d. Treatment. The neuromuscular and cardiac toxicity of hypermagnesemia can be acutely but transiently antagonized by giving intravenous calcium (5 to 10 mEq) to temporize while more definitive therapy is instituted.[94] All magnesium-containing preparations must be stopped. Urinary excretion of magnesium can be increased by expanding extracellular volume and inducing diuresis with a combination of saline and furosemide. In emergency situations and in patients with renal failure, magnesium may be removed by dialysis.

E. Phosphate

1. Physiologic considerations. Phosphorus, in the form of phosphate, exists in monovalent or divalent forms ($H_2PO_4^-$ or $H_2PO_4^{2-}$). Of total body phosphorus, 90% exists in bone, 10% is intracellular, and the remain-

---

Box 22-10 Hypomagnesemia: acute treatment

Intravenous Mg*: 8-16 mEq bolus over 1 hr, followed by 2-4 mEq/L as continuous infusion
Intramuscular Mg*: 10 mEq q 4-6 hr

From Prough DS, Mathru M: Acid-base, fluids, and electrolytes. In Barash PG, Cullen BF, Stoelting RK, eds: *Clinical anesthesia*, Philadelphia, 1997, Lippincott-Raven.
*MgSO$_4$: 1 g = 8 mEq Mg. MgCl$_2$: 1 g = 10 mEq Mg.

der, less than 1%, is found in the extracellular fluid. The normal serum phosphate concentration ranges from 2.7 to 4.5 mg/dl in adults. Absorption occurs in the duodenum and jejunum and is largely unregulated.

Control of phosphate concentration is achieved by altered renal excretion and redistribution within the body compartments. Phosphate is freely filtered at the glomerulus and its concentration in the glomerular ultrafiltrate is similar to plasma. The filtered phosphate is then reabsorbed in the proximal tubule, where it is cotransported with sodium.[95] Phosphate reabsorption in the kidney is regulated primarily by PTH, dietary intake, and insulin-like growth factor.[95] Phosphate excretion is increased by volume expansion and decreased by respiratory alkalosis.

Because phosphate provides the primary energy bond in adenosine triphosphate (ATP) and creatine phosphate, severe phosphate depletion results in cellular energy depletion. Phosphorus is an essential element of second messenger systems, including cAMP and phosphoinositides, and a major component of nucleic acids, phospholipids, and cell membranes. As part of 2,3-diphosphoglycerate, phosphate is important for offloading oxygen from the hemoglobin molecule. Phosphorus also functions in protein phosphorylation and acts as a urinary buffer.

2. Hypophosphatemia

a. Pathophysiology. Hypophosphatemia is characterized by low concentrations of phosphate-containing cellular components, including ATP, 2,3-diphosphoglycerate, and membrane phospholipids. Serious life-threatening organ dysfunction may occur when the serum phosphate concentration falls below 1 mg/dl.

b. Clinical features. Neurologic manifestations of hypophosphatemia include paresthesias, myopathy, encephalopathy, delirium, seizures, and coma.[96] Hematologic abnormalities include dysfunction of erythrocytes,

platelets, and leukocytes. Muscle weakness and malaise are common. Respiratory muscle failure and myocardial dysfunction are problems of particular concern in perioperative patients.[97,98]

Common in postoperative or traumatized patients, hypophosphatemia (phosphate less than 2.5 mg/dl) is caused by three primary abnormalities in phosphate homeostasis: an intracellular shift of phosphate, an increase in renal losses, and a decrease in GI absorption. Carbohydrate-induced hypophosphatemia (i.e., the refeeding syndrome,[99] mediated by insulin-induced cellular phosphate uptake) is the type most commonly encountered in hospitalized patients. Hypophosphatemia also may occur as catabolic patients become anabolic, and during medical management of DKA. Acute alkalemia, which may reduce serum phosphate to 1 mg/dl, increases intracellular consumption of phosphate by increasing the rate of glycolysis. Respiratory alkalosis probably explains the hypophosphatemia associated with gram-negative bacteremia and salicylate poisoning. Excessive renal losses account for the hypophosphatemia associated with hyperparathyroidism, hypomagnesemia, hypothermia, diuretic therapy, and renal tubular defects in phosphate absorption. Excessive GI loss of phosphate is most commonly secondary to the use of phosphate-binding antacids or to malabsorption syndromes.

c. Diagnosis. Measurement of urinary phosphate aids in differentiating hypophosphatemia resulting from renal losses from that caused by excessive GI losses or redistribution of phosphate into cells. Extrarenal causes of hypophosphatemia cause avid renal tubular phosphate reabsorption, reducing urinary excretion to less than 100 mg/day.

d. Treatment. Patients who have severe (less than 1 mg/dl) or symptomatic hypophosphatemia require intravenous phosphate administration (Table 22-4).[99] In

Table 22-4. Repletion of moderate or severe hypophosphatemia in patients with normal renal function

Setting	Route/dosage	Salt form	Volume/diluent
Moderate 1-2.2 mg/dl	Oral 16-20 mmol/dose, 2-3 times/day	Potassium when serum $[K^+] < 4$ mEq/L, otherwise sodium, when available	May be added to enteral formula ($\geq$500 ml)
Moderate with IV access 　Recent onset without symptoms 　Recent onset with symptoms 　Prolonged or numerous causes	Intravenous 0.08 mmol/kg (2.5 mg/kg) 0.1 mmol/kg (3.1 mg/kg) 0.16 mmol/kg (5 mg/kg)	Potassium when serum $[K^+] < 4$ mEq/L, otherwise sodium	D_5W,* 250-1000 ml by infusion pump
Severe 　<1 mg/dl and >0.5 mg/dl 　<0.5 mg/dl 　or 　$\leq$1 mg/dl	Intravenous 0.25 mmol/kg (7.75 mg/kg) 0.5 mmol/kg (15 mg/kg) 0.32 mmol/kg (9.92 mg/kg)	Potassium when serum $[K^+] < 4$ mEq/L, otherwise sodium	D_5W, 250-500 ml by infusion pump

From Brooks MJ, Melnik G: *Pharmacology* 51:713, 1995.
*Unless patient is glucose intolerant.
D_5W, 5% dextrose in water; *[K⁺]*, potassium concentration.

chronically hypophosphatemic patients, the estimated dose should be infused over 12 hours. For moderately hypophosphatemic adult patients suffering from critical illness, the use of 15 mmol boluses (465 mg) mixed with 100 ml 0.9% sodium chloride and given over a 2-hour period safely repletes phosphate.[100] The dose is then adjusted as indicated by the serum phosphate concentration because the cumulative deficit cannot be predicted accurately. Oral therapy can be substituted for parenteral phosphate once the serum phosphate concentration exceeds 2 mg/dl. Continued therapy with phosphate supplements is required for 5 to 10 days in order to replenish body stores. Insulin infusions lower plasma phosphate concentration, probably through increased uptake into skeletal muscle cells.

3. Hyperphosphatemia

a. Pathophysiology. Hyperphosphatemia is caused by three basic mechanisms: inadequate renal excretion, increased movement of phosphate out of cells, and increased phosphate or vitamin D intake. Renal excretion of phosphate remains adequate until the GFR falls below 25 ml/min. Rhabdomyolysis, sepsis, and rapid cell lysis from chemotherapy can cause hyperphosphatemia, especially if renal function is impaired.

b. Clinical features. The clinical features of hyperphosphatemia (phosphate greater than 5 mg/dl) relate primarily to the development of hypocalcemia and ectopic calcification.

c. Diagnosis. Measurements of BUN, SCr, GFR, and urinary phosphate are helpful in the differential diagnosis of hyperphosphatemia. Normal renal function accompanied by high phosphate excretion (more than 1500 mg/day) indicates an oversupply of phosphate. An elevated BUN, elevated SCr, and low GFR suggest impaired renal phosphate excretion. Normal renal function and phosphate excretion less than 1500 mg/day suggest increased phosphate reabsorption (i.e., hypoparathyroidism).

d. Treatment (see Table 22-1). Hyperphosphatemia is corrected by eliminating the cause and correcting the associated hypocalcemia. The serum concentration is reduced by restricting intake, increasing urinary excretion with saline and acetazolamide (500 mg every 6 hours), and increasing GI losses by enteric administration of aluminum hydroxide (30 to 45 ml every 6 hours). Aluminum hydroxide absorbs phosphate that has been secreted into the gut lumen and increases phosphate loss, even if none is ingested. Hemodialysis and peritoneal dialysis are effective in removing phosphate in patients who have renal failure.

II. ACID-BASE DISORDERS AND TREATMENT

Metabolic and respiratory acid-base disturbances are common consequences of preoperative medications, intraoperative and postoperative anesthetic and analgesic drugs, and blood loss and fluid replacement. Severe acid-base abnormalities contribute to morbidity and mortality. Treatment may be required preoperatively, intraoperatively, or postoperatively to reverse the acid-base effects of diseases or treatments and to limit complications. The following reviews the pathogenesis, major complications, physiologic compensatory mechanisms, and treatment of the four simple acid-base disorders: metabolic alkalosis, metabolic acidosis, respiratory alkalosis, and respiratory acidosis.

A. Overview of acid-base equilibrium

The conventional approach to describing acid-base equilibrium is the Henderson-Hasselbalch equation:

$$pH = 6.1 + \log \frac{[HCO_3^-]}{0.03(PaCO_2)} \quad (22\text{-}5)$$

where 6.1 is the pK_a of carbonic acid, and 0.03 is the solubility coefficient in blood of carbon dioxide (CO_2). Because the concentration of bicarbonate ($[HCO_3]$) is largely regulated by the kidneys whereas $PaCO_2$ is controlled by the lungs, the emphasis on acid-base interpretation for the past 80 years has been to examine disorders in terms of metabolic disturbances (i.e., those in which $[HCO_3^-]$ is primarily increased or decreased) and respiratory disturbances (i.e., those in which $PaCO_2$ is primarily increased or decreased).

One factor complicating acid-base interpretation has been the use of pH, the negative logarithm of the hydrogen ion concentration ($[H^+]$), to define the acidity or alkalinity of solutions or blood. Back-converting pH to $[H^+]$ results in a simpler alternative to the Henderson-Hasselbalch equation, the Henderson equation, as follows:

$$[H^+] = \frac{24 \times PaCO_2}{[HCO_3^-]} \quad (22\text{-}6)$$

In this equation, the relationship between the three major variables measured or calculated in blood gas samples is evident. Conversion of pH to $[H^+]$ can be accomplished by knowing that the $[H^+]$ is 40 mmol/L at a pH of 7.4, that an increase in pH of 0.10 pH units reduces $[H^+]$ to 0.8 times the starting $[H^+]$ concentration, that a decrease in pH of 0.10 pH units increases the $[H^+]$ by a factor of 1.25, and that small changes (i.e., less than 0.05 pH units) produce approximately a 1 mmol/L increase in $[H^+]$ for each 0.01 decrease in pH or a decrease in $[H^+]$ of 1 mmol/L per 0.01 increase in pH.

Conventional acid-base interpretation is suitable for clinical use but overemphasizes the role of hydrogen and bicarbonate ions in determining pH. A more exacting approach to acid-base interpretation, originally proposed by Stewart[101] and reviewed by Eicker,[102] distinguishes between the independent and dependent variables that define pH. In this approach, the only independent variables are $PaCO_2$, the strong ion difference (SID), and the concentration of proteins. The strong ions are those that are highly dissociated and are present in large concentrations, including Na^+, K^+, Cl^-, and lactate. Proteins, which are less dissociated, are not strong ions. The SID, calculated as ($Na^+ + K^+ - Cl$), under normal circumstances is approximately 42 mEq/L. By using a series of equations, acid-base status can be described more precisely using the Stewart approach.

However, this review uses the conventional approach based on arterial blood gases, in part because of the greater mathematical complexity of the Stewart approach and in part because there is little evidence that the clinical interpretation or treatment of common acid-base disturbances is handicapped by the simple constructs of the conventional Henderson-Hasselbalch or Henderson equations.

1. Metabolic alkalosis. Metabolic alkalosis usually is characterized by an alkalemic pH (greater than 7.45) and hyperbicarbonatemia (more than 27 mEq/L). The pathophysiology of metabolic alkalosis has been divided into generating and maintenance factors (Table 22-5).[103] Generating factors include nasogastric suction and diuretic administration. The maintenance of metabolic alkalosis depends on a continued stimulus for the reabsorption of HCO_3^- from the distal renal tubules. Renal hypoperfusion, perhaps better categorized as decreased effective arterial volume, and hypokalemia are major maintenance factors.

Metabolic alkalosis is associated with a wide variety of effects on serum electrolytes and on cardiac and pulmonary physiology. Alkalemia decreases serum potassium and ionized calcium[104] and, through induction of hypokalemia, may precipitate cardiac arrhythmias and potentiate the toxicity of digoxin. Compensatory hypoventilation (hypercarbia) in response to metabolic alkalosis is variable (Box 22-11) and may be exaggerated,[105] especially in patients who have chronic obstructive pulmonary disease or who have received narcotics. Alkalemia may contribute to the development of atelectasis through a combination of increased bronchial tone and decreased ventilatory effort. A leftward shift in the oxyhemoglobin dissociation curve may make oxygen less available to the tissues, as may alkalemia-induced decreased cardiac output.

If arterial blood gases have not been obtained, assessment of serum electrolytes can suggest metabolic alkalosis in patients who have risk factors such as vomiting, nasogastric suction, or chronic diuretic use. The serum electrolyte determination includes a direct measurement of total CO_2 content (usually abbreviated on electrolyte reports as CO_2). Because most CO_2 in the blood is carried in the form of HCO_3^-, the measurement of total CO_2 should exceed the calculation (from simultaneous arterial blood gases) of $[HCO_3^-]$ by about 1 mEq/L; that is, if the calculated $[HCO_3^-]$ on an arterial blood gas sample is 24 mEq/L, the "CO_2" on the serum electrolytes should be approximately 25 mEq/L. If either measurement exceeds normal by more than 4 mEq/L, one or both of two disturbances is possible: the patient has a primary metabolic alkalosis

---

Box 22-11 Rules for predicting respiratory compensation (hypoventilation) in response to metabolic alkalosis

$PaCO_2$ increases approximately 0.5 to 0.6 mm Hg for each 1.0-mEq/L increase in $[HCO_3^-]$.
The last two digits of the pH should equal the $[HCO_3^-]$ + 15.

From Prough DS, Mathru M: Acid-base, fluids, and electrolytes. In Barash PG, Cullen BF, Stoelting RK, eds: *Clinical anesthesia*, Philadelphia, 1997, Lippincott-Raven.
PaCO₂, Arterial carbon dioxide pressure; *[HCO₃⁻]*, bicarbonate concentration.

Table 22-5. Generation and maintenance of metabolic alkalosis

Generation	Example	Maintenance
Loss of acid from extracellular space		
Loss of gastric fluid	Vomiting; nasogastric drainage	↓ EAV
Urinary loss of acid; continued Na⁺ delivery to the distal tubule in presence of hyperaldosteronism	Primary aldosteronism	K⁺ depletion + aldosterone excess
	Diuretic administration	↓ EAV + K⁺ depletion
Excessive HCO_3^- loads		
Absolute		
NaHCO₃	NaHCO₃ administration	↓ EAV
Metabolic conversion of salts of organic acid anions to HCO_3^-	Lactate, acetate, citrate administration	↓ EAV
Relative		
Alkaline loads in renal failure	Alkali administration to patients with renal failure	Renal failure
Posthypercapnic state	Abrupt correction of chronic hypercapnia	↓ EAV

From Prough DS, Mathru M: Acid-base, fluids, and electrolytes. In Barash PG, Cullen BF, Stoelting RK, eds: *Clinical anesthesia*, Philadelphia, 1995, Lippincott-Raven.
EAV, Effective arterial volume; *Na⁺*, sodium; *K⁺*, potassium; *HCO₃⁻*, bicarbonate; *NaHCO₃*, sodium carbonate.

or has conserved HCO_3^- in response to chronic hypercarbia.

Recognition of hyperbicarbonatemia on a preoperative serum electrolyte determination justifies arterial blood gas analysis and should alert the anesthesiologist to the possibility that the metabolic alkalosis is maintained by hypovolemia or hypokalemia, either of which could complicate the perioperative course. For example, Table 22-6 illustrates changes in arterial blood gases and electrolytes with chronic diuretic administration.

If an arterial blood gas sample confirms the presence of metabolic alkalosis, perioperative iatrogenic respiratory alkalosis should be avoided because the combination of two primary alkaloses may cause severe enough alkalemia to produce cardiovascular depression, arrhythmias, and the other complications. Table 22-7 illustrates the effects of hyperventilation on the arterial blood gases from the previous example. Acute decreases in Pa_{CO_2} produce predictable effects on pH and $[HCO_3^-]$ (Box 22-12).

At times, it may be necessary to treat metabolic alkalosis before surgery or to modify intraoperative fluid management. In general, treatment of metabolic alkalosis can be divided into etiologic and nonetiologic therapy. Etiologic therapy consists of measures such as expansion of intravascular volume to increase renal perfusion (effective arterial volume) or the administration of potassium to reverse hypokalemia. Theoretically, because hypoproteinemia can cause a mild metabolic alkalosis (Fig. 22-14),[106-108] infusion of albumin should

help to restore $[HCO_3^-]$ to normal. However, $[HCO_3^-]$ elevations secondary to hypoproteinemia are unlikely to be clinically important and there is no established role for using albumin to treat metabolic alkalosis. Nonetiologic therapy of metabolic alkalosis includes the administration of $[H^+]$ (in the form of ammonium chloride, arginine hydrochloride, or 0.1 N hydrochloric acid), the administration of acetazolamide (a carbonic anhydrase inhibitor that causes renal HCO_3^- wasting), or acid dialysis.[109] Of these, in an acute situation associated with high risk secondary to metabolic alkalosis, 0.1 N hydrochloric acid most rapidly corrects metabolic alkalosis. However, dilute hydrochloric acid must be given into a central vein; peripheral infusion causes severe tissue damage. For intraoperative fluid therapy of a patient with

Table 22-6. Development of metabolic alkalosis secondary to chronic diuretic administration

	Baseline	Chronic diuresis
pH	7.40	7.47
Pa_{CO_2}	40 mm Hg	45 mm Hg
$[HCO_3^-]$	24 mEq/L	32 mEq/L
"CO_2"	25 mEq/L	33 mEq/L
$[Cl^-]$	105 mEq/L	97 mEq/L
$[Na^+]$	140 mEq/L	140 mEq/L
$[K^+]$	4 mEq/L	2.8 mEq/L

Pa_{CO_2}, Arterial carbon dioxide pressure; $[HCO_3^-]$, bicarbonate concentration; "CO_2," total carbon dioxide on serum electrolyte analysis; $[Cl^-]$, chloride concentration; $[Na^+]$, sodium concentration; $[K^+]$, potassium concentration.

Table 22-7. Metabolic alkalosis plus intraoperative hyperventilation

	Metabolic alkalosis	Intraoperative hyperventilation
pH	7.47	7.62
Pa_{CO_2}	45 mm Hg	30 mm Hg
$[HCO_3^-]$	32 mEq/L	29 mEq/L
"CO_2"	33 mEq/L	30 mEq/L

Pa_{CO_2}, Arterial carbon dioxide pressure; $[HCO_3^-]$, bicarbonate concentration; "CO_2," total carbon dioxide.

Box 22-12 Rules for $[HCO_3^-]$ and pH changes in response to acute and chronic decreases in Pa_{CO_2}

If Pa_{CO_2} acutely decreases by 10 mm Hg
  pH will increase 0.10
  $[HCO_3^-]$ will decrease 2 mEq/L
If hypocarbia is sustained
  pH will nearly normalize
  $[HCO_3^-]$ will decrease 5-6 mEq/L for each chronic 10–mm Hg decrease in Pa_{CO_2}*

*Hospitalized patients rarely develop compensation for chronic hypocarbia because of stimuli that enhance distal tubular reabsorption of sodium.
$[HCO_3^-]$, Bicarbonate concentration; Pa_{CO_2}, arterial carbon dioxide pressure.

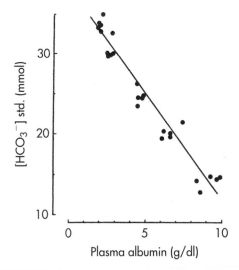

Fig. 22-14. Bicarbonate concentration ($[HCO_3^-]$) as a function of in vitro modification of plasma albumin concentration. Note that a normal albumin concentration (~4 g/dl) is associated with a $[HCO_3^-]$ of approximately 24 mmol; a decrease to ~2 g/dl is associated with an $[HCO_3^-]$ of approximately 30 mmol. *std.*, Value standardized to a P_{CO_2} of 40 mm Hg. (From Rossing TH, Maffeo N, Fencl V: *J Appl Physiol* 61:2260, 1986.)

metabolic alkalosis, 0.9% saline theoretically is preferable to lactated Ringer's solution. Saline tends to generate a hyperchloremic acidosis (i.e., reducing $[HCO_3^-]$),[110] whereas lactate provides additional substrate for hepatic generation of HCO_3^-.

2. Metabolic acidosis. Metabolic acidosis, characterized by an acidemic pH (less than 7.35) and hypobicarbonatemia (less than 21 mEq/L), results from abnormal external loss of HCO_3^- or buffering by endogenous HCO_3^- of endogenous or exogenous acids. By calculating the anion gap, two types of metabolic acidosis may be distinguished, based on whether the calculated anion gap is normal or increased (Table 22-8).[111] The term *anion gap* refers to the fact that routine electrolyte determinations commonly measure a greater proportion of total serum cations than of anions. The commonly measured cation, $[Na^+]$, usually exceeds by approximately 9 to 13 mEq/L the total concentration of the anions, $[Cl^-]$ and $[HCO_3^-]$. In situations such as diarrhea, biliary drainage, and renal tubular acidosis, in which HCO_3^- is lost externally, the anion gap—that is, $[Na^+] - ([Cl^-] + [HCO_3^-])$—is normal (less than 13 mEq/L). The anion gap also remains normal in hyperchloremic acidosis associated with perioperative infusion of 15 ml/kg/hr of 0.9% saline for surgical procedures lasting 3 to 4 hours (Table 22-9).[110] An increased anion gap (more than 13 mEq/L) results from one of three pathophysiologic states (lactic acidosis, ketoacidosis, or uremia) or to ingestion of toxic quantities of substances such as aspirin, ethylene glycol, and methanol. In these clinical circumstances, the anion gap increases because HCO_3^- ions are used to buffer hydrogen ions from the excess production of metabolic acids, whereas serum $[HCO_3^-]$ is replaced by the associated anion.

The clinical responses to acidemia are diverse and important. If pH is sufficiently reduced, myocardial contractility may be reduced,[112] pulmonary vascular resistance may increase,[112] systemic vascular resistance may decrease,[113] and there may be an impaired response of the cardiovascular system to endogenous or exogenous catecholamines.[114] The severity of the pH reduction in metabolic acidosis is usually offset by compensatory hyperventilation.[115] Inadequate compensatory hyperventilation in response to metabolic acidosis is usually an ominous finding and is physiologically equivalent to respiratory acidosis. Patients who fail to compensate for acute metabolic acidosis may require intubation and mechanical ventilation until the metabolic acidosis is effectively treated, unless there is a simple, reversible reason for failed compensation (e.g., excessive opioid administration). If a patient with metabolic acidosis requires mechanical ventilation, either in the intensive care unit or during surgery, minute ventilation should be adjusted to replicate physiologically appropriate ventilatory compensation until the primary process can be corrected; otherwise, pH may decrease severely (Table 22-10).

The anesthetic implications of metabolic acidosis are proportional to the physiologic severity of the underlying process. Although patients with hyperchloremic metabolic acidosis may be healthy, those with lactic acidosis, ketoacidosis, uremia, or toxic ingestions will be chronically or acutely ill. Occasionally, on physical examination metabolic acidosis may be suspected because of compensatory hyperventilation and hyperpnea. The serum electrolytes will demonstrate a decreased "CO_2." The anion gap should be evaluated. Arterial blood gases may be indicated to quantify the severity of metabolic acidosis and to assess the adequacy of compensation. Preoperative assessment should evaluate renal function, pulmonary status, and evidence of hypovolemia or hypoperfusion. If metabolic acidosis is secondary to shock, direct arterial pressure monitoring and, occasionally, pulmonary arterial catheterization may be indicated.

Table 22-9. Changes from preoperative to postoperative values

	Saline ($n = 15$)	Plasmalyte 148 ($n = 15$)
Sodium (mEq/L)	+1.8 (1.3)	+0.6 (1.8)
Potassium (mEq/L)	−0.05 (0.50)	−0.15 (0.45)
Chloride (mEq/L)	+6.9 (2.3)*	+0.6 (1.2)*
Chloride (24 hr) (mEq/L)	+1.5 (2.3)	−1.3 (2.4)
Standard bicarbonate (mEq/L)	−4 (2)*	−0.7 (1.0)*
Base excess	−5 (2.1)*	−1.2 (1.1)*

From McFarlane C, Lee A: *Anaesthesia* 49:779, 1994.
*$p < 0.01$. Values are mean (SD). Plasmalyte 148 contains 140 mEq/L sodium, 98 mEq/L chloride, and 27 mEq/L acetate (which is hepatically metabolized to bicarbonate).

Table 22-8. Differential diagnosis of metabolic acidosis

Elevated anion gap	Normal anion gap
Diseases	Saline infusion
Uremia	Renal tubular acidosis
Ketoacidosis	Diarrhea
Lactic acidosis	Carbonic anhydrase inhibition
Toxins	Ureteral diversions
Methanol	Early renal failure
Ethylene glycol	Hydronephrosis
Salicylates	

Table 22-10. Inadequate intraoperative ventilatory compensation for metabolic acidosis

	Spontaneous ventilation	Mechanical ventilation
pH	7.29	7.13
$PaCO_2$	29 mm Hg	49 mm Hg
$[HCO_3^-]$	14 mEq/L	16 mEq/L

$[HCO_3^-]$, Bicarbonate concentration.
Note: In the presence of metabolic acidosis, an otherwise innocuous increase in arterial carbon dioxide pressure *($PaCO_2$)* may create severe acidemia.

If time permits, preoperative correction of the primary processes that have generated metabolic acidosis should be accomplished. During anesthesia and surgery, patients with metabolic acidosis secondary to hypoperfusion may have exaggerated hypotensive responses to drugs and positive pressure ventilation. As noted earlier, sudden cessation of ventilatory compensation for the metabolic acidosis may result in severe acidemia. During anesthesia, measurement of the gradient between $PaCO_2$ and end-tidal CO_2 facilitates continuous monitoring of the adequacy of ventilatory compensation. Intermittent measurement of arterial blood gases provides feedback about the efficacy of treatment of the underlying metabolic process.

The treatment of metabolic acidosis consists of the treatment of the primary pathophysiologic process (i.e., hypoperfusion, hypoxia) and, if pH is severely decreased, administration of $NaHCO_3$. A commonly used calculation of an initial dose of $NaHCO_3$ is as follows:

$$NaHCO_3 \ (mEq/L) = \frac{Wt \ (kg) \times 0.3 \times (24 \ mEq/L - Actual \ HCO_3)}{2} \quad (22\text{-}7)$$

where 0.3 is the assumed HCO_3^- distribution space, and 24 mEq/L is the normal value for $[HCO_3^-]$ on arterial blood gas determination. The calculation markedly underestimates dosage in severe metabolic acidosis.

If $NaHCO_3$ is infused, arterial blood gases should be measured again after approximately 5 minutes. In infants and children, an appropriate initial dose is 1 to 2 mEq/kg of body weight. Hyperventilation, though an important compensatory response to metabolic acidosis, is not definitive therapy for metabolic acidosis.

One continuing controversy is the use of $NaHCO_3$ to treat acidemia induced by lactic acidosis. Certainly, the best treatment for lactic acidosis is restoration of adequate tissue oxygenation. However, when pH is less than 7.25, the conventional approach has been to administer $NaHCO_3$ to improve pH, based on the concept that alkalinization should improve systemic hemodynamics and enhance responsiveness to catecholamines. However, few data support the use of $NaHCO_3$ to treat lactic acidosis. In experimental animals, administration of $NaHCO_3$ transiently increased mean arterial blood pressure while increasing pH[116]; however, intracellular pH did not improve. Moreover, there was no substantial difference between $NaHCO_3$, carbicarb (a combination of sodium carbonate and $NaHCO_3$), and equimolar sodium chloride.[116] This suggests that the primary effect on hemodynamics may result from the administration of a hypertonic salt solution. In animals with hypoxic acidosis, carbicarb improved pH and cardiac index more than did $NaHCO_3$; $NaHCO_3$ increased $PaCO_2$ because the buffering of $[H^+]$ by HCO_3^- produced H_2CO_3, which dissociated to H_2O and CO_2.[117]

Although several studies have demonstrated that bicarbonate therapy is safe in critically ill patients and in perioperative patients,[118-120] no study has demonstrated that it improves outcomes. In critically ill patients with lactic acidosis, there were no important differences between the effects of 0.9 mol $NaHCO_3$ and 0.9 mol sodium chloride.[121] The effects on cardiac output and arterial pressure were similar, despite increases in pH, $[HCO_3^-]$, and $PaCO_2$ after administration of sodium bicarbonate. It is important to note that $NaHCO_3$ did not increase the clinical cardiovascular response to catecholamines and reduced plasma ionized calcium.[121] Although other buffers and metabolic interventions have been used to treat lactic acidosis, neither carbicarb[120] nor dichloroacetate[122] has improved clinical outcome. Although many clinicians continue to administer $NaHCO_3$ to patients with persistent lactic acidosis and ongoing deterioration,[123] it is unlikely that the treatment is efficacious.

The buffer tris-hydroxymethyl aminomethane (THAM) is effective at reducing $[H^+]$ and does not generate CO_2 as a byproduct of buffering[124]; however, there is no generally accepted indication for THAM.

3. Respiratory alkalosis. Usually characterized by an alkalemic pH (greater than 7.45) and always characterized by hypocarbia ($PaCO_2$ less than 35 mm Hg), respiratory alkalosis describes an increase in minute ventilation to a level greater than that required to excrete the metabolic production of CO_2. Hyperventilation may be secondary to pain, anxiety, hypoxemia, central nervous system disease, or metabolic disturbances (e.g., hepatic encephalopathy or sepsis). Consequently, the development of spontaneous respiratory alkalosis in a previously normocarbic patient requires evaluation. Rules describing acute and chronic changes in pH and $[HCO_3^-]$ in response to acute and chronic decreases in $PaCO_2$ are described in Box 22-12.

Alkalemia secondary to respiratory alkalosis or metabolic alkalosis may produce hypokalemia, hypocalcemia, cardiac arrhythmias, bronchoconstriction, and hypotension, and may potentiate the toxicity of cardiac glycosides. In addition, rapid changes in $PaCO_2$ alter cerebral blood flow. Acutely doubling minute ventilation reduces $PaCO_2$ from 40 mm Hg to 20 mm Hg and halves cerebral blood flow. Conversely, if minute ventilation is halved acutely, $PaCO_2$ and cerebral blood flow also double. The acute changes in cerebral blood flow accommodate within 8 to 24 hours, associated with a return of cerebrospinal fluid $[HCO_3^-]$ toward normal.[125,126] Subsequent changes in $PaCO_2$, after accommodation of the cerebrospinal fluid $[HCO_3^-]$ to chronic hypocapnia or hypercapnia, again acutely change cerebral blood flow.

Patients who have been chronically spontaneously hyperventilating or who have been therapeutically hyperventilated require intraoperative maintenance of a similar $PaCO_2$. Acute hyperventilation may be useful in neurosurgical procedures to reduce brain bulk and to control intracranial pressure (ICP) during emergency surgery for noncranial injuries associated with acute closed-head trauma. In those situations, intraoperative monitoring of arterial blood gases, correlated with capnography, facilitates control of $PaCO_2$. However, acute profound hypocapnia (less than 20 mm Hg) may produce electroencephalogram evidence of cerebral ischemia.

4. Respiratory acidosis. Respiratory acidosis, usually characterized by a low pH (less than 7.35) and always characterized by hypercarbia ($PaCO_2$ greater than 45 mm Hg), occurs when minute ventilation is insufficient to eliminate CO_2 production without an increased capillary-alveolar CO_2 gradient. Respiratory acidosis may be either acute, without compensation by renal $[HCO_3^-]$ retention, or chronic, with $[HCO_3^-]$ retention offsetting the decrease in pH. Respiratory acidosis occurs because of a decrease in minute alveolar ventilation $(_A)$, an increase in production of carbon dioxide (CO_2), or both, from the following equation:

$$Pa_{CO_2} = K(V_{CO_2})/V_A \qquad (22\text{-}8)$$

where K = constant. (Of course, rebreathing of exhaled, carbon dioxide-containing gas may also increase Pa_{CO_2}.) A reduction in V_A may be caused by an overall decrease in minute ventilation (V_E) or an increase in the amount of wasted ventilation (V_D), according to the following equation:

$$V_A = V_E - V_D \qquad (22\text{-}9)$$

Decreases in V_E may result from central ventilatory depression by drugs or central nervous system injury, increased work of breathing, or airway obstruction or neuromuscular dysfunction. Increases in V_D occur with severe chronic obstructive pulmonary disease, pulmonary embolism, and most acute forms of respiratory failure. V_{CO_2} may be increased by sepsis, high-glucose parenteral feeding, or fever.

Patients with chronic hypercarbia resulting from intrinsic pulmonary disease require careful preoperative evaluation. The ventilatory restriction imposed by upper abdominal or thoracic surgery may be a particular risk to patients who chronically are unable to excrete V_{CO_2} at a normal Pa_{CO_2}. Administration of narcotics and sedatives, even in small doses, may cause hazardous ventilatory depression. During preoperative evaluation, the anesthesiologist should consider direct arterial pressure monitoring and frequent intraoperative blood gas determinations, as well as postoperative pain management. End-tidal CO_2 may substantially underestimate Pa_{CO_2}. Intraoperatively, a patient with chronic hypercapnia should be ventilated to maintain a normal pH. An abrupt increase in minute ventilation may result in profound alkalemia, and the associated complications, because the chronic elevation in $[HCO_3^-]$ will remain after Pa_{CO_2} is abruptly reduced (analogous to the addition of hyperventilation to metabolic alkalosis). Postoperatively, prophylactic ventilatory support may be required for selected patients with chronic hypercarbia. Epidural narcotic administration is one potential alternative that may provide adequate postoperative analgesia without undue depression of ventilatory drive.

The treatment of respiratory acidosis depends on the acuity of the process. Acute respiratory acidosis may require mechanical ventilation unless a simple etiologic factor (e.g., narcotic overdose or residual muscular blockade) can be treated quickly. Bicarbonate administration rarely is indicated unless severe metabolic acidosis is also present or unless mechanical ventilation is ineffective in reducing acute hypercarbia. In contrast, chronic respiratory acidosis is rarely managed with ventilation. Rather, efforts are made to improve pulmonary function to permit more effective elimination of carbon dioxide. During acute exacerbations of chronic hypercapnic respiratory failure, patients may be treated at extremely high levels of Pa_{CO_2}, allowing renal compensation to maintain pH compensation but occasionally receiving $NaHCO_3$.

B. Rapid bedside analysis of acid-base status

Prompt, effective management of perioperative acid-base disturbances requires the ability to make a correct diagnosis. Rapid interpretation of a patient's acid-base status involves the integration of three sets of data: arterial blood gases, electrolytes, and history. The following stepwise approach facilitates interpretation (Box 22-13).

1. Is the pH life-threatening, requiring immediate intervention? Certain data require immediate attention. Respiratory acidosis with a pH less than 7.1 suggests the need for intubation and ventilatory support, whereas a metabolic acidosis with a similar pH suggests the need for appropriate etiologic intervention and perhaps alkalinizing therapy. A pH greater than 7.55 may require emergent treatment if it is associated with acute complications such as cardiac arrhythmias.
2. Is the pH acidemic (pH less than 7.35) or alkalemic (pH greater than 7.45)? The pH usually indicates one primary process (i.e., acidosis produces acidemia, alkalosis produces alkalemia). Note that the suffix "-osis" indicates a primary process that, if unopposed, will produce the corresponding pH change. The suffix "-emia" refers to the pH. A compensatory process is not considered an "-osis." Of course, a patient may have mixed "-oses," that is, more than one primary process.
3. Could the acid-base status be explained by only an acute increase or decrease in Pa_{CO_2}? In other words, are the arterial blood gases consistent with (though not necessarily diagnostic of) a simple acute respiratory alkalosis or acidosis. Box 22-12 summarizes the changes in pH and $[HCO_3^-]$ associated with acute hyperventilation. For example, an acute decline in Pa_{CO_2} from 40 mm Hg to 30 mm Hg would increase pH from 7.40 to 7.50 and de-

---

Box 22-13 Sequential approach to acid-base interpretation

1. Is the pH life-threatening, requiring immediate intervention?
2. Is the pH acidemic or alkalemic?
3. Could the entire arterial blood gas picture represent only an acute increase or decrease in Pa_{CO_2}?
4. If the answer to Question 3 is "No," is there evidence of a chronic respiratory disturbance or an acute metabolic disturbance?
5. Are appropriate compensatory changes present?
6. Is an anion gap present?
7. Do the clinical data fit the acid-base picture?

Pa_{CO_2}, Arterial carbon dioxide pressure.

Box 22-14 Relationships between pH, $[HCO_3^-]$, and acute and chronic hypercapnia

If $PaCO_2$ acutely increases by 10 mm Hg
  pH will decrease 0.05
  $[HCO_3^-]$ will increase 1 mEq/L
If $PaCO_2$ chronically increases by 10 mm Hg
  pH will return toward normal
  $[HCO_3^-]$ will increase 4 mEq/L

$[HCO_3^-]$, Bicarbonate concentration; *$PaCO_2$*, arterial carbon dioxide pressure.

Box 22-15 Rules for respiratory compensation of metabolic acidosis

$PaCO_2 = [HCO_3^-] \times 1.5 + 8.0$
The last two digits of the pH equal $[HCO_3^-] + 15$

$PaCO_2$, Arterial carbon dioxide pressure; *$[HCO_3^-]$*, bicarbonate concentration.

crease the calculated $[HCO_3^-]$ from 24 mEq/L to 22 mEq/L. Box 22-14 summarizes the changes in pH and $[HCO_3^-]$ associated with acute hypoventilation.

4. The answer "No" to Question 3 prompts the next question: Is there evidence of a chronic respiratory disturbance or of an acute metabolic disturbance? If the magnitude of the pH and $[HCO_3^-]$ changes are not consistent with a simple acute respiratory disturbance, a chronic respiratory problem (more than 24 hours) should be considered. The rules for a chronic respiratory disturbance are listed in Box 22-12. Note that the pH becomes nearly normal with compensation. The patient's history or previously obtained laboratory results may provide clues as to whether the respiratory changes are acute or chronic. If neither an acute respiratory change nor a chronic compensatory change can explain the entire blood gas picture, then a primary metabolic disturbance may also be present.

5. Are appropriate compensatory changes present? Boxes 22-11 and 22-15 list the rules for compensation that should occur in response to metabolic alkalosis and acidosis, respectively. Note that respiratory compensation for metabolic acid-base disturbances occurs rapidly. Several general rules describe compensation. First, overcompensation is rare. Second, inadequate or excessive compensation suggests an additional primary disturbance. Third, hypobicarbonatemia associated with an increased anion gap is not compensatory. Finally, the rules describing the expected relationships between pH, $[H^+]$, and $[HCO_3^-]$ describe a logarithmic relationship. The more the pH deviates from 7.40, the less accurate the rules become.

6. Is an increased anion gap present? The electrolytes and anion gap should be assessed unless the acid-base status is clearly explained by recent pathophysiologic or therapeutic events (e.g., metabolic acidosis in a patient undergoing emergency surgery for a ruptured abdominal aortic aneurysm or intentional respiratory alkalosis in a patient undergoing craniotomy). Metabolic acidoses associated with a high anion gap require specific interventions, thus necessitating a correct diagnosis. Failure to consider the presence or absence of an increased anion gap may result in an erroneous diagnosis and failure to initiate appropriate treatment.

7. Do the clinical data fit the acid-base picture? This question may at first seem out of sequence. Although diagnostic testing usually is obtained because of a suspicion of a specific disorder, arterial blood gases are often obtained for monitoring. Failure to consider whether clinical findings are consistent with an acid-base interpretation may lead to serious errors in clinical management.

C. Example

A 55-year-old man has received 3 days of nasogastric suction for partial small bowel obstruction. Before nasogastric suction, he had severe nausea and emesis persisting for 48 hours. Arterial blood gases are as follows: pH 7.40, $PaCO_2$ 40 mm Hg, and $[HCO_3^-]$ 24 mEq/L. Serum electrolytes are as follows: $[Na^+]$ 140 mEq/L, $[Cl^-]$ 94 mEq/L, and CO_2 25 mEq/L. What are the answers to the questions in Box 22-13?

1. The pH of 7.40 is normal and requires no immediate intervention.
2. The pH is neither acidemic nor alkalemic.
3. The $PaCO_2$ of 40 mm Hg is normal.
4. Based on the arterial blood gases, there is no metabolic disturbance or chronic respiratory disturbance.
5. Based on the arterial blood gases, no compensatory processes are present.
6. The anion gap is 21 mEq/L. Despite a normal pH, $PaCO_2$, and $[HCO_3^-]$, the patient has a severe metabolic acidosis. Because the $[HCO_3^-]$ is normal, another process that increases $[HCO_3^-]$ must be offsetting the expected reduction in $[HCO_3^-]$ associated with metabolic acidosis.
7. A history of vomiting and nasogastric suction should suggest the possibility of primary metabolic alkalosis; however, if vomiting were sufficiently severe to produce hypovolemic shock and lactic acidosis, the previously increased $[HCO_3^-]$ concentration would be reduced as it buffered endogenous H^+ (Table 22-11).

This sequence illustrates the clinically important concept that the final pH, $PaCO_2$, and $[HCO_3^-]$ represent the result of several vectors that influence acid-base equilibrium. Complex disturbances can be interpreted only by using a thorough, stepwise approach.

Table 22-11. Metabolic alkalosis with subsequent lactic acidosis

	Normal	Metabolic alkalosis secondary to vomiting and nasogastric suction	Superimposed metabolic acidosis secondary to hypoperfusion
pH	7.40	7.50	7.40
$Paco_2$	40 mm Hg	46 mm Hg	40 mm Hg
$[HCO_3^-]$	24 mEq/L	35 mEq/L	24 mEq/L
Na^+	140 mEq/L	140 mEq/L	140 mEq/L
Cl^-	105 mEq/L	94 mEq/L	94 mEq/L
CO_2	25 mEq/L	36 mEq/L	25 mEq/L
Anion gap	10 mEq/L	10 mEq/L	21 mEq/L

$Paco_2$, Arterial carbon dioxide pressure; $[HCO_3^-]$, bicarbonate concentration, Na^+, sodium; Cl^-, chloride; CO_2, carbon dioxide.

III. SUMMARY

Disorders of electrolytes and acid-base status occur commonly in surgical patients. Reasons include chronic underlying diseases, previous medical treatment, hemorrhage, infusion of intravenous fluids, physiologic changes accompanying acute surgical illness, and substitution of mechanical ventilation for spontaneous ventilation. If sufficiently severe, abnormalities of electrolytes and acid-base status may increase the likelihood of perioperative mortality and morbidity. Consequently, one key responsibility of anesthesiologists is prompt diagnosis and effective treatment of abnormalities in the concentrations of sodium, potassium, calcium, magnesium, phosphate, hydrogen ion, bicarbonate, and $Paco_2$.

REFERENCES

1. Teitelbaum I, Kleeman CR, Berl T: The physiology of the renal concentrating and diluting mechanism. In Narins RG, ed: *Clinical disorders of fluid and electrolyte metabolism*, New York, 1994, McGraw-Hill, p 101.
2. Fried LF, Palevsky PM: Hyponatremia and hypernatremia. In Saklayen MG, ed: *The Medical Clinics of North America: renal disease*, Philadelphia, 1997, WB Saunders, p 585.
3. Abramow M, Beauwens R, Cogan E: Cellular events in vasopressin action, *Kidney Int* 21:S56, 1987.
4. Fushimi K, Uchida S, Hara Y, et al: Cloning and expression of apical membrane water channel of rat kidney collecting tubule, *Nature* 361:549, 1993.
5. Harris HW Jr, Strange K, Zeidel ML: Current understanding of the cellular biology and molecular structure of the antidiuretic hormone-stimulated water transport pathway, *J Clin Invest* 88:1, 1991.
6. Levin AR, Gardner DG, Samson WK: Natriuretic peptides, *N Engl J Med* 339:321, 1998.
7. Schrier RW: Pathogenesis of sodium and water retention in high-output and low-output cardiac failure, nephrotic syndrome, cirrhosis, and pregnancy. Parts 1 and 2, *N Engl J Med* 319:1065, 1988.
8. Laragh JH: The endocrine control of blood volume, blood pressure and sodium balance: atrial hormone and renin system interactions, *J Hypertens* 4(suppl 2):S143, 1986.
9. Needleman P, Greenwald JE: Atriopeptin: a cardiac hormone intimately involved in fluid, electrolyte, and blood-pressure homeostasis, *N Engl J Med* 314:828, 1986.
10. Conte G, Bellizzi V, Cianciaruso B, et al: Physiologic role and diuretic efficacy of atrial natriuretic peptide in health and chronic renal disease, *Kidney Int* 51:S28, 1997.
11. Anderson RJ, Chung HM, Kluge R, et al: Hyponatremia: a prospective analysis of its epidemiology and the pathogenetic role of vasopressin, *Ann Intern Med* 102:164, 1985.
12. Tierney WM, Martin DK, Greenlee MC, et al: The prognosis of hyponatremia at hospital admission, *J Gen Intern Med* 1:380, 1986.
13. Berl T: Treating hyponatremia: damned if we do and damned if we don't, *Kidney Int* 37:1006, 1990.
14. Lien YH, Shapiro JI, Chan L: Effects of hypernatremia on organic brain osmoles, *J Clin Invest* 85:1427, 1990.
15. Moran SM, Jamison RL: The variable hyponatremic response to hyperglycemia, *West J Med* 142:49, 1985.
16. Rothenberg DM, Berns AS, Ivankovich AD: Isotonic hyponatremia following transurethral prostate resection, *J Clin Anesth* 2:48, 1990.
17. Campbell HT, Fincher ME, Sklar AH: Severe hyponatremia without hypoosmolality following transurethral resection of the prostate (TURP) in end stage renal disease, *Am J Kidney Dis* 12:152, 1988.
18. Hahn RG: The transurethral resection syndrome, *Acta Anaesthesiol Scand* 35:557, 1991.
19. Chung H, Kluge R, Schrier RW, et al: Postoperative hyponatremia: a prospective study, *Arch Intern Med* 146:333, 1986.
20. Gomola A, Cabrol S, Murat I: Severe hyponatraemia after plastic surgery in a girl with cleft palate, medial facial hypoplasia and growth retardation, *Paediatr Anesth* 8:69, 1998.
21. Arieff AI: Postoperative hyponatraemic encephalopathy following elective surgery in children, *Paediatr Anesth* 8:1, 1998.
22. Akaishi T, Sakuma Y: Estrogen-induced modulation of hypothalamic osmoregulation in female rats, *Am J Physiol* 258:R924, 1990.
23. Stone JD, Crofton JT, Share L: Sex differences in central adrenergic control of vasopressin release, *Am J Physiol* 257:R1040, 1989.
24. Arieff AI, Kozniewska E, Roberts TP, et al: Age, gender, and vasopressin affect survival and brain adaptation in rats with metabolic encephalopathy, *Am J Physiol* 268:R1143, 1995.
25. Fraser CL, Arieff AI: Fatal central diabetes mellitus and insipidus resulting from untreated hyponatremia: a new syndrome, *Ann Intern Med* 112:113, 1990.
26. Steele A, Gowrishankar M, Abrahamson S, et al: Postoperative hyponatremia despite near-isotonic saline infusion: a phenomenon of desalination, *Ann Intern Med* 126:20, 1997.
27. Ayus JC, Arieff AI: Postoperative hyponatremia, *Ann Intern Med* 126:1005, 1997.
28. Hirshberg B, Ben-Yehuda A: The syndrome of inappropriate antidiuretic hormone secretion in the elderly, *Am J Med* 103:270, 1997.
29. Cornforth BM: SIADH following laparoscopic cholecystectomy, *Can J Anaesth* 45:223, 1998.
30. Mulloy AL, Caruana RJ: Hyponatremic emergencies, *Med Clin North Am* 79:155, 1995.
31. Al-Mufti H, Arieff AI: Hyponatremia due to cerebral salt-wasting syndrome: combined cerebral and distal tubular lesion, *Am J Med* 77:740, 1984.
32. Kroll M, Juhler M, Lindholm J: Hyponatremia in acute brain disease, *J Intern Med* 232:291, 1992.

33. Wijdicks EFM, Ropper AH, Hunnicutt EJ, et al: Atrial natriuretic factor and salt wasting after aneurysmal subarachnoid hemorrhage, *Stroke* 22:1519, 1991.

34. Yamaki T, Tano-oka A, Takahashi A, et al: Cerebral salt wasting syndrome distinct from the syndrome of inappropriate secretion of antidiuretic hormone (SIADH), *Acta Neurochir* 115:156, 1992.

35. Ayus JC, Arieff AI: Symptomatic hyponatremia: making the diagnosis rapidly, *J Crit Illness* 5:846, 1990.

36. Karmel KS, Bear RA: Treatment of hyponatremia: a quantitative analysis, *Am J Kidney Dis* 21:439, 1994.

37. Sterns RH, Riggs JE, Schochet SS Jr: Osmotic demyelination syndrome following correction of hyponatremia, *N Engl J Med* 314:1535, 1986.

38. Laureno R, Karp BI: Myelinolysis after correction of hyponatremia, *Ann Intern Med* 126:57, 1997.

39. Soupart A, Decaux G: Therapeutic recommendations for management of severe hyponatremia: current concepts on pathogenesis and prevention of neurologic complications, *Clin Nephrol* 46:149, 1996.

40. Brunner JE, Redmond JM, Haggar AM, et al: Central pontine myelinolysis and pontine lesions after rapid correction of hyponatremia: a prospective magnetic resonance imaging study, *Ann Neurol* 27:61, 1990.

41. Pradhan S, Jha R, Singh MN, et al: Central pontine myelinolysis following "slow" correction of hyponatremia, *Clin Neurol Neurosurg* 97:340, 1995.

42. Miller GM, Baker HL Jr, Okazaki H, et al: Central pontine myelinolysis and its imitators: MR findings, *Radiology* 168:795, 1988.

43. Sarnaik AP, Meert K, Hackbarth R, et al: Management of hyponatremic seizures in children with hypertonic saline: a safe and effective strategy, *Crit Care Med* 19:758, 1991.

44. Adrogué HJ, Madias NE: Aiding fluid prescription for the dysnatremias, *Intensive Care Med* 23:309, 1997.

45. Vassar MJ, Fischer RP, O'Brien PE, et al: A multicenter trial for resuscitation of injured patients with 7.5% sodium chloride: the effect of added dextran 70, *Arch Surg* 128:1003, 1993.

46. Mattox KL, Maningas PA, Moore EE, et al: Prehospital hypertonic saline/dextran infusion for post-traumatic hypotension. The USA Multicenter Trial, *Ann Surg* 213:482, 1991.

47. Young RSK, Truax B: Hypernatremic hemorrhagic encephalopathy, *Ann Neurol* 5:588, 1979.

48. Ayus JC, Armstrong DL, Arieff AI: Effects of hypernatraemia in the central nervous system and its therapy in rats and rabbits, *J Physiol* 492:243, 1996.

49. Phillips PA, Rolls BJ, Ledingham JGG, et al: Reduced thirst after water deprivation in healthy elderly men, *N Engl J Med* 311:753, 1984.

50. Rowe JW, Shock NW, DeFronzo RA: The influence of age on the renal response to water deprivation in man, *Nephron* 17:270, 1976.

51. Seckl JR, Dunger DB, Lightman SL: Neurohypophyseal peptide function during early postoperative diabetes insipidus, *Brain* 110:737, 1987.

52. Griffin KA, Bidani AK: How to manage disorders of sodium and water balance: five-step approach to evaluating appropriateness of renal response, *J Crit Illness* 5:1054, 1990.

53. Strange K: Regulation of solute and water balance and cell volume in the central nervous system, *J Am Soc Nephrol* 3:12, 1992.

54. Feig PU: Hypernatremia and hypertonic syndromes, *Med Clin North Am* 65:271, 1981.

55. McManus ML, Churchwill KB, Strange K: Regulation of cell volume in health and disease, *N Engl J Med* 333:1260, 1995.

56. Chanson P, Jedynak CP, Dabrowski G, et al: Ultralow doses of vasopressin in the management of diabetes insipidus, *Crit Care Med* 15:44, 1987.

57. Cobb WE, Spare S, Reichlin S: Neurogenic diabetes insipidus: management with dDAVP (1-desamino-8-D arginine vasopressin), *Ann Intern Med* 88:183, 1978.

58. Rabinowitz L: Aldosterone and potassium homeostasis, *Kidney Int* 49:1738, 1996.

59. Swedner KJ, Goldin SM: Active transport of sodium and potassium ions: mechanism, function, and regulation, *N Engl J Med* 302:777, 1980.

60. Mandal AK: Hypokalemia and hyperkalemia. In Saklayen MG, ed: *The Medical Clinics of North America: renal disease,* Philadelphia, 1997, WB Saunders, p 611.

61. Vitez TS, Soper LE, Wong KC, et al: Chronic hypokalemia and intraoperative dysrhythmias, *Anesthesiology* 63:130, 1985.

62. Hirsch IA, Tomlinson DL, Slogoff S, et al: The overstated risk of preoperative hypokalemia, *Anesth Analg* 67:131, 1988.

63. Weiner ID, Wingo CS: Hypokalemia: consequences, causes, and correction, *J Am Soc Nephrol* 8:1179, 1997.

64. Gorden P: Glucose intolerance with hypokalemia: failure of short-term potassium depletion in normal subjects to reproduce the glucose and insulin abnormalities of clinical hypokalemia, *Diabetes* 22:544, 1973.

65. Gennari FJ: Hypokalemia, *N Engl J Med* 339:451, 1998.

66. Rimmer JM, Horn JF, Gennari FJ: Hyperkalemia as a complication of drug therapy, *Arch Intern Med* 147:867, 1987.

67. Kuvin JT: Electrocardiographic changes of hyperkalemia, *N Engl J Med* 338:662, 1998.

68. Wrenn KD, Slovis CM, Slovis BS: The ability of physicians to predict hyperkalemia from the ECG, *Ann Emerg Med* 20:1229, 1991.

69. Kemper MJ, Harps E, Müller-Wiefel DE: Hyperkalemia: therapeutic options in acute and chronic renal failure, *Clin Nephrol* 46:67, 1996.

70. Zaloga GP, Chernow B, Cook D, et al: Assessment of calcium homeostasis in the critically ill surgical patient: the diagnostic pitfalls of the McLean-Hastings nomogram, *Ann Surg* 202:587, 1985.

71. Edelson GW, Kleerekoper M: Hypercalcemia crisis, *Med Clin North Am* 79:79, 1995.

72. Rutecki GW, Whittier FC: Recognizing hypercalcemia: the "3-hormone, 3-organ rule," *J Crit Illness* 13:59, 1998.

73. Adler AJ, Ferran N, Berlyne GM: Effect of inorganic phosphate on serum ionized calcium concentration in vitro: a reassessment of the "trade-off hypothesis," *Kidney Int* 28:932, 1985.

74. Rutledge R, Sheldon GF, Collins ML: Massive transfusion, *Crit Care Clin* 2:791, 1986.

75. Lebowitz MR, Moses AM: Hypocalcemia, *Semin Nephrol* 12:146, 1992.

76. Guise TA, Mundy GR: Evaluation of hypocalcemia in children and adults, *J Clin Endocrinol Metab* 80:1473, 1995.

77. Sutters M, Gaboury CL, Bennett WM: Severe hyperphosphatemia and hypocalcemia: a dilemma in patient management, *J Am Soc Nephrol* 7:2055, 1996.

78. Zaloga GP, Strickland RA, Butterworth JFIV, et al: Calcium attenuates epinephrine's β-adrenergic effects in postoperative heart surgery patients, *Circulation* 81:196, 1990.

79. Mathru M, Rooney MW, Goldberg SA, et al: Separation of myocardial versus peripheral effects of calcium administration in normocalcemic and hypocalcemic states using pressure-volume (conductance) relationships, *Anesth Analg* 77:250, 1993.

80. Davis KD, Attie MF: Management of severe hypercalcemia, *Crit Care Clin* 7:175, 1991.

81. Ryzen E, Martodam RR, Troxell M, et al: Intravenous etidronate in the management of malignant hypercalcemia, *Arch Intern Med* 145:449, 1985.

82. Gucalp R, Ritch P, Wiernik PH, et al: Comparative study of pamidronate disodium and etidronate disodium in the treatment of cancer-related hypercalcemia, *J Clin Oncol* 10:134, 1992.

83. Chan FKW, Koberle LMC, Thys-Jacobs S, et al: Differential diagnosis, causes, and management of hypercalcemia, *Curr Probl Surg* 34:449, 1997.

84. Flink EB: Nutritional aspects of magnesium metabolism, *West J Med* 133:304, 1980.

85. Whang R, Hampton EM, Whang DD: Magnesium homeostasis and clinical disorders of magnesium deficiency, *Ann Pharmacother* 28:220, 1997.

86. Wong ET, Rude RK, Singer FR, et al: A high prevalence of hypomagnesemia and hypermagnesemia in hospitalized patients, *Am J Clin Pathol* 79:348, 1983.

87. Whang R, Ryder KW: Frequency of hypomagnesemia and hypermagnesemia: requested vs routine, *JAMA* 263:3063, 1990.

88. Salem M, Munoz R, Chernow B: Hypomagnesemia in critical illness: a common and clinically important problem, *Crit Care Clin* 7:225, 1991.

89. Chernow B, Bamberger S, Stoiko M, et al: Hypomagnesemia in patients in postoperative intensive care, *Chest* 95:391, 1989.

89a. Murray MJ, Coursin DB, Pearl RG, et al, eds: *Critical care medicine: perioperative management,* Philadelphia, 1997, Lippincott-Raven, p. 228.

90. Harris MNE, Crowther A, Jupp RA, et al: Magnesium and coronary revascularization, *Br J Anaesth* 60:779, 1988.

91. Teo KK, Yusuf S, Collins R, et al: Effects of intravenous magnesium in suspected acute myocardial infarction: overview of randomised trials, *BMJ* 303:1499, 1991.

92. Tzivoni D, Banai S, Schuger C, et al: Treatment of torsade de pointes with magnesium sulfate, *Circulation* 77:392, 1988.

93. James MFM, Beer RE, Esser JD: Intravenous magnesium sulfate inhibits catecholamine release associated with tracheal intubation, *Anesth Analg* 68:772, 1989.

94. van Hook JW: Hypermagnesemia, *Crit Care Clin* 7:215, 1991.

95. Murer H, Werner A, Reshkin S, et al: Cellular mechanisms in proximal tubular reabsorption of inorganic phosphate, *Am J Physiol (Cell Physiol)* 260:C885, 1991.

96. Peppers MP, Geheb M, Desai T: Hypophosphatemia and hyperphosphatemia, *Crit Care Clin* 7:201, 1991.

97. Aubier M, Murciano D, Lecocguic Y, et al: Effect of hypophosphatemia on diaphragmatic contractility in patients with acute respiratory failure, *N Engl J Med* 313:420, 1985.

98. O'Connor LR, Wheeler WS, Bethune JE: Effect of hypophosphatemia on myocardial performance in man, *N Engl J Med* 297:901, 1977.

99. Brooks MJ, Melnik G: The refeeding syndrome: an approach to understanding its complications and preventing its occurrence, *Pharmacology* 15:713, 1995.

100. Rosen GH, Boullata JI, O'Rangers EA, et al: Intravenous phosphate repletion regimen for critically ill patients with moderate hypophosphatemia, *Crit Care Med* 23:1204, 1995.

101. Stewart PA: Independent and dependent variables of acid-base control, *Respir Physiol* 33:9, 1978.

102. Eicker SW: An introduction to strong ion difference, *Vet Clin North Am Food Anim Pract* 8:45, 1990.

103. Sabatini S, Arruda JAL, Kurtzman NA: Disorders of acid-base balance, *Med Clin North Am* 62:1223, 1978.

104. Riley LJ Jr, Elson BE, Narins RG: Acute metabolic acid-base disorders, *Crit Care Clin* 5:699, 1987.

105. Goldring RM, Cannon PJ, Heinemann HO, et al: Respiratory adjustment to chronic metabolic alkalosis in man, *J Clin Invest* 47:188, 1968.

106. Rossing TH, Maffeo N, Fencl V: Acid-base effects of altering plasma protein concentration in human blood in vitro, *J Appl Physiol* 61:2260, 1986.

107. Figge J, Mydosh T, Fencl V: Serum proteins and acid-base equilibria: a follow-up, *J Lab Clin Med* 120:713, 1992.

108. Figge J, Rossing TH, Fencl V: The role of serum proteins in acid-base equilibria, *J Lab Clin Med* 117:453, 1991.

109. Ponce P, Santana A, Vinhas J: Treatment of severe metabolic alkalosis by "acid dialysis," *Crit Care Med* 19:583, 1991.

110. McFarlane C, Lee A: A comparison of Plasmalyte 148 and 0.9% saline for intra-operative fluid replacement, *Anaesthesia* 49:779, 1994.

111. Badrick T, Hickman PE: The anion gap: a reappraisal, *Am J Clin Pathol* 98:249, 1992.

112. Opie LH, Kadas T, Gevers W: Effect of pH on the function and glucose metabolism of the heart, *Lancet* 2:551, 1963.

113. Wildenthal K, Mierzwiak DS, Myers RW: Effects of acute lactic acidosis of left ventricular performance, *Am J Physiol* 241:1352, 1968.

114. Stokke DB, Andersen PK, Brinklov MM, et al: Acid-base interactions with noradrenaline-induced contractile response of the rabbit isolated aorta, *Anesthesiology* 60:400, 1984.

115. Albert MS, Dell RB, Winters RW: Quantitative displacement of acid-base equilibrium in metabolic acidosis, *Ann Intern Med* 66:312, 1967.

116. Beech JS, Nolan KM, Iles RA, et al: The effects of sodium bicarbonate and a mixture of sodium bicarbonate ("carbicarb") on skeletal muscle pH and hemodynamic status in rats with hypovolemic shock, *Metabolism* 43:518, 1994.

117. Rhee KH, Toro LO, McDonald GG, et al: Carbicarb, sodium bicarbonate, and sodium chloride in hypoxic lactic acidosis: effect on arterial blood bases, lactate concentrations, hemodynamic variables, and myocardial intracellular pH, *Chest* 104:913, 1993.

118. Mathieu D, Neviere R, Billard V, et al: Effects of bicarbonate therapy on hemodynamics and tissue oxygenation in patients with lactic acidosis: a prospective, controlled clinical study, *Crit Care Med* 19:1352, 1991.

119. Mark NH, Leung JM, Arieff AI, et al: Safety of low-dose intraoperative bicarbonate therapy: a prospective, double-blind, randomized study, *Crit Care Med* 21:659, 1993.

120. Leung JM, Landow L, Franks M, et al: Safety and efficacy of intravenous carbicarb in patients undergoing surgery: comparison with sodium bicarbonate in the treatment of mild metabolic acidosis, *Crit Care Med* 22:1540, 1994.

121. Cooper DJ, Walley KR, Wiggs BR, et al: Bicarbonate does not improve hemodynamics in critically ill patients who have lactic acidosis: a prospective, controlled clinical study, *Ann Intern Med* 112:492, 1990.

122. Stacpoole PW, Wright EC, Baumgartner TG, et al: A controlled clinical trial of dichloroacetate for treatment of lactic acidosis in adults, *N Engl J Med* 327:1564, 1992.

123. Kaehny WD, Anderson RJ: Bicarbonate therapy of metabolic acidosis, *Crit Care Med* 22:1525, 1994.

124. Nahas GG, Sutin KM, Fermon C, et al: Guidelines for the treatment of acidaemia with THAM, *Drugs* 55:191, 1998.

125. Severinghaus JW, Mitchell RA, Richardson BW, et al: Respiratory control at high altitude suggesting active transport regulation of CSF pH, *J Appl Physiol* 18:1155, 1963.

126. Christensen MS: Acid-base changes in cerebrospinal fluid and blood, and blood volume changes following prolonged hyperventilation in man, *Br J Anaesth* 46:348, 1974.

Chapter 23

Complications of Blood Transfusion

Randall Goskowicz

The administration of a blood product is indicated to resolve a deficit in a blood component. Even without considering the complications associated with blood transfusion, the administration of blood is a costly therapy, both monetarily and in terms of the metabolic cost of the assimilation of cellular elements, foreign proteins, electrolytes, and toxic preservative components. Complications arise as a result of the administration of blood products, some of which, despite the best preventative measures, may be fatal. Clearly, just as for any other therapy, the administration of blood products may proffer significant benefit, but it always involves significant risk. The indications for the administration of blood products are discussed elsewhere; this chapter specifically addresses the risks of blood transfusion. On one hand, the administration of blood has never been as safe as it is now, as more complications are recognized, characterized, and systematically prevented. On the other hand, the complete elimination of risk is impossible. For example, despite laboratory methods that have provided human immunodeficiency virus (HIV) testing that is far greater than 99% sensitive, the risk of contracting HIV remains 1 in 493,000 units. This risk was estimated in 1992 to result in approximately 18 to 27 infected donations in the United States each year, whereas the institution of p24 antigen testing in 1996 was expected to decrease this exposure by 25%.[1,2] It is incumbent on anesthesiologists, who administer more blood than any other specialists in medicine, to appreciate the complications of blood transfusion and to be able to articulate these risks to colleagues and patients. Only when blood is administered with the same appreciation for its risks and benefits as, for example, muscle relaxants will the transfusion of each and every unit of blood be fully justified.

I. IMMUNOLOGICALLY MEDIATED COMPLICATIONS

The etiology, characteristics, incidence, and mortality of the immunologically mediated complications are summarized in Table 23-1.

A. Red blood cell–mediated complications

Hemolytic transfusion reactions are immune reactions mediated by antigens present on the red blood cell (RBC) membrane. Hemolytic transfusion reactions are a major source of fatality from the transfusion of blood products. In a review of transfusion-related deaths over the decade spanning 1976 to 1985, Sazama[3] noted 355 fatalities in the United States. Excluding deaths related to infectious disease, 158 out of 256 deaths resulted from acute hemolysis and another 26 resulted from delayed hemolysis (Table 23-2).

Table 23-1. Major immune-mediated transfusion reactions

Type	Cause	Characteristics	Incidence per unit	Mortality
Acute hemolytic transfusion reaction	Recipient Ab versus donor RBC Ag	Hemolysis, hemoglobinuria, hypotension, DIC, renal failure, fever	1 in 25,000	6%-10%
Delayed hemolytic transfusion reaction	Recipient Ab versus donor RBC Ag	Fever, jaundice, decreasing hemoglobin	1 in 2500	Rare
Febrile nonhemolytic transfusion reaction	Recipient Ab versus donor granulocyte Ag; stored cytokines	Fever >38° C, chills, rigors, hypotension, headache, tachycardia, rare dyspnea	1 in 200	None reported
Transfusion-related acute lung injury	Donor Ab versus recipient leukocyte Ag; stored cytokines	Dyspnea/noncardiogenic pulmonary edema 1-6 hr after transfusion, chills, fever, hypotension	Between 1 in 2400 and 1 in 5000	5%-10%
Platelet-related febrile reaction	Recipient Ab versus donor platelet Ag; cytokines	Fever >38° C, rare dyspnea, platelet destruction	? 1 in 200 or less	None reported
Posttransfusion purpura	Recipient Ab versus donor platelet PL^{A1} Ag	Thrombocytopenia, purpura, petechiae, platelet refractory state, fever	Rare, never following FFP administration	Rare with therapy
Allergic reactions	Recipient Ab versus donor Ag	Typically mild (hives) although potentially severe (hypotension and bronchospasm)	Urticarial: 1 in 200 Anaphylaxis: 1 in 150,000	Urticarial: rare Anaphylaxis secondary IgA deficiency: 20%
TA-GVHD	Donor lymphocytes versus host tissues	Fever, rash, liver and gut dysfunction, bone marrow suppression	200 cases in literature	90%-100%

Ab, Antibody; *RBC,* red blood cell; *Ag,* antigen; *DIC,* disseminated intravascular coagulation; *FFP,* fresh frozen plasma; *TA-GVHD,* transfusion-associated graft versus host disease.

1. Acute hemolytic transfusion reactions. Acute hemolytic transfusion reactions (AHTRs) are the immunologic sequelae of the binding of donor RBC antigens by recipient antibodies. By far, the most common cause of AHTRs is the transfusion of the wrong unit of blood to a given patient because of clerical error.[3] Once clerical error has been excluded, the incidence of AHTR falls significantly. It is estimated that despite cross-matching there is one incompatible unit of blood transfused out of every 33,000 units of RBCs.[4] The American College of Pathologists found 843 AHTRs in the United States over a 5-year period, of which 6% resulted in fatalities.[5] The severity of the reaction is determined by the subclass of antibody involved and the number of immune complexes formed.[6] For example, complexes may form between recipient RBC antigens and donor antibodies or between the antigens and antibodies of incompatible donated units (interunit reactions), but these interactions rarely result in symptoms. Although there are over 300 recognized RBC surface antigens, most (83%) of the fatalities from acute hemolytic reactions involve only the antigens from ABO blood grouping, and a few additional minor antigen groups (e.g., the Rh, Kell, Kidd,

Table 23-2. Cause of transfusion-associated deaths in order of reported frequency, 1976-1985

Number	Cause
158	Acute hemolysis
42	Non-A, non-B hepatitis
31	Acute pulmonary edema
26	Hepatitis B
26	Bacterial contamination
26	Delayed hemolysis
15	Not associated
12	Donation of blood product
8	Anaphylaxis
5	External hemolysis
3	AIDS*
1	RBCs not deglycerolized
1	Graft versus host disease
1	Record unavailable

Modified from Sazama K: *Transfusion* 30:583, 1990.
*Early in acquired immunodeficiency syndrome (AIDS) epidemic.

and Duffy groups) are responsible for most of the remaining AHTRs.[3]

The most common symptom of an AHTR in a nonanesthetized patient is fever, occurring in 74% of the cases described by Pineda, Brzica, and Taswell.[7] Chills are also noted approximately half of the time, with additional occasional symptoms of a vague sense of uneasiness, lower back pain, chest pain, dyspnea, or generalized flushing. These symptoms are often masked in the anesthetized patient, and the only signs present may be hemoglobinuria, transient hypertension followed by profound hypotension, or shock. In severe cases, disseminated intravascular coagulation (DIC) may present concomitantly with diffuse oozing from catheter sites and wound edges.

The pathophysiology of an AHTR involves the binding of donor RBCs by recipient antibodies, which, in the case of the immunoglobulin G (IgG) subclass, are capable of both fixing complement and binding to the effector cells of the immune system or, in the case of the IgM subclass, capable only of fixing complement.[8] The fixing of complement results in cell lysis if the complement cascade goes to completion, and otherwise results in the binding of antibody-antigen complexes by macrophages with extravascular cell lysis. Intravascular lysis results in free hemoglobinemia and sanguinous urine. Extravascular lysis results in hyperbilirubinemia as free hemoglobin

is metabolized. Regardless of whether the complement cascade goes to completion, the activation of the complement cascade results in the elaboration of complement fragments with the release of histamine and serotonin and resultant vasodilation, hypotension, bronchospasm, and cutaneous flushing. A decrease in blood pressure is associated with the release of endogenous catecholamines with a decrease in splanchnic and renal blood flow. The latter, along with direct vasoconstriction from various cytokines, is principally responsible for renal failure, although the presence of red cell stroma and free hemoglobin in the renal tubules may also contribute. In addition to the complement cascade, the role of numerous cytokines (tumor necrosis factor, monocyte chemoattractant factor, and interleukins) in the pathogenesis of AHTR has recently been appreciated (Fig. 23-1 and Table 23-3). The presence of antibody-coated RBCs elicits the release of interleukins and tumor necrosis factor from monocytes, which results in hypotension, fever, and DIC.[9]

The diagnosis of an AHTR during anesthesia is usually first suggested by the presence of hemoglobinuria with or without hemodynamic instability, although bronchospasm may rarely be a presenting sign. The severity of the transfusion reaction and the duration of the sequelae appear to be proportionate to the volume of blood infused and the quantity of antibody and antigen in com-

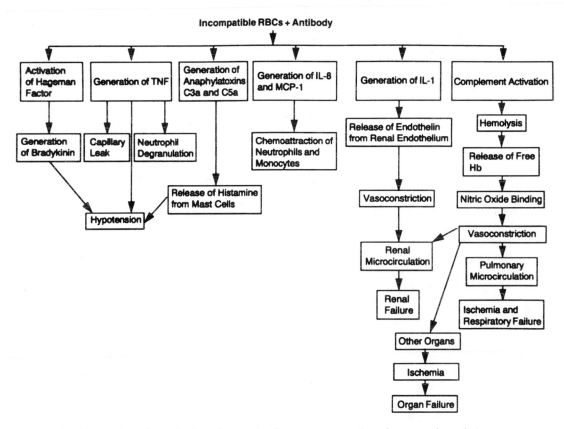

Fig. 23-1. Hemodynamic alterations and inflammatory sequelae of an acute hemolytic transfusion reaction. *Hb,* Hemoglobin; *IL,* interleukin; *MCP,* monocyte chemoattractant protein; *TNF,* tumor necrosis factor. (From Capon SM, Goldfinger D: *Transfusion* 35:513, 1995.)

plex. Therefore when a reaction is suspected, it is imperative to stop the transfusion immediately, even as the diagnostic evaluation continues.

Confirmation of a hemolytic transfusion begins with notification of the blood bank of a potential reaction. The blood bank will then reevaluate all suspect units of blood to ensure that a systematic error has not occurred that could result in a reaction in another patient. Concomitantly, measures are taken to confirm quickly that the patient in question is receiving compatible blood. A recent analysis of the causes of hemolytic reactions demonstrated that the majority of transfusion reactions are the result of human error.[3] A similar analysis identified the operating room as the site of error in 14% of cases, usually because blood was given to the wrong patient. Although most bedside errors were the responsibility of the administering nurse, the anesthesiologist working in the operating room was the most common source of physician error.[10] The evaluation in the operating room should therefore begin with a complete reassessment of the patient's identification and the labeling on the blood unit. An anticoagulated blood sample should then be sent off to the laboratory along with the intact and uncontaminated unit of blood. The specimen will be used to retype and cross the patient's blood against the unit of blood received, to assess for free hemoglobin, and to test for antibody-coated RBCs (direct antiglobulin test). In the event of an AHTR, at least one of these tests should be positive. There may be an absence of free hemoglobin if the amount of hemolysis has been limited and sufficient haptoglobin is present to quickly bind free hemoglobin, transporting the hemoglobin to the liver for breakdown. The administration of more than 20 ml of incompatible blood is usually enough to fully saturate serum haptoglobin. There may also be a negative serum antiglobulin test if all antibody-coated RBCs have been sequestered by the reticuloendothelial system. If, despite an initial negative evaluation, an AHTR is strongly suspected, a decrease in the post-transfusion versus pretransfusion haptoglobin concentrations may confirm the diagnosis. Additional tests suggestive of an AHTR include the lack of an appropriate rise in hemoglobin concentrations with transfusion and the presence of hemosiderinuria and methemoglobin-albumin complexes in the urine.[11,12] The evaluation of a suspected AHTR varies somewhat by institution, and it is imperative to enlist the assistance of the blood bank specialist when a reaction is suspected.

The presence of significant symptoms (e.g., fever, dyspnea, urticaria, or hemoglobinuria) in the demonstrated absence of an AHTR suggests that another type of transfusion reaction may be ongoing. See Box 23-1 for the differential diagnosis for these symptoms.

The treatment for an AHTR consists of stopping the transfusion, initiating supportive care to maintain the blood pressure with a systolic at 100 mm Hg or above, promoting a diuresis of at least 1.5 ml/kg/hr with the administration of fluid and furosemide, and monitoring for severe sequelae of an AHTR, such as DIC, renal failure, and severe shock. Dopamine is a logical choice as a pressor to maintain blood pressure and renal blood flow because of both its prominent dopa and its β-adrenergic effects at doses less than 8 μg/kg/min. If the blood pressure does not improve, higher doses may be needed to further evoke the α-adrenergic effects of dopamine, although this may have a net effect of reducing renal blood flow. Diuresis should be promoted vigorously with the use of furosemide, which, at a dose of 1 mg/kg and unlike mannitol, increases renal cortical perfusion and may decrease the risk of renal failure. Alkalinization of the urine by the administration of sodium bicarbonate solution has been advocated in the past because alkalin-

Table 23-3. Mediators of the systemic inflammatory response and their biologic effects

Mediator	Hemodynamic effects	Coagulation effects	Other effects
TNF	Hypotension	Increase tissue factor activity and decrease thrombomodulin expression by endothelial cells	Fever, capillary leak
IL-1	Hypotension, endothelin release	Increase tissue factor activity and decrease thrombomodulin expression by endothelial cells	Fever, leukocytosis; stimulate other cytokine production
IL-6			Stimulate T-cell proliferation and immunoglobulin production
IL-8			Neutrophil chemoattraction
MCP-1			Monocyte chemoattraction
Complement		Thromboplastin release by WBCs	Activate phagocytes, stimulate cytokine production
Nitric oxide	Vasodilation		
Endothelin	Vasoconstriction		
Leukocyte adhesion molecules			Attract WBCs

From Capon SM, Goldfinger D: *Transfusion* 35:513, 1995.
TNF, Tumor necrosis factor; *IL*, interleukin; *MCP*, monocyte chemoattractant protein; *WBC*, white blood cell.

Box 23-1 Determination of transfusion reaction type by presenting symptom

Fever or chills
Immediate
  Acute hemolytic transfusion reaction
  Bacterial contamination of blood product
  Febrile nonhemolytic reaction
  Platelet-related febrile reaction
  Transfusion-related acute lung injury
Delayed
  Delayed hemolytic transfusion reaction
  Transfusion-acquired infection (e.g., malaria, HIV, EBV, CMV)
  Transfusion-associated graft versus host disease
  Posttransfusion purpura

Hemolysis (may present as hemoglobinuria)
Acute hemolytic transfusion reaction (D)
Delayed hemolytic transfusion reaction (D)
Bacterial contamination (gram-negative bacteremia) (D, R)
Protozoal infection (malaria or babesiosis) (D, R)
Mechanical trauma to RBCs
  Thermal injury
    Overheating (>40° C) (D)
    Freezing or partial freezing (D)
  Osmotic injury
    Sterile water for bladder irrigation during cystoscopy (R)
    Reconstitution of RBCs with nonisotonic solutions (D)
    Use of inadequately deglycerolized RBCs (D)

Shearing injury
  High-pressure infusion (D)
  Mechanical valves, vascular grafts, hematomas (D, R)
  Extracorporeal circulation (D)
  Small catheter size (D)
Drug-induced hemolysis
  Penicillin, quinidine, α-methyldopa (D, R)
Disease-mediated hemolysis
  Hemolytic anemias: G6PD deficiency, autoimmune anemias, sickle cell anemia (D, R)
  Paroxysmal nocturnal hemoglobinuria (R)
  Hemolytic uremic syndrome (D, R)
  Thrombotic thrombocytopenic purpura (D, R)
  Sepsis with disseminated intravascular coagulation (D, R)
  Microangiopathic hemolytic anemia (D, R)

Dyspnea
Anaphylactic reaction
Acute hemolytic transfusion reaction
Transfusion-related acute lung injury
CHF/volume overload
Adult respiratory distress syndrome
Febrile nonhemolytic transfusion reaction with pulmonary manifestations

Urticaria
Urticarial transfusion reaction

Adapted from Welborn JL, Hersch J: *Postgrad Med* 90:125, 1991; Cooper CL: Complications of transfusion therapy. In Lake CL, Moore RA, eds: *Blood: hemostasis, transfusion, and alternatives in the perioperative period,* New York, 1995, Raven; Beauregard P, Blajchman MA: *Transfus Med Rev* 8:184, 1994.
HIV, Human immunodeficiency virus; *EBV,* Epstein-Barr virus; *CMV,* cytomegalovirus; *D,* lysis of donor cells; *R,* lysis of recipient cells; *RBCs,* red blood cells.

izatión increases hemoglobin solubility and may limit the precipitation of hemoglobin in distal renal tubules. The efficacy of this practice has not been proven. Fluid administration should be pursued cautiously in the presence of oliguria or anuria that persists despite the initial aggressive administration of fluid. The use of central monitoring to assess cardiac output and central cardiac filling pressures may be indicated to avoid iatrogenic fluid overload. In extreme cases, dialysis may be necessary to reverse electrolyte and fluid imbalances.

After renal failure, the next most common cause of morbidity and mortality from an AHTR results from DIC. The management of DIC is highly controversial. One view supports the administration of heparin to limit procoagulant elements of the coagulation cascade and thereby limit the formation of disseminated clot. The opposing view instead suggests the use of supportive therapy to replace consumed clotting factors and platelets and limit the diffuse hemorrhage that is often the end point of DIC. There are no data to support either mode of therapy, although in the surgical setting where vascular integrity is violated, the latter strategy, which focuses on prevention of hemorrhage, is more

commonly applied.[11] DIC is a frequent sequel to AHTR, so that early and frequent assessments of coagulation status via prothrombin time/partial thromboplastin time (PT/PTT), platelet count, fibrinogen concentration, fibrin degradation products, and thromboelastogram are often necessary. Ongoing blood loss as a result of surgical hemorrhage and hemorrhagic diathesis may result in the need for blood products even as the treatment of an AHTR is ongoing. In this case, type O Rh-negative RBCs and platelets and type AB fresh frozen plasma (FFP) should be used.[12] If the patient is known to have specific RBC antibodies, it will be necessary to provide RBCs that lack the corresponding specific RBC antigens. Because of complexities such as this, it is imperative that the blood bank specialist be consulted in the care of these patients.

Because the antibodies that initiate an AHTR are almost always readily identifiable, AHTRs should be virtually completely preventable. The compulsive verification of patient-unit matching should prevent virtually all AHTRs.

2. Alloimmunization and delayed hemolytic transfusion reactions. Alloimmunization is the sensitization of the recipient to donor antigens, whether from RBCs, platelets, leukocytes, or plasma proteins, with the formation of alloantibody that coats donor RBCs but fails to result in hemolysis. The major clinical consequence of alloimmunization to RBC antigens is that it tends to prolong the type and screen process for patients receiving multiple consecutive RBC transfusions. Alloimmunization occurs at a rate of approximately 1% per unit transfused.[13] In a study by Vichinsky et al,[14] of 107 patients who underwent transfusion for sickle cell anemia, 30% of patients produced antibodies to foreign RBC proteins (alloantibodies). Most patients who ultimately developed alloantibodies did so after 3 units. The presence of an alloantibody does not guarantee that a patient will subsequently have a delayed hemolytic transfusion reaction (DHTR) involving that antibody. In the study by Vichinsky et al,[14] a group of multiply transfused patients developed alloantibodies 30% of the time but had evidence of DHTR only 13% of the time.

A DHTR occurs in a patient who has been previously sensitized to a foreign antigen (i.e., during pregnancy or from a previous transfusion) but whose antibody concentration is too low to be detectable by standard antibody detection screens. If the patient is then reexposed to the foreign antigen, the patient may develop a hemolytic response that is delayed by up to 30 days because of the time required for the patient's immune system to generate a high enough titer to manifest a response. The frequency of DHTRs is not precisely known because most reactions are mild and are clinically unrecognized. Ness et al[15] estimated the rate of DHTRs to be approximately 1 out of 854 multiply transfused patients. Although DHTRs may result in mortality, death is much more common from AHTRs; in Sazama's study[3] the number of deaths caused by DHTRs was 26, whereas 6 times that number died from AHTRs (see Table 23-2).

The nature of the alloantibody involved determines the nature of the DHTR. Antibodies capable of rapid hemolysis (e.g., antibodies to the Duffy and Kidd antigens) results in rapid intravascular hemolysis occurring between 5 and 10 days after the transfusion. These patients occasionally present with fever and chills immediately after transfusion, followed 2 to 4 days later by malaise, fever, chills, and progressive anemia. For antibodies not capable of producing intravascular hemolysis, signs and symptoms are limited to hyperbilirubinemia, with hemolysis occurring in the extravascular space. As seen in Table 23-4, a variety of antigens have been implicated in fatal DHTRs.

Once a DHTR is suspected, the diagnosis may be difficult to confirm. Often, the number of surviving antibody-coated RBCs may be very low, although a direct antiglobulin test should still be positive. Establishing the identity of the culprit antibody is important to prevent future reactions, although this may prove difficult. The titer of the antibody fluctuates depending on the stage of the reaction. After the reaction has resolved, titers usually decrease to low, often undetectable concentrations once again. Although typically it is simply a difficulty of detection of the antibody, the diagnosis of

Table 23-4. Antibodies responsible for delayed hemolytic transfusion reactions

Antibody	Percentage of reactions
Anti-E (Rh)	34
Anti-jKa (Kidd)	30
Anti-Fy (Duffy)	14
Anti-K (Kell)	13
Anti-MNSs	4
Anti-C, Lu, Ce, U, Co	<5

Modified from Nicholls MD: *Anaesth Intens Care* 21:15,1993.

malaria or babesiosis should be entertained in the patient with evidence of hemolysis in the absence of an identifiable antibody and with a negative direct antiglobulin test. Other causes of hemolysis (e.g., from mechanical sources) are noted in Box 23-1.

The management of a DHTR is the same as that for an AHTR: primarily supportive, with vigilance for severe sequelae. After stabilization, the patient should be informed of his or her increased risk of reaction following transfusion and should carry medical alert documents. This is particularly true for patients who possess an antibody that is not readily identifiable. If the patient does not carry alerting documents, prevention of a DHTR is very difficult because the antibody responsible for the reaction is typically undetectable. Maintenance of a high degree of suspicion may result in early diagnosis when a DHTR occurs and may reduce resultant morbidity.

B. Leukocyte-mediated complications

Transfused leukocytes are the cause of both the febrile nonhemolytic transfusion reaction (FNTR) and transfusion-related acute lung injury (TRALI).

1. Febrile nonhemolytic transfusion reactions. An FNTR is defined as an increase of temperature of at least 1° C in association with the transfusion of a unit of RBCs or whole blood in the absence of an identifiable cause.[16] FNTRs are the most common of all transfusion reactions, occurring at a rate of 1 in 200 units transfused.[17,18] FNTRs are not associated with lasting morbidity unless they are accompanied by pulmonary symptoms.

The primary symptom of an FNTR is an increase in temperature of at least 1° C. Symptoms that may accompany the fever include chills, rigors, hypotension, headache, tachycardia, a feeling of uneasiness, flushing, nausea, and vomiting. Symptoms typically have an onset 45 minutes after the transfusion begins, lasting 1 or 2 hours. Although the symptoms are usually physiologically well tolerated, patients with a tenuous cardiovascular status may develop shock. The symptoms of a typical FNTR are often indistinguishable from those of acute sepsis (i.e., from the transfusion of a contaminated unit of blood) or from those of an AHTR.

Pulmonary symptoms may rarely accompany an FNTR with hypoxia, dyspnea, and noncardiogenic pulmonary edema. This type of reaction may be similar to TRALI, and is discussed in the section on TRALI later in this chapter.

Febrile reactions occurring after the administration of platelets probably are caused by a different mechanism than are FNTRs. Platelet-associated febrile reactions are discussed in the section on platelet-mediated complications later in this chapter.

The pathophysiology of the FNTR is not fully elucidated. FNTRs tend to occur in recipients who have antibodies directed against leukocyte antigens, including human leukocyte antigens (HLA) and granulocyte-specific antigens, which react against leukocytes transfused in donor RBC units.[6] Which antigens are specifically involved, and the possibility that surface antigens from other cellular elements (such as platelets and lymphocytes) play a role in the FNTR, is debatable. In a recent study, 24 cases of FNTR were reviewed and it was noted that 71% of patients had demonstrable antileukocyte antibodies, and the remainder did not. Although the most severe reactions were associated with the presence of antibodies, not all patients with a history of FNTRs have demonstrable antibodies.[19] It appears that between 0.25 and 2.5×10^9 leukocytes are required to produce a reaction, whereas a unit of RBCs contains 4×10^9 leukocytes.[6] A modest fractional decrease in the number of leukocytes per unit of RBCs is probably adequate to eliminate the risk of an FNTR. The elaboration of interleukin-1 and other cytokines released by donor leukocytes and recipient macrophages results in the elevation in temperature that occurs with an FNTR.[20,21]

A fever in the context of a transfusion is most often caused by some underlying factor (e.g., medication, infection, or inflammation), and not by the transfusion per se. Inexpensive assays are now available that detect anti-HLA antibodies within 1 day of testing and are often helpful in excluding an FNTR. The initial evaluation of a fever following transfusion consists of stopping the transfusion while comprehensively ruling out other possible causes of transfusion-associated fever (see Box 23-1), including an AHTR or bacterial contamination of the administered unit of blood. Blood bank personnel should be consulted when an FNTR or any other transfusion reaction is suspected.

After stopping the transfusion and while ruling out other causes of fever, the management of an FNTR consists of supportive care. The patient should be treated with antipyretics and surface cooling for comfort. The use of antihistamines is not efficacious. Meperidine may be indicated in low doses to suppress rigors.

Multiparous women and patients who have received multiple transfusions are at a higher risk for FNTRs because antibody production is induced by prior exposure to foreign leukocyte antigens. Fifty-five percent of multiparous women are positive for antileukocyte antibodies.[12] Several measures may significantly decrease the risk of an FNTR by removing leukocytes, including filtration and apheresis. Because only one in eight patients who have had an FNTR ever encounter one again,[22] it is debatable whether these measures are worth the additional cost.[23] If a patient has a compelling history for an FNTR and a positive assay for anti-HLA antibodies, then leukoreduced blood may be used after the first incidence of an FNTR.

2. Transfusion-related acute lung injury. TRALI is a syndrome of respiratory distress, pulmonary edema, and hypoxia occurring 1 to 6 hours after transfusion of plasma-containing blood products. The respiratory symptoms of TRALI are often accompanied by chills, fever, and hypotension. There is probably more than one mechanism for the production of TRALI, although the most common involves the reaction between leukoagglutinating antibodies present in particular units of donor plasma that react with recipient leukocytes. Any plasma-containing blood product (whole blood, FFP, platelets, RBCs, or cryoprecipitate) can cause TRALI, although most reactions are associated with the infusion of whole blood, FFP, or RBCs. TRALI is estimated to occur in one in 2400 patients receiving at least one unit of blood.[24] TRALI has an associated mortality of 5% to 10% (see Table 23-1).[25]

The pathophysiology of TRALI probably results from recipient leukoagglutinating antibodies that react with donor neutrophils or a reaction by substances produced and stored in blood product units, including activated complement fragments, cytokines,[26] or aggregated leukocytes ("leukoemboli").[16] In most cases of TRALI, the presence of antileukocyte antibodies can be demonstrated in the serum of the donor that correspond to HLA antigens expressed by the recipient. When specific antibodies to patient leukocytes are not identified, TRALI is thought to be secondary to the effects of substances produced by cellular elements during storage. A respiratory distress syndrome that is clinically indistinguishable from TRALI may also be seen following the transfusion of granulocytes, although the mechanism of this reaction is thought to be similar to that for an FNTR, involving recipient antileukocyte antibodies and donor leukocytes.[27] Regardless of whether the culprit antibody is produced by the donor (as in an FNTR) or by the recipient (as in TRALI), the interaction of leukocytes with antileukocyte antibodies involves the common pathogenesis of aggregation of leukocytes with the accumulation of these aggregates in the pulmonary vasculature. The aggregated leukocytes generate adhesive molecules that facilitate leukocyte transmigration into the interstitial space between the alveolar epithelium and the capillary endothelium. Once sequestered, granulocytes release toxic substances,[6] resulting in capillary leakage and the noncardiogenic pulmonary edema characteristic of TRALI.[28] A recent study suggests that the patient's underlying condition may contribute to the pathogenesis of TRALI. Silliman et al[29] studied patients with TRALI compared with control patients with a history of febrile or urticarial transfusion reactions. They noted that every patient with TRALI had a history of underlying clinical factors, such as infection, cytokine administration, recent surgery, or massive transfusion. They suggest that patients with underlying clinical conditions may be predisposed to the development of TRALI.[29,30] At this time, the role of predisposing factors in the development of TRALI remains the subject of investigation.

The differential diagnosis of respiratory distress following a transfusion includes volume overload, AHTR,

TRALI, severe FNTR with pulmonary symptoms, anaphylaxis, and adult respiratory distress syndrome (ARDS) from some other cause (see Box 23-1). As noted, TRALI is rare, and the evaluation should seek to rule out volume overload, a far more common complication especially at extremes of age and in patients with chronic anemia. The evaluation often involves placement of a pulmonary artery catheter to demonstrate a low to normal central venous pressure and pulmonary artery capillary wedge pressure, consistent with noncardiogenic pulmonary edema. Most patients with TRALI have an antileukocyte antibody identified in the donor blood unit that will react to the patient's HLA type.[25] Diagnosis in patients without such evidence cannot be distinguished from ARDS, and the diagnosis is often made in retrospect based on a generally milder course seen with TRALI, and on the basis of the clinical context.[12] Whenever TRALI is suspected it is imperative to notify the blood bank immediately so that other blood components from the same donor can be diverted from administration to another patient.

The management of TRALI is primarily supportive, with supplemental oxygen and mechanical ventilation as needed. Furosemide and corticosteroids are widely used, although their efficacy has not been established rigorously. The usual course is rapid recovery within 2 to 4 days.[31] In one particularly severe case, extracorporeal membrane oxygenation was used successfully for a patient for whom mechanical ventilation was insufficient.[32]

Because TRALI results from the transfusion of blood products with antileukocyte antibodies, prevention consists of avoiding units of blood containing these antibodies. Multiparous women and patients who have undergone multiple transfusions are most likely to develop these antibodies. Popovsky[31] recommends the routine diversion of blood components that contain large fractions of plasma (i.e., components other than RBCs) from women donors who have had three or more pregnancies. A more recent compromise position adopted by the American Association of Blood Banks (AABB) has been to restrict blood products from donors who have produced an antibody that has been demonstrated to have resulted in TRALI. Because TRALI is donor-specific for a given recipient, the administration of other blood products after a reaction should not be problematic.

C. Platelet-mediated complications

The transfusion of platelets may result in both platelet-related febrile reactions (PRFRs) and posttransfusion purpura (PTP). Also briefly included in Box 23-2 is the differential for other causes of less than expected increases in platelet counts following platelet administration (i.e., the platelet refractory state).

1. Platelet-related febrile reactions. A PRFR is characterized by a rise in temperature of more than 1° C following the infusion of platelets in the absence of an alternative explanation. These reactions are probably similar pathophysiologically to the classic FNTR, in which the antileukocyte antibodies of blood transfusion recipients react with donor leukocytes. In fact, many

---

> **Box 23-2** Causes of the platelet refractory state
>
> Fever
> Infection
> Splenomegaly
> Coagulopathy
>   Disseminated intravascular coagulation
> Immunologic reaction
>   HLA antibody–mediated
>   Antiplatelet antibodies
>   ABO incompatibility
>   Autoantibodies
>   Drug-induced platelet-reactive antibodies
> Cardiopulmonary bypass
> Graft versus host disease
> Antibiotic therapy
> Brisk hemorrhage

---

cases of FNTR are probably caused by a reaction between antiplatelet antibodies in the recipient and transfused platelets, although securing a definitive diagnosis in these cases is often impossible because the antibody responsible for the reaction often is not identified. Platelets have been implicated as the source of antigen in many cases of FNTR in which a specific antileukocyte antibody has not been identified.[21] In this case, the culprit antibody is probably to HLA antigens shared by both platelets and leukocytes.

FNTRs occurring secondary to specific platelet antigens may result in the destruction of donated platelets, manifested by a failure of the recipient to achieve the expected rise in platelet count after a platelet transfusion. In this scenario, alternative causes of a platelet refractory state should also be considered (see Box 23-2).

Some febrile reactions probably are not caused by antibody-antigen interactions but may be the result of the infusion of cytokines stored in the platelet concentrates.[33] Older platelets have been associated with a rate of reaction twice that of younger platelet units, probably related to the accumulation of cytokines over time.[34]

The management of a posttransfusion fever, whether caused by leukocytes, platelets, or cytokines, remains the same: The transfusion is stopped while more serious conditions, such as bacterial contamination, or an AHTR are considered. The treatment of a patient who sustains repeated febrile episodes after the transfusion of platelets may be difficult, particularly if the patient is severely thrombocytopenic. The patient may be administered HLA-matched leukocyte-reduced donor platelets that have been obtained via apheresis, which should result in a less than 50% chance of fever or platelet destruction.

2. Posttransfusion purpura. PTP is a rare, potentially fatal syndrome, the cardinal element of which is the destruction of both transfused and native recipient platelets 5 days to 2 weeks after the transfusion of platelet-containing blood products.[35] Blood products that may trigger PTP include platelet concentrates, packed RBCs, whole blood, and fresh plasma, although it is not seen after the administration of previously frozen plasma. PTP occurs most often in multiparous women, but may also be seen in patients who have been exposed to platelets via a blood transfusion in the past.

Patients with PTP are typically febrile and may complain of shaking chills. However, PTP is distinguished by the presence of severe unexplained thrombocytopenia and petechiae of the skin, mucous membranes, and gingival surfaces. Significant internal hemorrhage may occur, including often fatal intracranial hemorrhage. A less severe reaction that is limited to fever and occurs after the transfusion of platelets may be a form of FNTR. PTP differs from a platelet-related FNTR in that the latter results in the destruction solely of transfused platelets, whereas the former involves destruction of native and transfused platelets, accounting for the severe thrombocytopenia seen in PTP.

The pathophysiology of PTP is complex. Most patients with PTP are phenotypically homozygous for an uncommon allele of the platelet PL antigen system, known as PL^{A2}. This allele is present in less than 2% of the population, depending on race. When exposed to the PL^{A1} antigen, usually during pregnancy, these patients develop an anti-PL^{A1} antibody approximately 6% of the time.[36] Subsequent exposures induce an anamnestic response with the formation of complement-fixing anti-PL^{A1} antibodies and the destruction of transfused platelets. The conundrum of PTP is why the patient's own platelets, which should not express foreign antigens, are destroyed along with nonnative platelets. A complete review of the mechanism for this process is available.[35] Briefly, hypotheses include the binding of PL^{A1}-antibody complexes to native platelets with subsequent platelet destruction, the patient's own platelets acquiring the phenotype of the destroyed transfused platelets (i.e., the jumping antigen theory), and the formation of an autoantibody versus the patient's own platelets.

Although the PL alloantigen system appears to be the most commonly responsible for PTP, other antigen systems, such as the Bak, Pen, and Br systems, have also been implicated. Of these, all but the Bak system have one allele that is expressed more than 98% of the time. The fact that the vast majority of the population is one phenotype accounts for the rarity of antiplatelet reactions.

The diagnosis of PTP is primarily clinical, although it may be clinched by demonstrating the presence of a high-titer complement-fixing antibody directed against a platelet antigen present in a previously transfused unit of blood. Given the rarity of PTP, the possibility of other potential causes of thrombocytopenia must be pursued. PTP is thought to be underdiagnosed, probably because it is confused with other potential sources of thrombocytopenia. Because the course of therapy may be significantly affected by early treatment, the vigorous and timely assessment of thrombocytopenia is important. The differential diagnosis for a patient presenting with a fever 1 week after a transfusion includes a DHTR, a transfusion-acquired infection (e.g., malaria), transfusion-associated graft versus host disease (TA-GVHD), and

PTP (see Box 23-1). A cardinal sign of PTP is the failure to achieve an expected rise in the platelet count after the transfusion of platelets. The differential diagnosis for platelet refractoriness is listed in Box 23-2.

PTP usually is a self-limiting disorder, although the severity and duration of symptoms may be attenuated by therapy; the course lasts up to 3 weeks in untreated patients, whereas with treatment patients have responded within 2 to 4 days. The most commonly used therapy is intravenous immunoglobulin (IVIG), an agent commonly used in autoimmune disorders.[37] Alternative therapy includes plasmapheresis and high-dose corticosteroids. The former must be carried out via large-bore intravenous catheters, the placement of which in a thrombocytopenic patient may carry significant risk. Corticosteroids are less often efficacious, although they may be beneficial when other modalities have failed.[38] Despite the often severely low concentrations of platelets endured by patients with PTP, the transfusion of platelets usually fails to provide an expected rise in the platelet count and may result in a severe systemic reaction. Even PL^{A1} antigen-negative platelets have failed to survive during the period of maximal thrombocytopenia.[39] Because patients may continue to hemorrhage throughout PTP, RBC transfusion may be required. If so, washed RBCs should be used, although even platelet- and leukocyte-depleted RBCs have resulted in systemic reactions.[40,41]

Patients at risk for PTP include multiparous women and those who have been previously exposed to platelet antigens via blood transfusion. However, given the phenotypic homogeneity of platelet antigens, the frequency of PTP is very low. At this time, there are no advocates for the systematic testing of platelet phenotype in at-risk patients, particularly because PTP has occurred despite the administration of platelet-depleted blood products.

D. Protein-mediated complications

The protein-mediated complications of blood transfusion are allergic in nature, and are among the most common transfusion reactions. Allergic reactions may be either anaphylactic, in which case they are mediated by IgE antibodies, or immediate generalized (anaphylactoid) reactions, in which case they are not mediated by IgE. Most allergic reactions are immediate generalized reactions (IGRs) of a mild type, although rare reactions involving anti-IgA antibodies may be severe. Protein-mediated complications may follow the transfusion of any blood product component, including FFP.[12]

Certain patient populations may be a higher risk for allergic reactions. It has been suggested that the transfusion of blood products from atopic donors may result in a higher incidence of allergic reactions in recipients by the passive transmission of IgE. However, a recent study found a firmer association between the degree of atopy in the recipient, as measured by the concentrations of IgE antibodies, and the incidence of allergic reactions. It was concluded that atopic recipients tend to have allergic transfusion reactions and that donor screening is unlikely to be beneficial in avoiding reactions.[42]

1. Immediate generalized reactions. There are several grades of IGRs, from the mild form manifested by an urticarial rash, to a moderate form manifested by the presence of mild hypotension with respiratory distress, to profound hypotension, bronchospasm, and cardiac arrest in the most severe cases. Most allergic reactions are IGRs of a mild type, resulting only in a rash and urticaria and occurring commonly, in approximately 1% to 3% of all transfusions. Provided that a patient's symptoms are confined to an urticarial rash with no fever, the administration of blood may continue after the administration of an antihistamine.

The pathophysiology of IGRs involves the cross-linking of IgE antibodies, which have already become bound to mast cells, with transfused antigen. There follows a release of mediators that are the same as with an anaphylactic reaction (i.e., histamine, prostaglandins, leukotrienes, and various kinins). Although various blood proteins are often responsible for an IGR, other sources must be considered, such as the coadministration of a drug such as penicillin, additives from blood processing, and products elaborated by cells in storage that are transmitted passively during transfusion.

Therapy of IGRs involves verbal reassurance of the patient along with the administration of antihistamines. More severe reactions may require the administration of supplemental oxygen, fluid, and vasopressors, including epinephrine. Prophylaxis with antihistamines and steroids should be considered for patients with a history of significant IGRs. RBCs that have been washed to remove plasma proteins may be administered to patients who have had a moderate to severe reaction despite prophylactic treatment with antihistamines and steroids.

2. Anaphylactic reactions. The cause of most anaphylactic reactions is the same as that for allergic reactions: the reaction by the donor to a foreign protein. The pathophysiology, management, and prevention of these reactions are the same as for allergic reactions. Another cause of severe anaphylactic reactions may be the transfusion of IgA to a patient who has a deficiency of IgA or who is homozygous for an IgA immunotype. Approximately 1 in 700 people have a complete deficiency of IgA. Of these patients, 20% to 60% develop anti-IgA antibodies, and only 20% of those with antibodies have a clinically significant reaction to IgA. Overall, anti-IgA–mediated reactions are rare, occurring in 1 of every 25,000 to 50,000 transfusions.[12] Aside from those with a congenital isolated absence of IgA, patients with common variable immune deficiency receiving frequent γ-globulin injections may also develop anti-IgA antibodies.

Symptoms of an anti-IgA reaction are typically severe, with the immediate onset of pain, nausea, dyspnea, and severe hypotension. The differential diagnosis includes an acute massive hemolytic reaction, although a negative direct Coombs test rules this out. Management of an anaphylactic reaction is supportive and may involve the use of vasopressors, definitive airway management, and mechanical ventilation. Because the cause of an anaphylactic reaction is rarely determined, prevention involves limiting exposure of the patient to foreign proteins by the comprehensive washing of RBCs before transfusion.

E. T-Lymphocyte–mediated complications: transfusion-associated graft versus host disease

Graft versus host disease (GVHD) is the clinical manifestation of a reaction of donor lymphocytes against host tissues that occurs most often in the setting of bone marrow transplantation (BMT). This section discusses a rare, often fatal subtype of GVHD that occurs after transfusion of blood: transfusion-associated graft versus host disease (TA-GVHD). Although only 200 cases have been described in the literature, a 90% fatality rate has earned this entity significant interest.[43]

The pathophysiology of TA-GVHD involves the reaction of donor lymphocytes against recipient tissue. Sufficient numbers of viable donor lymphocytes may be found in virtually any blood product except for FFP, frozen deglycerolized RBCs, cryoprecipitate, and factor concentrates. In most patients, such reactions are prevented because the recipient's immune system recognizes transfused lymphocytes as foreign and immediately destroys these lymphocytes—the host versus graft response. Patients unable to mount an antigraft response are most likely to develop TA-GVHD. Billingham[44] defines three requirements for the development of TA-GVHD: There must be HLA differences between the host and the donor, there must be immunocompetent cells in the graft, and the host must be unable to reject immunocompetent donor lymphocytes.

The manifestations of TA-GVHD principally involve the skin, gut, bone marrow, and liver. The initial presentation is of a fever, rash, diarrhea, and elevated liver function tests, including transaminases and bilirubin. As the syndrome progresses, the rash spreads from the trunk to the extremities as liver function tests and gastrointestinal symptoms become incapacitating (Fig. 23-2). This phase is accompanied by bone marrow suppression with pancytopenia, with most patients succumbing to infectious complications within 3 weeks after initial presentation.

Patients most commonly afflicted with TA-GVHD are immunocompromised patients who receive blood that is not HLA compatible. Such patients fail to destroy the donated lymphocytes, which then initiate an immune reaction against the host.

Immunocompetent patients may also suffer from TA-GVHD when the host fails to eliminate the donated lymphocytes. This occurs most commonly when a recipient who is heterozygous for a particular HLA antigen receives blood that is homozygous for one of the host's HLA antigens. In this case, the host fails to recognize the donated lymphocytes as foreign while the donated cells initiate a TA-GVHD reaction against HLA antigens that they recognize as foreign.[45] Sufficient sharing of HLA antigens is most commonly seen when patients receive blood from close relatives or when the genetic heterogeneity within a given population is limited (e.g., in Japan).[46]

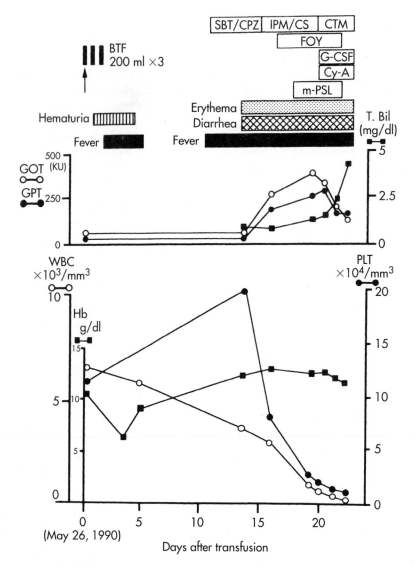

Fig. 23-2. Clinical findings and laboratory abnormalities in patients with transfusion-associated graft versus host disease. *BTF,* Blood transfusion; *CTM,* cefotiam; *Cy-A,* cyclosporine A; *FOY,* gabexate mesilate; *G-CSF,* granulocyte colony-stimulating factor; *GOT,* glutamic-oxaloacetic transaminase; *GPT,* glutamic-pyruvic transaminase; *Hb,* hemoglobin; *IPM/CS,* imipenem-cilastatin; *m-PSL,* methyl prednisolone; *PLT,* platelets; *SBT/CPZ,* sulbactam-cefoperazone; *T. Bil,* total bilirubin; *WBC,* white blood cell. (From Kobayashi H, Kitano K, Kishi E, et al: *Am J Hematol* 43:51, 1993.)

The diagnosis of TA-GVHD is often difficult because this rare entity may not be considered, particularly when other causes (e.g., infections, drug reactions) may present in a similar fashion. Characteristic findings of TA-GVHD are most often revealed on skin biopsy, although suggestive findings are often noted on liver and bone marrow biopsy. A more definitive diagnosis may be obtained by demonstrating the presence of donor lymphocytes in the transfusion recipient. Several methods have been described to aid in the HLA typing of the host and recipient cells, including polymerase chain reaction (PCR)–based HLA typing.[47] These tests must be interpreted in the appropriate clinical context, as in some scenarios (e.g., after liver or bone marrow transplantation) in which chimerism of lymphocytes may appropriately result in the presence of both donor and recipient lymphocytes.[48,49]

Management of TA-GVHD has been uniformly disappointing. Immunosuppressive therapies that have been successful in GVHD following BMT have not proven effective in TA-GVHD. Apparently no factors are predictive of cure, including how soon in the course of the disease treatment is initiated.

The greatest risk for the development of TA-GVHD is among immunosuppressed patients. Although there are case reports of TA-GVHD occurring in the context of virtually every type of immunosuppression, patients with acquired immunodeficiency syndrome (AIDS) have not been reported to have contracted TA-GVHD. There is speculation that the AIDS disease process may itself prohibit TA-GVHD and that the diagnosis of TA-GVHD is missed because symptoms are attributed to other coexisting diseases. The risk of TA-GVHD among various patient populations is noted in Box 23-3.

As noted earlier, immunocompetent patients who develop TA-GVHD usually have received blood from a close relative or from another member of their own genetically homogeneous population. Transfusions from parents and children, followed by second-degree relatives, followed by siblings, present the greatest risk.[50] It has been suggested that a number of the cases of TA-GVHD that have been associated with immunocompromise secondary to malignancy actually may have resulted from the fact that patients received nonirradiated directed donations from family members. Therefore the contribution of related donations, which can result in TA-GVHD regardless of immune status, may be underappreciated. The risk of TA-GVHD from receiving blood from within one's genetically homogeneous population has also been quantified. The risk of administering blood from an HLA homozygote to a patient with shared HLA heterozygosity in Japan is 1 in 312, whereas in Europe among white males it is 1 in 1024.[51] Most cases of TA-GVHD in Japan in immunocompetent patients receiving unrelated donor blood have involved the most common HLA haplotype in the country.[52] Although the risk of TA-GVHD among Japanese is higher than among other groups, the rate of TA-GVHD is disproportionately higher, suggesting that other factors, such as reporting or disease recognition, may increase the rate of TA-GVHD in this population. It is hypothesized that a critical number of lymphocytes of a given viability must be transfused in order to trigger a TA-GVHD reaction.[53] The prominent use in Japan of fresh blood, which contains a higher concentration of viable lymphocytes,[54] may explain the higher incidence of TA-GVHD in this population.

The principal means of preventing TA-GVHD is via the irradiation of blood with 2000 to 3500 cGy. The AABB currently mandates the use of blood irradiated with 2500 cGy for all patients at significant risk for developing TA-GVHD.[55] Although there is no comprehensive agreement on which patients are at significant risk, the risk stratification proposed by Shivdasani and Anderson (see Box 23-3) is a reasonable guide. Gamma irradiation effectively inactivates almost all T-lymphocytes in a unit of blood, reducing the number of cells able to respond to mitogen stimulus by several $\log_{10}$ factors. Despite the use of irradiation to substantially decrease the number of viable lymphocytes, there have been three cases of TA-GVHD after the administration of irradiated blood.[56,57] Side effects of irradiation include hyperkalemia, decreased platelet viability, and decreased RBC survival but are not usually clinically significant.[43,58] Other methods to decrease the number or viability of transfused lymphocytes via the use of lymphocyte filters have resulted in TA-GVHD in two cases.

Box 23-3 Risk groups for transfusion-associated graft versus host disease

Patient groups at significant risk
Bone marrow transplant patients
Congenital immunodeficiency syndromes
Intrauterine transfusions
Transfusions from blood relatives
Premature newborns
Neonates receiving exchange transfusions
Patients receiving human leukocyte antigen–matched platelet transfusions
Patients with Hodgkin's disease

Patient groups in which occasional case reports suggest some increased risk
Hematologic malignancies other than Hodgkin's disease
    Acute leukemia
    Non-Hodgkin's lymphoma
Solid organ transplant recipients
Solid tumors treated with chemotherapy or radiation therapy
    Neuroblastoma
    Glioblastoma
    Rhabdomyosarcoma
    Immunoblastic sarcoma

No defined increased risk compared with general population
Full-term neonates
Patients with acquired immunodeficiency syndrome
Patients receiving immunosuppressive therapy

From Shivdasani RA, Anderson KC: Graft-versus-host disease. In Petz LD, Swisher SN, Kleinman S, et al, eds: *Clinical practice of transfusion medicine*, ed 3, New York, 1996, Churchill Livingstone.

Box 23-4 Reported clinical outcomes from the immunomodulatory effects of blood transfusion

Improved organ allograft survival
Recurrence of malignancy
Susceptibility to postoperative infection
Prevention of recurrent abortion
Suppression of inflammatory bowel disease

Modified from Klein HG: Immunomodulation caused by blood transfusion. In Petz LD, Swisher SN, Kleinman S, et al, eds: *Clinical practice of transfusion medicine*, ed 3, New York, 1996, Churchill Livingstone.

F. Transfusion-related immunomodulation

The transfusion of blood has multiple immunologic consequences. Of these, the immunomodulating effect of blood transfusion is certainly the most subtle, but it may have multiple clinical consequences (Box 23-4). Despite a large number of studies, there is significant controversy over the magnitude of the effects of blood transfusion, the mechanisms of immunomodulation, and how these effects may affect clinical practice.

Blood transfusions modulate immune function in a number of ways, including the development of Fc receptor blocking factors, lymphocyte activation, changes in lymphocyte subpopulations, and down-regulation of antigen-presenting cells.[59] Whether or how these changes result in clinical effects is unclear. Several reviews of the physiology of the immune system and possible mechanisms of transfusion-related immunomodulation have recently been published.[60-62]

That blood transfusion results in a dose-dependent increase in renal allograft survival appears certain. Opelz et al[63] in 1973 established that blood transfusion before renal transplantation was associated with prolonged renal allograft survival (Fig. 23-3). Later studies demonstrated a similar effect for cardiac allografts. Improvements in immunosuppressive drug regimens have made the benefit of pretransplant blood transfusion more difficult to discern. There has also been some suggestion that changes in the processing of RBCs, which have resulted in significantly fewer leukocytes and less plasma per unit of RBCs, may account in part for the diminished effect of RBC transfusions on allograft survival.[64,65] Some transplant centers continue to use pretransplant blood transfusion in some patients undergoing renal transplantation.

The association between the transfusion of blood and cancer recurrence is far from clear. Over 40 studies have been published on the relationship between transfusion and cancer recurrence. A comprehensive analysis of these studies must account for multiple variables in each study, such as sample size, study design, tumor type, and transfusion dose.[66] Meta-analysis of the best data has been performed by Vamvakas and Moore,[67] who conclude that any effect of blood transfusion on cancer recurrence is a small effect and that such an effect could be established only with a randomized controlled experiment. At this time, a causal association between blood transfusion and cancer recurrence is debatable.

The role of blood transfusion on perioperative infection is controversial. Principal difficulties with studies attempting to establish a link between transfusion and infection include defining *infection* and accounting for surgical variability. Attempts to control for the acts of transfusion by randomizing allogeneic transfusion with autologous transfusion may be confounded by the assumption that patients capable of autologous donation are intrinsically healthier, although the need for transfusion is a marker for underlying illness. Twenty retrospective and four prospective studies have been published, and difficulties with methodology plague each one. However, the majority seem to associate preoperative blood transfusion with perioperative infection. Vamvakas

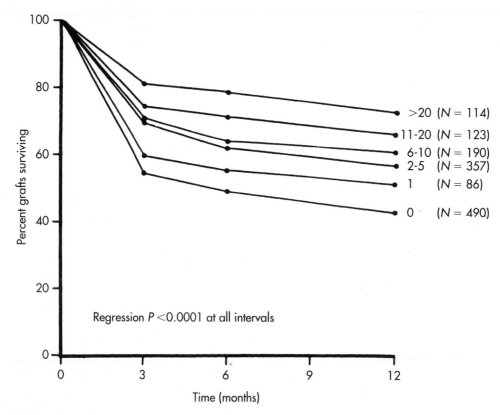

Fig. 23-3. Renal allograft survival in months as a function of prior allogeneic blood transfusions. Patients are grouped by the number of units received; numbers in parentheses indicate the number of patients in each group. (From Opelz G, Terasaki PI: *N Engl J Med* 299:799, 1978.)

and Moore[68] reviewed the accumulated data and concluded that there is no unequivocal study demonstrating the association between blood transfusion and infection.

Taylor and Faulk[69] describe three patients with a history of multiple spontaneous abortions who received buffy coat–rich plasma from unrelated donors and subsequently successfully conceived. This initiated a series of studies evaluating the efficacy of blood transfusion as a means of inhibiting spontaneous abortion. The outcome of these studies may have been influenced by a placebo effect from the administration of blood products. Although Mowbray et al[70] were able to demonstrate a significant decrease in spontaneous abortion associated with the infusion of allogeneic leukocytes from patients' spouses and intravenous immune globulin, respectively, another study using albumin as a placebo was not able to demonstrate an effect.[71] The positive influence of antenatal counseling and support on pregnancy rates[72] was not controlled for in many studies, so the effect of transfusion on pregnancy rates cannot be confirmed.

Blood transfusion may decrease the rate of recurrence of Crohn's disease. The most impressive association between blood transfusion and a decreased recurrence of Crohn's disease was a retrospective study from 1989 in which patients who received a blood transfusion at the time of bowel resection had a recurrence rate of 19%, compared with 59% among those who were not transfused.[73] Subsequent studies have failed to show this association. Some surgeons continue to transfuse patients preferentially for Crohn's disease.

II. NONIMMUNOLOGICALLY MEDIATED COMPLICATIONS

There are two general categories of nonimmunologically mediated complications associated with blood transfusion: those caused by an accelerated *rate* of blood transfusion, such as hypocalcemia, and those secondary to the transfusion of a large *quantity* of blood, such as volume overload.

A. Rate-related complications

Recent advances in blood warmer and infusion catheter technology have permitted the administration of euthermic blood to patients at rates exceeding 1 L/min. The use of these technologies has obviated concerns over the risk of hypothermia from blood transfusion while it has exacerbated the risk from hyperkalemia, hypocalcemia, and acute acidosis.

1. Ionized hypocalcemia. Ionized hypocalcemia, defined as a serum concentration of less than 1.1 mmol/L, is an unusual complication, occurring almost exclusively in the setting of the rapid transfusion of blood to trauma victims or neonates.

Hypocalcemia is manifested primarily in the cardiovascular system with a decrease in blood pressure and pulse pressure, an increase in ventricular filling pressure, and a prolongation in the QT interval on the electrocardiogram (ECG).[74-76] With very low concentrations of ionized calcium, bizarre or inverted T waves may develop, followed by severe arrhythmias (Fig. 23-4).[77] Patients

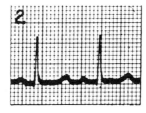
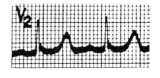
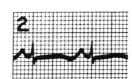
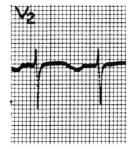

Fig. 23-4. Electrocardiographic effects of hypocalcemia. *Top,* Total serum calcium concentration of 7 mg/dl. *Bottom,* Total serum calcium concentration of 4.2 mg/dl. (From Marriott HJL: *Practical electrocardiography,* ed 7, Baltimore, 1983, Williams & Wilkins.)

with a history of heart failure or who are taking β-adrenergic blocking agents may manifest signs of hypocalcemia at higher Ca^{++} concentrations and more severely than other patients.[78]

Ionized hypocalcemia following blood transfusion occurs as a result of citrate toxicity. Citrate is added to stored blood in order to bind Ca^{++} and thereby inhibit the coagulation cascade. The severity of ionized hypocalcemia depends on the rate of citrate administration and the rate of citrate elimination and calcium mobilization from body tissues (Box 23-5).

The effect of citrate infusion on ionized calcium concentrations is rate dependent. Calcium is present in three forms in human serum: as ionized calcium, as protein-bound calcium, and as ligand-bound calcium. When citrate is infused at a low rate, the amount of ligand-bound calcium increases, the amount of protein-bound calcium decreases, and the amount of ionized calcium remains stable. Only when a higher rate of citrate infusion is reached does the ionized calcium concentration begin to decrease.[79]

The rate at which citrate-containing blood products must be administered in order to result in ionized hypocalcemia has been studied by Denlinger et al,[75] who found that among normovolemic, normothermic, otherwise healthy patients, hypocalcemia is prominent and persistent only when the rate of whole blood infusion surpasses approximately 1 unit of blood in every 5 minutes (Fig. 23-5). The rate at which toxicity occurred in this study was approximately 1 ml/kg/min, although this was achieved with the administration of whole blood with a low citrate concentration. The amount of citrate per unit of blood varies depending on the preservative

Box 23-5 Factors affecting the development of symptomatic blood transfusion–associated ionized hypocalcemia

Rate of citrate administration

Rate of administration of blood products
Type of blood product (e.g., fresh frozen plasma, red blood cells)
Blood product storage media (e.g., CPDA-1, AS-3)

Rate of citrate elimination

Rate of citrate metabolism (primarily hepatic)
  Temperature (hypothermia)
  Hepatic function
Rate of citrate excretion (primarily renal)

Rate of calcium mobilization from peripheral body stores

Ionized magnesium concentration
Parathyroid function
Peripheral tissue perfusion

and the blood product used. A unit of RBCs preserved with AS-1 solution contains 176 mg citrate and blood preserved in AS-3 contains 596 mg citrate. Units of FFP preserved in CPDA-1 contain 840 mg per unit.[80] Although a rate of 1 ml/kg/min is often quoted as the threshold for the development of ionized hypocalcemia, the use of different blood products and the patient's condition may result in hypocalcemia at a lower rate of infusion.

Hypocalcemia is also affected by the rate of elimination of infused citrate. The elimination of infused citrate is primarily via enzymatic metabolism to isocitrate and HCO_3^- in the liver in a temperature-dependent process. There may also be a role for the renal excretion of excess citrate, which may be blunted in patients with renal insufficiency.

The reequilibration of calcium from the peripheral tissues depends on magnesium concentrations, parathormone concentrations, and peripheral tissue perfusion. Decreased magnesium concentrations both inhibit the release of parathormone[81] and enhance the movement of Ca^{++} from extracellular fluid into bone,[82] resulting in decreased Ca^{++} concentrations. Furthermore, the treatment of hypomagnesemia with magnesium sulfate may further decrease Ca^{++} concentrations, as sulfate binds Ca^{++} and decreases free Ca^{++} concentrations.[83] In general, a finding of sustained ionized hypocalcemia should

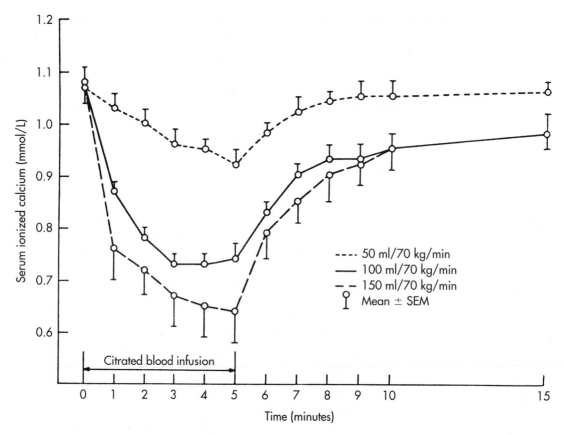

Fig. 23-5 The effect of increasing rates of infusion of citrate-containing blood products on the serum ionized calcium concentration. (From Denlinger JK, Nahrwold ML, Gibbs PS, et al: *Br J Anaesth* 48:995, 1976.)

provoke a search for hypomagnesemia; hypocalcemia may be refractory to therapy until hypomagnesemia is treated, preferably with magnesium chloride.

The maintenance of normocalcemia also depends on the mobilization of calcium from peripheral body stores via a parathormone-dependent process that may be severely inhibited in states of diminished tissue perfusion.[84] There is indirect evidence that good perfusion is critical for the maintenance of normal Ca^{++} concentrations. Drop and Laver[79] studied critically ill patients, evaluating the response of ionized hypocalcemia to an infusion of calcium. They noted that the administration of calcium alone was not sufficient to normalize ionized calcium concentrations and that some patients required isoproterenol infusions before their calcium concentrations would normalize. This study has been interpreted to suggest that adequate perfusion of tissues may be more important than CaCl administration per se in normalizing calcium concentrations, perhaps by facilitation of the reequilibration of calcium from peripheral body stores. It also suggests that although the administration of banked blood initially may result in a decrease in calcium concentrations from the effect of citrate, the ultimate restoration of volume will eventually permit a return of normal calcium homeostasis.

The appearance of signs attributable to hypocalcemia, including a decrease in blood pressure and pulse pressure with an increase in ventricular filling pressure in the presence of a prolonged QT interval on the ECG, warrants the measurement of ionized calcium. The diagnosis of ionized hypocalcemia is simplified by the availability of a fast and accurate blood test. Once it has been established that the patient is hypocalcemic, treatment depends on the degree of concomitant hypoperfusion, hypothermia, and renal and liver dysfunction.[79] The treatment of ionized hypocalcemia often begins with the administration of calcium chloride in a dose of 5 to 10 mg/kg, although repeated doses or continuous infusions may be necessary. Calcium gluconate is equally effective for the treatment of ionized hypocalcemia even in the complete absence of hepatic function, provided it is administered in doses three times larger on a per kilogram basis to account for the difference in molar equivalency of calcium when complexed with gluconate.[85] The presence of refractory hypocalcemia should prompt an assessment of the magnesium concentration that, if low, should be treated with the administration of magnesium chloride. Hypocalcemia should also prompt an evaluation of tissue perfusion, which should be augmented with the administration of fluid or inotropes when necessary. The overtreatment of hypocalcemia may result in hypercalcemic arrhythmias. Given the ready availability of Ca^{++} concentrations, there is no role for the protocol-driven administration of calcium with the administration of blood.

Certain patient populations, in whom metabolism or excretion of citrate or the reequilibration of calcium is impaired, would be expected to manifest hypocalcemia at rates of infusion of less than 1 ml/kg/min (Box 23-6). These patients include trauma victims, neonates, and the critically ill. Trauma patients are at additional risk

---

Box 23-6 Patient groups at increased risk for symptomatic ionized hypocalcemia

Trauma victims
Hypoperfused (hypovolemic) patients
Hypothermic patients
Functionally anhepatic patients
Premature infants
Neonates with intrauterine growth retardation
Newborns of diabetic mothers
Otherwise normal patients undergoing rapid transfusion
Patients with underlying heart failure
Patients taking β-adrenergic blocking agents

---

because, in addition to receiving blood at a rapid rate of infusion, they may have diminished liver function, hypothermia, and decreased tissue perfusion. Premature infants, neonates with intrauterine growth retardation, and newborns of diabetic mothers all have an increased incidence of hypocalcemia after blood transfusion. In these patient populations, the principal pathology lies with a diminished release of calcium from peripheral stores, because of either diminished parathormone release or the presence of a smaller calcium depot. Neonatologists often use calcium infusions to maintain ionized calcium concentrations during the administration of blood to their patients.[86]

In addition to trauma patients and neonates, the critically ill may be particularly prone to the development of ionized hypocalcemia because they often have low ionized calcium concentrations, even in the absence of shock or massive transfusions.[87] Some intensivists advocate the routine monitoring of ionized calcium concentrations in this population with even minor transfusions.

2. Hyperkalemia and hypokalemia

a. Hyperkalemia. As recently as 1982, the risk of hyperkalemia as a consequence of the administration of blood was regarded as a myth.[88] Large-bore catheters and rapid infusion devices permit the rapid transfusion of blood, which has been associated with hyperkalemic cardiac arrest.[89] A renewed appreciation for this complication has resulted in the publication of several studies, which are reviewed here.

The electrophysiologic effects of hyperkalemia are the most serious. An increased extracellular K^+ concentration increases the resting myocardial membrane potential, which decreases the speed of depolarization of myocardial fibers and decreases the rate of spontaneous depolarization in pacemaker cells. These effects result in progressive peaking of the T wave and widening of the QRS complex, culminating in asystole (Fig. 23-6).[89] Secondary effects of hyperkalemia include a decrease in cardiac output, which may have significant hemodynamic consequences.

Key factors in the development of hyperkalemia after blood transfusion include the amount of K^+ in each unit of RBCs, the rate of administration, and the patient population. K^+ accumulation in the plasma of stored RBC

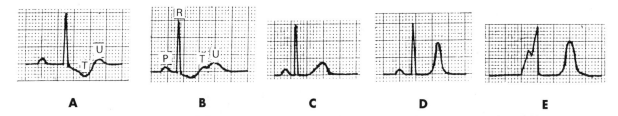

Fig. 23-6. Electrocardiographic effects of hypokalemia and hyperkalemia. **A,** K^+ concentration of 2.5 mEq/L. **B,** K^+ concentration of 3.5 mEq/L. **C,** K^+ concentration of 4 mEq/L, normal ECG. **D,** K^+ concentration of 7 mEq/L. **E,** K^+ concentration of 8.5 mEq/L. (From Goldman MJ: *Principles of clinical electrocardiography,* ed 12, Los Altos, Calif, 1986, Lange.)

Table 23-5. Levels of serum constituents for blood stored in citrate phosphate dextrose adenine (CPDA-1) and AS-1 media over time

Day	0	1	3	7	14	21	28	35	42
CPDA-1									
pH	6.94	6.91	6.84	6.80	6.72	6.62	6.50	6.40	6.37
K^+ (mEq/L)	4.7	10	17	30	43	56	66	72	71
CPD-ADSOL (AS-1)									
pH	6.97	6.92	6.85	6.77	6.53	6.47	6.40	6.32	6.32
K^+ (mEq/L)	2.1	5.7	11	18	28	39	42	47	53

From Jeter EK, Gadsden RH, Cate J IV: *Ann Clin Lab Sci* 21:177, 1991.

units is caused by the transmembrane movement of K^+ out of RBCs into the extracellular fluid in response to an increasingly acidic environment. Different RBC preservatives affect both the degree of acidity and the amount of potassium accumulation in the extracellular plasma (Table 23-5).[90] Units of blood nearing expiration may have plasma K^+ concentrations as high as 100 mEq/L.[91] Because the plasma volume in a unit of blood is 60 ml, the total amount of K^+ in a unit nearing expiration is approximately 1.5 to 7 mEq.

Along with an elevated K^+ concentration, a rapid rate of administration predisposes to the development of hyperkalemia. Upon administration, donated RBCs respond to an environment with far lower acidity by taking up K^+ into the cell. However, this process may require several days to complete.[92] The K^+ from the plasma of the transfused unit that is not immediately taken up into the transfused RBCs must be assimilated by the recipient's tissues. The uptake of K^+ by recipient tissue is favored by alkalosis, β-adrenergic agonists, and the presence of insulin, and is finite in capacity. At extremely high rates of administration of K^+-rich fluid, the processes of K^+ clearance may not pertain because there is inadequate time for the clearance of excess K^+ by these mechanisms. Brown et al[91] noted that in these circumstances, the redistribution of K^+ follows single-compartment kinetics in which K^+ distributes only within the plasma compartment. Furthermore, they advanced the concept that the relative rate of flow of K^+-rich perfusate compared to the patient's overall cardiac output is the key determinant of hyperkalemic toxicity. In fact, if K^+ flow rates are sufficiently high, the concentration of K^+ reaching the myocardium may be high enough to act as iatrogenic cardioplegia. This mecha-

nism is most relevant among neonates, in whom it is physically possible to rapidly inject volumes of blood that are proportionately large compared to the patient's cardiac output.

Several studies have attempted to estimate the rate at which the administration of blood may result in hyperkalemia. Linko and Saxelin[93] noted hyperkalemia after the administration of blood at a rate of more than 0.3 ml/kg/min.

Although Linko and Saxelin correlated the rate of blood administration with the incidence of hyperkalemia, Wall and Pavlin showed no such correlation, and suggested that individual patient factors may account for the variable appearance of hyperkalemia at different rates of administration. Patient risk factors for the development of hyperkalemia include renal insufficiency, crush injuries, acidosis, and total body hypoperfusion. Patients with a high total body K^+ content, such as patients with renal insufficiency or a crush injury, begin with less of a safety margin when K^+ is administered. In addition, these patients may have a decreased capacity to assimilate administered K^+. Acidosis predisposes to the development of hyperkalemia by causing a shift of K^+ out of the cell.[94] A decrease in pH of 0.1 may increase K^+ concentrations by 0.5 to 2 mEq/L.[95] Acidosis also results in hyperkalemia by a direct inhibition of K^+ secretion in the distal renal tubules.[96]

Inadequate or decreasing tissue perfusion has been stressed by some authors as a key risk factor in K^+ toxicity. Brown et al[91] note that poor perfusion may limit the assimilation of K^+ by the body and that a stable rate of blood infusion in a patient with a decreasing cardiac output increases the relative proportion of flow that is K^+ rich. Hyperkalemia by itself diminishes cardiac output,

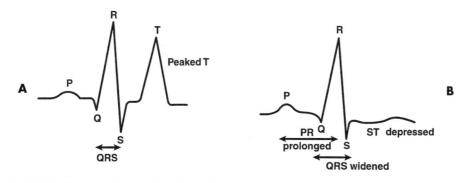

Fig. 23-7. Electrocardiographic effects of hypomagnesemia. Note prolongation of the QRS interval, peaking of the T wave, and ultimate prolongation of the PR interval. **A,** Moderate hypomagnesemia. **B,** Severe hypomagnesemia. (From Seelig M: *Ann N Y Acad Sci* 162:906, 1969.)

which may have a feedforward effect in promoting cardiac arrest.[97] In addition to the factors noted earlier, the effects of other electrolytes (calcium, magnesium), the presence of hypothermia, and the acid-base status at the level of the myocardiocyte also must be considered. It is likely that the interplay of multiple factors determines the incidence and severity of hyperkalemia in the transfused patient.

The appearance of peaked T waves on the ECG is worrisome and usually necessitates the initiation of therapy to decrease the plasma K^+ concentration. This initially consists of a calcium chloride bolus at 10 mg/kg, a sodium bicarbonate bolus at 0.5 mEq/kg, and the initiation of hyperventilation. The therapeutic aim is to cause alkalemia, which results in a shift of K^+ to the intracellular compartment, although the administration of bicarbonate, separately from alkalosis, has an effect on decreasing plasma K^+ concentrations.[98] Insulin (administered with 50% dextrose) stimulates the assimilation of K^+ by the body, and furosemide is administered to encourage renal K^+ elimination. Some have also used magnesium administration in this context, based in part on a report showing that hypermagnesemia had prevented hyperkalemic ECG changes in four patients despite the presence of hyperkalemia.[99]

Certain patient populations may benefit from measures to decrease the amount of K^+ in units of transfused blood. Some neonatologists either wash RBCs or request the freshest RBCs for administration to their patients. Another clinician has advocated the use of a single unit of RBCs for transfusion, even up to the expiration date of the unit, arguing that this practice limits donor exposures to the neonate. Concerns over hyperkalemia are limited by slow administration of blood with careful monitoring.[100]

b. Hypokalemia. Hypokalemia is probably a more common complication of blood transfusion than hyperkalemia, particularly if plasma K^+ concentrations are corrected for concomitant acidosis.[101] As for hyperkalemia, the effects of hypokalemia are most apparent on the ECG and include a diminished T wave followed by loss of the T wave and appearance of a U wave (see Fig. 23-6). Hypokalemia is most often noted after the need for transfusion resolves. The appearance of hypokalemia is partially caused by the active reuptake by transfused

RBCs of K^+, but also by the metabolism of each millimole of transfused citrate to 3 mEq of HCO_3^-. The resulting alkalosis results in a further movement of K^+ into the cells.[102] Ongoing renal elimination and tissue assimilation of K^+ also act to decrease K^+ concentrations.[103] Although it is known that the effects of hypomagnesemia may resemble the effects of hypokalemia, and that a low magnesium concentration may predispose for the development of hypokalemia, the role of transfusion-associated hypomagnesemia in the pathogenesis of hypokalemia has not been studied rigorously. A failure of hypokalemia to respond to treatment should prompt an evaluation of the magnesium concentration.

Many clinicians avoid treating hypokalemia in the operating room unless electrocardiographic evidence of hypokalemia is apparent because the unnecessary administration of K^+ invites catastrophic hyperkalemia with arrhythmias. The correction of perturbations of plasma K^+ concentrations must be guided by frequent plasma K^+ concentrations.

3. Hypomagnesemia. There has been an increasing interest in the development of hypomagnesemia in the setting of blood transfusion. Hypomagnesemia is defined by a total serum magnesium (Mg) concentration of less than 0.6 mmol/L. The Mg concentration is affected by the concentration of albumin, which binds 25% to 30% of serum Mg. Hypoalbuminemia may falsely lower Mg concentrations; the correction formula is Mg (corrected) = Mg + 0.05 (40 − albumin g/L).[104]

Hypomagnesemia has been associated with prolonged QT intervals, torsade de pointes, sudden death, tachyarrhythmias, ventricular fibrillation refractory to defibrillation, hypotension, and seizures.[83] In particular, there have been reports of the development of hypomagnesemia after massive blood transfusion.[105,106] The effects of hypomagnesemia on cardiac conduction result from the role of magnesium ions (Mg^{++}) in the normal function of sodium-potassium–dependent ATPase, which maintains normal intracellular concentrations of K^+. The similarity between some of the electrophysiologic effects of hypomagnesemia (PR interval prolongation and ST segment depression) and hypokalemia have been suggested to be caused by the central role of Mg^{++} in the maintenance of normal transmembrane gradients of K^+ in the cardiac cell (Fig. 23-7).[107] The role of hypomagnesemia in increasing the risk of digitalis toxicity further supports a link between Mg^{++} and K^+.[108]

The pathophysiology of hypomagnesemia in the setting of a blood transfusion is thought to be caused by the binding of Mg^{++} by citrate in a manner similar to the binding of Ca^{++} by citrate.[109] The amount of citrate or rate of infusion necessary for significant hypomagnesemia to occur is not known, although one study suggests that the Mg^{++} concentration does not decrease as much as the calcium concentration after the administration of citrate.[110] Further studies are necessary before a reasonable estimate of a toxic rate of blood administration can be established.

Hypomagnesemia may significantly decrease the concentrations of both Ca^{++} and K^+. Hypomagnesemia is known to inhibit the release of parathormone[81] while enhancing the movement of Ca^{++} from extracellular fluid into bone,[111] both of which decrease Ca^{++} concentrations. Furthermore, hypocalcemia may accompany hypomagnesemia during the administration of citrate. The treatment of hypomagnesemia with magnesium sulfate may further decrease Ca^{++} concentrations because sulfate binds Ca^{++} and decreases free Ca^{++} concentrations.[83] In general, a finding of hypocalcemia should provoke a search for hypomagnesemia as well, with the understanding that hypocalcemia may be refractory to therapy until hypomagnesemia is treated, preferably with magnesium chloride. Hypomagnesemia also augments renal losses of K^+, so hypokalemia may be refractory to therapy unless hypomagnesemia is treated.[112]

The management of hypomagnesemia involves the administration of magnesium chloride (MgCl) intravenously. The administration of magnesium sulfate may decrease Ca^{++} because of the binding of Ca^{++} by sulfate.[113] Hypomagnesemia may be prevented in critically ill patients by the administration of 1 to 2 g MgCl daily. Guidelines for the acute treatment of hypomagnesemia are not readily available, although the administration of 1 to 2 g intravenously with close monitoring of the Mg concentration appears to be a safe approach. Chernow et al[83] note that a patient with normal renal function may excrete 40 to 60 g Mg per day, whereas the common use and sustained therapeutic experience with the use of Mg in patients with preeclampsia attest to a wide therapeutic margin of safety.[83]

Certain patient populations are at increased risk for the development of clinically significant hypomagnesemia, most notably those with low baseline concentrations of Mg. These include patients with gastrointestinal losses of Mg, pancreatitis, alcoholism, renal insufficiency, and various endocrinopathies, including hyperparathyroidism and hyperthyroidism. Various drugs may also diminish Mg, including diuretics, gentamycin, and cardiac glycosides.[83] A reasonable strategy for preventing hypomagnesemia is to assess an Mg concentration if there is a significant likelihood of the administration of large amounts of blood, particularly if the patient has risk factors for preexisting hypomagnesemia.

4. Acid-base effects. Upon initial processing for storage, RBCs are placed in an acidic, citrate-rich medium with a pH of approximately 6.94 (see Table 23-5). Over the ensuing 42 days of storage, the pH progressively decreases to a nadir of approximately 6.3 just before blood unit expiration. The progressive decline in pH is because RBCs, lacking the cellular machinery for aerobic metabolism, must generate ATP via a glycolytic process that results in the elaboration of lactic acid.[114] As part of this process, CO_2 production results in a buildup of CO_2 within gas-impermeable storage bags.[115] Despite this acid load, however, the infusion of a unit of RBCs is typically assimilated efficiently without resulting in acidosis. In fact, most of the citrate in a unit has been metabolized within 2 hours, and the patient soon manifests a metabolic alkalosis. The initial process of assimilation of electrolytes and the restoration of RBCs to their normal ionic concentrations is an energy-requiring process.[116] In the setting of hypovolemia and acute trauma, this process may be delayed and the normal process of resolution of acidosis and onset of alkalosis may be delayed. Certain groups of patients may not assimilate the acid load as rapidly. These include patients with a decreased cardiac output, who may have decreased pulmonary perfusion and diminished ability to excrete CO_2. Similarly, any lung injury that inhibits CO_2 excretion may stall assimilation.[101]

The paradox of the administration of RBCs in an acidic solution for the resuscitation of a hypoperfused state marked by metabolic acidosis is that although volume resuscitation is imperative for the resolution of hypovolemia and lactic acidosis, the short-term effect is to worsen acidosis. The rate of blood transfusion required to produce metabolic acidosis has not been studied in a controlled fashion, although Linko and Saxelin[93] noted this effect among patients transfused at rates exceeding 1.2 ml/kg/min. The abrupt infusion of a potassium-rich solution may worsen the effects of rapid transfusion because both hyperkalemia and acidosis may decrease cardiac output, which may further limit assimilation. However, the fundamental problem in such situations is the underlying degree of volume deficit. The administration of blood products is necessary in this situation and ultimately contributes to the resolution of acidosis.[117,118] It has been suggested that an ongoing metabolic acidosis after the administration of RBCs in some patients results more from the severity of their injury and depth of hypoperfusion, not the rapid administration of RBCs per se.

The management of acidosis during ongoing blood loss involves the restoration of euvolemia, with the careful titration of blood products as tolerated by the patient. Bicarbonate administration is of limited benefit in the absence of adequate ventilation. For an established metabolic acidosis, however, bicarbonate may be transiently helpful. Augmentation of cardiac output with inotropic agents to improve tissue perfusion may be of benefit. Vigilance for and treatment of concomitant electrolyte disturbances that may predispose to arrhythmias is imperative in this setting.

5. Hypothermia. Hypothermia has been defined as a temperature of less than 35° C. The adverse effects of hypothermia are well established and include impairments of the stress response and immune system, impaired drug clearance, impaired metabolism of citrate, hypovolemia caused by cold diuresis, exacerbation of lactic acidosis, cardiac arrhythmias, and coagulopathy.[119] Among trauma patients in particular, several effects of hypothermia are synergistic. Trauma patients are often cold and acidotic upon admission, and often have a depressed myocardial function as a result.[117] These patients are then exposed to cold fluids and a cold environment, which further depresses their cardiac function and increases lactic acidosis, both of which worsen coagulopathy. Worsening coagulopathy often results in the administration of more blood products, with attendant risks, including hypothermia. It is not surprising that several studies have demonstrated an increased risk of mortality among patients who have become hypothermic.[117,118,120,121] Other risks of hypothermia have also been established, including the increased risk of postoperative shivering and discomfort,[122] wound infection,[123] and increased risk of intraoperative myocardial ischemia.[124]

The development of hypothermia after the administration of unwarmed blood products depends on the rate at which the blood is administered versus the ability of the patient to generate sufficient heat to maintain body temperature. The warming of a single unit of RBCs from 4° C to 37° C requires approximately 10 kcal of energy. Though not a staggering energy loss, this represents 10 kcal that the patient will expend on heat generation instead of on other required functions. Outcome data on wound infection and overall death rate suggest that the energy burden of assimilating cold blood is not without cost. It is tempting to limit the use of blood warming techniques to instances when a high rate of administration of blood is used. However, maintaining normothermia during surgery or resuscitation can be an ordeal, and every reasonable means to maintain temperature should be pursued. Current technology permits the administration of blood warmed to 37° C at a rate of up to 1500 ml/min using a countercurrent technique.[119] In locations where blood warmers are impractical, an alternative method of warming blood that involves mixing RBCs with saline at 70° C has been described.[125] One significant concern with this method is the risk of developing massive hemolysis; this technique has not been embraced by the AABB or the Food and Drug Administration (FDA). Iserson and Huestis[119] recently reviewed currently available blood warming technologies and concluded that it is possible to fully resuscitate a patient with virtually any survivable rate of hemorrhage while maintaining normothermia.

The treatment of a patient who has become hypothermic is often difficult. All fluids should be warmed, and forced air heaters should be used to maintain a layer of warm air next to the patient's skin. When forced air warmers are impractical or unavailable, warming the entire surgical room is a helpful interim measure. Lavage of body cavities with warmed fluids may be helpful, although severe hypothermia requires core rewarming via the use of cardiopulmonary bypass with a high flow heat exchanger.

B. Volume-related complications

Volume-related complications are those that increase in likelihood with the transfusion of an increasing number of units of blood. Complications falling in this category have received great attention recently. Trauma associated with the use of high-power weapons has led to increasingly aggressive resuscitation of victims, with the administration of ever-increasing blood volumes. The advent of AIDS has heightened awareness of the risk of contracting infectious disease from the transfusion of blood. New data have become available on the development of coagulopathies in the setting of massive blood transfusion. It is incumbent on the practicing anesthesiologist to become articulate in communicating the risk of these complications to patients and colleagues and to learn to avoid them when possible.

1. Dilutional coagulopathy

a. Dilutional thrombocytopenia. Dilutional thrombocytopenia (DT) has been variously defined as a decrease in platelet count to less than 50,000 to 100,000 per μl through the transfusion of platelet-poor blood products or crystalloid. As such, DT is not strictly a complication of blood transfusion, but is a predictable sequel to the fluid resuscitation of patients with major hemorrhage. The fact that many patients with DT are also predisposed to coagulopathies from other causes (e.g., hypothermia or factor deficiency) often makes it difficult to confirm DT as the cause of a bleeding diathesis.

The replacement of a patient's blood volume with products, which are essentially devoid of platelets, predictably dilutes the patient's platelet pool.[126] Hiippala, Myllyla, and Vahtera[127] studied the rate of decline of platelet count and coagulation factor concentration in patients undergoing abdominal or urologic surgery and estimated that a patient's platelet count will go below 50,000/μl after the replacement of approximately 230% of the patient's calculated blood volume (CBV) with RBCs (Fig. 23-8). Because approximately 12 units of RBCs correspond to the red cell mass of a 70-kg patient, significant DT is expected after approximately 27 units of RBCs have been administered to a 70-kg patient.

Although DT caused by blood transfusion is a mathematical inevitability, the presence of DT does not predict the need for platelet replacement therapy. In fact, there are no tests that correlate platelet number or function with bleeding diathesis. Harrigan et al[128] in 1982 studied massively transfused patients and noted that despite having low platelet counts and prolonged bleeding times, none of the patients studied had a clinically apparent coagulopathy. Other studies have confirmed a lack of utility of the bleeding time as a qualitative test of platelet function.[129,130] Thromboelastography has been assessed as a means of correlation between platelet number or function and the presence of a coagulation deficit, although it does not appear to be specific enough to reliably predict the need for platelet transfusion in all populations. The decision to administer platelets is based on both the presence of a platelet count of less than 100,000/μl and a clinically apparent hemorrhagic diathesis. To achieve an increase in platelet count of approxi-

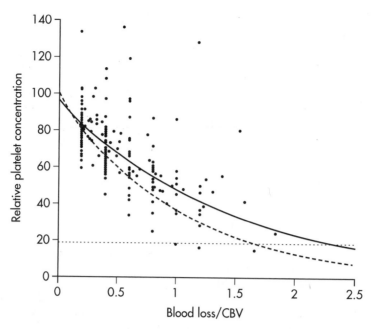

Fig. 23-8. Relative platelet concentration versus blood replacement in calculated blood volumes *(CBV)*. The relative platelet concentration decreases to less than 50,000 platelets/μl after a replacement of approximately 2.3 CBV. (From Hiippala ST, Myllyla GJ, Vahtera EM: *Anesth Analg* 81:360, 1995.)

mately 100,000/μl, the patient should receive one unit of single-donor platelet concentrate for each 10 kg of body weight. Many blood banks are now recommending the use of single-donor apheresis platelet units, which contain the equivalent of 5 to 8 regular platelet units and have the added advantage of exposing the recipient to only one donor.

Not all clinicians are prepared to wait for clinically apparent coagulopathy before administering platelets. Some have advocated the administration of platelets based on the clinical scenario alone (i.e., that the patient has lost approximately two blood volumes). Because of laboratory delays, many such decisions are made without the benefit of a platelet count. This preemptive approach may decrease the risk of hemorrhage and perhaps even the overall use of blood products if the administered platelets have a net effect of limiting blood product administration. The alternative approach of waiting for clinically apparent hemorrhage before administering platelets limits the wastage of platelets but may also increase the overall blood loss and administration of blood products. Either way, treatment must be based on clinical judgment. A blind, protocol-driven administration of platelets is both wasteful of products and fails to decrease blood loss. In a study by Tuman et al,[131] thromboelastography (TEG) was used to evaluate the potential for hemorrhage among patients suffering blood losses of up to 80% of their CBV. Among patients suffering a blood loss of 80% CBV, only 50% appeared to have a platelet deficit that required therapy. If these patients had been treated according to protocol, half would have received blood products unnecessarily. Furthermore, Reed et al[132] demonstrated that neither coagulopathy nor mortality was affected by the prophylactic treatment of trauma pa-

tients with platelets or coagulation factors. The decision to replace platelets is made more challenging by the knowledge that other causes of hemorrhage often exist in patients receiving large blood transfusions, such as DIC, preexisting platelet defects, and hypothermia.[133] In the absence of a readily available index of the adequacy of platelet number or function, the clinician is forced to use clinical judgment and the sense of DT as an inevitable process associated with the replacement of two or more blood volumes in order to guide therapy.

Certain populations may have an increased risk of developing DT earlier in the course of therapy. These patients are those with a low baseline platelet count (e.g., secondary to idiopathic thrombocytopenic purpura) or function (e.g., secondary to uremia or cardiopulmonary bypass) and those with destruction of platelets (e.g., secondary to DIC). Such patients require more frequent monitoring in order to stay ahead of platelet dilution.

b. Dilution of clotting factors. Dilution of clotting factors (DCF) is defined as a decrease in the number of clotting factors caused by the transfusion of factor-poor blood products or crystalloid. Unlike DT, in which all blood products are devoid of platelets, only packed RBCs are significantly devoid of coagulation factors. Whole blood contains stable concentrations of all factors but factors V and VIII, which gradually decrease to 15% and 50% of normal, respectively, over 21 days of storage. Only 5% and 30% of factors V and VIII are required for normal clotting, so the transfusion of whole blood does not result in clinically significant dilution of factors.[134] DCF occurs in patients resuscitated with RBCs or crystalloid.

Hiippala, Myllyla, and Vahtera[127] studied the dilution of platelets and factors and noted that the fibrinogen was the most vulnerable of the factors measured, with a concentration of 1 g/L being reached after the replacement of 142% of the CBV (Fig. 23-9). The fact that other factors decrease more slowly was ascribed to a variable release of factors stored in endogenous sources, although the mechanism of this has not been confirmed or defined.[127] Although these data are helpful in preparing for hemorrhage, few clinicians have factor concentrations at their disposal during blood transfusion. PT and PTT have been recommended to guide factor replacement therapy. Unfortunately, the predictive value of PT and PTT for coagulopathy is debatable. Crosby[133] notes that PT and PTT have both a poor positive predictive value and poor sensitivity as indicators of bleeding tendency. Murray et al[135] note that increases in PT and PTT commonly accompanied the loss of more than 50% of the CBV, and that when the PT and PTT were prolonged to greater than 1.5 times normal, a subjective increase in surgical bleeding was observed in their study. Prolongation of PT and PTT cannot be considered a reliable predictor of coagulopathy.

Although prolongation of PT and PTT commonly accompanies ongoing hemorrhage, the cause is not always simply DCF. Massively transfused patients, particularly those with a history of prolonged hypotension, ongoing hypothermia, or antecedent acidosis, often develop consumptive coagulopathies that take the form of disseminated intravascular coagulopathy.[117,118] Although the development of DCF after blood transfusion is often predictable, the coagulopathy may be refractory to the administration of factors alone if it is due to causes other than DCF alone.

Current recommendations are to administer FFP for the treatment of DCF only if the PT and PTT are prolonged to 1.5 times normal, and then only in the presence of a clinical coagulopathy. Problems with this approach include variability in the assessment of the surgical field and the inevitable laboratory delays in returning PT and PTT results. New technologies that allow the rapid (i.e., 5-minute) assessment of PT and PTT in the operating room may make the treatment of DCF less cumbersome. As for DT, there is no role for the prophylactic administration of FFP for the treatment of DCF. Many such protocols advocate the administration of FFP after every several units of red cells. This is especially unnecessary because data suggest that when blood loss is confined to less than one blood volume, patients often exhibit a hypercoagulable state.[131] For patients with larger blood loss, data show no benefit to prophylactic administration of FFP.[136]

Certain populations may be at increased risk for DCF, notably those with a preexisting coagulopathy caused by vitamin K deficiency, Coumadin therapy, or hepatic insufficiency. As noted earlier, trauma patients may develop coagulopathies secondary to acidosis, hypoperfusion, or hypothermia, and these patients may be expected to manifest coagulopathies earlier in the course of dilution.

2. Volume overload. Volume overload may result from the administration of large quantities of blood or from the excessively rapid administration of blood. Over-

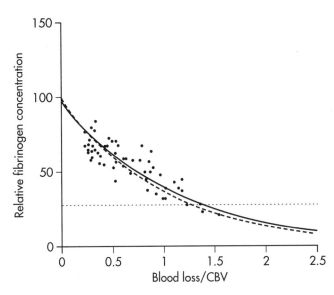

Fig. 23-9. Relative fibrinogen concentration versus blood replacement in calculated blood volumes *(CBV)*. The relative fibrinogen concentration decreases to less than 1 g/L after a replacement of approximately 1.4 CBV. (From Hiippala ST, Myllyla GJ, Vahtera EM: *Anesth Analg* 81:360, 1995.)

load presents as congestive heart failure, with increased left heart filling pressures, pulmonary edema, tachypnea, and tachycardia. Although in theory any patient may develop volume overload, patients at highest risk are those with a history of respiratory and circulatory compromise, the elderly, and the very young. Additionally, patients with a long history of compensated anemia with increased circulating blood volume may develop symptoms of congestive heart failure with the administration of limited amounts of blood.[137] Recommendations are to transfuse blood at a slow rate of approximately 2 ml/kg/hr if possible and to maintain vigilance for overload in high-risk populations. The use of component therapy (i.e., RBCs) for the treatment of anemia instead of whole blood may further decrease risk. The concomitant administration of furosemide with blood may limit symptoms in hypervolemic patients. Treatment of volume-overloaded patients presenting with dyspnea includes supportive therapy while ruling out other elements of the differential diagnosis, including TRALI, anaphylactic reaction, AHTR, ARDS, and an FNTR with pulmonary manifestations (see Box 23-1).[12]

3. Iron overload. Each unit of RBCs contains approximately 200 mg iron. For patients suffering ongoing hemorrhage, this dose of iron is assimilated easily. For patients with chronic anemic conditions (e.g., congenital hemolytic anemia, aplastic anemia, sickle cell anemia, and thalassemia) who do not have ongoing blood loss, the accumulation of iron may be significant. Iron accumulates in the heart, liver, and endocrine organs, and the patient may eventually develop myocardial failure with arrhythmias, diabetes, or hepatic insufficiency. It is estimated that transfusion hemosiderosis may result after the administration of as few as 100 units of RBCs.[137]

Oral iron chelation therapy is efficacious in the prevention of hemosiderosis, and has been proven successful in treating some of the manifestations of established hemosiderosis.[138]

4. Microaggregates. Microaggregates (MAs) are composed primarily of degenerating platelets along with granulocyte debris and fibrin strands and measure somewhat larger than 40 μm in diameter. MAs form rapidly during blood storage, with increasing number and size of MAs over time. MAs are distinguished from larger "macroaggregates," which are clots of RBCs in solution and are removed by 170-μm filters, which are a standard part of a blood administration tubing set.

Once administered via intravenous infusion, MAs are removed by the lung vascular bed.[133] The infusion of MAs can be significantly limited by filtration with an MA filter (MAF). Two different MAF types are available. The screen type, composed of woven polyester, intercepts MAs, and the depth type of filter, composed of polyurethane foam, removes MAs by absorption.[139] MAs are also infused via the arterial route during cardiopulmonary bypass. Special high-flow, low-impedance filters are available for the removal of MAs from the arterial limb of a cardiopulmonary bypass machine.

Some studies conducted in the early 1970s on massive trauma victims from the Vietnam conflict suggested that intravenous MAs may play a role in augmenting lung injury and may result in ARDS.[140] Not all studies were able to demonstrate a correlation between the amount of blood transfused and the degree of MA embolization, or in the incidence of ARDS following massive transfusion.[141-143] Subsequent investigators drew a firmer association between the degree of overall injury and the incidence of ARDS, and suggested that the amount of blood transfused was just a covariable with the degree of injury.[144] The incidence of ARDS associated with massive trauma is declining, which may be explained by the use of different resuscitation techniques that feature more rapid and comprehensive fluid resuscitation. At this time there is no clear consensus on the role of MAs in the pathogenesis of ARDS. The use of MAFs may be con-

traindicated in the setting of massive transfusion because these filters may result in significant impedance to flow.

Aside from their use in preventing ARDS, MAFs have been advocated to limit the incidence of febrile reactions, which are mediated by platelets and leukocytes.[133] However, there has been no controlled evaluation of MAFs for this indication. The only clear consensus regarding the use of MAFs has been to limit the perfusion of the arterial circulation with MAs while perfusing with a cardiopulmonary bypass circuit.

5. Infectious diseases. In 1992, Dodd[145] estimated that 3 in 10,000 blood recipients contract serious or fatal transfusion-transmitted infectious disease. This figure compares favorably to an estimated rate of 60 out of 10,000 hospitalized patients who have died as a result of accidental or preventable causes other than their underlying diseases. Despite a low rate of serious infectious complications, the transmission of infectious agents via the transfusion of blood is perceived by the lay public as the principal risk of blood transfusion. A recently published estimate of the rate of infection from blood transfusion is noted in Table 23-6, and the infectious risk of the important infectious agents by blood component type is shown in Table 23-7. The continued transmission of infections via blood transfusion despite blood screening procedures may occur in one of three ways.[146] The

Table 23-6. The risk of infection transmission per unit of blood transfused in the United States

Human immunodeficiency virus	1 in 493,000
Hepatitis A	1 in 1,000,000*
Hepatitis B	1 in 63,000
Hepatitis C	1 in 103,000
Human T-cell lymphotropic virus	1 in 641,000
Aggregate risk for these agents	1 in 34,000

Modified from Schreiber G, Busch M, Kleinman S, et al: *N Engl J Med* 334:1685, 1996.
*Data from Giacoia GP, Kasprisin DO: *South Med J* 82:1357, 1989.

Table 23-7. Infectious risk of some infectious agents by blood component type

Infectious agent	Whole blood and red blood cells	Platelets	Fresh frozen plasma cryoprecipitate	Coagulation factor concentrates	Immune globulin	Plasma protein fraction and albumin
Human immunodeficiency virus 1/2	Yes	Yes	Yes	No	No	No
Human T-cell lymphotropic virus I/II	Yes	Yes	No	No	No	No
Hepatitis	Yes	Yes	Yes	No	No*	No
Cytomegalovirus	Yes†	Yes†	No	No	No	No
Bacteria	Yes	Yes	Yes	No	No	No
Malaria	Yes	Yes	No	No	No	No
Syphilis	Yes	Yes	No	No	No	No
Parvovirus B19	Yes	Yes	Yes	Yes	No	No

*There are few cases of hepatitis C transmission in the United States, prevented now by viral inactivation and polymerase chain reaction screening.
†Prevented by leukocyte-reduced blood components.

first is that the donor donates blood too early in the infectious process to have detectable infectivity, during an interval called the window period. For example, it is estimated that the window period of HIV infection with current testing methods is 22 days.[147] An estimate of the window period associated with the detection of viral infections (with currently available technology) is presented in Table 23-8. A second means of contracting disease despite screening procedures is via the transmission of an agent, such as hepatitis C virus (HCV), that may exist in a chronic carrier state despite a negative screening test. Last, human error may contribute to the transmission of disease in the event of faulty reporting of a blood unit's infectivity. For these reasons, it is probably not possible to develop a blood supply that is free of the risk of transmitting infectious disease. Anesthesiologists, as practitioners who often prescribe blood, should be aware of the risks of transfusion-transmitted infections and be able to articulate these risks to colleagues and the public.

Table 23-8. Estimates of the window periods associated with the detection of viral infections with currently available technology

	Length of window period (days)	
Virus	Estimate	Range
Human immuno-deficiency virus	22	6-38
Hepatitis B	59	37-87
Hepatitis C	82	54-192
Human T-cell lymphotropic virus	51	36-72

Modified from Schreiber GB, Busch MP, Kleinman SH, et al: *N Engl J Med* 334:1685, 1996.

a. Viral infections

(1) HEPATITIS B VIRUS. Hepatitis B virus (HBV) is a DNA virus of the class Hepadnaviridae that is the etiologic agent responsible for serum hepatitis. In addition, HBV DNA may become integrated into host DNA, an event that may be the cause of many as 25% to 33% of the 1000 cases of primary hepatocellular carcinoma in the United States each year.[148] The clinical course of HBV infection is well described and may be followed by serologic markers of infection, immunologic response, and either resolution or progression to a chronic carrier state. Acute infection is characterized by the detection of hepatitis B surface antigen (HBsAg) (Fig. 23-10). Over the ensuing 3 months, either antibodies against HBsAg will be detected, indicating convalescence, or HBsAg and antibodies to HB core antigen (anti-HBcAg) will persist, indicating a chronically infected state (Fig. 23-11).

During acute infection, the HBV may circulate at concentrations of up to 10^7 particles/ml. Therefore even minute amounts of blood may transmit infection. The most efficient mode of infection with HBV is via blood-to-blood contact, although the virus may be transmitted via birth contact or transmucosal infection. It is estimated that up to 30% of needlestick injuries that are contaminated with HBV may result in infection. Case reports of infection resulting from cross-country running involving scratches from vegetation and subsequent communal bathing emphasize the extreme infectivity of HBV.[149] Patients who have detectable HBsAg are considered infectious. Retrospective studies of patients infected with HBV have demonstrated several possible outcomes of infection. Seventy percent of patients have an asymptomatic, self-limiting course. Another 20% have a self-limiting course after either mild or severe symptoms of icterus, fatigue, anorexia, and nausea. One percent of patients have a fulminant course, with an 85% mortality rate. In addition to acute infection, a subpopulation of patients goes on to develop chronic infection;

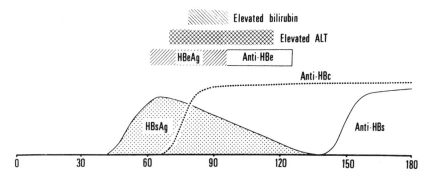

Fig. 23-10. Serologic and biochemical events in acute hepatitis B infection. Note that the patient may have a complete absence of both hepatitis B surface antigen *(HBsAg)* and antibody to hepatitis B surface antigen *(anti-HBs)* after approximately 135 days even though actively infected. The presence of antibody to hepatitis B core antigen *(anti-HBc)* confirms the diagnosis in this situation. *ALT,* Alanine aminotransferase; *Anti-HBe,* antibody to hepatitis B envelope antigen; *HBeAg,* hepatitis B envelope antigen. (From Dodd RY: Hepatitis. In Petz LD, Swisher SN, Kleinman S, et al, eds: *Clinical practice of transfusion medicine,* ed 3, New York, 1996, Churchill Livingstone.)

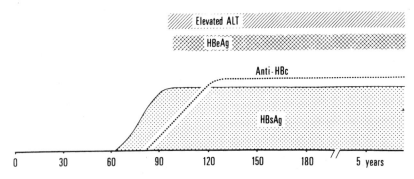

Fig. 23-11. Serologic and biochemical events in chronic hepatitis B infection/hepatitis B surface antigen *(HBsAg)* carrier state. *ALT,* Alanine aminotransferase; *Anti-HBc,* antibody to hepatitis B core antigen; *HBeAg,* hepatitis B envelope antigen. (From Dodd RY: Hepatitis. In Petz LD, Swisher SN, Kleinman S, et al, eds: *Clinical practice of transfusion medicine,* ed 3, New York, 1996, Churchill Livingstone.)

Table 23-9. Implementation of policies to reduce the risk of transfusion-transmitted infection

Intervention	Date
Testing for HBsAg	July 1972
Exclusive use of nonpaid donors	September 1975
Exclusion of individuals at high risk for AIDS	March 1983
Redefining high-risk behavior (includes homosexual men with >1 partner before 1979)	December 1984
Testing for antibody to HIV	Spring 1985
Redefining high-risk sexual behavior (includes homosexual men with >1 partner before 1977)	September 1985
Permit donors to confidentially exclude their donations from being transfused	October 1986
Testing for alanine aminotransferase	Late 1986
Testing for anti-HBc	Spring 1987
Testing for HTLV-I	November 1988
Testing for anti-HCV	Summer 1990
Second-generation tests for anti-HCV	March 1992
Testing for HIV-2	June 1992
Testing for HIV p24 antigen	March 1996

From Berry AJ, Whitsett CF: Infectious risks of transfusions. In Lake CL, Moore RA, eds: *Blood: hemostasis, transfusion, and alternatives in the perioperative period,* New York, 1995, Raven.
HBsAg, Hepatitis B virus surface antigen; *AIDS,* acquired immunodeficiency syndrome; *HIV,* human immunodeficiency virus; *anti-HBc,* antibody to hepatitis B virus core antigen; *HTLV-I,* human T-cell lymphotropic virus type I; *anti-HCV,* antibody to hepatitis C virus; *HIV-2,* human immunodeficiency virus type 2.

the likelihood of this course is greatest among neonates (75% to 90%) and children (25%).[148] Ten percent of adult patients go on to a chronic carrier state; about half of them have a chronic persistent hepatitis, which is a mostly asymptomatic, nonprogressive form. The other half develop chronic active hepatitis, which goes on to cirrhosis within 10 years. Patients who are of greatest risk to pass on hepatitis through transfusion are those who have not experienced symptoms of hepatitis and yet are still infectious. These patients include those with chronic persistent hepatitis and those who donate blood while in the window period, when they are infectious without manifesting any outward evidence of infection or serologic markers for infection. The window period for HBV detection is currently estimated to be 59 days,[150] although PCR-based testing (perhaps available within the next several years) may result in a reduction of the window period by up to 25 days (see Table 23-8).[1] Blood from blood donors who are within the window period

accounts for the majority of the cases of transfusion-associated HBV infection.

It is estimated that 300,000 new cases of HBV infection occur per year in the United States, with approximately 750,000 to 1 million infectious HBV carriers.[151] Approximately 1.4% of the new cases of HBV infection are associated with a recent blood transfusion, although only a fraction of these are thought to be causally related.[152] The overall incidence of HBV seropositivity in the United States is 5.7%, with the highest incidence being among patients undergoing hemodialysis, male prisoners, and clients in institutions for the developmentally disabled.[153]

The first line of defense against the risk of transfusion-transmitted HBV is an extensive blood donor selection protocol. The temporal sequence of implementation of screening criteria to reduce the risk of transfusion-transmitted HIV, HBV, and HCV is presented in Table 23-9. Donor screening selects for a population that is least likely to carry HBV, and considerably enhances the negative predictive value of serologic testing. The second line of defense against transfusion-transmitted HBV is the use of serologic testing. Currently, blood donated in the United States is tested for both HBsAg and anti-HBcAg. HBsAg is assessed by enzyme immunoassay (EIA), whereas antibody to core antigen is detected by the use of an inhibition assay based on a solid-phase antibody to HBcAg.[154] The detection of anti-HBcAg has been used as an adjunct to HBsAg testing because some donors may have been infected recently and may have a low concentration of HBsAg without having achieved a protective concentration of HBsAb (see Fig. 23-10). A small proportion of chronic carriers of HBV may also be infectious despite having an undetectably low titer of HBsAg. Anti-HBcAg has been found to be helpful in identifying these people.[155] With the use of both exclusion criteria and serologic testing, the risk of HBV infection is estimated to be approximately 1 in 63,000 per unit of blood transfused.[1] There is some speculation that the risk of transfusion-transmitted HBV infection has been eliminated in the United States, just as a recent report has noted no serologic evidence for transfusion-transmitted HBV in Canada.[145] The American Red Cross reports less than 100 cases of posttransfusion HBV infection per year. However, this incidence is consistent with the rate of HBV infection for the population at large, suggesting that the cases of transfusion-transmitted HBV infection may simply reflect the occurrence of infection in the population regardless of transfusion.[149]

HBsAb appears to confer protection from infection with HBV. Therefore prophylaxis has centered on the administration of HBsAb (passive immunization) or the stimulation of an immune response by the administration of a vaccine containing inactivated HBsAg (active immunization). Hepatitis B immune globulin (HBIG) has been recommended for the prevention of HBV infection after high-risk exposures (e.g., after a needle-stick injury to health care personnel and for infants of HBsAg-positive mothers). A recombinant form of the HBV vaccine has been shown to be efficacious in many patient populations, particularly in the newborn infants of HBsAg-positive mothers. By the administration of HBV vaccine to all newborns as part of a routine vaccination program, vertical transmission of HBV is expected to be limited significantly.

(2) HEPATITIS A VIRUS. Hepatitis A virus (HAV) is an RNA picornavirus that is responsible for approximately 50% of the hepatitis that occurs in the United States each year. The clinical course is acute and self-limited, with no chronic carrier state and a mortality of 0.2%.[156] The disease is characterized by four phases: the incubation phase of 25 days, the prodromal phase of 2 to 10 days, the hepatitis phase of 4 to 6 weeks, and the convalescent phase. A brief viremia may develop during the end of the asymptomatic phase and the beginning of the prodromal phase, and this is the period during which an asymptomatic donor may transmit the disease by blood transfusion. There are several case reports of the transmission of HAV in this fashion.[157,158] Hepatic inflammation does

not occur until after symptoms begin in the prodromal phase, so that surrogate testing for infection using alanine aminotransferase is not helpful in detecting infectious donors. After a prodromal phase characterized by fever, chills, malaise, and arthralgias, the true symptomatic phase may set in, with anorexia, nausea, vomiting, abdominal tenderness, and jaundice. The laboratory diagnosis of HAV infection is based on an enzyme immunoassay for anti-HAV IgM. IgG anti-HAV antibodies subsequently develop.[154]

The prevalence of HAV in the population despite the absence of obvious hepatic symptoms demonstrates the often asymptomatic nature of HAV infection. Approximately 20% of U.S. residents have antibodies to HAV by age 20, and 50% by age 50.[159] Seroprevalence of HAV varies considerably by location in the United States, although the overall rate of seropositivity in the donor population is 20%. Given the lack of a carrier state and the brief window period between the onset of infectivity and the onset of symptoms in donors, it is not surprising that the risk of HAV transmission by blood transfusion is less than 1 in 1 million (see Table 23-6).[160] Despite a low apparent risk of HAV transmission, surveillance continues because the rate of seroprevalence among intravenous drug users in the United States is increasing, perhaps signaling an increase in the seroprevalence of HAV in the United States.[161] HAV vaccines are becoming available and may be used in the near future for populations at risk.[162]

(3) HEPATITIS C VIRUS. Following the characterization of HBsAg and implementation of testing for HAV and HBV in the late 1970s, it was recognized that up to 95% of all transfusion-related hepatic infections were not secondary to either HAV or HBV. It was not until 1989 that the etiologic agent for 85% of all non-A, non-B hepatitis (NANBH) was identified as HCV. HCV is an RNA virus that is similar to previously described flaviviruses, although it is considered to be in a class of its own.[149] Infection with HCV is characterized in only 25% of infections by a mild degree of hepatic inflammation with a mean incubation period of 15 weeks. The delay until the development of measurable anti-HCV is estimated at 82 days (see Table 23-8). The majority of HCV morbidity is the result of chronic hepatic inflammation. Seventy percent of those infected develop chronic liver dysfunction, and 60% develop histologic evidence of cirrhosis.[163] Up to 20% of patients with NANBH studied over 20 years developed hepatic failure, many of whom were infected with HCV.[164] The recent characterization of this illness and lack of longitudinal data make long-term prognosis uncertain. Some studies suggest that like HBV infection, HCV infection may result in hepatocellular carcinoma.[165,166]

The diagnosis of HCV infection is based on a change in the EIA for antibodies to HCV (anti-HCV) from negative to positive in the setting of hepatitis. A confirmatory, possibly more accurate test for detecting HCV infection is the recombinant immunoblot assay (RIBA).[167] Efforts are under way to develop a quantitative EIA, additional non-EIA confirmatory tests, and a EIA that is specific for anti-HCV IgM. At this time it is impossible to distinguish clearly a chronic HCV carrier state from more recent infection.[154]

Because the majority of the cases of NANBH before 1994 were actually HCV infections, researchers have been able to make some inferences about the causes of HCV. In 1992 there were 6010 cases of NANBH, for an incidence of 3.36 per 100,000, of which probably 85% were caused by HCV.[168] Because of underreporting and asymptomatic infection, the actual rate of HCV may be up to 10 per 100,000. The major risk factor for NANBH was the use of injection drugs with shared needles. Only 4.3% of cases of NANBH were associated with transfusion.[169] Subsequent studies suggest a seroprevalence of anti-HCV of approximately 1% in the U.S. blood donor population. Principal transmission is via the parenteral route, with sexual transmission being a rare and inefficient mode of transmission.[170] The infectivity of HCV is less than that of HBV, with only 3% of health care workers contracting the disease after needlestick exposures, as opposed to a 30% rate for a similar exposure to HBV.[171] Patients who are positive for anti-HCV are assumed to be infectious because the majority of HCV infections are chronic. These patients are advised to refrain from donating blood, but changes in their sexual practices probably are not necessary.[151]

The risk of HCV transmission by transfusion has declined steadily as more accurate assays for HCV have become available. Before 1986, the risk of HCV infection per unit was 0.45%. Surrogate testing for NANBH by alanine aminotransferase and anti-HBcAg concentrations resulted in a decline to 0.19%, and the introduction of anti-HCV testing further diminished the risk to 0.06% per unit.[170,172] Subsequent improved testing has resulted in a lower estimated risk of 1 in 103,000 per unit of blood transfused as of 1996.[1] Patients who are infectious for HCV without testing positive by second-generation EIA may be chronic carriers who lack the HCV antibody or may be donating blood in the window period, when the patients are infectious but have not yet developed an antibody to HCV. The window period for the detection of HCV with currently available tests is 82 days[173-175] (see Table 23-8). New testing modalities based on PCR technology may further decrease the window period by as many as 59 days, potentially reducing the risk of infection by 72%.[1]

The continued practice of surrogate testing for HCV via the use of alanine aminotransferase (ALT) and anti-HBcAg is currently under debate.[173] The AABB no longer requires the use of an ALT concentration, but it is still required in Europe. Proponents argue that an elevated ALT may be the only sign of infection with HCV or another non-A, non-B, non-C hepatitis. Pending improved testing for HCV and the characterization of other sources of hepatitis, surrogate testing will probably continue, even if not required by the AABB.

The development of a vaccine against HCV has been unsuccessful because the virus appears to exhibit shifting antigenic presentation. The apparent lack of fully protective antibodies may explain both the common chronicity of HCV infection and difficulties in developing a vaccine.

(4) NON-A, NON-B, NON-C HEPATITIS. With the realization in 1990 that up to 10% of what had previously been known as NANBH was not caused by HCV, the unwieldy term *non-A, non-B, non-C hepatitis* (NANBNCH) was coined. There appear to be two different types of NANBNCH: an enterically transmitted hepatitis E virus (HEV), epidemiologically similar to HAV, and a parenterally transmitted form. HEV is found primarily in countries with poor sanitation and is transmitted as a waterborne pathogen. The mortality rate of HEV is approximately 0.2% to 1%, except among pregnant women, in whom the mortality approaches 20% in the third trimester.[154] HEV is not parenterally transmitted, and therefore not a significant cause of posttransfusion hepatitis.

There is currently significant debate over the existence of a parenterally transmitted NANBNCH in the United States. Various causes have been examined. One possible etiologic agent is the hepatitis G virus (HGV) or its variant, GB virus C (GBV-C), both of which are RNA flaviviruses. Recent data suggest that these agents are found in 1.7% of volunteer blood donors in the United States, and that less than 50% of patients administered infectious blood subsequently test positive for this agent. Most patients infected with these agents do not develop chronic hepatitis, and the significance of infection is currently debated.[176,177] Aside from HGV, some hepatologists have suggested that CMV may be partially responsible for posttransfusion hepatic inflammation.[178] It is also possible that NANBNCH is not caused by an infectious agent at all. A study from Canada noted that the incidence of NANBNCH was the same in patients transfused with allogeneic and autologous blood.[179] NANBNCH may simply represent a nonspecific hepatic inflammation occurring in the postoperative period. Clinical data suggest that the episodes of NANBNCH are mild and self-limited. As other potential causes are evaluated or ruled out over the next several years, the nature of NANBNCH may become clearer.

(5) HEPATITIS D VIRUS. Hepatitis D virus (HDV), or delta particle, is another source of hepatic inflammation. HDV is a defective RNA virus that requires the presence of HBV in order to replicate. HDV may be transmitted with HBV as a coinfection, or it may be subsequently transmitted to a patient chronically infected with HBV as a superinfection. Evidence of HDV infection is via detection of the antibody to HDV. HDV infection is often associated with fulminant hepatitis when contracted as a coinfection, but when contracted as a superinfection it often presents with rapidly progressive chronic disease.[180] The epidemiology of HDV is similar to that for HBV, with 5% of HBV carriers worldwide also being infected with HDV.[154]

The risk of transfusion-transmitted HDV infection is limited by excluding blood that is infectious for HBV.

(6) HUMAN IMMUNODEFICIENCY VIRUS. AIDS was first characterized in 1981 after a cluster of homosexual men and injection drug abusers became afflicted with *Pneumocystis carinii* infections and unusually invasive Kaposi's sarcoma. HIV, of which there are two major

recognized strains, has been implicated as the cause of AIDS. HIV, a lentivirus from the retrovirus family, replicates by transcribing genetic information from its RNA genome into the host DNA genome via the enzyme reverse transcriptase, using cellular machinery to produce proteins necessary for viral replication.[181]

The clinical course of AIDS is one of progressive immunodeficiency as a result of depletion primarily of helper T lymphocytes, ultimately resulting in death secondary to immunocompromise with overwhelming opportunistic infection. Of the 230,179 patients with AIDS reported to the Centers for Disease Control (CDC) as of June 1992, more than 66% have died.[182] The diagnosis of HIV infection is now based on screening by recombinant DNA and peptide antigen-based enzyme immunoassays that are sensitive for both HIV-1 and HIV-2. These assays have a specificity greater than 99.5%.[183] Confirmation of infection is via Western blot, which is based on HIV-1 viral lysate. A Western blot for HIV-2 is expected to be licensed shortly.[181] Other assays involving PCR technology and highly specific HIV-associated antigens are also being developed.

The epidemiology of HIV is typical of an infectious disease with a prolonged clinical incubation period (estimated to be approximately 8 years for HIV).[184] The first infected patients to be identified were homosexual and bisexual men who were infected in the 1970s but who did not show evidence of infection until 1981. AIDS was first described among recipients of blood and blood components in 1982, although retrospective analysis demonstrates that there was a significant risk of transfusion-associated (TA) HIV-1 infection in San Francisco as early as 1978.[185] The risk of TA HIV-1 infection rose in San Francisco until 1982, peaking at 1.1% per unit transfused (Fig. 23-12). The decline in the risk of TA HIV-1 infection beginning in 1983 reflected in large part the self-deferral of approximately 90% of infected people from the donation of blood during that time. The subsequent development of tests to detect HIV-1 decreased the risk substantially further. The pattern of disease transmission among hemophiliacs followed a similar pattern of infection, with peak risk of infection occurring by October 1982.[186]

The CDC evaluated the temporal risk of HIV-1 infection from transfusion during the period from 1982 to 1991. They noted 4619 cases of TA HIV infection, or 2% of the 222,418 cases of AIDS in the United States.[187] The rate of diagnosis of AIDS peaked in 1987 and remained stable, whereas the rate of HIV infection peaked earlier, in 1984, at 714 cases per year (Fig. 23-13). Since that time, the rate of infection has fallen off considerably, to approximately 43 patients per year.

The decrease in TA HIV infection after 1984 reflects the use of multiple measures of protection to limit the spread of HIV in the U.S. population. These measures include self-deferral by people at risk for exposure to

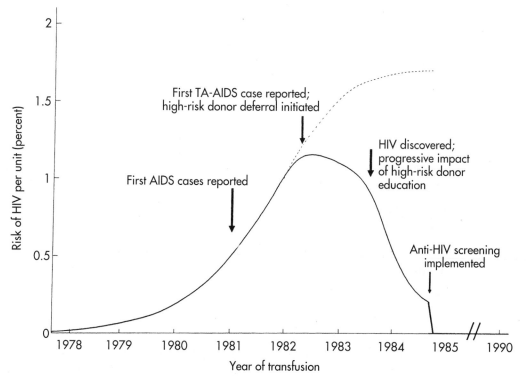

Fig. 23-12. Risk of human immunodeficiency virus *(HIV)* infection from transfusion in San Francisco before anti-HIV screening. *TA-AIDS,* Transfusion-acquired acquired immunodeficiency syndrome. (From Busch MP: Retroviral infections. In Petz LD, Swisher SN, Kleinman S, et al, eds: *Clinical practice of transfusion medicine,* ed 3, New York, 1996, Churchill Livingstone.)

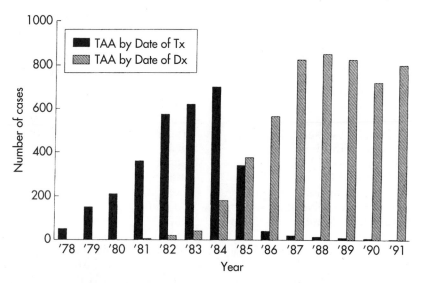

Fig. 23-13. Distribution of 5038 transfusion-associated cases of acquired immunodeficiency syndrome (AIDS) as of June 1992. *Dx,* Diagnosis; *TAA,* transfusion-acquired AIDS; *Tx,* transfusion. (From Busch MP: Retroviral infections. In Petz LD, Swisher SN, Kleinman S, et al, eds: *Clinical practice of transfusion medicine,* ed 3, New York, 1996, Churchill Livingstone.)

HIV, and serologic testing for HIV (see Fig. 23-12). Also, in the event of a possible TA HIV infection, the donor of the implicated unit of blood is tested for possible asymptomatic infection. With the continued spread of HIV among the heterosexual populace, the utility of exclusion of donors based on sexual practices may diminish.[183] The proportion of AIDS cases attributed to heterosexual transmission has increased from a cumulative rate of 4% in 1988 to 7% in 1994.[188]

Among those transfused with a unit of HIV-positive blood, the rate of infection is 89.5%.[189] Units of RBCs older than 26 days and those that had been washed before administration had a lower risk of infectivity.[190] Reducing the risk of HIV infection by reducing the number of leukocytes in transfused units has been evaluated but is not fully effective. Further studies have demonstrated that no population of blood recipients is immune from HIV infection if given a large enough inoculum over successive occasions.

The most recent estimation of risk of TA HIV infection is approximately 1 in every 493,000 units transfused (see Table 23-6).[1] This risk was estimated in 1992 to result in approximately 18 to 27 infected donations in the United States each year, and the institution of p24 antigen testing in 1996 was expected to decrease this exposure by 25%.[1,2] The rate of HIV-2 infection in the United States is estimated to be less than 1 in 10 million because HIV-2 is prominent only in portions of Africa. The continued transmission of HIV despite serologic testing probably results from the donation of blood during the window period, when donors are infected with HIV but have a negative HIV screening test. The window period of HIV infection with currently available testing is estimated to be 22 days (see Table 23-8 and Fig. 23-14). The development of an assay capable of detecting HIV infection earlier while preserving the current very high

rate of specificity is ongoing. The use of p24 antigen testing (started in March 1996) and both DNA and RNA PCR testing may further decrease the window period for detection by 6 to 11 days.[1] Despite increasingly sensitive detection techniques, it is unlikely that the U.S. blood supply will ever be completely free of HIV.

(7) HUMAN T-CELL LYMPHOTROPIC VIRUS TYPE I AND II. HTLV-I and HTLV-II are classified as type C oncornaviruses of the retrovirus family. Oncornaviruses are typically lymphoproliferative and are capable of producing cellular transformation and malignancy. Two diseases have been associated with HTLV-I: adult T-cell leukemia/lymphoma (ATL/L) and HTLV-I–associated myelopathy/tropical spastic paraparesis (HAM/TSP).[183] The link between ATL/L and HTLV-I was made in Japan in 1984.[191] ATL/L is characterized by abnormal lymphocytes, generalized lymphadenopathy, hepatomegaly, hepatic dysfunction, splenomegaly, bone lesions, and hypercalcemia.[192] Most patients are 40 to 60 years old and reside in a specific region in Japan where HTLV-I is endemic, suggesting a prolonged latency period of ATL/L after infection at birth. The incidence of ATL/L among those infected with HTLV-I is estimated to be 2% to 4%. The median survival after diagnosis with ATL/L is poor, averaging only 11 months.

The link between HTLV-I and tropical spastic paraparesis was made in 1985 among a population in the Caribbean where HTLV-I is endemic.[193] HAM/TSP is characterized by progressive chronic spastic paraparesis, lower limb weakness, urinary incontinence, impotence, sensory disturbance, low back pain, lower extremity hyperreflexia, and impaired vibration sense. It is considered to be an immune-mediated disease with a latency period of 3 years after transfusion and an incidence of 1% among those infected with HTLV-I. Corticosteroids and danazol are often effective in improving symptoms.

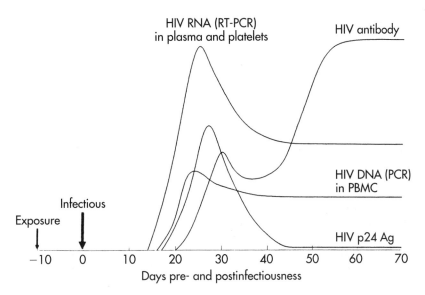

Fig. 23-14. Sequence of virologic events during primary human immunodeficiency virus *(HIV)* infection. Hematologic dissemination consistent with an infectious blood donation (defined as day 0) occurs 1 to 2 weeks after HIV exposure. Viremia is first detectable by polymerase chain reaction *(PCR)* for HIV RNA in platelets or plasma on days 14 to 16, with viral RNA and p24 antigen concentrations peaking between days 20 and 30. Infected peripheral blood mononuclear cells *(PBMC)* with detectable HIV DNA are detected after free virus at stable low concentrations at days 17 to 20. Earliest detectable antibody to HIV appears between days 20 and 25, with an early IgM spike followed by high titer IgG. Seroconversion induces the clearance of viremia to set points that correlate with the long-term outcome of disease and with a high probability of secondary transmission of the virus. (From Busch MP: *Vox Sang* 67[suppl 1]:S13, 1994.)

HTLV-II has not been linked definitively with a disease process, although there are several reports of a myelopathy similar to HAM/TSP occurring in HTLV-II–infected patients.[194] Although HTLV-II probably carries a lower risk of subsequent illness than HTLV-I, the former is endemic to Native American populations of the southwestern United States, Mexico, and Central America, and also among intravenous drug abusers in the United States, and so may have greater implications for physicians in the United States.

The decision to screen for HTLV-I and HTLV-II in the U.S. blood supply was made after a study in 1986 determined that the incidence of HTLV-I seropositivity among blood donors in the United States was 0.025%, suggesting that approximately 2800 new infections were occurring as the result of blood transfusion in the United States annually.[195] In 1988 the FDA recommended that all blood donations be screened for antibodies to HTLV-I by EIAs. The HTLV-I EIA is based on HTLV-I lysates that, though sensitive, have a poor positive predictive value when used to screen a population with a low incidence of disease. The HTLV-I EIA is often successful at detecting HTLV-II activity as well, although a more sensitive and specific assay is being sought. Recent data suggest that up to 22% of patients infected with HTLV-II are missed by the current HTLV-I EIA.[196] A Western blot is available to confirm the presence of HTLV-I or HTLV-II.[183]

The efficiency of transmission of infection via blood transfusion is less for HTLV-I and HTLV-II than for HIV, probably because HTLV is transmitted only by cellular components of blood. Furthermore, units of blood over the age of 14 days have limited infectivity.[183] The overall transmission of HTLV-I by cellular blood components is 45% to 63%.[197] The incidence of HTLV-II transmission by blood transfusion is probably similar to that for HTLV-I.[198] Retrospective analysis of HTLV infectivity suggested a risk of HTLV-I and HTLV-II transmission by blood transfusion before EIA testing of 1 in 5,000 per unit.[199] Subsequent testing of blood donors revealed that the risk of infection is decreased by an order of magnitude with the use of EIA testing, resulting in an overall risk of HTLV-I and HTLV-II infection from a blood transfusion of approximately 1 in 50,000 in the United States.[145] Other observers have combined more recent data to estimate the risk of HTLV-I or HTLV-II infection from the transfusion of blood at approximately 1 in 641,000 units transfused.[1] There are no apparent attempts to develop a vaccine for HTLV at this time.

(8) EPSTEIN-BARR VIRUS. Epstein-Barr virus (EBV) is a DNA virus classified as a herpesvirus. The majority of EBV infections occur asymptomatically in school-age children, transmitted by oropharyngeal secretions. When infection occurs in adulthood as mononucleosis it may be characterized by fever, pharyngitis, tonsillitis, lym-

phadenopathy, and lymphocytosis. Rare hepatomegaly and splenomegaly may occur.[200] EBV has also been suggested as the etiologic agent of chronic fatigue syndrome, which is characterized by repeated bouts of pharyngitis, weakness, fatigue, myalgias, and lymphadenopathy.[201] EBV has also been implicated in Burkitt's lymphoma, nasopharyngeal carcinoma, lymphoma in transplant recipients, and a pneumonitis in patients with AIDS. Patients at greatest risk for symptomatic infection with EBV are severely immunosuppressed BMT recipients, and even in this population the course of disease is mild. Most BMT recipients develop symptoms as the result of reactivation of latent virus, although approximately 10% of BMT recipients are seronegative and are thus at risk for primary EBV infection from transfusion. The mildness of disease in this population suggests that the passive transmission of anti-EBV antibodies with their infected transfusion may be somewhat protective.

EBV is ubiquitous in the U.S. population, with over 90% of blood donors testing positive for antibodies to EBV. The transmission of EBV by blood transfusion was first documented in 1969, resulting in a mononucleosis-like syndrome several weeks after transfusion.[202] Subsequent investigators have suggested that the infections might have been caused by CMV transmission. Given the mild course of EBV illness even among the severely immunocompromised, there is currently no recommendation to avoid EBV-positive blood for EBV-negative recipients.[200]

(9) CYTOMEGALOVIRUS. Cytomegalovirus (CMV) is a DNA herpesvirus that, like other herpesviruses, may cause symptoms following primary infection, following reactivation after a prolonged latent phase, or with reinfection with a second strain of the virus.[200] CMV exposure is common, with 30% to 100% of adults being seropositive. The primary infection of CMV in an immunocompetent adult infrequently results in a mild mononucleosis-type syndrome. The transmission of CMV via blood transfusion was first studied in the 1960s, although studies concluded that the risk of transmission of this agent through blood transfusion to a seronegative adult was only 19%. Of these patients, only 1.6% developed clinically apparent infections.[203] Because most of the population is already seropositive for CMV, the transmission of CMV does not appear to be a significant health risk to immunocompetent adults.

The majority of concern over CMV transmission has subsequently focused on various immunocompromised recipient populations: BMT recipients, solid organ transplant recipients, patients infected with HIV, intrauterine fetuses of seronegative mothers, and low-birthweight neonates born to seronegative mothers. In these immunocompromised patient groups, infection may lead to serious consequences, including pneumonitis, hepatitis, gastroenteritis, retinitis, and disseminated disease. Not all immunocompromised patients carry the same risk of infection, and measures to avoid CMV infectious blood products should be altered accordingly (Box 23-7). The risk of mortality from CMV varies by patient population, with the greatest risk being to BMT recipients contract-

ing CMV pneumonitis, in whom the fatality rate is 50%. Other patient populations have a much lower risk of mortality, usually in the 2% to 5% range.[204]

There are two laboratory tests for CMV. The most commonly used is the enzyme-linked immunosorbent assay (ELISA), which is used for the screening of blood and for the assessment of recipients. The ELISA identifies antibodies against CMV antigens. The ELISA is poorly predictive for infectivity: Only 19% of CMV positive patients are infectious. A negative ELISA does not preclude infectivity, as 1% to 3.5% of CMV-negative patients are infectious.[205] Finally, a positive ELISA is not predictive for recent infection in a patient who has viral symptoms, although a recent rise in the CMV titer may suggest infection with a new strain of CMV or reactivation of virus. For the purpose of diagnosing recent infection, CMV viral culture is used. Limitations of this technique have included a growth period of up to 6 weeks. Newer techniques that augment tissue culture infection may return results over as little as 72 hours. Despite its limitations, ELISA is a faster test and is most commonly used for screening blood before it is administered to patients at risk for significant infection and for

---

Box 23-7 Patients at risk for transfusion-transmitted cytomegalovirus (CMV) infection

Patients for whom the risk is well established
CMV-seronegative pregnant women
Premature infants (<1200 g) born to CMV-seronegative mothers
CMV-seronegative recipients of allogeneic bone marrow transplants from CMV-seronegative donors
CMV-seronegative patients with evidence of infection with HIV-1
Intrauterine transfusions

Patients for whom the risk is less well established but sufficient to merit consideration
CMV-seronegative patients receiving tissue transplants (renal, heart, liver, lung) from CMV-seronegative donors
CMV-seronegative patients who are potential candiates for bone marrow transplantation (allogeneic or autologous)
CMV-seronegative autologous bone marrow transplant recipients
CMV-seronegative patients undergoing splenectomy
CMV-seronegative recipients of bone marrow from CMV-seropositive donors

Patients for whom the risk is not established
CMV-seropositive recipients of bone marrow transplants
Full-term neonates
CMV-seropositive recipients of solid organ allografts (e.g., heart, kidney)

From Sayers MH: Cytomegalovirus and other herpesviruses. In Petz LD, Swisher SN, Kleinman S, et al, eds: *Clinical practice of transfusion medicine*, ed 3, New York, 1996, Churchill Livingstone.
CMV, Cytomegalovirus; *HIV*, human immunodeficiency virus.

determining CMV serologic status in pregnant patients, neonates, and transplant candidates.

Given the risk of transmitting CMV infection from even CMV-seronegative donors and the high prevalence of CMV in the blood pool, alternatives to the administration of CMV-negative blood have been sought to limit the risk of infection from blood transfusion. Because transfusion-associated (TA) CMV infection is restricted to cellular blood components containing leukocytes,[206] leukoreduction, by means of selective filtration of leukocytes, has been recently advocated as a means of limiting infectious risk.[207] This method cannot remove all infectious leukocytes from a donor unit of blood. However, because the risk of infection is related to both the amount of infectious inoculum and the degree of immunocompromise in the recipient, leukoreduction is often effective for limiting risk. The AABB has recently embraced this technology, although some institutions that use leukoreduction continue to avoid the administration of CMV-seropositive blood in the highest-risk recipients.[208,209]

(10) OTHER VIRUSES

(A) PARVOVIRUS B19. Parvovirus B19 is the etiologic agent for fifth disease (erythema infectiosum), transient aplastic crisis and severe anemia in patients with preexisting chronic hemolytic anemia, and intrauterine infection with fetal death.[210-212] Parvovirus B19 is transmitted via respiratory secretions and also parenterally via blood products. Between 30% and 60% of adults are seropositive for antibody to parvovirus B19.[213] Transmission is most common with pooled products such as clotting factor concentrates because the virus is not easily inactivated by the usual heat and detergent methods of viral inactivation.[214]

(B) HUMAN HERPESVIRUS 6. Human herpesvirus 6 (HHV6) was formerly known as human B lymphotropic virus (HBLV) until it became apparent that HHV6 has tropism for T lymphocytes and other blood cells. Primary HHV6 infection commonly occurs in childhood as roseola (exanthem subitum), resulting in a fever and maculopapular rash. Rarely, hepatic inflammation may also occur.[215] A majority of children have been infected with HHV6 by 3 years of age.[200]

Patients at greatest risk for infection or reactivation of virus are BMT recipients.[216] In this group, HHV6 infection has been associated with a pneumonitis and poor graft function.[217,218] Reactivation of previous infection is considered to be the principal source of infection in these patients. There is no clear consensus at this time whether the HHV6-seronegative patients should receive only HHV6-seronegative blood products. This may be difficult to implement because 80% to 88% of blood donors are HHV6 seropositive.[219] Larger studies to delineate the significance of HHV6 infection are under way.

b. Transfusion-associated sepsis. Transfusion-associated sepsis (TAS) occurs very rarely, although with a high mortality rate. The precise number of TAS cases is not known, but in 1991, 6 of 46 transfusion-associated deaths, or 7.3%, were caused by TAS.[220] The overall rate of TAS appears to be increasing. The etiologic agent involved varies by blood product. The most common organisms contaminating RBCs are *Yersinia enterocolitica* and various *Pseudomonas* species. *Y. enterocolitica* is the most pathogenic, with seven out of the eight fatalities in the United States from bacterial contamination from 1986 to 1991 being caused by *Y. enterocolitica.*[221] Platelet products are most commonly contaminated with *Staphylococcus aureus, Staphylococcus epidermidis,* or diphtheroids.[211] The most common symptoms associated with TAS are fever, chills, hypotension, nausea, headache, and dyspnea.[222] In severe cases, congestive heart failure, DIC, renal failure, and death may occur.[221] Symptoms after the administration of contaminated platelets typically develop within an hour; symptoms may not develop until hours or days following transfusion with contaminated RBC units. Despite therapy with multiple antibiotics, the mortality is high.[223] The factors affecting patient outcome with TAS are noted in Box 23-8.

Contamination of RBC units may occur by the donation of blood from a bacteremic donor or during the subsequent processing of blood. The growth of most bacteria is inhibited by cold storage temperatures, although several, such as *Y. enterocolitica,* thrive even at low temperatures. Unlike for many viruses, there is no feasible laboratory screening test for bacterial contamination. Interview screening is also not useful. Although 50% of *Y. enterocolitica* bacteremic donors have a recent history of gastrointestinal distress, so do 13% of the remaining donors.[224] Although *Y. enterocolitica* is the organism most often implicated with TAS, contamination on a per unit basis is rare. In one study, over 100,000 units of RBCs were cultured without finding a single incident of *Yersinia* contamination. Bacterial contamination of RBC units may also occur during venipuncture or subsequent processing of blood. Most organisms encountered will not survive cold storage, although during postcold processing (e.g., RBC deglycerolization of frozen RBCs) or the washing of cells, bacteria may be introduced.[211]

Although the outcome of TAS is often fatal, the overall risk of death from TAS is very low, approximately 1 in 9 million units of RBCs.[225]

Box 23-8   Factors affecting patient outcome with transfusion of bacterially contaminated blood products

V   Virulence of the organism

I   Immune status and general condition of the recipient

C   Concentration and bolus dosage of bacteria transfused

T   Timely recognition and therapeutic intervention

I   Intensity of patient monitoring, inpatient versus outpatient

M   Medicines the patient is receiving (i.e., antibiotics)

From Krishnan LA, Brecher ME: *Hematol Oncol Clin North Am* 9:167, 1995.

Contamination of platelet units is more likely than contamination of RBCs overall, and also more likely to result in death. Twenty-one of the 29 fatalities from TAS from 1986 to 1991 were caused by platelet transfusion (see Table 23-2).[3] The incidence of contamination of platelets probably is as great as 1 in 1000.[226] The incidence of platelet contamination may be much greater than for RBC units because platelets are stored at 22° C, whereas RBCs are stored at 4° C. Most of the organisms cultured are typical skin flora, including *Staphylococcus epidermidis* and *Bacillus cereus*. Organisms implicated in mortality are usually split between gram-positive and gram-negative organisms, including *Staphylococcus, Klebsiella, Serratia,* and *Streptococcus*. The source of contamination is thought to be inadequate sterilization of skin before venipuncture during donation, or possibly the passage of a skin plug from needle puncture into the platelet unit. The rate of TAS from platelet units is increasing, perhaps because of the increased use of platelets and longer storage times. Despite these factors, the risk of death following a platelet transfusion is still extremely low, approximately 1 in 1 million.[225]

Several strategies have been suggested to decrease the risk of TAS. These include increased donor screening, a reduction in blood storage times, bacteriologic screening of blood products, and processing of blood to remove bacteria. The storage time for platelets has already been decreased from 7 to 5 days, largely because of concerns over the risk of bacterial contamination. Evaluation of a practical means of performing rapid bacteriologic screening of blood products before administration is under development. As a practical matter, each unit of blood should be inspected for evidence of contamination, which may include a purple or black discoloration and the presence of gas or clots. In addition, blood should be transported promptly and used immediately after it leaves refrigeration. Methods of blood warming should be in-line and should immediately precede blood administration. Any patient manifesting signs of sepsis after a blood transfusion should be treated with broad-spectrum antibiotics, and the possibility of TAS should be investigated. Any case of suspected sepsis should be reported to the blood bank immediately so that they may remove other contaminated components from the same donor.

c. Other bacterial and protozoal infections. Although a large number of organisms other than those discussed earlier may be transmitted by the transfusion of blood, this rarely occurs in the United States. Because of the low incidence of these infections, this section is treated with a cursory overview, with appropriate references noted for further review.

(1) SYPHILIS. Syphilis is transmitted by *Treponema pallidum,* a spirochete with fastidious growing conditions.[211] Because *T. pallidum* does not survive beyond 120 hours at 4° C, this organism is passed on only via platelets and fresh blood products.[227] Blood donations are currently screened for syphilis with a rapid phase reactant (RPR) or a hemagglutinin assay. These tests are less than ideal because they either lack sensitivity and specificity or diagnose donors in whom the disease has already been treated. The frequency of positive tests is approximately 1 in 1000 to 2000.[228] The FDA is considering halting routine testing for syphilis, although some have advocated its continued use as a surrogate test for HIV infection. Transfusion-related syphilis is a more significant problem in developing countries, where refrigeration may be absent and fresh blood is often used.[229]

(2) MALARIA. Malaria is caused by various species of the genus *Plasmodium* and usually presents between 1 week to 1 month after transfusion with RBCs, with fever and hemolysis. The rate of transfusion-transmitted malaria in the United States is approximately 0.25 cases per million units of blood. The rate in developing countries where malaria is endemic is probably far greater. The principal weapon for limited transfusion-associated malaria infection is donor screening. Currently the AABB recommends permanently excluding any donor with a history of clinically apparent malaria, any immigrant from endemic areas for a period of 3 years, and any person traveling from the United States who has traveled to an endemic area for a period of 1 year.[211] Studies have demonstrated that the transmission of malaria would be eliminated in 80% of cases of documented transmission in the United States if the appropriate donor screening had been applied and the donors had answered screening questions accurately.[3,230] Although systematic testing of blood for a *Plasmodium* antigen has been adopted in Europe and India, there is no role for this practice in the United States at this time because the low rate of disease in the United States substantially reduces the predictive value of antigen testing.

(3) BABESIOSIS. Babesiosis is caused by the organism *Babesia microti,* a protozoan carried by the tick *Ixodes dammini*. Endemic areas of the United States include Minnesota, Wisconsin, Connecticut, and the islands off of the coast of the northeastern United States. The illness incubates from 2 to 8 weeks after the infecting bite and most often results in asymptomatic illness. Symptoms may include fever, headaches, shaking chills, thrombocytopenia, and hemolytic anemia. An increasing titer of anti-Babesia IgG or visualization of the parasite on a blood smear confirms the diagnosis. The overall rate of death is low, except among splenectomized or immunocompromised patients.[231] Infection is transmitted only by RBC-containing units, including RBCs, deglycerolized frozen RBCs, and platelets. Because *B. microti* is a hardy organism, infection may be transmitted by blood units as old as 35 days. Current methods of screening will exclude donors who are anemic or febrile. Patients who have been formally diagnosed with babesiosis are permanently deferred from blood donation. No other screening questions or laboratory tests have proven useful.[232] The rate of transfusion-transmitted babesiosis is rare, with only 10 reported cases in the last 15 years.

(4) CHAGAS'S DISEASE. Chagas's disease is caused by *Trypanosoma cruzi,* which is transmitted by the reduviid bug and is endemic to Latin America. In Brazil, for example, up to 20,000 cases of transfusion-transmitted

Chagas's disease occur per year.[233] Previously not considered to be a threat to the U.S. blood supply, the continued migration of infected people from endemic areas makes Chagas's disease of some concern. Chagas's disease is transmitted in RBCs, platelets, WBCs, FFP, and cryoprecipitate. Chagas's disease classically presents 3 to 6 weeks after initial contact, with an antibiotic-resistant fever, hepatomegaly and splenomegaly, pericardial effusion, and myocarditis. Diagnosis is via identification of the organism in a buffy-coat smear. Many infected people may remain asymptomatic for months or years, and it is estimated that up to 100,000 such people are in the United States at this time.[234] A high prevalence of infected donors in Washington, D.C., led to testing of donors for *T. cruzi* using an unlicensed immunofluorescence technique that found that 5% of immigrants from endemic areas were seropositive for *T. cruzi*.[235] Currently, no effective laboratory screening test is available, although one is under development. Current recommendations are to defer prospective donors from endemic areas until an effective test is available. Three cases of transfusion-transmitted Chagas's disease have been documented, although it is likely that many more have occurred.[233] The current AABB standard is to permanently defer people with a history of Chagas's disease. Serologic testing is available but is notoriously nonpredictive in populations where the disease rate is low.[231]

(5) LYME DISEASE. Lyme disease is caused by *Borrelia burgdorferi*, a spirochete that, like *B. microti*, is carried by the tick *Ixodes dammini*. This illness is endemic to the upper Midwest, including Wisconsin, Minnesota, Michigan, and Illinois, in California, and in the northeast.[231] Diagnosis is based on a characteristic constellation of symptoms including arthralgias and fever following a tick bite, which is often accompanied by a characteristic rash that spreads outward from the bite site. In the absence of the appropriate history and rash, the disease is notoriously difficult to diagnose, and no screening laboratory test is available. Fortunately, most prospective blood donors with active spirochetemia are symptomatic and would be deferred from donation on the basis of their symptoms. The organism is hardy, and live organisms have been found in 6-week-old RBCs, 6-day-old platelets, and 45-day-old FFP. There has never been a documented case of *Borrelia* transmitted by transfusion. There are two cases in which blood donated by asymptomatic donors was transfused to patients with no apparent subsequent infection.[236] The AABB has recommended accepting blood from asymptomatic donors with a history of infection if they have received antibiotic therapy. No other screening is considered necessary.[232]

(6) OTHER PATHOGENS. Many other organisms may be transmitted by blood transfusion, although the rate of infection is generally so low that they are not considered significant health risks to the U.S. population. Diseases transmitted include African trypanosomiasis, filariasis, leishmaniasis, toxoplasmosis, brucellosis, and rickettsial infection. Of these, *Leishmania tropica* recently received attention since the development of visceral leishmaniasis in seven members of the military in the Persian Gulf during the Gulf War.[237] Blood donations were deferred from people traveling to this area from August 1990 until the ban was lifted in December 1993. None of the potentially infectious donors were subsequently diagnosed with infection, and transfusion-transmitted leishmaniasis infection is considered to be a rare event.[238] For additional reading on other possible transfusion-transmitted pathogens, the reader is referred to more comprehensive sources.[211]

ACKNOWLEDGMENT

The author would like to thank Dr. Thomas Lane, director of transfusion services at the University of California, San Diego Medical Center, for his review of this manuscript.

REFERENCES

1. Schreiber GB, Busch MP, Kleinman SH, et al: The risk of transfusion-transmitted viral infections, *N Engl J Med* 334:1685, 1996.
2. Centers for Disease Control and Prevention: U.S. Public Health Service guidelines for testing and counseling blood and plasma donors for human immunodeficiency virus type 1 antigen, *MMWR* 45(RR-2):1, 1996.
3. Sazama K: Reports of 355 transfusion-associated deaths: 1976 through 1985, *Transfusion* 30:583, 1990.
4. Linden JV, Paul B, Dressler KP: A report of 104 transfusion errors in New York State, *Transfusion* 32:601, 1992.
5. Simon T: Proficiency Testing Program. *CAP Survey 1991,* Northfield, Ill, 1991, College of American Pathologists.
6. Rosse WF: Untoward consequences of transfusion. In *Clinical immunohematology: basic concepts and clinical applications,* Boston, 1990, Blackwell Scientific, p 389.
7. Pineda AA, Brzica SM Jr, Taswell HF: Hemolytic transfusion reaction. Recent experience in a large blood bank, *Mayo Clin Proc* 53:378, 1978.
8. Beauregard P, Blajchman MA: Hemolytic and pseudo-hemolytic transfusion reactions: an overview of the hemolytic transfusion reactions and the clinical conditions that mimic them, *Transfus Med Rev* 8:184, 1994.
9. Capon SM, Goldfinger D: Acute hemolytic transfusion reaction, a paradigm of the systemic inflammatory response: new insights into pathophysiology and treatment, *Transfusion* 35:513, 1995.
10. Honig CL, Bove JR: Transfusion-associated fatalities: review of Bureau of Biologics reports 1976-1978, *Transfusion* 20:653, 1980.
11. Jenner PW, Holland PV: Diagnosis and management of transfusion reactions. In Petz LD, Swisher SN, Kleinman S, et al, eds: *Clinical practice of transfusion medicine,* ed 3, New York, 1996, Churchill Livingstone, p 905.
12. Cooper CL: Complications of transfusion therapy. In Lake CL, Moore RA, eds: *Blood: hemostasis, transfusion, and alternatives in the perioperative period,* New York, 1995, Raven, p 319.
13. Lostumbo MM, Holland PV, Schmidt PJ: Isoimmunization after multiple transfusions, *N Engl J Med* 275:141, 1966.
14. Vichinsky EP, Earles A, Johnson RA, et al: Alloimmunization in sickle cell anemia and transfusion of racially unmatched blood, *N Engl J Med* 322:1617, 1990.
15. Ness PM, Shirey RS, Thoman SK, et al: The differentiation of delayed serologic and delayed hemolytic transfusion reactions: incidence, long-term serologic findings, and clinical significance, *Transfusion* 30:688, 1990.
16. Adverse effects of blood transfusion. In Walker RH, ed: *Technical manual of the American Association of Blood Banks,* ed 11, Bethesda, Md, 1993, American Association of Blood Banks.
17. Snyder EL: Prevention of HLA alloimmunization: role of leukocyte depletion and UV-B irradiation, *Yale J Biol Med* 63:419, 1990.

18. Goldfinger D, Lowe C: Prevention of adverse reactions to blood transfusion by the administration of saline-washed red blood cells, *Transfusion* 21:277, 1981.

19. Brubaker DB: Clinical significance of white cell antibodies in febrile nonhemolytic transfusion reactions, *Transfusion* 30:733, 1990.

20. Mintz PD: Febrile reactions to platelet transfusions, *Am J Clin Pathol* 95:609, 1991.

21. Dzik WH: Is the febrile response to transfusion due to donor or recipient cytokine? *Transfusion* 32:594, 1992.

22. Kevy SV, Schmidt PJ, McGinniss MH, et al: Febrile, nonhemolytic transfusion reactions and the limited role of leukoagglutinins in their etiology, *Transfusion* 2:7, 1962.

23. Dzieczkowski JS, Barrett BB, Nester D, et al: Characterization of reactions after exclusive transfusion of white cell-reduced cellular blood components, *Transfusion* 35:20, 1995.

24. Weber JG, Warner MA, Moore SB: What is the incidence of perioperative transfusion-related acute lung injury? *Anesthesiology* 82:789, 1995.

25. Popovsky MA, Chaplin HC Jr, Moore SB: Transfusion-related acute lung injury: a neglected, serious complication of hemotherapy, *Transfusion* 32:589, 1992.

26. Heddle NM, Klama LN, Griffith L, et al: A prospective study to identify the risks associated with acute reactions to platelet and red cell transfusions, *Transfusion* 33:794, 1993.

27. Ward HN: Pulmonary infiltrates associated with leukoagglutinin transfusion reactions, *Ann Intern Med* 73:689, 1970.

28. Swank DW, Moore SB: Roles of the neutrophil and other mediators in adult respiratory distress syndrome, *Mayo Clin Proc* 64:1118, 1989.

29. Silliman CC, Paterson AJ, Dickey WO, et al: The association of biologically active lipids with the development of transfusion-associated acute lung injury: a retrospective study, *Transfusion* 37:719, 1997.

30. Florell SR, Velasco SE, Fine PG: Perioperative recognition, management, and pathologic diagnosis of transfusion-related acute lung injury, *Anesthesiology* 81:508, 1994.

31. Popovsky MA, Moore SB: Diagnostic and pathogenetic considerations in transfusion-related acute lung injury, *Transfusion* 25:573, 1985.

32. Worsley MH, Sinclair CJ, Campanella C, et al: Non-cardiogenic pulmonary oedema after transfusion with granulocyte antibody containing blood: treatment with extracorporeal membrane oxygenation, *Br J Anaesth* 67:116, 1991.

33. Stack G, Snyder EL: Cytokine generation in stored platelet concentrates, *Transfusion* 34:20, 1994.

34. Muylle L, Wouters E, DeBock R, et al: Reactions to platelet transfusion: the effect of the storage time of the concentrate, *Transfus Med* 2:289, 1992.

35. McCrae KR, Herman JH: Posttransfusion purpura: two unusual cases and a literature review, *Am J Hematol* 52:205, 1996.

36. Blanchette VS, Chen L, de Friedberg ZS, et al: Alloimmunization to the PLA1 platelet antigen: results of a prospective study, *Br J Haematol* 74:209, 1990.

37. Becker T, Panzer S, Maas D, et al: High-dose intravenous immunoglobulin for post-transfusion purpura, *Br J Haematol* 61:149, 1985.

38. Puig N, Sayas MJ, Montoro JA, et al: Post-transfusion purpura as the main manifestation of a trilineal transfusion reaction, responsive to steroids: flow cytometric investigation of granulocyte and platelet antibodies, *Ann Hematol* 62:232, 1991.

39. Gerstner JB, Smith MJ, Davis KD, et al: Posttransfusion purpura: therapeutic failure of PLA1-negative platelet transfusion, *Am J Hematol* 6:71, 1997.

40. Godeau B, Fromont P, Bettaieb A, et al: Relapse of posttransfusion purpura after transfusion with frozen-thawed red cells, *Transfusion* 31:189, 1991.

41. Kalish RI, Jacobs B: Post-transfusion purpura: initiation by leukocyte-poor cells in a polytransfused woman, *Vox Sang* 53:169, 1987.

42. Wilhelm D, Kluter H, Klouche M, et al: Impact of allergy screening for blood donors: relationship to nonhemolytic transfusion reactions, *Vox Sang* 69:217, 1995.

43. Shivdasani RA, Anderson KC: Graft-versus-host disease. In Petz LD, Swisher SN, Kleinman S, et al, eds: *Clinical practice of transfusion medicine*, ed 3, New York, 1996, Churchill Livingstone, p 931.

44. Billingham RE: The biology of graft-versus-host reactions, *Harvey Lect* 62:21, 1966.

45. Shivdasani RA, Haluska FG, Dock NL, et al: Brief report: graft-versus-host disease associated with transfusion of blood from unrelated HLA-homozygous donors, *N Engl J Med* 328:766, 1993.

46. Shivdasani RA, Anderson KC: HLA homozygosity and shared HLA haplotypes in the development of transfusion-associated graft-versus-host disease, *Leuk Lymphoma* 15:227, 1994.

47. Hayakawa S, Chishima F, Sakata H, et al: A rapid molecular diagnosis of posttransfusion graft-versus-host disease by polymerase chain reaction, *Transfusion* 33:413, 1993.

48. Schlitt HJ, Kanehiro H, Raddatz G, et al: Persistence of donor lymphocytes in liver allograft recipients, *Transplantation* 56:1001, 1993.

49. Bertheas MF, Lafage M, Levy P, et al: Influence of mixed chimerism on the results of allogeneic bone marrow transplantation for leukemia, *Blood* 78:3103, 1991.

50. Kanter MH: Transfusion-associated graft-versus-host disease: do transfusions from second-degree relatives pose a greater risk than those from first-degree relatives? *Transfusion* 32:323, 1992.

51. Takahashi K, Juji T, Miyamoto M, et al: Analysis of risk factors for post-transfusion graft-versus-host disease in Japan. Japanese Red Cross PT-GVHD Study Group, *Lancet* 343:700, 1994.

52. Otsuka S, Kunieda K, Kitamura F, et al: The critical role of blood from HLA-homozygous donors in fatal transfusion-associated graft-versus-host disease in immunocompetent patients, *Transfusion* 31:260, 1991.

53. von Fliedner V, Higby DJ, Kim U: Graft-versus-host reaction following blood transfusion, *Am J Med* 72:951, 1982.

54. Suzuki K, Akiyama H, Takamoto S et al: Transfusion-associated graft-versus-host disease in a presumably immunocompetent patient after transfusion of stored packed red cells, *Transfusion* 32:358, 1992.

55. Widmann FK, ed: *Standards for blood banks and transfusion services*, ed 15, Bethesda, Md, 1993, American Association of Blood Banks.

56. Lowenthal RM, Challis DR, Griffiths AE, et al: Transfusion-associated graft-versus-host disease: report of an occurrence following the administration of irradiated blood, *Transfusion* 33:524, 1993.

57. Sproul AM, Chalmers EA, Mills KI, et al: Third party mediated graft rejection despite irradiation of blood products, *Br J Haematol* 80:251, 1992.

58. Strauss RG: Routinely washing irradiated red cells before transfusion seems unwarranted, *Transfusion* 30:675, 1990.

59. Brunson ME, Alexander JW: Mechanisms of transfusion-induced immunosuppression, *Transfusion* 30:651, 1990.

60. Landers DF, Hill GE, Wong KC, et al: Blood transfusion–induced immunomodulation, *Anesth Analg* 82:187, 1996.

61. Klein HG: Immunomodulation caused by blood transfusion. In Petz LD, Swisher SN, Kleinman S, et al, eds: *Clinical practice of transfusion medicine*, ed 3, New York, 1996, Churchill Livingstone, p 59.

62. Dzik S, Blajchman MA, Blumberg N, et al: Current research on the immunomodulatory effect of allogeneic blood transfusion, *Vox Sang* 70:187, 1996.

63. Opelz G, Sengar DP, Mickey MR, et al: Effect of blood transfusion on subsequent kidney transplants, *Transplant Proc* 5:253, 1973.

64. Triulzi D, Heal J, Blumberg N: Transfusion-induced immunomodulation and its clinical consequences. In Nance SJ, ed: *Transfusion medicine in the 1990s*, Bethesda, Md, 1990, American Association of Blood Banks, p 1.

65. Landers DF, Hill GE, Wong KC, et al: Blood transfusion-induced immunomodulation, *Anesth Analg* 82:187, 1996.

66. Klein HG: Immunomodulation caused by blood transfusion. In Petz LD, Swisher SN, Kleinman S, et al, eds: *Clinical practice of transfusion medicine*, ed 3, New York, 1996, Churchill Livingstone, p 59.

67. Vamvakas E, Moore SB: Perioperative blood transfusion and colorectal cancer recurrence: a qualitative statistical overview and meta-analysis, *Transfusion* 33:754, 1993.

68. Vamvakas EC, Moore SB: Blood transfusion and postoperative septic complications, *Transfusion* 34:714, 1994.

69. Taylor C, Faulk WP: Prevention of recurrent abortion with leucocyte transfusions, *Lancet* 2:68, 1981.

70. Mowbray JF, Gibbings C, Lidell H, et al: Controlled trial of treatment of recurrent spontaneous abortion by immunisation with paternal cells, *Lancet* 1:941, 1985.

71. Heine O, Mueller-Eckhardt G: Intravenous immune globulin in recurrent abortion, *Clin Exp Immunol* 97(suppl 1):39, 1994.

72. Stray-Pedersen B, Stray-Pedersen S: Etiologic factors and subsequent reproductive performance in 195 couples with prior history of habitual abortion, *Am J Obstet Gynecol* 148:140, 1984.

73. Williams JG, Hughes LE: Effect of perioperative blood transfusion on recurrence of Crohn's disease, *Lancet* 2:1524, 1989.

74. Denlinger JK, Nahrwold ML: Cardiac failure associated with hypocalcemia, *Anesth Analg* 55:34, 1976.

75. Denlinger JK, Nahrwold ML, Gibbs PS, et al: Hypocalcaemia during rapid blood transfusion in anesthetized man, *Br J Anaesth* 48:995, 1976.

76. Scheidegger D, Drop LJ: The relationship between duration of Q-T interval and plasma ionized calcium concentration: experiments with acute, steady-state (Ca++) changes in the dog, *Anesthesiology* 51:143, 1979.

77. Marriott HJL: *Practical electrocardiography,* ed 7, Baltimore, 1983, Williams & Wilkins.

78. Ladbrook J, Wynn V: Citrate intoxication, *Br J Med* 2:523, 1958.

79. Drop LJ, Laver MB: Low plasma ionized calcium and response to calcium therapy in critically ill man, *Anesthesiology* 42:300, 1975.

80. Dzik WH, Kirkley SA: Citrate toxicity during massive transfusion, *Transfus Med Rev* 2:76, 1988.

81. Rude RK, Oldham SB, Sharpe CF Jr, et al: Parathyroid hormone secretion in magnesium deficiency, *J Clin Endocrinol Metab* 47:800, 1978.

82. Juan D: Hypocalcemia: differential diagnosis and mechanisms, *Arch Intern Med* 139:1166, 1979.

83. Chernow B, Smith J, Rainey TG, et al: Hypomagnesemia: implications for the critical care specialist, *Crit Care Med* 10:193, 1982.

84. Silberstein LE, Naryshkin S, Haddad JJ, et al: Calcium homeostasis during therapeutic plasma exchange, *Transfusion* 26:151, 1986.

85. Martin TJ, Kang Y, Robertson KM, et al: Ionization and hemodynamic effects of calcium chloride and calcium gluconate in the absence of hepatic function, *Anesthesiology* 73:62, 1990.

86. Kliegman RM, Wald MK: Problems in metabolic adaptation: glucose, calcium, and magnesium. In Klaus MH, Fanaroff AA, eds: *Care of the high-risk neonate,* ed 3, Philadelphia, 1986, WB Saunders, p 220.

87. Wilson RF, Soullier G, Antonenko D: Ionized calcium levels in critically ill surgical patients, *Am Surg* 45:485, 1979.

88. Zauder HL: Massive transfusion, *Int Anesthesiol Clin* 20:157, 1982.

89. Jameson LC, Popic PM, Harms BA: Hyperkalemic death during use of high-capacity fluid warmer for massive transfusion, *Anesthesiology* 73:1050, 1990.

90. Jeter EK, Gadsden RH, Cate J IV: Effects of irradiation on red cells stored in CPDA-1 and CPD-ADSOL (AS-1), *Ann Clin Lab Sci* 21:177, 1991.

91. Brown KA, Bissonnette B, MacDonald M, et al: Hyperkalaemia during massive blood transfusion in paediatric craniofacial surgery, *Can J Anaesth* 37(4 pt 1):401, 1990.

92. Valeri CR, Hirsch NM: Restoration in vivo of erythrocyte adenosine triphosphate, 2,3 diphosphoglycerate, potassium ion, and sodium ion concentrations following the transfusion of acid-citrate-dextrose–stored human red blood cells, *J Lab Clin Med* 73:722, 1969.

93. Linko K, Saxelin I: Electrolyte and acid-base disturbances caused by blood transfusions, *Acta Anaesthesiol Scand* 30:139, 1986.

94. Adler S, Fraley DS: Potassium and intracellular pH, *Kidney Int* 11:433, 1977.

95. Perez GO, Oster JR, Vaamonde CA: Serum potassium concentration in acidemic states, *Nephron* 27:233, 1981.

96. Mahnensmith R, Thier SO, Cooke CR, et al: Effect of acute metabolic acidemia on renal electrolyte transport in man, *Metabolism* 28:831, 1979.

97. Scheller MS, Mazzei WJ, Zornow MH, et al: A comparison of the effects of central versus peripheral bolus injections of potassium chloride on aortic root potassium concentrations in swine, *J Cardiothorac Anesth* 3:172, 1989.

98. Fraley DS, Adler S: Correction of hyperkalemia by bicarbonate despite constant blood pH, *Kidney Int* 12:354, 1977.

99. Kraft LF, Katholi RE, Woods WT, et al: Attenuation by magnesium of electrophysiologic effects of hyperkalemia in human and canine heart, *Am J Cardiol* 45:1189, 1980.

100. Liu EA, Mannino FL, Lane TA: Prospective, randomized trial of the safety and efficacy of a limited donor exposure transfusion program for premature neonates, *J Pediatr* 125:92, 1994.

101. Wilson RF, Binkley LE, Sabo FM Jr, et al: Electrolyte and acid-base changes with massive blood transfusions, *Am Surg* 58:535, 1992.

102. Carmichael D, Hosty T, Kastl D, et al: Hypokalemia and massive transfusion, *South Med J* 77:315, 1984.

103. Rudolph R, Boyd CR. Massive transfusion: complications and their management, *South Med J* 83:1065, 1990.

104. Kroll MH, Elin RJ: Relationships between magnesium and protein concentration in serum, *Clin Chem* 31:244, 1985.

105. McLellan BA, Reid SR, Lane PL: Massive blood transfusion causing hypomagnesemia, *Crit Care Med* 12:146, 1984.

106. Kulkarni P, Bhattacharya S, Petros AJ: Torsades de pointes and long QT syndrome following major blood transfusion, *Anaesthesia* 47:125, 1992.

107. Burch GE, Giles TD: The importance of magnesium deficiency in cardiovascular disease, *Am Heart J* 94:649, 1977.

108. Seller RH, Cangiano J, Kim KE, et al: Digitalis toxicity and hypomagnesemia, *Am Heart J* 79:57, 1970.

109. Killen DA, Grogan EL II, Gower RE, et al: Response of canine plasma-ionized calcium and magnesium to the rapid infusion of acid-citrate-dextrose (ACD) solution, *Surgery* 70:736, 1971.

110. Lieberman N, Plevak D, Moyer T, et al: Is it important to measure magnesium concentrations during and immediately after liver transplantation? *Transplant Proc* 25:1826, 1993.

111. Juan D: Hypocalcemia: differential diagnosis and mechanisms, *Arch Intern Med* 139:1166, 1979.

112. Shils ME: Experimental human magnesium depletion, *Medicine* 48:61, 1969.

113. Eisenbud E, LoBue CC: Hypocalcemia after therapeutic use of magnesium sulfate, *Arch Intern Med* 136:688, 1976.

114. Benson RE, Isbister JP: Massive blood transfusion, *Anaesth Intensive Care* 8:152, 1980.

115. Rutledge R, Sheldon GF, Collins ML: Massive transfusion, *Crit Care Clin* 2:791, 1986.

116. Sohmer PR, Scott RL: Metabolic burden of massive transfusion, *Prog Clin Biol Res* 108:273, 1982.

117. Ferrara A, MacArthur JD, Wright HK, et al: Hypothermia and acidosis worsen coagulopathy in the patient requiring massive transfusion, *Am J Surg* 160:515, 1990.

118. Harke H, Rahman S: Haemostatic disorders in massive transfusion, *Bibl Haematol* 46:179, 1980.

119. Iserson KV, Huestis DW: Blood warming: current applications and techniques, *Transfusion* 31:558, 1991.

120. Jurkovich GJ, Greiser WB, Luterman A, et al: Hypothermia in trauma victims: an ominous predictor of survival, *J Trauma* 27:1019, 1987.

121. Steinemann S, Shackford SR, Davis JW: Implications of admission hypothermia in trauma patients, *J Trauma* 30:200, 1990.

122. Kurz A, Sessler DI, Narzt E, et al: Postoperative hemodynamic and thermoregulatory consequences of intraoperative core hypothermia, *J Clin Anesth* 7:359, 1995.

123. Kurz A, Sessler DI, Lenhardt R: Perioperative normothermia to reduce the incidence of surgical-wound infection and shorten hospitalization. Study of Wound Infection and Temperature Group, *N Engl J Med* 334:1209, 1996.

124. Frank SM, Beattie C, Christopherson R, et al: Unintentional hypothermia is associated with postoperative myocardial ischemia. The Perioperative Ischemia Randomized Anesthesia Trial Study Group, *Anesthesiology* 78:468, 1993.

125. Iserson KV, Knauf MA, Anhalt D: Rapid admixture blood warming: technical advances, *Crit Care Med* 18:1138, 1990.

126. Marsaglia G, Thomas ED: Mathematical consideration of cross circulation and exchange transfusion, *Transfusion* 11:216, 1971.

127. Hiippala ST, Myllyla GJ, Vahtera EM: Hemostatic factors and replacement of major blood loss with plasma-poor red cell concentrates, *Anesth Analg* 81:360, 1995.

128. Harrigan C, Lucas CE, Ledgerwood AM, et al: Primary hemostasis after massive transfusion for injury, *Am Surg* 48:393, 1982.

129. Lind SE: The bleeding time does not predict surgical bleeding, *Blood* 77:2547, 1991.

130. Petz LD: Platelet transfusions. In Petz LD, Swisher SN, Kleinman S, et al, eds: *Clinical practice of transfusion medicine,* ed 3, New York, 1996, Churchill Livingstone, p 359.

131. Tuman KJ, Spiess BD, McCarthy RJ, et al: Effects of progressive blood loss on coagulation as measured by thromboelastography, *Anesth Analg* 66:856, 1987.

132. Reed RL II, Ciavarella D, Heimbach DM, et al: Prophylactic platelet administration during massive transfusion: a prospective, randomized, double-blind clinical study, *Ann Surg* 203:40, 1986.

133. Crosby ET: Perioperative haemotherapy. I. Indications for blood transfusion, *Can J Anaesth* 39:695, 1992.

134. Miller RD: Transfusion therapy, In Miller RD, ed: *Anesthesia,* ed 4, New York, 1994, Churchill Livingstone, p 1619.

135. Murray DJ, Pennell BJ, Weinstein SL, et al: Packed red cells in acute blood loss: dilutional coagulopathy as a cause of surgical bleeding, *Anesth Analg* 80:336, 1995.

136. Murray DJ, Olson J, Strauss R, et al: Coagulation changes during packed red cell replacement of major blood loss, *Anesthiology* 69:839, 1988.

137. Jenner PW, Holland PV: Diagnosis and management of transfusion reactions. In Petz LD, Swisher SN, Kleinman S, et al, eds: *Clinical practice of transfusion medicine,* ed 3, New York, 1996, Churchill Livingstone, p 905.

138. Gabutti V, Piga A: Results of long-term iron-chelating therapy, *Acta Haematologica* 95:26, 1996.

139. Calhoun L: Blood product preparation and administration, In Petz LD, Swisher SN, Kleinman S, et al, eds: *Clinical practice of transfusion medicine,* ed 3, New York, 1996, Churchill Livingstone, p 305.

140. Moseley RV, Doty DB: Death associated with multiple pulmonary emboli soon after battle injury, *Ann Surg* 171:336, 1970.

141. Collins JA: The causes of progressive pulmonary insufficiency in surgical patients, *J Surg Res* 9:685, 1969.

142. Collins JA, Gordon WC Jr, Hudson TL, et al: Inapparent hypoxemia in casualties with wounded limbs: pulmonary fat embolism? *Ann Surg* 167:511, 1968.

143. Martin AM Jr, Simmons RL, Heisterkamp CA III: Respiratory insufficiency in combat casualties. I. Pathologic changes in the lungs of patients dying of wounds, *Ann Surg* 170:30, 1969.

144. Snyder EL, Hezzey A, Barash PG, et al: Microaggregate blood filtration in patients with compromised pulmonary function, *Transfusion* 22:21, 1982.

145. Dodd RY: The risk of transfusion-transmitted infection, *N Engl J Med* 327:419, 1992.

146. Kleinman S, Busch MP: General overview of transfusion-transmitted infections. In Petz LD, Swisher SN, Kleinman S, et al, eds: *Clinical practice of transfusion medicine,* ed 3, New York, 1996, Churchill Livingstone, p 809.

147. Busch MP, Lee LL, Satten GA, et al: Time course of detection of viral and serological markers preceding human immunodeficiency virus type 1 seroconversion: implications for screening of blood and tissue donors, *Transfusion* 35:91, 1995.

148. Berry AJ, Whitsett CF: Infectious risks of transfusions. In Lake CL, Moore RA, eds: *Blood: hemostasis, transfusion, and alternatives in the perioperative period,* New York, 1995, Raven, p 289.

149. Dodd RY: Transfusion-transmitted hepatitis virus infection, *Hematol Oncol Clin North Am* 9:137, 1995.

150. Mimms LT, Mosley JW, Hollinger FB, et al: Effect of concurrent acute infection with hepatitis C virus on acute hepatitis B virus infection, *BMJ* 307:1095, 1993.

151. Centers for Disease Control: Public Health Service inter-agency guidelines for screening donors of blood, plasma, organs, tissues, and semen for evidence of hepatitis B and hepatitis C, *MMWR* 40(RR-4):1, 1991.

152. Centers for Disease Control: *Hepatitis surveillance report no 55,* Atlanta, 1994, Centers for Disease Control and Prevention, p 1.

153. McQuillan GM, Townsend TR, Fields HA, et al: Seroepidemiology of hepatitis B virus infection in the United States, 1976 to 1980, *Am J Med* 87(suppl 3A):5S, 1989.

154. Dodd RY: Hepatitis. In Petz LD, Swisher SN, Kleinman S, et al, eds: *Clinical practice of transfusion medicine,* ed 3, New York, 1996, Churchill Livingstone, p 847.

155. Hoofnagle JH, Seefe LB, Bales ZB, et al: Type B hepatitis after transfusion with blood containing antibody to hepatitis B core antigen, *N Engl J Med* 298:1379, 1978.

156. Purcell RH: Hepatitis viruses: changing patterns of human disease, *Proc Natl Acad Sci U S A* 91:2401, 1994.

157. Noble RC, Kane MA, Reeves SA, et al: Posttransfusion hepatitis A in a neonatal intensive care unit, *JAMA* 252:2711, 1984.

158. Sherertz RJ, Russell BA, Reuman PD: Transmission of hepatitis A by transfusion of blood products, *Arch Intern Med* 144:1579, 1984.

159. Lemon SM: Type A viral hepatitis: new developments in an old disease, *N Engl J Med* 313:1059, 1985.

160. Giacoia GP, Kasprisin DO: Transfusion-acquired hepatitis A, *South Med J* 82:1357, 1989.

161. Centers for Disease Control: Hepatitis A among drug abusers, *MMWR* 37:297, 1988.

162. Westblom TU, Gudipati S, DeRousse C, et al: Safety and immunogenicity of an inactivated hepatitis A vaccine: effect of dose and vaccination schedule, *J Infect Dis* 169:996, 1994.

163. Aledort LM: Consequences of chronic hepatitis C: a review article for the hematologist, *Am J Hematol* 44:29, 1997.

164. Koretz RL, Abbey H, Coleman E, et al: Non-A, non-B posttransfusion hepatitis: looking back at the second decade, *Ann Intern Med* 199:110, 1993.

165. Tsukuma H, Hiyama T, Tanaka S, et al: Risk factors for hepatocellular carcinoma among patients with chronic liver disease, *N Engl J Med* 328:1797, 1993.

166. Tong MJ, El-Farra NS, Reikes AR, et al: Clinical outcomes after transfusion-associated hepatitis C, *N Engl J Med* 332:1463, 1995.

167. Conry-Cantilena C, VanRaden M, Gibble J, et al: Routes of infection, viremia, and liver disease in blood donors found to have hepatitis C virus infection, *N Engl J Med* 344:1691, 1996.

168. Centers for Disease Control: *Hepatitis surveillance report no. 55,* Atlanta, 1994, Centers for Disease Control and Prevention, p 1.

169. Alter HJ, Hadler SC, Judson FN, et al: Risk factors for acute non-A, non-B hepatitis in the United States and association with hepatitis C virus infection, *JAMA* 264:2231, 1990.

170. Donahue JG, Nelson KE, Munoz A, et al: Antibody to hepatitis C virus among cardiac surgery patients, homosexual men, and intravenous drug users in Baltimore, Maryland, *Am J Epidemiol* 134:1206, 1991.

171. Kiyosawa K, Sodeyama T, Tanaka E, et al: Hepatitis C in hospital employees with needlestick injuries, *Ann Intern Med* 115:367, 1991.

172. Kleinman S, Alter H, Busch M, et al: Increased detection of hepatitis C virus (HCV)-infected blood donors by a multiple-antigen HCV enzyme immunoassay, *Transfusion* 32:805, 1992.

173. Busch MP, Korelitz JJ, Kleinman SH, et al: Declining value of alanine aminotransferase in screening of blood donors to prevent posttransfusion hepatitis B and C infection, *Transfusion* 35:903, 1995.

174. Lelie PN, Cuypers HT, Reesink HW, et al: Patterns of serological markers in transfusion-transmitted hepatitis C virus infection using second-generation HCV assays, *J Med Virol* 37:203, 1992.

175. Kleinman S, Busch MP, Korelitz JJ, et al: The incidence/window period model and its use to assess the risk of transfusion-transmitted human immunodeficiency virus and hepatitis C virus infection, *Transfus Med Rev* 11:155, 1997.

176. Cheung RC, Keeffe EB, Greenberg HB: Hepatitis G virus: is it a hepatitis virus? *West J Med* 167:23, 1997.

177. Roth WK, Waschk D, Marx S, et al: Prevalence of hepatitis G virus and its strain variant, the GB agent, in blood donations and their transmission to recipients, *Transfusion* 37:651, 1997.

178. Alter HJ: You'll wonder where the yellow went: a 15-year retrospective of posttransfusion hepatitis. In Moore SB, ed: *Transfusion-transmitted viral disease*, Arlington, Va, 1987, American Association of Blood Banks, p 53.

179. Blajchman MA, Bull SB, Feinman SV: Post-transfusion hepatitis: impact of non-A non-B hepatitis surrogate tests, *Lancet* 345:21, 1995.

180. Purcell RH: Hepatitis viruses: changing patterns of human disease. *Proc Natl Acad Sci U S A* 91:2401, 1994.

181. Busch MP: Retroviral infections. In Petz LD, Swisher SN, Kleinman S, et al, eds: *Clinical practice of transfusion medicine*, ed 3, New York, 1996, Churchill Livingstone, p 822.

182. Transfusion-transmitted viruses. In Walker RH, ed: *Technical manual of the American Association of Blood Banks,* ed 11, Bethesda, Md, 1993, American Association of Blood Banks.

183. Williams AE, Sullivan MT: Transfusion-transmitted retrovirus infection, *Hematol Oncol Clin North Am* 9:115, 1995.

184. Medley GF, Anderson RM, Cox DR, et al: Incubation period of AIDS in patients infected via blood transfusion, *Nature* 328:719, 1987.

185. Busch MP, Young MJ, Samson SM, et al: Risk of human immunodeficiency virus (HIV) transmission by blood transfusions before the implementation of HIV-1 antibody screening, *Transfusion* 31:4, 1991.

186. Kroner BL, Rosenberg PS, Aledort LM, et al: HIV-1 infection incidence among persons with hemophilia in the United States and western Europe, 1978-1990, *J Acquir Immune Defic Syndr* 7:279, 1994.

187. Selik RM, Ward JW, Buehler JW: Trends in transfusion-associated acquired immune deficiency syndrome in the United States, 1982 through 1991, *Transfusion* 33:890, 1993.

188. United States Public Health Service: Statistics from the Centers for Disease Control and Prevention, *AIDS* 8:399, 1994.

189. Donegan E, Stuart M, Niland JC, et al: Infection with human immunodeficiency virus type 1 among recipients of antibody-positive blood donations, *Ann Intern Med* 113:733, 1990.

190. Donegan E, Lenes BA, Tomasulo PA, et al: Transmission of HIV-1 by components type and duration of shelf storage before transfusion, *Transfusion* 30:851, 1990.

191. Seiki M, Eddy R, Shows TB, et al: Non-specific integration of the HTLV provirus genome into adult T-cell leukaemia cells, *Nature* 309:640, 1984.

192. Centers for Disease Control and Prevention and USPHS Working Group: Guidelines for counseling persons infected with human T-lymphotropic virus type I (HTLV-I) and type II (HTLV-II), *Ann Intern Med* 118:448, 1993.

193. Jacobson S, Raine CS, Mingioli ES, et al: Isolation of an HTLV-I-like retrovirus from patients with tropical spastic paraparesis, *Nature* 331:540, 1988.

194. Jacobson S, Lehky T, Nishimura M, et al: Isolation of HTLV-II from a patient with chronic, progressive neurological disease clinically indistinguishable from HTLV-I-associated myelopathy/tropical spastic paraparesis, *Ann Neurol* 33:392, 1993.

195. Williams AE, Fang CT, Slamon DJ, et al: Seroprevalence and epidemiologic correlates of HTLV-I infection in US blood donors, *Science* 240:643, 1988.

196. Hjelle B, Wilson C, Cyrus S, et al: Human T-cell leukemia virus type II infection frequently goes undetected in contemporary US blood donors, *Blood* 81:1641, 1993.

197. Kamihira S, Nakasima S, Oyakawa Y, et al: Transmission of human T-cell lymphotropic virus type I by blood transfusion before and after mass screening of sera from seropositive donors, *Vox Sang* 52:43, 1987.

198. Donegan E, Lee H, Operskalski EA, et al: Transfusion transmission of retroviruses: human T-lymphotropic viruses types I and II compared with human immunodeficiency virus type 1, *Transfusion* 34:478, 1994.

199. Nelson KE, Donahue JG, Munoz A et al: Transmission of retroviruses from seronegative donors by transfusion during cardiac surgery: a multicenter study of HIV-1 and HTLV-I/II infections, *Ann Intern Med* 117:554, 1992.

200. Sayers MH: Cytomegalovirus and other herpesviruses. In Petz LD, Swisher SN, Kleinman S, et al, eds: *Clinical practice of transfusion medicine,* ed 3, New York, 1996, Churchill Livingstone, p 875.

201. Dubois RE, Seeley JK, Brus I, et al: Chronic mononucleosis syndrome, *South Med J* 77:1376, 1984.

202. Gerber P, Walsh JH, Roseblum EN, et al: Association of EB-virus infection with the post-perfusion syndrome, *Lancet* 1:593, 1969.

203. Bayer WL, Tegtmeier GE, Barbara JA: The significance of non-A, non-B hepatitis, cytomegalovirus and the acquired immune deficiency syndrome in transfusion practice, *Clin Hematol* 13:253, 1984.

204. Bowden RA: Transfusion-transmitted cytomegalovirus infection, *Hematol Oncol Clin North Am* 9:155, 1995.

205. Tegtmeier GE: Cytomegalovirus infection as a complication of blood transfusion, *Semin Liver Dis* 6:82, 1986.

206. Hersman J, Meyers JD, Thomas ED, et al: The effects of granulocyte transfusions on the incidence of cytomegalovirus infection after allogeneic marrow transplantation, *Ann Intern Med* 96:149, 1982.

207. Lane TA, Anderson KC, Goodnough LT, et al: Leukocyte reduction in blood component therapy, *Ann Intern Med* 117:151, 1992.

208. American Association of Blood Banks: *Leukocyte reduction for the prevention of transfusion-transmitted cytomegalovirus,* bulletin #97-2, Bethesda, Md, 1997, American Association of Blood Banks, p 1.

209. Bowden RA, Slichter SJ, Sayers M, et al: A comparison of filtered leukocyte-reduced and cytomegalovirus (CMV) seronegative blood products for the prevention of transfusion-associated CMV infection after marrow transplant, *Blood* 86:3598, 1995.

210. Transfusion-transmitted viruses. In Walker RH, ed: *Technical manual of the American Association of Blood Banks,* ed 11, Bethesda, Md, 1993, American Association of Blood Banks.

211. Berry AJ, Whitsett CF: Infectious risks of transfusions. In Lake CL, Moore RA, eds: *Blood: hemostasis, transfusion and alternatives in the perioperative period,* New York, 1995, Raven, p 289.

212. Skupski DW, Wolf CFW, Bussel JB: Fetal and perinatal transfusion. In Petz LD, Swisher SN, Kleinman S, et al, eds: *Clinical practice of transfusion medicine,* ed 3, New York, 1996, Churchill Livingstone, p 607.

213. Centers for Disease Control and Prevention: Risks associated with human parvovirus B19 infection, *MMWR* 38:81, 1989.

214. Lefrere JJ, Mariotti M, Thauvin M: B19 parvovirus DNA in solvent/detergent-treated anti-haemophilia concentrates, *Lancet* 343:211, 1994.

215. Tajiri H, Nose O, Baba K, et al: Human herpesvirus-6 infection with liver injury in neonatal hepatitis, *Lancet* 335:863, 1990.

216. Yoshikawa T, Suga S, Asano Y, et al: Human herpesvirus-6 infection in bone marrow transplantation, *Blood* 78:1381, 1991.

217. Carrigan DR, Drobyski WR, Russler SK, et al: Interstitial pneumonitis associated with human herpesvirus-6 infection after marrow transplantation, *Lancet* 338:147, 1991.

218. Burd EM, Knox KK, Carrigan DR: Human herpesvirus-6–associated suppression of growth factor–induced macrophage maturation in human bone marrow cultures, *Blood* 81:1645, 1993.

219. Saxinger C, Polesky H, Eby N, et al: Antibody reactivity with HBLV (HHV-6) in US populations, *J Virol Methods* 21:199, 1988.

220. Regulatory affairs: fatality statistics, *AABB News Briefs,* 14:B-2, August 1992.

221. Update: *Yersinia enterocolitica* bacteremia and endotoxin shock associated with red blood cell transfusions: United States, 1991, *MMWR* 40:176, 1991.

222. Morduchowicz G, Pitlik SD, Huminer D, et al: Transfusion reactions due to bacterial contamination of blood and blood products, *Rev Infect Dis* 13:307, 1991.

223. Goldman M, Blajchman MA: Blood product-associated bacterial sepsis, *Trans Med Rev* 5:73, 1991.

224. Grossman BJ, Kollins P, Lau PM, et al: Screening blood donors for gastrointestinal illness: a strategy to eliminate carriers of *Yersinia enterocolitica, Transfusion* 31:500, 1991.

225. Krishnan LA, Brecher ME: Transfusion-transmitted bacterial infection, *Hematol Oncol Clin North Am* 9:167, 1995.

226. Centers for Disease Control: Bacterial contamination of platelet pools: Ohio, 1991, *MMWR* 41:36, 1992.

227. van der Sluis JJ, ten Kate FJ, Vuzevski VD, et al: Transfusion syphilis, survival of *Treponema pallidum* in stored donor blood. II. Dose dependence of experimentally determined survival times, *Vox Sang* 49:390, 1985.

228. Does it make sense for blood transfusion services to continue the time-honored syphilis screening with cardiolipin antigen? *Vox Sang* 41:183, 1981.

229. De Schryver A, Meheus A: Syphilis and blood transfusion: a global perspective, *Transfusion* 30:844, 1990.

230. Nahlen BL, Lobel HO, Cannon SE, et al: Reassessment of blood donor selection criteria for United States travelers to malarious areas, *Transfusion* 31:798, 1991.

231. Benson K: Bacterial and parasitic infections. In Petz LD, Swisher SN, Kleinman S, et al, eds: *Clinical practice of transfusion medicine,* ed 3, New York, 1996, Churchill Livingstone, p 891.

232. *Recommendations regarding babesiosis and potential transmission by blood transfusion,* Arlington, Va, 1989, American Association of Blood Banks.

233. Schmunis GA: *Trypanosoma cruzi,* the etiologic agent of Chagas' disease: status in the blood supply in endemic and nonendemic countries, *Transfusion* 31:547, 1991.

234. Kirchhoff LV: American trypanosomiasis (Chagas' disease): a tropical disease now in the United States, *N Engl J Med* 329:639, 1993.

235. Skolnick A: Deferral aims to deter Chagas' parasite, *JAMA* 265:173, 1991.

236. Halkier-Sorensen LH, Kragballe K, Nedergaard ST, et al: Lack of transmission of *Borrelia burgdorferi* by blood transfusion, *Lancet* 1:550, 1990.

237. Magill AJ, Grogl M, Gasser RA Jr, et al: Viscerotropic leishmaniasis caused by *Leishmania tropica* in soldiers returning from Operation Desert Storm, *N Engl J Med* 328:1383, 1993.

238. Grogl M, Daugirda JL, Hoover DL, et al: Survivability and infectivity of viscerotropic *Leishmania tropica* from Operation Desert Storm participants in human blood products maintained under blood bank conditions, *Am J Trop Med Hyg* 49:308, 1993.

Chapter 24

Causes and Consequences of Maternal-Fetal Perianesthetic Complications

Brian K. Ross

H.S. Chadwick

January 19, 1847, marked the beginning of a new era in the field of anesthesiology and specifically in the management of the pain of labor and delivery. On that date, James Young Simpson administered ether for delivery in an obstetric patient with a deformed pelvis.[1] At that time physicians felt no need to relieve the pain of childbirth because they believed it to be a normal component of a physiologic process; in fact, many viewed the agonies of childbirth as an indicator of safety. This, in addition to the opposition by the early church to obstetric anesthesia, slowed acceptance of obstetric anesthesia by the medical community. It was not until nearly a decade later that opposition to labor analgesia began to fade as the result of John Snow's administration of chloroform to Queen Victoria of England for childbirth. With the Queen's approval of "that blessed chloroform," pain relief became acceptable, even respectable. It was recognized even from its inception, however, that obstetric anesthesia carried with it considerable risk of complications, many of which could be devastating. Aspiration and death were common results of obstetric anesthesia.

Since its early beginnings, obstetric anesthesia has had a long and tedious course in establishing itself as a genuine subspecialty. Despite the work of dedicated physi-

cians such as Bonica, Crawford, Marx, Shnider, and Ostheimer, who practiced and taught the art and science of obstetric anesthesia, this subspecialty did not attract interest equal to that of other areas. All too often obstetric anesthesia was provided by nonanesthesiologists.[2] It is interesting to note that even a routine noncomplicated surgery in an operating theater was often attended by one surgeon, one or two assistants, scrub and circulating nurses, and a fully trained anesthesiologist. At the same time, however, for the birth of a baby there may be one physician, one nurse, and inadequate or haphazard anesthesia coverage. Many obstetric suites had to make do with older-generation anesthesia machines and monitors no longer considered suitable for nonobstetric anesthesia. Anesthesiology-provided epidural services and dedicated full-time anesthesia coverage were the exception rather than the rule for labor and delivery. When anesthesia service was available, it often was provided by anesthesia personnel with little training or interest in the special problems of the obstetric patient.

With the escalation of medical liability crises, particularly in obstetrics and anesthesiology, the medical community has been forced to focus attention on the quality of care provided to obstetric patients. In an effort to improve the quality of care for obstetric patients we must take every opportunity to identify and understand the price one pays for providing obstetric anesthesia. This chapter hopes to point out the expected consequences of labor and delivery analgesia and anesthesia while identifying and explaining the complications associated with obstetric anesthesia. In this way we learn from experience and improve the safety and efficacy of anesthetic care.

Available information for the study of complications can be derived from national maternal mortality statistics, clinical audits, case reports, and a variety of experimental studies. When looking at such data one must always remember that data collected from individual sites may not be applicable to all venues. The data may come from centers of excellence where the standards of practice, skill of the staff, and the patient population served may be unique to that institution. Certainly the proportion of trainees to fully trained staff has dramatic impact on the incidence of complications. Moreover, complication rates tend to rise and fall as practice techniques change or improve. How the data are collected also influences complication incidences. Recollections are not reliable. Poor documentation and recording of even the most basic information by anesthesiologists makes data collection even more difficult. This problem was highlighted in a study by Brown and Russell[3] that was designed to discover the extent of use of general, epidural, and spinal anesthesia for elective and emergency cesarean section. Although only the simplest information was requested, 65% of the respondents were unable to respond even in part. One must appreciate how much more difficult it is to discover the frequency of complications, when even denominator data do not exist. To obtain meaningful information about complication rates one must rely on carefully designed prospective audits in which attention to completeness is foremost. With this in mind, the authors will use the available literature in an attempt to shed some light on the frequency of naturally occurring and iatrogenic complications in the field of obstetric anesthesia.

One source of data to which anesthesiologists should pay particular attention is the Closed Claims Project established by the American Society of Anesthesiologists (ASA).[4] We have dedicated a section of this chapter exclusively to this information. The data from this project are an accumulation of insurance claims closed against anesthesiologists since the project's inception in 1985. The importance of these data to anesthesiologists is that they highlight the injuries that result in complaints by patients. The ASA Closed Claims Project provides an ongoing source of information about liability risks in obstetric anesthesia.[5]

I. CHANGES IN OBSTETRIC ANESTHESIA PRACTICE

One of the critical elements in avoiding complications of obstetric anesthesia is making available qualified, fully trained anesthesiologists. A study commissioned by the Committee on Obstetric Anesthesia of the ASA and the Liaison Committee for Obstetrics and Gynecology of the American College of Obstetricians and Gynecologists in 1981 provided a description of anesthesia practices in labor and delivery units across the United States.[2] A decade and a half ago anesthesiologists were available full-time in only 21% of all hospitals, and on nights and weekends in only 15%. Even in the larger hospitals, obstetricians provided a significant portion of the regional anesthesia used for labor and delivery. The most commonly used forms of pain relief during labor were parenteral narcotics, barbiturates, tranquilizers, or a combination thereof. Nearly 50% of all cesarean sections were performed under general anesthesia and only 44% of these were done under the direction of an anesthesiologist. During this same time, 25% percent of newborn resuscitations were performed by staff other than pediatricians or anesthesiologists. The study concluded that the availability of obstetric anesthesia personnel must be improved if the quality of care were to be improved and the complications of obstetric anesthesia reduced.

In 1992, a full decade later, the 1981 survey was repeated by Hawkins et al.[6] The study contrasts the characteristics of the obstetric anesthesia work force and the types of obstetric analgesia and anesthesia delivered in 1981 versus 1992. In 1992, epidural analgesia for labor was performed more often by or under the direction of an anesthesiologist (Table 24-1). Fewer than 5% of epidural anesthetics for labor were administered by obstetricians, compared to 30% in 1981. Likewise, obstetricians are no longer providing their own anesthesia for cesarean sections, with 96% of the anesthetics in the larger obstetric units being delivered by or directed by anesthesiologists. Concerns about medicolegal liability may have been the primary reasons obstetricians no longer provide their own anesthesia for cesarean sections. Overall, the type and availability of obstetric analgesia and anesthesia have improved, but there continues to be room for considerable improvement in staffing patterns. There has been an increased availability of regional techniques in the provision of labor analgesia and cesarean section anesthesia in the past decade (Table 24-2). Far fewer parturients receive no analgesia, and the use of epidural analgesia for labor has more than doubled. Anesthesiologists have been made aware of the increased risks involved in general anesthesia for the parturient because of airway difficulties and aspiration. The use of general anesthesia for cesarean delivery decreased from 35% in 1981 to 12% in 1992 in the largest services, and from 46% to 22% in the smallest services, a major improvement. The percentage of women receiving regional anesthesia for cesarean births increased, with the use of epidural anesthesia approximately doubling. Changes that have occurred in obstetric anesthesia practice are generally positive, but more active participation by anesthesiologists, especially in the smallest delivery services, is still needed.

II. MATERNAL MORTALITY

The *Report on Confidential Enquiries into Maternal Mortality in England and Wales* provides one of the

Table 24-1. Personnel providing epidural analgesia for labor and anesthesia for cesarean section, 1981 and 1992

	Hospitals with 1500 births		Hospitals with 500-1499 births		Hospitals with <500 births	
	1981	1992	1981	1992	1981	1992
Labor						
Anesthesiologist*	70%	95%	61%	79%	35%	42%
Independent CRN†	4%	4%	8%	16%	10%	55%
Obstetrician	26%	0%	31%	5%	46%	3%
Cesarean section						
Anesthesiologist*	90%	96%	81%	88%	51%	41%
Independent CRNA†	7%	4%	15%	12%	36%	59%
Obstetrician	3%	0%	4%	0%	9%	0%

From Hawkins JL, Gibbs CP, Orleans M, et al: *Anesthesiology* 87:135, 1997.
*Personally performed or medically directed resident or CRNA.
†Not medically directed by an anesthesiologist.
CRNA, Certified registered nurse anesthetist.

Table 24-2. Types of analgesia provided for patients in labor and anesthesia provided for patients undergoing cesarean section, 1981 and 1992

	Hospitals with 1500 births		Hospitals with 500-1499 births		Hospitals with <500 births	
	1981	1992	1981	1992	1981	1992
Labor						
None	27%	11%	33%	14%	45%	33%
Parenteral	52%	48%	53%	60%	37%	48%
Paracervical	5%	2%	5%	4%	6%	7%
Spinal	0%	4%	0%	4%	0%	4%
Epidural	22%	51%	13%	33%	9%	17%
Cesarean section						
Epidural	29%	54%	16%	45%	12%	29%
Spinal	33%	35%	35%	40%	37%	49%
General	35%	12%	45%	15%	46%	22%

From Hawkins JL, Gibbs CP: Orleans M, et al: *Anesthesiology* 87:135, 1997.

most comprehensive and accurate sources of information concerning maternal mortality. Each maternal death is reviewed carefully by an obstetric assessor and since 1973 by an anesthetic assessor (if an anesthetic was given). The cause of death is determined and classified using the ICD-9 (International Classification of Diseases, 9th Division) scheme. These reports have been compiled for 3-year periods beginning in 1952. Maternal death usually is defined as the death of a woman while pregnant or within 42 days of termination of pregnancy from any cause related to or aggravated by the pregnancy or its management but not from accidental or incidental causes. This arbitrary time limit has been shown to miss as many as 17% of deaths from maternal causes.[7] For this reason, recent authors have extended the time period to 90 days[8,9] or even 1 year.[10,11]

Although maternal mortality, defined as the number of maternal deaths per 100,000 (or 10,000) live births, has decreased dramatically in the last 50 years, deaths of pregnant women continue to be an important public health concern. Women continue to experience preventable pregnancy-related deaths,[12] and certain groups of women continue to be at greater risk of death. Older parturients and parturients of the black race, who were at increased risk of pregnancy-related death some 50 years ago, remain at greater risk today. For example, the cause-specific pregnancy-mortality ratio for cardiomyopathy was 5.9 times greater in black women than in white women, and the mortality from anesthesia was 6.6 times greater for black women.[13]

The maternal mortality in the United States was reported as 83 per 100,000 live births in 1950, but by 1984 it had declined to 7.8 per 100,000.[8] The mortality rate continued to make a small decline in 1987 to 7.2 but increased to 10 in 1990.

One of the first comprehensive presentations of maternal mortality in the United States was reported in 1985 by Kaunitz et al.[11] Data for the years 1974 to 1978 were compiled from various sources, including maternal death certificates identified by the National Center for Health Statistics and state health departments and from state maternal mortality reports. The leading causes of death, excluding those associated with abortive outcomes, were pulmonary embolism of all types, hypertensive disease of pregnancy, obstetric hemorrhage, obstetric infection, cerebrovascular accidents, and anesthetic complications. The data from England and Wales for 1976 to 1978 are similar except that anesthetic complications were responsible for 12.4% of maternal deaths, compared to the 4% reported by Kaunitz et al (Table 24-3). Kaunitz et al[11] speculated that because of medicolegal concerns, some anesthetic-related deaths may have been attributed to other (unavoidable) causes, such as amniotic fluid embolism. Although anesthesia is by no means the leading cause, it clearly ranks among the main causes of maternal death.

The most recent comprehensive data on material mortality in the United States are from Berg et al.[13] Data were compiled from the Centers for Disease Control and Prevention's Pregnancy-Related Mortality Surveillance System. The leading causes of pregnancy-related death are now hemorrhage, embolism, and hypertensive disorders of pregnancy (Fig. 24-1). Death from anesthesia is the sixth leading cause of pregnancy-related mortality in the United States. The cause-specific pregnancy-related mortality ratio for deaths from anesthesia decreased 47%,

Table 24-3. Major causes of maternal deaths in the United States and in England and Wales*

| | United States | | England and Wales | | | | | |
| | 1974–1978 | | 1976–1978 | | 1979–1981 | | 1982–1984 | |
	No.	%	No.	%	No.	%	No.	%
Embolism								
Thrombotic	271	10.9	43	19.8	23	12.9	25	18.1
Amniotic	189	7.6	11	5.1	18	10.1	14	10.1
Hypertensive disease of pregnancy	421	17.0	29	13.4	36	20.2	25	18.1
Obstetric hemorrhage	331	13.4	24	11.1	14	7.9	9	6.5
Obstetric infection	199	8.0	15	6.9	8	4.5	2	1.4
Anesthesia	98	4.0	27	12.4	22	12.4	18	13.0

Data from Kaunitz AM, Hughes JM, Grimes DA, et al: *Obstet Gynecol* 65:605, 1985; Turnbull A, Tindall VR, Beard RW, et al: *Report on confidential enquiries into maternal deaths in England and Wales 1982-1984*, London, 1989, Her Majesty's Stationary Office.
*The major causes of maternal deaths in the United States and England are shown. The actual numbers and percentages of all maternal deaths are indicated. Some figures in the data from London and Wales differ from previously published data because of reclassification of some deaths in the most recently published report.

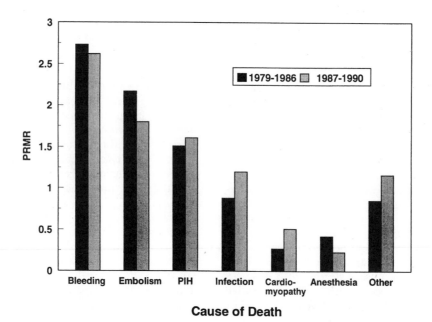

Fig. 24-1. Cause-specific pregnancy-related mortality ratio *(PRMR)* for 1979 to 1986 and 1987 to 1990, United States. *PRMR*, Pregnancy-related deaths per 100,000 live births. (From Berg CJ, Atrash HK, Koonin LM, et al: *Obstet Gynecol* 88:161, 1996.)

whereas the ratio for deaths from cardiomyopathy increased by approximately 70% and the ratio for deaths from infection increased by 36%. It appears we have made some progress in the delivery of obstetric anesthesia care.

It is informative and worthwhile to look in detail at the causes of obstetric deaths associated with anesthesia. Hawkins et al[14] characterized the obstetric anesthesia deaths in the United States by specific causes, the relationships of these deaths to the type of anesthetic, and the type of obstetric procedure for the time period 1979 to 1990. Anesthesia-related deaths (at least 82%) occur primarily during cesarean section. The cause of anesthetic death was directly related to the type of anesthetic administered (Table 24-4). Airway management issues, which included aspiration, induction or intubation problems, inadequate ventilation, and respiratory failure, were associated with 52% of the deaths in which general anesthesia was administered. Regional anesthesia was being administered in about 25% of the anesthesia-related deaths. Most deaths (70%) occurred in women receiving epidural anesthesia; the remainder were associated with spinal anesthesia. These deaths usually were the result of local anesthetic toxicity or an inadvertent high spinal or epidural. The type of anesthesia resulting in maternal deaths changed during the 12-year study period. After 1984 there was an abrupt decrease in deaths due to regional anesthesia, and the number of deaths associated with general anesthesia remained nearly unchanged (Fig. 24-2). The latter finding is discouraging given the marked decrease in the use of general anesthesia in the last decade. However, the increased relative risk of general anesthesia over regional anesthesia may be the result of the fact that regional anesthesia is being used for lower-risk elective procedures. General anesthesia is often used in emergency situations, in patients for whom regional anesthesia is difficult to administer (morbid obesity), or when regional anesthesia is contraindicated (coagulopathy or preeclampsia), a hypothesis supported

by Endler et al as well.[8] The rapid decline in maternal mortality has been attributable to fewer deaths because of infection, hemorrhage, and preeclampsia.

Mortalities related to anesthesia have tended to parallel the overall decline in maternal mortality.[15] Although the percentage of deaths attributable to anesthesia in England and Wales has trended upward since 1952 (Table 24-5),[16] the actual number of deaths from anesthesia reported in the *Report on Confidential Inquiries into Maternal Deaths in England and Wales* has declined since 1952. Thus given the increase in number of anesthetics administered for cesarean section, labor, and legal abortion, one must conclude that there has been an impressive reduction in the overall risk of anesthetic-related maternal death.[16]

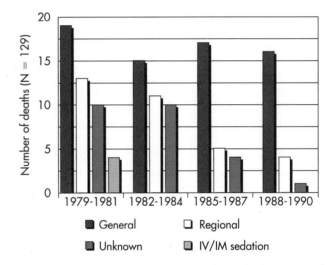

Fig. 24-2. Anesthesia-related maternal deaths by types of anesthesia, United States, 1979 to 1990. *IV/IM,* Intravenous/intramuscular. (From Hawkins JL, Koonin LM, Palmer SK, et al: *Anesthesiology* 86:277, 1997.)

Table 24-4. Causes of anesthesia-related deaths during obstetric deliveries: United States, 1979-1990

Causes of death	General anesthesia (*n* = 67)	Regional anesthesia (*n* = 33)	IV/IM sedation (*n* = 4)	Unknown anesthesia (*n* = 25)	Total No.	Total %
Airway problems						
Aspiration	33%	—	25%	24%	29	23
Induction/intubation problems	22%	—	—	—	15	12
Inadequate ventilation	15%	—	50%	16%	16	12
Respiratory failure	3%	—	—	—	2	2
Cardiac arrest during anesthesia	22%	6%	—	52%	30	23
Local anesthetic toxicity	—	51%	—	—	17	13
High spinal/epidural	—	36%	—	—	12	9
Overdosage	—	—	25%	—	1	1
Anaphylaxis	—	—	—	4%	1	1
Unknown	5%	6%	—	4%	6	5
Total*	100%	100%	100%	100%	129	100

From Hawkins JL, Koonin LM, Palmer SK, et al: *Anesthesiology* 86:277, 1997.
*Percentages may not add to 100.00 because of rounding.
IV, Intravenous; *IM,* intramuscular; —, no deaths reported in this category.

The leading causes of anesthetic deaths have changed over the years. Deaths caused by severe hypotension associated with spinal anesthesia have decreased, and now most deaths are associated with the induction of general anesthesia.[16-18] In recent years, difficult tracheal intubation has superseded inhalation of gastric contents as the leading cause of anesthesia-related maternal mortality.[19,20] This change may be attributable to the routine use of tracheal intubation, cricoid pressure, and antacid prophylaxis with general anesthesia in obstetrics. In the report from England and Wales covering the years 1982 to 1984, 10 of 18 deaths directly attributed to anesthesia were related to difficult intubation. Seven deaths were attributed to pulmonary aspiration, and two of these were precipitated by difficult intubation.[20] Other less common causes of death include misuse of drugs and difficulty with anesthesia equipment. In the 1982-1984 report, all anesthetic-related deaths were judged to be caused by some form of substandard care. One specifically noted factor was the frequency with which inexperienced anesthesiologists are involved in such cases. Several other risk factors that often are associated with anesthetic fatalities have been identified. In a review of anesthesia-related maternal mortality in Michigan for the years 1972 to 1984, 12 of 15 deaths were associated with the induction of general anesthesia under emergent conditions and an equal number were associated with obesity; in over half the cases hypertensive disease was a risk factor.[8]

III. CLOSED CLAIMS DATA

In 1985 the ASA Committee on Professional Liability began a study of insurance company files involving closed claims against anesthesiologists (see Chapter 31). In 1991 the subset of files involving obstetric anesthesia was analyzed and compared with the set of nonobstetric claims.[4] Although retrospective case review studies such as this can provide useful information about liability risk, they cannot provide information on the relative frequency of various complications because neither the total number of injuries nor the total number of anesthetics administered is known. The most recent analysis of the obstetric-related data was published in 1996, with a total ASA closed claims database of 3533 files.[5]

The most common injuries for which a file was opened were maternal death (19% of all obstetric claims), newborn brain injury (19%), and headache (15%) (Table 24-6). The anesthesiologists who reviewed the files be-

Table 24-5. Maternal deaths caused by anesthesia in England and Wales

Years	Maternal mortality per 100,000 total births	Number of deaths caused by anesthesia	Percentage of all deaths caused by anesthesia
1961-1963	26	28	4.0
1964-1966	20	50	8.7
1967-1969	16	50	10.9
1970-1972	13	37	10.4
1973-1975	11	31	13.2
1976-1978	11	30	13.2
1979-1981	11	22	12.2

Modified from Morgan M: *Br J Anaesth* 59:842, 1987.

Table 24-6. Most common injuries in the obstetric anesthesia files*

	Total obstetric files (*n* = 434)	Regional anesthesia (*n* = 290)	General anesthesia (*n* = 133)	Cesarean section (*n* = 310)	Vaginal delivery (*n* = 124)
Maternal death	19% (83)	11% (31)‡	39% (52)	23% (71)‡	10% (12)
Newborn brain damage	19% (82)	18% (51)	21% (28)	17% (52)	24% (30)
Headache	15% (64)	21% (61)‡	2% (2)	10% (32)‡	26% (32)
Maternal nerve damage	10% (43)	13% (38)‡	4% (5)	10% (30)	10% (13)
Pain during anesthesia	9% (37)	12% (36)‡	0% (0)	11% (35)‡	2% (2)
Back pain	8% (36)	12% (36)‡	0% (0)	6% (18)†	15% (18)
Maternal brain damage	7% (32)	6% (17)	11% (14)	9% (29)‡	2% (3)
Emotional distress	7% (31)	8% (23)	6% (8)	7% (23)	6% (8)
Newborn death	6% (27)	6% (16)	6% (8)	6% (18)	7% (9)
Aspiration pneumonitis	5% (20)	1% (2)‡	14% (18)	5% (16)	3% (4)

From Chadwick HS: *Int J Obstet Anesth* 5:258, 1996 (*n* = 3533).
*The most common injuries in the obstetric files are shown in order of decreasing frequency. Percentages are based on the total files in each group. Some files indicated more than one injury and are represented more than once. In some files the type of anethetic was not recorded. Files involving brain damage include only patients who were alive when the file was closed.
†$p < 0.05$.
‡$p < 0.01$.

lieved that only 46% of the newborn brain injuries and 26% of the newborn deaths were in any way related to anesthetic care. When cases involving a claim for newborn injury only were excluded, the most common injuries were maternal death (23%), headache (18%), and nerve damage (12%) (Table 24-7). The high proportion (47%) of claims for minor injuries such as headache, pain during anesthesia, backache, and emotional distress illus-

trate that in the obstetric setting, even minor side effects and complications may result in litigation.

Much can be learned from analyzing the critical events that lead to the injuries resulting in an insurance company file being opened. In both the obstetric and nonobstetric files, damaging events related to the respiratory system were most common (Table 24-8). Difficult tracheal intubation and pulmonary aspiration were the most common of such events in the obstetric files. This finding is consistent with reports that these events are the leading causes of anesthetic-related maternal mortality. Convulsions, most caused by local anesthetic toxicity, were much more common in the obstetric claims (9%) than in the nonobstetric claims (2%) and are the single most common event leading to an injury in the obstetric claims. It is reassuring that the number of these claims has fallen off significantly since 1984. This is probably because of greater awareness of problems with systemic local anesthetic toxicity (especially bupivacaine toxicity) in parturients, the importance of appropriate monitoring, use of test doses, fractionating local anesthetic injections, and the recommendation to avoid bupivacaine 0.75% in obstetrics.

The obstetric files constitute 12% of the ASA closed claims database and accounted for 11% of the total number of payments made but 14% of the total dollars expended. Although the expenditure per claim was greater for the obstetric cases, the disproportion was not striking. For cases in which payments were made, the median payments were greater in the obstetric group (Table 24-9). This is not surprising because there are two patients at risk and because the average age of parturients and their infants is lower than that of patients in the nonobstetric files. Although there were fewer claims involving general anesthesia, they resulted in more severe

Table 24-7. Maternal injuries compared to similar injuries in the nonobstetric files*

	Maternal injury files (n = 356)	Non-obstetric files (n = 3099)
Maternal/patient death	23% (83)‡	36% (1111)
Headache	18% (64)‡	2% (50)
Maternal/patient nerve damage	12% (43)†	17% (523)
Pain during anesthesia	10% (37)‡	1% (27)
Back pain	10% (34)‡	1% (37)
Maternal/patient brain damage	9% (32)†	13% (403)
Emotional distress	9% (31)‡	4% (115)
Aspiration pneumonitis	6% (20)†	2% (58)

From Chadwick HS: *Int J Obstet Anesth* 5:258, 1996 (n = 3533).
*The most common maternal injuries in the obstetric anesthesia files are shown in order of decreasing frequency. Percentages are based on the total files in each group. Some files, especially those with a fatal outcome, had more than one injury and are represented more than once. Cases involving brain damage include only patients who were alive when the file was closed
†$p < 0.05$.
‡$p < 0.01$.

Table 24-8. Most common damaging events in the obstetric anesthesia files*

	Nonobstetric files (n = 3099)	Obstetric files (n = 434)	Obstetric regional (n = 290)	Obstetric general (n = 133)
Respiratory system	30% (914)†	18% (80)	6% (16)†	47% (63)
Difficult intubation	6% (181)	7% (30)	0.5% (1)†	22% (29)
Aspiration	2% (52)	4% (17)	1% (2)†	11% (15)
Esophageal intubation	6% (178)†	2% (10)	1% (2)	6% (8)
Inadequate ventilation/oxygenation	9% (266)†	2% (9)	2% (6)	2% (2)
Bronchospasm	1% (43)	2% (7)	1% (2)	4% (5)
Premature extubation	1% (42)	1% (3)	0% (0)	2% (3)
Airway obstruction	3% (82)†	0.5% (2)	1% (2)	0% (0)
Inadequate FIO₂	0.5% (5)	0.5% (2)	0.5% (1)	1% (1)
Convulsions	2% (45)†	9% (34)	12% (30)†	3% (4)
Equipment problems	10% (315)†	6% (27)	8% (23)	3% (4)
Cardiovascular system	9% (287)†	4% (18)	4% (13)	3% (4)
Wrong drug/dose	4% (113)	3% (13)	2% (6)	5% (7)

From Chadwick HS: *Int J Obstet Anesth* 5:258, 1996 (n = 3533).
*The most common damaging events in the obstetric files are illustrated in order of decreasing frequency. Percentages are based on the total files in each group. Specific damaging events were not identified in all cases. Some files indicated more than one damaging event, although only the most significant is listed. Statistical comparisons are made between obstetric and equivalent nonobstetric files as well as between obstetric regional and nonobstetric general anesthetics.
†$p < 0.01$.

Table 24-9. Payment data*

	Nonobstetric files (n = 3099)	Obstetric files (n = 434)	Obstetric regional (n = 290)	Obstetric general (n = 133)
No payment	33% (1018)†	39% (171)	44% (129)‡	28% (37)
Payments made	59% (1814)†	52% (224)	45% (130)‡	66% (88)
Median payment	$100,000‡	$200,000	$77,500‡	$345,426
Range	$15-$23.2 million	$675-$6.8 million	$675-$6.8 million	$750-$6 million

From Chadwick HS: *Int J Obstet Anesth* 5:258, 1996 (*n* = 3533).
*Payment frequency and dollar amounts (not adjusted for inflation) are illustrated. Percentages are based on the total number of files in each group and do not sum to 100% because of missing data. Statistical comparisons are made between payment distributions for obstetric and nonobstetric claims and for obstetric regional and obstetric general anesthetics. Claims with no payments were excluded for calculations of median payment and range.
†$p < 0.05$.
‡$p < 0.01$.

injuries and higher payments than the claims involving regional anesthesia.

IV. MATERNAL COMPLICATIONS

A. Maternal pathophysiology and pharmacology

Pregnancy, in and of itself, is accompanied by many physiologic alterations that increase the risk of maternal complications. In some instances complications may be difficult to ascribe to a specific cause that is anesthetic related or attributable to inherent risks associated with pregnancy. The anesthesiologist who provides care for obstetric patients must be aware of the physiologic alterations of pregnancy, the medical risks associated with pregnancy and delivery, and the risks associated with anesthetic interventions and how these are modified in the pregnant patient.

1. Bleeding. Obstetric hemorrhage ranks as the leading cause of maternal mortality.[13] Conditions associated with an increased risk of bleeding include abruptio placentae, placenta previa, prior cesarean delivery (especially if associated with an anterior placenta), uterine atony, uterine rupture, retained placenta, and coagulation disorders. Although obstetric hemorrhage is not considered an anesthetic complication, when anesthetic care is involved, the anesthesiologist must share responsibility for assessing risk of hemorrhage, ensuring availability of blood and blood products, and establishing a mechanism to recruit additional help if needed. Primary responsibility for ensuring adequate venous access and appropriate replacement of fluids and blood components must be assumed by the anesthesiologist. In the presence of coagulopathy, the anesthesiologist must consider the risks associated with regional anesthetic procedures, central venous catheter insertion, and potential for unexpected bleeding with obstetric procedures.

2. Embolism. Pulmonary embolism is the second leading cause of maternal mortality, with thromboembolism being most common.[13] The hypercoagulability associated with pregnancy and the sluggish venous blood flow in the pelvis and lower extremities predispose the parturient to deep venous thrombosis and thromboembolism.[21] Massive pulmonary embolism of any type results in sudden hypotension and cardiac collapse. Smaller embolic events can present with a variety of nonspecific signs and symptoms including dyspnea, tachypnea, hypoxemia, cough, and rales. Amniotic fluid embolism is considered to be a rare and usually fatal complication of pregnancy[22]; respiratory distress, cyanosis, and cardiovascular collapse may occur rapidly. Unlike with other forms of embolism, disseminated intravascular coagulation is believed to accompany amniotic fluid embolism.[22] If a central venous or pulmonary artery catheter is in place, it may be possible to confirm the diagnosis by recovering fetal squamous cells, fat from vernix caseosa, or lanugo hair. Some authors believe that embolism of fetal or placental tissue may be much more common than previously believed.[23,24] Air embolism, once believed to be a very rare complication in obstetrics, has been detected using precordial Doppler monitoring in 11% to 52% of cesarean deliveries.[25,26] Malinow et al[26] found that chest pain and dyspnea were closely associated with evidence of air embolism. Because of the nonspecific nature of signs, symptoms, and results of diagnostic tests, it may not always be clear whether a pulmonary or cardiac problem was the result of an embolic event or some other cause. Acute cardiac failure, pulmonary aspiration, and drug reactions may mimic pulmonary embolism. In the event of death, an autopsy may be necessary to confirm the diagnosis.

3. Tocolysis. Modern tocolytic agents such as the β-mimetics (terbutaline and ritodrine) and magnesium sulfate allow obstetricians to manage preterm labor or temporarily stop labor for maternal or fetal indications. These drugs can have potent physiologic effects that may complicate anesthetic management. Although it is the β_2 effect that is responsible for inhibition of uterine activity, all commonly used β-mimetic tocolytic agents have some β_1 activity. Schneider, Jonas, and Tejani[27] studied 32 women receiving ritodrine as therapy for preterm labor and found cardiac symptoms in 31%, significant arrhythmias in 10% to 20%, and electrocardiogram (ECG) changes consistent with ischemia in 10% to 20%.[27] Pulmonary edema has also been associated with the use of tocolytics.[28] The pathophysiologic processes involved are not clear, but risk factors include preeclampsia, multiple gestation, preexisting cardiac or pulmonary disease, and signs of infection. Anesthesiologists should look for decreasing hematocrit without bleeding, dyspnea, tachypnea, wheezing, and cough. Particular consideration should be given to appropriate monitoring, careful fluid balance, and choice of anesthetic agents.[29] Halothane should be avoided because of its propensity to sensitize the heart to epinephrine-induced premature ventricular beats.

4. Pregnancy-induced hypertension. Pregnancy-induced hypertension (PIH) affects up to 30% of pregnancies in some populations[30,31] and is the third leading cause of maternal mortality in the United States.[13] Most of these deaths occur in patients with preeclampsia or eclampsia, which affects about 7% of all pregnancies.[32] Preeclampsia is characterized by the triad of hypertension, proteinuria, and generalized edema, usually occurring after the twentieth week of gestation. The proximate cause of death in half of these cases is intracranial hemorrhage or cerebral edema.[33] Despite the prevalence of this disease, little is known about its cause. The peripartum period is the time of greatest risk for the parturient.

Preeclampsia involves many pathophysiologic alterations that can pose particular problems for the anesthesiologist. Coagulation problems are common and can include decreased platelet count, abnormal platelet function, and decreased fibrinogen.

Thrombocytopenia occurs in 18% of women with preeclampsia,[34] and even those without thrombocytopenia may have prolonged bleeding times.[34,35] Preeclampsia is the most common cause of consumptive coagulopathy in the obstetric population, but usually it is not severe.[36] The anesthesiologist must pay particular attention to the risks associated with regional anesthetic procedures as well as risks of hematoma associated with placement of central venous and pulmonary artery catheters.

Hypertension, by definition a hallmark of preeclampsia, may be severe and can present problems in anesthetic management. Of particular concern is the potential for an exaggerated hypertensive response to tracheal intubation. This could lead to intracranial hemorrhage, the leading cause of mortality in preeclamptic women,[33] transtentorial herniation in the presence of cerebral edema,[37] or pulmonary edema caused by acute left ventricular failure.[38]

Another characteristic of preeclampsia is generalized edema often accompanied by intravascular volume depletion and hemoconcentration. Sympathetic blockade associated with regional anesthesia can quickly lead to hypotension and fetal distress. For this reason, some recommend against the use of epidural anesthesia in patients with preeclampsia or eclampsia.[39] However, others have pointed out the advantages of epidural analgesia, particularly in preeclamptic women. These include maternal analgesia without the need for systemic depressant drugs, reduced maternal catecholamine concentrations,[40] improved placental blood flow,[41] and the ability to facilitate obstetric procedures. Careful attention must be given to restoring adequate intravascular fluid volume before and during onset of epidural block. This process must be undertaken with great care because of the risk of precipitating pulmonary edema[42] or cerebral edema.[37,43] However, epidural analgesia can be used safely, even in many severely preeclamptic patients, by careful titration of intravascular volume and epidural local anesthetic.[44] In some patients this may require a central venous or pulmonary artery pressure catheter in addition to the usual monitors.

5. Aortocaval compression. Aortocaval compression, although not a complication of anesthetic care, can modify actions of anesthetics to increase the likelihood of adverse outcomes. Supine hypotension syndrome in pregnancy was first described in 1953.[45] Ten percent to 15% of patients at term develop hypotension, tachycardia (or bradycardia), and sometimes nausea when they are supine. Although only a minority of patients become hypotensive, up to 90% have decreased venous return and decreased cardiac output because of compression of the inferior vena cava by the gravid uterus.[46] Most patients are able to compensate for the decrease in cardiac output by increasing systemic vascular resistance. When this compensatory mechanism is attenuated, as with epidural block, the result can be unexpected and profound hypotension. Because uterine perfusion is in large measure pressure dependent, even modest degrees of hypotension may not be well tolerated by the fetus.[47] Even in the absence of hypotension, the increased systemic vascular resistance or direct compression of the aorta by the uterus may result in decreased uterine perfusion and may adversely affect fetal well-being. Maintaining laboring women in the supine position is associated with a progressive decrease in fetal blood pH. We continue to be amazed at how often, even in the modern tertiary care center, the effects related to aortocaval compression are allowed to occur and go unrecognized by trained health care professionals.

B. Complications associated with general anesthesia

The majority of anesthetic deaths in the obstetric population are associated with general anesthesia. The two main causes of these deaths are failure to intubate the trachea and inhalation of gastric contents.

1. Aspiration of gastric contents. Aspiration of gastric contents is the only cause of maternal death that has not declined in the last 20 years,[48] accounting for 6% to 22% of the anesthetic-related deaths in nonpregnant patients and 28% to 36% of maternal deaths.[49]

Pregnancy increases the threat of aspiration. Gastric emptying is decreased after the thirty-fourth week of pregnancy because of mechanical displacement of the gastroesophageal junction and pylorus and the combined effects of increased plasma progesterone concentration[50] and decreased plasma concentrations of the hormone motilin,[51] which result in slowed gastric motility. Gastric motility is also slowed by the pain of labor, fear, apprehension, and the use of opioids for treating labor pain. Roberts and Shirley[52] found that 25% of women undergoing cesarean section may be at risk for aspiration of acid gastric contents, regardless of the interval between the last meal and the onset of labor.

Antacids increase gastric fluid pH and should reduce the risk of acid-aspiration injury. However, Gibbs et al[53] demonstrated that dilute solutions of particulate antacids introduced in the lungs of dogs produce acute pulmonary injury comparable to that produced by instillation of acid. Recent studies using 0.3 molar sodium citrate, a nonparticulate antacid, have demonstrated it to be effective for increasing gastric pH.[54,55] A disadvantage of sodium citrate is its brief duration of effectiveness (2 to 3 hours), necessitating its use shortly before induction of anesthesia.

Blocking gastric histamine (H_2) receptors reduces gastric volume and acidity without adversely affecting the neonate.[56,57] However, there has been concern that the pharmacokinetic interaction between H_2 antagonists and local anesthetics might lead to inhibition of local anesthetic metabolism, resulting in local anesthetic toxicity.[58,59] This concern applies less to ranitidine than to cimetidine, and less to bupivacaine than to lidocaine. Dailey et al[60] suggest that the cimetidine-lidocaine interaction may not be as clinically important as was first believed. Nonetheless, ranitidine may be the preferred H_2 blocker because its duration of action exceeds that of cimetidine and it is less likely to interfere with hepatic metabolism.

Emptying the stomach has been suggested to be useful in the prevention of pulmonary aspiration. However, Brock-Utne et al[61] found that, in addition to being unpleasant, gastric suction by means of a large-bore tube does not guarantee an empty stomach or decrease the number of patients at risk from acid aspiration. Metoclopramide may be a useful adjunct to decrease the risk of aspiration because it increases lower esophageal sphincter tone, speeds gastric emptying, and does not adversely affect the neonate.[62,63] At least 15 minutes is required for metoclopramide to reduce gastric volume.[64]

In summary, an H_2-receptor antihistamine combined with a nonparticulate antacid, such as sodium citrate, seems to be most effective at minimizing the risk of acid aspiration.[65] Remember that no drug or combination of drugs removes completely the risk of acid aspiration.

2. Difficult or failed intubation. Difficulty with tracheal intubation during anesthetic induction is a life-threatening situation. There is little doubt that the trachea of obstetric patients may be more difficult to intubate than that of their nonobstetric counterparts. The parturient, especially the preeclamptic, may have pharyngeal and laryngeal edema.[66,67] The airway mucosa is hyperemic and prone to bleeding. Large breasts may impair proper laryngoscope positioning for visualization of the cords and hamper proper application of cricoid pressure. Improperly applied cricoid pressure can distort or displace laryngeal anatomy or occlude the esophagus inadequately. Additionally, the thorax may be lifted into an unusual position by a hip wedge. Finally, there is a tendency to attempt tracheal intubation before the muscle relaxant has taken full effect.

Difficult tracheal intubation, often unexpected, has been identified as one of the most common contributory factors to anesthetic-related maternal deaths. The risk of failed intubation in the obstetric population has been reported to be as great as 1 in 300 undergoing cesarean section.[68] A number of attempts have been made to predict patients in whom tracheal intubation will subsequently prove to be difficult.[69,70] Moving even just a few patients from the unanticipated difficult airway category to the anticipated difficult airway category would reduce the risk of injury to the parturient significantly. One of the few studies of risk analysis of factors related to difficult intubation in the obstetric patient was performed by Rocke et al.[71] Factors identified as predictive were Mallampati class, short neck, receding mandible, and protruding maxillary incisors. It would behoove all obstetric anesthesia practitioners to review this report carefully.

To minimize the complications of failed intubation, the entire labor and delivery staff should be familiar with a failed tracheal intubation protocol. There are no hard and fast rules as to the techniques and steps one should use. New devices that have been found to be useful during difficult intubations and with which anesthesiologists should become familiar are the woven endotracheal tube introducer (Eschmann stylet)[72] and a jet ventilating device that may allow oxygenation or ventilation through a cricothyroid or cricotracheal membrane puncture (Sanders device).[73] Probably the single most popular device that has taken over the management of the unanticipated difficult obstetric airway is the laryngeal mask airway (LMA).[74,75] Placement of the LMA in patients in whom intubation or ventilation is not possible can be life-saving. Cricoid pressure may need to be released momentarily while the LMA is being placed, but it should be reestablished and maintained until the surgery is over and the mother is awake.

The parturient is prone to rapid desaturation because of increased oxygen consumption and reduced oxygen reserve caused by a reduced functional residual capacity.[76] Keep in mind that options may be limited because of the foreshortened time interval from apnea to desaturation. Preoxygenation is a standard technique for minimizing hypoxemia during induction. The use of pulse oximetry has led some to believe that 4 vital capacity breaths are as efficacious as 3 minutes of preoxygenation before induction.[77,78] Recent studies looking at denitrogenation as an end point of preoxygenation have shown that 8 to 10 vital capacity breaths or 3 full minutes of normal ventilation with the anesthetic system fully "charged" with oxygen are required for adequate denitrogenation.[65,79] There are few situations, even in obstetrics, that are so critical that even 30 seconds cannot be devoted to thorough denitrogenation before induction of anesthesia. In the event of inability to intubate the trachea, bag-mask ventilation with correctly applied cricoid pressure must be initiated promptly and a decision made whether to continue with the procedure or awaken the patient. Fig. 24-3 is an example of an algorithm used in the event of a failed tracheal intubation in the obstetric patient.

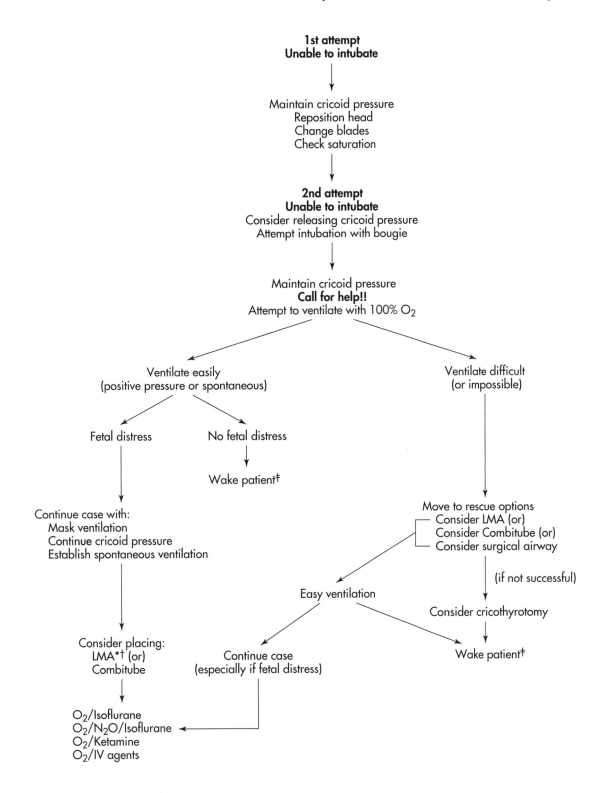

1st attempt
Unable to intubate

↓

Maintain cricoid pressure
Reposition head
Change blades
Check saturation

↓

2nd attempt
Unable to intubate
Consider releasing cricoid pressure
Attempt intubation with bougie

↓

Maintain cricoid pressure
Call for help!!
Attempt to ventilate with 100% O₂

Ventilate easily
(positive pressure or spontaneous)

Ventilate difficult
(or impossible)

Fetal distress   No fetal distress

Wake patient‡

Continue case with:
   Mask ventilation
   Continue cricoid pressure
   Establish spontaneous ventilation

Move to rescue options
   Consider LMA (or)
   Consider Combitube (or)
   Consider surgical airway

(if not successful)

Easy ventilation   Consider cricothyrotomy

Consider placing:
   LMA*† (or)
   Combitube

Continue case
(especially if fetal distress)

Wake patient‡

O₂/Isoflurane
O₂/N₂O/Isoflurane
O₂/Ketamine
O₂/IV agents

*May consider placing an endotracheal tube through the LMA; this maneuver must be practiced ahead of
   time.
†With the advent of the LMA, blind nasal intubation is not advocated.
‡After awake, consider fiberoptic intubation or regional anesthesia.

Fig. 24-3. Algorithm for managing a difficult intubation. *LMA*, laryngeal mask airway.

Related to the problem of difficult tracheal intubation is unrecognized esophageal intubation. The signs of esophageal intubation should be obvious, but anesthesiologists continue to be misled. Signs such as bilateral breath sounds, fogging of the endotracheal tube, and absence of sounds over the epigastrium are time-honored indications of proper endotracheal tube placement. However, the continuing presence of carbon dioxide in exhaled gas is the only absolute diagnostic test of correct placement of the endotracheal tube.[80,81] Every obstetric anesthetizing location must be equipped with a device for detecting exhaled carbon dioxide. These detectors can be as sophisticated as mass spectrometry or infrared capnography, or as simple as qualitative CO_2 detectors. Chemical indicators capable of detecting CO_2 in one or two breaths have become available (Fenem Airway Management Systems, New York).[82] Box 24-1 summarizes suggested precautions to be taken to minimize complications from the induction of general anesthesia in the parturient.

3. Awareness during general anesthesia. Maternal awareness is a concern that must be addressed when general anesthesia is used. The incidence of awareness in the obstetric population can vary from 7% to as high as 25%.[83-85] Anesthesiologists lack a generally accepted indicator of anesthetic adequacy, so estimating anesthetic depth is a daily challenge for anesthesiologists. This is particularly true in settings in which one wants to minimize anesthetic exposure, such as childbirth. Although vital signs are used clinically to monitor patients status during anesthesia, hemodynamic responses alone are often not adequate because many poorly predictive factors contribute to hemodynamic responses. Movement to skin incision has classically been used to judge anesthetic potency and depth, but obstetric anesthetic practice often involves the use of neuromuscular blocking agents. A recently introduced anesthetic depth monitor appears to have considerable potential in predicting anesthetic depth and recovery from anesthesia and thus may find a place in obstetric anesthesia. The bispectral analysis (BIS) of the electroencephalogram (EEG) is a signal-processing technique that has been proposed as a pharmacodynamic measure of anesthetic effects on the central nervous system (CNS).[86,87] Previous studies have demonstrated that BIS monitoring can be used to assess the hypnotic effects of anesthetics (Table 24-10).[88] Additional studies suggest that routine use of BIS monitoring can provide an early indication of change in anesthetic requirement and thus may result in improved anesthetic titration and better interpretation of the patient's analgesic state, and may allow a more rapid emergence from anesthesia.[89-92] However, there is still question as to whether BIS will provide an adequate indication of awareness during anesthesia.[93] The role of BIS in obstetric anesthesia is still to be clarified, but this device may eventually be shown to be a useful adjunct to our anesthetic monitors.

A major conflict arises when a general anesthetic is provided to the parturient to render her unconscious

---

Box 24-1   Suggested precautions for the induction of general anesthesia in the parturient

Familiarization with a failed intubation protocol for all delivery room personnel
Careful evaluation of the patient's airway, if difficult, consider:
   Awake tracheal intubation
   Regional anesthesia
Routine prophylaxis with a nonparticulate antacid; consider H_2-blocker, metoclopramide
Rapid sequence induction of anesthesia with properly applied cricoid pressure (Sellick's maneuver)
Immediate verification of proper endotracheal tube replacement by:
   Electronic end-tidal CO_2 monitor
   Fenem CO_2 detector
Assessment to rule out right main-stem endobronchial intubation
Awake tracheal extubation

---

and at the same time have minimal effects on the uterus and infant. There are three periods during which maternal awareness is likely to occur: during or shortly after tracheal intubation (usually an implication of inadequate dose of induction agent), at the time of delivery (an implication that an insufficient anesthetic agent has been provided), and during the insertion of the final skin sutures or staples (insufficient anesthesia in an attempt to provide rapid awakening).

The ideal induction agent has not been found for the obstetric patient. Thiopental in a dose of 4 mg/kg has been found to be safe for the mother and reliable at producing amnesia during induction.[94] However, because thiopental readily crosses the placenta, there are concerns of neonatal depression. Methohexital provides adequate early amnesia but confers no advantage over thiopental in its neonatal effects.[95] Ketamine in doses of 1 mg/kg has been shown to be an alternative to thiopental in reducing early maternal awareness with little or no neonatal depression.[96] A new induction agent, propofol, has recently been released in the United States. Fetal well-being, as judged by Apgar scores and cord blood gases, was not different from that of infants whose mothers underwent thiopental induction.[97] Propofol appears to efficacious and safe.

Minimizing drug-induced depression of the neonate can result in a high incidence of maternal awareness. Moir demonstrated that lack of maternal awareness could be ensured with an inspired mixture of 0.5% halothane in 50% oxygen and 50% nitrous oxide without harm to the neonate.[98] Similar results have been noted with equipotent concentrations of other potent inhaled anesthetics.[83] The incidence of awareness varies inversely with the concentration of nitrous oxide and the volatile anesthetic.[84] It is now apparent that a small amount of volatile anesthetic (0.5 minimum alveolar concentration) and nitrous oxide

Table 24-10. Bispectral analysis (BIS) range guidelines

BIS	Clinical endpoints and sedation ranges	Clinical situation
100	Awake/light to moderate sedation	Awake or resting state. Sedated for special procedures. Response to vigorous stimulation during surgery. Emergence from general anesthesia.
70	Light hypnotic state Very low probability of recall	Short surgical procedures requiring deep sedation or light anesthesia. Results from a multicenter study demonstrated that when the BIS was <70 there was very low probability of recall.*
60	Moderate hypnotic state Unconscious	Maintenance range during surgical procedures. Results from a multicenter study demonstrated that when the BIS was <60, subjects were unconscious.*
40	Deep hypnotic state	Barbiturate coma. Profound hypothermia. Burst suppression.
0	EEG suppression	

From *An overview of the clinical uses of the bispectral index,* Natick, Mass, Aspect Medical Systems.
*Ranges are based on results from several studies including a multicenter study of the BIS involving the administration of four commonly used anesthetics: propofol, midazolam, alfentanil, and isoflurane. *Anesthesiology* 86:836, 1997. References on file at Aspect.
Note: Anesthesia has many components. The BIS reflects the level of consciousness. To assess responsiveness, the degree of surgical stimulation and level of analgesia must be taken into consideration.
Note: BIS values and ranges assume that the EEG is free of artifacts that can affect its performance.

(50%) reaching the fetus during the interval between induction of anesthesia and delivery is of little or no consequence to the ultimate well-being of the infant.[99] The maternal stress response, likely to be evoked by awareness, may lead to reduced uteroplacental perfusion and is potentially much more harmful to the infant.[100]

4. Uterine atony. Uterine atony occurs in approximately 2% to 5% of all vaginal deliveries.[101] In a report by Gibbs of 501 consecutive maternal deaths in Texas, postpartum uterine atony was the leading cause of death in the parturient.[102] The risk of uterine atony is increased with high parity, multiple births, polyhydramnios, large infants, retained placenta, and general anesthesia. Local anesthetics have not been associated with uterine atony.

The volatile anesthetics produce a dose-related decrease in uterine contractility and tone, thereby increasing the risk of postpartum bleeding.[103] However, increased blood loss has not been consistently demonstrated with low-dose halothane (0.1% to 0.8%), enflurane (0.5% to 1.5%), or isoflurane (0.75%).[104,105] The uterine relaxation induced by low-dose volatile anesthetics can be overcome with intravenous oxytocin after delivery.[106] Fear of uterine atony should not preclude the use, at least initially, of volatile anesthetics during general anesthesia for cesarean section. If after delivery there is evidence of uterine atony, the volatile anesthetic can be discontinued, nitrous oxide concentration increased to 70%, and an opioid and benzodiazepine added to ensure maternal anesthesia and amnesia.

C. Complications associated with regional anesthesia

1. Global concerns. Two national surveys indicate that most of the anesthetic interventions for obstetric patients in this country involve regional anesthesia.[2,6] Not surprisingly, many complications have been associated with the use of regional anesthesia. Many complications are common to both spinal and epidural techniques, whereas others usually are associated with the particular type of regional anesthetic.

a. Hypotension. The most common causes of maternal death associated with regional anesthesia are mismanagement of hypotension and local anesthetic toxicity. Hypotension is undoubtedly the most common complication seen with spinal or epidural anesthesia in the parturient. One of the major reasons for hypotension is decreased venous return to the heart because of partial occlusion of the inferior vena cava by the gravid uterus.[46,107,108] Hypotension may be worsened by obvious or occult peripartum blood loss. In the face of a regional block, acute intravascular volume changes may be poorly tolerated because the normal physiologic compensatory mechanisms are blocked by sympathectomy.

Maternal organ systems will tolerate moderate degrees of hypotension. However, because the uterus is essentially a nonautoregulating organ,[109] uterine blood flow decreases linearly with decreased perfusion pressure. Because of this, the placenta may be inadequately perfused while the parturient remains asymptomatic. It is difficult to predict at what maternal blood pressure fetal asphyxia will develop. It appears that uteroplacental anatomy, baseline maternal blood pressure, and duration of hypoperfusion are all critical. Fetal bradycardias, acidosis, and low Apgar scores have been reported with maternal systolic blood pressures of less than 100 mm Hg for periods of 5 to 15 minutes.[47,110,111] Clinical experience has shown that signs of fetal distress often occur at systolic blood pressures greater than 100 mm Hg in hypertensive patients. On the other hand, fetuses of mothers who normally have systolic blood pressures of less than 100 mm Hg seem to tolerate this without difficulty.

Patients with PIH are at particular risk of becoming hypotensive with regional anesthesia. Reduced intravascular volume, which may be less than 80% of normal pregnant values,[112] predisposes these patients to significant hypotension with the onset of even partial sympathectomy. The risk of fetal distress is further compounded by the fact that these patients often have abnormal placental vasculature and uteroplacental insufficiency. Any intervention that may decrease maternal blood pressure, such as antihypertensive therapy or regional block, must be initiated in a slow, controlled fashion with attention to intravascular volume status.[44] Fetal heart rate monitoring, when available, should be used by the anesthesiologist in conjunction with more routine monitors to gauge the effects of anesthetic intervention.

To prevent potential complications to mother or fetus, the anesthesiologist must take all necessary steps to avoid hypotension in the obstetric patient. This includes avoiding aortocaval compression, providing adequate fluid preloading, and using vasopressor therapy when necessary. Ephedrine has been shown to have the least detrimental effect on uterine perfusion and is considered to be the vasopressor of choice in obstetric patients.[113] As a rule, a systolic blood pressure of 100 mm Hg should be used as a lower limit in previously normotensive patients. In the hypertensive patient, any sudden decrease in blood pressure greater than 20% should be treated. A recent clinical study in which low-risk patients were treated in accordance with this usual rule demonstrated that changes in maternal blood pressure were not correlated with any signs of fetal distress.[114]

b. High segmental blockade. Higher-than-anticipated blocks can be a cause of complications in the obstetric patient. The most common complication associated with high block is hypotension. If hypotension is severe, loss of consciousness will occur, resulting in loss of protective airway reflexes. Nausea and vomiting are commonly associated with hypotension and in the presence of depressed airway reflexes may lead to pulmonary aspiration of gastric contents. If neuraxial block extends into the cervical segments, respiratory insufficiency can result from intercostal and diaphragmatic paralysis.

There is controversy regarding local anesthetic requirement of pregnant patients having epidural or spinal anesthesia.[115] It is generally believed that the epidural and subarachnoid requirements of the parturient are approximately one third those of nonpregnant women.[116-118] In the case of epidural blocks this may be attributable to wider spread of anesthetic solution because of epidural venous engorgement. Similarly, spinal cerebrospinal fluid volume may be reduced, resulting in greater spread of anesthetic solution administered into the lumbar subarachnoid space. Recently, several studies have indicated that peripheral neuronal tissue in gravid animals and humans may be more sensitive to the effects of local anesthetics.[119,120] Although there is some controversy about the local anesthetic requirements for pregnant patients, it is evident from clinical experience that there is great variability in the extent of block achieved with usual doses of local anesthetic in parturients. It behooves the practitioner to be aware of potentially decreased anesthetic requirements and to take a conservative approach.

c. Neurologic injury
(1) NEUROPATHIES IN THE PERIPARTUM PERIOD. Among complications of childbirth, neurologic injury can result from both obstetric and anesthetic causes. Neurologic injuries were once a well-recognized consequence of childbirth, but the current preference of cesarean delivery over a potentially difficult vaginal delivery has resulted in pelvic entrapment neuropathies becoming much less common.[121] Regional anesthesia always carries some risk of neurologic injury; therefore a postpartum neurologic deficit in a patient having a regional anesthetic will inevitably focus suspicion on the anesthetic. The obstetric anesthesiologist must therefore be able to distinguish among symptoms of preexisting disease, symptoms attributable to pregnancy or delivery, and complications related to the anesthetic. Postpartum neurologic complications are much more likely to arise from obstetric or natural causes than from peripartum regional anesthesia. The incidence of neurologic complications after regional anesthesia is estimated at 1 in 11,000[122] to 1 in 20,000,[123] well below the 1 in 3000 that may be expected in parturients not having an anesthetic.[124]

Any form of neuritis may occur in pregnancy. Several excellent articles review both the common neuropathies of pregnancy and those associated with the administration of anesthesia in the parturient.[124-128] Although most neuropathies have unknown causes, some are attributable to unsuspected trauma, excessive weight gain, fluid retention during pregnancy, the hormonal changes of pregnancy, and underlying medical conditions often aggravated by pregnancy. Peripartum polyneuropathies are usually the result of pregnancy and are seldom seen as a result of anesthetic trespass. The differential diagnosis in patients with diffuse peripheral polyneuropathy is no different from that in the nonpregnant patient and includes metabolic disease, collagen vascular disease, and medications.

Mononeuropathies are the most troubling of the neuropathies for the obstetric anesthesiologist because they often mimic complications of general or regional anesthesia. Any of the cranial nerves can be affected. The brachial plexus may be compressed between the clavicle and first rib from the increased weight of the breasts and abdomen combined with sagging of the shoulder. Sensory loss, pain, and shoulder wasting may ensue. Neuropathy of the ulnar nerve, sometimes in association with median nerve involvement, has been described in the peripartum period. Full recovery usually occurs after delivery. Median neuropathy at the wrist (carpal tunnel syndrome), the most common mononeuropathy in the upper extremity, occurs in at least 7% of parturients.[129]

Neuropathy of the lateral femoral cutaneous nerve (meralgia paresthetica, meaning "paresthetic thigh pain") was first described by Burnhart and Roth in 1895.[129] Mild sensory loss to touch and pinprick with occasional hyperesthesia may develop; because this nerve is purely sensory, no motor impairment is seen. During pregnancy, symptoms usually begin in the last trimester.[130] The lateral femoral cutaneous nerve has a very long course and thus may be stretched by the increased weight and exaggerated lordosis of pregnancy.[131] The exact cause of damage to the nerve is unknown, but injury may occur inside the pelvic wall, as it passes beneath the inguinal ligament, or at the fascia lata. Symptoms may be permanent but most often resolve within 3 months after delivery. The femoral nerve may be injured during vaginal delivery, cesarean section, hysterectomy, or other lower abdominal procedures.[132,133] This nerve is vulnerable to compression from retractors positioned against the greater psoas muscle, from hemorrhage into the iliopsoas muscle, and from trauma as it leaves the abdomen adjacent to the femoral artery. The prognosis is good in most cases; however, on occasion there may be pain and persistent weakness for several months. Neuropathy of the obturator nerve is rare but may be caused by a difficult labor, hematoma, or compression from the fetal head or high forceps. Sciatic neuropathy may occur during pregnancy, particularly during the last trimester as the sacral plexus is compressed by the fetus.[134] Pain is sometimes severe enough to warrant bed rest. Permanent injury is rare, and symptoms clear quickly after delivery. The lateral peroneal nerve may be compressed as it crosses the fibular head by poorly positioned leg supports, resulting in foot drop.[126] Alternative theories for this nerve lesion include compression of the lumbosacral trunk, particularly after prolonged labor and midforceps delivery in women with platypelloid pelvises. Foot drop, in these circumstances, should be unilateral and on the same side as the infant's brow. Prognosis is good for complete resolution of this injury. Radiculopathies caused by a combination of physical effects of pregnancy (effect of relaxin on joint ligaments) and trauma (changing posture and weight associated with pregnancy) also are common. Radicular symptoms have been observed to appear during pregnancy in 39% of parous females with surgically proved lumbar disk protrusions,[135] most often involving the L5-S1 disk. Symptoms may occur at any time during pregnancy, labor, delivery, or the early postpartum period. Motor weakness may be severe.

Bladder dysfunction is common in the obstetric patient. Although bladder symptoms are common during pregnancy, nervous system lesions causing these symptoms are rare. Prolonged pressure on the pelvic nerves by the fetal head in the second stage of labor or during a difficult delivery can lead to partial denervation of the bladder, resulting in a hypotonic, distended bladder, with frequency and postvoid residual volume.

Backache often is attributed to spinal or epidural anesthesia. Grove[136] reports the incidence of backache after nonepidural vaginal deliveries to be 40% in patients with spontaneous deliveries and 25% in patients with instrumented deliveries. Crawford[137] reports an incidence of 45% in parturients treated with epidural anesthesia, which is only slightly greater than that in parturients not receiving epidural anesthesia in Grove's study.[136] It appears that the incidence of backache in the parturient is 30% to 40% regardless of whether regional or general anesthesia is used. The cause is probably related to ligamentous strain from pregnancy.

(2) ANESTHETIC-ASSOCIATED NEUROPATHIES. Nerve injury associated with general anesthesia in obstetrics can and does occur (see Table 24-6).[138] These injuries are not discussed here because they are covered elsewhere in this text. The complications from regional anesthesia are also not discussed in detail because they are covered in Chapters 3 and 4. However, the symptom complexes associated with obstetric anesthesia are discussed briefly.

Serious complications associated with epidural/spinal blockade in obstetrics are exceedingly rare.[139] Prolonged neural blockade attributable to local anesthetic action must be considered with any of the local anesthetic agents used for spinal or epidural anesthesia. However, prolonged neural blockade (greater than 48 hours) has been reported only after repeated epidural injections of 0.5% bupivacaine for labor.[140-142] Extended blockade in obstetric patients has been attributed to accumulation of highly lipid-soluble agents. The block usually resolves without long-lasting untoward effects.

Trauma to nerve pathways from spinal or epidural needles and catheters is extremely rare.[122,143] Obstetric factors are probably four to six times more likely than regional blockade to cause neuropathology.[144,145] Nerve root trauma is particularly unlikely if styletted catheters are not used.[146] If nerve roots are injured, symptoms may occur over the segment or segments involved, and symptoms usually resolve spontaneously. Sensory roots are more often affected than motor roots are. Nerve root injury is more common after spinal than after epidural anesthesia. Trauma to the spinal cord can be avoided if dural puncture or epidural placement is caudal to the conus medullaris (L1-L2). Nerve root trauma usually is heralded by severe lancing pain with needle placement, which, if elicited, should result in immediate withdrawal of the needle. Epidural and intrathecal catheters have been suspected of causing trauma to spinal roots. There is little objective evidence in the literature of trauma caused by an epidural catheter. The use of intrathecal catheters, particularly of the microcatheter design (26 to 32 gauge), at one time was quite common. Intrathecal catheters may be more likely to damage the spinal cord and roots of the cauda equina. In addition to the possibility of direct trauma, a recent article by Rigler et al[147] details four cases of cauda equina syndrome occurring after continuous spinal anesthesia using microcatheters. They postulate that the combination of maldistribution and a high dose of local anesthetic resulted in neurotoxic injury.[147] In addition, breakage of microcatheters has been reported. The risk of neurologic injury and loss of catheter tips with the use of subarachnoid catheters should not be treated lightly.

The anesthesiologist should have an organized and thorough approach to the patient presenting with neurologic symptoms. Questions that are helpful to ask include the following: What is the nature of the symptom (sensory, motor, both; unilateral, bilateral)? What is the location of the suspected lesion? Can it be explained on an anatomic and physiologic basis? Are there related medical conditions that might explain the symptoms? Are there circumstances surrounding the pregnancy, labor, and delivery that might be the cause of the suspected lesion (that is, protracted labor, difficult or instrument delivery, cesarean section, and use of retractors)? Were there any difficulties during the anesthetic that might explain the lesion? A careful physical examination should document sensory and motor deficits as either segmental or peripheral. The results of the history and physical examination will dictate the need for additional consultation and diagnostic tests.

d. Regional anesthesia in patients with coagulopathy. Coagulopathy has been considered an absolute contraindication to regional anesthesia in the obstetric patient.[148] This is especially true for labor analgesia, where there may be no clear medical indication for the procedure other than the relief of pain associated with a normal physiologic process. The risk of epidural, subdural, or subarachnoid hematoma with neuraxial block seems obvious, although it is difficult to quantify such risk. Hematomas may occur spontaneously even in the absence of risk factors.[149] Neuraxial hematoma formation has been reported as occurring after lumbar puncture, often in association with anticoagulation therapy.[150] However, no case reports can be found in which a regional anesthetic procedure in an obstetric patient with coagulopathy resulted in neurologic injury as a result of hematoma formation.[151] This may be because regional anesthetics are avoided in such patients or because such cases have not been reported in the literature.

Anesthetic interventions in obstetrics often are required on an urgent or emergent basis, often before laboratory results and coagulation studies are available. Retrospective studies indicate that a significant number of parturients have received epidural anesthetics with platelet counts being considerably below normal.[151,152] This can be a particular problem in preeclamptic patients who, in addition to thrombocytopenia, often have a defect in platelet function, which can prolong bleeding time.[35] None of the studies just mentioned have found neurologic injury as a result of neuraxial hematoma, even in the obstetric patient at risk. A review of the ASA closed claims database, containing over 250 closed claims involving obstetric anesthesia for the years 1976 to 1990, found no claims related to neuraxial hematoma formation. Although neuraxial hematoma is a devastating complication requiring immediate surgical decompression, the incidence appears to be very low. Prudence dictates avoiding regional procedures in parturients with abnormal coagulation parameters; however, in cases

where conduction anesthesia offers particular advantages, the benefits may outweigh the potential risks.[44,151]

e. Regional anesthesia in patients with infection. The potential for spreading infection to the neuraxis has been the main contraindication of regional anesthetic techniques in patients with active infections. Skin infections over the site of needle insertion might allow spread of infection to the epidural space or to the subarachnoid space. Vascular trauma during regional procedures may allow bloodborne organisms to seed infection in the epidural or subarachnoid space, resulting in epidural abscess or meningitis.

Epidural abscesses have usually been the result of osteomyelitis or spontaneous hematogenous spread, and the risks associated with epidural anesthesia seem to be very low.[153] Most cases related to regional anesthesia were reported in the early days of caudal anesthesia for labor.[154] Meningitis after regional anesthesia also is rare, although three cases were reported recently in association with epidural anesthesia. One case may have involved the introduction of bloodborne bacteria into the cerebrospinal fluid during unintentional subarachnoid puncture or during subsequent blood patching.[155] The second case involved an uncomplicated epidural anesthetic for labor and delivery, with subsequent meningitis caused by a bacterium common in dental caries.[156] In the third case, introduction of bacteria from the skin surface may have been the likely cause of meningitis.[156] In another recent case report, meningitis was described as occurring after obstetric spinal anesthesia for removal of a retained placenta.[157] In that case it was not clear whether the cause was chemical irritation or a partially treated bacterial infection. Although such cases are very rare, the potential for neuraxial infection, introduced either from the skin or from organisms in the blood, must be considered.

The use of regional anesthesia in patients with chorioamnionitis is controversial.[158,159] Because these patients often have positive blood cultures, the risk of seeding infection is a possibility. However, some anesthesiologists will initiate regional anesthetics in parturients with amnionitis if antibiotic therapy is being given and they are not grossly septic. This practice has not resulted in reports of epidural abscess or meningitis.

Similar concerns about spreading infection by needle trauma have been raised in pregnant patients with herpes infections. Herpes simplex virus type 2 (HSV-2) is an increasingly common infection in women of childbearing age. In the greater Seattle area, approximately 30% of women of childbearing age are seropositive for HSV-2, and 8% to 10% have symptoms consistent with recurrent outbreaks.[159a] Approximately 30% to 50% of women with a history of recurrent HSV-2 infections deliver by cesarean section.[160] Regional anesthesia seems to be safe in patients with recurrent HSV-2 infections,[21,161] perhaps because these recrudescences are not associated with viremia. However, because primary infections are associated with viremia and often severe generalized symptoms such as fever, lymphadenopathy, and headache, it is advisable to avoid regional anesthesia in patients with primary infections.

f. Pain and emotional injury. Examination of obstetric anesthesia closed claims files reveals that 47% of the injuries claimed were for headache, backache, pain during anesthesia, and emotional injury (see Table 24-7).[4] These problems rarely are considered to be significant anesthetic complications, but it is clear that many women are distressed sufficiently to initiate legal action. Most of these cases involved anesthesia for cesarean section, and most of the anesthetics involved were regional techniques. Obstetric patients may be at greater risk for some of these complications (such as postdural puncture headache [PDPH]) by virtue of age, gender, and the popularity of regional anesthesia in this setting. However, even allowing for a greater risk of such complications, there appear to be a disproportionate number of claims for minor injury in obstetric anesthesia compared to nonobstetric anesthesia. The reasons for this are not clear; however, postpartum emotional lability and depression[162,163] or unrealistic expectations may play a role. Birthing educators should include preparation for unexpected operative delivery, and anesthesiologists should compassionately but accurately describe the procedures and experiences that a woman may encounter during anesthesia for obstetric procedures.

2. Spinal anesthesia. In addition to the general concerns of regional anesthesia in the obstetric patient just outlined, two deserve particular emphasis with relation to spinal anesthesia. These are the risks of hypotension and PDPH.

a. Hypotension. As discussed previously, hypotension is of particular concern in the obstetric patient because of the need to maintain adequate uterine perfusion pressure. Spinal anesthesia can result in sudden and profound hypotension, especially in the hypovolemic patient, because of the rapidity with which sympathetic block develops. Intravascular volume status may be difficult to assess in the presence of occult hemorrhage (such as abruptio placentae) or in the patient with PIH. In such circumstances, the rush to provide an emergently needed anesthetic with a spinal block may result in maternal or fetal death. A review of all maternal deaths in Michigan directly related to anesthesia between 1972 and 1984 found that at least three and perhaps all four deaths in patients with spinal anesthetics were related to hypotension. Two of these patients had PIH.[8]

b. Postdural puncture headache. PDPH is a well-known complication of procedures in which the dura mater of the spinal cord is perforated. The rate of accidental dural puncture following epidural placement is on the order of 0.5% to 1%.[164,165] However, headache is also a common symptom in the early postpartum period, even in the absence of anesthesia. The incidence of postpartum headache may be as high as 30% to 40% at the end of the first postpartum week, but in many cases its cause is unknown.[166,167] Pregnancy can modify the course of several headache syndromes, so the incidence and severity of headache can be increased during the peripartum period. Box 24-2 lists causes of postpartum headache sometimes confused with PDPH.[168] When a headache occurs after spinal or epidural anesthesia, it must be considered a potentially serious complication and must be differentiated from other causes of headache in the postpartum period. Table 24-11 lists the clinical features found to be most useful in differentiating PDPH from other peripartum headaches.[166,169] However, the most distinguishing characteristic of a PDPH is its dependence on the position of

---

Box 24-2 Differential diagnosis for headache in the parturient

Acute migraine
Cluster headache
Tension (psychogenic) headache
Chronic paroxysmal hemicrania
Meningitis
Cortical vein thrombosis
Pseudotumor cerebri
Tumor
Preclampsi and eclampsia
Subarachnoid hemorrhage

Table 24-11. Clinical features of postdural puncture and postpartum headache

	Postdural puncture headache	Postpartum headache
Onset	Within first 5 days after dural puncture (90% within 3 days)	Between 3 and 6 days postpartum
Duration	Usually 2 or 3 days, seldom longer than 1 week	May last 12 hours
Characteristics	50% frontal 25% occipital 25% diffuse Severity dependent on patient position Throbbing in nature	Primarily bifrontal Patient position unimportant Continuous in nature
Associated symptoms	Blurred or double vision Photophobia Dizziness, tinnitus decreased hearing Nausea and vomiting Unresponsive to minor analgesics	Vision rarely affected Mild photophobia No auditory component Mild nausea and vomiting Responds to minor analgesics Previous family history common

the patient. Headache severity is always maximal when the patient is in the upright position and diminishes significantly, if not completely, when the patient is in the horizontal position. The caution of Bonica[170] continues to be applicable today: "A headache should not be attributed to spinal puncture unless it is brought on or aggravated by assuming the erect position and relieved by assuming the horizontal position or flexion and extension of the head."

The problem of PDPH is better avoided than treated. Obstetric anesthesiologists who want to include spinal anesthesia in their practices should be familiar with the factors that have been implicated in influencing the development of PDPH. These have been the subject of a number of reviews and include needle size (increasing incidence with larger diameter of needle), needle bevel orientation (higher incidence with perpendicular insertion to the longitudinal orientation of dural fibers), angle-of-needle approach to the dura (decreased incidence with more acute angle of approach), needletip design (lower incidence with pencil-point or conical-point needles), number of dural punctures (higher incidence with increased number of dural punctures), gender (higher incidence in women), age (higher incidence in younger patients), and prior PDPH (higher incidence in patients with a history of PDPH).[169,171] The obstetric patient is at particular risk of developing PDPH because these patients are young and female, and many experience a period of bearing down that appears to increase the headache incidence.[172] However, this latter finding has not been observed universally.[173]

PDPH usually occurs 1 to 5 days after dural puncture and characteristically persists for 3 to 5 days. On rare occasions the headache can last for months.[174,175] Because a PDPH is self-limiting and often disappears within 1 week,[169] initial treatment can be conservative. However, the incapacitating nature of this headache significantly impairs mother-infant bonding and the parturient's ability to care for her newborn. Analgesics (such as acetaminophen, codeine) may provide some relief until the headache resolves. Bed rest is advisable, because of the postural nature of the symptoms, but does not reduce the incidence of headache.[176,177] Prolonged bed rest may actually be contraindicated in the postpartum period because of the risk of deep venous thrombosis. In an effort to return the cerebrospinal fluid pressure to normal, fluids (3000 ml/day) by mouth or intravenously and abdominal binders have been recommended.[178] Epidural saline solution by bolus injection or continuous infusion has been shown in some studies to be effective in controlling the symptoms of PDPH.[172,179,180]

Caffeine has been used in managing PDPH. The cerebral vasoconstrictor activity of caffeine has been credited for the relief of symptoms in 80% of patients.[181] It has been shown to be an effective and inexpensive treatment both in intravenous and oral forms.[182-184] A typical treatment regimen is 500 mg caffeine sodium benzoate given over 4 hours by intravenous infusion or 300 mg caffeine given orally. One disadvantage of caffeine is that it may result in only temporary relief of symptoms.

The most effective treatment of PDPH appears to be the closure of the dural rent with the injection of autologous blood into the epidural space, "the epidural blood patch." The discovery of the efficacy of the epidural blood patch (EBP) in the treatment of PDPH by DiGiovanni and Dunbar in 1970[185] was a terrific boon to patients and anesthesiologists. EBP has been shown to be efficacious in 95% to 100% of patients.[186,187] There has been much discussion regarding the optimum volume of blood to use,[187-189] the level at which the blood patch should be performed,[190] and the optimal timing of the procedure after dural puncture. In one study, EBP within 24 hours had a failure rate of 71%, compared to 4% if performed after 24 hours.[189] However, in another study, prophylactic EBP was effective at preventing a significant number of PDPH.[191] Epidural blood patches have been shown to be effective months after dural puncture.[181,192] However, current practice at many institutions is to perform an epidural blood patch 24 to 48 hours after the onset of symptoms. Ten to 15 ml of autologous, nonheparinized blood is injected into the epidural space near the level of the suspected dural rent. Because epidural blood patches are simple, effective, and free of serious complications, there is little reason to delay treatment, particularly when headache is severe. However, the injection of blood into the epidural space is commonly associated with backache and mild signs of meningeal irritation. Potential complications, though very rare, include epidural infection, obliteration of the extradural space, and nerve root compression. Subarachnoid injection of blood can potentially result in adhesive arachnoiditis.

c. Transient neurologic symptoms. Since its first use in 1948, lidocaine has enjoyed widespread efficacy and success as an intrathecal agent for spinal anesthesia. Phillips et al[193] reported lidocaine's impressive safety in a prospective study of 10,440 patients. However, in 1991 case reports began to appear implicating 5% hyperbaric lidocaine in the development of cauda equina syndrome when used via microcatheters for continuous spinal anesthesia.[147,194] From the flurry of investigative reports that followed, three features seem to be inextricably associated with these neurologic complications: The resultant blocks were "patchy" and restricted to sacral distributions, lidocaine doses used (greater than 100 mg) far exceeded the usual doses used for single-injection spinal anesthesia, and maldistribution of the local anesthetic because of improper use of the microcatheter appeared to play an important role. In 1992 microcatheters were withdrawn from the North American market and the controversy surrounding 5% hyperbaric lidocaine seemed to be at an end.

In the wake of the microcatheter controversy, in 1993, yet another controversy surrounding 5% hyperbaric lidocaine surfaced. Schneider et al[195] reported four documented and six anecdotal instances of lumbosacral radiculopathy following single-dose subarachnoid injection of 5% hyperbaric (7.5% dextrose) lidocaine for various surgeries in the lithotomy position. The symptom complex has since become known as transient neurologic symptoms (or transient radicular irritation [TRI]) and is characterized by transient lumbosacral monoradicular cramping back, buttock or lateral thigh, and calf pain. The onset of these symptoms usually follows a symptom-free period and resolves completely within 3 to 14 days. The initial response to this report was to assume that what was being observed was guilt by association; that is, our sensitivity to such symptoms was heightened by the unfortunate circumstances surrounding the use of the microcatheters. However, since this initial report there have been numerous studies describing a similar complex of symptoms.[196,197] Hampl et al[198] observed the incidences of transient neurologic symptoms in a prospective, blinded, nonrandomized study in 270 gynecologic patients. About one-third of the patients who received 5% lidocaine complained of transient neurologic symptoms, whereas no patients in the group of patients receiving 0.5% hyperbaric bupivacaine complained of these symptoms. Similar randomized and nonrandomized studies confirmed these results.[199,200] Most recent studies report an incidence of transient neurologic symptoms in the range of 16% to 37%.[198,200] The lithotomy position has been suggested to be a potential contributory factor in the neurologic sequelae following the administration of 5% hyperbaric lidocaine for spinal anesthesia.

Animal studies have confirmed that hyperbaric 5% lidocaine and 0.5% tetracaine can cause neurotoxicity with irreversible nerve blockade, whereas 1.5% lidocaine or 0.75% bupivacaine may cause a prolonged blockage that is reversible.[201,202] The latter studies, in which the blockade was delayed but reversible did demonstrate evidence of neurotoxicity under histologic examination.[203] These changes may be indicative of the potential mechanism of transient neurologic symptoms.

In 1995, ASTRA distributed a "Dear Doctor" letter to practicing anesthesiologists acknowledging the reports of transient neurologic symptoms and revising their package insert, making the following recommendations:

- 5% lidocaine should be diluted with an equal volume of cerebrospinal fluid or preservative-free saline before injection.
- A maximum of 100 mg of lidocaine should be used for spinal anesthesia.
- The spinal needle should be removed and replaced if inadequate spread of anesthesia requires an additional dose.
- Spinal needles of sufficient gauge should be used to ensure adequate withdrawal of cerebrospinal fluid through the needle before and after anesthetic administration.

Some practitioners advocate the abandonment of 5% hyperbaric lidocaine altogether.[204] The authors believe that one must approach the use of 5% hyperbaric lidocaine with caution, particularly if the patient is to be in the lithotomy position. For short obstetric procedures (i.e., cervical cerclage in lithotomy) one could choose 1.5% hyperbaric lidocaine, which is now commercially available. For cesarean section, where the duration of surgery may be quite short, one might choose 0.75% hyperbaric bupivacaine.

As a final note, it now appears that transient neurologic symptoms may be associated not just with lidocaine but may be present following use of other anesthetics as well. Recent studies have reported TRI following administration of spinal bupivacaine,[205] tetracaine,[206] and most recently 4% mepivacaine.[207]

3. Epidural anesthesia

a. Unsatisfactory block. Although rarely considered a true complication of epidural anesthesia in obstetrics, unsatisfactory or inadequate block has been reported to have an incidence of 6% to 15%.[208] Doughty[209] found that catheter manipulation was required in 18.6% of patients before satisfactory analgesia was achieved. The importance of the problem is demonstrated by the ASA Closed Claims Study, in which 9% of obstetric anesthesia malpractice claims alleged inadequate anesthesia (see Table 24-6). One of the most common causes of inadequate block is catheter malposition. In some cases the malpositioning problem may be attributable to migration of the catheter out of an intervertebral foramen because of insertion of an excessive length of catheter.[210] Placing the catheter no more than 3 to 4 cm into the epidural space seems to be associated with more reliable blocks.

Another mechanism has been proposed to explain some cases of patchy blocks. Dalens, Bazin, and Haberer,[211] using mixtures of local anesthetic and radiographic contrast solution, found that the technique of using air for the loss of resistance creates air bubbles in the epidural space, which physically displace local anesthetic solutions and may result in patchy blocks or skipped segments.

Studies of epidural anatomy using advanced imaging techniques and epiduroscopy have confirmed the existence of a dorsal median septum (plica mediana dorsalis) in the lumbar epidural space.[212,213] Using contrast epidurography and wide-range gray-scale computed tomography, Savolaine et al[213] demonstrated dorsolateral transverse membranes in addition to the plica mediana dorsalis. These structures subdivide the epidural space and may impede the symmetric spread of local anesthetic solutions. The current trend of using continuous epidural infusions of very-low-concentration local anesthetic solutions (often combined with opioids) may compound the problem of asymmetric blocks. In a study reported by Mogensen et al,[214] half of the patients receiving 0.125% bupivacaine infusions for postoperative analgesia had a primarily unilateral block.

b. Uterine rupture. Some obstetricians have raised the concern that epidural anesthesia may block the pain associated with uterine rupture and delay diagnosis, thereby increasing maternal and fetal morbidity or mortality.[215,216] Because of the growing trend for encouraging a trial of labor in patients with prior cesarean sections, this concern must be considered. As pointed out by Chestnut,[217] pain is neither a specific nor a sensitive sign of uterine scar rupture. Among 32 patients with rupture of a previously scarred uterus, Golan, Sandbank, and Rubin[216] report that 47% were completely asymptomatic and 75% were not associated with unusual pain.

Fetal heart rate monitoring may provide the best indication of uterine rupture.[218] Rupture of a previously unscarred uterus is usually a more catastrophic event, which may be associated with continuous abdominal pain. It is unlikely that this type of pain would go unrecognized with typical low-dose epidural analgesia for labor. Nonetheless it is our opinion that epidural analgesia for labor is not advisable in patients at risk for uterine rupture (such as prior uterine instrumentation, grand multiparity, oxytocin stimulation of labor) unless fetal heart rate and intrauterine pressure are monitored continuously.

Concern has also been raised that the process of flexing the torso of a parturient during epidural placement, particularly in the sitting position, may result in abnormal intraabdominal pressures, which could result in uterine rupture.[216,219] The small number of cases in which an association was claimed between the flexed position during epidural placement and uterine rupture seems unconvincing. In those cases, evolving uterine rupture could have been the cause of the pain necessitating epidural analgesia.[217] A recent study of intrauterine pressures in patients having epidural catheters placed found no increase in maximum intraamniotic pressure during flexion, in either the sitting or the lateral decubitus positions.[220]

c. Unintentional subdural block. The subdural space is a potential space between the dura and the arachnoid membranes. Several reports have confirmed the unintentional catheterization of this potential space as well as delayed subdural migration of an epidural catheter.[221-224] Typically, the onset of block is similar to that of epidural anesthesia, and for this reason test doses to rule out subarachnoid block will not allow detection of a subdural injection.[222] However, the extent of block produced from a given volume of local anesthetic is usually much greater with subdural injection. It is not uncommon to have spread of block to the cervical level with 6 to 10 ml of local anesthetic solution.[222,223] When small volumes of water-soluble contrast media are injected into the subdural space, they spread rapidly over a large number of segments, usually cephalad. Subdural blocks may be patchy or asymmetric.[223] To avoid this complication, one should initiate epidural blocks slowly with incremental doses, taking particular care to notice any signs of unexpected high concentrations during onset of the block. Subdural blocks should be managed in the same way as high spinal blocks, with support of blood pressure, ventilation, and protection of the airway as necessary. Recently, the subdural administration of morphine was reported in the treatment of a patient with cancer pain.[225] The authors noted a greatly reduced dose requirement compared to that required by the epidural route, suggesting the potential for respiratory depression with unintentional subdural morphine administration.

d. Unintentional subarachnoid block. Unintentional dural puncture during epidural placement is a common complication with a reported frequency of 1.6% to 2.9%[221]; however, the frequency can vary widely depending on the skill and experience of the practitioner. It is

usually recognized at the time of occurrence and has a high likelihood of resulting in subsequent PDPH. Unrecognized injection of local anesthetic into the subarachnoid space through an epidural needle or catheter is a much less common, though potentially fatal, complication. If large volumes of local anesthetic are injected, the result is sudden and massive spinal blockade (total spinal) characterized by severe hypotension, loss of consciousness, and apnea. To avoid catastrophic consequences, one must secure the airway immediately and establish ventilation. Blood return to the heart must be facilitated by a left-lateral, head-down position and rapid intravenous fluid administration. Vasopressors should be used as required to restore adequate perfusion pressure. To decrease high subarachnoid pressure and minimize potential neurotoxic effects from a large volume of subarachnoid local anesthetic, some authors have recommended draining cerebrospinal fluid.[226]

e. Systemic local anesthetic toxicity. Systemic local anesthetic toxicity has been one of the main causes of maternal mortality associated with epidural anesthesia. CNS and cardiovascular toxic reactions have long been recognized as complications of local anesthetic overdose or, more commonly, unintentional intravascular injection. However, before the widespread use of long-acting amide local anesthetics such as bupivacaine, these reactions rarely led to fatal cardiac arrest. In 1979, Albright[227] reported six cases of cardiac arrest after bupivacaine or etidocaine injections. Albright speculated that the long-acting amide local anesthetics may be more cardiotoxic and that resuscitation from cardiac arrest induced by these agents may be more difficult. Since then, he has collected at least 44 cases of maternal cardiac arrest, 30 of which have been fatal.[228] Data from the ASA Closed Claims Study indicate that convulsion was the single most common critical event that led to serious complications among the obstetric-related claims.[4] Of 19 convulsions in the group of obstetric claims, 17 probably were attributable to local anesthetic toxic reactions with epidural anesthesia. In 10 of these 17 cases, epinephrine was not used in the test dose, and in the remaining 7 insufficient data were available to know whether epinephrine-containing test doses were used. Bupivacaine was the local anesthetic used in 15 of the 17 cases. In the remaining 2 cases the anesthetic was not specified. Two of the 19 convulsions appeared to be eclamptic seizures. Eighty-three percent of the convulsions resulted in neurologic injury or death to the mother, newborn, or both.

Many factors influence the toxicity of local anesthetic agents. One important factor is the relative potency of the anesthetic. Numerous studies indicate that the seizure-producing potential is directly related to anesthetic potency.[229,230] The relationship between anesthetic potency and cardiovascular toxicity is less clear. Liu et al,[231] using cumulative doses of lidocaine or bupivacaine in anesthetized and ventilated dogs, concluded that the cardiotoxicity was similar to the intrinsic potency of the drugs when hypotension and asystole were used as the end point. Since then, other studies using a variety of animal models have demonstrated that bupivacaine has a greater potential for causing arrhythmias.[232-236] Bupivacaine is different from other local anesthetics (such as lidocaine) in that it can induce cardiac arrhythmias such as ventricular tachycardia and fibrillation. Other local anesthetics typically produce progressive conduction block with widened QRS complexes and eventual asystole. Research has been directed toward explaining these observations, but the answers are not clear. Clarkson and Hondeghem[237] propose that differential binding properties of local anesthetic at the sodium channel may explain the greater arrhythmogenic potential of bupivacaine. Others emphasize the role of the CNS in explaining the potential for bupivacaine, but not lidocaine, to induce cardiac arrhythmias.[238,239]

Factors that may lower the cardiotoxic threshold for bupivacaine are hyperkalemia,[240] pregnancy,[235] and hypoxia and acidosis.[241] Morishima et al[235] showed that the pregnant sheep is more sensitive to the cardiotoxic effects of bupivacaine than the nonpregnant sheep. This sensitivity appears to be attributable to decreased plasma protein binding for bupivacaine in the pregnant animal.[242] When ventilation is supported during experimental infusions of local anesthetics, the margin of safety between CNS toxicity and cardiovascular collapse is much wider than when ventilation is not supported. Moore et al[243,245] demonstrated significant acidosis and hypoxia within 30 seconds after the onset of local anesthetic–induced convulsions in humans. In the event of a local anesthetic convulsion, it is imperative to rapidly initiate effective ventilation and oxygenation to prevent cardiovascular collapse. Animal studies show that it is possible to resuscitate animals after massive bupivacaine infusions[233,245] and that it is not more difficult to resuscitate after bupivacaine-induced arrest than after lidocaine-induced cardiac arrest.[233] However, it may be much more difficult to resuscitate a pregnant patient than a nonpregnant patient because of partial occlusion of the inferior vena cava by the gravid uterus.[246] For this reason, emergent delivery should be performed if resuscitation efforts are not quickly successful. Cases in which resuscitation was not accomplished until after emergent delivery of the infant have been reported.[247]

With the link between bupivacaine and cardiotoxicity established, there was a perceived need for a new, long-acting amide local anesthetic, particularly in the area of obstetrics. Bupivacaine's cardiotoxicity appears to be enhanced by pregnancy.[235,248] A new drug is available to the obstetric anesthesiologist; this is ropivacaine. Generally speaking, amide local anesthetics exist as S and R stereoisomers, with the S isomer having a longer duration of action and lower systemic toxicity. With recent technological advances, single-isomer local anesthetic formations are becoming available for clinical use. Ropivacaine is a homolog of mepivacaine and bupivacaine. The commercially available formulation of ropivacaine is only in the form of an S isomer. Animal studies show that ropivacaine has less CNS and cardiovascular toxicity than does bupivacaine.[249-251] In human volunteers ropivacaine caused fewer CNS symptoms and was less toxic than bupivacaine (as defined by the doses and plasma concentrations that were tolerated).[252] After epidural administration for cesarean section, the elimination half-life of ropivacaine was shorter than that of bupivacaine.[253] In contrast to findings for bupivacaine, progesterone does not increase myocardial sensitivity to ropivacaine.[254] Finally, the block produced by ropivacaine is similar to that of bupivacaine for labor analgesia and cesarean section.[255,256] Ropivacaine appears to be a suitable alternative to bupivacaine, particularly for use in obstetric anesthesia. However, as with any other agent, we should continue to adhere to meticulous technique and fractional dosing.

Since the unfortunate problems with bupivacaine and the editorial by Albright,[227] the anesthesia community has become increasingly aware of the potential problems with local anesthetic toxicity in general and bupivacaine cardiotoxicity in particular. In 1983 the Food and Drug Administration issued a warning against the use of bupivacaine 0.75% in obstetrics.[257] Since then, we have become aware of only one or two deaths from bupivacaine toxic reactions.[257a] Of course, local anesthetic systemic toxic reactions are better avoided than treated. To this end, the practice of not injecting more than 5 ml of anesthetic solution at one time and the use of an effective test dose have surely improved the safety of epidural anesthesia in obstetrics.

Aspiration of blood from an epidural needle or catheter is an unreliable sign of intravascular placement. To minimize the chances of unintentional intravascular injection, we advocate the use of a test dose. The test dose in obstetric patients should fulfill a number of criteria: It must contain a marker to identify an intravascular injection of anesthetic, the changes seen with the test injection should be distinguishable from the cyclic changes seen during active labor, the marker must not be toxic to the mother or fetus, and the test dose should be easy to perform. The most commonly used marker for detecting intravascular injection has been epinephrine since Moore and Batra[258] reported that 15 μg epinephrine, when injected intravascularly, resulted in a 30-beats/min increase in heart rate within 20 to 45 seconds. However, opponents have suggested that epinephrine, if given intravenously, might have deleterious effects on uterine blood flow, thus leading to fetal distress.[259,260] In addition, heart rate changes seen with intravenous epinephrine might be difficult to distinguish from the 20% to 30% changes that may occur with uterine contractions.[261,262] Although these concerns are real, there are few case reports in the obstetric literature linking epinephrine test doses with adverse outcomes, whereas there are reports of large numbers of patients benefiting from the advantages of the epinephrine test dose.[263] Epinephrine test doses should be used with caution, or perhaps not at all, in patients with uteroplacental insufficiency or in those who have a potential for an exaggerated response to intravenous epinephrine (as with PIH).[264] Some patients, such as those being treated with β-adrenergic–receptor blockers, may develop hypertension and bradycardia, not tachycardia, in response to epinephrine.[265,266] One can avoid complications by identifying these patients before an epinephrine test dose is administered. Alternatives to the epinephrine test dose have been proposed: a bolus of plain local anesthetic solution,[267,268] isoproterenol,[269] or air.[270] However, significantly more validation of these techniques is necessary before one can recommend replacing the epinephrine test dose. Regardless of the type of test dose one chooses, there is no substitute for close observation of the patient by someone trained to detect adverse signs and symptoms of local anesthetic toxicity.

f. Neurotoxicity. Neurotoxicity from clinically used concentrations of local anesthetics is extremely rare. Drug manufacturers go to great lengths to ensure that their products cause minimal local tissue reaction. Nonetheless, it is clear that virtually all local anesthetics in sufficiently high concentration will cause injury to nerve tissue.[271,272] Case reports have linked neurologic injury from spinal anesthesia with various local anesthetics,[273] although it has not always been clear whether the local anesthetic or a contaminant was the cause. One of the most serious sequelae is adhesive arachnoiditis. This condition involves a gradual proliferation of the arachnoid, resulting in scarring and obliteration of the subarachnoid space. The signs and symptoms of the resulting cauda equina syndrome may be progressive over months or years and usually involve weakness and numbness in the lower extremities, with bowel, bladder, and sexual dysfunction.

In recent years the local anesthetic most often linked with neurotoxicity has been 2-chloroprocaine. This agent has been very popular in obstetrics because of its rapid onset, short duration of action, and very low systemic toxicity. In most of the reported cases of neurologic injury it appears that the local anesthetic was unintentionally injected subarachnoid,[274] although this may not always have been the case.[275] A considerable amount of research has been directed at determining whether the cause of neurotoxicity was the drug itself or the antioxidant sodium bisulfite with which the local anesthetic was formulated to minimize oxidation. Some laboratory[276] and animal studies[277] indicate that the sodium bisulfite was the most likely cause of neurotoxicity. However, other studies indicate that the drug itself may be more neurotoxic than other commonly used local anesthetics.[278] Presumably because of the concern regarding sodium bisulfite, the manufacturers substituted EDTA as the antioxidant in commercially available 2-chloroprocaine. The drug continues to be available to the practitioner, but due care should be exercised in its use. Reports indicate that the epidural use of the newly formulated 2-chloroprocaine containing EDTA may be associated with severe spasmodic back pain.[279,280] Recently the manufacturers have taken EDTA out of the formulation in the hope that back pain might be avoided. A very recent report appears to support this contention.[281] However, some of the authors' recent experience indicates that back pain continues to be a problem in the absence of EDTA.

One should use all local anesthetics as directed without exceeding the recommended concentration or total dose. Before injection of significant volumes of local anesthetic, a test dose should be given to rule out subarachnoid as well as intravascular placement. In addition, it is advisable to use disposable equipment whenever possible to minimize the risk of introducing contaminants, such as detergents or cleaning solutions, during regional anesthetic procedures.

g. Drug administration errors. Errors in drug or blood product administration are responsible for a small but consistent number of anesthesia-related maternal complications and deaths.[4,20,282] The *Report on Confidential Enquiries into Maternal Deaths in England and Wales* for the last two triennia indicate that approximately 5% of anesthetic-related deaths may be attributable to such errors.[10,20] It is likely that many more errors do not result in obvious complications and go unreported. Contributing to the occurrence of such errors is the emergent nature of many obstetric procedures, as well as lack of attention and judgment because of sleep deprivation. Some drug administration errors have included the injection of thiopental, diazepam, or potassium chloride into the epidural space.[283-285] In most of these cases patients have recovered without permanent sequelae. The popularity of continuous epidural infusions for labor analgesia increases the likelihood of errors involving the infusion apparatus.[285] To minimize the chances of infusing magnesium, oxytocin, or other drugs into the epidural space, epidural infusion devices should be uniquely different from those used to infuse intravenous medications. Connecting tubing should not have injection ports, and epidural catheters should be labeled clearly. All medication errors are avoidable and indefensible; they remind us of the constant need to maintain vigilance and attention to detail.

h. Back pain. Back pain is a common complaint of the parturient and one identified in the ASA Closed Claims Project as commonly resulting in payment (see Table 24-6). A prospective audit demonstrated that about 50% of women have back pain some time during pregnancy.[286,287] Low back pain is a nonspecific complaint reported more commonly by younger or unmarried mothers and those with a history of back pain before pregnancy. Because two out of three women may have backache immediately after delivery, it is important to distinguish between this and sacroiliac strain, a more severe persistent pain arising from sacroiliac dysfunction. Localized tenderness at the epidural or spinal insertion site is not an unexpected report, but this complaint usually is transient and is the only type of back pain for which the anesthesiologist should take responsibility. Numerous prospective surveys have shown no link between regional analgesia in labor and new postpartum backache.[286,288] All have failed to find a link between epidural anesthesia and back pain when looking at such factors as duration of analgesia, difficulty of needle or catheter insertion, and motor blockade.[289-291] However, anesthesiologists should be aware that despite the lack of association, many parturients and their caregivers prefer to blame regional anesthesia for their back complaints.

4. Spinal opioid complications. Spinally injected opioids have been used in the obstetric population since Wolfe and Nichols first described the use of epidurally injected fentanyl in postcesarean patients.[292] Since then the use of spinal opioids in obstetrics has continued to grow. Numerous studies have demonstrated the superiority of epidural compared to intramuscular or intravenous opioid administration for providing postcesarean analgesia.[293-295] The efficacy of epidural opioids, when used alone, for providing labor analgesia has been disappointing.[296,297] However, various combinations of low-dose local anesthetic and opioids have proved to be effective for managing labor pain. These combinations appear to act synergistically to provide analgesia[298] but minimize the undesirable side effects of either agent alone. Chestnut et al[299] found that a continuous infusion of bupivacaine 0.0625% with fentanyl 0.0002% provided analgesia comparable to that of bupivacaine 0.125% alone, but with significantly less motor block. The advantage of this is that patients have more mobility, are easier to care for, and can push effectively. However, spinal opioids are associated with several side effects and potential complications. The most common side effects are pruritus, nausea and vomiting, and urinary retention. More serious problems are the potential for oral herpesvirus recrudescence and the most feared complication, respiratory depression.

Pruritus is undoubtedly the most common side effect seen with epidurally injected morphine. The reported incidence in obstetric patients varies from 60% to 90%.[300] Obstetric patients may be more sensitive to both the analgesic effects and the side effects of epidural morphine.[301] In one study in which postcesarean patients were given a mean dose of 4.3 mg epidural morphine, the incidence of pruritus was 70%. In 43% the itching was mild and no treatment was required, in 22% treatment was effective, and in 6% symptoms were troubling despite treatment with diphenhydramine 25 mg intramuscularly or naloxone 0.1 mg intravenously.[302] The incidence of pruritus may be less with other opioids, such as fentanyl and meperidine,[295,303] and may not be seen at all with agonist-antagonist opioids such as butorphanol.[304]

Nausea and vomiting are common in obstetric patients, although most studies indicate a higher incidence in women treated with epidural (or intrathecal) morphine than in those given narcotic or nonnarcotic analgesics intravenously or intramuscularly. The mechanism of neuraxial opioid-induced nausea and vomiting may involve direct stimulation of the chemoreceptor trigger zone in the medulla. The incidence has been reported to be as high as 53% in obstetric patients after epidural morphine, but more commonly the reported incidence is in the range of 16% to 25%.[300] Treatment of nausea and vomiting associated with epidural opioids consists of conservative doses of metoclopramide (5 to 10 mg intravenously), droperidol (0.625 mg intravenously), or transdermal scopolamine.[305]

The mechanism responsible for urinary retention with spinal opioids is poorly understood but is believed to involve a direct effect of the opioid at the sacral spinal cord. Obstetric patients commonly have voiding difficulty because of genitourinary trauma associated with vaginal or cesarean delivery. Surprisingly, urinary retention rarely has been cited as a clinically significant problem associated with neuraxial opioid analgesia in obstetric patients. One of the reasons for this problem may be the common practice of catheterizing the bladder of patients during labor and the use of indwelling catheters for 12 to 24 hours after cesarean delivery.

A new complication of epidural morphine in postcesarean patients has become apparent in the past few years. Two retrospective studies suggest that parturients given epidural morphine may be more susceptible to recrudescence of oral herpes infections.[306,307] A recent prospective study compared the incidence of oral herpes outbreaks in postcesarean patients given morphine epidurally or intramuscularly. Fourteen of the 96 women in the epidural group (14.6%) developed herpetic lesions, whereas none in the intramuscular group suffered a recurrence.[308] Postulated mechanisms for this phenomenon include local trauma associated with scratching in response to facial pruritus, or a direct stimulation of virion reactivation in the trigeminal ganglia by morphine. The severity of some of these outbreaks raises the concern for potential transmission of infection to the newborn. If recurrent oral herpetic lesions have been a problem for a woman, it may be advisable to avoid giving neuraxial opioids.

Respiratory depression is potentially the most serious complication of neuraxial opioid administration. Case reports describing respiratory depression appeared soon after spinal opioids were introduced into clinical practice. Large retrospective and prospective studies have estimated the incidence in the general surgical population at 0.25% to 0.9%.[309,310] Most cases of respiratory depression have occurred within 8 hours of drug administration and probably are attributable to direct depression of brainstem respiratory centers by opioid spread within the cerebrospinal fluid. Low respiratory rates and somnolence have only rarely been reported in obstetric patients. It has been postulated that the parturient may be particularly resistant to ventilatory depression because of the increased respiratory drive that occurs during pregnancy.[311] However, depressed CO_2 response slopes have been documented in postcesarean patients after epidural morphine or butorphanol.[304] In a prospective study of 1000 cesarean section patients given 5 mg morphine for postoperative pain control, Leicht et al[312] found four patients with respiratory rates of less than 10 breaths per minute. Two of these patients were given naloxone, although only one was documented to have true respiratory depression. These data are the best available in this patient population and indicate that the incidence of respiratory depression may be as high as 0.2%.

It has been suggested that the use of more lipophilic opioids such as fentanyl may be safer than morphine because the drug would be absorbed rapidly in the lumbar spinal cord, making it unavailable to cause respiratory depression by cephalad spread in the cerebrospinal fluid.[313] However, in a recent case report, 100 μg epidural fentanyl, given during cesarean section, resulted in severe respiratory depression.[314] It is clear that the use of neuraxial opioids in all patients must be performed with great vigilance. Respiratory rate alone is a poor indicator of ventilatory depression.[315,316] Somnolence may be a more reliable indicator and should be specifically evaluated.[317] The use of neuraxial opioids in obstetrics should be predicated on an organizational structure that ensures knowledgeable staff and the ability to provide the necessary monitoring for as long as indicated.[318]

V. FETAL COMPLICATIONS

Adverse fetal outcome is one of the most common causes for liability claims involving obstetric anesthesia. Although in half of such claims anesthetic care may have been completely appropriate,[4] the importance of ensuring fetal well-being while providing maternal anesthesia cannot be overemphasized. Protecting the fetus from complications of anesthesia necessitates maintaining adequate uterine perfusion, optimizing fetal oxygenation, and limiting the use of drugs in the mother that may cause newborn depression. The importance of avoiding aortocaval compression and hypotension has been discussed. Supplemental oxygen should be administered to laboring women if there is any question of fetal distress because this has been shown to improve neonatal oxygenation.[319]

All systemic medications commonly used during labor for anxiolysis and analgesia readily cross the placenta and can cause neonatal depression. Meperidine may produce neonatal depression as a function of both the dose given and the time interval between maternal administration and delivery of the infant, with the second hour after administration being the most worrisome.[320] Morphine in doses of 5 to 10 mg intramuscularly or 2 to 3 mg intravenously has a duration of 4 to 6 hours and in equianalgesic doses produces more respiratory depression than meperidine does.[321] Fentanyl is a highly lipid-soluble, rapid-acting opioid. In doses of 25 to 50 μg intravenously or 50 to 100 μg intramuscularly, fentanyl has a duration of action of 60 to 120 minutes, respectively. In one study, fentanyl (1 μg/kg) was administered intravenously just before cesarean delivery and did not produce adverse effects on neonatal Apgar scores, neurobehavioral scores, or blood gas values.[322] Fentanyl might therefore be a reasonable adjunct to labor analgesia or cesarean section anesthesia. Butorphanol (Stadol) and nalbuphine (Nubain) are two synthetic agonist-antagonist opioid analgesics. Both cross the placenta and have depressant effects on the newborn, similar to those seen with meperidine.[323,324] Benzodiazepines sometimes are used for the treatment of maternal anxiety before delivery of the infant. Both diazepam and midazolam have the potential for causing neonatal respiratory depression; however, low doses of diazepam (2.5 to 10 mg) intravenously have been used with minimal neonatal effects.[325] Despite these findings, it is best to avoid CNS–depressant drugs in obstetric patients until after delivery of the infant.

A potential hazard of general anesthesia in obstetrics is that of neonatal depression. Large doses of thiopental (8 mg/kg) can result in neonatal depression.[326] However, single doses of 4 mg/kg will not expose the fetal brain to high concentrations of thiopental and will not result in significant neonatal depression.[327] Ketamine in doses of 0.2 to 0.5 mg/kg was not found to cause newborn depression[328] and when given in doses of 1 mg/kg intravenously for induction of general anesthesia, it resulted in slightly better neurobehavioral scores than when thiopental was used.[329] Etomidate has a rapid onset and short duration of action and has also been used in obstetrics. The maternal-to-fetal base excess differences and clinical status of the newborn were found to be superior to that when thiopental was used.[330] Etomidate carries with it the concern for adrenal suppression. In the neonate this is not a significant problem when etomidate is used as the induction agent for elective cesarean section.[331] Midazolam provides no real benefit over thiopental as an induction agent for elective cesarean section.[332] Midazolam was shown to have no advantage in Apgar scores, time to first cry, and need to provide supplemental oxygen to the newborn. There were no real differences in neurobehavioral scores; however, general body tone, response to changes in body temperature, and arm recoil were somewhat depressed compared to those in neonates whose mothers were given thiopental. Use of propofol, the newest induction agent, for elective cesarean section at a dose of 2.8 mg/kg has been shown to result in lower 1- and 5-minute Apgar scores. The lower scores were attributable to somnolence and hypotonus. CNS depression was evidenced by significantly lower neurobehavior scores.[333] Propofol will require further study before one can recommend its use as an induction agent, particularly in the setting of fetal distress.

The controversy over general and regional anesthesia for cesarean section continues to draw attention from obstetric anesthesiologists. Since Virginia Apgar reported her conclusions in 1957,[334] it generally has been believed that neonates are more vigorous after cesarean section under regional anesthesia than under general anesthesia. Early studies found that neonatal depression (measured by Apgar scores) resulted from the use of potent halogenated agents for cesarean section.[335] Neonatal depression may be related to the duration of anesthesia before delivery, as reported by Stenger, Blechner, and Prystowsky[336] and Finster and Poppers.[337] What is probably of greater importance is the uterine incision-to-delivery interval. Depressed infants in deliveries in which the uterine incision-to-delivery intervals have exceeded 90 seconds have been reported.[338,339] It is now evident that with prudent use of low-dose halogenated agents, left uterine displacement, supplemental oxygen, and expeditious delivery (particularly short uterine incision-to-delivery intervals), general anesthesia does not result in significant newborn depression.[40,340,341] A recent comparison of the effects of general and regional anesthesia for elective cesarean section demonstrated no difference in neurobehavioral responses of newborn infants.[342] It is currently unclear whether regional or general anesthesia confers any advantage to the fetus in distress. Well-conducted regional or general anesthetics appear to be equally safe.[343]

Regional anesthesia in obstetrics is not without potential neonatal or fetal complications. The most common complications are attributable to placental hypoperfusion. Epidural anesthesia is preferred over subarachnoid blocks by many anesthesiologists because the block level is more easily controlled, sympathectomy occurs less rapidly, and hypotension is easier to prevent. However, subarachnoid anesthesia exposes the fetus to less anesthetic drug, thus minimizing potential toxic effects. No clear answer exists as to which method of regional anesthesia is superior with respect to the fetus. In addition, the best agent to use for regional anesthesia continues to be debated.[344] Despite potential problems with cardiotoxicity, bupivacaine continues to be used extensively in obstetrics. Its long duration of action and superior sensory-to-motor blocking properties offer particular advantages in obstetric anesthesia.

Some neonatal complications are associated with particular regional anesthetic techniques. Paracervical blocks were at one time popular in obstetrics for providing pain relief during labor. However, depending on the local anesthetic used, dose, and preexisting fetal condition, fetal bradycardia and fetal death have been reported to have an incidence of 2% to 70%.[326,345] Because of this, paracervical blocks rarely are used today. Caudal anesthesia continues to be popular in some anesthetic practices. Placement of the caudal needle must be performed with care, and a rectal examination should be performed to exclude the possibility of accidental puncture of the fetal presenting part. Sinclair et al[346] report fetal local anesthetic toxicity as a consequence of direct fetal injection during caudal anesthesia.

The administration of neuraxial opioids, both as sole agents and as adjuncts, for labor or delivery has become exceedingly popular. Subarachnoid sufentanil and more recently fentanyl have been associated with significant fetal bradycardias.[347-350] The mechanism of this bradycardia is still unknown but appears not to be related to maternal hypotension, but rather has been associated with the occurrence of a significant increase in uterine tone and contractions. More studies must be completed before the mechanism is clearly understood. However, these reports should make us all mindful that all agents administered during labor and delivery must be used with caution and vigilance.

It is clear that the perinate may be influenced by anesthetic effects on placental perfusion, placental transfer of depressant drugs, and anesthetic effects on the course of labor. However, small amounts of systemic medication or properly conducted general or regional anesthesia should have no significant effect on the course of labor or infant well-being.

VI. SUMMARY

The care of obstetric patients can be challenging for the anesthesiologist. Often obstetric patients are not well informed and not well prepared for anesthetic interventions. Care often is required emergently, with little time for proper assessment and examination of the patient. Maternal physiologic and pathologic conditions may further complicate anesthetic management. Perhaps for these, as well as other reasons, anesthesia-related complications remain one of the leading causes of maternal mortality. It is incumbent on us to do all we can in an attempt to eliminate adverse consequences of anesthetic care.

REFERENCES

1. Wallace DH, Sidawi JE: Complications of obstetrical anesthesia. In *Obstetrical anesthesia. Supplement No 3 to the 20th edition of Williams obstetrics*, Norwalk, Conn, 1997, Appleton & Lange, p 1.
2. Gibbs CP, Krischer J, Peckham BM, et al: Obstetric anesthesia: a national survey, *Anesthesiology* 65:298, 1986.
3. Brown G, Russell I: A survey of anaesthesia for caesarean section, *Int J Obstet Anesth* 4:214, 1995.
4. Chadwick HS, Posner K, Caplan RA, et al: A comparison of obstetric and nonobstetric anesthesia malpractice claims, *Anesthesiology* 74:242, 1991.
5. Chadwick HS: An analysis of obstetric anesthesia cases from the American Society of Anesthesiologists closed claims project database, *Int J Obstet Anesth* 5:258, 1996.
6. Hawkins JL, Gibbs CP, Orleans M, et al: Obstetric anesthesia work force survey, 1981 versus 1992, *Anesthesiology* 87:135, 1997.
7. Rochat RW, Rubin GL, Selik R, et al: Changing the definition of maternal mortality: a new look at the postpartum interval, *Lancet* 1:831, 1981.
8. Endler GC, Mariona FG, Sokol RJ, et al: Anesthesia-related maternal mortality in Michigan, 1972 to 1984, *Am J Obstet Gynecol* 159:187, 1988.
9. Lehmann DK, Mabie WC, Miller JMJ, et al: The epidemiology and pathology of maternal mortality: Charity Hospital of Louisiana in New Orleans, 1965-1984, *Obstet Gynecol* 69:833, 1987.
10. Turnbull AC: Report on confidential enquiries into maternal deaths in England and Wales, 1979-1981, London, 1986, Her Majesty's Stationary Office.
11. Kaunitz AM, Hughes JM, Grimes DA, et al: Causes of maternal mortality in the United States, *Obstet Gynecol* 65:605, 1985.
12. Sachs B, Brown D, Driscoll S, et al: Maternal mortality in Massachusetts: trends and prevention, *N Engl J Med* 316:66, 1987.
13. Berg CJ, Atrash HK, Koonin LM, et al: Pregnancy-related mortality in the United States, 1987-1990, *Obstet Gynecol* 88:161, 1996.
14. Hawkins JL, Koonin LM, Palmer SK, et al: Anesthesia-related deaths during obstetric delivery in the United States, 1979-1990, *Anesthesiology* 86:277, 1997.
15. Bassell GM, Marx GF: Anesthesia-related maternal mortality. In Shnider SM, Levinson G, eds: *Anesthesia for obstetrics*, ed 2, Baltimore, 1987, Williams & Wilkins, p 325.
16. Morgan M: Anaesthetic contribution to maternal mortality, *Br J Anaesth* 59:842, 1987.
17. Greiss FCJ, Anderson SG: Elimination of maternal deaths from anesthesia, *Obstet Gynecol* 29:677, 1967.
18. Klein MD, Clahr J: Factors in the decline of maternal mortality, *JAMA* 168:237, 1958.
19. Marx GF, Berman JA: Anesthesia-related maternal mortality, *Bull N Y Acad Med* 61:323, 1985.
20. Turnbull AC, Tindall VR, Beard RW, et al: Report on confidential enquiries into maternal deaths in England and Wales, 1982-1984, London, 1989, Her Majesty's Stationary Office.
21. Ramanathan S, Sheth R, Turndorf H: Anesthesia for cesarean section in patients with genital herpes infections: a retrospective study, *Anesthesiology* 64:807, 1986.
22. Morgan M: Amniotic fluid embolism, *Anaesthesia* 34:20, 1979.
23. Plauche WC: Amniotic fluid embolism, *Am J Obstet Gynecol* 147:982, 1983 (letter).

24. Ross M, Nowicki K, Rangarajan NS: Asymptomatic pulmonary embolism during pregnancy, *Obstet Gynecol* 37:131, 1971.

25. Karuparthy VR, Downing JW, Husain FJ, et al: Incidence of venous air embolism during cesarean section is unchanged by the use of a 5 to 10 degree head-up tilt, *Anesth Analg* 69:620, 1989.

26. Malinow AM, Naulty JS, Hunt CO, et al: Precordial ultrasonic monitoring during cesarean delivery, *Anesthesiology* 66:816, 1987.

27. Schneider EP, Jonas E, Tejani N: Detection of cardiac events by continuous electrocardiogram monitoring during ritodrine infusion, *Obstet Gynecol* 71:361, 1988.

28. Wheeler AS, Patel KF, Spain J: Pulmonary edema during beta-2-tocolytic therapy, *Anesth Analg* 60:695, 1981.

29. Dailey PA: Anesthesia for preterm labor. In Shnider SM, Levinson G: *Anesthesia for obstetrics,* Baltimore, 1987, Williams & Wilkins, p 243.

30. Pritchard JA, MacDonald PC, Gant NF: Hypertensive disorders in pregnancy. In Pritchard JA, MacDonald PC, Gant NF, eds: *Williams obstetrics,* ed 17, Norwalk, Conn, 1985, Appleton-Century-Crofts, p 539.

31. Easterling TR, Benedetti TJ, Schmucker BC: Maternal cardiac output in preeclamptic pregnancies: a longitudinal study, meeting of the Society of Perinatal Obstetricians, New Orleans, abstract:4, 1989.

32. Gutsche BB, Cheek TG: Anesthetic considerations in preeclampsia-eclampsia. In Shnider SM, Levinson G, eds: *Anesthesia for obstetrics,* ed 2, Baltimore, 1987, Williams & Wilkins, p 225.

33. Hibbard LT: Maternal mortality due to acute toxemia, *Obstet Gynecol* 42:263, 1973.

34. Ramanathan J, Sibai BM, Vu T, et al: Correlation between bleeding times and platelet counts in women with preeclampsia undergoing cesarean section, *Anesthesiology* 71:188, 1989.

35. Kelton JG, Hunter DS, Neame PB: A platelet function defect in preeclampsia, *Obstet Gynecol* 65:107, 1985.

36. Weiner CP: The obstetric patient and disseminated intravascular coagulation, *Clin Perinatol* 13:705, 1986.

37. Donaldson JO: Eclampsia and other causes of peripartum convulsions. In Donaldson JO, ed: *Neurology of pregnancy,* Philadelphia, 1978, WB Saunders.

38. Fox EJ, Sklar GS, Hill CH, et al: Complications related to the pressor response to endotracheal intubation, *Anesthesiology* 47:524, 1977.

39. Pritchard JA, Pritchard SA: Standardized treatment of 154 consecutive cases of eclampsia, *Am J Obstet Gynecol* 123:543, 1975.

40. Abboud T, Artal R, Sarkis R, et al: Sympathoadrenal activity, maternal, fetal, and neonatal responses after epidural anesthesia in the preeclamptic patient, *Am J Obstet Gynecol* 144:915, 1982.

41. Jouppila P, Jouppila R, Hollmen A, et al: Lumbar epidural analgesia to improve intervillous blood flow during labor in severe preeclampsia, *Obstet Gynecol* 59:158, 1982.

42. Benedetti TJ, Kates R, Williams V: Hemodynamic observations in severe preeclampsia complicated by pulmonary edema, *Am J Obstet Gynecol* 152:330, 1985.

43. Benedetti TJ, Quilligan EJ: Cerebral edema in severe pregnancy-induced hypertension, *Am J Obstet Gynecol* 137:860, 1980.

44. Lechner RB, Chadwick HS: Anesthetic care of the patient with preeclampsia, *Anesth Clin North Am* 8:95, 1990.

45. Howard BK, Goodson JH, Mengert WF: Supine hypotensive syndrome in late pregnancy, *Obstet Gynecol* 1:371, 1953.

46. Kerr MG, Scott DB, Samuel E: Studies of the inferior vena cava in late pregnancy, *BMJ* 1:532, 1964.

47. Zilianti M: Fetal heart rate and pH of fetal capillary blood during epidural analgesia in labor, *Obstet Gynecol* 36:881, 1970.

48. Moir D: Anaesthesia and maternal deaths, *Scott Med J* 24:187, 1979.

49. Tomkinson J, Turnbull A, Robson G, et al: Report on confidential enquiries into maternal deaths in England and Wales, 1976-1978, London, 1982, Her Majesty's Stationary Office.

50. Csapo A: Progesterone "block," *Am J Anat* 98:273, 1956.

51. Christofide ND, Ghatei MA, Bloom SR, et al: Decreased plasma motilin concentrations in pregnancy, *BMJ* 285:1453, 1982.

52. Roberts RB, Shirley MA: The obstetrician's role in reducing the risk of aspiration pneumonitis, *Am J Obstet Gynecol* 124:611, 1976.

53. Gibbs CP, Schwartz DJ, Wynn JW, et al: Antacid pulmonary aspiration in the dog, *Anesthesiology* 51:380, 1979.

54. Gibbs CP and Banner TC: Effectiveness of Bicitra as a preoperative antacid, *Anesthesiology* 61:97, 1984.

55. Dewan DM, Floyd HM, Thistlewood JM, et al: Sodium citrate pretreatment in elective cesarean section patients, *Anesth Analg* 64:34, 1985.

56. Thompson EM, Loughran PG, McAuley DM, et al: Combined treatment with ranitidine and saline antacids prior to obstetric anaesthesia, *Anaesthesia* 39:1086, 1984.

57. Gillett GB, Watson JD, Langford RM: Ranitidine and single-dose antacid therapy as prophylaxis against acid aspiration syndrome in obstetric practice, *Anaesthesia* 39:638, 1984.

58. Freely J: Increased toxicity and reduced clearance of lidocaine by cimetidine, *Ann Intern Med* 96:592, 1982.

59. Knapp AB, Maguire W, Keren G, et al: The cimetidine-lidocaine interaction, *Ann Intern Med* 98:174, 1983.

60. Dailey PA, Hughes SC, Rosen MA, et al: Effect of cimetidine and ranitidine on lidocaine concentrations during epidural anesthesia for cesarean section, *Anesthesiology* 69:1013, 1988.

61. Brocke-Utne JG, Rout C, Moodley J, et al: Influence of preoperative gastric aspiration on the volume and pH of gastric contents in obstetric patients undergoing cesarean section, *Br J Anaesth* 62:397, 1989.

62. Brocke-Utne JG, Dow TGB, Welman S, et al: The effect of metoclopramide on the lower oesophageal sphincter in late pregnancy, *Anaesth Intensive Care* 6:26, 1978.

63. Bylsma-Howell M, Riggs KW, McMorland GH, et al: Placental transport of metoclopramide: assessment of maternal and neonatal effects, *Can Anaesth Soc J* 30:487, 1983.

64. Wyner J, Cohen SE: Gastric volume in early pregnancy: effect of metoclopramide, *Anesthesiology* 57:209, 1982.

65. Carmichael FJ, Cruise CJE, Crago RR, et al: Preoxygenation: a study of denitrogenation, *Anesth Analg* 68:406, 1989.

66. Brock-Utne JG, Downing JW, Seedat F: Laryngeal oedema associated with preeclamptic toxaemia, *Anaesthesia* 32:556, 1977.

67. MacKenzie AI: Laryngeal oedema complicating obstetric anaesthesia, *Anaesthesia* 33:271, 1978.

68. Lyons G: Failed intubation: six year's experience in a teaching maternity unit, *Anaesthesia* 40:75, 1985.

69. Mallampati S, Gatt S, Gugino L, et al: A clinical sign to predict difficult tracheal intubation: a prospective study, *Can J Anaesth* 32:429, 1985.

70. Cormack R, Lehave J: Difficult tracheal intubation in obstetrics, *Anaesthesia* 39:1105, 1984.

71. Rocke D, Murray W, Rout C, et al: Relative risk analysis of factors associated with difficult intubation in obstetric anesthesia, *Anesthesiology* 77:67, 1992.

72. Kidd J, Dyson A, Latto I: Successful difficult intubation: use of the gum elastic bougie, *Anaesthesia* 43:437, 1988.

73. Benumof JL, Scheller JJ: The importance of transtracheal jet ventilation in the management of the difficult airway, *Anesthesiology* 71:769, 1989.

74. Springer D, Jahr J: The laryngeal mask airway: safety, efficacy, and current use, *Am J Anesth* 22:65, 1995.

75. Brimacombe J, Berry A: The laryngeal mask airway for obstetric anaesthesia and neonatal resuscitation, *Int J Obstet Anesth* 3:211, 1994.

76. Archer GW, Marx GF: Arterial oxygen tension during apnoea in parturient women, *Br J Anaesth* 46:358, 1974.

77. Gambee AM, Hertzka RE, Fisher DM: Preoxygenation techniques: comparison of three minutes and four breaths, *Anesth Analg* 66:468, 1987.

78. Norris MC, Dewan DM: Preoxygenation for cesarean section: a comparison of two techniques, *Anesthesiology* 62:827, 1985.

79. Russell GN, Smith CL, Snowdon SL, et al: Pre-oxygenation and the parturient patient, *Anaesthesia* 42:346, 1987.

80. Birmingham PK, Cheney FW, Ward RJ: Esophageal intubation: a review of detection techniques, *Anesth Analg* 65:886, 1986.

81. Guggenberger H, Lenz G, Federle R: Early detection of inadvertent oesophageal intubation: pulse oximetry vs. capnography, *Acta Anaesthesiol Scand* 33:112, 1989.

82. Strunin L, Williams T: The FEF end-tidal carbon dioxide detector, *Anesthesiology* 71:621, 1989.

83. Juul J, Lie B, Nielsen SF: Epidural analgesia vs general anesthesia for cesarean section, *Acta Obstet Gynecol Scand* 67:203, 1988.

84. Crawford JS: Awareness during operative obstetrics under general anaesthesia, *Br J Anaesth* 43:179, 1971.

85. Lyons G, MacDonald R: Awareness during cesarean section, *Anaesthesia* 46:62, 1991.

86. Sigl JC, Chamoun NC: An introduction to bispectral analysis for the EEG, *J Clin Monit* 10:392, 1994.

87. Sebel PS, Lang E, Rampil IJ, et al: A multicenter study of bispectral electroencephalogram analysis for monitoring anesthetic effect, *Anesth Analg* 84:891, 1997.

88. Leslie K, Sessler DI, Smith WD, et al: Prediction of movement during propofol/nitrous oxide anesthesia: performance of concentration, electroencephalographic, pupillary, and hemodynamic indicators, *Anesthesiology* 84:52, 1996.

89. Glass PSA, Sebel PS, Rosow CE, et al: Improved propofol titration using the bispectral index (BIS), *Anesthesiology* 85:A351, 1996.

90. Payne FB, Sebel PS, Glass PSA, et al: Bispectral index (BIS) monitoring allows faster emergence from propofol/alfentanil/N_2O anesthesia, *Anesthesiology* 85:A1056, 1996.

91. Bloom M, Greenwald S, Day R: Analgesics decrease arousal response to stimulation as measured by changes in bispectral index, *Anesthesiology* 85:A481, 1996.

92. Plaud B, Billard V, Debaene B: BIS predict inadequate level of anesthesia during sevoflurane administration, *Anesthesiology* 87:A326, 1997.

93. Wagner K, Schneider G, Werner C, et al: Bispectral EEG analysis may not indicate awareness during propofol/alfentanil anesthesia, *Anesthesiology* 85:A473, 1996.

94. Hodgkinson R, Bhatt M, Kim SS, et al: Neonatal neurobehavioral tests following cesarean section under general and spinal anesthesia, *Am J Obstet Gynecol* 132:670, 1978.

95. Morgan M, Holdcroft A, Whitwam JG: Comparison of thiopentone and methohexitone as induction agents for caesarean section, *Anaesth Intensive Care* 8:431, 1980.

96. Schultetus RR, Hill CR, Dharamraj CM, et al: Wakefulness during cesarean section after anesthetic induction with ketamine, thiopental, or ketamine and thiopental combined, *Anesth Analg* 65:723, 1986.

97. Moore J: A comparison between propofol and thiopentone as induction agents in obstetrics anaesthesia, *Anaesthesia* 44:753, 1989.

98. Moir DD: Anaesthesia for caesarean section: an evaluation of a method using low concentrations of halothane and 50 percent of oxygen, *Br J Anaesth* 42:136, 1970.

99. Crawford JS, Lewis M, Davies P: Maternal and neonatal responses related to the volatile agent used to maintain anaesthesia at caesarean section, *Br J Anaesth* 57:482, 1985.

100. Morishima HO, Pedersen H, Finster M: Influence of maternal psychological stress on the fetus, *Am J Obstet Gynecol* 131:286, 1978.

101. Newton M: Postpartum hemorrhage, *Am J Obstet Gynecol* 94:711, 1966.

102. Gibbs CE, Locke WE: Maternal deaths in Texas, 1969 to 1973: a report of 501 consecutive maternal deaths from the Texas Medical Association's Committee on Maternal Health, *Am J Obstet Gynecol* 126:687, 1976.

103. Munson ES, Embrom WJ: Enflurane, isoflurane, and halothane and isolated human uterine muscle, *Anesthesiology* 46:11-14, 1977.

104. Stallabrass P: Halothane and blood loss at delivery, *Acta Anaesthesiol Scand* 25(suppl):376, 1966.

105. Thirion AV, Wright RG, Messer CP, et al: Maternal blood loss associated with low dose halothane administration for cesarean section, *Anesthesiology* 69:A693, 1988.

106. Marx GF, Kim YI, Lin C, et al: Postpartum uterine pressures under halothane or enflurane anesthesia, *Obstet Gynecol* 51:695, 1978.

107. Kerr MG: Cardiovascular dynamics in pregnancy and labour, *Br Med Bull* 24:19, 1968.

108. Bieniarz J, Crottogini JJ, Curuchet E, et al: Aortocaval compression by the uterus in late human pregnancy, *Am J Obstet Gynecol* 100:203, 1968.

109. Griess FC Jr: Pressure-flow relationship in the gravid uterine vascular bed, *Am J Obstet Gynecol* 96:41, 1966.

110. Hon EH, Reid BL, Hehre FW: The electronic evaluation of fetal heart rate. II. Changes with maternal hypotension, *Am J Obstet Gynecol* 79:209, 1960.

111. Moya F, Smith B: Spinal anesthesia for cesarean section: clinical and biochemical studies of effects on maternal physiology, *JAMA* 179:609, 1962.

112. Bletka M, Hlavaty V, Trnkova M, et al: Volume of whole blood and absolute amount of serum proteins in the early stage of late toxemia of pregnancy, *Am J Obstet Gynecol* 106:10, 1970.

113. Ralston DH, Shnider SM, deLorimier AA: Effects of equipotent ephedrine, metaraminol, mephentermine and methoxamine on uterine blood flow in the pregnant ewe, *Anesthesiology* 40:354, 1974.

114. Lechner RB, Droste S, Chadwick HS: Lumbar epidural analgesia and changes in the fetal heart rate pattern: a blinded study of 139 patients, *Anesthesiology* 71:A853, 1989.

115. Grundy EM, Zamora AM, Winnie AP: Comparison of spread of epidural anesthesia in pregnant and nonpregnant women, *Anesth Analg* 57:544, 1978.

116. Shnider SM, Levinson G: Obstetric analgesia. In Miller RD: *Anesthesia,* ed 2, New York, 1986, Churchill Livingstone, p 1688.

117. Bromage PR: *Epidural analgesia,* Philadelphia, 1978, WB Saunders, p 522.

118. Cheek TG, Gutsche BB: Maternal physiologic alterations during pregnancy. In Shnider SM, Levinson G, eds: *Anesthesia for obstetrics,* Baltimore, 1987, Williams & Wilkins, p 3.

119. Flanagan HL, Datta S, Lambert DH, et al: Effect of pregnancy on bupivacaine-induced conduction blockade in the isolated rabbit vagus nerve, *Anesth Analg* 66:123, 1987.

120. Butterworth JF, Walker FO, Lysak SZ: Pregnancy increases median nerve susceptibility to lidocaine, *Anesthesiology* 72:962, 1990.

121. Reynolds F: Maternal sequelae of childbirth, *Br J Anaesth* 75:515, 1995.

122. Usubiaga JE: Neurological complications following epidural anesthesia, *Int Anesthesiol Clin* 13:1, 1975.

123. Hellman K: Epidural anaesthesia in obstetrics: a second look at 26,127 cases, *Can Anaesth Soc J* 12:398, 1965.

124. Hill EC: Maternal obstetric paralysis, *Am J Obstet Gynecol* 83:1452, 1962.

125. Massey EW, Cefalo RC: Neuropathies of pregnancy, *Obstet Gynecol Surv* 34:489, 1979.

126. Massey E: Mononeuropathies in pregnancy, *Semin Neurol* 8:193, 1988.

127. Brown JT, McDougall A: Traumatic maternal birth palsy, *J Obstet Gynaecol Br Empire* 64:431, 1957.

128. Philip BK: Complications of regional anesthesia for obstetrics, *Reg Anesth* 8:17, 1983.

129. Massey EW, Cefalo RC: Managing the carpal tunnel syndrome in pregnancy, *Contemp Obstet Gynecol* 9:39, 1977.

130. Rhodes P: Meralgia paraesthetica in pregnancy, *Lancet* 2:831, 1957.

131. Pearson MG: Meralgia paraesthetica with reference to its occurrence in pregnancy, *J Obstet Gynecol Br Empire* 64:427, 1957.

132. Donaldson JO, Wirz D, Mashman J: Bilateral postpartum femoral neuropathy, *Conn Med* 49:496, 1985.

133. Adelman U, Goldberg GS, Puckett JD: Postpartum bilateral femoral neuropathy, *Obstet Gynecol* 42:845, 1973.

134. Whittaker WG: Injuries to the sacral plexus in obstetrics, *Can Med Assoc J* 79:62, 1958.

135. O'Connell J: Lumbar disk protrusions in pregnancy, *J Neurol Neurosurg Psychiatry* 23:138, 1960.

136. Grove LH: Backache, headache, and bladder dysfunction after delivery, *Br J Anaesth* 45:1147, 1973.

137. Crawford JS: Lumbar epidural block in labour: a clinical analysis, *Br J Anaesth* 44:66, 1972.

138. Silva M, Mallinson C, Reynolds F: Sciatic nerve palsy following childbirth, *Anaesthesia* 51:1144, 1996.

139. Scott D, Hibbard B: Serious complications associated with epidural/spinal blockade in obstetrics, *Int J Obstet Anesth* 4:133, 1995.

140. Bromage PR: An evaluation of bupivacaine in epidural analgesia for obstetrics, *Can Anaesth Soc J* 16:46, 1969.
141. Cuerden C, Buley R, Downing JW: Delayed recovery after epidural analgesia for labour, *Anaesthesia* 32:773, 1977.
142. Pathy GV, Rosen M: Prolonged block with recovery after extradural analgesia for labour, *Br J Anaesth* 47:520, 1975.
143. Vandam LD, Dripps RD: A long-term follow-up of 10,098 spinal anesthetics. II. Incidence and analysis of minor sensory neurological defects, *Surgery* 38:463, 1955.
144. Tubridy N, Redmond J: Neurological symptoms attributed to epidural analgesia in labour: an observational study of seven cases, *Br J Obstet Gynaecol* 103:832, 1996.
145. Holdcroft A, Gibbard FB, Hargrove RL, et al: Neurological complications associated with pregnancy, *Br J Anaesth* 75:522, 1995.
146. Yoshii W, Rottman R, Rosenblatt R: Epidural catheter induced traumatic radiculopathy in obstetrics: one center's experience, *Reg Anesth* 19:132, 1994.
147. Rigler ML, Drasner K, Krejcie TC, et al: Cauda equina syndrome after continuous spinal anesthesia, *Anesth Analg* 72:275, 1991.
148. Shnider SM, Levinson G, Ralston DH: Regional anesthesia for labor and delivery. In Shnider SM, Levinson G, eds: *Anesthesia for obstetrics,* Baltimore, 1987, Williams & Wilkins, p 119.
149. Dawson BH: Paraplegia due to spinal epidural haematoma, *J Neurol Neurosurg Psychiatry* 26:171, 1963.
150. Owens EL, Kasten GW, Hessel EA II: Spinal subarachnoid hematoma after lumbar puncture and heparinization: a case report, review of the literature, and discussion of anesthetic implications, *Anesth Analg* 65:1201, 1986.
151. Rasmus KT: Unrecognized thrombocytopenia and regional anesthesia in parturients: a retrospective review, *Obstet Gynecol* 73:943, 1989.
152. Rolbin SH, Abbott D, Musclow E, et al: Epidural anesthesia in pregnant patients with low platelet counts, *Obstet Gynecol* 71:918, 1988.
153. Baker AS, Ojemann RG, Swartz MN, et al: Spinal epidural abscess, *N Engl J Med* 293:463, 1975.
154. Bromage PR: *Epidural analgesia,* Philadelphia, 1978, WB Saunders, p 682.
155. Berga S, Trierweiler MW: Bacterial meningitis following epidural anesthesia for vaginal delivery: a case report, *Obstet Gynecol* 74:437, 1989.
156. Ready LB, Helfer D: Bacterial meningitis in parturients after epidural anesthesia, *Anesthesiology* 71:988, 1989.
157. Roberts SP, Petts HV: Meningitis after obstetric spinal anaesthesia, *Anaesthesia* 45:376, 1990.
158. Bromage PR: Neurologic complications of regional anesthesia for obstetrics. In Shnider SM, Levinson G, eds: *Anesthesia for obstetrics,* Baltimore, 1987, Williams & Wilkins, p 321.
159. Behl S: Epidural analgesia in the presence of fever, *Anaesthesia* 40:1240, 1985.
159a. Brown ZA: Personal communication, 1990.
160. Brown ZA, Berry S, Vontver LA: Genital herpes simplex virus infections complicating pregnancy: natural history and peripartum management, *J Reprod Med* 31:420, 1986.
161. Crosby ET, Halpern SH, Rolbin SH: Epidural anaesthesia for Caesarean section in patients with active recurrent genital herpes simplex infections: a retrospective review, *Can J Anaesth* 36:701, 1989.
162. Hopkins T, Marcus M, Campbell S: Post-partum depression: a critical review, *Psychol Bull* 95:498, 1984.
163. Thirkettle JA, Knight RG: The psychological precipitants of transient postpartum depression: a review, *Curr Psychol Res Rev* 4:143, 1985.
164. Gleeson C, Reynolds F: Accidental dural puncture rate in UK obstetric practice, *Int J Obstet Anesth* 6:203, 1997.
165. Stride P, Cooper G: A 20-year survey from the Birmingham Maternity Hospital, *Anaesthesia* 42:1110, 1993.
166. Stein G, Morton J, Marsh A, et al: Headaches after childbirth, *Acta Neurolog Scand* 69:74, 1984.
167. Pitt B: Maternity blues, *Br J Psychiatry* 122:431, 1973.
168. Reik L: Headaches in pregnancy, *Semin Neurol* 8:187, 1988.
169. Gielen M: Postdural puncture headache (PDPH): a review, *Reg Anesth* 14:101, 1989.
170. Bonica JJ: *Principles and practice of obstetric analgesia and anesthesia,* Philadelphia, 1967, FA Davis, p 721.
171. Lybecker H, Moller JT, Max O, et al: Incidence and prediction of postdural puncture headache: a prospective study of 1021 spinal anesthesias, *Anesth Analg* 70:389, 1990.
172. Okell RW, Sprigge JS: Unintentional dural puncture: a survey of recognition and management, *Anaesthesia* 42:1110, 1987.
173. Ravindran RS, Viegas OJ, Tasch MD, et al: Bearing down at the time of delivery and the incidence of spinal headache in parturients, *Anesth Analg* 60:524, 1981.
174. Abouleish E: Epidural blood patch for the treatment of chronic post–lumbar-puncture cephalgia, *Anesthesiology* 49:291, 1978.
175. Abouleish E, de la Vega S, Blendinger I, et al: Long-term follow-up of epidural blood patch, *Anesth Analg* 54:459, 1975.
176. Jones RJ: The role of recumbency in the prevention and treatment of postspinal headache, *Anesth Analg* 53:788, 1974.
177. Carbaat PA, van Crevel H: Lumbar puncture headache: controlled study on the preventive effect of 24 hours bed rest, *Lancet* 2:1133, 1981.
178. Moore DC: *Anesthetic techniques for obstetrical anesthesia and analgesia,* Springfield, Ill, 1964, Charles C Thomas.
179. Baysinger CL, Menk EJ, Harte E, et al: The successful treatment of dural puncture headache after failed epidural blood patch, *Anesth Analg* 65:1242, 1986.
180. Usubiaga JE, Usubiaga LE, Brea LM, et al: Effect of saline injections on epidural and subarachnoid space pressures and relation to postspinal anesthesia headache, *Anesth Analg* 46:293, 1967.
181. Jarvis AP, Greenawalt JW, Fagraeus L: Intravenous caffeine for postdural puncture headache, *Anesth Analg* 65:316, 1986 (letter).
182. Sechzer PH, Abel L: Post-spinal anesthesia headache treated with caffeine: evaluation with demand method part I, *Curr Ther Res* 24:307, 1978.
183. Baumgarten RK: Should caffeine become the first-line treatment for postdural puncture headache? *Anesth Analg* 66:913, 1987.
184. Camann WR, Murray RS, Mushlin PS, et al: Effects of oral caffeine on postdural puncture headache: a double-blind, placebo-controlled trial, *Anesth Analg* 70:181, 1990.
185. DiGiovanni AJ, Dunbar BS: Epidural injections of autologous blood for postlumbar-puncture headache, *Anesth Analg* 1970:268, 1970.
186. Brownridge P: The management of headache following accidental dural puncture in obstetric patients, *Anaesth Intensive Care* 11:4, 1983.
187. Ostheimer GW, Palahniuk RJ, Shnider SM: Epidural blood patch for post-lumbar-puncture headache, *Anesthesiology* 41:307, 1974.
188. Crawford JS: Experiences with epidural blood patch, *Anaesthesia* 35:513, 1980.
189. Loeser EA, Hill GE, Bennett GM, et al: Time vs success rate for epidural blood patch, *Anesthesiology* 49:147, 1978.
190. Szeinfeld M, Ihmeidan IH, Moser MM, et al: Epidural blood patch: evaluation of the volume and spread of blood injected into the epidural space, *Anesthesiology* 64:820, 1986.
191. Cheek TG, Banner R, Sauter J, et al: Prophylactic extradural blood patch is effective: a preliminary communication, *Br J Anaesth* 61:340, 1988.
192. Wilton NCT, Globerson JH, DeRosayro AM: Epidural blood patch for postdural puncture headache: it's never too late, *Anesth Analg* 65:895, 1986.
193. Phillips OC, Ebner H, Nelson AT, et al: Neurologic complications following spinal anesthesia with lidocaine: a prospective review of 10,440 cases, *Anesthesiology* 30:284, 1969.
194. Ross BK, Coda B, Heath CH: Local anesthetic distribution in a spinal model: a possible mechanism of neurologic injury after continuous spinal anesthesia, *Reg Anesth* 17:69, 1992.
195. Schneider M, Ettlin T, Kaufman M, et al: Transient neurologic toxicity after hyperbaric subarachnoid anesthesia with 5% lidocaine, *Anesth Analg* 76:1154, 1993.
196. Sjostrom S, Blass J: Severe pain in both legs after spinal anesthesia with hyperbaric 5% lignocaine solution, *Anaesthesia* 49:700, 1994.

197. Pinczower G, Chadwick H, Woodland R, et al: Bilateral leg pain following lidocaine spinal anaesthesia, *Can J Anaesth* 42:217, 1995.
198. Hampl K, Schneider M, Ummenhofer W, et al: Transient neurological symptoms after spinal anesthesia, *Anesth Analg* 81:1148, 1995.
199. Tarkkila P: Transient radicular irritation after spinal anaesthesia with hyperbaric 5% lidocaine, *Br J Anaesth* 74:328, 1995.
200. Pollock J, Neal J, Stephenson C, et al: Prospective study of the incidence of transient radicular irritation in patients undergoing spinal anesthesia, *Anesthesiology* 84:1361, 1996.
201. Lambert LA, Lambert DH, Strichartz GR: Irreversible conduction block in isolated nerves by high concentrations of local anesthetics, *Anesthesiology* 80:1082, 1994.
202. Drasner K, Sakura S, Chan V, et al: Persistent sacral sensory deficit induced by intrathecal local anesthetic infusion in the rat, *Anesthesiology* 80:847, 1994.
203. Sakura S, Chan V, Ciriales R, et al: Intrathecal infusion of lidocaine in the rat results in dose-dependent, but not concentration-dependent, sacral root injury, *Anesthesiology* 79:A851, 1993.
204. deJong RH: Last round for a "heavyweight?" *Anesth Analg* 78:3, 1994.
205. Tarkkila P, Huhtala J, Tuominen M, et al: Transient radicular irritation after bupivacaine spinal anesthesia, *Reg Anesth* 21:26, 1996.
206. Sumi M, Sakura S, Kosaka Y: Intrathecal hyperbaric 0.5% tetracaine as a possible cause of transient neurologic toxicity, *Anesth Analg* 82:1076, 1996.
207. Lynch J, zur Nieden M, Kasper S, et al: Transient radicular irritation after spinal anesthesia with hyperbaric 4% mepivacaine, *Anesth Analg* 85:872, 1997.
208. Brownridge PR, Taylor G, Ralston DH: Neural blockade for obstetrics and gynecology. In Cousins MJ, Bridenbaugh PO, eds: *Neural blockade in clinical anesthesia and management of pain,* Philadelphia, 1980, JB Lippincott, p 480.
209. Doughty A: Lumbar epidural analgesia-the pursuit of perfection, with special reference to midwife participation, *Anaesthesia* 30:741, 1975.
210. Bromage PR: *Epidural analgesia,* Philadelphia, 1978, WB Saunders, p 226.
211. Dalens B, Bazin J, Haberer J: Epidural bubbles as a cause of incomplete analgesia during epidural anesthesia, *Anesth Analg* 66:679, 1987.
212. Blomberg R: The dorsomedian connective tissue band in the lumbar epidural space of humans: an anatomical study using epiduroscopy in autopsy cases, *Anesth Analg* 65:747, 1986.
213. Savolaine ER, Pandya JB, Greenblatt SH, et al: Anatomy of the human lumbar epidural space: new insights using CT-epidurography, *Anesthesiology* 68:217, 1988.
214. Mogensen T, Dirkes W, Bigler D, et al: No tachyphylaxis during postoperative continuous epidural 0.125% bupivacaine infusion, *Reg Anesth* 13:117, 1988.
215. O'Driscoll K: An obstetrician's view of pain, *Br J Anaesth* 47:1053, 1975.
216. Golan A, Sandbank O, Rubin A: Rupture of the pregnant uterus, *Obstet Gynecol* 56:549, 1980.
217. Chestnut DH: Uterine rupture and epidural anesthesia, *Obstet Gynecol* 66:295, 1985.
218. Elkins T, Onwuka E, Stovall T, et al: Uterine rupture in Nigeria, *J Reprod Med* 30:195, 1985.
219. Plauche WC, Von Almen W, Muller R: Catastrophic uterine rupture, *Obstet Gynecol* 64:792, 1984.
220. Parker L, Dewan DM: *Epidurals and uterine rupture: does acute anteflexion alter intraamniotic pressure?* Madison, Wis, 1990, Society for Obstetrical Anesthesia and Perinatology, p E-29.
221. Boys JE, Norman PF: Accidental subdural analgesia: a case report, possible clinical implications and relevance to "massive extradurals," *Br J Anaesth* 47:1111, 1975.
222. Lee A, Dodd KW: Accidental subdural catheterization, *Anaesthesia* 41:847, 1986.
223. Manchanda VN, Murad SHN, Shilyansky G, et al: Unusual clinical course of accidental subdural local anesthetic injection, *Anesth Analg* 62:1124, 1983.
224. Hartrick CT, Pither C, Pai U, et al: Subdural migration of an epidural catheter, *Anesth Analg* 64:175, 1985.
225. Brown G, Atkinson GL, Standiford SB: Subdural administration of opioids, *Anesthesiology* 71:611, 1989.
226. Shnider SM, Levinson G, Ralston DH: Regional anesthesia for labor and delivery. In Shnider SM, Levinson G, eds: *Anesthesia for obstetrics,* ed 2, Baltimore, 1987, Williams & Wilkins, p 115.
227. Albright GA: Cardiac arrest following regional anesthesia with etidocaine or bupivacaine, *Anesthesiology* 51:285, 1979.
228. Albright GA, Stevenson DK: Local anesthetics. In Albright G, Ferguson IJ, Joyce IT, eds: *Anesthesia in obstetrics,* ed 2, Boston, 1986, Butterworth, p 115.
229. deJong RH, Ronfeld RA, DeRosa RA: Cardiovascular effects of convulsant and supraconvulsant doses of amide local anesthetics, *Anesth Analg* 61:3, 1982.
230. Liu PL, Feldman HS, Giasi R, et al: Comparative CNS toxicity of lidocaine, etidocaine, bupivacaine, and tetracaine in awake dogs following rapid intravenous administration, *Anesth Analg* 62:375, 1983.
231. Liu P, Feldman HS, Covino BM, et al: Acute cardiovascular toxicity of intravenous amide local anesthetics in anesthetized ventilated dogs, *Anesth Analg* 61:317, 1982.
232. Rosen MA, Thigpen JW, Shnider SM, et al: Bupivacaine-induced cardiotoxicity in hypoxic and acidotic sheep, *Anesth Analg* 64:1089, 1985.
233. Chadwick HS: Toxicity and resuscitation in lidocaine- or bupivacaine-infused cats, *Anesthesiology* 63:385, 1985.
234. Kotelko DM, Shnider SM, Dailey PA, et al: Bupivacaine-induced cardiac arrhythmias in sheep, *Anesthesiology* 60:10, 1984.
235. Morishima HO, Pedersen H, Finster M, et al: Bupivacaine toxicity in pregnant and nonpregnant ewes, *Anesthesiology* 63:134, 1985.
236. Sage DJ, Feldman HS, Arthur GR, et al: The cardiovascular effects of convulsant doses of lidocaine and bupivacaine in the conscious dog, *Reg Anesth* 10:175, 1985.
237. Clarkson CW, Hondeghem LM: Mechanism for bupivacaine depression of cardiac conduction: fast block of sodium channels during the action potential with slow recovery from block during diastole, *Anesthesiology* 62:396, 1985.
238. Heavner JE: Cardiac dysrhythmias induced by infusion of local anesthetics into the lateral cerebral ventricle of cats, *Anesth Analg* 65:133, 1986.
239. Thomas RD, Behbehani MM, Coyle DE, et al: Cardiovascular toxicity of local anesthetics: an alternative hypothesis, *Anesth Analg* 65:444, 1986.
240. Avery T: The influence of serum potassium on cerebral and cardiac toxicity of bupivacaine and lidocaine, *Anesthesiology* 61:134, 1984.
241. Sage DJ, Feldman HS, Arthur GR, et al: Influence of lidocaine and bupivacaine on isolated guinea pig atria in the presence of acidosis and hypoxia, *Anesth Analg* 63:1, 1984.
242. Santos AC, Pedersen H, Harmon T, et al: Does pregnancy alter the systemic toxicity of local anesthetics? *Anesthesiology* 70:991, 1989.
243. Moore DC, Crawford RD, Scurlock JE: Severe hypoxia and acidosis following local anesthetic-induced convulsions, *Anesthesiology* 53:259, 1980.
244. Moore DC, Thompson GE, Crawford RD: Long-acting local anesthetic drugs and convulsions with hypoxia and acidosis, *Anesthesiology* 56:230, 1982.
245. Kasten GW, Martin ST: Successful cardiovascular resuscitation after massive intravenous bupivacaine overdosage in anesthetized dogs, *Anesth Analg* 64:491, 1985.
246. Kasten GW, Martin ST: Resuscitation from bupivacaine-induced cardiovascular toxicity during partial inferior vena cava occlusion, *Anesth Analg* 65:341, 1986.
247. DePace NL, Betesh JS, Kotler MN: Postmortem cesarean section with recovery of both mother and offspring, *JAMA* 248:971, 1982.
248. Moller RA, Datta S, Fox J, et al: Effects of progesterone on the cardiac electrophysiologic action of bupivacaine and lidocaine, *Anesthesiology* 76:604, 1992.

249. Feldman H, Arthur G, Covino B: Comparative systemic toxicity of convulsant and supraconvulsant doses of ropivacaine, bupivacaine and lidocaine in the conscious dog, *Anesth Analg* 70:80, 1989.

250. Reiz S, Haddmark S, Johansson G, et al: Cardiotoxicity of ropivacaine: a new amide local anaesthetic agent, *Acta Anaesthesiol Scand* 33:93, 1898.

251. Feldman H, Arthur G, Pitkanen M, et al: Treatment of acute systemic toxicity after the rapid intravenous injection of ropivacaine and bupivacaine in the conscious dog, *Anesth Analg* 73:373, 1991.

252. Scott D, Lee A, Fagan D, et al: Acute toxicity of ropivacaine compared with that of bupivacaine, *Anesth Analg* 69:563, 1989.

253. Datta S, Camann W, Bader A, et al: Clinical effects and maternal fetal plasma concentrations of epidural ropivacaine versus bupivacaine for cesarean section, *Anesthesiology* 82:1346, 1995.

254. Moller R, Covino B: Effect of progesterone on cardiac electrophysiologic alterations produced by ropivacaine and bupivacaine, *Anesthesiology* 77:735, 1992.

255. Stienstra R, Jonker T, Bourdrez R, et al: Ropivacaine 0.25% versus bupivacaine 0.25% for continuous epidural analgesia in labor: a double-blind comparison, *Anesth Analg* 80:285, 1995.

256. Griffin R, Reynolds F: Extradural anaesthesia for caesarean section: a double-blind comparison of 0.5% ropivacaine with 0.5% bupivacaine, *Br J Anaesth* 74:512, 1995.

257. FDA Drug Bulletin: Adverse reactions with bupivacaine. In *FDA Drug Bulletin*, Rockville, Md, 1983, US Department of Health and Human Services, p 23.

257a. Albright: Personal communication, 1990.

258. Moore DC, Batra MS: The components of an effective test dose prior to epidural block, *Anesthesiology* 55:693, 1981.

259. Hood DD, Dewan DM, James FMI: Maternal and fetal effects of epinephrine in gravid ewes, *Anesthesiology* 64:610, 1986.

260. Chestnut DH, Weiner CP, Martin JG, et al: Effect of intravenous epinephrine on uterine artery blood flow velocity in the pregnant guinea pig, *Anesthesiology* 65:633, 1986.

261. Cartwright PO, McCarroll SM, Antzaka C: Maternal heart rate changes with a plain epidural test dose, *Anesthesiology* 65:226, 1986.

262. Leighton BL, Norris MC, Sosis M, et al: Limitations of epinephrine as a marker of intravascular injection in laboring women, *Anesthesiology* 66:688, 1987.

263. Moore DC, Batra MS, Bridenbaugh LD, et al: Maternal heart changes with a plain epidural test dose: validity of results open to question, *Anesthesiology* 66:854, 1987.

264. Talledo OE, Chesley LC, Zuspan FP: Renin-angiotensin system in normal and toxemic pregnancies. III. Differential sensitivity to angiotensin II and norepinephrine in toxemia of pregnancy, *Am J Obstet Gynecol* 100:218, 1968.

265. Hom M, Johnson P, Mulroy M: Blood pressure response to an epinephrine test dose in beta-blocked subjects, *Anesthesiology* 67:A268, 1987.

266. Popitz-Berges F, Datta S, Ostheimer GW: Intravascular epinephrine may not increase heart rate in patients receiving metoprolol, *Anesthesiology* 68:815, 1988.

267. Grice SC, Eisenach JC, Dewan DM, et al: Evaluation of 2-chloroprocaine as an effective intravenous test dose for epidural analgesia, *Anesthesiology* 67:A627, 1987.

268. Roetman KJ, Eisenach JC: Evaluation of lidocaine as an intravenous test dose for epidural anesthesia, *Anesthesiology* 69:A669, 1988.

269. Leighton BL, DeSimone CA, Norris MC, et al: Isoproterenol is an effective marker of intravenous injection in laboring women, *Anesthesiology* 71:206, 1989.

270. Leighton BL, Gross JB: Air: an effective indicator of intravenously located epidural catheters, *Anesthesiology* 71:848, 1989.

271. Meyers RR, Kalichman MW, Reisner LS, et al: Neurotoxicity of local anesthetics, *Anesthesiology* 65:119, 1986.

272. Ready LB, Plumer MH, Haschke RH, et al: Neurotoxicity of intrathecal local anesthetics in rabbits, *Anesthesiology* 63:364, 1985.

273. Marx GF: Maternal complications of regional analgesia, *Reg Anesth* 6:104, 1981.

274. Reisner LS, Hochman BN, Plumer MH: Persistent neurologic deficit and adhesive arachnoiditis following intrathecal 2-chloroprocaine injection, *Anesth Analg* 59:452, 1980.

275. Ravindran RS, Bond VK, Tasch MD, et al: Prolonged neuronal blockade following regional analgesia with 2-chloroprocaine, *Anesth Analg* 59:447, 1980.

276. Gissen AJ, Datta S, Lambert D: The chloroprocaine controversy. II. Is chloroprocaine neurotoxic? *Reg Anesth* 9:135, 1984.

277. Wang BC, Hillman DE, Spielholz NI, et al: Chronic neurological deficits and Nesacaine-CE: an effect of the anesthetic, 2-chloroprocaine, or the antioxidant, sodium bisulfite? *Anesth Analg* 63:445, 1984.

278. Meyers RR, Kalichman MW, Reisner LS, et al: Neurotoxicity of local anesthetics: altered perineurial permeability, edema, and nerve fiber injury, *Anesthesiology* 64:29, 1986.

279. Fibuch EE, Opper SE: Back pain following epidurally administered Nesacaine-MPF, *Anesth Analg* 69:113, 1989.

280. Ackerman III WE: Back pain after epidural Nesacaine-MPF, *Anesth Analg* 70:224, 1990.

281. Drolet P, Veillette Y: Back pain following epidural anesthesia with 2-chloroprocaine (EDTA-free) or lidocaine, *Reg Anesth* 22:303, 1997.

282. Chopra V, Bovill JG, Spierdijk J: Accidents, near accidents and complications during anaesthesia: a retrospective analysis of a 10-year period in a teaching hospital, *Anaesthesia* 45:3, 1990.

283. Tessler MJ: Inadvertent epidural administration of potassium chloride: a case report, *Can J Anaesth* 35:631, 1988.

284. Forestner JE, Raj PP: Inadvertent epidural injection of thiopental: a case report, *Anesth Analg* 54:406, 1975.

285. Lin D, Becker K, Shapiro HM: Neurologic changes following epidural injection of potassium chloride and diazepam: a case report with laboratory correlations, *Anesthesiology* 65:210, 1986.

286. Russell R, Dundas R, Reynolds F: Long-term backache after childbirth: prospective search for causative factors, *BMJ* 312:1384, 1996.

287. Ostgaard H, Andersson G: Postpartum low-back pain, *Spine* 17:53, 1992.

288. Macarthur A, Macarthur C, Weeks S: Epidural anesthesia and long term back pain after delivery: a prospective cohort study, *BMJ* 311:1336, 1995.

289. Loughnan B, Carli F, Romney M, et al: The influence of epidural analgesia on the development of new backache in primiparous women: report of a randomized controlled trial, *Int J Obstet Anesth* 6:203, 1997.

290. MacArthur C, Lewis M: Anaesthetic characteristics and longterm backache after obstetric epidural anaesthesia, *Int J Obstet Anesth* 5:8, 1996.

291. Clark V, McQueen M: Factors influencing backache following epidural analgesia in labour, *Int J Obstet Anesth* 2:193, 1993.

292. Wolfe MJ, Nicholas ADG: Selective epidural analgesia, *Lancet* 2:150, 1979.

293. Cohen SE, Woods WA: The role of epidural morphine in the postcesarean patient: efficacy and effects on bonding, *Anesthesiology* 58:500, 1983.

294. Rosen MA, Hughes SC, Shnider SM, et al: Epidural morphine for the relief of postoperative pain after cesarean delivery, *Anesth Analg* 62:666, 1983.

295. Brownridge P, Frewin DB: A comparative study of techniques of postoperative analgesia following caesarean section and lower abdominal surgery, *Anaesth Intensive Care* 13:123, 1985.

296. Hughes SC, Rosen MA, Shnider SM, et al: Maternal and neonatal effects of epidural morphine for labor and delivery, *Anesth Analg* 63:319, 1984.

297. Writer WDR, James FM III, Wheeler AS: Double-blind comparison of morphine and bupivacaine for continuous epidural analgesia in labor, *Anesthesiology* 54:215, 1981.

298. Akerman B, Arwestrom E, Post C: Local anesthetics potentiate spinal morphine anticociception, *Anesth Analg* 67:943, 1988.

299. Chestnut DH, Owen CL, Bates JN, et al: Continuous infusion epidural analgesia during labor: a randomized, double-blind comparison of 0.0625% bupivacaine/0.0002% fentanyl versus 0.125% bupivacaine, *Anesthesiology* 68:754, 1988.

300. Chadwick HS, Ross BK: Analgesia for post–cesarean delivery pain, *Anesthesiol Clin North Am* 7:133, 1989.

301. Writer WDR, Hurtig JB, Edelist G, et al: Epidural morphine prophylaxis of postoperative pain: report of a double-blind multicentre study, *Can Anaesth Soc J* 32:330, 1985.

302. Chadwick HS, Ready LB: Intrathecal and epidural morphine sulfate for postcesarean analgesia: a clinical comparison, *Anesthesiology* 68:925, 1988.

303. Naulty JS, Datta S, Ostheimer GW, et al: Epidural fentanyl for postcesarean delivery pain management, *Anesthesiology* 63:694, 1985.

304. Abboud TK, Moore M, Zhu J, et al: Epidural butorphanol or morphine for the relief of post-cesarean section pain: ventilatory response to carbon dioxide, *Anesth Analg* 66:887, 1987.

305. Kotelko DM, Rottman RL, Wright WC, et al: Transdermal scopolamine decreases nausea and vomiting following cesarean section in patients receiving epidural morphine, *Anesthesiology* 71:675, 1989.

306. Gieraerts R, Navalgund A, Vaes L, et al: Increased incidence of itching and herpes simplex in patients given epidural morphine after cesarean section, *Anesth Analg* 66:1321, 1987.

307. Crone LL, Conly JM, Clark KM, et al: Recurrent herpes simplex virus labialis and the use of epidural morphine in obstetric patients, *Anesth Analg* 67:318, 1988.

308. Crone LL, Conly JM, Storgard C, et al: Herpes labialis in parturients receiving epidural morphine following cesarean section, *Anesthesiology* 73:208, 1990.

309. Stenseth R, Sellevold O, Breivik H: Epidural morphine for postoperative pain: experience with 1085 patients, *Acta Anaesthesiol Scand* 29:148, 1985.

310. Gustafsson LL, Schildt B, Jacobsen K: Adverse effects of extradural and intrathecal opiates: report of a nationwide survey in Sweden, *Br J Anaesth* 54:479, 1982.

311. Korbon GA, James DJ, Verlander JM, et al: Intramuscular naloxone reverses the side effects of epidural morphine while preserving analgesia, *Reg Anesth* 10:16, 1985.

312. Leicht CH, Hughes SC, Dailey PA, et al: Epidural morphine for analgesia after cesarean section: a prospective report of 1000 patients, *Anesthesiology* 65:A366, 1986.

313. Bromage PR: The price of intraspinal narcotic analgesia: basic constraints, *Anesth Analg* 60:461, 1981.

314. Brockway MS, Noble DW, Sharwood-Smith GH, et al: Profound respiratory depression after extradural fentanyl, *Br J Anaesth* 64:243, 1990.

315. Ready LB, Oden R, Chadwick HS, et al: Development of an anesthesiology-based postoperative pain management service, *Anesthesiology* 68:100, 1988.

316. Rawal N, Wattwil M: Respiratory depression after epidural morphine: an experimental and clinical study, *Anesth Analg* 63:8, 1984.

317. Ready LB, Chadwick HS, Wild LM: Additional comments regarding an anesthesiology-based postoperative pain service, *Anesthesiology* 69:139, 1988.

318. Ready LB, Wild LM: Organization of an acute pain service: training and manpower, *Anesth Clin North Am* 7:229, 1989.

319. Ramanathan S, Gandhi S, Arismendy J, et al: Oxygen transfer from mother to fetus during cesarean section under epidural anesthesia, *Anesth Analg* 61:576, 1982.

320. Shnider SM, Moya F: Effects of meperidine on the newborn infant, *Am J Obstet Gynecol* 89:1009, 1964.

321. Way WL, Costley EC, Way EL: Respiratory sensitivity of the newborn infant to meperidine and morphine, *Clin Pharmacol Ther* 6:454, 1965.

322. Eisele JH, Wright R, Rogge P: Newborn and maternal fentanyl levels at cesarean section, *Anesth Analg* 61:179, 1982.

323. Quilligan EJ, Keegan KA, Donahue MJ: Double-blind comparison of intravenously injected butorphanol and meperidine in parturients, *Int J Obstet Gynecol* 18:363, 1980.

324. Miller RR: Evaluation of nalbuphine hydrochloride, *Am J Hosp Pharm* 37:942, 1980.

325. Rolbin SH: Diazepam during cesarean section: effects on neonatal Apgar scores, acid-base status, neurobehavioural assessment and maternal and fetal plasma norepinephrine levels, Society of Obstetrical Anesthesia and Perinatology, abstract 447, 1977.

326. Shnider SM: Paracervical block anesthesia in obstetrics, *Am J Obstet Gynecol* 107:619, 1970.

327. Finster M: Plasma thiopental concentrations in the newborn following delivery under thiopental-nitrous oxide anesthesia, *Am J Obstet Gynecol* 95:621, 1966.

328. Akamatsu TJ, Bonica JJ, Rehmet R: Experiences with the use of ketamine for parturition. I. Primary anesthetic for vaginal delivery, *Anesth Analg* 53:284, 1974.

329. Hodgkinson R, Marx GF, Kim SS, et al: Neonatal neurobehavioral tests following vaginal delivery under ketamine, thiopental and extradural anesthesia, *Anesth Analg* 56:548, 1977.

330. Downing JW, Buley RJR, Brock-Utne JG, et al: Etomidate for induction of anaesthesia at caesarean section: comparison with thiopentone, *Br J Anaesth* 51:135, 1979.

331. Reddy BK, Pizer B, Bull PT: Neonatal serum cortisol suppression by etomidate compared with thiopentone, for elective caesarean section, *Eur J Anaesthesiol* 5:171, 1988.

332. Ravlo O, Carl P, Crawford ME, et al: A randomized comparison between midazolam and thiopental for elective cesarean section anesthesia. II. Neonates, *Anesth Analg* 68:234, 1989.

333. Celleno D, Capogna G, Tomassetti M, et al: Neurobehavioral effects of propofol on the neonate following elective caesarean section, *Br J Anaesth* 62:649, 1989.

334. Apgar V, Holaday DA, James LS, et al: Comparison of regional and general anesthesia in obstetrics, *JAMA* 165:2155, 1957.

335. Benson RC, Shubeck F, Clark WM, et al: Fetal compromise during elective cesarean section, *Am J Obstet Gynecol* 91:645, 1965.

336. Stenger VG, Blechner JN, Prystowsky H: A study of prolongation of obstetric anesthesia, *Am J Obstet Gynecol* 103:901, 1969.

337. Finster M, Poppers PJ: Safety of thiopental used for induction of general anesthesia in elective cesarean section, *Anesthesiology* 29:190, 1968.

338. Datta S, Ostheimer GW, Weiss JB, et al: Neonatal effect of prolonged anesthetic induction for cesarean section, *Obstet Gynecol* 58:331, 1981.

339. Crawford JS, Davies P: Status of neonates delivered by elective caesarean section, *Br J Anaesth* 54:1015, 1982.

340. Warren TM, Datta S, Ostheimer GW, et al: Comparison of the maternal and neonatal effects of halothane, enflurane, and isoflurane for cesarean delivery, *Anesth Analg* 62:516, 1983.

341. Crawford JS, Burton M, Davies P: Anaesthesia for section: further refinements of a technique, *Br J Anaesth* 45:726, 1973.

342. Kangas-Saarela T, Koivisto M, Jouppila R, et al: Comparison of the effects of general and epidural anaesthesia for cesarean section on the neurobehavioural responses of newborn infants, *Acta Anaesthesiol Scand* 33:313, 1989.

343. Marx GF, Luykc WM, Cohen S: Fetal-neonatal status following caesarean section for fetal distress, *Br J Anaesth* 56:1009, 1984.

344. Kuhnert BR, Kennard MJ, Linn PL: Neonatal neurobehavior after epidural anesthesia for cesarean section, *Anesth Analg* 67:64, 1988.

345. Rosefsky JB, Petersiel ME: Perinatal deaths associated with mepivacaine paracervical-block anesthesia in labor, *N Engl J Med* 278:530, 1968.

346. Sinclair JC, Fox HA, Lentz JF, et al: Intoxication of the fetus by a local anesthetic: a newly recognized complication of maternal caudal anesthesia, *N Engl J Med* 273:1173, 1965.

347. Cohen S, Cherry C, Holbrook R, et al: Intrathecal sufentanil for labor analgesia: sensory changes, side effects, and fetal heart rate changes, *Anesth Analg* 77:1155, 1993.

348. Honet J, Arkoosh V, Norris M, et al: Comparison among intrathecal fentanyl, meperidine, and sufentanil for labor analgesia, *Anesth Analg* 75:734, 1992.

349. Clarke V, Smiley R, Finster M: Uterine hyperactivity after intrathecal injection of fentanyl for analgesia during labor, *Anesthesiology* 81:81, 1994.

350. Friedlander J, Fox H, Cain C, et al: Fetal bradycardia and uterine hyperactivity following subarachnoid administration of fentanyl during labor, *Reg Anesth* 22:378-381, 1997.

Chapter 25

Anesthesia Complications Occurring Primarily in the Very Young

Jennifer E. O'Flaherty
Frederic A. Berry

The very nature of anesthesia practice is to carefully review any potential or actual bad outcome and, when possible, to determine causation. In this way, the art and science of anesthesia can continually be advanced. Sometimes a situation or condition that was originally believed to be a result of negligent medical practice turns out to be another of Mother Nature's twists. An example of this is the infant with cerebral palsy. It was and often still is believed by some that cerebral palsy is caused primarily by preventable birth asphyxia and therefore there must have been negligence on the part of the anesthesiologist and obstetrician.[1] Recent studies have documented the lack of significant adverse antenatal events in the majority of mothers who delivered infants who later were found to have cerebral palsy.[2,3] What, then, is the cause of this devastating problem? A recent study on the causes of cerebral palsy pointed out that there is evidence that exposure to placental or maternal infection may be associated with cerebral palsy.[4] As the authors point out, the signs commonly attributed to birth asphyxia (i.e., low Apgar scores, resuscitation, and neonatal seizures) also occur in this situation. Assuming negligence as the cause of these signs is obviously inappropriate and represents negligence in itself. Obstetric and anesthetic care in the United States has steadily improved over the years, but the frequency of cerebral palsy has remained steady.[5]

Unfortunately, the legal profession with the assistance of the medical profession has pursued and won many medicolegal suits for children with cerebral palsy when there was no evidence of negligence. These "expert" opinions by physicians should be subject to the same analysis and accountability as any scientific paper. However, at present there is little accountability in this field. There are many plaintiffs' experts, among them academic anesthesiologists who travel the country giving irresponsible opinions about medical negligence cases, to the severe detriment of the medical profession as well as the unfortunate patients and their families.

It is hoped that this chapter will provide the anesthesiologist with an understanding of some of the complications that occur in the very young. It is also the goal of this chapter to provide the anesthesiologist with information so that the pitfalls can be avoided wherever possible, but also so that they can recognize that certain unavoidable complications will occur regardless of the degree of skill and care, and that a bad outcome is not equivalent to negligent care.

I. THE NEWBORN

A newborn is defined as an infant in the first 24 hours of life. This is the period of transition or adaptation in which the dependent fetus becomes the more independent newborn. The fetus depends on the umbilical circulation for nutrition, oxygenation, and metabolism. At birth, there is adaptation of all the various organ systems, a process that is mainly completed within the first 72 hours but goes on for approximately the first month of life. It is evident that the condition of the infant at birth is related to both the condition of the mother and the maternal-fetal circulation. Changes in the maternal-fetal circulation that may result in fetal damage may not be evident during the pregnancy and become manifest only in the neonatal period or in the several months thereafter. Meconium staining or aspiration is an example of a condition that may be present at birth but whose cause may have been present for a much longer period of time. Meconium aspiration is discussed in greater detail later. Cerebral palsy is an example of a condition in which there may have been long-term asphyxia of the infant, resulting in cerebral palsy, but the infant may appear normal at birth.

Various catastrophic events may occur at the time of delivery. These catastrophic events may be attributable to the preexisting medical condition of the mother, such as toxemia with seizure activity, or they may be attributable to the process of anesthesia, that is, the inability to intubate or the aspiration of gastric contents. The effect on the fetus is directly determined by the duration of the problem and the ability to resuscitate the mother. In general, if there is an acute problem with the mother, resulting in either hypotension or hypoxia, the fetus is left in utero until the mother can be resuscitated and then the mother can resuscitate the fetus. Reversibility depends on the cause of the asphyxia, the length of time it has existed, and the rapidity with which the infant is resuscitated.

A. Maternal fluid therapy with dextrose

The use of regional anesthesia has led to routine prehydration of the mother because in some parturients the resulting sympathectomy has resulted in hypotension. This is the reason why it is recommended that before epidural anesthesia, particularly for cesarean section, 1 to 2 L of balanced salt solution be administered. Dextrose should not be routinely included in this fluid because it was shown years ago that when a bolus of dextrose and salt solution was administered before delivery, some of the infants developed an acidosis that became evident shortly after birth. The acidosis was found to be caused by hypoglycemia. The mechanism for the hypoglycemia is that dextrose crossing the placenta stimulates the fetus's pancreas to release insulin in order to regulate the blood concentration of glucose. After birth, the extra supply of dextrose from the mother was discontinued, and the insulin released by the pancreas in some newborn infants resulted in hypoglycemia and acidosis.

B. Meconium aspiration

Considerable controversy has developed in the last several years about the treatment of the infant delivered from a mother in whom there has been either meconium staining of the amniotic fluid or the frank passage of meconium.[6-8] Intrauterine hypoxia can cause the fetus to pass meconium. If the hypoxia occurs in the immediate time of the delivery, the meconium often is thick and tenacious. This form of meconium mechanically obstructs the airway and must be removed by endotracheal suction. Various techniques have been described to accomplish this. On the other hand, meconium staining of the amniotic fluid may be a result of either a short or long period of hypoxia that occurred before the period of labor and delivery. Depending on the length of time that the meconium has been present in the amniotic fluid, there will be varying degrees of meconium staining of the infant's skin and fingernails. At times the reason for the interruption of the maternal placental oxygen flow has been corrected and the meconium-stained infant will have a normal Apgar score at birth. At other times, however, the reason for the decreased oxygen delivery may still be present and the Apgar score may be low at birth. If there is chronic intrauterine hypoxia, the fetus is susceptible to developing increased amounts of muscle in the blood vessels of the lung, with the result that the newborn infant may develop a condition known as persistent pulmonary hypertension.[9] These infants may have low Apgar scores at birth, need extensive resuscitation, and, depending on the degree of persistent pulmonary hypertension with its right-to-left shunt, have varying degrees of respiratory failure. As soon as this condition is identified and it becomes evident that the normal resuscitative and supportive techniques are not successful, these infants may be candidates for extracorporeal membrane oxygenation (ECMO) or nitric oxide. Even with that, they may well have a fatal outcome if they have severe pulmonary hypertension. It must be obvious from this discussion that it is difficult to tell immediately at birth what the various ramifications of meconium staining of the amniotic fluid or the infant are. Infants who have the meconium aspiration syndrome and who require intubation and ventilation when studied later in childhood are often found to have long-term pulmonary sequelae. The problems include airway hyperreactivity, elevated closing volumes, and hyperinflation.

In recent years, opinion about the management of meconium aspiration has changed. Many infants who have meconium staining are born with Apgar scores of 7 to 9. In the past, it was recommended that even these infants be intubated and suctioned. However, recent studies have strongly suggested that the risk-to-benefit ratio of this approach must be reevaluated.[6,7] In the prospective study of the routine suctioning of meconium-stained infants, regardless of Apgar score, there was a 2% incidence of iatrogenic pulmonary and laryngeal disorders. Although no mortality was reported, there was significant morbidity. Esophageal perforation has been reported as a result of the routine suctioning of a meconium baby with an Apgar score of 8.[10] Therefore it is time that we appreciated that meconium staining and the presence of meconium indicate an entire spectrum of disease. In some infants, there is chronic and acute hypoxia with a low Apgar score, and the infant needs immediate intubation, suctioning, and resuscitation. In some infants the airway may be obstructed by tenacious meconium that must be suctioned from the airway. In other infants with normal Apgar scores, the presence of meconium is a marker for a hypoxic episode that has long since passed. There is no benefit and potential harm in the routine suctioning and tracheal intubation of these infants.

II. THE NEONATE

The neonate is defined as an infant in the first 30 days of life. This is the time during which most life-threatening congenital anomalies become evident. These include craniofacial syndromes, congenital heart defects, congenital diaphragmatic hernia (CDH), tracheoesophageal fistula (TEF), anterior abdominal wall defects, and myelomeningocele. The most common cause of mortality in the first 30 days of life is prematurity. The second most common cause of mortality and morbidity in the first 30 days of life is congenital defects. Some infants have the problems of both prematurity and a congenital defect. Fortunately, of the congenital defects, only gastroschisis requires immediate therapy, so a period of stabilization can be achieved in most cases before surgery. Because additional congenital anomalies occur more often in infants with one congenital anomaly, renal, neurologic, and cardiac evaluations should be undertaken in any infant in whom surgery is contemplated. In congenital anomalies such as a TEF, the major risk of death and illness in an infant greater than 2 kg is not from the surgical condition itself, but from congenital heart disease. In general, congenital heart defects are found in approximately 20% of the infants with CDH, TEF, and omphalocele.

At present, few newborns require emergency surgical procedures. In most circumstances, if the local surgical team does not believe itself capable of treating the neonate, arrangements can be made for transport to a facility that is capable of providing care. The major issue would be stabilization of the infant and then safe, rapid transport to a tertiary facility.

A. Specific congenital anomalies

1. Craniofacial syndromes and cervical spine anomalies. It is beyond the scope of this chapter to list all po-

tential complications, or the actual complications that have been reported, with the various genetic syndromes. However, several examples are given to show the complexity of the problems and the enormous challenges the anesthesiologist may face. One of the problems with these genetic disorders is that they occur rarely and either may not be recognized initially or may not have known perioperative complications. However, some syndromes have well-defined perioperative implications.

The most common cause of difficult intubation in neonates with craniofacial syndromes is micrognathia. Well-recognized syndromes that commonly involve micrognathia include achondrogenesis, cri du chat, Edwards (trisomy 18), Patau (trisomy 13), Goldenhar, Rubinstein-Taybi, Smith-Lemli-Opitz, Treacher Collins, and the Pierre Robin sequence. The Pierre Robin sequence is the classic illustration of micrognathia, in which there is a primary defect in mandibular development in utero before the ninth week of gestation. The resulting severe micrognathia may lead to airway obstruction in the neonate, even without general anesthesia or sedation, and may make direct visualization of the glottis extremely difficult because there is no space in which to displace the tongue. A variety of alternative intubation techniques have been suggested, including the laryngeal mask airway (LMA),[11-13] digitally assisted intubation,[14] fiberoptic nasal intubation,[15,16] retrograde tracheal intubation,[17] laryngoscopy with the Bullard laryngoscope,[18] and blind nasal intubation in the prone position with hyperextension of the neck.[19] Other causes of difficult intubation in neonates with craniofacial syndromes include facial asymmetry, small mouth opening, and macroglossia. In the case of facial asymmetry, the glottis may be visualized more easily by displacing the tongue to the side that is larger. Cleft lip or palate, although often associated with craniofacial syndromes, do not usually pose additional concerns for the anesthesiologist.

Genetic syndromes with cervical spine involvement may present several challenges to the anesthesiologist. A short neck or fused vertebrae can prevent easy direct laryngoscopy secondary to an inability to extend the head. This is very likely to occur in the Klippel-Feil malformation sequence (1 in 42,000 births)[20,21] and in achondroplasia (1 in 15,000 births).[22,23] Rather than cervical spine fusion and immobility, some patients with genetic syndromes are at risk for cervical spine instability, which may result in compression of the spinal cord with varying degrees of disability. In the Klippel-Feil sequence there is a risk of hypermobility at the cervical level where motion at the interspace is maintained. Down syndrome, occurring in approximately 1 in 1000 births, is the most common single disorder that may involve atlantoaxial instability.[24,25] In Down syndrome the problem is ligamentous laxity of the transverse ligaments. Normally the connective tissue helps to stabilize the cervical spine; however, in this syndrome there is abnormal connective tissue. Subluxation narrows the diameter of the cervical canal and may cause spinal cord compression. Approximately 12% to 32% of all children with Down syndrome have laxity of the connective tissue, resulting in atlantoaxial instability, depending on the definition of instability and the age of the cohort.[26] There is also a high incidence of bony abnormality of the atlas and axis (6%), which may increase the potential for instability. Of the children with atlantoaxial instability, approximately 10% become symptomatic sometime during their lifetime. The earliest age at which this instability has been reported is 3 years. Unfortunately, radiographic criteria of atlantoaxial instability are not predictive of a tendency to subluxation. Most patients who develop atlantoaxial subluxation had neurologic signs or symptoms preceding the subluxation. Because radiographic evidence of atlantoaxial instability does not correlate with risk of subluxation and cord injury, many are advocating a careful preoperative neurologic examination and further workup (radiographs, neurosurgical consult) only in patients who are symptomatic.[27] There are ongoing studies of the natural history of this problem, but the anesthesiologist needs to be aware of this potential and maintain the head in as neutral a position as possible in the perioperative period. The predisposition to subluxation may be increased by the loss of muscle tone and manipulation of the head that occurs during general anesthesia and laryngoscopy. There have been case reports of spinal cord injury caused by atlantoaxial subluxation in patients with Down syndrome undergoing general anesthesia.[28-30]

2. Hypoplastic left heart syndrome. Fortunately, hypoplastic left heart syndrome is a rare congenital defect, occurring in 1 in 6000 live births; however, it accounts for 15% of all neonatal deaths from congenital heart disease.[31] Hypoplastic left heart syndrome in its most common form consists of an underdeveloped left ventricle, mitral valve, and aortic root. Until recently hypoplastic left heart syndrome was a lethal defect, with a mortality approaching 95% within the first month of life. In 1980, Norwood first described a surgical technique for palliation of hypoplastic left heart syndrome. Since then, modifications have resulted in a three-staged surgical palliation that ultimately allows the right ventricle to act as the systemic chamber and produces separation of the pulmonary and systemic blood flows with a Fontan procedure. Refinements in operative technique have led to improved survival of these patients. The 5-year actuarial survival for patients undergoing the staged Norwood procedure is between 60% and 70%, and the oldest survivors are now in their young teens.[32,33]

Instead of the palliative repair of the Norwood procedure, some advocate definitive repair with heart transplantation. Results of transplantation are comparable to those of surgical palliation in terms of survival[34]; however, transplantation involves several other concerns. There is a shortage of suitable donors, and the mortality of infants waiting for a donor heart is high. Also, heart transplantation and immunosuppression have been associated with accelerated atherosclerosis, leading to increased mortality beginning in the teen years. Considering the continually improving success of surgical management of hypoplastic left heart syndrome, it is now clear that terminal care is not the only option for these patients.

The long-term neurodevelopmental outcome for these patients has not yet been determined because survival has until recently been severely limited. However, both congenital and acquired neurologic abnormalities have been documented in these patients. There is a 29% incidence of major or minor anatomic central nervous system abnormalities in infants with hypoplastic left heart syndrome.[35] These abnormalities include agenesis of the corpus callosum, micrencephaly, ocular defects, and an immature cortical mantle. Acquired neuropathologic lesions were detailed in a study of 40 infants with hypoplastic left heart syndrome, all of whom expired and had a detailed postmortem neuropathologic examination.[36] Forty-five percent of the infants had combinations of hypoxic-ischemic lesions and intracranial hemorrhage. The major associated findings in infants with cerebral necrosis included hyperglycemia and low diastolic blood pressures during surgery with cardiopulmonary bypass and hypothermic circulatory arrest. Although acidosis and hypercapnia were not associated with significant problems, hyperglycemia was. This report suggests that the acquired brain lesions in some of these infants may have resulted from augmentation by hyperglycemia of the effects of hypoxia on the central nervous system.

3. Congenital diaphragmatic hernia. The incidence of CDH is between 1 in 2000 to 1 in 5000 live births. A developmental defect in the posterolateral diaphragm, usually on the left side (more than 90% of cases), is associated with herniation of abdominal viscera into the thorax, abnormal fetal lung development, and other abnormalities such as pulmonary hypertension, surfactant deficiency, and sometimes cardiac left ventricular hypoplasia.[37] A small percentage of the patients with CDH who die have such severe pulmonary hypoplasia as to not be able to survive extrauterine life, but the great majority of infants with CDH who die have adequate pulmonary size but have alveoli that are not adequately recruited, have alveoli that are iatrogenically damaged by aggressive ventilation if normocapnia is strictly adhered to, or have persistent right-to-left shunting of blood and persistent hypoxemia. Patients with CDH have abnormal pulmonary vasculature and increased sensitivity to the stimuli of pulmonary vasoconstriction.[38] Pulmonary hypertension and the resultant increase in pulmonary vascular resistance in CDH have led to persistent right-to-left shunting of blood through the ductus arteriosus and the foramen ovale. This results in a vicious cycle of hypercarbia, acidosis, and progressive hypoxemia, and may end in death. A portion of the persistent pulmonary hypertension in CDH may be caused by a relatively noncompliant lung secondary to inadequate recruitment of alveoli.

Examination of the amniotic fluid in infants with CDH suggests a deficiency of lung surfactant.[39] Exogenous surfactant therapy has been advocated as treatment even in instances where the lecithin/sphingomyelin ratio is normal because examination has shown qualitative as well as quantitative deficiencies in surfactant.[40] There is also evidence to indicate that treatment with inhaled nitric oxide, a selective pulmonary vasodilator, might improve oxygenation and survival in infants with CDH.[41]

Many patients with CDH will have a "honeymoon" period during which there is adequacy of gas exchange, hemodynamic stability, and stability of respiratory mechanics. Often these patients subsequently deteriorate, especially after repair of CDH. It has been demonstrated that stabilization of these neonates with delayed surgical repair of the hernia leads to increased survival and decreased morbidity.[42,43] The ideal time to repair the diaphragmatic hernia is unknown, but it may be after echocardiographic evidence of normal pulmonary artery pressures has been maintained for at least 24 hours. If conventional mechanical ventilation does not stabilize the neonate with CDH, then an alternative method such as high-frequency oscillatory ventilation or jet ventilation should be considered.

In the mid-1980s, ECMO was introduced as a means of treating patients with reversible failure of oxygenation and ventilation before or after repair of the diaphragmatic hernia. Obviously, patients whose pulmonary hypoplasia is so severe as to not permit extrauterine survival will not benefit in the long run from ECMO. ECMO provides total cardiorespiratory support and allows for a period of lung rest during which both pulmonary hypertension and parenchymal injury improve. Surgical repair of the diaphragmatic hernia while the patient is on ECMO has the advantage that postoperative decline in pulmonary function can be controlled and recurrent pulmonary hypertension can be treated. The major disadvantage is lack of hemostasis in a heparinized patient in whom surgical site bleeding and perioperative intracranial hemorrhage have been reported.

The mortality for infants born with CDH remained constant at about 50% until very recently. With recent improvements in neonatal critical care and preoperative stabilization, delayed surgery, and the use of ECMO in selected cases, the survival rate for CDH is reported to be as high as 90%.[42-44] However, long-term studies have identified multiple additional problems in patients who survive CDH. Coexisting morbidities include hearing loss, vision impairment, seizures, developmental delay, and problems of failure to thrive.[45] A very recent study suggests that delays in neurologic development are more common in infants surviving CDH who required ECMO than in those who did not. The difference in neurologic outcome may be related to the severity of the presenting illness or may be related to effects of ECMO that are as yet unidentified.[46]

4. Tracheoesophageal fistula. The infant with TEF may have associated esophageal atresia, prematurity and respiratory distress syndrome (RDS), or congenital heart disease (20% incidence). Without associated congenital heart disease, the survival of the neonate with TEF is 90% to 100%. Morbidity remains high, however, and is related to aspiration pneumonitis (when gastric contents are aspirated via the fistula), ineffective ventilation (when ventilatory gases are lost through the fistula into the stomach), and hemodynamic compromise (when a grossly distended stomach impedes venous return to the

heart). Aspiration pneumonitis is responsible for up to 50% of the morbidity in patients before surgical ligation.[47] After surgical repair of the TEF, morbidity is related to anastomotic leakage or stricture formation.[48] Premature infants with RDS and TEF represent an enormous challenge for the management team. In these patients especially, the stomach is much more compliant than the lungs, with the result that positive-pressure ventilation may be ineffective in ventilating the lungs but effective in the expansion of the stomach, which predisposes the infant to regurgitation and aspiration. Distention of the stomach with gas also elevates the diaphragm and may inhibit ventilation and decrease venous return. For these reasons, these infants are often treated with immediate separation of the gastrointestinal and respiratory tracts through emergency ligation of the TEF. A definitive repair can then be performed later when conditions have improved.[49] The availability of surfactant has decreased the complexity and improved the clinical outcome in at least some of these patients with concomitant TEF and RDS.[50]

In the infant with TEF, the anesthesiologist is faced with the problem of placing the tip of the endotracheal tube below the fistula. Most fistulas originate in the membranous posterior part of the lower trachea and connect into the distal end of the esophagus. Excessive positive-pressure ventilation may fill the stomach with gas, setting up the potential for regurgitation, aspiration, and reduced ventilation. Therefore the placement of the endotracheal tube below the fistula is a useful technique in the treatment of these infants. It appears that the easiest technique to achieve this placement is to pass the endotracheal tube into one mainstem bronchus, as evidenced by chest movement and breath sounds, and then slowly withdraw the tube until there are bilateral breath sounds and chest movement. Alternatively, if a gastrostomy tube is in place, the end of the gastrostomy tube can be placed under a water seal. After intubation, gentle positive pressure will force gas flow through the fistula and bubble out through the gastrostomy tube. The endotracheal tube is then advanced until the bubbling stops. At this point the distal end of the tube should be beyond the fistula. If the patient has a gastrostomy tube, it should always be open and left at the head of the table beside the anesthesiologist so that it cannot be obstructed. A patent gastrostomy tube is very useful for decompressing the stomach if gastric distention occurs with ventilation. However, gastrostomy tubes are no longer routinely used in patients with TEF before definitive repair.[51]

Another management technique for isolating the gastrointestinal and respiratory tracts is the passage of a Fogarty catheter down the trachea and into the fistula under direct visualization through a rigid bronchoscope. Traditionally this has been advocated for sick neonates with severe RDS or pneumonitis, but has more recently been advocated for all neonates with TEF. Surgical repair may follow.[47]

5. Anterior abdominal wall defects: gastroschisis and omphalocele. Gastroschisis is a developmental aberration in which there is a full-thickness defect in the abdominal wall, almost invariably located to the right of an intact umbilical cord. The incidence of gastroschisis is approximately 0.7 per 10,000 births. It has been hypothesized that gastroschisis results from a defect in differentiation of the somatopleural mesenchyme, an in utero rupture of a hernia of the umbilical cord, or an intrauterine interruption of the blood supply to the anterior abdominal wall.[52,53] The result is a hernia of the abdominal contents that is not covered by any membrane. The potential for loss of fluid and heat and the development of infection is great. The incidence of associated congenital anomalies with gastroschisis is very low. An omphalocele is an embryologic defect, probably a defect in the process of body infolding. The incidence of omphalocele is approximately 1 in 5000 live births. The incidence of omphalocele is 20 times greater in stillborns than in live-borns, showing that there is increased risk of early fetal death with this anomaly. The normal division by the diaphragm of the thoracoabdominal cavity from a single cavity into a double cavity occurs at approximately 6 to 10 weeks of fetal life. At this point, the intestines herniate into the umbilical cord while the diaphragm develops. By the 11th week of fetal life, all of the bowel should return to its final place within the abdomen. With an omphalocele there is a defect in the abdominal wall that includes muscle, fascia, and skin. Thus varying amounts of bowel remain in their extraabdominal location, covered only by peritoneum and amnion. The incidence of associated visceral malformations is 50% to 70%, of chromosomal abnormalities is 30%, and of congenital heart defects is approximately 20% to 30%.[53] The incidence of respiratory insufficiency is also high in omphalocele. Often, the ultimate prognosis depends largely on the presence and nature of the associated anomalies.

Prenatal diagnosis of abdominal wall defects through maternal α-fetoprotein screening and high-resolution ultrasound has meant that the majority of these patients are diagnosed in utero. Though traditionally associated with open neural tube defects, elevated maternal α-fetoprotein concentrations also are associated with abdominal wall defects, more often with gastroschisis than with omphalocele. The majority of these infants are then delivered by cesarean section, although there is ongoing debate as to whether the mode of delivery (vaginal versus abdominal) has any impact on outcome. The real advantage of prenatal diagnosis is that delivery may then occur in a center with adequate perinatal and pediatric surgical care.

Postnatal treatment of the patient with gastroschisis involves keeping the exposed bowel moist with saline-soaked gauze and placing the infant in a sterile bag to minimize evaporative losses and infection. These precautions are unnecessary in patients with an omphalocele because the bowel is covered by a membrane. In either case, a nasogastric tube should be placed to prevent bowel distention. Gastroschisis patients will need intravenous antibiotics and intravenous fluid to replace the significant fluid losses from the exposed bowel. Because of the associated extreme risk of infection and the stag-gering losses of fluid, the defect in gastroschisis requires immediate surgical closure. Primary surgical closure of either defect is preferred because there is a lower incidence of sepsis, bowel obstruction, fistulae formation, and need for more surgeries. However, in some cases the abdominal wall defect is so large and the amount of extruded viscera is so great that primary closure is impossible or the resultant intraabdominal tension is too high. This increased intraabdominal pressure may be transmitted to the blood vessels of the lower extremities, reducing venous return and causing edema of the lower extremities. Increased intraabdominal pressure may also result in a reduction of blood flow to the abdominal organs, most often manifesting as bowel necrosis or as renal failure secondary to renal ischemia. Finally, increased intraabdominal pressure may elevate the diaphragm and interfere with ventilation. In these cases it is necessary to create a silo by covering the defect with Silastic mesh and suturing the edges of the mesh to the intact abdominal fascia. This is followed by staged reduction in the size of the silo over the next 7 to 14 days until the abdominal contents can be restored fully to the abdomen and the defect can be closed by fascia to fascia approximation. It has been shown that intraabdominal pressures greater than 20 to 25 cm of water necessitate the placement of a silo. Perioperatively, all of these infants should remain intubated and paralyzed to allow maximal abdominal muscle relaxation in order to accommodate the returned viscera. Recent successes in delayed fascial closure have emphasized that avoidance of increased intraabdominal pressure improves the overall prognosis for these patients.[54]

6. Myelomeningocele. Myelomeningocele is a neural tube disorder characterized by a dorsal vertebral defect and herniation of variable amounts of meninges, cerebrospinal fluid, cauda equina, or residual spinal cord. There is usually some degree of neurologic compromise below the level of the lesion. The incidence is 1 in 400 births in previously unaffected families and may rise to 1 in 20 after the birth of an affected infant. Primary prevention of neural tube defects has been shown to occur with maternal ingestion of at least 0.4 mg per day of folic acid at the time of conception. Recent evidence suggests that the risk of neural tube defects, even in families with one infant with myelomeningocele, can be reduced by up to 70% in women with adequate intake of folic acid.[55]

Eighty percent of myelomeningoceles are in the lumbar or sacral region. Maternal serum α-fetoprotein screening and high-resolution ultrasound have significantly increased the prenatal diagnosis of this defect. It is important that these patients be identified prenatally so that they may be delivered by cesarean section. Trauma during vaginal delivery can exacerbate the neurologic compromise associated with myelomeningocele or cause rupture of the meningeal covering, leading to an increased risk of infection. Nearly 100% of patients with myelomeningocele have a hindbrain malformation known as the Arnold-Chiari malformation, which results in caudal displacement of the lower brainstem. This may lead to herniation of the caudal vermis through the foramen magnum, kinking of the medulla and upper cervical cord, and subsequent disruption of the vascular supply to the brainstem and compromise of the lower cranial nerves. Eighty to 90% of these patients develop hydrocephalus, often in the first several months after birth, requiring shunting of the cerebrospinal fluid in order to prevent detrimental increases in intracranial pressure.

Eighty to 90% of patients with myelomeningocele have neurogenic bladder dysfunction, requiring repeated bladder catheterization and surgical procedures. The repeated exposure to latex products is believed by many to be the cause of the well-recognized high incidence of latex allergy in these children. There is a relationship between the degree of exposure (number of operations) and the development of immunoglobulin E (IgE) antibodies to latex.[56,57] This allergy has led to anaphylaxis in the operating room.[58,59] Because patients with myelomeningocele are at risk for multiple exposures to latex, many practitioners now advocate primary prevention by avoidance of latex-containing products perioperatively in all patients with myelomeningocele, whether or not they have demonstrated an allergy to latex. For patients with a history of latex allergy, there has been controversy over whether to provide allergy prophylaxis before a planned surgical procedure. To clarify this issue, a recent study examined 267 procedures in 162 children previously identified as latex allergic. These patients did not receive premedication with antihistamines or steroids. Of the 267 procedures there was only one instance of allergic reaction (anaphylaxis) in a patient who was inadvertently exposed to a latex-containing product (an epidural catheter syringe with a latex stopper). Thus for children who are latex allergic, it appears that a latex-free environment is sufficient in preventing perioperative anaphylaxis and that premedication with allergy-modifying medications is unnecessary.[60] As the issue of latex allergy gains publicity, manufacturers are likely to make it easier to identify latex-containing products and easier to obtain products that are latex-free.

B. Extracorporeal membrane oxygenation

ECMO is a technique of supportive therapy that has been in widespread use in this country for over 10 years. Since its introduction, ECMO has had a much higher rate of success in neonates (overall survival rate approximately 80%) than in older pediatric patients or adults (overall survival rate approximately 50%). Its primary use in infants has been for respiratory failure that occurs with meconium aspiration syndrome or RDS; however, it may be used in any type of respiratory failure. There has been a recent decline in the use of neonatal ECMO because many patients are being successfully treated at the referral hospital with surfactant, high-frequency oscillatory ventilation, and nitric oxide rather than being referred for ECMO.[61]

The object of ECMO is to allow the lung to rest while minimizing barotrauma and alveolar hyperoxia. The period of ECMO varies from hours to days. Originally the technique involved cannulization of the right internal jugular vein as the vessel that would provide the blood supply for the pump oxygenator and cannulization of the right internal carotid artery for the return of oxygenated blood to the infant. Alternatively, ECMO can be accomplished via a venovenous circuit, in which a double-lumen catheter is placed in the right atrium to drain deoxygenated blood and return oxygenated blood. Venovenous ECMO results in a mixture of deoxygenated and oxygenated blood in the right atrium. While on ECMO, the infant's lungs should remain inflated with an FIO_2 of 30% at 5 cm of positive end-expiratory pressure (PEEP). As the infant's lungs and PaO_2 improve, he or she is slowly weaned from ECMO by decreasing the ratio of extracorporeal blood flow to that of the infant's cardiac output.

Several problems are associated with ECMO. These include heparinization and the consequent dangers of intracranial bleeding and ligation of the internal carotid artery. The infants who receive ECMO are all critically ill, so it is difficult to tell whether instances of neurologic damage or bad outcome are a result of ECMO or of the initial insult. However, certain post-ECMO observations are being made, including changes in the retina, changes in the pattern of cerebral circulation, structural changes in the brain, seizures, and developmental delay.[62,63] Technical advances that may help prevent neurologic complications with ECMO include venovenous rather than venoarterial bypass, cephalic venous drainage to help maintain normal cerebral blood flow, and reconstruction of the carotid artery after ECMO. The long-term benefit of carotid artery reconstruction is unclear at this time.[64]

The pharmacokinetics of drugs commonly administered to patients on ECMO are not well understood. The ECMO circuit tubing, the membrane oxygenator, and the heat exchanger provide a large surface area that has the potential to bind drugs. In effect, the ECMO circuit results in an increase in the neonate's volume of distribution and potentially reduces the bioavailability of drugs such as fentanyl, morphine, and the barbiturates. To make matters more complicated, it appears that newer circuits bind drugs more avidly than do circuits that have been in clinical use for a while. Temperature also seems to affect binding of drugs to the circuit components. Therefore it is very difficult to determine adequate dosing of drugs except by following serum drug concentrations. The route of administration for a drug also influences its pharmacokinetics. Drugs may be administered intravenously directly to the neonate, or may be administered through any number of infusion ports in the ECMO circuit. Drugs administered directly to the ECMO circuit may bind extensively to the circuit until saturation is reached, or pool in the venous reservoir, particularly at low flows, thus significantly decreasing the dose of drug that reaches the patient.[65]

C. Prenatal cocaine exposure and its effects on the infant

The use of cocaine by Americans has increased dramatically over the past two decades, with an estimated 20 to 30 million Americans having used cocaine at some point in their lives and approximately 5 million using cocaine on a regular basis.[66] Many users are women of childbearing age. The prevalence of cocaine use in the obstetric population is approximately 10%. Identifying the cocaine user has been extremely difficult because self-reporting has been shown to be extremely unreliable.[67] The anesthesiologist must maintain a high level of suspicion. The single most important predictor of cocaine use in pregnancy has been shown to be lack of prenatal care.[68] Cocaine is an amino alcohol base that is structurally similar to synthetic local anesthetics such as lidocaine. Cocaine prevents the reuptake of neurotransmitters such as epinephrine, norepinephrine, dopamine, and serotonin at nerve terminals. This leads to increased concentrations of these neurotransmitters and an exaggerated responsiveness or supersensitivity that can affect the central nervous and cardiovascular systems. There is increased motor activity, hyperthermia, and a host of cardiovascular effects, including hypertension, tachycardia, and vasoconstriction. Because cocaine is metabolized by serum and hepatic cholinesterases, there may be sustained high blood concentrations of cocaine in pregnant women secondary to the well-documented decrease in serum cholinesterase activity during pregnancy. Experiments in animals have shown the maternal-to-fetal ratio of plasma cocaine to be approximately 3:1. The lower plasma concentrations in the fetus may result from placental metabolism of cocaine or decreased placental blood flow secondary to the vasoconstricting effects of cocaine.[69] Surprisingly, fetal cocaine exposure has not been associated with any specific pattern of teratogenesis.[70,71] Breastfeeding may provide the neonate with an additional route of exposure to cocaine.

Intracranial hemorrhage and seizures occur more commonly in cocaine-using parturients. The cause of intracranial bleeding probably is secondary to an acute increase in systemic blood pressure after cocaine use and subsequent rupture of an aneurysm. Cocaine use has also been associated with myocardial ischemia and infarction, arrhythmias, and valvular abnormalities in pregnant women. It is important for the anesthesiologist and the obstetrician to be able to distinguish between hypertension associated with cocaine use and hypertension associated with preeclampsia or eclampsia. There is an increased incidence of spontaneous abortion among cocaine users. Cocaine users are also at increased risk of having preterm labor, placental abruption, and stillbirth. Interestingly, the increased risk of placental abruption occurs even in patients whose use of cocaine was limited to the first trimester, suggesting that the mechanism of this increased risk is disruption of placental adherence to the uterine wall secondary to cocaine-induced vasoconstriction. Finally, cocaine use has also been associated with the development of thrombocytopenia, and it may be prudent to obtain a platelet count in known users before deciding on a regional anesthetic technique.[71]

There is an increased incidence of prematurity, inhibited intrauterine growth, and microcephaly in babies born to cocaine-using mothers, presumably because of uteroplacental insufficiency from cocaine-induced vaso-

constriction. There is also an increased risk of various developmental defects in the fetus, which include cavitary central nervous system lesions; facial abnormalities such as cleft lip; limb-reduction defects; other skeletal defects; cardiac anomalies such as pulmonary stenosis, transposition of the great vessels, and hemopericardium; vascular anomalies; genitourinary anomalies; and intestinal atresia or infarction.[71] The exact cause of this spectrum of developmental problems is not fully understood, but the underlying pathogenesis is likely to be vascular disruption.[72] Vascular disruption probably is secondary to the vascular effects of cocaine, which lead to uterine, placental, or fetal vasoconstriction. Disruption of the blood supply may lead to altered morphogenesis of the developing structures. For example, disruption of blood flow to the fetal heart may interfere with the development of a specific region of the heart. Disruption of blood flow has been shown to be a cause of limb reduction defects. Disruption of the superior mesenteric artery early in fetal life may lead to intestinal atresia, and if it occurs later in fetal life, it may result in bowel infarction.

Depending on when the mother last used cocaine, the infant might also undergo a neonatal abstinence syndrome. These infants exhibit hyperflexion and prolonged periods of scanning eye movements, excessive irritability, and tachypnea. Neurobehavioral follow-up on cocaine-exposed infants shows an increased risk of delayed fine and gross motor skills, hypotonia, irritability, abnormal reflexes, electroencephalographic abnormalities, and seizures.[71,73,74] There may be an increased risk of sudden infant death syndrome (SIDS) in infants exposed to cocaine in utero, but an association has not yet been established clearly.[75] Renal dysfunction has also been reported in neonates exposed to cocaine in utero and may have implications for drug selection in these patients.

The cardiovascular changes found in newborns exposed to cocaine in utero may have important implications for the anesthesiologist. Increased heart rates and systemic blood pressures have been documented in cocaine-exposed newborns. Van de Bor, Walther, and Ebrahimi[76] recently studied 15 full-term newborn infants whose mothers had a history of cocaine use during pregnancy. Table 25-1 displays the data. The cocaine-exposed infants had higher arterial blood pressures and lower cardiac outputs and stroke volumes, consistent with a transplacental passage of catecholamines or of cocaine, which then resulted in increased concentrations of circulating catecholamines. Of particular interest to the anesthesiologist is that by day 2 the differences between the cocaine and the control groups had completely disappeared. It appears from these data that if an infant of a cocaine-using mother is born with a congenital anomaly requiring surgery, that surgery should be postponed until at least the second postnatal day, unless the surgery is emergent, in order to allow the effects of cocaine to abate.

III. THE PREMATURE INFANT

A premature birth is defined in terms of gestational age and weight.[77] Gestational age is measured from concep-

Table 25-1. Cardiac function in cocaine-exposed and control full-term newborn infants on the first and second day of life

	Day 1			Day 2		
	Cocaine-exposed group ($n = 15$)	Control group ($n = 22$)	P value	Cocaine-exposed group ($n = 15$)	Control group ($n = 22$)	P value
Cardiac output (ml/kg/min)	183 ± 12	235 ± 13	<.05	222 ± 10	240 ± 8	NS
Stroke volume (ml/kg)	1.3 ± 0.1	1.9 ± 0.1	<.005	1.6 ± 0.1	1.8 ± 0.1	NS
Heart rate (beats/min)	142 ± 11	133 ± 20	NS	140 ± 11	134 ± 12	NS
Arterial blood pressure (mm Hg)	60 ± 2	41 ± 2	<.001	55 ± 1	56 ± 2	NS

From van de Bor M et al: *Pediatrics* 85:31, 1990.
Results are given as means ± SD; P values were obtained from Student's test for unpaired observations; *NS*, not significant.

tion until birth, and the premature infant is an infant born at less than 37 weeks gestational age and weighing less than 2.5 kg. Prematurity is one of the leading causes of infant mortality and morbidity. The reasons for it are multiple and are not discussed here. Medical technology has brought about an increased survival of these very small infants, many of whom have catastrophic short-term and long-term medical problems. The group of premature infants who have the highest risk for a devastating outcome are those with a birthweight below 1500 g, and they are defined as extremely-low-birthweight infants.[78,79] These are the premature infants who usually require prolonged intubation, ventilation, resuscitation, and other measures. The percentage who end up with visual disturbances, mental retardation, seizures, and other major medical problems is often as high as 30% to 40% of the survivors. Unfortunately, quality of life has not been part of the formula for the treatment of these infants, and outcome studies in these infants reveal that technology for survival has far exceeded our ability to provide a meaningful life. Nonetheless, the anesthesiologist is faced with the anesthetic treatment of these infants. This discussion is concerned primarily with the complications that may accompany the anesthetic treatment of the premature infant for surgery. The most common surgical procedures are for the treatment of the retinopathy of prematurity and inguinal hernias. A common concern is postoperative apnea. An unresolved question is at what postconceptual age these patients can be treated in an ambulatory surgery unit.

A. Retinopathy of prematurity

In the last 40 years, the clinical picture and treatment of infants with retinopathy of prematurity has undergone major change.[80-82] It was recognized in the early and mid-1950s that the unrestricted use of oxygen in the premature infant was associated with a very high incidence of retinopathy of prematurity. After this, very restrictive policies were developed limiting the use of oxygen in the newborn infant. At that time, the analysis of blood gases was in its infancy and attempts to correlate arterial oxygen values with retinopathy of prematurity proved to be formidable and fruitless. However, one

thing did become evident with the restrictive management of oxygen administration to newborns. Up until this point, there had been a progressive decrease in the mortality and morbidity of infants. After the restrictive oxygen policies, there was a leveling off and in some countries an increase in the incidence of central nervous system damage that was attributed to the restrictive use of oxygen.[83] Over the ensuing years, attempts were made to determine a safe level of oxygenation, as determined by transcutaneous oxygen values and later by the pulse oximetry. One study did support an association between the incidence and severity of the retinopathy of prematurity and the duration of exposure to transcutaneously measured arterial oxygen concentrations greater than 80 mm Hg. The duration of exposure was quite prolonged (hours per day for up to 4 weeks). Their study also found that the more immature the infant and the sicker the infant, the higher the incidence of the retinopathy of prematurity, regardless of intensive attempts to evaluate and control the administration of oxygen.[82] Therefore the development of retinopathy of prematurity does not necessarily represent a breach of care.

This leaves the anesthesiologist in a quandary. There has never been any documentation that the short time of an anesthetic is sufficient for the development of the retinopathy of prematurity. There are differences of opinion as to how the anesthesiologist should attempt to control the oxygen saturation of the premature infant. One opinion is that attempts should be made to control oxygenation by monitoring the oxygen saturations and keeping them between approximately 90% and 95%. The other opinion is that the short period of anesthesia is insignificant and that hypoxia is much more of a danger than the retinopathy of prematurity. There appears to be no consensus on this issue. The current policy of these authors is to add either air or nitrous oxide, depending on the surgical situation, to the inspired oxygen concentration so that the pulse oximeter reads below 100. However, on some occasions, even with the premature breathing essentially room air, the saturation may still be 99 to 100. When the premature infant is unstable and there are problems with either circulation or maintaining the saturation at a stable level, then the FIO_2 is increased to 100% as needed until the condition stabilizes, regardless of the oxygen saturation.

B. Prematurity and incidence of inguinal hernia

Hernias that appear in infants under 1 year of age have a natural course different from that of hernias that appear after a year. The incarceration rate of hernias in infants under 1 year of age approaches 31%, compared to a 15% to 18% incidence in hernias that appear after 1 year of age.[84] In addition, the incidence of hernias in premature infants is much higher than the incidence of hernias in full-term infants.[85] One of the best studies to document the problems of the premature infant and hernia repair is that of Rescorla and Grosfeld.[84] They report a series of 100 infants who were operated on by the time they were 2 months of age; 30% of these infants were premature, 42% had a history of RDS, and 16% had been ventilated for this condition. A congenital heart defect was found in 19%. Of these infants, 31% had an incarcerated hernia and 9% were found to have an intestinal obstruction. Two percent of the infants had a gonadal infarction. It becomes evident that the infant who develops a hernia while in the premature nursery is at high risk for developing an urgent or emergent surgical problem. For that reason, these infants must be operated on within a reasonable period of time after discovery of the hernia, rather than waiting or being discharged home to grow until some arbitrary age or weight in the hopes that there will be no supervening incarceration or intestinal obstruction.

C. Periventricular-intraventricular hemorrhage

There is no question that the premature infant runs a much higher risk of developing periventricular-intraventricular hemorrhage (PV-IVH). Also, it is believed that newborn infants, regardless of gestational age, who have suffered from acute hypoxia have decreased autoregulation.[86] Decreased autoregulation results in a condition in which cerebral blood flow is pressure passive, and any increases in blood pressure increase cerebral blood flow and the potential for PV-IVH. At any rate, some of the manipulations performed by the anesthesiologists have the potential to induce hypertension, particularly if these manipulations are done in the unanesthetized state. This includes manipulations such as the starting of intravenous fluids and awake intubation. Also, the use of some anesthetic techniques, such as an opioid-pancuronium combination, can result in hypertension. Recent studies in a group of premature infants who were observed for PV-IVH have provided some insight into the incidence and natural history of PV-IVH and some of the factors that might possibly be associated with it.[87] These studies were performed because it was suggested in the pediatric literature that increases in blood pressure, which often occur with intensive care procedures, were believed to be implicated in the pathogenesis of PV-IVH.

What is the bottom line for the anesthesiologist? Because it appears that there is some correlation between peak systolic pressures and the development of PV-IVH,

at least in the first several days of life, it appears that, when possible, all procedures (that is, intubations) should be done with sedation or anesthesia unless the infant is so critically ill that the risk would exceed the benefits. The general belief is that all procedures must be thought of in a risk-benefit fashion. For example, if an infant is vomiting and has the risk of aspiration during induction and intubation, an awake intubation should be considered, but a rapid sequence induction and intubation may be as safe depending on the circumstances. On the other hand, if there are no compelling reasons for an awake intubation, the infant deserves the same consideration as older patients and should receive the appropriate anesthesia or sedation. Just because a premature infant can be overpowered is not a reason to withhold appropriate anesthetic techniques for both comfort and blood pressure control.[88]

D. The premature nursery graduate and associated medical problems

It follows that with the increasing number of premature infants who survive there is an increasing number of premature nursery graduates. They present medical problems in three different areas: chronic lung disease, subglottic stenosis, and apnea.

1. Chronic lung disease. Any infant who has been intubated and ventilated is a candidate for chronic lung disease.[89] The majority of the infants who have this problem are premature infants who were born with a deficiency of surfactant, resulting in RDS. The results of various studies indicate that there usually is an immediate improvement in lung function and outcome with surfactant treatments. The infants who receive surfactant have a lower incidence of pulmonary interstitial emphysema and pneumothorax than do control infants. Very-low-birthweight infants with bronchopulmonary dysplasia (BPD) have a higher rate of mental retardation and poorer motor outcome than those who do not develop BPD.[90]

However, there still will be infants who have chronic lung disease. This chronic lung disease presents as a spectrum of clinical problems. In the infant with mild disease, there may be only increased secretions and mild reactive airway disease. At the far end of the spectrum is the child with severe BPD and severe reactive airway disease who is oxygen dependent. There is a significant mortality among these infants. The important issue for the anesthesiologist is to be able to identify the infant with chronic lung disease. Severe chronic lung disease is identified easily. Many of these infants are on chronic diuretic therapy, and the diuretics should be continued in the perioperative period. Mild respiratory disease and mild reactive airway disease in a premature infant may be difficult for the anesthesiologist to identify because the patient may be asymptomatic and may become symptomatic only with the airway manipulation of anesthesia and surgery. The red flag for the possibility of residual lung disease is a history of intubation and ventilation. If the infant is growing normally, is feeding normally, and has had minimal respiratory infections or symptoms, in all likelihood he or she will not have any problems. However, if the infant has frequent episodes of coughing, recurrent respiratory tract infections, and so on, there is a high index of suspicion that this infant will present some clinical challenges. Infants with residual airway disease present with varying degrees of bronchospasm, increased secretions, and decreased compliance. Infants with moderate to severe degrees of residual lung disease must be treated as inpatients, whereas those who have mild residual disease can be treated expectantly as outpatients. These infants benefit from anticholinergics to reduce secretions and dilate large airways. Because of reactive airway disease, they are prone to problems with laryngospasm, bronchospasm, and secretions and are best treated with an endotracheal tube, except in the shortest anesthetic procedures. In addition, they should remain intubated until awake. Infants with mild residual lung disease might slip through preoperative screening and develop problems with bronchospasm or laryngospasm during induction and intubation. Topical Xylocaine 3 mg/kg at intubation reduces the laryngeal reactivity. In other infants the troubles occur at the end of surgery. Premature extubation of these infants often results in a tumultuous postoperative course. For that reason, any infant who appears to be having any degree of reactive airway disease should be left intubated until awake with active protective airway reflexes. This period of postoperative intubation can be smoothed over by the administration of intravenous anticholinergics as well as 1 to 1.5 mg/kg of intravenous lidocaine at the end of surgery. This dose can be repeated one time in 5 minutes. It is the practice of these authors to use supplementary regional or local anesthesia whenever possible in infants and children. This strategy minimizes or eliminates the need for intraoperative narcotics, reduces or eliminates the need for muscle relaxants and subsequent reversal agents, and decreases the need for inhaled anesthetics so that the infant recovers his or her airway reflexes rapidly after surgery and can be extubated in a timely fashion.

2. Subglottic stenosis. In 1981, Jones et al[91] reported on a group of premature infants who had been intubated and ventilated for respiratory problems, 20% of whom subsequently developed subglottic stenosis after discharge. At the time of discharge from the premature nursery, they were believed to be asymptomatic and without airway difficulty. The subglottic stenosis became evident only when the infants acquired a respiratory infection. The increased secretions and edema from the airway infection, when added to the previously unrecognized subglottic stenosis, caused the infants respiratory embarrassment, which eventually led to the diagnosis of subglottic stenosis. Reactive airway disease may be blamed for these respiratory findings. Tachypnea, retractions, and wheezing are all signs of both reactive airway disease and subglottic stenosis, and in infants who have been intubated and ventilated the anesthesiologist needs to keep in mind that the patient may have one or both of these conditions. The first time that the anesthesiologist may become aware that an infant has unrecognized subglottic stenosis is when endotracheal intubation is at-

tempted. If an infant cannot be intubated with the normal-size endotracheal tube and the next smaller size endotracheal tube cannot be passed or there is no air leak, the presence of subglottic stenosis should be suspected. At that point, the anesthesiologist is faced with a quandary. If this is emergency surgery that cannot be delayed, an endotracheal tube must be used even if it is small and the infant is ventilated for the surgical procedure. Extubation may be possible at the end of surgery with the use of dexamethasone (Decadron) and racemic epinephrine. If the surgery is elective, postponement until the airway can be evaluated fully seems to be the most conservative approach. If a pediatric surgeon familiar with airway disease is immediately available, an evaluation of the airway can be made and then a judgment made as to whether to proceed with the surgery.

3. Apnea. Apnea is a common finding in the premature infant and is believed to be caused by an immature respiratory center. The incidence of apneic episodes is inversely correlated with conceptual age. As premature infants approach the conceptual age of 44 to 48 weeks, the incidence of apnea decreases rapidly to almost nil.[92] One of the problems with the various studies is the definition of apnea. Brief apnea is defined as a respiratory pause of less than 15 seconds, not associated with bradycardia, whereas prolonged or potentially life-threatening apnea is defined as a respiratory pause of 15 seconds or longer or less than 15 seconds if accompanied by bradycardia. Bradycardia is defined in this situation as a heart rate of less than 100 beats/min for at least 5 seconds. There has been a concern that the administration of anesthetics and other depressants might increase the incidence of apnea in premature infants. Many studies have been done in premature infants at the various conceptual ages. It is important to use the term *conceptual age,* which is defined as the age from the time of conception until the current age. It is the gestational age plus postnatal age.

An unresolved issue is at what postconceptual age (PCA) to allow superficial and hernia surgery to be done on an ambulatory basis. There are two current opinions. One is that infants under 50 weeks of PCA should be admitted for all surgery and should be monitored overnight for apnea and bradycardia. Infants over 50 weeks of PCA can be treated as ambulatory patients with no special precautions. The second opinion is that all patients under 60 weeks of PCA must be admitted and monitored and that these infants can be treated as ambulatory patients only when they are older than 60 weeks of PCA.[93] A recent study, which was a combined analysis of eight studies that had previously been done, evaluated the risk of apnea as it was related both to PCA and gestational age.[94] The final conclusions of the study were that the limitations of the study and of the analysis were such that the decision about what is an acceptable risk for postoperative apnea rests with each institution and each physician. It is these authors' practice to admit premature infants with a PCA of 50 weeks or less for surgery and, if they are older than that, to consider them for ambulatory surgery. However, if they have postoperative apneic episodes of more than a transient nature, then they are admitted and monitored.

There is also a difference of opinion about whether the choice of anesthesia makes any difference in the outcome. Several studies suggest that regional anesthesia is the preferred technique in high-risk infants. However, it is well known that the administration of sedatives to an infant with regional anesthesia causes an incidence of apnea that is similar to that seen with general anesthesia. In addition, both spinal anesthesia and caudal anesthesia have an incidence of complications significant enough that the choice of technique is not simple.

Some surgeons do not like to operate on infants with only regional anesthesia and because no studies indicate that one technique (general or regional) has superior advantages over the other, it is inappropriate for the anesthesiologist to insist that the surgeon operate using an anesthetic technique that he or she is not comfortable with.

IV. COMPLICATIONS OF ANESTHETIC TECHNIQUES IN INFANTS

Any discussion of anesthetic techniques in infants must consider the current trend in regional anesthesia, which has been touted by some to be extremely safe and to avoid many of the difficulties associated with postoperative apnea. Certainly the learning curve plays a significant part in the incidence of complications as the anesthesiologist acquires the necessary skills in mastering each anesthetic technique. This is not to suggest that the anesthesiologist should be proficient only in general anesthesia. The requirements of anesthesia practice are such that the anesthesiologist must continually adapt new techniques and drugs to his or her practice.

A. General anesthesia

Most anesthesiologists are more comfortable using general anesthesia for infants, particularly for high-risk infants. Regional or local anesthesia can be added for intraoperative and postoperative analgesia. The major complications with general anesthesia in the infant are associated with the establishment and maintenance of the airway and the period of extubation and recovery from the anesthetic. Some anesthesiologists do an awake intubation to establish the airway in the small infant, but this is becoming less common. The complications in the premature infant and in the asphyxiated infant have been discussed previously. Other complications associated with awake intubation include trauma to the airway and hypoxia. The degree of hypoxia was not fully appreciated until the advent of the pulse oximeter. However, anyone who has performed or watched an awake intubation in the small infant can appreciate the struggle, which is accompanied by coughing, breath holding, and desaturation. Insufflation of oxygen, either with the laryngoscope or by another technique, may reduce but may not circumvent the problem because it results from the fact that the infant is breath-holding or coughing and not ventilating.

B. Complications of neuromuscular blockers

One of the most serious and difficult to recognize complications of neuromuscular blockers is an anaphylactoid or anaphylactic reaction. Anaphylaxis under anesthesia may present differently than in the awake patient. Usually three systems are involved in anaphylaxis: the cardiovascular system, the respiratory system, and the skin. However, during anesthesia only one of these systems may be involved, or there may be delayed recognition of the other systems. One of the most common presentations of anaphylaxis is an initial tachycardia followed by severe hypotension. Alternatively, the respiratory system may be the only system involved in anaphylaxis, with a resulting decrease in compliance and a decrease in oxygenation. The differential diagnosis includes an obstructed endotracheal tube, a circuit problem, or a machine problem. The recent recognition of latex anaphylaxis has greatly heightened the interest and awareness of anesthesiologists in this problem. The treatment is epinephrine, starting with 5 to 10 µg/kg and increasing the dose as needed to stabilize the blood pressure and reduce the bronchospasm. High dosages of epinephrine may be needed.

Another potential problem with neuromuscular blockers is that as they produce relaxation the infant's airway may become obstructed and he or she may develop postobstructive pulmonary edema.[95] It is a paradox that the upper airway muscles relax and the airway becomes obstructed but the infant still has sufficient negative intrathoracic pressure to generate pulmonary edema. Hypoxia in this situation increases the likelihood that pulmonary edema will develop. The treatment is to leave the patient intubated with PEEP until the oxygen saturation normalizes.

C. To intubate or not to intubate? Potential complications

The question often arises in the small infant who is going to have a short procedure (under 30 minutes): Does the patient need to be intubated? There is no question that the very skilled clinician usually can manage even the most difficult airway with a mask or an LMA, but the clinician who rarely treats such infants might not have the skills to use these techniques. For that reason, most clinicians intubate most infants under 6 months for most surgical procedures. The exception to this is an examination under anesthesia that is going to require 5 or 10 minutes or hernia repair with a fast and skilled surgeon. In the older infant, airway management is considerably easier, and with the use of the precordial stethoscope, pulse oximeter, and capnograph, an ongoing assessment of the success in airway management is immediately available. If there is any question about airway management, particularly if documented by the various monitors, endotracheal intubation is the technique of choice. The LMA has proven to be useful as a bridging or definitive airway in infants with difficult airways. The LMA is finding a place in the routine anesthetic treatment of these infants, but this change has been accompanied by a loss of skill in laryngoscopy and endotracheal intubation.

D. Timing of extubation and postoperative ventilation: avoiding premature extubation

One of the most difficult judgment calls for the anesthesiologist is when to remove the endotracheal tube. If the condition of the infant is marginal, or there is any question about whether the infant will be able to maintain protective reflexes or ventilation, the endotracheal tube should be left in place and the infant sent to the recovery room or directly to the pediatric or newborn intensive care unit. Many of the complications of anesthesia in the infant are related to the issue of the timing of extubation.

If the infant is healthy enough, with appropriate anesthetic planning he or she can be extubated at the end of the procedure in the operating room with protective reflexes intact or taken to the postanesthesia care unit (PACU), where a decision can be made in an unhurried fashion about the appropriate time for extubation. If after a reasonable period the infant still is not ready for extubation, he or she is transferred to the intensive care unit and care is transferred to the medical staff of the intensive care unit. The final group of infants are those who are expected to need postoperative ventilatory support. The anesthetic in this case is tailored to maintain a degree of sedation and paralysis at the end of the surgery so that the infant may be more safely transported to the intensive care unit, where the care is transferred from the anesthesiologist to the intensive care medical staff. It is usually anticipated that these infants will be extubated in a matter of hours or days.

How does the anesthesiologist avoid the complication of premature extubation, which can include airway obstruction, hypoxia, pulmonary edema, bradycardia, and delayed awakening because of inability to adequately ventilate? The key is that the infant should be extubated when awake, with protective airway reflexes intact and the neuromuscular system optimal. One of the ways to minimize the amount of muscle relaxant, as well as minimize the intraoperative administration of narcotics, is to use various forms of local infiltration or regional anesthesia for the surgical procedure. This allows the anesthesiologist to use a lighter level of anesthesia so that the infant recovers airway reflexes quickly and can be extubated sooner. Postoperative narcotics can be titrated in slowly in the PACU. Signs that the infant is ready for extubation are opening of the eyes, crying, coughing, swallowing, and reaching for the endotracheal tube. Even with the most diligent care, airway obstruction after extubation cannot always be avoided, and the clinician must be prepared to reintubate the infant. In some infants, there is always some degree of doubt whether reintubation will be successful. These infants should be extubated in the PACU in an unhurried manner, with equipment and personnel at the bedside.

E. Complications of regional anesthesia

1. Epidural (caudal) anesthesia. Regional anesthesia has been highly touted as a very safe technique for infants.[96] However, some special factors make the infant more susceptible to complications in certain areas. One of the most popular and effective regional anesthetic techniques in the infant is caudal epidural anesthesia. However, it should be remembered that the dural sac in the infant may end as low as the S3 level, whereas in the older child and adult the dural sac ends at the S1 level. The technique described is to penetrate the sacrococcygeal ligament at the sacral hiatus and then advance the needle a short distance into the caudal canal. It is obvious in the small infant that great care must be taken as to how far the needle is advanced. Many clinicians do not advance the needle, but use the technique of penetrating the sacrococcygeal ligament, which has a distinctive feel; the loss of resistance as the anesthetic is injected indicates that the needle is in the epidural space. The needle is not advanced, thereby reducing the chance of complications from either intradural or intravascular administration. Aspiration should be done very gently, and some clinicians suggest detaching the syringe from the needle or extension tubing and determining whether there is intravascular needle placement. High negative aspiration pressure on the syringe may collapse the vein and minimize the chance of return of blood. Another precaution to minimize the possible effects of an intravascular injection are to put epinephrine in the solution at a concentration of 5 μg/ml of anesthetic and to divide the dose into thirds and inject each third, wait 20 to 30 seconds, and then continue. A recent report on the detection of intravascular injection of local anesthetics in children revealed that there was a 5.6% incidence of intravascular injection with a large number of pediatric epidural blocks.[97] The incidence of intravascular injections was 3.8% with a straight needle and 6.7% when the epidural was done with a catheter. The important findings in the study were as follows. In approximately 15% of the patients, the intravascular injection was detected by the aspiration of blood. Seventy-five percent had an increase in heart rate of more than 10 beats/min, but of more importance was the fact that when electrocardiogram (ECG) strips were analyzed, 83% of the intravascular injection patients had T-wave amplitude increases greater than 25%. The anesthetic used was 0.25% bupivacaine with epinephrine 1:200,000. The other important issue emphasized in this study was the importance of dividing the dose by incremental injection, as suggested earlier. Despite extreme care and negative aspiration, total spinal anesthesia has been reported in an infant after a carefully performed caudal epidural block. Another potential complication with caudal anesthesia is the fact that the posterior bony plate of the sacrum is very soft and it is quite easy for the caudal needle to penetrate the bone and terminate in the bone marrow. This complication can be minimized by using a No. 22 short-bevel needle and by both aspiration and awareness that the ease of injection of the solution is a sign of correct needle placement for a caudal epidural injection. As with a lumbar epidural, if the solution cannot be easily administered, the needle must be relocated.

An infrequent but potentially devastating complication of epidural anesthesia in infants is the occurrence of a venous air embolism when the technique involves using air for the loss of resistance. Because of this danger, most anesthesiologists recommend using either saline or the anesthetic solution in the loss of resistance technique. We prefer to use the local anesthetic solution.

Another potential complication of postoperative pain management with continuous epidural catheters is the potential for overdose with central opioids or with the local anesthetic solution. Recent recommendations for epidural bupivacaine infusions after a loading dose of 2 to 2.5 mg/kg are an infusion rate not to exceed 0.25 mg/kg per hour for neonates and an infusion rate not to exceed 0.5 mg/kg per hour in older infants and children.[98] The major risk with epidural infusions of bupivacaine is the development of seizures, whereas the major risk with epidural opioids is respiratory depression.

2. Spinal anesthesia. Spinal anesthesia is another regional anesthetic technique that has become very popular, particularly in the high-risk infant. However, some differences between infants and older patients must be appreciated. One of these is the fact that it takes a very large dose of the spinal anesthetic to accomplish anesthesia, and the second is that, even with the large dose, the duration of the block is shorter than that found in the adult. As an example, the dose of tetracaine in an infant is 0.5 mg/kg. In a 70-kg adult, this would represent a dose of 35 mg and would last much longer than it does in an infant. This large dose of tetracaine provides only 60 minutes of anesthesia for the infant. Therefore one of the problems of spinal anesthesia in the infant is the short duration of the block, which may not be appreciated until the infant begins to move and the various adjuncts must be added. Usually this requires the administration of intravenous sedation, which in premature infants results in an incidence of postoperative apnea similar to that of general anesthesia. In some institutions, intravenous access is not obtained until after the spinal anesthetic is administered. The reason for this is that the veins of the lower extremities are then more easily cannulated after the regional anesthetic is given and that sympathectomy rarely causes pressure changes in infants. However, precious time may be required for intravenous access. Gaining intravenous access after the induction of epidural anesthesia is a different matter. Intravenous access is strongly recommended before epidural anesthesia. The most feared complication of epidural anesthesia is intravascular injection. The way to treat intravascular injection is the use of intravenous medications such as epinephrine, calcium, and sodium bicarbonate. If an intravascular injection occurs without the presence of intravenous access, it is much more difficult to treat.

Another complication of spinal anesthesia is the occurrence of a high spinal block. Surprisingly, high spinal block is not associated with significant cardiovascular changes (i.e., hypotension) in the infant. There are at least two theories as to why this occurs and it may be a combination of these. Dohi, Naito, and Takahashi[99] suggest that the reason for the lack of vasodilation is that there is relative immaturity of the sympathetic nervous system so that there is minimal vasodilation. However, Oberlander et al[100] believe that there is a decrease in parasympathetic activity and modulation of the heart rate and that this effect results in the absence of significant cardiovascular change with the sympathectomy of a high spinal or epidural anesthetic. The anesthesiologist must be aware that this lack of cardiovascular change can be a double-edged sword. One of the signs of a total spinal or a very high epidural anesthetic in the older child and adult is that there is a decrease in blood pressure, and this may be one of the early warning signs of trouble. This decrease is not found in an infant, and the first sign of total spinal block may be interference with ventilation, as reported by Warner et al.[95] The first sign of trouble was desaturation followed by evidence of paralysis. This report also demonstrates that potential complications of anesthetic management are associated with the positioning of infants. Some surgeons request that cautery be used. This requires the placement of a ground plate. Some surgeons lift the feet and torso of the infant and place the Bovie pad on the upper back of the infant, thereby flexing the entire body on the neck. This maneuver may cause the spinal anesthetic to migrate cephalad and cause respiratory insufficiency. Removal of the pad at the end of surgery can also cause difficulty if the infant has just been extubated and is attempting to regain control of his or her airway. If the infant is then lifted by the feet and rotated on the neck to remove the pad, this step can interfere with ventilation and may cause regurgitation. Therefore the Bovie pad should be placed on the upper chest, buttocks, or leg, or the infant rolled gently onto his or her side to remove the Bovie pad.

These various complications emphasize the importance of close monitoring with a precordial stethoscope and a pulse oximeter regardless of whether regional anesthesia or general anesthesia is being used. One must always be aware that Murphy's law is the constant companion of the anesthesiologist. The next point to remember is that the anesthesiologist must always believe the monitors until the patient and the monitors have been checked.

F. Always believe the monitors

If there is one theme that the anesthesiologist must remember when dealing with small infants and children, it is that you must always believe the monitors. If any abnormal values appear on a monitor or if it is thought that the monitor is not functioning, the infant must be checked for ventilation and circulation. This check should include an analysis of the anesthetic mixtures, the ventilation, feeling the pulse, and so on. Also, if there is any question, the surgeon should be informed. We have reviewed many medical malpractice cases in which monitors were ignored for several minutes because they were believed to be inaccurate. Then it was discovered after the blood pressure cuff had been moved or the ECG patches replaced or a new oximeter probe attached that the problem was actually in the patient. There is no question that the equipment must be checked if the values appear to be wrong, but this is done after the ventilation and circulation of the patient have been checked.

Whenever there are unexpected findings on the monitor, first the patient should be checked, then the surgeon informed, and then the monitors checked.

G. Sudden onset of hypotension or bradycardia

The complication of sudden-onset hypotension or bradycardia has undergone an etiologic reevaluation in the past several years because of the pulse oximeter and the ability to monitor end-tidal gases. Previously, the sudden appearance of hypotension or bradycardia was often attributed to progressive hypoxia that had been missed by the nonvigilant anesthesiologist. Many plaintiff's experts traveled the country espousing such a view. The pulse oximeter has revealed several things. First of all, progressive hypoxia does not lead to the sudden appearance of bradycardia or hypotension. Severe hypoxia results in alterations in the heart rate or rhythm as well as the blood pressure before severe bradycardia and hypotension. In other words, the sudden onset of bradycardia or hypotension is suggestive of a severe cardiovascular collapse attributable to a rare but profound vagal response, an anaphylactic or anaphylactoid reaction, air embolism, or hyperkalemia. On occasion there may also be a volume deficit that by itself is tolerated but may be difficult to treat and reverse when complicated by one of these events. The signs of an anaphylactoid or anaphylactic reaction and the percentage of patients involved are listed in Table 25-2. The classic triad of anaphylaxis is involvement of the skin, respiratory system, and cardiovascular system. One can readily appreciate from the table that not all three systems need to be involved for such a diagnosis to be made; isolated bronchospasm or hypotension can occur. When it does, it often is associated with a high morbidity.

The evaluation and treatment of bradycardia with or without severe hypotension involves the clinician evaluating the vital signs, immediately terminating anesthesia, and notifying the surgeon. Bradycardia in the infant is usually defined as a heart rate under 100. If the heart rate drops from 120 to 100, then it seems appropriate to administer atropine in a dose of 0.02 mg/kg, which can be repeated. On the other hand, if the heart rate changes suddenly (i.e., within seconds or a minute) from 120 to 60, this indicates a severe problem. Vagal stimulation can cause this change, and release of the traction on the viscera or whatever else is stimulating the vagus may or may

not result in the heart rate returning to normal. This is a different situation than when the heart rate decreases slowly and there is time to evaluate the situation. The reason is that the young infant is dependent on heart rate for cardiac output and when the heart rate drops below 100, cardiac output drops dramatically and there is rapid onset of ischemia. Atropine is not the drug of choice in this situation because in all probability the peripheral circulation is inadequate and it takes time for atropine to become effective. The treatment of the acute onset of hypotension or bradycardia is epinephrine 5 to 10 μg/kg intravenously. If there is any question about the adequacy of the peripheral circulation, external cardiac massage must be instituted to maintain or increase the circulation. The remainder of the treatment consists of turning off all anesthetics, ventilating with 100% oxygen, expanding the vascular volume with a balanced salt solution or blood, informing the surgeon, and seeking the cause of the problem. The patient may well need additional doses of epinephrine or an epinephrine infusion in the case of anaphylaxis.

H. Complications of fluid management associated with glucose control

The two major potential complications in glucose control are those of hypoglycemia and hyperglycemia.

1. Hypoglycemia. One of the difficulties in understanding the control of glucose in the infant and older child is a definition of hypoglycemia. Several papers give multiple glucose ranges. A quotation from one paper brings the problem into focus: "Albert Aynsley-Green returned to the clinical problem of defining neonatal hypoglycemia and illustrated the current dilemma by citing various definitions ranging from 18 to 72 mg/dl glucose from 36 pediatric textbooks and from 178 British pediatricians, the majority of whom used levels of less than 36 mg/dl in full-term infants and less than 20 mg/dl in premature small-for-gestational-age babies as their definition of hypoglycemia."[101] Years ago, the issue of hypoglycemia was rarely a problem for the anesthesiologist because great quantities of glucose were given to all infants. An appreciation of the potential problems of hyperglycemia has resulted in a closer look at the risks and benefits of glucose in patients.

In several situations the metabolic status of the baby and the issue of hypoglycemia may be a potential problem for the anesthesiologist. We know that premature infants who are small for gestational age, infants of diabetic mothers, and infants with heart failure all have the potential to become hypoglycemic. As a general rule, it would be useful to know what their blood glucose concentrations are before anesthesia and surgery. It has been well documented, at least in normal older infants and children, that the blood glucose concentrations remain stable or increase during the period of anesthesia and surgery. The glucometer has a 20% error range at low glucose concentrations. If there is a question, then the glucose must be checked by the standard glucose testing. If an infant has had problems with hypoglycemia, a constant infusion of glucose during the perioperative period

Table 25-2. Signs of an anaphylactic or anaphylactoid reaction

Signs	Patients involved (%)
Tachycardia	94
Circulatory collapse	92
Widespread flush, edema	79
Bronchospasm	39
Cardiac arrest	14
Bradycardia	6
Arrhythmias	4

will prevent the potential problems of hypoglycemia. This is usually given in a constant infusion in a dose of 5 to 7 mg/kg/min. Infants who have been on hyperalimentation or dextrose 10% should have the infusion continued during the perioperative period.

2. Hyperglycemia: the dangers of glucose and cerebral ischemia. Over the past several years, there has been an enormous interest in the association between the administration of glucose and its effects on the outcome after cerebral ischemia.[102] In several of the experimental studies that have been performed, the animals who did not receive glucose but who suffered an ischemic episode appeared to recover normally, whereas those who had received glucose during the period of ischemia and resuscitation had much worse neurologic outcomes.[103] This is extremely important for the anesthesiologist because occasionally there may be unavoidable episodes of ischemia of the central nervous system secondary to ventilatory or circulatory problems. It appears that if intravenous glucose is administered during this period or in the immediate recovery period, the glucose may adversely affect the outcome. The suggested mechanism is that the intravenous glucose, though it may not greatly increase blood glucose, may well increase brain glucose. In the face of ischemia sufficient to trigger anaerobic metabolism, the presence of increased brain glucose results in a greater production of lactic acid in the central nervous system, which results in a decrease in the brain pH, which has been shown to aggravate neuronal injury.[103] In the normal patient, it is prudent to administer glucose-free solutions.

V. COMPLICATIONS OF SUCCINYLCHOLINE
A. Hyperkalemia

In 1992, the Food and Drug Administration's attention was drawn to reports by the Malignant Hyperthermia Association of the United States and the North American Malignant Hyperthermia Registry that a number of cardiac arrests had occurred in apparently healthy children given succinylcholine as a part of a routine anesthetic, usually for a minor surgical procedure.[104] The mortality rate for these events reported between 1990 and 1993 was 40%.[105] The reports prompted an investigation into the cause of these cardiac arrests. Hyperkalemia was demonstrated in a number of cases and suspected in a number of others. In the vast majority of patients tested, Duchenne muscular dystrophy (DMD) or other myopathy was subsequently diagnosed. This hyperkalemia is distinct from, and should not be confused with, malignant hyperthermia (MH).

DMD is the most common muscular dystrophy in children. It is inherited as X-linked recessive, and thus is evident only in males. Even though the usual onset of the symptoms of DMD is sometime during the second to third year of life, the underlying neuromuscular disease may come to the attention of the anesthesiologist at an earlier age. Alterations within the muscle cell in patients with DMD result in a flux of potassium when succinylcholine is administered. This flux of potassium may result in varying degrees of hyperkalemia, which may

lead to significant arrhythmia or asystole.[104,105] Previously, anesthesiologists avoided using succinylcholine in any infant with a family history of DMD or a physical examination indicative of a myopathy. However, in approximately 30% of children with DMD there is no family history of the disease. These recent reports indicate that there are a number of children whose myopathy is undetected, but who are nonetheless at risk for hyperkalemic arrest after the administration of succinylcholine. In November 1993, the Burroughs Wellcome Company changed the Anectine (succinylcholine chloride) package insert to state, "Except when used for emergency tracheal intubation or in instances where immediate securing of the airway is necessary, succinylcholine is contraindicated in children and adolescent patients."[106] There has been ongoing controversy as to whether the use of succinylcholine should be contraindicated in female infants and children, because the majority of congenital myopathies occur only in males, and whether the use of succinylcholine should be contraindicated in children beyond the age of 2 or 3 years, because a careful history and physical examination should reveal evidence of a myopathy by that age.

B. Myalgias

Another complication of succinylcholine, which may be mitigated by pretreatment, is that of myalgias. Succinylcholine, particularly in infants and small children, results in damage to the muscle cell, as evidenced by increased concentrations of creatinine phosphokinase (CPK) and by myoglobinemia and in some cases myoglobinuria. This is a normal response to succinylcholine. It can be minimized or prevented by pretreatment with a nondepolarizing muscle relaxant. This pretreatment results in a pronounced reduction in the concentrations of CPK and a considerable reduction in myalgias. Infants who are not of walking age will be little bothered by the myalgias, but infants and children of walking age should be pretreated, even though our ability to evaluate this problem in these patients is difficult. For older children and adults the problem of myalgia is so common that the clinician should always plan to use pretreatment before succinylcholine.[107]

C. Masseter spasm

Recent studies concerning the normal response of the masseter muscle to succinylcholine have caused us to completely reevaluate the issue of masseter spasm.[108,109] These studies reveal that the normal response of the masseter muscle to succinylcholine is an increase in tone. As seen in Fig. 25-1, this increase in tone is maximal at the time when the fasciculations and the nerve twitch have terminated. Attempts to perform laryngoscopy at this point occur at a time when the masseter muscle has its maximal tone. A small but significant number of patients have sufficient masseter muscle tone (1 in 100) so as to make it difficult to open the mouth.[109] This may well explain some of the previous reports of masseter spasm. What has also been found in these studies is that low dosages of succinylcholine delay the time of onset of the

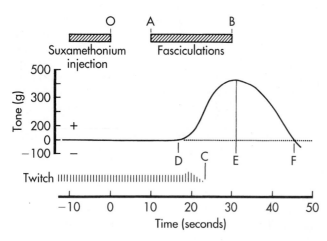

Fig. 25-1. Normal response of the masseter muscle to succinylcholine. *A* and *B*, Period of observed facial muscle fasciculation. *C*, Cessation of muscle twitch from ulnar nerve stimulation. *D*, Onset of increased muscle tone. *E*, Maximum muscle tone. *F*, Offset of increased muscle tone. (From Leary NP, Ellis FR: *Br J Anaesth* 64:488, 1990.)

increase in masseter muscle tone. Therefore to avoid the complication of masseter spasm, two techniques are suggested: waiting 20 seconds until fasciculations have stopped and using a larger dose of succinylcholine: 2 mg/kg in infants and children and 1.5 mg/kg in adults.

D. Malignant hyperthermia

MH is a pharmacogenetic disease characterized by a hypermetabolic state. The primary biochemical aberration occurs in skeletal muscle, where intracellular concentrations of calcium become abnormally high. Increased intracellular calcium forces cells into a hypermetabolic state that can lead to increased oxygen consumption, increased carbon dioxide and heat production, and respiratory acidosis. As adenosine triphosphate (ATP) stores become exhausted, the muscle contraction-relaxation cycle arrests in the contraction phase, producing muscular rigidity. Finally, as ATP stores are completely used up, cell integrity is jeopardized and cells begin to leak potassium, calcium, CPK, and myoglobin. A severe metabolic acidosis results. Up to 70% of untreated cases end in death. With treatment, the case fatality rate has dropped to 7%. Fortunately, MH is rare, occurring in approximately 1 in 220,000 general anesthetics.[110] More than half of the reported cases of MH occur in children. There is a family history of MH in approximately 25% of cases. It is difficult to determine the youngest age at which MH has occurred in infants. One paper reported a possible MH reaction in a 7-week-old infant.[111] MH probably is a genetically heterogeneous disorder in humans. Unfortunately, this means that a simple DNA-based diagnostic test for MH susceptibility is unlikely to be developed in the near future.[112]

There is still no universally accepted definition of MH.[113] Diagnosis of MH depends on clinical signs such as increased end-tidal carbon dioxide, tachycardia, tachypnea, muscle rigidity, sweating, fever, and acidosis.

An unexplained increase in end-tidal carbon dioxide is often the most sensitive sign of developing MH. Fever is more often a late sign. Caffeine-halothane muscle contracture testing has been used since the early 1970s for the diagnosis of MH susceptibility and is still the gold standard. Unfortunately, this test is invasive and expensive. It requires a fresh muscle sample, which necessitates that the patient travel to one of the 10 centers in North America that still perform this test. In most cases it is easier to treat the patient with a suspicious personal or family history as being MH susceptible and administer a local, regional, or nontriggering general anesthetic. The only certain triggers of MH are the volatile agents and succinylcholine, and they are avoided easily. If MH is suspected during the administration of an anesthetic, one must abort the surgical procedure as soon as possible, discontinue the use of triggering agents, hyperventilate with 100% oxygen, provide active cooling and supportive care, and administer intravenous Dantrolene 2.5 to 3 mg/kg. Dantrolene is a direct skeletal muscle relaxant that works by inhibiting the release of calcium from the sarcoplasmic reticulum, and has been a life-saving agent in cases of MH.

Several papers have strongly suggested that masseter spasm is highly correlated with the development of MH and point out that a high percentage of patients with masseter spasm have a muscle biopsy that is positive for MH susceptibility.[114,115] In fact, a recent study found that 59% of patients (41 of 70) referred for muscle biopsy because they experienced masseter muscle rigidity after succinylcholine were indeed MH susceptible, although only 12% of those (5 of 41) developed clinical signs of MH.[116] On the other hand, the reported incidence of masseter spasm (as high as 1 in 100 general anesthetics in one study)[117] is much greater than the reported incidence of MH (approximately 1 in 220,000 general anesthetics). This tremendous discrepancy suggests the need for another explanation for the significance of masseter spasm. In many cases it appears that masseter spasm is not a significant indicator of MH but may well be a normal finding. This is still a point of controversy; as a result, the clinician is faced with two diametrically opposed positions on what to do with the patient who develops increased masseter muscle tone after succinylcholine administration. One approach is to consider masseter muscle spasm to be strongly associated with the development of MH and to discontinue the anesthetic, or at least switch to a nontriggering anesthetic, and observe the patient carefully for developing signs of MH.[116,118] The other approach, which we follow, is to recognize that increased masseter muscle tone after succinylcholine is common in children and may not be an indicator of MH susceptibility but may occur normally with the administration of succinylcholine.[119-121] The anesthetic may be continued safely, although these patients should be monitored carefully for developing signs of MH.

VI. SUMMARY

The anesthesiologist dealing with infants is walking through a minefield of various potential complications and bad outcomes, some of which are preventable and some, regardless of effort, are nonpreventable. Preparation to avoid or identify these complications includes continuing medical education, consultation with colleagues, careful monitoring of the patient, and luck. The one caveat, particularly in infants, is always to believe the monitors.

ACKNOWLEDGMENT
The editorial assistance of Robert Bland is greatly appreciated.

REFERENCES

1. Hey E: Fetal hypoxia and subsequent handicap: the problem of establishing a causal link. In Chamberlain GVP, Orr CJB, Sharp F, eds: *Litigation and obstetrics and gynecology,* London, 1985, Royal College of Obstetricians and Gynecologists.
2. Torfs CP, Vandenberg B, Oechsli FW, et al: Prenatal and perinatal factors in the etiology of cerebral palsy, *J Pediatr* 116:615, 1990.
3. Perlman JM: Intrapartum hypoxic-ischemic cerebral injury and subsequent cerebral palsy: medicolegal issues, *Pediatrics* 99:851, 1997.
4. Grether JK, Nelson KB: Maternal infection and cerebral palsy in infants of normal birth weight, *JAMA* 278:207, 1997.
5. Freeman JM, Nelson KB: Intrapartum asphyxia and cerebral palsy, *Pediatrics* 82:240, 1988.
6. Linder N, Aranda JV, Tsur M, et al: Need for endotracheal intubation and suction in meconium-stained neonates, *J Pediatr* 112:613, 1988.
7. Wiswell TE, Tuggle JM, Turner BS: Meconium aspiration syndrome: have we made a difference? *Pediatrics* 85:715, 1990.
8. Katz VL, Bowes WA: Meconium aspiration syndrome: reflections on a murky subject, *Am J Obstet Gynecol* 166:171, 1992.
9. Murphy JD, Vawter GF, Reid LM: Pulmonary vascular disease in fetal meconium aspiration, *J Pediatr* 104:758, 1984.
10. Topsis J, Kinas HY, Kandall SR: Esophageal perforation: a complication of neonatal resuscitation, *Anesth Analg* 69:532, 1989.
11. Baraka A: Laryngeal mask airway for resuscitation of a newborn with Pierre-Robin syndrome, *Anesthesiology* 83:645, 1996.
12. Markakis DA, Sayson SC, Schreiner MS: Insertion of the laryngeal mask airway in awake infants with the Robin sequence, *Anesth Analg* 75:822, 1992.
13. Hansen TG, Joensen H, Henneberg SW, et al: Laryngeal mask airway guided tracheal intubation in a neonate with the Pierre Robin syndrome, *Acta Anaesth Scand* 39:129, 1995.
14. Sutera PT, Gordon GJ: Digitally assisted tracheal intubation in a neonate with Pierre Robin syndrome, *Anesthesiology* 78:983, 1993.
15. Howardy-Hansen P, Berthelsen P: Fiberoptic bronchoscopic nasotracheal intubation of a neonate with Pierre Robin syndrome, *Anaesthesia* 43:121, 1988.
16. Scheller JG, Schulman SR: Fiberoptic bronchoscopic guidance for intubation of a neonate with Pierre Robin syndrome, *J Clin Anesth* 3:45, 1991.
17. Yonfa AE, Klein E, Mackall LL: Retrograde approach to nasotracheal intubation in a child with severe Pierre Robin syndrome: a case report, *Anesthesiol Rev* 10:29, 1983.
18. Baraka A, Muallem M: Bullard laryngoscopy for tracheal intubation in a neonate with Pierre-Robin syndrome, *Paediatr Anaesth* 4:111, 1994.
19. Populaire C, Lundi JN, Pinaud M, et al: Elective tracheal intubation in the prone position for a neonate with Pierre Robin syndrome, *Anesthesiology* 62:214, 1985.
20. Naquib M, Farag H, Ibrahim AE, et al: Anaesthetic considerations in Klippel-Feil syndrome, *Can Anaesth Soc J* 33:66, 1986.
21. Daum REO, Jones DJ: Fiberoptic intubation in Klippel-Feil syndrome, *Anaesthesia* 43:18, 1988.
22. Kalla GN, Fening E, Obiaya MO: Anaesthetic management of achondroplasia, *Br J Anaesth* 58:117, 1986.
23. Berkewitz I, Raja S, Bener K, et al: Dwarfs: pathophysiology and anesthetic implications, *Anesthesiology* 73:739, 1990.
24. Msall ME, Reese ME, DiGaudio K, et al: Symptomatic atlantoaxial instability associated with medical and rehabilitative procedures in children with Down syndrome, *Pediatrics* 85:447, 1990.
25. Davidson RG: Atlantoaxial instability in individuals with Down syndrome: a fresh look at the evidence, *Pediatrics* 81:857, 1988.
26. Mitchell V, Howard R, Facer E: Down's syndrome and anaesthesia, *Paediatr Anaesth* 5:379, 1995.
27. Litman RS, Zerngast BA, Perkins FM: Preoperative evaluation of the cervical spine in children with trisomy-21: results of a questionnaire study, *Paediatr Anaesth* 5:355, 1995.
28. Litman RS, Perkins FM: Atlantoaxial subluxation after tympanomastoidectomy in a child with trisomy 21, *Otolaryngol Head Neck Surg* 110:584, 1994.
29. Moore RA, McNicholas KW, Warren SP: Atlanto-axial subluxation with spinal cord compression in a child with Down's syndrome, *Anesth Analg* 66:89, 1987.
30. Williams JP, Somerville GM, Miner ME, et al: Atlanto-axial subluxation and trisomy-21: another perioperative complication, *Anesthesiology* 67:253, 1987.
31. Morris CD, Outcalt J, Menashe VD: Hypoplastic left heart syndrome: natural history in a geographically defined population, *Pediatrics* 85:977, 1990.
32. Kern JH, Hayes CJ, Michler RE, et al: Survival and risk factor analysis for the Norwood procedure for hypoplastic left heart syndrome, *Am J Cardiol* 80:170, 1997.
33. Bove EL, Lloyd TR: Staged construction for hypoplastic left heart syndrome: contemporary results, *Ann Surg* 224:387, 1996.
34. Bardo K, Turrentine MW, Sun K, et al: Surgical management of hypoplastic left heart syndrome, *Ann Thorac Surg* 62:70, 1996.
35. Glauser TA, Rorke LB, Weinberg PM, et al: Congenital brain anomalies associated with the hypoplastic left heart syndrome, *Pediatrics* 85:984, 1990.
36. Glauser TA, Rorke LB, Weinberg PM, et al: Acquired neuropathologic lesions associated with the hypoplastic left heart syndrome, *Pediatrics* 85:991, 1990.
37. Karamanoukian HL, O'Toole SJ, Glick PL: "State-of-the-art" management strategies for the fetus and neonate with congenital diaphragmatic hernia, *J Perinatol* 16:540, 1996.
38. Shochat SJ: Pulmonary vascular pathology in congenital diaphragmatic hernia, *Pediatr Surg Int* 2:331, 1987.
39. Hisanga S, Shimokawa H, Kashiwabara Y, et al: Unexpected low lecithin/sphingomyelin ratio associated with fetal diaphragmatic hernia, *Am J Obstet Gynecol* 27:905, 1984.
40. Glick PL, Leach CL, Besner GE, et al: Pathophysiology of congenital diaphragmatic hernia. III. Surfactant replacement for the high risk neonate with congenital diaphragmatic hernia, *J Pediatr Surg* 28:1, 1992.
41. Hennenberg SW, Jepsen S, Anderson PK, et al: Inhalation of nitric oxide as a treatment of pulmonary hypotension in congenital diaphragmatic hernia, *J Pediatr Surg* 6:853, 1995.
42. Frenckner B, Ehren H, Granholm T, et al: Improved results in patients who have congenital diaphragmatic hernia using preoperative stabilization, extracorporeal membrane oxygenation, and delayed surgery, *J Pediatr Surg* 32:1185, 1997.
43. Reickert CA, Hirshl RB, Schumacher R, et al: Effect of very delayed repair of congenital diaphragmatic hernia on survival and extracorporeal life support use, *Surgery* 120:766, 1996.
44. Reickert CA, Hirschl RB, Atkinson JB, et al: Congenital diaphragmatic hernia survival and use of extracorporeal life support at selected level III nurseries with multimodality support, *Surgery* 123:304, 1998.
45. Lund DP, Mitchell J, Kharasch V, et al: Congenital diaphragmatic hernia: the hidden mortality, *J Pediatr Surg* 29:258, 1994.
46. McGahren J, Krishna M, Rodgers BM: Neurologic outcome is diminished in survivors of congenital diaphragmatic hernia requiring extracorporeal membrane oxygenation, *J Pediatr Surg* 32:1216, 1997.
47. Reeves ST, Burt N, Smith CD: Is it time to reevaluate the airway management of tracheoesophageal fistula? *Anesth Analg* 81:866, 1995.

48. Tsai JY, Berkery L, Wesson DE, et al: Esophageal atresia and tracheoesophageal fistula: surgical experience over two decades, *Ann Thorac Surg* 64:778, 1997.

49. Beasley SW, Myers NA, Auldist AW: Management of the premature infant with esophageal atresia and hyaline membrane disease, *J Pediatr Surg* 27:23, 1992.

50. de Lorimier AA: Letter to editor, *J Pediatr Surg* 28:1082, 1993.

51. Shaul DB, Schwartz MZ, Marr CC, et al: Primary repair without routine gastrostomy is the treatment of choice for neonates with esophageal atresia and tracheoesophageal fistula, *Arch Surg* 124:1188, 1989.

52. Hoyme HE, Higginbottom MC, Jones JL: The vascular pathogenesis of gastroschisis: intrauterine interruption of the omphalomesenteric artery, *J Pediatr Surg* 98:228, 1981.

53. Paidas MJ, Crombleholme TM, Robertson FM: Prenatal diagnosis and management of the fetus with an abdominal wall defect, *Semin Perinatol* 18:196, 1994.

54. Krasna IH: Is early fascial closure necessary for omphalocele and gastroschisis? *J Pediatr Surg* 30:23, 1995.

55. Wald NJ: Folic acid and neural tube defects: the current evidence and implications for prevention, *Ciba Found Symp* 181:192, 1994.

56. Pittman T, Kiburz J, Gabriel K, et al: Latex allergy in children with spina bifida, *Pediatr Neurosurg* 22:96, 1995.

57. Porri F, Pradal M, Lemiere C, et al: Association between latex sensitization and repeated latex exposure in children, *Anesthesiology* 86:599, 1997.

58. Gerber AC, Jorg W, Zbinden S, et al: Severe intraoperative anaphylaxis to surgical gloves: latex allergy, an unfamiliar condition, *Anesthesiology* 71:800, 1989.

59. Holzman RS: Latex allergy: an emerging operating room problem, *Anesth Analg* 76:635, 1993.

60. Holzman RS: Clinical management of latex-allergic children, *Anesth Analg* 85:529, 1997.

61. Wilson JM, Bower LK, Thompson JE, et al: ECMO in evolution: the impact of changing patient demographics and alternative therapies for ECMO, *J Pediatr Surg* 31:1116, 1996.

62. Lazar EL, Abramson SJ, Weinstein S, et al: Neuroimaging of brain injury in neonates treated with extracorporeal membrane oxygenation: lessons learned from several examinations, *J Pediatr Surg* 29:186, 1994.

63. Patrias MC, Rabinowicz IM, Klein MD: Ocular findings in infants treated with extracorporeal membrane oxygenator support, *Pediatrics* 82:560, 1988.

64. Levy MS, Share JC, Fauza DO, et al: Fate of the reconstructed carotid artery after extracorporeal membrane oxygenation, *J Pediatr Surg* 30:1046, 1995.

65. Noerr B: ECMO and pharmacotherapy, *Neonatal Network* 15:23, 1996.

66. Abelson HI, Miller JD: A decade of trends in cocaine use in the household population, *National Institute on Drug Abuse Research Monograph Series* 61:35, Rockville, Md, 1985, National Institutes of Health.

67. Zuckerman B, Amaro H, Cabral H: Validity of self reporting of marijuana and cocaine use among pregnant adolescents, *J Pediatr* 115:812, 1989.

68. McCalla S, Minkoff HL, Feldman J, et al: Predictors of cocaine use in pregnancy, *Obstet Gynecol* 79:641, 1992.

69. Spear LP, Frambes NA, Kirstein CL: Fetal and maternal brain and plasma levels of cocaine and benzoylecgonine following chronic subcutaneous administration of cocaine during gestation in rats, *Psychopharmacology* 97:427, 1989.

70. Madden JD, Payne TF, Miller S: Maternal cocaine abuse and effect on the newborn, *Pediatrics* 77:209, 1986.

71. Kain ZN, Rimar S, Barash PG: Cocaine abuse in the parturient and effects on the fetus and neonate, *Anesth Analg* 77:835, 1993.

72. Hoyne HE, Jones KL, Dixon SD, et al: Prenatal cocaine exposure and fetal vascular disruption, *Pediatrics* 85:743, 1990.

73. Doberczak TM, Shanzer S, Senie RT, et al: Neonatal neurologic and electroencephalographic effect of intrauterine cocaine exposure, *J Pediatr* 113:354, 1988.

74. Belcher HME, Wallace PM: Neurodevelopmental evaluation of children with intrauterine cocaine exposure, *Pediatr Res* 29:206A, 1991.

75. Chasnoff IJ: In-utero cocaine exposure increases risk of SIDS, *Pediatr News* 21:22, 1987.

76. van de Bor M, Walther FJ, Ebrahimi M: Decreased cardiac output in infants of mothers who abused cocaine, *Pediatrics* 85:30, 1990.

77. Berry FA, Badgwell JM: Anesthesia for the ex-premature and ex-extracorporeal membrane oxygenated infant. In Badgwell JM, ed: *Clinical pediatric anesthesia*, Philadelphia, 1997, Lippincott-Raven, p 195.

78. McCormick MC: The outcomes of very low birth weight infants: are we asking the right questions? *Pediatrics* 99:869, 1997.

79. O'Shea TM, Klinepeter KL, Goldstein DJ, et al: Survival and developmental disability in infants with birth weights of 501 to 800 grams, born between 1979 and 1994, *Pediatrics* 100:982, 1997.

80. Keith CG, Doyle LW: Retinopathy of prematurity in extremely low birth weight infants, *Pediatrics* 95:42, 1995.

81. Flynn JT, Bancalari E, Snyder ES, et al: A cohort study of transcutaneous oxygen tension and the incidence and severity of retinopathy of prematurity, *N Engl J Med* 326:1050, 1992.

82. Phelps DL: Retinopathy of prematurity, *N Engl J Med* 326:1078, 1992 (editorial).

83. Bolton DPG, Cross KW: Further observations on cost of preventing retrolental fibroplasia, *Lancet* 1:445, 1974.

84. Rescorla FJ, Grosfeld JL: Inguinal hernia repair in the perinatal period and early infancy: clinical considerations, *J Pediatr Surg* 19:832, 1984.

85. Peevy KJ, Speed FA, Hoff CJ: Epidemiology of inguinal hernia in preterm neonates, *Pediatrics* 77:246, 1986.

86. Lou HC, Lassen NA, Friis-Hansen B: Impaired autoregulation of cerebral blood flow in the distressed newborn infant, *J Pediatr* 94:118, 1979.

87. Perry EH, Bada HS, Ray JD, et al: Blood pressure increases, birth weight-dependent stability boundary, and intraventricular hemorrhage, *Pediatrics* 85:727, 1990.

88. Berry FA, Gregory GA: Do premature infants require anesthesia for surgery? *Anesthesiology* 67:291, 1987.

89. Rojas MA, Gonzalez A, Bancalari E, et al: Changing trends in the epidemiology and pathogenesis of neonatal chronic lung disease, *J Pediatr* 126:605, 1995.

90. Singer L, Yamashita T, Lilien L, et al: A longitudinal study of developmental outcome of infants with bronchopulmonary dysplasia and very low birth weight, *Pediatrics* 100:987, 1997.

91. Jones R, Bodnar A, Roan Y, et al: Subglottic stenosis in newborn intensive care unit graduates, *Am J Dis Child* 135:367, 1981.

92. Liu LMP, Coté CJ, Goudsouzian NG, et al: Life-threatening apnea in infants recovering from anesthesia, *Anesthesiology* 59:506, 1983.

93. Kurth CD, Spitzer AR, Broennle AM, et al: Postoperative apnea in preterm infants, *Anesthesiology* 66:483, 1987.

94. Coté CJ, Zaslavsky A, Downes JJ, et al: Postoperative apnea in former preterm infants after inguinal herniorrhaphy, *Anesthesiology* 82:809, 1995.

95. Warner LO, Martino JD, Davidson PJ, et al: Negative pressure pulmonary oedema: a potential hazard of muscle relaxants in awake infants, *Can J Anaesth* 37:580, 1990.

96. Giaufré E, Balens B, Gombert A: Epidemiology and morbidity of regional anesthesia in children: a one-year prospective survey of the French-Language Society of Pediatric Anesthesiologists, *Anesth Analg* 83:904, 1996.

97. Fisher QA, Shaffner DH, Yaster M: Detection of intravascular injection of regional anaesthetics in children, *Can J Anaesth* 44:592, 1997.

98. Berde CB: Convulsions associated with pediatric regional anesthesia, *Anesth Analg* 75:164, 1992.

99. Dohi S, Naito H, Takahashi T: Age-related changes in blood pressure and duration of motor block in spinal anesthesia, *Anesthesiology* 50:319, 1979.

100. Oberlander TF, Berde CB, Lam KH, et al: Infants tolerate spinal anesthesia with minimal overall autonomic changes: analysis of heart rate variability in former premature infants undergoing hernia repair, *Anesth Analg* 80:20, 1995.

101. Cornblath M, Schwartz R, Aynsley-Green A, et al: Hypoglycemia in infancy: the need for a rational definition, *Pediatrics* 85:834, 1990.
102. Wass CT, Lanier WL: Glucose moderation of ischemic brain injury: review and clinical recommendations, *Mayo Clin Proc* 71:801, 1996.
103. D'Alecy LG, Lundy EF, Barton KJ, et al: Dextrose containing intravenous fluid impairs outcome and increases death after eight minutes of cardiac arrest and resuscitation in dogs, *Surgery* 100:505, 1986.
104. Rosenberg H, Gronert GA: Intractable cardiac arrest in children given succinylcholine, *Anesthesiology* 77:1054, 1992.
105. Larach MG, Rosenberg H, Gronert GA, et al: Hyperkalemic cardiac arrest during anesthesia in infants and children with occult myopathies. *Clin Pediatr* 36:9, 1997.
106. Badgwell JM, Hall SC, Lockhart C: Revised label regarding use of succinylcholine in children and adolescents. II, *Anesthesiology* 80:243, 1994.
107. Findlay GP, Spittal MJ: Rocuronium pretreatment reduces suxamethonium-induced myalgia: comparison with vecuronium, *Br J Anaesth* 76:526, 1996.
108. Van der Spek AFL, Fang WB, Ashton-Miller JA, et al: The effects of succinylcholine on mouth opening, *Anesthesiology* 67:459, 1987.
109. Leary NP, Ellis FR: Masseteric muscle spasm as a normal response to suxamethonium, *Br J Anaesth* 64:488, 1990.
110. Ording H: Incidence of malignant hyperthermia in Denmark, *Anesth Analg* 64:700, 1985.
111. Wilhoit RD, Brown RE, Bauman LA: Possible malignant hyperthermia in a 7-week-old infant, *Anesth Analg* 68:688, 1989.
112. Ball SP, Johnson KJ: The genetics of malignant hyperthermia, *J Med Genet* 30:89, 1993.
113. Hopkins PM, Halsall PJ, Ellis FR: Diagnosing malignant hyperthermia susceptibility, *Anaesthesia* 49:373, 1994.
114. Flewellen EH, Nelson TE: Halothane-succinylcholine induced masseter spasm: Indicative of malignant hyperthermia susceptibility? *Anesth Analg* 63:693, 1984.
115. Rosenberg H, Fletcher JE: Masseter muscle rigidity and malignant hyperthermia susceptibility, *Anesth Analg* 65:161, 1986.
116. O'Flynn RP, Shutack JG, Rosenberg H, et al: Masseter muscle rigidity and malignant hyperthermia susceptibility in pediatric patients, *Anesthesiology* 80:1228, 1994.
117. Schwartz L, Rockoff MA, Koka BV: Masseter spasm with anesthesia: incidence and implications, *Anesthesiology* 61:772, 1984.
118. Rosenberg H: Management of patients in whom trismus occurs following succinylcholine, *Anesthesiology* 68:654, 1988 (reply to letter).
119. Gronert GA: Management of patients in whom trismus occurs following succinylcholine, *Anesthesiology* 68:653, 1988 (letter).
120. Berry FA, Lynch C III: Succinylcholine and trismus, *Anesthesiology* 70:161, 1989 (letter).
121. Littleford JA, Patel LR, Bose D, et al: Masseter muscle spasm in children: implications of continuing the triggering anesthetic, *Anesth Analg* 72:151, 1991.

Injury to the Anesthesiologist

Jay B. Brodsky

All health care workers are exposed to hazards in the workplace.[1,2] Anesthesiologists are at particular risk for a number of physical, chemical, biologic, and psychosocial dangers. This chapter reviews the occupational health hazards that the practicing anesthesiologist faces daily.

I. OCCUPATIONAL EXPOSURE

A. Waste anesthetic gases

Some of the drugs we use in the practice of anesthesiology may have subtle, long-range effects on our health and that of our co-workers. The one potential environmental health hazard that is almost unique to our specialty is exposure to waste anesthetic gases.

1. Reproductive hazards. How dangerous is exposure to waste anesthetic gases? Although this question was posed over three decades ago, we still do not have a definitive answer.

Most studies have focused on the association between waste anesthetic agents, fertility, and pregnancy. Interest in this subject began with a survey of working conditions in the Soviet Union published in 1967.[3] This was the first of many retrospective studies to report that pregnancies among female anesthesiologists often ended in spontaneous abortion. The author proposed that this unexpected finding was attributable to some factor or factors in the workplace, with stressful working condi-

tions and chronic exposure to trace amounts of anesthetics as the most plausible causes.

Since publication of this small uncontrolled study, numerous larger epidemiologic surveys have considered the problem of anesthetic practice and pregnancy outcome. Many[4-8] but not all[9,10] have reported an increased risk of spontaneous abortion for women who work in an environment where trace concentrations of anesthetic gases are present. Although the actual cause of the reproductive complications has not been and probably never will be identified absolutely, chronic exposure to waste gases may be an important factor.

Exposure to clinical concentrations of inhaled anesthetics consistently causes toxic effects on experimental animals, possibly because these agents exert physiologic depressant effects on respiratory and cardiovascular function of the mother.[11] When animals are exposed to trace concentrations of those same gases (that is, concentrations without physiologic effects), the results have been less dramatic. Only nitrous oxide is consistently teratogenic, even at a concentration as low as 0.1% (1000 ppm).[11,12] This concentration of nitrous oxide is often present in the ambient air of modern "scavenged" operating rooms,[13] and without gas scavenging, peak concentrations of nitrous oxide in the air of operating rooms can exceed 9000 ppm.[14,15]

Among anesthetics, nitrous oxide is unique because it inactivates the vitamin B_{12}–dependent enzyme methionine synthetase.[16] Exposure to even a low concentration of nitrous oxide reduces the production of methionine, which in turn interrupts the conversion of uridine to thymidine. Rapidly dividing tissues are most affected because methionine synthetase is essential for normal DNA production. It is possible that interference with vitamin B_{12} function may account for the high incidence of infertility and undesirable reproductive outcomes in men and women chronically exposed to nitrous oxide.[17]

The epidemiologic studies that have associated occupational exposure to anesthetic gases and adverse reproductive outcome have been justly criticized because they usually compared anesthesiologists and nurses exposed to a variety of anesthetic agents with control groups of physicians and nurses working outside the operating room environment.[18-20]

Because of controversy regarding the interpretation of these studies, the American Society of Anesthesiologists (ASA) commissioned a group of epidemiologists and biostatisticians to evaluate the health problems attributed to waste anesthetic gases. Their full report was submitted to the ASA in 1982[21] and an abridged version was published in 1985.[22]

This report found that the risk of spontaneous abortion for pregnant physicians and nurses working in the operating room was 30% greater than that for the control population. The relative risk for congenital anomalies in the children of operating room personnel was 20% higher. These conclusions were reached after 17 articles relevant to the issue were considered and all but six were rejected. Because of design shortcomings, even the results from these six best studies were considered inconclusive, and the true reproductive risk, if any, from anesthetic exposure remains unknown.

It is now well established that work-related stress can have a significant negative effect on pregnancy outcome.[23] This raises the question whether the greater incidence of spontaneous abortions in pregnant anesthesiologists and operating room nurses is caused by waste gas exposure or by their stressful occupations.

The single major epidemiologic study that eliminated many of the shortcomings of other similar studies, and perhaps answers the question of waste gas exposure versus stress as the cause of undesirable pregnancy outcomes, was not included in the reviews of health and reproductive outcomes after trace gas exposure.

Unlike anesthesiologists, dental professionals are a unique group to study because dentists doing essentially the same kind of work may or may not use inhaled anesthetics. Of the dentists that use anesthetics, the majority use only nitrous oxide. In the National Dental Study, Cohen et al[24] compared nitrous oxide–exposed dental workers with similar controls, that is, dentists and their assistants who worked under the same job stresses, who worked with the same materials, but who were not exposed to any inhaled anesthetics, including nitrous oxide.

This study reported that both paternal and maternal exposure to nitrous oxide was associated with a signifi-cantly higher rate of spontaneous abortions than in unexposed controls. Women directly exposed to nitrous oxide at work had a doubling in their miscarriage rate. Paternal exposure was not associated with a higher rate of congenital abnormalities; however, congenital abnormalities were more common in the children of female dental assistants directly exposed to nitrous oxide.

Because of experimental evidence that pregnant animals exposed to as little as 1000 ppm nitrous oxide have increased rates of fetal loss, it is easier to explain a toxic reproductive effect for female dental assistants directly exposed to nitrous oxide. How do we explain the increased spontaneous abortion rates for wives of male anesthesiologists and dentists?

The sperm or semen of exposed men may be damaged by nitrous oxide. Male rats breathing 20% nitrous oxide develop abnormal sperm and testicular damage within 2 weeks, some as soon as 3 days.[25] Male rats exposed to 10% nitrous oxide for 1 hour had a pronounced reduction in testicular methionine synthetase activity, which required up to 72 hours for that enzyme activity to return to normal.[26]

A study of male anesthesiologists found no differences in sperm morphology or sperm count among anesthesia residents at the start of their training and after 1 year of exposure to anesthetics.[27] However, each of the residents in this study had worked in modern operating rooms with gas scavenging, so their exposure to waste gases presumably was minimal.

The controversy continues as to whether female anesthesiologists and operating room nurses have an increased incidence of undesirable reproductive outcomes.

Most recently, Maran, Knill-Jones, and Spence[10] surveyed all female physicians who graduated medical school in the United Kingdom between 1977 and 1984.[10] Details of medical specialty and work practices and medical and obstetric histories were obtained from more than 9000 respondents. This study reported that female anesthesiologists did not have an increased risk of infertility. In addition, they found no correlation between maternal occupation, hours working in the operating room, the use of waste gas–scavenging equipment, and the incidence of spontaneous abortions or congenital abnormalities in live-born children.

It is now believed that occupational exposure to nitrous oxide by medical and dental personnel during its routine use as an anesthetic is unlikely to produce adverse reproductive outcomes. An important exception may be B_{12}-deficient workers or those routinely exposed to very high nitrous oxide levels.[28]

2. Neurologic and other organ toxicity. Besides its effects on the reproductive system, in clinical concentrations nitrous oxide under experimental conditions is also toxic to the hematologic, immune, and nervous systems in both animals and humans.[16] There is indirect evidence that occupational exposure to lower concentrations of nitrous oxide may also be a health hazard for humans.

For example, a study of 21 dentists habitually exposed to nitrous oxide found that bone marrow function was depressed in 3 of the 21, and 2 of these 3 had abnormal white cells in the periphery.[29] The National Dental Study reported greater rates of liver disease, kidney disease, and neurologic disease among dental professionals using nitrous oxide.[24]

The most striking finding of the National Dental Study was the difference in neurologic complaints between nitrous oxide–exposed people and the unexposed controls.[30] Dentists heavily exposed to nitrous oxide complained of numbness, tingling, and muscle weakness four times as often as unexposed dentists. The combination of halogenated agents and nitrous oxide did not increase the incidence of these problems, an indication that the symptoms were associated with nitrous oxide exposure only.

Layzer[31,32] described a polyneuropathy characterized by numbness, paresthesia, or clumsiness in the extremities, which he called nitrous oxide neuropathy. With continued exposure to nitrous oxide, the disease progresses to severe weakness, gait disturbances, loss of sphincter control, and impotence. Although many of Layzer's patients abused nitrous oxide for recreational purposes, two had been exposed only during its routine clinical use.

Nitrous oxide neuropathy is identical to the neuropathy of pernicious anemia. Monkeys develop neuropathy only if they are fed a vitamin B_{12}–deficient diet for 5 years.[33] However, the same monkeys breathing 15% nitrous oxide develop neuropathy after several weeks.[34] Nitrous oxide, even chronic exposure at low concentrations, oxidizes B_{12}, in turn reducing methionine synthetase activity.[35] Because low concentrations of B_{12} result in pernicious anemia, there is a biochemical basis for the neurologic complications of occupational exposure to nitrous oxide identified in the National Dental Study.

Since Layzer's initial reports, additional cases of severe myeloneuropathy and macrocytic anemia associated with low serum concentrations of vitamin B_{12} after prolonged exposure to nitrous oxide have been reported.[36] In one case, the use of methionine seemed to arrest the progression of the disease and accelerate recovery. At present we still do not know what level of exposure (concentration and duration) is needed for nitrous oxide to be neurotoxic to humans.

Waste gas exposure can have more subtle effects. In a series of studies Bruce et al[37,38] exposed volunteers to 500 ppm nitrous oxide for 4 hours with different trace concentrations of halothane.[37,38] They reported significant decreases in performance during several audiovisual tasks and short-term memory tests in the exposed groups. Others have been unable to duplicate these findings,[39] and studies of volunteers in unscavenged operating rooms have failed to detect impairment in psychomotor performance even when the concentration of nitrous oxide exceeded 2000 ppm.[40] There is still no convincing evidence that exposure to a subclinical concentration of anesthetic agents have any effects on cognition. However, the speculation remains that if anesthetics can render a patient completely unconscious at one concentration, lower concentrations of those same agents might impair the thought processes of exposed personnel.

3. Anesthetic standards and practices. Information on long-term exposure to anesthetic agents in humans has come from epidemiologic surveys. However, these surveys cannot prove a cause-and-effect relationship because they are not controlled scientific experiments. At best they are useful in assessing adverse environmental factors, one of which may be exposure to anesthetic gases. Additionally, problems with inadequate response rates, possible responder bias and inaccurate recall of events, failure to verify medical data, and lack of comparable control groups are serious limitations of the studies of health and reproductive hazards in the operating room.[18,20,41]

Conditions in the operating room have changed since the data from many of the earlier epidemiologic surveys were collected. Equipment maintenance programs, monitoring for gas leaks, changes in anesthetic practices, and scavenging of waste anesthetic gases are now universally practiced in the United States.[42-44] These efforts have resulted in a 90% reduction in exposure to waste anesthetic gases when compared to the concentrations present when the various health surveys were conducted.[42] Thus the potential for health and reproductive problems from waste anesthetic gas exposure probably has been reduced significantly.

However, exposure of anesthesiologists and other operating room personnel to waste anesthetic gases continues to occur because of unrecognized leaks.[13] The major source of environmental contamination is from leakage during mask anesthetic techniques. Equipment leakage also occurs from high-pressure fittings and exhalation valves and when the vaporizers are filled. Even with controlled ventilation and active scavenging, the potential for nitrous oxide contamination persists, especially during pediatric surgery.[45]

With a mask anesthetic technique, concentrations of nitrous oxide can exceed 1500 ppm.[13] Using a laryngeal mask airway (LMA) rather than a conventional mask greatly reduces exposure to nitrous oxide in the anesthesiologist's breathing zone.[46]

The National Institute of Occupational Safety and Health (NIOSH) recommended as a standard the routine use of scavenging and control measures to keep maximal concentrations of nitrous oxide less than 25 ppm and halogenated agents less than 5 ppm.[47] These concentrations were chosen because they were believed to be technically achievable, although NIOSH realized that a safe concentration could not be defined. Unfortunately, reduction of gas exposure to these concentrations has been difficult to achieve in actual clinical practice.[48,49] Using a low-leakage anesthesia machine, high room ventilation rates, a functioning scavenging system, avoidance of mask ventilation, and strict control of endotracheal tube cuff pressure, concentrations of nitrous oxide still could not be kept below NIOSH threshold values.[50]

The National Dental Study was probably the best designed of the epidemiologic surveys.[24] Its findings, combined with those of animal studies demonstrating significant toxic effects of nitrous oxide, suggest that long-term exposure to nitrous oxide may have serious health consequences. However, there is still no firm evidence that exposure to trace concentrations of any anesthetic gas is a health hazard to humans, but there is no proof that it is not. Until a cause-and-effect relationship is proved or disproved, it seems prudent to minimize unnecessary waste gas exposure in the workplace.

Many questions remain unanswered about the consequences of chronic exposure to waste anesthetic agents. Are the effects in the workplace similar to the experimental findings seen in the laboratory? Is there a real health risk for anesthesiologists and nurses working in an environment where exposure to these gases occurs daily? Should health care workers be informed of the potential risk before being exposed to waste anesthetic gases?

Whereas concern over waste gas exposure has diminished among a new generation of anesthesiologists who have been trained to use scavenging systems, occupational exposure has become an important issue in the postanesthesia care unit (PACU).[51] PACU nurses work in close proximity to patients during the early stages of recovery from anesthesia, and it is during this time that patients exhale the highest concentrations of anesthetic gases. Therefore concern over the legal implications and the possibility of government regulation of exposure to waste anesthetic gases in areas other than the operating room persists.[52]

Everyone agrees that the real health risks of workplace exposure to anesthetic gases can be determined conclusively only by a large-scale prospective study. Unfortunately, such a study has never been and probably never will be undertaken. The almost universal practice of waste gas scavenging and the more recently recognized problems of stress and chemical substance abuse among anesthesiologists have directed our attention away from the problem of waste gas exposure to potentially more serious occupational health issues. However, anesthesiologists must remain concerned about the potential hazards of waste gas exposure, especially to nitrous oxide. The potential adverse health effects of nitrous oxide have led some anesthesiologists to question its continued use.[53]

B. Infections

Because of our close contact with patients, many of whom have contagious diseases, anesthesiologists are vulnerable to contracting viral and bacterial infections.[54,55] Exposure can range from the benign and common (rhinovirus) to the extremely rare and dangerous (Creutzfeldt-Jakob virus).[56] More recently, exposure to drug-resistant tuberculosis has once again become a potentially serious occupational risk in the operating room.[57]

Although exposure to most infectious agents presents no significant threat to the immunocompetent anesthesiologist, two viruses—human immunodeficiency virus (HIV) and hepatitis B virus (HBV)—are potentially lethal and are of great concern to us all.

1. Acquired immunodeficiency syndrome. HIV, the retrovirus that causes acquired immunodeficiency syndrome (AIDS), has also been called human T-cell lymphotropic virus, type III (HTLV-III) and lymphadenopathy-associated virus (LAV).[58,59] AIDS is associated with a broad spectrum of diseases, including problems with the pulmonary, neurologic, and gastrointestinal systems, the skin and mucosal surfaces, lymph nodes, and the retina. Any body organ or system can be involved.

HIV is most often spread through infected blood, vaginal secretions, and semen, and usually is transmitted by sexual contact, needle sharing, and transfusion of contaminated blood products, and from mother to newborn in the perinatal period. HIV is not transmitted by casual contact.[60] Live HIV has been isolated from blood, semen, urine, saliva, vaginal secretions, bone marrow, lymph nodes, spleen, cerebrospinal fluid, and tears of infected patients.

Patients in high-risk groups include homosexual or bisexual men, heterosexual intravenous drug users, and hemophiliacs and other recipients of blood products. Others considered at high risk are sex partners of patients with AIDS and infants of HIV-positive mothers. The percentage of patients infected with HIV who have no identified risk factor is 3% to 4%. Because it is impossible to identify all patients as HIV seropositive without specific screening tests, during the past decade it has become necessary to treat every patient as potentially infected with HIV or other bloodborne pathogens.[61]

Few diseases have created greater anxiety among the health care workers than AIDS. The Centers for Disease Control (CDC) defines a health care worker as a person whose activities involve contact with patients or patients' blood or body fluids. As a group, anesthesiologists are among the health care workers potentially at greatest risk for HIV exposure.

What are the risks that an anesthesiologist will contact AIDS from a patient? In 1987, of the 32,395 adults identified to the CDC as having AIDS, 1875 (5.8%) were health care workers.[62] Of the HIV-positive health care workers, 95% belonged to a high-risk (homosexual, intravenous drug abuser) group. For the remaining 5% the means of transmission was initially undetermined, but after careful review of follow-up information, more than half of these workers were reclassified when recognized risk factors were identified.

By 1993, 284,840 AIDS cases had been reported to the CDC and at that time it was estimated that more than 1.5 million people were infected with HIV in the United States alone.[63] Of these, the CDC had documented 46 health care workers in the United States who acquired HIV infection at work. An additional 97 HIV-positive health care workers were identified, but the route of infection could not be documented.

Of documented occupational transmission, 89% followed percutaneous exposure to HIV-infected blood or body fluid. The remaining patients were infected by mucocutaneous exposure.

The greatest risk is from needlestick injuries rather than contact of infected blood or body fluid with intact skin or mucous membranes. HIV seroconversion is most likely to occur after deep percutaneous injury from a large, hollow needle. Although gloves can reduce the volume of blood transferred during a needlestick injury, a large blood-filled needle is still capable of transmitting sufficient virus to produce infection after piercing a latex glove.

Data in 1987 of health care workers showed that only 6 of 2000 documented accidental exposures to HIV resulted in seroconversion.[62] In another prospective evaluation of health care workers with documented percutaneous or mucous membrane exposure to body fluids or blood from HIV-infected patients, seroconversion did not occur in any of 74 workers with nonpercutaneous exposures.[64] In 3 of 351 percutaneous exposures to infected blood, seroconversion did occur. In each instance the worker had a small break in the skin, and in one some blood also splattered into the mouth.

The overall risk of HIV seroconversion after a single exposure to HIV-infected blood is currently believed to be between 0.3% and 0.4% for percutaneous exposure and less than 0.1% for mucous membrane and skin exposures.[65,66] The latent period between exposure and infection to seropositivity in health care workers exposed to HIV is 90 to 180 days.[67]

Although many prospective studies have claimed that the risk of occupationally acquired HIV infection is very low,[64,68-72] documented infection from patients does occur.[62] The growing number HIV-positive patients increases the chances that more health care workers will be exposed and become infected.[73] No one knows the real incidence of HIV infection in the general population, and it varies greatly by geographic location. For example, 10 years ago more than 4% of patients presenting at an inner-city emergency department, when tested, had unrecognized HIV infection.[74] These numbers are increasing. More recently, of 2523 patients tested at the Johns Hopkins Hospital, 612 (24%) were infected with at least one or a combination of HIV, HBV, or hepatitis C virus (HCV).[75]

Although approximately 6% of the labor force in the United States is defined as health care workers, this group comprised less than 5% of AIDS cases reported to the CDC. The incidence of AIDS and HIV infection in health care workers has remained stable at about 5% for more than a decade.[76,77] In nearly every case of HIV-infected health care workers, nonoccupational lifestyle factors were believed to be responsible for the infection.

The incidence of HIV seropositivity among anesthesiologists is unknown. Up to now, there has been only one report of an anesthesiologist becoming infected at work. The annual risk of occupational HIV infection is proportional to the annual number of needlestick injuries by an individual, the statistical risk of infection after a single HIV-infected needlestick injury, and the prevalence of HIV-infected patients in the population.[78]

The risk of needlestick injury for anesthesiologists is estimated to be 1.3 per year, the risk of seroconversion from needlestick exposure is 0.3% to 0.4%, and the prevalence of HIV in the population is 0.32% to 23.6%, depending on location. Therefore the calculated range for risk of an anesthesiologist over a 30-year period (assuming no change in HIV prevalence or benefit from protective measures) ranges from 0.05% to 4.5% or from 0.002% to 0.129% per year. This range is so large because the incidence of HIV infection differs so greatly in different locations.

Despite the low risk, documented cases of AIDS transmission from patients to health care workers underscore the need for strict adherence to the infection control guidelines issued by the CDC.

If exposure to blood or other fluids does occur, the patient should be approached for consent for HIV testing. The legal issues involved in ascertaining a patient's HIV status are complex and vary from state to state. In general, the physician must obtain and document specific informed consent in order to test a patient for HIV.

If the patient is already known to have AIDS or AIDS-related condition (ARC), refuses testing, or is tested positive for HIV, the exposed worker should be informed and tested serially for evidence of infection. Testing shortly after the incident will help rule out prior infection.

CDC guidelines recommend that health care workers who perform invasive procedures know their HIV status and, if positive, that they do not perform exposure-prone procedures. The AIDS crisis is unique in the way it has been politicized. Some people are concerned that a hospital might prevent an HIV-positive anesthesiologist from practicing. Although there have been frequent attempts to require mandatory HIV testing of physicians, there has never been a known case of an anesthesiologist transmitting HIV to a patient. In fact, with the exception of the infamous Florida dentist believed to have infected six of his patients, there are no other documented instances of a health care worker infecting a patient with HIV.

The CDC estimates that the probability of HIV transmission from an infected surgeon to a patient during an invasive procedure is extremely low, ranging from 1 in 42,000 to 1 in 420,000 operations. Both the CDC and the ASA regard the practice of anesthesiology as presenting a much lower infection risk to the patient.

The projected cost to a large hospital for testing the blood of health care workers is about $250,000 annually.[79] In theory, this would prevent 0.02663 transmissions, or cost up to $91,000,000 per transmission prevented.

There is no scientific evidence, current government effort, or economic reason to impose routine HIV testing of anesthesiologists for the purpose of protecting patients. Both the Rehabilitation Act (1973) and the Americans with Disabilities Act (1990) preclude treatment discrimination of HIV-infected patients and protect health care workers against disability-based discrimination in employment.

2. Hepatitis. Although HIV has become a major concern, the risk of similar exposure to hepatitis has often been ignored. The loss of quality-adjusted life expectancy is almost identical for a physician contracting HIV or HBV infection.[80]

HBV is probably the most serious occupational health danger facing anesthesiologists. Whereas worldwide very few health care workers (from non–high-risk groups) have contracted AIDS through occupational exposure, more than 20% of anesthesiologists have serologic markers denoting previous exposure to HBV.

The two common human hepatitis viruses—hepatitis A virus (HAV) and HBV—have been well described, whereas two others, HCV and hepatitis D virus (HDV, delta virus), have more recently been identified.[81,82]

There is minimal risk to the anesthesiologist of parenteral transmission of HAV because of the absence of a chronic carrier state. HAV is spread predominantly by the fecal-oral route, although it can be transmitted from contact with gastrointestinal fluids.[83] If contamination occurs, serum immune globulin should be taken within 2 weeks of exposure.

Formerly the diagnosis of non-A, non-B (NANB) hepatitis required negative HAV and HBV serology and the exclusion of a history of exposure to hepatotoxic drugs.[84] Recently HCV has been isolated and identified as a major cause of NANB hepatitis.[82] The diagnosis of HCV now can be definitely established serologically. HCV transmission after percutaneous exposure to blood at work has been documented.[85] Although no vaccine is available for HCV, remission can be induced with α-interferon. Precautions against HCV are similar to those for HBV.[86]

HDV depends on HBV for replication, and although no specific vaccine is available, HBV vaccine or hepatitis B immunoglobulin (HBIG) given as a prophylaxis or after exposure can prevent both HBV and HDV infection.

The major threat to the anesthesiologist is HBV. Approximately 9000 to 18,000 of the 300,000 people in the United States infected annually with HBV are health care workers.[85] Of these, approximately 450 require hospitalization and 200 die from acute or chronic HBV infection.[87]

Anesthesia personnel are among the highest-risk group for HBV because occupational exposure results primarily from handling blood and blood products.[88-90] The risk of HBV exposure begins during residency training and continues throughout the professional career of the anesthesiologist.[91] Using assays for HBV antigens as evidence of prior or current infection, serologic markers for HBV are present in 20% to 49% of anesthesiologists, an incidence five times greater than the rate for the general public.[87,90,92] Similarly high rates of HBV seropositivity have been reported among Canadian[93,94] and European anesthesiologists.[95-97]

About one fourth of people positive for HBV antigen develop clinical hepatitis; for the remainder the HBV infection resolves without significant hepatic damage. Fewer than 1% of patients with HBV develop fulminant hepatitis, but it is associated with a 60% mortality.

Unlike HIV, where 100% of infected patients become carriers, 6% to 10% of people infected with HBV become chronic carriers. Not only do carriers have the potential to infect others, but also about 25% of the HBV carriers develop chronic active hepatitis, which often progresses to cirrhosis. The risk of hepatocellular carcinoma is 200 times greater in HBV carriers than among noncarriers. Over a thousand patients die of HBV-related hepatocellular carcinoma each year in the United States.

As with HIV, certain populations have a high prevalence of HBV. These include all patients with liver disease, patients undergoing hemodialysis or those who have had a renal transplant, patients with leukemia, all immunosuppressed patients, intravenous drug abusers, homosexual men, and immigrants from Southeast Asia. Although fewer than 10% are carriers, all HBV-positive patients and their secretions must be considered infectious.

In the United States from 1979 to 1989 the prevalence of new acute HBV cases increased by 37%, and by 1993 it was estimated that 1.25 million people in this country were HBV positive.[98] About 0.1% of the general population are asymptomatic HBV carriers, and between 1% and 1.5% of all hospital patients are seropositive for HBV. Thus an anesthesiologist treating 100 patients per month is likely to encounter an HBV-positive person at least once a month.

Unfortunately, because many patients with serum markers for HBV have no clinical history of hepatitis and are not members of any recognized high-risk group, occupational exposure risk is usually greatest from patients not suspected of being carriers.[99] Therefore wearing gloves and taking special precautions only when working with a patient from a high-risk group does not prevent exposure to HBV.

Even in light of the increasing prevalence of HIV and HBV in the patient population, only 88% of anesthesiologists responding to a questionnaire reported that they complied with CDC guidelines when presented with an HIV- or HBV-infected patient.[100] Even fewer (24.7%) adhered to those guidelines when the patient's status was unknown and the patient was considered at low risk. Among respondents the majority reported a needlestick injury within the preceding 12 months but fewer than half sought treatment after the injury. These surprising findings were similar to a study that reported that among house staff only 30% of needlestick injuries are reported.[101]

Reasons for not reporting needlestick injuries include lack of time, ignorance of risk, unfamiliarity with the reporting mechanism, concern about breaches in confidentiality, and potential professional discrimination.

Although contact with blood probably is the most important risk factor, every body secretion from a carrier is potentially dangerous. If any exposure occurs, such as a skin puncture with a dirty needle, HBIG should be administered immediately. If the patient is known to be antigen positive and the exposed health care worker is antigen negative, administration of HBIG within 48 hours of exposure followed by the first dose of an HBV vaccine within 7 days is recommended.[102]

For high-risk groups, such as anesthesiologists, HBV vaccine should be administered simultaneously with HBIG because this will initiate lasting immunity.

There is a potential risk of catching AIDS from HBIG because it is prepared from plasma, and viral inactivation may not be complete or effective. There have also been reports of HBV and HCV transmitted through HBIG.

HBV vaccine is the only effective way to prevent infection. All personnel exposed to patients or blood products should be immunized. Anesthesiologists should be vaccinated during residency. It is estimated that only 30% to 40% of susceptible medical personnel in the United States have been vaccinated. This is surprising because the vaccine is safe, immunogenic, and effective in preventing HBV infection. In fact, the vaccine is so safe and effective that the CDC now recommends universal HBV vaccination for infants.[103] New Occupational Safety and Health Administration (OSHA) regulations require all employers to offer the appropriate HBV vaccination series and postexposure follow-up treatment and testings to employees with occupational exposure to blood and other potentially infectious materials.

Anesthesiologists with prior exposure to HBV should be tested first for the presence of antibodies and then vaccinated if necessary. New house staff should receive the vaccine without prior serologic testing. The vaccine is given as a series of three intramuscular injections at 0, 1, and 6 months.[76] Follow-up serologic testing should be performed 6 to 8 weeks after the last dose to ensure that adequate levels of antibody have developed. A seroconversion rate of 85% to 95% is reported. Revaccination produces adequate antibody titers in only 30% to 50% of those who initially failed to respond to vaccination.

Table 26-1 gives the current recommendations for anesthesia personnel who have been stuck with a needle.

If antibody concentrations to HBV were tested within the past year and are known to be positive, nothing has to be done. Anyone who was antibody positive to HBV in the past but who has not been tested in several years should be rechecked for seropositivity. If there is a long delay in obtaining the results, it is advisable to take an HBIG or a booster shot. Anyone previously vaccinated who did not seroconvert should receive HBIG and a full course of the vaccine.

Although it has been recommended that everyone exposed to blood be tested annually for antibody status, adults with normal immune status do not require such frequent routine serologic testing. After vaccination, protection against clinical or viremic HBV lasts more than 5 years.

The side effects of HBV vaccine are minor, the most common problem being soreness in the arm at the site of inoculation. Although it is less painful to receive the vaccination in the buttocks, there may be a suboptimal response for those vaccinated at this site.[104] There are no adverse effects to receiving the vaccine in HBV carriers or immunosuppressed patients.

One reason many anesthesiologists resisted being vaccinated has been concern that the original vaccine (Engerix-B[r]), introduced in 1982, might transmit HIV. This vaccine is prepared from plasma. The concern has persisted even though the HIV virus, and all other known human viruses, are killed by the steps involved in the preparation of HBV vaccine. Extensive studies found no evidence that HIV was transmitted by the plasma-derived vaccine.[105] There have been no reports of AIDS after HBV vaccination in people who did not belong to a high-risk behavior group. This vaccine is considered safe even though several cases of Guillain-Barré syndrome occurred after vaccination.

A second vaccine (Recombivax HB[r]), prepared with recombinant DNA technology from noninfectious material, was introduced in 1986.[105-107] Because only a portion of the HBV viral genome that codes for the surface coat of HBV is present, no potentially infectious viral DNA (such as HIV) can be produced. No human or animal plasma or other derivatives are used in the preparation of this vaccine. It appears to be almost equivalent in its immunogenicity and protective action to the older, plasma-derived vaccine.[108,109] This vaccine offers increased safety, immunogenicity, and lower cost with absolutely no risk of HIV exposure.[107]

The responses of 919 health care workers at a university hospital at risk for occupational exposure to patients' blood were studied to examine the factors involved in acceptance or refusal of HBV vaccine.[110] People with knowledge of the disease (physicians, nurses) were more

Table 26-1. Recommendations for postexposure prophylaxis for percutaneous or mucosal exposure to hepatitis B

Exposed person	Treatment when source is		
	HBsAg positive	HbsAg negative	Unknown
Unvaccinated	HBIG 1× and initiate HB vaccine	Initiate HB vaccine	Initiate HB vaccine
Previously vaccinated, known responder	Test exposed for anti-HBs 1. If adequate, no treatment 2. If inadequate, HB vaccine booster dose	No treatment	No treatment
Known nonresponder	HBIG 2× or HBIG 1× plus HB vaccine	No treatment	If known high-risk source, treat as if source were HBsAg positive
Response unknown	Test exposed for anti-HBs If inadequate, HBIG 1× plus vaccine booster If adequate, no treatment	No treatment	Test exposed for anti-Hbs 1. If inadequate, HB vaccine booster dose 2. If adequate, no treatment

HB, Hepatitis B; *HBsAG*, HB surface antigen; *HBIG*, HB immune globulin (dose 0.06 ml/kg intramuscularly).

likely to complete the vaccination series. Refusal was related primarily to concern over the possibility of side effects from the vaccine. Younger physicians (house staff) and those with increased exposure to blood (operating room–based anesthesiologists and surgeons) were the most likely to complete the vaccination course.

   3. *Prevention of bloodborne infections.* The CDC has published practice recommendations to prevent the transmission of bloodborne infections in the health care setting.[64,85,111] The ASA Committee on Occupational Health of Operating Room Personnel republished these recommendations.[112] Because HBV is more infectious than HIV, recommendations to prevent the former also prevent the latter. Anesthesiologists must adhere rigorously to these precautions to minimize their risk of exposure.

   The foremost dictum is that every patient must be considered potentially infected, either with HIV, HBV, or other bloodborne pathogens.

   Accidental needlesticks and cuts account for most incidents of percutaneous exposure to blood and represent the major risk for HBV and HIV infection.[70] Anesthesiologists have a high incidence of needlesticks in their practice.[113] Of the health care workers who become infected with HIV in the workplace, the majority do so after needlestick exposure. Although analysis of needlestick injuries and cuts with sharp instruments indicate that the risk of infection is extremely low, all sharp items must be considered potentially infective and handled with care. Needles should not be recapped, bent, broken, removed from syringes, or manipulated by hand. Recapping needles is the most common cause of inadvertent skin puncture. Contaminated disposable syringes and needles and other sharp items should be placed immediately after use in puncture-resistant containers located in the anesthesia work area.

   Barriers should be placed between the potential source of infection and the anesthesiologist. Gloves must always be readily available and should be worn at all times, but especially when in contact with blood, blood products, body fluids, or any item soiled with these fluids. Because gloves will not prevent penetrating injuries, care must always be exercised with uncapped needles. The routine use of gloves alone did not reduce the incidence of HBV infection in new anesthesia residents.

   Gloves should be worn when in contact with mucous membranes or the nonintact skin of all patients. It is a common practice to double-glove when the diagnosis HIV or HBV is known. Gloves should be changed between patient contacts.

   Protective eyewear should be worn in situations in which blood or saliva can be spread. Standard surgical masks do not adequately protect against blood-bearing aerosols, which can contaminate the mucous membranes of the eyes, nose, or mouth. Masks and goggles and glasses should be used for procedures that are likely to produce droplets of blood or body fluids. Surgical masks that combine face protection and a plastic eye shield are available. The eye shield is treated with an antifogging agent similar to that used on ski goggles, and the mask contains a fluid repellent so that splattered fluids bead up on the mask surface.

   Gowns or aprons should be worn to protect against splashes of blood or body fluids during procedures. Disposable gowns do not completely prevent cutaneous exposure of contaminated blood.[114] Clothing should be changed as soon as possible if soiled.

   Prevention of exposure to saliva by using mouthpieces, resuscitation bags, and other ventilation devices during cardiopulmonary resuscitation is recommended. Mouth-to-mouth breathing should be avoided whenever possible.

   Health care workers with exudative skin lesions or dermatitis should refrain from direct patient care until the skin condition resolves. Anesthesiologists with chapped hands, open cuts, or abrasions must protect the involved skin areas. Hands must be washed immediately if they come into contact with blood or other fluids, as well as before and after any patient care procedure. After inadvertent percutaneous or mucous membrane exposure to blood or body fluids, the affected area should be thoroughly washed immediately.

   A major difference between HIV and HBV exposure is that the latter can be prevented by vaccination. Both the HBV vaccines currently available are safe and effective. All anesthesiologists should be immunized against HBV unless they are serologically positive from previous exposure. There is no vaccination for HIV.

   Every hospital should develop protocols for handling accidental exposure in the workplace, and all injuries or exposures should be reported. After an exposure (such as a needlestick, contamination of mucosa or conjunctiva, open wound or skin abrasion, or splash) the health care worker should be tested for HIV and HBV.

   The safety and effectiveness of short-term zidovudine (AZT) administration after accidental percutaneous exposure to HIV-positive blood is unknown.[115] Earlier data suggested that AZT postexposure prophylaxis could reduce the risk of HIV transmission after occupational exposure to HIV-infected blood by as much as 79%.[116] However, 4 of 1103 health care workers with percutaneous exposure to HIV-infected blood seroconverted and 1 of these became infected with HIV despite immediate use of AZT after exposure.[117]

   The drug has unpleasant side effects that include nausea, malaise, insomnia, myalgias, diaphoresis, fever, anorexia, and headache. Between 30% and 50% of exposed health care workers did not complete the planned course of AZT therapy because of these side effects.[117,118]

   It is believed that when the blood serologic status is unknown, the likelihood of seroconversion is a function of the local prevalence of HIV infection. Because the benefits of AZT do not clearly outweigh the risk when that prevalence is less than 20%,[119] one probably should not administer AZT.

   Two new drugs, lamivudine (3TC; 150 mg twice daily) and indinavir (IDV; 800 mg twice daily), have recently become available. Protocols for use of these drugs in a variety of different exposure scenarios have been devised by the CDC[66] (Table 26-2).

Table 26-2. Centers for Disease Control recommendations for chemoprophylaxis after occupational exposure to human immunodeficiency virus (HIV) (1996)

Type of exposure	Source material*	Antiviral prophylaxis	Antiretroviral regimen
Percutaneous	Blood		
	Highest risk	Recommend	ZDV, 3TC, IDV
	Increased risk	Recommend	ZDV, 3TC, +/− IDV
	No increased risk	Offer	ZDV, 3TC
	Potentially infected fluid or tissue	Offer	ZDV, 3TC
	Other body fluid	Do not offer	
Mucous membrane	Blood	Offer	ZDV, 3TC, +/− IDV
	Fluid with visible blood; fluid, tissue	Offer	ZDV, +/−3TC
	Other body fluids	Do not offer	
Open skin†	Blood	Offer	ZDV, 3TC, +/−IDV
	Fluid	Offer	ZDV, +/−3TC
	Other fluids	Do not offer	

*Highest risk, Deep injury with large-diameter hollow needle from high HIV titer blood; large volume of blood; *increased risk,* exposure to large volume of blood or blood with high HIV titer; *no increased risk,* neither exposure to large volume of blood nor blood with a high HIV titer (e.g., solid needle from source patient with asymptomatic HIV infection); *infectious fluid* includes semen, vaginal secretions, cerebrospinal, synovial, peritoneal, pericardial, and amniotic fluids.
†For skin exposure without increased risk, drug toxicity outweighs the benefit of postexposure chemoprophylaxis.
ZDV, Zidovudine (AZT, 200 mg three times daily); *3TC,* lamivudine (150 mg twice daily); *IDV,* indinavir (800 mg three times daily); if IDV not available, use saquinavir 600 mg three times daily).

These newer agents can be started as late as 36 hours following exposure. Lamivudine is generally well tolerated in combination with AZT and is not associated with adverse effects other than those associated with AZT alone. Indinavir does cause nephrolithiasis in as many as 10% of patients.

After administration of general anesthesia to a patient known to be HIV or HBV positive, the anesthesia machine and other nondisposable equipment should be cleaned. HIV is very weak and does not readily survive outside the body. It is easily killed by many common disinfectants, including household bleach. Techniques that produce high-level disinfection (those that are tuberculocidal) should be used routinely for processing equipment that comes into contact with mucous membranes (laryngoscope blades, breathing circuits) because they are effective in eliminating HBV and HIV. Items that enter sterile cavities (needles, endotracheal tubes) require sterilization before use and optimally should be used only once. Equipment in contact with intact skin (blood pressure cuffs) need not be cleaned after use unless it is contaminated with blood or body fluids. Blood and body fluid spills should be cleaned as soon as possible using soap and water because HBV is a hardy virus that may remain infectious for at least 1 week in dried blood on an environmental surface.[120] After this, an appropriate disinfectant or germicide can be used. With patients known to be HIV or HBV positive, disposable equipment including soda lime, esophageal stethoscopes, endotracheal tubes, and laryngoscope blades should be used whenever possible and then discarded.

4. Herpes. The herpes simplex virus (HSV) can infect oral mucosa (HSV I and II) or the genital area (HSV II). Oral HSV is quite common in adults, and the fingers of anesthesiologists can be inoculated by direct contact with saliva from infected patients. Because of the frequency of hand washing in the operating room, fingers often are traumatized around the nail bed area, predisposing the anesthesiologist to herpetic whitlow.[121-123]

The infection begins at the site where the skin integrity has been broken. There is itching and pain, followed by the appearance of a vesicle surrounded by erythema. Generalized symptoms of malaise, fever, and lymphadenopathy may also occur. The infection is usually self-limiting, lasting up to 3 weeks. The antiviral drug acyclovir can be used to treat the primary infection.

The infected anesthesiologist represents a risk of cross-infection to the patient and therefore should be very cautious with any local cutaneous lesions on his or her hands. Gloves, now routinely used to protect against HBV and HIV, prevent contamination by HSV as well.[124]

C. Environmental exposure

1. Chemical. Methylmethacrylate, the acrylic cement used to secure surgically implanted prostheses to bone, is supplied in two components, a liquid and a powder, which are mixed together before use.

Potentially toxic vapors are released during mixing. Rats exposed to these vapors develop severe liver damage, tracheal mucosal inflammation, and other side effects.[125] Factory workers producing methylmethacrylate have a high incidence of abnormal blood chemistry values (glucose, blood urea nitrogen, albumin, cholesterol, and bilirubin) and respiratory, genitourinary, and cutaneous problems.[126,127]

In humans, severe dyspnea, wheezing, coughing, and rhinorrhea have been reported after occupational contact with methylmethacrylate vapor.[128-130] A systemic reaction including hypertension, dyspnea, and generalized erythroderma has also been reported in an operating room nurse after exposure to methylmethacrylate.[131] Methylmethacrylate monomers are known to affect the nervous, cardiovascular, cutaneous, gastrointestinal, and respiratory systems.

Although OSHA set a maximum 8-hour exposure to methylmethacrylate at 100 ppm, a NIOSH study found evidence of harmful effects at half that concentration.[132]

Methylmethacrylate should always be mixed so that the fumes are vented outside the operating room. Scavenging devices, which can reduce the vapor concentration by as much as 75%, also should be used.[133]

2. Radiation. We are all familiar with the potential dangers of long-term exposure to ionizing radiation. Unfortunately, invisibility and absence of an immediate effect of radiation often give rise to complacency among nonradiologic personnel such as anesthesiologists, who are often exposed to radiation at work.

Examinations performed outside the radiology department are more likely to be hazardous than those performed within because protection is never as complete as in the specialized department.[134]

Several studies have attempted to measure the amount of radiation exposure by anesthesiologists. In one study, measuring chambers were placed in various locations in the operating and radiology suites during procedures requiring the presence of an anesthesiologist.[135] The measured radiation was only a small fraction of the amount of whole body exposure per week considered permissible. In a second study, 10 anesthesiologists wore radiation dosimeters at work.[136] Their average radiation exposure during the 10-week study period was well below the acceptable limit. But most of the exposure occurred during the first week of the study; thereafter individual and average values all tended to decrease sharply and then level out. The investigators believed that wearing the dosimeter made the anesthesiologists more conscious of the radiation hazard and thus more cautious.

In a more recent study, anesthesiologists wore standard radiation safety film badges in the operating room and in the radiology department at a pediatric hospital.[137] The badges were sensitive to cumulative doses of radiation greater than 10 mrem. In the operating rooms exposure was less than 10 mrem/month. However, in the cardiac catheterization unit dosimetric readings ranged from 20 to 180 mrem/month. The higher level of exposure exceeded guidelines for nonradiation workers. This study concluded that there was no need for routine dosimetric monitoring of anesthesiologists working in the operating room, but for anesthesiologists often working in fluoroscopy areas such as the cardiac catheterization laboratory, routine monitoring with a dosimeter should be considered.

Special efforts should be taken to avoid manipulating patients during examinations. Any radiation that does not pass directly from the source through the patient to the recording material is hazardous because x rays are reflected from surfaces, causing a scattering effect. Unless their immediate presence is essential, anesthesiologists should leave the room. If one must stay in the room with the patient, a minimal distance of 3 feet is recommended, with exposure decreasing sharply as distance is increased. Six feet of air provides the protection equivalent to 9 inches of concrete or 2.5 mm of lead.[134] Aprons and other lead-rubber protective devices are not always completely protective, and any cracks in the apron can completely destroy any protection.

Radiation exposure should be kept to the absolute minimum because there probably is no threshold below which radiation is completely harmless.[138]

3. Latex allergy. Over the past decade there has been a steadily increasing demand for latex gloves, prompted by the adaptation of universal precautions to protect against bloodborne infection. The widespread use of latex gloves has created a new occupational health concern for anesthesiologists: latex allergy.[139]

Latex allergy was not recognized as a problem until 1979.[140] Since then there has been an exponential increase in the number of reports of latex allergy.[141] Of the 1100 severe latex allergic reactions reported to the Food and Drug Administration between 1988 and 1992, more than two thirds of the reported cases were in health care workers. These included 15 deaths from anaphylaxis. It is estimated that 5% to 10% of health care workers have some manifestation of latex sensitivity.[142] The incidence may be even higher in certain groups of health care workers.[143,144]

There are three basic types of latex allergic reactions.[145] The most common is a nonimmunologic irritant contact dermatitis of the hand. The problem presents with dryness, pruritus, fissuring, and cracking of the skin, followed by redness, swelling, exudation, and crusting. Chronic exposure can lead to lichenification, scaling, and hyperpigmentation. In health care workers the lesion usually involves the hands.[146]

The two immunologic-mediated reactions are an immediate (type I) hypersensitivity reaction and a delayed (type IV) reaction.[147]

The majority (80%) of reactions are delayed type IV reactions. The allergy is usually to the chemical additives that are used during the manufacturing process to maintain the integrity of the gloves and not to the latex itself, whereas the immediate type I hypersensitivity reaction is to proteins in the rubber. The extent of allergic reactions ranges from minor reactions to anaphylaxis and death.

Several factors are associated with an increased risk of latex allergy. Sensitization to latex increases with the number of exposures.[148] Most latex reactions result from exposure to examining or surgical gloves. Health care workers are the largest at-risk group, with women having a higher prevalence than men. Frequent use of disposable gloves, history of atopic disease, and hand dermatitis are the major risk factors.[149]

Symptoms can be nonspecific and mimic other problems. Often the presentation appears as rhinoconjunctivitis (tearing, red puffy eyes, nasal congestion, sneezing), asthma (chest tightness, coughing, wheezing), or a hoarse voice. Gastrointestinal complaints can also occur. The sensitivity can present as a rash, pruritus, or burning of the hands.[150]

There is no cure other than treatment of the symptoms and latex avoidance. Delay in diagnosis can lead to progression of symptoms, with increasingly more severe reactions. Latex allergy is indicated by a temporal relationship of symptoms to working hours combined with one of several skin tests now available.[151]

There are multiple exposure routes. The allergen can enter the body by direct dermal contact, absorption through open skin, mucocutaneous exposure, and even inhalation. In fact, airborne latex allergens account for the majority of exposures by health care workers.

Medical gloves, especially powdered gloves, are the major contributor of latex airborne allergens. The concentration of allergen varies between different commercial gloves brands. Even among the same brand concentration of allergens can vary tremendously from manufactured lot to lot.

Latex aeroallergen concentrations vary in different sites within the hospital, with concentrations greatest where powdered latex gloves are used most commonly.[152] Anesthesiologists have the highest exposure compared with other health care workers who wear gloves in their work.

Several practical steps can be taken to reduce or even avoid latex allergen exposure.

The use of nonpowdered, low-allergen latex gloves, synthetic gloves, or vinyl gloves reduces or eliminates airborne latex allergens. Glove manufacturers should label their products to indicate their composition, including the presence of chemical additives and the allergen content.

Intact skin is an effective barrier. Open sores and cuts should be covered with bandages before a latex glove is donned. Washing and drying the hands after every glove change decreases the allergen load. Water-based hand lotions should also be available at the scrub sink and used by anyone using latex gloves.

Indirect contact has been implicated in several reports. A physician's wife developed symptoms of latex allergy from glove powder on her husband's hands.[153] Her symptoms disappeared when strict hand-washing procedures were implemented. Health care workers should also avoid wearing scrub suits home after working in the operating room because indirect exposure from aeroallergens has caused latex allergy in children and spouses.

Finally, personnel such as anesthesiologists with severe symptomatic occupational latex allergy may have to consider changing jobs.[154]

4. Magnetic fields. Magnetic resonance (MR) studies have become an important diagnostic tool. Anesthesiologists often are exposed to magnetic rays during studies involving pediatric or uncooperative patients. More recently, open MR units have been created to allow direct surgical access during studies.[155] MR imaging does not require ionizing radiation, but high-strength MR imaging requires several kilowatts of radiofrequency power. This has elicited concern about exposure risks to the anesthesiologist who must stay in close physical contact with the patient in the scanner.

Studies of microwave radiation have shown that exposure can limit neuroendocrine responses in laboratory animals.[156] The magnetic field in normal work MR units is usually less than 1 millitesla (mT).[157] This is much less than the whole-body limit recommended by the American Conference of Government and Industrial Hygienists (60 mT) or the International Commission on Non-Ionizing Radiation Protection (200 mT). However, the actual risk to the anesthesiologist, particularly if his or her presence is frequently required in an active radiology department, is unknown.[158]

MR is known to be dangerous in certain special circumstances. People with pacemakers or implanted stimulators, ferromagnetic vascular clips, or any other ferromagnetic metal must avoid these strong magnetic fields. Orthopedic prostheses do not pose a hazard.

The noise generated by MR imagers has caused temporary hearing loss.[159] Although studies in animals suggest that exposure to MR imaging is safe, the effects of exposure of the pregnant health care worker remain unknown.[160]

5. Lasers. Use of light amplification by stimulated emission of radiation (laser) technology has grown over the past decade, with a variety of different lasers being used in the operating room. The immediate health hazard to the anesthesiologist is eye injury from either direct exposure or reflected radiation. Burn injuries to the cornea, retina, and optic nerve have been reported. Protective eyewear, designed for the specific wavelength of the laser being used, must be worn.

The vapors and cellular debris (the plume) resulting from the laser are potentially harmful.[161] The plume may contain live bacteria or intact viral DNA, the HIV virus being the most notable.[162-166] The smoke has been shown to be mutagenic and can contain particles small enough to penetrate deep within the respiratory tract. Most surgical masks do not trap the small particles released, so care must be taken not to inhale the material. Vaporized debris should be scavenged with an efficient evacuator system to prevent plumes of laser fragments from polluting the operating room environment.[167]

6. Noise. The U.S. government defines hazardous noise as levels that reach 90 adjusted decibels (dBA) for 8 hours per day.[134,168] The time for permissible levels is halved for every increase of 5 dBA, so 95 dBA exposure is permissible for 4 hours. Measured noise levels in operating rooms often exceed 90 dBA.[169] The noise levels in our operating rooms have greatly increased with the proliferation of monitors and surgical equipment. Monitor alarms are intended to be loud and disruptive. Noise pollution decreases work performance and may reduce vigilance.[170] It is believed that during long, complicated operative procedures normal fatigue levels are increased by the presence of these noises, which actually lessens the competence of the anesthesiologist. At higher levels workers show signs of irritability. Loud sounds stimulate the hormonal stress response and have been associated with blood pressure elevation.

7. Light. Under certain conditions surgical light can strike the cornea at levels that exceed accepted safety standards.[171] There is a potential for retinal damage to operating room staff from close exposure to these lights.

II. PERSONAL STRESS
A. Physical hazards

At one time or another, every anesthesiologist experiences some physical injury at work. A partial list of potential physical hazards in the hospital environment includes conjunctivitis from the splash of solutions, slippery floors (especially around scrub sinks), airborne contaminants from improperly functioning air-conditioning systems, electric shock from poorly grounded equipment, and punctures and skin lacerations from needlesticks and from breaking glass ampules.[168] Such minor injuries as skin punctures now assume far more importance with the risk of exposure to HIV and HBV.

The 1967 study of working conditions in Russian operating rooms drew attention to health problems other than the reproductive hazards already discussed.[3] The majority of anesthesiologists interviewed for that study experienced headaches, backaches, fatigue, frequent upper respiratory tract infections, and other complaints.

One of these complaints, "anesthesiologist's back," is recognized as a major occupational problem. It was once described as the "most prevalent noninfectious occupational morbidity" for anesthesia personnel.[172] Over 70% of the anesthesiologists interviewed experienced either back pain or radiculopathy. Back pain has been attributed to strain from lifting and transferring patients or from poor posture during patient monitoring.

However, there may be another cause for this problem. Acute back problems that do not resolve promptly or improve within 2 weeks may be caused by significant behavioral factors that impede recovery.[173] These factors can include interpersonal, economic, or occupational stress. Several studies have directly related both physical and mental stress in the workplace to the prevalence of sciatica and low back pain.[174,175] Therefore the high incidence of back pain experienced by anesthesiologists can be associated with the increase in job-related stress now occurring in our specialty.

B. Substance abuse
1. Drugs and alcohol

a. Definition. A variety of terms are used in discussing substance abuse and chemical dependency[176] (Box 26-1).

Drug or substance abuse is said to occur when drug or alcohol use interferes with a person's health or economic and social function. Drug addiction is characterized by progressive and compulsive use of drugs despite destructive consequences. These operational definitions indicate a difference in degree between abuse and addiction. The crossover point between these two conditions is not sharp but includes loss of voluntary control of drug use and denial of any problems relating to such use.

Physical dependence involves pharmacologic tolerance and a characteristic withdrawal syndrome upon discontinuance of chronic drug use. Unlike addiction, dependency can be produced in anyone given the appropriate drug.

b. Etiology. Addiction to opioids is a major occupational health problem for anesthesiologists.[177] Addictive disease may occur only in susceptible people. Susceptibility may be hereditary, resulting in a neurochemical de-

---

Box 26-1 Definitions of chemical dependency terms

Abuse: Substance abuse is a situation in which drugs or alcohol interfere with one's health or economic or social function.

Addiction: A chronic disorder characterized by the compulsive use of a substance resulting in physical, psychologic, or social harm to the user; use continues despite the harm incurred.

Advocacy: Written and verbal support of the recovering individual by treatment professionals to federal, state, and hospital authorities.

Cross-tolerance: Tolerance, originally produced by long-term administration of one drug, toward a second drug not previously administered.

Physical dependence: A physiologic state of adaptation to a drug or alcohol, usually characterized by the development of tolerance to the drug's effects and the emergence of a withdrawal syndrome during prolonged abstinence.

Psychologic dependence: The emotional state of craving a drug, either for its positive effect or to avoid negative effects associated with its absence.

Recovery: A process of overcoming both physiologic and psychologic dependence on a drug.

Rehabilitation: The restoration of an optimum state of health by medical, psychologic, social, and peer group support for a chemically dependent person.

Relapse: Recurrence of alcohol- or drug-dependent behavior in a person who has previously achieved and maintained abstinence for a significant time beyond the period of detoxication.

Sobriety: Generally, the state of complete abstinence from alcohol of other drugs of abuse in conjunction with a satisfactory quality of life.

---

rangement.[178,179] The amount of drug exposure necessary for addictive disease to develop depends on the specific drug, the circumstances of exposure, and the person's susceptibility. The synthetic opioids used in the practice of anesthesiology have an extremely high addictive potential. The more potent the drug, the faster the onset of addiction when a person chooses to self-administer that drug. When exposed to a critical combination of drugs and external conditions, susceptible people become dependent on chemicals.

c. Clinical manifestations. Often, the first sign is withdrawal from outside interests because all activities, such as working, sleeping, and socializing, revolve around the use of drugs (Box 26-2). As the illness continues, the entire focus of the addict's life is dedicated to the acquisition and use of drugs. Drug use continues compulsively, despite adverse consequences and eventual isolation and deterioration of personal relationships at home and at work. The addict's personality often acquires the traits of fear, guilt, emotional lability, and loss of self-esteem.[180] There may be frequent unexplained illnesses and multiple job changes in an attempt to thwart discovery of the addictive illness.[181]

Box 26-2 Signs and symptoms of addiction in anesthesiologists*

Personal

Personal hygiene and dressing habits decline.
Personality and behavior change (wide mood swings; often depression, anger, and irritability alternating with periods of euphoria).
Withdraws from family.
Has violent outbursts.
Experiences sexual dysfunction.
Neglects social commitments, isolates self.

Professional

Prefers to work alone (to divert drugs for personal use); refuses lunch and coffee relief; often offers to relieve others.
Often requests bathroom relief (site for drug administration).
Volunteers for extra cases, often for procedures in which large amounts of narcotics are available (e.g., cardiac surgery).
Often at hospital when off duty, volunteers for extra call (stays close to drug supply to prevent withdrawal).
Difficult to find between cases (takes short naps after using drugs).
Requests increasing amounts of opioids for patients; requests inappropriately high doses for operation being performed.
Charting is increasingly sloppy and unreadable; falsifies records.
May insist on administering opioids personally to his or her patients in the postanesthesia care unit; patients may complain of pain out of proportion to the amount of opioid charted on anesthesia record.
May wear long-sleeved gowns to hide needle tracks.
Narcotic addicts often have pinpoint pupils; may display evidence of withdrawal (diaphoresis, tremors).
Weight loss and pale skin are common.
Addicts often are found comatose or dead (if undetected).

*Even when several signs are present the observer should never assume that a colleague is chemically dependent or directly confront the suspected addict.

Addicted anesthesiologists isolate themselves from their peers by working alone, often on long cases, to facilitate their access to drugs. They may volunteer to relieve other anesthesiologists because it gives them an opportunity to divert drugs for their own use.

Changes in behavior often are noted. Mood swings at work are common, with periods of irritability, anger, euphoria, and depression.

Although the association seems logical, there are no published reports to demonstrate that impaired physicians are more likely to commit malpractice than nonimpaired physicians. Typically the professional life of the person is the last to be affected by addiction.[182]

At higher doses anesthetic drugs of abuse are potentially lethal. In a review of 180 case reports of substance abuse by residents in anesthesiology, there were 13 (7%) instances in which the initial presentation of the problem

was death from overdose.[183] The extreme potency of the opioids used may explain why anesthesiologists become chemically dependent and suffer from premature deaths from overdose and suicide.[184] In a study of drug abuse in anesthesiology residency programs, of 334 confirmed cases of substance abuse, follow-up study was possible in 235 cases. Thirty subjects (12.8%) died of drug overdose.[185,186] Even higher mortalities were reported by others.[187]

d. Prevalence. Chemical dependency and drug addiction have reached epidemic proportions in American society, and the medical profession certainly is not immune.[188-192] In fact, alcohol and drug dependency are more common among physicians than among the general population, and as a group, anesthesiologists are at a particularly high risk of developing this illness.[180,193-195]

Although anesthesiologists make up less than 4% of physicians in the United States, they are overrepresented in treatment groups of chemically dependent physicians, accounting for over 10% of physicians in treatment.[180,196,197] The largest group of physicians treated in the Medical Association of Georgia Impaired Physicians Program (MAG-IPP) has been anesthesiologists.[198,199] More recent data from the Medical Board of California's Diversion Program listed 31 of the 206 physicians active in the program as anesthesiologists.[200] This high participation rate may be partly a function of the zeal with which our specialty has addressed the problem to the extent that we are better than others at recognizing addicted colleagues and referring them to appropriate treatment facilities. One poll found a substance-abuse prevalence rate of 2% among all anesthesia residents.[183] A questionnaire was sent to the 260 graduates over a 30-year period of one anesthesia residency program; 183 anesthesiologists responded.[201] Of those, 29 (15.8%) identified themselves as being substance dependent. Nineteen were alcohol impaired, 6 were drug impaired, and 4 were dependent on both drugs and alcohol.

e. Epidemiology. Speculation abounds as to positive causative factors. It has been suggested that physicians with an addictive potential or personality choose anesthesiology as a career in order to satisfy their needs. Alternatively, the specialty of anesthesiology may provide the environment that drives a susceptible individual to addictive disease. The most often-cited environmental factors include excessive job stress and the ready availability of drugs.[202]

The majority of drug-addicted physicians have a family history of substance abuse.[201,203] However, 85% of anesthesia residents in the MAG-IPP reported that one reason they were attracted to anesthesia was easy drug access. In fact, nearly 8% chose anesthesia as a specialty after they had become addicted.

As job stress or fatigue becomes overwhelming, they may start out experimenting with anesthetic drugs under the guise of "therapeutic optimism."[204,205] In this mind set, the anesthesiologists believe that they can self-administer the anesthetic drugs to desired effect in the same manner in which they dispense it to their patients, never considering that they may become addicted. Obvious in this progression is the ease of access to highly addictive drugs. Because many of the drugs used in anesthesia practice require only small amounts for their therapeutic effect, diverting nontraceable amounts of these drugs is easy.[201]

Impaired anesthesiologists, compared with other anesthesiologists in practice, tend to be younger, with residents and fellows significantly overrepresented. Outside the academic environment it may be easier for addicted anesthesiologists to isolate themselves and avoid detection because their clinical activities rarely are evaluated by their colleagues.

Compared to other physicians, addicted anesthesiologists are more likely to abuse two or more substances. With the easy availability of opioids, exclusive abuse of alcohol alone is rare. Previously, the drugs of choice were fentanyl and demerol, but sufentanil has replaced the latter.

Only older anesthesiologists in the various diversion programs are more likely to abuse alcohol. Parenteral (intravenous or intramuscular) abuse is far more likely than oral use. Not unexpectedly, compared to personnel in other specialties, anesthesiologists are more likely to abuse drugs at work.

f. Prevention. The best prevention for chemical dependency begins with education early in the training program. Counseling and information regarding substance abuse and related material should be added to every residency curriculum. Most anesthesia residency programs now have at least one lecture on substance abuse, and many departments have a substance abuse program or committee and offer special seminars concerning substance abuse to physicians and their spouses.

To discourage abuse and to identify anesthesiologists who may be diverting drugs from the workplace, many anesthesia departments have now adopted changes in the ways in which they account for the use of these drugs.[206-208] For example, at my institution, at the start of each work day the operating room satellite pharmacy releases a locked box to each resident containing controlled substances. Any partially used ampules or syringes are returned with the unused drugs at the completion of the work schedule. On a random basis, boxes are selected and returned syringes are examined by refractometry. If the results of the test are not appropriate, all items returned by that person are examined for a period of 2 weeks. The objective is to distinguish between an occasional labeling or measurement error and a consistent pattern. All materials with an unexpected response to refractometry are saved and submitted for gas chromatographic analysis. The confidential reports are reported to the department chairperson.

g. Treatment. Understanding the problem and recognizing that a colleague needs help are in the best interests of that person and his or her patients. There is a critical need for anesthesiologists to be ready at all times to deal with emergencies, and prolonged use of addictive substances impairs cognitive and perceptual functions.[209] Unfortunately, many anesthesiologists remain poorly informed about impairment and addiction and are therefore reluctant or unable to recognize and respond to a colleague afflicted with this disease. As a result, the

---

Box 26-3 American Society of Anesthesiologists Policy Statement on Chemical Dependence (1991)

1. Chemical dependence is a medical disease.
2. Untreated or relapsing chemical dependence is incompatible with safe clinical performance of anesthesia.
3. It shall be the duty of all members of the department of anesthesia to share their concerns about chemical dependence, in themselves or other members of the department, in confidence, with the designated resource person.
4. The Chief of Anesthesia or designee shall act as a confidential resource person on chemical dependence.
5. The Chief of Anesthesia, with appropriate consultation, will judge whether any member of the department is suffering from untreated or relapsing chemical dependence.
6. All members of the department of anesthesia, as a condition of staff privileges, agree to accept the Chief of Anesthesia's decision on the diagnosis of chemical dependence.
7. Should the Chief of Anesthesia judge that a member of the department is suffering from active chemical dependence, the member shall immediately be placed on leave of absence.
8. Should it be determined that the departmental member is not suffering from chemical dependence, this diagnosis shall be expunged from his/her record and he/she shall be allowed to return to work without prejudice.
9. All members of the department should obtain medical insurance coverage for treatment of chemical dependence.
10. Return from medical leave for chemical dependence shall be governed by departmental Chemical Dependence Re-Entry Policy.
11. Departmental policy on chemical dependence in no way supersedes departmental or institutional policy governing intoxication on duty or conviction of a felony.
12. The name of the resource person for chemical dependence for the department (and his or her telephone and pager numbers) should be available to everyone.

---

chemically dependent physician often remains untreated as the disease progresses, often to a fatal outcome.

The American Medical Association maintains that chemical dependency should be treated as an illness and that the patient (that is, the impaired physician) is entitled to the same legal rights and medical treatment opportunities afforded patients with other illnesses. On the other hand, in order to protect patients and the public, physicians are required to report to the appropriate regulatory body credible evidence of impairment that affects the competence of their colleagues. Thus we all have an obligation to refer colleagues with suspected chemical dependency for diagnosis and treatment. The ASA policy statement on chemical dependence is shown in Box 26-3.

The first step in the process involves confronting the addicted anesthesiologist. This should not be done on a one-on-one basis because of the difficulty in breaking down the barrier of denial. Rather, information regarding suspected drug abuse or addiction should be collected and corroborated by as many people as possible and presented in a structured forum known as intervention. The setting varies depending on the circumstances but should always be performed in an empathic and nonjudgmental manner.

It is common for the intervention team to face massive denial, anger, threats, and hostility. Involvement of the family and close associates may help break down the denial and achieve the objective of referring the addicted anesthesiologist to a specialist facility for diagnosis and to initiate treatment. However, the anesthesiologist may elect to leave the department, seek drugs from alternate sources, or consider suicide.

Treatment is usually based on the recovery model of Alcoholics Anonymous. There is no cure for addiction, but appropriate treatment and follow-up observation can restore the chemically dependent physician to health and a productive life free of drugs. This process of change is called recovery, and recovery is a life-long process. During treatment patients identify the factors that trigger drug use and develop coping skills. Self-help group interactions are beneficial. Lack of understanding and support by peers seriously compromises the chances for long-term recovery.

Successful treatment is a multidisciplinary effort. Detoxification, monitored abstinence, intensive education, and behavior modification through self-help groups and psychotherapy are usually achieved by in-patient treatment early in recovery. Specific blocking drugs (disulfiram [Antabuse] for alcohol; naltrexone [Trexan] for opiates) often are used. Methadone is never used. Naltrexone is particularly valuable for anesthesiologists, and naltrexone therapy is usually a prerequisite for return to work.

h. Reentry. Before 1980, the most common approach to drug addiction in anesthesiology was to redirect the recovering addicted anesthesiologist into another specialty because returning to the operating room was believed to be analogous to allowing a recovering alcoholic bartender to tend bar.[181] However, several studies have reported that for all physicians, completion of long-term therapy can have a favorable outcome. Of the first 334 chemically dependent physicians to complete a 4-month residential and 20-month aftercare program at MAG-IPP, 93% were in recovery and practicing medicine 2.5 to 10 years after treatment.[210] The overall death rate from addictive disease for these physicians was 1%. Fifty-five of 56 anesthesiologists who completed the MAG-IPP program were in recovery and were practicing medicine. Of those who returned to anesthesia, 90% (36 of 40) successfully did so; the other 4 switched specialties. Of the 9 anesthesiologists who did not complete treatment, 4 died of their addictive disease.[210]

Based on statistics such as these,[196,210,211] the ASA Committee on Occupational Health of Operating Room Personnel concluded in their 1986 publication that "following adequate therapy and follow-up, it appears that the prognosis for long-term recovery and return to (anesthesia) practice . . . should be encouraged and supported."[212]

But a limited number of follow-up studies reveal that chemically dependent anesthesiologists may have a different prognosis from that of other physicians. Results of a survey sent to the 159 anesthesiology training programs in the United States indicate that drug rehabilitation followed by redirection into another specialty may be a more prudent course for the anesthesiology trainee who abuses parenteral drugs.[183] Of 113 residents who reentered anesthesia training, the success rate (completion of anesthesia residency training and maintenance of a drug-free state during clinical practice) among parenteral opioid abusers was only 34% (27 of 79), compared to a rate of 70% among the nonopioid abuser group. There were 14 cases of suicide or lethal overdose among trainees who were allowed to reenter anesthesia programs. Death as the initial relapse symptom occurred in 13 of the 79 (16%). Ward, Ward, and Saidman[186] report that 70% of addicted anesthesiologists following rehabilitation were lost to medicine and at least 10% died of addictive disease. These chilling statistics have caused many to reevaluate the wisdom of allowing former substance abusers to return to anesthesia training.

Still, the majority of residency programs allow residents with a history of substance abuse to reenter their programs. Proponents of this approach argue that anesthesiologists in recovery prove to be a useful resource in the identification and referral of other addicted residents to treatment facilities. Also, the possibility of reentry into clinical practice offers a powerful incentive for seeking treatment.[213] The annual report (1990) of the ASA Committee on Occupational Health of Operating Room Personnel states that an exception should be made for early anesthesia trainees (junior residents), who should be directed into another specialty rather than be given an opportunity to reenter an anesthesia training program.

If the impaired physician is allowed to reenter his or her department, structured plans must be formalized to facilitate safe and smooth reintegration back into the department. Everyone must have a clear understanding of what is to be involved in the physician's ongoing recovery program, and a written contract is mandatory. Clear and direct lines of communication must be maintained, and all parties involved (the physician, his or her colleagues, the hospital, and his or her patients) must be safeguarded.[214] Many of the doubts and concerns about the impaired physician can be allayed through staff education.

The contract outlining the recovering addict's responsibilities should include an agreement to abstain from self-administration of mood-altering substances, and a plan of action should be developed should a relapse occur. All medications must be prospectively approved by a physician familiar with the disease of addiction and the individual patient's history. A physician should be assigned to monitor compliance with the terms of the reentry contract.

The monitor should meet with the recovering addict at regular intervals and be responsible for organizing collection of urine and blood samples. The recovering physician must participate in a program of random, unannounced, witnessed urine and blood screening tests.

The hospital-based impaired physicians' committee should serve as the liaison between the returning physician and all the groups interested in monitoring his or her practice. This advocacy group can also monitor the recovery of the addicted anesthesiologist. All states now have licensing boards or regulatory agencies with Impaired Professionals Programs (IPPs) for cooperative action with hospital or department committees.

Individual or group therapy is also advised, along with periodic contact with the impaired physicians' committee and physician advocate.

If the returning physician has been out of practice for any length of time, participation in retraining or refresher courses should be encouraged. Undue stress at work must be avoided, with adequate time off and vacation. Finally, it is in everyone's best interest to record and document the physician's clinical performance, the results of the urine screening tests, attendance at therapy sessions, and other positive actions.

Frequent random drug screening is important. A major problem in identification and follow-up observation of addicted physicians is that most of the commercially available urine and blood screening tests currently used to detect recent drug use do not accurately measure fentanyl, sufentanil, or alfentanil.[215] Furthermore, unless the person has already been identified as chemically dependent and is in recovery, most physicians will not voluntarily submit to routine urine and blood screening. It is possible that unscheduled, random urine screening of all anesthesiologists, along with tighter control of narcotics, could help control the problem.

2. Inhaled anesthetics. In the past, inhaled agents were widely used for recreational purposes. Historically, "ether frolics or jags" and "laughing gas parties" existed long before either of these agents was used during surgery. The clinical application of these gases (that is, the start of anesthesiology as a specialty) began when people noticed the absence of reactions to painful injuries while their friends were under the influence of these agents.

Deaths from nitrous oxide, halothane, and ether sniffing are still reported, usually as a result of associated hypoxia.[216] The inhaled anesthetic of choice is "laughing gas," partly because for many years nitrous oxide was believed to be free of any morbidity. We now recognize that recreational abuse of nitrous oxide is not innocuous but can be associated with several health problems, including neuropathy.

C. Stress

Stress is defined as any factor that causes bodily or mental tension by placing demands on a person. Like most physicians, anesthesiologists are exposed to a multitude of physical, psychologic, and emotional demands that affect both our own health and our ability to provide medical care to our patients.[217,218]

Anesthesiologists work continuously in situations in which a mistake or error in judgment can result in patient death or injury. Often, the only time an anesthesiologist receives publicity is when a patient care disaster occurs. There may be a relationship between high levels of drug and alcohol abuse among anesthesiologists and the effects of stress and fatigue.[204]

Some occupational sources of stress are unavoidable, but others can be modified and controlled. Jackson[219] cites an example of one of the many subtle stresses facing anesthesiologists. Historically, the preanesthetic visit on the night before surgery allowed the anesthesiologist to meet and evaluate the patient. The initial evaluation of many high-risk patients now occurs minutes before the induction of anesthesia. Much of the stress we experience each work day comes from the uncertainty, the depersonalization, the inconvenience, and the uncontrollability of our work practices, as exemplified by the hurried preanesthetic process.

1. Professional burnout. Besides the obvious hazards and stresses related to direct patient care already discussed, there are other demands from patients, colleagues, and the institution that may not be met and often lead to physical and emotional deterioration. Although most of us cope satisfactorily with work-related stresses, the incidence of substance abuse and suicide among our colleagues illustrates the failure of many others to compensate.

Production pressure, sometimes mistaken for increased efficiency in the operating room, has certainly increased the work-related stress experienced by anesthesiologists. This pressure may have deleterious effects on both the physician and the patient. In a questionnaire of California anesthesiologists, Gaba, Howard, and Jump[220] noted that almost half the respondents felt that increased production pressure had resulted in unsafe actions by anesthesiologists.

Professional burnout is emotional exhaustion caused by such stress. Symptoms include physical exhaustion, emotional detachment, boredom and cynicism, impatience, irritability, and a feeling of not being appreciated. The last often leads to paranoia, disorientation, psychosomatic complaints, and depression.[221]

Burnout should be suspected if a colleague demonstrates increased absenteeism, decreasing enthusiasm, declining performance, and lack of focus and communication. Unless the sufferer learns to relax (both mentally and physically), exercises to work off stress, or develops new interests or even changes his or her career, the outcome can be quite serious.

2. Fatigue. Anesthesiologists often work long hours and suffer considerable sleep loss. There are often financial incentives to work longer and harder. There is always pressure from many sources to be more efficient (that is, to provide more service with fewer physicians). Although efficiency may be defined by cost considerations and is greatest with a heavy work load, effectiveness is highest with a moderate work load.[222] When reasonable limits are exceeded, stress and fatigue are inevitable.

Work efficiency decreases with sleep deprivation.[223,224] Studies performed on medical house officers acutely and chronically deprived of sleep demonstrate impairment in efficiency, with difficulty in thinking and learning.[225-227] Performance among anesthesiologists was lower at the end of a long shift than at the beginning of the shift when they were refreshed.[228] The reduction in cognitive function associated with fatigue may contribute to potentially dangerous incidents in the operating room.[229] Decreased work satisfaction and poor self-concept have also been described with heavy work loads.[215] Marital and sexual dysfunction has also been attributable to fatigue from work.[230,231] Excessive sleep deprivation and prolonged and uninterrupted stressful work not only fatigues the person, but also can cause personality alterations, cognitive and behavioral deterioration, and eventual progression to emotional and physical illness as well as professional burnout.[232]

We have an obligation to modify whatever factors are controllable so as not to jeopardize our own health and that of our patients. Fatigue is one factor that can be controlled.

Several state legislatures have considered the problems of sleep deprivation among physicians. Most attempts to set standards for maximum work hours have been arbitrary, often without objective data to support them. However, because inadequate or irregular sleep patterns do increase the risks of errors,[233] voluntary guidelines for anesthesiologists are recommended. Limiting work hours to reasonable levels and the provision of adequate numbers of physicians to alleviate particularly heavy demands are essential.

The following suggestions are guidelines that limit working hours to numbers less than those that have been shown to produce performance deficits.[204]

- Any anesthesiologist involved with a procedure lasting more than 3 hours should be relieved for short periods every 2 hours.
- No anesthesiologist should regularly work more than a 16-hour work day without a full 12-hour recovery period.
- No anesthesiologist should be on call for more than 24 hours without a full 24-hour recovery period.
- Anesthesiologists must say no to unreasonable work demands.

Other stress factors also can be addressed.[234] There must be flexibility and adaptability in covering case loads. More challenging cases and work exposure to difficult surgeons should be a distributed fairly among the group. An adequate amount of vacation time should be available.

There must be some mechanism for the anesthesiologist who becomes fatigued or physically ill, or who has demanding administrative responsibilities, to be covered by his or her colleagues. Cases with suboptimal outcomes should be discussed in a nonthreatening manner.

D. Personal health

All deaths among members of the ASA over a four-decade period were examined and the causes compared with the Metropolitan Life Insurance standardized tables for deaths among similar-aged men.[235-237]

Deaths rates among anesthesiologists from 1930 to 1946 were similar to those in the period 1947 to 1956 but greater than those from 1957 to 1971, an indication that exposure to the fluorinated anesthetic agents introduced in the mid-1950s may not be an important health hazard influencing the mortality of anesthesiologists.[237]

Coronary artery and other vascular diseases accounted for more than half the deaths; however, the rate was less than the expected death rate for controls. Likewise, although malignancies were the next highest cause of death, the incidence of cancer was lower than expected. In fact, all categories of death attributable to illness were lower than in the control group, often by as much as 30%. Similar reductions in the rate of cancer among anesthesiologists have been reported in Great Britain.[10,238]

These studies reveal a single surprising finding: The third highest cause of death among anesthesiologists has been suicide. Suicide is discussed in the next section.

The overall mortality experience for both American and British anesthesiologists has been shown to compare favorably with that of other physicians.[10,235-238] However, these retrospective questionnaire surveys are notoriously inaccurate.[18] Therefore a prospective study of consultant anesthetists in England was attempted.[239] It investigated the records in the National Health Service for rates of early retirement among anesthesiologists because of permanent ill health and deaths while they were still employed. The control group consisted of consultants in four other hospital specialty groups.

Approximately two thirds of all consultants in the five specialty groups during the period of 1966 to 1983 were included in this study. Retirement because of ill health among male anesthetists was approximately twice that of other physicians. The number of early retirements for any reason was also greater than that for other specialties. The numbers of deaths while they were actively employed was also higher. The values in these categories were also higher for female anesthetists, but the numbers were too small for analysis. Unfortunately, no information on the nature of the health problems or causes of death were made available. The two usual explanations for the apparent excesses in morbidity among anesthesiologists are exposure to waste anesthetic gases and stress and fatigue.

A third possibility is that the results were attributable to selection rather than environmental factors. It is possible that physicians with a predisposition to poor health are attracted to anesthesiology. This is unlikely because ASA studies have demonstrated a lower mortality for anesthesiologists than for the general population.[236] The major causes of mortality among male American anesthesiologists less than 55 years of age are drug overdose and suicide.

More subtle health hazards have also been suggested.[240,241] For example, studies in the Soviet Union and Great Britain report increased rates for liver disease, lumbar disk disease, peptic ulcer disease, hypertension, headaches, insomnia, and reproductive problems.[3,241] Presumably, occupational stress, chemical abuse, and exposure to anesthetic gases may all contribute to these generalized, nonspecific health findings.

E. Suicide

Medicine is a demanding and stressful profession, with high rates of alcoholism, drug abuse, and suicide. Suicide among professionals (physicians, dentists, lawyers) occurs more often than in the general population.[242] For example, suicide is reported to be two to three times more common and is the leading cause of premature death among all physicians.[243] Presumably because of the pressures of work and fatigue, substance abuse, or declining health, suicide is more common among physicians and their spouses.[244]

Anesthesiologists commit suicide more often than other specialists, with the possible exception of psychiatrists. Anesthesiologists have a suicide rate of 44 to 55 per 100,000. This is twice the rate for surgeons and three to five times the rate for pediatricians. Suicide accounted for 19 of 211 (9%) of deaths in one ASA study of causes of death among American anesthesiologists.[245] The retrospective surveys of deaths during the 1950s to 1970s found that suicides accounted for more than 6% of all deaths, four times more than expected from mortality statistics.[235,236] Furthermore, other deaths reported as accidents may have been suicides, an indication that the actual rate may be even greater.

Fourteen of the 19 suicide deaths in the most recent ASA study were among anesthesiologists less than 55 years of age. A high incidence of suicide has also been reported among anesthesia residents still in training.[246] For anesthesiologists 65 to 75 years of age, the suicide rate was 15 times greater than expected,

Involvement in a malpractice suit has been implicated in cases of suicide.[247] A subpopulation of an already high-risk specialty is the anesthesiologist involved in litigation. An anesthesiologist being sued suffers tremendous emotional stress and anxiety. A study of 192 suits over an 11-year period involving 185 of the approximately 400 anesthesiologists in the State of Washington revealed 4 suicides (2.2%), a suicide attempt in 1 of every 45 anesthesiologists being sued.[248,249]

Litigation is just one contributing cause. Long work hours, demanding patients and peer pressures, overwork, and fatigue are believed to be major factors in physician suicide and are often offered by chemically addicted physicians as the conscious reason for their use of drugs.[250]

The association of substance abuse and suicide has not been examined fully. Suicide attempts are known to be common among physicians with recognized drug-related problems.[251] Chemical dependency on narcotics is believed to be a new phenomenon. Before the 1970s alcohol was the major drug of dependency. It is interesting that although the suicide rate among anesthesiologists was high during the period 1930 to 1946, it was

nearly equal to that of other physicians, particularly during the Depression years (1930 to 1940), when the white male death rate for suicide was high.[237] Accidental drug overdose may play a role in the dramatic increase in deaths listed as suicide in more recent years.[187]

F. The impaired anesthesiologist

Many of the problems discussed in this chapter lead to a common end point: the impaired physician. A physician is considered impaired when he or she is unable to be a healthy family or community member or to practice medicine safely. Impairment can be attributable to advancing age, physical or psychiatric disability, emotional problems, or substance abuse. Substance abuse and chemical dependency are believed to be the leading causes of impairment among anesthesiologists. To compound the situation, these problems usually occur at a time when the person is most productive.

In general the medical profession has policed its own members by disciplining members compromised by mental or physical illness, chemical dependence, or lack of diligence in keeping current. Physicians are required to report to the appropriate body credible evidence of impairment that affects the competence of their colleagues. We all have an obligation to urge colleagues with physical or mental illnesses or with chemical dependency to seek treatment.

REFERENCES

1. DiBenetto DV: Occupational hazards of the health care industry: protecting health care workers, *AAOHN J* 43:131, 1995.
2. Bojanowski LM: Safety among health-care workers in the NHS, *Br J Hosp Med* 57:47, 1997.
3. Vaisman AI: Work in operating theaters and its effects on the health of anaesthesiologists, *Eksp Khir Anestesiol* 12:44, 1967 (in Russian).
4. Cohen EN, Bellville JW, Brown BW Jr: Anesthesia, pregnancy, and miscarriage: a study of operating room nurses and anesthetists, *Anesthesiology* 35:343, 1971.
5. Knill-Jones RP, Rodriques LV, Moir DD, et al: Anaesthetic practice and pregnancy: a controlled survey of women anaesthetists in the United Kingdom, *Lancet* 1:1326, 1972.
6. Rosenberg P, Kirves A: Miscarriages among operating theatre staff, *Acta Anaesthesiol Scand* 53(suppl):37, 1973.
7. Knill-Jones RP, Newman BJ, Spence AA: Anaesthetic practice and pregnancy: controlled survey of male anaesthetists in the United Kingdom, *Lancet* 2:807, 1975.
8. American Society of Anesthesiologists: Occupational disease among operating room personnel: a national study. Report of an ad hoc committee on the effect of trace anesthetics on operating room personnel, *Anesthesiology* 41:321, 1980.
9. Axelsson G, Rylander R: Exposure to anaesthetic gases and spontaneous abortion: response bias in a postal questionnaire study, *Int J Epidemiol* 11:250, 1982.
10. Maran NJ, Knill-Jones RP, Spence AA: Infertility among female hospital doctors in the UK, *Br J Anaesth* 76:581, 1996 (letter).
11. Lane GA, Nahrwold ML, Tait AR, et al: Anesthetics as teratogens: nitrous oxide is fetotoxic, xenon is not, *Science* 210:899, 1980.
12. Vieira E, Cleaton-Jones P, Austin JC, et al: Effects of low concentrations of nitrous oxide on rat fetuses, *Anesth Analg* 59:175, 1980.
13. Barker JP, Abdelatti MO: Anaesthetic pollution: potential sources, their identification and control, *Anaesthesia* 52:1077, 1997.
14. Corbett TH: Retention of anesthetic agents following occupational exposure, *Anesth Analg* 52:614, 1973.

15. Harrington JM: The health of anaesthetists, *Anaesthesia* 42:131, 1987 (editorial).
16. Brodsky JB, Cohen EN: Adverse effects of nitrous oxide, *Med Toxicol* 1:362, 1986.
17. Buckley DN, Brodsky JB: Nitrous oxide and male fertility, *Reprod Toxicol* 1:93, 1988.
18. Vessey MP: Epidemiological studies of the occupational hazards of anaesthesia: a review, *Anaesthesia* 33:430, 1978.
19. Mazze RI, Lecky JH: The health of operating room personnel, *Anesthesiology* 62:226, 1985.
20. Tannenbaum TN, Goldberg RJ: Exposure to anesthetic gases and reproductive outcome: a review of the epidemiologic literature, *J Occup Med* 27:659, 1985.
21. Colton T: *Evaluation of the epidemiologic evidence for occupational hazards of anesthetic gases,* Park Ridge, Ill, 1982, American Society of Anesthesiologists.
22. Buring JE, Hennekens CH, Mayrent SI, et al: Health experiences of operating room personnel, *Anesthesiology* 62:325, 1985.
23. Gabbe SG, Turner LP: Reproductive hazards of the American lifestyle: work during pregnancy, *Am J Obstet Gynecol* 176:826, 1997.
24. Cohen EN, Gift HC, Brown BW, et al: Occupational disease in dentistry and chronic exposure to trace anesthetic gases, *J Am Dent Assoc* 101:21, 1980.
25. Kripke BJ, Kelman AD, Shah NK, et al: Testicular reaction to prolonged exposure to nitrous oxide, *Anesthesiology* 44:104, 1976.
26. Brodsky JB, Baden JM, Serra M, et al: Nitrous oxide inactivates methionine synthetase activity in the rat testis, *Anesthesiology* 61:66, 1984.
27. Wyrobek AJ, Brodsky JB, Gordon L, et al: Sperm studies in anesthesiologists, *Anesthesiology* 55:527, 1981.
28. Louis-Ferdinand RT: Myelotoxic, neurotoxic and reproductive adverse effects of nitrous oxide, *Adv Drug React Toxicol Rev* 13:193, 1994.
29. Sweeney B, Bingham RM, Amos RJ, et al: Toxicity of bone marrow in dentists exposed to nitrous oxide, *BMJ* 291:567, 1985.
30. Brodsky JB, Cohen EN, Brown BW, et al: Exposure to nitrous oxide and neurologic disease among dental professionals, *Anesth Analg* 60:297, 1981.
31. Layzer RB: Myeloneuropathy after prolonged exposure to nitrous oxide, *Lancet* 2:1227, 1978.
32. Layzer RB, Fishman RA, Schafer JA: Neuropathy following abuse of nitrous oxide, *Neurology* 28:504, 1978.
33. Agamanolis DP, Chester EM, Victor M, et al: Neuropathology of experimental vitamin B_{12} deficiency in monkeys, *Neurology* 26:905, 1976.
34. Scott JM, Dinn JJ, Wilson P, et al: Pathogenesis of subacute combined degeneration: a result of methyl group deficiency, *Lancet* 2:334, 1981.
35. Nunn JF, Sharer N: Inhibition of methionine synthetase by trace concentrations of nitrous oxide, *Br J Anaesth* 53:1099, 1981.
36. Stacy CB, Di Rocco A, Gould RJ: Methionine in the treatment of nitrous-oxide-induced neuropathy and myeloneuropathy, *J Neurol* 239:401, 1992.
37. Bruce DL, Bach MJ, Arbit J: Trace anesthetic effects on perceptual, cognitive and motor skills, *Anesthesiology* 40:453, 1974.
38. Bruce DL, Bach MJ: Effects of trace anaesthetic gases on behavioural performance of volunteers, *Br J Anaesth* 48:871, 1976.
39. Smith G, Shirley AW: A review of the effects of trace concentrations of anaesthetics on performance, *Br J Anaesth* 50:701, 1978.
40. Gambill AF, McCallum RN, Henrichs TF: Psychomotor performance following exposure to trace concentrations of inhalation anesthetics, *Anesth Analg* 58:475, 1979.
41. Ferstandig LL: Trace concentrations of anesthetic gases: a critical review of their disease potential, *Anesth Analg* 57:328, 1978.
42. Whitcher CE, Cohen EN, Trudell JR: Chronic exposure to anesthetic gases in the operating room, *Anesthesiology* 35:348, 1971.
43. Lecky JH: The mechanical aspects of anesthetic pollution control, *Anesth Analg* 56:769, 1977.
44. Whitcher C, Piziali RL: Monitoring occupational exposure to inhalation anesthetics, *Anesth Analg* 56:778, 1977.
45. Chang WP, Kau CW, Hseu SS: Exposure to anesthesiologists to nitrous oxide during pediatric anesthesia, *Ind Health* 35:112, 1997.
46. Fullekrug B, Pothmann W, Werner C, et al: The laryngeal mask airway: anesthetic gas leakage and fiberoptic control of positioning, *J Clin Anesth* 5:357, 1993.
47. National Institute for Occupational Safety and Health: *Criteria for a recommended occupational exposure to waste anesthetic gases and vapors,* HEW (NIOSH) pub no 77-140, Washington, DC, 1977, US Government Printing Office.
48. Tran N, Elias J, Rosenberg T, et al: Evaluation of waste anesthetic gases, monitoring strategies, and correlations between nitrous oxide levels and health symptoms, *Am Ind Hyg Assoc J* 55:36, 1994.
49. Schuyt HC, Verberk MM: Measurement and reduction of nitrous oxide in operating rooms, *J Occup Environ Med* 38:1036, 1996.
50. Hoerauf KH, Koller C, Taeger K, et al: Occupational exposure to sevoflurane and nitrous oxide in operating room personnel, *Int Arch Occup Environ Health* 69:134, 1997.
51. Austin PR, Austin PJ: Measurement of nitrous oxide concentrations in a simulated post anesthesia care unit environment, *J Perianesth Nurs* 11:259, 1996.
52. Huffman LM: Regulations, standards, and guidelines protecting PACU healthcare workers, *J Perianesth Nurs* 11:231, 1996.
53. Eger EI: Should we not use nitrous oxide? In Eger EI, ed: *Nitrous oxide,* New York, 1985, Elsevier.
54. du Moulin GC, Hedley-Whyte J: Hospital-associated viral infections and the anesthesiologist, *Anesthesiology* 59:51, 1983.
55. Schlech WF III: The risk of infection in anaesthetic practice, *Can J Anaesth* 35:S846, 1988.
56. Sepkowitz KA: Occupationally acquired infections in health care workers. Part II, *Ann Intern Med* 125:917, 1996.
57. Doyle AJ: Tuberculosis: preventing occupational transmission to health care workers, *AAOHN J* 43:475, 1995.
58. Barre-Sinoussi F, Cherman JC, Rey F, et al: Isolation of a T-lymphotropic retrovirus from a patient at risk for acquired immune deficiency syndrome (AIDS), *Science* 220:868, 1983.
59. Gallo RC, Salahuddin SZ, Popovic M, et al: Frequent detection and isolation of cytopathic retroviruses (HTLV-III) from patients with AIDS and at risk for AIDS, *Science* 224:500, 1984.
60. Friedland GH, Saltzman BR, Rogers MF, et al: Lack of transmission of HTLV-III/LAV infection to household contacts of patients with AIDS or AIDS-related complex with oral candidiasis, *N Engl J Med* 314:344, 1986.
61. Baker JL, Kelen GD, Sivertson KT, et al: Unsuspected human immunodeficiency virus infection in critically ill emergency patients, *JAMA* 257:2609, 1987.
62. Centers for Disease Control: Update: human immunodeficiency virus infections in health-care workers exposed to blood of infected patients, *MMWR* 36:285, 1987.
63. Centers for Disease Control: Impact of the expanded AIDS surveillance case definition in AIDS case reporting, *MMWR* 42:308, 1993.
64. Centers for Disease Control: Recommendations for prevention of HIV transmission in health-care settings, *MMWR* 36(suppl 2S):3S, 1987 (published in *JAMA* 258:1293, 1987).
65. Henderson DK, Fahey BJ, Willy M, et al: Risk for occupational transmission of human immunodeficiency virus type 1 (HIV-1) associated with clinical exposure: a prospective evaluation, *Ann Intern Med* 113:740, 1990.
66. Centers for Disease Control: Update: provisional public health service recommendations for chemoprophylaxis after occupational exposure to HIV, *MMWR* 45:468, 1996.
67. Marcus R: Surveillance of health care workers exposed to blood from patients infected with the human immunodeficiency virus, *N Engl J Med* 319:1118, 1988.
68. Gerderding JL, Bryant-LeBlanc CE, Nelson K, et al: Risk of transmitting the human immunodeficiency virus, cytomegalovirus, and hepatitis B virus to health care workers exposed to patients with AIDS and AIDS-related conditions, *J Infect Dis* 156:1, 1987.
69. McCray E: Occupational risk of acquired immunodeficiency syndrome among health care workers, *N Engl J Med* 314:1127, 1986.

70. Centers for Disease Control: Update: acquired immunodeficiency syndrome and human immunodeficiency virus infection among health-care workers, *MMWR* 37:229, 1988.
71. Weiss SH, Saxinger WC, Rechtman D, et al: HTLV-III infection among health care workers: association with needle-stick injuries, *JAMA* 254:2089, 1985.
72. Henderson DK, Shah AJ, Zak BJ, et al: Risk of nosocomial infection with human T-cell lymphotropic virus type III/lymphadenopathy-associated virus in a large cohort of intensively exposed health care workers, *Ann Intern Med* 104:644, 1986.
73. Howard RJ: Human immunodeficiency virus testing and the risk to the surgeon of acquiring HIV, *Surg Gynecol Obstet* 171:22, 1990.
74. Kelen GD, Fritz S, Qaqish B, et al: Unrecognized human immunodeficiency virus infection in emergency department patients, *N Engl J Med* 318:1645, 1988.
75. Kelen GD, Green GB, Purcell RH, et al: Hepatitis B and hepatitis C in emergency department patients, *N Engl J Med* 326:1399, 1992.
76. Weiss SH: Risks and issues for the health care worker in the human immunodeficiency virus era, *Med Clin North Am* 81:555, 1997.
77. Chamberland ME, Petersen LR, Munn JP, et al: Human immunodeficiency virus infection among health care workers who donate blood, *Ann Intern Med* 121:269, 1994.
78. Buergler JM, Kim R, Thisted RA, et al: Risk of human immunodeficiency virus for surgeons, anesthesiologists, and medical students, *Anesth Analg* 75:118, 1992.
79. Chavey WE, Cantor SB, Clover RD, et al: Cost-effectiveness analysis of screening health care workers for HIV, *J Fam Pract* 38:249, 1994.
80. Owens DK, Nease RF Jr: Occupational exposure to human immunodeficiency virus and hepatitis B virus: a comparative analysis of risk, *Am J Med* 92:503, 1992.
81. Jacobson IM, Dienstag JL, Werner BG, et al: Epidemiology and clinical impact of hepatitis D virus (delta) infection, *Hepatology* 5:188, 1985.
82. Williams AE, Dodd RY: The serology of hepatitis C virus in relation to post-transfusion hepatitis, *Ann Clin Lab Sci* 20:192, 1990.
83. Sherertz RJ, Russel BA, Reuman PD: Transmission of hepatitis A by transfusion of blood products, *Arch Intern Med* 144:1579, 1984.
84. Tabor E: The three viruses of non-A, non-B hepatitis, *Lancet* 1:743, 1985.
85. Hepatitis C virus: guidance on the risks and current management of occupational exposure. PHLS Hepatitis Subcommittee. Communicable Disease Report. *CDR Rev* 3:R135, 1993.
86. Browne RA, Chernesky MA: Viral hepatitis and the anaesthetist, *Can Anaesth Soc J* 31:279, 1984.
87. Denes AE, Smith JL, Maynard JE, et al: Hepatitis B infections in physicians: results of a nationwide seroepidemiologic survey, *JAMA* 239:210, 1978.
88. Berry AJ, Greene ES: The risk of needlestick injuries and needlestick transmitted diseases in the practice of anesthesiology, *Anesthesiology* 77:1007, 1992.
89. Berry AJ, Isaacson IJ, Hunt MD, et al: The prevalence of hepatitis B viral markers in anesthesia personnel, *Anesthesiology* 60:6, 1984.
90. Berry AJ, Isaacson IJ, Kane MA, et al: A multicenter study of the prevalence of hepatitis B viral serologic markers in anesthesia personnel, *Anesth Analg* 63:738, 1984.
91. Berry AJ, Isaacson IJ, Kane MA, et al: A multicenter study of the epidemiology of hepatitis B in anesthesia residents, *Anesth Analg* 64:672, 1985.
92. Fyman PN, Hartung J, Weinberg S, et al: Prevalence of hepatitis B markers in the anesthesia staff in a large inner-city hospital, *Anesth Analg* 63:433, 1984.
93. Malm DN, Mathias RG, Turnbull KW, et al: Prevalence of hepatitis B in anaesthesia personnel, *Can Anaesth Soc J* 33:167, 1986.
94. Chernesky MA, Browne RA, Rondi P: Hepatitis B virus antibody prevalence in anaesthetists, *Can Anaesth Soc J* 31:239, 1984.
95. Siebke JC, Degré M: Prevalence of viral hepatitis in the staff in Norwegian anaesthesiology units, *Acta Anaesthesiol Scand* 28:549, 1984.
96. Carstens J, Macnab GM, Kew MC: Hepatitis-B virus infection in anaesthetists, *Br J Anaesth* 49:887, 1977.
97. Janzen J, Tripatzis I, Wagner V, et al: Epidemiology of hepatitis B surface antigen (HBsAg) and antibody to HBsAg in hospital personnel, *J Infect Dis* 137:261, 1978.
98. Wisnom CJ, Lee RJ: Increased seroprevalence of hepatitis B in dental personnel necessitates awareness of revised pediatric hepatitis B vaccine recommendations, *J Public Health Dent* 53:231, 1993.
99. Linnemann CC Jr, Hegg ME, Ramundo N, et al: Screening hospital patients for hepatitis B surface antigen, *Am J Clin Pathol* 67:257, 1977.
100. Tait AR, Tuttle DB: Prevention of occupational transmission of human immunodeficiency virus and hepatitis B virus among anesthesiologists: a survey of anesthesiology practice, *Anesth Analg* 79:623, 1994.
101. Mangione CM, Gerberding JL, Cummings SR: Occupational exposure to HIV: frequency and rates of underreporting of percutaneous and mucocutaneous exposures by medical housestaff, *Am J Med* 90:85, 1991.
102. Centers for Disease Control, Immunization Practices Advisory Committee: Postexposure prophylaxis of hepatitis B, *MMWR* 33:285, 1984.
103. Centers for Disease Control: Hepatitis B virus: a comprehensive strategy for eliminating transmission in the United States through universal childhood vaccination, *MMWR* 40:1, 1991.
104. Centers for Disease Control: Suboptimal response to hepatitis B vaccine given by injection into the buttock, *MMWR* 34:105, 1985.
105. Francis DP, Feorino PM, McDougal S, et al: The safety of the hepatitis B vaccine: inactivation of the AIDS virus during routine vaccine manufacture, *JAMA* 256:869, 1986.
106. Scolnick EM, McLean AA, West AJ, et al: Clinical evaluation in healthy adults of a hepatitis B vaccine made by recombinant DNA, *JAMA* 251:2812, 1984.
107. Brown SE, Stanley C, Howard CR, et al: Antibody responses to recombinant and plasma-derived hepatitis B vaccines, *BMJ* 292:159, 1986.
108. Okada N, Eldred L, Cohn S, et al: Comparative immunogenicity of plasma and recombinant hepatitis B virus vaccines in homosexual men, *JAMA* 260:3635, 1988.
109. Goilav C, Prinsen H, Piot P: Protective efficacy of a recombinant DNA vaccine against hepatitis B in male homosexuals: results at 36 months, *Vaccine* 8(suppl):S50, 1990.
110. Doebbeling BN, Ferguson KJ, Kohout FJ: Predictors of hepatitis B vaccine acceptance in health care workers, *Med Care* 34:58, 1996.
111. Centers for Disease Control: Recommendations for preventing transmission of infection with human T-lymphotropic virus type III/lymphadenopathy-associated virus in the workplace, *MMWR* 34:681, 1985.
112. Berry AJ: Practice advisory: prevention of blood-borne infections (hepatitis B and AIDS), *American Society of Anesthesiologists Newsletter,* July 1988.
113. Mathieu A: Acquired immune deficiency syndrome, hepatitis and herpes: risks and implications for anesthesia personnel, *Semin Anesth* 6:231, 1987.
114. Lovitt SA, Nichols RL, Smith JW, et al: Isolation gowns: a false sense of security? *Am J Infect Control* 20:185, 1992.
115. Henderson DK: Postexposure chemoprophylaxis for occupational exposure to human immunodeficiency virus type 1: current status and prospects for the future, *Am J Med* 91:312S, 1991.
116. Centers for Disease Control: Case-control study of HIV seroconversion in health-care workers after percutaneous exposure to HIV-infected blood: France, United Kingdom, and United States, January 1988–August 1994, *MMWR* 39, 1994.
117. Tokars JI, Marcus R, Culver DH, et al: Surveillance of HIV infection and zidovudine use among health care workers after occupational exposure to HIV-infected blood, The CDC Cooperative Needlestick Group, *Ann Intern Med* 118:913, 1993.

118. Schmitz SH, Scheding S, Volitis D, et al: Side effects of AZT prophylaxis after occupational exposure to HIV-infected blood, *Ann Hematol* 69:135, 1994.

119. Sacks HS, Rose DN: Zidovudine prophylaxis for needlestick exposure to human immunodeficiency virus: a decision analysis, *J Gen Intern Med* 5:132, 1990.

120. Bond WW, Favero MS, Petersen NJ, et al: Survival of hepatitis B virus after drying and storage for one week, *Lancet* 1:550, 1981 (letter).

121. Orkin FK: Herpetic whitlow: occupational hazard to the anesthesiologist, *Anesthesiology* 33:671, 1970.

122. Rosato FE, Rosato EF, Plotkin SA: Herpetic paronychia: an occupational hazard of medical personnel, *N Engl J Med* 283:804, 1970.

123. Juel-Jensen BE: Herpetic whitlows: an occupational risk, *Anaesthesia* 28:324, 1973.

124. DeYoung GG, Harrison AW, Shapley JM: Herpes simplex cross infection in the operating room, *Can Anaesth Soc J* 15:394, 1968.

125. Chan PC, Eustis SL, Huff JE, et al: Two-year inhalation carcinogenesis studies of methyl methacrylate in rats and mice: inflammation and degeneration of nasal epithelium, *Toxicology* 52:237, 1988.

126. Cromer J, Kronoveter K: *A study of methylmethacrylate exposure and employee health,* DHEW pub no 77-119 (NIOSH), Washington, DC, 1976, US Government Printing Office.

127. Jeidrychowski W: Styrene and methyl methacrylate in the industrial environment as a risk factor of chronic obstructive lung disease, *Int Arch Occup Environ Health* 51:151, 1982.

128. Pickering CA, Bainbridge D, Birtwistle IH, et al: Occupational asthma due to methyl methacrylate in an orthopaedic theatre sister, *BMJ* 292:1362, 1986.

129. Lee CM: Unusual reaction to methyl methacrylate monomer, *Anesth Analg* 63:371, 1984 (letter).

130. Schwettmann RS, Casterline CL: Delayed asthmatic response following occupational exposure to enflurane, *Anesthesiology* 44:166, 1976.

131. Scolnick B, Collins J: Systemic reaction to methylmethacrylate in an operating room nurse, *J Occup Med* 28:196, 1986.

132. National Institute for Occupational Safety and Health: Recommendations for occupational safety and health standards, *MMWR* 35:33S, 1976.

133. Taylor G: A scavenging device for venting methylmethacrylate monomer vapor, *Anesthesiology* 41:612, 1974.

134. Barker D: Protection and safety in the x-ray department, *Radiography* 44:45, 1978.

135. Keen RI: The radiation hazard to anaesthetists, *Br J Anaesth* 32:224, 1960.

136. Linde HW, Bruce DL: Occupational exposure of anesthetists to halothane, nitrous oxide and radiation, *Anesthesiology* 30:363, 1969.

137. Henderson KH, Lu JK, Strauss KJ, et al: Radiation exposure of anesthesiologists, *J Clin Anesth* 6:37, 1994.

138. Lamberton LF: An examination of the clinical and experimental data relating to the possible hazard to the individual of small doses of radiation, *Br J Radiol* 31:229, 1958.

139. Holzman RS: Latex allergy: an emerging operating room problem, *Anesth Analg* 76:635, 1993.

140. Nutter AF: Contact urticaria to rubber, *Br J Dermatol* 191:597, 1979.

141. Slater JE: Latex allergy, *J Allergy Clin Immunol* 94:139, 1994.

142. Turjanmaa K: Incidence of immediate allergy to latex gloves in hospital personnel, *Contact Dermatitis* 17:270, 1987.

143. Lagier F, Vervloet D, Lhermet I, et al: Prevalence of latex allergy in operating room nurses, *J Allergy Clin Immunol* 90:319, 1992.

144. Fisher AA: Allergic contact reactions in health personnel, *J Allergy Clin Immunol* 90:729, 1992.

145. Truscott W, Roley L: Glove-associated reactions: addressing an increasing concern, *Dermatol Nurs* 7:283, 1995.

146. Arellano R, Bradley J, Sussman G: Prevalence of latex sensitization among hospital physicians occupationally exposed to latex gloves, *Anesthesiology* 77:905, 1992.

147. Sussman GL, Beezzhold DH: Allergy to latex rubber, *Ann Intern Med* 122:43, 1995.

148. Porri F, Pradal M, Lemiere C, et al: Association between latex sensitization and repeated latex exposure in children, *Anesthesiology* 86:599, 1997.

149. Hunt LW, Fransway AF, Reed CE, et al: An epidemic of occupational allergy to latex involving health care workers, *J Occup Environ Med* 37:1204, 1995.

150. Charous BL, Hamilton RG, Yunginger JW: Occupational latex exposure: characteristics of contact and systemic reactions in 47 workers, *J Allergy Clin Immunol* 94:12, 1994.

151. Heese A, van Hintzenstern J, Peters KP, et al: Allergic and irritant reactions to rubber gloves in medical health services, *J Am Acad Dermatol* 25:831, 1991.

152. Swanson MC, Bubak ME, Hunt LW, et al: Quantification of occupational latex aeroallergens in a medical center, *J Allergy Clin Immunol* 94:445, 1994.

153. Karanthansis P, Cooper A, Zhou K, et al: Indirect latex exposure causes urticaria/anaphylaxis, *J Allergy Clin Immunol* 91:526, 1994 (letter).

154. Kam PCA, Lee MSM, Thompson JF: Latex allergy: an emerging clinical and occupational health problem, *Anaesthesia* 52:570, 1997.

155. Fried MP, Hsu L, Topulos GP, et al: Image-guided surgery in a new magnetic resonance suite: preclinical considerations, *Laryngoscope* 106:411, 1996.

156. Kido DK, Morris TW, Erickson JL, et al: Physiologic changes during high field strength MR imaging, *AJR* 148:1215, 1987.

157. Jonsson P, Barregard L: Estimated exposure to static magnetic fields for the staffs of NMR-units, *Occup Med* 46:17, 1996.

158. Patteson SK, Chesney JT: Anesthetic management for magnetic resonance imaging: problems and solutions, *Anesth Analg* 74:121, 1992.

159. Brummett RE, Talbot JM, Charuhas P: Potential hearing loss resulting from MR imaging, *Radiology* 169:539, 1988.

160. Prasad N, Wright DA, Ford JJ, et al: Safety of 4-T MR imaging: study of effects on developing frog embryos, *Radiology* 174:251, 1990.

161. Nezhat C, Winer WK, Nezhat F, et al: Smoke from laser surgery: is there a health hazard?, *Lasers Surg Med* 7:376, 1987.

162. Baggish MS, Baltoyannis P, Sze E: Protection of the rat lung from the harmful effects of laser smoke, *Lasers Surg Med* 8:248, 1988.

163. Byrne PO, Sisson PR, Oliver PD, et al: Carbon dioxide laser irradiation of bacterial targets in vitro, *J Hosp Infect* 9:265, 1987.

164. Garden JM, O'Banion MK, Shelnitz LS, et al: Papillomavirus virus in the vapor of carbon dioxide laser–treated verrucae, *JAMA* 259:1199, 1988.

165. O'Grady KF, Easty AC: Electrosurgery smoke: hazards and protection, *J Clin Eng* 21:149, 1996.

166. McKinley IB Jr, Ludlow MO: Hazards of laser smoke during endodontic therapy, *J Endodontics* 20:558, 1994.

167. Goldman L: Proposal to develop a detailed safety program for general/laser surgical patients infected with AIDS, *Lasers Surg Med* 19:351, 1996.

168. DePaolis MV, Cottrell JE: Miscellaneous hazards: radiation, infectious diseases, chemical and physical hazards, *Int Anesthesiol Clin* 19:131, 1981.

169. Shapiro RA, Berland T: Noise in the operating room, *N Engl J Med* 287:1236, 1972.

170. Davenport WG: Vigilance and arousal: effects of different types of background stimulation, *J Psychol* 82:339, 1972.

171. Fox RA, Henson PW: Potential ocular hazard from a surgical light source, *Australas Phys Eng Sci Med* 19:12, 1996.

172. Bause GS, Black RG: Anesthesiologist's back: epidemiology of a major occupational disease, *Anesth Analg* 65:S13, 1986.

173. Gillette RD: Behavioral factors in the management of back pain, *Am Fam Physician* 53:1313, 1996.

174. Heliovaara M, Makela M, Knekt P, et al: Determinants of sciatic and low-back pain, *Spine* 16:608, 1991.

175. Ahlberg-Hulten GK, Theorell T, Sigala F: Social support, job strain and musculoskeletal pain among female health care personnel, *Scand J Work Environ Health* 21:435, 1995.

176. Rinaldi RC, Steindler EM, Wilford BB, et al: Clarification and standardization of substance abuse terminology, *JAMA* 259:555, 1988.

177. Silverstein JH, Silva DA, Iberti TJ: Opioid addiction in anesthesiology, *Anesthesiology* 79:354, 1993.

178. Donovan JM: An etiologic model of alcoholism, *Am J Psychiatry* 143:1, 1986.

179. Cadoret RJ, Troughton E, O'Gorman TW, et al: An adoption study of genetic and environmental factors in drug abuse, *Arch Gen Psychiatry* 43:1131, 1986.

180. Spiegelman WG, Saunders L, Mazze RI: Addiction and anesthesiology, *Anesthesiology* 60:335, 1984.

181. Serry N, Bloch S, Ball R, et al: Drug and alcohol abuse by doctors, *Med J Aust* 160:402, 1994.

182. Talbott GD, Wright C: Chemical dependency in health care professionals, *State Art Rev Occup Med* 2:581, 1987.

183. Menk EJ, Baumgarten RK, Kingsley CP, et al: Success of reentry into anesthesiology training programs by residents with a history of substance abuse, *JAMA* 263:3060, 1990.

184. Gallegos KV, Browne CH, Veit FW, et al: Addiction in anesthesiologists: drug access and patterns of substance abuse, *Q Rev Biol* 14:116, 1988.

185. Ward CF, Saidman LJ: Controlled substance abuse: a survey of training programs, 1970-1980, *Anesthesiology* 55:345, 1981.

186. Ward CF, Ward GC, Saidman LJ: Drug abuse in anesthesia training programs, a survey: 1970 through 1980, *JAMA* 250:922, 1983.

187. Gravenstein JS, Kory WP, Marks RG: Drug abuse by anesthesia personnel, *Anesth Analg* 62:467, 1983.

188. Keeve JP: Physicians at risk: some epidemiologic considerations of alcoholism, drug abuse, and suicide, *J Occup Med* 26:503, 1984.

189. American Medical Association Council on Mental Health: The sick physician: impairment by psychiatric disorders, including alcoholism and drug dependence, *JAMA* 223:684, 1973.

190. Bissell L, Jones RW: The alcoholic physician: a survey, *Am J Psychiatry* 133:1142, 1976.

191. McAuliffe WE, Wechsler R, Rohman S, et al: Psychoactive drug use by young and future physicians, *J Health Soc Behav* 25:34, 1984.

192. McAuliffe WE, Rohman S, Santangelos S, et al: Psychoactive drug use among practicing physicians and medical students, *N Engl J Med* 315:805, 1986.

193. Wallot H, Lambert J: Drug addiction among Quebec physicians, *Can Med Assoc J* 126:927, 1982.

194. Brewster JM: Prevalence of alcohol and other drug problems among physicians, *JAMA* 255:1913, 1986.

195. Lutsky I, Hopwood M, Abram SE, et al: Use of psychoactive substances in three medical specialties: anesthesia, medicine and surgery, *Can J Anaesth* 41:561, 1994.

196. Gualtieri AC, Consentino JP, Becker JS: The California experience with the diversion program for impaired physicians, *JAMA* 249:226, 1983.

197. Herrington RE, Benzer DG, Jacobson GR, et al: Treating substance use disorders among physicians, *JAMA* 247:2253, 1982.

198. Farley WJ, Talbott GD: Anesthesiology and addiction, *Anesth Analg* 62:465, 1983 (editorial).

199. Talbottt GD, Gallegos KV, Wilson PO, et al: The Medical Association of Georgia's Impaired Physicians Program: review of the first 1000 physicians: analysis of specialty, *JAMA* 257:2927, 1987.

200. Medical Board of California: *The Medical Board's Diversion Program,* January 1995.

201. Lutsky I, Hopwood M, Abram SE, et al: Psychoactive substance abuse among American anesthesiologists: a 30-year retrospective study, *Can J Anaesth* 40:915, 1993.

202. Goodwin DW, Davis DH, Robins LN: Drinking amid abundant illicit drugs: the Vietnam case, *Arch Gen Psychiatry* 32:230, 1975.

203. Flaherty JA, Richman JA: Substance use and addiction among medical students, residents, and physicians, *Psychiatr Clin North Am* 16:1898, 1993.

204. Parker JB: The effects of fatigue on physician performance: an underestimated cause of physician impairment and increased patient risk, *Can J Anaesth* 34:489, 1987.

205. McCue JD: The effects of stress on physicians and their medical practice, *N Engl J Med* 306:458, 1982.

206. Shovick VA, Mattei TJ, Karnack CM: Audit to verify use of controlled substances in anesthesia, *Am J Hosp Pharm* 45:1111, 1988.

207. Adler GR, Potts FE, Kirby RR, et al: Narcotic control in anesthesia training, *JAMA* 253:3133, 1985.

208. Lecky JH, Aukburg SJ, Conahan TJ, et al: A departmental policy addressing chemical substance abuse, *Anesthesiology* 65:414, 1986.

209. Robinson EL, Fitzgerald JS, Gallegos KQ: Brain functioning and addiction: what neuropsychologic studies reveal, *J Med Assoc Ga* 74:74, 1985.

210. Talbott GD, Richardson AC Jr, Mashburn JS, et al: The Medical Association of Georgia's Disabled Doctors Program: a 5-year review, *J Med Assoc Ga* 70:545, 1981.

211. Morse RM, Martin MA, Swenson WM, et al: Prognosis of physicians treated for alcoholism and drug dependence, *JAMA* 251:743, 1984.

212. American Society of Anesthesiologists: *Questions and answers about chemical dependency and physician impairment,* Park Ridge, Ill, July 1986, American Society of Anesthesiologists.

213. Corsino BV, Morrow DH, Wallace CJ: Quality improvement and substance abuse: rethinking impaired provider policies, *Am J Med Qual* 11:94, 1996.

214. Ackerman TF: Chemically dependent physicians and informed consent disclosure, *J Addict Dis* 15:25, 1996.

215. Stiller RL, Scierka A, Davis PJ, et al: A method to increase recovery of fentanyl from urine, *J Toxicol Clin Toxicol* 27:101, 1989.

216. Chadly A, Marc B, Barres D, et al: Suicide by nitrous oxide poisoning, *Am J Forensic Med Pathol* 10:330, 1989.

217. Green A, Duthie HL, Young HL, et al: Stress in surgeons, *Br J Surg* 77:1154, 1990.

218. Richardsen AM, Burke RJ: Occupational stress and work satisfaction among Canadian women physicians, *Psychol Rep* 72:811, 1993.

219. Jackson SH: Stress in the life of the anesthesiologist, *Bull Calif Soc Anesth* 39:2, 1990.

220. Gaba DM, Howard SK, Jump B: Production pressure in the work environment: California anesthesiologists' attitudes and experiences, *Anesthesiology* 81:488, 1994.

221. Ansell EM: Professional burn-out: recognition and management, *J Am Assoc Nurse Anesth* 49:135, 1981.

222. Binner PR, Potter A, Halpern J: Workload levels, program costs, and program benefits: an output value analysis, *Adm Ment Health* 3:156, 1976.

223. Friedman RC, Bigger JT, Kornfeld DS: The intern and sleep loss, *N Engl J Med* 285:201, 1971.

224. Morgan BB Jr, Brown BR, Alluisi EA: Effects on sustained performance of 48 hours continuous work and sleep loss, *Hum Factors* 16:406, 1974.

225. Goldman LI, McDonough MT, Rosemond GP: Stresses affecting surgical performance and learning. I. Correlation of heart rate, electrocardiogram, and operation simultaneously recorded on videotapes, *J Surg Res* 12:83, 1972.

226. Friedman RC, Kornfeld DS, Bigger TJ: Psychological problems associated with sleep deprivation in interns, *J Med Educ* 48:436, 1973.

227. Leighton K, Livingston M: Fatigue in doctors, *Lancet* 1:1280, 1983 (letter).

228. Narang V, Laycock JR: Psychomotor testing of on-call anaesthetists, *Anaesthesia* 41:868, 1986.

229. Cooper JB, Newbower RS, Kitz RJ: An analysis of major errors and equipment failures in anesthesia management: considerations for prevention and detection, *Anesthesiology* 60:34, 1984.

230. Yogev S, Harris S: Women physicians during residency years: workload, work satisfaction and self-concept, *Soc Sci Med* 17:837, 1983.

231. Vaillant GE, Sobowale NC, McArthur C: Some psychologic vulnerabilities of physicians, *N Engl J Med* 287:372, 1972.

232. Friedmann J, Globus G, Huntley A, et al: Performance and mood during and after gradual sleep reduction, *Psychophysiology* 14:245, 1977.

233. Mitler MM, Carskadon MA, Czeisler CA, et al: Catastrophes, sleep, and public policy: consensus report, *Sleep* 11:100, 1988.

234. McCue JD: The effects of stress on physicians and their medical practice, *N Engl J Med* 306:458, 1982.

235. Bruce DL, Eide KA, Linde HW: Causes of death among anesthesiologists: a 20-year study, *Anesthesiology* 29:565, 1968.

236. Lew EA: Mortality experience among anesthesiologists, 1954-1976, *Anesthesiology* 51:195, 1979.

237. Linde HW, Mesnick PS, Smith NJ: Causes of death among anesthesiologists: 1930-1946, *Anesth Analg* 60:1, 1981.

238. Doll R, Peto R: Mortality among doctors in different occupations, *BMJ* 1:1433, 1977.

239. McNamee R, Keen RI, Corkill CM: Morbidity and early retirement among anaesthetists and other specialists, *Anaesthesia* 42:133, 1987.

240. Spence AA, Cohen EN, Brown BW, et al: Occupational hazards for operating room–based physicians: analysis of data from the United States and the United Kingdom, *JAMA* 238:955, 1977.

241. Spence AA, Knill-Jones RP: Is there a health hazard in anaesthetic practice? *Br J Anaesth* 50:713, 1978.

242. Olkinuora M, Asp S, Juntunen J, et al: Stress symptoms, burnout and suicidal thoughts in Finnish physicians, *Soc Psychiatry Psychiatr Epidemiol* 25:81, 1990.

243. Rose KD, Rosow I: Physicians who kill themselves, *Arch Gen Psychiatry* 29:800, 1973.

244. Sakinofsky I: Suicide in doctors and wives of doctors, *Can Fam Physician* 26:837, 1980.

245. Bruce DL, Eide KA, Smith NJ, et al: A prospective survey of anesthesiologist mortality, 1967-1971, *Anesthesiology* 41:71, 1974.

246. Helliwel PJ: Suicide amongst anaesthetists-in-training, *Anaesthesia* 38:1097, 1983.

247. Wohl S: Death by malpractice, *JAMA* 255:1927, 1986.

248. Solazzi RW, Ward RJ: Analysis of anesthetic mishaps: the spectrum of medical liability cases, *Int Anesthesiol Clin* 22:43, 1984.

249. Birmingham PK, Ward RJ: A high-risk suicide group: the anesthesiologist involved in litigation, *Am J Psychiatry* 142:1225, 1985 (letter).

250. Bressler B: Suicide and drug abuse in the medical community, *Suicide Life Threat Behav* 6:170, 1967.

251. Crawshaw R, Bruce JA, Eraker PL, et al: An epidemic of suicide among physicians on probation, *JAMA* 243:1915, 1980.

PART THREE

Surgical Complications That Might Be Attributed to Anesthesia

Chapter 27

Cardiothoracic Surgery

Medhat S. Hannallah

I. **Complications Presenting Mainly with Respiratory Dysfunction**
  A. Respiratory Dysfunction Caused by the Surgery Itself
    1. Effect of lung resection
    2. Effect of cardiac surgery
  B. Right-to-Left Shunting After Lung Resection Through a Patent Foramen Ovale
  C. Unilateral Reexpansion Pulmonary Edema
  D. Pulmonary Torsion
  E. Tracheobronchial Disruption
    1. Tracheal disruption
    2. Bronchial disruption
  F. Contralateral Pneumothorax
  G. Phrenic Nerve Palsy
    1. During open heart surgery
    2. During noncardiac thoracic surgery
II. **Complications Presenting Mainly with Hemodynamic Instability**
  A. Myocardial Ischemia
  B. Cardiac Arrhythmias Following Thoracotomy

C. Hemorrhage
    1. Following thoracic surgery
    2. Following cardiovascular surgery
  D. Mediastinal Shift Following Pneumonectomy
  E. Cardiac Herniation Following Pneumonectomy
  F. Inadvertent Transection of the Pulmonary Artery Catheter
  G. Complications of Intercostal Nerve Block Performed by the Surgeon Under Direct Vision During Thoracotomy
III. **Complications Presenting Mainly with Neurologic Deficits**
  A. Upper-Extremity Neuropathy
    1. Following open heart surgery
    2. Following thoracotomy
  B. Spinal Cord Ischemia
    1. Paraplegia following thoracotomy
    2. Paraplegia following aortic aneurysm repair
  C. Vagus and Recurrent Laryngeal Nerve Injury
  D. Horner's Syndrome
  E. Subarachnoid-Pleural Fistula Following Thoracotomy

Perioperative complications occurring in the course of cardiothoracic surgery often are difficult to distinguish from those caused by complications of anesthetic techniques and anesthetic agents. Respiratory dysfunction, hemodynamic instability, or neurologic deficits that occur during and after cardiothoracic surgery are as likely to be a complication of surgery as of anesthesia. Therefore awareness of these surgical complications and their different presentations should help the anesthesiologist in early diagnosis and therapy.

The cardiothoracic surgical complications presented in this chapter are classified according to their primary clinical presentations. However, overlap in these presentations often occurs. The important category of complications related to cardiopulmonary bypass (CPB) is discussed in detail in Chapter 13.

I. COMPLICATIONS PRESENTING MAINLY WITH RESPIRATORY DYSFUNCTION

A. Respiratory dysfunction caused by the surgery itself

1. Effect of lung resection. Resection of pulmonary tissue results in a decrease in the cross-sectional area of the pulmonary vasculature.[1,2] The resulting increase in right ventricular (RV) afterload can have a major impact on cardiopulmonary function. Van Mieghan and

Demedts[1] compared pulmonary function before and after uncomplicated lung resection with the patients acting as their own controls. They found that resection of pulmonary tissue caused a decrease in vital capacity of 15% after lobectomy and 35% to 40% following pneumonectomy. After operation the compliance per unit lung volume was reduced, implying that the lung had become stiffer. Maximum effort tolerance decreased after pneumonectomy with a normal pulmonary artery (PA) pressure at rest and an increase in PA pressure and pulmonary vascular resistance on effort. This indicated loss of the normal physiologic decrease in pulmonary vascular resistance during effort and was explained by the limited reserve in distention and recruitment of the vascular bed after removal of a significant part of the pulmonary tissue.

Van Mieghan and Demedts[1] also showed that cardiac output and stroke volume during effort decreased after lung resection, resulting in an increase in peripheral arterial blood pressure and peripheral vascular resistance. These hemodynamic changes were similar but less pronounced after lobectomy than after pneumonectomy. The authors also showed that arterial oxygen saturation on effort decreased after pneumonectomy, possibly because of the absolute decrease in diffusing capacity. Carbon dioxide elimination, on the other hand, was maintained during exercise, indicating that the ventilatory capacity in the remaining lung was sufficient. Reed, Spinale, and Crawford[2] performed serial measurements of RV performance after pulmonary resection and identified significant RV dilation indicative of RV dysfunction after routine pulmonary resection. RV end-diastolic volume increased on the first and second postoperative days, and by the second postoperative day RV ejection fraction was significantly lower than preoperative baseline values and those of the early postoperative period.

These changes usually are well tolerated by most patients who undergo major lung resection. Nonetheless, every effort should be made preoperatively to distinguish patients with compromised pulmonary function, who will not tolerate the changes associated with lung resection and who are therefore at increased risk of developing respiratory failure postoperatively. Preoperative xenon-133 regional ventilation and perfusion studies in conjunction with overall pulmonary function tests usually are reliable in calculating predicted postresection lung function and in determining whether the patient is likely to tolerate the planned resection.[3] However, intraoperative surgical complications such as bleeding into the bronchus or injury to a major pulmonary vessel leading to an unanticipated need to perform more extensive resection can seriously increase the operative risk. In addition, trauma and compression of the remaining lung tissue or prolonged lung collapse during surgery can significantly impair postoperative lung function and may tip the balance against a patient with a borderline function, thus precipitating postoperative respiratory failure.

Patients who have undergone pneumonectomy are reported to be at increased risk of serious pulmonary edema.[4,5] The risk is higher following right-sided pneumonectomy because the right lung has approximately 55% of the lung mass and lymphatic pump capacity. As a result, only 45% of the capillaries and lymphatic system remain to carry the blood flow and filtered fluid back to the circulation after right-sided pneumonectomy.[5] Monitoring fluid therapy using the Swan-Ganz balloon-tipped catheter is therefore important in the perioperative management of these patients. However, it is important to realize that after pneumonectomy pulmonary capillary wedge pressure (PCWP) may reflect a falsely low value.[4] Wittnich et al[4] observed postpneumonectomy patients in whom pulmonary edema developed, but whose PCWP was near normal. In an attempt to explain this finding, they performed canine experiments that demonstrated that after pneumonectomy, inflation of the balloon of the Swan-Ganz catheter to obtain PCWP can result in considerable occlusion of the remaining cross-sectional area of the pulmonary circulation. This occlusion acutely increased the RV afterload, resulting in reduced cardiac output and reduced left atrial pressure (LAP). Although the PCWP under these circumstances still accurately reflected LAP, these values were artificially lowered by the balloon inflation, so they resulted in a falsely low PCWP reading.

Finally, the thoracotomy incision itself has a major potentially deleterious effect on postoperative pulmonary

function.[6] The resulting postoperative pain causes splinting of the chest wall, compression of the lungs, and a decrease in the functional residual capacity (FRC). The splinting also prevents coughing and deep breathing, which promotes retention of secretions and atelectasis that, in turn, further decrease the FRC. The decrease in the FRC below the closing volume of the lungs and the atelectasis result in postoperative hypoxemia and predispose to infection. These complications can be reduced effectively by appropriate postoperative pain control.[7] Because of its negative impact on pulmonary function, avoidance of thoracotomy, using the more limited thoracoscopic approach whenever possible, is advantageous, particularly in the high-risk patient.[8]

2. Effect of cardiac surgery. Abnormalities of chest wall function associated with a median sternotomy in cardiac patients do not usually cause major respiratory dysfunction.[9] However, cardiac surgical patients who have the internal mammary artery harvested for their coronary artery bypass graft (CABG) may have more pulmonary problems postoperatively because they are more susceptible to developing pleural effusions secondary to pleural trauma or hemorrhage.[10]

Postoperative atelectasis is common in patients after cardiac surgery.[11] The atelectasis is often worse in the left than in the right lower lobe (Fig. 27-1). This may be related to retraction of the left lower lobe during surgery, postoperative gastric distention, or possibly transient paresis of the left hemidiaphragm. The incidence of atelectasis in general was found to be higher the greater the number of CABGs, the longer the operative and the CPB time, when the pleural space was entered, when a right atrial drain and a cardiac insulating pad were not used, and with a lower body temperature.[11]

B. Right-to-left shunting after lung resection through a patent foramen ovale

Dyspnea after major lung resection usually is attributable to loss of alveolar volume and restriction of the pulmonary vascular bed, whereas dyspnea and hypoxemia after lung resection occur on rare occasions in patients without pulmonary hypertension as a result of right-to-left shunt through a patent foramen ovale.[12-17] This syndrome is most commonly described following right-sided pneumonectomy. Characteristically, the resulting dyspnea and hypoxemia appear late in the postoperative period and are produced by assumption of an erect position and relieved by a recumbent one (platypnea and orthostatic cyanosis). Nonetheless, Holtzman et al[14] reported a postpneumonectomy patient who developed the syndrome immediately after operation and in whom symptoms were not affected by position.

The mechanism of the right-to-left shunt is thought to be mediastinal distortion after the right-sided pneumonectomy. The inferior vena cava remains fixed in position, but the right atrium is shifted to the right, thus favoring opening of a foramen ovale.[12] The postural nature of the syndrome is thought to be a result of accentuation of mediastinal distortion in the upright position, with further shift of the right atrium and widening of the ori-

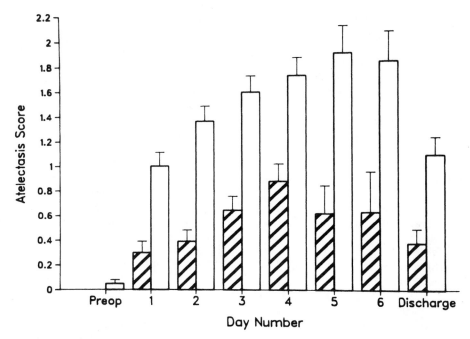

Fig. 27-1. Atelectasis scores for right *(hatched bars)* and left *(open bars)* lungs preoperatively, on postoperative days 1-6, and on discharge. (From Wilcox P, Baile E, Hards J, et al: *Chest* 93:693, 1988.)

fice of the patent foramen ovale. The fact that the syndrome has also been described after left-sided pneumonectomy[15] and lobectomy[16,17] suggests that factors other than mechanical alteration in right atrial configuration might be at play, such as a change in the relationship between right and left ventricular compliance with the right ventricle and the right atrium becoming less compliant than the left.[13,15]

Because the incidence of probe-patent foramen ovale in adults is about 25%,[18] this syndrome should be suspected in any patient with abnormal shunting and hypoxemia after major lung resection. Two-dimensional or transesophageal echocardiography can be very helpful in confirming the diagnosis.[12,15,16] Cardiac catheterization is indicated if surgical closure of the patent foramen ovale is considered. Surgical closure usually offers immediate dramatic improvement in oxygenation.

C. Unilateral reexpansion pulmonary edema

Unilateral reexpansion pulmonary edema (RPE) is a rare complication that occurs when a chronically collapsed lung is rapidly reexpanded by evacuation of large amounts of air or fluid, usually with application of high negative intrapleural pressure.[19-27] Rapid reexpansion of a collapsed lung or sudden increase in negative intrapleural pressure causes a rapid increase in pulmonary capillary pressure and blood flow. This increase can lead to fluid transudation across the capillary and alveolar membranes and result in an increase in pulmonary extravascular water.[28] Occasionally it is only a roentgenographic phenomenon, without clinical manifestations.[21] However, in most cases RPE presents with mild or severe cardiorespiratory insufficiency and can be fatal in up to 20% of cases.[19]

Factors that have been implicated in the pathogenesis of this condition include the following:

- Chronicity of collapse: RPE usually occurs when lung collapse has been present for more than 3 days. However, RPE can develop regardless of the duration of the collapse.[24,25]
- Technique of lung reexpansion: The rapidity of reexpansion is a major contributing factor in the development of RPE.[26] The rate of expansion appears to be more critical than the method of lung inflation or the level of negative pressure applied, which explains the fact that RPE has occurred without suction and after reinflation of the lung by positive-pressure ventilation.[19]
- Increased pulmonary vascular permeability[27]: Factors implicated as a cause of the increased pulmonary vascular permeability include hypoxic injury to the capillary and alveolar membranes, mechanical damage, and decreased surfactant. Pulmonary blood flow is reduced by atelectasis, and the resulting hypoxia may cause vascular damage directly or indirectly as a result of oxygen-derived free radicals generated by reperfusion of previously hypoxic lung tissues. Mechanical stress to blood vessels during reexpansion may also contribute to increased vascular permeability. Finally, loss of tissue surfactant has been documented in atelectatic lungs after 24 hours of induced pneumothorax and may contribute to the development of atelectasis and increased vascular permeability.

Slow evacuation of air or fluid from the pleural space by underwater seal drainage alone or by repeated aspiration of less than 1000 ml of fluid or air may aid in preventing

RPE as well as the reexpansion hypotension that sometimes occurs concomitantly.[23]

Because RPE generally is self-limited, the aim of treatment is to ensure that adequate oxygenation and circulation are provided until it resolves.[19] In the patient with only roentgenographic evidence of pulmonary edema and no hypoxemia, no specific treatment is necessary. Mild hypoxemia often is corrected by supplemental nasally administered oxygen. When severe hypoxemia is present, often accompanied by expectoration of large amounts of frothy sputum, intubation and mechanical ventilation with positive end-expiratory pressure are required. Hypotension and low cardiac output must be managed by volume replacement and inotropic agents, as guided by invasive hemodynamic monitoring.

D. Pulmonary torsion

Pulmonary torsion is rotation of a segment, a lobe, or an entire lung on its bronchovascular pedicle.[29] If untreated, the involved lung parenchyma usually will progress to infarction and gangrene. For gangrene to occur, interruption of both the bronchial and pulmonary circulations is required.[30]

Pulmonary torsion may occur following blunt chest trauma,[31,32] nonpulmonary thoracic procedures,[33-35] and pulmonary resections.[29,30,36-38] The risk of torsion of a whole lung following a nonpulmonary procedure increases with division of the inferior pulmonary ligament to improve surgical exposure.[33-35] Oddi et al[33] suggest that the capability of the double-lumen tube to deflate the lung completely during dissection might be another factor that increases the hazard of lung torsion during nonpulmonary procedures. Postresection torsion most commonly involves the right middle lobe following a right upper lobectomy.[36-38] For this to occur, the oblique fissure must be complete, and no sutures or adhesions can exist between the middle and lower lobes. Right lower lobe torsion after right upper lobe resection is the next most common complication.[39] Lobar torsion has also been reported involving the left upper lobe following lower lobectomy[29] and left lower lobe following upper lobectomy.[30,39]

Pulmonary torsion often occurs with nonspecific signs and symptoms, so a high index of suspicion is required to make this diagnosis. Presenting features include chest pain and a clinical picture of sepsis or shock. An early air leak may cease suddenly as torsion occludes the airway. Hypoxemia may be present, but may not be profound because both ventilation and perfusion are impaired by torsion.[29,33] Breath sounds over the affected area may be absent or diminished. Chest roentgenograms may show opacification of the twisted pulmonary tissue and a change in the position of an opacified lobe or pulmonary vasculature on serial chest radiographs.[40] The vascular markings may be seen extending laterally from the hilum and sweeping superiorly in a concave-upward fashion, rather than downward in the normal anatomic direction of the vasculature. Other radiographic findings include lobar air trapping and bronchial cutoff or distortion. Bronchoscopy may reveal bronchial obstruction that ad-

mits the bronchoscope with pressure but recurs when the bronchoscope is withdrawn.[38]

Prevention of torsion requires an understanding of the factors that contribute to its occurrence. During hilar dissection, care should be taken to avoid direct injury to remaining pulmonary vessels. As the interlobar or intersegmental fissure is developed, the position of the remaining lung should be noted to prevent intraoperative torsion. If the remaining lobes or segments are unusually mobile, they should be sutured lightly together. During nonpulmonary surgery the lung should be retracted very carefully after division of the inferior pulmonary ligament.

Immediate exploratory thoracotomy and detorsion is required to salvage the involved lobe. This is most important in patients whose preoperative pulmonary function demonstrates inability to tolerate a pneumonectomy. However, if it is already infarcted, removal of the affected lung is required to avoid infectious complications.

E. Tracheobronchial disruption

1. Tracheal disruption. The trachea is one of the mediastinal structures subject to injury during intrathoracic surgery. Renna[41] reported a case of tracheal rupture caused by median sternotomy for cardiac surgery. As soon as the sternotomy was completed, there was a sudden decrease in the tidal volume effectively given to the patient, indicating a leak somewhere in the circuit. The cuff of the endotracheal tube was deflated, and attempts to reinflate it were unsuccessful, suggesting that the endotracheal tube cuff was damaged. At the same time, air bubbles could be seen coming out of the trachea under direct vision of the operating field. The trachea was repaired with interrupted sutures, and the endotracheal tube was changed. The operation then continued uneventfully, and the patient made good recovery.

Haddow and Tays[42] reported another case of tracheal injury similarly presenting as endotracheal tube cuff leak. The injury occurred during open heart surgery as a result of mediastinal dissection using electrocautery. The hole was found in the part of the trachea situated superior to the innominate vein approximately 2 cm inferior to the suprasternal notch. As in the first case, the tracheal tear was successfully repaired.

2. Bronchial disruption. Bronchial disruption following lung resection results in a bronchopleural fistula (BPF). This complication was more common before the decline in the incidence of pulmonary tuberculosis. A particularly high risk of developing BPF existed in patients undergoing pulmonary resection who had endobronchial tuberculous disease and a preoperative positive sputum.[43,44] Other factors implicated in the formation of a BPF following lung resection include an excessively long stump that accumulates excessive secretions; overzealous dissection of the parabronchial tissue, thus compromising the bronchial blood supply; failure to provide tissue cover of a previously irradiated or diseased bronchus; and the technique of bronchial stump closure.[45] The incidence of fistula formation seems to be much higher when the bronchial stump is closed with interrupted sutures than when the stump is closed by stapling.[46]

A BPF typically manifests 1 to 2 weeks following resection but can occur at any time.[47] It often is associated with an infected pleural space. If this infection becomes chronic, it will lead to pleural space and mediastinal fibrosis. A late BPF arising in such a complicated fibrotic postpneumonectomy space is not likely to lead to mediastinal shift. An early postoperative BPF following pneumonectomy, on the other hand, may have a dramatic presentation because the mediastinum is mobile and predisposes to contralateral shift and compromise of the remaining lung function.

Bronchopleural fistula may present acutely, with sudden expectoration of potentially infected material from the pleural space caused by airway communication.[47] Flooding the airways may lead to acute respiratory compromise. Patients who develop a BPF may also present acutely with tension pneumothorax. Subacutely, patients may present with an insidious deterioration marked by fever and minimally productive cough.

If chest tubes are not in place, a chest tube should be inserted as soon as the diagnosis of a lobar stump fistula is made.[45] Patients developing a BPF following pneumonectomy are at great risk of spillage of contaminated pleural fluid into the remaining lung.[45] Therefore they should be positioned with the operated side down immediately, and a chest tube must be inserted into the pleural space. No suction should be applied to the drainage system because harmful mediastinal shift will occur. The decision to reoperate depends on the general condition of the patient, the presence of empyema, the condition of the bronchial tissues adjacent to the stump, and in the case of a lobar stump fistula, the functional ability of the patient to withstand additional resection.[45] Conservative therapy with tube drainage is indicated in the presence of empyema or significant necrosis or inflammation of the bronchial stump in a patient who is not likely to withstand completion pneumonectomy. Surgical repair of the fistula has to include coverage of the repair site by viable tissue that will provide additional blood supply for healing. If the repair fails, thoracoplasty or muscle flap closure of the fistula and the pleural space may be needed. Advances in critical care management may provide an alternative to the surgical approaches in patients with BPF who are poor operative candidates.[47]

F. Contralateral pneumothorax

Contralateral pneumothorax during thoracic surgery could result from damage to the contralateral pleura.[48] It can occur during thoracotomy for lung resection or for nonpulmonary surgery and during open heart surgery. If tension pneumothorax develops, the resulting mediastinal shift and compression of the great vessels and opposite lung will lead to hypoxemia, increased difficulty in ventilation of the lungs, and circulatory collapse.

Other nonsurgical causes of this serious complication include central venous cannulation and barotrauma caused by using high airway pressures during ventilation or by complications resulting from the use of double-lumen endobronchial tubes.

A high index of suspicion should be maintained about pneumothorax if there is any intraoperative or postoperative respiratory embarrassment. A chest radiograph can confirm the diagnosis. A chest drain is indicated for symptomatic patients and for large pneumothoraces. Tension pneumothorax is a medical emergency. There may not be time to wait for a chest radiograph or for formal insertion of a chest drain. Once the diagnosis of tension pneumothorax is suspected, a large-bore intravenous cannula should be inserted through the chest wall, preferably in the second intercostal space in the midclavicular line. This usually is followed by a dramatic improvement in the patient's condition and allows for unhurried insertion of a chest drain.

G. Phrenic nerve palsy

1. During open heart surgery. The incidence of phrenic nerve palsy after open heart surgery has been widely estimated as between 10% and 73%.[11,49-52] The most common cause is direct hypothermia from the application of iced saline slush to the pericardial sac for topical cold cardioplegia. Esposito and Spencer[50] demonstrated a 73% incidence of phrenic nerve damage in a control group of patients in whom no attempt was made to shield the phrenic nerve from direct exposure to ice. In a second group of patients a pericardial insulation pad was used to prevent contact of the iced slush with the phrenic nerve. Phrenic nerve palsy occurred in only 17% of these patients. Another postulated cause of phrenic nerve palsy after open heart surgery is primary stretch of the nerve, which may occur during retraction of the sternum or during prolonged pericardial stretch.[49]

Phrenic nerve lesion following open heart surgery usually is unilateral. It affects mainly the left phrenic nerve, resulting in persistent paralysis of the left hemidiaphragm. Isolated right phrenic nerve palsy following open heart surgery has also been described.[52] When suspected, a phrenic nerve lesion can be demonstrated as elevation of the corresponding hemidiaphragm on an inspiratory chest roentgenogram. Paradoxic diaphragmatic motion on fluoroscopy confirms the diagnosis.

Unilateral diaphragmatic paralysis usually is asymptomatic despite the fact that it decreases vital capacity and forced expiratory volume by about 20%.[53] The role of phrenic nerve palsy as a cause of respiratory complications following open heart surgery is controversial. Esposito and Spencer[50] blame phrenic nerve palsy for being responsible for severe life-threatening respiratory complications following open heart surgery. Wilcox et al,[11] on the other hand, concluded that because the incidence of phrenic nerve palsy is low following open heart surgery, other factors must explain the high incidence of atelectasis following this surgery. Markand et al[52] reached a similar conclusion following a prospective study of the incidence of respiratory complications and phrenic nerve palsy, as documented by nerve conduction studies, following open heart surgery. The incidence of left lower lobe atelectasis or infiltrates in the patients studied was found to be 98%, whereas the incidence of documented diaphragmatic dysfunction in these patents was only 11%.

Bilateral phrenic nerve palsy following open heart surgery is a rare but potentially serious complication. Werner and Geiringer[49] reported a patient who developed this complication despite the use of a cardiac insulation pad. The patient required total ventilatory support for 3 months and partial ventilatory support for an additional 3 months. Chandler et al[54] described five patients who developed bilateral diaphragmatic paralysis as a complication of local cardiac hypothermia during open heart surgery. All patients complained of severe orthopnea, exertional dyspnea, and daytime somnolence for months before the paralysis finally resolved. One patient required 4 months of mechanical ventilatory support before her recovery.

2. During noncardiac thoracic surgery. The phrenic nerve lies superficially beneath the mediastinal pleura. It can be damaged through involvement with malignant disease and is also liable to be damaged during pulmonary resection performed via thoracotomy[55] or thoracoscopy.[8] Phrenic nerve damage should therefore be suspected when a patient with no apparent pulmonary compromise cannot be weaned from the ventilator postoperatively.[55]

Bilateral phrenic nerve palsy is a recognized complication of extracardiac procedures performed to treat congenital cardiovascular anomalies in infants and small children.[56] Although most of these patients can be treated conservatively by endotracheal intubation and mechanical ventilation, tracheostomy or diaphragmatic plication occasionally is needed. Bilateral phrenic nerve palsy resulting in respiratory failure has also been described following bilateral first rib excision performed for bilateral thoracic outlet syndrome.[57]

II. COMPLICATIONS PRESENTING MAINLY WITH HEMODYNAMIC INSTABILITY
A. Myocardial ischemia

Patients undergoing cardiothoracic surgery are at high risk of developing perioperative myocardial ischemia because of the nature of their underlying disease and because of the stress of surgery itself.[58,59] Perioperative surgical complications and variations of the surgical technique can further increase that risk. For example, the incidence of myocardial infarction following CABG surgery has been shown to increase with prolonged cross-clamp time and with prolonged CPB.[59] Myocardial ischemia during CABG surgery could also result from trauma to the coronary arteries from clamps or sutures, from forcing the grafts into a position that compromises their blood flow during closure of the pericardium, or from accidental injury to the grafts during reopening of the chest. Lifting or manipulation of the heart and compression of the heart or the great vessels during intrathoracic surgery are common causes of significant reduction in cardiac output and of serious arrhythmias, both of which can precipitate myocardial ischemia. Vigilance on the part of the anesthesiologist and recognition of these events can therefore save the patient from a potentially serious injury or from an unnecessary intervention to treat an otherwise reversible condition.

Tumor embolization during dissection around the hilum of the lung has been reported to cause radial artery occlusion.[60] A similar mechanism can lead to embolization of various debris or gas bubbles into the coronary or other blood vessels supplying vital organs and predispose to ischemic injury of these organs.

B. Cardiac arrhythmias following thoracotomy

Cardiac arrhythmia has long been a recognized complication of thoracic surgery.[61-66] It occurs most commonly on the second or third postoperative day, with a reported incidence ranging from 2.7% to 30%. Cardiac arrhythmias following thoracotomy are almost exclusively atrial in nature. Mowry and Reynolds[63] found the frequency of their occurrence to be 73% for atrial fibrillation, 23% for atrial flutter, and 5% for supraventricular tachycardia. The loss of sinus rhythm and the rapid ventricular rate adversely affects cardiac output, with a resulting decrease in coronary, renal, and cerebral blood flow. In addition to the increased morbidity, a significant increase in mortality has been reported in association with arrhythmias following pulmonary surgery,[64,66] particularly pneumonectomy.[65]

Several predisposing factors have been found to increase the incidence of arrhythmias following lung resection. Mowry and Reynolds[63] studied 574 such patients and found that the incidence of atrial arrhythmias increased with the increase in the magnitude of the resection, being 3.1% after lobectomy and 19.4% after pneumonectomy. The incidence of arrhythmias was significantly higher after left-sided pneumonectomy (22.7%) than after right-sided pneumonectomy (14.2%). Advancing age and the presence of preexisting cardiovascular disease also predisposed patients to a higher incidence of postoperative arrhythmias. Krowka et al[65] suggest that right-sided heart distention secondary to increased pulmonary vascular resistance or fluid overload is a possible cause of arrhythmias following lung resection. The authors demonstrated an increased incidence of arrhythmias following pneumonectomy in patients who developed postoperative radiographic evidence of interstitial pulmonary edema or perihilar infiltrates. However, the exact relationship between right-sided heart distention and postpneumonectomy arrhythmias remains to be determined. Other proposed causes of arrhythmias after thoracotomy include hypoxemia, postoperative hyperadrenergic condition, vagal irritation, intrapericardial dissection, and previous thoracic irradiation.

Shields and Ujiki[64] prospectively demonstrated the efficacy of perioperative digitalization in reducing the incidence of arrhythmias in a series of 123 thoracotomy patients. The incidence of postoperative arrhythmias was 2.7% for digitalized patients and 14% in nondigitalized patients. The authors therefore recommended routine digitalization before thoracotomy. Mowry and Reynolds,[63] on the other hand, recommend limiting preoperative digitalization to patients at a high risk of developing arrhythmias, namely older patients undergoing pneumonectomy. Others[67,68] advise against routine digitalization.

Aggressive management of arrhythmias after thoracotomy is needed.[67] Before initializing antiarrhythmic therapy, it is important to consider possible precipitating or aggravating factors for the arrhythmia, such as hypoxia, administration of sympathomimetic agents, anemia, fever, pain, or anxiety, and to evaluate the hemodynamic consequences of the arrhythmia. The therapeutic goal can then be defined, which can be suppression of the arrhythmia, slowing of the ventricular rate, or simply correction of a possible precipitating mechanism and observation of the natural course of the arrhythmia. In addition to digitalis, agents that can be used for the prevention and treatment of atrial arrhythmias following thoracotomy include β-blockers, amiodarone, adenosine, and calcium-channel blockers such as verapamil and diltiazem. Direct current cardioversion may be needed to terminate persistent arrhythmias.

C. Hemorrhage

1. Following thoracic surgery. Bleeding following thoracic surgery is almost always from the systemic circulation (e.g., from the intercostal or bronchial vessels or from branches of the azygous system).[55] Bleeding from the low-pressure pulmonary circulation is rare. Although it is a low-pressure system, hemorrhage from the pulmonary vessels, when it occurs, can be massive because the system carries a high flow and because bleeding occurs into a low-pressure, high-volume space. Hemorrhage from raw surfaces is more common after pneumonectomy than after lobectomy because following lobectomy the opposition of the remaining lobes of lung against the chest wall and mediastinum may greatly diminish bleeding from these surfaces.

In a series of 1428 pulmonary resections, Peterffy and Henze[69] reported 113 hemorrhagic episodes; 30% occurred after pneumonectomy, 66% after lobectomy, and 6% after segmentectomy. Emergency thoracotomy was required in 37 patients (2.6%). Six of the patients died, four as the result of hemorrhage. In another three patients, massive bleeding (from the PA in two and from a systemic vessel in one) was found to be the cause of death at autopsy. Thus the overall incidence of mortality related to uncontrolled bleeding was less than 0.1%.

When chest tubes are in place, an output of blood of more than 200 ml/hr for 4 to 6 hours indicates massive bleeding.[55] However, lesser output may result from clot formation within the pleural space or in the drainage system. The reliance on the amount of drainage to determine the blood loss can therefore be misleading. High hematocrit in chest tube drainage, progressive lowering of the patient's hematocrit, signs of hypovolemia, or signs of tension hemithorax are other manifestations of significant bleeding.[6]

2. Following cardiovascular surgery. Bleeding following cardiovascular surgery is significantly influenced by the patient's underlying disease and by the nature of the surgery itself. Other factors that can predispose the patient to excessive bleeding include massive blood transfusion, anticoagulation, and the complex and heterogenous hemostatic defects that can result from CPB.[70]

Bleeding into the pericardium following cardiac surgery can give rise to pericardial tamponade, which interferes with normal cardiac filling and can seriously reduce cardiac output. The classic diagnostic finding is elevation and equalization of the filling pressures.[71] Right atrial, pulmonary capillary wedge, left atrial, and ventricular diastolic pressures approach each other and reflect the increased intrapericardial pressure. Pericardial tamponade can be a life-threatening emergency that requires immediate reexploration.

D. Mediastinal shift following pneumonectomy

Mediastinal shift following pneumonectomy may cause displacement of the heart, the great vessels, the trachea, and the major bronchi. If excessive, it can lead to severe hemodynamic and respiratory compromise.

The postpneumonectomy pleural space usually is closed without drainage unless excessive bleeding occurs or infection is likely.[72] Efforts can be made to adjust the pressure in the operated hemithorax to be slightly negative, thus maintaining the mediastinum in a neutral position.[72] This adjustment can be made simply by thoracocentesis and removal of air until the trachea is in the midline, as determined by examining its position in relation to the suprasternal notch or by a chest radiograph. However, care must be exercised to avoid removing excessive amounts of air from the operated hemithorax because this can lead to a significant shift of the mediastinum toward that side. For this reason, continuous suction should not be applied to the drainage tube if one is used after a pneumonectomy. Alternatively, intermittent controlled drainage by periodic unclamping of the drainage tube can be used.

An early mediastinal shift toward the remaining lung often results from atelectasis and loss of volume in that lung. Aggressive physiotherapy, bronchoscopy, and suctioning are indicated in that case.[55] However, excessive suctioning of the remaining lung should be avoided. Mediastinal shift toward the remaining lung can also result from accumulation of blood or malignant effusions,[73] tension chylothorax,[74] or tension pneumothorax in the operative side. The latter may indicate infection in the pleural cavity with possible bronchopleural fistula.

A rare specific syndrome affecting mostly infants and young children has been described that is characterized by excessive mediastinal shift occurring late following a right-sided pneumonectomy or occasionally a left-sided pneumonectomy in the presence of a right aortic arch.[75] The mediastinal shift leads to counterclockwise rotation of the heart and displacement of the great vessels and the trachea, with stretching and narrowing of the left mainstem bronchus and compression of the left pulmonary vessels. Patients with severe airway obstruction may require surgery for mediastinal repositioning with or without prostheses. Patients who still show severe malacic obstruction of the airway after mediastinal repositioning may require tracheal and bronchial resection.

E. Cardiac herniation following pneumonectomy

The intrapericardial approach to radical pneumonectomy, introduced in 1946, allows easier access to major vessels for ligation and permits more extensive excision of the tumor.[76] However, herniation of the heart through the pericardial defect is a serious potential risk of this technique.[77-86]

The deleterious effects of cardiac herniation result from cardiac malposition with subsequent torsion of the great vessels, obstruction of the outflow tracts of the heart, and strangulation of the prolapsed ventricles by the borders of the pericardial defect[82] (Fig. 27-2). The severe hemodynamic disturbances in right-sided herniation result mainly from cardiac malposition. The counterclockwise rotation of the dextropositioned heart results in a gross degree of torsion of the atriocaval junction and in ventricular outflow tract obstruction.[82] On the other hand, the effects of left-sided herniation on the circulation result more from compression of the ventricular muscle by the edges of the pericardial defect. Increasing edema and congestion of the herniated heart caused by the constricting edges of the defect aggravate the condition. Damage to the myocardium results in ischemic electrocardiographic changes, widening complexes, and arrhythmias.[82]

The presence of a medium or large defect in a pericardial cavity free of adhesions is a prerequisite for cardiac herniation to occur. The actual herniation can be precipitated by events that increase intrapleural pressure in the nonsurgical hemithorax, such as coughing or hyperinflating the remaining lung, or that decrease intrapleural pressure in the surgical hemithorax, such as applying suction to the chest drains[84] (see Fig. 27-2). Cardiac herniation following intrapericardial pneumonectomy usually occurs at the end of the operation with repositioning the patient, particularly with the surgical side down. It rarely occurs after the first 24 hours because of the rapid development of adhesions between the heart and the parietal pericardium.[84] However, one case has been reported as late as 28 hours postoperatively.[86]

If cardiac herniation is suspected, a chest radiogram generally is diagnostic in right-sided herniation. However, left-sided herniation may be appreciated only on a lateral chest film demonstrating the posterior displacement of the heart. Thoracoscopy has also been used as an aid to diagnose left-sided cardiac herniation.[83]

Several approaches have been advocated to prevent this complication, including wide excision of the pericardium, closure of all pericardial defects, and suturing the edge of the pericardial defect to the adjacent myocardium.[45] All large right-sided pericardial defects must be closed.[45] However, when repairing a pericardial defect, it is important to ensure that the repaired pericardial sac is not tight because a tight pericardial sac can result in hemodynamic compromise.[87] In contrast, for left-sided defects, wide excision of the pericardium can avoid this complication. Because the heart normally is positioned in the left thorax, displacement alone will not result in hemodynamic compromise unless the heart is strangulated through a small pericardial defect.[45]

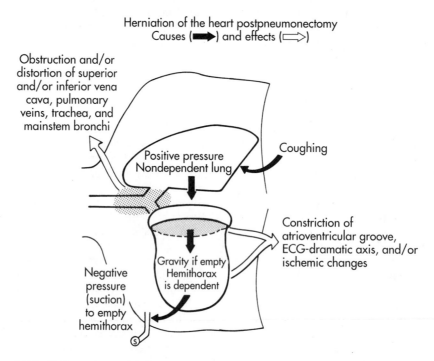

Fig. 27-2. Following a transpericardial radical pneumonectomy, the heart may herniate through a pericardial defect into the empty hemithorax. The solid arrows indicate the factors that can cause herniation of the heart. The open arrows indicate the effects of this complication. (From Benumof JL, ed: *Anesthesia for thoracic surgery,* ed 2, Philadelphia 1995, WB Saunders.)

Once the diagnoses of cardiac herniation is made, initial treatment consists of placing the patient in the lateral decubitus position with the nonsurgical side down and decreasing mean airway pressure. Injecting air into the surgical hemithorax also may be helpful. The return of normal vital signs allows a safer return to the operating room and surgical closure of the pericardium. If conservative measures fail to produce hemodynamic stability, immediate thoracotomy and reduction of the heart and great vessels are indicated.

F. Inadvertent transection of the pulmonary artery catheter

Pulmonary artery catheterization is associated with many potential complications, including arrhythmias, infection, pulmonary infarction, and PA rupture.[88] Inadvertent transection of a pulmonary artery catheter (PAC) is another rare but potentially serious complication associated with the use of PACs during cardiothoracic surgery.

Cohen, Neustein, and Kirschner[89] reported a case of inadvertent transection of the tip of the PAC, including the balloon, by the surgical stapler during a left-sided pneumonectomy (Fig. 27-3, A). Following stapling of the left PA, the PA pressure suddenly rose, and the waveform became flat and presented an occlusion pattern, while the central venous pressure tracing maintained its normal configuration. Because the distal end of the PAC was fixed to the staple line, attempting to pull it out could have resulted in major bleeding from laceration of the left PA. Alternatively, a vascular clamp was placed proximally across the neck of the PA stump, and two guide ligatures were placed at the edge of the stump to achieve control of the vessel. The staple line together with the portion of the PAC fixed to it were then transected (Fig. 27-3, B). By slight release of the vascular clamp, it was then possible to withdraw the remainder of the PAC (Fig. 27-3, C). The vascular clamp was immediately reapplied and the left PA stump was sutured.

Digital palpation of the PA by the surgeon may not detect the PAC because the catheter is small relative to the size of the PA or because of distorted anatomy.[89] The PAC usually floats to the right PA.[90] However, in some cases it does float to the left PA, particularly if there is limitation of the PA blood flow to the right lung, as there may be in the presence of lung disease, or if the patient is placed in the right lateral decubitus position while the PAC is inserted.[90] Therefore unless the position of the PAC is determined by radiograph or transesophageal echocardiography, no assumption should be made of its location and the catheter should be withdrawn before the PA is clamped.

In another reported case,[91] the main PA containing the PAC was included in the aortic cross-clamp in the course of an aortic valve replacement. In the subsequent repair of the aortotomy, following separation from CPB, the PA was noted to be caught in the suture line. CPB had to be reinitiated to allow pulmonary arteriotomy and release and removal of the PAC.

G. Complications of intercostal nerve block performed by the surgeon under direct vision during thoracotomy

Because the dural sheath can extend through the intervertebral foramen around the medial 2 to 3 cm of an intercostal nerve, it is possible to inject local anesthetics directly into the subarachnoid space through one of the dural sleeves when the needle tip is directed subcostally just lateral to a transverse process when intercostal nerve block is performed by the surgeon under direct vision during thoracotomy.[92,93] The resulting total spinal anesthesia leads to immediate profound hypotension and subsequent delayed emergence from anesthesia and regain of motor function.

A similar clinical presentation may also result from accidental intravascular injection of a large amount of local anesthetic during performance of the intercostal nerve block.[92] Because of the proximity of each intercostal nerve to its corresponding artery and vein throughout much of their course subcostally, the potential for this complication is significant. Signs of cardiovascular collapse would not be associated with convulsive skeletal muscle movements if neuromuscular blockade were present intraoperatively.

III. COMPLICATIONS PRESENTING MAINLY WITH NEUROLOGIC DEFICITS
A. Upper-extremity neuropathy

1. Following open heart surgery. Upper-extremity neuropathy following cardiac surgery could result from injury to the brachial plexus, the ulnar nerve at the elbow, or both.[94] Morin et al[94] encountered a 6% incidence of upper-extremity neuropathy among 958 patients who underwent median sternotomy. Among 38 of the patients who underwent motor and sensory conduction studies, the injury was localized to the level of the elbow in 13, to the brachial plexus in 10, and to both locations in 6. A very high incidence of 37.7% of upper-extremity neuropathy was reported in a well-designed prospective study of 53 patients who had cardiac surgery using median sternotomy and who had detailed sensory and motor testing performed on their upper extremities before and after surgery.[95] Other studies reported widely variable incidences of upper-extremity neuropathy following cardiac surgery.[96-102] This could be explained partly by the fact that different criteria were used to define the complication in these studies and that some data were collected prospectively and others were collected retrospectively.

Several mechanisms have been proposed to explain the occurrence of upper-extremity neuropathy following cardiac surgery. These include stretch of the brachial plexus during sternal retraction,[96] injury of the plexus by posterior first rib fracture,[97,98] local pressure on the plexus by the first rib during sternal retraction,[100] and traumatic cannulation of the internal jugular vein.[101] Previous neuropathies and long CPB runs also were found to predispose to such injury.[95]

Ulnar nerve damage during open heart surgery can result from nerve compression at the elbow.[103] Nonethe-

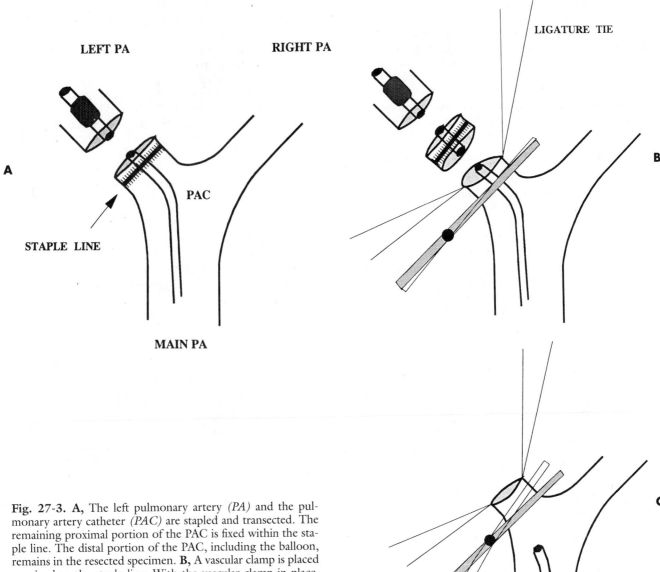

LEFT PA

RIGHT PA

A

PAC

STAPLE LINE

MAIN PA

LIGATURE TIE

B

C

VASCULAR CLAMP OPEN

Fig. 27-3. A, The left pulmonary artery *(PA)* and the pulmonary artery catheter *(PAC)* are stapled and transected. The remaining proximal portion of the PAC is fixed within the staple line. The distal portion of the PAC, including the balloon, remains in the resected specimen. **B,** A vascular clamp is placed proximal to the staple line. With the vascular clamp in place, the staples fixing the PAC to the left PA stump are resected. **C,** A suture ligature is applied on both sides of the distal PA stump to maintain control of the vessel while the vascular clamp is opened briefly to allow withdrawal of the PAC. The vascular clamp is then reapplied for definitive repair of the left PA stump. (From Cohen E, Neustein S, Kirschner P: *J Cardiothorac Vasc Anesth* 7:337, 1993.)

less, factors other than general anesthesia and intraoperative positioning have been found to be associated with perioperative ulnar neuropathies. These factors include prolonged hospitalization and being a man at the extremes of body habitus.[104]

The association between median sternotomy and brachial plexus injury was first described in five patients by Kirsh et al[96] in 1971. Based on cadaver studies, the authors postulated that the mechanism of injury in their patients was stretch of the brachial plexus during sternal retraction. Because the plexus is fixed by the prevertebral fascia to the transverse processes medially and by the ax-

illary fascia laterally, any force that tends to increase the distance between these points can cause a stretch injury to the nerves. The authors therefore recommended avoiding too wide separation of the sternal halves during surgery, which, they observed, markedly reduced the incidence of nerve damage in their practice.

Baisden, Greenwald, and Symbas[97] postulate that posterior first rib fracture occurring during sternal retraction was responsible for brachial plexus injury following open heart surgery. The authors found that although occult rib fractures were difficult to detect on routine chest roentgenograms, the fractures were readily detectable on bone scans. Using such a sensitive diagnostic tool, rib fractures were found to occur commonly and at multiple levels in patients who had undergone median sternotomy. However, only posterior first rib fractures were associated with brachial plexus injury. Vander Salm, Cereda, and Cutler[98] performed an autopsy study that demonstrated fractured first ribs penetrating the brachial plexus in 11 of 15 patients whose sternum was opened with the sternal retractor placed in a cephalad location, but in none in 15 patients whose sternum was opened with the retractor displaced two intercostal spaces caudally. However, in a follow-up study,[99] the authors failed to show a correlation between the presence of rib fractures and the occurrence of neurologic symptoms.

Treasure et al[100] observed that in their patients hand weakness and numbness in the distribution of C_8-T_1 was common after median sternotomy. They hypothesized that the neurologic deficit was caused by local pressure by the first rib during sternal retraction, which produced local ischemia of the lower trunk of the brachial plexus. Hanson et al[101] also observed that 85% of the brachial plexus injury following open heart surgery involved the lower trunk or C_8-T_1 nerve roots, but they postulated that traumatic cannulation of the internal jugular vein might be the major mechanism of the plexus injury. However, this hypothesis was refuted by others.[102]

Symptoms of brachial plexus injury following open heart surgery range from mild dysesthesias and numbness in an ulnar or C_8-T_1 distribution to severe burning pain involving the entire arm.[101] Motor signs range from mild clumsiness of a hand to marked weakness of the intrinsic hand muscles. Although the symptoms occasionally produce long-term disability, in most instances it resolves within 2 to 3 months.[92,93,101]

Based on available data, the risk of brachial plexus injury during open heart surgery can be reduced by avoidance of wide retraction of the sternum and of high placement of the sternal retractors. Arm and neck positions that tend to stretch the plexus also should be avoided.[105] Because ulnar nerve compression at the elbow contributes significantly to the incidence of upper-extremity neuropathy following open heart surgery, every effort should be made to thoroughly pad the elbow to protect it against compression during surgery.

2. Following thoracotomy. The potential for brachial plexus and ulnar nerve stretch or compression is very significant during thoracotomy performed in the lateral decubitus position. Brachial plexus compression after thoracotomy has also resulted from a malpositioned chest tube.[106] The tube was placed high in the mediastinum, and the symptoms were immediately relieved on withdrawal of the chest tube approximately 5 cm.

B. Spinal cord ischemia

Epidural and intrathecal anesthesia and analgesia are increasingly used in patients undergoing cardiac, thoracic, and major vascular surgery.[107-109] Spinal cord injury is a feared complication of these techniques that could result either from direct injury during epidural needle placement in the thoracic area or from compression by

an epidural hematoma in an anticoagulated patient. Nonetheless, when evaluating a patient who develops spinal cord ischemia following cardiothoracic or vascular surgery, it is important to be aware that this rare complication could also be surgically induced.

1. Paraplegia following thoracotomy. Iatrogenic paraplegia can develop after a routine thoracotomy. In most of the described cases there was persistent bleeding from the intercostal vessels at the posterior end of the incision between the ribs, and the complication was felt to be caused by the technique used for hemostasis. In one report of three patients who developed paraplegia following posterolateral thoracotomy incisions, the underlying mechanism for the spinal cord ischemia was believed to be placement of an absorbable hemostatic gauze made of oxidized regenerated cellulose (Surgicel) in the posterior angle of the incision.[110,111] Although the surgeons were careful not to pack or compress the gauze into the angle between the ribs or push it into the intercostal foramen, in each case, when an exploratory laminectomy was finally performed, the oxidized cellulose was found in the spinal canal. Because the material is known to swell considerably, it was believed that the gauze must have migrated from the posterior angle of the thoracotomy into the spinal canal through the intervertebral foramen, causing spinal cord compression. Delay in making the diagnosis resulted in permanent neurologic damage in all three patients. The involved physicians were criticized for failure to remember that paraplegia had a local cause and that the operative procedure could have caused it, and for their delay in involving the neurosurgeons.

In another reported case of postpneumonectomy paraplegia, the spinal cord ischemia was caused by an epidural hematoma without any attempts at epidural catheter placement.[112] Oxidized regenerated cellulose was also thought to have caused this complication by blocking the egress of bleeding from the T_5 posterior left intercostal artery. During the procedure, when bleeding could not be controlled by conventional means, the surgeon applied Surgicel to induce hemostasis. Postoperatively, a motor and sensory neurologic deficit below the T_5 level was present. An emergency laminectomy was performed, and an acute thrombus was found anterior to the spinal cord that extended from the T_5 to the T_7 level, with obvious cord compression. Although the laminectomy was performed within 2 hours after completion of the pneumonectomy, the patient did not recover any sensory or motor function.

Mathew and John[113] reported another case of paraplegia caused by spinal cord infarction that occurred during left-sided pneumonectomy. The authors felt that the ischemia in their patient resulted from interference with the blood supply of the spinal cord through the radicular arteries at the fourth thoracic segment, which is known to be a watershed area of blood supply and hence vulnerable to ischemia. A major source of blood supply of the spinal cord is the arteria radicularis magna of Adamkiewicz, which is always found among the lower thoracic or upper lumbar roots, usually on the left. The authors theorized that an intercostal artery that gave origin to a major radicular artery might have been damaged during thoracotomy, thus accounting for the cord ischemia. Therefore they recommended particular caution in avoiding damage to the left lower intercostal vessels during thoracotomy.

2. Paraplegia following aortic aneurysm repair. The risk of ischemic spinal cord injury during operations on the descending thoracic and thoracoabdominal aorta is significant.[114] The incidence can be as high as 41% in patients with a dissecting aneurysm involving most of the descending thoracic and abdominal aorta. Several factors, alone or in combination, contribute to the development of spinal cord ischemia during aortic aneurysm surgery.[115] These include perioperative hypotension; aortic clamping, particularly high-level clamping without the use of a shunt or bypass; increased cerebrospinal fluid (CSF) pressure; and sacrifice of important intercostal arteries. A number of adjunctive techniques have been used during surgical procedures on the descending thoracic and thoracoabdominal aorta in an attempt to reduce or eliminate spinal cord ischemia.[115] These include maintenance of adequate distal flow and perfusion pressure with a shunt or some form of bypass, monitoring of spinal cord function using somatosensory or motor evoked potential, hypothermia, reimplantation of intercostal and lumbar arteries, CSF drainage, and the use of pharmacologic agents such as steroids, barbiturates, calcium-channel blockers, oxygen free radical scavengers, and papaverine. Unfortunately, none of those techniques have proven to be completely effective. An important reason for this is the failure of these techniques to reliably and noninvasively localize the level of origin of arteries from the aorta that are critical to the spinal cord circulation.[115]

C. Vagus and recurrent laryngeal nerve injury

Unilateral vagus nerve injury can lead to postoperative gastrointestinal atony. Esposito and Spencer[50] encountered clinical symptoms of gastric ileus in 8% of nondiabetic patients who developed phrenic nerve palsy during open heart surgery. The symptoms included early satiety, poor appetite, and nausea with occasional vomiting. Massively distended stomach was confirmed by upright chest roentgenograms. The authors hypothesized that this syndrome may possibly represent hypothermic injury to the thoracic vagi.

If the vagus nerve is damaged high in the chest proximal to the origin of the recurrent laryngeal nerve, manifestations of recurrent laryngeal nerve palsy will result. However, the recurrent laryngeal nerve is more likely to be injured directly during mediastinal lymph node dissection in patients with lung cancer[116] and during mediastinoscopy[117] or thoracoscopy.[8] Because the right recurrent laryngeal nerve leaves the vagus nerve higher up in the mediastinum than the left recurrent laryngeal nerve, injury of the latter is more common.

Unilateral recurrent laryngeal nerve injury leads to paralysis of the ipsilateral vocal cord. The patient may present with a weak and hoarse voice or with the more severe symptoms of partial airway obstruction and aspiration.

D. Horner's syndrome

Horner's syndrome can result from injury to the sympathetic chain, especially the ansa hypoglossus as it loops down on the subclavian artery.[45] It can also be caused by injury to the stellate ganglion during line placement in the neck. The syndrome usually is transient and manifests with ipsilateral ptosis and dilation of the pupil. Lack of tears on the affected side may cause a dry and irritated cornea.

E. Subarachnoid-pleural fistula following thoracotomy

Subarachnoid-pleural fistula occurs most often in association with traumatic injuries of the thoracic spine[118-121] and with posterior chest wall resections. However, two reports[122,123] have described the complication following elective thoracotomy. These fistulas probably occurred as a traction injury to the dural sleeve of an intercostal nerve as the surgeons were gaining exposure through a posterolateral thoracotomy.

If the dural tear is not detected and closed at the time of operation, it allows free escape of CSF into the pleural cavity postoperatively. The fistula also allows air from a pneumothorax to enter the subarachnoid space and cause headache, obtundation, and focal neurologic deficits.[122,123] Meningitis is a threat as long as the fistula remains open.

If a patient who develops subarachnoid-pleural fistula following thoracotomy also happens to have an indwelling epidural catheter for postoperative pain control, some of the symptoms caused by the fistula, namely headache and meningism, can be blamed easily on the epidural. Awareness of the potential for this rare complication is therefore important.

REFERENCES

1. Van Mieghan W, Demedts M: Cardiopulmonary function after lobectomy or pneumonectomy for pulmonary neoplasm, *Respir Med* 83:199, 1989.
2. Reed CE, Spinale FG, Crawford FA: Effect of pulmonary resection on right ventricular function, *Ann Thorac Surg* 53:578, 1992.
3. Wahi R, McMurtrey M, DeCaro L, et al: Determinants of perioperative morbidity and mortality after pneumonectomy, *Ann Thorac Surg* 48:33, 1989.
4. Wittnich C, Trudel J, Zidulka A, et al: Misleading "pulmonary wedge pressure" after pneumonectomy: its importance in postoperative fluid therapy, *Ann Thorac Surg* 42:192, 1986.
5. Zeldin RA, Normandin D, Landtwing D, et al: Postpneumonectomy pulmonary edema, *J Thorac Cardiovasc Surg* 87:359, 1984.
6. Benumof JL: Early serious complications specifically related to thoracic surgery. In Benumof JL, ed: *Anesthesia for thoracic surgery,* ed 2, Philadelphia, 1995, WB Saunders, p 696.
7. Benumof JL: Management of postoperative pain. In Benumof JL, ed: *Anesthesia for thoracic surgery,* ed 2, Philadelphia, 1995, WB Saunders, p 756.
8. Jancovici R, Lang-Lazdunski L, Pons F, et al: Complications of video-assisted thoracic surgery: a five-year experience, *Ann Thorac Surg* 61:533, 1996.
9. Julian OC, Lopez-Belio M, Dye WS: The median sternal incision in intracardiac surgery with extracorporeal circulation: a general evaluation of its use in heart surgery, *Surgery* 42:753, 1957.

10. Kollef MH, Peller T, Knodel A, et al: Delayed pleuropulmonary complications following coronary artery revascularization with internal mammary artery, *Chest* 94:68, 1988.

11. Wilcox P, Baile E, Hards J, et al: Phrenic nerve function and its relationship to atelectasis after coronary artery bypass surgery, *Chest* 93:693, 1988.

12. Berry L, Bradue S, Hogan J: Refractory hypoxemia after pneumonectomy: diagnosis by transesophageal echocardiography, *Thorax* 47:60, 1992.

13. Dlabal PW, Stutts B, Jenkins D, et al: Cyanosis following right pneumonectomy: importance of patent foramen ovale, *Chest* 81:370, 1992.

14. Holtzman H, Lippmann M, Nakhjauan F, et al: Postpneumonectomy interatrial right-to-left shunt, *Thorax* 35:307, 1980.

15. La Bresh KA, Pietro D, Coates E, et al: Platypnea syndrome after left pneumonectomy, *Chest* 79:605, 1981.

16. Vacek JL, Foster J, Quinton R, et al: Right-to-left shunting after lobectomy through a patent foramen ovale, *Ann Thorac Surg* 39:576, 1985.

17. Springer RM, Gheorghiade M, Chakko S, et al: Platypnea and interatrial right-to-left shunting after lobectomy, *Am J Cardiol* 51:1802, 1983.

18. Hagen P, Scholz D, Edwards W: Incidence and size of patent foramen ovale during the first 10 decades of life, *Mayo Clin Proc* 59:17, 1984.

19. Mahfood S, Hix W, Aaron B, et al: Reexpansion pulmonary edema, *Ann Thorac Surg* 45:340, 1988.

20. Desiderio DP, Meister M, Bedford RF: Intraoperative re-expansion pulmonary edema, *Anesthesiology* 67:821, 1987.

21. Bernstein A: Reexpansion pulmonary edema, *Chest* 77:708, 1980.

22. Matsumiya N, Dohi S, Kimura T, et al: Reexpansion pulmonary edema after mediastinal tumor removal, *Anesth Analg* 73:646, 1991.

23. Khoo ST, Chen FG: Acute localized pulmonary edema, *Anaesthesia* 43:486, 1988.

24. Ravin CE, Dahmash NS: Reexpansion pulmonary edema, *Chest* 77:709, 1980.

25. Sherman S, Ravikrishnan KP: Unilateral pulmonary edema following reexpansion of pneumothorax of brief duration, *Chest* 77:714, 1980.

26. Marland AM, Glauser FL: Hemodynamic and pulmonary edema protein measurements in a case of reexpansion pulmonary edema, *Chest* 81:250, 1982.

27. Sprung CL, Loewenherz J, Baier H, et al: Evidence for increased permeability in reexpansion pulmonary edema, *Am J Med* 71:497, 1981.

28. Sewell RW, Fewel J, Grover F, et al: Experimental evaluation of reexpansion pulmonary edema, *Ann Thorac Surg* 26:126, 1978.

29. Kucich VA, Villarreal JR, Schwartz DB: Left upper lobe torsion following lower lobe resection, *Chest* 95:1146, 1989.

30. Kelly MV, Kyger ER, Miller WC: Postoperative lobar torsion and gangrene, *Thorax* 32:501, 1977.

31. Dougherty DC: Traumatic torsion of the lung, *N Engl J Med* 256:385, 1957.

32. Selmonosky CA, Flege JB, Ehrenhaft JL: Torsion of a lung due to blunt thoracic trauma, *Ann Thorac Surg* 4:166, 1967.

33. Oddi MA, Traugott R, Will R, et al: Unrecognized intraoperative torsion of the lung, *Surgery* 89:390, 1981.

34. Fisher CF, Ammar T, Silvoy G: Whole lung torsion after a thoracoabdominal esophagogastrectomy, *Anesthesiology* 87:162, 1997.

35. Goskowicz R, Harrell JH, Roth DM: Intraoperative diagnosis of torsion of the left lung after repair of a disruption of the descending thoracic aorta, *Anesthesiology* 87:164, 1997.

36. Chambers RF, Sweeney DF: Gangrenous sequestration of remaining lobe following lobectomy, *Ann Thorac Surg* 5:156, 1968.

37. Schuler JG: Intraoperative lobar torsion producing pulmonary infarction, *J Thorac Cardiovasc Surg* 65:951, 1973.

38. Pinstein ML, Winer-Muram H, Eastridge C, et al: Middle lobe torsion following right upper lobectomy, *Radiology* 155:580, 1985.

39. Livaudais W, Cavanaugh DG, Geer TM: Rapid postoperative thoracotomy for torsion of the left lower lobe: case report, *Mil Med* 145:698, 1980.

40. Felson B: Lung torsion: radiographic findings in nine cases, *Radiology* 162:631, 1987.

41. Renna M: A novel complication of sternotomy for cardiac surgery, *J Cardiothorac Vasc Anesth* 8:133, 1994.

42. Haddow GR, Tays R: Tracheal injury: a cause for unexplained endotracheal cuff leak during mediastinal dissection, *Anesth Analg* 84:684, 1997.

43. Malave G, Foster E, Wilson J, et al: Bronchopleural fistula: present-day study of an old problem, *Ann Thorac Surg* 11:1, 1971.

44. Hankins JR, Miller J, Attar S, et al: Bronchopleural fistula: thirteen-year experience with 77 cases, *J Thorac Cardiovasc Surg* 76:755, 1978.

45. Piccione W, Faber LP: Management of complications related to pulmonary resection. In Waldhausen JA, Orringer MB, eds: *Complications in cardiothoracic surgery*, St Louis, 1991, Mosby, p 336.

46. Forrester-Wood CP: Bronchopleural fistula following pneumonectomy for carcinoma of the bronchus, *J Thorac Cardiovasc Surg* 80:406, 1980.

47. Baumann MH, Sahn SA: Medical management and therapy of bronchopleural fistula in the mechanically ventilated patient, *Chest* 97:721, 1990.

48. Gabbott DA, Carter JA: Contralateral tension pneumothorax during thoracotomy for lung resection, *Anaesthesia* 45:229, 1990.

49. Werner RA, Geiringer SR: Bilateral phrenic nerve palsy associated with open-heart surgery, *Arch Phys Med Rehabil* 71:1000, 1990.

50. Esposito RA, Spencer FC: The effect of pericardial insulation on hypothermic phrenic nerve injury during open-heart surgery, *Ann Thorac Surg* 43:303, 1987.

51. Wheeler WE, Rubis L, Jones C, et al: Etiology and prevention of topical cardiac hypothermia-induced phrenic nerve injury and left lower lobe atelectasis during cardiac surgery, *Chest* 88:680, 1985.

52. Markand ON, Moorthy S, Mahomed Y, et al: Postoperative phrenic nerve palsy in patients with open-heart surgery, *Ann Thorac Surg* 39:68, 1985.

53. Fackler CD, Perret GE, Bedell GN: Effect of unilateral phrenic nerve section on lung function, *J Appl Physiol* 23:923, 1967.

54. Chandler KW, Rozas C, Kory R, et al: Bilateral diaphragmatic paralysis complicating local cardiac hypothermia during open heart surgery, *Am J Med* 77:243, 1984.

55. Aghdami A, Keenan RL: Complications of thoracic surgery. In Kaplan JA, ed: *Thoracic anesthesia*, ed 2, New York, 1991, Churchill Livingstone, p 709.

56. Hong-Xu Z, D'Agostino R, Piteick P, et al: Phrenic nerve injury complicating closed cardiovascular surgical procedures for congenital heart disease, *Ann Thorac Surg* 39:445, 1985.

57. Rosett RL: An unusual cause of postoperative respiratory failure, *Anesthesiology* 66:695, 1987.

58. Nagusaki F, Flehinger BJ, Martini N: Complications of surgery in the treatment of carcinoma of the lung, *Chest* 82:25, 1982.

59. Roberts AJ: Perioperative myocardial infarction and changes in left ventricular performance related to coronary artery bypass graft surgery, *Ann Thorac Surg* 35:219, 1983.

60. Oxorn DC: Suspected tumor embolism as a cause of arterial line dysfunction, *Can J Anaesth* 35:440, 1988.

61. Baily CC, Betts RH: Cardiac arrhythmias following pneumonectomy, *N Engl J Med* 299:356, 1943.

62. Currens JH, White PD, Churchill EE: Cardiac arrhythmias following thoracic surgery, *N Engl J Med* 299:360, 1943.

63. Mowry FM, Reynolds EW: Cardiac rhythm disturbances complicating resectional surgery of the lung, *Ann Intern Med* 61:688, 1964.

64. Shields TW, Ujiki GT: Digitalization for prevention of arrhythmias following pulmonary surgery, *Surg Gynecol Obstet* 126:743, 1968.

65. Krowka MJ, Pairolero P, Trastek V, et al: Cardiac dysrhythmias following pneumonectomy: clinical correlates and prognostic significance, *Chest* 91:490, 1987.

66. Von Knorring J, Lepantalo M, Lindgren L, et al: Cardiac arrhythmias and myocardial ischemia after thoracotomy for lung cancer, *Ann Thorac Surg* 53:642, 1992.

67. Van Mieghem W: The complications of thoracic surgery: prophylaxis and treatment of arrhythmias, *Acta Cardiol* 50:381, 1995.

68. Lindgren L, Lepantalo M, Von Knorring J, et al: Effect of verapamil on right ventricular pressure and atrial tachyarrhythmia after thoracotomy, *Br J Anaesth* 66:205, 1991.

69. Peterffy A, Henze A: Hemorrhagic complications during pulmonary resection, *Scand J Thorac Cardiovasc Surg* 17:283, 1983.
70. Dyke CM, Sobel M: Hemorrhagic and thrombotic complications of cardiac surgery. In Baue AE, ed: *Glenn's thoracic and cardiovascular surgery,* ed 6, Stanford, Conn, 1996, Appleton & Lange, p 1793.
71. Reddy S, Curtiss E, O'Toole J, et al: Cardiac tamponade: hemodynamic observations in man, *Circulation* 58:265, 1978.
72. Hartz RS, Joob AW: General principles of postoperative care. In Shields TW, ed: *General thoracic surgery,* ed 4, Philadelphia, 1994, Williams & Wilkins, p 341.
73. Pope AR, Joseph JH: Pleuroperitoneal shunt for pneumonectomy cavity malignant effusion, *Chest* 96:686, 1989.
74. Karwande SV, Wolcott MW, Gay WA: Postpneumonectomy tension chylothorax, *Ann Thorac Surg* 42:585, 1986.
75. Grillo HC, Shepard J, Mathisen D, et al: Postpneumonectomy syndrome: diagnosis, management, and results, *Ann Thorac Surg* 54:638, 1992.
76. Allison PR: Intrapericardial approach to the lung root in the treatment of bronchial carcinoma by dissection pneumonectomy, *J Thorac Cardiovasc Surg* 15:99, 1946.
77. Yacoub MH, Williams WG, Ahmad A: Strangulation of the heart following intrapericardial pneumonectomy, *Thorax* 23:261, 1968.
78. Gates GF, Sette RS, Cope JA: Acute cardiac herniation with incarceration following pneumonectomy, *Radiology* 94:561, 1970.
79. Wright MP, Nelson C, Johnson A, et al: Herniation of the heart, *Thorax* 25:656, 1970.
80. Levin PD, Faber LP, Carleton RA: Cardiac herniation after pneumonectomy, *J Thorac Cardiovasc Surg* 61:104, 1971.
81. McKlveen JR, Urgena RB, Rossi NP: Herniation of the heart following radical pneumonectomy: a case report, *Anesth Analg* 5:680, 1972.
82. Deiraniya AK: Cardiac herniation following intrapericardial pneumonectomy, *Thorax* 29:545, 1974.
83. Rodgers BM, Moulder PV, DeLaney A: Thoracoscopy: new method of early diagnosis of cardiac herniation, *J Thorac Cardiovasc Surg* 78:623, 1979.
84. Cassorla L, Katz JA: Management of cardiac herniation after intrapericardial pneumonectomy, *Anesthesiology* 60:362, 1984.
85. Weinlander CM, Abel MD, Piehler JM: Spontaneous cardiac herniation after pneumonectomy, *Anesth Analg* 65:1085, 1986.
86. Baaijens PF, Hasenbos M, Lacquet L, et al: Cardiac herniation after pneumonectomy, *Acta Anaesthesiol Scand* 36:842, 1992.
87. Wall RT, Pass HI, McDonald HD: Unusual presentation and novel solution for hemodynamic compromise during thoracic surgery, *Anesthesiology* 66:566, 1987.
88. Shah KB, Rao T, Laughin S, et al: A review of pulmonary artery catheterization in 6245 patients, *Anesthesiology* 61:271, 1984.
89. Cohen E, Neustein SM, Kirschner PA: Inadvertent transection of a pulmonary artery catheter during thoracic surgery, *J Cardiothorac Vasc Anesth* 7:337, 1993.
90. Parlow JL, Milne C, Cervenko FW: Balloon flotation is more important than flow direction in determining the position of flow-directed pulmonary artery catheter, *J Cardiothorac Vasc Anesth* 6:20, 1992.
91. Eguaras MG, Luch M, Valdivia J, et al: An unusual complication of Swan-Ganz catheter use, *Tex Heart Inst J* 19:149, 1992.
92. Gallo JA, Lebowitz P, Battit G, et al: Complications of intercostal nerve blocks performed under direct vision during thoracotomy: a report of two cases, *J Thorac Cardiovasc Surg* 86:628, 1983.
93. Benumof JL, Semenza J: Total spinal anesthesia following intercostal nerve blocks, *Anesthesiology* 43:124, 1975.
94. Morin JE, Long R, Elleker M, et al: Upper extremity neuropathies following median sternotomy, *Ann Thorac Surg* 34:181, 1982.
95. Seyfer AE, Grammer N, Bogumill G, et al: Upper extremity neuropathies after cardiac surgery, *J Hand Surg* 10A:16, 1985.
96. Kirsh MM, Magee K, Gago O, et al: Brachial plexus injury following median sternotomy incision, *Ann Thorac Surg* 11:315, 1971.
97. Baisden CE, Greenwald LV, Symbas PN: Occult rib fractures and brachial plexus injury following median sternotomy for open-heart operations, *Ann Thorac Surg* 38:192, 1984.
98. Vander Salm TJ, Cereda JM, Cutler BS: Brachial plexus injury following median sternotomy, *J Thorac Cardiovasc Surg* 80:447, 1980.
99. Vander Salm TJ, Cutler BS, Okike ON: Brachial plexus injury following median sternotomy: part II, *J Thorac Cardiovasc Surg* 83:914, 1982.
100. Treasure T, Garnett R, O'Connor J, et al: Injury of the lower trunk of the brachial plexus as a complication of median sternotomy for cardiac surgery, *Ann R Coll Surg Engl* 62:378, 1980.
101. Hanson MR, Breuer A, Furlan A, et al: Mechanism and frequency of brachial plexus injury in open-heart surgery: a prospective analysis, *Ann Thorac Surg* 36:675, 1983.
102. Tomlinson DL, Hirsch I, Kodali S, et al: Protecting the brachial plexus during median sternotomy, *J Thorac Cardiovasc Surg* 94:297, 1987.
103. Wey JM, Guinn GA: Ulnar nerve injury with open-heart surgery, *Ann Thorac Surg* 39:358, 1985.
104. Warner MA, Warner ME, Martin JT: Ulnar neuropathy: incidence, outcome, and risk factors in sedated or anesthetized patients, *Anesthesiology* 81:1332, 1994.
105. Clausen EG: Postoperative "anesthetic" paralysis of the brachial plexus: a review of the literature and report of nine cases, *Surgery* 12:933, 1942.
106. Mangar D, Kelly D, Holder D, et al: Brachial plexus compression from a malpositioned chest tube after thoracotomy, *Anesthesiology* 74:780, 1991.
107. Chaney MA: Intrathecal and epidural anesthesia and analgesia for cardiac surgery, *Anesth Analg* 84:1211, 1997.
108. Tuman KJ, McCarthy R, March R, et al: Effect of epidural anesthesia and analgesia on coagulation and outcome after major vascular surgery, *Anesth Analg* 73:696, 1991.
109. Yeager MP, Glass D, Neff R, et al: Epidural anesthesia and analgesia in high risk surgical patients, *Anesthesiology* 66:729, 1987.
110. Walker WE: Paraplegia associated with thoracotomy, *Ann Thorac Surg* 50:178, 1990.
111. Short HD: Paraplegia associated with the use of oxidized cellulose in posterolateral thoracotomy incisions, *Ann Thorac Surg* 50:288, 1990.
112. Perez-Guerra F, Holland JM: Epidural hematoma as a cause of postpneumonectomy paraplegia, *Ann Thorac Surg* 39:282, 1985.
113. Mathew NT, John S: Iatrogenic ischaemic paraplegia, *Med J Aust* 2:29, 1970.
114. Crawford ES, Crawford JL, Safi HJ, et al: Thoracoabdominal aortic aneurysms: preoperative and intraoperative factors determining immediate and long-term results of operations in 605 patients, *J Vasc Surg* 3:389, 1986.
115. Laschinger JC, Izumoto H, Kouchoukos NT: Evolving concepts in prevention of spinal cord injury during operations on the descending thoracic and thoracoabdominal aorta, *Ann Thorac Surg* 44:667, 1987.
116. Bollen EC, van Duin CJ, Theunissen PH, et al: Mediastinal lymph node dissection in resected lung cancer: morbidity and accuracy of staging, *Ann Thorac Surg* 55:961, 1993.
117. Ashbaugh DG: Mediastinoscopy, *Arch Surg* 100:568, 1970.
118. Bramwit DN, Schmelka DD: Traumatic subarachnoid-pleural fistula, *Radiology* 89:737, 1967.
119. DePinto D, Payne T, Kittle CF: Traumatic subarachnoid-pleural fistula, *Ann Thorac Surg* 25:477, 1978.
120. Higgins CB, Mulder DB: Traumatic subarachnoid-pleural fistula, *Chest* 61:189, 1972.
121. Overton MC, Hood RM, Farris RG: Traumatic subarachnoid-pleural fistula: case report, *J Thorac Cardiovasc Surg* 51:729, 1966.
122. Frantz PT, Battaglini JW: Subarachnoid-pleural fistula: unusual complication of thoracotomy, *J Thorac Cardiovasc Surg* 79:873, 1980.
123. Labadie EL, Hamilton R, Lundell O, et al: Hypoliquorrheic headache and pneumocephalus caused by thoraco-subarachnoid fistula, *Neurology* 27:993, 1977.

Chapter 28

Complications Related to Abdominal Surgery with an Emphasis on Laparoscopy

Girish P. Joshi

The field of abdominal surgery, which comprises a significant portion of all major surgical procedures, has been radically changed with the introduction of laparoscopy. Recent advances in robotic and video technology have made the use of laparoscopic procedures more widely applicable. With the evolution of laparoscopy, a substantial number of abdominal procedures are being performed using this approach, including cholecystectomy, appendectomy, inguinal hernia repair, vagotomy, hiatal hernia repair, colectomy, Nissens fundoplication, splenectomy, and nephrectomy. The complications that might occur during open abdominal surgery include cardiovascular and pulmonary dysfunction, fluid and electrolyte abnormalities, hemorrhage requiring blood component transfusion, hypothermia, and renal and liver dysfunction. These complications are discussed in other chapters.

Compared with the traditional open abdominal approach, the laparoscopic approach is associated with less postoperative pain, shorter hospital stay, fewer overall adverse events, more rapid return to normal activity, and significant cost savings. The advantages of laparoscopic surgery have led to a trend toward performing these procedures in older and sicker patients with significant co-existing cardiopulmonary disease.[1] However, it is important that the benefits of laparoscopic procedures be weighed against associated complications. A thorough knowledge of potential perioperative complications is necessary to provide optimal patient care. The focus of this chapter is on complications associated with laparoscopic surgical procedures.

Complications unique to laparoscopic surgery include those related to creation of pneumoperitoneum, patient positioning, and surgical instrumentation. Intraperitoneal carbon dioxide (CO_2) insufflation and changes in patient position during laparoscopic surgery have several hemodynamic, pulmonary, and endocrine effects.[2] In addition, a number of surgical complications, including acute hemorrhage, bowel and bladder perforation, gas embolization, subcutaneous emphysema, pneumothorax, and pneumomediastinum, may occur during the laparoscopic procedure.[3-5] Postoperative complications include pulmonary impairment, pain, nausea and vomiting, wound infection, peritonitis, delayed hemorrhage, incisional hernia, and metastases at the trocar insertion sites.

I. INCIDENCE OF PERIOPERATIVE COMPLICATIONS

The majority of data regarding the incidence of complications related to laparoscopic surgery are derived from the gynecologic surgery literature. The incidence of minor complications reported from gynecologic laparoscopic procedures ranges from 1% to 4%, and the incidence of major complications ranges from 0.3% to 2.8%.[6,7] The overall mortality rates from laparoscopy have decreased significantly over the past three decades. A review of 100,000 cases from 1951 to 1968 revealed a mortality of 1 per 1000 cases,[8] whereas recent reviews report a mortality of 0.5 to 2 per 10,000 gynecologic laparoscopic procedures.[9,10] A study from the Centers for Disease Control indicated that anesthetic complications may account for approximately one third of the reported deaths associated with laparoscopic tubal ligation.[9] Recently, Steiner et al[11] reported a reduction in the overall mortality rate for cholecystectomy from 0.84% in 1989 to 0.56% in 1992.

It is important to note that the majority of gynecologic laparoscopic procedures are diagnostic or minor operative procedures performed in young and healthy patients. Nongynecologic laparoscopic procedures, by comparison, are more extensive and performed in older and sicker patients. Therefore the complication rate with general surgical laparoscopic procedures may be greater than that reported in the gynecologic surgery literature. In addition, the incidence of complications is greatly influenced by the training, experience, skill, and judgment of the surgeon performing the procedure. A survey found that the complication rate for surgeons who had performed fewer than 100 laparoscopic procedures was almost four times greater than for surgeons with more experience.[12] Because these procedures are new, there is an initial learning curve, which may result in a greater incidence of complications.

Limited data are becoming available with regard to general surgical laparoscopic procedures. A series of more than 1100 laparoscopic cholecystectomies had no operative deaths and a total complication rate of 5.2%.[13] Another survey of more than 1500 laparoscopic cholecystectomies reported one death (0.07%) and a morbidity of 5.1%.[14] These data compare favorably with the complication rates reported for open cholecystectomy.[15] Data from 11 studies (more than 3000 laparoscopic cholecystectomies) show that the complication rate with laparoscopic procedures was one sixth that reported after open cholecystectomy.[16] Similarly, Steiner et al[11] report 33% lower overall operative mortality with laparoscopic cholecystectomy than with open cholecystectomy. In a recent national survey of 77,604 laparoscopic cholecystectomies reported by Deziel et al,[17] over one half of the operative deaths were attributed to technical complications of the laparoscopic procedure. In particular, attention has been focused on the incidence of associated bile duct injuries.

II. SURGICAL TECHNIQUE

The first step in laparoscopy is establishment of pneumoperitoneum to allow surgical exposure and manipulation of abdominal contents. Most laparoscopists use the Veress needle, inserted through a small subumbilical incision, for initial access into the peritoneal cavity. An electronic variable-flow insufflator, which automatically terminates flow at a preset intraabdominal pressure (IAP), usually between 12 and 15 mm Hg, is used to achieve pneumoperitoneum. A trocar is then inserted in place of the Veress needle, and a video laparoscope is inserted through the trocar. Multiple trocars are then placed under direct vision for placement of various instruments necessary for dissection.

The ideal insufflating gas would be colorless, nonexplosive, physiologically inert, and readily soluble in plasma. Because air supports combustion and can cause significant cardiopulmonary disturbances with inadvertent embolization, it is no longer considered appropriate. Nitrous oxide (N_2O) has been used because it is better tolerated hemodynamically,[18] but it too supports combustion.[19] To avoid the problems related to CO_2 absorption, nitrogen,[20] helium,[21] and argon[22] have been investigated. Although these inert gases provide hemodynamic stability, they have a lower blood gas solubility than CO_2, so venous gas embolism would be more serious. Even the use of the argon beam coagulator in laparoscopy can lead to significant intraperitoneal accumulation of argon, which can result in gas embolism.[23]

III. COMPLICATIONS RELATED TO PNEUMOPERITONEUM
A. Cardiovascular function

Laparoscopic surgery is associated with several hemodynamic changes that may result from the effects of anesthetic technique, positioning, mechanical and neuroendocrine effects of pneumoperitoneum, and the effects of absorbed CO_2. However, the role of these factors may be difficult to distinguish. The extent of hemodynamic changes depends on the patient's preoperative status, the surgical technique including the IAP attained, the volume of CO_2 absorbed, and the anesthetic technique including the ventilatory technique.

Although major cardiovascular complications associated with laparoscopic procedures are rare, there have been reports of arrhythmias, severe hypotension, and even cardiac arrest.[24,25] Approximately one third of all the intraoperative complications are caused by cardiovascular dysfunction. The incidence of acute cardiovascular collapse during gynecologic laparoscopy was estimated to be 1 in 2000, with a mortality of 1 in 10,000 in the early 1970s, falling to 1 in 100,000 by the end of the 1970s.[26,27] Importantly, most cases of the cardiac arrest occurred during induction of pneumoperitoneum.[26] The differential diagnosis of sudden cardiovascular collapse during laparoscopy is shown in Box 28-1.

Box 28-1 Differential diagnosis of sudden cardiovascular collapse during laparoscopy

Profound vasovagal reaction
Gas embolism
Hemorrhage
Cardiac arrhythmia
Pneumothorax
Excessive intraabdominal pressure
Myocardial infarction
Anesthetic drug-related

1. Hemodynamic changes in healthy patients. During gynecologic laparoscopic procedures, the creation of pneumoperitoneum and assumption of the lithotomy position with a steep head-down tilt have several hemodynamic consequences. However, the hemodynamic changes have been found to be insignificant with lower (less than 20 mm Hg) IAP.[28-30] It must be noted that gynecologic procedures usually require a short duration of insufflation and are performed on young and otherwise healthy patients.

With the laparoscopic approach being extended to gastrointestinal and urologic surgical procedures that require longer periods of CO_2 insufflation than the gynecologic procedures, significant hemodynamic changes have been reported. In a series of 15 healthy patients undergoing laparoscopic cholecystectomy, Joris et al[31] report that induction of anesthesia and reverse Trendelenburg positioning before CO_2 insufflation caused a 35% to 40% reduction in cardiac index (CI), as determined by pulmonary artery catheter (Fig. 28-1). The CI decreased by another 50% (from the preinduction values) after creation of pneumoperitoneum (IAP = 15 mm Hg). However, the CI returned to preinduction values within 15 minutes, suggesting a biphasic effect. The biphasic changes in CI have also been reported in other studies with both single and serial measurements.[32,33] Using continuous impedance cardiography, Westerband et al[32] observed a 30% reduction in CI with creation of pneumoperitoneum. During laparoscopic Nissen fundoplication, the surgical disruption of the esophageal hiatus can cause increased mediastinal and pleural pressure, resulting in significant reduction in cardiac output.[34]

However, other investigators did not observe a significant decrease in cardiac output in healthy patients.[35,36] Girardis et al[36] measured CI and systemic vascular resistance index (SVRI) using radial artery pressure profile analysis. The CI was not influenced by the increase in IAP or accumulation of plasma CO_2. Cunningham et al[37] claimed that left ventricular function, as determined by transesophageal echocardiographic estimation of ejection fraction, was preserved following CO_2 insufflation and patient position changes, despite decrease in the left ventricular end-diastolic area (a measure of preload). Possibly, insufflation performed in the supine position (rather than head-down position) might have avoided the decrease in cardiac output.[2] The differences in the anesthetic technique, the degree of IAP and head-up position, and the methods used to evaluate the hemodynamic variables may also be responsible for the discrepancies in the findings of various studies.

Induction of pneumoperitoneum is also associated with an increase in both systemic vascular resistance (SVR) and mean arterial pressure (MAP).[31,38] Similar to changes in CI, there was partial restoration of SVR within 15 minutes after CO_2 insufflation.[31] Although the reduction in CI paralleled the time course of increase in SVR, the cause-effect relationship between CI and SVR

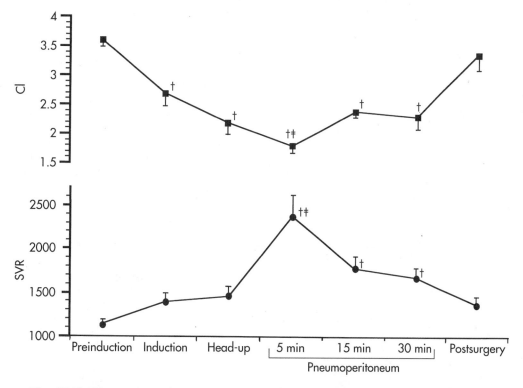

Fig. 28-1. Changes in cardiac index *(CI)* and systemic vascular resistance *(SVR)* in healthy patients undergoing laparoscopic cholecystectomy. Values are mean ± SEM. †p <0.05 versus preinduction; ‡p <0.05 versus head-up position. (Modified from Joris JL, Noirot DP, Legrand MJ, et al: *Anesth Analg* 76:1067, 1993.)

is unclear. A linear correlation was found between changes in the SVR and increases in the plasma concentrations of renin and aldosterone.[38] Similarly, the plasma concentrations of vasopressin increased significantly after pneumoperitoneum and paralleled the time course of increases in SVR values.[39] The increase in SVR may also result from compression of the abdominal arteries by increased IAP. The increase in SVR represents an increase in the afterload of the heart, which may increase the myocardial wall tension and thus the myocardial oxygen demand.[37] However, despite the acute hemodynamic changes during laparoscopic cholecystectomy, O'Leary et al[38] did not observe any myocardial ischemia as suggested by ECG ST segment changes.

Assessment of left ventricular preload is complex. In clinical practice, estimation of left ventricular volume and pressure measurements are used as approximations of left ventricular preload. However, correlation between volume and pressure is not linear. The central venous pressure (CVP) and pulmonary artery occlusion pressure (PAOP) increase significantly with induction of pneumoperitoneum.[31,32] However, the observed increase in the cardiac filling pressures (as determined by pulmonary artery catheter) is questioned because pneumoperitoneum increases intrathoracic pressures and decreases thoracic compliance. This may result in false increases in CVP and PAOP. Therefore it is suggested that transmural pressures should be used to estimate the left ventricular filling volumes.[18]

Gannedahl et al[40] evaluated the hemodynamic changes with pneumoperitoneum (IAP = 11 to 13 mm Hg) while patients were placed in different body positions (15- to 20-degree tilts). These investigators used both pulmonary artery catheters and transesophageal echocardiography to determine the various hemodynamic variables (Table 28-1). They observed an increase in echocardiographic volume indices of preload (end-diastolic area) and increase in PAOP (Fig. 28-2).[40] However, there was no correlation between the magnitude of changes in the PAOP values and the changes in end-diastolic area.[40] Interestingly, after establishment of pneumoperitoneum, the filling volume (end-diastolic

area) was significantly greater than preinsufflation values, irrespective of posture.[40] In other words, pneumoperitoneum counteracts the reduction in the cardiac filling volumes observed in the head-up position. Cunningham et al[37] did not observe any changes in end-diastolic area during pneumoperitoneum, but the end-diastolic area values observed in their patients were higher than those reported as normal.[40] In addition, differences in study design, anesthetic technique, and IAP may also explain the conflicting findings.

Kelman et al[29] report that with moderate increase in IAP (less than 20 mm Hg), the transmural cardiac filling pressures and cardiac output increased. This may be a result of an increase in the intravascular volume from compression of the abdominal organs (liver and spleen) caused by the increased IAP.[35,41] Furthermore, the increased sympathetic output from hypercarbia and neurohormonal responses may also be contributing factors.[2,31] This would explain the increase in echocardiographic volume indices of preload (end-diastolic area).[40] The lack of changes in the end-systolic area and fractional area shortening observed by Gannedahl et al[40] suggest that myocardial contractility is maintained during laparoscopic surgery.

The reported changes in heart rate during laparoscopic procedures are variable. The incidence of arrhythmias during laparoscopy is approximately 14%.[42] Bradyarrhythmias, including bradycardia, atrioventricular dissociation, nodal rhythm, and asystole have been attributed to a vagal response secondary to the Veress needle or trocar insertion and mesenteric traction from pneumoperitoneum. Tachyarrhythmia may be caused by hypercarbia resulting from systemic absorption of CO_2 and the neuroendocrine response to pneumoperitoneum.

Increased IAP associated with pneumoperitoneum can result in reduction in splanchnic and renal perfusion.[43] Bongrad et al[44] report a positive correlation between the duration and extent of increased IAP and decrease in bowel mucosal oxygen tension. Reduction in urine output during laparoscopic procedures has been reported.[45,46] The diminished urine output is attributed to the compression of renal vessels and increased plasma

Table 28-1. Hemodynamic measurements before and during pneumoperitoneum (PP) during laparoscopic cholecystectomy in healthy patients

	Supine	Head-down	Head-up	Supine with PP
Heart rate (beats/min)	61 ± 7	53 ± 4	66 ± 9	66 ± 16
MAP (mm Hg)	69 ± 7	76 ± 7	64 ± 9	91 ± 11
CVP (mm Hg)	6.2 ± 2.9	10.2 ± 3.5	0.8 ± 3.5	10.9 ± 2.7
PAOP (mm Hg)	9.8 ± 1.0	13.6 ± 1.5	4.0 ± 3.8	13.0 ± 2.7
MPAP (mm Hg)	14.1 ± 1.5	17.4 ± 1.2	8.5 ± 3.5	18.4 ± 3.7
CI (L/min/m²)	2.2 ± 0.3	2.2 ± 0.3	2.1 ± 0.6	2.0 ± 0.4
SVR (dynes/sec/cm⁵)	1310 ± 302	1381 ± 313	1419 ± 342	1795 ± 444

Modified from Gannedahl P, Odeberg S, Brodin LA, et al: *Acta Anaesthesiol Scand* 40:160, 1996.
Values are mean ± SD. *ns,* Not significant; *MAP,* mean arterial pressure; *CVP,* central venous pressure; *PAOP,* pulmonary artery occlusion pressure; *MPAP,* mean pulmonary artery pressure; *CI,* cardiac index; *SVR,* systemic vascular resistance.

renin activity. Plasma renin activity increases after creation of pneumoperitoneum.[38,45] The urinary N-acetyl-β-D-glucosaminidase (NAG) excretion increased in patients undergoing laparoscopic cholecystectomy, suggesting transient renal dysfunction. The urinary excretion of NAG, a lysosomal enzyme, sensitively and noninvasively indicates potential renal tubular damage. Because renal function often is impaired in the elderly and in patients with generalized atherosclerosis, there may be a greater risk of renal impairment during prolonged laparoscopic surgery in these groups. Koivusalo et al[43] report that the decreased urine output during laparoscopic surgery returned to normal approximately 60 minutes after deflation of the abdomen.

2. Hemodynamic changes in patients with cardiovascular dysfunction. Significant hemodynamic changes have been reported during laparoscopic procedures in patients with cardiopulmonary dysfunction.[47,48] However, these changes were considerably more extensive in patients with significant comorbidities than in healthy patients. The CI decreased by approximately 60% to 65% after CO_2 insufflation (IAP = 15 mm Hg) and remained less than the baseline value until deflation of the abdomen (Table 28-2).[47] A biphasic response, observed in healthy patients, was not observed in this patient population. This may be related to the severity of the cardiac dysfunction. Three of the 17 patients included in this study required administration of nitroglycerin to maintain the MAP pressure less than 100 mm Hg or an SVR value less than 2000 dynes/sec/cm^5, and one patient required administration of dobutamine to maintain the CI of more than 2 L/min/m^2. Other investigators have also recommended perioperative administration of a nitroglycerin infusion (0.5 to 1 μg/kg/min) in patients

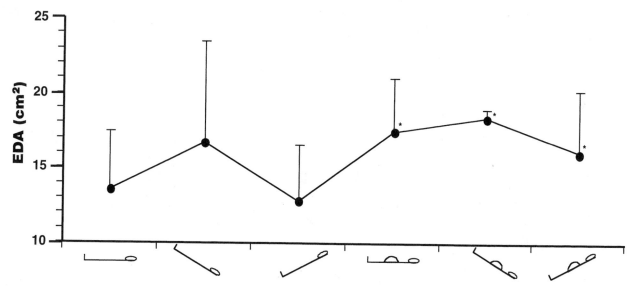

Fig. 28-2. Effects of pneumoperitoneum and position changes on end-diastolic area *(EDA)* in healthy patients undergoing laparoscopic cholecystectomy. The EDA increased significantly ($p < 0.04$) following creation of pneumoperitoneum irrespective of patient position. Values are mean ± SD. *$p < 0.05$ versus preinsufflation. (Modified from Gannedahl P, Odeberg S, Brodin LA, et al: *Acta Anaesthesiol Scand* 40:160, 1996.)

Head-down with PP	Head-up with PP	Before PP vs. after PP	Supine vs. head-down	Supine vs. head-up	Head-down vs. head-up
53 ± 3	70 ± 8	ns	$p < 0.01$	ns	$p < 0.001$
87 ± 8	84 ± 13	$p < 0.001$	ns	ns	ns
15.9 ± 4.6	3.1 ± 2.6	$p < 0.001$	$p < 0.002$	$p < 0.001$	$p < 0.001$
18.3 ± 4.1	6.6 ± 3.0	$p < 0.001$	$p < 0.001$	$p < 0.001$	$p < 0.001$
20.0 ± 6.1	10.8 ± 2.5	$p < 0.004$	ns	$p < 0.001$	$p < 0.001$
2.0 ± 0.2	1.8 ± 0.3	ns	ns	ns	ns
1577 ± 344	2047 ± 430	$p < 0.001$	ns	ns	ns

Table 28-2. Measured and derived data at various time points during laparoscopic cholecystectomy in patients with severe cardiac dysfunction

	T_1	T_2	T_3	T_4
Heart rate (beats/min)	81 ± 17	73 ± 16	77 ± 15	75 ± 14
MAP (mm Hg)	96 ± 20	72 ± 15**	101 ± 18*	84 ± 17
CI (L/min)	2.7 ± 0.7	2.1 ± 0.7	1.9 ± 0.7*	1.9 ± 0.5**
CVP (mm Hg)	10 ± 5	10 ± 3	18 ± 5**	15 ± 5*
PAOP (mm Hg)	15 ± 9	12 ± 4	21 ± 7*	17 ± 7
SVR (dynes/sec/cm⁵)	1575 ± 688	1499 ± 620	2152 ± 880*	1781 ± 735
PVR (dynes/sec/cm⁵)	174 ± 78	232 ± 167	269 ± 110	246 ± 139

From Hein HAT, Joshi GP, Ramsay MAE, et al: *J Clin Anesth* 9:261, 1997.
Values are mean ± SD. *$p < 0.05$ versus T_1; **$p < 0.05$ versus T_2.
T_1, Before induction of anesthesia; T_2, 5 minutes after induction of anesthesia but before incision; T_3, 5 minutes after peritoneal CO_2 insufflation and reverse Trendelenburg position and left lateral tilt; T_{4-8}, every 10 minutes after reverse Trendelenburg position; T_9, after exsufflation and return to supine position; T_{10}, 10 minutes after attaining supine position; *MAP*, mean arterial pressure; *CI*, cardiac index; *CVP*, central venous pressure; *PAOP*, pulmonary artery occlusion pressure; *SVR*, systemic vascular resistance; *PVR*, pulmonary vascular resistance.

Table 28-3. Measured and derived data at various time points during laparoscopic cholecystectomy in cardiac transplant recipients

	T_1	T_2	T_3	T_4
Heart rate (beats/min)	97 ± 13	89 ± 11	93 ± 13	92 ± 11
MAP (mm Hg)	115 ± 18	86 ± 20*	114 ± 21	97 ± 21*
CI (L/min/m²)	3.2 ± 0.9	2.3 ± 0.5*	2.6 ± 0.6	2.7 ± 0.7
CVP (mm Hg)	11 ± 7	10 ± 3	17 ± 5**	16 ± 4**
PAOP (mm Hg)	13 ± 4	11 ± 3	16 ± 4**	17 ± 4**
SVR (dynes/sec/cm⁵)	1571 ± 603	1485 ± 473	1728 ± 642	1361 ± 435
PVR (dynes/sec/cm⁵)	85 ± 60	150 ± 91*	175 ± 65*	148 ± 46*

From Joshi GP, Hein HA, Ramsay MA, et al: *Anesthesiology* 85:929, 1996.
Values are mean ± SD. *$p < 0.05$ versus T_1; **$p < 0.05$ versus T_2.
T_1, Before induction of anesthesia; T_2, 5 minutes after induction of anesthesia but before incision; T_3, 5 minutes after peritoneal CO_2 insufflation and reverse Trendelenburg position and left lateral tilt; T_{4-8}, every 10 minutes after reverse Trendelenburg position; T_9, after exsufflation and return to supine position; T_{10}, 10 minutes after attaining supine position; *MAP*, mean arterial pressure; *CI*, cardiac index; *CVP*, central venous pressure; *PAOP*, pulmonary artery occlusion pressure; *SVR*, systemic vascular resistance; *PVR*, pulmonary vascular resistance.

with cardiac dysfunction to avoid the changes in SVR and the related decrease in CI during laparoscopic cholecystectomy.[49]

Feig et al[50] evaluated the hemodynamic changes occurring during various laparoscopic procedures in patients with underlying cardiac or pulmonary disease. The hemodynamic variables were optimized preoperatively to achieve SVR values of less than 1200 dynes/sec/cm⁵ and CI values more than 2.1 L/min/m² using intravenous fluid administration, nitrates, or β-agonists. Despite optimal preoperative hemodynamic status, pharmacologic intervention (with nitroglycerin) was required in 9 of the 15 patients. In addition, the abdominal insufflation pressure had to be decreased from 15 to 10 mm Hg in 4 of the 15 patients studied.[50] However, this study was limited because it included varied types of laparoscopic surgical procedures including abdominal-perineal resection, hemicolectomies, and colostomy closures that were performed using variable patient positions (i.e., head-up or head-down tilt). In addition, meaningful trends in hemodynamic changes could not be determined because there were fewer data collection points.

Safran, Sgambati, and Orlando[48] describe mixed venous oxygen saturation (SvO_2) changes during laparoscopy in patients with severe cardiac dysfunction. The investigators observe that, when compared with patients in whom the SvO_2 increased, reduction in SvO_2 values was associated with larger reductions in CI, higher MAP, and reduced oxygen delivery. In addition, the hemodynamic changes observed with reduction in SvO_2 appeared to be related to decreased venous return and hypovolemia. These investigators suggest that continuous SvO_2 monitoring can be used to identify hemodynamic tolerance to laparoscopic procedure in high-risk patients.

Dhoste et al[51] evaluated the hemodynamic and ventilatory changes during laparoscopic cholecystectomy in elderly patients (age greater than 75 years) with significant comorbidities (ASA physical status III). Following induction of pneumoperitoneum, CI increased by 19% and the SVR did not change. In addition, the SvO_2 was greater during pneumoperitoneum. The indexed oxygen delivery (DO_2i) increased and the indexed oxygen consumption (VO_2i) remained stable, suggesting an improvement in cardiovascular status. These investigators

T$_5$	T$_6$	T$_7$	T$_8$	T$_9$	T$_{10}$
76 ± 12	74 ± 13	72 ± 12	71 ± 11	74 ± 11	78 ± 16
87 ± 13	86 ± 14	82 ± 16	87 ± 13	85 ± 17	93 ± 23
1.8 ± 0.4**	1.7 ± 0.5**	1.8 ± 0.6**	1.7 ± 0.4**	2.2 ± 0.5	2.3 ± 0.5
15 ± 4*	15 ± 4*	13 ± 4	13 ± 3	11 ± 4	11 ± 5
16 ± 5	17 ± 6	15 ± 7	15 ± 6	15 ± 6	16 ± 8
1864 ± 558	1973 ± 843	1838 ± 656	1956 ± 555	1568 ± 561	1659 ± 795
262 ± 162	241 ± 146	211 ± 140	232 ± 145	228 ± 115	206 ± 117

T$_5$	T$_6$	T$_7$	T$_8$	T$_9$	T$_{10}$
91 ± 13	89 ± 13	91 ± 12	91 ± 13	96 ± 15	90 ± 15
96 ± 15*	97 ± 13*	93 ± 14*	94 ± 17*	99 ± 15*	93 ± 16*
2.7 ± 0.9	2.7 ± 0.8	2.6 ± 0.7	3.0 ± 0.9	3.4 ± 1.2	3.4 ± 1.5
15 ± 5**	14 ± 6	13 ± 5	13 ± 5	11 ± 3	9 ± 3
16 ± 5**	16 ± 5**	15 ± 5**	14 ± 5	14 ± 5	13 ± 4
1419 ± 499	1440 ± 405	1457 ± 434	1284 ± 439	1198 ± 322	1198 ± 420
148 ± 39*	140 ± 31	121 ± 51	135 ± 36	123 ± 39	121 ± 30

also observe that the preload (as determined by right ventricular end-diastolic volume index) remained unchanged during pneumoperitoneum. They conclude that laparoscopic cholecystectomy is well tolerated by this patient population provided head-up tilt is moderate (10 degrees) and the IAP is maintained below 12 mm Hg.

Cholecystectomy often is required in cardiac transplant recipients because of an increased incidence of cholelithiasis caused by use of cyclosporine for immunosuppression. Joshi et al[52] evaluated the hemodynamic changes associated with pneumoperitoneum and patient positioning during laparoscopic cholecystectomy in 11 cardiac transplant recipients. In contrast to the observations in healthy patients and in patients with cardiopulmonary dysfunction, the CI (as determined by pulmonary artery catheter) did not change significantly during the laparoscopic procedure in these patients (Table 28-3). Furthermore, there were no significant changes in SVR. The investigators postulate that the differences in the hemodynamic responses in this population may be caused by persistent denervation of the heart and subsequent pathophysiologic changes in the cardio-

vascular system following orthotopic cardiac transplantation.[53,54] Because the cardiac plexus is divided during cardiac transplantation, the posttransplantation cardiac function profile is different from that of patients with normal innervated hearts. It is possible, but remains to be demonstrated, that neurohumoral responses during laparoscopic cholecystectomy in posttransplant patients may be different from those observed in healthy patients. Furthermore, a lack of Valsalva response to pneumoperitoneum and a 15% increase in circulating blood volume after cardiac transplantation may explain the maintenance of cardiac output.[55]

The adverse effects of increased IAP and hypercarbia caused by pneumoperitoneum can be avoided by the use of an abdominal wall lift device. With this device, insufflation with low volumes of CO_2 (2 to 6 L) are required and the abdominal pressure is maintained between 1 and 4 mm Hg.[56] Lindgren, Koivusalo, and Kellokumpu[57] report that, compared with conventional pneumoperitoneum, use of an abdominal wall lift device for laparoscopic cholecystectomy was associated with higher pulmonary compliance, lower CVP and femoral venous pressures, and decreased postoperative side effects including nausea, vomiting, and shoulder pain, and provided a faster recovery. Furthermore, changes in hemodynamic and neuroendocrine responses were minimal compared with those observed with conventional CO_2 insufflation.[45] Similarly, a totally gasless technique for laparoscopic cholecystectomy resulted in smaller hemodynamic and pulmonary changes and higher urine output.[58] However, the surgical view obtained with the use of the gasless technique may not be optimal.

B. Pulmonary function

Changes in pulmonary function with pneumoperitoneum are compounded by those caused by changes in positioning and anesthesia.[59] Elevation of the diaphragm caused by pneumoperitoneum may be associated with reduction in lung volumes, including functional residual capacity. Several investigators report a decrease in the pulmonary compliance during laparoscopic surgery.[60-62] In patients undergoing laparoscopic procedures with 15-degree head-down tilt, the total pulmonary compliance decreased by 40% and there was only a partial return to preinsufflation values after deflation.[61] However, in patients undergoing laparoscopic cholecystectomy with 20-degree head-up tilt, the total pulmonary compliance decreased by 20% and it returned to preinsufflation values immediately after deflation of the abdomen.[61]

In patients undergoing laparoscopy, the lung and chest wall elastance and resistance increased when the patients were in head-down position.[63] Although the lung elastance and resistance values also increased in the head-up position, these values were lower than those observed in the head-down position. Furthermore, these increases in lung elastance and resistance correlated positively with body weight and body mass index.[63] Elevations of lung impedance increase alveolar pressure, which may increase the risk of lung injury, whereas increases in chest wall impedance increase intrathoracic pressures, which may reduce venous return to the heart and thus decrease the cardiac output. In addition, the increase in minute ventilation necessary to maintain normocarbia further increases the peak airway pressures.[60,62]

Increased IAP and upward displacement of the diaphragm can cause alveolar collapse and ventilation-perfusion mismatching, resulting in hypoxemia and hypercarbia. The differential diagnosis of increased arterial CO_2 concentrations during laparoscopic surgery is shown in Box 28-2. In healthy patients whose lungs were being mechanically ventilated, the arterial-to-end-tidal CO_2 ($ETCO_2$) gradient did not change significantly during pneumoperitoneum in gynecologic laparoscopy and laparoscopic cholecystectomy.[64-66] Girardis et al[36] report that pneumoperitoneum (IAP less than 15 mm Hg) did not produce significant changes in pulmonary gas exchange. Brampton and Watson[67] report that monitoring of $ETCO_2$ during laparoscopy could be used to reflect arterial CO_2 tension, except during creation of pneumoperitoneum. However, other investigators report an increase in the arterial-to-$ETCO_2$ gradient.[68-70] The discrepancies between various studies may reflect differ-

---

Box 28-2 Differential diagnosis of increased arterial carbon dioxide concentrations during laparoscopy

Carbon dioxide absorption
Increased dead space ($\dot{V}/\dot{Q}$ mismatch)
   Abdominal distention
   Position of the patient
   Mechanical ventilation
   Reduced cardiac output
Carbon dioxide embolism
Pneumothorax, pneumomediastinum, pneumopericardium
Subcutaneous emphysema

---

ences in anesthetic and ventilatory technique, IAP, and changes in patient positioning.

The changes in pulmonary function with pneumoperitoneum may become significant in obese patients and in patients with pulmonary disease. The arterial-to-$ETCO_2$ gradient was moderately higher in the elderly[51] and in patients with cardiopulmonary dysfunction.[64] Therefore the $ETCO_2$ may not reflect arterial CO_2 tension in this patient population. In addition, significant acidosis was observed in patients with cardiopulmonary dysfunction.[64] These authors suggest that preoperative arterial blood gas analysis would be appropriate in patients with significant cardiopulmonary dysfunction undergoing laparoscopic procedures. In addition, these patients may require careful intraoperative arterial blood gas monitoring.

A recent study reports that after deflation of the abdomen, it may require approximately 45 minutes for the CO_2 concentrations to return to preinsufflation values.[36] Therefore patients with impaired ventilation after general anesthesia or those with significant cardiopulmonary disease may be adversely affected by hypercapnia in the immediate postoperative period.[71] In addition, significant impairment of diaphragmatic contractile function has been documented after laparoscopic cholecystectomy, which may present an additional hazard in patients with diaphragmatic dysfunction.[72] Respiratory failure has been reported after laparoscopic cholecystectomy in a patient with chronic hemidiaphragm paralysis resulting from neck surgery and irradiation.[73] Upward displacement of the paralyzed hemidiaphragm following creation of pneumoperitoneum can cause pulmonary atelectasis, which may not be clinically apparent intraoperatively because of positive-pressure ventilation. However, with resumption of spontaneous ventilation patients may become hypoxemic and require positive-pressure ventilation until the collapsed lung reexpands.

Hypoxemia can occur during laparoscopic surgery. The differential diagnosis of hypoxemia during laparoscopic surgery is shown in Box 28-3. Cunningham and Schlanger[74] report a case of significant intraoperative hypoxemia during laparoscopic cholecystectomy in a patient with sickle cell anemia. The authors postulate that hypoxemia may have resulted from ventilation-perfusion

Preexisting conditions
  Cardiopulmonary dysfunction
  Morbid obesity
Hypoventilation
  Patient position
  Pneumoperitoneum
  Tracheal tube obstruction
  Inadequate ventilation
Intrapulmonary shunting
  Reduced functional residual capacity (pneumoperitoneum induced)
  Endobronchial intubation
  Pneumothorax
  Emphysema (subcutaneous or mediastinal)
  Pulmonary aspiration of gastric contents
Reduced cardiac output
  Hemorrhage (trocar injury)
  Inferior vena cava compression
  Impaired venous return (pneumoperitoneum)
  Arrhythmia (hypercarbia or inhaled anesthetics)
  Myocardial depression (drug induced or acidosis)
  Decreased cardiac output (pneumoperitoneum induced)
  Carbon dioxide embolism

Modified from Cunningham AJ, Schlanger M: *Anesth Analg* 75:838, 1992.

mismatching and intrapulmonary shunting secondary to decreased lung volumes and extensive interstitial lung disease, coupled with a further decrease in functional residual capacity induced by the creation of a pneumoperitoneum. These authors suggest that preoperative pulmonary function testing including arterial blood gas analysis should be performed in patients with pulmonary dysfunction as determined on clinical examination. Furthermore, if laparoscopy is performed, a radial artery cannula for monitoring of arterial blood gas analysis should be considered. If refractory hypoxemia or high airway pressures occur during the surgery, there should be a low threshold for recommending conversion from a laparoscopic to an open procedure.

C. Carbon dioxide absorption

During insufflation, CO_2 is administered at 6 L/min to maintain an IAP of approximately 12 to 15 mm Hg. Diffusion of CO_2 from the peritoneal cavity to the blood leads to increased CO_2 concentration in the blood. The increased concentration of CO_2 may be managed by increasing the minute ventilation by 10% to 15%.[68] However, Tan, Lee, and Tweed[75] report that a 20% to 30% increase in minute ventilation was necessary to maintain normocarbia during laparoscopy. Some investigators suggest that hyperventilation should be commenced before CO_2 insufflation in an effort to decrease the tissue storage of CO_2 and thus avoid significant hypercarbia. However, patients with impaired cardiopulmonary function and restricted CO_2 clearance may retain CO_2,

resulting in a clinically significant respiratory acidosis despite aggressive ventilatory or pharmacologic interventions.[64]

Interestingly, absorption of CO_2 was not influenced significantly by the duration of intraperitoneal insufflation[76] and was not linearly related to IAP.[77] Pulmonary elimination of CO_2 during laparoscopy was reported to be biphasic. There was an initial rapid increase in CO_2 elimination, which reflects rapid peritoneal absorption. The CO_2 absorption reached a maximum at a low IAP and did not increase significantly despite further increases in IAP, which may be caused by compression of peritoneal vessels.[77] However, arterial CO_2 concentrations increased even after the CO_2 absorption had reached a plateau. This may be related to impaired CO_2 elimination from an increase in dead space resulting from elevated intrathoracic pressure and a reduction in cardiac output caused by increased IAP.

It has been shown that CO_2 pneumoperitoneum can have different physiologic impacts in different laparoscopic procedures.[78] This may depend on intraperitoneal or extraperitoneal insufflation. Although CO_2 absorption reached a plateau within 10 minutes after initiation of intraperitoneal insufflation (e.g., during cholecystectomy), it continued to increase slowly throughout extraperitoneal CO_2 insufflation (e.g., during pelviscopy).[76] Furthermore, the increases in $ETCO_2$ concentration and pulmonary elimination of CO_2 were more marked during extraperitoneal insufflation than during intraperitoneal insufflation.[76]

Hypercarbia resulting from CO_2 insufflation has direct and indirect hemodynamic effects.[79] The direct effects of increased CO_2 concentration include peripheral vasodilation and depression of myocardial contractility. The indirect effects of CO_2 include activation of the central nervous system and sympathoadrenal system, which increases myocardial contractility and causes tachycardia and hypertension. Exogenous CO_2 increases SVR and CI during mechanical ventilation, suggesting that the indirect effects of CO_2 seem to dominate.[80] The absorbed CO_2 can have deleterious effects in patients with preexisting cerebrovascular, pulmonary, or cardiovascular diseases. Hypercarbia is a major concern in a patient with increased intracranial pressure. During laparoscopy, the blood flow velocity through the middle cerebral artery can increase by as much as 50%, probably because of hypercarbia. Pulmonary vasoconstriction caused by direct effects of hypercarbia may be deleterious in patients with pulmonary hypertension or right ventricular ischemia or infarction. Life-threatening hypercapnia, respiratory acidosis, and cardiopulmonary collapse associated with laparoscopic cholecystectomy have been reported.[24,81-84]

D. Gas embolism

Significant CO_2 embolism is a rare but potentially lethal complication of laparoscopic surgery. Profound hypotension, cyanosis, and asystole have been described following CO_2 embolism.[85-94] The incidence of gas embolism during laparoscopy is difficult to ascertain because the criteria for diagnosis of gas embolism vary considerably.

Using precordial Doppler, Wadhwa et al[95] did not observe any gas embolism in 100 patients undergoing gynecologic laparoscopic procedures. However, Derouin et al[96] reported that minor CO_2 embolism (as diagnosed by transesophageal echocardiography) occurred commonly during laparoscopic cholecystectomy. However, these emboli did not cause any significant cardiopulmonary instability.

Gas embolism occurs when an open vein has a lower pressure than the surrounding pressure. The most common cause of clinically apparent CO_2 embolism is inadvertent intravascular placement of the Veress needle. Because CO_2 is more soluble in the blood than N_2O or air, a greater volume of CO_2 embolism can be tolerated. The lethal dose of CO_2 gas embolism is significantly greater than that of air (25 ml/kg versus 5 ml/kg, respectively). A large amount of CO_2 must enter the vessels rapidly (more than 1 L/min) before significant gas embolism can occur. The rapid absorption of CO_2 facilitates dissolution of the foam and results in rapid reversal of hemodynamic impairment. Embolic episodes most commonly occurred during creation of pneumoperitoneum and gallbladder dissection.[96] During CO_2 insufflation, gas embolism can occur through a tear in a vessel in the abdominal wall or on the peritoneum. The embolic episodes decreased after completion of pneumoperitoneum because increased IAP may have collapsed the injured vessel. During the dissection of gallbladder, gas embolism can occur from the vascular openings on the surface of the liver, which are kept patent by the surrounding parenchyma. Pulmonary air embolism after inadvertent puncture by the air-cooled laser has been reported during laparoscopic laser cholecystectomy.[91]

The presenting signs of gas embolism during laparoscopy include sudden cardiovascular collapse, hypoxemia, tachycardia or other arrhythmias, and pulmonary edema. In addition, a "mill wheel" murmur may be auscultated with a precordial or esophageal stethoscope. A sudden increase in the $ETCO_2$ during laparoscopy may be indicative of gas embolism. However, the $ETCO_2$ may also decrease because of cardiovascular collapse. Cyanosis of the head and neck resulting from inflow obstruction to the right side of the heart may also occur. Neurologic impairment may result from anoxic damage or paradoxic embolism through a probe-patent foramen ovale.

Adequate monitoring and a high index of suspicion result in early detection and prevention of serious sequelae of CO_2 embolism. If gas embolism is suspected, CO_2 insufflation should be discontinued and the abdomen deflated. The patient should be turned to the left lateral decubitus with head-down position to allow the gas to rise into the apex of the right ventricle and prevent entry into the pulmonary artery. Because of similar solubilities of N_2O and CO_2 in blood, there should not be significant diffusion of N_2O into or out of the CO_2 bubbles. Discontinuation of N_2O allows administration of 100% oxygen, and hyperventilation results in rapid CO_2 elimination. In addition to aggressive cardiopulmonary resuscitation, a central venous catheter should be placed to aspirate the gas. Hyperbaric oxygen and cardiopulmonary bypass have also been used to treat gas embolism successfully.[92,93]

IV. COMPLICATIONS RELATED TO INSTRUMENTATION
A. Extraperitoneal insufflation

Insertion of the Veress needle is performed without endoscopic visual control. Therefore a potential exists for incorrect placement of the needle and injury to the underlying structures. The locations in which the needle may be placed erroneously include the subcutaneous tissue, preperitoneal space, viscus, or vascular space. Inadvertent gas insufflation in the omentum, mesentery, or retroperitoneum can also occur.

Subcutaneous or preperitoneal insufflation caused by incorrect positioning of the Veress needle or trocar or leakage around the trocar occurs in approximately 0.5% of cases, although most of the complications are minor. Insufflation of CO_2 above the abdominal fascia causes subcutaneous emphysema, which is identified by palpating crepitus over the abdominal wall. Extensive subcutaneous emphysema may extend into the chest wall and the neck. Subcutaneous emphysema in the neck and face may also be caused by gas tracking up from the pneumothorax or pneumomediastinum. Because there is a continuum of fascial planes between the cervical tissues and the mediastinum,[97] subcutaneous gas in the neck may lead to pneumomediastinum or pneumothorax.[81,98-100] Tension pneumothorax has been reported following trocar insertion and CO_2 insufflation.[101] Intraperitoneal CO_2 can enter the mediastinum or the thorax through a congenital defect in the diaphragm.[102] A tear may occur in the visceral peritoneum, allowing retroperitoneal dissection of CO_2 into the mediastinum. Pneumothorax caused by pneumoperitoneum usually occurs on the left side but can be bilateral.[100] There also have been reports of pneumopericardium during laparoscopy.[103-105] It is proposed that pneumopericardium may occur when the CO_2 is forced through the inferior vena cava into the mediastinum and the pericardium[103] or when CO_2 tracks through the defect in the membranous portion of the diaphragm, which has a communication in the embryo between the pericardial and the peritoneal cavities.[105]

When subcutaneous emphysema occurs, the area for diffusion increases and CO_2 absorption into the blood may increase substantially, which may lead to significant hypercapnia and respiratory acidosis.[84,106,107] Excessive changes in airway pressure and increases in $ETCO_2$ may be early signs of CO_2 extravasation.[98,107] Significant pneumothorax can lead to cardiopulmonary impairment requiring immediate placement of a chest tube.[102] Although expansion of a CO_2-filled space with N_2O is not a serious problem, N_2O should be discontinued immediately after CO_2 extravasation outside the peritoneal cavity is suspected. In most cases no specific intervention may be necessary and the subcutaneous emphysema may resolve soon after the abdomen is deflated.[81] In some cases, however, it may be necessary to deflate the abdomen temporarily to allow elimination of CO_2, followed by reinsufflation with lower IAP to prevent further extravasation of CO_2. A chest radiograph should be obtained in patients with cervical emphysema to rule out pneumothorax or pneumoperitoneum. The potential complications related to the insertion of the Veress needle may be avoided by placement of the first trocar through a minilaparotomy incision.[108] In addition, the secondary trocars should be placed under direct vision.

B. Vascular injuries

Although many precautions usually are taken, serious and even fatal vascular complications can occur during instrumentation. Vascular injuries are the second most common surgical complications reported in gynecologic laparoscopy. In gynecologic literature, the overall incidence of vascular injuries was 0.64%; however, 80% of these were in the mesosalpinx. Insertions of the Veress needle or trocar into major vessels including the aorta, common iliac vessels, and inferior vena cava have been reported.[109-111] Injury to the common iliac artery requiring allograft repair has been described in a patient undergoing gynecologic laparoscopy.[112] Laceration of mesenteric vessels by the Veress needle or the trocar resulting in mesenteric hematoma has also been reported.[113] Injury to major vessels can be diagnosed easily by the return of blood from the Veress needle or the trocar. However, in some cases the bleeding may be concealed if the injury is confined to the retroperitoneal space. Strict adherence to basic principles of Veress needle and trocar insertion and identification of patients at risk should avoid major vascular injuries. Upon diagnosis of vessel damage, the Veress needle or the trocar should be left in situ to avoid further bleeding and to help identify the site of injury. Movement of the needle or trocar could extend the tear in the vessel. Immediate laparotomy should be performed to control the bleeding and repair the injury.

Injuries to the vessels in the abdominal wall (e.g., superficial and deep epigastric vessels) are becoming increasingly common because of the use of multiple trocars.[114] Injury to dilated abdominal wall veins, especially paraumbilical or recannulized umbilical veins in patients with portal hypertension, may result in significant hemorrhage. Transillumination of the abdominal wall with an endoscope to identify superficial abdominal wall vessels and placement of trocars lateral to the rectus sheath and above the internal ring should minimize the injury to the epigastric vessels. Most abdominal wall bleeding resolves without intervention, but if bleeding persists, hemostasis can be achieved with sutures, ligation, or tamponade with a Foley catheter balloon.[115] Stretch of the vascular adhesions by the expansion of pneumoperitoneum can cause a tear in the vessel and lead to hemorrhage. Hemorrhage may occur during laparoscopic cholecystectomy because of disruption, division, or avulsion of the cystic or hepatic artery. Conversion to an open procedure for uncontrollable hemorrhage has been reported in up to 1.9% of laparoscopic cholecystectomies.[5] Concealed bleeding caused by vessel injury may present in the postoperative period as a fall in hematocrit

values, hematoma formation, or excessive postoperative pain. Postoperative hemorrhage requiring transfusion or reexploration is reported to occur with a frequency of approximately 0.5%.[5]

C. Gastrointestinal injuries

Perforations of the stomach and the intestines are common visceral injuries.[116,117] In addition, lacerations of the liver, spleen, and colonic mesentery have also been reported.[118] The incidence of bowel injury during laparoscopy is approximately 0.1%, with a mortality rate of approximately 5%; however, many of these injuries probably go unrecognized or unreported.[119] The risk factors for bowel injuries during Veress needle or trocar insertion include previous abdominal surgery, metastatic disease, gastric distention during induction of anesthesia, and gastric distention associated with the use of a mask or the LMA. Electrocautery and lasers may cause thermal injuries to the viscera and abdominal vessels. Most thermal injuries heal without intervention. However, failure to recognize the injuries can result in significant morbidity and mortality.[117,120] Gastric decompression before placement of Veress needle should minimize stomach injuries. Because perforation of the bowel is commonly caused by adhesions of the viscera to the anterior abdominal wall, placement of the trocar using a minilaparotomy should be considered in patients with previous abdominal surgery. If the Veress needle perforates the bowel and no leakage of the enteric contents is observed, conservative management can be undertaken. However, bowel injury by the trocar must be repaired either laparoscopically or through a laparotomy.

D. Urinary tract injuries

Injuries to the bladder can occur either during placement of the Veress needle or the trocar or during surgical dissection. However, injuries to the bladder and the ureter are rare, with a reported incidence of 2 per 10,000 cases. Previous abdominal surgery and congenital anomaly of the lower urinary tract may increase the risk of urinary tract injuries. This author is aware of a bladder injury during surgical dissection in a patient undergoing laparoscopically assisted vaginal hysterectomy. The bladder injury was suspected because of sudden deflation of the abdomen, pneumaturia (gas bubbles in the urinary bag), and hematuria. Prevention and recognition of urinary tract injuries are critical because early identification may decrease the severity of the complication. Decompression of the bladder by placement of a urinary catheter has been recommended to avoid these injuries.

V. COMPLICATIONS RELATED TO ANESTHETIC TECHNIQUE
A. Airway management

General anesthesia with tracheal intubation remains the preferred technique for laparoscopic procedures. Tracheal intubation ensures airway protection and allows control of ventilation to maintain normocarbia. Although many authors have described the use of spontaneous breathing during gynecologic laparoscopic procedures, it could be disadvantageous during CO_2 insufflation, particularly in patients in a steep head-down position.[121] Some practitioners have used the laryngeal mask airway (LMA) to maintain the airway during brief gynecologic laparoscopic procedures. However, the LMA does not provide a seal against pulmonary aspiration of gastric contents. In addition, positive-pressure ventilation through the LMA may cause gastric distention and increase the possibility of regurgitation of gastric contents. Concern has been expressed that patients undergoing laparoscopic procedures are at an increased risk of regurgitation and possible aspiration of gastric contents because of increased IAP from pneumoperitoneum, as well as lithotomy and head-down position and external pressure on the abdomen by the surgeon.[122] On the other hand, raised IAP increases the lower esophageal sphincter pressure, so the barrier pressure actually increases, thereby reducing the possibility of regurgitation.[123]

A recent study using pH probes failed to demonstrate regurgitation during gynecologic laparoscopy with intermittent positive-pressure ventilation using an LMA.[124] Scott[125] reports no cases of pulmonary aspiration in a series of 5000 patients undergoing pelvic laparoscopy during which patients breathed spontaneously through a face mask. Goodwin, Rowe, and Ogg[126] evaluated the use of the LMA as part of a spontaneous breathing technique during gynecologic laparoscopy. The authors conclude that the technique is safe for brief laparoscopic procedures. A survey of more than 10,000 anesthetics reported uneventful use of the LMA with positive-pressure ventilation in patients undergoing gynecologic laparoscopic procedures without clinical evidence of regurgitation or aspiration of gastric contents.[127] Although the LMA may prove to be a satisfactory alternative to tracheal tube in low-risk patients, it should be avoided in obese patients, those with hiatal hernias, and those steep head-down position, and when large volumes of insufflating gas are used.

Inadvertent endobronchial intubation may result from frequent positional changes during the laparoscopic procedure.[128] In addition, creation of the pneumoperitoneum may result in cephalad movement of the carina and subsequent endobronchial intubation. Therefore the position of the tracheal tube should be reassessed after creation of the pneumoperitoneum and position changes.

B. Nitrous oxide

Nitrous oxide is widely used in anesthesia because of its analgesic properties and its ability to reduce the requirements of expensive volatile and intravenous anesthetic drugs. However, its use is controversial during laparoscopic surgery because of the concerns regarding its ability to diffuse into the bowel lumen, causing distention and impaired surgical access. Gas volume in the intestinal lumen has been found to increase by up to 200% in 4 hours when N_2O was administered to dogs.[129] Furthermore, patients receiving N_2O during colonic surgery had greater bowel distention, impaired operating condi-

tions, and significantly prolonged bowel dysfunction compared with those receiving air.[130] However, Taylor et al[131] could not find any difference in surgical conditions during laparoscopic cholecystectomy procedures lasting 70 to 80 minutes with or without the use of N_2O. Importantly, bowel distention did not increase with time and the surgeons could not differentiate the patients in whom N_2O was used from those in whom N_2O was not used. Interestingly, most published studies in the anesthesia literature on gynecologic laparoscopy have used N_2O. Although some data suggest that N_2O can increase the incidence of postoperative nausea, there is no convincing reason to avoid N_2O during laparoscopic procedures because of its emetic properties.[132,133]

When N_2O is used as a part of a balanced anesthetic technique, it diffuses into the peritoneal cavity. As laparoscopic surgical techniques become more complex and with the increasing use of lasers and electrocautery, the chance of bowel perforation and release of highly volatile bowel gases (methane and hydrogen) into the peritoneal cavity increases. If the N_2O in the peritoneal cavity reaches high concentrations that could support combustion of these bowel gases, an explosion hazard could exist. Neuman et al[134] evaluated the concentrations of N_2O in the peritoneal cavity and concluded that it is possible to achieve N_2O concentrations that can support combustion of bowel gas. These authors recommend that if a bowel perforation is recognized, the peritoneal cavity should be vented and purged with CO_2, and N_2O removed from the anesthetic mixture. If the N_2O concentration is reduced or eliminated during laparoscopic surgery, this hazard can be minimized or eliminated. Omitting N_2O from the anesthesia regimen may be an option in elderly patients with cardiopulmonary dysfunction or when there are surgical difficulties.

C. Intraoperative opioids

Opioids administered as part of a balanced anesthetic technique can cause spasm of the choledochoduodenal sphincter. The increases in intrabiliary pressure after administration of equianalgesic doses of fentanyl, morphine, meperidine, and pentazocine were 99.5%, 52.7%, 61.3%, and 15.1%, respectively.[135] These increases may result in unnecessary exploration of the common bile duct because the cholangiographic findings of sphincter spasm may be indistinguishable from those produced by a stone impacted in the distal common bile duct. Jones et al[136] found a 3% incidence of failure of contrast material to reach the duodenum in patients receiving fentanyl 10 µg/kg. However, the spasm could be reversed in all cases by the administration of glucagon 2 mg. Furthermore, small incremental doses of opioids are unlikely to cause significant biliary spasm.

VI. POSTOPERATIVE COMPLICATIONS
A. Postoperative pulmonary function

Patients undergoing upper abdominal surgery are at a greater risk of pulmonary complications than those undergoing lower abdominal surgery. The adverse effects of upper abdominal surgery on postoperative pulmonary function have been reviewed extensively.[137] The pulmonary complications include atelectasis, retained secretions, aspiration, infection, impaired pulmonary function, pleural effusion, and thromboembolism. The factors responsible for postoperative pulmonary impairment include preoperative pulmonary status, site of surgical incision, extent of transected abdominal muscles, residual anesthetic effects, diaphragmatic dysfunction, and postoperative pain. Complications are particularly common in patients with predisposing factors such as obesity, cigarette smoking, chronic pulmonary disease, and old age. Despite major advances in prevention and treatment of recognized pulmonary complications after abdominal surgery, morbidity remains 20% to 25%.[138] The vital capacity, which is critical for effective coughing, is decreased by 40% to 50% and the FRC is reduced by 70% to 80% after upper abdominal surgery. This reduction in lung volumes remained for 7 to 14 days after surgery.[139] The mortality in patients with significant postoperative pulmonary complications is approximately 3% to 5%.[138]

The most likely causes of pulmonary impairment in the postoperative period are diaphragmatic dysfunction (caused by stretching from pneumoperitoneum and CO_2 irritation) and inadequate pain relief. It is suggested that minimal incision discomfort following laparoscopic surgery (compared with open abdominal surgery) diminishes postoperative pulmonary complications.[140-143] The reductions in forced vital capacity, forced expiratory volume in 1 second, and forced expiratory flow were significantly lower after laparoscopic cholecystectomy than after open cholecystectomy.[140] Several initial studies report a lower incidence of pulmonary complications after laparoscopic surgery than after open surgery (5% versus 25%).[138,140,144]

B. Postoperative pain

It has been suggested that laparoscopic procedures are associated with less postoperative pain or lower analgesic requirements than are open abdominal procedures. Dubois, Berthelot, and Levard[1] report reduced postoperative pain after laparoscopic surgery. Other investigators report a similar degree of postoperative pain with both open and laparoscopic cholecystectomy, but opioid requirements and duration of pain were less after laparoscopic surgery.[141,143] The pain after open abdominal procedures is mainly parietal in origin (abdominal wall), whereas the pain after laparoscopic procedures is mainly visceral in origin.[145] Nevertheless, laparoscopic procedures can still result in considerable discomfort, thereby delaying return to normal activities.[146] The cause of postoperative pain after laparoscopic procedures is multifactorial. Shoulder pain secondary to diaphragmatic irritation is a common occurrence after laparoscopy.[147] Furthermore, the nature of the surgical technique also influences the incidence and degree of postoperative pain. During laparoscopic tubal ligation, electrocauterization resulted in less discomfort than spring-loaded clips, and both techniques were less painful than tubal rings.[148]

Numerous clinical studies indicate that postoperative pain is not always treated effectively. This has increased

awareness of the importance of effective pain management after ambulatory surgery. Multimodal analgesia techniques involving the use of opioids, nonsteroidal antiinflammatory drugs (NSAIDs), and local anesthetics are becoming increasingly popular.[149] Multimodal analgesic techniques provide improved analgesia with fewer side effects and faster recovery and discharge.[150]

Local anesthetic techniques are becoming increasingly popular adjuvants to general anesthesia because they provide significant perioperative analgesia. Subcutaneous infiltration of the surgical wound (laparoscopy portals) with local anesthetics can decrease postoperative pain and systemic analgesic requirements. Topical application with bupivacaine or etidocaine at the tubal ligation site was found to be beneficial in alleviating postoperative discomfort.[151] Similarly, infiltration of the mesosalpinx with 0.5% bupivacaine or 1% etidocaine significantly decreased postoperative pain and cramping after tubal ligation.[152-154]

Intraperitoneal instillation of local anesthetics is another simple and effective technique for providing pain relief during the early postoperative period. Intraperitoneal administration of 80 ml 0.5% lidocaine or 0.125% bupivacaine with epinephrine was effective in reducing the intensity of pain after gynecologic surgery.[155] However, intraperitoneal local anesthetics in low concentrations (less than 0.5%) were not effective for treating pain after laparoscopic cholecystectomy.[145,156] Recent clinical studies found that administration of 15 ml of 0.5% bupivacaine under direct vision into the hepatodiaphragmatic space, near and above the hepatoduodenal ligament and above the gallbladder area before and after surgery, provided effective pain relief and decreased the analgesic requirements after laparoscopic cholecystectomy.[157,158]

The use of NSAIDs has become more widespread with reports of their opioid-sparing effects. Preemptive use of NSAIDs has been shown to be effective in reducing postoperative pain. When oral naproxen was administered before laparoscopic surgery, postoperative pain scores, opioid requirements, and the time to discharge were significantly reduced.[159] Compared with placebo or fentanyl 75 μg intravenously, oral ibuprofen (800 mg) and naproxen (500 mg) suppositories were associated with superior analgesia and less nausea in the late recovery period and after discharge from the outpatient facility.[160] Use of ketorolac decreased the analgesic requirements but did not reduce the incidence of nausea or improve postoperative ventilatory function.[161] Interestingly, neither oral hydrocodone-acetaminophen combination nor oral ketorolac proved to be very effective after outpatient laparoscopic tubal ligation, possibly because of the high incidence of postoperative nausea and vomiting in this patient population.[162]

The aim of an analgesic technique should be not only to decrease the pain score but also to facilitate earlier mobilization and reduce perioperative complications.[163] There should be increased emphasis on prevention rather than treatment of postoperative pain. Regular dosing with pain medications provides better analgesia than does administration of these drugs on an as-needed basis. Finally, multimodal or balanced analgesia techniques are effective, with fewer side effects and faster recovery.

C. Postoperative nausea and vomiting

Patients undergoing laparoscopic surgery are at a greater risk for postoperative nausea and vomiting (PONV), which may delay recovery and discharge. Intraperitoneal insufflation and bowel manipulation increase the incidence of PONV, and pelvic surgery and female gender are additional risk factors. Prophylactic administration of antiemetic medications such as droperidol 0.625 mg or ondansetron 2 to 4 mg intravenously may decrease the incidence of PONV in patients undergoing laparoscopy.

D. Other morbidity

A variety of minor but troublesome side effects, including sore throat, fatigue, dizziness, and visual disturbances, also may occur after laparoscopic surgery. One of the most common complaints after laparoscopic surgery is muscle pains, which can limit the patient's ability to return to normal activities.[164] These myalgias originally were thought to result from the use of succinylcholine. However, eliminating this drug did not prevent muscle pain following laparoscopic surgery.[165]

High IAP (more than 20 mm Hg) can cause inferior vena caval compression, resulting in pooling of blood in the lower extremities and a decrease in venous return to the heart. With increased IAP, the femoral venous pressures increased[57,166] and flow velocity decreased,[167] which may increase the potential for deep vein thrombosis and pulmonary embolism. However, the mortality from pulmonary embolism after laparoscopic cholecystectomy (0.016%)[168] was lower than that after conventional surgery (0.8%).[169] Perhaps minimal tissue trauma and early ambulation associated with laparoscopic procedures reduce postoperative venous stasis. The lithotomy and head-down positions impede flow and result in venous stasis. Prolonged surgery in the lithotomy position may cause a compartment syndrome.

Because laparoscopic cholecystectomy requires head-up position, restraining straps are placed across the thighs to prevent the patient from sliding down the operating table, which may cause compression of nerves and postoperative neuropathy.[170] Therefore a foot board to absorb the patient's weight should be used routinely in procedures requiring head-up positioning.

E. Postoperative surgically related complications

Infections of the wound and peritoneum, although rare and minor, can occur in elderly, obese, diabetic, and immunocompromised patients. Postoperative fever and abdominal tenderness are the initial signs of infection or bowel perforation. Delayed bleeding from the operative site may present as abdominal pain, abdominal distention, falling hematocrit values, hemodynamic instability, or oliguria. Management of delayed bleeding depends on its source and the degree of hemodynamic instability. A CT scan of the abdomen may be useful in identifying the site and extent of the hematoma. In addition, a radiolabeled red cell study can identify the presence of

bleeding. An incisional hernia can develop at the trocar insertion sites, possibly caused by inadequate reapproximation of the wound, premature suture disruption, or infection. A rare complication of laparoscopy is dissemination of malignancy at trocar insertion sites.[171] Seeding along the tracks of an instrument has been reported with primary cancers of the colon, stomach, ovary, and biliary tract. Unrecognized bladder perforation may lead to azotemia, particularly when it is associated with ascites and hyponatremia.

VII. LAPAROSCOPIC SURGERY IN SPECIAL POPULATIONS
A. Pregnant patients

Elective abdominal surgery during pregnancy has been discouraged because of perceived risks of inducing premature birth or causing abortion. In cases where surgery is unavoidable (e.g., appendicitis or cholecystitis), open abdominal surgery has been performed with minimal fetal mortality or morbidity.[172,173] Women with suspected ectopic pregnancy have been exposed to laparoscopy in the first trimester and have progressed to normal term gestations.[174] Early reports considered pregnancy an absolute contradiction to nonobstetric laparoscopic surgery.[175,176] However, numerous recent clinical reports of successful laparoscopic surgery in pregnant women imply that previous concerns were unwarranted.[177-191] This finding has led many practitioners to believe that laparoscopic surgery is safe during pregnancy and may offer benefits to the patient.[192]

Although the cardiopulmonary changes during laparoscopic surgery in nonpregnant patients have been well documented, the changes in pregnant patients have not been described. Concern has been raised regarding the effect of hypercarbia on fetal acid-base balance and placental gas exchange, as well as effects of increased IAP on the uterine blood flow.[193] In pregnant ewes, CO_2 pneumoperitoneum increased the placental vascular resistance by 32% and decreased the placental blood flow by 61%.[193] Seventy-seven percent of the decrease in placental blood flow resulted from decreases in perfusion pressure, and 23% of the change was attributed to the increase in placental vascular resistance. Although the fetal arterial pressure increased by 16% and fetal venous pressure increased by 70%, there was no net change in fetal perfusion pressure. Fetal organ flows, vascular resistance, pH, and blood gas values also were unaffected by insufflation. Fetal hypercarbia should not occur if maternal CO_2 concentrations are maintained within normal limits. However, preliminary data in pregnant animals suggest that respiratory acidosis occurs during pneumoperitoneum despite increase in minute ventilation and normal ET_{CO_2}.[194] Furthermore, in some patients arterial CO_2 concentrations may be significantly underestimated by ET_{CO_2} values because the arterial-to-ET_{CO_2} gradient is increased in pregnant women.

Continuous transabdominal fetal heart rate monitoring is possible from approximately 18 weeks' gestation. However, many practitioners choose not to use fetal heart rate monitoring until the fetus is of viable age because little can be done to alter the course of surgery in the event of intraoperative fetal distress. On the other hand, in the event of fetal distress during laparoscopy, regardless of the gestational age, reducing abdominal insufflation pressure or deflation of the abdomen, adjusting the ventilation to normalize CO_2 concentration, or changing the patient position to optimize hemodynamics may improve the fetal environment. A transvaginal ultrasound probe, with a technician counting the fetal heart rate manually, has been used to monitor fetal heart rate during laparoscopic surgery.[182]

Laparoscopic surgery has been performed safely, without any adverse maternal or fetal outcome, in the first, second, and third trimesters of pregnancy. However, laparoscopy in the first trimester remains controversial because little is known about the effects of abdominal insufflation and CO_2 absorption on the developing fetus. Appendectomy and cholecystectomy have been performed using the laparoscopic approach as early as 8 weeks' gestation.[179,195] Because fetal organogenesis is complete by the beginning of the second trimester, it is the preferred time for surgical intervention. In addition, compared with the third trimester, the uterus does not restrict surgical access, nor is it as vulnerable to trauma during instrumentation, and the incidence of premature labor is less during the second trimester. Insufflation of CO_2 into the uterine cavity of patients undergoing tubal ligation after termination of pregnancy (12 to 14 weeks) has been reported.[196] Therefore an open technique for trocar placement is advocated in pregnant patients. A recent review of a small series of pregnant women undergoing laparoscopic surgery reported a significant fetal mortality and recommend avoiding the laparoscopic approach in this patient population.[177] Patients in the third trimester of pregnancy should not undergo laparoscopic surgery.[197] However, additional clinical and laboratory investigations are necessary to evaluate fetal risk associated with laparoscopic surgery.

The important goal of anesthesia in the pregnant patient is the maintenance of adequate uterine blood flow. Left lateral tilt (to avoid caval compression), limited IAP (12 mm Hg or lower), limited head-down or head-up tilt (10 degrees), fetal monitoring, and use of tocolytic agents when appropriate have been suggested to improve outcome after laparoscopic surgery. Many authors recommend arterial blood gas analysis to monitor arterial CO_2 concentrations in pregnant women undergoing laparoscopic surgery.

B. Pediatric patients

The development of sophisticated video equipment and scaled-down endosurgical instruments has made laparoscopic surgery practicable in the pediatric population. There is increasing interest in performing conventional procedures in pediatric surgery via the laparoscopic approach, the main areas being the intraabdominal testis, appendectomy, cholecystectomy, and pyloromyotomy. However, there is little information on the complications associated with these procedures in this group.

The differences in the abdominal anatomy of a child make the safe insertion of instruments more challenging. The liver in a child normally extends 1 to 3 cm below the right costal margin, and the spleen tip often is palpable in the left upper abdomen. A nasogastric tube should be used to decompress the stomach because it has a more horizontal orientation across the abdomen. Similarly, placement of a urinary catheter is essential because the bladder extends into the abdomen. It is important to note that the presence of an unrecognized patent processus vaginalis or hernial sac, not an uncommon feature in an infant, can lead to a painful scrotal emphysema.

The smaller peritoneal cavity in children requires smaller gas volumes for adequate insufflation. IAPs of 15 to 30 mm Hg were associated with a progressively decreasing CI in piglets.[198] In addition, IAPs greater than 15 mm Hg have been reported to decrease renal, hepatic, and intestinal blood flow in neonatal lambs.[199] Therefore low IAPs (5 to 11 mm Hg) are recommended in the pediatric population,[200] in contrast to adults, in whom IAPs are maintained around 15 mm Hg. However, there are no studies evaluating the cardiopulmonary changes in children.

Another concern in small children is the possibility of hypothermia caused by insufflation with CO_2 at room temperature. The core temperature has been reported to decrease with CO_2 insufflation during laparoscopic cholecystectomy.[45] The use of an uncuffed tracheal tube in small children is also of concern because increased intrathoracic pressures caused by pneumoperitoneum might lead to increased leak and inadequate ventilation. In addition, there is an increased risk of pulmonary aspiration caused by lack of a tracheal seal. With increased experience with laparoscopic procedures in healthy children, these procedures are now performed in children with cardiopulmonary dysfunction.[201]

VIII. MESENTERIC TRACTION SYNDROME

Traction on the abdominal mesentery and bowel manipulation is a common cause of intraoperative hemodynamic changes, particularly during major vascular surgery.[202-204] The intensity of these hemodynamic changes is variable and occasionally may be prolonged and severe.[205] The cause of this response is contradictory. It was suggested that mesenteric traction causes an afferent sympathetic stimulation that results in vasodilation of the splanchnic system and venous pooling in the splanchnic capacitance vessels.[206] However, Jacobson[207] demonstrated a constriction rather than dilation of the splanchnic vasculature upon splanchnic nerve stimulation. Seltzer et al[202] observed an increase in cardiac output and decrease in SVR, suggesting that the reduction in MAP was secondary to reduction in SVR and not caused by decreased venous return. In addition, these investigators noted flushing of the skin in the area around the head and neck during mesenteric traction. It was noted that patients receiving aspirin or ibuprofen did not have significant hemodynamic changes or increase in prostacyclin concentrations.[203,204,208] Furthermore, the time sequence between the onset of traction and the hemodynamic and cutaneous response suggested a hormonal mechanism. Local production of prostacyclin may be causative because endothelial cells lining blood vessels and the intestinal mucosa contain enzymes capable of synthesizing prostaglandins.[209]

Recent studies have documented that the cause of this hypotension is vasodilation secondary to prostacyclin (PGI_2) release from the mesentery and the bowel.[203,204,210] A significant correlation between increase in concentrations of 6-keto-prostaglandin-$F_{1\alpha}$ (a prostacyclin metabolite) and hemodynamic changes has been reported.[204,210] Hudson et al[211] compared the transabdominal and retroperitoneal approaches for aortic surgery and found that significant reduction in SVR and higher concentrations of 6-keto-prostaglandin-$F_{1\alpha}$ occurred after bowel exploration in the transabdominal group. The peak changes in 6-keto-prostaglandin-$F_{1\alpha}$ concentrations and maximum reduction in SVR occurred 10 minutes after the onset of manipulation of the abdominal contents and resolved after 30 minutes. Prophylactic administration of cyclooxygenase inhibitors (e.g., ibuprofen) has been shown to prevent the prostacyclin release and the associated hemodynamic changes.[210] However, prophylactic treatment with ibuprofen has not been adopted because of concerns regarding ibuprofen's effect on platelet aggregation, and the renal function also may be responsible. In addition, the hemodynamic changes usually are of short duration, and are treated effectively with fluid administration. In patients with persistent hypotension following mesenteric traction, administration of intravenous ketorolac may be efficacious.[212]

IX. SUMMARY

The frontiers of laparoscopic surgery have extended from gynecologic procedures to general surgical techniques. As new applications for laparoscopy continue to emerge, it is important for anesthesiologists to be familiar with the possible complications associated with the various laparoscopic procedures. Only by an appreciation of the potential complications of a procedure can we minimize their overall incidence.

The effects of pneumoperitoneum with CO_2 are complex and may combine direct mechanical compressive effects, neurohumoral responses, and changes induced by the absorbed CO_2. The cardiopulmonary changes associated with pneumoperitoneum are influenced by the degree of tilt, the patient's age, weight, and associated comorbidities (i.e., cardiac and pulmonary function), anesthetic drugs administered, and ventilatory technique. The hemodynamic changes associated with laparoscopy include reduction in CI and increase in SVR and MAP. The pulmonary changes associated with pneumoperitoneum include reduction in lung volumes and increase in peak airway pressure. In addition, the minute ventilation must be increased to maintain normocarbia. The induction of pneumoperitoneum in the horizontal position (rather than in head-up position) may decrease the severity of these hemodynamic changes. In addition, the cardiopulmonary response to laparoscopy may be avoided by limiting the degree of IAP (to 10 mm Hg)

and head-up tilt (to 10 degrees), particularly in patients with severe cardiopulmonary dysfunction.

Although it has been suggested that patients with severely impaired cardiopulmonary function should have invasive hemodynamic monitors (e.g., arterial and central venous pressure measurements), the role of these measurements remains to be determined. However, because $ETCO_2$ is a poor guide to $PaCO_2$ during laparoscopy in sick patients, monitoring of serial $PaCO_2$ concentrations may be desirable. Some patients may require pharmacologic intervention with nitroglycerin or β-adrenergic agonists. If pharmacologic interventions remain inadequate in maintaining the hemodynamic status of the patient, it may be necessary to deflate the peritoneum temporarily. After cardiopulmonary stabilization, cautious slow reinsufflation may then be attempted. However, with persistent signs of significant cardiopulmonary impairment, it may be necessary to convert to an open procedure. Further studies are necessary to assess the feasibility and safety of newer laparoscopic procedures.

REFERENCES

1. Dubois F, Berthelot G, Levard H: Laparoscopic cholecystectomy: historical perspective and personal experience, *Surg Laparosc Endosc* 1:52, 1991.
2. Wahba RWM, Beique F, Kleiman SJ: Cardiopulmonary function and laparoscopic cholecystectomy, *Can J Anaesth* 42:51, 1995.
3. Nord HJ: Complications of laparoscopy, *Endoscopy* 24:693, 1992.
4. Capelouto CC, Kavoussi LR: Complications of laparoscopic surgery, *Urology* 42:2, 1993.
5. Crist DW, Gadacz TR: Complications of laparoscopic surgery, *Surg Clin North Am* 73:265, 1993.
6. Peterson HB, Hulka JF, Phillips JM: American Association of Gynecologic Laparoscopists' 1988 membership survey on operative laparoscopy, *J Reprod Med* 35:587, 1990.
7. Riedel HH, Lehmann-Willenbrock E, Conrad P, et al: German pelviscopic statistics for the years 1978-1982, *Endoscopy* 18:219, 1986.
8. Mintz M: Risks and prophylaxis in laparoscopy: a survey of 100,000 cases, *J Reprod Med* 18:269, 1977.
9. Peterson HB, De Stefano F, Rubin GL, et al: Deaths attributable to tubal sterilization in the United States, 1977 to 1981, *Am J Obstet Gynecol* 146:131, 1983.
10. Hulka JF, Peterson HB, Phillips JM: American Association of Gynecologic Laparoscopists' 1988 membership survey on laparoscopic sterilization, *J Reprod Med* 35:584, 1990.
11. Steiner CA, Bass EB, Talamini MA, et al: Surgical rates and operative mortality for open and laparoscopic cholecystectomy in Maryland, *N Engl J Med* 330:403, 1994.
12. Phillips J, Keith D, Keith L, et al: Survey of gynecological laparoscopy for 1974, *J Reprod Med* 15:45, 1975.
13. Cuschieri A, Dubois F, Mouiel J, et al: The European experience with laparoscopic cholecystectomy, *Am J Surg* 161:385, 1991.
14. The Southern Surgeons Club: A prospective analysis of 1518 laparoscopic cholecystectomies, *N Engl J Med* 324:1073, 1991.
15. Scher KS, Scott-Conner CE: Complications of biliary surgery, *Am Surg* 53:16, 1987.
16. Holohan TV: Laparoscopic cholecystectomy, *Lancet* 338:801, 1991.
17. Deziel DJ, Millikan KW, Economou SG, et al: Complications of laparoscopic cholecystectomy: a national survey of 4292 hospitals and an analysis of 77,604 cases, *Am J Surg* 165:9, 1993.
18. Ivankovitch AD, Miletich DJ, Albrecht RF, et al: Cardiovascular effects of intraperitoneal insufflation with carbon dioxide and nitrous oxide in the dog, *Anesthesiology* 42:281, 1975.

19. Gunatilake DE: Case report: fatal intraperitoneal explosion during electrocoagulation via laparoscopy, *Int J Gynaecol Obstet* 15:353, 1978.
20. Eisenhauer DM, Saunders CJ, Ho HS, et al: Hemodynamic effects of argon pneumoperitoneum, *Surg Endosc* 8:315, 1994.
21. McMahon AJ, Baxter JN, Murray W, et al: Helium pneumoperitoneum for laparoscopic cholecystectomy: ventilatory and blood gas changes, *Br J Surg* 81:1033, 1994.
22. Mann C, Boccara G, Grevy V, et al: Argon pneumoperitoneum is more dangerous than CO_2 pneumoperitoneum during venous gas embolism, *Anesth Analg* 85:1367, 1997.
23. Croce E, Azzola M, Russo R, et al: Laparoscopic liver tumour resection with the argon beam, *Endosc Surg Allied Technol* 2:186, 1994.
24. Brantley III JC, Riley PM: Cardiovascular collapse during laparoscopy: a report of two cases, *Am J Obstet Gynecol* 159:735, 1988.
25. Shifran JL, Adlestein L, Finkler NL: Asystolic cardiac arrest: a rare complication of laparoscopy, *Obstet Gynecol* 79:840, 1992.
26. Cognat M, Gerald D, Vigneaud A: Le risque d'arret cardiaque au cours de la coelioscopie: etude a partir de 50,000 coelioscopies et d'une experimentation animale, *J Gynecol Obstet Biol Reprod* 7:925, 1976.
27. Semm K: Statistical survey of gynecological laparoscopy pelviscopy in Germany, *Endoscopy* 11:101, 1979.
28. Marshall RL, Jebson PJR, Davie IT, et al: Circulatory effects of carbon dioxide insufflation of the peritoneal cavity for laparoscopy, *Br J Anaesth* 44:680, 1972.
29. Kelman GR, Swapp GH, Smith I, et al: Cardiac output and arterial blood gas tension during laparoscopy, *Br J Anaesth* 44:1155, 1972.
30. Smith I, Benzie RJ, Gordon NL, et al: Cardiovascular effects of peritoneal insufflation of carbon dioxide for laparoscopy, *BMJ* 3:410, 1971.
31. Joris JL, Noirot DP, Legrand MJ, et al: Hemodynamic changes during laparoscopic cholecystectomy, *Anesth Analg* 76:1067, 1993.
32. Westerband A, Van De Water JM, Amzallag M, et al: Cardiovascular changes during laparoscopic cholecystectomy, *Surg Gynecol Obstet* 175:535, 1992.
33. Liu S-Y, Lieghton T, Davis I, et al: Prospective analysis of cardiopulmonary responses to laparoscopic cholecystectomy, *J Laparoendosc Surg* 1:241, 1991.
34. Talamini MA, Mendoza-Sagaon M, Gitzelmann CA, et al: Increased mediastinal pressure and decreased cardiac output during laparoscopic Nissen fundoplication, *Surgery* 122:345, 1997.
35. Odeberg S, Ljungqvist O, Svenberg T, et al: Haemodynamic effects of pneumoperitoneum and the influence of posture during anaesthesia for laparoscopic surgery, *Acta Anaesthesiol Scand* 38:276, 1994.
36. Girardis M, Broi UD, Antonutto G, et al: The effect of laparoscopic cholecystectomy on cardiovascular function and pulmonary gas exchange, *Anesth Analg* 83:134, 1996.
37. Cunningham AJ, Turner J, Rosenbaum S, et al: Transoesophageal echocardiographic assessment of haemodynamic function during laparoscopic cholecystectomy, *Br J Anaesth* 70:621, 1993.
38. O'Leary E, Hubbard K, Tormey W, et al: Laparoscopic cholecystectomy: hemodynamic and neuroendocrine responses after pneumoperitoneum and changes in position, *Br J Anaesth* 76:640, 1996.
39. Joris J, Lamy M: Neuroendocrine changes during pneumoperitoneum for laparoscopic cholecystectomy, *Br J Anaesth* 70:A33, 1993 (abstract).
40. Gannedahl P, Odeberg S, Brodin LA, et al: Effects of posture and pneumoperitoneum during anaesthesia on the indices of left ventricular filling, *Acta Anaesthesiol Scand* 40:160, 1996.
41. Diamant M, Benumof JL, Saidman LJ: Hemodynamics of increased intra-abdominal pressure: interaction with hypovolemia and halothane anesthesia, *Anesthesiology* 48:23, 1978.
42. Myles PS: Bradyarrhythmias and laparoscopy: a prospective study of heart rate changes with laparoscopy, *Aust N Z J Obstet Gynaecol* 31:171, 1991.
43. Koivusalo A-M, Kellokumpu I, Ristkari S, et al: Splanchnic and renal deterioration during and after laparoscopic cholecystectomy: a comparison of carbon dioxide pneumoperitoneum and the abdominal wall lift method, *Anesth Analg* 85:886, 1997.
44. Bongrad F, Pianim N, Dubecz S, et al: Adverse consequences of increased intra-abdominal pressure on bowel tissue oxygenation, *J Trauma* 39:519, 1995.
45. Koivusalo A-M, Kellokumpu I, Scheinin M, et al: Randomized comparison of the neuroendocrine response to laparoscopic cholecystectomy using either conventional or abdominal wall lift techniques, *Br J Surg* 83:1532, 1996.
46. Chiu A, Chang L, Birkett D, et al: The impact of pneumoperitoneum, and gasless laparoscopy on the systemic and renal hemodynamics, *J Am Coll Surg* 181:397, 1995.
47. Hein HAT, Joshi GP, Ramsay MAE, et al: Hemodynamic changes during laparoscopic cholecystectomy in patients with severe cardiopulmonary disease, *J Clin Anesth* 9:261, 1997.
48. Safran D, Sgambati S, Orlando RI: Laparoscopy in high-risk cardiac patients, *Surg Gynecol Obstet* 176:548, 1993.
49. Iwase K, Takenaka H, Yagura A, et al: Hemodynamic changes during laparoscopic cholecystectomy in patients with heart disease, *Endoscopy* 24:771, 1992.
50. Feig BW, Berger DH, Dougherty TB, et al: Pharmacologic intervention can reestablish baseline hemodynamic parameters during laparoscopy, *Surgery* 116:733, 1994.
51. Dhoste K, Lacoste L, Karayan J, et al: Haemodynamic and ventilatory changes during laparoscopic cholecystectomy in the elderly ASA III patients, *Can J Anaesth* 43:783, 1996.
52. Joshi GP, Hein HA, Ramsay MA, et al: Hemodynamic response to anesthesia and pneumoperitoneum in orthotopic cardiac transplant recipients, *Anesthesiology* 85:929, 1996.
53. Regitz V, Bossaller C, Strasser R, et al: Myocardial catecholamine content after heart transplantation, *Circulation* 82:620, 1990.
54. Clark DA, Schroeder JS, Griepp RB, et al: Cardiac transplantation in man: review of first three year's experience, *Am J Med* 54:563, 1973.
55. Tamburino C, Corcos T, Feraco E, et al: Hemodynamic parameters one and four weeks after cardiac transplantation, *Am J Cardiol* 63:635, 1989.
56. Banting S, Shimi S, Van der Velpen G, et al: Abdominal wall lift, *Surg Endosc* 7:57, 1993.
57. Lindgren L, Koivusalo A, Kellokumpu I: Conventional pneumoperitoneum compared with abdominal wall lift for laparoscopic cholecystectomy, *Br J Anaesth* 75:567, 1995.
58. Koivusalo A-M, Kellokumpu I, Scheinin M, et al: A comparison of gasless mechanical and conventional carbon dioxide pneumoperitoneum methods for laparoscopic cholecystectomy, *Anesth Analg* 86:153, 1997.
59. Wilcox S, Vandam LD: Alas, poor Trendelenburg and his position! A critique of its uses and effectiveness, *Anesth Analg* 65:574, 1988.
60. Bardoczky GI, Engelman E, Levartlet M, et al: Ventilatory effects of pneumoperitoneum monitored with continuous spirometry, *Anaesthesia* 48:309, 1993.
61. Oikkonen M, Tallgren M: Changes in respiratory compliance at laparoscopy: measurements using side stream spirometry, *Can J Anaesth* 42:495, 1995.
62. Makinen MT, Yli-Hankala A: The effect of laparoscopic cholecystectomy on respiratory compliance as determined by continuous spirometry, *J Clin Anesth* 8:119, 1996.
63. Fahy BG, Barnas GM, Flowers JL, et al: The effects of increased abdominal pressure on lung and chest wall mechanics during laparoscopic surgery, *Anesth Analg* 81:744, 1995.
64. Wittgen CM, Andrus CH, Fitzgerald SD, et al: Analysis of the hemodynamic and ventilatory effects of laparoscopic cholecystectomy, *Arch Surg* 126:997, 1991.
65. Puri GD, Singh H: Ventilatory effects of laparoscopy under general anaesthesia, *Br J Anaesth* 68:211, 1992.
66. Bures E, Fusciardi J, Lanquetot H, et al: Ventilatory effects of laparoscopic cholecystectomy, *Acta Anaesthesiol Scand* 40:566, 1996.
67. Brampton WJ, Watson RJ: Arterial to end-tidal carbon dioxide tension difference during laparoscopy: magnitude and effect of anesthetic technique, *Anaesthesia* 45:210, 1990.

68. Wahba RW, Mamazza J: Ventilatory requirements during laparoscopic cholecystectomy, *Can J Anaesth* 40:206, 1993.
69. Fitzgerald SD, Andrus CH, Baudendistel LJ, et al: Hypercarbia during carbon dioxide pneumoperitoneum, *Am J Surg* 163:186, 1992.
70. Ciofolo MJ, Clergue F, Seebacher J, et al: Ventilatory effects of laparoscopy under epidural anesthesia, *Anesth Analg* 70:357, 1990.
71. Kazama T, Ikeda K, Kato T, et al: Carbon dioxide output in laparoscopic cholecystectomy, *Br J Anaesth* 76:530, 1996.
72. Erice F, Fox GS, Salib YM, et al: Diaphragmatic function before and after laparoscopic cholecystectomy, *Anesthesiology* 79:966, 1994.
73. Sadovnikoff N, Maxwell LG: Respiratory failure after laparoscopic cholecystectomy in a patient with chronic hemidiaphragm paralysis, *Anesthesiology* 87:996, 1997.
74. Cunningham AJ, Schlanger M: Intraoperative hypoxemia complicating laparoscopic cholecystectomy in a patient with sickle hemoglobinopathy, *Anesth Analg* 75:838, 1992.
75. Tan PL, Lee TL, Tweed WA: Carbon dioxide absorption and gas exchange during pelvic laparoscopy, *Can J Anaesth* 39:677, 1992.
76. Mullet CE, Viale JP, Sagnard PE, et al: Pulmonary CO_2 elimination during surgical procedures using intra- or extraperitoneal CO_2 insufflation, *Anesth Analg* 76:622, 1993.
77. Lister DR, Rudston-Brown B, Warriner B, et al: Carbon dioxide absorption is not linearly related to intraperitoneal carbon dioxide insufflation pressures in pigs, *Anesthesiology* 80:129, 1994.
78. Liem MS, Kallewaard JW, deSmet AM, et al: Does hypercarbia develop faster during laparoscopic herniorrhaphy than during laparoscopic cholecystectomy? Assessment with continuous blood gas monitoring, *Anesth Analg* 85:1995.
79. Rasmussen JP, Dauchot PJ, De Palma RG, et al: Cardiac function and hypercarbia, *Arch Surg* 113:1196, 1978.
80. Cullen D, Eger E: Cardiovascular effects of carbon dioxide in man, *Anesthesiology* 41:345, 1974.
81. Kalhan SB, Reaney JA, Collins RL: Pneumoperitoneum and subcutaneous emphysema during laparoscopy, *Cleve Clin J Med* 57:639, 1990.
82. Holzman M, Sharp K, Richards W: Hypercarbia during carbon dioxide gas insufflation for therapeutic laparoscopy: a note of caution, *Surg Laparosc Endosc* 1:11, 1992.
83. Shantha TR, Harden J: Laparoscopic cholecystectomy: anesthesia-related complications and guidelines, *Surg Laparosc Endosc* 1:173, 1991.
84. Kent III RB: Subcutaneous emphysema and hypercarbia following laparoscopic cholecystectomy, *Arch Surg* 126:1154, 1991.
85. Clarke CC, Weeks DB, Gudson JP: Venous carbon dioxide embolism during laparoscopy, *Anesth Analg* 56:650, 1977.
86. Root B, Levy MN, Pollack EA: Gas embolism death after laparoscopy delayed by "trapping" in the portal circulation, *Anesth Analg* 57:232, 1978.
87. Yacoub OF, Cardona IJ, Coveler LA, et al: Carbon dioxide embolism during laparoscopy, *Anesthesiology* 57:533, 1982.
88. Shulman D, Aronson HB: Capnography in the early diagnosis of carbon dioxide embolism during laparoscopy, *Can Anaesth Soc J* 31:455, 1984.
89. de Plater RM, Jones IS: Non-fatal carbon dioxide embolism during laparoscopy, *Anaesth Intensive Care* 17:359, 1989.
90. Ostman PL, Pantle-Fisher FH, Faure EA, et al: Circulatory collapse during laparoscopy, *J Clin Anesth* 2:129, 1990.
91. Greville AC, Clements EA, Erwin DC, et al: Pulmonary air embolism during laparoscopic laser cholecystectomy, *Anaesthesia* 46:113, 1991.
92. McGrath RB, Zimmerman JE, Williams JF, et al: Carbon dioxide embolism treated with hyperbaric oxygen, *Can J Anaesth* 36:586, 1989.
93. Diakun TA: Carbon dioxide embolism: successful resuscitation with cardiopulmonary bypass, *Anesthesiology* 74:1151, 1991.
94. Beck DH, McQuillan PJ: Fatal carbon dioxide embolism and severe haemorrhage during laparoscopic salpingectomy, *Br J Anaesth* 72:243, 1994.
95. Wadhwa RK, McKenzie R, Wadhwa SR, et al: Gas embolism during laparoscopy, *Anesthesiology* 48:74, 1978.
96. Derouin M, Couture P, Boudreault D, et al: Detection of gas embolism by transesophageal echocardiography during laparoscopic cholecystectomy, *Anesth Analg* 82:119, 1996.
97. Maunder RJ, Pierson DJ, Hudson LD: Subcutaneous and mediastinal emphysema, pathophysiology, diagnosis, and management, *Arch Intern Med* 144:1447, 1984.
98. Hasel R, Arora SK, Hickey DR: Intraoperative complications of laparoscopic cholecystectomy, *Can J Anaesth* 40:459, 1993.
99. Bard PA, Chen L: Subcutaneous emphysema associated with laparoscopy, *Anesth Analg* 71:101, 1990.
100. Doctor NH, Hussain Z: Bilateral pneumothorax associated with laparoscopy: a case report of a rare hazard and review of the literature, *Anaesthesia* 28:75, 1973.
101. Whiston RJ, Eggers KA, Morris RW, et al: Tension pneumothorax during laparoscopic cholecystectomy, *Br J Surg* 78:1325, 1991.
102. Gabbott DA, Dunckley AB, Roberts FL: Carbon dioxide pneumothorax occurring during laparoscopic cholecystectomy, *Anaesthesia* 47:587, 1992.
103. Nicholson RD, Berman ND: Pneumopericardium following laparoscopy, *Chest* 76:605, 1979.
104. Herrerias J, Ariza A, Garrido M: An unusual complication of laparoscopy: pneumopericardium, *Endoscopy* 12: 254-5, 1991.
105. Knos GB, Sung YF, Toledo A: Pneumopericardium associated with laparoscopy, *J Clin Anesth* 3: 56-9, 1991.
106. Hall D, Goldstein A, Tynan E, et al: Profound hypercarbia late in the course of laparoscopic cholecystectomy: detection by continuous capnometry, *Anesthesiology* 79:173, 1993.
107. Pearce DJ: Respiratory acidosis and subcutaneous emphysema during laparoscopic cholecystectomy, *Can J Anaesth* 41:314, 1994.
108. Hasson HM: A modified instrument and method for laparoscopy, *Am J Obstet Gynecol* 110:886, 1971.
109. McDonald PT, Rich NM, Collins GJ, et al: Vascular trauma secondary to diagnostic and therapeutic procedure: laparoscopy, *Am J Surg* 135:651, 1978.
110. Katz M, Beck P, Tancer ML: Major vessel injury during laparoscopy: anatomy of two cases, *Am J Obstet Gynecol* 135:544, 1979.
111. Peterson HB, Greenspan JR, Ory HW: Death following puncture of the aorta during laparoscopic sterilization, *Obstet Gynecol* 59:133, 1982.
112. Baadsgard SE, Bille S, Egeblad K: Major vascular injury during gynecologic laparoscopy: report of a case and review of published cases, *Acta Obstet Gynaecol Scand* 68:283, 1989.
113. Esposito JM: Hematoma of the sigmoid colon as a complication of laparoscopy, *Am J Obstet Gynecol* 117:581, 1973.
114. Pring DW: Inferior epigastric hemorrhage: an avoidable complication of laparoscopic clip sterilization, *Br J Obstet Gynaecol* 90:480, 1983.
115. Green LS, Loughlin KR, Kavoussi LR: Management of epigastric vessel injury during laparoscopy, *J Endourol* 6:99, 1992.
116. Reynolds RC, Fauca AL: Gastric perforation, an anesthesia-induced hazard in laparoscopy, *Anesthesiology* 38:84, 1973.
117. Thompson BH, Wheeless CRJ: Gastrointestinal complications of laparoscopy sterilization, *Obstet Gynecol* 41:669, 1973.
118. Dancygier H, Jacob RA: Splenic rupture during laparoscopy, *Gastrointest Endosc* 29:63, 1983 (letter).
119. Yuzpe AA: Pneumoperitoneum needle and trocar injuries in laparoscopy, a survey on possible contributing factors and prevention, *J Reprod Med* 35:485, 1990.
120. Salzstein EC, Schwartz SF, Levinson CJ: Perforation of the small intestine secondary to laparoscopic tubal cauterization, *Ann Surg* 177:34, 1973.
121. Vegfors M, Engborg L, Gupta A, et al: Changes in end-tidal carbon dioxide during gynecologic laparoscopy: spontaneous versus controlled ventilation, *J Clin Anesth* 6:199, 1994.
122. Duffy BL: Regurgitation during pelvic laparoscopy, *Br J Anaesth* 51:1089, 1979.
123. Jones MJ, Mitchell RW, Hindocha N: Effect of increased intra-abdominal pressure during laparoscopy on the lower esophageal sphincter, *Anesth Analg* 68:63, 1989.

124. Bapat PP, Verghese C: Laryngeal mask airway and the incidence of regurgitation during gynecological laparoscopies, *Anesth Analg* 85:139, 1997.

125. Scott DB: Regurgitation during laparoscopy, *Br J Anaesth* 52:559, 1980 (letter).

126. Goodwin APL, Rowe WL, Ogg TW: Day case laparoscopy: a comparison of two anaesthetic techniques using laryngeal mask during spontaneous breathing, *Anaesthesia* 47:892, 1992.

127. Verghese C, Brimacombe JR: Survey of laryngeal mask airway usage in 11,910 patients: safety and efficacy for conventional and nonconventional usage, *Anesth Analg* 82:129, 1996.

128. Burton A, Steinbrook RA: Precipitous decrease in oxygen saturation during laparoscopic surgery, *Anesth Analg* 76:1177, 1993.

129. Eger E II, Saidman LJ: Hazards of nitrous oxide anesthesia in bowel obstruction and pneumothorax, *Anesthesiology* 26:61, 1965.

130. Scheinin B, Lindgren L, Scheinin TM: Perioperative nitrous oxide delays bowel function after colonic surgery, *Br J Anaesth* 64:154, 1990.

131. Taylor E, Feinstein R, White PF, et al: Anesthesia for laparoscopic cholecystectomy. Is nitrous oxide contraindicated? *Anesthesiology* 76:541, 1992.

132. Erkola O: Nitrous oxide: laparoscopic surgery, bowel function, and PONV, *Acta Anaesthesiol Scand* 38:767, 1994.

133. Sukhani R, Lurie J, Jabamoni R: Propofol for ambulatory gynecologic laparoscopy: does omission of nitrous oxide alter postoperative emetic sequelae and recovery? *Anesth Analg* 78:831, 1994.

134. Neuman GG, Sidebotham G, Negoianu E, et al: Laparoscopy explosion hazards with nitrous oxide, *Anesthesiology* 78:875, 1993.

135. Radnay PA, Brodman E, Mankikar D, et al: The effect of equianalgesic doses of fentanyl, morphine, meperidine, and pentazocine on common bile duct pressure, *Anaesthetist* 29:26, 1980.

136. Jones RM, Detmer M, Hill AB, et al: Incidence of choledochoduodenal sphincter spasm during fentanyl-supplemented anesthesia, *Anesth Analg* 60:638, 1981.

137. Wahba RWM: Perioperative functional residual capacity, *Can J Anaesth* 38:384, 1991.

138. Hall C, Tarala RA, Hall L, et al: A multivariate analysis of the risk of pulmonary complications after laparotomy, *Chest* 99:923, 1991.

139. Craig DB: Postoperative recovery of pulmonary function, *Anesth Analg* 60:46, 1981.

140. Frazee RC, Roberts JW, Okeson GC, et al: Open versus closed laparoscopic cholecystectomy: a comparison of postoperative pulmonary function, *Ann Surg* 214:651, 1991.

141. Joris J, Cigarini I, Legrand M, et al: Metabolic and respiratory changes after cholecystectomy performed via laparotomy and laparoscopy, *Br J Anaesth* 69:341, 1992.

142. Rademaker BM, Ringers J, Odoom JA, et al: Pulmonary function and stress response after laparoscopic cholecystectomy: comparison with subcostal incision and influence of thoracic epidural analgesia, *Anesth Analg* 75:381, 1992.

143. Putensen-Himmer G, Putensen C, Lammer H, et al: Comparison of postoperative respiratory function after laparoscopic or laparotomy for cholecystectomy, *Anesthesiology* 77:675, 1992.

144. Ponsky JL: Complications of laparoscopic cholecystectomy, *Am J Surg* 161:393, 1991.

145. Joris J, Thiry E, Paris P, et al: Pain after laparoscopic cholecystectomy: characteristics and effect of intraperitoneal bupivacaine, *Anesth Analg* 81:379, 1995.

146. Frazer RA, Hotz SB, Hurtig JB, et al: The prevalence and impact of pain after day-care tubal ligation surgery, *Pain* 39:189, 1989.

147. Edwards ND, Barclay K, Catling SJ, et al: Day case laparoscopy: a survey of postoperative pain and an assessment of the value of diclofenac, *Anaesthesia* 46:1077, 1991.

148. Chi I-C, Cole LP: Incidence of pain among women undergoing laparoscopic sterilization by electrocoagulation, the spring-loaded clip, and the tubal ring, *Am J Obstet Gynecol* 135:397, 1979.

149. Dahl JB, Rosenberg J, Dirkes WE, et al: Prevention of postoperative pain by balanced analgesia, *Br J Anaesth* 64:518, 1990.

150. Michaloliakou C, Chung F, Sharma S: Preoperative multimodal analgesia facilitates recovery after ambulatory laparoscopic cholecystectomy, *Anesth Analg* 82:44, 1996.

151. McKenzie R, Phitayakorn P, Uy NT, et al: Topical bupivacaine and etidocaine analgesia following fallopian tube banding, *Can J Anaesth* 36:510, 1989.

152. Baram D, Smith C, Stinson S: Intraoperative etidocaine for reducing pain after laparoscopic tubal ligation, *J Reprod Med* 35:407, 1990.

153. Kaplan P, Freund R, Squires J, et al: Control of immediate postoperative pain with topical bupivacaine hydrochloride for laparoscopic Falope ring tubal ligation, *Obstet Gynecol* 76:798, 1990.

154. Van Ee R, Hemrika DJ, De Blok S, et al: Effects of ketoprofen and mesosalpinx infiltration on postoperative pain after laparoscopic sterilization, *Obstet Gynecol* 88:568, 1996.

155. Narchi P, Benhamou D, Fernandez H: Intraperitoneal local anesthetic for shoulder pain after day-case laparoscopy, *Lancet* 338:1569, 1991.

156. Rademaker BM, Kalkman CJ, Odoom JA, et al: Intraperitoneal local anaesthetics after laparoscopic cholecystectomy: effects on postoperative pain, metabolic responses and lung function, *Br J Anaesth* 72:263, 1994.

157. Pasqualucci A, de Angelis V, Contardo R, et al: Preemptive analgesia: intraperitoneal local anesthetic in laparoscopic cholecystectomy: a randomized, double-blind, placebo-controlled study, *Anesthesiology* 85:11, 1996.

158. Mraovic B, Jurisic T, Kogler-Majeric V, et al: Intraperitoneal bupivacaine for analgesia after laparoscopic cholecystectomy, *Acta Anaesthesiol Scand* 41:193, 1997.

159. Comfort VK, Code WE, Rooney ME, et al: Naproxen premedication reduces postoperative tubal ligation pain, *Can J Anaesth* 4:349, 1992.

160. Rosenblum M, Weller RS, Conard PL, et al: Ibuprofen provides longer lasting analgesia than fentanyl after laparoscopic surgery, *Anesth Analg* 73:250, 1991.

161. Liu J, Ding Y, White PF, et al: Effects of ketorolac on postoperative analgesia and ventilatory function after laparoscopic cholecystectomy, *Anesth Analg* 76:1061, 1993.

162. White PF, Joshi GP, Carpenter RL, et al: A comparison of oral ketorolac and hydrocodone-acetaminophen for analgesia after ambulatory surgery: arthroscopy versus laparoscopic tubal ligation, *Anesth Analg* 85:37, 1997.

163. Joshi GP: Postoperative pain management, *Int Anesthesiol Clin* 32:113, 1994.

164. Smith I, Ding Y, White PF: Muscle pain after outpatient laparoscopy: influence of propofol versus thiopental and enflurane, *Anesth Analg* 76:1181, 1993.

165. Tang J, Joshi GP, White PF: Comparison of rocuronium and mivacurium to succinylcholine during outpatient laparoscopic surgery, *Anesth Analg* 82:994, 1996.

166. Beebe D, McNevin M, Belani K, et al: Evidence of venous stasis after abdominal insufflation for laparoscopic cholecystectomy, *Surg Gynecol Obstet* 176:443, 1993.

167. Goodale RL, Beebe DS, McNevin MP, et al: Hemodynamic, respiratory, and metabolic effects of laparoscopic cholecystectomy, *Am J Surg* 166:533, 1993.

168. Scott TR, Zucker KA, Bailey RW: Laparoscopic cholecystectomy: a review of 12,397 patients, *Surg Laparosc Endosc* 2:191, 1992.

169. Collins R, Scrimgeour A, Yusuf S, et al: Reduction in fatal pulmonary embolism and venous thrombosis by perioperative administration of subcutaneous heparin, *N Engl J Med* 318:1162, 1988.

170. Johnston RV, Lawson NW, Nealson WH: Lower extremity neuropathy after laparoscopic cholecystectomy, *Anesthesiology* 77:835, 1992 (letter).

171. Cava A, Roman J, Gonzalez Quintela A, et al: Subcutaneous metastasis following laparoscopy in gastric adenocarcinoma, *Eur J Surg Oncol* 16:63, 1990.

172. Mazze RI, Kallen B: Reproductive outcome following anesthesia and operation during pregnancy: a registry of 5405 cases, *Am J Obstet Gynecol* 161:1178, 1989.

173. Mazze RI, Kallen B: Appendectomy during pregnancy: a Swedish registry of 778 cases, *Obstet Gynecol* 77:835, 1991.

174. Samuellson S, Sjovall A: Laparoscopy in suspected ectopic pregnancy, *Acta Obstet Gynecol Scand* 51:31, 1972.

175. Gadacz TR, Talamini MA: Traditional versus laparoscopic cholecystectomy, *Am J Surg* 161:336, 1991.

176. Talamini MA: Controversies in laparoscopic cholecystectomy: contraindications, cholangiography, pregnancy, and avoidance of complications, *Baillieres Clin Gastroenterol* 7:881, 1993.

177. Amos JD, Schorr SJ, Norman PF, et al: Laparoscopic surgery during pregnancy, *Am J Surg* 171:435, 1996.

178. Steinbrook RA, Brooks DC, Datta S: Laparoscopic cholecystectomy during pregnancy: review of anesthetic management, surgical considerations, *Surg Endosc* 10:511, 1996.

179. Shaked G, Twena M, Charuzi I: Laparoscopic cholecystectomy for empyema of gallbladder during pregnancy, *Surg Laparosc* 4:65, 1994.

180. Costantino GN, Vincent GJ, Mukalian GG, et al: Laparoscopic cholecystectomy in pregnancy, *J Laparoendosc Surg* 4:161, 1994.

181. Edelman DS: Alternative laparoscopic technique for cholecystectomy during pregnancy, *Surg Endosc* 8:794, 1994.

182. Hart RO, Tamadon A, Fitzgibbons RJJ, et al: Open laparoscopic cholecystectomy in pregnancy, *Surg Laparosc Endosc* 3:13, 1993.

183. Jackson SJ, Sigman HH: Laparoscopic cholecystectomy in pregnancy, *J Laparoendosc Surg* 3:35, 1993.

184. Pucci RO, Seed RW: Case report of laparoscopic cholecystectomy in the third trimester of pregnancy, *Am J Obstet Gynecol* 165:401, 1991.

185. Rusher AH, Fields B, Henson K: Laparoscopic cholecystectomy in pregnancy: contraindicated or indicated? *J Ark Med Soc* 89:383, 1993.

186. Soper NJ, Hunter JG, Petrie RH: Laparoscopic cholecystectomy during pregnancy, *Surg Endosc* 6:115, 1992.

187. Weber AM, Bloom GP, Allan TR, et al: Laparoscopic cholecystectomy during pregnancy, *Obstet Gynecol* 78:958, 1991.

188. Arvidsson D, Gerdin E: Laparoscopic cholecystectomy during pregnancy, *Surg Laparosc Endosc* 3:193, 1991.

189. Eldering SC: Laparoscopic cholecystectomy in pregnancy, *Am J Surg* 165:625, 1993.

190. Morrell DG, Mullins JR, Harrison PB: Laparoscopic cholecystectomy during pregnancy in symptomatic patients, *Surgery* 112:856, 1992.

191. Schorr RT: Laparoscopic cholecystectomy and pregnancy, *J Laparoendosc Surg* 3:291, 1993.

192. Reedy M: Laparoscopy during pregnancy, *SLS Rep* 3:3, 1994.

193. Barnard JM, Chaffin D, Droste S, et al: Fetal response to carbon dioxide pneumoperitoneum in pregnant ewe, *Obstet Gynecol* 85:669, 1995.

194. Galan HL, Reedy MB, Bean JD, et al: Maternal and fetal effects of laparoscopic insufflation, *Anesthesiology* 81:A1159, 1994.

195. Schreiber JH: Laparoscopic appendectomy in pregnancy, *Surg Endosc* 4:100, 1990.

196. Barnet MB, Liu DT: Complications of laparoscopy during early pregnancy, *BMJ* 23:1974 (letter).

197. NIH Consensus Development Panel: Gallstones and laparoscopic cholecystectomy, *Surg Endosc* 7:271, 1993.

198. Lynch FP, Ochi T, Scully M, et al: Cardiovascular effects of increased intra-abdominal pressure in newborn piglets, *J Pediatr Surg* 9:621, 1974.

199. Masey SA, Koehler RC, Buck JR, et al: Effect of abdominal distention on central and regional hemodynamics in neonatal lambs, *Pediatr Res* 19:1244, 1985.

200. Walsh MT, Vetter TR: Anesthesia for pediatric laparoscopic cholecystectomy, *J Clin Anesth* 4:406, 1992.

201. Tobais JD, Holcomb GW: Anesthetic management for laparoscopic cholecystectomy in children with decreased myocardial function: two case reports, *J Pediatr Surg* 32:743, 1997.

202. Seltzer JL, Ritter DE, Starsnic MA, et al: The hemodynamic response to traction on the abdominal mesentery, *Anesthesiology* 63:96, 1985.

203. Seltzer JL, Goldberg ME, Larijani GE, et al: Prostacyclin mediation of vasodilation following mesenteric traction, *Anesthesiology* 68:514, 1988.

204. Gottlieb A, Skrinska VA, O'Hara P, et al: The role of prostacyclin in the mesenteric traction syndrome during abdominal aortic reconstructive surgery, *Ann Surg* 209:363, 1989.

205. Greek CRJ, Couper NB: Prolonged hypotension secondary to mesenteric traction during a transabdominal aneurysm, *J Cardiothorac Anesth* 3:341, 1989.

206. Batchelder BM, Cooperman LH: Effects of anesthetics on splanchnic circulation and metabolism, *Surg Clin North Am* 55:787, 1975.

207. Jacobson ED: Control of the splanchnic circulation, *Yale J Biol Med* 50:301, 1977.

208. Utsunomiya T, Krausz MM, Dunham B, et al: Maintenance of cardiodynamics with aspirin during abdominal aortic aneurysmectomy, *Ann Surg* 194:602, 1981.

209. Balaa MA, Powell DW: Prostaglandin synthesis by enterocyte microsomes of rabbit small intestine, *Prostaglandins* 31:609, 1986.

210. Hudson JC, Wurm WH, O'Donnell TFJ, et al: Ibuprofen pretreatment inhibits prostacyclin release during abdominal exploration in aortic surgery, *Anesthesiology* 72:443, 1990.

211. Hudson JC, Wurm WH, O'Donnell TF, et al: Hemodynamics and prostacyclin release in the early phases of aortic surgery: comparison of transabdominal and retroperitoneal approaches, *Vasc Surg* 7:190, 1988.

212. Latson TW, Reinhart DJ, Allison PM, et al: Ketorolac tromethamine may be efficacious in treating hypotension from mesenteric traction, *J Cardiothorac Vasc Anesth* 6:456, 1992.

Chapter 29

Perioperative Embolic Complications

Levon M. Capan
Sanford M. Miller

Surgery and related interventional procedures are important factors in the development of embolic events. These potentially fatal and highly morbid complications not only challenge the anesthesiologist's perioperative diagnostic and therapeutic skills, but also may have medicolegal implications such as the differentiation of fatal massive embolism from preventable causes of perioperative death or determination of the appropriateness of prophylactic measures in a given patient.[1] Although the occurrence rates of some types of perioperative embolic complications have been reported, the overall incidence of surgery-related embolism has not been determined. However, it is well known that it is less common than other anesthetic complications, especially during the intraoperative period. The type, frequency, and timing of perioperative embolism are related primarily to the procedure performed, but other factors, such as the patient's clinical condition and the extent, appropriateness, and timing of preventive measures, may also play important roles.

Surgery may result in venous or arterial embolism by blood clot, fat, gas, tissue, or foreign substances. The causes, pathogenesis, clinical presentation, and management differ depending on the site of the embolism and the material embolized. For example, the primary pathophysiologic process in pulmonary embolism (PE) involves obstruction of the pulmonary artery (PA) or its major branches if the embolized material consists of clot or tumor, whereas fat and amniotic fluid affect primarily the lung microvasculature, often producing a clinical picture similar to that of acute respiratory distress syndrome (ARDS). Thus the clinical aspects of each type of surgically induced embolism are discussed separately. Primary importance is given to thromboembolism because of its frequent occurrence. Issues that are common for other embolic phenomena also are discussed in the venous thromboembolism section.

I. VENOUS AND PARADOXICAL EMBOLISM

The vast majority of perioperative embolic complications are caused by material developing in or entering the venous system and traversing the peripheral and central veins to the right heart and the PAs. As discussed later, the mechanisms by which emboli lodge in the venous system vary depending on the type of embolizing material and the procedure causing the complication. Under certain conditions emboli may enter the left heart via cardiac septal defects or intrapulmonary arteriovenous channels, resulting in paradoxical embolism to the systemic circulation. Because of the excellent filtering capability of the lung, small quantities of embolized material within the venous system generally do not produce clinically important deleterious effects if paradoxical embolism does not occur.

A. Paradoxical embolism

As suggested by Johnson,[2] three conditions are necessary for paradoxical embolism to occur: presence of embolizing material in the venous system, an abnormal anatomic communication between the right and left sides of the

heart, and an intracardiac pressure gradient promoting right-to-left shunting. Of course, clinical, angiographic, or pathologic evidence of arterial embolism should be present to establish this diagnosis. Even then, unless the passage of emboli through a septal defect into the left heart is actually observed with two-dimensional (2-D) echocardiography,[3] the diagnosis remains presumptive in most cases. Thus other causes of systemic emboli, such as atrial fibrillation, left-sided thrombi, or valvular vegetations should be ruled out before the diagnosis of paradoxical embolism is entertained.

Thrombi and air are the substances most often involved in paradoxical embolism; septic vegetations from the tricuspid valve, fat, tumor, and amniotic fluid also may produce systemic emboli. Although interventricular defects and pulmonary arteriovenous shunts can allow passage of embolizing substances,[4,5] the vast majority of paradoxical emboli pass through interatrial communications. Patent foramen ovale (PFO) is the most common lesion, with an incidence of 27.3% (range 25% to 35%) in postmortem examination of an unselected population.[6] Because of the lower sensitivity of imaging techniques, echocardiographic studies demonstrate an incidence of about 10%.[7,8] In 98% of the population the size of the defect is less than 10 mm (mean size 4.9 mm, range 1 to 19 mm).[6] Furthermore, most PFOs are only potentially patent (probe patent) and open only when there is a significant interatrial pressure gradient. In an interesting study, Hausmann, Mugge, and Daniel[9] demonstrated that patients with PFO in whom a cerebral ischemic event was thought to be caused by paradoxical embolism had wider foramina and greater right-to-left shunting than those with PFO whose ischemia was from other causes. Although the high frequency of interatrial communication and the low incidence of paradoxical embolism preclude establishing a definite cause-and-effect relationship between the two, a higher incidence of PFO has been demonstrated in patients with embolic ischemia that could not be explained by any other cause.[6,10,11]

Another abnormality that may permit right-to-left shunting in up to 90% of cases is atrial septal aneurysm; it has been identified in 1% of autopsy and 0.2% of echocardiographic studies. It involves bulging of the fossa ovalis depending on the pressure interaction between the atria. Echocardiographic criteria of this lesion include a greater than 10-mm protrusion of all parts of the atrial septum from the central plane, greater than 15-mm excursion of the septum during the cardiac cycle, and greater than 15-mm diameter for the base of the aneurysm.[6,12] Patients with atrial septal aneurysm have a higher incidence of PFO (33%) than the normal population (27.3%); the occurrence of atrial septal defects and atrial thrombi also is higher, increasing the likelihood of systemic embolism. Of the 195 patients with atrial septal aneurysm in one study, 38 had atrial septal defect, 65 PFO, and 3 sinus venosus defect.[12]

A right-to-left shunt is the final prerequisite for an embolus to cross an interatrial defect. Major acute PE with associated PA and right heart hypertension can produce a fixed pressure gradient between the atria during all phases of the cardiac cycle and thus promote paradoxical embolism. A correlation between the severity of pulmonary thromboembolism (PTE) and the frequency of right-to-left shunting via a PFO has been shown even in hemodynamically stable patients without preexisting cardiopulmonary disease.[13] Transient reversal of the interatrial pressure gradient during the cardiac cycle also has the potential to cause paradoxical embolism. In susceptible patients, a small amount of right-to-left shunting normally occurs during the onset of ventricular contraction and in early diastole.[14] In the presence of a large septal defect, this can lead to entry of an embolus into the left side of the heart. Studies in patients with atrial septal defects using oximetric analysis, dye dilution, fiberoptic catheters, intracardiac Doppler, and transthoracic echocardiography (TTE) have all demonstrated varying degrees of right-to-left shunting.[6] Patient position is also likely to affect the direction of flow between the atria. Left lateral decubitus and erect postures place the left atrium in a relatively dependent position, facilitating right-to-left shunt.[6] However, there are more serious causes of right-to left shunting during the perianesthetic period. Agitation, straining, bucking, and coughing in spontaneously breathing patients may cause the right atrial pressure (RAP) to exceed that of the left atrium and potentially lead to paradoxical embolism.[15] In normal subjects, Valsalva maneuver or straining may cause a decrease in volume and increase in pressure of the right atrium; increased intrathoracic pressure limits the venous return and thus cardiac filling. In patients with atrial septal defects, the right atrium is filled from the left side; thus changes in intrathoracic pressure cause little change in atrial filling. However, during the release phase of the Valsalva maneuver, a sudden volume increase in the right atrium can lead to right-to-left shunting.[6]

Intrathoracic pressure increases during positive-pressure ventilation but usually not to the levels produced by a Valsalva maneuver. The effect of positive-pressure ventilation on the pressure gradient between the right and left atria probably depends on the peak airway pressure, on the patient's position, and on whether positive end-expiratory pressure (PEEP) is applied. Unless an airway pressure of 20 cm H_2O is sustained for at least 5 seconds, ventilation with zero end-expiratory pressure does not seem to cause right-to-left shunt, but shunting may occur during the release phase when 20 cm H_2O PEEP is added to a high tidal volume.[16,17] Do lower levels of PEEP facilitate interatrial right-to-left shunting? Studies performed to explore the mechanism of venous air embolism (VAE) in sitting neurosurgical patients have found conflicting results. In the study of Perkins and Bedford,[18] of 11 patients only 2 had RAP exceeding pulmonary capillary wedge pressure (PCWP) initially; the corresponding number was 7 after institution of 10 cm H_2O PEEP. The studies by Pearl and Larson[19] in dogs and by Zasslow et al[20] in humans demonstrated that up to 10 cm H_2O PEEP did not cause any change in the PCWP-RAP gradient because the increased intrathoracic pressure affects both atria. Indirect measurement of the left atrial pressure through PCWP, and measuring PCWP

and RAP during end-expiration instead of immediately after releasing PEEP when the gradient is most likely to be positive,[21] precludes extrapolation of these findings into clinical practice. It probably is prudent to avoid PEEP whenever the likelihood of paradoxical embolism exists, unless it is essential to improve oxygenation.

The disastrous potential consequences of paradoxical embolism necessitate effective prophylaxis. Several general aspects must be addressed: preventing the development and circulation of embolic material, recognizing patients with interatrial defects preoperatively and planning for surgery appropriately, monitoring for paradoxical embolism during the operative procedure, preventing right-to-left shunt, and treating the complications of systemic embolism. Prevention is discussed in the specific sections of this chapter.

B. Imaging of interatrial communications before surgery

Echocardiography (M-mode, 2-D transthoracic, and phased array 2-D transesophageal) and Doppler techniques have revolutionized the diagnosis of interatrial septal abnormalities. Currently the best window to the septum is 2-D transesophageal echocardiography (TEE). Evaluation of the interatrial septum requires the use of an echogenic contrast medium; agitated saline, gelatin, or albumin that contains microbubbles of air can be used for this purpose. The technique involves asking the patient to strain or perform a Valsalva maneuver and then injecting the contrast intravenously over a 2- to 3-second period just before the release of the strain. Appearance of contrast in the left atrium within one to four beats of injection indicates interatrial communication; transpulmonary passage requires a longer time. This technique has been used before craniotomy in sitting position,[8] but it can be used in other clinical settings that carry a high risk of paradoxical embolism.

Transcranial Doppler (TCD) is another study that has been used to detect right-to-left shunting. Because it is noninvasive and requires minimal or no sedation, patients may perform a stronger Valsalva maneuver than during TEE and thus produce a greater interatrial gradient. TCD has been used alone and in combination TEE. Using predetermined criteria (i.e., more th microbubbles in the middle cerebral artery within 10 seconds of contrast injection), a preliminary study found this technique both sensitive and specific. Using oxypolygelatin for contrast in conjunction with the Valsalva maneuver provided better results than saline and cough.[22] The contrast TCD appears to be slightly more reliable than the contrast TEE and is able to recognize both minimal and massive interatrial shunts.[23] Combining the two techniques increases the rate of PFO detection.[23] In many centers the presence of interatrial defect is an important factor in the decision to avoid the sitting position for posterior fossa surgery in favor of a position with less likelihood of VAE.

As mentioned previously, the ability of contrast TEE and TCD to identify PFO is not absolute. Thus intraoperative paradoxical embolism may occur even if this lesion is excluded with one or both of these tests. Contrast TEE can be performed after induction of anesthesia using provocative maneuvers including ventilation with PEEP (20 cm H_2O) and high (1200 ml) tidal volumes.[17] This test appears to be more effective in diagnosing PFO than Valsalva in spontaneously breathing subjects or release of sustained inspiratory pressure in anesthetized patients.[17] In some situations intraoperative TEE can be helpful not only in recognizing right-to-left shunt, but also in demonstrating the entrance of embolic material into the left ventricle.[3,24] Once a PFO is recognized, paradoxical embolization may be prevented by anticoagulation, thrombolysis, or surgical thrombectomy and closure of the defect, depending on the clinical circumstances.[24-26] Once systemic embolization occurs, treatment is limited to prevention of further embolic events by chronic anticoagulation and, in selected patients, by surgical repair of the interatrial defect.[27] In cerebral air embolism, hyperbaric O_2 treatment may be effective if it is applied within a few hours after the embolic event.[28]

II. THROMBOEMBOLISM

Thromboembolism is the most common postoperative embolic complication; it is rare during the preoperative and intraoperative periods. The overall prevalence of venous thromboembolism in the United States is estimated to be 600,000 cases per year.[29] Only about 260,000 patients are treated medically because more than half of the embolic events are asymptomatic. In addition, many patients who present with typical signs and symptoms do not have the disease.[29] The overall annual mortality directly related to this complication is estimated to be between 50,000 and 100,000, representing 5% to 10% of all deaths in U.S. hospitals.[29] Major surgery is an important risk factor for the development of thromboembolism. Although the fraction of thromboembolic events caused by surgery is not known, a deep vein thrombosis (DVT) registry in a major tertiary-care hospital demonstrated that in almost half of the patients, DVT developed within 6 months of surgery; orthopedic, general abdominal, neurosurgical, thoracic, and cardiovascular procedures had the highest risk.[30] Major urologic, gynecologic, and trauma surgery is also considered to carry a high risk for thromboembolism.[31-33]

The overall potential risk of thromboembolism in general surgical, orthopedic, and urologic procedures is 14.5% for DVT, 2% for nonfatal PTE, and 0.7% for fatal PTE.[31] The corresponding figures for individual surgical specialties are shown in Table 29-1.[34-37] These figures are from patients who received the standard prophylaxis

Table 29-1. Approximate potential and generally achievable rates of thromboembolic complications after different types of surgery

Surgical specialty	DVT rate (%)	Nonfatal PTE rate (%)	Fatal PTE rate (%)	Reference
General surgery				
Potential	12 (8.3-13.9)	0.65 (0.54-0.84)	0.46 (0.024-0.84)	31
Achievable	5 (2.4-6.2)	0.34 (0.21-0.62)	0.11 (0.04-0.26)	31
Elective orthopedic surgery				
Potential	36	6.8-8.5	1.6	31
Achievable	17	6.8-8.5	0	31
Emergency orthopedic surgery				
Potential	49	0-1	2.3	31
Achievable	26	0-1	1.6	31
Vascular surgery				
Potential	16-18	1	0	37
Achievable	10	0.7	0	36
Urologic surgery				
Potential	30	1.13	0.57	31
Achievable	10	0	0	31
Neurosurgery				
Potential	29-43	5.7	3	34
Achievable	5.6	0.2	0.07	35
Major trauma				
Potential	58 (Proximal vein 18)	2-5	0.5-3	32
Achievable	6-15	1-1.5*	0.1-0.2*	33

*Estimated figures after prophylactic Greenfield filter placement.
DVT, Deep vein thrombosis; *PTE,* pulmonary thromboembolism.

used in the 1970s and 1980s. With modern preventive measures, thromboembolic complications have decreased by about 50% to 70%. Table 29-2 shows the specific procedures performed by each surgical specialty that carry an increased risk of perioperative thromboembolism. Additional procedures may rarely be complicated by thromboembolism. For example, despite the commonly observed hypocoagulable state, PTE may develop during orthotopic liver transplantation because of a combination of factors, such as the use of aprotinin and fresh frozen plasma and inferior vena cava obstruction by the large native liver.[38,39] Likewise, PTE may occur after lung transplantation as a result of promotion of clot formation at a stenotic PA anastomosis.[40] Apart from the type, the length of surgery is also a predisposing factor; an operating room time greater than 150 minutes was found to be an independent risk factor in general surgical patients.[41]

Some additional interventional maneuvers can induce thromboembolism. Central venous (CV) catheters account for almost all secondary upper-extremity DVT, which represents 1% to 2% of all DVT; PTE occurs in 12% of these cases.[42] Femoral vein catheterization may also cause DVT, rarely in adults but often in children (35%), especially in infants and newborns.[43] Inflation and deflation of extremity tourniquets or placement of Esmarch bandages may detach an already formed venous clot and lead to intraoperative embolization.[44] Positioning of the legs for lithotomy position may have the same effect. A left ventricular (LV) assist device or centrifugal pump used to support a failing heart also may cause thromboembolic complications.[45]

Patient-related factors also play a major role in the development of perioperative thromboembolism. These may be subdivided into those involving the general makeup of the patient and those related to his or her disease state. Of these, some have greater and others less impact. Usually their effects are additive, and more than one risk factor is commonly present in the patient with thromboembolism.[41] Patient-related risk factors include age greater than 40, previous thromboembolic event, preoperative hospital stay of 6 days or longer, immobility, more than one unit preoperative transfusion, presence of leg ulcer, and a previous major orthopedic event.[41] Less influential but still important factors are pregnancy, puerperium, estrogen therapy, use of oral contraceptives, obesity, and possibly lower-extremity varicose veins. Diseases that increase the likelihood of thromboembolism include malignancy, particularly of the stomach or the ovary, congestive heart failure, nephrotic syndrome, recent myocardial infarction, inflammatory bowel disease, and inherited hematologic disorders that induce hypercoagulability and altered procoagulant or anticoagulant mechanisms.

Of the blood dyscrasias,[46,47] deficiencies in antithrombin III, protein C and protein S, and heparin factor II result in inability to inhibit coagulation. A recently identified thrombophilia is caused by resistance to activated protein C, which is related to a mutation in factor V (Leiden factor V). As a result of this mutation, factor V cannot be inhibited by activated protein C.[46,48] The increased incidence of thromboembolism seen after certain operations may be related partly to blood dyscrasias. For example, in the Fontan procedure, which is performed for tricuspid atresia and involves anastomosing the right atrium or vena cava to the PA, PTE is a common complication; protein C, protein S, and factor VII may contribute to the development of this complication and indicate anticoagulant treatment for these children.[49] Because normal clotting is achieved by a balance between coagulation and fibrinolysis, decreased fibrinolytic function can also lead to a hypercoagulable state. Dysfibrinogenemias and hypoplasminogenemias or dysplasminogenemias are the primary abnormalities causing dysfibrinolysis. Of more than 100 dysfibrinogenemias described, only about 10% cause recurrent thromboembolic complications; the rest are associated with bleeding problems.[46] Dysplasminogenemias are caused by inherited deficiencies of plasminogen, defective release of tissue plasminogen activator (t-PA) from the vascular endothelium, elevated plasma concentrations of t-PA inhibitors, and a deficiency of contact factor (factor XII) that may induce failure of fibrinolysis activation.[46,50] Other conditions do not directly affect hemostasis or fibrinolysis but have an impact on these functions: hyperhomocystinemia, disorders caused by increased lipoprotein A, and modifications of histidine-rich glycoprotein.[46,47,51]

Except for resistance to activated protein C, only 2% of the general population and 13% of the subjects develop-

Table 29-2. Surgical procedures with increased likelihood of perioperative thromboembolism

General surgery	Open surgery of:
	Stomach
	Biliary tree
	Colon
	Pancreas
Urology	Pelvic surgery
	Open prostatectomy
	Cystectomy
Neurosurgery	Craniotomy
Trauma surgery	Spinal cord injuries
	Head injury
	Multiple trauma
	Pelvic fracture
	Hip fracture
	Lower-extremity long
	bone fracture
Vascular surgery	Abdominal aneurysmectomy
	Lower-extremity arterial
	reconstructive surgery
	Lower-extremity amputation
Orthopedic surgery	Hip replacement
	Knee replacement
Cardiac surgery	Valve surgery
	Repair of some congenital
	defects (Fontan procedure)
Transplant surgery	Lung transplant*

*At the site of pulmonary vascular anastomosis.

ing thromboembolism have these blood dyscrasias.[52] The incidence may be as high as 20% when the first episode of thromboembolism occurs before the age of 45, there is a family history of thrombosis, and thrombosis occurs spontaneously and recurrently.[52] The prevalence of activated protein C resistance, which is the most common inherited procoagulant disorder, is estimated as 3% to 7% in the general population, and, like other inherited deficiencies of coagulation inhibitors, it may be present in up to 45% of patients developing thromboembolism.[53] The presence of more than one type of blood dyscrasia increases the likelihood of thromboembolism[51]; multiple protein deficiencies are present in about 1% of patients with venous thromboembolism.[52] Detection of these inherited disorders in only a portion of patients with thromboembolism suggests the presence of a triggering mechanism. Because these effects may be triggered by surgery or childbirth and because there is a close association between venous thrombosis and inherited coagulation abnormalities, some clinicians suggest screening for these defects before surgery in patients with a family history of thromboembolism and, if positive, administering anticoagulants.[47]

Venous thromboembolism is rare in children and neonates; the incidence in Canada and the Netherlands for the 0- to 14-year-old group is 0.6 to 0.7 per 100,000 per year with no mortality.[54] The corresponding figures for the 15- to 24-year-old group are an incidence of 20.2 and a mortality of 0.3 per 100,000.[54] Usually one or more predisposing factors can be identified; venous catheterization, surgery, or trauma is the triggering event,[43,54] and genetic or acquired coagulation abnormalities are common underlying conditions. Although large extremity and torso veins are predominantly involved, during the first year of life renal vein thrombosis can occur; the cause is not well known but is believed to be an intrauterine disorder.[54] A careful family history and assays for the lupus anticoagulant, antithrombin-III, protein C, protein S, and the factor V Leiden mutation should be part of the evaluation of infants and children with venous thrombosis.

A. Pathophysiology

Venous thromboemboli traverse the systemic veins, the right heart chambers, and the pulmonary arterial tree. Lower-extremity veins are the source of more than 95% of instances; upper extremity, renal, hepatic, and mesenteric veins rarely are involved. Embolization of thrombi from the right heart can occur in the presence of atrial fibrillation, congestive heart failure, indwelling foreign bodies, tricuspid endocarditis, or rarely after myocardial contusion.[55] Thrombophlebitis is most common in the veins of the calf; fortunately, clots from this site rarely migrate to the pulmonary circulation. On the other hand, thrombi from more proximal regions, such as the femoral and iliac veins and the vena cava, often embolize to the lungs. At least 40% of patients with DVT have ventilation-perfusion ($\dot{V}/\dot{Q}$) scan or chest roentgenographic evidence of PTE, even though they may be asymptomatic, suggesting that the two conditions are in-

separable and should be considered one disease.[56] Intuitively, the embolic risk of a venous thrombus that has a long tail unattached to the vein wall and is moving freely with the blood flow should be greater than that of an obstructive clot. However, this may not be the case if early anticoagulant therapy is initiated.[57] Like the high incidence of PTE after proximal DVT, the incidence of DVT in patients with PTE is almost 80%.[58]

There is little doubt that postoperative venous thrombi are initiated by venous stasis, endothelial injury, or a hypercoagulable state. Stasis facilitates thrombosis by prolonging the interaction of coagulation factors with the stimulus, initiating clotting at the site of activation. Stasis usually results from prolonged immobilization, which produces a decreased massaging effect of the muscles on the extremity veins. There is a decrease in venous blood flow of as much as 50%, which starts during induction of general anesthesia and continues into the postoperative period.[59] Venous stasis may also occur as a result of surgical procedures in the vicinity of the large lower-extremity veins. For example, manipulation of the femoral shaft during hip replacement surgery may cause cessation of femoral venous blood flow.[60]

The undamaged endothelial surface normally promotes fibrinolysis by synthesis and secretion of t-PA and inhibits binding of coagulation factors such as thrombin through the effects of intracellular thrombomodulin and heparin sulfate. Endothelial injury inhibits these effects and promotes venous thrombosis by permitting contact between the blood and collagen in the underlying basement membrane, thus activating the coagulation cascade directly and by platelet adhesion. It is probably difficult to produce endothelial damage even when surgery is in the vicinity of the lower extremity veins. However, lower-extremity venous dilation, which may reach 28% intraoperatively and increase to 57% with a moderate fluid infusion, may tear the endothelial lining and cause clotting activation.[61,62] A preliminary study indicates that administration of fluids, especially saline, plasma, and Haemaccel, with resulting hemodilution, promotes venous thrombosis by inducing a hypercoagulable state.[63] The mechanism of this phenomenon is not known and requires further study. Nevertheless, hypercoagulation caused by the various factors we have discussed plays a major role in the pathophysiology of thromboembolism. Apart from this, surgery itself may cause an increase in fibrinogen, platelets, and platelet adhesiveness and a decrease in fibrinolysis that may last from 3 to 21 days postoperatively.[64,65]

Recent research on the pathogenesis of venous thrombosis has focused on its synergistic interaction with an inflammatory response,[66] which may also play a role in postthrombotic chronic venous insufficiency. The development of thrombus is the initial stimulus for inflammation of the vein wall. Small endothelial disruptions and procoagulant activity facilitate the development of clot in the valves and venous junctions, and subsequent activation of neutrophils and platelets. The process is further amplified by the attachment of neutrophils and platelets to the basement membrane and by further generation of procoagulant and inflammatory mediators. Following this, thrombin is released and fibrin is formed by complex development on platelet phospholipid surfaces. In the final phase, additional neutrophils, monocytes, and platelets adhere to the clot,

increasing its size. During this process activated leukocytes migrate into the vein wall from the venous lumen and the adventitia. Leukocyte extravasation is governed by a cytokine/chemokine gradient in the vein wall (Fig. 29-1).

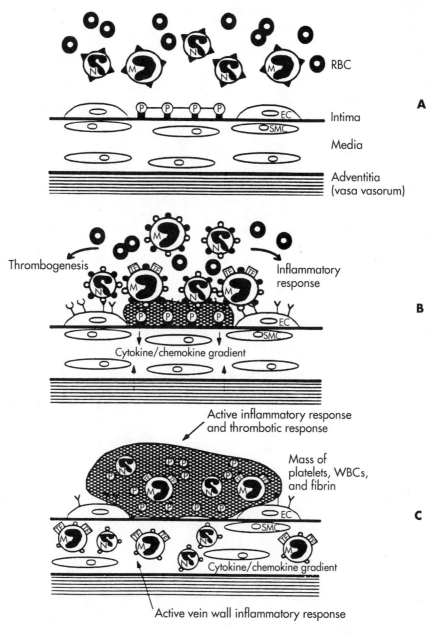

Fig. 29-1. Pathogenesis of deep vein thrombosis. **A,** Endothelial cell *(EC)* disruption allows adhesion of platelets *(P)* to the subendothelial surface. Squares represent fibrinogen between subendothelial space and platelets. In the lumen blood cells are circulating normally. *M,* Monocyte; *N,* neutrophil; *RBC,* red blood cell; *SMC,* smooth muscle cell; triangles represent L-selectin. **B,** Neutrophils and monocytes are stimulated and destroy L-selectin. They are now bound to P-selectin (solid circles) or endothelial cells and platelets. Tissue factor *(TF)* is formed on the surface of monocytes. Fibrin clot forms on the surface of activated platelets. Leukocytes gradually extravasate into the vein wall because of a cytokine/chemokine gradient. **C,** Fibrin clot is matured and contains platelets, leukocytes, and fibrin. Active inflammatory and thrombotic response occurs at the vein wall interface. The same reaction later takes place in the vein wall itself. (From Wakefield TW, Strieter RM, Prince MR, et al: *Cardiovasc Surg* 5:6, 1997.)

B. Mechanisms of hemodynamic and gas exchange abnormalities

Most available information about acute hemodynamic and gas exchange abnormalities in PTE comes from animal studies. These results should be extrapolated to humans only with great caution.

1. Hemodynamic abnormalities. The severity of hemodynamic and respiratory abnormalities after PTE is determined primarily by the extent of the vascular occlusion. In experimental animals reflex factors and humoral agents such as serotonin, histamine, and prostaglandin may play a role in the development of functional pulmonary and cardiovascular changes, but their contribution to human PTE is not clear.[67] However, hypoxia- or acidosis-induced pulmonary vasoconstriction can augment pulmonary vascular resistance and pressure.[68] Acute reduction of the patency of the pulmonary vascular bed causes an increase in mean pulmonary artery pressure (PAP), which in turn results in increased right ventricular (RV) work if adequate cardiac output is maintained. Because of the large reserve capacity of the pulmonary circulation, acute obstruction of up to 30% of the vascular cross-sectional area is not likely to cause a significant rise in total pulmonary vascular resistance or a sustained elevation of PAP in a patient with no preexisting cardiopulmonary disease.[69] The relationship between the degree of occlusion and the total pulmonary vascular resistance is approximately hyperbolic (Fig. 29-2)[70]: a mean PAP of 22 mm Hg corresponds to a 30% occlusion and 36 mm Hg corresponds to a 50% occlusion of the vascular bed.[69] It should be noted that the mean PAP will not exceed 40 mm Hg in patients without prior cardiopulmonary disease, even with pulmonary vascular occlusion well above 50%[69]; at this pressure the thin-walled

right ventricle (RV) begins to fail. In patients with chronic cardiopulmonary disease, including chronic PTE, which occurs in about 0.1% of patients after acute PTE, the correlation between the extent of pulmonary vascular occlusion, pulmonary vascular resistance, and PAP no longer exists. Furthermore, in patients with chronic RV hypertrophy, a mean PAP greater than 40 mm Hg can be generated, and depression of the cardiac output may occur with a smaller degree of obstruction than in previously healthy patients.[67,69,70]

Recently, new dimensions have been added to the understanding of the pathophysiology of acute pulmonary hypertension.[68] Conventionally, pulmonary vascular resistance is calculated as PAP minus LV filling pressure divided by cardiac output. This formula assumes that the effective pulmonary outflow pressure in West zone III of the lung is the same as the LV filling pressure. In addition, the pulmonary vascular resistance is defined with a single pressure-flow coordinate; an accurate description of the pulmonary vascular pressure-flow relationship would require measurements of pressure at several flow rates (i.e., cardiac outputs). Of course, this is difficult in the clinical setting. Nevertheless, when evaluation was performed in animals using multicoordinate vascular flow plots, it was found that the pressure-flow relationship is linear over a range of flow rates (Fig. 29-3)[68,71] The slope of the curve seen in Fig. 29-3 represents the incremental resistance of the pulmonary vascular tree (pressure change per unit flow change), whereas extrapolation of

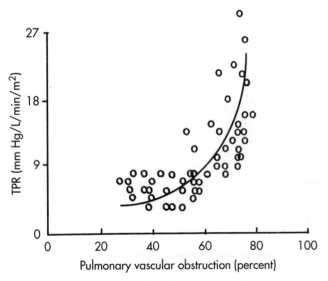

Fig. 29-2. Hyperbolic correlation between pulmonary vascular obstruction and total pulmonary vascular resistance *(TPR)* in acute pulmonary thromboembolism. Note that TPR begins to rise only after 30% to 40% of the pulmonary vasculature is obstructed. (From Azarian R, Wartski M, Collignon MA, et al: *J Nucl Med* 38:980, 1997.)

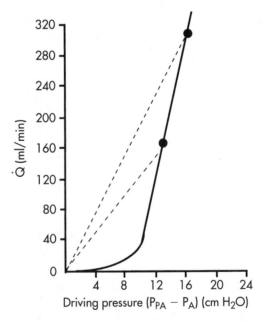

Fig. 29-3. Relationship between pulmonary blood flow ($\dot{Q}$) and driving pressure in zone 2 conditions. The slope of the solid line represents incremental resistance of the pulmonary vasculature. Extrapolation of the curve to a no-flow condition is the closing pressure. Dotted lines represent pressure-flow relationship of two points on the curve (see text for explanation). P_{PA}, Pulmonary arterial pressure; P_A, alveolar (airway) pressure. (From Graham R, Skoog C, Macedo W, et al: *J Appl Physiol* 54:1277, 1983.)

this curve to zero flow defines the closing pressure, that is, the effective vascular outflow pressure. Thus pulmonary hypertension may result from an increase in incremental resistance or an increase in effective closing pressure; the latter may exceed LV filling pressure in West zone III and alveolar pressure in West zone II. The clinical implication of this is that vasoactive agents used during resuscitation may have effects on the individual components of the pulmonary vascular resistance. In fact, data obtained from animals suggest that elevated PAP after PTE is mainly the result of increased mean pulmonary vascular closing pressure and usually not of increased incremental resistance.[72] This may be the reason that some vasoactive and inotropic agents produce better responses than others during resuscitation.[71]

With a pulmonary vascular obstruction that is severe enough to produce a substantial increase in RV afterload, several events take place in both the right and left sides of the heart.[67,73] RV myocardial wall tension and thus its oxygen consumption increase. This leads to decreased ventricular performance and dilation of its free wall and leftward shifting of the septum. Distention of the RV results in acute tricuspid regurgitation. The ejection fraction and stroke volume of the RV are therefore decreased.[67] This, coupled with decreased LV stroke volume, which is affected by the decreased end-diastolic volume resulting from the septal shift, produces a profound diminution of cardiac output and systemic blood pressure. This situation of decreased cardiac output and systemic blood pressure in the presence of increased RV end-diastolic pressure defines RV failure.[68] Reduced cardiac output further aggravates the already altered hemodynamic and oxygenation variables by several mechanisms. It results in a decrease in coronary perfusion. Right coronary artery perfusion, which normally takes place during both systole and diastole, is restricted to diastole by the acute RV distention. With decreased cardiac output the blood supply to the RV is further diminished. Furthermore, reduced cardiac output results in decreased mixed venous P_{O_2}, augmenting the arterial desaturation caused by the PTE-induced $\dot{V}/\dot{Q}$ mismatch. If these events are permitted to continue, RV infarction, shock, and death may ensue. A schematic description of the possible hemodynamic events after PTE is depicted in Fig. 29-4.

2. Gas exchange abnormalities. Several factors influence gas exchange following PTE. Not all of these are present in a given patient, nor do they all act in the same direction. Thus the blood gas response varies from patient to patient depending on the factors involved and their specific effects.[74] It follows that although blood gas abnormalities are present in a majority of patients with acute PTE, they are poor indicators of the extent of pulmonary vascular obstruction.[75]

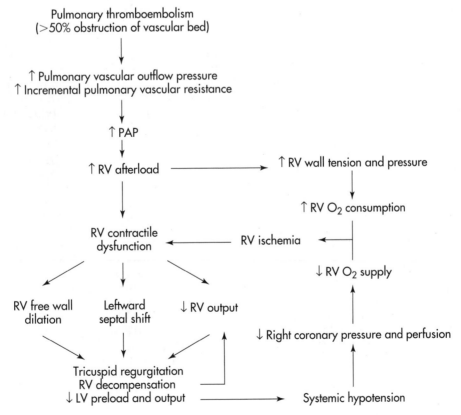

Fig. 29-4. Mechanism of hemodynamic abnormalities after significant pulmonary thromboembolism (PTE). *LV,* Left ventricle; *PAP,* pulmonary artery pressure; *RV,* right ventricle. (Modified from Lualdi JC, Goldhaber SZ: *Am Heart J* 130:1276, 1995.)

Hypoxemia and hypocapnia are the classical findings in spontaneously breathing patients following acute PTE. In awake patients breathing room air, PaO_2 is less than 80 mm Hg in 85% to 90% and less than 60 mm Hg in 30% of instances during the acute phase of an embolic event.[74] The alveolar-arterial O_2 gradient increases in 80% to 95% of patients.[74,75] Hypocapnia, although perhaps not as universal as hypoxemia, is also common and is accompanied by respiratory alkalosis; $PaCO_2$ is less than 37 mm Hg in 80% and less than 26 mm Hg in 20% of spontaneously breathing patients with acute PTE.[74] Hypercapnia may occur in some patients if the reflex hyperventilation is inadequate. The kinetics of CO_2 have been studied recently in experimental animals during the acute phase of single-lung PA occlusion.[76] Elevation of $PaCO_2$ with retention of tissue CO_2 results primarily from decreased exhaled CO_2 volume caused by increased alveolar dead space. Although the increased $PaCO_2$ brings the exhaled CO_2 volume back to baseline within about an hour, the end-tidal CO_2 remains low because of the large dead space. Thus the end-tidal CO_2 concentration in mechanically ventilated patients with acute PTE (at least within the 1- to 2-hour period after the event) does not indicate the variation in the exhaled CO_2 volume or the $PaCO_2$.[76] Although rare, progressive hypercapnia refractory to maximal spontaneous reflex hyperventilation or supramaximal minute volume during mechanical ventilation may occur. These patients may not respond rapidly enough to anticoagulant or thrombolytic therapy and may be candidates for emergency pulmonary embolectomy.

Both nonpulmonary and pulmonary mechanisms produce gas exchange abnormalities in acute PTE. Extrapulmonary factors are involved only occasionally; they include reduced cardiac output, right-to-left intracardiac shunt, and RV failure. Within the lung, $\dot{V}_A/\dot{Q}$ inequality is involved in the majority of cases.[74] Intrapulmonary shunting is a less common but often coexistent factor. Low PvO_2, diffusion impairment, and increased dead space (V_D/V_t) may also be involved in hypoxemia and hypocapnia, but less often than the other pulmonary factors.[74]

$\dot{V}_A/\dot{Q}$ abnormalities may vary widely in severity, even among different regions of the lung in the same patient. Thus the effect of $\dot{V}_A/\dot{Q}$ abnormality on PaO_2 depends on whether high or low $\dot{V}_A/\dot{Q}$ units are predominant and whether small or large segments are involved. For example, complete occlusion of a small lung unit with normal $\dot{V}_A/\dot{Q}$ does not alter oxygenation significantly. However, even a 50% occlusion of a major segment with a normally high $\dot{V}_A/\dot{Q}$ may result in significant hypoxemia because blood flow may be shunted from the embolized region to normal segments, converting them to low $\dot{V}_A/\dot{Q}$ units.[74] The low $\dot{V}_A/\dot{Q}$ in this area can be normalized by increasing ventilation, a homeostatic mechanism that usually occurs and is also responsible for hypocapnia. Nevertheless, this hyperventilation is not always capable of normalizing the PaO_2 because the ventilation of both hypoperfused and hyperperfused regions is increased and any $\dot{V}_A/\dot{Q}$ mismatch remains.[77]

Shunt may develop by several mechanisms after PTE. The most common are postembolic atelectasis and infarction.[74,77] Atelectasis following vascular occlusion may develop from alveolar duct or small airway obstruction, or from surfactant loss. Other causes of increased shunt include opening of pulmonary arteriovenous anastomoses or intracardiac septal defects, and pulmonary edema. PTE is also likely to cause changes in pulmonary mechanics; breathing pattern; reflex responses such as hypoxic pulmonary vasoconstriction and hypocapnic bronchoconstriction; and humoral responses, including a release of serotonin, which stimulates bronchoconstriction.[74,77] For example, PE causes an increase in airway resistance and a fall in both dynamic and static compliance, which may increase $\dot{V}_A/\dot{Q}$ mismatch and shunt.[77] Likewise, according to experimental work, hypoxic pulmonary vasoconstriction is partially inhibited in PTE and thus may not effectively prevent gas exchange abnormalities. Even when a shunt involves a small segment, hypoxic vasoconstriction in normal areas of the lung caused by decreased FIO_2 can result in severe deterioration of gas exchange, probably by shifting blood flow from these regions to the low $\dot{V}_A/\dot{Q}$ areas.[78]

C. Clinical management

Proper management of venous thromboembolism can make a significant difference in the patient's outcome. More than one half of deaths from PTE occur within the first hour, usually because of massive occlusion of the main PA and its branches.[79] It was estimated in the 1970s that in more than 60% of the patients surviving the first hour, clinical management was inappropriate; their mortality was approximately 30%.[79] When the patient was appropriately treated, the mortality was between 5% and 10%.[79] With proper continued management, an even lower death rate (2.5%) has been reported.[80] In the survivors of this study, including both medical and surgical patients, the recurrence rate was 8.3%; 45% of these died within 1 year. It should be emphasized that after initial management, the possibility of long-term recurrence depends mainly on readily recognizable factors; surgery and trauma carry the lowest long-term risk, compared to other factors such as malignancy.[81] Thus appropriate initial diagnosis, with treatment that is usually continued for about 3 to 6 months, is particularly important in the surgical population.

1. Diagnosis. Anesthesiologists are likely to be presented with all possible clinical scenarios of venous thromboembolism. However, diagnosis is particularly important in the following phases of anesthetic care:

1. Preoperatively, to recognize proximal DVT in order to take preventive measures against embolic complications or to postpone surgery
2. Before induction of a general anesthetic or after administration of regional anesthesia, to recognize an acute embolism and thus to postpone surgery, treat the acute condition, and proceed with definitive diagnostic measures
3. Intraoperatively, to diagnose and treat PTE if it occurs

4. Four to 5 days postoperatively, to recognize both DVT and PTE and to perform any necessary diagnostic and therapeutic measures

a. Diagnosis of proximal deep vein thrombosis. To a certain extent, the clinical manifestations are related to the type of venous thrombosis. In the rare form, phlegmasia cerulea dolens, thrombophlebitis is massive; all of the main venous channels and their collaterals are blocked. The limb is massively swollen, distally mottled, and bluish in color. This syndrome usually occurs in cachectic terminal cancer patients, and eventually leads to gangrene of the extremity because of cessation of arterial flow from spasm produced by the virtually total venous outflow obstruction. The remaining two types, occlusive and nonocclusive DVT, are not as obvious clinically.[82] The typical findings—pain, tenderness, and extremity swelling—may be minimal. In fact, the majority of venous thrombi are clinically silent, probably because they do not produce complete obstruction, collateral channels form, and many of the patients are supine in bed, which partly or completely alleviates swelling.[82] Clinical suspicion proves positive in only a small minority of patients.[82] Many conditions can mimic this complication, including muscular contusions or rupture, popliteal cyst, popliteal aneurysm, myositis, cellulitis, and arthritis.

Thus in most instances, initiation of treatment requires confirmation by objective tests. The diagnostic gold standard is venography. A persistent filling defect, lack of venous opacification, abrupt interruption of the flow of contrast in a vein, and flow diversion with opacification of collateral branches are the principal positive findings. However, this examination requires administration of large doses of contrast medium, which in 2% to 3% of patients can cause thrombosis; it is costly and often is not feasible in critically ill patients because of the need for transport to the radiology suite. For this reason, noninvasive studies are used first. Currently venography is performed when the results of noninvasive examinations are doubtful or technically limited, or when thrombosis of upper-body veins such as the innominate or superior vena cava is suspected.

The most clinically useful noninvasive tests are impedance plethysmography and real-time B-mode ultrasonography with or without Doppler flow detection. Both of these tests detect proximal (above the knee) venous thrombosis best, which is clinically acceptable because most clots that embolize to the lungs originate from this site. Both have high sensitivity and specificity in detecting symptomatic proximal thrombi,[82] although the accuracy of ultrasonography exceeds that of impedance plethysmography.[83] Unfortunately, neither test is satisfactory for screening asymptomatic patients[82,84] Dressings, casts, and open extremity wounds also render performance of these tests difficult. The problems in detecting asymptomatic thrombi with these techniques are probably related to their small size and nonocclusive nature. Nevertheless, the accuracy of these examinations is enhanced by repetition and comparison of results, to the extent that serially obtained negative findings justify withholding anticoagulant therapy. Thrombi usually can be visualized by real-time B-mode ultrasonography, but the most important positive finding is inability to collapse the vein with gentle pressure applied over the probe. The test is easy to perform and can be done in the operating room by a physician with experience in vascular ultrasonography by connecting a 7.5-MHz vascular probe to an echocardiography unit. Compression ultrasonography is less useful in regions proximal to the axilla and the inguinal ligament because of difficulty in compressing veins in these areas.

Diagnosis of DVT in pregnancy poses two major problems.[85] First, utmost consideration should be given to avoiding fetal radiation exposure. Thus venography, if necessary, may have to be limited. Second, in the third trimester of pregnancy, the gravid uterus may itself cause venous outflow obstruction, leading to a false positive result.

Several other tests have been introduced during recent years to improve the accuracy or safety of diagnosis.[82] Computed tomography can identify thrombosed veins in the abdomen and pelvis that cannot be detected by ultrasound or impedance plethysmography. Magnetic resonance venography, although not yet suitable for routine use, has a high diagnostic accuracy rate. Radionuclide venography also is being developed for this purpose.

b. Diagnosis of pulmonary thromboembolism in the awake patient. Most episodes of PTE are undiagnosed or unsuspected because the signs and symptoms are mild or may imitate other conditions. Thus the most important step in diagnosis is a high index of suspicion. Thereafter, the diagnostic strategy involves interpretation of the presenting signs, symptoms, and routine diagnostic tests, which often establish the need for more specific examinations. The clinical features of PTE are so diverse and are so often characteristic of so many other clinical conditions that isolated signs may have only minimal diagnostic value. On the other hand, signs, symptoms, ECG findings, and the plain chest radiograph can help greatly in indicating the presence of this syndrome.

The clinical severity of PTE varies from subclinical to profound shock and rapid death, probably depending on the extent of the vascular occlusion. Symptomatic PTE is classified into three categories when the patient survives beyond the first 2.5 hours. Although these categories have different names in the literature, they appear to describe the same entities[86,87]: pulmonary infarction syndrome (minor), isolated dyspnea syndrome (moderate or submassive), or circulatory collapse syndrome (major, catastrophic, or massive). The fulminant form usually leads to early death. Using data from the Prospective Investigation of Pulmonary Embolism Diagnosis (PIOPED),[88] Stein and Henry[86] recently demonstrated that pleuritic pain, hemoptysis, rales, and tachycardia occurred more often in the pulmonary infarct syndrome than in the other two categories. Dyspnea was the predominant symptom in the isolated dyspnea syndrome. Cough, leg swelling, leg pain, tachypnea, and an increased pulmonary component of the second heart sound were common, but occurred with similar frequencies in all three syndromes. Nonspecific clinical signs, such as arrhythmias, fever, unexplained heart failure, mental confusion, bronchospasm, or even seizures may infrequently be the presenting clinical features of PTE.

(1) ECG. ECG findings are nonspecific and are more likely to be absent (almost half of patients) in pulmonary infarction syndrome than in the other two categories. Right bundle-branch block is more likely to occur in the presence of hemodynamic instability than in stable patients. The most common ECG abnormality is ST-segment and T-wave changes, which are present in almost half of the patients in each category. A recent report suggests that T-wave inversion may assist in defining the severity of embolic obstruction. This sign is common in patients with extensive PTE and usually disappears within a few days. Its persistence suggests continuation of the embolic process.[89]

(2) CHEST RADIOGRAPH. On the chest roentgenogram, atelectasis, pulmonary parenchymal abnormalities, and pleural effusion are more likely to occur in the pulmonary infarction syndrome than in the other two types. Elevation of the diaphragm may be a manifestation of atelectasis. Cardiomegaly is likely to occur in patients with hemodynamic instability. Enlargement of the PAs and radiolucency caused by decreased vascularization distal to the arterial obstruction (Westermark's oligemic area) also may be noted. While helping to differentiate between the different forms of PTE, the chest roentgenogram can also aid in the detection of other diseases that may mimic the syndrome: aspiration, atelectasis, pneumonia, pneumothorax, pulmonary edema, cardiac tamponade, pulmonary contusion, and unsuspected neoplasm.

Although hypoxia is a common occurrence in PTE, patients with pulmonary infarction syndrome are more likely to have normal room air PaO_2 than those with isolated dyspnea syndrome or circulatory collapse. Clearly, a normal PaO_2 does not rule out PTE. Although clinical features alone can by no means make or eliminate the diagnosis, clinical evaluation increases the overall diagnostic probability when combined with the results of lung scanning. This test is an important step toward definitive diagnosis.

(3) LUNG SCANNING. Perfusion scanning, performed by intravenous injection of isotope-labeled human albumin macroaggregates, is the essential part of the lung scan. An external photoscanner records the distribution of albumin in the pulmonary vascular distribution. Ventilation scanning, which is obtained by recording the alveolar distribution of inhaled and exhaled radioactive aerosols with a gamma camera, is needed in some but not all instances depending on the results of the perfusion scan. The size and pattern of perfusion defects and matching or mismatching of these with the chest roentgenogram or ventilation scan are used to establish the probability of diagnosis. Large perfusion defects that do not match the ventilation pattern are more likely to be caused by PTE than by other cardiopulmonary disorders. In a large-scale prospective investigation, the PIOPED study[88] demonstrated that a scan highly positive by predetermined criteria established the presence of PTE with high probability: The diagnosis was verifiable in 86% of cases demonstrated by pulmonary angiography. The diagnosis also can be ruled out with reasonable certainty if the scan findings are normal or near normal, although in the PIOPED study this group, representing 14% of the total, had a 4% incidence of PTE on pulmonary angiogram.[88] The major diagnostic problem for the lung scan is that the results in most patients with suspected PTE correspond to low- or intermediate-probability criteria for the actual presence of the disease, necessitating pulmonary angiography, which has its own limitations.[88,90] In the PIOPED study 72% of the patients had low- and intermediate-probability scans; of these only 21% had angiographically proven PTE.[88]

(4) PULMONARY ANGIOGRAPHY. Pulmonary angiography is considered positive if there is a constant intraluminal filling defect or cutoff of arteries.[87] Although often observed in patients with PTE, areas of oligemia and asymmetry of blood flow are not specific and may also occur in patients with chronic lung disease.[87] Angiography may also permit an estimation of the severity of the disease. For example, massive embolism is generally present when more than 50% of the pulmonary arterial tree is occluded or shows defects.[87] To minimize the volume of radiopaque material used and to obtain hemodynamic data before contrast injection, selective angiography can be performed using pigtail or balloon flotation catheters inserted via an antecubital or femoral vein. Unfortunately, angiography is not available at all times in all hospitals; it necessitates transport of critically ill patients with its inherent risks; and it is associated with a small (0.5%) but significant rate of complications, some of which may be major, such as contrast media reactions, myocardial injury, cardiac perforation, serious arrhythmias, and cardiac arrest. Thus for the past several years, substantial effort has been directed to the exploration of noninvasive diagnostic techniques. Development of these studies will probably require several years; during this time, pulmonary angiography, although with gradually decreasing frequency, will probably continue to be used for definitive diagnosis of PTE.

(5) METHODS TO AVOID PULMONARY ANGIOGRAPHY, WITH EMPHASIS ON ECHOCARDIOGRAPHY. As mentioned earlier, combining the probabilities estimated from clinical evaluation and lung scanning may improve diagnostic accuracy in most but not all instances[58,88,90] (Table 29-3) and permit treatment without further testing. This may be the case when a high-probability lung scan coexists with a high or intermediate degree of clinical suspicion. In fact, a recent report suggests that in this situation there may not be a need for a ventilation scan[90]; a perfusion scan that shows a wedge-shaped defect, combined with a clinical evaluation that indicates a very likely or possible presence of PTE, predicts a positive diagnosis in 99% of patients.[90] However, this combination occurs in only 10% to 30% of patients with abnormal perfusion scans; clearly the majority of patients require additional diagnostic tests.

A positive result on examination of the lower extremity for proximal DVT in patients suspected of PTE may avoid a pulmonary angiogram. This may be particularly useful in the immediate preoperative period. These find-

Table 29-3. The likelihood of pulmonary thromboembolism diagnosed with a combination of clinical evaluation and lung scan data

Clinical probability	Lung scan probability	Likelihood of pulmonary thrombo-embolism (%)
High or very likely	High	96-99
Intermediate or possible	High	80-92
Low or unlikely	Low	2-6
Low or unlikely	High	50-55
High or very likely	Intermediate or low	30-39

Data from Hull RD, Hirsh J, Carter CJ, et al: *Ann Intern Med* 98:891, 1983; Miniati M, Pistolesi M, Marini C, et al: *Am J Respir Crit Care Med* 154:1387, 1996; Saltzman HA, Alavi A, Greenspan RH: *JAMA* 263:2753, 1990.

ings may warrant anticoagulant treatment, or a vena cava filter in preoperative patients, without an angiography because the therapy of both DVT and PTE is the same. In fact, this approach may also eliminate the need for lung scans in many suspected patients. Of course, negative results cannot rule out PTE.

As mentioned earlier, compression ultrasonography is a more sensitive test for DVT than impedance plethysmography. Although some studies have demonstrated 61% sensitivity and 97% specificity in the diagnosis of DVT in patients presenting to the emergency department with suspected PTE,[91] a recent prospective investigation failed to demonstrate a significant benefit of this approach.[92] Compression ultrasonography may avoid about 14% of lung scans and 9% of pulmonary angiographies, but 13% of patients would be treated unnecessarily. If the test were used only in patients with nondiagnostic lung scans, 9% of angiographies would be unnecessary but 26% of patients would be treated unnecessarily. In contrast to the results of previous studies, the overall sensitivity of compression ultrasonography in *asymptomatic* patients with PTE was only 29%. This finding was attributed to the dislodgment of small, less organized, soft thrombi from their venous origin to the lungs.

Measurement of the blood concentration of D-dimer, the particle cleaved from clotted (cross-linked) fibrin, provides another noninvasive diagnostic approach. This test is more specific than fibrin degradation products (FDP) for detection of thrombosis, because it signals only the breakdown of cross-linked fibrin, whereas FDP can be a product of fibrin or fibrinogen. High concentrations of both products in the blood are strong evidence of intravascular coagulation but do not necessarily establish the diagnosis of PTE. A high D-dimer concentration is virtually useless as an indicator of PTE, but a concentration less than 500 mg/L strongly suggests the absence of intravascular clotting and thus decreases the need for angiography.[93,94] The accuracy of the test relies heavily on an intact fibrinolytic mechanism; otherwise, D-dimer and FDP concentrations are low despite in-

travascular coagulation. For the test to be reasonably reliable, D-dimer should be measured using enzyme-linked immunosorbent assay (ELISA), which requires time and is not well suited to emergency situations. Although the latex agglutination technique is rapid, it is not as accurate as ELISA. Overall the D-dimer test may be useful for screening, but its role in critically ill hospitalized patients is not yet sufficiently determined.

Two techniques may eventually replace pulmonary angiography for noninvasive definitive diagnosis: spiral computed tomography (SCT) and TTE or TEE. SCT is obtained by a continuously rotating CT scanner. A high volume (up to 140 ml) of contrast material is injected at a high rate (3 to 6 ml/sec) to provide adequate vascular contrast. The procedure is completed within a few minutes, and only about 30 seconds of breath holding is required. This technique achieves between 90% and 100% sensitivity and 96% to 100% specificity.[95,96] With this method even distal partially or completely obstructing pulmonary filling defects can be detected, although lesions of the main, lobar, or segmental PAs are seen best, whereas subsegmental vessels are difficult to visualize. Possible limitations of SCT are the following: Interlobar lymph nodes may be misinterpreted as PE, the lingula and horizontally aligned vessels in the right middle lobe may be inadequately scanned, and peripheral areas of the upper and lower lobes may not be visualized adequately. Contrast-enhanced electron beam CT, another variant, also appears useful in diagnosing acute PTE, but additional data are needed before its clinical usefulness can be established.

Echocardiography is the most useful tool for many anesthesiologists in the diagnosis of PTE, not only because it is available and permits timely evaluation in the operating room or the postanesthesia unit, but also because these physicians have experience in using the device and interpreting its results. TTE or TEE can demonstrate RV overload, hypokinesis, and dilation. Of course, these findings are not specific for acute PTE; they may be present in patients with pulmonary hypertension, septal defects, or anomalous pulmonary venous return. However, these results may serve as important clues when an acute event suggests PTE clinically.[97] Echocardiography also helps in ruling out other acute cardiac events such as papillary muscle rupture with acute mitral regurgitation, tamponade, and ventricular septal rupture[97] and can be helpful in selecting appropriate therapy for hemodynamically unstable patients during resuscitation.[98] On the other hand, the RV may not show dysfunction in a significant proportion of patients with extensive acute PTE. Thus the ability to visualize clots in the right heart[99] (embolism in transit) and the PA or its branches gains importance.

The TTE probe (2.5 to 5 MHz) is placed on the right sternal border and moved along the sternum until the best view is found. TEE is superior to the transthoracic approach; the omniplane probe (5 MHz) provides the best results, but the biplane probe may be used if it is not available. The probe is introduced into the esophagus in its neutral position and after a four-chamber view is obtained, it is withdrawn 2 to 3 cm to the basal view. Rotation of the omniplane transducer from 0 to 110 degrees allows complete visualization of the pulmonary outflow tract, pulmonic valve, main PA, and right PA to the right pulmonary veins. The left PA can be visualized only at its origin from the main PA. If only a single-plane probe is available, the best view of the aortic valve (Mercedes sign) is obtained, and then the probe is flexed to its extreme position. This maneuver allows visualization of the pulmonary outflow tract, the main PA, its bifurcation, and the right and left pulmonary arteries. In each of these approaches, the flow can be measured with the color Doppler, and a reliable estimate of the pulmonary pressure may be obtained by recording the Doppler flow velocity in the RV outflow tract. The RV systolic pressure, which is the same as the PA systolic pressure, can be measured using the tricuspid regurgitation signal recorded by a continuous-wave Doppler. The peak velocity of the regurgitation jet, which is proportional to the right heart systolic atrioventricular pressure gradient, serves to estimate systolic PA pressure according to the following equation[100]:

$$\text{Pulmonary artery systolic pressure} = 4V^2 + \text{Central venous pressure}$$

During morphologic examination of the pulmonary vessels, any structures that protrude from the vessel wall into the lumen, have distinct borders, and interfere with blood flow can be considered to be thrombi.[97] Intraluminal masses that move separately from adjacent structures are also unequivocally thrombi[97] and suggest the presence of an acute event.[101] Linear, immobile, and poorly defined structures within a vessel are not necessarily clots.[97]

Functional abnormalities of the RV usually require the presence of at least 30% obstruction of the pulmonary arterial bed. The echocardiographic signs of acute RV pressure overload include an RV end-diastolic diameter greater than 27 mm, an LV end-diastolic dimension less than 36 mm, a dilated right PA (greater than 11.4 mm), tricuspid regurgitation with peak velocity of the regurgitation jet between 2.7 and 3.5 m/sec, RV hypokinesis, leftward deviation of the interventricular septum, decreased right-to-left ventricular diameter ratio, paradoxical systolic septal motion, and septal flattening.[87,102] The latter may also occur in chronic cor pulmonale. Differentiation between acute and chronic cor pulmonale can be made by echocardiographic observation of the inferior vena cava: Dilation during inspiration is evidence of acute cor pulmonale, whereas collapse suggests chronic RV overload.[87] Not all of these signs are present in all patients with PTE, but their number increases as the severity of embolism increases.

The diagnostic characteristics of TEE are shown in Table 29-4. In general, this examination offers a reasonable possibility of immediate confirmation of PTE, depending on both morphologic and functional changes.[96,101] Because of its low negative predictive value, however, it cannot be relied on to rule out PTE in doubtful cases. Also, it appears to be inferior to other noninvasive methods for detecting subsegmental and hemodynamically insignificant PE. Intravascular ultrasound is in development; it has been shown to detect pulmonary thrombi with reasonable accuracy.[103] Improvement in catheter design may render this technique useful.

c. Diagnosis of pulmonary thromboembolism in the anesthetized patient. The diagnosis of PTE during general anesthesia poses special challenges because the classic signs and symptoms are obscured, the patient's clinical indicators may be produced by various other intraoperative events, and most of the specific radiologic tests cannot be performed. Thus symptomatic treatment or resuscitation often must precede definitive diagnosis.

PTE may occur during any phase of general anesthesia, including induction, limb manipulation, the intraoperative period, and recovery. The treatment may be different for those who develop the complication before the beginning of surgery; if hemodynamically unstable, these patients may benefit from systemic thrombolysis.[104] Thus early determination of the cause of any hemodynamic instability is imperative.

Hypotension, alterations in heart rate, decreased arterial oxygen tension and often saturation, and an abrupt drop in end-expiratory CO_2 concentration with increase in $P(a\text{-}ET) CO_2$ gradient are the classical intraoperative signs, although the absence of some of these does not eliminate the possibility of PTE. For example, using data from the PIOPED trial, Stein et al[75,105] demonstrated that in spontaneously breathing patients, a normal PaO_2 or $P(A\text{-}a)O_2$ gradient could not exclude PTE. In another report, PTE was silent and not associated with hypotension or hypoxemia; increased $P(a\text{-}ET)CO_2$ gradient was the only sign.[106] In severe PTE, however, oxygenation is almost always altered, and hypercapnia unresponsive even to maximal minute ventilation may also occur.[107] Jugular venous distention, arrhythmias, electromechanical dissociation, ST-segment depression, and right bundle-branch block may also be present in some patients. Many acute intraoperative events present with a similar clinical picture: severe hemorrhage, inferior vena cava compression, anaphylaxis, increased vagal tone or release of vasoactive mediators secondary to visceral traction, myocardial ischemia or infarction, cardiac tamponade, and pneumothorax. In patients monitored with a

Table 29-4. Diagnostic characteristics of transesophageal echocardiography for pulmonary thromboembolism according to two series

Authors	Sensitivity (%)	Specificity (%)	Positive predictive value (%)	Negative predictive value (%)
Wittlich, Erbel, Eichler, et al[101]	97	89	91	96
Prusczyk, Torbicki, Pacho, et al[96]	80	100	100	52.9

PA or right atrial (RA) catheter, a sudden increase in PAP and central venous pressure (CVP) may be noted; the PCWP remains low. Elevated mean PAP (up to 40 mm Hg) and CVP in the face of increased pulmonary vascular resistance and hypotension rules out hypovolemia and limits the diagnostic possibilities to myocardial ischemia, acute right heart failure, and reactive pulmonary hypertension. Intraoperative TEE is invaluable in differentiating among these possibilities. Rapid diagnosis may be made by demonstrating the morphologic and functional signs of PTE described earlier, and other cardiac pathology may be ruled out.[104,108]

2. Treatment. To a great extent, treatment and prophylaxis of DVT can be considered preventive measures against PTE. The primary therapy for DVT is anticoagulation. Additional therapeutic maneuvers may be neces-

sary, depending on the presentation of the disease. Anticoagulation may begin before a definitive diagnosis is established, when risk factors such as injury, postoperative state, systemic infection, or immobility are present. Even if a clot cannot be identified in these circumstances, the treatment administered can be prophylactic. Any of the available anticoagulant agents (unfractionated heparin, low-molecular-weight heparin, or warfarin) can be used for this purpose. Unfractionated heparin may be administered at four dosage schedules, depending on the level of anticoagulation required: minidose, low dose, medium dose, and high dose. These are adjusted for low-risk prophylaxis, high-risk prophylaxis, and treatment. Two treatment regimens generally are described for warfarin: low intensity and high intensity. Table 29-5 describes the guidelines for each of these regimens,

Table 29-5. Guidelines for various levels of heparin and warfarin anticoagulation

Anticoagulant	Route of administration	Approximate loading dose	Approximate maintenance dose	Target coagulation level
Heparin				
Prophylaxis				
Minidose	SC		5000 U q 8-12 hr	None
Low-dose	IV	3000-5000 U	1000 U/hr	aPTT 3-5 sec above normal
Treatment				
Medium-dose	IV	10,000 U	2000 U/hr	aPTT twice normal
High-dose	IV	20,000 U	5000 U/hr	aPTT maximum (~150 sec)
Low-molecular-weight heparin				
Low-risk prophylaxis*				
Dalteparin	SC		2500 U qd	None
Enoxaparin	SC		2000 U (20 mg) qd	None
Nadroparin	SC		3100 U qd	None
Tinzaparin	SC		3500 U qd	None
Ardeparin	SC		—	—
Danaparoid	SC		750 U bid	None
High-risk prophylaxis†				
Dalteparin	SC		5000 U qd	None
Enoxaparin	SC		4000 U (40 mg) qd	None
Nadroparin	SC		60 U/kg qd	None
Tinzaparin	SC		50 U/kg qd	None
Ardeparin	SC		50 U/kg bid	None
Danaparoid	SC		750 U bid	None
Treatment				
Dalteparin	SC		100 U/kg bid	None
Enoxaparin	SC		100 U/kg bid	None
Nadroparin	SC		90 U/kg bid	None
Tinzaparin	SC		175 U/kg bid	None
Ardeparin	SC		—	—
Warfarin‡				
Low-intensity	PO§	10 mg	2.5-7.5 mg	INR 2.0-3.0 (PT 1.3-1.5 times normal)
High-intensity	PO§	10-20 mg	5-10 mg	INR 3.0-4.5 (PT 1.5-2.0 times normal)

*Uncomplicated general surgery.
†Abdominal pelvic surgery for cancer or in patients with previous episode of venous thromboembolism, hip or knee replacement, hip or pelvic fractures, acute spinal injury, or multiple trauma.
‡Response to warfarin is variable and requires close monitoring. The loading dose is within the range between maintenance and twice the maintenance dose.
§IV dose same as PO.
SC, Subcutaneous; *IV,* intravenous; *aPTT,* activated partial thromboplastin time; *PO,* per os; *INR,* international normalized ratio; *PT,* prothrombin time.

which can be used not only for treatment and prophylaxis of DVT, but for pulmonary and systemic arterial embolism as well. The dosages of intravenous unfractionated heparin (which is more reliable than the subcutaneous route) and of oral warfarin should be adjusted to the activated partial thromboplastin time (aPTT) and international normalized ratio (INR) or prothrombin time (PT). The INR is preferable to the PT; there is no discrepancy between values obtained by different laboratories on the same blood samples. A wide variation in PT may be seen because of the different types of thromboplastin that may be used.[109,110] Generally, an INR of 2.0 to 3.0 corresponds to a PT 1.3 to 1.5 times normal; an INR of 3.0 to 4.5 is equivalent to a PT 1.5 to 2.0 times normal.[110] Although there is no difference in therapeutic benefit between low- and high-intensity warfarin treatment, bleeding complications occur more often with the latter.[111] Thus, except in the most severe thromboembolic complications, warfarin therapy should maintain low therapeutic INRs.

During heparin therapy, the hematocrit and platelet count are probably more important than the aPTT. When heparin-induced bleeding causes a drop in hematocrit sufficient to necessitate transfusion, the treatment should be discontinued or at least readjusted to a low dose. Heparin-induced thrombocytopenia may be mild or severe.[112] Although the former usually is inconsequential, the latter, for reasons that are unclear, can result in severe intravascular thrombotic complications and end-organ damage as a result of platelet-fibrin clots. Recovery of the platelet count usually occurs with discontinuation of heparin. Danaparoid, a heparinoid formed by dermatan sulfate, heparin sulfate, and chondroitin sulfate, can also be used in heparin-induced thrombocytopenia.[113]

Low-molecular-weight-heparins (LMWHs) are administered subcutaneously and offer the advantage of not requiring laboratory monitoring. They differ from unfractionated heparins primarily in that their antithrombin III activity on factor Xa is two to four times greater than their antithrombin activity on factor IIa.[114,115] Compared to unfractionated heparin, LMWHs also exhibit less binding to plasma protein and endothelium, better bioavailability at small doses, less inhibition of platelet function, no increase in vascular permeability, and non–dose-dependent clearance.[114,115] Consequently, these agents have a more predictable anticoagulant effect of longer duration and seem to cause hemorrhagic complications less often than does unfractionated heparin.[114,115] Therapeutically, they are at least as safe and effective as unfractionated heparin,[116,117] and currently they are about 10% less expensive.[118] Generally, their anticoagulant effect peaks about 3 to 4 hours after injection and gradually declines to 50% of the maximum after 12 hours.[115] Thus increased bleeding from surgery or trauma will occur if administration is not timed properly. Large doses should precede surgery by about 12 hours; low doses can be given within 1 to 2 hours of a planned procedure (see Table 29-5).[114]

Unlike LMWHs, and to a certain extent unfractionated heparin, tight control of warfarin dosage is essential because of a greater likelihood of bleeding. Many drugs interact with the effects of warfarin; some lead to an increased and others to a decreased response. If bleeding occurs, it should be treated with intravenous vitamin K_1 oxide and, in severe cases, with fresh frozen plasma to increase the concentrations of vitamin K–dependent coagulation factors.

As mentioned earlier, deep vein thrombophlebitis may present in one of three forms: nonocclusive, occlusive, and phlegmasia cerulea dolens. If anticoagulation is not contraindicated by surgery within the previous 5 to 10 days or by a preexisting bleeding disorder, medium-dose unfractionated heparin treatment is sufficient for the first two forms, whereas phlegmasia cerulea dolens is best treated with a high-dose regimen. Low-intensity warfarin may be administered simultaneously with or 3 to 4 days after heparin administration if the patient can eat and if anticoagulation is planned for more than a week. Heparin can be discontinued when warfarin produces an INR value between 2.0 and 3.0. Upper-extremity thrombophlebitis is treated with medium-dose heparin. Additional thrombolytic therapy may be considered for both upper- and lower-extremity thrombophlebitis if pain and swelling do not respond promptly to anticoagulation.[119] If anticoagulation is contraindicated, low-molecular-weight dextran can be used with some benefit in any form of venous thrombosis. The following measures may also be required: elevation of the limb with or without elastic compression for lower-extremity occlusive or nonocclusive thrombosis; fluid replacement, and in some instances thrombectomy, for phlegmasia cerulea dolens; and removal of an intravascular catheter followed by culture of any clot and broad-spectrum antibiotic therapy for septic thrombophlebitis of the upper or lower extremity.

3. Prophylaxis. Prophylaxis of DVT, which, as mentioned earlier, is also prevention of PTE, is the most effective measure to reduce morbidity and mortality from this cause. An institutional policy for prophylaxis, with periodic auditing of how it is implemented, may be useful in achieving good results. Although this aspect of care traditionally has been considered the primary responsibility of surgeons, anesthesiologists also need to be involved for several reasons. First, determining which patients are at high risk of venous thromboembolism and evaluating the appropriateness of preoperative prophylaxis are important functions of the anesthesiologist. Second, preventive measures may affect the choice between general and regional anesthesia. Finally, critical care anesthesiologists may have to manage prophylaxis themselves during the early postoperative period.

The available data on the prevention of venous thromboembolism are substantial and somewhat confusing because of the multitude of techniques and perioperative clinical situations and their interactions. For example, all general surgical procedures do not carry the same risk and thus require different prophylactic regimens (Table 29-6). Likewise, a prophylactic technique that is satisfac-

Table 29-6. Recommended prophylactic measures for each level of perioperative thromboembolic risk in general surgical patients

Low risk	Moderate risk	High risk	Very high risk
Uncomplicated minor surgery in patients younger than 40 years with no clinical risk factors	Major surgery in patients older than 40 years with no other clinical risk factors	Major surgery in patients older than 40 years who have additional risk factors	Major surgery in patients older than 40 years plus previous venous thromboembolic or malignant disease, orthopedic surgery or hip fracture, stroke, or spinal cord injury
No specific measure necessary	GCS, LDUH (q 12 h), and IPCS	LDUH (q 8 hr), LMWH, and IPCS	LMWH, oral anticoagulants, IPCS (with LDUH or LMWH), and ADH

Data from Clagett GP, Anderson FA, Heit J, et al: *Chest* 108:312S, 1995; Salzman EN, Hirsh J: Prevention of venous thromboembolism. In Colman RN, Hirsh J, Marder VJ, et al, eds: *Hemostasis and thrombosis: basic principles and clinical practice,* ed 3, Philadelphia, 1994, JB Lippincott. *GCS,* Graduated compression stockings, also called elastic stockings; *LDUH,* low-dose unfractionated heparin; *IPCS,* intermittent pneumatic compression stockings; *LMWH,* low-molecular-weight heparin; *ADH,* adjusted-dose heparin.

tory for a general surgical patient may not necessarily be beneficial for a given orthopedic operation; in fact, as discussed later in this chapter, a technique that may be efficacious for one orthopedic procedure may be ineffective for another. Finally, the hemorrhagic complications of anticoagulant therapy may be more hazardous in neurosurgery than for any other surgical procedures. Additionally, a large number of patients are required for any study to convincingly demonstrate the efficacy of a particular technique. Thus, rather than surveying the large number of existing papers, we describe the findings of five recent meta-analyses that review most of the significant data on the prevention of thromboembolism.[120-124]

There are two general prophylactic strategies. Surveillance of patients with duplex studies at regular intervals and using preventive measures only when there are positive findings appears attractive. However, this approach is cumbersome and often unreliable because, as discussed earlier, ultrasonography is only moderately sensitive in asymptomatic patients with DVT, who represent 60% to 80% of high-risk patients.[82,84,122,123] The second approach involves routine use of prophylaxis and appears to be more practical and cost-effective.[122,123] Prophylactic measures counteract various phases of the development, propagation, and embolization of venous thrombi (Fig. 29-5). Selection should be based on risk assessment, the proven efficacy of a specific regimen in a given clinical setting, and the risk of complications.

There are two categories of preventive measures: pharmacologic, including various anticoagulant agents, and mechanical, which aims to counteract stasis of lower-extremity blood flow and (although this is a controversial issue) may increase fibrinolytic activity.[125,126] Pharmacologic regimens include subcutaneous fixed low-dose unfractionated heparin (LDUH) (5000 IU every 8 to 12 hours), unfractionated heparin at a dose adjusted to keep aPTT at the upper limit of normal, LMWH at a dose specified in Table 29-5, oral warfarin (see Table 29-5), dextran, aspirin, or another nonsteroidal antiinflammatory drug (NSAID), and the recently introduced agents

hirudin and its analog, hirulog. These latter drugs are antithrombin-III–independent selective bivalent thrombin inhibitors and can inactivate clot-bound thrombin.[122] A 65–amino-acid peptide, hirudin is produced by the salivary glands of the medicinal leech; currently it is synthesized using recombinant DNA technology. The usual dose is 15 mg subcutaneously twice daily. Hirulog is given as 1 mg/kg subcutaneously three times a day. Both agents appear to be safe.[122]

Dextrans act in several ways: They reduce platelet aggregation, improve regional blood flow, and facilitate breakdown of thrombi by increasing fibrinolysis and altering clot structure. Both dextran 40 and 70 are effective in reducing thromboembolism, but they have disadvantages: increased risk of bleeding, allergic reactions, and the need for intravenous access.[120] The efficacy of the antiplatelet agents, aspirin and the NSAIDs, in reducing the incidence of DVT is doubtful at best.[120]

As is widely known among anesthesiologists, spinal and epidural anesthesia decrease the short-term incidence of DVT and PTE after emergency hip surgery, elective hip replacement, and other forms of surgery by about 30% to 50% compared to general anesthesia.[120] This effect may be related to a decrease in platelet adhesion, aggregation, and release resulting from a direct effect of the anesthetic agents, a reduction in blood viscosity secondary to the fluid loading necessitated by induced vasodilation, a decreased activation of clotting factors, and early patient mobilization after surgery. It is not known whether neuraxial opioid analgesia produces the same effect, whether there is any long-term benefit to extending the duration of the epidural anesthetic infusion, or whether any additional decrease in risk can be obtained by concomitant use of other prophylactic measures.

Mechanical methods have a special place in the prevention of perioperative thromboembolic complications because they are not associated with bleeding. The most effective of these techniques is early ambulation. Although intermittent pneumatic compression stockings

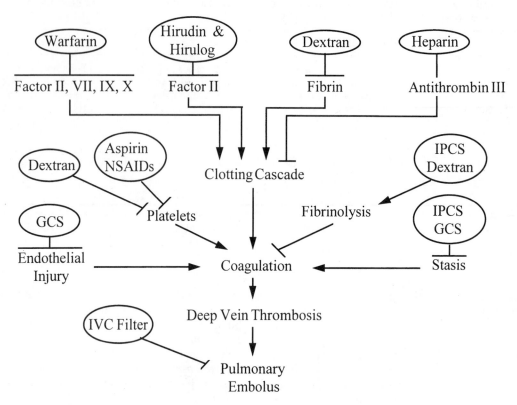

Fig. 29-5. Prophylactic measures *(flat-ended lines)* blocking thromboembolism at various phases of development. Arrows indicate stimulation. *GCS,* Graduated compression stockings; *IPCS,* intermittent pneumatic compression stockings; *NSAIDs,* nonsteroidal antiinflammatory drugs. (Modified from Kibel AS, Loughlin KR: *J Urol* 153:1763, 1995.)

(IPCS) and graduated compression stockings (GCS) are the traditional forms of mechanical protection, other methods have been introduced recently: plantar compression and passive leg movement.[125] IPCS exert their effect by increasing blood return from the lower extremities by 180% to 240% and (although this is controversial) by stimulating fibrinolysis.[125,126] GCS work by increasing the venous blood velocity by 20% and by preventing overdistention of the veins, thereby avoiding endothelial damage and thrombus formation.[124] Although studies have shown a reduction in incidence of DVT with IPCS and GCS comparable to that associated with heparin prophylaxis, others have failed to demonstrate this effect.[124] These devices have an important preventive role, but in high-risk patients they can be relied on only in combination with other antithrombotic agents. Even in this setting, their beneficial effects have not been proven.[120] GCS should not be used in patients with lower-extremity ischemia. Likewise, if GCS are too tight, they may promote rather than prevent venous thrombosis.

Table 29-6 provides guidelines for selection of prophylactic methods in general surgical patients with various levels of risks.[121,127] As mentioned earlier, various prophylactic protocols may be effective in different surgical procedures during the perioperative period. The

following information should suggest the most acceptable method in each clinical setting.

a. Orthopedic surgery. In elective hip replacement surgery, postoperative subcutaneous LMWH (see Table 29-5 for dose of each agent), low-intensity warfarin initiated preoperatively or immediately following surgery to achieve an INR between 2.0 and 3.0, and unfractionated heparin started preoperatively at a dose adjusted to an aPTT at the upper limit of normal are equally effective.[121,122] LMWH probably is preferable because it is easy to administer and does not require laboratory monitoring. However, even with this agent, there is a significant incidence of DVT (15%).[122] Subcutaneous hirudin (15 mg twice daily) and hirulog (1 mg/kg three times daily) appear to be more effective than LMWH in preliminary studies and may ultimately be the agents of choice.[122] Spinal and epidural anesthesia probably are preferable to general anesthesia because they reduce the prevalence of postoperative venous thromboembolism.[122] IPCS and GCS may also be helpful. Antiplatelet agents and LDUH are of limited value in hip replacement.[122]

For knee replacement surgery the most effective prophylaxis can be obtained by subcutaneous LMWH postoperatively or by IPCS. (GCS are ineffective.)[121,122] LMWH and IPCS are comparably effective in this setting[121]; combined use may be more effective than either alone. It should be emphasized that even with these measures, there is a high prevalence of DVT; hirudin or hirulog may be more effective in this situation as well.

Despite an increased likelihood of bleeding complications in emergency hip surgery, subcutaneous LMWH or oral warfarin adjusted to an INR between 2.0 and 3.0 is the prophylaxis of choice.[121] Antiplatelet agents and LDUH have little beneficial effect. IPCS or GCS should be applied as an adjunct measure whenever possible, even though their role has not been determined conclusively. There is evidence to suggest that development of DVT occurs during the first 8 to 12 days and becomes symptomatic afterward, usually after the patient is discharged from the hospital. Thus continuation of prophylaxis through the 2 weeks following surgery is essential.[122] A longer duration of anticoagulant therapy should be based on the underlying risks of thromboembolism. Prophylactic use of an inferior vena cava filter rarely is needed in orthopedic patients. Its use is limited to patients at high risk for thromboembolism who have ongoing bleeding that precludes the use of anticoagulant therapy.[121]

b. General surgery. A strategy for the prophylaxis of DVT in general surgery patients is summarized in Table 29-6. No treatment beyond early mobilization is required in low-risk patients.[121] Patients at moderate risk may benefit from IPCS and GCS started during surgery and retained throughout the postoperative period. LDUH (5000 IU subcutaneously), administered 2 hours before and 12 hours after surgery, is also effective in these patients. For high-risk patients, LDUH is given every 8 hours and has a protective effect equivalent to that of LMWH. This regimen should be replaced by IPCS in patients who may be prone to wound hematomas. In very-high-risk general surgical patients, prophylaxis includes heparin (LDUH or LMWH), dextran, and IPCS. Heparin should be started preoperatively, and dextran and IPCS intraoperatively.[121] Warfarin rarely is used in general surgery because it is cumbersome, requires monitoring, and should be started preoperatively, although it may be indicated in selected very-high-risk patients. Its dose should be adjusted to achieve an INR between 2.0 and 3.0.[121] Aspirin or other NSAIDs are not recommended for this purpose in general surgery.[121]

c. Elective neurosurgery. The fear of intracranial bleeding has led clinicians to concentrate on mechanical prophylaxis in elective neurosurgery. The recommended technique is IPCS with or without GCS, beginning at the onset of the procedure, although these devices leave many patients at risk of thromboembolism.[121,122] LDUH alone or combined with mechanical devices is an acceptable alternative and may be considered in high-risk patients.[121] Although further studies are needed, recent trials of LMWH also show promising results in this group of patients.[122]

In acute spinal cord injury, DVT and PTE occur mainly during the first 2 weeks. The limited existing data suggest that LMWH is superior to adjusted-dose heparin, although both can be used.[121,122] Warfarin prophylaxis may also be effective. Used alone, LDUH, IPCS, and GCS have not been shown to have significant beneficial effects, although they may be helpful if they are used in combination or with other methods.[121]

d. Multiple trauma. Patients with multiple trauma, especially those who are elderly, who require surgery, who have lower-extremity fractures or spinal cord injury, or who have received multiple transfusions, are at very high risk of thromboembolic complications. Warfarin and LMWH appear to cause a greater decrease in the incidence of DVT and PTE in these patients than does LDUH. However, LMWH is associated with a higher incidence of bleeding than is LDUH. Thromboembolic complications are common even when LMWH is used; obviously, a better prophylactic technique is required for these patients.[121,122]

In general, early ambulation is the most effective method of prophylaxis and should be used for all patients, including those who are at low risk of venous thromboembolism, when antithrombotic drugs cannot be justified. In medium-risk patients, the combination of mechanical methods with anticoagulant treatment is appropriate. High-risk patients provide an absolute indication for anticoagulant prophylaxis. Of the available anticoagulants, LMWH appears to be preferable to the others, not necessarily because of greater effectiveness, but because of its ease of administration. The selection between heparins and warfarin is based primarily on the duration of treatment required; heparin is preferred for short-term (up to 5 days) and warfarin for long-term management. These drugs may be given according to a range of protocols: preoperative initiation with postoperative continuation, initiation 24 hours after surgery, or postoperative initiation of both heparin and Coumadin, followed by Coumadin alone after 3 to 4 days. None of the available prophylactic techniques can reliably eliminate the possibility of DVT. Thus high-risk patients undergoing surgery may need to be examined with preoperative duplex ultrasound in order to ensure prevention of perioperative PTE.

D. Treatment of pulmonary thromboembolism

There are two aspects to the treatment of PTE: acute hemodynamic and ventilatory support and definitive treatment with anticoagulants, thrombolysis, or surgery.

1. Hemodynamic and ventilatory support. Hypotension, transient or persistent, is the most common hemodynamic sign of clinically significant acute PTE. Intraoperatively, a decrease in blood pressure is more likely to result from other causes, such as hypovolemia, overdose of anesthetic agents, anaphylaxis, myocardial ischemia, compression or traction on great vessels, cardiac tamponade, or tension pneumothorax or hemothorax. Hypotension from any cause may be modified by the effects of the patient's baseline cardiovascular status, anesthetics, and positive-pressure ventilation, making differential diagnosis difficult. As mentioned earlier, TEE may be an extremely useful tool in this setting.[104,108] The hemodynamic response to volume loading, which is the first measure taken against hypotension, depends on the magnitude of RV afterload.[68] In patients with severe pulmonary hypertension and an enlarged RV, rapid fluid administration may augment RV distention, increasing its O_2 consumption, decreasing its perfusion, and thus producing ischemia and failure. On the other hand, in patients with less severe pulmonary hypertension, volume expansion may increase RV preload and output. Especially if aggressive, fluid therapy may require placement of a PA catheter with serial measurements of PAP and PCWP and cardiac output determination in order to enable appropriate titration. However, when there is leftward septal shift and altered LV geometry, the resultant elevation in PCWP may result in premature reduction or discontinuation of fluid administration. Monitoring the ventricular size and contractility with TEE may be helpful in these circumstances.

As mentioned earlier, increased pulmonary vascular resistance leads to an increase in pulmonary and decreased systemic arterial pressures. This phenomenon may result from elevation of pulmonary vascular closing pressure, incremental vascular resistance, or both.[68] Thus it is not surprising that, as demonstrated in animal studies, the efficacy of vasoactive agents in improving hemodynamic abnormalities may vary depending on the underlying mechanism of the hemodynamic abnormality.[68]

Epinephrine (100- to 500-μg bolus, followed by a continuous infusion of 0.1 to 1 μg/kg/min) often is administered for severe hypotension that persists despite an initial fluid challenge. The α-effects (vasoconstriction) of this agent, combined with its β-activity (inotropic), improve the perfusion and contractility of the RV.[128] When the hemodynamic abnormality is less severe, dobutamine infusion (8 to 10 μg/kg/min) may be considered.[129] This drug improves hemodynamics because of its inotropic and pulmonary vasodilating activity, although through its β-effects, it may cause or increase systemic hypotension. In animals, dopamine can also increase cardiac output after PTE; this effect occurs at high doses, which also produce profound tachycardia.[130] α-Adrenergic agents are useful in the treatment of systemic shock resulting from acute RV failure after PTE. In this regard, norepinephrine, because of its combined α- and β-adrenergic effects, is preferable to the pure α-adrenergic activity of neosynephrine.[68] The improvement of RV function with α-adrenergic agents results primarily from augmentation of coronary perfusion by elevation of systemic blood pressure; this effect usually is sufficient to compensate for their potentially deleterious pulmonary vasoconstrictive effects. Isoproterenol should in theory improve hemodynamics in this setting because it produces pulmonary vasodilation in addition to its inotropic activity. However, it actually caused further deterioration when administered to animals in shock from massive PTE, probably as a result of systemic vasodilation and consequent RV ischemia.[68] Nevertheless, isoproterenol's beneficial effects may predominate in mildly hypotensive patients, and cardiac output may improve.[68] The phosphodiesterase inhibitors amrinone and milrinone also have inotropic and pulmonary and systemic vasodilating

properties, but unlike isoproterenol, they have been shown to improve altered hemodynamics in animals after PTE. Although these drugs have not been tested systematically in humans, an isolated case report describes improvement in hemodynamics and oxygenation with amrinone.[131] This improvement is surprising because in the past these agents have been shown to decrease oxygenation by increasing pulmonary shunting and blunting hypoxic pulmonary vasoconstriction.[68]

None of the systemic pulmonary vasodilating agents (nitroglycerin, sodium nitroprusside, hydralazine, prostaglandin E_1) are likely to be beneficial because they all produce systemic vasodilation and diminish mean arterial pressure and coronary perfusion.[68] They may also increase right-to-left shunting in the lung. Therefore they should not be used in hypotensive patients; when the blood pressure is normal, they should be administered with caution and with adequate fluid therapy. On the other hand, inhaled vasodilators are selective and may improve RV function by reducing pulmonary vascular resistance. Aerosolized prostacyclin (30 to 50 ng/kg/min) and nitric oxide (10 to 20 ppm) can be used in this fashion. Experience with inhaled prostacyclin is limited. On the other hand, results from animal experiments and recent experience with patients suggest that by selective reduction of PAP, inhaled nitric oxide may improve hemodynamics and oxygenation in acute PTE.[132,133] It should be emphasized that the increase in pulmonary perfusion from nitric oxide may increase shunting and produce decreased oxygenation.[134] Thus to determine the overall effect of this treatment, monitoring of RV function by TEE, or of pulmonary hemodynamics and cardiac output, may be necessary.[134] Nitric oxide may inhibit platelet aggregation and thus may cause bleeding, especially in those receiving anticoagulant and thrombolytic treatment.[133] Likewise, the possibility of a rebound increase in PAP after discontinuation of the agent implies that it should be used only with utmost caution,[133] and only in severely ill patients who are not responding to other therapeutic modalities or who present contraindications to such therapy.

Hypoxemia should be treated actively, not only to avoid its well-known deleterious systemic effects, but also to counteract the pulmonary vasoconstriction it induces. Increasing PaO_2 to greater than 100 mm Hg may be sufficient to achieve this objective. PEEP ventilation should be titrated carefully because impeding venous return and reducing RV preload may result in severe hemodynamic deterioration.

2. Definitive treatment of pulmonary thromboembolism. The devastating consequences of hemorrhagic complications associated with the use of anticoagulants and thrombolytics in the immediate perioperative period make some modification of the standard treatment of PTE necessary. The vast majority of emboli occur several days after surgery and thus may permit the safe use of anticoagulants, although thrombolytics should be withheld for at least 10 days postoperatively. In fact, because postoperative PTE usually occurs within 2 weeks of surgery, thrombolytic therapy is highly unlikely to be of benefit at all. On the other hand, there may be an indication for these agents when PTE produces severe hemodynamic and pulmonary abnormalities in the immediate preoperative period. Because heparin produces a substantial decrease in recurrence of and mortality from PTE,[135] it has been considered the standard treatment of this complication. Its use in treatment of surgical patients, although not clearly defined, depends mainly on four factors: the severity of the embolism, the timing of the embolic event with relation to the surgery or injury, the presence of potential bleeding sites, and preexisting coagulation abnormalities.

a. Heparin. The severity of the embolism is a factor in deciding on the heparin dose and determining whether it should be administered before or after diagnostic results are obtained. To our knowledge, there are no reliable data about the safe times for initiation of heparin after surgery. Nevertheless, clinicians empirically estimate that 24 hours are needed for clots in severed vessels to gain adequate strength, even though heparin's effects on fibrin deposition and fibrinolysis can affect even older clots.[136] Some wounds are more likely than others to bleed with anticoagulant treatment; thus the surgeon's opinion as to the initiation of heparin therapy is important. Furthermore, certain preexisting lesions (e.g., central nervous system [CNS] injuries, retroperitoneal tumors) are likely to bleed, with catastrophic consequences. Preexisting coagulation abnormalities, whether caused by disease states or drugs, may also potentiate the hemorrhagic effects of heparin, as may advanced age. Caution should therefore be exercised during therapeutic heparin use in these patients.

Patients with PTE require higher doses of heparin than those with DVT, probably because of a shorter half-life and increased clearance of the agent.[137] Thus the effects of heparin should be monitored initially by aPTT every 4 to 6 hours and then daily to maintain a value between 1.5 and 2.5 times control. With this measure alone, the risk of recurrence of PTE and bleeding complications is likely to be minimized.

Moderate-dose heparin therapy (see Table 29-5) may be initiated while confirmatory diagnostic tests are performed; when there is a possibility of minor thromboembolism in a patient who presents with transient tachypnea, mild blood gas changes, premature beats, or tachyarrhythmia; and when there is substantial risk of embolism and no contraindication to anticoagulation. Alternatively, the diagnosis may be assumed and treatment continued without diagnostic tests as long as the risk is present. If PTE is suspected but is unlikely, or if anticoagulation may be risky, diagnostic tests (D-dimer, FDP, and noninvasive vascular studies) should be ordered. If the results are negative, no anticoagulant treatment, except perhaps prophylaxis, is indicated. If one or more diagnostic tests yield positive results, confirmation with pulmonary angiography should be obtained and followed by initiation or continuation of moderate- or high-dose heparin (see Table 29-5).

When the patient exhibits transient hypotension, tachycardia or other arrhythmias, tachypnea, a significant decrease in PaO_2 and $PaCO_2$, apprehension, and signs of pulmonary infarction, moderate- or high-dose heparin (see Table 29-5) can be started if PTE is the likely cause. If PTE is unlikely or anticoagulation seems risky, an attempt may be made to establish the diagnosis by pulmonary angiography or noninvasive peripheral venous studies. If the diagnosis is not confirmed but the patient is at risk for thromboembolism and anticoagulation is not contraindicated, low- or moderate-dose heparin should be administered (see Table 29-5). If the diagnosis is confirmed and anticoagulation is not contraindicated, moderate-dose heparin should be given to hemodynamically stable patients, and high-dose therapy is administered to those who are unstable.

LMWH has proven efficacy in DVT and does not require monitoring for dose adjustment. Recently it has been compared with intravenous unfractionated heparin in a European multicenter study. A fixed once-daily subcutaneous dose of 175 anti–factor Xa U/kg of tinzaparin was as effective and safe as unfractionated heparin (50 IU/kg bolus followed by 500 IU/kg/day infusion) in patients with submassive PTE.[138]

As in DVT, anticoagulation with oral warfarin can be started within the first 5 days of heparin therapy. Heparin should be continued for at least 4 to 6 days to give time for depletion of vitamin K–dependent factors with long biologic half-lives. Recurrence of venous thromboembolism can be prevented in most instances by maintaining the INR between 2.0 and 3.0, which corresponds to a PT between 1.3 and 1.5 times control. Oral anticoagulation usually is continued for 3 to 6 months, but may be administered for a longer period and even indefinitely if uncontrollable major risk factors are present.

b. Thrombolytic therapy. As mentioned earlier, thrombolytic therapy is contraindicated within 10 to 15 days of surgery. Other contraindications are organ biopsy, puncture of incompressible vessels, lumbar puncture, first and last trimester of pregnancy, delivery, serious trauma, prolonged cardiopulmonary resuscitation, an active intracranial process, gastrointestinal or genitourinary bleeding within 3 months, a hemorrhagic disorder, aortic aneurysm, and thrombi within the left side of the heart.[87] In the very rare situation in which perioperative thrombolytic therapy is used, the objective is to promote rapid resolution of PE and thus to normalize the PAP in order to treat or prevent a potentially fatal RV dysfunction.[139] Additionally, an intravenous thrombolytic may also lyse the original peripheral venous thrombi and thus prevent further embolization.

Of the three available thrombolytics, streptokinase may be neutralized by antibodies already present as a result of previous streptococcal infections. To overcome the effects of these antibodies, a loading dose of streptokinase should be administered before initiation of the infusion. Streptokinase may deplete circulating plasminogen after a few hours; thus it can be infused for only 6 to 8 hours per day, followed by heparin infusion until the next dose. Like streptokinase, urokinase lacks fibrin specificity and produces a systemic lytic state. Both of these enzymes are superior to heparin in improving hemodynamics, pulmonary circulation on angiography, and lung scans.[87] However, mortality and the incidence of early recurrence of PTE are not likely to be better with thrombolytic therapy than with heparin.[87]

t-PA, which is produced with recombinant DNA technology, theoretically should be somewhat more specific for fibrin clot than streptokinase and urokinase. This agent lyses the clot locally and, by the time it reaches the systemic circulation, is largely deactivated by circulating t-PA inhibitor. Nevertheless, in practice t-PA behaves like urokinase.

Several administration schedules are described for thrombolytics (Table 29-7). The therapeutic regimen approved by the U.S. Food and Drug Administration (FDA) can provide marked hemodynamic improvement, although the onset of effect is slow, requiring at least 12 hours of infusion. Therapeutic regimens that can provide rapid lysis over a period of 2 hours are more popular (see Table 29-7). A weight-adjusted bolus dose of urokinase or t-PA (see Table 29-7) may provide rapid improvement of hemodynamics with fewer bleeding complications, although further trials are needed to prove the efficacy and safety of this technique. Injection of urokinase directly into the clot has also been described; 2200 IU/kg/hr is administered via a PA catheter for up to 24 hours until lysis of the thrombus is complete (see Table 29-7). This method, which includes simultaneous administration of heparin 500 IU/hr via a peripheral vein, is said to be less likely to be associated with bleeding complications in surgical patients than other techniques of thrombolysis.[40,140] The efficacy and safety of this method must be demonstrated with randomized studies.

The incidence of bleeding during thrombolytic therapy is many times higher than with anticoagulants and depends on both the dosage and the duration of treatment. With careful administration of thrombolytics, the incidence of major hemorrhage is less than 5% and that of intracranial bleeding is about 1% to 2%.[141,142] Hemorrhage occurs not only because of thrombolysis at sites of vascular injury, but also because of a systemic lytic state resulting from the formation of plasmin, which produces fibrinogenolysis and destruction of other coagulation proteins such as factors V and VIII.

Monitoring of thrombolytic therapy serves two purposes: to obtain information about therapeutic effect and to predict and thus prevent bleeding. Improvements in hemodynamics and in the results of pulmonary angiography and scanning suggest that treatment is successful. Furthermore, an increase in the D-dimer concentration indicates breakdown of cross-linked fibrin. To avoid bleeding, plasma fibrinogen should be maintained above 0.2 g/dl to ensure that the native clotting mechanism is not exhausted. Lower fibrinogen concentrations should alert the physician to discontinue thrombolytic therapy.[140] Heparin is commonly administered during thrombolytic therapy. Thus the thrombin time, a previously useful monitor, currently is of no value. It should be emphasized that bleeding after thrombolytic therapy can be minimized by establishing a diagnosis before attempting treatment and by critically evaluating the risk of hemorrhage against the severity of the embolic process, especially in the presence of a major contraindication such as surgery.[87]

c. Embolectomy. Embolectomy is an alternative to thrombolysis for acute treatment of patients with massive thromboembolism. Either catheter or surgical techniques may be used. These are more useful than thrombolysis for surgical patients. The catheter techniques are

Table 29-7. Half-life and dosing schedules of thrombolytic agents in pulmonary thromboembolism

Agent	Half-life (minutes)	Type of administration	Dose
Streptokinase	80	FDA approved	Loading dose: 250,000 IU over 30 min Maintenance dose: 1,000,000 IU/hr for 24 hr
Urokinase	15	FDA approved	Loading dose: 2000 IU/lb over 10 min Maintenance dose: 2000 IU/lb over 12-24 hr or Loading dose: 4000 IU/lb over 10 min Maintenance dose: 4000 IU/lb over 12 hr
		Short-term	Loading dose: 1 million IU over 10 min Maintenance dose: 2 million IU over 110 min
		Bolus lysis	15,000-20,000 IU/lb over 10 min
		Direct PA injection	Loading dose: 2200 IU/kg into the PA clot Maintenance: 2200 IU/kg/hr PA infusion until clot is lysed
Tissue plasminogen activator (Alteplase)	4	FDA approved	100 mg as a continuous IV infusion over 2 hr or Loading dose: 10 mg as a bolus Maintenance dose: 90 mg over 2 hr
		Bolus lysis	0.6 mg/lb administered over 2 min

Data from Janata-Schwatczek K, Weiss K, Riezinger I, et al: *Semin Thromb Hemost* 22:33, 1996; Lualdi JC, Goldhaber SZ: *Am Heart J* 130:1276, 1995; Molina JE, Hunter DW, Yedlicka JW, et al: *Am J Surg* 163:375, 1992.
PA, Pulmonary artery; *IV,* intravenous.

suction catheter embolectomy,[143] catheter-directed clot fragmentation with or without local fibrinolysis,[144] and high-speed rotational catheter thrombolysis.[73] Surgical embolectomy is associated with a prohibitively high mortality rate of as much as 40%.[145] Thus it is used only in rare instances, such as massive PTE associated with severe hypotension and hypoxemia or CO_2 accumulation despite maximal minute volumes with mechanical ventilation. Data from experimental animals suggest that the end-tidal CO_2 tension increases immediately after removal of clot from a PA. However, it remains high and does not reflect $PaCO_2$ for at least an hour after release of the occlusion. It is VCO_2/breath (CO_2 elimination in each breath) that accurately reflects CO_2 elimination,[107] although this value has not been measured clinically.

Patients presenting with catastrophic PTE with cardiac arrest, shock, bradyarrhythmia, and other grave signs should receive cardiopulmonary resuscitation and massive doses of heparin in addition to tracheal intubation, mechanical ventilation with 100% O_2, and inotropic support. High-dose heparin therapy may be continued if the patient survives emergency treatment. It should be emphasized that open or closed cardiac massage may be ineffective because complete obstruction of the PA with saddle embolus does not permit filling of the left heart. In these situations TEE may be helpful in showing the effectiveness of resuscitation. In severe cases unresponsive to resuscitation, pulmonary embolectomy may be necessary.

3. Prophylaxis of pulmonary embolism.
The best way to avoid venous thromboembolism is to prevent clot formation in midsized and large systemic veins, especially in patients who are elderly or immobilized, who have sustained major surgical or traumatic injuries, or who have a history of a spontaneous thrombotic event. Techniques to prevent development of venous thrombosis have already been discussed: surveillance with duplex studies, early ambulation, elastic stockings, low-molecular-weight dextran, intermittent pneumatic compression of the calf muscles, and anticoagulation. All of these measures also apply to prevention of PTE both before and after DVT has been diagnosed. However, these measures may be unreliable or impossible to use in certain instances. In these circumstances, a prophylactic vena cava filter provides the best protection against perioperative PTE. A vena cava filter may be indicated in patients with contraindications to anticoagulation (brain or spinal cord lesion, trauma or surgery, or a previous bleeding episode), serious side effects of anticoagulation (heparin allergy, bleeding, thrombocytopenia), or recurrence of PTE despite anticoagulation. It may also be indicated for prophylaxis in extremely high-risk patients in unusual circumstances (e.g., severe pelvic fractures, paradoxical embolism, or uncontrolled septic thromboembolism).[87,146]

The Greenfield filter, made of a special combination of metals, can be folded into a cannula introduced via a jugular or femoral vein.[146,147] After release from the cannula and because of the memory of the metal, the device takes its preformed shape of a cage or umbrella and attaches to the wall of the vena cava by protruding hooks.

If a femoral vein is used, phlebography should be performed first in order to document the absence of clot along its route. The filter is expected to remain in place permanently. Nevertheless, complications may occur, such as dislocation or entry of a hook into an adjacent organ. Although the filter is reliable in the vast majority of cases, clot occasionally may propagate through the device and embolize.[146,147]

4. Anesthetic considerations.
Apart from recognition, treatment, and prevention of perioperative thromboembolism, several other clinical issues may involve the anesthesiologist. Many patients who present for surgery are already receiving anticoagulants and thus require management of these agents before and after surgery. The second consideration is the use of regional anesthesia in the anticoagulated patient. Finally, there is the problem of selection of anesthetic agents and techniques for a procedure following an acute thromboembolic event.

a. Management of anticoagulation during the perioperative period.
Most patients who have had PTE within the past 3 to 6 months are receiving oral warfarin. Interruption of this treatment in the perioperative period in order to prevent bleeding is associated with an increased risk of thromboembolism. Assuming that the agent is discontinued 4 days preoperatively and restarted shortly after surgery and that the patient's INR during treatment is between 2.0 and 3.0, the risk of thromboembolism has been shown to be equivalent to the absence of anticoagulation for 1 day before and 1 day after surgery.[148] Although the risk of 1 day's loss of anticoagulation is no different from normal in nonsurgical patients, it becomes substantial in the early postoperative period because surgery increases the short-term incidence of recurrence 100-fold.[148]

The risk of recurrent thromboembolism depends on the timing of the original event. Within 1 month of an acute episode, the recurrence rate is about 40%; after the second month it decreases to 10%. Anticoagulant therapy decreases these rates by 80%. On the other hand, if heparin is used in the immediate postoperative period, the risk of bleeding is high: approximately 3% following 2 days of intravenous heparin administration.[148] Nevertheless, the likelihood of postoperative bleeding from heparin is much lower than the risk of recurrent thromboembolism, especially in the first month after an acute episode. As calculated by Kearon and Hirsh,[148] perioperative heparin treatment will prevent 7162 out of 10,000 recurrent thromboembolic events in the first month, 1328 of 10,000 in the second month, and 332 of 10,000 after the third month following an acute episode. In contrast, the risk of major bleeding with use of heparin during this period is 300 per 10,000. Thus it has been calculated that 559 per 10,000, 93 per 10,000, and 13 per 10,000 patients will be saved from death or disability during the first, second, and later months following an acute episode.

With the preceding facts in mind, Kearon and Hirsh[148] recommend the following anticoagulation protocol for patients with previous thromboembolism. Given the high chance of recurrence, surgery should be avoided within the first month following an acute event. When surgery is urgent, intravenous heparin is given before and after the procedure whenever the INR is less than 2.0. Before surgery aPTT is monitored and maintained at a therapeutic level, so heparin can be cleared from the blood by discontinuing its administration 6 hours before surgery. Postoperatively, heparin should not be given for at least 12 hours if there is any evidence of bleeding from surgical or puncture wounds. After this time, heparin is administered by infusion rather than by bolus, and the aPTT is measured about 12 hours after therapy is restarted. Within the first month of an acute episode, or if there is a major risk of bleeding from heparin, a vena cava filter may be appropriate. Preoperative intravenous heparin may be unnecessary for patients who have been receiving warfarin for more than 1 month, but postoperative heparin is indicated until the INR is brought to 2.0 with warfarin. All of these patients should also receive mechanical prophylaxis: GCS or IPCS. For patients on warfarin who require emergency surgery, switching to heparin is not possible despite its short onset and elimination times; these patients may have to be treated with fresh frozen plasma or vitamin K.

b. Regional anesthesia in the anticoagulated patient. Patients who are receiving prophylactic or therapeutic anticoagulants for thromboembolism may require regional anesthesia. Neural injury caused by bleeding after a superficial nerve block is unlikely because a hematoma is readily visible and often preventable by external compression. On the other hand, neurologic dysfunction from hematoma after spinal or epidural anesthesia may have grave consequences.[115] These are rare complications, occurring in 0.5 per 100,000 spinal and 0.7 per 100,000 epidural anesthetics. Blocks of deep nerves, such as the sciatic, may also be complicated by bleeding and subsequent limb paralysis. Vandermeulen, van Aken, and Vermylen[149] describe 61 cases of neuraxial blockade–induced spinal hematomas between 1906 and 1994. In 1995 Dahlgren and Tornebrandt[150] reported on three spinal hematomas following 8501 subarachnoid and 9232 epidural anesthetics between 1991 and 1994. A recent FDA Public Health Advisory informed U.S. anesthesiologists that more than 30 spinal hematomas had occurred after subarachnoid and epidural blocks between May 1993 and November 1997; this number had reached 40 by April 15, 1998.[151] The common feature in all of these patients was hemostatic abnormality, generally induced by anticoagulants. In the oldest series 68% of the patients had received heparin[149]; in the second, all three patients were anticoagulated[150]; and in the FDA report, all 40 patients had been taking LMWH.[151]

It appears that the potential for development of spinal hematoma varies depending on the timing of the regional anesthesia in relation to the last dose of anticoagulant, and on the type and dosage of the agent used. Spinal hematoma is very unlikely as long as heparin is not given for at least 1 hour after the spinal or epidural puncture, the patient does not have a preexisting coagulation disorder, and the degree of anticoagulation is monitored carefully. The epidural catheter should be removed when the heparin activity is lowest.[149] In addition, some au-

thors believe in postponing surgery if blood returns from the needle or catheter; this obviously is a safe but impractical measure.[152,153]

The risk of spinal bleeding is also low in patients receiving subcutaneous unfractionated heparin if the needle placement or catheter removal is delayed for at least 4 hours following the last dose of heparin and the aPTT is monitored in patients with liver disease and long-term thromboembolism.[115] Oral warfarin prophylaxis also appears to be safe even if it is started immediately after surgery[154]; it takes about 3 days for the PT to become elevated and about 6 days to establish the effective patient/control PT ratio of 1.3 to 1.5. By this time the catheter will have been removed. Removal of spinal catheters in anticoagulated patients is probably as critical a factor as placement; in Vandermeulen, van Aken, and Vermylen's series[149] of the 32 patients with spinal hematomas who had indwelling catheters, 15 developed the hematoma immediately following catheter removal. A gradually increasing level of an oral anticoagulant permits timely removal of the catheter before the establishment of the desired therapeutic effect. Nevertheless, as with heparin, anticoagulant activity must be monitored carefully because of significant patient variability in response to these agents.[154,155] Preoperative antiplatelet agents are unlikely to increase the risk of bleeding after central regional anesthesia.[156] However, it has been suggested that their use in patients receiving heparin or Coumadin may increase the risk of spinal hematoma.[153]

The FDA warning about the use of neuraxial blockade in patients receiving LMWH reduced the confidence inspired by earlier European reports[157] about the safety of regional anesthesia in this setting. A careful look at the patients who developed spinal hematoma discloses several risk factors: epidural anesthesia, especially using an indwelling catheter; placement or removal of the epidural catheter shortly after a dose of LMWH; initiation of prophylaxis preoperatively or immediately after surgery; old age; concomitant administration of intravenous heparin, dextran, antiplatelet agents, or LMWH; and traumatic or repeated epidural or spinal puncture.[115] Guidelines for the management of regional anesthesia in patients receiving perioperative LMWH have been published recently by Horlocker and Heit[115] and Haljamae.[158] Apart from the general principle of balancing the risk of spinal hematoma against the benefits of regional anesthesia for a specific patient, they recommend avoiding concomitant administration of medications affecting hemostasis, using a single-dose spinal rather than an epidural anesthetic whenever possible, placing the needle at least 12 hours after the last dose of LMWH, delaying a subsequent dose for at least 2 hours after needle placement, and delaying administration of the agent postoperatively in patients who have already been receiving the agent preoperatively. If prophylaxis is to be initiated postoperatively, they recommend leaving the epidural catheter overnight and administering the first dose of LMWH 2 hours after the catheter is removed. Clearly, a catheter should not be removed earlier than 12 hours following a dose of LMWH. Neurologic function should be monitored carefully in the early postoperative period; early detection and intervention is the key to prevention of permanent paralysis. Monitoring of neurologic function includes observing numbness, weakness, or bowel and bladder dysfunction; back pain, a common symptom of epidural hematoma, is uncommon in this population, probably because of intraoperative opioids.

E. Use of anesthetic agents in pulmonary thromboembolism

In acute PTE the highest priority is to provide maximum alveolar O_2 tension in order to alleviate hypoxic pulmonary vasoconstriction. Maintenance of myocardial contractility is also important if RV failure is to be avoided in the face of elevated pulmonary resistance. Thus administration of anesthetics should be discontinued. Although it can be argued that pulmonary vasodilation from inhaled anesthetics may decrease the significance of their myocardial depressant activity, in experimental studies of PTE, isoflurane has been shown to cause hemodynamic deterioration through severe al-

teration of RV performance.[159] Intravenous anesthetics have fewer deleterious effects on hemodynamics than inhaled anesthetics.[159] Nitrous oxide may elevate pulmonary hypertension and increase pulmonary vascular resistance in the presence of acute PTE.[160] In addition, its myocardial depressant effect may result in severe hemodynamic deterioration. Clearly anesthetics should be avoided in acute PTE; if their use is essential, their dosage should be titrated carefully.

III. VENOUS AIR EMBOLISM

Although most often associated with neurosurgical procedures in the sitting position, VAE may be seen in a wide variety of procedures, both surgical and diagnostic. In some of these procedures the embolizing gas may be nitrogen, argon, or oxygen, although the clinical effects generally are similar. Venous air or gas embolism has been reported in neurosurgery in lateral, supine, and prone positions (Fig. 29-6 and Table 29-8); in head and neck surgery[161]; in hip replacement; in cesarean sections,[162,163] hysteroscopy, and endometrial ablation with

Table 29-8. Incidence of air embolism in various positions

Position	No. of patients	Detectable air embolism		Amount of air aspirated (ml)	Gradient (cm)
		No. of cases	Percent		
Sitting	400	100	25.0	2-500	20-65
Lateral	60	5	8.3	3-200	5-18
Supine	48	7	14.6	2-150	5-18
Prone	10	1	10.0	45	7.5
Totals	518	113			

From Albin MS, Carroll RG, Maroon JC: *Neurosurgery* 3:380, 1978.

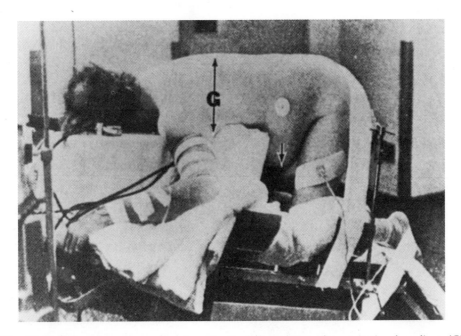

Fig. 29-6. Patient in prone position in a Hasting's frame. Note the gravitational gradient *(G)* between the spinous process and the heart. (From Albin MS, Ritter RR, Pruett CE, et al: *Anesth Analg* 73:346, 1991.)

or without use of insufflating gas[164,165]; in open prostatectomies[166,167]; in cardiopulmonary bypass[168]; as a complication of CV catheter or transvenous pacemaker placement[169]; after pulmonary barotrauma[170]; during cryosurgery of bone tumors[171]; in orthotopic liver transplantation during dissection of the native liver, unclamping of graft vessels, or as a result of venovenous bypass dysfunction[172-174]; and in many other situations[175] such as during use of argon coagulator,[176] hydrogen peroxide irrigation or pulsed lavage of open wounds,[177,178] intraosseous air injection,[179] administration of fluids with devices that permit rapid flow rates at warm temperature, and direct reinfusion of recovered blood from the collection chamber of the autotransfusion device.[180] Fortunately, symptomatic VAE is infrequent; however, entrainment of large quantities of air may result in major problems and may be fatal.

A. Etiology

The common factor in VAE is a negative gradient between veins exposed to the atmosphere and the venous pressure.[175,181] This explains why the sitting position is the major source of concern for the possibility of clinically significant air entrainment. In the sitting patient, the gradient between the incision and the heart may be as much as 25 cm (Fig. 29-7). At the same time, both the diploic veins and the dural sinuses are held open by connective tissue and, unlike most other veins, cannot collapse as a result of negative pressure (Fig. 29-8).

Both the quantity of air and the rate at which it enters the venous system are important factors in its clinical significance. The generally accepted values, based on both animal studies and clinical experience, are as follows. Early symptoms (gasp, hypotension) may be produced by rapid entrainment of approximately 1 ml/kg of air; 4

to 7 ml/kg is fatal. Slow infusions of less than 0.15 ml/kg/min generally are well tolerated because the lungs are able to excrete air from the pulmonary capillaries at these rates. Thresholds for the various changes seen in dogs are shown in Fig. 29-9.[182] Spillover of air from the lungs into the systemic circulation occurs in most dogs at doses of air greater than 0.35 ml/kg/min.[4] Infusion rates greater than 1.8 ml/kg/min are fatal in dogs, and probably in humans as well.[182]

B. Symptoms, signs, and diagnosis

This discussion emphasizes the findings in the sitting position because this is the most important source of air embolism in the operating room.

1. Transesophageal echocardiography. The earliest clinical evidence of air embolism may be obtained by TEE. This can show single bubbles and indicate to some extent the rapidity and severity of air entrainment. Unfortunately, the equipment is expensive and generally requires a dedicated person to view the display on a full-time basis.[175] In addition, it is too sensitive because such a small amount of air will not produce problems. Furthermore, the probe may produce esophageal ulceration or glottic injury as a result of prolonged pressure on the pharyngeal and esophageal mucosa when the neck is flexed, as for posterior craniectomy.[183,184]

TTE or TEE may be of value preoperatively in diagnosing patent or probe-patent foramen ovale and therefore in finding the patients at highest risk of paradoxical embolism.[185] In addition, TEE is the only study that can demonstrate air in the left side of the heart.[183,184,186,187] Thus it is valuable for recognition of paradox as it is happening. However, symptomatic paradoxical embolism is a rare occurrence during posterior fossa surgery. It has been described in patients with no indication of PFO on

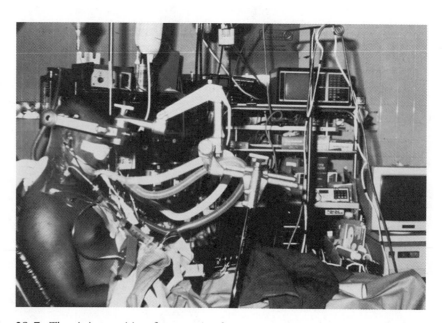

Fig. 29-7. The sitting position for posterior fossa surgery. This position creates the largest gradient between the incision and the heart, and thus the greatest risk of air embolism, of any type of surgery.

TEE, possibly because of the limitations of the technique or because air may also filter into the systemic circulation through the lungs.[4,5,188-191] For these reasons, there is controversy about the cost-benefit value of TEE, both as a routine preoperative test and for intraoperative monitoring.[183,192]

2. Transthoracic Doppler ultrasonography. The Doppler is one of the most valuable monitors for air in seated patients. It is noninvasive and, when properly placed, is capable of recognizing as little as 0.25 ml of air entering the right atrium. It is most useful in the sitting and supine positions because proper placement may be difficult when the patient is lateral or prone. The device works by transmitting an ultrasonic beam and sensing the echoes as the beam is reflected from the various moving surfaces in the chest. Thus it is sensitive to the motion of the cardiac walls and valves and to the presence of any density interface in its path.

In order to detect air embolism, the Doppler probe is placed over the right atrium, generally at the right bor-

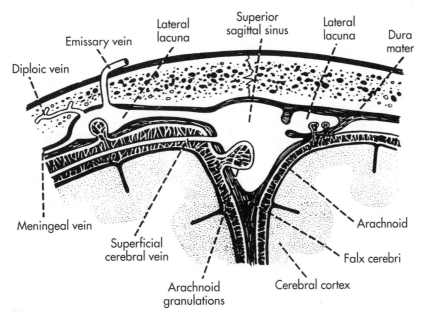

Fig. 29-8. The venous drainage of the cranium. The dural sinuses and the diploic veins are unable to collapse because they are held open by fibrous tissue connections to surrounding structures. (From Burt AM: *Textbook of neuroanatomy,* Philadelphia, 1992, WB Saunders.)

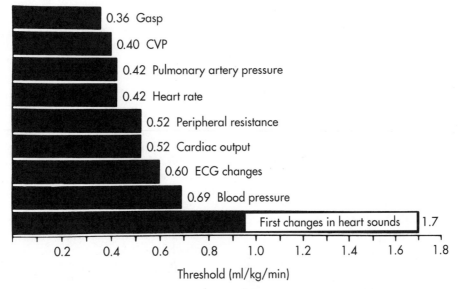

Fig. 29-9. Rates of air entrainment to produce various signs in dogs. *CVP,* Central venous pressure; *ECG,* electrocardiographic. (From Adornato DC, Gildenberg PL, Ferrario CM, et al: *Anesthesiology* 49:120, 1978.)

der of the sternum between the third and seventh ribs. The probe is moved until the best sound is obtained and then taped firmly into position. Proper placement is assured by rapid injection of about 5 ml of saline solution or a small amount of air through the CV catheter. The normal cardiac sounds are replaced, at least transiently, by the grinding sounds characteristic of air in the atrium. If a good signal cannot be obtained at the right side of the sternum, the left side may be tried. It is most important to test the position of the probe in this location because there is a possibility that it may overly the ventricle.

As mentioned, the monitor is sensitive to minimal quantities of air; as little as 0.25 ml may be detected with careful attention. Unfortunately, anything that induces turbulence in the blood flow will sound the same.[193] Thus recognition of an embolism with this monitor is a subjective matter, and there is also no way of measuring the quantity of air entrained. In addition, air embolism may occur without producing any signal on the Doppler, especially if the entrainment of air is slow. For these reasons, the device should not be used as the sole monitoring aid for air embolism. In most situations, a CV catheter and capnography are also needed to provide useful information.

3. Capnography. A significant decrease in the end-tidal P_{CO_2} (ET_{CO_2}) is seen with embolization of 15 to 25 ml of air into the pulmonary circulation, a result of the increase in physiologic dead space caused by ventilation of uncirculated regions of the lung.[175] When the Doppler does not detect the presence of air, this may be the first sign of an embolic event. Although other problems, such as water in the analysis cell, may produce this finding, one must assume that it is the result of an embolus in any patient at risk until proven otherwise. Capnography is less capable of indicating when embolism ceases because the P_{CO_2} does not return to normal until the air is excreted from the lungs. This usually requires 15 to 20 minutes.

4. End-tidal nitrogen. Provided that air is not used as an anesthetic carrier gas, appearance of N_2 in end-tidal gas during mechanical ventilation should suggest air embolism, even though a leak in the breathing circuit may result in a similar finding. End-tidal N_2 monitoring probably provides earlier recognition of VAE than ET_{CO_2}, especially when air entry to the venous circulation occurs at a slow rate.[194] A sudden drop in ET_{CO_2} occurs in these circumstances only when a significant decrease in cardiac output and an increase in PAP occurs as a result of a large amount of air within the pulmonary circulation, whereas end-tidal N_2 appears with air entry rate as slow as 1 ml/kg/min. In fact, at the time of ET_{CO_2} decrease a paradoxical decrease in end-tidal N_2 concentration also occurs. This may be related to hypotension, low cardiac output, and an increased number of ventilated but not perfused alveoli.[194]

5. Central venous catheter. Proof of entrainment of air into the venous circulation is found most definitely by the ability to withdraw air bubbles from the superior vena cava. A CV line therefore is a requirement in the seated patient. The multiorifice (Bunegin-Albin) cath-

eter is probably the best for this purpose because it may be able to access a larger proportion of the entrained air than a standard catheter. Placement is important. The tip of a single-lumen catheter is optimally positioned at the junction of the superior vena cava and the right atrium. A Bunegin-Albin catheter is best positioned with its distal end in the right atrium about 2 cm beyond the vena caval junction. This can be ensured by a chest radiograph or, perhaps better, by ECG, using the saline-filled catheter as one of the leads. As the catheter is passed, the P wave, initially deflected downward, becomes equally biphasic at the level of the sinus node, which is the end point.

It should be emphasized that the CV line is primarily for diagnosis. Air passes rapidly through the superior vena cava, and thus is past the end of the catheter by the time its presence is suspected. Although entrainment may be continuous, air can be withdrawn into a syringe only intermittently, so much of it is not retrieved. However, as we have noted, the presence of bubbles in blood withdrawn from the CV line is diagnostic of air embolism, and the best indication that entrainment has stopped is that air is no longer obtained.

6. Pulmonary artery pressure. A significant elevation in both systolic and diastolic PAP is seen with 20 to 25 ml of air in the pulmonary vasculature. Thus this is a sensitive indicator of the complication and, unlike the Doppler probe, is both objective and quantitative. In addition, it may be possible to remove some of the air in the pulmonary circulation with the catheter. For these reasons, some authors recommend a PA catheter in all sitting patients.[195] Unfortunately, the narrow lumens of the Swan-Ganz catheter imply that aspiration of embolized air may be too slow to be useful. Furthermore, withdrawal from the distal end of the catheter is useful only if the embolus involves the particular artery in which the catheter is located. It seems that the PA catheter is not as useful as a single-lumen CV line in the sitting patient.

7. Arterial blood pressure. An arterial line is a standard aspect of the monitoring of most major neurosurgery. Because of the possibility of brainstem effects on the blood pressure, it is required in any posterior fossa procedure. A sudden decrease in blood pressure is the first clinical sign of air embolism and is seen with 50 to 60 ml of entrained air. By the time this occurs, the patient must be treated urgently because arrhythmias and possibly cardiovascular collapse may follow in short order.

8. Electrocardiogram. Adornato et al[182] described the cardiopulmonary changes during slow air infusion in dogs. The first ECG change was peaked P waves, followed by ST-segment depression. Like the alterations in the arterial pressure, these are late and nonspecific signs and obviously cannot be relied on for diagnosis by themselves.

9. Heart sounds. In the classical literature, the earliest indication of an air embolism is a transient sharpening of the second heart sound. This probably was a finding in experimental animals. It is difficult to imagine how it would have been possible to hear this with a precordial stethoscope in a noisy operating room. By the time the more obvious changes in heart sounds occur, the patient is in severe trouble. Adornato described a drumlike sound, which was not heard until significant cardiovascular decompensation had occurred. The mill-wheel murmur is an indicator of air in the pulmonic valve, and thus of massive quantities of air in the circulation. The final sign was once described as "shaking a plastic bag half filled with air and half with water." By the time this sign is present, the patient probably is beyond help.

Fortunately, in situations other than the sitting position, air embolism is both less common and usually less severe. However, because the patient rarely is monitored with the same intensity as for posterior fossa surgery, major entrainment of air may occur without being recognized until the blood pressure falls. The only good monitor in these cases is the capnograph. Thus in any operation in which the incision is above the heart, a fall in the ETCO$_2$ should be considered to be the result of an air embolism unless another cause is found.

C. Management

In procedures that do not involve the pressure gradients characteristic of the sitting position, air embolism may be prevented by maintaining the patient's blood volume. Albin et al[181] report three cases of extensive spine fusions in the prone position. The procedures were both long and bloody, and it is likely that the blood volume and thus the CVP were permitted to fall to the point at which there was a negative venous pressure at the operative site. Severe air embolism resulted, and all three patients died.

During endometrial ablation,[165] cryosurgery of bone tumors,[171] and use of the argon coagulator,[176] prevention involves allowing adequate exhaust of gases developing within closed spaces. Hydrogen peroxide application to open wounds and intraosseous air injection should be abandoned because they are associated with a high likelihood of massive VAE.[79,177] During perioperative autotransfusion, recovered blood should always be transferred to a reinfusion bag before it is returned to the patient.[180]

To many people, the first thought in the treatment of air embolism is to change the patient's position. However, when the patient is sitting in head pins and the posterior fossa is open, this would be a very difficult maneuver. Several effective measures can be taken before moving the patient is necessary. The first three should be essentially simultaneous; fortunately, they are capable of controlling the majority of embolic events.

1. Inform the surgeon. In most cases the entry of air can be stopped by flooding or packing the wound. The site of entrainment usually can then be found by careful inspection.

2. Withdraw from the central venous catheter. A 35- or 60-ml syringe is attached via a stopcock to the central line. As discussed, the diagnosis can be established by the appearance of small air bubbles in the syringe. Blood may be withdrawn and reinjected (discarding the air, of course) until no more bubbles are seen. The question may be legitimately raised as to the wisdom of reinjecting blood from an ordinary syringe. We have never seen a problem from this maneuver. To be safer, 1000 units of heparin may be added to the intravenous solution and periodically used to flush the syringe and tubing. If large quantities of air are retrieved, it is best to withdraw as much as possible as rapidly as possible. In this case blood may be taken from the central line and returned via a peripheral vein while aspiration continues with a second syringe. Obviously, much of the entrained air will still escape the catheter, but it is possible that enough will be retrieved to avert serious consequences.

3. Discontinue nitrous oxide. The size of embolized air bubbles is increased by absorption of nitrous oxide. For this reason, use of the agent in any surgery with a risk of air embolism is controversial. Some anesthesiologists believe that N$_2$O should be avoided altogether in these procedures,[196] whereas others believe that its use either does not change the severity of the embolism or at least provides an early warning of open vessels because emboli are detectable more quickly.[197] It seems obvious that minimizing the size of the bubbles is a desirable end, and certainly one should avoid N$_2$O when possible in these situations. On the other hand, our own practice commonly includes the use of sensory and motor evoked potentials (SEP and MEP) during posterior fossa surgery, often combined with facial nerve monitoring. In these cases, muscle relaxants and halogenated anesthetics are contraindicated because MEPs are unobtainable when they are used. Our anesthetic technique therefore consists of propofol and fentanyl infusions combined with N$_2$O and O$_2$. Thus N$_2$O is a valuable addition to the hypnosis and analgesia provided by the intravenous agents. When air is detected in these cases, N$_2$O is discontinued and we maintain the patient with the infusions alone or add a halogenated agent and forgo MEP monitoring.

4. Jugular vein pressure. Manually occluding the jugulars increases the venous pressure in the head and thus produces bleeding from any open veins, which generally makes any obscure site of air entry obvious. This simple measure also is very effective when the previous maneuvers do not stop the embolization. Fortunately, the surgeon almost always can localize the site of air entry fairly quickly when the jugulars are occluded because it is impractical to perform this maneuver for a prolonged period of time.

5. Positive end-expiratory pressure. Theoretically, PEEP is also capable of increasing the cerebral venous pressure and thus decreasing the entrainment of air.[198,199] Unfortunately, this has not been demonstrated. Studies have shown no change in the quantity or rate of air entrainment when PEEP is used.[18,200] In addition, the use of PEEP in a patient who already has pulmonary artery occlusion and elevated CVP may precipitate severe hypotension and also increase the likelihood of right-to-left shunt and paradoxical embolism in a patient with a PFO.[18,19,184,201] Although whether an increase in the right-to-left atrial pressure gradient actually occurs with PEEP is a controversial issue,[20] it is prudent to avoid PEEP in this situation.

6. *Position.* As noted, it may be difficult to change the position of a patient in the middle of surgery. If all other methods of controlling air entry fail, however, the wound should be packed quickly and the site of incision should be positioned below the heart by whatever means necessary, in order to stop further entrainment of air. In the sitting patient, this may require detaching the patient from the head frame and lowering the head of the table. In rare circumstances, the operation may have to be continued or concluded with the patient prone. The ideal, and commonly recommended, position may be left lateral decubitus and Trendelenburg, which may help move air out of the RV outflow tract,[202] although recent studies in dogs[203,204] cast doubt on the effectiveness of positional change.

7. *Resuscitation.* Once the blood pressure starts to fall, supportive measures are required. Fluid administration in order to raise the CVP, vasopressors, and cardiac massage are used as indicated. The latter maneuver may help break up air bubbles in the right heart chambers and mobilize air out of the heart and great vessels and into the lungs, from which it can be eliminated.[202,205]

IV. CARBON DIOXIDE EMBOLISM

Embolization of carbon dioxide is a complication of laparoscopic surgery and generally results from direct injection of the gas into an injured vessel. Fortunately, although they may be lethal, clinically significant emboli are uncommon. The reported incidence in 1976 was 15 in 113,253 gynecologic laparoscopies.[206] CO_2 embolism may be even less common in pelvic procedures today because lower pressures are now used to inflate the peritoneal cavity. It seems likely that the risk of this complication is higher in laparoscopic cholecystectomy, although its incidence has not yet been analyzed. Subclinical embolism is undoubtedly considerably more common. Derouin et al[207] observed gas embolism with TEE in 11 of 16 patients during laparoscopic cholecystectomy. Other procedures may also be associated with CO_2 embolization: carbon dioxide arteriography,[208] hysteroscopy,[209,210] arthrography,[211] and endometrial ablation.[212]

The rate of excretion of CO_2 from the lungs is much faster than that of air, so it may be expected that a larger quantity may be needed to produce clinical problems. In a study on pigs, Mann et al[213] found that the threshold for hypotension was approximately 4 ml/kg body weight. However, the rapid rate of injection characteristic of insufflation (1 to 8 ml/sec) implies that clinical embolism may occur very rapidly, and hypotension and a mill-wheel murmur may be the first indications of the complication.

Although the earliest indications of CO_2 embolism may be obtained with TEE or the precordial Doppler,[213,214] these are rarely used during laparoscopic surgery. Diagnosis of this complication thus depends on careful observation of the patient's signs. The initial indication of an acute embolism is a fall in the ET_{CO_2}; obstruction of the pulmonary veins is a more significant factor than increased output of the gas. Hypotension, hypoxemia, arrhythmias, and alteration in heart sounds, including a mill-wheel murmur, commonly follow shortly thereafter.[215]

Treatment is similar to that for air embolism.[216] The procedure should be stopped, and gas injection and nitrous oxide administration should be discontinued. Hyperventilation assists in excretion of CO_2, and a CV catheter should be inserted in an effort to aid in aspiration of the gas. Change in position, though easier than when the patient is sitting, may not be effective; indeed, it may be counterproductive, particularly in cerebral embolization, where it may increase intracranial pressure without dislodging the emboli.[216] Of course, resuscitation is required for cardiopulmonary collapse.

V. FAT EMBOLISM

This pathologic entity is characterized by occlusion of multiple blood vessels with fat globules that are too large to pass through the capillaries. Because fat globules are fluid and thus deformable, complete vascular occlusion is rare and, if it occurs, short-lasting.[217] Anesthesiologists are likely to deal with this complication, especially if they are involved in the care of patients with skeletal trauma. Fat can be detected in pulmonary arterial samples of up to 70% of patients with long-bone or pelvic fractures, especially if the PA catheter is wedged.[218] On the other hand, fat embolism syndrome (FES), a clinical picture that exhibits a wide spectrum of severity, occurs much less often; the reported perioperative incidence ranges from 0% to 20% but generally is between 3.5% and 5%.[219] Statistical data about *intraoperative* FES are not available, but in institutions where long-bone and pelvic fractures are managed with early operative fixation, this rate is about 0.2% to 0.4%.[219]

A. Etiology

Common perioperative causes of fat embolism are listed in Table 29-9. In long-bone fractures, movement of unstable bone fragments and reaming of the medullary cavity produce increased intramedullary pressure and thus promote entrance of marrow contents into torn venous channels that remain open even in shock because they are attached to the cancellous bone.[220] Open fractures are less likely to cause fat embolism and FES because, unlike in closed injuries, there may be some medullary decompression.[221] Conversely, substantial elevation of intramedullary pressure, often to more than 500 mm Hg, may occur with reaming of the bone during total hip or knee arthroplasty.[222] In total knee arthroplasty, insertion of the alignment guide and femoral and tibial prostheses into the marrow cavities may be responsible for an increased likelihood and severity of fat embolization. Venting or evacuating the intramedullary canal before instrumentation may alleviate this problem. Use of a tourniquet may prevent egress of fat into the systemic circulation, at least until the cuff is released.

The type and location of the fracture may play a role in the development of fat embolism; fractures of the femoral shaft and pelvis and multiple fractures appear to increase the incidence and severity of this complication,

Table 29-9. Possible etiologic factors and mechanisms in the development of perioperative fat embolism

Etiologic factors	Mechanisms
Traumatic factors	
Fractures (long bone, pelvis)	Entry of bone marrow contents into disrupted medullary vessels
Burns	Entry of subcutaneous fat into disrupted vessels
Subcutaneous adipose tissue injuries	Entry of subcutaneous fat into disrupted vessels
Surgery	
Intramedullary nailing	Elevated intramedullary pressure and disruption of medullary vessels
Total hip arthroplasty, total knee arthroplasty	Elevated intramedullary pressure from insertion of prosthesis and cement, and destruction of medullary vessels
Nontraumatic factors	
Procedures	
Cardiopulmonary resuscitation	Fracture of ribs and sternum by external cardiac massage
Cryosurgery of bone	Elevation of intramedullary pressure by edema in the medullary cavity resulting from cryosurgical damage to cell membranes
Intraosseous fluid and drug administration	Entry of fat droplets into medullary vessels
Liposuction	Entry of subcutaneous fat into disrupted vessels
Intraoperative autotransfusion	Transfusion of fat-containing blood obtained during hip arthroplasty
Lymphangiography	Proximal lymphatic obstruction causing intravascular passage of lipid-soluble contrast medium
Hysterosalpingography	Lymphatic and venous intravasation of oil-soluble contrast media injected into uterine cavity
Drugs	
Lipid emulsions	Alteration in the stability of the emulsion resulting in agglutination and production of lipid-fibrin emboli

Modified from Capan LM, Miller SM, Patel KP: *Anesthesiol Clin North Am* 11:25, 1993.

probably because larger amounts of fat are released into the circulation.[223] Other causes of fat embolism include burns, liposuction, and extensive soft tissue trauma (see Table 29-9), although FES develops rarely if at all after these injuries.[219,224] Nontraumatic causes of fat embolism are extremely rare (see Table 29-9). Among these, intraosseous fluid and drug administration may produce fat embolism, but FES is unlikely.[220] Intraoperative autotransfusion can cause fat embolism if the blood contains a large amount of fat, as in hip arthroplasty.[225] Fat embolism after hyperalimentation probably results from agglutination of lipid emulsion and combination of these particles with fibrin.[226] Lipids in healthy adults are cleared at a maximum rate of 3.8 g/kg body weight/day. Fat overload may occur if more than this amount is administered. Thus lipid emulsion therapy should be monitored by frequent measurement of the plasma triglyceride concentration and visual evaluation of plasma turbidity.[226,227]

B. Pathophysiology

Despite many theories, the pathophysiology of FES has not been elucidated firmly. Nevertheless, the mechanical and biochemical theories have gained acceptance and deserve to be mentioned.[219] The mechanical theory holds that FES is a result of increased intramedullary pressure, which forces marrow into injured venous sinusoids and thus into the general circulation, resulting in obstruction of pulmonary and systemic capillaries. The diameter of the smallest pulmonary capillaries is about 7 mm. Thus the fat globules that occlude pulmonary vessels are larger than this, whereas obstruction of organ vasculature does

not occur in lipemia because the lipid particles are smaller. Cor pulmonale may develop following obstruction of pulmonary vessels if adequate compensatory vasodilation does not occur. Fat globules also may gain access to the brain, kidney, myocardium, or other organs because increased RA and RV pressures may result in the passage of fat globules through a cardiac septal defect, a probe-patent foramen ovale, pulmonary-bronchial anastomoses, or pulmonary capillaries. Clinically, fulminant FES exhibits these features: acute cor pulmonale develops shortly after skeletal injury or surgery, and severe edema may develop in systemic organs.[228,229]

According to the biochemical theory, fat globules in the pulmonary or systemic circulation originate from lipids normally present in the blood. Physicochemical alteration of these substances can cause FES by toxicity or obstruction.[230] Toxicity is caused primarily by free fatty acids (FFA) that affect pneumocytes and pulmonary capillary endothelium, producing a clinical picture similar to that of ARDS.[231] Toxic FFAs may be produced in the lung by the action of pulmonary lipase on neutral embolic fat[231] or directly from body fat in response to stress-induced catecholamines.[232] The obstructive mechanism causes FES by the coalescence of 1-mm-diameter chylomicrons into 10- to 40-mm globules, triggered by the release of mediators at the fracture site.[219] These newly formed fat globules then obstruct the pulmonary or other organ vasculature.[230]

Neither the mechanical nor the biochemical theory provides a totally satisfactory explanation for the development of FES. Thus attempts have been made to explain its genesis by a combined theory in which obstruction of capillaries by fat or marrow is the initiating event. In one view, embolized fat originates from both traumatized fat depots and coalescence of blood lipids. In the most widely accepted view, a few hours after an initial obstructive process, FFAs exert their toxic effects on the initially embolized organs.[219] Again, the sequence of events that produces FES is poorly understood. For this reason, some authors believe that FES is actually the same entity as ARDS.[233]

C. Diagnosis

There are differences between awake and anesthetized patients in the clinical presentation of FES. The latter are discussed in the section on anesthetic considerations. In unanesthetized patients FES may present in three degrees of severity: subclinical, nonfulminant subacute, and fulminant acute.[219] These variants are distinguished by the time of onset of symptoms after injury and by the severity of the clinical picture (Table 29-10). The subclinical and nonfulminant subacute forms develop at least 12 hours after trauma, whereas the fulminant form is characterized by rapid progression of clinical symptoms that begin within a few hours following injury and, in many cases, may be fatal or result in neurologic or pul-

monary sequelae.[219] Manipulation of the pelvis and the long bones of the lower extremity by closed reduction, traction, methylmethacrylate application, insertion of prostheses, or even repair with plates can precipitate any of these degrees of FES within several days after injury.[234-237]

In the subclinical form, symptoms are either nonspecific (tachycardia, tachypnea, or fever) or absent. Hypoxemia (room air PaO_2 less than 80 mm Hg) occurs in 50% to 90% of patients after lower-extremity injuries and generally is attributed to fat embolism. Hypocapnia and thrombocytopenia (platelet count less than 200,000/μl) often are present.[219] Classically, the nonfulminant subacute form is characterized by the presence of some or all of the three major indicators: respiratory distress, diffuse nonspecific cerebral signs, and petechial rash. Several other nonspecific signs and symptoms may be present: tachycardia; fever; retinal signs, including exudates, cotton-wool spots, edema, hemorrhage, or intravascular fat globules; lipuria; and jaundice. Respiratory insufficiency or failure, manifested by the symptoms shown in Table 29-10, often gives the clinical picture of ARDS. Interestingly, however, there are anecdotal reports of FES without pulmonary abnormalities.[238]

Table 29-10. Clinical forms of fat embolism syndrome

Clinical form	Occurrence after injury (%)	Onset after injury	Clinical presentation	Mortality rate (%)
Subclinical	>60	12-72 hr	Nonspecific or absent symptoms (tachycardia, tachypnea, fever) Moderate hypoxemia (PaO_2 <80 mm Hg in room air) Moderate elevation of $AaDO_2$ (>20 mm Hg in room air) Moderate hypocapnia ($PaCO_2$ ≤30 mm Hg during spontaneous breathing) Moderate decrease of platelet count (<200,000/μl)	0
Nonfulminant subacute (classic form)	Single fracture, 1-5 Multiple fracture, 5-10	12-96 hr	Dyspnea, tachypnea Fever Tachycardia Petechiae Cerebral signs Hypoxemia (PaO_2 <60 mm Hg in room air) Anemia Thrombocytopenia and coagulation abnormalities Lung opacities on chest radiograph	0-5
Fulminant*	<0.2	Few hours	Acute cor pulmonale Frank pulmonary edema Moderate to severe hypotension Cerebral signs Severe hypoxemia Acidosis	>50

From Capan LM, Miller SM, Patel KP: *Anesthesiol Clin North Am* 11:25, 1993.
*Because of rare occurrence, reliable incidence and mortality statistics are not available.
AaDO₂, Alveolo-arterial oxygen difference.

Neurologic signs are nonspecific, nonlateralizing CNS manifestations of diffuse encephalopathy: acute confusion, stupor, coma, decerebrate rigidity, and convulsions. Focal neurologic signs are so uncommon in FES that their occurrence after trauma should arouse the suspicion of head or spinal cord injury. A change in affect, behavior, or consciousness after a lower-extremity fracture suggests the possibility of FES. The CNS signs are the result of both hypoxemia and embolization of cerebral vessels with fat. Cerebral edema, caused by hypoxemia, embolic ischemia, and toxic FFA-induced cerebrovascular disruption, probably contributes to the neurologic deterioration more often than is generally thought.

Petechiae are pathognomonic for FES, but depending on the report, they appear in 25% to 95% of patients with this complication.[219] The rash usually appears late, between 12 and 96 hours after injury, and occupies the upper portion of the body, including the chest, neck, upper arms, axillae, shoulders, oral mucous membranes, and conjunctivae; petechiae probably are localized to the upper part of the body because fat, which is lighter than blood, floats. Thrombocytopenia does not appear to play a role in the development of petechiae; occlusion and distention of dermal capillaries by fat globules and increased endothelial fragility are responsible for this sign.[219]

The fulminant acute form of FES is an accelerated and more severe variant of the classic subacute type (see Table 29-10). It is rare, and although it can occur spontaneously after a skeletal injury, it often develops shortly after closed reduction of a fracture, manipulation of a deformed hip, reaming of the femur for insertion of an intramedullary prosthesis, or application of cement. Clinically it may present with acute cor pulmonale, pulmonary edema, various severe nonspecific cerebral signs, hemodynamic instability, coagulopathy, or pyrexia. No laboratory, radiologic, or electrocardiographic findings are pathognomonic for FES; they are either too sensitive or lack specificity. Nevertheless, a room air PaO_2 value less than 60 mm Hg following skeletal injury in a patient with no other pulmonary pathology suggests FES.[239] However, the absence of hypoxemia in the presence of other signs and symptoms cannot exclude the diagnosis. Furthermore, hypoxemia is present in many patients with lower-extremity fractures who show no evidence of FES. Most patients with FES develop respiratory alkalosis initially, because of tachypnea and hyperventilation, but $PaCO_2$ may rise later as respiratory failure progresses.

Measurement of blood lipids, including triglyceride, phospholipids, cholesterol and FFAs, and serum lipase, is not helpful for diagnosis.[219] Neither is cytologic examination of blood, urine, or sputum.[219] On the other hand, it has been shown that in trauma patients, the diagnosis of FES can be established if more than 5% of the cells retrieved by bronchoalveolar lavage contain fat globules.[240] However, the results of more recent studies do not confirm the value of this test.[241-244] These investigators found that fat globules were common in pulmonary washings from trauma and nontrauma patients without FES.[241,242,244] It has been suggested that bronchoalveolar lavage can be diagnostic for posttraumatic

FES if the threshold for lipid-laden macrophages is 30% instead of 5%.[243] Other laboratory findings include a drop in hematocrit level to less than 30% within 24 to 48 hours in about 75% to 80% of patients and coagulation abnormalities reflected by thrombocytopenia, increased platelet aggregation, prolonged prothrombin and activated thromboplastin times, and appearance of FDP and D-dimer in the plasma.[219] The plasma fibrinogen concentration shows a biphasic pattern; it decreases initially, but a rebound hyperfibrinogenemia ensues within 3 to 5 days.[219] Disseminated intravascular coagulation (DIC) may occur, especially during the fulminant form of FES, but this is rare. Neither the change in hematocrit nor the coagulation abnormalities are specific for FES.

Typical abnormalities on the chest radiograph include diffuse, evenly distributed flakelike shadows and increased interstitial and alveolar densities (snowstorm appearance).[219] Infiltrates are usually patchy, bilateral, and symmetric, and involve the perihilar and basilar areas, sparing the apices. Cardiomegaly, pulmonary vascular congestion, and pleural effusion are absent. Enlargement of the right heart may be detected if cor pulmonale develops. None of these findings is specific for FES; in addition, they occur in only 30% to 50% of affected individuals and lag 12 to 24 hours behind clinical symptoms.[219] CT scan of the lung may have greater diagnostic value than the chest radiograph; multiple mottled subsegmental defects suggest FES. The use of ventilation-perfusion scans has been suggested, especially in equivocal cases of FES with normal or borderline chest radiographic findings or a questionable clinical presentation.[245] Subsegmental (mottled) perfusion defects, although nonspecific, may be suggestive of FES.[246]

In cerebral FES diffuse edema and hemorrhagic infarcts in the cerebral deep white matter, basal ganglia, corpus callosum, and cerebellar hemispheres may be demonstrated on CT scan of the brain by absence of cortical sulci, compression of the lateral ventricles, and presence of lesions. Magnetic resonance imaging (MRI) appears to be more sensitive in detecting FES-induced brain lesions[247]; the findings include hypointense signals on T1-weighted images and hyperintense signals on T2-weighted images.[248] Other tests that can be used for this purpose are single-photon emission computed tomography (SPECT) and TCD; both of these nonspecific tests show low cerebral blood flow in the acute stage.[247] The electrocardiogram usually is normal, unless cor pulmonale, acute myocardial ischemia, or extensive pulmonary involvement is present.

Because there are no specific signs, symptoms, or laboratory findings, FES remains primarily a diagnosis of exclusion. Table 29-11 indicates the diseases and complications that should be considered in differential diagnosis. In the multiple-trauma patient, the manifestations of associated injuries may mask FES and mislead the clinician.[249] Of all the clinical findings, petechiae are the most reliable and probably the only sign that permits a definitive diagnosis.[219] Acute hypoxia is another prominent sign, but by itself it is not diagnostic of FES.

Five schemes developed over the past 25 years, mostly for research purposes, may aid in the recognition of the

Table 29-11. Diseases and complications that may be confused with fat embolism syndrome

System	Clinical findings	Diseases or complications
Pulmonary	Respiratory distress Pulmonary edema Increased AaDo$_2$ Hypoxemia Hypocarbia Hypercarbia	Aspiration pneumonitis Thromboembolism Air embolism Pulmonary contusion Pulmonary sepsis Cardiogenic pulmonary edema Neurogenic pulmonary edema Postobstruction pulmonary edema Tracheobronchial secretions Diffuse atelectasis
Cardiovascular	Hypotension Tachycardia Arrhythmia Pulmonary edema Increased AaDo$_2$ Hypoxemia	Hypovolemia Shock from any origin Hemorrhage Myocardial infarction Myocardial contusion Isolated or global pump failure Anaphylactic or anaphylactoid reactions

Neurologic	Confusion
	Disorientation
	Agitation
	Seizure
	Stupor
	Focal neurologic findings
	Failure to recover from anesthesia
	Elevated intracranial pressure
		Head injury
		Embolic phenomena (air, clot, arteriosclerotic plaque)
		Encephalopathy
		  Metabolic
		  Toxic
		  Infectious
		  Neoplastic
		Delirium tremens
		Psychiatric disorders
		Decompression sickness
		Anesthetic complications

Hematologic	Anemia Clotting abnormalities Oozing Thrombocytopenia Prolonged prothrombin time, activated partial thromboplastin time	Hemorrhage Dilutional coagulopathy Disseminated intravascular coagulation Fibrinolysis Preexisting coagulopathy

From Capan LM, Miller SM, Patel KP: *Anesthesiol Clin North Am* 11:25, 1993.
AaDo$_2$, Alveolo-arterial oxygen difference.

syndrome. Gurd and Wilson's[250] criteria require the presence of at least one of three major clinical features (petechial rash, respiratory insufficiency, or cerebral involvement), four of five minor signs (pyrexia, tachycardia, retinal changes, jaundice, or renal signs), and fat macroglobulinemia. Lindeque et al[239] include blood gas findings in their diagnostic protocol, which they claim not only permits instant diagnosis, but also circumvents the problem of underdiagnosis; using their scheme, they were able to diagnose twice as many cases of FES as would be found by Gurd and Wilson's criteria. Their positive indicators are sustained Pao$_2$ less than 60 mm Hg, sustained Paco$_2$ greater than 55 mm Hg, pH less than 7.3, sustained respiratory rate greater than 35 breaths/min despite adequate sedation, and increased work of breathing. At least one of these findings in a patient with long-bone fracture establishes the diagnosis of FES. Murray and Racz[251] consider the presence of tachycardia, tachypnea, pyrexia, and CNS manifestations with arterial hypoxemia as the diagnostic indicators. Schonfeld

et al[252] include seven signs, each of which is assigned a score: petechiae (score = 5), diffuse alveolar infiltrates (4), Pao$_2$ less than 70 mm Hg (3), confusion (1), fever higher than 38° C (1), heart rate greater than 120 beats/min (1), and respiratory rate greater than 30/min (1). A cumulative score greater than 5 is considered diagnostic. The most recent scheme was proposed by Vedrienne, Guillaume, and Gagnieu,[244] who included pulmonary infiltrates, neurologic and electroencephalographic findings, petechiae, platelet count, retinal changes, serum lipids, and long-bone or pelvis fracture. They assigned a score of 0 for absence of any abnormality, 1 for mild abnormality, and 2 for severe abnormality. A cumulative score of at least 8 is needed for a positive diagnosis.

D. Surgical and anesthetic considerations

The perioperative management of FES involves prevention, mostly by the surgeons, and prompt recognition and intervention by the anesthesiologist.

1. Prevention. Prevention of FES is possible during several phases of management. The decision to reduce and stabilize a fracture within a few hours following the injury probably is the most effective prophylactic measure. Indeed, in multiple trauma, fixation of long-bone and pelvic fractures during the initial procedure simultaneously with or shortly after surgery for thoracoabdominal or brain injuries decreases not only the occurrence of FES[218,253,254] but also the overall rate of pulmonary and septic complications. Patients treated in this manner require a shorter period of postoperative ventilation, develop fever and positive blood cultures less often, and have shorter stays in the intensive care unit (ICU).[218,254,255] Although some clinicians argue against early intramedullary rodding of long-bone fractures and claim that it may increase the risk of pulmonary complications in patients with multiple trauma and those with lung contusion,[256,257] there is little support for this idea.[234,249,253,254]

Whether early fixation should be performed when the evaluation suggests the presence of FES is not clear. One of our patients who showed signs of FES preoperatively developed an exacerbation of the complication intraoperatively, with the end result of severe brain damage. A similar scenario resulted in the death of a 60-year-old woman during closed fracture reduction.[258] Additional intraoperative fat emboli may overwhelm the compensatory ability of the pulmonary circulation. In our experience, postponing surgery for a few days does not always improve the prognosis, but it may reduce the frequency and severity of unfavorable events that may arise from the combination of FES, anesthesia, and surgery.[219] In any event, the occurrence of severe and persistent hemodynamic, metabolic, and gas exchange abnormalities; cardiac rhythm disturbances; or acute pulmonary edema during fixation of long-bone fractures or arthroplasty requires restricting further surgery to the shortest possible procedure and, after hemodynamic and metabolic stabilization, transferring the patient to the postanesthesia care unit for definitive assessment and treatment.[219] The rationale for curtailing surgery in these circumstances is that the clinical picture may be caused by PTE, which requires placement of a Greenfield vena cava filter, and that if the signs are indeed caused by FES, not only are further showers of emboli possible but cerebral complications, especially brain edema, cannot be assessed and treated adequately.[219]

Certain surgical techniques may limit the possibility of fat embolization and thus of the "cement implantation syndrome" during prosthesis insertion in total hip or knee arthroplasties. This time-limited syndrome is characterized by pulmonary hypertension, oxygen desaturation, hypotension, and rarely cardiac arrest at the time of cement and prosthesis insertion. The elevated PAP may last for up to 24 hours. The syndrome probably results from pulmonary embolization of bone marrow contents or intramedullary debris, rather than from methylmethacrylate toxicity,[259,260] because intravenous injection of several times the quantity of cement released during arthroplasty is unlikely to produce these symptoms.[261] Many patients develop postoperative cerebral signs such

as confusion or stupor, which may be mistakenly attributed to the effects of anesthesia. Although embolic occlusion of pulmonary vessels by fat and other bone marrow contents is now considered the primary cause of the syndrome, the activity of reflex or humoral mechanisms, the compliance of the pulmonary vasculature, and the patient's preoperative cardiovascular status may have a role in determining the severity of pulmonary hypertension. Thus the relationship between the quantity of fat in the lung and the degree of PAP change is not linear.[262] Prevention of this complication involves reducing the amount of material embolized during surgery. Surgical measures to achieve this goal include the use of high-pressure, high-volume pulsatile lavage of the femoral shaft before insertion of the prosthesis,[263] venting of the marrow cavity to limit the rise in pressure during cement and prosthesis insertion,[259] the use of a noncemented prosthesis in the patient with cardiovascular compromise,[259,264,265] and avoiding certain types of long-stemmed prostheses.[259,266] Extreme care should be exercised during revision arthroplasty[267] and surgery for pathologic fractures[259]; the risk of embolism is increased in these patients.

2. Recognition and intervention. The clinical presentation of FES in anesthetized patients differs from that seen in conscious patients; CNS symptoms are masked by general anesthesia, and other signs, except those characterizing the fulminant type, may be overlooked easily. Monitoring of hemodynamic status, oxygenation, and end-tidal CO_2; TEE; observing the temporal relationship of symptoms with surgical events such as insertion of the intramedullary prosthesis or methylmethacrylate; and the patient's response to treatment are the mainstays of diagnosis. The most common manifestations are sudden hypotension, tachycardia, bradycardia, arrhythmia, decreased lung compliance, hypoxemia, and pulmonary edema. Other signs include severe unexplained surgical bleeding or oozing from multiple sites secondary to DIC. Failure to regain consciousness after anesthesia may be the only cerebral sign. Continuous arterial pressure monitoring confers advantages because the hemodynamic consequences of FES may develop suddenly and measurement of serial blood gases is essential, especially during surgical instrumentation. A significant decline in arterial O_2 tension may not be detected by pulse oximetry if high inspired O_2 concentrations are used. Furthermore, when hypotension and peripheral vasoconstriction ensue, the pulse oximeter may cease working.

End-tidal CO_2 monitoring may not be as sensitive in detecting marrow embolism as it is in other types of PE. In a dog model, Byrick et al[268] demonstrated that CO_2 decreased only slightly despite a consistent increase in PA pressure. The lack of response may be caused by obstruction of only the small pulmonary vessels by the microemboli, leaving larger vessels intact to participate in gas exchange. However, it is not clearly known whether these animal studies can be extrapolated to humans, although a recent report documented intraoperative pulmonary fat embolism without a change in end-tidal CO_2.[269]

TEE is extremely sensitive to the presence of marrow particles in the right heart during surgical manipulation of the affected bone.[234-236,270] Entry of these "flakes" into the left heart through a PFO or via the pulmonary vessels also may be detected.[235,236,270] The rate of fluid infusion should be reduced during periods when fat embolism may occur; rapid administration of fluids produces a similar echocardiographic image. In contrast to the impressive sensitivity of echocardiography in detecting fat embolism, there is little correlation between the quantity or size of the embolic particles and hemodynamic or oxygenation changes.[270] Although some relationship has been demonstrated between a high degree of atrial opacification and clinically significant hemodynamic instability,[265] a wide range of echocardiographically detected embolic intensity is devoid of any clinical impact.[269,270] On the other hand, embolism-induced segmental wall motion abnormalities, RV dilation, septal flattening or shift, and the resulting alteration in LV geometry are likely to be associated with significant hemodynamic and oxygenation abnormalities. Although routine use of intraoperative TEE for detection of fat embolism during high-risk procedures cannot be recommended at this time, this device may be useful especially in patients with limited cardiopulmonary reserve.

The basic hemodynamic abnormality in FES is similar to that of other scenarios of pulmonary hypertension; RV strain and failure my produce right heart dilation, septal shift, and decreased LV size and cardiac output.[262] The low $P\overline{v}O_2$ caused by the decrease in cardiac output may contribute to hypoxemia. Under these circumstances, the ability to increase the heart rate is essential to maintain the cardiac output and oxygen delivery.[262] Patients who cannot increase their pulse because of preexisting cardiac disease, pacemaker dependency, β-blocking agents, deep inhalation anesthesia, or a high-level epidural or spinal anesthesia are likely to develop major hemodynamic abnormalities.[262]

During anesthesia the use of direct arterial and CV monitoring (right atrial or PA) may help in the recognition of the adverse cardiopulmonary effects of FES in susceptible patients on a timely basis. In addition, the CV line can be used to administer vasoactive agents (vasopressors, inotropes) during an acute episode; it can also help to regulate fluid resuscitation, which may be beneficial or harmful depending on the degree of septal shift. Large increases in CVP suggest reduction of fluid therapy. Because the impact of an embolic event depends on the response of the cardiovascular system, use of depressant anesthetics when the embolism occurs may have deleterious effects. Animal studies show greater hemodynamic stability and improved outcome after hip arthroplasty under fentanyl anesthesia than with inhalation agents.[271] Finally, the use of a high inspired O_2 concentration shortly before, during, and after skeletal instrumentation not only compensates for embolism-induced hypoxemia but also may maintain low PAP by counteracting hypoxic pulmonary vasoconstriction.

Absence of recovery from anesthesia or agitation without recovery of consciousness following high-risk lower-extremity surgery may be caused by FES. Attributing these events to prolonged effects of anesthetics and administering sedative or opioid agents to treat restlessness may easily result in further delay in recognition of the syndrome. Although sedation of agitated patients is indicated after neurologic examination, CT or MRI evaluation of the brain should be performed early in the postoperative period. Diffuse brain edema in this setting is consistent with FES and calls for measures to control the intracranial pressure.

E. Treatment

Alcohol infusion, aprotinin, and high-dose corticosteroid treatment have been used without proven efficacy.[219] High-dose corticosteroid therapy also is used prophylactically. Supportive therapy with aggressive ventilatory care, fluids, inotropes, and intracranial pressure management remains the mainstay of treatment.[219]

VI. AMNIOTIC FLUID EMBOLISM

Embolic complications are the leading causes of maternal mortality in the United States, accounting for 17% of pregnancy-related deaths, which during the period between 1980 and 1985 surpassed those caused by hypertension (12%), hemorrhage (9%), ectopic pregnancy (10%), stroke (8%), anesthesia (7%), cardiomyopathy (4%), and infection (3.5%).[272] Amniotic fluid embolism (AFE), a devastating complication of pregnancy characterized by alterations in oxygenation, hemodynamics, and coagulation, is fortunately rare, but it accounts for 9% of all maternal mortality and about 60% of deaths caused by PE.[273] With steadily improving obstetric care and thromboembolism prophylaxis, it is likely that mortality from these causes will further decrease and render AFE the leading cause of death during pregnancy. Although some improvement in recognition and management of AFE has occurred in recent years, the syndrome remains unpredictable, unpreventable, and without specific treatment, resulting in high mortality and permanent neurologic morbidity. Excluding some anecdotal reports describing high survival rates in a small number of patients studied,[274,275] the mortality from this syndrome, which has a reported incidence between 1 in 8000 and 1 in 80,000 pregnancies, is about 60% to 70%, with neurologically intact maternal and fetal survival rates of only 15% and 39%, respectively.[276]

A. Pathogenesis and pathophysiology

It is the traditional belief that advanced maternal age, multiparity, meconium staining of the amniotic fluid, large or dead fetus, vaginal delivery, and increased uterine tone or tetany caused either spontaneously or by administration of oxytocin are risk factors for AFE. However, analysis of a large number of cases could not find any association between AFE and tumultuous labor, use of oxytocin, route of delivery, or increased fetal size.[276,277] On the other hand, meconium in the amniotic fluid at the time of embolism and preexistent fetal death do appear to be risk factors for development of severe AFE syndrome.[276,278] In most instances the syndrome develops during labor. In the remaining patients it develops during or shortly after vaginal or cesarean delivery. In addition, AFE has been described during first- or second-trimester termination of pregnancy, uncomplicated second-trimester pregnancy, evacuation of missed abortion at 18 weeks, blunt abdominal trauma, placental abruption at 28 weeks, uterine rupture, lower uterine segment laceration, third-trimester amniocentesis, and insertion of a uterine pressure catheter, and up to 1.5 hours after delivery.[279] It is speculated that late development of this complication reflects release of amniotic fluid into the general circulation after pooling in the uterine vessels. Return of venous tone, as in recovery from spinal anesthesia or movement of the patient, is conjectured to be another factor in late amniotic fluid mobilization.[280] It appears that a facilitating factor, whether abnormal insertion of the placenta, tears in the uterus, or an intrauterine procedure, must also be present. Thus in order for this complication to occur, there must be rupture of membranes and uterine veins. Yet AFE does not develop in all instances in which amniotic fluid enters the circulation, probably because of an inadequate quantity of fluid or absence of substances that can produce the syndrome.[279]

Embolic amniotic fluid contains fat from vernix caseosa, squamous cells from the fetal skin, mucin from the fetal intestine, and trophoblastic cells. These elements can be identified with special staining techniques in blood samples obtained from the PA and occasionally from the systemic blood. However, squamous and trophoblastic cells also may be recovered from asymptomatic patients. Thus presence of these cells in the maternal blood cannot be considered a marker of AFE syndrome.[281] It may be that these patients represent a separate group with subclinical disease, as seen in fat embolism, or that squamous cells enter the circulation from another source (e.g., during venipuncture).

Clark et al[275,276] have added new dimensions to the understanding of the mechanisms of hemodynamic alterations in AFE syndrome. They reject pure mechanical obstruction as the sole cause of this disorder and propose that the primary abnormality is functional, involving the heart and the pulmonary vasculature. The first reaction to AFE is sudden, severe, transient pulmonary hypertension with hypoxemia, which has been demonstrated in animals[278] but not in humans, probably because it disappears by the time PA catheterization is completed. Obstruction of pulmonary vessels may play a role in this response, but the simultaneous increase in systemic pressure suggests that vasoconstriction secondary to a fetal antigen or vasoactive substances such as leukotrienes, thromboxane, prostaglandins, or bradykinin is more significant. This initial response probably is responsible for the inability to resuscitate and the early deaths of some patients. Following this phase there is LV or global cardiac dysfunction with secondary pulmonary hypertension. This has been confirmed in at least two anecdotal reports using echocardiography.[282,283] Thus, unlike other

types of PE, RV strain, failure, and cor pulmonale are unlikely causes of the hemodynamic alterations in AFE syndrome. Clark et al[276] describe this hypotensive phase as anaphylactoid syndrome of pregnancy and draw attention to marked similarities between AFE syndrome and anaphylactic and septic shock. Nevertheless, patients with AFE syndrome do not exhibit other signs of anaphylaxis such as skin rash or bronchospasm. The cause of the myocardial depression is not clear; it may be related to myocardial depressant factors in the amniotic fluid.[284] Pulmonary edema is a common occurrence in AFE syndrome. It may be related to left heart failure, fluid overloading, and capillary leak secondary to activation of vasoactive inflammatory mediators. In fact, ARDS, which is responsible for the majority of the late deaths, often develops, suggesting the contribution of the latter mechanism. It has been suggested that arachidonic acid metabolism is intimately involved in the overall etiology and pathophysiology of the AFE syndrome; amniotic fluid contains arachidonic acid pathway enzymes and metabolites such as PGE_2 and PGF_{2a}, which are known to produce cardiorespiratory effects similar to those occurring in the syndrome.[279]

Coagulopathy develops in about half the patients with AFE syndrome[277,285] and may be life threatening in 10%.[286] A tissue factor that can initiate coagulation has been identified in amniotic fluid,[287] and in vitro studies have shown that it can aggregate platelets, activate the complement cascade and factor X, and release factor III. The thromboplastic effect of amniotic fluid and trophoblastic tissue probably is the primary mechanism of the DIC that typically occurs in AFE syndrome.[286]

Cerebral dysfunction in AFE may be caused by three mechanisms: direct effect of low PaO_2 and low cardiac output, transpulmonary passage of amniotic fluid into the systemic circulation, and passage of amniotic fluid through a PFO.[288] Of these, hypoxemia probably is the most important factor. Transpulmonary passage, which has already been shown for fat in animals,[219] is even more likely to occur with amniotic fluid. In most instances, passage through a foramen ovale requires elevation of right atrial and ventricular pressures to produce blood flow to the left heart. Because right-sided failure or cor pulmonale is uncommon in AFE (except in the initial period of pulmonary hypertension), this mechanism probably is uncommon.

B. Clinical manifestations and diagnosis

The clinical presentation of AFE is variable; not all patients develop the dramatic classic picture of abrupt dyspnea and hypotension followed by rapid progression to cardiopulmonary arrest, with manifestations of severe coagulopathy if time permits. Almost half of patients die within the first hour. Of those who survive, 25% to 70% develop pulmonary edema. In Morgan's series,[277] the initial symptoms in almost 50% of patients involved the respiratory system, hypotension or arrhythmia occurred in 25%, hemorrhage in 15%, and unconsciousness and convulsions in 10%. Brief preliminary symptoms of anxiety, agitation, shivering, cough, and vomiting often occur. Cyanosis almost invariably is present; hypoxemia is the result of pulmonary shunting, decreased cardiac output, increased peripheral oxygen extraction, and probably some right-to-left cardiac shunting in the presence of a probe-patent foramen ovale during the initial period of pulmonary hypertension. Under general anesthesia, hypotension, hypoxemia, arrhythmia, pulmonary edema, and generalized bleeding are the usual presenting symptoms. Occasionally the syndrome develops over a period of several hours with some dyspnea and coagulopathy but without the acute features described earlier.

There is no reliable test for definitive antemortem diagnosis of AFE. Recovery of squamous epithelial cells in the blood samples obtained from the pulmonary capillaries via a wedged Swan-Ganz catheter[289] can support the clinical impression but cannot establish the diagnosis. Demonstration[290] of these elements in pulmonary catheter aspirates from asymptomatic women in labor suggests that small amounts of fetal debris normally enter the maternal circulation without producing symptoms. Fat, hair, or mucin in PA blood also strengthen the possibility of AFE, but their presence still is not absolutely reliable.[279] New noninvasive tests designed to detect fetal material in the maternal plasma indirectly have been used in only a small number of patients, so their reliability has not yet been determined. One of these uses the monoclonal antibody TKH-2 to demonstrate increased concentrations of sialyl-Tn antigen in the serum; this indicates entry of meconium or fetal intestinal mucin into the maternal circulation.[291] In another test, zinc coproporphyrin, an indicator of meconium, can be detected in the maternal plasma.[292] Fetal debris found postmortem in the maternal pulmonary circulation is a more certain indicator than antemortem demonstration, and many pathologists consider it sufficient for definitive diagnosis. The ability to examine concentrated fetal material in histologic sections of lung tissue using special stains to identify squames, fetal intestinal mucin, fat, and lanugo hair make pathologic diagnosis reliable. Recently the monoclonal antibody TKH-2 has been used for histologic diagnosis of AFE and found to be even more reliable than these techniques.[293]

The lack of a definitive test necessitates vigorous exclusion of other clinical possibilities. In the differential diagnosis of AFE syndrome, the following should be considered: total spinal or high epidural anesthesia, an intravenous bolus or overdose of local anesthetic, allergic reactions, inadequate inspired O_2, hemorrhagic shock, placental abruption, PTE, air embolism, acute myocardial infarction, aspiration of gastric contents, sepsis, cardiomyopathy, cerebral embolus, ruptured intracranial aneurysm, and eclampsia.[286,288] The demonstration of initial pulmonary hypertension or, subsequently, of moderately increased PAP, increased wedge pressure, and decreased cardiac output could be useful, but this type of monitoring almost always is initiated after the diagnosis is made. Likewise, TEE could theoretically be useful to exclude thromboembolism and demonstrate LV failure that might be from AFE syndrome.

C. Management

There is no specific therapy for the AFE syndrome; aggressive supportive treatment after prompt diagnosis is the strategy of management.[279,285,286] This involves administering the highest possible concentration of inspired O_2 both before and after intubating the trachea. If hypoxemia persists despite mechanical ventilation with 100% O_2, PEEP can be titrated. If they are used, the doses of sedative/hypnotic agents given before tracheal intubation should be reduced; ketamine (0.5 to 1 mg/kg) and succinylcholine (1 mg/kg) are the preferred agents.

An arterial line should be established to monitor the response to the efforts to improve the cardiac output and tissue perfusion with fluids and pharmacologic agents. In the presence of LV failure and pulmonary hypertension, administration of large volumes of fluids may result in pulmonary edema. Nevertheless, judicious fluid administration is essential to improve venous return and cardiac filling. This will enable sympathomimetic and inotropic agents (ephedrine, 5 to 10 mg bolus doses; epinephrine, 4 to 24 μg/min; norepinephrine, 2 to 4 μg/min; dopamine, 2 to 40 μg/kg/min; dobutamine, 2 to 40 μg/kg/min) to improve cardiac output. Once adequate circulation is established, pulmonary edema can be treated with diuretics. A PA catheter should be placed as early as possible during treatment; Clark et al[275] demonstrated 100% survival in five patients in whom fluid and inotropic therapy was guided with central hemodynamic monitoring. Central monitoring also helps in managing ARDS, which may develop later.

An intraaortic balloon pump has been used in patients with persistent hypotension and documented LV failure despite fluid and inotropic therapy.[279] Pulmonary arterial embolectomy with a good outcome has also been described in a mother with AFE syndrome. However, it is not clear whether AFE was responsible for the hemodynamic abnormality in this patient; the material removed from the PA contained squamous cells but in a thromboembolus.[294] Persistent hypoxia may occur when ARDS develops after the acute event. Parenteral pulmonary vasodilators may be beneficial in these instances, but they may be associated with hypotension and increased shunting from vasodilation in the face of alveolar exudation. Successful use of inhaled aerosolized prostacyclin (30 to 40 ng/kg/min), a selective pulmonary vasodilator, has been described in a patient with ARDS after AFE syndrome.[295] This route of administration may have minimal hypotensive effects because the short half-life of the drug limits its systemic activity. Furthermore, the agent is preferentially distributed to the ventilated parts of the lung, producing its maximal vasodilatory effect in regions with good ventilation and thus improving ventilation/perfusion matching. Nitric oxide also may be used for this purpose, but it requires specialized equipment that is not needed for prostacyclin.[132,133]

Compression of the inferior vena cava by the pregnant uterus may prevent venous return; vigilance in maintaining manual uterine shift is essential. Emergency delivery of the fetus may be considered not only to improve the effectiveness of maternal chest compression during cardiac arrest, but also to increase the chance of fetal survival. Clark et al[276] showed a 100% neonatal survival rate, with only 33% neurologic deficit, if the cardiac arrest to delivery interval was less than 15 minutes. A longer period was associated with substantially decreased survival and an increased rate of neurologic abnormalities in surviving neonates. Of course, continuous fetal monitoring should be performed during the entire time of treatment.

Coagulopathy is best treated with fresh frozen plasma, cryoprecipitate, platelets, and packed red cells. Serial coagulation profiles, including PT, aPTT, platelet count, fibrinogen, FDP, and fibrin D-dimer, should be obtained, along with clinical follow-up to monitor the effectiveness of treatment and the progress of the disease. Bleeding in AFE syndrome may result not only from DIC but also from placental insertion abnormalities and uterine atony. Recognition and prompt treatment of these conditions is of utmost importance. Uterine atony is treated by infusion of oxytocin or intramuscular 15-methyl-PGF_{2a} (Hemabate, 0.25 mg).

VII. TUMOR EMBOLISM
A. Venous emboli

These emboli rarely are diagnosed premortem, although they are not uncommon. In 366 patients dying of carcinoma of breast or stomach, hypernephroma, or choriocarcinoma, Winterbaur and Elfenbein[296] found pulmonary tumor emboli in 26%. The reason that so many of these emboli are not diagnosed clinically is not clear; possibly most are simply asymptomatic, and the symptoms in others may be so nonspecific as to be attributed to another type of embolism or a different pathologic process altogether. The proportion of patients with tumor emboli who have symptoms is unknown, although about half of the 33 symptomatic patients in Winterbaur's series exhibited clinical indications of PE.

Tumor emboli occur in a wide range of sizes, from microscopic to large enough to occlude one or both main pulmonary arteries.[297,298] Pathologically, they consist of nests of malignant cells encased in thrombi; because the cells are isolated from the circulation, they eventually degenerate, unlike true metastases. Thus the indicators of tumor emboli result from the fact that they are emboli rather than that they are tumors.[297] They include respiratory distress and decreased breath sounds, tachycardia, and jugular venous distention.

The characteristic laboratory findings are of a severe nonspecific subacute embolic process.[299] PaO_2 is reduced, commonly to less than 50 mm Hg, probably from increased intrapulmonary shunting (from opening of arteriovenous shunts, reperfusion of atelectatic regions, and localized pulmonary edema) as well as $\dot{V}/\dot{Q}$ mismatch. The RV systolic and PAP may be very high and occasionally are higher than the systemic arterial pressure.[300] The chest radiograph usually is normal despite this severe pathology in the lungs.[297,299] Cardiac enlargement, pulmonary arterial prominence, and infiltrates are seen only occasionally; indeed, a normal chest film in the presence

of dyspnea and hypoxia indicates an embolic process and rules out lymphatic spread (i.e., metastasis) of the primary tumor as a cause of the patient's symptoms. $\dot{V}/\dot{Q}$ scans typically show normal ventilation associated with numerous small, subsegmental, peripheral perfusion defects. Pulmonary angiography is a high-risk procedure in the face of hypoxia and pulmonary hypertension and may result in fatal cardiac failure. Therefore this procedure is contraindicated in these patients.[300]

It should be noted that all these findings are nonspecific. Usually the only way to differentiate tumor emboli from other subacute emboli (thrombus, amniotic fluid, fat, foreign body, septic, parasitic) is by open lung biopsy.

B. Arterial emboli

The majority of arterial tumor emboli originate from intracardiac neoplasms; those arising from other sources are extremely rare. Most of the latter arise from advanced pulmonary carcinoma, primary vascular tumors, or direct tumor invasion of an arterial wall.[300]

Intracavitary tumors of the heart are uncommon; about 70% are benign, and about half of these are myxomas, of which the majority are located in the left atrium. Typically, myxomas are both pedunculated and friable and embolize in 24% to 36% of patients with these tumors.[301] Significantly, about half of these emboli are to the brain; thus stroke is a common, and occasionally the first, clinical manifestation of a cardiac tumor.

The symptoms of arterial tumor emboli depend on the site embolized and vary from lower-extremity vascular insufficiency to stroke. Patients with cerebral emboli usually die from the combined effects of stroke and cachexia from the primary tumor. Emboli in the arteries of the extremities may be removed by embolectomy. Excision of a primary cardiac tumor requires open-heart surgery and possibly valve replacement or repair of the septum.[300]

C. Anesthetic considerations

Management of anesthesia in the patient with pulmonary tumor embolism must take into account both the emboli and the primary malignancy. Therefore the major considerations are to maintain oxygenation and cardiac function and to provide sufficient blood volume to maintain oxygen delivery without precipitating right heart failure.[300]

Local or regional anesthesia probably is the best choice in appropriate procedures, such as embolectomy or placement of a vena caval filter. If general anesthesia is required for major surgery, both arterial and Swan-Ganz catheters generally are necessary so that the patient's cardiac and volume status can be closely monitored. It should be noted that if the tip of the PA catheter is in an impaired region of the lung, the wedge pressures do not reflect left atrial function.

If the patient is cachectic, the blood volume as a function of the body weight is unpredictable. In addition, fat and muscle mass and serum albumin are decreased, and there may also be alterations in the serum proteins. If the patient has been receiving chemotherapy, the hepatic enzymes may be induced. All of these factors make the patient's requirements for medications unpredictable. Thus all anesthetic agents should be administered with great care.[300]

Probably the best way to maintain the patient's cardiovascular status is an opioid technique following induction with either a benzodiazepine or etomidate.[300] Nitrous oxide probably is safe if pulmonary vascular resistance is not markedly elevated and if its use permits a high enough inspired oxygen concentration to maintain the patient's PaO_2. The halogenated agents should be used carefully; isoflurane generally is safe at low doses, but higher doses may cause myocardial depression. Obviously, the patient's fluid requirements should be controlled carefully; hypotension is treated with a fluid challenge and inotropes as necessary.

Chemotherapy presents unique problems in these patients.[302,303] Indeed, the embolic episode may be precipitated by the tumor necrosis produced by chemotherapeutic agents. Anemia, leukopenia, and thrombocytopenia are common results of bone marrow suppression and must be evaluated appropriately and treated preoperatively if necessary. Some agents, especially Cytoxan, may decrease plasma pseudocholinesterase. Prolonged apnea may follow administration of succinylcholine, which probably should be avoided. Other agents, notably methotrexate and bleomycin, may produce direct pulmonary injury and further complicate the problems produced by the embolic process. ARDS is common after surgery in patients who have received these drugs, even if they have been given 6 to 12 months preoperatively. This may be related to oxygen sensitivity because limiting the FIO_2 to 0.25 seems to prevent the complication. Cisplatin may cause renal tubular damage; fluid administration and possibly mannitol may prevent it. Doxorubicin, daunorubicin, and cisplatin produce diffuse and occasionally severe cardiomyopathy, resulting in a low-voltage electrocardiogram and a decreased ejection fraction. The patient requires preoperative digitalization and scrupulous attention to intraoperative fluid management.

VIII. INFECTIOUS EMBOLI

Septic emboli are uncommon and often unrecognized. Although they may arise in any part of the body, the most common sites are the pelvis, the tricuspid and pulmonic valves, the abdomen, the veins of the extremities, and the skin and subcutaneous tissues.[304] Valvular endocarditis is common in intravenous drug abusers as a result of the use of contaminated needles and syringes. Foreign bodies may be involved. For instance, an infected venous catheter or a pacemaker wire may be a direct source of emboli, or it may produce septicemia, which in turn may result in bacterial endocarditis involving one or both valves of the right heart. Vegetations may then detach and embolize to the lungs.

A. Gram-positive emboli

Most septic emboli involve *Staphylococcus aureus:* 85% of cases of endocarditis in addicts, 50% of pulmonary abscesses following vascular cannulation, and most tonsillar abscesses and skin infections are caused by this organism, as are many wound infections.[305] Streptococci and enterococci are more often associated with pelvic thrombophlebitis, abdominal abscesses, and childbirth. These emboli produce areas of pneumonia that coalesce rapidly to form a pulmonary abscess.

Symptomatically, the patient exhibits shaking chills and a high fever in addition to the usual signs of PE: dyspnea, chest pain, cough, hemoptysis, and tachycardia. On auscultation, the lungs may be normal, or there may be altered breath sounds and inspiratory rales.[305] There may at times be frank consolidation and pleural effusion. The leukocyte count is elevated, and bacteremia may or may not be present. On chest radiograph, there may be a single abscess or multiple abnormalities involving one or both lungs.[305]

B. Gram-negative emboli

Escherichia coli, Klebsiella, and *Proteus* are the organisms most often involved in abdominal infections. They usually cause diffuse or lower-lobe pneumonitis by hematogenous spread from the source of the infection. Gram-negative septicemia may exhibit a fulminant course that progresses rapidly to septic shock.[305]

Clinically, there may be scantily productive cough, dyspnea, and fever, but very few other signs that cannot be attributed to the primary infection. Physical findings generally are confined to the lower lobes of the lungs and include inspiratory rales and dullness to percussion. The chest radiograph usually shows patchy lower-lobe infiltrates. Sputum stains are positive for gram-negative rods, and there is a preponderance of gram-negative organisms on sputum culture. Leukocytosis may or may not be present.

C. Anaerobic emboli

Microaerophilic streptococci and anaerobes such as fusobacteria and *Bacteroides* may complicate bowel perforation; these organisms may also be involved in pelvic inflammatory disease, septic abortions, and pelvic vein thrombosis, as well as oral infections and tonsillitis. PE may originate in any of these sources.[305]

Anaerobic PE may produce severe symptoms: cough, dyspnea, shaking chills, pleural pain, high fever, and prostration. Cough may be nonproductive or there may be foul-smelling sputum, a diagnostic indicator of anaerobic pulmonary infection. Auscultation may disclose few signs, or there may be large areas of rales and altered breath sounds, a pleural friction rub, and signs of pleural effusion. The chest radiograph shows patchy infiltrates that increase rapidly in size, eventually forming abscesses. If a pleural effusion is present, gas may be seen above the fluid. Anemia may develop rapidly, and icterus from liver damage and hemolysis is common. Anaerobic culture of blood and pleural fluid (which has a putrid odor in 50% of cases) will establish the diagnosis.

D. Treatment

Every effort should be made to find the source of the infection, from careful history and physical examination to radiography, ultrasonography, or bone scanning. No therapy for septic PE can be successful until the primary infection is removed; this may involve incision and drainage of an abscess, removal of a foreign body, ligation or excision of infected veins, or open-heart surgery for replacement of an infected valve. Most pulmonary abscesses respond to antibiotics; pleural effusions should be drained surgically.[300]

In addition to the pulmonary derangements resulting from the embolic process, severe problems may be produced by the patient's pneumonia and further exacerbated by the hypermetabolism resulting from fever.[305] Of course, appropriate treatment of the infection and of septic shock is required; these issues are beyond the scope of this chapter.[306] However, it should be noted that the risk of ARDS is enormous. These patients should be intubated and ventilated at the first sign of respiratory difficulty.

E. Anesthetic considerations

In addition to the general principles of management for PE, certain problems are unique to the septic patient, particularly one who is in septic shock.[300] As is well known, certain antibiotic agents interact with muscle relaxants, especially colistin, kanamycin, the streptomycins, tetracyclines, and polymyxin B. Prolonged apnea may result when one of these agents is used in the anesthetized patient.[307] Although these effects may be reversible with calcium salts in some cases, it is probably best to leave the patient intubated and ventilated until the effects of the neuromuscular blockers dissipate. Febrile patients should be cooled preoperatively because increased oxygen demand and CO_2 production may increase the risk of hypoxia.

In appropriate circumstances, regional anesthesia may be the best choice in the stable patient. However, axillary and femoral blocks should be avoided if there is lymphadenopathy or lymphadenitis in the involved region. Spinal and epidural anesthesia also should not be used if the infected area is in the back, or in the presence of septicemia.[300,307]

If the patient is in septic shock, every effort should be made to stabilize his or her condition preoperatively, although surgery should not be unduly delayed because the downhill course will not be reversed until the source of infection is treated.[306] The patient will generally have been intubated and ventilated preoperatively. Arterial and PA catheters should be inserted if they are not already in place. General anesthesia may present formidable difficulties. Probably the safest is a high-dose fentanyl-oxygen technique following a careful ketamine or midazolam induction. If the patient is in severe shock, these induction agents may produce marked hypotension and thus should not be used. If the patient is in deep coma, no anesthetic agents may be needed. Oxygen and a muscle relaxant may be all that is required and, indeed, all the patient can tolerate.[306,307]

IX. FOREIGN BODY EMBOLI

Foreign bodies are uncommon sources of emboli, and generally present few problems for the anesthesiologist.

It is usually the primary problem rather than the embolism itself that represents the major risk to the patient. For instance, if a CV catheter breaks off and is carried to a PA, the event is significant not so much because of the obstruction to the vessel as because of the illness that led to insertion of the catheter in the first place.[300]

Several types of foreign bodies may embolize. Medically inserted catheters and wires are among the more significant.[308] The incidence of these has decreased because through-the-needle catheters (Intracaths) are no longer used. At present, the most common iatrogenic emboli result from severing of a catheter while cutting a fixation suture and from fatigue of the catheter material.[309,310] Embolism of guidewires and pacemaker electrodes generally is the result of mishandling. Bullets and other missiles rarely embolize.[311] Both the sources and the destinations of foreign bodies vary widely, and the problems they produce are equally variable.[312]

Arterial foreign body emboli may be removed with a transvascular grasping device under local anesthesia or by direct cut-down to a peripheral vessel, and therefore present no special problems to the anesthesiologist. Intracardiac emboli should be extracted, by open-heart surgery if necessary, in order to prevent further migration, interference with a valve, or myocardial instability.[309,310] On the other hand, asymptomatic emboli to pulmonary, cerebral, or pelvic arteries are probably best left in place because their removal may cause more problems than it solves.[313] Most venous emboli can be left in place, although the possibility of morbidity is high (25%) relative to the complications of their extraction.

Other emboli may result from the methylmethacrylate used for total hip prostheses or neuroradiologic embolization,[314] and from substances used to dilute abused intravenous drugs, such as talc, starch, and sawdust. Methylmethacrylate emboli rarely are of clinical significance. The degree of pulmonary impairment associated with intravenous drug abuse is widely variable, but in rare cases, granulomatosis may be severe enough to produce major complications.[315]

In general, anesthesia is not a particular problem in the patient with a foreign body embolism.[300] Most patients are young, and many procedures need only local anesthesia. Furthermore, few of these procedures are urgent; the patient's condition can be optimized preoperatively. If the patient is a drug abuser with significant pulmonary dysfunction, anesthetic management and perioperative respiratory support should be the same as for any patient with chronic obstructive pulmonary disease.

X. ARTERIAL EMBOLISM

Improved prophylaxis of rheumatic heart disease, a decreasing incidence of congenital heart disease, and more effective therapy for acquired atherosclerotic and valvular heart disease have resulted in a decreased incidence of arterial embolism in the past decade. The need for surgical management of the complications of arterial embolism is also less, partly because of decreased occurrence and probably partly because they are managed more commonly with anticoagulant and thrombolytic agents.[316,317] Nevertheless, perioperative embolic arterial complications do occur and tax the decision-making capabilities of anesthesiologists.

In the perioperative period, arterial embolization can be caused by any of the substances involved in venous embolism. However, thromboembolism probably is the most common. Arterial embolism may result from passage of thrombus, fat, air, or amniotic fluid through a septal defect. Transpulmonary passage is also possible for fat, air, and amniotic fluid.[5,191] Air may also enter the arterial circulation accidentally during cardiopulmonary bypass or during irrigation of arterial lines. Thoracic injuries, whether penetrating or blunt, can lead to entry of alveolar air into the pulmonary veins and then to the left heart and systemic circulation during mechanical ventilation.[318] A similar phenomenon may occur during resection of tracheal tumors with the YAG laser (Marc Tissot, personal communication, August 1998). During laser surgery, air in the trachea may enter the veins of the tumor and may proceed to the left side of the heart and systemic circulation via the bronchial veins. Prevention involves applying the laser in short bursts and ventilating the lungs with small tidal volumes and low airway pressures. If a TEE is used, air may be noted in the left heart. Surgically produced debris may also move from body cavities into the circulation and cause infarcts in various organs with significant clinical manifestations.[319]

The principal source of arterial thromboembolism is the heart and, less often, the great vessels. Cardiac disorders such as atrial fibrillation, myocardial infarction, congestive heart failure, valvular disease, or artificial valves promote thrombus formation.[148,320,321] If cardiac evaluation, including an ultrasound examination, yields negative results, the large blood vessels, especially an abdominal aortic aneurysm, should be suspected as a source. Ultrasonography, abdominal CT scan, and aortography all are capable of demonstrating aortic thrombi. The thoracic aorta is also an important source of arterial embolism.[322] Protruding mobile or ulcerated atherosclerotic plaques are the most commonly embolized substances from the aorta.[322] These are formed from fibrinous material, calcium fragments, cholesterol crystals, and thrombi; they all have embolic potential. Arterial embolism also can occur in the absence of any of these mechanisms. For example, bacteremic infections with or without endocarditis can produce embolic stroke or myocardial infarction, probably by activating the coagulation system.[323]

In the heart, thrombi resulting from atrial fibrillation and atrial myxomata typically are located in the left atrium or the left atrial appendage.[320] More than half of the thrombi that originate in the heart, and 33% to 75% of all cases of arterial emboli, are associated with atrial fibrillation.[321] Cardiac thrombi secondary to myocardial infarction usually are located in the left ventricle. Acute transmural anterior wall myocardial infarction is notorious for promoting intracardiac thrombus, probably because of apical involvement and a larger size than is typical of infarcts in other areas.[321] Valvular vegetations can occur on the mitral or aortic valves. Emboli resulting from valve infections usually are small and therefore produce microvascular effects. However, fungal and some types of bacterial endocarditis can produce large vegetations that may occlude major arteries if they embolize. Sterile intracardiac thrombi (marantic endocarditis), usually seen in chronically ill patients, may also dislodge. Left atrial myxomas and other pedunculated friable cardiac tumors also have embolization potential.[300,301,321]

The brain is the destination of 66% of all arterial emboli from the heart, probably because the innominate and left carotid arteries are the first vessels thrombus encounters after the aorta.[320] The remaining 34% of thrombi embolize to the viscera and the extremities, most commonly to the mesenteric and renal arteries. Emboli originating in aortic arch lesions are more likely to be directed to the left side of the brain and the extremities rather than the right brain because they usually originate distal to the innominate artery.[321]

A. Pathophysiology

The mechanism of formation of intracardiac thrombus varies depending on the underlying disorder. In atrial fibrillation and myocardial infarction, stasis of blood caused by atrial or ventricular wall akinesis or hypokinesis results in thrombus formation. Ventricular thrombi usually develop within the first week after myocardial infarction. Thrombus forms on diseased or artificial cardiac valves primarily because of the loss of endothelial integrity, which permits platelet aggregation, leading to fibrin-platelet complex formation and deposition.[321]

The release of thrombi into the circulation is facilitated by several factors, most importantly by a small area of attachment to the cardiac wall, mobility of the thrombus, and vigorous contractions of the myocardium.[321] Isolation from the circulation because of akinesis or hypokinesis encourages thrombus formation but mitigates against systemic embolization. For example, LV aneurysms, which form 3 months or more after infarction, are very likely to contain thrombi, but embolize infrequently because there is minimal blood flow around the thrombus. In contrast, thrombi in patients with idiopathic dilated cardiomyopathy are highly likely to embolize because they often have limited areas of attachment to the ventricular wall and overlie a normally contracting myocardium. This prevents organization of the thrombus at its edges, leaving it friable and more likely to fragment into the bloodstream.[321]

Atherosclerotic plaques may be raised and detached from the arterial wall by blood flow or more commonly by trauma or intravascular instrumentation. These plaques, which contain fibrinous material, calcium fragments, cholesterol crystals, and thrombi, embolize as a diffuse shower involving several organs. The signs and symptoms of this type of embolism are more subtle than those of cardiac origin because the small fragments lodge in arteries with internal diameters of only 50 to 200 mm. Apart from atheromatous plaques, arteries may harbor adherent mural thrombi made of fibrin and platelets. Stenotic lesions, intravascular thrombosis at suture sites of previous grafts, and vessel wall aneurysms may also contain mural thrombi, which usually are small but occasionally may be quite large.

Perioperative arterial embolization usually occurs in the postoperative period. Dehydration, abnormal cardiovascular dynamics such as ventricular wall motion abnormalities and arrhythmias, and the normal perioperative hypercoagulable state may be responsible for thrombus formation on a previously asymptomatic and unsuspected lesion such as an ulcerating atheroma. The underlying risk is an important predictor of perioperative embolization, although the predictive ability of different risk factors varies. For example, the presence of atrial fibrillation generally is a far greater indicator of risk than carotid atherosclerotic disease. Thus an embolic stroke in the presence of carotid disease requires a search for other possible sources in addition to the obvious carotid plaque.[321]

B. Clinical issues

Anesthesiologists may need to deal with three clinical issues in the patient with arterial embolism.

1. Operative management. Patients who require surgery for arterial embolism are likely to have systemic abnormalities such as cardiac ischemia, myocardial infarction, arrhythmias, stroke, sepsis, metabolic imbalance, or other major illnesses. The source of embolism should be ascertained in these patients because it is likely that the underlying etiology may necessitate alterations in anesthetic management. Cardiac ischemic disease, thyrotoxicosis, valvular heart disease, and arrhythmias are some of the possible causes. If there is no obvious embolic source, a cardiac origin should be ruled out first even in the absence of clinical evidence of heart disease. If there is no cardiac source, a vascular origin is likely, implying that significant atherosclerotic disease is present.

Acute arterial embolism may occur in peripheral, visceral, coronary, and cerebral arteries. Surgery is indicated in patients with embolism to extremity and certain visceral arteries.

a. Embolism to extremity arteries. Evaluation of the limb is essential because not all patients with peripheral arterial embolism are candidates for surgery. If the limb is viable on initial examination, the chance for operative success is reasonably good even when a significant amount of time has elapsed since the embolic event. Based on clinical assessment, patients can be divided into three categories: viable limb, limb with threatened viability, and irreversibly nonviable limb.[324] The viable limb is characterized by intact capillary return, normal motor and sensory function, and audible arterial and venous Doppler signals. The limb with threatened viability exhibits slow capillary return. Motor and sensory functions are diminished but not lost, and the venous Doppler signal is audible although the arterial is not. A limb in this condition is likely to be salvaged if treated promptly. An irreversibly nonviable limb is characterized by absent capillary return, mottled skin, profound paralysis and sensory loss, and inaudible arterial and venous Doppler signals.[324]

There is time to assess a viable limb with an emergency arteriogram. If an occlusion suggestive of embolic origin is identified and the patient's general condition permits, embolectomy is indicated.[325] If a thrombus is more likely or the risk of surgery is prohibitive, thrombolytic therapy can be administered. Direct infusion of urokinase into the affected artery at a rate of 4000 IU/min for 4 hours, then at 2000 IU/min for up to 48 hours, appears to be as effective as immediate surgery.[326] If thrombolytic therapy is contraindicated, anticoagulation with medium- to high-dose heparin (see Table 29-5) should be given. The patient with a limb of threatened viability must be taken to the operating room emergently, and embolectomy must be performed. There is no time for an arteriogram. If the completion arteriogram is satisfactory, anticoagulation with heparin should be instituted.[327]

Nonviable limbs carry a high risk of operative mortality because of the reperfusion syndrome, characterized by metabolic acidosis, elevated serum creatinine, and hyperkalemia, which produce arrhythmias, hypotension, rhabdomyolysis, and renal failure. Edema and necrosis in skeletal muscle actually worsen after reperfusion because of accumulation of free radicals and leukocyte activation.[321] Reperfusion syndrome may occur in some patients who are assessed as having viable or threatened limbs but whose extremities actually are nonviable. Active monitoring of hemodynamics, acid-base status, and electrolytes, and prompt treatment, if necessary, are indicated. Insulin and glucose are administered for hyperkalemia, bicarbonate is given for metabolic acidosis and to prevent myoglobin precipitation in renal tubules, and fluids and vasopressors are infused to treat hemodynamic alterations and to establish an adequate urine output. The therapy for a patient with a nonviable extremity is high-dose heparin anticoagulation (see Table 29-5) for 2 to 3 days, to allow sharp demarcation of the ischemic region from the rest of the limb. This permits successful amputation at the lowest possible level. Moderate- or high-dose heparin therapy may also be indicated for other patients before embolectomy for two reasons. The first is to determine the viability of the limb; this will improve as collateral flow is mobilized.[328] Second, heparin treatment minimizes the possibility of recurrent embolism.[329]

The Fogarty catheter is used for embolectomy, which usually can be performed under local anesthesia.[328] Regional anesthesia often is contraindicated because most patients arrive in the operating room anticoagulated. Immediate preoperative heparinization appears to improve the limb salvage rate.[328] Invasive monitoring, at least an arterial line, is necessary because many of these patients are critically ill, with serious cardiac abnormalities. Intraoperative completion angiography is essential; as many as 30% of patients have residual thrombus.[330] Radiocontrast material may be associated with various problems: anaphylactic or anaphylactoid reactions, alterations in cardiac conduction and contractility, changes in pulmonary function, and vagally mediated bradycardia and hypotension.[331]

Arterial thrombosis may be misdiagnosed as arterial embolism. The former requires more involved surgery such as thromboendarterectomy, arterial patching, or even a bypass procedure, which usually cannot be performed under local anesthesia. Clinically, the differentiation of embolism from thrombosis is based on history and physical examination. As compared to arterial thrombosis, arterial embolism is characterized by a more sudden onset, more severe symptoms, and minimal or no preexisting vascular disease. On examination the opposite limb usually is normal, chronic skin changes are absent, and ischemia is profound because collateral circulation is inadequate.[321]

b. Visceral embolism. Surgery is indicated for embolism to the mesenteric and sometimes to the renal arteries. The earliest symptom of mesenteric artery embolism is severe pain, although physical examination of the abdomen typically reveals minimal or no positive findings.[332] This feature often results in delay in diagnosis, and thus in surgical treatment. A high index of suspicion is the key to the diagnosis. An angiogram may be performed early based on this suspicion or in patients in whom a nonocclusive cause, such as low cardiac output or shock-induced mesenteric thrombosis, is a possibility. Although an angiogram can differentiate between the two, mesenteric thrombosis carries a much grimmer prognosis than does mesenteric embolism. Up to 80% of patients with emboli can survive without significant residual defects if surgery is performed before more than 50% of the intestine has become irreversibly damaged.[321] Surgical repair involves mesenteric embolectomy or autogenous vein aortomesenteric bypass in the early stage and intestinal resection in the late stages. Intraoperative assessment of the viability of the intestine is based on evaluation of its color. Thus a second-look laparotomy within 24 hours is recommended to detect missed necrotic bowel and to evaluate the results of surgery.[332] In selected patients, local intraarterial thrombolytic therapy after a diagnostic angiography may prove successful.[333]

After the early stages mesenteric infarction is associated with serious systemic effects. Edematous and necrotic mucosa renders the intestinal wall permeable to bacteria and fluid, resulting in bacterial peritonitis, sepsis, septic shock syndrome, and massive fluid shifts. Gastrointestinal bleeding may occur and cause a decrease in hematocrit. Before this event, however, the hematocrit may increase because of severe dehydration. Metabolic acidosis is common. Antibiotic coverage and beat-to-beat arterial and CV monitoring of volume status therefore are mandatory during surgery. A PA catheter should be inserted because most patients are elderly and have cardiovascular compromise, not only as a preexisting condition but also as a result of sepsis.

As a general principle, the source of the embolus should be determined and the underlying condition should be corrected if possible. Postoperative low- or moderate-dose heparin (see Table 29-5) should be initiated within 24 to 48 hours if there is no active bleeding. Heparin can be continued for 2 to 3 days; then warfarin is given for long-term prophylaxis.

Mesenteric embolism also may be caused by atherosclerotic plaques. Their small size usually causes submucosal occlusion with multiple small infarcts in the bowel. Massive infarction or perforation is rare. However, atypical gastrointestinal symptoms may arise. Perhaps some of the intestinal problems that occur after cardiopulmonary bypass result from atheromatous microembolization.

Renal artery embolism is manifested by sudden onset of flank pain with or without microscopic hematuria. Definitive diagnosis requires CT scanning, renal arteriography, or both. If no blood flow to the kidney can be demonstrated by these tests, treatment with moderate-dose heparin anticoagulation (see Table 29-5), catheter infusion of a thrombolytic agent, or surgery, including embolectomy, aortorenal bypass, or nephrectomy, may be indicated. Unless embolization is bilateral, hypertension is unlikely.

2. Management of procedure-related arterial embolism. Table 29-12 lists procedures that may cause arterial embolism. Many of these are not performed in the operating room. Left heart catheterization may be com-

Table 29-12. Procedures that may cause arterial embolism

Procedure	Type of embolism
Cardiopulmonary bypass for open heart surgery	Atherosclerotic plaque, debris, air, thrombus
Thoracic aortic aneurysm repair	Atherosclerotic plaque, debris, air, thrombus
Carotid endarterectomy	Atherosclerotic plaque, debris, thrombus, air
Coronary rotational atherectomy	Atherosclerotic plaque, thrombus
Percutaneous balloon mitral valvuloplasty	Atherosclerotic plaque, thrombus
Centrifugal pump for postcardiotomy ventricular failure	Thrombus
Endovascular repair of abdominal aortic aneurysm	Atherosclerotic plaque, thrombus
Adult venous reservoir* in cardiopulmonary bypass circuits	Air
Ventricular assist device implantation	Thrombus
Intraaortic balloon pump placement	Thrombus
Transjugular intrahepatic portosystemic shunt with coil embolization	Thrombus
Therapeutic embolization with various materials	Material used, thrombus
Left heart catheterization	Air, debris
Cardioversion	Thrombus
Procedures that can be complicated by pulmonary embolism	Thrombus, fat, air, amniotic fluid, or other material by paradoxical embolism

*Medtronic Maxima hard-shell reservoir.

plicated by dislodgment of a protruding aortic atheroma.[322] If these complications are identified by TEE, catheterization of the brachial artery may prevent damage to the intimal surfaces of the femoral and iliac arteries and the aorta, reducing the potential for embolization.[322] During percutaneous balloon mitral valvuloplasty, embolization of valvular debris and intracardiac thrombus can be prevented by echocardiographic assessment of the valve and anticoagulation before the procedure.[334] Ventricular assist devices are used in patients with severe ventricular dysfunction. Systemic thromboembolism may occur if blood stasis is permitted in the ventricle.[335] Placement of the atrial cannula tip through the mitral valve prevents formation of cardiac thrombus. TEE helps in proper positioning of the cannula. Anticoagulation also is essential.[335] During high-speed rotational atherectomy, debris may travel distally and produce clinically significant morbidity or occasionally mortality.[336]

a. Carotid endarterectomy. In the operating room carotid endarterectomy often is complicated by cerebral embolism of air and debris.[337] Ulcerated plaques with associated thrombus are likely to embolize during dissection and cannot be identified reliably by preoperative color duplex ultrasonography.[338] Intraoperative TCD monitoring can detect potentially dangerous embolization and permit modification of the surgical technique.[337,338] Distal microembolization of debris is also possible during repair of abdominal aortic aneurysms, especially with the endovascular technique.[339]

b. Cardiopulmonary bypass. Systemic air embolism is a significant threat during open-heart surgery. Air bubbles may form when venous blood enters a reservoir containing a low volume of fluid.[340] Thus reservoirs should not be operated with less than 1000 ml of fluid content.[340] Retained intracardiac air may be ejected into the arterial circulation during cardiac surgery. Thus careful removal by the surgeons is necessary before declamping of the aorta and separation from bypass. This complication is more likely to occur after valve replacement than after coronary artery bypass surgery.[341] The first step is to mobilize the air from the pulmonary veins. Next, for removal of mobilized air, a properly placed left atrial vent is essential; a continuous ascending aorta-to-venous shunt has also been used. The absence of residual air should be demonstrated objectively; 2-D or M-mode TEE of the left atrium and ventricle is satisfactory. Another technique for removal of retained air in the pulmonary vein involves raising the reservoir of the cardiopulmonary bypass pump to increase movement of blood from the pulmonary vein into the left atrium; a vent connected to variable suction in this location removes the air. Continuous monitoring of ET_{CO_2} and PAP may be useful for ensuring complete removal of air. It has been suggested that ET_{CO_2} greater than 25 mm Hg and mean PAP over 90% of the prebypass level indicates satisfactory air removal.[342] Reducing the cerebral blood flow by hyperventilation during filling of the heart may also reduce the volume of air reaching the brain.

Although there is no consensus about how to manage pH and P_{CO_2} during cardiopulmonary bypass, it appears that the incidence of postoperative neuropsychologic disturbances is less with α-stat mode, possibly because it aids in preservation of cerebral autoregulation and reduction in embolization to the cerebral circulation by decreasing cerebral blood flow.[343] With pH-stat management, pH and Pa_{CO_2} values are corrected for the patient's core temperature, whereas in α-stat mode no attempt at correction is made.

c. Thoracic aneurysm repair. Atheroembolism from manipulation of the ascending aorta is another cause of end-organ ischemia and postoperative stroke or neuropsychologic dysfunction.[344] Approximately 50% of cerebral complications after repair of thoracic aortic aneurysms are caused by embolism.[345] Advanced age, aortic arch lesions, and atherosclerotic aneurysm are important risk factors.[345] Placement of an intraaortic balloon pump in patients with protruding aortic atheromas can lead to cerebral embolism; TEE may detect these events.[322] Prevention of cerebral ischemia involves several measures. Preoperative assessment of the aorta by chest roentgenogram and cardiac catheterization and intraoperative evaluation with TEE with or without epiaortic ultrasound to detect aortic atheromatous disease may indicate the need for surgical measures to prevent release of aortic plaques.[346,347] TCD monitoring also may contribute to reducing the incidence of cerebral embolization; the timing and number of emboli can be identified with this device.[348] A temperature between 32° and 34° C when embolization occurs may offer some brain protection. However, rewarming during separation from bypass may exacerbate ischemic damage; rapid and intense rewarming should be avoided. The site of temperature monitoring may influence rewarming; monitoring at the nasopharynx may prevent hyperthermia and possibly attendant neurologic damage.[349]

d. Cardioversion. Cardioversion for atrial fibrillation may be complicated by arterial thromboembolism. Although it is performed to improve hemodynamics and avoid anticoagulation, this procedure is associated with a stroke risk of 1.5% per treatment (range 0% to 7%) and probably an even greater rate of systemic embolism.[320] Cardioversion for chronic atrial fibrillation is more likely to be complicated by embolism than that for acute disease, although it has been demonstrated that atrial fibrillation for as little as 3 days may be associated with atrial thrombus formation.[350] Arterial thromboembolism after cardioversion typically occurs on the third day, but it may be present as early as the first day and as late as 2 to 3 weeks following the procedure. The mechanism of the complication is the release of thrombus from the underlying atrial wall after resumption of atrial contractile activity. The delay in embolization is caused by atrial stunning; atrial mechanical activity lags a few days behind the appearance of P waves on the ECG.[320]

Prevention involves 3 weeks of warfarin treatment (INR = 2.0 to 3.0) before and 4 weeks after cardioversion if atrial fibrillation has been present for longer than 2 days.[320] Postcardioversion anticoagulation is recommended because there is a possibility of recurrence of the arrhythmia and increased coagulability during the period of atrial stunning induced by the procedure.[320] Atrial fibrillation in patients with mitral stenosis, an LV ejection fraction less than 40%, and spontaneous echo contrast (SEC) in the left atrium suggests the presence of left atrial thrombus.[320] Spontaneous echo contrast, which is referred to as swirl, smoke, or rouleaux formation, is the appearance of stagnant blood in the left atrium on echocardiography. TEE provides reasonably good visualization of thrombus in the atrium and its appendage. A transthoracic echocardiogram is unlikely to diagnose thrombus in the atrial appendage reliably.[351] It has been suggested that the decision to anticoagulate the patient can be based on the finding of TEE; anticoagulation would not be required if thrombus were not visualized. This approach appears promising, but its value has not yet been conclusively demonstrated. The preliminary results of a multicenter study investigating this issue suggest that screening of atrial thrombus with TEE before instituting anticoagulation is safer, with fewer bleeding complications and less need for emergent cardioversion.[352]

3. Perioperative treatment of patients receiving thromboembolism prophylaxis. Surgery may be indicated in patients who have had previous episodes of thromboembolism or are at risk of developing the complication, and who are thus receiving prophylaxis. As we have discussed, conditions associated with a high likelihood of thromboembolic complications are previous venous thromboembolism, atrial fibrillation, a mechanical heart valve, and a history of arterial thromboembolism within 1 month.[148] These patients receive long-acting anticoagulation (warfarin), and discontinuing the drug during the perioperative period may result in arterial thromboembolism. Fortunately, in contrast to venous thromboembolism, it is only the cessation of warfarin and not the surgical procedure that increases the embolic risk.[148] The risk of perioperative arterial thromboembolism associated with each of these conditions varies. Even the same condition presenting under different circumstances may have different risks.[320] Management of anticoagulation before and after elective surgery in these situations has been of recent interest; treatment is based on the risk of recurrent thromboembolism in each condition. Recommendations for patients with a history of venous thromboembolism have already been presented. This section deals only with conditions that carry the risk of arterial thromboembolism.

Patients with atrial fibrillation, a condition that produces a seventeenfold increase in stroke rate if it is associated with rheumatic valvular disease and a fivefold increase if the origin is nonvalvular, demonstrate an annual cerebral thromboembolism rate between 1% and 18%.[320,353] This variation is related to the clinical presentation of the arrhythmia. Indeed, coexistent hypertensive heart disease, diabetes mellitus, history of transient ischemic attack (TIA) or stroke, age above 65, congestive heart failure, and angina or myocardial infarction increase the chance of stroke in nonrheumatic atrial fibrillation.[320] Likewise, echocardiographic findings such as

left atrial thrombus, LV wall abnormalities, and possibly the finding of SEC indicate an increased risk of arterial embolism.[320] Based on the number of these coexisting risk factors, patients with atrial fibrillation can be subdivided into high-, moderate-, and low-risk categories, with 12% to 15%, 5% to 8%, and about 1% incidence of stroke without warfarin prophylaxis, respectively (Table 29-13). Warfarin treatment decreases this rate substantially in the high- and moderate-risk category but has little effect in low-risk patients (see Table 29-13). Most low-risk patients are not treated with warfarin, but if they have been, discontinuation for a few days before and after surgery is unlikely to result in arterial thromboembolic events. However, patients with moderate- and high-risk atrial fibrillation may be vulnerable even with brief perioperative cessation of warfarin. Unfortunately, there are few studies examining the management of anticoagulation or the risk of stopping warfarin during the perioperative period in these patients. Two recent reviews have addressed this issue and proposed some guidelines for perioperative management of anticoagulation not only for atrial fibrillation but also for patients with prosthetic valves and recent arterial embolism.[148,320] The following recommendations are based on their proposals.

Patients with atrial fibrillation and multiple risk factors undergoing major surgery require anticoagulation throughout the perioperative period. In hospitalized patients this involves stopping warfarin 3 to 5 days before surgery. Heparin treatment is aimed at an aPTT of approximately twice normal, which correlates with a hep-

Table 29-13. Annual rate of cerebral thromboembolism in atrial fibrillation

Risk category	Annual percentage of stroke
High risk* without warfarin prophylaxis	12-15
High risk* with warfarin prophylaxis	4-8
Moderate risk† without warfarin prophylaxis	5-8
Moderate risk† with warfarin prophylaxis	1-2
Low risk‡ with or without warfarin prophylaxis	<1

Clinical risk factors: congestive heart failure, hypertension, diabetes mellitus, stroke/TIA.
Echocardiographic risk factors: left atrial thrombus, left ventricular dysfunction, or possibly spontaneous echo contrast.

Modified from Hanson EW, Lowson SM: *Anesth Analg* 87:217, 1998.
*High risk: two or three clinical risk factors or stroke/transient ischemic attack (TIA) within the last year.
†Moderate risk: one clinical risk factor, one or two echocardiographic risk factors, or stroke/TIA > 1 year.
‡Low risk: age <65 yr, no clinical risk factor.

arin blood concentration of 0.2 to 0.4 IU/ml by protamine titration assay. Heparin is discontinued 6 hours before surgery. The aPTT immediately preoperatively should be less than 1.5 times normal and the PT within 120% of normal (INR = 1.5) for the surgery to proceed. Another approach is to continue warfarin until 24 to 48 hours preoperatively. If PT is greater than 120% of normal on the day of surgery, intravenous or subcutaneous vitamin K (1 mg) or fresh frozen plasma can be given to normalize it. Although the patient's stay in the hospital may be reduced with this strategy, the response to vitamin K is not predictable, and fresh frozen plasma is associated with the risks of transfusion. For emergency surgery, however, it is the only choice to reverse the effects of warfarin. Intravenous heparin should be restarted about 24 hours after surgery once the risk of active bleeding becomes minimal.[320] Another recommendation is not to restart heparin postoperatively,[148] but this approach may be associated with the danger of thromboembolism in high-risk patients with atrial fibrillation. In those with moderate- or low-risk atrial fibrillation, warfarin treatment can be safely stopped for up to 5 days before major surgery and restarted postoperatively. For minor surgery with minimal likelihood of bleeding (e.g., cataract operations, dental extraction), anticoagulation does not have to be discontinued perioperatively.

The recommendations for patients with prosthetic valves are again based on underlying risk of thromboembolism. It is well known that mechanical mitral valves carry a high annual rate of thromboembolism (17%), whereas the risk in patients with an aortic valve is less than 6%.[320] Thus the recommendations for patients with these valves are similar to those for high-risk and low- to moderate-risk atrial fibrillation, respectively. Acute arterial embolism within 1 month of any planned surgery carries a high risk (15%) of peripheral thromboembolism if the patient does not receive anticoagulant treatment, which reduces the incidence by 66%.[148] Thus it is prudent to avoid elective surgery for 1 month after an arterial embolic event. If surgery cannot be delayed, warfarin should be replaced with intravenous heparin preoperatively. Postoperatively, heparin should be resumed as soon as hemostasis is adequate.[148]

It follows, then, that anticoagulation can be safely discontinued perioperatively if the annual risk of arterial thromboembolism for the patient's specific clinical condition is less than 6%. Conversely, heparin should be administered until and shortly following surgery if the annual rate of arterial thromboembolism exceeds this value.

REFERENCES

1. Parker-Williams J, Vickers R: Major orthopaedic surgery on the leg and thromboembolism, *BMJ* 303:531, 1991 (editorial).
2. Johnson BI: Paradoxical embolism, *J Clin Pathol* 4:316, 1951.
3. Falk V, Walther T, Krankenberg H, et al: Trapped thrombus in a patent foramen ovale, *Thorac Cardiovasc Surg* 45:90, 1997.
4. Butler BD, Hills BA: Transpulmonary passage of venous air emboli, *J Appl Physiol* 59:543, 1985.
5. Bedell EA, Berge KH, Losasso TJ: Paradoxic air embolism during venous air embolism: transesophageal echocardiographic evidence of transpulmonary air passage, *Anesthesiology* 80:947, 1994.
6. Schwartzman DS, Attubato MJ, Feit F: Interatrial septum and its role in systemic embolism, *Anesthesiol Clin North Am* 10:795, 1992.
7. Wilmshurst PT, de Belder MA: Patent foramen ovale in adult life, *Br Heart J* 71:209, 1994.
8. Guggiari M, Lechat PH, Garen-Colonne C, et al: Early detection of patent foramen ovale by two-dimensional contrast echocardiography for prevention of paradoxical air embolism during sitting position, *Anesth Analg* 67:192, 1988.
9. Hausmann D, Mugge A, Daniel WG: Identification of patent foramen ovale permitting paradoxic embolism, *J Am Coll Cardiol* 26:1030, 1995.
10. Lechat P, Mas J, Lascault G, et al: Prevalence of patent foramen ovale in young patients with cerebrovascular accident, *N Engl J Med* 318:1148, 1988.
11. Petty GW, Khandheria BK, Chu C-P, et al: Patent foramen ovale in patients with cerebral infarction. A transesophageal echocardiographic study, *Arch Neurol* 54:819, 1997.
12. Mugge A, Daniel WG, Angermann C, et al: Atrial septal aneurysm in adult patients: a multicenter study using transthoracic and transesophageal echocardiography, *Circulation* 91:2785, 1995.
13. Miller RL, Das S, Anandarangam T, et al: Relation between patent foramen ovale and perfusion abnormalities in acute pulmonary embolism, *Am J Cardiol* 80:377, 1997.
14. Levin AR, Spoch MS: Atrial pressure flow dynamics in atrial septal defect (secundum type), *Circulation* 37:476, 1968.
15. Moorthy SS, Dierdorf SF: Significance of atrial septal aneurysm: report of a case, *J Clin Anesth* 8:595, 1996.
16. Cucchiara RF, Seward JB, Nishimura RA, et al: Identification of patent foramen ovale during sitting position craniotomy by transesophageal echocardiography with positive airway pressure, *Anesthesiology* 63:107, 1985.
17. Papadopoulos G, Brock M, Eyrich K: Intraoperative contrast echocardiography for detection of a patent foramen ovale using a provocation test and ventilation with PEEP respiration, *Anaesthesist* 45:235, 1996.
18. Perkins NAK, Bedford RF: Hemodynamic consequences of PEEP in seated neurological patients: implications for paradoxical air embolism, *Anesth Analg* 63:429, 1984.
19. Pearl RG, Larson P: Hemodynamic effects of positive end-expiratory pressure during continuous venous air embolism in the dog, *Anesthesiology* 64:724, 1986.
20. Zasslow MA, Pearl RG, Larson CP, et al: PEEP does not affect left atrial-right atrial pressure difference in neurosurgical patients, *Anesthesiology* 68:760, 1988.
21. Black S, Cucchiara RF, Nishimura RA, et al: Parameters affecting occurrence of paradoxical air embolism, *Anesthesiology* 71:235, 1989.
22. Albert A, Muller HR, Hetzel A: Optimized transcranial Doppler technique for the diagnosis of cardiac right-to-left shunts, *J Neuroimaging* 7:159, 1997.
23. Devuyst G, Despland PA, Bogousslavsky J, et al: Complementarity of contrast transcranial Doppler and contrast transesophageal echocardiography for the detection of patent foramen ovale in stroke patients, *Eur Neurol* 38:21, 1997.
24. Plotkin IM, Fox JA, Aranki S, et al: Usefulness of transesophageal echocardiography in the diagnosis and surgical management of a paradoxical embolus extending through a patent foramen ovale, *Anesth Analg* 84:1166, 1997 (letter).
25. Zerio C, Canterin FA, Pavan D, et al: Spontaneous closure of a patent foramen ovale and disappearance of impending paradoxical embolism after fibrinolytic therapy in the course of massive pulmonary embolism, *Am J Cardiol* 76:422, 1995.
26. Caes FL, van Belleghem YV, Missault LH, et al: Surgical treatment of impending paradoxical embolism through patent foramen ovale, *Ann Thorac Surg* 59:1559, 1995.
27. Ruchat P, Bogousslavsky J, Hurni M, et al: Systematic surgical closure of patent foramen ovale in selected patients with cerebrovascular events due to paradoxical embolism: early results of a preliminary study, *Eur J Cardiothorac Surg* 11:824, 1997.
28. Bitterman H, Melamed Y: Delayed hyperbaric treatment of air embolism, *Israel J Med Sci* 29:22, 1993.

29. Anderson FA, Wheeler HB: Venous thromboembolism: risk factors and prophylaxis, *Clin Chest Med* 16:235, 1995.

30. Piccioli A, Prandoni P, Goldhaber SZ: Epidemiologic characteristics, management, and outcome of deep venous thrombosis in a tertiary-care hospital: the Brigham and Women's Hospital DVT registry, *Am Heart J* 132:1010, 1996.

31. Collins R, Scrimgeour A, Yusuf S, et al: Reduction in fatal pulmonary embolism and venous thrombosis by perioperative administration of subcutaneous heparin, *N Engl J Med* 318:1162, 1988.

32. Geerts WH, Code KI, Jay RM, et al: A prospective study of venous thromboembolism after major trauma, *N Engl J Med* 331:1601, 1994.

33. Geerts WH, Jay RM, Code KI, et al: A comparison of low-dose heparin with low-molecular-weight heparin as prophylaxis against venous thromboembolism after major trauma, *N Engl J Med* 335:701, 1996.

34. Swann KW, Black PM: Deep vein thrombosis and pulmonary emboli in neurosurgical patients: a review, *J Neurosurg* 61:1055, 1984.

35. Flinn WR, Sandager GP, Silva MB, et al: Prospective surveillance for perioperative venous thrombosis: experience in 2643 patients, *Arch Surg* 131:472, 1996.

36. Fletcher JP, Batiste P: Incidence of deep vein thrombosis following vascular surgery, *Int Angiol* 16:65, 1997.

37. Reilly MK, McCabe CJ, Abbott WM, et al: Deep venous thrombophlebitis following aortoiliac reconstructive surgery, *Arch Surg* 117:1210, 1982.

38. Manji M, Isaac JL, Bion J: Survival from massive intraoperative pulmonary thromboembolism during orthotopic liver transplantation, *Br J Anaesth* 80:685, 1998.

39. Sopher M, Braunfeld M, Shackleton C, et al: Fatal pulmonary embolism during liver transplantation, *Anesthesiology* 87:429, 1997.

40. Bousamra M II, Mewissen MW, Batter J, et al: Pulmonary artery thrombolysis and stenting after a bilateral sequential lung transplantation, *J Heart Lung Transplant* 16:678, 1997.

41. Flordal PA, Bergqvist D, Burmark US, et al: Risk factors for major thromboembolism and bleeding tendency after elective general surgical operations, *Eur J Surg* 162:783, 1996.

42. Kooij JDB, van der Zant FM, van Beek EJR, et al: Pulmonary embolism in deep venous thrombosis of the upper extremity: more often in catheter-related thrombosis, *Neth J Med* 50:238, 1997.

43. Talbott GA, Winters WD, Bratton SL, et al: A prospective study of femoral catheter-related thrombosis in children, *Arch Pediatr Adolesc Med* 149:288, 1995.

44. Parmet JL, Berman AT, Horrow JC, et al: Thromboembolism coincident with tourniquet deflation during total knee arthroplasty, *Lancet* 341:1057, 1993.

45. Curtis JJ, Walls JT, Schmaltz RA, et al: Use of centrifugal pumps for postcardiotomy ventricular failure: technique and anticoagulation, *Ann Thorac Surg* 61:296, 1996.

46. Bick RL, Pegram M: Syndromes of hypercoagulability and thrombosis: a review, *Semin Thromb Hemost* 20:109, 1994.

47. Thomas DP, Roberts HR: Hypercoagulability in venous and arterial thrombosis, *Ann Intern Med* 126:638, 1997.

48. Ridker PM, Hennekens CH, Lindpaintner K, et al: Mutation in the gene coding for coagulation factor V and the risk of myocardial infarction, stroke, and venous thrombosis in apparently healthy men, *N Engl J Med* 332:912, 1995.

49. Jahangiri M, Shore D, Kakkar V, et al: Coagulation factor abnormalities after the Fontan procedure and its modifications, *J Thorac Cardiovasc Surg* 113:989, 1997.

50. Schulman S, Wiman B: Significance of hypofibrinolysis for the risk of recurrence of venous thromboembolism: Duration of Anticoagulation (DURAC) trial study group, *Thromb Haemost* 75:607, 1996.

51. Ridker PM, Hennekens CH, Selhub J, et al: Interrelation of hyperhomocystinemia, factor V Leiden, and risk of future venous thromboembolism, *Circulation* 95:1777, 1997.

52. Mateo J, Oliver A, Borrell M, et al: Laboratory evaluation and clinical characteristics of 2132 consecutive unselected patients with venous thromboembolism: results of Spanish multicentric study on thrombophilia (EMET* Study), *Thromb Haemost* 77:444, 1997.

53. Bertina RM, Reitsma PH, Rosendaal FR, et al: Resistance to activated protein C and factor V Leiden as risk factors for venous thrombosis, *Thromb Haemost* 74:449, 1995.

54. Rosendaal FR: Thrombosis in the young: epidemiology and risk factors. A focus on venous thrombosis, *Thromb Haemost* 78:1, 1997.

55. Timberlake GA, McSwain NE: Thromboembolism as a complication of myocardial contusion: a new capricious syndrome, *J Trauma* 28:535, 1988.

56. Moser KM, Fedullo PF, LitteJohn JK, et al: Frequent asymptomatic pulmonary embolism in patients with deep venous thrombosis, *JAMA* 271:223, 1994.

57. Pacouret G, Alison D, Pottier J-M, et al: Free-floating thrombus and embolic risk in patients with angiographically confirmed proximal deep venous thrombosis, *Arch Intern Med* 157:305, 1997.

58. Hull RD, Hirsh J, Carter CJ, et al: Pulmonary angiography, ventilation lung scanning, and venography for clinically suspected pulmonary embolism with abnormal perfusion lung scan, *Ann Intern Med* 98:891, 1983.

59. Tripolitis AJ, Bodily KC, Blackshear WM Jr, et al: Venous capacitance and outflow in the postoperative patient, *Ann Surg* 190:634, 1979.

60. Warwick D, Martin AG, Glew D, et al: Measurement of femoral vein blood flow during total hip replacement, *J Bone Joint Surg* 76-B:918, 1994.

61. Coleridge-Smith PD, Hasty JH, Scurr JH: Venous stasis and vein lumen changes during surgery, *Br J Surg* 77:1055, 1990.

62. Comerota AJ, Stewart GJ, Alburger PD, et al: Operative venodilation: a previously unsuspected factor in the cause of postoperative deep vein thrombosis, *Surgery* 106:301, 1989.

63. Ruttman TG, James MFM, Viljoen JF: Haemodilution induces a hypercoagulable state, *Br J Anaesth* 76:412, 1996.

64. Gallus AS, Hirsh J, Gent M: Relevance of preoperative and postoperative blood tests to postoperative leg-vein thrombosis, *Lancet* 2:805, 1973.

65. Mansfield AO: Alteration in fibrinolysis associated with surgery and venous thrombosis, *Br J Surg* 59:754, 1972.

66. Wakefield TW, Strieter RM, Prince MR, et al: Pathogenesis of venous thrombosis: a new insight, *Cardiovasc Surg* 5:6, 1997.

67. Dries DJ, Mathru M. Cardiovascular performance in embolism, *Anesthesiol Clin North Am* 10:755, 1992.

68. Layish DT, Tapson VF: Pharmacologic hemodynamic support in massive pulmonary embolism, *Chest* 111:218, 1997.

69. McIntyre KM, Sasahara AA: The hemodynamic response to pulmonary embolism in patients without prior cardiopulmonary disease, *Am J Cardiol* 28:288, 1971.

70. Azarian R, Wartski M, Collignon MA, et al: Lung perfusion scans and hemodynamics in acute and chronic pulmonary embolism, *J Nucl Med* 38:980, 1997.

71. Graham R, Skoog C, Macedo W, et al: Dopamine, dobutamine and phentolamine effects on pulmonary vascular mechanics, *J Appl Physiol* 54:1277, 1983.

72. Ducas J, Prewitt RM: Pathophysiology and therapy of right ventricular dysfunction due to pulmonary embolism, *Cardiovasc Clin* 17:191, 1987.

73. Lualdi JC, Goldhaber SZ: Right ventricular dysfunction after acute pulmonary embolism: pathophysiologic factors, detection, and therapeutic implications, *Am Heart J* 130:1276, 1995.

74. Dantzker DR: Effects of pulmonary embolism on the lung, *Anesthesiol Clin North Am* 10:781, 1992.

75. Stein PD, Goldhaber SZ, Henry JW: Alveolar-arterial oxygen gradient in the assessment of acute pulmonary embolism, *Chest* 107:139, 1995.

76. Breen PH, Mazumdar B, Skinner SC: How does experimental pulmonary embolism decrease CO_2 elimination? *Respir Physiol* 105:217, 1996.

77. D'Angelo E: Lung mechanics and gas exchange in pulmonary embolism, *Haematologica* 82:371, 1997.

78. Delcroix M, Mélot C, Vermeulen F, et al: Hypoxic pulmonary vasoconstriction and gas exchange in acute canine pulmonary embolism, *J Appl Physiol* 80:1240, 1996.

79. Dalen JE, Alpert JS: Natural history of pulmonary embolism, *Prog Cardiovasc Dis* 17:257, 1975.

80. Carson JL, Kelley MA, Duff A, et al: The clinical course of pulmonary embolism, *N Engl J Med* 326:1240, 1992.
81. Prandoni P, Lensing AWA, Prins MR: The natural history of deep-vein thrombosis, *Semin Thromb Hemost* 23:185, 1997.
82. Weinmann EE, Salzman EW: Deep-vein thrombosis, *N Engl J Med* 331:1630, 1994.
83. Heijboer H, Büller HR, Lensing AWA, et al: A comparison of real time compression ultrasonography with impedance plethysmography for the diagnosis of deep-vein thrombosis in symptomatic outpatients, *N Engl J Med* 329:1365, 1993.
84. Wells PS, Lensing AWA, Davidson BL, et al: Accuracy of ultrasound for the diagnosis of deep vein thrombosis in asymptomatic patients after orthopedic surgery, *Ann Intern Med* 122:47, 1995.
85. Douketis JD, Ginsberg JS: Diagnostic problems with venous thromboembolic disease in pregnancy, *Haemostasis* 25:58, 1995.
86. Stein PD, Henry JW: Clinical characteristics of patients with acute pulmonary embolism stratified according to their presenting syndromes, *Chest* 112:974, 1997.
87. Janata-Schwatczek K, Weiss K, Riezinger I, et al: Pulmonary embolism. II Diagnosis and treatment, *Semin Thromb Hemost* 22:33, 1996.
88. Saltzman HA, Alavi A, Greenspan RH: Value of the ventilation/perfusion scan in acute pulmonary embolism: results of the prospective investigation of pulmonary embolism diagnosis, *JAMA* 263:2753, 1990.
89. Ferrari E, Imbert A, Chevalier T, et al: The ECG in pulmonary embolism. Predictive value of negative T waves in precordial leads: 80 case reports, *Chest* 111:537, 1997.
90. Miniati M, Pistolesi M, Marini C, et al: Value of perfusion lung scan in the diagnosis of pulmonary embolism: results of the Prospective Investigative Study of Acute Pulmonary Embolism Diagnosis (PISA-PED), *Am J Respir Crit Care Med* 154:1387, 1996.
91. Perrier A, Bounameaux H, Morabia A, et al: Diagnosis of pulmonary embolism by a decision analysis based strategy including clinical probability, D-dimer and ultrasonography: a management study, *Arch Intern Med* 156:531, 1996.
92. Turkstra F, Kuijer PMM, van Beek EJR, et al: Diagnostic utility of ultrasonography of leg veins in patients suspected of having pulmonary embolism, *Ann Intern Med* 126:775, 1997.
93. Perrier A, Desmarais S, Goehring C, et al: D-dimer testing for suspected pulmonary embolism in outpatients, *Am J Respir Crit Care Med* 156:492, 1997.
94. van Beek EJR, Schenk E, Michel BC, et al: The role of plasma D-dimer concentration in the exclusion of pulmonary embolism, *Br J Haematol* 92:725, 1996.
95. Remy-Jardin MJ, Remy J, Deschildre F, et al: Diagnosis of acute pulmonary embolism with spiral CT: comparison with pulmonary angiography and scintigraphy, *Radiology* 200:699, 1996.
96. Pruszczyk P, Torbicki A, Pacho R, et al: Noninvasive diagnosis of suspected severe pulmonary embolism: transesophageal echocardiography versus spiral CT, *Chest* 112:722, 1997.
97. Pruszczyk P, Torbicki A, Kuch-Wocial A, et al: Transesophageal echocardiography for definitive diagnosis of haemodynamically significant pulmonary embolism, *Eur Heart J* 16:534, 1995.
98. van Der Wouw P, Koster R, Delemarre BJ, et al: Diagnostic accuracy of transesophageal echocardiography during cardiopulmonary resuscitation, *J Am Coll Cardiol* 30:780, 1997.
99. Fisman DN, Malcolm ID, Ward ME: Echocardiographic detection of pulmonary embolism in transit: implications for institution of thrombolytic therapy, *Can J Cardiol* 13:685, 1997.
100. Jardin F, Dubourg O, Bourdarias J-P: Echocardiographic pattern of acute cor pulmonale, *Chest* 111:209, 1997.
101. Wittlich N, Erbel R, Eichler A, et al: Detection of central pulmonary artery thromboemboli by transesophageal echocardiography in patients with severe pulmonary embolism, *J Am Soc Echocardiogr* 5:514, 1992.
102. Kasper W, Geibel A, Tiede N, et al: Die Echocardiographie in der diagnostik der lungenembolie, *Herz* 14:82, 1989.
103. Tapson VF, Davidson CJ, Kisslo KB, et al: Rapid visualization of massive pulmonary emboli utilizing intravascular ultrasound, *Chest* 105:888, 1994.
104. Marti RA, Ricou F, Tassonyi E: Life-threatening pulmonary embolism at induction of anesthesia: utility of transesophageal echocardiography, *Anesthesiology* 81:501, 1994.
105. Stein PD, Goldhaber SZ, Henry JW, et al: Arterial blood gas analysis in the assessment of suspected acute pulmonary embolism, *Chest* 109:78, 1996.
106. Taniguchi S, Irita K, Sakaguchi Y, et al: Arterial to end-tidal CO_2 gradient as an adjunct to unmasking silent pulmonary embolism, *Lancet* 348:1451, 1996 (letter).
107. Breen PH, Mazumdar B, Skinner S: Carbon dioxide elimination measures resolution of experimental pulmonary embolus in dogs, *Anesth Analg* 83:247, 1996.
108. Wilson WC, Frankville DD, Maxwell W, et al: Massive intraoperative pulmonary embolus diagnosed by transesophageal echocardiography, *Anesthesiology* 81:504, 1994.
109. Ansell JE: Imprecision of prothrombin time monitoring of oral anticoagulation, *Am J Clin Pathol* 98:237, 1992.
110. Ts'ao C: The use and limitations of the INR system, *Am J Hematol* 47:21, 1994.
111. Hirsh J, Poller L, Deykin D, et al: Optimal therapeutic range for oral anticoagulants, *Chest* 95(suppl 2):5S, 1989.
112. Silver D, Kapsch DN, Tsoi EK: Heparin induced thrombocytopenia, thrombosis and hemorrhage, *Ann Surg* 198:301, 1983.
113. Chong BH, Ismail F, Cade J, et al: Heparin-induced thrombocytopenia: studies with a new low molecular weight heparinoid, Org 10172, *Blood* 73:592, 1989.
114. Weitz JI: Low-molecular-weight heparins, *N Engl J Med* 337:688, 1997.
115. Horlocker TT, Heit JA: Low molecular weight heparin: biochemistry, pharmacology, perioperative prophylaxis regimens, and guidelines for regional anesthetic management, *Anesth Analg* 85:874, 1997.
116. Hull RD, Raskob GE, Pineo GF, et al: Subcutaneous low-molecular-weight heparin compared with continuous intravenous heparin in the treatment of proximal vein thrombosis, *N Engl J Med* 326:975, 1992.
117. The Columbus Investigators: Low-molecular-weight heparin in the treatment of patients with venous thromboembolism, *N Engl J Med* 337:657, 1997.
118. Hull RD, Raskob GE, Rosenbloom D, et al: Treatment of proximal vein thrombosis with subcutaneous low-molecular-weight heparin vs intravenous heparin: an economic perspective, *Arch Intern Med* 157:289, 1997.
119. Hirsh J, Turpie AG: Use of plasminogen activators in venous thrombosis, *World J Surg* 9:25, 1990.
120. Bullingham A, Strunin L: Prevention of postoperative venous thromboembolism, *Br J Anaesth* 75:622, 1995.
121. Clagett GP, Anderson FA, Heit J, et al: Prevention of venous thromboembolism: American College of Chest Physicians (ACCP) consensus conference on antithrombotic therapy, *Chest* 108:312S, 1995.
122. Agnelli G, Sonaglia F: Prevention of venous thromboembolism in high risk patients, *Haematologica* 82:496, 1997.
123. Verstraete M: Prophylaxis of venous thromboembolism, *BMJ* 314:123, 1997.
124. Kibel AS, Laughlin KR: Pathogenesis and prophylaxis of postoperative thromboembolic disease in urological pelvic surgery, *J Urol* 153:1763, 1995.
125. Christen Y, Wustchert R, Weimer D, et al: Effects of intermittent pneumatic compression on venous hemodynamics and fibrinolytic activity, *Blood Coagul Fibrinolysis* 8:185, 1997.
126. Jacobs DG, Piotrowski JJ, Hoppensteadt DA, et al: Hemodynamic and fibrinolytic consequences of intermittent pneumatic compression, *J Trauma* 40:710, 1996.
127. Salzman EW, Hirsh J: Prevention of venous thromboembolism. In Colman RW, Hirsh J, Marder VJ, et al, eds: *Hemostasis and thrombosis: basic principles and clinical practice,* ed 3, Philadelphia, 1994, JB Lippincott, p 1332.
128. Boulain T, Lanotte R, Legras A, et al: Efficacy of epinephrine therapy in shock complicating pulmonary embolism, *Chest* 104:300, 1993.
129. Jardin F, Genevray B, Brun-Ney D, et al: Dobutamine: a hemodynamic evaluation in pulmonary embolism shock, *Crit Care Med* 13:1009, 1985.
130. Mathru M, Venus B, Smith R, et al: Treatment of low cardiac output complicating acute pulmonary hypertension in normovolemic goats, *Crit Care Med* 14:120, 1986.

131. Spence TH, Newton WD: Pulmonary embolism: improvement in hemodynamic function with amrinone therapy, *South Med J* 82:1267, 1989.

132. Böttiger BW, Motsch J, Dörsam J, et al: Inhaled nitric oxide selectively decreases pulmonary artery pressure and pulmonary vascular resistance following acute massive pulmonary microembolism in piglets, *Chest* 110:1041, 1996.

133. Capellier G, Jacques T, Balvay P, et al: Inhaled nitric oxide in patients with pulmonary embolism, *Intensive Care Med* 23:1089, 1997.

134. Tulleken JE, Zitlstra JG, Evers K, et al: Oxygen desaturation after treatment with inhaled nitric oxide for obstructive shock due to massive pulmonary embolism, *Chest* 112:296, 1997 (letter).

135. Pollak EW, Sparks FC, Barker WF: Pulmonary embolism: an appraisal of therapy in 516 cases, *Arch Surg* 107:66, 1973.

136. Kessler CM: Anticoagulation and thrombolytic therapy, *Chest* 95(suppl):245, 1989.

137. Hirsh J, van Aken WG, Gallus AS, et al: Heparin kinetics in venous thrombosis and pulmonary embolism, *Circulation* 53:691, 1976.

138. Simmoneau G, Sors H, Charbonnier B, et al: A comparison of low-molecular-weight heparin with unfractionated heparin for acute pulmonary embolism, *N Engl J Med* 337:663, 1997.

139. Goldhaber SZ, Haire WD, Feldstein ML, et al: Alteplase versus heparin in acute pulmonary embolism: randomized trial assessing right ventricular function and pulmonary perfusion, *Lancet* 314:507, 1993.

140. Molina JE, Hunter DW, Yedlicka JW, et al: Thrombolytic therapy for postoperative pulmonary embolism, *Am J Surg* 163:375, 1992.

141. Marder VJ, Sherry S: Thrombolytic therapy: current status, *N Engl J Med* 318:1585, 1988.

142. Kanter DS, Mikkola KM, Patel SR, et al: Thrombolytic therapy for pulmonary embolism: frequency of intracranial hemorrhage and associated risk factors, *Chest* 111:1241, 1997.

143. Greenfield LJ, Proctor MC, Williams DM, et al: Long term experience with transvenous catheter pulmonary embolectomy, *J Vasc Surg* 18:450, 1993.

144. Stock KW, Jacob AL, Schnabel KJ, et al: Massive pulmonary embolism: treatment with thrombus fragmentation and local fibrinolysis with recombinant human tissue plasminogen activator, *Cardiovasc Intervent Radiol* 20:364, 1997.

145. Meyer G, Tamisier D, Sors H, et al: Pulmonary embolectomy: a 20-year experience at one center, *Ann Thorac Surg* 51:232, 1991.

146. Rohrer MJ, Scheidler MG, Wheeler HB, et al: Extended indications for placement of an inferior vena cava filter, *J Vasc Surg* 10:44, 1989.

147. Fink JA, Jones BT: The Greenfield filter as the primary means of therapy in venous thromboembolic disease, *Surg Gynecol Obstet* 172:253, 1991.

148. Kearon C, Hirsh J: Management of anticoagulation before and after elective surgery, *N Engl J Med* 336:1506, 1997.

149. Vandermeulen EP, van Aken H, Vermylen J: Anticoagulants and spinal-epidural anesthesia, *Anesth Analg* 79:1165, 1994.

150. Dahlgren N, Tornebrandt K: Neurological complications after anaesthesia: a follow-up of 18,000 spinal and epidural anesthetics performed over three years, *Acta Anaesthesiol Scand* 39:872, 1995.

151. Horlocker TT, Wedel DJ: Spinal and epidural blockade and perioperative low molecular weight heparin: smooth sailing on the Titanic, *Anesth Analg* 86:1153, 1998 (editorial).

152. Rao TL, El-Etr AA: Anticoagulation following placement of epidural and subarachnoid catheters: an evaluation of neurologic sequelae, *Anesthesiology* 55:618, 1981.

153. Ruff RL, Dougherty JH: Complications of lumbar puncture followed by anticoagulation, *Stroke* 12:879, 1981.

154. Horlocker TT, Wedel DJ, Schlichting JL: Postoperative epidural analgesia and oral anticoagulant therapy, *Anesth Analg* 79:89, 1994.

155. Wu CL, Perkins FM: Oral anticoagulant prophylaxis and epidural catheter removal, *Reg Anaesth* 21:517, 1996.

156. Horlocker TT, Wedel DJ, Offord KP: Does preoperative antiplatelet therapy increase the risk of hemorrhagic complications associated with regional anesthesia? *Anesth Analg* 70:631, 1990.

157. Bergqvist D, Lindblad B, Matzch T: Low molecular weight heparin for thromboprophylaxis and epidural/spinal anaesthesia: is there a risk? *Acta Anaesthesiol Scand* 36:605, 1992.

158. Haljamae H: Thromboprophylaxis, coagulation disorders and regional anesthesia, *Acta Anaesthesiol Scand* 40:1024, 1996.

159. Ewalenko P, Brimiouille S, Delcroix M, et al: Comparison of the effects of isoflurane with those of propofol on pulmonary vascular impedance in experimental embolic pulmonary hypertension, *Br J Anaesth* 79:625, 1997.

160. Schulte-Sasse U, Hess W, Tarnow J: Pulmonary vascular responses to nitrous oxide in patients with normal and high pulmonary vascular resistance, *Anesthesiology* 57:9, 1982.

161. Hybels RL: Venous air embolism in head and neck surgery, *Laryngoscope* 90:946, 1980.

162. Lew TWK, Tay DHB, Thomas E: Venous air embolism during cesarean section: more common than previously thought, *Anesth Analg* 77:448, 1993.

163. Younker D, Rodriguez V, Kavanaugh J: Massive air embolism during cesarean section, *Anesthesiology* 65:77, 1986.

164. Mushkat Y, Luxman D, Nachum Z, et al: Gas embolism complicating obstetric or gynecologic procedures, *Eur J Obstet Gynecol* 63:97, 1995.

165. Hebbard PD: Venous embolism of diathermy evolved gases complicating endometrial ablation using glycine irrigant, *Anaesth Intensive Care* 26:112, 1998.

166. Razvi HA, Chin JL, Bhandari R: Fatal air embolism during radical retropubic prostatectomy, *J Urol* 151:433, 1994.

167. Albin MS, Ritter RR, Reinhardt R, et al: Venous air embolism during radical retropubic prostatectomy, *Anesth Analg* 74:151, 1992.

168. Stoney WS, Alford WC, Burrus GR, et al: Air embolism and other accidents using pump oxygenators, *Ann Thorac Surg* 29:336, 1980.

169. Kimura BJ, Chaux GE, Maisel AS: Delayed air embolism simulating pulmonary thromboembolism in the intensive care unit: role of echocardiography, *Crit Care Med* 22:1884, 1994.

170. Bricker MB, Morris WP, Allen SJ, et al: Venous air embolism in patients with pulmonary barotrauma, *Crit Care Med* 22:1692, 1994.

171. Schreuder HWB, van Beem HBH, Veth RPH: Venous gas embolism during cryosurgery for bone tumors, *J Surg Oncol* 60:196, 1995.

172. Souron V, Fletcher D, Goujard E, et al: Venous air embolism during orthotopic liver transplantation in a child, *Can J Anaesth* 44:1187, 1997.

173. Khoury GF, Mann ME, Porot MJ, et al: Air embolism associated with veno-venous bypass during orthotopic liver transplantation, *Anesthesiology* 67:848, 1987.

174. Prager MC, Gregory GA, Ascher NL, et al: Massive venous air embolism during orthotopic liver transplantation, *Anesthesiology* 72:198, 1990.

175. Albin MS, Carroll RG, Maroon JC: Clinical considerations concerning detection of venous air embolism, *Neurosurgery* 3:380, 1978.

176. Veyckemens F, Michel I: Venous gas embolism from an argon coagulator, *Anesthesiology* 85:443, 1996 (letter).

177. Despond O, Fiset P: Oxygen venous embolism after use of hydrogen peroxide during lumbar discectomy, *Can J Anaesth* 44:410, 1997.

178. Sides CA: Pulsed saline lavage causing venous air embolism in a patient with Paget's disease, *Br J Anaesth* 76:330, 1996.

179. Rusheen JM, Hsu D, Lee C, et al: Venous air embolism during surgical manipulation of a femoral cyst, *Anesthesiology* 72:200, 1990.

180. Linden JV, Kaplan HS, Murphy MT: Fatal air embolism due to perioperative blood recovery, *Anesth Analg* 84:422, 1997.

181. Albin MS, Ritter RR, Pruett CE, et al: Venous air embolism during lumbar laminectomy in the prone position, *Anesth Analg* 73:346, 1991.

182. Adornato DC, Gildenberg PL, Ferrario CM, et al: Pathophysiology of intravenous air embolism in dogs, *Anesthesiology* 49:120, 1978.

183. Cucchiara RF, Nugent M, Seward JB, et al: Air embolism in upright neurosurgical patients: detection and localization by two-dimensional echocardiography, *Anesthesiology* 60:353, 1984.

184. Cucchiara RF, Seward JB, Nishimura RA, et al: Identification of patent foramen ovale during sitting position craniotomy by transesophageal echocardiography with positive airway pressure, *Anesthesiology* 63:107, 1985.

185. Schwarz G, Fuchs G, Weihs W, et al: Sitting position for neurosurgery: experience with preoperative contrast echocardiography in 301 patients, *J Neurosurg Anesthesiol* 6:83, 1994.

186. Furuya H, Okumura F: Detection of paradoxical air embolism by transesophageal echocardiography, *Anesthesiology* 60:374 1984.

187. Furuya H, Suzuki T, Okumura F, et al: Detection of air embolism by transesophageal echocardiography, *Anesthesiology* 58:124, 1983.

188. Gottdiener JS, Papademetriou V, Noargiacomo A, et al: Incidence and cardiac effects of systemic venous air embolism: echocardiographic evidence of arterial embolism via noncardiac shunt, *Arch Intern Med* 148:795, 1988.

189. Marquez J, Sladen A, Gendell H, et al: Paradoxical air embolism without an intracardiac septal defect, *J Neurosurg* 55:997, 1981.

190. Tommasino C, Rizzardi R, Beretta L, et al: Cerebral ischemia after venous air embolism in the absence of intracardiac defects, *J Neurosurg Anesth* 8:30, 1996.

191. Thackray NM, Murphy PM, McLean RF, et al: Venous air embolism accompanied by echocardiographic evidence of transpulmonary air passage, *Crit Care Med* 24:359, 1996.

192. Petrozza PH: Preoperative echocardiography and the sitting position, *J Neurosurg Anesth* 6:71, 1994.

193. Palmon SC, Moore LE, Lundberg J, et al: Venous air embolism: a review, *J Clin Anesth* 9:251, 1997.

194. Sprung J, Whalley D, Schoenwald PK, et al: End-tidal nitrogen provides an early warning of slow, ongoing venous air embolism, *Anesthesiology* 85:1203, 1996.

195. Marshall WK, Bedford RF: Use of a pulmonary-artery catheter for detection and treatment of venous air embolism, *Anesthesiology* 55:131, 1980.

196. Kytta J, Tanskanen P, Randell T: Comparison of the effects of controlled ventilation with 100% oxygen, 50% oxygen in nitrogen, and 50% oxygen in nitrous oxide on responses to venous air embolism in pigs, *Br J Anaesth* 77:658, 1996.

197. Lossaso TJ, Muzzi DA, Dietz NM, et al: Fifty percent nitrous oxide does not increase the risk of venous air embolism in neurosurgical patients operated upon in the sitting position, *Anesthesiology* 77:21, 1992.

198. Muravchick S, DeLisser E, Welch F: The use of PEEP to identify the source of cardiopulmonary air embolism, *Anesthesiology* 49:294, 1978.

199. Voorhees RM, Fraser RAR, van Poznak A: Prevention of air embolism with positive end expiratory pressure, *Neurosurgery* 12:503, 1983.

200. Toung T, Ngeow YK, Long DL, et al: Comparison of the effects of positive end-expiratory pressure and jugular venous compression on canine cerebral venous pressure, *Anesthesiology* 61:169, 1984.

201. Black S, Cucchiara RF, Nishimura RA, et al: Parameters affecting occurrence of paradoxical air embolism, *Anesthesiology* 71:235, 1989.

202. Alvaran SB, Toung JK, Graff TE, et al: Venous air embolism: comparative merits of external cardiac massage, intracardiac aspiration, and left lateral decubitus position, *Anesth Analg* 57:166, 1978.

203. Geissler HJ, Allen SJ, Mehlhorn U, et al: Effect of body repositioning after venous air embolism, *Anesthesiology* 86:710, 1997.

204. Mehlhorn U, Burke EJ, Butler BD, et al: Body position does not affect the hemodynamic response to venous air embolism in dogs, *Anesth Analg* 79:734, 1994.

205. Ericsson JA, Gottlieb JD, Sweet RB: Closed-chest cardiac massage in the treatment of air embolism, *N Engl J Med* 270:1353, 1964.

206. Philips J, Keith D, Hulka J, et al: Gynecologic laparoscopy in 1975, *J Reprod Med* 16:105, 1976.

207. Derouin M, Couture P, Boudreault D, et al: Detection of gas embolism by transesophageal echocardiography during laparoscopic cholecystectomy, *Anesth Analg* 82:119, 1996.

208. Rundback J, Shah PM, Wong J, et al: Livedo reticularis, rhabdomyolysis, massive intestinal infarction, and death after carbon dioxide angiography, *J Vasc Surg* 25:337, 1997.

209. Finkiotis G: Hysteroscopy: a review, *Obstet Gynecol Surg* 49:273, 1994.

210. Corson SL, Brooks PG, Soderstrom RM: Gynecologic endoscopic gas embolism, *Fertil Steril* 65:529, 1996.

211. Nishanian EV, Goudsouzian NG: Carbon dioxide embolism during hip arthrography in an infant, *Anesth Analg* 86:299, 1998.

212. Kelly M, Mathews HML, Weir P: Carbon dioxide embolism during laser endometrial ablation, *Anaesthesia* 52:62, 1997.

213. Mann C, Boccara G, Fabre JM, et al: The detection of carbon dioxide embolism during laparoscopy in pigs: a comparison of transesophageal Doppler and end-tidal carbon dioxide monitoring, *Acta Anaesthesiol Scand* 41:281, 1997.

214. Couture P, Boudreault D, Derouin M, et al: Venous carbon dioxide embolism in pigs: an evaluation of end-tidal carbon dioxide, transesophageal echocardiography, pulmonary artery pressure, and precordial auscultation as monitoring modalities, *Anesth Analg* 79:867, 1994.

215. Moskop RJ Jr, Lubarsky DA: Carbon dioxide embolism during laparoscopic cholecystectomy, *South Med J* 87:414, 1994.

216. Weissman A, Kol S, Peretz BA: Gas embolism in obstetrics and gynecology, *J Reprod Med* 41:103, 1996.

217. Sevitt S: The significance and pathology of fat embolism, *Ann Clin Res* 9:173, 1977.

218. Lozman J, Deno C, Feustel PJ, et al: Pulmonary and cardiovascular consequences of immediate fixation or conservative management of long-bone fractures, *Arch Surg* 121:992, 1986.

219. Capan LM, Miller SM, Patel KP: Fat embolism, *Anesthesiol Clin North Am* 11:25, 1993.

220. Orlowski JP, Carmen JJ, Petras RE, et al: The safety of intraosseous infusions: risks of fat and bone marrow emboli to the lungs, *Ann Emerg Med* 18:1062, 1989.

221. Duis HJT, Nijsten MWN, Klasen JH, et al: Fat embolism in patients with isolated fracture of the femoral shaft, *J Trauma* 28:383, 1988.

222. Duncan JAT: Intraoperative collapse or death related to the use of acrylic cement in hip surgery, *Anaesthesia* 44:149, 1989.

223. Needham AP, McLean AS, Stewart DE: Severe cerebral fat embolism, *Anaesth Intensive Care* 24:502, 1996.

224. Fourme T, Vieillard-Baron A, Loubières Y, et al: Early fat embolism after liposuction, *Anesthesiology* 89:782, 1998.

225. Henn-Beilharz A, Hoffmann R, Hempel V, et al: Origin of deemulsified fat in autotransfusion for elective hip surgery, *Anaesthesist* 39:88, 1990.

226. Kitchell CC, Balogh K: Pulmonary lipid emboli in association with long-term hyperalimentation, *Hum Pathol* 17:83, 1986.

227. Haber LM, Hawkins EP, Seilheimer DK, et al: Fat overload syndrome: an autopsy study with evaluation of the coagulopathy, *Am J Clin Pathol* 89:223, 1988.

228. Hagley SR: Fulminant fat embolism syndrome, *Anaesth Intensive Care* 11:162, 1983.

229. Hagley SR, Lee FC, Blumbergs PC: Fat embolism syndrome with total hip replacement, *Med J Aust* 145:541, 1986.

230. Levy D: The fat embolism syndrome, *Clin Orthop* 261:281, 1990.

231. Peltier LF: Fat embolism. III. The toxic properties of neutral fat and free fatty acids, *Surgery* 40:665, 1956.

232. McNamara JJ, Molot M, Dunn R, et al: Lipid metabolism after trauma: role in the pathogenesis of fat embolism, *J Thorac Cardiovasc Surg* 63:968, 1972.

233. Gossling HR, Pellegrini VD Jr: Fat embolism syndrome: a review of the pathophysiology and physiological basis of treatment, *Clin Orthop* 165:68, 1982.

234. Pell ACH, Christie J, Keating JF, et al: The detection of fat embolism by transesophageal echocardiography during reamed intramedullary nailing, *J Bone Joint Surg* 75B:921, 1993.

235. Propst JW, Siegel LC, Schnittger I, et al: Segmental wall motion abnormalities in patients undergoing total hip replacement: correlations with intraoperative events, *Anesth Analg* 77:743, 1993.

236. Christie J, Robinson CM, Pell ACH, et al: Transcardiac echocardiography during invasive intramedullary procedures, *J Bone Joint Surg* 77B:450, 1995.

237. Schemitsch EH, Jain R, Turchin DC, et al: Pulmonary effects of fixation of a fracture with a plate compared with intramedullary nailing, *J Bone Joint Surg* 79A:984, 1997.

238. Jacobs S, Al Thagafi MYA, Biary N, et al: Neurological failure in a patient with fat embolism demonstrating no lung dysfunction, *Intensive Care Med* 22:1461, 1996.

239. Lindeque BG, Schoeman HS, Domisse GF, et al: Fat embolism and the fat embolism syndrome: a double blind therapeutic study, *J Bone Joint Surg* 69A:128, 1986.

240. Chastre J, Fagon JY, Soler P, et al: Bronchoalveolar lavage for rapid diagnosis of the fat embolism syndrome in trauma patients, *Ann Intern Med* 113:583, 1990.

241. Roger N, Xaubet A, Agusti C, et al: Role of bronchoalveolar lavage in the diagnosis of fat embolism syndrome, *Eur Respir J* 8:1275, 1995.

242. Stanley JD, Hanson RR, Hicklin GA, et al: Specificity of bronchoalveolar lavage for the diagnosis of fat embolism syndrome, *Am Surg* 60:537, 1994.

243. Mimoz O, Edouard A, Beydon L, et al: Contribution of bronchoalveolar lavage to the diagnosis of posttraumatic pulmonary fat embolism, *Intensive Care Med* 21:973, 1995.

244. Vedrienne JM, Guillaume C, Gagnieu MC: Bronchoalveolar lavage in trauma patients for fat embolism syndrome, *Chest* 102:1323, 1997.

245. Park HM, Ducret RP, Brindley DC: Pulmonary imaging in fat embolism syndrome, *Clin Nucl Med* 11:521, 1986.

246. Skarzynski JJ, Slavin JD Jr, Spencer RP, et al: Matching ventilation/perfusion images in fat embolization, *Clin Nucl Med* 11:40, 1986.

247. Satoh H, Kurisu K, Ohtani M, et al: Cerebral fat embolism studied by magnetic resonance imaging, transcranial Doppler sonography, and single photon emission computed tomography: case report, *J Trauma* 43:345, 1997.

248. Citerio G, Bianchini E, Beretta L: Magnetic resonance imaging of cerebral fat embolism: a case report, *Intensive Care Med* 21:679, 1995.

249. Bulger EM, Smith DG, Maier RV, et al: Fat embolism syndrome: a 10-year review, *Arch Surg* 132:435, 1997.

250. Gurd AR, Wilson RI: The fat embolism syndrome, *J Bone Joint Surg* 56B:408, 1974.

251. Murray DA, Racz GB: Fat embolism syndrome (respiratory insufficiency syndrome): a rationale for treatment, *J Bone Joint Surg* 56A:1338, 1974.

252. Schonfeld SA, Ploysongsang Y, Di Lisio R, et al: Fat embolism prophylaxis with corticosteroids: a prospective study of high-risk patients, *Ann Intern Med* 99:438, 1983.

253. Svenningsen S, Nesse O, Finsen V, et al: Prevention of fat embolism syndrome in patients with femoral fractures: immediate or delayed operative fixation? *Ann Chir Gynaecol* 76:163, 1987.

254. Behrman SW, Fabian TC, Kudska KA, et al: Improved outcome with femur fractures: early versus delayed fixation, *J Trauma* 30:792, 1990.

255. Seibel R, La Duca J, Hassett JM, et al: Blunt multiple trauma (ISS 36), femur traction, and the pulmonary failure–septic state, *Ann Surg* 202:283, 1985.

256. Pape H, Auf'm'kolk M, Paffrath T, et al: Primary intramedullary femur fixation in multiple trauma patients with associated lung contusion: a cause of posttraumatic ARDS? *J Trauma* 34:540, 1993.

257. Talucci RC, Manning J, Lampard S, et al: Early intramedullary nailing of femoral shaft fractures: a cause of fat embolism syndrome, *Am J Surg* 146:107, 1983.

258. O'Toole DP, Gilroy D, Bali IM: Fulminant fat embolism associated with closed fracture reduction, *Ulster Med J* 55:86, 1986.

259. Byrick RJ: Cement implantation syndrome: a time limited embolic phenomenon, *Can J Anaesth* 44:107, 1997 (editorial).

260. Pietak S, Holmes J, Matthews R, et al: Cardiovascular collapse after femoral prosthesis surgery for acute hip fracture, *Can J Anaesth* 44:198, 1997.

261. Mc Laughlin RE, Di Fazio CA, Hakala M, et al: Blood clearance and acute pulmonary toxicity of methylmethacrylate in dogs after simulated arthroplasty and intravenous injection, *J Bone Joint Surg* 55A:1621, 1973.

262. Murphy P, Edelist G, Byrick RJ, et al: Relationship of fat embolism to hemodynamic and echocardiographic changes during cement arthroplasty, *Can J Anaesth* 44:1293, 1997.

263. Byrick RJ, Bell RS, Kay JC, et al: High-volume, high-pressure pulsatile lavage during cemented arthroplasty, *J Bone Joint Surg* 71A:1331, 1989.

264. Orsini EC, Byrick RJ, Mullen BM, et al: Cardiopulmonary function and pulmonary microemboli during arthroplasty using cemented or non-cemented components, *J Bone Joint Surg* 69A:822, 1987.

265. Ereth MH, Weber JG, Abel MD, et al: Cemented versus noncemented total hip arthroplasty: embolism, hemodynamics, and intrapulmonary shunting, *Mayo Clin Proc* 67:1066, 1992.

266. Patterson BM, Healey JH, Cornell CN, et al: Cardiac arrest during hip arthroplasty with a cemented long-stem component, *J Bone Joint Surg* 73A:271, 1991.

267. Urban MK, Sheppard R, Gordon MA, et al: Right ventricular function during revision total hip arthroplasty, *Anesth Analg* 82:1225, 1996.

268. Byrick RJ, Kay CJ, Mullen JB: Capnography is not as sensitive as pulmonary artery pressure monitoring in detecting marrow embolism, *Anesth Analg* 68:94, 1989.

269. Lafont ND, Kostucki WM, Marchand PH, et al: Embolism detected by transesophageal echocardiography during hip arthroplasty, *Can J Anaesth* 41:850, 1994.

270. Lafont ND, Kalonji MK, Barre J, et al: Clinical features and echocardiography of embolism during cemented hip arthroplasty, *Can J Anaesth* 44:112, 1997.

271. Guest CB, Byrick RJ, Mazer CD, et al: Choice of anaesthetic regimen influences haemodynamic response to cemented arthroplasty, *Can J Anaesth* 42:928, 1995.

272. Koonin LM, Atrash HK, Lawson HW, et al: Maternal mortality surveillance, United States, 1979-1986, *MMWR CDC Surveill Summ* 40:1, 1991.

273. Kaunitz AM, Hughes JM, Grimes DA, et al: Causes of maternal mortality in the United States, *Obstet Gynecol* 65:605, 1985.

274. Choi DMA, Duffy BL: Amniotic fluid embolism, *Anaesth Intensive Care* 23:741, 1995.

275. Clark S, Cotton D, Ganik B, et al: Central hemodynamic alterations in amniotic fluid embolism, *Am J Obstet Gynecol* 158:1124, 1988.

276. Clark SL, Hankins GDV, Dudley DA, et al: Amniotic fluid embolism: analysis of the national registry, *Am J Obstet Gynecol* 172:1158, 1995.

277. Morgan M: Amniotic fluid embolism, *Anaesthesia* 34:20, 1979.

278. Hankins GDV, Snyder RR, Clark SL, et al: Acute hemodynamic and respiratory effects of amniotic fluid embolism in the pregnant goat model, *Am J Obstet Gynecol* 168:1113, 1993.

279. Gillie MH, Hughes SC: Amniotic fluid embolism, *Anesthesiol Clin North Am* 11:55, 1993.

280. Margarson MP: Delayed amniotic fluid embolism following cesarean section under spinal anesthesia, *Anaesthesia* 50:804, 1995.

281. Kuhlman K, Hidvegi D, Tamura RK, et al: Is amniotic fluid material in the central circulation of peripartum patients pathologic? *Am J Perinatol* 2:295, 1985.

282. Girard P, Mal H, Laire J, et al: Left heart failure in amniotic fluid embolism, *Anesthesiology* 64:262, 1986.

283. Dib N, Bajwa T: Amniotic fluid embolism causing severe left ventricular dysfunction and death: case report and review of the literature: catheterization and cardiovascular diagnosis, *Cathet Cardiovasc Diagn* 39:177, 1996.

284. Richards DS, Carter LS, Corke B, et al: The effect of human amniotic fluid on the isolated perfused rat heart, *Am J Obstet Gynecol* 158:210, 1988.

285. Burrows A, Khoo SK: The amniotic fluid embolism syndrome: 10 years experience at a major teaching hospital, *Aust NZ J Obstet Gynaecol* 35:245, 1995.

286. McDougall RJ, Duke GJ: Amniotic fluid embolism syndrome: case report and review, *Anaesth Intensive Care* 23:735, 1995.
287. Lockwood C, Bach R, Guha A: Amniotic fluid contains tissue factor, a potent initiator of coagulation, *Am J Obstet Gynecol* 165:1335, 1991.
288. Noble WH, St-Amand J: Amniotic fluid embolus, *Can J Anaesth* 40:971, 1993.
289. Masson R: Amniotic fluid embolism, *Clin Chest Med* 13:657, 1992.
290. Clark SL, Pavlova Z, Greenspoon J, et al: Squamous cells in the maternal pulmonary circulation, *Am J Obstet Gynecol* 154:104, 1986.
291. Kobayashi H, Ohi H, Terao T: A simple noninvasive, sensitive method for diagnosis of amniotic fluid embolism by monoclonal antibody TKH-2 that recognizes NeuAc alpha 2-6 GalNAc, *Am J Obstet Gynecol* 168:848, 1993.
292. Kanayama N, Yamazaki T, Naruse H, et al: Determining zinc coproporphyrin in maternal plasma: a new method for diagnosing amniotic fluid embolism, *Clin Chem* 38:526, 1992.
293. Kobayashi H, Ooi H, Hayakawa H, et al: Histological diagnosis of amniotic fluid embolism by monoclonal antibody TKH-2 that recognizes NeuAc alpha 2-6 GalNAc epitope, *Hum Pathol* 28:428, 1997.
294. Esposito RA, Grossi EA, Coppa G, et al: Successful treatment of postpartum shock caused by amniotic fluid embolism with cardiopulmonary bypass and pulmonary artery thromboembolectomy, *Am J Obstet Gynecol* 163:572, 1990.
295. Van Heerden PV, Webb SAR, Hee G, et al: Inhaled aerosolized prostacyclin as a selective pulmonary vasodilator for the treatment of severe hypoxaemia, *Anaesth Intensive Care* 24:87, 1996.
296. Winterbaur RH, Elfenbein IB, Ball WC: Incidence and clinical significance of tumor embolization of the lungs, *Am J Med* 45:271, 1968.
297. Schriner RW, Ryu JH, Edwards WD: Microscopic pulmonary tumor embolism causing subacute cor pulmonale: a difficult antemortem diagnosis, *Mayo Clin Proc* 66:143, 1991.
298. Zakowski MF, Edwards RH: Wilm's tumor presenting as sudden death due to tumor embolism, *Arch Pathol Lab Med* 114:605, 1990.
299. Chan CK, Hutcheon MA, Hyland RH, et al: Pulmonary tumor embolism: critical review of clinical, imaging, and hemodynamic features, *J Thorac Imaging* 2:4, 1987.
300. Miller SM: Tumor, infectious, and foreign body emboli, *Anesthesiol Clin North Am* 11:79, 1993.
301. Talley JD, Wenger NK: Atrial myxoma: overview, recognition, and management, *Compr Ther* 13:12, 1987.
302. Howland WS, Goldiner PL: Physiologic management of the cancer patient during surgery, *Curr Probl Cancer* 3:11, 1978.
303. Selvin BLL: Cancer chemotherapy: implications for the anesthesiologist, *Anesth Analg* 60:425, 1981.
304. Griffith GL, Maull KI, Satchatello CR: Septic pulmonary embolism, *Surg Gynecol Obstet* 144:105, 1977.
305. Louria DB: Embolic infections of the lungs. In Baum GL, Wolinsky E, eds: *Textbook of pulmonary diseases,* ed 3, Boston, 1983, Little, Brown, p 501.
306. Kaufman B: Management of septic shock. In Capan LM, Miller SM, Turndorf H, eds: *Trauma: anesthesia and intensive care,* Philadelphia, 1991, JB Lippincott, p 801.
307. Caldwell TB: Infectious diseases. In Katz J, Benumof JL, Kadis LB, eds: *Anesthesia and uncommon diseases,* ed 3, Philadelphia, 1990, WB Saunders, p 698.
308. Grabenwoeger F, Bardach G, Dock W, et al: Percutaneous extraction of centrally embolized foreign bodies: a report of 16 cases, *Br J Radiol* 61:1014, 1988.
309. Lybecker H, Andersen C, Hansen MK: Transvenous removal of intracardiac catheter fragments, *Acta Anaesthesiol Scand* 33:565, 1989.
310. Roye GD, Breazeale EE, Byrnes JPM, et al: Management of catheter emboli, *South Med J* 89:714, 1996.
311. Michelassi F, Pietrabissa A, Ferrari M: Bullet emboli to the systemic and venous circulation, *Surgery* 107:239, 1990.
312. Schurr M, McCord S, Croce M: Paradoxical bullet embolism, *J Trauma* 40:1034, 1996.
313. Massad M, Slim MS: Intravascular missile embolism in childhood, *J Pediatr Surg* 25:1292, 1990.
314. Pelz DM, Lownie SP, Fox AJ, et al: Symptomatic pulmonary complications from liquid acrylate embolization of brain arteriovenous malformations, *Am J Neuroradiol* 16:19, 1995.
315. Siegel H: Human pulmonary pathology associated with narcotic and other addictive drugs, *Hum Pathol* 3:55, 1972.
316. Sylvester PA, Davies AH, Holgate A, et al: The role of thrombolysis in the management of thromboembolic disorders: a four-year review, *Eur J Vasc Endovasc Surg* 9:459, 1995.
317. Hess H, Mietaschk A, von Bilderling P, et al: Peripheral arterial occlusions: local low-dose thrombolytic therapy with recombinant tissue-type plasminogen activator (rt-PA), *Eur J Vasc Endovasc Surg* 12:97, 1996.
318. Saada M, Goarin J-P, Riou B, et al: Systemic gas embolism complicating pulmonary contusion: diagnosis and management using transesophageal echocardiography, *Am J Respir Crit Care Med* 152:812, 1995.
319. Walley VM, Peters HJ, Veinot JP, et al: The clinical and pathologic manifestations of iatrogenically produced mesothelium-rich fragments of operative debris, *Eur J Cardiothorac Surg* 11:328, 1997.
320. Hanson EW, Lowson SM: Atrial fibrillation and thromboembolism, *Anesth Analg* 87:217, 1998.
321. Nacht A: Arterial embolism, *Anesthesiol Clin North Am* 11:103, 1993.
322. Kronzon I, Tunick PA: Atheromatous disease of the thoracic aorta: pathologic and clinical implications, *Ann Intern Med* 126:629, 1997.
323. Valtonen V, Kuikka A, Syrjanen J: Thromboembolic complications in bacteraemic infections, *Eur Heart J* 14(suppl K):20, 1993.
324. Rutherford RB, Flanigan DP, Gupta SK, et al: Suggested standards for reports dealing with lower extremity ischemia, *J Vasc Surg* 4:80, 1986.
325. Neuzil DF, Edwards WH Jr, Mulherin JL, et al: Limb ischemia: surgical therapy in acute arterial occlusion, *Am Surg* 63:270, 1997.
326. Ouriel K, Veith FJ, Sasahara AA: Thrombolysis or peripheral arterial surgery: phase I results, Topas Investigators, *J Vasc Surg* 23:64, 1996.
327. Rutherford RB: Acute limb ischemia: clinical assessment and standards for reporting, *Semin Vasc Surg* 5:4, 1992.
328. Burgess NA, Scriven MW, Lewis MH: An 11-year experience of arterial embolectomy in a district general hospital, *J R Coll Surg Edinb* 39:93, 1994.
329. Blaisdell FW, Steele M, Allen RE: Management of acute lower extremity arterial ischemia due to embolism and thrombosis, *Surgery* 84:822, 1978.
330. Quinones-Baldrich WJ, Saleh S: Acute arterial occlusion. In Moore WS, ed: *Vascular surgery,* Philadelphia, 1991, WB Saunders, p 578.
331. Goldberg M: Systemic reactions to intravascular contrast material, *Anesthesiology* 60:46, 1984.
332. McKinsey JF, Gewertz BL: Acute mesenteric ischemia, *Surg Clin North Am* 77:307, 1997.
333. Kwauk ST, Bartlett JH, Hayes P, et al: Intraarterial fibrinolytic treatment for mesenteric arterial embolus: a case report, *Can J Surg* 39:163, 1996.
334. Demirtas M, Usal A, Birand A, et al: A serious complication of percutaneous mitral valvuloplasty: systemic embolism. How can we decrease it? Case history, *Angiology* 47:285, 1996.
335. Resano F, Goldstein SA, Boyce SW: Thromboembolic complications in a peripartum cardiomyopathy patient supported with the Abiomed BVS-5000 ventricular assist device, *ASAIO J* 42:240, 1996.
336. Duong van Huyen JP, Fornes P, Iliou MC, et al: Fatal coronary embolization following rotational atherectomy, *Histopathology* 29:73, 1996.
337. Gaunt ME, Martin PJ, Smith JL, et al: Clinical relevance of intraoperative embolization detected by transcranial Doppler ultrasonography during carotid endarterectomy: a prospective study of 100 patients, *Br J Surg* 81:1435, 1994.

338. Gaunt ME, Brown L, Hartshorne T, et al: Unstable carotid plaques: preoperative identification and association with intraoperative embolization detected by transcranial Doppler, *Eur J Vasc Endovasc Surg* 11:78, 1996.

339. Thompson MM, Smith J, Ross Naylor A, et al: Microembolization during endovascular and conventional aneurysm repair, *J Vasc Surg* 25:179, 1997.

340. Mitchell SJ, Willcox T, McDougal C, et al: Emboli generation by the Medtronic Maxima hard-shell adult venous reservoir in cardiopulmonary bypass circuits: a preliminary report, *Perfusion* 11:45, 1996.

341. Oka Y, Inoue T, Hong Y, et al: Retained intracardiac air: transesophageal echocardiography for definition of incidence and monitoring removal by improved techniques, *J Thorac Cardiovasc Surg* 91:329, 1986.

342. Hoka S, Okamoto H, Yamaura K, et al: Removal of retained air during cardiac surgery with transechocardiography and capnography, *J Clin Anesth* 9:457, 1997.

343. Murkin JM: The role of CPB management in neurobehavioral outcomes after cardiac surgery, *Ann Thorac Surg* 59:1308, 1995.

344. Roach GW, Kanchuger M, Mangano CM, et al: Adverse cerebral outcomes after coronary bypass surgery, *N Engl J Med* 335:1857, 1996.

345. Okita Y, Takamoto S, Ando M, et al: Predictive factors for postoperative cerebral complications in patients with thoracic aortic aneurysm, *Eur J Cardiothorac Surg* 10:826, 1996.

346. Marschall K, Kanchuger M, Kessler K, et al: Superiority of transesophageal echocardiography in detecting aortic arch atheromatous disease: identification of patients at increased risk of stroke during cardiac surgery, *J Cardiothorac Vasc Anesth* 8:5, 1994.

347. Davila-Roman VG, Phillips KJ, Daily BB, et al: Intraoperative transesophageal echocardiography and epiaortic ultrasound for assessment of atherosclerosis of the thoracic aorta, *J Am Coll Cardiol* 28:942, 1996.

348. O'Dwyer C, Prough DS, Johnston WE: Determinants of cerebral perfusion during cardiopulmonary bypass, *J Cardiothorac Vasc Anesth* 10:54, 1996.

349. Nathan HJ: The management of temperature during hypothermic cardiopulmonary bypass. I. Canadian survey, *Can J Anaesth* 42:669, 1995.

350. Stoddard MF, Dawkins PR, Prince CR, et al: Left atrial appendage thrombus is not uncommon in patients with acute atrial fibrillation and a recent embolic event: a transesophageal echocardiographic study, *J Am Coll Cardiol* 25:452, 1995.

351. Husain AM, Alter M: Transesophageal echocardiography in diagnosing cardioembolic stroke, *Clin Cardiol* 18:705, 1995.

352. Klein AL, Grimm RA, Black IW, et al: Cardioversion guided by transesophageal echocardiography: the ACUTE Pilot Study—a randomized, controlled trial, *Ann Intern Med* 126:200, 1997.

353. Wolf PA, Dawber TR, Thomas HE Jr, et al: Epidemiologic assessment of chronic atrial fibrillation and risk of stroke: the Framingham study, *Neurology* 28:973, 1978.

PART FOUR

Medicolegal Considerations

Chapter 30

Assessment of Anesthetic Risk

John Peder Erickson
Michael F. Roizen

Patients have always wanted to know what may happen to them perioperatively. Now they are demanding to know. They are not interested in statistics, comorbidities, risk adjustment, or whether a perioperative event is caused by anesthesia, surgery, or their medical conditions. They simply want to know what may happen during and after an operation and how likely it is to happen to them. Payors also are demanding to know. Because of this demand, the once dormant field of assessing anesthetic risk has taken on a new and broader perspective.[1] Within the next 5 years, anesthesiologists may be expected to know and to provide information about perioperative risks, not only for their own patients, but also for other patients as well. To provide these data, it is necessary to understand the various methods by which risk is assessed.

Assessment of anesthetic risk was alluded to as early as 1915.[2] Its present popularity derives from its use in cost-containment, quality assurance, and litigation.[3-5] Payors have tried to cut their costs by sending patients to practitioners with better outcomes (and fewer complications), linking payment to quality of care. The result is that hospitals and physicians try to prove to payors that they provide good care, and payors try to deny access or reduce payment for poor outcomes.[6] Similarly, litigation would not proceed without bad outcomes. The patient tries to prove that the bad outcome was caused by poor care; the hospital and physician try to prove that the bad outcome was inevitable because of the severity of the pa-

tient's disease. Even in quality assurance when litigation is not involved, it is necessary to account for the inherently greater risk of a bad outcome for patients in poor health. Of two patients undergoing knee arthroscopy, the 65-year-old with a 90% stenosis of his left main coronary artery will have a greater risk for perioperative myocardial infarction than will a healthy 28-year-old.

There are circumstances unique to anesthesiology that both simplify and make more complex the task of assessing anesthetic risk. Anesthesiologists generally have provided a service with other physicians (surgeons, obstetricians, radiologists) in a limited number of physically similar locations (operating room, recovery room). Recently our practice has expanded to include intensive care units (ICUs), postoperative pain services, pain clinics, and preoperative consultation clinics. Thus at times it is difficult to determine whether a specific outcome was caused by anesthetic factors, surgical factors, or both. Additionally, the causal link between surrogate or perioperative outcomes (such as postoperative nausea or myocardial ischemia) and global outcomes (such as death or myocardial infarction) is unclear.[7]

Lastly, anesthetic risk has a different weight than does surgical risk. The risk of anesthesia is now far less than the risk of almost any operative or nonoperative procedure for which it is administered. It is rare for a patient to refuse anesthesia or for a surgeon to refuse to perform a procedure because of anesthetic risk. Because this is true, anesthetic risk is often thought of as nonexistent.

Relevant literature provides some information needed to assess risk, such as randomized, controlled, prospective studies.[8-10] One typical example is the Coronary Artery Surgery Study, which evaluated perioperative cardiac outcomes after coronary artery bypass surgery.[11] Such studies are useful for determining world records of perioperative results (most good outcomes and fewest bad outcomes) and estimates of specific risks in a small number of circumstances. Because of the large number of variables in clinical medicine, these estimates may or may not be applicable to your patients in seemingly similar circumstances. This issue was demonstrated in a striking fashion in Maine after a series of studies on therapy for benign prostatic hypertrophy. Actual perioperative mortality and rate of reoperation after transurethral resection of the prostate were 3 and 20 times greater, respectively, than expected from review of the urologic literature.[12]

Assessing anesthetic risk for a specific group of patients requires more than the results of available randomized clinical trials. It also requires information about outcomes and risk factors for those specific patients. In this chapter we deal with assessment of risk for your patients, regardless of whether you are an individual anesthesiologist or a member of a group of anesthesiologists or health care organizations with sites where anesthesia is administered.

I. HISTORY OF RISK ASSESSMENT IN ANESTHESIA

As early as 1915 Codman pointed out that in order to improve patient care, hospitals had to determine their results, analyze them to find strengths and weaknesses, compare them with those of other hospitals, and promote members of the medical staff on the basis of the results they achieved with patients (Box 30-1).[1] In 1924 Ward suggested the need to follow results in hospitalized patients.[13]

There were several attempts to identify and in some cases quantify undesirable outcomes related to anesthetic care in the post–World War II years.[14] Unfortunately, measuring outcomes was a field that lay dormant until the late 1960s, when Donabedian presented a framework for the measurement of health care.[15]

But these good beginnings were sidetracked. Eventually peer review and professional standards review organizations (PSROs) were set up by Congress in the 1970s and early 1980s to evaluate health care and to ensure that all providers were meeting minimum standards.[16] From the 1950s, the Joint Commission on Accreditation of Hospitals (JCAH) had always stressed evaluation of the structural variables of health care: staff, buildings, and equipment. Such evaluations resulted in an impressive push to get buildings, equipment, and paperwork in order for scheduled inspections but had less impact on the outcome of care. The JCAH changed its name to the JCAHO (Joint Commission on Accreditation of Healthcare Organizations) in the mid-1980s and since then

---

Box 30-1 Risk assessment timeline

1915	Measurement of results of medical care proposed
1924	Follow-up of hospitalized patients proposed
1950s	JCAHO founded
1960s	Framework for evaluation of health care quality developed
1970s	Professional standards review organizations formed
1980s	Agenda for Change (JCAHO) and Effectiveness in Healthcare Initiative (HCFA)
1986	National Practitioner Database mandated
1988	HCFA released yearly hospital morbidity and mortality data
1990	New York State releases cardiac morbidity and mortality data
1993	HCFA stopped the yearly release of hospital morbidity and mortality data
2000+	How do we use outcome data to improve health care?

JCAHO, Joint Commission for the Accreditation of Healthcare Organizations; *HCFA,* Health Care Financing Administration.

---

has attempted to use outcome measurements to evaluate the patient care provided by the organizations it certifies.[17] In the late 1980s, the Health Care Financing Administration (HCFA) accelerated the process of measuring outcomes by releasing aggregate morbidity and mortality data about Medicare patients.[18] The Health Care Quality Improvement Act of 1986 mandated creation of a national database for problems of licensure and hospital privileges.[19] In 1990, New York State released the first results from the Cardiac Surgery Reporting System.[20] By the end of the decade, every physician was aware of the need to assess risk in medicine; even the lay press carried stories on quality in medicine.[21] Risk assessment had become a politically and economically sensitive topic.

Despite this heightened sensitivity, HCFA stopped publishing hospital morbidity and mortality data in 1993 because of difficulties in risk adjustment and an underwhelming response from the public. The decision was made to release either good data or no data at all. The beneficial changes in the practice of medicine and the feared legal abuses stemming from the release of these data never materialized. It is unclear why release of data by the HCFA was so much more successful conceptually than practically.[22]

II. WHAT IS RISK ASSESSMENT?

Risk is the degree of likelihood that an undesirable event will occur. The field of risk assessment in medicine is broad in scope but as yet insufficiently developed to allow one to assess risk comprehensively. The science of risk assessment crosses many disciplines, including medicine, biology, mathematics, politics, economics, law, psychology, sociology, and philosophy. The use of risk assessment is different for different individuals and organizations. Patients are interested in different risks than are physicians, who in turn make different use of risk assessment than do insurers. Risk assessment itself encompasses three related but dissimilar activities: risk estimation, risk evaluation, and risk management.

A. Risk estimation

Risk estimation involves quantifying risk. The most effective way to do this is to understand the science behind the risk in question. Unfortunately, the scientific basis for individual risks related to anesthesia in particular and medicine in general is not completely understood; if it were, each risk probably would be eliminated. The use of randomized, controlled, prospective data to which the scientific method can be applied is the next best alternative. Thus clinical trials are of great value, despite the difficulty of completing them, for many medical questions. However, clinical outcomes for anesthesiology are difficult to study because of the many variables that affect outcome. Often the available clinical studies are limited by not being controlled for physician, institution, socioeconomic class, or patient comorbidity.

The third best approach is to use data that are retrospective, uncontrolled, and nonrandomized (past experience). These data can be effective as long as their limits are appreciated; predictions cannot be made as reliably as with the results of a controlled, blinded scientific study.[23] On the other hand, this retrospective, epidemiologic approach is used by various tumor registries, and data from a large segment of the world can be analyzed.

Another example of data gathered in this way is found in the Coronary Artery Surgery Registry compiled by the National Heart, Lung and Blood Institute. Data from more than 24,000 patients who had coronary artery bypass surgery between 1974 and 1979 were recorded. From many pieces of information collected for each patient, estimates of the incidence of various perioperative events can be made. Because the number of patients is so large and the time period so long, most physicians should be able to achieve better results than those reported because many improvements in medical care have been made since 1979 (such as cardioplegia and better care in the ICU). Thus one can assume that if adverse events at the hands of a physician are not equal to or less than those reported, that physician's results may be inferior. Two examples of events reported are perioperative myocardial infarction and congestive heart failure, for which incidence can be determined for different preoperative groups (that is, for patients with uncompensated heart failure, unstable angina, or uncontrolled arrhythmias).[11]

Although not so reliably predictive of future risk, experience is useful for predicting risk in the hands of the group from whom the data were drawn. A nonmedical example of the application of this approach to predicting risk is provided by Lloyd's of London. Using accurate records of shipping losses to estimate probabilities of future losses, Lloyd's of London has survived as an insurer for over 300 years. On the other hand, the financial difficulties suffered by Lloyd's in the 1980s illustrate the problems inherent in not having sufficient information. In the 1960s and 1970s, U.S. court decisions held insurers liable for asbestos and other pollution-linked damages, even though when these risks were insured decades earlier, these activities were not only legal, but sanctioned by the U.S. government. Limitations of a retrospective method are that, unlike the results of a scientific study, data can be interpreted in more than one way; retrospective data usually are not as complete as data from randomized, clinical trials, and past data will not help one to assess new risks.

Other methods of quantifying risk are useful in situations in which no or limited data exist, such as nuclear plant meltdowns or the long-term effects of air pollution. In these cases, risk estimation involves extrapolation from current knowledge using mathematical methods to deal with incomplete data. Although these non–data-based methods are much less accurate for prediction than are data-based methods, they are at least usable from a financial point of view because of the law of large numbers; that is, even though the odds of your house burning down in a 100-year period may be almost 100%, the odds of all houses burning down in any single year are much less. Although the law of large numbers is useful for dealing with financial risk, it is of little use to patients for determining what to do next.

B. Risk evaluation

Risk evaluation involves determining whether a patient's risk category and medical condition reduce or increase reported risk rates for adverse outcomes. This process is more subjective than estimation of risk because risk evaluation is highly dependent on circumstances. Risk adjustment is the part of risk evaluation of most interest to anesthesiologists who want to separate bad outcomes caused by patient disease or factors over which no one has control from those caused by poor care.

C. Risk management

Preventing undesirable events, decreasing their severity, and minimizing the damage in the event of their occurrence is called risk management. This aspect of risk assessment is the most important because measuring and evaluating risk are meaningless if nothing is done about the problem.

Despite attempts to base risk assessment on a scientific foundation, political, social, and economic agendas play major roles. Because of these agendas, risk assessment tends to be undertaken with goals that may not always be objective or scientific.[24,25] Payors want to prove care was bad or, more subtly, render a hospital and physicians unable to prove care was good. Similarly, physicians want to prove to regulators and colleagues that they give good care. These powerful biases also must be considered in the process of risk assessment.[26]

III. ESTIMATING ANESTHETIC RISK

Estimating anesthetic risk requires identifying potential risks, determining the relevant ones (for our purposes, those caused by anesthesia), collecting the necessary data, and calculating the estimates.

A. Identifying risks

Identifying risks is the easiest part of estimating risk. Long lists of good and bad perioperative outcomes can be found in books dealing with anesthetic and surgical complications.[8,9] Relevant outcomes sometimes are called indicators. The difficult task is to identify the relevance and significance of any given risk. The JCAHO has spent several years with limited success trying to identify the key indicators that reflect good or poor care in a reliable and robust way.

When informing the patient of potential risk, it is important not to restrict consideration only to risks caused by anesthesia. As of now, all risk is bad; there are no "best" risks or indicators to be guided by in choosing the most desirable anesthesiologist. The absence of serious adverse outcomes is desirable. But is absence of stroke better than absence of death or myocardial infarction? On the other hand, temporary or transient bad outcomes are of less relevance than permanent or severe bad outcomes.

B. Collecting the data

Collecting the data is the most costly part of estimating anesthetic risk because of the time and effort required. The cost is further increased by the tendency to continue collecting data that over time prove to be of little value. Collection continues because it is assumed that all data must have value. The difficulty is reeducating the data collectors and changing the database to eliminate the collection of valueless data. Additionally, the collection of relevant data can easily perturb the risk measures that will be determined. Data collected for one purpose (such as billing) may have unknown biases when the data are used for a completely different purpose (determining risks of bad outcomes). Finally, it is possible that the cost of data collection may be greater than the value of risk assessment obtained (especially if nothing can be done to decrease the risk).

The easiest way to collect data is to get it from someone else who already has it. If the cardiology department keeps track of the incidence of congestive heart failure and myocardial infarctions in your hospital, getting this information may be easier than trying to compile your own list of the patients who had congestive heart failure or infarctions. The next easiest way is to find the randomized clinical trials in the literature that contain the data and draw the appropriate conclusions. The drawbacks of such data have already been discussed. The population may not be the same as your patient population, rendering the conclusions inappropriate for your patients. The experience of the caregivers involved may be different from the experience of those at your institution.

Using billing information is another way to collect information useful for estimating anesthetic risk. Procedure and diagnostic codes (CPT* and ICD-9† codes, respectively), types of monitors used (arterial catheters, transesophageal echocardiography), and medications delivered (nitroglycerin, epinephrine) are examples of information collected for billing from which conclusions may be drawn about outcomes. But these data have several limitations. Because reimbursement for some CPT and ICD-9 codes is greater than for others, systematic errors in favor of the more highly reimbursed procedures may be present. Billing codes can have a moderately high error rate (as much as 10% to 15% for hospital discharge coding) or be unavailable until after the patient is discharged, which may be too late. Even if readily available, billing information may not answer all questions about the risk of anesthesia. This concern was exemplified in a study of carotid endarterectomy, gastrointestinal endoscopy, and coronary angiography; the authors concluded that appropriateness of care could not be predicted from easily available information about patients, physicians, and hospitals.[27] Because bureaucracies that are part of the billing process are comfortable with and well served by coding schemes, physicians must deal with this information in order to be reimbursed for their services. It would be an advantage if anesthesiologists could influence the process so that variables relevant to anesthetic risk, perioperative risk, and risk adjustment were included.[28] One study of outcome after coronary artery bypass graft surgery found that adding only three variables to data already collected accounted for 90% of the difference in mortality between institutions, as opposed to 36% of the difference with risk adjustment by Medicare without these three variables.[29]

Another way of obtaining information on risk is to review insurance records, as was done in the American Society of Anesthesiologists (ASA) Closed Claims Study.[30,31] This method may uncover the cause of risks, but one often does not know the population from which the numbers were drawn (for example, do the participating insurers insure 20% or 80% of the people who give anesthesia in the United States?). The data obtained with this method also are not practical for risk assessment by individual anesthetists for their patients because the data come only from closed malpractice claims and therefore apply to a small, select population. This approach also is very time-consuming. On the other hand, such data are useful for risk management because they allow anesthesiologists to learn from the mistakes of others.

---

*CPT is the five-digit code assigned to procedures performed on patients. The codes are taken from the AMA's *Physician's Current Procedural Terminology,* available in book form and on magnetic tapes from the AMA Order Department, 535 N. Dearborn Street, Chicago, IL 60610.
†ICD-9 is short for ICD-9-CM (International Classification of Diseases, 9th revision, Clinical Modification). These are the six- to eight-character codes assigned to diagnoses of disease as approved by the United States Center for Health Statistics. The codes are available in book form and on disk or tape from Health Care Knowledge Resources, P.O. Box 971, Ann Arbor, MI 48106, and from the American Medical Association. The medical coding division of 3M also has an automated coding package.

Despite the availability of different sources of data for risk assessment, several obstacles stand in the way of using them successfully. Interestingly enough, one of the obstacles is anesthesiologists themselves. Not unique to our specialty are the unwritten medical mores that good doctors do not inquire about the results of the care other doctors give to patients.[32] Pressure against this mentality comes from the fact that peer review is ineffective if peers are shut off from information about each other's outcomes. Moore provided an apt analogy to describe the current system for the regulation of the quality of open-heart surgery:

Imagine a country served by hundreds of small airlines, each of which kept its safety record a tightly held secret. Flight safety was under the total control of the pilots of each airline, and their deliberations and actions, if any, were legally secret in many states. The accepted doctrine was that the pilot is the captain of the ship, and ordinarily is the sole judge of what is safe. About the only way to get rid of an unsafe pilot was through a vote of the pilots of that airline. If a crash occurred, a total news blackout was imposed to maintain public confidence. The airlines varied widely in how thoroughly they investigated crashes, if at all, and the secret inquiries were normally headed by the pilot's closest colleagues.

Large differences in safety records developed among the many airlines. However, the air traveler rarely got access to such information. Even when accident records were occasionally revealed, industry spokesmen insisted that routes, weather, and aircraft were so different that comparisons were meaningless. Other than paying the airfare of all elderly passengers, the federal government had practically no role in airline safety. Most of us would consider this a bizarre and homicidal way to run an airline industry. However, it accurately describes the much riskier business of hospital care for heart patients.[21]

The specter of Big Brother and fears of litigation are quite legitimately raised in defense of this behavior. The release of aggregate Medicare data on mortality and morbidity by the HCFA and the demand by third-party payors to see evidence of quality of care have so far not resulted in the realization of either of these fears.[3] However, the reason these concerns are somewhat moot is less that the issue has been forced by making data public but rather that neither the public nor anyone else can determine how to use the data. It is also interesting to note the range of discussion of outcome-related issues in the free-wheeling forum provided on the Internet. Although plaintiffs' attorneys are aware of these discussion groups and probably have accessed them at times, no instances have emerged in which legal advantage was gained by monitoring these discussions. It is possible that the Internet will provide a venue to conduct peer review that is both globally effective and individually anonymous. Although in the future patients may refuse to go to a physician whose results are not available for audit, at this time a recommendation by another individual or physician carries more weight than numeric data.

Other obstacles to data collection are the huge volume of information and the current impossibility of organizing everything that may be needed at some future time. One way to circumvent these obstacles is to get information periodically about perioperative events that are

---

Box 30-2 Relevant information for analysis of outcomes

Identifying information
  Name
  Medical record number
  Date of procedure
Date and time (time course)
  Occurrence of the outcome
  Discovery of the outcome
  Therapy for the outcome
  Resolution of the outcome
Severity of the outcome
Duration of the problem
Conclusion about the cause and subsequent actions taken

---

fairly common (nausea, perioperative delays). Some outcomes can be recorded automatically, such as the measurements on monitors in the operating room. Others are as readily detected postoperatively as at the time they occur, such as deaths and cardiac arrests, both brought to the attention of other departments in a hospital anyway. Still other events can be detected by postoperative visits, phone calls, or postcards to be returned by patients.[33] Computers have facilitated the storage of large volumes of information, but they still do not resolve the problems of the accuracy of the data collected and how to use the data for risk adjustment.

Whatever collection method is used, complete information is much more useful than incomplete information. One of the advantages of the ASA Closed Claims Study was that a reviewer made a complete summary of the relevant events in each case.[31] Such a summary allows for future reexamination of the data unhampered by incomplete information. Recording and tracking only indicators is of limited usefulness because such information is incomplete. It is important, then, not to store an indicator code alone but to include sufficient information so that what happened can be reconstructed later. Keats suggested a list of the information that should be included for outcome (Box 30-2).[31]

IV. EVALUATING ANESTHETIC RISK

Quantitative evaluation of anesthetic risk is a desirable goal. Use of computerized analysis of billing data is even more desirable.[34] However, it is currently impossible to achieve because our understanding of and information about many perioperative outcomes are incomplete. Even if the information were complete, the evaluation of risk requires that a judgment be made about the significance of any risk. In the past 20 years, this judgment was made by physicians, based almost exclusively on scientific data and often without adequate consideration of the preferences of their patients. The judgment about the significance of any risk depends on the judge, and the patient, physician, payor, hospital administrator, and politician have overlapping but somewhat different views in this regard.

Another difficulty in managing risk is determining with whom or what outcomes and risk adjusters are associated. Do bad results follow the physician from hospital to hospital, or do bad results stay with the hospital even though the physicians and other personnel associated with, but not necessarily the cause of, incidents have left the institution?

Another factor that complicates the issue of risk evaluation is the concept of rescue.[35] Is an institution better or worse than another if it has the same patient survival rate, with a high incidence of poor results during the period of care but an excellent record in treating these poor results? For example, is the risk at two hospitals the same if the survival after a given operation is the same and patient satisfaction is equal, but one hospital has a tenfold greater incidence of postoperative cardiac arrest with all arrests being treated successfully? It seems less desirable to depend on appropriate, timely, and complex interventions to repeatedly rescue patients from complications that may have been prevented. It has also been suggested that the difference between good hospitals or physicians and bad ones is how well they handle problems and how well they prevent them. Theoretically, the effect of rescues should be governed by economics because the cost of a rescue should be greater than the cost of prevention. It is unclear whether this is the case in the real world.

Recently the importance of patient preferences in risk evaluation of medical therapy has been given long overdue attention. Investigators in Maine examined the therapy for benign prostatic hypertrophy over a 4-year period. Although it was not exactly a new discovery, it was observed that patients had a wide range of tolerance for symptoms indicative of prostatic obstruction. In elegant calculations, the investigators showed that the value patients placed on additional years of life determined the level of symptoms they would tolerate before agreeing to undergo surgery.[36] For example, a patient who knows he has a 10% chance of impotence or incontinence after transurethral resection of the prostate may prefer watchful waiting and symptoms of obstruction to these two outcomes if the procedure itself does not prolong life expectancy. In such a situation, accurate data about outcomes are critical because a decision harmful to the patient may be made if risks are understated or benefits overstated.

The Medical Outcomes Study is another investigation that reveals the relationship between patient preferences and outcome. The intent of this observational study of clinicians and patients in Boston, Chicago, and Los Angeles was to determine whether variation in outcomes could be explained by variation in the clinician and the system providing care.[37] The investigators also considered outcomes of the chronically ill beyond medical improvement (e.g., blood pressure reduction), including social functioning, general health perception, and satisfaction with care (e.g., the patient's response to questions such as "Do you feel well?" "Do you look forward to getting out of bed?"). One of the early reports demonstrated significant decrements in measures of these three nonmedical outcomes in patients afflicted with hypertension, diabetes, congestive heart failure, myocardial infarction, angina, arthritis, and chronic lung, gastrointestinal, or back problems.[38] Heart disease and gastrointestinal disorders had the greatest overall impact on outcomes; hypertension had the least. Patients with more than one condition had greater decrements in nonmedical outcomes than those with only one condition. Both of these excellent studies point to the importance of the patient's view in the evaluation of medical risk. We can safely assume that this view pertains to anesthetic risk as well.

A. Risk adjustment

The most popular aspect of research in evaluating anesthetic risk is risk adjustment. Risk adjustment involves correcting outcome data for the effects of coexisting diseases in patients. Outcomes must be adjusted because sicker patients have worse outcomes than healthy patients. Risk adjustment helps in separating bad outcomes unrelated to anesthesia, such as death in a patient brought to the operating room with a gunshot wound that destroyed the midbrain, from outcomes related to anesthesia, such as death from esophageal intubation in a healthy 19-year-old with normal airway anatomy undergoing shoulder arthroscopy.

Unfortunately, risk adjustment can be misused.[39,40] The most common misuse of risk adjustment is to defend bad outcomes: "We do sicker patients." In some cases, the reason for higher rates of bad outcomes may be justified, but not in all. Intentionally or unintentionally, the cause of bad outcomes may be obscured by risk adjustment. The death of a 75-year-old patient during an endotracheal tube change after a procedure for a ruptured abdominal aortic aneurysm can be explained away on the basis of high perioperative risk for that patient. On the other hand, risk adjustment can be used to place blame where the cause is not known. If the same 19-year-old just mentioned dies intraoperatively without a discernible cause, one attributed to anesthesia may be assigned incorrectly.

Attempting to identify in advance patients whose cost of care will be greater is an administrative misuse of risk adjustment, as are attempts to use risk adjustment to predict outcome. Risk indicators are tools to measure outcome and to adjust it for the effects of patient disease, not tools to predict outcome or length of stay. For example, diagnosis-related groups are used by some hospitals as guidelines for discharging their patients. Because payment is not greater for a diagnosis-related group even when costs are greater, some hospitals see the opportunity to increase profitability by discharging patients when insurance ends instead of cutting the costs of delivering care. Encouragement to cut costs for care delivery was the reason for the establishment of diagnosis-related groups.

Risk adjustment methods abound.[14,41-43] The observation that there are many different methods and approaches is the best evidence that a single, best method has yet to be created. Risk adjustment schemes are easy to create but difficult to validate. Their growth has been fueled by the financial rewards and prestige given to those whose plan is officially adopted by organizations such as Medicare or the JCAHO. The caveat in the application of such plans is that there is no single best way to adjust outcomes for multiple preexisting medical conditions, even for outcomes related to an isolated circumstance such as delivery of anesthesia.

On the other hand, adjusters that are applied to a specific situation encompassing a few variables often are successful. Examples are the Apgar score for neonates and the Glasgow coma scale for assessment of the extent of head injury. Both are measurements taken in specific clinical situations. The Apgar score is determined within 5 minutes after birth, and the Glasgow coma scale is used only for patients with acute head injury. Each also measures the function of only a few physiologic systems: the Apgar score for the heart, lungs, and brain, and the Glasgow coma scale for one organ, the injured brain. This narrow scope eliminates the need to determine appropriate weighting of the various measurements used by a given risk adjuster.

Contrast these methods with the popular approach of searching retrospectively for statistically significant associations between outcomes and risk factors. Were numerically significant risk factors the cause of a given outcome or merely associated with it? Causal factors can be weighted equally because, by definition, each potentially caused the outcome. On the other hand, factors merely associated with an outcome have different weights. Consider the risk factors for perioperative myocardial infarction in an emergent coronary artery bypass graft performed on a patient with systemic atherosclerosis. The existence of atherosclerosis systemically may mean that a patient's coronary arteries are also affected but not necessarily that the patient will suffer an infarction perioperatively. An emergency coronary artery bypass procedure performed on a patient suffering infarction is a risk factor directly linked to perioperative myocardial infarction.

There is no evidence that complex risk adjustment methods are more successful than simple ones. One of the simplest unofficial ways to judge risk for mortality of hospitalized patients is to observe whether they walked into the hospital or were carried in. It appears that five to seven risk adjusters provide stratification as effectively as would a larger number of variables.[44] This fact is not surprising because when too many risk adjusters are used, the adjusters become less than completely independent. Note in Table 30-1 how much can be inferred from the small number of risk adjusters displayed. Also, every patient becomes unique, which defeats the purpose of creating generalized categories of risk. (An analogy exists with the rating of mutual funds. With many categories over long time periods, most funds are in the top five in at least one category and time period.)

Although volume appears to have a beneficial effect on outcome, there is also no evidence that volume of data alone provides a greater advantage in risk adjustment. Several databases of hospital outcomes and risk variables have been constructed that include data from millions

Table 30-1. An example of risk stratification with up to nine factors

Factor	Information
Procedure	Repair abdominal aortic aneurysm
Sex	Male
Age	65 Years
Urgency	Urgent, not emergent
Organ function	
Neurologic	Normal
Cardiac	Coronary artery bypass graft (4 years ago)
Vascular	Peripheral vascular disease
Pulmonary	Normal
Renal	Creatinine = 2.1

of patients.[45,46] Currently the users of these large databases do not enjoy a clinical advantage in cost saving and quality of care over their competitors for contracts from payors.

To adjust anesthetic risk in a clinical setting, the most useful factors to consider are age, procedure, diagnosis, and end-organ impairment. It is not so much systemic disease as end-organ damage from disease that affects outcome. The diabetic patient with coronary artery disease is at increased risk for postoperative myocardial infarction because of arterial occlusion, not because of the metabolic derangements of diabetes.[47]

In the next section we review some methods of risk adjustment that are relevant to anesthesiology.[48]

B. Risk adjustment methods

1. Aldrete score. The Aldrete score is used to categorize the postoperative condition of patients in the recovery room.[49] This score has limited usefulness for risk adjustment because the same low numbers can represent widely different clinical conditions and measurement is taken only at a specific time in the perioperative course of events. Given the score, one still must examine the patient's medical record. The Aldrete score is an example of a risk adjustment method restricted to a limited clinical situation.

2. Apgar score. Although not directly applicable to assessing anesthetic risk, the Apgar score is among the oldest risk adjustment systems. Devised by an anesthesiologist in 1953, it provides an effective and reliable method to assess the overall status of newborns. The Apgar score measures a limited part of the spectrum of medical illness. The lesson to be learned from this evaluation method is that risk should be assessed for patients from homogeneous groups with respect to age, end-organ function, and procedure and include parts of the perianesthetic spectrum rather than all of it.[50]

3. American Society of Anesthesiologists assessment of physical status. The ASA assessment of physical status has been in existence for more than 50 years.[51] Although not developed as a tool for risk adjustment, the score does exactly that for 40% to 60% of all anesthetized patients. It is best at separating the perfectly healthy (ASA physical status 1) and the deathly ill (ASA physical status 5) from the rest of the surgical population. It is also fairly good at separating the less than healthy (ASA physical status 2) from the critically ill (ASA physical status 4). It is less accurate for determining risk for patients of ASA physical status 3 because criteria for evaluation are comprehensive and not limited to specific organ failures. A patient with congestive heart failure and coronary artery disease in ASA physical status 3, for example, might be at greater risk for perioperative myocardial infarction than for respiratory arrest. The opposite might be true for a premature infant with an ASA physical status 3.

The designation E (emergency) in the ASA physical status score is even less useful. Patients classified E vary greatly, and perhaps the lack of attention practitioners can give to the other medical problems of emergency patients makes their outcomes appear worse than those of other patients. Categories that would differentiate the following are needed: patients who go directly to the operating room upon arrival at the hospital; patients who have surgery within the hour, 12 hours, or 24 hours; and patients for whom a procedure is delayed one or more days without ill effect. The outcomes of a so-called emergency group that includes both the critically ill and those who have waited as much as a day or two before surgery may appear worse than the outcomes of an otherwise comparable group of patients undergoing elective surgery. This inaccurate pooling may be the basis for support in the literature for effect of emergency status on outcome. Apart from these difficulties with the E category, grouping patients together with respect to their ASA physical status is a simple, moderately sensitive, and moderately specific endeavor.

4. Acute Physiology and Chronic Health Evaluation (APACHE II, III, IV). The acute physiology and chronic health evaluation (APACHE) was developed for an ICU setting by a physician in an anesthesia department.[52] It is based on the assumption that the physiologic measurements obtained in the course of a critically ill patient's stay in an ICU yield an accurate assessment of the severity of that patient's illness. APACHE has been more of a conceptual success to date than a commercial success. It takes 12 measures: heart rate, mean blood pressure, respiratory rate, temperature, Glasgow coma scale, hematocrit, white blood cell count, serum potassium, serum sodium, serum creatinine, arterial pH, and arterial PaO_2. Each measure is then assigned a weight that has been determined empirically. The maximum score is 71, with increasing age counting for up to 6 points and chronic illness or emergency presentation up to 5 points. Higher totals denote more severe illness.

Although the APACHE method of assessment may not be entirely applicable in anesthesia, its organ-based approach probably is the most effective way to handle risk adjustment for anesthetized patients in some situations because many undesirable perioperative outcomes are determined more by impaired organ function than by disease processes. On the other hand, it is of little use in

adjusting for risks related to human error or the malfunctioning of complex systems. For assessment of long-term risk, which tends to be related more to the disease process than to an acute physiologic disorder, the organ-based approach is not so effective.

5. Glasgow coma scale. The Glasgow coma scale is a scoring system to rate the severity of injury to the central nervous system.[53] It is of limited usefulness to anesthesiologists because almost all of our patients are awake and conscious preoperatively and postoperatively. It also illustrates the success of risk adjustment methods that are restricted to a part of the clinical spectrum.

6. Goldman cardiac risk scale. The Goldman cardiac risk scale is a popular method for rating the severity of cardiovascular disease.[54] It has the advantage of being restricted to evaluation of one part of the clinical spectrum: patients with cardiac disease undergoing noncardiac surgery. That the Goldman scale has not become the risk adjuster for perioperative cardiac outcomes is evidence of the difficulty of accurately weighting multiple risk factors with variable degrees of cause-and-effect linkage when creating a multifactorial index for risk adjustment.

7. HealthQuiz. HealthQuiz* has been under development since 1987. It was initially begun as an attempt to automate the process of selecting laboratory tests and to ensure thorough history taking. HealthQuiz was also used to assess perioperative risk with algorithms based on patterns of answers to some of the 134 questions asked by the machine. Patients' responses to some questions are valuable only in conjunction with responses to others, although all the questions are necessary for the algorithm. In statistical terms, these questions influence prediction through high-order interactions, which often go undetected by classic multivariate methods such as logistic regression and discriminant analysis. In the last decade, new multivariate techniques, such as recursive partitioning, have been developed specifically to discover such interactions. These methods are also called classification and regression trees because they provide the predictive capability of multiple regression by direct construction of a decision tree instead of through a linear model.[55]

HealthQuiz has been a tremendously successful concept. Efforts toward development of a commercial product helped contribute to an enormous decrease in the amount of preoperative testing performed in the United States each year. Clinically, HealthQuiz suffers from procedural limitations, such as the time it takes for patients to complete all responses to questions (well over 5 minutes). Some patients are physically, mentally, or psychologically unable to use the device without assistance. Because of these factors, the commercial and clinical uses of HealthQuiz for risk adjustment in anesthesiology have not been as successful as the concept itself.

---

*Dr. Roizen developed this video preoperative health questionnaire at the University of Chicago to help ameliorate the problem of inefficient preoperative assessments and test selection methods. If the product is successful, Dr. Roizen will benefit financially.

8. Judgment. Judgment is used regularly for risk assessment, but as a general method it is unreproducible and unreliable.

9. Classifications of angina by the New York Heart Association and the Canadian Cardiovascular Society. These classifications provide yet another example of the relative success of risk adjusters for limited clinical circumstances.[47]

10. American Society of Anesthesiologists/Vitez severity scale. The ASA/Vitez severity scale for risk adjustment in anesthesia is the first to take into account the severity as well as the course of adverse outcomes.[56] It differentiates events such as death and stroke, which are irreversible or severe, from hypotension and transient hypoxia, which are neither severe nor irreversible. It also separates irreversible events from those that take months to resolve or those of a transient nature. The main drawback to this method is the secrecy that has surrounded the evaluation process so far. Effective evaluation is best served by openness. There is no advantage to having only a few individuals aware of potential problems, something not encouraged in the evaluation of risk. When objective criteria are available for the evaluation process, this method may be excellent for adjusting outcomes so that a unified rating system for outcomes can be used to assess performance.

11. Diagnosis-related groups. Diagnosis-related groups (DRGs) provide the basis for the prospective payment system used by Medicare to determine hospital payments. Although DRGs have been criticized for not classifying patients into homogeneous groups, this deficiency is more a result of inadequacies in the ICD-9-CM coding process than in the DRG plan.[57] DRGs were developed from the best clinical and financial information available at the time. Their use for risk adjustment by anesthetists is limited because DRGs deal with treatment of disease processes rather than end-organ failure. But because DRGs are the basis for hospital reimbursement, we need to be aware of their existence.

12. Quality-adjusted life-years (QALYs). A successful outcome of medical care is more than just cure of a disease. Also important are the cost of the cure and the kind of life a patient will lead afterward. Expensive cures may be clinical successes but therapeutic failures if a patient's quality of life is worse afterward. For several years, economists and decision analysts have tried to incorporate the intangible factors surrounding quality of life into a number that would quantify subjective factors.

One result has been the QALY. The methods used to calculate quality-adjusted life-years are still under development, but the product of the calculation is a number assigned to a therapy that includes both expected outcomes and quality of life. The usefulness of the QALY is its potential to direct society's health care resources toward treatments that result in the greatest improvement for the most people at the lowest cost. The concept is appealing, but ethical problems arise when clinical decisions for individual patients are based on summaries of community opinions that do not consider patients' preferences. The disadvantages of the widespread application of QALYs have been discussed at length elsewhere; that the method includes criteria other than purely medical considerations in its assessment of outcome is an advantage.[58]

13. The Intubation Difficulty Scale. This recently proposed addition to the collection of risk adjustment methods divides the process of intubation into its component parts to facilitate future intubation attempts. It appears to be another example of a successful risk adjustment method directed at a limited segment of the clinical field. However, further testing and evaluation are needed before its true clinical utility can be determined.[59]

The current state of the art of risk adjustment is best summed up by the observation that the Food and Drug Administration would not have approved any risk adjustment method if the method first had to meet the standards of efficacy required for approval of drugs and medical devices.[45]

V. MANAGING ANESTHETIC RISK

What to do about identified risks is the most difficult and important aspect of risk assessment in anesthesiology. This question is complicated further by the fact that the impetus for risk management to date has been almost exclusively financial considerations.[60] Financial motives introduce a bias toward resolving problems with a high cost-benefit potential and away from factors that have a low cost-benefit potential. Enjoyment of life cannot be calculated in dollar value, so efforts may be directed away from solutions that would increase quality of life.

The simplest way to deal with the risk of anesthesia is not to administer an anesthetic. No bad anesthetic outcome is suffered from an anesthetic that is not given. In other areas of medicine, preventing disease is almost always cheaper, faster, and safer than treating the results of disease. Public health measures aim at preventing infectious disease or lessening the risk of coronary artery disease by warning of the added risk for smokers or those with untreated hypertension or high-cholesterol diets. However, our patients usually do not choose anesthesia; rather they decide to undergo procedures for which anesthesia is necessary.

A variation on the idea of not administering anesthesia is limiting the types of patients a specific anesthetist may anesthetize. Either because some patients are too sick for a particular anesthesiologist to handle or because an anesthesiologist has had bad results or no experience with the intended techniques, there may be certain patients and anesthesiologists who should not interact. For example, should anesthesiologist 7 in the Texas heart study, if he or she is unable to improve, be allowed to continue to anesthetize patients with cardiovascular disease?[61] Today, this suggestion may seem outlandish. But if payment becomes linked to outcome, it may suddenly seem fiscally sound and acceptable.

Another approach to managing anesthetic risk is to track selected outcomes across the range of all practitioners and institutions, that is, identify the "bad apples" and stop them from practicing anesthesia. This is the JCAHO approach, and it has the advantage of accumulating much data so that statistical analysis can be applied to the problem. Yet because such identification is performed by an external entity, it creates a counterproductive inspector-inspected relationship.[62] If 90% of anesthesiologists' energies are devoted to impressing an inspector, they will not be used for improving care. When anesthesiologists become adept at performing for inspectors, JCAHO will be forced to expend energy on auditing inspections. The result is an endless escalation of effort to catch or avoid being caught, which siphons resources away from patient care. It is a highly optimistic hope that the "new" concentration on indicators garnered from the efforts of external regulation will lead to improvement in care because this is something that has not happened for the past several decades.

Sanctioning official standards is another approach to risk management.[63-65] Those who use this approach assume that if correct behavior is identified, mandated, and carried out, good outcomes will result. Unfortunately, human behavior is the most difficult factor to change under any circumstances. It is much more effective to change the system so that potential damage from unwanted behaviors is minimized. Also, if standards follow (rather than precede) changes in practice, they may well codify what already happens instead of leading to positive change. Furthermore, if standards are used against physicians or hospitals in court, the whole process will be rendered ineffective. On the other hand, discussions and strong statements about the imposition of standards may have led some hospitals to improve equipment availability, thus allowing a higher quality of care to be delivered. Because of the attention given by the JCAHO and the HCFA to outcomes, more anesthesiologists now take a greater interest in outcomes than they did before.

As was stated in the introduction to this chapter, within 5 years patients and payors may demand to see outcome data. Ironically, when the first edition of this book appeared, we predicted that patients and payors would demand to see outcome data within 5 years. It may be that until patients actually pay for their health care with their own after-tax dollars instead of their employers' pretax dollars, the demand for outcome data may remain limited. After more than a decade of research into risk adjustment, it is apparent that adjusting risks for severity of illness is not simple. It is analogous to prospectively identifying the best mutual fund or predicting the Super Bowl winner. In one case, past performance is no guarantee of future success and in the other instance, endless analysis of seemingly relevant statistics does not guarantee a successful assessment. Yet we look to the past for guidance because we have nowhere else to look. At this time, going to doctors and hospitals with long histories of delivering health care successfully is as good a way as any of getting good care, but there is no perfect way to analyze these histories to assess, predict, or guarantee the quality of that care.

The most important aspect of risk assessment is the effort to correct action in the face of incomplete and imperfect data. Although attempts should be made to collect accurate and complete data, completeness and accuracy are not always possible. Numerous ways to adjust information for severity of illness exist, all useful but none optimal. Simple risk adjustment methods can be as effective as complicated ones for certain groups of patients. Currently the cornerstones of adjustment for anesthetic risk are age, procedure, and end-organ impairment. Patient satisfaction is also being explored, as is the quality of the patient's life. Risk assessment is also an integral part of the focus of disease management and evidence-based medicine.[66] Regardless of what method we use, we must continue to improve the ways we measure how well we take care of patients, we must inform each patient of the risk of having undesirable perianesthetic outcomes, and we must work toward reducing that risk. This is the ultimate clinical utility of risk assessment.

REFERENCES

1. Brook RH, Kamberg CJ, McGlynn EA: Health system reform and quality, *JAMA* 276:476, 1996.
2. Codman EA: *A study in hospital efficiency,* Boston, undated (c. 1916), Thomas Todd Co.
3. Roper WL, Winkenwerder W, Hackbarth GM, et al: Effectiveness in health care: an initiative to evaluate and improve medical practice, *N Engl J Med* 319:1197, 1988.
4. Greenfield S: The state of outcome research: are we on target? *N Engl J Med* 320:1142, 1989.
5. Angell M, Kassirer JP: Quality and the medical marketplace: following the elephants, *N Engl J Med* 335:883, 1996 (editorial).
6. Grumet GW: Health care rationing through inconvenience: the third party's secret weapon, *N Engl J Med* 321:607, 1989.
7. Fisher DM: Surrogate end points: are they meaningful? *Anesthesiology* 81:795, 1994 (editorial).
8. Ross AF, Tinker JH: Anesthesia risk. In Miller RD, ed: *Anesthesia,* ed 3, New York, 1990, Churchill Livingstone.
9. Brown DL, ed: *Risk and outcome in anesthesia,* Philadelphia, 1988, JB Lippincott.
10. Gravenstein N, ed: *Manual of complications during anesthesia,* Philadelphia, 1991, JB Lippincott.
11. Foster ED, Davis KB, Carpenter JA, et al: Risk of noncardiac operation in patients with defined coronary disease: the Coronary Artery Surgery Study (CASS) registry experience, *Ann Thorac Surg* 41:42, 1986.
12. Fisher ES, Wennberg JE: Administrative data in effectiveness studies: the prostatectomy assessment. In Heithoff KA, Lohr KN, eds: *Effectiveness and outcomes in health care,* Washington, DC, 1990, National Academic Press.
13. Ward GG: The value and need of more attention to end-results and follow-up in hospitals today, *Bull Am Coll Surg* 8:29, 1924.
14. Blumberg MS: Risk adjusting health care outcomes: a methodologic review, *Med Care Rev* 43:351, 1986.
15. Donabedian A: *The definition of quality and approaches to its assessment,* Ann Arbor, Mich, 1980, Health Administration Press.
16. Dans PF, Wiener JP, Otter SE: Peer review organizations: promises and potential pitfalls, *N Engl J Med* 313:1131, 1985.
17. *Agenda for change: update* (newsletter), Chicago, 1988, Joint Commission on Accreditation of Healthcare Organizations.
18. Hartz AJ, Krakauer H, Kuhn EM, et al: Hospital characteristics and mortality rates, *N Engl J Med* 321:1720, 1989.
19. Iglehart JK: Health policy report: Congress moves to bolster peer review: the Health Care Quality Improvement Act of 1986, *N Engl J Med* 316:960, 1987.
20. Green J, Wintfeld N: Report cards on cardiac surgeons: assessing New York State's approach, *N Engl J Med* 332:1229, 1995.
21. Moore TJ: *Heart failure: a critical inquiry into American medicine and the revolution in heart care,* New York, 1989, Random House.
22. Voelker R: Why has "historic" public disclosure of hospital performance data attracted so little attention? *JAMA* 273:689, 1995.
23. Bailar JC III: The promise and problems of meta-analysis, *N Engl J Med* 337:559, 1997.

24. Johnston R: The characteristics of risk assessment research. In Conrad J, ed: *Society, technology and risk assessment,* New York, 1980, Academic Press.
25. Mazur A: Societal and scientific causes of the historical development of risk assessment. In Conrad J, ed: *Society, technology and risk assessment,* New York, 1980, Academic Press.
26. Winterfeldt DV: Four theses on the application of risk assessment methods. In Conrad J, ed: *Society, technology and risk assessment,* New York, 1980, Academic Press.
27. Brook RH, Park RE, Chassin MR, et al: Predicting the appropriate use of carotid endarterectomy, upper gastrointestinal endoscopy, and coronary angiography, *N Engl J Med* 323:1173, 1990.
28. Musen MA: The strained quality of medical data, *Methods Inf Med* 28:123, 1989.
29. Pine M, Smith D, Roizen MF, et al: National norms and your surgical mortality rates: how anesthesia records help, *Anesthesiology* 71:A919, 1989 (abstract).
30. Brunner EA: Analysis of anesthetic mishaps: the National Association of Insurance Commissioners' Closed Claims Study, *Int Anesthesiol Clin* 22:17, 1984.
31. Keats AS: The closed claims study, *Anesthesiology* 73:199, 1990 (editorial).
32. Beck WC, Meyer KK: Should surgeons know their colleagues' wound infection rates? *Infect Surg* 6:361, 1988.
33. Cohen MM, Duncan PG: Postoperative follow-up and quality of care, *Semin Anesth* 7:270, 1988.
34. Soumerai SB, Lipton HL: Computer-based drug-utilization review: risk, benefit, or boondoggle? *N Engl J Med* 332:1641, 1995.
35. Silber JH, Williams SV, Krakauer H, et al: Hospital and patient characteristics associated with death after surgery: a study of adverse outcomes and failure to rescue, *Med Care* 30:615, 1992.
36. Barry MJ, Mulley AG Jr, Fowler FJ, et al: Watchful waiting vs immediate transurethral resection for symptomatic prostatism: the importance of patients' preferences, *JAMA* 259:3010, 1988.
37. Tarlov AR, Ware JE Jr, Greenfield S, et al: The medical outcomes study: an application of methods for monitoring the results of medical care, *JAMA* 262:925, 1989.
38. Stewart AL: Functional status and well-being of patients with chronic conditions, results from the Medical Outcomes Study, *JAMA* 262:907, 1989.
39. Perrow C: *Normal accidents: living with high-risk technologies,* New York, 1984, Basic Books.
40. Iezzoni LI: The risks of risk adjustment, *JAMA* 278:1600, 1997.
41. Laupacis A, Sackett DL, Roberts RS: An assessment of clinically useful measures of the consequences of treatment, *N Engl J Med* 318:1728, 1988.
42. Stein RE, Gortmaker SL, Perrin EC, et al: Severity of illness: concepts and measurements, *Lancet* 2:1506, 1987.
43. McMahon LF Jr, Billi JE: Measurement of severity of illness and the Medicare prospective payment system: state of the art and future directions, *J Gen Intern Med* 3:482, 1988.
44. Jones RH, Hannan EL, Hammermeister KE, et al: Identification of preoperative variables needed for risk assessment of short-term mortality after coronary artery bypass graft surgery, *J Am Coll Cardiol* 28:1478, 1996.
45. Jencks SF: Issues in the use of large data bases for effectiveness research. In Heithoff KA, Lohr KN, eds: *Effectiveness and outcomes in health care,* Washington, DC, 1990, National Academic Press.
46. Iezzoni LI, ed: *Risk adjustment for measuring health outcomes,* Chicago, 1994, Health Administration Press.
47. Roizen MF: Anesthetic implications of concurrent diseases. In Miller RD, ed: *Anesthesia,* ed 4, New York, 1994, Churchill Livingstone.
48. Iezzoni LI: Risk adjustment for medical effectiveness research: an overview of conceptual and methodological considerations, *J Investig Med* 43:136, 1995.
49. Aldrete JA, Kroulik D: A postanesthetic recovery score, *Anesth Analg* 49:924, 1970.
50. Apgar V: A proposal for a new method of evaluation of the newborn infant, *Anesth Analg* 32:260, 1953.
51. New classification of physical status, *Anesthesiology* 24:111, 1963.
52. Knaus WA: APACHE II: a severity of disease classification system, *Crit Care Med* 13:818, 1985.
53. Shapiro H, Drummond J: Neurosurgical anesthesia and intracranial hypertension. In Miller RD, ed: *Anesthesia,* ed 3, New York, 1990, Churchill Livingstone.
54. Mangano DT, Goldman L: Preoperative assessment of patients with known or suspected coronary artery disease, *N Engl J Med* 333:1750, 1995.
55. Breiman L: *Classification and regression trees,* Belmont, Calif, 1984, Wadsworth.
56. Vitez TS: A model for quality assurance in anesthesiology, *J Clin Anesth* 2:280, 1990.
57. Mullin RL: Diagnosis-related groups and severity: ICD-9-CM, the real problem, *JAMA* 254:1208, 1985.
58. LaPuma J, Lawlor EF: Quality-adjusted life-years: ethical implications for physicians and policymakers, *JAMA* 263:2917, 1990.
59. Adnet F, Borron SW, Racine SX, et al: The Intubation Difficulty Scale (IDS): proposal and evaluation of a new score characterizing the complexity of endotracheal intubation, *Anesthesiology* 87:1290, 1997.
60. Couch NP, Tilney NL, Rayner AA, et al: The high cost of low-frequency events, *N Engl J Med* 304:634, 1981.
61. Slogoff S, Keats AS: Does perioperative myocardial ischemia lead to postoperative myocardial infarction? *Anesthesiology* 62:107, 1985.
62. Berwick DM: Continuous improvement as an ideal in health care, *N Engl J Med* 320:53, 1989.
63. Eichorn JH: Prevention of intraoperative anesthesia accidents and related severe injury through safety monitoring, *Anesthesiology* 70:572, 1989.
64. Orkin FK: Practice standards: the Midas touch or the emperor's new clothes? *Anesthesiology* 70:567, 1989.
65. Moss E: New Jersey enacts anesthesia standards, *Anesthesia Patient Safety Foundation Newsletter* 4:13, 1989.
66. Ellrodt G, Cook DJ, Lee J, et al: Evidence-based disease management, *JAMA* 278:1687, 1997.

Chapter 31

Current Spectrum of Anesthetic Injury

Karen L. Posner
Frederick W. Cheney

The professional liability crisis of affordability of the mid-1980s focused attention on the issue of patient injury from anesthesia. To improve patient safety, the American Society of Anesthesiologists (ASA) implemented several programs, one of which was the development of a national database of cases of anesthetic injury in the United States. Since 1985 the Committee on Professional Liability has been conducting a study of insurance company closed malpractice claims against anesthesiologists in order to identify major areas of loss and the contribution of substandard care to poor anesthetic outcome. This type of in-depth information about adverse anesthetic outcomes in the United States had not been available previously. The major objective of the Closed Claims Project is the development of strategies to reduce the risk of patient injury.

The ASA Closed Claims Project database is a standardized collection of case summaries of adverse anesthetic outcomes that were retrieved by practicing anesthesiologists from professional liability insurance company closed claims files.[1] As of January 1997, 3791 claims were collected from 35 insurance organizations throughout the United States.

To collect data, one or more anesthesiologists visit each insurance company office to review all files for claims against anesthesiologists. Claims for dental injury are excluded. A standardized data collection instrument is completed and a summary compiled for claims in which there is enough information to reconstruct the sequence of events, nature of the injury, and relationship between the actions of the care providers and the patient injury. Of the claims in the current database, 76% occurred between 1980 and 1990.

It should be recognized that there are major limitations to this sort of analysis. There is no information about the total number of patients at risk and no information about the incidence of an injury. Geographic balance is uncertain because the data obtained depend on which companies agree to participate in the study. Also, there is a selectivity of claims in that only those in which there is enough information in the file to reconstruct the sequence of events and nature of the injury are entered into the database.

However, a great deal of relevant information can still be gained, and as the data emerged, it became obvious they could be used in two major ways. First, broad areas have been identified in which changes in practice were suggested by high-incidence occurrence of a single mishap (such as esophageal intubation) and in which the usefulness of preventive measures such as capnography might be inferred. As the project continued into the 1990s, the data could be used to investigate the effects of such changes in practice. A second major way in which the data can be used is by in-depth study of specific types of injury that occurred without apparent cause. An important example is unexpected cardiac arrest during spinal anesthesia.[2] What follows is a summary of the major findings to date.

I. ADVERSE OUTCOMES AND INJURY
A. Overview

The database is broken down into two broad categories: complications or adverse anesthetic outcomes and damaging events. Damaging events are the specific incidents that lead to adverse outcomes. There are fewer damaging events than adverse outcomes because many complications occur without an apparent damaging event being identified during the perioperative period.

The most common adverse outcomes were death (34%), nerve damage (16%), and patient brain damage

(12%), accounting for nearly two thirds of all claims (Table 31-1). Less common adverse outcomes included airway trauma, emotional distress, eye injury, pneumothorax, newborn injury, headache, and stroke. Other less common outcomes are listed in Table 31-1. Some claims involved multiple complications, and in 2% of claims there was no obvious injury.

The damaging events or specific critical incidents leading to the adverse outcomes were predominantly respiratory, representing 1058, or 28%, of the total claims (Table 31-2). The next most common but by far less frequent damaging events leading to injury were those involving equipment (10%) and those of the cardiovascular system (9%) (see Table 31-2). The most common equipment problems involved anesthesia gas delivery systems, peripheral intravenous lines, and central lines (2% each). Administration of the wrong drug or dose was associated with 3% of claims. In 11% of all claims, no damaging event was noted. Adverse outcomes not usually associated with damaging events include nerve damage, headache, pain during regional anesthesia, awareness, myocardial infarction, and hepatic or renal failure.

B. Adverse respiratory system events and outcomes

Difficulties in management of the respiratory system were the most common cause of injury and also the most common cause of severe injury such as death and brain damage.[3,4] Three mechanisms of injury accounted for the majority of adverse respiratory events and nearly 20% of all claims: inadequate ventilation (289 claims, 8%), difficult tracheal intubation (231 claims, 6%), and esophageal intubation (189 claims, 5%) (Table 31-3). Inadequate ventilation, the most common respiratory mechanism, is a nonspecific incident category in which the patient's lungs were inadequately ventilated or oxygenated but the exact cause was not apparent from the records available. The remaining adverse respiratory events were produced by a variety of low-frequency mechanisms, including airway obstruction, bronchospasm, aspiration, premature and inadvertent extubation, and endobronchial intubation (see Table 31-3). Each of these low-frequency mechanisms represented less than 3% of the overall claims. Problems with anesthesia gas delivery equipment (anesthesia machine, vaporizer, ventilator, breathing circuit, supply tanks and lines, and supplemental O_2 tanks) were less common (2% of all claims) but led to serious injury in most cases.[5]

Death or permanent brain damage occurred in 85% of the respiratory-related claims, compared to only 30% of

Table 31-1. Adverse outcomes (incidence of 2% or greater) in claims reviewed by the American Society of Anesthesiologists Closed Claims Project

Outcome	Number of claims (n = 3791)	Percentage
Death	1277	34
Nerve damage	604	16
Brain damage (patient)	466	12
Airway trauma	239	6
Emotional distress	153	4
Eye damage	135	4
Pneumothorax	134	4
Newborn injury	130	3
Headache	120	3
Stroke	105	3
Aspiration pneumonia	89	2
Back pain	87	2
Awareness	75	2
Burns	71	2
Pain during surgery	66	2
Myocardial infarction	63	2
No obvious injury	90	2

Table 31-2. Damaging events in claims reviewed by the American Society of Anesthesiologists Closed Claims Project

Event	Number of claims (n = 3791)	Percentage
Respiratory system	1058	28
Equipment problems	379	10
Cardiovascular system	345	9
Wrong drug or dose	130	3
No event identified	423	11
Other specific events	399	11
Event of uncertain nature	1057	28

Table 31-3. Adverse respiratory system events in claims reviewed by the American Society of Anesthesiologists Closed Claims Project

Most common respiratory system events	Number of claims	Percentage of 3791
Inadequate ventilation	289	8
Difficult intubation	231	6
Esophageal intubation	189	5
Airway obstruction	91	2
Aspiration	77	2
Premature tracheal extubation	52	1
Bronchospasm	50	1
Unintentional tracheal extubation	42	1
Endobronchial intubation	21	1
Anesthesia gas delivery equipment problems		
Breathing circuit	28	1
Vaporizer	15	0.4
Ventilator	12	0.3
Anesthesia machine	5	0.1
Supply tanks, lines, supplemental O_2 tubing	12	0.3

nonrespiratory claims ($p \leq 0.05$). Death and permanent brain damage occurred in over 90% of the claims for inadequate ventilation and esophageal intubation and in 56% of claims for difficult intubation. In the difficult tracheal intubation category, many claims were for trauma to the airway. Most claims for anesthesia gas delivery equipment problems resulted in death or brain damage (76%).[5]

Claims for esophageal intubation were usually accompanied by detailed descriptions of the events and actions that accompanied this event.[3] Auscultation of breath sounds was documented in 59% of claims for esophageal intubation, although in many of these auscultation led to the erroneous conclusion that the endotracheal tube was located in the trachea when it was actually in the esophagus.[3]

Airway obstruction accounted for only 2% of claims, but most cases (87%) resulted in death or brain damage. Airway obstruction most often involved the upper airway, occurring during general anesthesia.[4] Bronchospasm generally occurred in patients with a history of asthma, chronic obstructive pulmonary disease, or smoking and was most common during induction and intubation during general anesthesia.[4] However, bronchospasm also occurred in many patients without these risk factors, and a number of claims involved regional anesthesia. Death or brain damage was a nearly universal outcome in bronchospasm claims (94%).

Risk factors in claims for aspiration were mask anesthesia, obstetric or emergency surgery, and airway management problems such as difficult or esophageal intubation.[4] The overall rate of claims for aspiration was low (3%) compared to that found in earlier studies,[6] possibly reflecting successful strategies for prevention and treatment of this problem. This is consistent with more recent findings that 64% of patients who aspirate during the perioperative period have no respiratory sequelae.[7]

Airway trauma may occur after difficult tracheal intubation, yet fewer than half of all airway trauma claims cited this mechanism. Most claims for airway trauma followed routine intubation and involved injury to the larynx, pharynx, or esophagus.[4]

Pneumothorax resulting from airway management problems was less common than needle-related pneumothorax, but the outcome in the former cases typically was poor (death or brain damage in two thirds).[4] Pneumothorax related to airway management involved such mechanisms as esophageal or tracheal perforation from airway instrumentation and barotrauma from misuse of anesthesia gas delivery equipment.[4]

The major lessons learned from this analysis were that, of the three major mechanisms of adverse respiratory events, esophageal intubation and inadequate ventilation should be preventable by better monitoring. This finding contributed to the adoption of end-tidal CO_2 monitoring for verification of endotracheal intubation and intraoperative use of pulse oximetry as standards by the ASA. The third major mechanism, difficult tracheal intubation, is less amenable to prevention by better monitoring. To prevent adverse outcomes from difficult tracheal

intubation, the ASA developed a guideline for management of the difficult airway.[8] The effect of pulse oximetry and CO_2 monitoring on liability is discussed later in this chapter. It is still too soon to evaluate the effectiveness of the difficult airway management algorithm in prevention of patient injury.

C. Adverse outcomes associated with obstetric anesthesia

Of the 3791 claims analyzed, 469 (12%) were for cases involving obstetric anesthesia[9] (Table 31-4). Among the obstetric claims, 334 (71%) involved cesarean section and 135 (29%) involved vaginal delivery.

It is surprising that the most common adverse outcome for which a claim was filed was newborn brain damage (91 claims, 19%). Only 41% of these injuries to the newborn were considered by the reviewers to be anesthesia related. In contrast, in 71% of all obstetric claims and 70% of nonobstetric claims anesthesia was considered as playing a major role in the injury. These data point out a possible high liability risk for obstetric anesthesiologists in that they tend to be sued for adverse newborn outcome regardless of whether the outcome was anesthesia related.

Maternal death accounted for nearly the same number of claims (88 claims, 19%) as newborn brain damage (see Table 31-4). The most common damaging events in obstetric claims were inadequate ventilation, difficult tracheal intubation, aspiration, and esophageal intubation (Table 31-5). This finding is consistent with reports that difficulty with tracheal intubation and pulmonary aspiration are the leading causes of anesthetic-related maternal

Table 31-4. Most common adverse outcomes among obstetric anesthesia claims reviewed by the American Society of Anesthesiologists Closed Claims Project

	Claims ($n = 469$)	Regional ($n = 315$)	General ($n = 144$)
Newborn brain damage	91 (19%)	56 (18%)	32 (22%)
Maternal death*	88 (19%)	32 (10%)	56 (39%)
Headache*	66 (14%)	63 (20%)	2 (1%)
Nerve damage	49 (10%)	43 (14%)	5 (3%)
Back pain*	41 (9%)	41 (13%)	0 (0%)
Pain during anesthesia*	39 (8%)	37 (12%)	1 (1%)
Maternal brain damage	35 (7%)	20 (6%)	14 (10%)
Emotional distress	33 (7%)	24 (8%)	9 (6%)
Newborn death	30 (6%)	17 (5%)	10 (7%)

*$p \leq 0.01$ between proportion of obstetric regional and obstetric general claims for this outcome.
The regional ($n = 315$) and general ($n = 144$) anesthesia subsets do not sum to the total ($n = 469$) because of claims with other techniques (no anesthesia, $n = 4$; both general and regional, $n = 3$) or missing data ($n = 3$).

morbidity and mortality.[10-12] Pulmonary aspiration of gastric contents was cited in 6% of the obstetric claims, as compared to only 3% of the nonobstetric claims ($p \leq 0.01$). However, in half the cases aspiration was associated with other problems such as difficult or esophageal intubation. All but two of the obstetric claims involving aspiration occurred in cases in which general anesthesia was used.

The high incidence of headache (see Table 31-4) among the obstetric claims (14% of total obstetric claims) relative to the incidence among nonobstetric claims (1% of total nonobstetric claims) was surprising. It is also surprising that relatively minor injuries such as headache, pain during anesthesia, back pain, and emotional injury combined to make up 31% of the total obstetric claims. This compares to an incidence of these injuries of only 6% in the nonobstetric claims. Claims for pain during cesarean section under regional anesthesia were quite common. Of the 206 claims involving cesarean section under regional anesthesia, 17% were for pain during surgery. It is not clear to what extent this reflects true differences in the frequency of such complications in obstetric patients or other factors, such as unrealistic expectations or general dissatisfaction with the care provided.

Regional anesthesia was used in approximately two thirds (67%) of the obstetric claims. This is in contrast to the nonobstetric claims, in which 76% received general anesthesia and only 17% received regional anesthesia. It is apparent that some damaging events and resultant injuries are much more common with certain anesthetic techniques (see Tables 31-4 and 31-5). Claims for maternal death and respiratory system–related adverse events were significantly more common in cases involving general anesthesia, whereas claims for headache, nerve injury, pain during anesthesia, and back pain were significantly more common in cases in which the primary anesthetic technique was regional anesthesia (see Tables 31-4 and 31-5). Some complications such as newborn brain damage, newborn death, and maternal brain damage were not significantly associated with either regional or general anesthesia (see Table 31-4).

The major lesson learned from analysis of obstetric claims is that in some respects the professional liability risk of obstetric anesthesia differs from that of nonobstetric anesthesia. Although adverse newborn outcome was often judged not to be related to anesthetic care, newborn brain damage was a leading cause of claims against obstetric anesthesiologists. As expected, some damaging events, such as aspiration and convulsions, were more common among the obstetric than the nonobstetric claims. However, not expected was that a great percentage of the obstetric claims were for relatively minor injuries such as headache, back pain, and emotional injury. A thorough discussion with patients before anesthesia concerning the

Table 31-5. Most common damaging events among the obstetric claims reviewed by the American Society of Anesthesiologists Closed Claims Project

	Claims ($n = 469$)	Regional ($n = 315$)	General ($n = 144$)
Respiratory system*	85 (18%)	16 (5%)	68 (47%)
Inadequate ventilation	10 (2%)	6 (2%)	3 (2%)
Difficult tracheal intubation*	32 (7%)	1 (<0.5%)	31 (22%)
Aspiration*	19 (4%)	2 (1%)	17 (12%)
Esophageal intubation	10 (1%)	2 (1%)	8 (6%)
Bronchospasm	7 (1%)	2 (1%)	5 (3%)
Inadequate FIO_2	2 (<0.5%)	1 (<0.5%)	1 (1%)
Airway obstruction	2 (<0.5%)	2 (1%)	0% (0)
Premature extubation	3 (1%)	0 (0%)	3 (2%)
Cardiovascular system	20 (4%)	14 (4%)	5 (3%)
Inappropriate fluid therapy	4 (1%)	3 (1%)	1 (1%)
Excessive blood loss	2 (<0.5%)	0 (0%)	2 (1%)
Intravascular injection of regional anesthesia	5 (1%)	5 (2%)	0 (0%)
Other cardiovascular event	9 (2%)	6 (2%)	2 (1%)
Other Events			
Convulsion†	34 (7%)	29 (9%)	5 (3%)
Equipment problems†	31 (7%)	27 (9%)	4 (3%)
Wrong drug or dose	12 (3%)	6 (2%)	6 (4%)
High regional block*	14 (3%)	14 (4%)	0 (0%)
No event identified	60 (13%)	40 (13%)	18 (13%)

*$p \leq 0.01$ and †$p \leq 0.05$ between proportion of obstetric regional and obstetric general anesthesia claims with this event noted.
The regional ($n = 315$) and general ($n = 144$) anesthesia subsets do not sum to the total ($n = 469$) because of claims with other techniques (no anesthesia, $n = 4$; both general and regional, $n = 3$) or missing data ($n = 3$).

risks of these minor injuries may prevent some of these claims.

D. Nerve injury

Claims for nerve injury were those in which there were clinical, anatomic, or laboratory findings consistent with damage to discrete elements of the spinal cord or peripheral nervous system. Nerve injury occurred in 604 patients, or 16% of the total 3791 claims (see Table 31-1). The distribution of nerve damage claims is shown in Table 31-6. General anesthesia was the primary technique in 58% and regional anesthesia was the primary technique in 38% of the 604 nerve injury claims. Of the 229 regional anesthetics, the most common techniques were subarachnoid block (38%), epidural block (27% lumbar, 4% caudal), and axillary block (15%). No obvious patterns were observed that would indicate an association between nerve injury and surgical procedure. Of the various common surgical positions, the prone and lithotomy positions were associated with claims for nerve damage. The proportion of nerve injury claims associated with the prone position (9%) was nearly twice that of nonnerve injuries (5%, $p \leq 0.01$), and lithotomy (12%) was also more common than in nonnerve injuries (8%, $p \leq 0.05$).

Ulnar neuropathy represented nearly one third of all nerve injuries and was by far the most common single nerve injury for which a claim was filed[13] (see Table 31-6). Claims for ulnar nerve damage differed from those for other nerves in that they were more often filed by males, the mechanism of injury itself was least often apparent in the claim file, and the injury was more likely to have occurred during general anesthesia than during regional anesthesia. Ulnar nerve injury occurred despite padding placed over the affected nerves in about 20% of the claims.[13] Symptoms of ulnar nerve injury first occurred 2 days or later after surgery in approximately 20% of the cases.[13]

The medicolegal review process provided very little insight into the mechanism by which ulnar neuropathy occurs after anesthesia. Despite intensive investigation, the mechanism of ulnar nerve injury was observed in the perioperative period in only 6% of the claims. The occurrence of ulnar nerve injury in the presence of padding over the affected nerve indicates that some mechanism of injury other than those commonly described in the literature may be operative.[13] One subsequent study found preoperative slowing of ulnar nerve conduction in patients with post–median sternotomy ulnar neuropathy.[14] The only substantive information gained from medicolegal review was that 74% of ulnar nerve claims were filed by male patients, as compared to about 40% male incidence for claims for other nerve injuries and for claims not involving nerve damage. These data are in agreement with other studies of perioperative nerve injuries[15-17] and are suggestive of an anatomic predisposition associated with the male body habitus.

Claims for injuries to the brachial plexus and lumbosacral nerve roots were the next most common after claims for ulnar nerve injury (see Table 31-6). Spinal cord injuries and isolated median and radial nerve injuries were much less common, as were injuries to femoral and sciatic nerves. The mechanism of injury was noted in about one fourth of the claims for brachial plexus injury and about one third of the claims for lumbosacral nerve root injury. Anesthetic-related causes of brachial plexus injury included the use of shoulder braces and head-down position, suspension of the patient's arm from a bar, other obvious malpositions, and regional anesthesia technique.[13] Most lumbosacral nerve root injuries having identifiable anesthetic cause (31%) were attributed to the administration of regional anesthesia and included technique-related mechanisms such as paresthesia or pain during placement of spinal or epidural needle or pain during injection of a local anesthetic.

The major lesson learned from analysis of nerve damage claims is that most anesthetic-related nerve injuries seem to occur without identifiable mechanism. Although the mechanism of nerve injury was noted in one quarter to one third of the cases of brachial plexus injury and lumbosacral nerve root injury, most ulnar nerve injuries occurred without any apparent mechanism. This is important not only for injury prevention but also for liability. The unclear mechanism of nerve injuries, especially in the ulnar nerve, may be a liability in itself because it leads to the presumption that the anesthesiologist must have done something wrong if the injury occurred in the perioperative period.[13]

E. Cardiac arrest during spinal anesthesia

During review of claims in the initial stages of the ASA Closed Claims Project, an unusual number of cardiac arrests in young healthy patients during spinal anesthesia that resulted in death or severe neurologic injury were identified.[2] In order to study this phenomenon in depth, the entire claim file was obtained and examined in detail. Fourteen such cases in which all records could be obtained were identified out of the first 900 claims. The patients were young (age 36 ± 15 years) and healthy (8 patients ASA physical status 1; 6 patients ASA physical status 2). Nine procedures were elective and five were

Table 31-6. Claims for nerve injury

Nerve	Number of claims	Percentage of 604
Ulnar	177	29
Brachial plexus	125	21
Lumbosacral nerve root	86	14
Spinal cord	64	11
Sciatic	31	5
Median	25	4
Radial	16	3
Femoral	14	2
Multiple nerves*	19	3
Other nerves*	47	8

*Includes phrenic, pudendal, perineal, seventh cranial, suprascapular, optic, and unspecified other nerves, each with a frequency of less than 1%.

emergencies. The sites of surgery were pelvic (8 cases), lower abdominal (2 cases), rectal (2 cases), and lower extremity (2 cases). Monitoring included blood pressure cuff in all cases, an electrocardiogram in 13, and a precordial stethoscope in 6 cases. Seven patients were sedated to the point of no spontaneous verbalization and 5 patients were verbalizing up to the time of arrest. In the sedated patients the doses of opioids and hypnotics were well within customary ranges. Six patients were receiving nasal oxygen before the arrest.

The major conclusions that can be reached from an in-depth analysis of these cases and subsequent reports[18-22] of cardiac arrest during spinal and epidural anesthesia are that the phenomenon occurs suddenly and appears to be circulatory in origin. The initial hypothesis was that the patients were oversedated, and such a condition led to hypoventilation with subsequent cardiac arrest from hypoxemia. Because half of the patients were verbalizing at the time of arrest and 40% were receiving nasal oxygen, it seemed unlikely that hypoxemia was the cause of cardiac arrest in all 14 patients.[2]

Subsequently reported cases with SpO_2 monitoring indicate good oxygen saturation immediately before sudden bradycardia and asystole.[18-22] Many of the patients were conversing when bradycardia and asystole occurred, and ECG readings support the sudden nature of this phenomenon. All patients were resuscitated without sequelae. It should be pointed out that these reported cases represent good outcomes, whereas the closed claims cases represent poor outcomes. The most likely mechanism of the asystole is sudden vagal predominance in the presence of high sympathetic blockade, which blocked the cardioaccelerator fibers. This is supported by a recent report[23] that describes sudden bradycardia and hypotension in three ASA 1 patients with blocks at the T4 to T6 level. The sudden bradycardia and hypotension were associated with an increase in vagal tone, as evidenced by measurements of spontaneous baroreflex activity.[23]

What factors led to the poor outcomes? First was disbelief of the caregiver that the heart rate could slow so rapidly. In many cases confirmatory diagnostic activity such as attempts to cycle the automatic blood pressure machine preceded pharmacologic treatment of the arrest. By the time atropine or ephedrine was administered intravenously there was no effective cardiac action to circulate the drugs. Sedation often delayed the diagnosis because the signs and symptoms of cerebral ischemia were obscured. Another factor leading to poor outcome was inadequate circulation to the brain and heart, engendered by closed-chest massage in the presence of the α-adrenergic receptor blockade induced by spinal anesthesia. Epinephrine usually was necessary before the return of a spontaneous heartbeat. Experimental study of dogs[24] has shown that spinal anesthesia decreases coronary perfusion pressure, reducing the efficacy of cardiopulmonary resuscitation (CPR). Epinephrine administration increases coronary perfusion pressure during CPR.[24]

The lesson learned from these cases is that sudden bradycardia and asystole do occur with spinal and epidural anesthesia in healthy patients. Early treatment of bradycardia with epinephrine should be carried out especially if conventional doses of atropine and ephedrine are not effective. If asystole occurs, a full resuscitation dose of epinephrine should be administered immediately upon recognition of the arrest in order to reverse the α-blockade and direct perfusion to the heart and brain. Prophylactic treatment of heart rates under 60 with vagolytic agents in patients with a high spinal level may be an effective preventive strategy.

II. TRENDS IN ANESTHETIC INJURY OVER TIME
A. Decline in death, brain damage, and respiratory events

Longitudinal study of anesthesia claims over the course of the Closed Claims Project suggests significant changes in patterns of patient injury as well as the causes of such injury.[25] Claims for death and brain damage have declined from representing 56% of all claims in the late 1970s to only 33% in the early 1990s ($p \le 0.05$, Fig. 31-1).[26] Adverse respiratory events have also decreased, from 35% of claims in the late 1970s to only 17% in the 1990s ($p \le 0.05$). As a cause of death and brain damage, respiratory events have declined from 56% in the 1970s to 38% in the 1990s. The most dramatic decrease involved claims for inadequate ventilation, which accounted for 22% of all death and brain damage claims in the 1970s but only 7% in the 1990s.[26] Cardiovascular causes of death and brain damage have increased from 14% to 22% over the same time period. Claims for nerve injury have remained nearly constant.

B. Pulse oximetry and end-tidal CO_2 monitoring in anesthetic injury

As of January 1, 1990, use of pulse oximetry (SpO_2) became an ASA standard for intraoperative monitoring. One year later, end-tidal CO_2 ($ETCO_2$) monitoring became a standard for verification of correct endotracheal tube placement. These standards were adopted with the expectation that they would improve patient safety. Because these monitoring devices first came into clinical use in the middle to late 1980s, the ASA Closed Claims database now contains claims in which SpO_2 or $ETCO_2$ monitoring was in use intraoperatively. Analysis of 1836 claims in which the adverse event occurred during the intraoperative period under general anesthesia provides some insight into the nature of the role of these monitors in patient outcome.

Among the 1836 intraoperative general anesthesia events leading to claims, there were 155 claims (8%) in which SpO_2 monitoring was used, 181 (10%) in which both SpO_2 and $ETCO_2$ were used, and 1471 (80%) in which neither was used intraoperatively. Respiratory system events were less commonly cited in claims with SpO_2 or $ETCO_2$ monitoring than in claims in which neither monitor was used (Fig. 31-2).[25] In contrast, events related to the cardiovascular system were more common in claims with SpO_2 or $ETCO_2$ monitoring than in claims with neither monitor in use (see Fig. 31-2).[25] This may

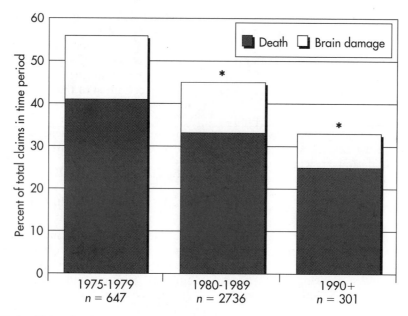

Fig. 31-1. Claims for death and brain damage as a proportion of all claims in the American Society of Anesthesiologists Closed Claims Project database. The proportion of death and brain damage claims has decreased in the 1980s and 1990s compared with 1975 to 1979. *$p < 0.05$ compared with 1975 to 1979. (From Cheney FW: *ASA Newsletter* 61:18, 1997.)

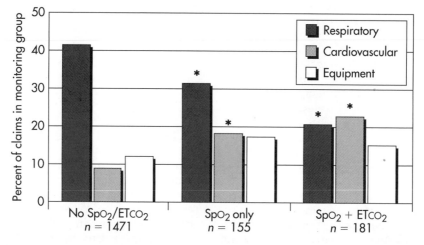

Fig. 31-2. Percentage of claims in each monitoring group that involved respiratory, cardiovascular, and equipment-related events. Only intraoperative general anesthesia claims were included. *$p < 0.05$ compared to the no-SpO_2/$ETCO_2$ group. (Modified from Cheney FW: *ASA Newsletter* 60:10, 1996.)

be a result of improved diagnosis of the mechanism of injury with SpO_2 or $ETCO_2$ data rather than a trend toward different causes of injury. The outcome in claims with SpO_2 or $ETCO_2$ monitoring was better than in claims with neither monitor in use: 45% death or brain damage in claims with SpO_2 or $ETCO_2$ monitoring and 58% in claims without.

Claims for respiratory events with SpO_2 or $ETCO_2$ monitoring in place were analyzed for factors leading to patient injury in spite of these monitors. There were cases of alarms switched off or disregarded. In some cases, monitor readings were misinterpreted as machine problems, delaying proper diagnosis. For example, esophageal intubations were not detected when $ETCO_2$ readings of zero were interpreted as machine failure or the monitor was ignored. Hypoxemia went undetected despite SpO_2 monitoring when the anesthesiologist focused on adjusting the probe, ignoring the patient's increasing cyanosis. Finally, there were multiple cases in which the pulse oximeter was in use during surgery but the damaging event occurred after its use was discontinued, either during transport or in the postanesthesia care unit.

III. SUMMARY

A review of 3791 anesthesia-related closed malpractice claims, most of which occurred between 1978 and 1990, revealed that the most common adverse outcomes were death (34% of claims), nerve damage (16% of claims), and brain damage (12% of claims). The leading causes of death and brain damage were respiratory in origin. Of the three leading respiratory damaging events, the incidence of adverse outcome from inadequate ventilation and esophageal intubation seems to be on the decline with the use of pulse oximetry and $ETCO_2$ monitoring. A strategy for the prevention of nerve injury was not apparent from this review, and more investigation into the pathophysiology of perioperative nerve injury is needed.

REFERENCES

1. Cheney FW, Posner K, Caplan RA, et al: Standard of care and anesthesia liability, *JAMA* 261:1599, 1989.
2. Caplan RA, Ward RJ, Posner K, et al: Unexpected cardiac arrest during spinal anesthesia: a closed claims analysis of predisposing factors, *Anesthesiology* 68:5, 1988.
3. Caplan RA, Posner KL, Ward RJ, et al: Adverse respiratory events in anesthesia: a closed claims analysis, *Anesthesiology* 72:828, 1990.
4. Cheney FW, Posner KL, Caplan RA: Adverse respiratory events infrequently leading to malpractice suits: a closed claims analysis, *Anesthesiology* 75:932, 1991.
5. Caplan RA, Vistica MF, Posner KL, et al: Adverse anesthetic outcomes arising from gas delivery equipment: a closed claims analysis, *Anesthesiology* 87:741, 1997.
6. Tiret L, Desmonts JM, Hatton F, et al: Complications associated with anaesthesia: a prospective survey in France, *Can Anaesth Soc J* 33:336, 1986.
7. Warner MA, Warner ME, Weber JG: Clinical significance of pulmonary aspiration during the perioperative period, *Anesthesiology* 78:56, 1993.
8. Caplan RA, Benumof JL, Berry FA, et al: Practice guidelines for management of the difficult airway: a report by the American Society of Anesthesiologists Task Force on Management of the Difficult Airway, *Anesthesiology* 78:597, 1993.
9. Chadwick HS, Posner K, Caplan RA, et al: A comparison of obstetric and nonobstetric anesthesia malpractice claims, *Anesthesiology* 74:242, 1991.
10. Hughes EC, Cochrane NE, Czyz PL: Maternal mortality study 1970-1975, *N Y State J Med* 76:2206, 1976.
11. Turnbull AC, Tindall VR, Robson G, et al: *Report on confidential enquiries into maternal deaths in England and Wales 1979-1981*, London, 1986, Her Majesty's Stationery Office.
12. Turnbull A, Tindall VR, Beard RW, et al: *Report on confidential enquiries into maternal deaths in England and Wales 1982-1984*, London, 1989, Her Majesty's Stationery Office.
13. Kroll DA, Caplan RA, Posner K, et al: Nerve injury associated with anesthesia, *Anesthesiology* 73:202, 1990.
14. Casscells CD, Lindsey RW, Ebersole J, et al: Ulnar neuropathy after median sternotomy, *Clin Orthop* 291:259, 1993.
15. Cameron MGP, Stewart OJ: Ulnar nerve injury associated with anaesthesia, *Can Anaesth Soc J* 22:253, 1975.
16. Dawson DM, Krarup C: Perioperative nerve lesions, *Arch Neurol* 46:1355, 1989.
17. Warner MA, Warner ME, Martin JT: Ulnar neuropathy. Incidence, outcome, and risk factors in sedated or anesthetized patients, *Anesthesiology* 81:1332, 1994.
18. Frerichs RL, Campbell J, Bassell GM: Psychogenic cardiac arrest during extensive sympathetic blockade, *Anesthesiology* 68:943, 1988.
19. Chester WL: Spinal anesthesia, complete heart block, and the precordial chest thump: an unusual complication and a unique resuscitation, *Anesthesiology* 64:600, 1988.
20. Gibbons JJ, Ditto FF III: Sudden asystole after spinal anesthesia treated with the "pacing thump," *Anesthesiology* 75:705, 1991.
21. Liguori GA, Sharrock NE: Asystole and severe bradycardia during epidural anesthesia in orthopedic patients, *Anesthesiology* 86:250, 1997.
22. Mackey DC, Carpenter RL, Thompson GE, et al: Bradycardia and asystole during spinal anesthesia: a report of three cases without morbidity, *Anesthesiology* 70:866, 1989.
23. Gratadour P, Viale JP, Parlow J, et al: Sympathovagal effects of spinal anesthesia assessed by the spontaneous cardiac baroreflex, *Anesthesiology* 87:1359, 1997.
24. Rosenberg JM, Wahr JA, Sung CH, et al: Coronary perfusion pressure during cardiopulmonary resuscitation after spinal anesthesia in dogs, *Anesth Analg* 82:84, 1996.
25. Cheney FW: The changing pattern of anesthesia-related adverse events, *ASA Newsletter* 60:10, 1996.
26. Cheney FW: Anesthesia patient safety and professional liability continue to improve, *ASA Newsletter* 61:18, 1997.

Chapter 32

The Cost of Adverse Outcome

Robert A. Caplan

I. WHY STUDY COST?

One of the major challenges in the analysis of health care is quantification: the task of finding numbers or values that offer a meaningful representation of a particular process or outcome. Quantitative measures provide a practical means for making comparisons, detecting changes, and evaluating relationships between risk and benefit.

Cost is an attractive measurement because it readily lends itself to numeric expression. The cost of a particular adverse outcome may be manifest in a variety of quantifiable ways, such as extra procedures or medications, extended length of hospital stay, days of rehabilitation, or delayed return to gainful employment. Even the less tangible cost of emotional suffering can be assessed by the use of structured surveys and rating systems.

To varying degrees of completeness and plausibility, many of the costs associated with adverse outcome can be measured in monetary units or dollars. In simplest terms, these dollars represent the expenses associated with rehabilitation or corrective treatments, or the losses resulting from the inability to work or obtain work-related benefits. An understanding of the dollar cost of adverse outcome can play an important role in risk management. Strategies for minimizing liability can be focused on the classes of injury that are associated with the highest dollar costs. This approach is appealing because it draws attention not only to rare and expensive events, but also to events of low cost that occur often enough to produce a significant aggregate impact.

This chapter is an examination of the cost of adverse outcomes from four perspectives. First, the basic economic factors that determine cost are explored. Second, specific factors that contribute to the cost of adverse anesthetic outcomes are examined in detail. Third, the dynamic relationship between the cost of adverse anesthetic outcomes and the cost of professional liability insurance is described. Finally, an overview of psychologic costs is presented.

II. THE COST OF ADVERSE OUTCOME
A. Estimating the damages of an adverse outcome

To provide a general foundation for understanding the dollar cost of adverse anesthetic outcomes, it is helpful to demonstrate the usual method for estimating the damages associated with an adverse anesthetic outcome. A hypothetical case of intraoperative death serves as a useful example.

> *Event description. In the late 1980s, a 51-year-old woman in otherwise excellent health was admitted for elective cholecystectomy. She died during anesthesia because of an unrecognized esophageal intubation. A detailed investigation indicated negligence on the part of the attending anesthesiologist, attributable to drug dependency and impaired vigilance.*

> *Socioeconomic setting. The patient was employed as a supervisor by a large corporation. She enjoyed her job and planned to work until 65 years of age. The patient was married for 30 years and was responsible for basic management of her household.*

Two types of damages are typically assessed: economic and noneconomic. Economic damages include actual expenses or anticipated dollar losses associated with the adverse outcome and its consequences. Typical examples of economic damages include hospital bills, fees for rehabilitation, projected costs of long-term care, lost wages, reduced earnings, and inability to have access to previous or anticipated services and benefits. Noneconomic damages are losses that cannot be measured directly or replaced by dollars but for which dollars will represent partial or symbolic compensation. Typical examples include pain, suffering, disfigurement, loss of companionship, and inability to enjoy previous avocations. In some cases, the symbolic purpose of noneconomic damages is to make an example of the case or serve as a form of punishment.[1]

For the case described here, a simple analysis of economic and noneconomic damages might proceed as follows:

1. Economic damages

a. Lost earnings. The patient's average salary during the 3 previous years of employment was $47,680 per year. Her yearly earnings generally increased at a rate that was equal to or slightly greater than the rate of inflation. Therefore the value of her earnings until 65 years of age can be estimated without discount as follows:

$$(65 - 51) \text{ years} \times \$47,680/\text{year} = \$667,520$$

b. Lost fringe benefits. In the metropolitan area where this patient lived, fringe benefits (such as vacation, medical and dental insurance) usually represented 6% of wages. The counterbalancing effect of inflation and yearly wage increases allows the value of lost fringe benefits to be estimated without discount as follows:

$$(65 - 51) \text{ years} \times \$47,680/\text{year} \times 0.06 = \$40,051$$

c. Lost pension benefit. The patient's life expectancy after retirement was estimated at 10 years. Her combined employment pension and Social Security benefit was estimated at $1,750 per month. The face value of this benefit is the product of the monthly benefit and the expected number of months of life after retirement ($210,000). However, these dollars would have been received in the future. If the lost pension benefit is paid as a lump sum in the present, a smaller amount will be required because the value of these present dollars, unlike a pension received in the future, is not eroded by inflation. If one assumes an average yearly inflation rate of 4%, this results in a downward adjustment or discount of approximately $107,705. Thus the lost pension benefit in present dollars is calculated as follows:

$$\$210,000 \text{ (face value)} - \$107,705 \text{ (discount)} = \$102,295$$

d. Loss of homemaking services. The average time spent on household care was estimated at 2 hours per day. The average agency rate for this service in the metropolitan area where the patient lived was $8.50 per hour. The recipient of homemaking services was the patient's husband, whose life expectancy was estimated at 21 years. Assuming, conservatively, that the requirement for homemaking service would remain fairly level over time and that the fee for this service would increase at a rate

equivalent to inflation, the present value of these services can be estimated without discount as follows:

$$2 \text{ hours/day} \times 365 \text{ days/year} \times 21 \text{ years} \times \$8.50/\text{hour} = \$130,305$$

e. Hospital and physician services. The patient died after 5 days of hospitalization in the intensive care unit. The total charge for hospital and physician services was $11,380. The patient's insurance policy provided for 70% coverage after a deductible of $500. The remaining bill was calculated as follows:

$$\$(11,380 - 500) \times 0.30 = \$3,264$$

2. Noneconomic damages.
The patient and her husband had a stable marriage and close relationships with their children and grandchildren. Both husband and wife enjoyed excellent health and had planned numerous activities for their retirement years. Although it is impossible to attach a dollar value to these losses, it is likely that a jury would respond generously to a request for compensation for the loss of companionship.

Investigation of this adverse outcome also revealed that members of the hospital staff and administration were aware that the responsible anesthesiologist had a recurrent history of drug abuse. Preventive action had not been pursued aggressively for a variety of reasons, including a close personal friendship between the chief of anesthesia and the impaired physician. This feature might lead a jury to respond generously to a request for punitive damages.

In the state where this patient lived, a tort reform law had placed a ceiling on the total amount of noneconomic damages. This ceiling was defined as 43% of the average annual wage for residents of the state, multiplied by the life expectancy of the patient. In this case, the ceiling was calculated as follows:

$$\$20,110 \times 0.43 \times 28 = \$242,124$$

The total estimate for economic and noneconomic damages in this case was $1,185,559 (Table 32-1). Al-

Table 32-1. Estimation of damages associated with an anesthesia-related death*

Item	Amount ($)
Economic damages	
Lost earnings	667,520
Lost fringe benefits	40,051
Lost pension benefits	102,295
Lost homemaking services	130,305
Hospital and physician fees	3,264
SUBTOTAL	943,435
Noneconomic damages	
Calculated ceiling	242,124
TOTAL	$1,185,559

*This estimate of the financial value of damages is based on a hypothetical case involving a 51-year-old employed woman who died as the result of an unrecognized esophageal intubation in the late 1980s. See text for a detailed description.

though this sum may seem surprisingly high, it could have been substantially greater if the patient had survived. For example, suppose this patient sustained hypoxic brain damage and required long-term institutional care or daily assistance from a skilled attendant. Chronic institutional care for a patient who requires assistance with all activities of daily life costs approximately $2,000 per month. Around-the-clock care from a live-in attendant costs about $3,000 per month. (These figures do not include associated medical treatment or special physical therapy.) If the patient's underlying medical status were robust, she might survive for 10 years, thereby increasing the estimated damages by $240,000 to $360,000. These calculations help demonstrate why adverse outcomes that lead to long-term institutional care for a child or young adult often result in total damages exceeding $3 million.

An important purpose of the preceding discussion is to illustrate the variety of assumptions that enter into the assessment of damages. Many of these are subject to negotiation. If both spouses have been employed, there may not be an economic need (from the standpoint of food, clothing, insurance, entertainment) to provide full future compensation for the wages and benefits of the deceased. This line of reasoning can be weakened by specific circumstances. For example, the family may be dependent on two sources of income to meet mortgage payments or pay college tuition fees. Or it may not be possible for the surviving spouse to single-handedly remain working, rear the children, and maintain a household.

Most claims are resolved by an adversarial process in which a plaintiff's attorney represents the injured party and a defense attorney represents the interests of the physician and the insurance carrier. In cases involving large damages, both sides usually hire an economist to calculate lost wages and benefits, discount rates, and consumption factors. The plaintiff's attorney customarily works on a contingency basis. If the injured party is successful in obtaining compensation for damages, the plaintiff's attorney usually receives 30% to 50% of the award. Additionally, the injured party must reimburse the plaintiff's attorney for the expenses of pursuing the case. For large awards, the overall reduction can be substantial. An analysis of almost 200 awards exceeding $1 million showed that the injured party ultimately recovered 43% of the original sum.[2] To ensure that the injured party receives adequate compensation, the plaintiff's attorney must take a generous approach to estimating damages. Noneconomic damages can play a particularly important role in this regard.

The basic goal of the insurance carrier is to minimize financial loss. When an adverse outcome is the result of negligent* care, the insurance carrier usually seeks an out-of-court settlement. In this situation, a settlement is often preferable to a trial because of the expensive nature

of a courtroom defense itself, plus the likelihood that the jury will award a substantial sum for economic and noneconomic damages. A settlement may be considered preferable to a trial even if the adverse outcome is not the result of negligence. This approach may be taken when a case has strong emotional elements that could sway the jury in favor of a generous award for the plaintiff.

The cost of a courtroom defense is substantial. A variety of basic services contribute to the expense (Table 32-2). The facts of a case are initially established by the process of discovery and deposition. Each deposition results in a charge for a court reporter and the associated costs of transcription and duplication. A simple deposition lasting 2 hours is associated with a fee of several hundred dollars. In a simple case, three to five witnesses and experts are often deposed before a trial. In a complicated case, many more depositions may be required.

Trial testimony by expert witnesses plays a critical role in courtroom proceedings. Expert witnesses typically charge $1,000 to $3,000 for a courtroom appearance. It is not unusual for the defense to call on two to five experts. In a complex case, it may be necessary to call on nationally recognized experts from distant cities. This introduces additional costs for travel. Defense attorneys charge an hourly rate in the range of $100 to $250 per hour. During a trial, the attorney may work 10 to 12 hours each day.

Charts, graphs, and medical illustrations play an important role in the courtroom because jury members may not be able to understand sophisticated medical concepts simply by listening to oral testimony. Visual aids result in charges ranging from $500 for a few simple displays to $5,000 for a complex set of illustrations.

Overall, the cost of a 1-week trial ranges from approximately $15,000 to $30,000. A complex 3-week trial may incur charges of $40,000 to $80,000. These figures vary considerably throughout the United States. The cost of defending a malpractice suit at trial in some large metropolitan areas can be two or three times greater than the amounts shown in Table 32-2. When the estimated damages are small, the insurance carrier and the plaintiff's attorney may both prefer an out-of-court settlement because the expense of litigation can severely diminish the economic advantage of victory on either side.

Table 32-2. Sample costs of defending a malpractice suit in court*

Item	1-Week trial ($)	3-Week trial ($)
Depositions (clerical fees)	1,000	2,000
Expert witness fees	8,000	20,000
Visual displays	1,000	3,000
Attorney fees	20,000	55,000
TOTAL COST	$30,000	$80,000

*Figures are based on approximate costs for the Northwest region of the United States in the mid-1990s. See text for a detailed description of each component.

---

*A discussion of negligence is beyond the scope of this chapter, but the interested reader can find an excellent description in a recent review by Cheney FW: Anesthesia and the law: the North American experience, *Br J Anaesth* 59:891, 1987.

B. Cost data from the ASA Closed Claims Project: specific factors

The American Society of Anesthesiologists Closed Claims Project is a structured evaluation of adverse anesthetic outcomes collected from 35 U.S. insurance carriers. A basic overview of the project is given in Chapter 31, and detailed descriptions of its methods have been published recently.[3-5] This section is an examination of cost data derived from cases in the Closed Claims database.

It is important to appreciate the temporal context of the Closed Claims database. Most cases in the database represent adverse outcomes that occurred in the 20-year period between 1975 and 1995. The interval between an adverse event and closure of its associated claim typically ranges from 3 to 5 years. Thus the cost data presented in this chapter represent payments made chiefly during the 1980s and the early 1990s.

All cost data are presented in original dollar amounts, without adjustment for inflation. Cost data represent either the amount of an out-of-court settlement or the amount of jury award. Transactional costs associated with investigation, analysis, or litigation of a claim are not included. Because these cost data do not conform to a normal distribution, median values and ranges are used for descriptive statistics.

The limitations of closed claims data are described in Chapter 31. In brief, these data were obtained from insurance carriers who agreed to participate in the Closed Claims Project. Thus we cannot be certain that this information provides a truly representative picture of financial liability. For similar reasons, it is difficult to compare closed claims data with liability statistics from other sources.

Legal factors that affect compensation are often in a state of flux. Tort reform laws, designed to control the rising costs of liability, were introduced beginning in the 1970s. Many of these laws subsequently underwent challenge, modification, or repeal.[6] Typical features of tort reform laws include limits on noneconomic damages, regulation of attorney fees, a shorter period for the statute of limitations, and the use of periodic or structured payments instead of lump-sum awards. The precise impact of these changes is difficult to define at any point in time.

1. The basic landscape of settlements and jury awards.

The amount of payment by settlement or jury award is known for approximately 90% of the cases in the Closed Claims database. This information reveals some of the basic features of the cost of adverse outcomes in anesthesia. In a recent analysis of 3791 claims (K. Posner, personal communication, 1998), payments ranged from $15 to $23,200,000. The amount of payment was $37,000 or less for one third of the cases, $100,000 or less for one half of the cases, and $375,000 or less for three fourths of the cases.

Large payments—defined as settlements or jury awards of $1 million or more—make up only 5% of the overall database. Within this group of large payments, 50% of the payments did not exceed $1,659,016, and 80% of the payments did not exceed $3,000,000. The frequency of large payments has not shown any significant increase from the early 1980s and through the mid-1990s.

2. Key relationships between cost and anesthesia care.

A large-scale analysis of cost data from the Closed Claims database was reported in 1989.[4] This investigation focused on 1004 cases in which a lawsuit was actually filed, encompassing 85% of the available database. Practicing anesthesiologists reviewed each case and used the concept of "reasonable and prudent practice at the time of the event" as a measure of the standard of care. There was sufficient information to permit a judgment of the standard of care in 869 cases. Overall, 46% of cases exhibited care that met standards, whereas 54% of cases exhibited substandard care. Adverse outcomes were rated using a standardized severity of injury scale[7] shown in Table 32-3. Scores of 1 to 5 indicate nondisabling injuries, scores of 6 to 8 indicate disabling injuries, and a score of 9 represents death. The median injury score was 7 (a severe, disabling injury).

Three principal features of cost emerged from this analysis. First, the frequency of payment was linked to standard of care but not to severity of injury. Second, the cost of claims was linked to both severity of injury and the standard of care. Third, adverse events that were judged preventable with better monitoring were associated with far more costly payments than those that were not considered preventable with better monitoring. Each feature is reviewed.

a. Likelihood of payment is a function of standard of care.

An important aspect of the cost of adverse outcomes is not just the magnitude of damages, but also the likelihood that payment will occur. Studies performed in the past two decades indicate that the overall likelihood of payment may be small if one considers the entire popu-

Table 32-3. Severity of injury scale*

Score	Examples
0	No obvious injury
1	Emotional injury: awareness, fright, pain during anesthesia
Temporary injury	
2	Insignificant: lacerations, contusions, no delay in recovery
3	Minor: fall in hospital, delay in recovery
4	Major: brain or nerve damage, unable to work
Permanent injury	
5	Minor: nondisabling damage to organs
6	Significant: loss of one eye or kidney, deafness
7	Major: paraplegia, blindness, loss of use of one limb
8	Grave: severe brain damage, quadriplegia, lifelong care
9	Death

From Brunner EA: *Int Anesthesiol Clin* 22:17, 1984.
*The severity of injury scale (SIS) is a standardized rating system for adverse outcomes. Descriptive categories are shown in boldface; specific examples are shown in light-face.

lation of adverse outcomes. The 1974 Medical Insurance Feasibility Study in California estimated that malpractice claims were filed by only 10% of all patients who were injured by negligent medical care.[8] This statistic was recently reaffirmed by the Harvard Medical Practice Study of patients hospitalized in 1984 in New York State.[9]

If an injured patient does file a suit, what is the likelihood that payment will occur? The Closed Claims database offers an opportunity to explore this question specifically for the specialty of anesthesiology. Payment was received in 62% of the lawsuits in the Closed Claims database, whereas no payment was received in 29% of cases. Payment data were missing in 9% of claims.

Severity of injury did not exert a significant effect on the frequency of payment (Fig. 32-1). Instead, standard of care was the determining factor. Cases that exhibited substandard care were associated with a higher incidence of payment than cases in which the standard of care was met ($p < 0.01$). If care was substandard, payment was received in at least 80% of cases. If the standard of care was met, patients received payment in approximately 40% of cases. These data indicate that the current tort-based system results in a pattern of compensation that favors the injured patient. However, one can readily appreciate that inequities exist for both the injured patient and the physician. Specifically, no compensation was obtained in 10% of the cases in which substandard care was delivered, whereas compensation was provided in 42% of cases where the physician met the appropriate standard.

Litigation under a tort-based system of law is currently the principal tool for resolution of malpractice claims, but it is not the only possible approach. Two other approaches are a fault-based system and a no-fault system. In a fault-based system, compensation depends on a finding of substandard care, with this determination presumably being made by peers. In a no-fault system, payment depends on a demonstration that the injury was caused by medical care, regardless of the relationship of care to the current standard of practice.

How might alternative compensation systems change the frequency of payment? Because the Closed Claims database contains information on standard of care as judged by peers, the presence and severity of injury, and the incidence of payment, it is possible to generate a comparative view (Table 32-4). The no-fault system produces the highest number of payments (980) because of a projected increase in claims paid in all three categories of injury. Rinaman[10] cautions that a no-fault system of compensation could cost approximately 4.5 times more than the current tort-based system, although a review by Manuel[11] suggests that the net expenditure might be less substantial. The fault-based system results in the lowest number of payments (467) in this analysis. The actual number of payments obtained under the tort-based system occupies an intermediate position (614). The projected reduction in payments under the fault-based system is attributable to a substantial decrease in the category of nondisabling injuries and a modest decrease in the category of disabling injuries. Although the tort-based and fault-based systems both show an identical

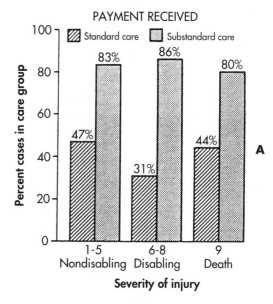

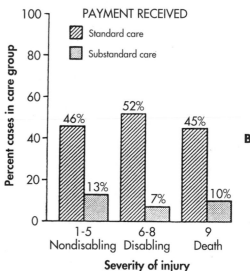

Fig. 32-1. Incidence of payment in malpractice suits from the Closed Claims database. **A,** Lawsuits in which payment was received. **B,** Lawsuits in which no payment was received. Cases exhibiting substandard care were associated with a higher incidence of payment than cases in which the standard of care was met ($p < 0.01$). There was no significant relationship between incidence of payment and severity of injury. Cases with missing data and lawsuits without injury are excluded. (From Cheney FW, Posner K, Caplan RA, et al: *JAMA* 261:1599, 1989.)

number of payments associated with death, this is just a coincidental finding because the two groups do not contain precisely the same cases.

At first glance, the fault-based system looks like an attractive alternative, but the result obtained from this analysis may be misleading. Because malpractice claims represent only a small fraction of the total set of adverse outcomes, the availability of an actual fault-based system ultimately might lead to more payments than a tort-based system. This question cannot be answered

Table 32-4. Number of claims paid under different systems of compensation*

Adverse outcome	Compensation system		
	Tort-based†	Fault-based‡	No-fault§
Nondisabling injury	201	82	365
Disabling injury	153	125	243
Death	260	260	372
TOTAL	614	467	980

From Cheney FW, Posner K, Caplan RA, et al: *JAMA* 261:1599, 1989.

*Modified from an analysis of 1006 lawsuits in the database of the Closed Claims Project. Lawsuits with a severity of injury score of 0 have been excluded.

†Entries represent the number of cases that actually resulted in payment, regardless of care.

‡Entries represent the number of cases in which payment would have occurred because of a determination of substandard care.

§Entries represent the number of cases in which payment would have occurred because of the presence of an injury.

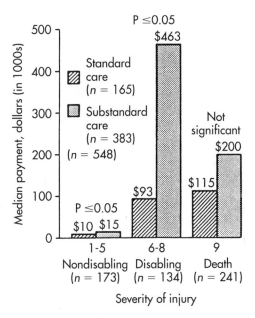

Fig. 32-2. Median payments associated with malpractice suits in the Closed Claims database. Cases with missing data and no payment are excluded. (From Cheney FW, Posner K, Caplan RA, et al: *JAMA* 261:1599, 1989.)

until there are better estimates of the proportion of injured patients who might access an alternative system of compensation and how the transactional costs would differ from the current tort-based approach. The potential importance of transactional costs merits particular attention. Current evidence indicates that less than half of the amount paid in professional liability premiums ultimately reaches patients in the form of financial compensation.[11]

b. Cost is a function of severity of injury and standard of care. The cost of adverse outcomes is linked to severity of injury (Fig. 32-2). Nondisabling injuries are associated with lower median payments, whereas disabling injuries and death are associated with higher median payments. As might be expected from the earlier discussion of the costs of long-term care, the highest median payments are associated with disabling injuries rather than death.

Standard of care produces an important interaction with the relationship between cost and severity of injury. In each of the three main categories of severity of injury, median payments are higher when care is judged substandard than in cases in which care meets the appropriate standard. This interaction is most pronounced for disabling injuries, in which the delivery of substandard care is associated with nearly a fourfold increase in median payments ($93,000 for standard care versus $463,000 for substandard care).

Table 32-5 presents a profile of costs for specific complications that occur with a frequency of 2% or greater in the Closed Claims database. Examination of the first three lines of this table leads to an important insight: Just two complications, death and permanent brain damage, account for almost half the cases. Both of these complications are associated with high severity of injury and, correspondingly, with high median payments. Although

this finding is not outwardly attractive, it does carry an important implication. If the more common claims are also the most expensive ones, strategies that successfully reduce the incidence of costly complications, even to a modest degree, are likely to make a significant impact on premium costs. The applicability of this concept has been emphasized by leading authorities in anesthetic risk management.[12,13]

Adverse outcomes involving the respiratory system account for approximately one third of all cases in the Closed Claims database. An in-depth investigation of 522 adverse respiratory events was recently conducted,[14] and an overview of the major findings has been presented in Chapter 31. Table 32-6 compares the cost of adverse respiratory outcomes with nonrespiratory complications. Several significant differences are evident. The median cost of adverse respiratory events ($200,000) is over five times as great as the median cost of nonrespiratory events ($35,000). This difference probably can be attributed to the fact that the most severe injuries, death and permanent brain damage, constitute 85% of the group of adverse respiratory events but only 30% of the nonrespiratory events. Another notable finding is the significantly higher frequency of payment for adverse respiratory events (72%) than for nonrespiratory events (51%). This difference probably reflects the high proportion of ratings of substandard care in the group of respiratory cases (76%) as opposed to the small proportion of substandard ratings in the nonrespiratory cases (30%). Adverse respiratory events represent a particularly urgent target for risk management efforts because the cost of these events is driven by three deleterious factors working in unison: frequency of occurrence, substandard care, and severity of injury.

Table 32-5. Cost profile of common adverse outcomes*

Adverse outcome	Percentage of claims ($n = 3001$)	Median payment ($)	Range of payment ($)
Death	35	200,000	250-6,336,738
Nerve damage	16	30,000	188-2,100,000
Brain damage	13	650,000	2,750-6,300,000
Airway trauma	6	25,000	15-1,150,000
Awareness/fright	4	18,000	390-9,000,000
Eye injury	3	21,250	25-1,000,000
Fetal/newborn injury	3	352,220	18,248-5,400,000
Headache	3	8,500	752-200,000
Pneumothorax	3	32,500	500-9,000,000
Aspiration	2	120,000	390-1,355,783

From Posner K: Personal communication, 1998.
*Cost of settlement or jury award for adverse outcomes representing 2% or more of 1541 cases in the ASA Closed Claims database.

Table 32-6. Comparison of cost for adverse outcomes associated with respiratory and nonrespiratory events*

	All respiratory events ($n = 522$)	All nonrespiratory events ($n = 1019$)
Outcome (% of cases)		
Death	66†	22
Permanent brain damage	19†	8
Other permanent injury	5†	25
Temporary injury	9†	39
No injury	1†	6
Payment		
Range	$1,000-6,000,000	<$1,000-5,400,000
Median	$200,000†	$35,000
Payment frequency (% of claims paid)	72†	51

From Caplan RA, Posner KL, Ward RJ, et al: *Anesthesiology* 72:828, 1990.
*Based on an analysis of 1541 cases from the ASA Closed Claims database. Care was judged to be substandard in 76% of the respiratory events and in 30% of the nonrespiratory events.
†$p <0.05$ compared to nonrespiratory events.

c. Cost is a function of monitoring and preventability. Can better monitoring lead to a reduction in the cost of adverse outcomes? The ASA Closed Claims database provides an intriguing clue. As part of the process of data collection, each closed claim was reviewed to determine which, if any, monitoring techniques might have prevented the adverse outcome, even if the monitoring technology was not available at the time of the incident. In making this judgment, the reviewing physicians assumed that the monitor would be used properly and the resultant data would be interpreted and acted upon in an appropriate manner. Significant interrater reliability for this type of judgment has been demonstrated previously.[5]

Tinker et al[15] conducted an analysis of monitoring in 1097 closed claims. This study indicated that better monitoring could have prevented the adverse outcome in 346 of the cases (31.5%). Most of the outcomes considered preventable with better monitoring were associated with respiratory system events (80%). The reviewers determined that a pulse oximeter, a capnometer, or a combination of these two monitors might have prevented the adverse outcome in 322 (93%) of the cases. Perhaps the most striking finding in this analysis was the relationship between preventable outcomes and cost. The median payment for adverse outcomes deemed preventable with better monitoring ($250,000) was 10 times greater than the median payment for cases that were not considered preventable ($22,500; $p < 0.01$).

Interpretation of these results must proceed cautiously. The reviewers were not asked to consider confounding factors such as equipment malfunction, diversion of attention, misinterpretation and misuse of data, or the impact of false positive and false negative results. Thus their judgments must be regarded as a near-maximum (and perhaps unattainable) estimate of the efficacy of better monitoring. Orkin[16] prepared an excellent overview of confounding factors. Keats[17] emphasizes that the net benefit of any new monitor or therapeutic approach cannot be defined accurately until large-scale studies determine whether the innovation is associated with significant side effects or harm. With noninvasive monitors such as the pulse oximeter and capnometer, the likelihood of direct physical harm is small, but one cannot arbitrarily exclude the possibility that errors in use or interpretation might be associated with significant long-term damage.

A related issue is the cost of prevention. Would a reduction in adverse outcomes attributable to better monitoring be accompanied by a reduction in insurance premiums sufficient to offset the expense of the monitors themselves? An exploratory analysis by Whitcher et al[18] provides an excellent overview of the principal considerations. One must be able to identify the preventable injuries and their cost, define the monitors required for prevention, provide an estimate of the reduction in injury and cost that will occur, and presume that market-

Table 32-7. Estimated cost per case for a pulse oximeter and capnometer*

Description	Oximeter	Capnometer
Purchase price	1,200	2,500
Two-year maintenance	240	500
TOTAL 2-YEAR COST	$1,440	$3,000
Patient uses over 2 years	2,000	2,000
COST PER PATIENT OVER 2 YEARS	$0.72	$1.50

*This analysis is based on three key assumptions: a 2-year recovery of the face value of the purchase price plus maintenance cost, a yearly maintenance cost equal to 10% of the purchase price, and 1000 patient-uses per year in the location where the device is situated.

place competition in the insurance industry is high enough to ensure that a significant proportion of the savings will pass through to the physician in the form of premium reductions. Using a 50% decrease in preventable injuries as the critical assumption, Whitcher's analysis suggests that oximetry and capnometry could indeed be incorporated in a cost-effective manner.

If one is uncertain about the efficacy of additional monitoring or the magnitude of premium reductions that might occur, it is helpful to consider the cost per case of a specific monitor. A useful way to approach this question is to calculate the cost per case that would be required to recover the purchase price plus the cost of maintenance over a specified period of time.[19] Table 32-7 displays this calculation for a midpriced pulse oximeter and capnometer in the mid-1990s. There are three key assumptions in this analysis (which can be altered to satisfy specific conditions): a 2-year period for recovery of the face value of the purchase price plus maintenance, a yearly maintenance estimate of 10% of the original purchase price, and 1000 uses per year in the anesthetizing location where the monitor is situated. The result is $2.22 per patient for the addition of a free-standing pulse oximeter and capnometer. A 2-year recovery period was chosen in this example as a hedge against rapidly changing technology (which could make a different device or approach more attractive), uncertain reimbursement factors, and unanticipated breakage or loss. Obviously the estimated cost declines if one can accept a longer period for recovery. For example, the combined cost per case decreases to $1.36 for a 5-year period and to $0.91 for a 7-year period. Such calculations can help practitioners and administrators explore attractive but incompletely defined benefits against the likelihood that the extra expense can be absorbed by local economic constraints.

C. The cost of professional liability insurance

The potential for anesthetic care to produce adverse outcomes of high cost creates a distinctive problem: A small number of anesthesia claims can make a disproportionately large contribution to the overall losses incurred by an insurance carrier. In past decades, this situation has played a major role in the high premium rates for anesthesiologists.

What happens if the incidence of high-cost outcomes changes? Because the process of setting future premiums relies strongly on past experience, the consequences of short-term fluctuations are dampened and the full effects of long-term trends are delayed. For high-cost outcomes, which can have a disproportionate impact on the financial status of an insurance carrier, there may be an added tendency to react swiftly when these events show an apparent increase and, conversely, to adopt a more cautious approach when the incidence appears to decline.

An appreciation of these basic factors can be gained from the changes in anesthesia liability insurance during the past two decades. The National Association of Insurance Commissioners undertook a study of medical claims that had been closed in the interval from 1975 to December 1978. Anesthesia claims represented only 3% of all claims but accounted for 11% of the total payout.[7] This finding succinctly illustrates the potential relationship between a small number of high-cost events and overall losses.

During the 1980s, this profile began to change. For the period between 1981 and 1985, St. Paul Fire and Marine Insurance Company, one of the nation's largest insurers of physicians, reported that anesthetic care produced 4.6% of all claims and accounted for approximately 7% of total losses.[13] By the late 1980s, St. Paul reported that anesthesia care was associated with 3.5% of all claims and only 3.6% of overall losses.[20] On a more focused geographic scale, Zeitlin[21] noted evidence of decreased anesthesia-related mortality in the Commonwealth of Massachusetts, and Eichhorn[22] reported a decrease in major anesthetic morbidity for the nine anesthesia departments affiliated with Harvard Medical School.

How has the insurance industry reacted to these changes? Recent reports indicate a favorable response.[18,20,23-25] The cost of a premium for a given specialty usually is linked to a relative rate factor or equivalent type of modifier. In general terms, a relative rate factor is determined by historical data on the loss per physician for a given specialty. Family practitioners who do not perform surgery often have the lowest relative rate factor, usually a value near 1.0. A base rate premium is multiplied by a specific relative rate factor to determine (along with other adjustments) the premium rate for each specialty. This approach distributes the cost of premiums among each specialty in approximate proportion to its expected losses. The changes in relative risk rating for anesthesiologists have generally been downward. For example, St. Paul lowered the relative rate factor for anesthesia from 6.0 to 4.0 in 1985 and to 2.05 in 1995. Controlled Risk Insurance Company (the insurance carrier for the Affiliated Harvard Hospitals) decreased the relative rate factor from 5.0 to 2.5 in 1995.[25] These changes in relative risk factors are roughly equivalent to a yearly premium reduction of $10,000.

Nationwide surveys of premium rates for anesthesiologists have been conducted in 1984, 1985, 1988, and

1990.[26-28] These surveys reflect data primarily from physician-owned insurance companies and St. Paul. Table 32-8 displays trends in the average cost of a 1-year claims-made policy with limits of $1,000,000/$3,000,000 (single claim/total annual claims). From 1984 to 1988, the average premium doubled from $16,165 to $32,339. The average 1990 rate of $25,637 is notable in that it represents a decrease of approximately 20% from the 1988 rate. Such data must be interpreted cautiously because not every state or carrier is represented.

A detailed display of the 1988 survey of professional liability insurance is shown in Table 32-9. This survey was conducted by the American Society of Anesthesiologists Committee on Professional Liability.[27] Questionnaires were sent to 40 physician-owned companies in the United States, and information was received from 38. Almost all companies (95%) offered claims-made policies. Over half of the companies (58%) offered a claims-made policy with liability limits of $1,000,000/$3,000,000. A notable feature of these data is the wide variation in rates. The average yearly premium for a mature claims-made policy with limits of $1,000,000/$3,000,000 was $105,550 in Florida but only $16,442 in Tennessee. Nearby states often exhibited large differences in rates: Compare Missouri ($74,809) and Kentucky ($28,494), or Arizona ($46,102) and Utah ($23,333). The factors contributing to these differences have not been studied in detail.

It is important to recognize that these changes are fragile. Although there is a strong perception that improved monitoring, especially for hypoxic events, has led to a decrease in highly adverse outcomes, definitive proof is still lacking.[16,17] Other forces contributing to reduced anesthesia losses may include diverse factors such as award limits created by tort reform, marketplace competition among insurers, better legal defense strategies, new anesthetic agents and techniques, improved preoperative management, aggressive postoperative care, and changes in medical training, education, and credentialing. The precise contribution of any one of these factors is difficult to assess. However, some generalizations are possible. The role of legal factors such as tort reform must be regarded as unpredictable because legislation enacted during one year may be modified or repealed later. Marketplace competition may result in some reductions, but this process is sharply limited by actuarial constraints. Prevention of adverse outcomes probably is the single most important and enduring factor that drives the reduction of premiums. Continuing efforts to

Table 32-8. Trends in annual premium rates for anesthesiologists*

Survey year	Average premium ($)	States represented
1984	16,165 ± 6,437	40
1985	18,693 ± 7,520	40
1988	32,339 ± 23,647	22
1990	25,637 ± 13,014	38

*Figures represent the average price of a 1-year claims-made policy with limits of $1,000,000/$3,000,000 (single claim/total annual claim). Data obtained primarily from physician-owned insurance companies and St. Paul Fire and Marine Insurance Company.[25-27]

Table 32-9. 1988 Survey of professional liability insurance

Insurance company (by state)	Annual rate ($)	Type of policy	Limits of liability
Alabama	20,934	MCM	1M/1M
Alaska	67,659	CM	1M/2M
Arizona	46,012	MCM	1M/3M
California Doctor's Co.*	16,803	MCM	1M/3M
California MIEC	21,260	MCM	1M/3M
California Norcal*	15,116	MCM	1M/3M
California SCPIE	22,976	CM	1M/3M
Colorado	21,448	MCM	1M/2M
Connecticut	33,561	MCM	1M/4M
District of Columbia	27,843	CM	1M/4M
Florida FPIC*	74,628	MCM	1M/3M
Florida Physicians*	105,550	MCM	1M/3M
Florida Physicians Protective*	75,584	MCM	1M/3M
Illinois	27,843	CM	1M/3M
Indiana	4,762	MCM	100K/300K
Iowa	29,043	MCM	1M
Kentucky	28,494	MCM	1M/3M
Louisiana	26,481	MCM	1M/1M
Maine	21,837	MCM	1M/3M
Maryland*	32,472	MCM	1M/3M
Michigan Physicians*	43,473	CM	1M/1M
Michigan PICOM*	41,869	MCM	1M/3M
Minnesota	16,836	MCM	1M/3M
Mississippi	17,472	MCM	1M/3M
Missouri Medico*	74,809	MCM	1M/2M
Missouri Wedgeworth	62,618	CM	1M/2M
New Mexico	15,446	Occurrence	100K/300K
New York*	27,402	MCM	1M/3M
North Carolina	12,386	MCM	1M/3M
Ohio	40,752	CM	1M/1M
Oklahoma	9,137	Occurrence	1M/1M
Oregon*	27,420	MCM	1M/3M
Pennsylvania*	12,001	MCM	200K/600K
Tennessee	16,442	MCM	1M/3M
Texas	19,151	MCM	1M/3M
Utah	23,333	MCM	1M/3M
Washington	20,575	MCM	1M/3M
Wisconsin	16,756	MCM	400K/1M

A detailed view of the range of insurance products and premium rates provided by physician-owned insurance companies. Data obtained by the American Society of Anesthesiologists Committee on Professional Liability.[27] *MCM*, Mature claims made; *M*, $1,000,000. *CM*, claims made; *K*, $1,000.
*Mean value for states in which rates vary by county.

understand the basic causes of adverse outcomes and validate the merits of specific preventive strategies are therefore essential. The basic features of this area of research are just now undergoing formal definition in the field of anesthesiology.[29,30]

D. Psychologic costs

A discussion of the cost of adverse outcomes would not be complete without acknowledging that these events can have a significant impact on the physician. During the past decade, Charles et al[31-33] have performed several quantitative studies of the physician's psychologic response to malpractice claims. In a recent survey of physicians whose malpractice claims progressed to trial, virtually all respondents (97%) acknowledged that the experience was associated with physical or emotional reactions.[32] Symptomatic reactions reported by more than 50% of the physicians included tension, depressed mood, frustration, anger, and insomnia. In addition, two behavioral responses were common: subsequent use of unnecessary tests (67%) and changes in record keeping (56%). The use of unnecessary tests is a particularly interesting finding because it demonstrates how adverse outcomes may produce undesirable economic effects that extend beyond the confines of professional liability insurance. One can also appreciate that symptomatic responses such as mood changes and insomnia might lead to economically significant decrements in work performance.

Solazzi and Ward[34] describe a particularly worrisome linkage between adverse outcomes and suicide. As part of an analysis of 192 anesthetic malpractice claims that occurred between 1971 and 1982, three suicides and one suicide attempt were discovered. One anesthesiologist killed himself a few weeks after giving an apparently routine caudal anesthetic that resulted in paraplegia. Another anesthesiologist committed suicide shortly after his case was dismissed in court. A third suicide occurred several weeks after a favorable award for the plaintiff. An attempted suicide took place while a physician was awaiting trial. Of course, the adverse outcomes and ensuing litigation process may not have been the only factors contributing to these events. A joint study by the American Medical Association and American Psychiatric Association revealed that physicians who ultimately succeed in taking their own lives often have preexisting histories of suicidal intent, drug abuse, and financial difficulties.[35] Perhaps the lesson to be conveyed is that adverse outcomes have the potential for triggering a life-threatening psychologic reaction.

Some insurance carriers, hospitals, and group practices now take a prospective approach to the psychologic impact of adverse outcomes. Physicians are informed of the availability of relevant reading materials, professional counseling, and one-to-one support from fellow colleagues who have experienced malpractice proceedings. Not much imagination is required to devise a sound economic rationale for such efforts. The knowledge and expertise of the defendant physician can be vital to the successful defense of a malpractice claim. It is far more likely that an emotionally stable, reassured physician will make a useful contribution to the defense process than one who is depressed, angry, or no longer extant.

III. SUMMARY

Adverse outcomes in anesthetic practice are associated with a wide range of damages. Although not all aspects of damage can be quantified with precision, many can be expressed in terms of dollar cost. This approach provides a workable basis to make comparisons, form aggregate estimates, and focus attention on classes of injury that are associated with the greatest losses.

Analysis of cost data from the Closed Claims Project indicates three principal relationships. Cases involving substandard care are more likely to result in payment than cases in which the physician meets the standard of care. The cost of settlement or jury award is greatest in cases characterized by both substandard care and disabling injury. Finally, adverse outcomes deemed preventable with better monitoring are associated with far higher payments than cases in which monitoring would not have contributed to prevention.

Severe anesthetic injuries are characterized by high economic damages. This feature creates the primary driving force for the high cost of professional liability insurance. Recent reports indicate a probable decline in the incidence of severe anesthetic injuries, along with a parallel but slower reduction in premium rates. These favorable trends can best be preserved by an improved understanding of the basic causes of adverse outcomes and continued efforts to measure the effectiveness of specific preventive strategies.

REFERENCES

1. Peters JD, Fineberg KS, Kroll DA, et al: *Anesthesiology and the law,* Ann Arbor, Mich, 1983, Health Administration Press.
2. Gibbs RF: *Legal perspectives on anesthesia,* 6:1, 1986 (comment).
3. Cheney FW: Anesthesia and the law: the North American experience, *Br J Anaesth* 59:891, 1987.
4. Cheney FW, Posner K, Caplan RA, et al: Standard of care and anesthesia liability, *JAMA* 261:1599, 1989.
5. Caplan RA, Posner K, Ward RJ, et al: Peer reviewer agreement for major anesthetic mishaps, *Qual Rev Bull* 14:363, 1988.
6. Walt D, Golin CB, eds: American Medical Association Special Task Force on Professional Liability and Insurance, *Professional liability in the '80s,* report no 2, Chicago, 1984, American Medical Association.
7. Brunner EA: The National Association of Insurance Commissioners' Closed Claims Study, *Int Anesthesiol Clin* 22:17, 1984.
8. Hiatt HH, Barnes BA, Brennan TA, et al: A study of medical injury and medical malpractice: an overview, *N Engl J Med* 321:480, 1989.
9. Brennan TA, Leape LL, Laird NM, et al: Incidence of adverse events and negligence in hospitalized patients: results of the Harvard Medical Practice study I, *N Engl J Med* 324:370, 1991.
10. Rinaman JC: The tort liability system: overview for the anesthesiologist. In Gravenstein JS, Holzer JF, eds: *Safety and cost containment in anesthesia,* Boston, 1988, Butterworth.
11. Manuel BM: Professional liability: a no-fault solution, *N Engl J Med* 322:627, 1990.
12. Holzer JF: Current concepts in risk management, *Int Anesthesiol Clin* 22:91, 1984.
13. Wood MD: Monitoring equipment and loss reduction: an insurer's view. In Gravenstein JS, Holzer JF, eds: *Safety and cost containment in anesthesia,* Boston, 1988, Butterworth.
14. Caplan RA, Posner KL, Ward RJ, et al: Adverse respiratory events in anesthesia: a closed claims analysis, *Anesthesiology* 72:828, 1990.

15. Tinker JH, Dull DL, Caplan RA, et al: Role of monitoring in prevention of anesthetic mishaps: a closed claims analysis, *Anesthesiology* 71:541, 1989.

16. Orkin FK: Practice standards: the Midas touch or the emperor's new clothes? *Anesthesiology* 70:567, 1989.

17. Keats AS: Anesthesia mortality in perspective, *Anesth Analg* 71:113, 1990.

18. Whitcher C, Ream AK, Parsons D, et al: Anesthetic mishaps and the cost of monitoring: a proposed standard for monitoring equipment, *J Clin Monit* 4:5, 1988.

19. Duberman SM, Bendixen HH: Concepts of fail-safe in anesthetic practice, *Int Anesthesiol Clin* 22:149, 1984.

20. Pierce EC: Anesthesiologists' malpractice premiums declining, *Anesthesia Patient Safety Foundation Newsletter* 4:2, March 1989.

21. Zeitlin GL: Possible decrease in mortality associated with anaesthesia: a comparison of two time periods in Massachusetts, USA, *Anaesthesia* 44:432, 1989.

22. Eichhorn JH: Prevention of intraoperative anesthesia accidents and related severe injury through safety monitoring, *Anesthesiology* 70:572, 1989.

23. Holzer JF: Risk manager notes improvement in anesthesia losses, *Anesthesia Patient Safety Foundation Newsletter* 4:2, March 1989.

24. McGinn PR: Practice standards leading to premium reductions, *Am Med News* p 28, Dec 2, 1988.

25. Pierce EC: The 34th Rovenstine lecture: 40 years behind the mask: safety revisited, *Anesthesiology* 84:965, 1996.

26. Cheney FW: Cost of malpractice insurance rises 17%, *American Society of Anesthesiologists Newsletter* 50:5, Feb 1986.

27. Wall RT, Cheney FW: The cost of professional liability insurance for anesthesiologists, *American Society of Anesthesiologists Newsletter* 52:7, Oct 1988.

28. Stuart M: The cost of medical malpractice insurance, rates across the United States for anesthesiologists, *Postgrad Year* 1:8, June 1990.

29. Gaba DM, Maxwell M, DeAnda A: Anesthetic mishaps: breaking the chain of accident evolution, *Anesthesiology* 66:670, 1987.

30. Allnutt MF: Human factors in accidents, *Br J Anaesth* 59:856, 1987.

31. Charles SC, Wilbert JR, Kennedy EC: Physicians' self-reports of reactions to malpractice litigation, *Am J Psychiatry* 141:563, 1984.

32. Charles SC, Wilbert JR, Franke KJ: Sued and nonsued physicians' self-reported reactions to malpractice litigation, *Am J Psychiatry* 142:437, 1985.

33. Charles SC, Pyskoty CE, Nelson A: Physicians on trial: self-reported reactions to malpractice trials, *West J Med* 148:358, 1988.

34. Solazzi RW, Ward RJ: The spectrum of medical liability cases, *Int Anesthesiol Clin* 22:43, 1984.

35. Council on Scientific Affairs: Results and implications of the AMA-APA physician mortality project: stage II, *JAMA* 257:2949, 1987.

Chapter 33

Risk Management and Quality Assurance

John H. Eichhorn

The twin concepts of risk management (RM) and quality assurance (QA) are integrally intertwined. RM was originally a creation of the insurance industry in an attempt to control payout on claims and thus financial loss. Quality assurance (used as a generic term with the recognition that it is the basis for programs generally known as quality improvement or quality management, each with or without *continual* or *total* as a prefix) usually is a multifactorial set of processes intended to optimize the quality of the medical care delivered. Clearly, optimal care is less likely to provoke malpractice claims and lawsuits, hence the intimate connection with RM. The QA process uses much of the same problem-solving algorithm as RM, and both programs have the same goal. The RM program sometimes can be considered an extension or broadening of the QA process into implementation of practical preventive and remedial measures regarding complications of anesthesia care. Recently, the patient safety movement within anesthesiology[1] has become prominent, and its goal of developing and implementing strategies specifically to minimize patient morbidity and mortality in anesthesia practice definitely interlocks with both RM and QA.

RM and QA relate to several other topics considered in this book. Evaluation of patient risk will reveal cases in which there is more than the usual probability of a complication. The insights gained will then lead to extra attention to issues of, for example, informed consent, record keeping, and plans for specific action in the event of an untoward incident. Epidemiology of complications reveals in what circumstances or with which patients certain complications may be most expected. Realization of these factors may lead to supplementation or alteration of the anesthetic plan, essentially a classic application of the concept of RM. An excellent general example is the epidemiologic discovery that unrecognized hypoventilation is the cause of the majority of intraoperative anesthesia-caused catastrophes. Over the last several years this discovery has led to the development and implementation of several strategies, functionally an application of the QA process, to minimize this documented risk. Specific discussion of what to do when sued (noting in particular that the probability exists that all anesthesia practitioners will be sued eventually, perhaps even multiple times) relates directly to the RM mechanism. Application of the RM and QA principles, especially those involving actions surrounding an adverse event, should make the subsequent response to a malpractice claim significantly easier for the defendant clinician.

I. RISK MANAGEMENT

RM in anesthesia is a comprehensive approach functionally involving all aspects of anesthesia care. RM is intended first to minimize the likelihood of anesthesia-caused or anesthesia-related complications (particularly the large fraction of these complications caused by human error). Second, both because of RM elements already in place before an adverse event and because of actions taken at the time of and after an untoward incident, RM will help minimize the impact of such an event on the patient, the anesthesia provider, and the medical care system.

Some of the elements of RM at first glance appear to be defensive in nature, particularly those regarding credentialing, equipment management, informed consent, record keeping, and response to an adverse event. Clearly, the overall goal of RM is optimal patient care. Correct and thorough application of the RM principles detailed in this chapter will help minimize complications and thus help optimize patient care. The other side of RM, after the primary efforts to promote the best-quality care, is its significant ability to help reduce liability exposure. Unfortunately, it is necessary to be aware of the medicolegal system and the facts of the so-called malpractice crisis periods of the 1970s and 1980s. Although there are strong suggestions that the medicolegal crunch of astronomically high settlements and awards, with consequent skyrocketing malpractice insurance premiums, has lessened in the 1990s,[2] it has been maintained that this is merely a cycle that will inevitably reverse itself.[3] In either case, it is legitimate to acknowledge that some attitudes and procedures in RM are influenced by the characteristics of the medicolegal system and the insurance industry and also by case precedents that have revealed characteristics that make more difficult the defense of anesthesia practitioners against unwarranted charges of malpractice. In theory, it is correct that the legal defensive issues (so-called defensive medicine) should not influence health care practices. However, the potentially devastating emotional and financial impact of a malpractice lawsuit on a practitioner—even a suit with no merit at all—is significant enough to justify awareness of and application of proven RM strategies intended to minimize the likelihood of malpractice claims.

Objective documentation and citable sources in the medical literature are less likely to be available when one is dealing with RM than when considering, for example, anesthetic complications directly involving physiology and pharmacology, such as whether isoflurane causes myocardial ischemia in patients with severe coronary artery disease through the steal phenomenon. In this chapter, relevant existing references are included, of course. However, there is also anecdotal reporting, including experiences of multiple, various anesthesia practitioners throughout the country. The topics covered here have been identified in some manner as the source of problems or solutions to problems within anesthesia practice. The purpose is to explain what issues are involved in each area of anesthesia RM and to offer suggestions (based on experience, where possible) on how best to deal with

these issues. Notice that these topics relate directly to the fundamental components of medical care (and many other endeavors) to which all elements ultimately can be reduced: structure, process, and outcome. Structure in medical care involves resources, including personnel, facilities, equipment (especially pertinent for anesthesia), and administration. Process involves how things are done, including the actual activities of patient care. The result of the interaction of these two is outcome (such as wellness, length of stay, dysfunction, morbidity, or mortality). Looking at features of clinical practice using this systematic approach helps facilitate RM approaches. Concerns about equipment clearly involve structure, whereas policy and procedure and most of the other identified areas of consideration concern process. The larger point is that everything considered eventually affects the outcome of anesthesia care.

A. Background

The terminology used in this area has been borrowed by the medical profession from business, industry, and other professions. Medical practitioners usually believe that they understand these terms well enough to communicate among themselves, but often this is not true. It is even more difficult when one is attempting to communicate with nonphysicians, such as hospital administrators, insurance company personnel, and regulatory and accrediting inspectors. Many medical practitioners still automatically associate RM with reams of apparently irrelevant paperwork demanded as fuel by a self-sustaining bureaucracy composed of nonmedical or quasimedical personnel. Overzealous emphasis early in the development of this still-young field on compiling statistics, doing audits, and filling out forms may have created a legacy of reluctance for involvement by anesthesia practitioners, more used to hands-on activity with rapid feedback. Nonetheless, it is vitally important for all concerned to realize that this type of activity not only is here to stay, but also has the potential to be enormously beneficial to the practice of anesthesia. Anesthesia providers must learn that this field has advanced significantly. It will continue to do so with the unhesitating, thoughtful involvement of those most interested (anesthesia practitioners themselves) in the reduction and eventual elimination of preventable anesthesia complications.

The concept of RM traditionally has been associated with the financial and economic side of business or professional activity. It started with the insurance industry recognizing risk: Certain activities predictably lead to a degree of loss. This risk then became the subject of efforts to plan to pay for the loss and to try to reduce the likelihood or magnitude of loss (and consequent cost). Thus an attempt was made to control or manage the known risk. Regarding anesthesia, clearly the data "demonstrate that anesthetic mishaps, although relatively few in number, present considerable risk of loss in the areas of hospital cost, human suffering, and the integrity of the medical profession" and, as a result, providers "have developed formal programs to systematically identify and control risks that may lead to patient injury or financial loss."[4] Financial loss usually means settlements and judgments associated with malpractice claims and suits. The emphasis of medical RM is correctly on the prevention of any loss-generating untoward incident or outcome. However, a key traditional component also is the effort to limit financial loss once an incident has occurred. A common impression is that the hospital or insurance company risk manager is the person to call as soon as an accident or injury is identified. Although this is true, there must be a shift in perception to the fact that prevention is primary and damage control (financial or otherwise), when needed, is a secondary part of the process.

Classic RM involves four steps: (1) identification of a problem (actual or potential injury or loss), (2) assessment and evaluation of the problem (determining the cause of injury or loss), (3) resolution of the problem (modification or elimination of the cause, by a change in practice, procedures, equipment, or behavior, and enforcement, with sanctions if necessary), and (4) a follow-up check on the resolution (to verify the desired result and to ensure continued effectiveness).

An example of minor injury but no financial loss involves a major medical center with a large volume of facial surgery. Through a combined mechanism of anesthetists' postoperative visits (and reports back to the clinical director of anesthesia), incident reports filed by floor nurses from the postoperative ward and a call from the surgeon doing most of these cases, it was established that a disproportionately large number of corneal abrasions were occurring during one type of operation. Investigative evaluation revealed that all anesthesia practitioners put lubricating ointment in the patient's eyes, which were then taped shut with paper tape. Some anesthetists used gauze pads, and some did not. All the patients sustaining corneal abrasions did not have gauze pads over their eyes. The resolution involved the issuance of a guideline, which was distributed in writing, discussed at a department-wide meeting and put in the procedure manual, stating that gauze pads should be used to cover the eyes of patients having that procedure. For follow-up evaluation, after several months, the surgeon was asked to confirm the impression that there had not been one identified corneal abrasion associated with the procedure since the new guideline was implemented.

In a larger-scale example, after notification from the malpractice insurer of perceived excessive anesthesia-caused losses, the Risk Management Committee of the Harvard Medical School Department of Anesthesia reviewed the available literature and all the anesthesia-related claims and incidents for the period 1976 to 1986 from the department's malpractice insurer. Considering the substantive identifiable problems discovered, the committee generated a list of subject categories into which problems and incidents were classified. In order of perceived magnitude, the list of identified areas associated with problems and incidents included (1) minimal monitoring during anesthesia (by far the most frequent issue) and in the postanesthetic recovery period, (2) anesthetizing locations outside traditional operating rooms, (3) equipment standards including preanesthetic equipment checkout, (4) equipment maintenance and servicing, (5) record keeping, and (6) preoperative and postoperative visits by anesthesia personnel. This list formed the basis of a program to devise strategies to improve clinical practice associated with each of the identified areas of attention. Because preventable intraoperative catastrophe accounted for the greatest cost, mandatory standards for intraoperative monitoring resulted.[5] At the time, this effort applied to one institution and seemed likely to be of general interest to most anesthesiologists, but it was first publicly offered and evaluated as an example of a new application of the RM process.[6] Further work along the same lines led to other standards concerning other topics on the original list of identified subject areas associated with problems and incidents.[7] After an appropriate interval, the follow-up component of the classic RM process led to an evaluation of the potential impact of the original Harvard monitoring standards.[8] Overall, this large-scale example shows the application of RM techniques that first stress prevention of untoward events and also include but go far beyond the traditional emphasis on financial loss.

In recent years, medical RM has received significantly greater attention. Among the reasons are the so-called malpractice crisis that has waxed and waned at various times from the mid-1970s until today, which heightened awareness of RM among anesthesia practitioners because of intense activity on the part of hospital administrations and malpractice insurance carriers; the major emphasis on cost containment in medical care, which has caused thorough critical review of many traditionally accepted practices with particular attention to outcome of care; and great emphasis by both regulators and the public on the quality of medical care, particularly on outcome, which has led to analysis of events at the most basic level in the medical care delivery system. These three factors tend to spotlight any adverse outcome of care, both specific instances and trends.

Adverse outcome of anesthesia care spans a spectrum. The most severe untoward results in anesthesia are rivaled in impact only by those in obstetrics. Anesthesia personnel must be constantly aware that anesthesia-related accidents have the potential to cause great harm. Until the late 1980s, anesthesiologists accounted for about 3% of American physicians and correspondingly generated about 3% of the number of malpractice claims filed. However, these claims accounted for about 11% of the total indemnity (dollars paid or set aside for future payment) for medical malpractice cases. Serious untoward results in anesthesia tend to have lasting impact (death or permanent injury), which is unfortunate and expensive. A comprehensive review of the causes of untoward outcome from anesthesia is beyond the scope of this chapter. They are discussed elsewhere in this book and in several classic reviews and papers.[9-17] Prominent in these discussions is the issue of preventability. Although there is debate about what fraction of adverse incidents might be prevented, it is an inescapable conclusion from study of the literature and from knowledge of current cases that a significant majority of major untoward results (anesthesia accidents) are preventable. There have been many thoughtful discussions on specific clinical strategies and practices for avoiding adverse outcome from anesthesia, including some labeled (probably incorrectly) as dealing with RM.[18] Discussion of specific monitoring equipment, anesthesia teaching techniques, and case analysis methods is valuable but is only one small component of a comprehensive RM program in anesthesia. Such a program must cover all relevant aspects of practice. Genuine RM in anesthesia must emphasize the creation of optimum conditions of structure and process and optimum preparation, awareness, and skill of the anesthesia practitioners. This will help to prevent complications and to minimize their impact when they occur.

B. Elements of risk management in anesthesia

1. Impact of managed care: new issues and threats. The enormous emphasis on cost cutting in medical care has created a new set of liability risks for physicians, including anesthesiologists. Patients (or their survivors) who believe justified medical care was denied or delayed because of administrative decisions involving issues of cost are suing both their health maintenance organizations (HMOs)/medical care organizations (MCOs) and the physicians who accepted the denials or delays of care that appear to have contributed to poor outcomes. Most of the first widely publicized cases involved refusal to cover diagnostic workups (e.g., for a breast lump) or treatments such as bone marrow transplants for patients with cancer (some enormous jury verdicts reported in the popular press). Of important note is that most MCOs originally were structured under federal laws intended to make them exempt from negligence claims, leaving the physician as the only "deep pocket" in sight. In 1997, Texas adopted a new law potentially making an MCO liable for the presumed adverse patient consequences of administrative denials or delays of care. Such new statutes do not absolve the physician of ultimate responsibility for the care rendered within a classically defined doctor-patient relationship, but do add a potential codefendant as the target of a lawsuit claiming medical malpractice.

Anesthesiologists are likely to face denial of MCO coverage of the cost of several different types of care initiated by anesthesiologists: desired diagnostic workup examinations (such as a cardiac echo) of worrisome preoperative findings, preoperative admissions to prepare chronically ill patients (such as a symptomatic asthmatic or chronic lung disease patient), invasive intraoperative monitoring (pulmonary artery catheter or TEE for a patient with severe arterial vascular disease and cardiac symptoms), postoperative admission to intensive care units (ICUs), and, particularly, postoperative admission to the hospital for monitoring and care of patients scheduled only for outpatient surgery. One step removed but involving similar ideas are peer review organizations (PROs), which seem to have evolved from guardians of the quality of care into watchdogs devoted almost exclusively to trying to limit the cost of health care services.[19]

Professional standards review organizations (PSROs) were established in 1972 as utilization review and QA overseers of the care of federally subsidized patients (Medicare and Medicaid). Despite their efforts to deal with quality of care, these groups largely were seen as being interested primarily in cost containment. A variety of negative factors led to the PSRO being replaced in 1984 with the PRO.[19] Each state has a PRO, most being associated with a state medical association. The objectives of a PRO include 14 statements related to hospital admissions (including the shifting of care to an outpatient basis as much as possible) and five related to quality of care (including the reduction of avoidable deaths and avoidable postoperative or other complications). The PROs comprise full-time support staff and physician reviewers paid as consultants or directors. Ideally, PRO monitoring will discover suboptimal care, and this will lead to specific recommendations for improvement in quality. There is a perception that the quality-of-care efforts are hampered by the lack of realistic objectives and that these PRO groups, like others before them, will largely or entirely function to limit the cost of health care services.[19] National physician groups such as the American Medical Association (AMA) are suspicious enough of the intentions of these groups to establish PRO monitoring programs.

Aside from the unrealized potential for quality improvement efforts, the most likely interaction between the local PRO and an anesthesia provider will involve a request for perioperative admission of a patient whose care is mandated to be outpatient surgery. This often is also an RM issue. For example, if the anesthesiologist believes that either preoperative admission for treatment to optimize cardiac, pulmonary, diabetic, or other medical status or postoperative admission for monitoring of labile situations such as uncontrolled hypertension will diminish clear anesthetic risk or risks for the patient, then an application to the PRO for approval of admission must be made and vigorously supported. All too often, however, such issues surface a day or two before the scheduled procedure in a preanesthesia screening clinic or even in a preoperative holding area outside the operating room on the day of surgery. This will continue to occur until anesthesiologists educate their surgeons about the types of associated medical conditions that may disqualify a proposed patient from the outpatient (ambulatory) surgical schedule. If adequate notice is given by the surgeon (e.g., at the time a case is scheduled for the operating room), the patient can be seen far enough in advance by an anesthesiologist to allow appropriate planning.

When the anesthesiologist first becomes aware of a patient with a complex medical problem 1 or 2 days preoperatively and some type of diagnostic or therapeutic intervention is indicated, the anesthesiologist can try to have the procedure postponed, if possible and reasonable, or he or she can undertake the time-consuming task of multiple telephone calls to obtain the surgeon's agreement and PRO approval and make the necessary arrangements. Because neither alternative is attractive, particularly from administrative and reimbursement perspectives, there may be a strong temptation to "let it slide" and try to deal with the patient as an outpatient even though this may be questionable from the RM viewpoint. Because anesthesia-related untoward outcome is generally rare, an adverse result is unlikely, yet the patient would be exposed to an avoidable risk. Because of both the workings of probability and the inevitable tendency to let progressively sicker patients slip by as the lax practitioners repeatedly "get away with it" and are lulled into a false sense of security, sooner or later an unfortunate outcome or preventable major complication or even death will occur.

The situation is even worse when the first contact with such a patient is immediately before the procedure on the day of surgery. There may be intense pressure from the patient, the surgeon, and even the operating room administrator and staff to proceed with a case for which the anesthesiologist believes the patient is poorly prepared, or even in danger. The arguments made regarding patient inconvenience and anxiety reflect valid concerns. However, these should not outweigh the best medical interests of the patient. Although this is a point in favor of evaluating all outpatients before the day of surgery, the anesthesiologist facing this situation on the day of operation should state clearly to all concerned the reasons for postponing the surgery, stressing the issue of avoidable risk, and then help with alternative arrangements (including dealing with the PRO, if necessary).

The other side of RM is that of liability exposure. Particularly regarding postoperative admission of ambulatory patients whose condition is unstable in some worrisome manner, it is an extremely poor defense against a malpractice claim to state that the patient was discharged home because the PRO deemed that operative procedure to be outpatient surgery. As bureaucratically annoying as it may be, it is a prudent RM strategy to admit the patient if any legitimate question exists, thus minimizing the chance for any complication, and later haggle with the PRO or the involved third-party payor, likely to be an HMO or an MCO with rigid cost-control protocols. Such situations are a classic application of the old idiom about a gram of prevention being worth a kilo of cure.

Inevitably, there will be frustration. However, the anesthesiologist must put the welfare of the patient first and push hard to do what is obviously reasonable. It is critical that the anesthesiologist scrupulously document all these efforts, even if they are denied by the MCO. Although not clearly established yet by legal precedents, this may help defend against any later negligence claim against the physician. These efforts to do what is clearly the right thing may even mean postponing a scheduled case (explaining the reasons to the irate surgeon, who also would be a defendant) or simply absorbing the cost of postoperative monitoring. Even though bad results are very rare, and almost always, one would probably "get away with it," anesthesiologists must not be pressured into doing what they know is unwise and even unsafe. In the event of an adverse outcome, there is no legal weight whatsoever in the defense of saying, "The HMO made me do what I knew was poor care (or even dangerous)."

The pervasive "production pressure" on anesthesiologists can degenerate into a form of economic credentialing: Anesthesiologists who seem to want too much preoperative diagnostic workup, are judged too slow between cases, or use too many expensive monitors and drugs may face loss of patients from an MCO or even privileges at a facility. Intense pressure to go fast, using as few people and resources as possible, will lead to cutting corners and danger to patients. Safe, reasonable care must prevail because citing, quoting, and even documenting this production pressure is no legal defense.

2. The credentialing process and clinical privileges. Most medical practitioners are scrupulously honest. Unfortunately, rare exceptions do occur. Cases have occurred in which physicians, nurses, or even untrained laypeople have forged credentials and lied on applications and in interviews and thus illegally obtained full licensure and privileges. Patients have been injured in a few extraordinary instances. Such cases have received widespread, often sensational publicity in the lay press and electronic media. Probably much less rarely, applicants for professional positions may have stretched the truth somewhat, either by exaggeration of past status and experience or by omitting key details with negative implications (such as investigations, license suspensions, major malpractice judgments, or even criminal prosecutions, including for patient abuse). Because of the few offenders with their widespread notoriety and because of the general rising expectations for the quality of care, the health care profession as a whole has significantly tightened up its credentialing procedures. With the radical changes in fundamental patient-doctor relationships in recent years, the pervasive public perception seems to be that the health care professionals are inadequately policed, particularly by their own mechanisms and organizations. Therefore intense public and political pressure has been placed on legislatures, regulatory and licensing agencies, and institutional administrators to identify fraudulent, criminal, and deviant health care providers and the incompetent or poor-quality practitioners who have frequent or severe enough poor results to attract attention. It is in this atmosphere that the RM implications become clear. It is reasonable to assume that the likelihood of complications will be less in the practice of those who are appropriately educated, trained, and experienced.

Unfortunately, it has become very important to consider legal doctrines such as vicarious liability and agency. Specific applicability varies from case to case and location to location. However, if an individual, group, or institution hires a practitioner or even simply approves a practitioner (as by securing or granting privileges), the individuals or institutions may be held liable along with that practitioner for the consequences of his or her actions. Of course, this is especially likely to be true if it is later discovered that something questionable in the offending practitioner's past had not come to light in the credentialing process. Accordingly, this process must be taken much more seriously than it was even a few years ago.

To the majority of practitioners who are completely honest, this emphasis on the credentialing process may seem annoying and unwieldy. Often it is inconvenient to have to arrange for transfer of certified copies of academic or training records from the distant past. However, the honest majority must recognize that such efforts are directed at protecting patients and the integrity of the profession. It is somewhat analogous to the annoyance caused by the metal detectors and baggage screening at airports, which are tolerated in the interest of the safety of all concerned.

a. Anesthesia department or group. Because of another type of legal case, some examples of which have been highly publicized, medical practitioners may be hesitant to give an honest evaluation (or even any evaluation at all) of people known to them who are seeking professional positions elsewhere. Obviously, someone writing a reference for a current or former co-worker should be honest. Adhering to clearly documentable facts is advisable. Stating a fact that is in the public record (such as a malpractice case lost at trial) does not justify an objection from the subject of the reference. Whether omitting such a fact is dishonest on the part of the reference writer is more uncertain. Including positive opinions and enthusiastic recommendations is no problem. Including facts that may be perceived as negative (such as the lost malpractice case and personal problems such as a history of treatment for substance abuse) and negative opinions are what some reference writers fear will provoke retaliatory lawsuits from the subject. As a result, many reference writers in these questionable situations confine their written material to brief and simple facts such as dates employed and position held.

Because a reference writer would not hesitate to include positive opinions, receipt of a reference that includes nothing more than dates worked and position held should raise suspicion that there may be more to the story. Receipt of such a reference about a person applying for a position should always lead to a telephone call (one that is not tape recorded by either party) to the writer. Such a telephone call may be advisable in all cases, regardless of what the written reference contains. Often, pertinent questions over the telephone can elicit much more candid information than might otherwise be available. In rare instances, there may be dishonesty through omission by the reference giver, even at this level. This may involve an individual, department or group, or institution that would like to get rid of the applicant. The applicant may have poor-quality practice, but the reference giver may be reluctant to approach licensing or disciplinary authorities (both because of the unpleasantness and out of concern about retaliatory legal action). The best way to avoid being victimized by this practice is to telephone an independent observer or source (such as a former employer or associate who no longer has a personal stake in the applicant's success) when any question exists. Because the ultimate goal is optimum patient care, the subjects applying for positions generally should not object to such calls being made. Discovery of a history of unsafe practices or of causing preventable anesthesia morbidity or mortality should raise doubts as to whether the applicant can be appropriately assigned, trained, and supervised to be maximally safe in the new environment.

All new personnel of all types in an anesthesia practice environment must be given a thorough orientation and checkout. Policy, procedures, and equipment may be unfamiliar to even the most thoroughly trained, experienced, and safe practitioner. This may occasionally seem tedious, but it is a critically important safety policy. A crisis situation caused by unfamiliarity with a new setting is not the optimal orientation session.

b. Hospital. Hospitals use checklists of requirements for the granting of medical staff privileges.[20,21] Verification of a valid license to practice, medical school graduation, residency training, board certification status, and prior disciplinary action is the responsibility of the hospital, facility, or institutional administrator or the medical staff executive department. Usually included, where applicable, are verification of prior hospital privileges and current malpractice insurance (often with minimum prescribed policy liability limits). Even though the state licensing mechanism should detect any discrepancies, it may be advisable for the institution to verify these basic credentials. Court decisions in which hospitals were found liable for negligence for failing to discover false statements on the application for privileges of a negligent physician[21] illustrate the hospital's key role in patient protection.

Many states now have reporting requirements that obligate health care facilities to inform the designated state authority (often the medical licensing body) of the occurrence of any of a list of circumstances involving practitioners. Certain major complications and adverse patient outcomes usually are included. Any peer review action, especially disciplinary findings and suspension, revocation, or modification of clinical privileges, along with knowledge of proved or suspected impairment, are always included. Obviously, in states with these laws, it is an integral component of the credentialing process (either granting or renewal of privileges) for the parties involved to check with the state mechanism for any relevant information concerning the applicant.

Potentially even more important is the National Practitioner Data Bank (NPDB). This federal mechanism is one of the responses to all the issues raised here. It is intended to prevent physicians from fleeing a series of adverse events in one state (or many states), concealing their history from another state's licensing authority, and then setting up shop in the new state. The NPDB depends on the reporting of information by all state licensing boards and all medical malpractice insurers. The information collected at the national level is available from the NPDB to peer review components of professional societies, health care facilities of all types, and state licensing boards and to plaintiffs' attorneys in certain limited circumstances involving claims against hospitals. This latter point is related in part to the fact that federal law requires hospitals to request information from the NPDB concerning each person appointed to the medical staff or granted clinical privileges. The states and the malpractice insurers report these types of information: indemnity payments made as a result of malpractice claims, adverse privilege actions taken by a health care entity, and licensure actions taken by state authorities. Practitioners themselves have the right to dispute the accuracy of entries in their NPDB files and to see their own files. In addition to the obvious RM benefits of hospitals checking this database as part of their credentialing process, it also will be wise for practitioners to verify that their own files are correct so as to prevent any inaccurate negative information from being circulated.

Periodic renewal of institutional clinical privileges also involves an obligation to evaluate and verify the competence of the subject practitioner. This process actually may be more important, albeit for different reasons, in the total scheme of health care delivery than the granting of initial privileges. However, renewals all too often are essentially automatic, receiving little attention and often depending solely on the department chairperson's recommendation. Again, statements on applications for renewal and any relevant peer review information must be checked judiciously. Groups of physicians or administrators responsible for evaluating hospital staff members and reviewing their privileges are appropriately concerned about retaliatory legal action by a staff member denied renewal. Such evaluating groups must be objective (with no political or financial motive) and as close to certain as possible, with documentation, that the staff person whose privileges would be revoked practices below standard and is a danger to patients. In such cases, evaluators are not only justified in revoking privileges, but obligated to do so or run the serious risk of being named additional codefendants in a subsequent malpractice action. Court decisions demonstrate that a hospital can be found liable if the incompetence of a staff member was known or should have been known and was not acted upon.[21] Furthermore, the hospital has an ethical obligation to protect the patients' best interests in such situations.

c. *State.* Specific requirements for medical licensing vary from state to state, but all states focus on the basic credentials of education, postgraduate training, and personal qualifications. For the reasons outlined earlier, more thorough verification of claimed credentials is performed. The inconvenience must be accepted as the cost of increased concern about the potential for harm from incompetent or dishonest practitioners.

A recent major development in state medical licensing is mandated continuing medical education (CME).[22,23] Many states specify the number of hours of CME credits that must be obtained, including distribution among categories. Documented CME credits within one's declared specialty may be mandated as well as specific requirements for study of RM and patient safety material. The effectiveness of such programs, especially as they relate to objective indices of patient care outcome, has not been evaluated thoroughly. An extension of this idea is the incipient movement to require current specialty

board certification as a condition of licensure. This proposal, however reasonable, seems unlikely to be adopted, even prospectively with a grandfather clause for those currently in practice.

Currently, the area of state involvement in RM issues receiving the most attention is discipline of incompetent, substance-dependent, and criminal physicians. Many states have reporting requirements specifying that any action taken against a practitioner by a group, department, or health care facility be reported to the state licensing or disciplining authority. In some circumstances, this would include discovery of or treatment for substance dependency. State boards often believe that an independent inquiry by an investigator not from the subject's own workplace can yield the most objective evaluation of fitness to practice. It is difficult to gauge the effectiveness of such efforts toward the laudable long-term goal of reducing preventable patient morbidity and mortality. However, in some cases, flagrantly unsafe practitioners have had medical licenses revoked. It is likely that state authorities will continue to increase activity in this area.

d. *Specialty boards and societies.* Of the 23 recognized medical specialty boards, 20 (as of this writing) require some type of periodic recertification of their diplomates. Many recertification programs are fairly new, such as the American College of Surgeons, which conducted its first examination in 1987, and it will likely be some time before a successful attempt is made to assess the impact of such programs on the quality of care or on patient care outcome. The American Board of Anesthesiology (ABA) has joined the majority of specialty boards in implementing formal recertification. For certifications earned before the year 2000, the original certification is considered permanent. For anesthesiologists who become board certified after 1999, their certificates will be valid for 10 years, and then the anesthesiologist is expected to take the recertifying examination. Any anesthesiologist certified before the year 2000 can voluntarily apply and take the new recertifying examination, earning a recertification certificate good for 10 years. Interestingly, the ABA is requiring that all oral board examiners be recertified.

Several specialty societies require relevant CME participation.[22,23] Although the American Society of Anesthesiologists (ASA) offers many extensive CME activities (some directly concerning RM), there is no formal requirement for participation as a condition of membership.

One extremely valuable program available through many state societies of anesthesiology and sometimes involving the ASA is the peer review assessment of an anesthesia group or department. When there are significant RM questions, a group or department may seek (or even be advised to seek) external input and advice from an objective team of volunteer peer reviewers sponsored by the appropriate professional society. In such cases, the suggestions from such a team (offered in a noncritical, nonthreatening manner) can help initiate or enhance RM activities.

e. Clinical privileges. The credentialing process leads ultimately to the granting of initial or renewal clinical privileges to practice in a given setting. The privilege-granting entity or person in a hospital (or facility with anesthesia services) almost always cannot fully evaluate the clinical credentials of an applicant for privileges in anesthesia and must rely on anesthesiologists, usually internal but sometimes outside the institution, for evaluation of clinical competence. How should this evaluation be made? The potential pitfalls of references were mentioned earlier. However, if an evaluator personally knows a co-worker or supervisor of an applicant, a judicious inquiry should produce valuable information. In the absence of this type of inside contact, questions often arise as how best to be certain of an applicant's competence. Most institutions have a mechanism of granting provisional privileges for some trial period, during which the clinical practice of the applicant is observed firsthand before a final decision on granting privileges is made. Before any offer of a position is extended, some institutions now ask an applicant to visit for a day or longer to assume the role of a trainee and render clinical care under the immediate, direct, one-to-one supervision of an evaluating staff member. The value of such programs remains to be seen.

A central issue today in the granting of clinical privileges, especially in procedure-oriented specialties, is whether to continue the common practice of approving blanket privileges. In effect, these privileges authorize the practitioner to attempt any treatment or procedure normally considered in the province of the applicant's medical specialty. Questions surrounding these considerations may have political and economic implications, such as which type of surgeon should be performing carotid endarterectomies or lumbar diskectomies. More important, however, is whether the practitioner being considered is really qualified to do everything covered by his or her specialty. Specifically, should the granting of privileges to practice anesthesia automatically approve the practitioner to handle pediatric cardiac cases, critically ill newborns (such as a 2-day-old baby with a diaphragmatic hernia), ablative pain therapy (such as an alcohol celiac plexus block under fluoroscopy), or high-risk obstetric cases? These questions raise the issue of procedure-specific or limited privileges. The RM considerations in this question are strong if practitioners who are not qualified or experienced enough are allowed, or even expected because of peer or scheduling pressures, to undertake major challenges for which they are not prepared. The likelihood of complications is increased, and the difficulty of defending the practitioner against a malpractice claim in the event of a catastrophe is significantly increased.

No clear answer is evident on the question of procedure-specific privileges. Ignoring issues of qualifications has clear negative potential. On the other hand, total adoption of such a system would soon result in an anesthesia department or group divided into many small "fiefdoms," with consequent atrophy of clinical skills outside one's specific area or areas. This is stifling for the practitioner and a disservice to the profession and its future. Each anesthesia department or group must address these issues. At the very least, the common practice of every applicant for new or renewal privileges checking off every line on the printed list of anesthesia procedures should be reviewed.

3. Policy, procedures, and standards of practice. Developing written policies and procedures often is perceived by medical practitioners as bureaucratic drudgery. This perception is less likely to be true for a practitioner who has turned to a detailed, carefully thought-out procedure manual during an actual or impending emergency and found the necessary information to approach a problem or even prevent an untoward outcome. The Joint Commission on Accreditation of Healthcare Organizations (JCAHO) requires a policy and procedure manual for anesthesia services within a hospital,[24] but this requirement should not be the driving force behind a potentially useful compendium.

a. Policy and procedure manuals. The first benefit of creating or updating a policy and procedure manual is that it forces the writers to focus on the topics. Multiple examples are possible, but all anesthesiologists are probably aware of at least one instance in which some long-standing routine in a hospital ("That's the way we've always done it") was finally reviewed as a manual was being updated for an impending JCAHO visit. The routine was found to be not only badly out of date and possibly inappropriate but also potentially dangerous. After the routine was changed, all involved noted the improvement and stated that the old way was "an accident waiting to happen." Such reviews should occur whenever needed but should be done at least annually and then particularly thoroughly every 3 years.

The major purpose of having such a written manual is to provide an instantly available source of suggestions, guidelines, recommendations, and standards for both the technical skills and the professional conduct of anesthesia practitioners. The necessary caveats remain that specific circumstances differ, and the involved practitioners will apply their judgment to the outlines provided in the manual.

A policy and procedure manual could probably include many examples of topics.[25] Combining these with an overview of the intended procedure, the manual logically is divided into two parts: organizational and procedural.

Included in the organizational component is the delineation of privileges and responsibilities of and expectations for all involved personnel: the chief or director of anesthesia, the clinical director (if different), deputy or division directors, attending staff physicians, resident and fellow physicians, other trainees, certified registered nurse anesthetists, physician assistants, monitoring technicians, equipment engineers or technicians, perfusionists, respiratory therapists, chest therapists, and any others. Immediately associated with this list should be a communications section with the verified addresses, telephone and pager numbers, and details of how to reach all personnel associated with the group or department. The intent is to minimize difficulty when help is being sought. Critically important is the delineation of call responsibilities (not a call schedule), a detailed list of what is expected of a staff member on one of the various levels of call with regard to presence in the institution at what hours, the telephone availability, pager availability, maximum permissible distance from the institution, and so on. Also included are the expectations from each call person. It is vital to have all such duties spelled out clearly, prospectively, in writing. Unfortunately, this factor often becomes a key element in the aftermath of an accident in which, it is charged, the appropriate personnel were not available or could not be found, particularly in the situation of a practice covering multiple hospitals with multiple persons on call and confusion as to precisely who must respond. The RM implications are clear: Qualified help should be available through an agreed-upon mechanism, which will help optimize care and reduce complications, and it would be extraordinarily unfortunate after a catastrophe for members of a department or group to be pointing fingers at each other, trying to shift responsibility for the emergency call that was not answered.

Also included in the organizational component of policy and procedure is a clear explanation of the orientation and checkout procedure for new personnel, CME requirements and opportunities, mechanism of evaluation of all personnel and of communication of this evaluation to them, disaster plans (or reference to a separate disaster manual or protocol), QA activities including membership of any standing committees responsible, and the format for statistical record keeping (number of procedures, types of anesthetics given, types of patients anesthetized, number and type of invasive monitoring, number and type of responses to emergency calls, and so on).

The procedural component of policy and procedure gives specific outlines of proposed courses of action for particular circumstances. Often there are copies of, references to, or paraphrases of the statements, guidelines, and standards appearing in the back of the ASA Directory of Members. Also included are references to or specific protocols for the areas mentioned in the JCAHO standards[24]: preanesthetic evaluation, immediate preinduction reevaluation, safety of the patient during the anesthetic period, release of the patient from any postanesthesia care unit (PACU), recording of all pertinent events during anesthesia, recording of postanesthesia visits, guidelines defining the role of anesthesia services in hospital infection control, and guidelines for safe use of general anesthetic agents. In addition, a partial list of other appropriate topics includes the following:

- Recommendations for preanesthesia apparatus checkout, as from the U.S. Food and Drug Administration (FDA)
- Guidelines for minimal monitoring (infant, child, adult, in the PACU)
- Procedure for transport of patients to the operating room, to the PACU, to the ICU
- Policy on ambulatory surgical patients (screening, use of regional anesthesia, discharge home)
- Policy on same-day admissions

- Policy on recovery room admission and discharge, including protocols and criteria
- Policy on ICU admission and discharge
- Policy on physicians responsible for writing orders in the PACU and the ICU
- Policy on informed consent
- Policy on the participation of patients in clinical research
- Guidelines for the support of cadaver organ donors and its termination
- Guidelines on environmental safety, including pollution with trace gases and electrical equipment inspection, maintenance, and hazard prevention
- Procedure for exchanging personnel during an anesthetic
- Procedure for the introduction of new equipment, drugs, or clinical practices
- Procedure for epidural and spinal opioid administration and subsequent patient monitoring (such as type, minimum time)
- Procedure for initial treatment of cardiac or respiratory arrest
- Policy on a patient's refusal of blood or blood products, including the mechanism to obtain a court order to transfuse
- Procedure for the management of malignant hyperthermia
- Procedure for the induction and maintenance of barbiturate coma
- Procedure for evaluation of suspected pseudocholinesterase deficiency

Individual departments or groups will add to the aforementioned suggestions as dictated by their specific needs. A thorough, carefully conceived policy and procedure manual is a valuable RM tool. Many of the components are intended to mandate or encourage practices that will prevent untoward events (such as unfamiliarity with a new anesthesia machine when called for an emergency case), help the management of crisis (such as malignant hyperthermia), and encourage communication in difficult situations (such as refusal of blood). Ideally, each staff member of a group or department would review the manual at least annually and sign off in a log indicating current familiarity with the policies and procedures.

b. Standards of practice. Many elements of policy and procedure could be considered local standards of practice. Some institutions actively avoid the term *standards* because of the potential medicolegal implications, especially if an untoward outcome occurs from practices carried out in a manner other than that contained in the policy and procedure manual. The medicolegal importance of the standard of care tends to reinforce the perception that, once promulgated, standards may dictate mandatory practice. Some departments deliberately promote this perception as part of RM efforts. As detailed earlier, the Harvard Medical School developed standards of practice for minimal intraoperative monitoring for its nine component hospital departments[5] and labeled them *standards* specifically to emphasize that the practices are perceived as so important as to be mandatory. The same type of thinking was involved when the ASA adopted as national policy "Standards for Basic Intra-operative Monitoring," which includes specifications for the presence of personnel during anesthetic administration and for continual evaluation of oxygenation, ventilation, circulation, and temperature.[25] Similarly, several other areas of anesthesia practice are covered by subsequent ASA standards.[25]

The minimal monitoring standards, for example, are process standards in that they prescribe actions and are met by carrying out these actions. At various levels (hospital, local, state, national), additional efforts at improving patient care are leading to promulgation of process standards or mandatory regulations. One of the more detailed examples is the body of regulations issued by the New Jersey State Department of Health in 1989.[26]

Another type of standard is that for outcome. Hypothetical examples include the statements that "the number of patients experiencing myocardial infarction intraoperatively or within 24 hours of operation should not exceed 0.5% of those anesthetized," or "the number of ambulatory surgical patients experiencing unplanned admission to the hospital for reasons related to the anesthesia should not exceed 1.0% of the outpatients anesthetized." Regulatory and accrediting agencies are moving toward the imposition of such standards. The JCAHO has gone through several versions of a proposed list of outcome indicators for anesthesia care. The overall intention is to encourage the identification of clinical practices that lead to adverse outcomes and their replacement with alternatives that will lead to meeting the standards. If realized, this sequence of events should have the additional RM benefit of reducing preventable morbidity and mortality.

4. Equipment: maintenance and records. Compared with human error, overt equipment failure is rare as a cause of critical incidents during anesthesia[9] or anesthesia-associated deaths,[27] although anesthesia apparatus problems have been well studied.[28-30] A widespread belief is that most equipment-related problems in anesthesia (aside from clear human error such as misuse or unfamiliarity) could be prevented by correct maintenance and servicing of the apparatus.

When there is a major equipment failure that, if undetected, would lead to patient harm, the monitoring procedures outlined in the preceding section should detect the development of an untoward situation. If one assumes an appropriate response from the anesthetist (which may even mean completely detaching the patient from the anesthetic-delivery system and ventilator and ventilating with a hand resuscitator bag until a new anesthesia machine can be secured), any adverse outcome to the patient should be avoided. However, occasionally, a patient is injured from equipment failure. Therefore efforts to minimize these equipment failures must be continued and even increased.

An excellent summary of a complete program for anesthesia equipment maintenance and service has been published.[31] A distinction is made between failure attributable to progressive deterioration of equipment, which should be preventable because it is observable and prompts appropriate action, and catastrophic failure, which often is not practical to try to predict. Emphasis is placed on preventive maintenance for mechanical parts and involves periodic performance checks every 4 to 6 months. Also provided is an annual safety inspection of each anesthetizing location covering 49 points and including the surrounding area and the immediate location, as well as the equipment itself. For equipment service, a description of a cross-reference system identifies the piece requiring service and the mechanism to secure the needed repair.

The general principles of equipment handling are straightforward. Before purchasing, the buyer must verify that a proposed piece of equipment meets all applicable standards, which usually is true for new equipment purchased directly from recognized major manufacturers. Stringent cost-containment measures may lead institutions or practices to consider purchasing used anesthesia equipment, and several dealers and brokers have established businesses for this purpose. Clearly, an extra measure of caution is required, particularly evaluating the age of used equipment and ensuring that it has the features that are considered mandatory by standard-setting agencies (e.g., vaporizer lockout and oxygen–nitrous oxide ratio protection devices on anesthesia machines).

On arrival at an institution, electrical equipment must be checked for absence of hazard (especially leakage current) and compliance with applicable electrical standards. Complex equipment, such as anesthesia machines and ventilators, should be assembled and checked out by a representative from the manufacturer or manufacturer's agent. There are potential adverse medicolegal implications of untrained personnel certifying a particular piece of equipment as functioning within specifications, even if they do it perfectly. It is also important to involve the representative, if necessary, in preservice and in-service training for those who will use the new equipment. Also, a sheet or section in the master equipment log must be created with the make, model, serial number, and in-house identification for each individual piece of capital equipment (anything with a serial number). This record not only allows immediate identification of any equipment involved in a future recall or product alert but also serves as the permanent repository of the record of every problem, problem resolution, maintenance, and servicing occurring until that particular piece is scrapped. This log must be kept up to date at all times. There have been rare but frightening examples of potentially lethal problems with anesthesia machines leading to product-alert notices requiring immediate identification of certain equipment and its service status.

The question of who should maintain and service anesthesia equipment has been widely debated and has significant RM implications. Some groups or departments rely on factory service representatives for all attention to capital equipment, whereas others engage independent service contractors, and still other (usually larger) departments have access to engineers or technicians in their institutions, their own departments, or a separate bioengineering or medical engineering department within the facility. Needs and resources differ. The single underlying tenet is simple: The person doing preventive maintenance and service must be qualified. Anesthesia practitioners may wonder how they can assess qualification. The best way is to unhesitatingly ask pertinent questions about the education, training, and experience of those involved, including asking for references and speaking to supervisors and managers responsible for those doing the work. Whether an engineering technician who spent a week at a course at a factory can perform the most complex repairs depends on a variety of factors that can be investigated by the practitioners ultimately using the equipment. Failure to be involved in this investigation exposes the practitioner to increased liability in the event of an untoward outcome associated with improperly maintained or serviced equipment.

Aside from preventive maintenance and servicing, adequate day-to-day clinical maintenance of equipment must be performed. In this era of emphasis on cost containment, anesthesia technicians are a popular target for budget cutters. It is false economy to reduce these personnel below the number needed to retrieve, clean, sort, disassemble, sterilize, reassemble, store, and distribute the equipment of daily anesthesia practice. Inadequate service in this area truly creates an accident waiting to happen. An improperly installed canister of carbon dioxide absorbent (e.g., a disposable canister placed in the absorber head still encased in the original plastic wrap, completely obstructing the flow of gas through the low-pressure side of the anesthesia machine) is only one of many possible sources of potential danger resulting from inadequate routine technical support.

Another difficult problem arises when anesthesia equipment becomes obsolete and should be replaced. Replacement of obsolete anesthesia machines and monitoring equipment is a key element of a risk modification program. Ten years has been cited as one estimate of the useful life of an anesthesia machine. Certainly, anesthesia machines exceeding 10 years of age may not meet the safety standards now in force for new machines and do not incorporate the new technology that advanced rapidly during the late 1980s and early to mid-1990s, much of which was intended to prevent untoward patient care incidents. Furthermore, such technology will most likely continue to advance at the same or even an accelerated rate in the future. To minimize their own potential liability, some anesthesia equipment manufacturers have refused to support (with parts and service) some of the oldest of their pieces (particularly gas machines) still in use. This reaction sends a strong message to practitioners that such equipment must be replaced as soon as possible.

If equipment fails, it must be removed from service and a replacement substituted. Groups or departments of anesthesia providers and the facilities in which they practice must have sufficient backup equipment to cover any reasonable incidence of failure. The equipment re-moved from service must be marked with a prominent label (so it is not mistakenly returned into service) containing the date, time, person discovering, and the details of the problem. The responsible personnel must be notified so that they can remove the equipment, make an entry in the log, and initiate the repair. As indicated later in the section on response to an adverse event, a piece of equipment involved or suspected in an anesthesia accident must be sequestered immediately and not touched by anybody, particularly not by any equipment service personnel. If a severe accident occurred, it may be necessary for the equipment in question to be inspected at a specific later time by a group of qualified representatives of the manufacturer, the service personnel, the plaintiff's attorney, the insurance companies involved, and the practitioner's defense attorney. Also, major equipment problems should be reported to the Medical Device Problem Reporting System of the U.S. FDA via the Device Experience Network (telephone 1-800-638-6725).[32] This system accepts voluntary reports from users and requires reports from manufacturers when there is knowledge of a medical device being involved in a serious incident. Application of all the principles outlined here should help minimize or even prevent equipment-related adverse outcomes of anesthesia.

5. Informed consent. It is a clear, underlying principle that every patient has the right to exercise control over his or her own body and must therefore consent to proposed treatments or procedures.[20] The issue of treatment in the absence of any consent at all (for whatever reason, but usually because of gross misunderstandings) involves potential claims by the patient of assault and battery. This is relatively rare and less likely to involve anesthesia providers than the issue of informed consent does. Informed consent is obtained by a discussion of the potential risks and benefits of a proposed treatment or procedure and any available alternatives and then ascertainment that the patient (or the patient's agent in the case of a child or an incompetent person) understands and agrees to what is being proposed.

There may still be some residual debate as to whether a separate informed consent is needed for the anesthesia for a planned surgical operation or whether consent to the operation implies consent for the anesthesia. In most centers now, anesthesia providers obtain a separate informed consent because wholly separate identifiable material risks are associated with the anesthetic independent of the surgery. It is inadequate to expect the surgeon to fully discuss the anesthetic and, particularly, any special implications for anesthesia of the patient's medical condition. Anesthesia providers do not perform surgery and cannot obtain a genuine informed surgical consent. Likewise, the surgeons are not anesthesiologists and simply do not have the training and experience to discuss the plans and risks of the anesthesia care.

In obtaining informed consent for anesthesia, the question arises as to what risks should be disclosed to the patient during the discussion. There must be a balance between giving enough information to allow a reasoned decision and frightening the patient with a long list of potential, extremely rare, severe complications, the latter making a trusting doctor-patient working relationship difficult. In the past, the standard was disclosure of risks that any reasonable physician would believe appropriate. This doctrine has been altered significantly over time to involve the "reasonable person" (patient) and now centers on the concept of material risk. A material risk "is one that the physician knows or ought to know would be significant to a reasonable person in the patient's position of deciding whether or not to submit to a particular medical treatment or procedure."[20] The landmark *Harnish* decision[33] stated that all risks must be disclosed to the patient in order to obtain informed consent. The equally important subsequent *Precourt* decision[34] added the qualification that there need not be disclosure of every conceivable, remotely possible complication of which severity or incidence is negligible. The decision stressed balancing the patient's right to know with fairness to physicians and avoiding "unrealistic and unnecessary burdens on practitioners."[35]

When the issue of informed consent for anesthesia arises, it usually involves questions about the occurrence of rare but devastating complications, such as severe neurologic damage or death. Whether the risk of these complications is considered negligible in a legal context remains to be determined. Therefore no firm guideline has been set as to whether it is wise to tell all patients that general anesthesia might lead to anoxic brain damage or death or that regional anesthesia could cause permanent paralysis. However, it is possible to state that all anesthesia procedures have some risks, including risks of injury and death, just like riding in a car or crossing the street. Most patients can identify with this analogy and are not threatened by it. Of course, questions about specific complications prompted by this statement should be answered. Statistics can be cited to give perspective. Again, patients understand when told that the risk of death or grave injury from an anesthetic for a healthy patient is far, far less than that from riding in an automobile during the normal course of a year. Any special risks attendant to the patient's medical or surgical condition should be discussed in more detail.

Consent is a state of mind achieved through the establishment of an understanding. It is not an act, such as the signing of one's name. Many anesthesia practitioners ask patients to sign a consent form that often includes a long list of potential complications and any specific additional risks for that particular patient. This is an accepted, reasonable practice. However, both the anesthetist and the patient must understand that no matter what the form says, it does not release the anesthetist from liability. The form is one way to document that an informed consent discussion took place, but it does not limit the patient's right to later make a claim in the event of an accident. Whether the form is used, a note is written out in the patient's chart, or both, there must be a clear record (created after the discussion) that a discussion took place and that informed consent was obtained. Verbal consent alone is not enough.

In certain life-threatening emergency circumstances, it may be necessary to administer anesthesia without consent. Case law recognizes this need, and the requirements outlined here are necessarily modified. In such an event, it is advisable to write a note in the chart as soon as possible about the necessity to go ahead and to notify the hospital administrator or counsel, or both, about the situation.

Obtaining genuine informed consent must not be a perfunctory bureaucratic irritation. It is an integral component of the anesthetist-patient relationship and forces discussion of important issues. Furthermore, today it is common for plaintiffs' attorneys to charge lack of informed consent in virtually any case of an unexpected poor patient outcome. Although the charge cannot be avoided, careful attention to the principles detailed here should eliminate concerns about inadequate informed consent for anesthesia care.

6. Record keeping. It would be difficult to begin to count the number of anesthesia malpractice cases that have been lost, even when there probably was no malpractice, because of inadequate, incomplete, or illegible anesthesia records. The anesthesia chart is the cornerstone of all information about an anesthetic case for RM purposes. The old dictum "If you didn't write it down, it didn't happen" is still applicable in a medicolegal sense. Even the best anesthetic care cannot be defended, or even referred to, if there is no clear record that such care took place. "If the record hardly exists . . . it is tantamount to an outright confession, in the eyes of the law, to careless practice."[36]

Documentation of the preanesthetic evaluation is all too often weak or inadequate in cases of malpractice claims against anesthesiologists. The guiding principles regarding what should be recorded are simple. The practitioner should document all the information necessary for another anesthesia provider to pick up the chart and quickly obtain a complete enough picture to safely and intelligently conduct the anesthetic. One good way to think of it is for the anesthesiologist doing the evaluation to project himself or herself into the role of picking up the chart and then include everything he or she would want to see. Furthermore, the preoperative evaluation should contain some evidence of the thinking associated with the evaluation. Assigning an ASA Physical Status value is a start. Recording any unusual or dangerous conditions and how these influence plans and risks is mandatory. In all cases, some type of statement about the anesthetic plan (or possible alternatives if the plan is not final, which is probably best if the person doing the preoperative evaluation is not going to be administering the anesthetic) is necessary. Again, it is unfortunate but true that the best possible care may not appear so in the record without some appropriate effort to document what went into that care. Even when thorough notes are written, they are of no help if they cannot be read. All notes must be dated and timed and made as legible as humanly possible.

A helpful review of the reasoning behind and the elements of the intraoperative anesthesia record[37] cites a study in which 95% of respondent anesthetists believed it important to keep anesthetic records and 74% included medicolegal protection among the reasons given for doing so. Aside from the potential legal uses, an excellent way of approaching the record is to try to do two things: Create a legible record of all pertinent events (required by JCAHO)[24] and have a compendium of all the salient features (history, allergies, chronic medications, acute medications, positioning, monitoring used, reasons for special monitoring, events, and the patient's responses to these and all factors) in as complete a manner as you would like to see them were you to be the next person, new to the patient, to give anesthesia. Virtually all facilities in which anesthesia is given have a preprinted form for accomplishing these goals. It must be legible, be as easy as possible to use, encourage completeness, and be reviewed frequently by those using it to see whether revision would improve it.

Electronic devices can be used in the maintenance of intraoperative anesthesia records. Noninvasive or invasive monitors may be connected to these computers so that vital signs, fractional inspired oxygen, expired volume and ventilation rate, arterial oxygen saturation, end-tidal CO_2, and, on some machines, volatile agent monitoring information are automatically recorded (with no possibility to edit in most models) at preset time intervals. Sensors that would automatically record gas flows, vaporizer settings, and infusions used are being developed. Other drugs and fluids given, blood lost, and events noted can be keyed in by the anesthetist (although alternatives such as a bar code reader, light pen, or even voice could be used). The computerized anesthesia record will automatically record the time of the entry, even if its operator states in the entry that an event or action took place at a different time. Studies on the efficacy and desirability of these automated records are under way. Proponents state that the technology allows more time to focus on the patient and that a genuinely complete record will give a truer picture of events and trends that should aid in evaluation of poor outcome, usually by demonstrating the absence of untoward intraoperative events and the wide range of normal vital signs that often is "smoothed out" on handwritten records. However, others state that automatic sampling may miss trends by picking up and recording transient major variations and even may record erroneous, grossly incorrect values caused by mechanical or electrical artifact, thus exposing the anesthesiologist to unjustified charges in the event of a poor outcome. Artifact rejection algorithms definitely have improved and continue to be an active area of research. Acceptance and use of the automated electronic anesthesia record will depend on the resolution of this typical risk-benefit ratio question and the ability to justify the significant capital cost of these instruments. Early enthusiasm by some practitioners for this technology was dampened by the ferocious cost-limiting and cost-reduction programs imposed by almost all health care facilities in the last few years. Proving an incremental financial benefit to justify the significant capital and maintenance costs of computerized anesthesia records is an ongoing issue that will continue to limit adoption of this technology.

In the use of any record keeping method for any anesthetic, a few basics are always true. Medications and vital signs should be recorded contemporaneously and should be entered first when there are many things to record, such as immediately after induction. Descriptive information, important as it is, can wait a moment. During the maintenance phase of the anesthetic, vital signs should be recorded at least every 5 minutes. Numeric values from instruments such as the pulse oximeter, capnograph, spirometer, mass spectrometer, and any other monitoring devices should be recorded at appropriate intervals. It is inadequate to note only that these or other devices were used. The generated information must be recorded both for reference (during or after the case) and to prove that the anesthetist was aware of what transpired during the anesthetic usage. Some routine patient monitors have a memory function that may or may not have printing abilities. It is important that practitioners know whether this is true for the particular monitor they are using. If the monitor has such a function and there is a questionable or overt untoward event and no effort is made to retrieve information from the memory function of the monitor, the practitioner faces an additional charge of suppression of relevant data that bears on any subsequent claim of malpractice. Particularly with the machines that can make a printout at the end of a case, debates within anesthesiology groups have occurred about the desirability or wisdom of generating such a printout and attaching it to the anesthesia record. Because in the majority of cases there is no problem, some practitioners argue that making a printout is superfluous, hence the emphasis on the ability to retrieve information when there is a patient care question. An experienced malpractice defense attorney would say in private that he wants that information if it strengthens his case and does not want it if the converse might be true. It is likely that having the information from the monitor's memory will be valuable no matter what it is because this detailed objective information can help point the way in planning a response to a charge of intraoperative anesthesia malpractice.

Postoperative documentation is critical in anesthesia RM. Aside from the fact that it is a JCAHO requirement to see patients in follow-up observation, it is simply good anesthesia care. It also broadens and deepens the relationship with the patient, which is necessarily transient, thus making less likely misunderstanding or misplaced hostility about the outcome of the surgery. Leaving a positive impression can be the key element in avoiding being named a codefendant in a malpractice action against the surgeon. More important, however, is the opportunity to discover any complications or issues with the patient. Most of these are minor and can be dealt with on the spot, thus eliminating any chance that they will grow out of proportion if neglected. It is reasonable to ask the patients what they remember about the operative experience (not directly whether they had recall during general anesthesia), whether they were hoarse, and whether the intravenous catheter and other equipment hurt, while also examining the chart and patient for more serious problems. Obviously, the patient's responses should be entered into a postoperative note along with some comment about current status (always including vital signs) and the anesthetist's assessment, such as "No apparent postanesthetic complications. Appears to be doing well."

If there is an adverse event, with or even without patient injury, a complete account of the facts and, when appropriate, an extremely careful outline of impressions and opinions should go on the chart as soon as possible. One important caution is that the entry thus made must not be influenced by the heat of the moment, guilt, the desire to imply blame or innocence on the part of any person, or the general disorganization that may accompany a significant event. It may be wise for one to seek advice from an objective person, perhaps a co-worker not involved in the case, while recording the account of the event. Great care is required in composing this summary note after an event involving potential or actual patient injury because that note will be scrutinized as intensely as if under a microscope for years to come. The single most important thing in all such cases is to never change the existing record. No matter what is on it, the actual record is better than an altered one. However excellent the anesthetic care may have been, alteration of an existing record guarantees the complete inability to defend against any charges, however unjustified they might be. If there is a need to explain, elaborate on, or fill in gaps in the record, it should be done as soon as practical by a dated and timed amendment note in the patient chart. Obviously, the contents of such a note must be thought out carefully. It may be advantageous for this note to be written in the presence of a genuinely objective witness.

Additional benefits in RM efforts accrue from complete and legible anesthetic records. Some of the necessary and desirable activities of RM and QA depend on the ability to retrieve and compile data about the anesthetic practice of both individuals and a group or department.

7. Meaningful morbidity and mortality conferences and continuing education. The JCAHO has a general requirement for all departments in a medical facility that there must be at least monthly meetings at which RM and QA activities are documented and reported. Most anesthesia departments, services, and groups have staff meetings, departmental conferences, or rounds at least monthly and use those occasions to satisfy the JCAHO meeting requirements. It is likely that some of these meetings satisfy the letter but not the spirit of the requirement. Presentations of departmental cases of unusual interest or cases in which there was a problem, followed by a thorough group review and discussion of the popular question, "What would you do differently next time?" are a good start. Likewise, staff meetings at which policy, procedure, equipment, and any associated problems are discussed also help. Inclusion of an open review of departmental statistics, including all complications, however trivial seeming, brings the effort closer to the intention of the requirement.

All the suggestions for meetings (whether called case conference presentations, morbidity and mortality rounds, or whatever) are intended to encourage a group of anesthesia providers to combine their thoughts and efforts for the common good: the minimization of untoward outcomes in their anesthesia practice. This is an opportunity for application of the classic RM process, in that future practice should be improved when the participants learn from present experience (failures and successes). The goal of minimizing future complications is obvious. Rapid devolution of a conference into a business meeting or pro forma meetings hurried through by a small fraction of the staff benefit no one and waste time. A case presentation needs interactive discussion to genuinely educate.

Formal CME must be approached with the same thoughtfulness to contribute to the quality of care and the avoidance of complications. Larger groups and departments usually run their own programs, using staff members to speak about areas of their interest and expertise and bringing in outside speakers to present reviews of basic material or news of recent developments or ongoing research. By no means should all the presentations deal directly with anesthesia. Not only could this get tedious for even the most committed audience, but also anesthesiologists need updated awareness of both the basics and the forefront of many other medical disciplines. Such meetings are excellent opportunities for surgeons to tell of advancements in their techniques. At the same time, there can be a give-and-take discussion regarding the interrelationship of anesthesia and the surgery in question. Allowing surgeon and anesthetist to see a situation from each other's perspective can only encourage beneficial cooperation.

Smaller departments or groups need to make deliberate efforts to ensure adequate opportunity for continuing education. This might involve securing access to an accredited CME program conducted by a large medical school department and then guaranteeing sufficient time for staff to participate. Also, an additional method involves providing time and in some circumstances financial support for staff to attend local, regional, or national CME programs (either specific workshops, symposia, and theme meetings or the CME components of professional society meetings). Most CME requirements for licensing or certification include some acknowledgment of individual reading. Every department, service, or group, regardless of size, needs a library facility of some sort, containing as many current textbooks, manuals, and journals as is practical for the number of people involved.

8. Response to an adverse event. Despite rigorous application of RM principles, it is likely that each anesthesiologist at least once in his or her professional life will be involved in a major anesthesia accident. Precisely because such an event is so rare, few are prepared for it. It is probable that the involved personnel will have no relevant experience. Although an obvious resource is a colleague who has had some exposure or experience, one may not be available.

The basic outline of an appropriate immediate response to an accident is straightforward and logical and has been outlined in detail.[38] Unfortunately, the principal personnel involved in a significant untoward event may react with such surprise or shock as to temporarily lose sight of logic. There have been cases of major accidents in an operating room in which the responsible anesthesiologist was so stunned on realizing what had happened that he or she became nonfunctional or, worse, left the room before help arrived.

At the moment anyone recognizes that a major anesthetic complication has occurred or is occurring, help must be called. A sufficient number of people to deal with the situation must be secured as quickly as possible. For example, if an esophageal intubation goes unrecognized long enough during the induction of general anesthesia to cause a cardiac arrest, the immediate need is for enough skilled personnel to conduct the resuscitative efforts, including making the correct diagnosis and replacing the tube into the trachea. Whether the anesthesiologist apparently responsible for the complication should direct the immediate remedial efforts depends on the person and the situation. In such a circumstance, it seems wise for a senior or supervising anesthesiologist to quickly evaluate the appropriateness of the behavior and actions of the involved party or parties and decide whether he, she, or they should be asked to step back and allow one of the responding personnel to give remedial care. Even in the heat of the moment, tact must be exercised.

In general, the primary anesthesia provider or providers should concentrate on continuing patient care. The anesthesiologist responsible for supervision of activities in that clinical area, having responded to the call for help, will become the incident supervisor. This person becomes responsible for administrative and investigative activities while the primary anesthesia provider or providers and others (as needed) care for the patient. The supervisor directs the process of immediate prevention of recurrence of the problem, event documentation, and ongoing investigation.

The primary anesthesia provider and any others involved must document relevant information. Never change any existing entries in the medical record. Write an amendment note if needed with careful explanation of why amendment is necessary, particularly stressing explanations of professional judgments involved. State only facts as they are known. Make no judgments about causes or responsibility. The same guidelines hold true for the filing of the incident report in the facility, which should be done as soon as is practical. Furthermore, all discussions with the patient or family should be documented carefully in the medical record.

In all circumstances, anesthesia equipment and supplies in use at the time of the untoward event, whether or not believed to be materially involved, should be sequestered under lock and key. Nothing can be altered or discarded. Equipment support personnel should be enlisted in this effort. There may be reluctance, for example, to take an anesthesia machine out of service. However, this type of action is mandatory until it is agreed upon by all involved that the equipment is not material to the accident investigation and can be inspected and returned to service or that it is material and plans are made for further investigation. A great many anesthesia malpractice cases have been lost because no one thought in time to save the endotracheal tube that was plugged with thick secretions, thus causing the impaired ventilation.

Immediately after a nonfatal accident, comprehensive evaluation and care of the patient should be carried out quickly and efficiently. Measures may be instituted to help limit anoxic brain damage. Close association and communication with the surgeon at that time and throughout subsequent events should be valuable. Furthermore, do not hesitate to call consultants immediately. Often a cardiologist, neurologist, neurosurgeon, or nephrologist can offer constructive suggestions that might improve the patient's prognosis. It is unfortunate when such requests are delayed and the consultant is later forced to state that "you might have had a better chance to save the _____ if only you had done _____ immediately after the incident 2 days ago."

As soon as this comprehensive care is under way, it is necessary for the personnel directly involved, often through the supervisor or anesthesia chief, to notify the facility administrator or risk manager. This person may, in turn, choose to notify the facility's malpractice insurance carrier. If different, the anesthetist's malpractice insurer should be called. Depending on the nature of the incident, the risk manager and the insurers may suggest becoming involved from the first contact with the family. If there is an involved surgeon of record, he or she probably will first notify the family, but the anesthetist and others (risk manager, insurance loss control officer or even legal counsel) might appropriately be included at the outset. Full disclosure of facts as they are best known with no confessions, opinions, speculation, or placing of blame is the best presentation throughout all dealings with the family and, when possible, the patient. Any attempt to conceal, withhold, or shade the truth will only confound an already difficult situation. Obviously, comfort and support should be offered, including, if appropriate, the services of facility personnel such as clergy, social workers, and counselors, particularly if there has been a death.[39]

The primary anesthesia provider and any others involved must document relevant information about the incident in the medical record. Never change any existing entries in the record. Write an amendment note if needed with careful explanation of why amendment is necessary, particularly stressing explanations of professional judgments involved. State only facts as they are known. Make no judgments about causes or responsibility and do not use judgmental terms. The same guidelines hold true for the filing of the incident report in the facility, which should be done as soon as is practical. Furthermore, all discussions with the patient or family should be documented carefully in the medical record. Also, although opinions may vary by location and among attorneys, the involved practitioners should make their own sets of more complete notes, including personal opinions and observations about competence and performance of all people involved, as soon as possible after the event. These will be extremely valuable 2 to 5 years later in preparing for testimony, but it is critical that these notes be immediately placed, at the time they are written, in the hands of the practitioners' attorneys, making them work product and thus preventing later discovery of the notes by anyone else.

Follow-up investigation after the immediate handling of the incident will involve the primary anesthesia provider or providers but should be directed by a senior supervisor, who may or may not be the same person as the incident supervisor on the scene at the time. The follow-up supervisor verifies the adequacy and coordination of ongoing care of the patient and facilitates communication among all involved, especially with the RM and QA personnel. Final decisions about the sequestered equipment must be made. If it is suggested that the equipment was involved in the accident, a plan is outlined (see p. 781). Last, it is necessary to verify that adequate postevent documentation is taking place.

Unpleasant as it is to contemplate, it is better to have a plan ahead of time and execute it in the event of an accident. Vigorous immediate intervention after an incident along the lines detailed here may improve the outcome for all concerned.

C. Summary

An anesthesia RM program should be a comprehensive compendium of efforts related to the topics outlined in this chapter. There is a necessary, significant intertwining of the two themes of quality of patient care and concern for liability exposure. Although many of the elements covered include medicolegal considerations specifically directed at avoidance or minimization of malpractice claims, the primary goal is optimum patient care. In all circumstances, doing everything possible to maximize the quality of care should help minimize the risks of complications. Minimizing these risks, in turn, minimizes the consequent risk of malpractice claims. It is not at all wrong to do some defensive thinking. It is important to address issues that have been found to be vulnerable points for anesthesia practitioners defending against malpractice claims, how to anticipate them, and how to best conduct care so as to minimize the risk of exposure to unjustified charges. However, thinking constantly oriented solely toward potential liability issues is unnecessary, inappropriate, and extremely taxing on the practitioner.

Because anesthesia practice is facilitative rather than specifically diagnostic or therapeutic, there is little tolerance for complications. An expectation has justifiably evolved that no patient should be harmed from anesthesia care. This attitude makes the medicolegal considerations for anesthesiologists probably more acute than for most other medical specialists. Distinguishing between a bad result attributable to the patient's disease and an iatrogenic injury can be difficult. Among the major benefits of an anesthesia RM strategy are the expectations that

the probability of both will be lower. Many now believe that there are fewer anesthesia incidents causing complications today, although this belief is debatable. However, some malpractice insurance companies have reduced premiums for all insured practitioners, and even more companies have dramatically reduced the risk classification and the resulting premiums specifically for anesthesiologists. Whether RM efforts like those outlined here have played a role in this encouraging change can never be proved definitively with hard statistics. Many insurance company officials and institutional risk managers believe that such efforts have contributed significantly to the improvement in claims experience. Because insurance actuaries are not by nature charitable people, the reductions in premiums must reflect reductions in insurance payout. Because of the nature of the legal profession today, it is highly unlikely that a large number of major complications or injuries are going unrecognized by the insurance system. These facts add up to an improvement in care, particularly anesthesia care. It is intuitively reasonable to believe that appropriately educated and trained, honest anesthesia practitioners doing work for which they are qualified under the guidance of sound thoughtful policy and procedure guidelines, using safe equipment, keeping complete legible records (about patients who understand and consent to their procedures), improving their practices through education, and being constantly aware of the appropriate response to an adverse incident, will give optimal care that minimizes the anesthetic risks to the patient and the medicolegal risks to the anesthesia practitioners themselves.

II. QUALITY ASSURANCE
A. Definition of *quality*

QA activities are intended to optimize the anesthesia care patients receive. The concept of QA arose from quality control efforts in manufacturing, intended to demonstrate that the finished product is complete, correct, and fully functional. This usually involves inspection, testing, or sampling. Anesthesiologists' product is the medical care rendered their patients. By analogy, QA involves inspecting and analyzing the care given.

The definition of *quality* in medical care and means of evaluating it have been discussed intensely. The outcome of care is the main focus, but many other aspects are also considered, including how QA data are used.[40,41] There have been debates as to whether only the practitioners' performance should be considered in assessing the quality of medical care, or whether the roles of the health care system and the actions of patients themselves should also be included.[42] Good- or acceptable-quality care can vary from patient to patient, depending on specific needs, which leads to suggestions that goals should be individualized, which may make screening quality for large numbers of patients more difficult.[43] However, a current popular definition of patient care quality revolves around the concept that medical care rendered to a patient should increase the likelihood of a desirable outcome for that patient and, simultaneously, reduce the probability of an undesirable outcome.

This concept of optimizing outcome is particularly pertinent to anesthesia care because surgical anesthesia is facilitative rather than therapeutic. A reasonable expectation has evolved among both the medical and public communities that anesthesia care should "first, do no harm." It has been suggested that the nature of intraoperative anesthesia care is uniquely amenable to the minimization of anesthesia-related adverse outcome. Furthermore, a well-conceived and well-implemented QA program can be a major component of this effort for all types of anesthesia-related care. Thus the key to anesthesia QA is patient outcome. There are several elements of care, each of which contributes eventually to patient outcome. Tracking, studying, and analyzing the results of anesthesia care create the basis for efforts to improve that care, which will then be reflected in improved patient outcome.

B. Elements of care and the problem process

Three relevant components make up most professional activities, including the delivery of medical care: structure, process, and outcome. Each is appropriately addressed by the QA process, even though the ultimate focus is on outcome.[42]

The classic example of a structural element in anesthesia is the apparatus. The practice of anesthesia depends heavily on equipment and supplies. Purchase of both and maintenance and servicing of the equipment are central to high-quality anesthesia care. Beyond questions about the adequacy of available equipment or its age, specific suggested programs for anesthesia equipment exist.[31] Included are issues of prepurchase evaluation, protocols for inspection of incoming equipment, preventive maintenance, electrical inspections, annual safety inspections, and thorough, documented orientation of all users to new equipment or supplies. All these issues are critical because of the medicolegal implications of the use of modern monitoring technologies such as pulse oximetry and capnography, for example. Likewise, a key component is thorough documentation of the entire history (maintenance, service, problems, failures) of pieces of capital equipment. These records can be an essential resource if an untoward patient outcome occurs while specific equipment is being used.

The element of *process* in anesthesia practice simply refers to how things are done. A good example of a QA issue is whether the ASA standards for basic intraoperative monitoring are being observed during administration of an anesthetic in a recognized anesthetizing location (main operating or off site). This could be the subject of a one-time investigation, a periodic audit, or a continual generic screen. There are many other possibilities. Is there a complete surgical workup on the chart before the patient arrives in the operating room? Is there a complete preanesthetic evaluation by a member of the anesthesia department? Was a complete report given on transfer to the PACU? Is there a postoperative evaluation? How many same-day-surgery procedures are canceled after the patients arrive for surgery? Many of these points involve documentation, and there can be concern

that this type of QA activity assesses writing ability rather than the quality of care. However, documentation has become critically important in medicine, particularly to the government regulators concerned with alleged fraud and abuse in the health care system. Also, from a liability standpoint, there are clear medicolegal instances in which "if you didn't write it down, you didn't do it." Therefore the process element in QA should focus on both the action and its documentation. Wide latitudes must be given in considering whether goals are accomplished. One practitioner doing QA evaluation might make a chart entry differently from what is written, but if the note is reasonably complete and communicative, the QA assessor is obligated to set aside issues of differences in style in favor of avoiding needless confrontation with the original author. In internal QA, rarely is the letter of the prescribed process nearly as important as the spirit of compliance. Sadly, recent developments apparently driven by financial considerations by third-party purchasers of health care, particularly government agencies, have led to demands for letter-perfect compliance with documentation regulations. Health care facilities are hiring administrators to be compliance officers and implementing elaborate compliance plans that are merely extensions of the traditional QA efforts but narrowly focused on documenting what was done and why for billing purposes.

Outcome issues in anesthesia care have received significant attention. The JCAHO has used various lists of outcome indicators and numeric criteria in the hospital/facility accreditation process. Because operative anesthesia care is facilitative rather than therapeutic, outcome often is viewed largely in terms of the presence or absence of complications. Complications can be as simple as deviations from prearranged plans (discharge home of a same-day-surgery patient at 5 PM rather than 2 PM) or as grave as death or profound central nervous system damage from unrecognized hypoventilation that caused hypoxemia and consequent cardiac arrest. Less extreme examples of outcome indicators include unplanned admissions to an ICU, unplanned extra stay in the hospital (such as after myocardial infarction, stroke, pulmonary edema, pneumonia), unplanned admission to the hospital of same-day-surgery patients and the reasons, remedial surgery or treatment necessitated by anesthesia care (e.g., drainage of a hematoma or insertion of a chest tube), reintubation in the PACU, and late hypoxemia discovered the night after surgery when the patient has returned to a regular room on a floor nursing unit.

Whether outcome is necessarily or even likely to be correlated with structure and process can be debated. A good outcome (e.g., the absence of complications from an anesthetic) may result from poor performance of a procedure with inadequate or inappropriate equipment. Most comprehensive QA programs incorporate the assumption that optimal outcome is more likely as result of correct process using appropriate equipment. There is a correct distinction between the organizational side and specific emphasis on outcome as the ultimate indicator. Evolution of this field has combined the two. Although it is possible for a system to consider only outcome and ignore structure and process, today most QA programs within health care address all three elements. Attempts to optimize structure and process will promote a friendly, efficient, cost-limited practice environment. Some years ago, there was inherent assumption that this optimization of structure and process would contribute to improved patient outcome. With the implementation of managed care and truly extraordinary emphasis on cost-cutting through limitation of personnel, services, medications, and support activities, it is again important to note that what may be optimum for those funding an activity may not necessarily be best for patient care. Accordingly, current emphasis should be on traditional patient outcome measures as the heart of the QA process, partly in reaction to the threat that excessive cost-cutting efforts may negatively affect quality.

Many detailed generic guidelines for QA programs are available, but the traditional construct consists of assessing quality by objective means (measurements, whenever possible) that are documented and then ensuring quality by reinforcing and rewarding what is perceived as high quality or, conversely, solving any problems discovered.[41] When, as a result of routine or targeted screening, known adverse events occur or it is suspected that quality is suboptimal, a problem can be said to exist, and this evokes what can be known as the problem process. This QA process invoked in response usually has four steps: problem identification, problem analysis and evaluation, problem resolution, and follow-up monitoring.

There may be debate about whether a single sentinel incident should trigger the full investigative activity of the problem process system. Clearly, if a major accident occurs, the process would apply. Short of that, however, one instance of one specific problem may indicate that a practitioner had a bad day. If such a problem does not recur, caused either by the individual practitioner or others in the department, those responsible for QA must decide whether the single instance warrants targeting a practitioner for an investigation that could lead to mandatory remedial action.

In general, the problem process is simple. Problem identification involves data acquisition and examination for patterns, trends, or specific incidents. There are many possible ways this can happen. Problem evaluation can be as simple as a case conference discussion within the department or as complex as seeking outside input from recognized experts, including even a formal peer review evaluation of the hospital or anesthesia department. Problem resolution, by definition, involves change. Some new policy, procedure, privilege, knowledge, or attitude will be applied to the identified problem. Follow-up is intended not only to verify that the problem has been resolved, but also to monitor for recurrence or mutation of the original issue.

C. Background

1. Theories. As noted, the concept of inspecting a finished product to see whether it has been made or processed correctly before it is offered for sale to ensure the quality of the product in the marketplace has existed for centuries. This process became more formalized with the creation of assembly lines in manufacturing facilities, particularly in automobile plants early in the twentieth century. The issue of whether to inspect carefully every replicate of product coming off the assembly line or rely on a sampling technique to reflect statistically what is happening has been debated and, in many contexts, still is. Such a question could be just as relevant to an anesthesia department or group organizing postanesthesia follow-up of patients who had ambulatory surgery the prior day. Multiple aspects of the application of QA concerns are outlined in detail in an excellent review.[44]

The modern quality movement is traced to W. Edwards Deming, who in 1950 became an adviser to Japanese industries rebuilding after World War II. He implemented a new type of program that evolved beyond QA product inspection into a total quality management system that involves intense involvement of front-line workers in helping corporate managers and officials improve the manufacturing process. He assumed that the workers wanted to do a good job and that when that did not occur, it was usually the fault of the system rather than the workers themselves. There is a heavy dose of philosophy of corporate life in Deming's "14 Points of Management Obligation"[45] that still has some application to any professional organization, including an anesthesiology group or department. Joseph Juran ("fitness to use"), Philip Crosby ("zero defects"), and Kauru Ishikawa ("total quality control") followed Deming, expanding and elaborating on the fundamental theme that optimum quality is the ultimate goal of any entity involved in producing goods or services and that there are myriad possible plans and systems to achieve this optimization. Although each proposed system differs in details, the underlying concepts involve vertical integration of ideas and intense cooperation at all personnel levels. Put as simply as possible, the goal was to move beyond the original QA mechanism that involved the simple identification of defective replicates on an assembly line (and assignment of blame for the problem) to a system approach, inspired and driven as much by the assembly line workers as by corporate management, that constantly analyzes structure, process, and outcome, making changes (improvements) to each element continually, all with the goal of optimal quality of the finished product. In anesthesia practice, the finished product is high-quality patient care. How the quality movement ideas apply to anesthesia practice is a valid consideration. There certainly must be an element of retrospective review of some (probably all) of the replicates of the product (cases completed) in a traditional QA mode, with the resulting data reviewed by both the practitioners involved and the responsible managers or officials of the practice group or department as well as of the facility or institution where the practice takes place. In addition, no one could argue against the potential value of a total quality management or continuous quality improvement effort in anesthesiology practice. Although the analogies to common practices in industrial manufacturing may not be quite as clear as with classic retrospective QA, extensive protocols for implementing such plans in various types of anesthesia practices have been published.[44]

2. Origins of quality assurance programs

a. Government influences. The concept of outside regulation is not new to practitioners of medicine. Since the eighteenth century, physicians sought to have licensing laws that differentiated between regularly and irregularly trained health care providers. In the late nineteenth and early twentieth century, medical organizations promoted licensing laws and other procedures to restrict the practice of medicine. These laws protected the public and the physicians. The public was protected from charlatans, and the physicians were protected from competition. At the same time that the medical profession promoted licensing laws, it also opposed any rules that interfered with licensed physicians practicing as they wanted.

Outside of state licensing laws, the first substantial laws leading to control of medical practice originated with movements for national health insurance. During the Depression, the federal government developed a serious interest in national health insurance. Opposition from the AMA was a key factor in eliminating health insurance from proposals for Social Security. However, as financial difficulties mounted, physicians found their practices suffering and sought to have government agencies pay for indigent health care. This medical welfare was envisioned to be only a short-term necessity. Although the AMA leadership encouraged its members to treat the poor without accepting payment from welfare agencies, the economic stress was too great for most doctors.

In the middle to late 1930s, the medical profession had changed its position from strong opposition to reluctant acceptance of certain types of health insurance. A key proviso to this acceptance was that practitioners maintain the right to choose their patients and set their fees. World War II forestalled national health insurance issues until the end of the 1940s. President Truman sponsored a national health plan that was opposed aggressively by the AMA. In 1949, playing on the fear of communism, the AMA launched a successful $1.5-million dollar campaign against Truman's plan.

The 1950s and 1960s were an era of vast economic growth in the United States. This growth did not apply equally to all classes, and disparities in medical care became more apparent. Care for the aged and the poor became popular causes, leading to the proposal for national health insurance. Originally Congress sought to avoid a confrontation with the AMA by calling for compulsory payment schedules for hospitals only and avoiding the question of physician fees. The AMA opposed the proposal and offered a voluntary plan that, startlingly, included a scheme for physician reimbursement. In 1965, Congress under a stimulus from President Johnson enacted a plan that combined elements of both congressional and AMA proposals: Medicare. The Medicare Bill contained three parts: Part A created a national insurance for hospital expenses, Part B created a national insurance for physician fees, and Medicaid increased federal support to states to help pay for medical care for the indigent.

Medicare infused enormous amounts of money into the health care system. Physicians and hospitals flourished because the Medicare reimbursement system paid "costs" and "usual, customary, and reasonable" fees. That is, to a certain extent the hospitals and physicians determined the fees. Unfortunately, the increase in health care dollars was coupled with a sense that the benefits to the public did not parallel the benefits to the doctors and hospitals. The focus of attention turned from the miracles of modern U.S. medicine to the abuses and faults of the profession, a theme that persists. It led in large measure to the creation and spread of the managed care industry, the 1994 Clinton proposal to revolutionize American medical care, and ongoing efforts by regulatory agencies to root out, stop, and punish fraud and abuse in U.S. health care financing.

b. Professional standard review organizations. The 1970s saw an increasing role of government in American medicine. With the enactment of Medicare and Medicaid, the federal government assumed responsibility for one of the most expensive programs in the history of government anywhere. Congress became increasingly alarmed at the escalating costs and abuses. Thus the primary impetus for government intrusion into the practice of medicine grew from economic concerns. In 1972, Congress passed amendments that created government reviews of physician practices. The Professional Standards Review Organizations Act was an attempt to oversee health care utilization. The vehicles for this utilization review were regional organizations directed by physicians. These PSROs were private groups under contract to the government.

The mission of PSROs was to identify unnecessary procedures so that the government would not pay for unwarranted medical services. PSROs were to develop local criteria for evaluating care provided to Medicare and Medicaid patients. Utilization review processes, which included "norms for care" for medical problems (such as normal length of stay for a cholecystectomy) were devised. Utilization review teams identified patients whose care fell outside the norms and reviewed those cases to determine whether care was appropriate. The penalty for falling outside the norm of care was denial of Medicare payment.

The AMA proposed that utilization reviews be conducted by physicians. The AMA's proposal was opposed from within and without. Inside the AMA, some objected to any peer review mandated by the government. Others believed that assessment of adequacy of health care should include representatives of the consumer group. Outside the profession, groups claimed that medical licensing boards and hospital medical review committees were ineffective in eliminating unacceptable care.

Operating as cost-containment units, the PSROs survived for about 10 years. PSRO decisions about appropriateness of care often were made by nurses and clerical personnel on the basis of paper reviews or telephone calls. There was little true peer review. In 1977, the

PSROs came under the control of the Health Care Finance Administration (HCFA, the organization that oversees the financing of Medicare). Increasing criticism and complaints about inconsistency in the performance of PSROs led to a plan for their elimination.

c. Peer review organizations. The 1980s saw attempts by the federal government to maintain financing of Medicare, a publicly popular program that was increasingly expensive. By 1982, the cost of providing a national health insurance had escalated to the point that it was feared that the Medicare Trust Fund would be bankrupted. In response, the Deficit Reduction Act of 1983 created the diagnosis-related groups (DRGs) system. Under this system, hospitals were paid a set amount for providing care to a Medicare patient based on the patient's diagnosis. It was up to the hospital to provide care for that patient within the limits of the fee set for that diagnosis. After this change in reimbursement, the HCFA again tried to encourage establishment of independent agencies to review the quality of care provided by institutions and individuals receiving Medicare reimbursements. These PROs were given government contracts to review care at health care facilities. In fact, the PROs were merely resurrected PSROs.

One of the charges to the PROs was to address quality of care issues: provision of necessary service, reduction of unnecessary procedures, and avoidance of complications and deaths. The PROs responded by outlining accepted practices, in effect making lists of what type of patient should be given what type of care. The HCFA went further, dictating that the PROs review each Medicare case looking for substandard care. As it happened, the directives were neither a major threat to physicians nor an effective means of ensuring QA. Few sanctions were imposed.

d. Medicare Program to Assure Quality. The limitations and problems with the PROs led to reevaluation of how to ensure QA for Medicare. In early 1990, the Institute of Medicine of the National Academy of Sciences published its proposal for the establishment of the Medicare Program to Assure Quality (MPAQ). MPAQ was to be built on the existing PRO structure, with a redirection of the PRO activity away from utilization review and toward quality of care. The goal was the development of strategies for collecting data, changing physician decision-making processes, and improving patient outcome. Efforts to develop this program continue.

e. Joint Commission for the Accreditation of Healthcare Organizations. One significant stimulus for the current interest and activity in medical QA came from the JCAHO. The JCAHO grew out of the American College of Surgery (ACS). In the early 1900s, the ACS became concerned about the level of health care delivered by U.S. hospitals. In 1912 the college surveyed 692 hospitals that contained 100 or more beds. Of these, 88% failed to meet basic standards of care set by the college. In an effort to improve hospital care, the college expanded its surveying activities. By the 1950s, hospital surveys had become such a large effort that the college sought a coalition with other professional organizations to manage the task. In December 1951, the AMA, the Canadian Medical Association (CMA), the American College of Physicians (ACP), and the American Hospital Association (AHA) agreed to help the ACS create an independent, nonprofit organization known as the Joint Commission for the Accreditation of Hospitals (JCAH).

In 1965, the role of the JCAH was escalated from voluntary to near mandatory when Congress made JCAH accreditation a mechanism for hospitals to be approved for participation in Medicare. In that same era, the JCAH expanded its activities to include a wide range of health care facilities (such as long-care facilities, psychiatric institutions, and outpatient centers) and changed from examining for minimal standards to examining for "optimal achievable standards." The power of the JCAH was extended as states incorporated JCAH accreditation into their requirements for licensure. In 1988, the JCAH changed its name to Joint Commission for the Accreditation of Health Care Organizations to reflect the change in the types of facilities that had developed.

In its current configuration, the JCAHO remains an organization directed primarily by physicians, who undertake the inspection and evaluation of health care facilities. The organization is headed by 22 commissioners: 7 from the AMA, 7 from the AHA, 3 from the ACP, 3 from the ACS, 1 from the American Dental Association, and 1 private citizen elected annually. The commissioners are advised by professional and technical advisory committees (PTACs). Committee members are chosen by professional societies on the basis of their expertise in a particular aspect of medical health care. It is through these committees that the ASA gains input into the JCAHO. Anesthesiologists appointed by the ASA president attend meetings with the JCAHO officers and advise the JCAHO as to how a department of anesthesia should be organized, what activities the anesthesia department should be involved in, and what steps an anesthesia department should take to protect the well-being of patients.

In the mid-1990s, the JCAHO underwent some stressful times, when widely publicized instances of poor medical practices occurred at hospitals that had passed JCAHO inspection. In response, the State of New York developed its own state-based review process, and the federal government decided to audit 10% of all JCAHO accreditation.

Using the power of its accreditation program, the JCAHO seeks to enforce the implementation of processes that it believes lead to better care. One of the most prominent processes is QA. QA was established as a required standard for approval as early as 1924, when the ACS prescribed that medical staffs should "review and analyze at regular intervals their clinical experience in the various departments of the hospital."

The process of QA acquired a more directed format in the 1970s when the JCAH began requiring medical audits. Medical audits started with the creation of a set of criteria by which one could infer proper care of the patient. Several randomly selected patient charts were reviewed in a retrospective fashion. The reviewers marked whether the criteria were present in the patient's record. The concept of audits was that elements of a medical record could be used to identify issues in medical care. Audits were perceived as less than ideal because the methodology focused attention on the record, not the care of the patient.

The JCAH made QA a major issue in 1982, when 62% of all cited violations related to failure to perform adequate QA. In 1984, the JCAHO attempted to establish a hospitalwide QA process with standardization of programs in all departments of a hospital. The device invented to accomplish this goal was generic or occurrence screening. Under the concept of occurrence screening, a department chose specific areas to investigate in an ongoing process. The premise behind occurrence screening was that a department could not possibly review every case but that activity in several important areas would reflect the overall care. The process did not work well. The staff often did not know which were the most important areas to investigate, the areas did not necessarily reflect overall care, and the staff still viewed QA as a bothersome bureaucratic process. There was little conviction that JCAHO QA processes provided insight into medical problems or improved practice, and the process became dominated by clerical personnel. Associated with the process was the designation of clinical indicators or sentinel events. Essentially, these were adverse events to be looked for on chart review. The detection of an indicator triggered a review of the chart to determine whether care had been adequate. The first pilot study to define indicators for anesthesia did not yield the desired results, partly because of the wide variability of anesthesia and hospital records. Nonetheless, a set of clinical indicators for anesthesia was devised, and departments of anesthesia were required to incorporate clinical indicators into their QA processes. Anesthesia groups and departments found themselves under a great deal of pressure to develop QA programs that adhered to the requirements of the JCAHO. The ASA had recognized the concept of QA in a landmark 1986 publication[46] that still has value. However, the ASA was surprised when in 1988 a workshop on QA attracted an overflow crowd. When the audience was asked how many were attending because of the JCAHO, nearly every hand was raised.

The criteria used by the JCAHO are published in its manual, which is available to hospitals and physicians. This manual stipulates the JCAHO standards for departments of a hospital seeking JCAHO accreditation. The standards for anesthesia services are created with consultation from representatives of various specialties. Although ASA representatives have input, the JCAHO maintains autonomy and does not necessarily heed or implement the ASA suggestions.

The philosophy of the JCAHO is that hospitals should be able to demonstrate quality improvement. That is, each department should be able to show that a problem of care was identified and resolved with resultant improvement in care. In general, JCAHO requirements have been largely process oriented and easily tested by documentation. Therefore one key to JCAHO approval involves recognizing what processes are required, implementing them, and then documenting that the processes are functioning. Documentation is key. Departments that are functioning according to JCAHO guidelines but have not adequately documented their organization (with printed and periodically revised rules, regulations, and bylaws) and activities (such as regular and acceptable minutes) have difficulty gaining approval.

The JCAHO requirements for an anesthesia department are generic enough to allow for multiple ways to achieve that requirement. Although flexibility is desirable, it brings with it the problem of vagueness. The decision as to whether a department's processes and documentation meet JCAHO standards is made by a JCAHO physician inspector during an extensive on-site examination. The physician inspector may or may not be knowledgeable about the pragmatic problems of providing anesthesia care. The inspector will judge the department according to the JCAHO manual. Thus where the manual is not specific, the inspector makes a subjective interpretation of the requirements and decides whether the department fulfills this interpretation. There have been situations in which individual inspectors have had ideas and criteria that differed from what is in the JCAHO manual, and this has occasionally produced some frustration on the part of the practitioners and facilities being inspected.

f. Medicare. The government attempts to influence quality of care through the Medicare program. To receive payments for Medicare patients, hospitals must have proof that the facility operates within an acceptable standard. Proof of adequate quality of care was either accreditation by a JCAHO survey or approval by a Medicare survey team. Medicare surveys parallel JCAHO surveys. Both require QA mechanisms to be in place. The HCFA organizes Medicare surveys but calls on outside agencies, often state health agencies, to perform the surveys. Medicare surveys differ from JCAHO surveys in that Medicare inspections are less peer review–oriented and more detailed than JCAHO surveys.

g. Managed care influences. The advent of managed care is a double-edged sword regarding QA efforts. Managed care is highly data driven, with particular emphasis on patient outcome statistics. Therefore managed care organizations strongly support and, in fact, mandate extensive QA activities that allegedly will amass a database that, in turn, will allow objective evaluations of which protocols and therapies are most effective and, especially, most cost-effective. Both traditional retrospective review of cases and prospective system-oriented continuous improvement schemes are relevant to the underlying efforts of managed care organizations to get health care to "do more with less" and, above all, less cost to the employers and government agencies purchasing the care for the consumers of the care. Accordingly, health care providers attempting to secure contracts for capitated payment for covered lives or guaranteed referrals of patient populations in discounted fee-for-service arrangements must stress their QA efforts and the resulting confirmatory data demonstrating both good patient outcome and cost efficiency. Commercial organizations advertising to groups of health care providers programs that will facilitate this effort sprang up quickly as the managed care industry grew in influence in the mid-1990s.

Health care consumer backlash to perceived denial of coverage for services, consultations, procedures, or medications and corner-cutting by assigned health care providers has led to another important application of the QA process oriented in almost an exactly opposite manner. Organizations of health care providers, be they national professional associations, state or local medical associations, or even practice groups themselves, have attempted to use QA efforts to suggest (or even "prove") that patient outcomes and their health in general have been adversely influenced by the stringent health care management (by cutback, delay, and denial) of managed care organizations. Statistical indications of poorer-quality patient outcomes demonstrated by a QA mechanism are potentially powerful evidence against the restrictions imposed by managed care organizations and are potentially useful in supporting government legislation or regulation controlling precisely what managed care organizations can do in achieving alleged cost-efficiency. This story is still being written. What is certain is that the strong interaction between QA mechanisms and the managed care industry will continue and probably grow over time.

D. Models and programs

1. *Audits, indicators, and criteria.* Traditional retrospective auditing of completed cases is most often associated with classic QA in a clinical group or department, including anesthesiology practices. Creation of a QA program involves assembling information and making many decisions. Are there existing QA mechanisms in other parts of the facility, area, or state that might apply or be adapted (in whole or part) to the anesthesiology organization seeking to implement a process? Regulations, lines and mechanisms of communication, and methods of reporting already may be set up. The new system in the anesthesiology organization may need to incorporate or at least interact with these existing constructs. Reporting requirements of the facility, state, and JCAHO must be considered. Furthermore, the organization's members must make decisions regarding what the database underlying the QA system will be. Setting up a coding mechanism and developing a program of descriptive data for entry that will cover every case done and every clinical activity within the organization can challenge a computer-facile department member or necessitate the services of a paid programmer. There are commercial program packages that advertise the ability to manage a QA system, and detailed departmental statistics often can be derived from or piggybacked onto computer programs used for billing.

Implementation of a QA program involves selection of indicators and establishment of performance criteria where necessary. Indicators are simply the events looked for when the database is reviewed and the resulting QA data are gathered. Criteria are the expected or acceptable rates or frequency of occurrence of these events.

An indicator often can be synonymous with the problems that are studied through the QA system (such as the frequency of anesthesia-caused or related complications), but indicators also may be positive (desirable functioning of a process and a good outcome, e.g., how many first cases each morning actually start on time). Usually, however, most of the classic indicators chosen involve complications or bad outcomes associated with anesthesia care. Several examples were provided earlier concerning structure, process, and outcome. Fig. 33-1 contains a sample of an audit form with a long list of anesthesia-related indicators. It is offered only as an illustrative example and is not necessarily a suggestion of required or even desirable indicators. Each department should develop its own list of indicators appropriate to the specific characteristics of the institution or facility. General indicators can be as simple as "cancellation of the case" or "more than two attempts needed to start an IV" or as grave as "intraoperative anesthesia-related death." Airway indicators might range from "chipped tooth" to "esophageal intubation" or "accidental extubation." Vital sign indicators include significant or dangerous deviations. Apparatus indicators could include "breathing system disconnection during mechanical ventilation." Organ system indicators include "myocardial ischemia," "aspiration," "postoperative nausea and vomiting," "significant atelectasis," "grossly abnormal blood gas values," or "neurologic change after anesthesia." These are merely illustrative examples. Considerable thought is required to establish a thorough but manageable list of indicators that an anesthesiology department wants to examine in its QA system. One specific indicator, such as failed regional blocks, might be studied intensely for a limited period after a problem is identified. The same indicator might or might not be part of a continuous, permanent list of indicators that are always being studied or tracked. This permanent list might have fewer than 10 indicators in one department and more than 100 in another. Creating the QA mechanism to track an indicator is initially more important than the number of indicators followed at any one time. It is obvious that major complications will immediately be widely known in most departments; therefore departments often focus their indicators on complications that might be missed or specific points identified as actual or potential problems.

The JCAHO at one time was involved with the idea of establishing indicators for generic screening within anesthesiology practices.[47] Extensive meetings and presentations were devoted in the early 1990s to attempts to establish a realistic list of important events that every anesthesiology organization should monitor constantly. The implication was that an excessive incidence of any of the listed indicators (exceeding the criterion threshold) was a problem that warranted the classic four-step problem process (identification, evaluation, resolution, and follow-up). One of the many editions of the list of

QUALITY ASSURANCE

Department of Anesthesiology

CLINICAL QUALITY ASSURANCE <u>PEER REVIEW</u> AUDIT

(Return form with anesthesia record to OR desk.

Do not make copies. Do not attach to patient record.)

Date _____   Preop: ☐ Complete
OR# _____   Other OR(s) attended _____   ☐ Completed in OR (e.g., labs)
Operation _____   (as posted)   ☐ Incomplete (explain below)
ASA Class _____   ☐ Made by another anesthetist
                                                  ☐ Plan changed (explain below)

Anesthetic   ☐ General   ☐ Regional   ☐ MAC
Anesthesiologist _____   Anesthesiology Resident _____
Surgeon _____   Surgery Resident _____
Recovery Room Nurse _____   Discharge: ☐ ONR ☐ ICU ☐ Ward ☐ Home

☐ NO UNTOWARD EVENTS (check below)   ☐ UNTOWARD EVENTS (check below)

OR RR   Airway   OR RR   Respiratory
__ __ Chipped tooth/loosened tooth   __ __ Postop ventilatory assistance
__ __ Stridor, laryngospasm, obstruction   (unplanned)
__ __ Failed rapid sequence induction __ __ Significant hypoxemia/hypercapnia
__ __ Nose bleed or other trauma of airway __ __ Pneumothorax
__ __ Inability to intubate by route __ __ Inappropriate bronchial intubation
         originally planned   __ __ Aspiration-respiratory distress
__ __ Esophageal intubation   syndrome
__ __ Lip trauma   __ __ Reintubation (other than accidental
__ __ Accidental extubation   extubation)
                                        __ __ Bronchospasm
        CV
__ __ Death   Miscellaneous
__ __ Cardiac arrest   __ __ Other (describe below)
__ __ Significant hypertension (sustained __ __ Hyperpyrexia >38° C
         >30% above preop systolic)   __ __ Hypothermia <34° C (uninduced)
__ __ Significant hypotension (sustained __ __ Wrong medication/dose given
         <30% below preop diastolic)   (describe below)
__ __ Significant bradycardia (30% below __ __ Drug reaction (allergic/adverse)
         preop or that associated with __ __ Intravascular line problem
         hypotension)   __ __ Delayed or erroneous lab report/other
__ __ Significant tachycardia (30% above __ __ Nausea and vomiting
         preop or that associated with __ __ Equipment failure (explain below)
         hypertension)   __ __ Pain medication delayed/inadequate
__ __ Myocardial ischemia/MI suspected
__ __ Congestive heart failure/pulmonary   Regional (including pain therapy)
         edema   __ __ Pain unresponsive to block
__ __ Dysrhythmia associated with one or __ __ Failed block, inadequate block
         more of the above   __ __ Toxic reaction
                                        __ __ Excessive block (high spinal)
        Discharge planning   __ __ Wet tap (epidural)
__ Unplanned outpatient admission
__ Unplanned transfer to ICU   Neurologic
__ Unplanned return to OR   __ __ Prolonged neuromuscular block
__ Unscheduled ONR   __ __ Prolonged sedation
__ >3 hr. stay in RR   __ __ Peripheral nerve injury
__ Delayed waiting for M.D. to evaluate __ __ Stroke
__ Delayed waiting for x-ray   __ __ Recall
__ Delayed waiting for room   __ __ Seizure
__ Delayed for medical reasons   __ __ Other damage (explain below)
__ Other delay (explain below)

For each of the above, describe briefly on back.

Fig. 33-1. Example of a list of anesthesia-related quality assurance indicators in a format that could serve as a generic screen case audit form. (Courtesy Jerry A. Cohen, MD, Department of Anesthesiology, University of Florida College of Medicine, Gainesville, Fla.)

JCAHO indicators is in Box 33-1. Inability of advisors and experts to agree on precisely which events should be indicators caused ongoing modifications and resulting delay and uncertainty regarding the use of the JCAHO indicator lists in actual practice. Furthermore, the JCAHO was anxious to validate the indicators by demonstrating statistically that the particular events listed as indicators were legitimate reflections of the quality of anesthesia care being delivered. The difficulties in achieving this validation and the consequent continued meetings, symposia, and discussions further hindered widespread application of one specific list of anesthesia events that would be accepted as the basis for traditional QA within anesthesiology practice.

Once indicators are chosen for a traditional QA program, it must be decided for which ones quantitative criteria should be established. These criteria functionally are group standards, but it is better from a medicolegal standpoint to avoid that particular label to minimize confusion with the concept of standard of care for one patient. Hypothetical criteria include "no more than 4% of

---

Box 33-1 Sample set of JCAHO anesthesia indicators (sentinel events)

Patients developing a central nervous system complication within 2 postprocedure days of procedures involving anesthesia administration

Patients developing a peripheral neurologic deficit within 2 postprocedure days of procedures involving anesthesia administration

Patients developing an acute myocardial infarction within 2 postprocedure days of procedures involving anesthesia administration

Patients with a cardiac arrest within 2 postprocedure days of procedures involving anesthesia administration

Intrahospital mortality of patients within 2 postprocedure days of procedures involving anesthesia administration

Patients with discharge diagnosis of fulminant pulmonary edema developed during procedures involving anesthesia administration or within 1 postprocedure day of conclusion

Patients diagnosed with an aspiration pneumonitis occurring during procedures involving anesthesia administration or within 2 postprocedure days of conclusion

Patients developing a postural headache within 4 postprocedure days following procedures involving spinal or epidural anesthesia administration

Patients experiencing a dental injury during procedures involving anesthesia care

Patients experiencing an ocular injury during procedures involving anesthesia care

Unplanned admission of patients to the hospital within 2 postprocedure days following outpatient procedures involving anesthesia

Unplanned admission of patients to an ICU within 2 postprocedure days of procedures involving anesthesia administration and with ICU stay greater than 1 day

---

same-day-surgery patients should require admission to the hospital for anesthesia-related causes," "there should be fewer than 2% accidental wet taps during attempts at epidural catheter placement," or "fewer than 0.5% of patients should require emergency reintubation in the PACU." Obviously, for many indicators of major complications, the desirable criterion will be "none." Some indicators do not lend themselves easily to absolute criteria. It may be difficult to specify an acceptable number of patients having diastolic blood pressure more than 30% below baseline if that is an indicator for tracking. In such cases, it is better to study the indicator, establish an average incidence for the department, and then evaluate the incidence over time to see whether it changes. This strategy is logical and should be acceptable to review and accrediting agencies when explained in this context. Once indicators and criteria are in place, a traditional retrospective QA program is ready to gather data.

2. Data gathering and screens (generic and focused). Among the most significant issues concerning a QA system are the sources of input data. There are many sources of potential problem identification, the most obvious being within the department: from word of mouth and cases discussed at rounds, incident reports, and, of course, the QA system itself. There may be other sources of problem identification inside the hospital (e.g., surgical colleagues and rounds, record room generic screens, or the nursing service) or outside the hospital (e.g., professional associates, meetings, literature). Most importantly, it must be determined whether a formal reporting mechanism to the departmental QA system will be used to record critical incidents (i.e., events that, if not recognized and corrected in time, would have led to untoward patient outcome). If so, assurances of anonymity or freedom from retribution must be built in or no events will be reported. Also, it must be determined whether every chart will be reviewed from a QA standpoint. This might appear cumbersome, but it need not be. If every chart is scanned, generic or occurrence screening can be performed. Generic screening is always a component of fully actualized traditional QA systems. Correctly constructed, it is the best source of initial clinical data input into a classic QA system.

A generic screen (also known as a QA or peer review audit) involves the review of each case, usually via the anesthesia record and associated notes and documents, to detect the appearance of the indicators described earlier. If one of the indicators is PACU admission longer than 4 hours, a chart reviewer (or, more likely now, a computer program looking at a facility's mainframe database) would check the PACU time and record all patients whose stays were longer than 4 hours. For indicators such as myocardial ischemia, if the data are collected by a chart reviewer, that person must be able to read "ST down, TNG started" on the anesthesia record and understand the implication of this entry and record it correctly in the QA data. Of course, for this type of generic screening, the information must be on the anesthesia record in the first place. Note that generic screening can identify a new or previously underappreciated problem that is then singled out for a separate intense study. Conversely, a problem can be identified by any mechanism and then studied separately or entered as an indicator in a generic screen to look for it prospectively. If it is studied separately, retrospectively, this becomes a focused screen in which a database is searched for a specific event, to establish both an occurrence rate and any pattern of associations that may exist. Occasionally, surprising findings result from focused screens that were triggered by an apparently coincidental or even insignificant stimulus. The identification of previously unsuspected problems that are subsequently addressed and solved is a gratifying result of this application of the QA process.

A key issue in data collection for QA involves the self-reporting mentality. Are anesthesia practitioners going to be honest in recording on the chart (or even a separate QA form) minor problems, complications, or near-accident situations that caused no identifiable harm? A central issue is completeness of the anesthesia record. If a practitioner working alone accidentally intubates the esophagus, immediately recognizes it, and then immediately correctly replaces the tube in the trachea, with no untoward effect at all, will this be recorded on the anesthesia record? Most anesthesiologists would agree that this should be recorded, but others might believe that this is quite common and benign, not worthy of mention. Personality issues are involved, and full discussion is impossible here. One important point, however, is how the QA data are used once they are collected. QA information can be used to create provider profiles, records of the number of times any specific person shows a QA indicator, whether it is a complication or an observation. Thus the fact that Practitioner X intubated the esophagus, however transiently, would be documented in his or her file. Some argue that this is valuable because if there is a pattern, then a practitioner can be advised and thus encouraged to seek further training or experience to overcome an apparent weakness or bad habit. Clearly, he or she must be informed in a friendly manner. However, if such QA provider profile information is used in any potentially adverse way, as in evaluation for promotion or salary increase or even for potential disciplinary action, there automatically would be incomplete recording or reporting of nonobvious problems or situations. There is no simple approach to this question, and it must be evaluated carefully in each facility or organization implementing a QA program.

An excellent example of a QA study involving several elements of this traditional QA process has been published.[48] A self-reporting form was completed by the immediate anesthesia providers when the patient was transferred to the PACU, and events that affected the patient's care, such as blood pressure changes, arrhythmia, intubation difficulty, hypoventilation, or hypovolemia were noted. One clear benefit was the enhancement of the transmission of information from the anesthetists to the PACU staff. Among more than 12,000 patients, 18% had at least one event (indicator) of note. The most common were hypotension and ar-

rhythmia. Increased information feedback to practitioners, based on the data, was instituted.

Throughout the QA process, those responsible for its administration must be certain that activities within the QA system are documented thoroughly. Nothing would be more frustrating to a departmental staff than cooperating with a QA process in which the generated data are not used. Not only must the department satisfy accreditation and reporting requirements, but the main purpose is also again to help optimize the care given. After the necessary analysis, the staff must be given regular, frequent, detailed feedback. If there are no indicators showing an incidence above the numeric criteria, the staff must be told that they are doing a good job. If problems are identified, the proposed solutions and QA follow-up should be discussed thoroughly. The group may not need to know the details of any situation involving only one person, but they should know that constructive QA activity is taking place. Input regarding problem identification must be cultivated. The program's success or failure depends on the responsiveness and communication of the responsible department leaders.

By far, the major stumbling block in QA programs is the front-line practitioner's resistance to completing forms. Occasionally, there may be an exceptional staff that universally cooperates, completing a generic screening form for every patient at the time of the case and completing it when the patient leaves the facility. More likely, compliance would be less than total. Although one or more members within an anesthesiology organization usually are willing or even eager to organize and administer the QA programs, sometimes a QA coordinator must be appointed. Sometimes the chief, director, or chairperson fills this role until the system is operating smoothly and proven unobtrusive; then a responsible person can be recruited. There must always be a physician in charge to review the data, make recommendations, and direct follow-up.

Acknowledgment of the frequent reality of staff attitudes about QA leads to a suggested method of organization. Maximum effort (through lectures, rounds, examples from leaders, personal encouragement, and exhortation) should be given to ensuring complete documentation of all aspects of care, particularly on the anesthesia record in the patient's chart. This then makes the medical chart the source of clinical input data for the anesthesia QA system, so that the staff are not expected to complete their own forms. The department can then train a nonprofessional person to collect and collate the QA raw data and prepare preliminary statistics for review by the departmental QA coordinator. The department size determines whether this activity can be accomplished by existing office staff or whether a new part-time or full-time person would be needed. Screening is labor intensive, and in a department with several thousand cases a year or more, a full-time person probably would be necessary. In this era of cost constraint, it may initially seem idealistic to suggest new personnel for this function. However, it can be clearly cost effective for the institution or anesthesia group to employ such a person, who may also double as a billing clerk. The QA system should function in an efficient, timely manner, with the employee dedicated to the task. This will please the staff, department, and institution. All reporting and review requirements will be met with a minimum of annoyance, and anesthesia practitioners' energy can be devoted to using the results to improve practice rather than to mere generation of statistics.

3. Alternatives in anesthesiology QA: the Las Vegas or Vitez model for judging clinical competence. In the late 1980s, the widespread interest in expanding QA activities beyond the traditional retrospective chart audit was present within American anesthesiology and an alternative approach was advanced.[49]

The model was based on three simple concepts:
- Competence must be decided by knowledgeable, unbiased peers who consider a wide range of evidence.
- The best indication of competence is outcome.
- Humans are inherently fallible, and the occurrence of an error, even one of great significance, does not necessarily indicate incompetence.

The model uses a semivoluntary system to collect information about anesthesia-related events. A short, general list of clinical indicators focuses attention on clinically significant occurrences, not unrelated happenings or theoretical problems:
- Cancellation of surgery
- Respiratory or cardiac arrest
- Soft-tissue injury to patient
- New neurologic abnormality (such as coma, seizure, paresis, paralysis)
- Inability to ventilate the lungs or intubate the trachea
- Reintubation of the trachea
- Sustained hypoxia
- Regurgitation or aspiration
- Difficulty of patient to breathe
- Unstable cardiac rhythm, heart rate, or blood pressure
- New myocardial ischemia or infarction
- Patient abandonment
- Death of the patient within 24 hours of surgery
- Any other event that may be related to anesthesia management

The list is distributed to anesthesia providers and personnel working in anesthetizing locations or in postoperative care units (such as PACU, postpartum unit, or ICU). Any of these events is reported to the anesthesia QA committee (AQAC) of the department of anesthesiology. This committee reviews cases and make recommendations to the department. The QA committee uses the hospital's QA department to process the occurrence report and prepare information about the case for review. One important step in this process is the use of copies of the record with names and identifying entries removed. In this manner, anonymity is built into the review system. The identity of the practitioner involved in the case is not to be disclosed to the committee or the department. To allow accounting of differences in clini-

cal case mix, institutional setting, and changes in performance over a period of time, codes and information identifying the practitioner, institution, date, type of surgery, and ASA physical status are entered into the database by the QA department.

A reviewer classifies each case according to a standard scheme, focusing on what actually happened to the patient. The first step in classifying an occurrence is to determine whether there was a clinically significant event that was related to equipment used, a decision made, or action taken by the anesthesiologist. Next, the reviewer determines the seriousness of the event, assigning an outcome score. Outcome scores translate description of an event (nominal data) to a number indicating severity (ordinal data):

0	No sequelae (such as reintubation of the trachea after esophageal intubation)
1-3	No harm to patient but escalation of care (such as ventilator required postoperatively because of improper use of relaxant)
4-6	Reversible damage to integrity of an organ (such as pulmonary edema from fluid overload)
7-9	Irreversible organ damage (such as myocardial infarction)
10	Death

This scoring system is important to the process because it transforms narrative and descriptive terms (nominal data) into numeric values (ordinal data), which can be used for more objective comparisons. The third step is for the reviewer to identify and classify any errors committed. Errors are classified by three categories: management area, nature of error, and genesis of error. Management area and nature of error describe what happened. Genesis of error describes why it happened. The categories and their subdivisions are shown here:

Management area: Airway, circulatory, neuromuscular blockade, regional

Nature of error: "None," an unavoidable circumstance; "Mechanical," failure of device; "Human," related to formulation or execution of a decision. Human errors are subdivided into three types. Judgmental errors occur when the action taken is the action intended. These are errors of faulty decision processes, such as administration of anesthesia by mask in a full-stomach situation. Technical errors occur when the action taken is not the action intended (such as a syringe swap). Such errors involve mistakes in the execution of a decision. Vigilance errors are errors associated with lack of adequate general attention (such as an intravenous infiltration). Judgmental errors are further classified by genesis:

Genesis of judgmental errors:
Inadequate knowledge
    Didactic
    Experience
Inadequate data; failure to seek data
Disregard data
    Failure to recognize pattern
    Failure to accept conclusion
Lack of alternative plan

The classification of errors is another key difference between this method and other QA processes. The basic concept that humans are inherently fallible leads to the theory that each practitioner may have a unique pattern of errors that defines his or her clinical performance. Even if different areas of management are involved, the same genesis of error may be repeated in all areas.

Error profiles are created from data collected by the AQAC. After approval of the department, AQAC findings are entered into the individual practitioners' files in the computer's database. As data accumulate, a picture emerges of the number, type, and frequency of errors made by individuals and the department as a whole. Reviews of the files are made periodically (as whenever a new error is made, at reappointment, annually) or whenever an incident generates concern about the abilities of a practitioner.

Just as athletes use videotapes to study and correct mistakes, error profiles are used to help individuals and the department identify important clinical issues and improve their performance. Without error profiles, it is impossible to know what must be repaired. Additionally, once error and outcome profiles are known, limits of acceptability can be set. Competence can be judged from the number, type, and severity of errors made because incompetent practitioners commit errors that are more numerous, less common, or more severe than those of competent members of the department.

Information from case reviews is used in error analysis. In error analysis, a profile of the practitioner is compared with the profile of the department. A profile contains six comparative elements and three minimal performance levels:

Comparative elements
- Frequency of anesthesia-related events
- Average negative outcome score
- Number of errors per event
- Area of clinical management
- Nature of errors
- Genesis of errors

Minimal expected performance levels
- Anesthetizes ASA physical status 1 and 2 patients without outcome score greater than 6
- Institutes appropriate life-sustaining actions in life-threatening situations
- Displays insight when involved in significant error

These minimal levels were determined by analysis of quality assessment data collected from four hospitals in the system where this program was created[49] and subsequent agreement among the practitioners. In dealing with serious illnesses, not every life-threatening situation was resolvable. However, the most unacceptable outcomes involved evidence that the practitioner had failed to recognize the severity of the problem or react appropriately. Accordingly, a standard was adopted that required evidence that the practitioner instituted appropriate life-sustaining actions in life-threatening situations. This minimal level acknowledges that even a competent practitioner may make a fatal error. However, the competent physician recognizes the gravity of

the situation and makes appropriate efforts to save the patient. Finally, lack of insight was a common and persuasive factor in decisions to restrict clinical activities. Thus a final standard decrees that when an appropriate peer review process judges an event to be related to anesthesia, the practitioner involved should pay heed to that judgment.

After establishing comparative and minimal levels, an individual's error profile is compared with the average error profile for the department. This comparison is used to make decisions about clinical performance. As reviews accumulate in the database, it becomes possible to identify which problems occur more frequently and which problems are more onerous for both the department and the individual provider. It is also possible to identify providers whose performance falls outside the acceptable realm. Comparisons with the group norm obviously are the place to start. Individual situations or practitioners that come under scrutiny because of the data gathered are handled in specific ways appropriate to the unique situation.

Although this model has facilitated QA in anesthesia, many problems still remain. First, detecting events that might be related to anesthesia is one of the most difficult problems facing QA systems. Computerized anesthesia record devices enhance detection methods. Computerized anesthesia record devices consist of computers capable of automatically recording signals from monitors (such as ECG, pressure transducers, gas analyzers) every 15 seconds. In addition, the anesthesiologist enters into the computer information such as events or drugs given. The computer database is then able to produce an accurate anesthesia record and reconstruct any event on a 15-second time scale. Such methodology will allow detection and accurate description of many more perioperative events than is currently possible.

Even with computerized data retrieval, many events (such as a broken tooth) are undetectable except by those caring for the patient. Therefore QA systems probably will always rely on the honesty and courage of the practitioner to report a possible error. Reporting by practitioners will improve as they realize that QA systems do not pose a threat to them. On the contrary, QA systems offer the most effective method to improve their clinical expertise.

A second area of difficulty is knowing exactly what happened. Determination of what happened is confounded by the lack of accurate details about events and the inexperience of peer reviewers. Details of an event often are indistinct because witnesses of any event often have conflicting and inaccurate descriptions of the occurrence. Memory for details fades with time; thus the longer the period of time between the occurrence and the search for information, the greater the loss and distortion of detail. Even when details have been recorded accurately, important parameters may not have been monitored. Computerized data retrieval systems will provide much more detail about clinical events. Still, many aspects of an occurrence will be known only to human witnesses. This means that QA systems must be able to identify and rapidly debrief people who have knowledge about the event.

A third problem for QA is case analysis. Case analysis is complicated by lack of knowledge about how a case review should be organized. One logical approach depends on the chronologic arrangement of events and information. As information is taken from the patient's record and arranged chronologically, the reviewer marks the bits of data that seem important to the event. After looking over the chronology, the reviewer then hypothesizes the mechanism by which the event occurred. The hypothesis is then tested against the facts of the case and the medical literature. Alternative hypotheses are tried to see whether they are consistent with the data.

Determining causation is also complicated by lack of information (such as no autopsy) and the presence of mitigating circumstances (concurrent diseases). These factors may obfuscate the assessment of the roles of anesthesia management in the event or injury. The model described earlier directs that under circumstances of uncertainty, QA decisions favor the practitioner, and the occurrence may be judged as not related to anesthesia care. As experience with formal case review grows, expert systems that will guide reviewers through case analysis will be developed. Over a period of time a library of peer review cases will aid in rapid analysis of recurrent events.

4. Anesthesia QA overview. Most groups of anesthesia practitioners will need some type of quality assessment and management system, whatever format it assumes, fueled by institutional, regulatory, and accrediting imperatives as well as an internal desire to optimize practice within the group. At a minimum, some type of retrospective review, either self-reported or by chart review (or, even better, both), will involve designation of indicators to be looked for, an evaluation of statistical trends of their appearance, as well as intense investigation of specific cases, particularly any in which there is a significant adverse outcome. Whether groups of anesthesia practitioners will expand their efforts into a model such as the one presented involving evaluation of specific practitioners' clinical competence will depend on desire, motivation, and resources of the group. Further expansion of the QA efforts into genuine continuous quality improvement systems may be desirable and laudable. The dedication and effort involved in coordinating review of the activity, performance, and opinions of every involved worker at every level and interface in any way related to the delivery of anesthesia care would be significant. The work would be formidable, but the possible beneficial return would be great. Results of such efforts would justifiably be the subject of presentations and publications that could be reviewed and could become the basis of recommendations presented in the next edition of this textbook.

Notable efforts have been made to incorporate the data gathered in QA systems into evaluations prompted by practitioners' applications for licenses and privileges. One of the most visible is the National Practitioners' Data Bank, a database into which entries are made of adverse actions involving any physician's license to practice or privileges at a given facility as well as of medicolegal lawsuits, claims, settlements, and judgments. The original purpose was national-level physician QA to prevent a practitioner who loses his or her license to practice in one state or a series of states from simply moving to a new state and starting practice again. The analogy to QA programs within a given state (as in New York[50]) administered by the state department of health, a state medical society, or even a state professional society is clear, as is the relationship to QA programs within given health care facilities or groups of practitioners. The potential benefit of using a QA database to look for an unusual number or severity of problems associated with one practitioner, or a persistent pattern of problems that come to the attention of the system, seems clear. Intelligent and thoughtful application of remedial suggestions or mandates (that are implemented and verified) clearly should help improve the quality of patient care, which is the ultimate goal of all QA efforts. Accordingly, information generated by a QA system at whatever level that is reasonably applied to the relicensing or recredentialing process should not threaten practitioners but, rather, should encourage them that genuine efforts to improve the quality of care are being made by all concerned.

III. SUMMARY

Delivery of optimal care is least likely to provoke malpractice claims and lawsuits, hence the intimate connection between QA efforts and RM. The basic QA process uses essentially the same problem-solving algorithm as RM and both programs have the same goal. The RM program can sometimes be considered an extension or broadening of the quality management process into implementation of practical preventive and remedial measures regarding complications of anesthesia care, always with an eye to the ultimate medicolegal implications. Presented here are the basics of both processes. Specific programs vary among facilities and groups of practitioners, incorporating local variations, conditions, traditions, and habits. However, it is universally true that application of the essential principles in whatever form will help improve and optimize the quality of care, which is clearly a desirable goal in itself and has the additional benefit of minimizing potential liability claims against the involved practitioners.

ACKNOWLEDGMENT

The author acknowledges the contribution of Dr Terry S. Vitez, author of the chapter on Quality Assurance from the first edition of the textbook. Pages 634-638 and 642-646 from the first edition were adapted with permission from Dr. Vitez for inclusion in this chapter.

REFERENCES

1. Morell RC, Eichhorn JH, eds: *Patient safety in anesthetic practice,* New York, 1997, Churchill Livingstone.
2. Eichhorn JH: Risk reduction. In Duncan P, ed: *Anesthetic risk and complications: problems in anesthesia,* vol 6, no 2, Philadelphia, 1992, Lippincott, p 278.
3. Keats AS: Anesthesia mortality in perspective, *Anesth Analg* 71:113, 1990.

4. Holzer JF: Analysis of anesthetic mishaps: current concepts in risk management, *Int Anesthesiol Clin* 22:91, 1984.
5. Eichhorn JH, Cooper JB, Cullen DJ, et al: Standards for patient monitoring during anesthesia at Harvard Medical School, *JAMA* 256:1017, 1986.
6. Hornbein TF: The setting of standards of care, *JAMA* 256:1040, 1986.
7. Eichhorn JH, Cooper JB, Cullen DJ, et al: Anesthesia practice standards at Harvard: a review, *J Clin Anesth* 1:56, 1988.
8. Eichhorn JH: Prevention of intraoperative anesthesia accidents and related severe injury through safety monitoring, *Anesthesiology* 70:572, 1989.
9. Cooper JB, Newbower RS, Long CD, et al: Preventable anesthesia mishaps: a study of human factors, *Anesthesiology* 49:399, 1978.
10. Hamilton WK: Unexpected deaths during anesthesia: wherein lies the cause? *Anesthesiology* 50:381, 1979.
11. Pierce EC Jr: Analysis of anesthetic mishaps: historical perspectives, *Int Anesthesiol Clin* 2:1, 1984.
12. Emergency Care Research Institute: Death during general anesthesia, *J Health Care Technol* 1:155, 1985.
13. Keenan RL: What is known about anesthesia outcome? In Eichhorn JH, ed: *Improving anesthesia outcome: problems in anesthesia*, vol 5, no 2, Philadelphia, 1991, Lippincott.
14. Lunn JN, ed: *Epidemiology in anesthesia*, London, 1986, Edward Arnold.
15. Cohen MM, Duncan PG, Pope WDB, et al: A survey of 112,000 anesthetics and one teaching hospital (1975-83), *Can Anaesth Soc J* 33:22, 1986.
16. Tinker JH, Dull DL, Caplan RA: Role of monitoring devices in prevention of anesthetic mishaps: a closed claims analysis, *Anesthesiology* 71:541, 1989.
17. Caplan RA, Posner KL, Ward RJ, et al: Adverse respiratory events in anesthesia: a closed claim analysis, *Anesthesiology* 72:828, 1990.
18. Pierce EC, ed: Risk management in anesthesia, *Int Anesthesiol Clin* 27(3):133, 1989.
19. Dans PE, Weiner JP, Otter SE: Peer review organizations: promises and potential pitfalls, *N Engl J Med* 313:1131, 1985.
20. Peters JD, Fineberg KS, Kroll DA, et al: *Anesthesiology and the law*, Ann Arbor, Mich, 1983, Health Administration Press.
21. Gilbert B: Relating quality assurance to credentials and privileges. In Chapman-Cliburn G, ed: *Risk management and quality assurance: issues and interactions* (a special publication of the *Quality Review Bulletin*), Chicago, Joint Commission on Accreditation of Hospitals, 1986, p 79.
22. Osteen AM, Gannon MI: Continuing medical education, *JAMA* 256:1601, 1986.
23. Wentz DK, Gannon MI, Osteen AM: Continuing medical education, *JAMA* 264:836, 1990.
24. Joint Commission on Accreditation of Healthcare Organizations: *AMH/97: Accreditation manual for hospitals,* Chicago, 1996, JCAHO.
25. American Society of Anesthesiologists: *Manual for anesthesia department organization and management,* Park Ridge, Ill, 1995, ASA.
26. Moss E: New Jersey enacts anesthesia standards. In Eichhorn JH, ed: *Anesthesia patient safety: a modern history, selections from the Anesthesia Patient Safety Foundation Newsletter,* Boston, 1996, Little Brown, p 138.
27. Lunn JN, Mushin WW: *Mortality associated with anaesthesia,* London, 1982, Nuffield Provincial Hospitals Trust.
28. Rendell-Baker L, ed: Problems with anesthetic and respiratory therapy equipment, *Int Anesthesiol Clin* 20(3):1, 1982.
29. Spooner RB, Kirby RR: Analysis of anesthetic mishaps: equipment-related anesthetic incidents, *Int Anesthesiol Clin* 22:133, 1984.
30. Cooper JB, Newbower RS, Kitz RJ: An analysis of major errors and equipment failures in anesthesia management: considerations for prevention and detection, *Anesthesiology* 60:34, 1984.
31. Duberman SM, Wald A: An integrated quality control program for anesthesia equipment. In Chapman-Cliburn G, ed: *Risk management and quality assurance: issues and interactions* (a special publication of the *Quality Review Bulletin*), Chicago, 1986, Joint Commission on Accreditation of Hospitals, p 105.
32. HHS pub no (FDA) 85-4196, 1985, Food and Drug Administration, Center for Devices and Radiologic Health, Rockville, Md 20857.
33. *Harnish v. Children's Hospital Medical Center,* 387 Massachusetts 152 (1982).
34. *Precourt v. Frederick,* 395 Massachusetts 689 (1985).
35. Curran WJ: Informed consent in malpractice cases: a turn toward reality, *N Engl J Med* 314:429, 1986.
36. Lunn JN: The role of the anaesthetic record. In Lunn JN, ed: *Epidemiology in anesthesia*, London, 1986, Edward Arnold, p 136.
37. Seed RGFL: Documentation. In Lunn JN, ed: *Epidemiology in anesthesia*, London, 1986, Edward Arnold, p 144.
38. Cooper JB, Cullen DJ, Eichhorn JH, et al: Administrative guidelines for response to an adverse anesthesia event, *J Clin Anesth* 5:79, 1993.
39. Bacon AK: Death on the table, *Anaesthesia* 44:245, 1989.
40. Schroeder SA: Outcome assessment 70 years later: are we ready? *N Engl J Med* 316:160, 1987.
41. Council on Medical Service: Guidelines for quality assurance, *JAMA* 259:2572, 1988..
42. Donabedian A: The quality of care: how can it be assessed? *JAMA* 260:1743, 1988.
43. Steffen GE: Quality medical care: a definition, *JAMA* 260:56, 1988.
44. Vitez TS, ed: Quality improvement systems and anesthesia, *Int Anesthesiol Clin* 30(2):1, 1992.
45. Deming WE: *Out of the crisis*, ed 2, Cambridge, 1996, MIT Center for Advanced Engineering Study.
46. Duberman S: *Quality assurance in the practice of anesthesiology*, Park Ridge, Ill, 1986, American Society of Anesthesiologists.
47. JCAHO: Development and application of indicators for continuous improvement in surgical and anesthesia care; measuring the quality of perioperative care, Oakbrook Terrace, Ill, 1991, JCAHO.
48. Cooper JB, Cullen DJ, Nemeskal R, et al.: Effects of information feedback and pulse oximetry on the incidence of anesthesia complications, *Anesthesiology* 67:686, 1987.
49. Vitez TS: A model for quality assurance in anesthesiology, *J Clin Anesth* 2:280, 1990.
50. Gellhorn A: Periodic physician recredentialing, *JAMA* 265:752, 1991.

Chapter 34

What to Do if Sued: An Analysis of the Allegation of Malpractice Brought Against an Anesthesia Provider

Nancy Jones Cummings

I. INTRODUCTION TO MEDICAL INJURY LITIGATION

Although insurance underwriters view anesthesiology as a high-risk specialty, a very small percentage of complications and adverse outcomes result in claims. In an analysis of the Harvard Malpractice Study published by the *New England Journal of Medicine*,[1] researchers found that very few cases of medical malpractice in hospitals resulted in claims and an even smaller percentage of verified instances of inadequate care resulted in patient recoveries.

Over the past 30 years fewer than 10% of medical liability lawsuits have reached trial. Physicians consistently prevail in a substantial majority (67%) of cases that are tried in the United States.[2] These statistics often are used by personal injury lawyers to suggest that the medical profession's concern with professional liability litigation is overstated. However, that interpretation fails to acknowledge either the intangible effects of the litigation system on the physician-patient relationship or the fact that, in a specific case, statistics are meaningless. Claims and lawsuits often are resolved by substantial payments that reflect the unpredictability of jury awards in sympathetic cases, even when the medical care is demonstrably appropriate. Research has demonstrated that knowledge of the severity of treatment and outcome often influ-

ences even objective medical reviewers' judgments of the appropriateness of care.[3]

In today's rapidly changing health care environment, a basic understanding of the malpractice litigation process can be a valuable asset for a physician. Familiarity with the litigation process can help a physician minimize the potential for treatment complications or patient concerns to lead to claims or lawsuits. And if litigation occurs, it can help a physician function effectively in a typically stressful time and contribute substantively to a successful resolution.

II. PRECURSORS TO LITIGATION

Claims and lawsuits often are preceded by patient inquiries, complaints, and requests for medical records. Although many patient inquiries, including requests for records, are entirely benign, physicians and their staffs should be sensitive and responsive to these indicators of dissatisfaction.

A. Record requests

Before a lawsuit begins, most commonly there is some indication of patient dissatisfaction. In most states patients have a right to receive copies of treatment records. There are some limited exceptions that may allow withholding portions of medical records when disclosure would endanger the patient or a third person. Physicians generally should provide copies of medical records when requested by a patient or a patient's attorney when the request includes a written authorization signed by the patient or a person empowered to act for the patient, such as a parent of a minor or a person designated in a medical power of attorney.

Physicians gain little by requesting an explanation for a patient's record request. An offer to prepare a report, narrative, or summary in response to a specific request for record copies may invite suspicion. Noncontemporaneous alteration, supplementation, or destruction[4] of records is almost always a liability-enhancing mistake. Physicians should obtain professional counsel before providing written or electronically recorded statements when it looks as if a patient complaint may result in a professional liability claim.

B. Claims and demands

Another common precursor to litigation is a patient's complaint to the physician or hospital, in the form of a claim or demand. A claim is an assertion that a claimant has been injured and is entitled to compensation. A demand is a statement of the amount of money or other consideration that the claimant requires in exchange for a release of the claim. Claims and demands may be verbal or written. A communication suggesting that a physician is legally responsible for patient injuries or economic losses fundamentally alters the physician-patient relationship. Although professional and ethical obligations to the patient remain in effect unless the physician-patient relationship is appropriately terminated, a claim or demand creates an adversarial legal relationship. Upon receipt of a claim or demand, a physician should contact his or her professional liability insurer and perhaps the risk manager in a hospital setting and obtain the assistance of counsel.

Many claims and demands are resolved without the payment of money or legal proceedings. However, the management of patient claims is a complex matter that requires analysis of medical issues and care to ensure that the physician's legal position is not undermined by well-intentioned but ineffective communications.

C. Percentage of medical malpractice cases that are tried

A small percentage of medical malpractice cases are tried. The Harvard Malpractice Study[4] calculated that the chance of a suit being filed by a patient with an identifiably negligent injury was 1 in 50. Of malpractice cases that are filed, 90% close without going to trial.

D. Communications after problems arise

Communications concerning complications and adverse outcomes should be informed, accurate, and courteous, and conveyed with sensitivity. The physician and staff should be supportive, without appearing apologetic or defensive. Patients occasionally misinterpret empathetic expressions as admissions of fault. Patients should be told that the physician will do everything reasonably possible to ensure the best medical outcome and that the relevant information will be shared as it becomes available.

Physicians should never express an opinion on cause or responsibility unless all pertinent information is available. Neither speculation nor criticism of other physicians or health care providers is appropriate during the critical early stages of postcomplication communications. The quality of communications between the patient and the physician at the time a problem arises often determines whether a claim or suit follows.

III. THE LITIGATION PROCESS

The pattern of litigation is predictable, but the pace of litigation is not.

A. Initiating a lawsuit

Most medical liability lawsuits are filed in state court. Although there are instances in which the federal courts may have jurisdiction (for instance, where a nonresident patient sues in the state where care was provided), medical injury claims generally are litigated in state courts. In most states liability may be imposed against a physician only when the evidence establishes that injury resulted from a physician's failure to satisfy the applicable standards of care. The standard of care must be established by competent medical evidence.

The term *standard of care* is a legal concept that has become incorporated into the lexicon of medicine. Despite wide variations in approaches to medical problems, lawyers expect physicians to identify the specific standard of care applicable to a claim or suit. Physicians often fall victim to the incorrect assumption that anything less than optimal care constitutes medical negligence.

Although there are many legal definitions for the term, the standard of care against which a physician is measured is a rule of reason, that is, a failure to exercise the degree of care expected of a reasonable prudent health care provider in the same or similar circumstances.[5] In most states, the applicable standard must be established by the testimony of a physician whose practice experience is similar to that of the defendant. Although physicians who testify on the standard of care issue are required to demonstrate familiarity with the standards of professional conduct applicable to the defendant's position, in most jurisdictions testifying experts are no longer required to practice in the same specific specialty or geographic location as the defendant.

A plaintiff must prove by a preponderance of evidence that a deviation occurred, that the deviation caused injury, and that money damages are appropriate to compensate the patient. Most medical injury litigation involves only claims for compensatory damages. Compensatory damages are the sum of money necessary to "make the plaintiff whole." On occasion, medical injury plaintiffs seek punitive or exemplary damages, which are intended to punish the defendant and deter future conduct. Punitive damage awards are rare, but they are assessed in approximately 6% of cases won by plaintiffs.[6]

A lawsuit typically is initiated when the patient files a complaint and the physician is served with a summons.

Once the complaint and summons have been received by the defendant, an answer must be filed within the time allowed, or a default judgment may be taken against the defendant. In most instances, a lawsuit names only the health care provider and provider organizations as defendants. In community property states, defendants' spouses sometimes are included in order to ensure the plaintiff's ability to recover damages from the entire "marital community" if insurance is unavailable or an award exceeds the limits of coverage available under the physician's insurance policy.

Upon receipt of a summons, complaint, or other notice of suit, the physician should immediately contact his or her professional liability insurer, health care organization risk manager, and attorney. In most instances, the professional liability insurer has the right to control most aspects of the litigation defense. The selection of counsel, right to consent to any settlement, and duty to cooperate with the insurer typically are discussed in the physician's insurance policy. In some instances a physician should consider retaining a personal attorney to monitor the defense and provide advice on insurance and professional regulatory matters, such as board licensing inquiries, that may not be covered by an insurance policy.

B. Attorneys and insurance company claims representatives

When a professional liability lawsuit is defended under a policy of insurance or through a health care organization's self-insurance program, involved physicians interact with defense lawyers, risk managers, and claim representatives. Professional liability insurance policies typically require the insurer to provide counsel to defend medical negligence lawsuits.[7] Although attorneys provided by the insurance company are paid by the insurer, the lawyer owes the same professional duty to the insured physician as he or she would owe to a client who independently retained his or her services.[8] Attorneys paid by an insurance company must be mindful of conflicts of interest that can arise from disputes between the insurance company and the insured physician. Most experienced insurance defense lawyers are adept at providing aggressive and effective representation without becoming entangled in conflicts of interest with the insurance company.[9] Occasionally, however, plaintiff attorney demands for settlement at amounts that exceed policy limits and other policy-related matters require the physician to obtain separate personal counsel. In some jurisdictions insurance companies are required to pay the cost of personal counsel.

Insurance company claim representatives and health care institution risk managers are very involved in litigated cases. Claim representatives represent the insurance company in arranging the retention of counsel, approving litigation strategies, and securing authority to settle cases. Risk managers are employed by health care organizations to oversee claims, insurance, and litigation. The risk manager interacts with insurance representatives, involved physicians, and their attorneys.

C. Splitting the litigation pie

Liability loss payments in the United States totaled $117 billion[10] in 1987, about 2.5% of the gross domestic product. Approximately one half of the dollars paid out each year for liability go to plaintiffs. In complicated litigation, more than one half goes to transaction costs, not to injured persons.

IV. THE DISCOVERY PROCESS

Discovery is the term used by lawyers to describe the procedures used to obtain information during the litigation process. Several vehicles are available for obtaining information. Interrogatories are written questions that are answered under oath. Depositions are oral question-and-answer sessions under oath. Requests for production of documents allow parties to obtain written and electronically recorded materials. When appropriate, an independent medical examination may be obtained and permission to enter property may be secured through the discovery process. Some states have disclosure requirements that supplement discovery. The discovery and disclosure processes are intended to facilitate the exchange of information relevant to the litigated issues. However, the scope of discovery is very broad, and information that may reasonably lead to the discovery of admissible evidence may be requested during the discovery process.[11]

V. DEPOSITIONS

A deposition is an out-of-court examination of a witness or party, taken under oath, before a court reporter. Testimony is taken by question and answer, as though in court, except that neither the judge nor a jury is present. Depositions are taken to gather information and preserve testimony. Transcripts of deposition testimony are used in court as affirmative evidence or for impeachment when a witness's trial testimony is inconsistent.

Parties and witnesses may be compelled by court order to attend depositions. Witnesses and parties are entitled to have an attorney present when their depositions are taken. Counsel should appear with the witness whenever the witness is a party in the litigation or there is a possibility that the witness may become a party. Depositions are critical components of the litigation process. Parties or key representatives of parties should prepare carefully for their deposition testimony[12]:

- Review the case in detail with your attorney.
- Assist your attorney in understanding relevant medical terminology and procedures.
- Make sure that you understand the litigation and deposition strategies.
- Review your medical records and the documents, reports, and literature provided by the attorney assigned to assist you.
- Be prepared to explain medical concepts and procedures in lay terms.

Depositions are used to preserve testimony and assess the deponent's demeanor as a witness. Courts are increasingly willing to allow the use of videotaped deposition testimony during discovery and trial presentations.

Table 34-1. Litigation expert versus treating physician

Expert	Treating physician
Specifically retained for forensic purposes	Not retained by any party to litigation
Expected to know all relevant medical records and literature	Expected to know only the records and information pertinent to the physician's involvement with the patient
Provides opinions on liability and causation	Provides factual testimony on care provided, information obtained, and prognosis
Paid for time in preparing and testifying	Generally reimbursed only for time spent in deposition or trial

Deponents should dress in a conservative, professional manner. Testimony should be courteous and even-tempered. Loss of composure or failure to take the proceedings seriously may materially compromise your position.

Deposition testimony must always be honest and responsive. However, a deposition is not an opportunity to make your case:

- Do not volunteer information.
- Do not speculate.
- Do not guess.

If a question is unclear, ask that it be repeated, rephrased, or clarified. Never answer a question that you do not understand. When questions relate to documents such as the medical record, ask to see the document to refresh your recollection and refer to it while testifying. If the lawyer representing you at the deposition objects, await the lawyer's instruction before answering. The grounds for objecting and refusing to answer in a deposition are very limited, but counsel representing a deponent should object to impermissible questions such as those seeking disclosure of privileged information and those that are manifestly beyond the permissible scope of discovery.

Because the outcome of medical injury litigation often is determined by the appearance, demeanor, and credibility of physician defendants and witnesses, deposition testimony is vital to the defense. Although the substance of a physician's testimony is important, the physician's attitude and the overall impression created often prove to be as significant as the testimony itself.[13]

VI. LITIGATION EXPERTS

In most instances a claim of professional negligence and a causal relationship between negligence and injury must be proven through expert testimony.[14] Expert testimony must establish a deviation from the applicable standard of care and a causal connection between this deviation and the plaintiff's injuries. Trial judges have broad latitude in deciding whether an expert has the requisite qualifications to testify. In physician professional negligence cases, testifying experts generally are physicians whose education, practice, and experience are capable of assisting a lay jury in evaluating trial issues.

Nondefendant physicians often are asked to consult with counsel on the medical aspects of litigated cases. Treating physicians generally are not required to offer opinions on standard of care in matters that are not di-

rectly related to their own treatment (Table 34-1). Nontreating experts are retained by the lawyers to consult on medical issues and offer trial testimony. In most instances, physicians who are parties in the lawsuit should have no direct contact with trial experts. Contact between defendant physicians and their experts may be seen as collusive when the matter is brought before a jury.

VII. PRETRIAL ISSUES AND ACTIVITIES
A. Multidefendant litigation

Medical liability litigation may involve multiple defendants, including physicians, nurses, hospitals, and other health care organizations. In some jurisdictions defendants are jointly and severally liable. That means that a successful plaintiff may collect the entire judgment from any one or combination of losing defendants. An increasing number of states have passed comparative fault legislation, which makes parties liable only for the specific percentage of liability assessed by a jury.[15] The relationship among codefendants in a lawsuit is delicate. In many instances, the interests of the parties are consistent. However, defense strategy sometimes dictates assessing fault against coparties. When that occurs, the potential for crossfire typically complicates the defense and may increase the plaintiff's potential recovery. Experienced defense lawyers, insurance representatives, and risk managers look for appropriate methods to minimize the crossfire hazard.

B. Pretrial motions

Motions are legal proceedings designed to obtain a court order resolving specific facets of a lawsuit. Motions may ask the court to modify the schedule of proceedings, add or delete parties, or resolve the myriad issues that arise during the course of litigation. A motion for summary judgment asks the court to rule in favor of the moving party on a substantive aspect of the case. A summary judgment motion may ask the court to dismiss the case in its entirety for lack of evidence on crucial elements of a claim. A motion may also ask the court to rule in favor of a plaintiff where a defense is insufficient for lack of evidence or failure to comply with the procedural requirements. Pretrial motions focus cases, dispose of collateral issues, and allow parties to influence the pace of litigation.

C. Pretrial conferences

Courts schedule pretrial conferences at various intervals during the litigation process. Pretrial conferences are used to clarify issues, limit discovery, and control scheduling and other issues. Defendant physicians typically do not attend these conferences.

D. Settlement and compromise of claims and suits

Settlements are compromises of cases that may take many forms. Settlement typically involves the payment of an agreed-upon sum of money in exchange for a release of claims. Settlements may involve a variety of negotiated terms and conditions. When professional liability insurance is involved, the right to settle is a matter of contract. Some insurance policies allow the insured physician to decide whether to settle. Other policies leave that decision to the insurance company's discretion.

A settlement conference is an opportunity to explore settlement in a structured setting presided over by a settlement judge or other experienced neutral facilitator. Courts often compel parties, their attorneys, and their insurance representatives to attend settlement conferences to make sure that the principals in the litigation receive all relevant information. Settlement conferences sometimes are helpful in arriving at solutions that would not be possible without the intervention of the settlement judge and an opportunity for the parties to participate directly and hear summaries of key evidence and argument.

The timing of a settlement varies with the dynamics of particular cases. In some instances, early settlements serve the interests of all concerned by resolving matters quickly, quietly, and with minimum cost and disruption. Most often, however, settlements result from clarification of liability and damage issues through the litigation process. A settlement on the eve of trial often is the result of aggressive litigation tactics that reduce excessive pretrial demands to more moderate figures that represent a reasonable compromise. A settlement at any stage is not a reflection on the quality of care provided by the involved physician. Settlements are entered to limit financial exposure and minimize the disruption imposed on the physician by our legal system.

A policy limit demand is a settlement proposal in which the plaintiff demands the payment of the entire policy limits available to a specific defendant. The demand typically includes a statement that the plaintiff will not negotiate a settlement within available policy limits beyond a specific deadline. If the insurance company refuses to pay the entire policy limits in accordance with the demand, the plaintiff's attorney often attempts to drive a wedge between the insured physician and the insurance company by offering a deal that protects the physician against a verdict in excess of policy limits while leaving the plaintiffs in a position to seek a larger sum from the insurance company. Although these types of proposals take many forms, most involve an agreement under which the physician cooperates in a proceeding that results in a verdict substantially greater than the available policy limits. The physician is required to assign whatever claims might exist against the insurance company for "insurance bad faith" in exchange for an agreement under which the doctor is protected from personal financial exposure. These types of arrangements create tension between the insured physician and the insurance company. The defense lawyer must tread carefully to avoid falling into a conflict of interest. Before entering this type of arrangement with the plaintiff, insured physicians should obtain personal counsel to get experienced advice.

The personal financial exposure imposed by professional liability litigation is a matter of serious concern to physicians. Appropriate professional liability insurance protection provides a cushion of financial security. Nevertheless, runaway verdicts are a foreseeable hazard in catastrophic injury litigation. Physicians should review their professional liability and other insurance policy limits regularly. The advice of experienced insurance and legal professionals can help minimize the risks of personal financial exposure. Although creative asset protection arrangements are advocated by some, the value and implications of asset protection, such as offshore trusts, require careful and informed consideration.

VIII. PREPARING FOR TRIAL

Trial preparation requires time, commitment, and mental toughness. A trial is an adversary proceeding in which the opposing party's objective is to establish a deviation from accepted standards of professional practice that can be compensated only through an award of substantial money damages. Trial preparation involves several stages, each of which offers its own challenge.

Despite the often tedious pace of litigation, firm trial dates are set eventually. Serious trial preparations should begin approximately 90 days before the trial date set by the court. The physician's initial trial preparation should begin with a review of the complaint filed by the plaintiff and the answer filed on behalf of each defendant. If other legal papers describe the claims and defenses more definitively, they should be reviewed with care. The second stage in trial preparation is a thorough review of all pertinent medical records. After becoming familiar with the medical records, the physician defendant should review the pertinent medical literature produced by the parties during the course of the litigation. With the advice of defense counsel, additional medical research may be conducted to resolve issues that emerge in the latter stages of the discovery process.

Having become thoroughly familiar with the legal issues, medical records, and pertinent literature, the physician defendant should begin a careful review of the depositions. Familiarity with the physician's own deposition is critical. If errors or omissions are discovered while reviewing the deposition, defense counsel should be advised so that appropriate steps may be taken to correct or clarify the record. Expert depositions should be reviewed with care, and any suggestions for bolstering helpful testimony and undermining the adverse parties' positions should be shared with defense counsel.

As the physician focuses on trial issues, it is important to make appropriate arrangements for practice coverage during the trial. The physician's personal involvement throughout the course of the trial is essential to ensure a strong substantive presentation and to demonstrate to the jury that the outcome is as important to the physician as it is to the plaintiff. Some professional liability insurance polices provide compensation for physicians during trial appearances. That subject should be explored well before the date set for trial.

Thirty to 60 days before trial, the physician should begin to focus on her or his personal presentation at trial. Defense counsel should be asked to schedule a meeting involving the physician and the insurance company representative to discuss trial plans and expectations. A specific schedule for testimony preparation should be set far enough ahead of trial to afford the physician a reasonable opportunity to practice for direct and cross-examination.

No trial is convenient. With adequate planning, major disruptions of family and professional life can be avoided. Physicians should expect the trial process to be tedious, frustrating, stressful, and occasionally depressing. Trials ebb and flow from day to day and witness to witness. Maintaining equilibrium and a positive outlook is important to a successful trial presentation.

Physicians must realize that they cannot control the course or outcome of a trial. They should nevertheless be assertive with their attorneys in demanding adequate planning, up-to-date information on trial and settlement developments, and an opportunity to make contributions to the trial presentation. Experienced trial lawyers usually anticipate and take steps to minimize the understandable frustration experienced by physicians who find themselves involved in professional liability trials.

IX. TRIALS

Personal injury cases typically are presented to a jury rather than a judge. States have differing standards on the composition of juries and the number of jurors whose votes are required to reach a verdict. In civil litigation, juries base their verdicts on the preponderance of the evidence. Proof "beyond a reasonable doubt," which is the evidentiary standard applicable in criminal cases, does not apply in civil litigation. Trials follow a set sequence in which the parties have an opportunity to select an impartial jury, summarize the evidence that is expected to be presented, present evidence, cross-examine adverse witnesses, submit motions seeking to dispose of issues before jury deliberations, submit instructions to be delivered to the jury by the judge, and argue the evidence as persuasively as possible. The plaintiff has the burden of proving each element of each claim by the preponderance of the evidence. Because they have the burden of persuasion, plaintiffs are given the opportunity to speak first and last in trial proceedings.

Physician defendants should be involved in all aspects of the trial. Jury selection often is aided by the insight that the physician defendant can bring to the process. The identification of issues and preparation for the examination and cross-examination of witnesses typically benefit from the thoughts and suggestions of the physician whose care is at issue in the lawsuit.

Points to emphasize in opening statement and closing argument generally are agreed upon by the entire defense team.

At the conclusion of the trial, the court provides instructions to the jury, which deliberates until a verdict is reached. Once the verdict is announced, the trial judge enters a final written judgment.

A defendant physician's attendance at trial generally is critical to a successful defense. Jurors must rearrange their daily lives to fulfill their civic duty for the justice system, and they have little tolerance for a defendant physician who claims his or her schedule won't permit the inconvenience of trial.

X. QUESTIONING JURORS

The jury system is premised on confidential jury deliberations. Stringent rules limit access by the parties, the court, and the media to the jury's deliberative process. When jurors or alternates are released, they may choose to speak with the parties or others. Under very limited circumstances, information provided by jurors may be used by the parties to impeach a verdict.

After a trial is concluded, the judge may permit the parties' attorneys to question the jurors. Insight can be gained about the jury's decision-making process. Experience has shown that jurors use many factors to assess credibility of witnesses, parties, and their attorneys in the courtroom. Posttrial interviews often confirm that physician defendants should dress conservatively and professionally at trial and be mindful that the jury and judge are observing their behavior and assessing their demeanor throughout the proceeding. Having a spouse or other supportive family member attend trial can be helpful for the physician. Even under the best circumstances, trials are difficult and stressful for defendants whose conduct is at issue.

XI. POSTTRIAL MATTERS

The jury's verdict does not end the lawyer's work in trial proceedings. Even after courtroom activities are concluded, posttrial matters typically continue for several weeks. Posttrial motions seeking relief from adverse decisions may be filed by either side. Applications for the award of costs (e.g., court fees, expert witness fees) and, under certain circumstances, attorneys' fees are resolved by the trial judge. After all posttrial matters are concluded, a final judgment is entered. Parties who are dissatisfied with the result of the trial may appeal the judgment. An appeal is made through written briefs and an oral argument to an appellate court. Juries do not hear appeals. The appellate court may sustain, modify, or reverse the trial court's rulings. If the case is reversed, the matter will be returned to the trial court for further proceedings, which may include the complete retrial under guidance provided by the appellate court decision.

Because appellate proceedings may consume an extended period of time, in most instances the party appealing a trial court decision is required to post a substantial supersedeas bond. The bond is intended to protect the prevailing party against economic losses resulting from the delay in realizing whatever benefits resulted from the trial court determination.

XII. THE RESIDUAL EFFECTS OF LITIGATION

A claim or lawsuit against a physician may have significant consequences regardless of outcome. Many states require prompt reporting to state licensing agencies of claims and suits against physicians. Licensing agencies review claims of medical negligence and determine whether disciplinary action is warranted. Professional liability insurers and credentialing bodies at hospitals and managed care organizations typically inquire about malpractice claims and suits as part of their ongoing quality assurance activities. Thus a physician whose care has been the subject of a claim or lawsuit should anticipate having to provide a detailed explanation of the matter well after the matter is resolved.

The Health Care Quality Improvement Act of 1986[16] established the National Practitioner Data Bank that assembles and maintains records on physician claims and professional disciplinary actions. Hospitals are required to query the data bank during their credentialing process. Other health care entities often query the data bank in connection with applications and renewals for privileges. Individuals, including personal injury lawyers, may also obtain access to data bank information.

Federal law requires prompt reporting to the data bank when payments are made on behalf of physicians to settle claims or lawsuits brought on behalf of a patient. Physicians are entitled to enter a response to data bank reports. There is a growing body of law dealing with data bank reports. In *Randall v. U.S.,*[17] an anesthesiologist sued to correct a data bank report. Although the physician's claims were dismissed because she had failed to participate in an administrative hearing, the court acknowledged that data bank reports carry a stigma that may warrant judicial intervention.

XIII. CONCLUSION

Iatrogenic injury claims continue to represent a serious challenge to anesthesia providers. The best defense to malpractice claims will always be prudent care and thoughtful communications with patients and their families. Unfortunately, under America's current system of justice, even consistently appropriate care and effective communications cannot immunize a physician from liability exposure.

When a physician's care becomes the subject of a claim or lawsuit, prudence dictates a careful and proactive team response in which experienced defense counsel and insurance or risk management representatives work together to obtain an appropriate resolution. The physician should be conversant with the litigation system and actively involved in all critical stages of the process. Although professional liability matters are never pleasant, an informed and involved physician can make an important contribution to the defense and resolution of claims and suits.

ACKNOWLEDGMENT

Grateful acknowledgment is given to Barry D. Halpern, Esq. of the Snell & Wilmer Law Firm, Phoenix, Arizona, for his generous and insightful contribution to this chapter.

REFERENCES

1. Brennan TA, Leape LL, Laiad NM: Incidence of adverse events and negligence in hospitalized patients: results of the Harvard Medical Practice Study 1, *N Engl J Med* 324:370, 1991.
2. American Bar Foundation: *Researching the law* 7(1):6, winter 1996.
3. Caplan RA, Posner KL, Cheney FW: Effect of outcome on physician judgment of appropriateness of care, *JAMA* 265:17, 1991.
4. Edmonds R: "Document Retention Policies and Spoliation of Evidence," For the Defense, 38(9), Sept 1996.
5. A.R.S. Section 12-563.
6. TIPS Committee News: *ABA tort and insurance practice section,* winter 1998, p 4.
7. Appleman C: *Insurance law and practice,* Section 4681 (1981).
8. Wittekind P: What physicians should expect from their insurer-retained attorneys in medical malpractice cases, *Surv Anesthesiol* 37:351, Dec 1993.
9. Bowdre KO: Conflicts of interest between insurer and insured: ethical traps for the unsuspecting defense counsel, *Am J Trial Advoc* 17:101, 1993; *Parsons v. Continental Nat. Am. Group,* 113 Ariz. 223, 550 P.2d 94 (1976).
10. A survey of the legal profession, *Economist,* July 18, 1992.
11. Rule 26(b)(1), Fed. R. Civ. P.
12. Halpern BD, Smith DH: *Deposition preparation handbook,* Phoenix, July 1994, Arizona Medical Association.
13. Ginsburg WH: Your courtroom attitude can break your malpractice case, *Physician's management,* Aug 1984.
14. Rule 702, Fed. Rules of Evidence; *Daubert v. Merrell Dow Pharmaceuticals, Inc.,* 113 S.Ct. 2786 (1993).
15. Uniform Contribution Among Tortfeasors Act, A.R.S. Sections 12-2506 et seq.
16. 42 U.S.C. Sections 11101(1), (2).
17. No. 92-96-CIV-3-BR (E.D.N.C. May 21, 1993), *aff'd* 30 F.2d 518 (4th Cir. 1994).

Index

Page numbers in *italics* indicate illustrations. Page numbers followed by *t* indicate tables.